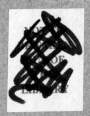

Topley & Wilson's

MICROBIOLOGY
AND MICROBIAL
INFECTIONS

First published in Great Britain 1929
Second edition 1936
Third edition 1946
Fourth edition 1955
Fifth edition 1964
Sixth edition 1975
Seventh edition 1983 and 1984
Eighth edition 1990
Ninth edition published in Great Britain 1998
by Arnold, a member of the Hodder Headline group,
338 Euston Road, London NW1 3BH

Co-published in the United States of America by
Oxford University Press, Inc.,
198 Madison Avenue, New York, NY 10016
Oxford is a registered trademark of Oxford University Press

British Library Cataloguing in Publication Data
A catalogue record for this book is available from the British Library

Library of Congress Cataloging-in-Publication Data
A catalog record for this book is available from the Library of Congress

ISBN 0 340 663189 (Volume 3) 1001164698
ISBN 0 340 614706 (Set)

Publisher:	Georgina Bentliff
Project Editor:	Sophie Oliver
Project Coordinator:	Melissa Morton
Production Controller:	Helen Whitehorn
Copy Editor:	Kathryn Bayly
Proofreader:	Elizabeth Weaver
Indexer:	Jan Ross

Typeset in 9.5/11pt New Baskerville by Photo·graphics
Printed and bound in Great Britain at The Bath Press, Avon

Topley & Wilson's

MICROBIOLOGY AND MICROBIAL INFECTIONS

NINTH EDITION

Leslie Collier
Albert Balows • **Max Sussman**

VOLUME 3

BACTERIAL INFECTIONS

VOLUME EDITORS
William J Hausler Jr • **Max Sussman**

A member of the Hodder Headline Group
LONDON • SYDNEY • AUCKLAND
Co-published in the USA by Oxford University Press, Inc., New York

Editor-in-Chief

Leslie Collier MD, DSc, FRCP, FRCPath
Professor Emeritus of Virology, The London Hospital Medical College, London;
formerly Director, Vaccines and Sera Laboratories, The Lister Institute of Preventive
Medicine, Elstree, Hertfordshire, UK

General Editors

Albert Balows AB, MS, PhD, ABMM
Professor Emeritus, Emory University School of Medicine and Georgia State
University; Former Director at The Center for Infectious Diseases, Centers for Disease
Control and Prevention, Atlanta, Georgia, USA

Max Sussman BSc, PhD, CBiol, FIBiol, FRCPath
Professor Emeritus of Bacteriology, Department of Microbiology, The Medical School,
Newcastle upon Tyne, UK

Volume Editors

William J Hausler Jr, AB, MA, PhD
Director Emeritus, State Hygienic Laboratory; Professor of Preventive Medicine,
College of Medicine; Professor of Oral Pathology, College of Dentistry; University of
Iowa, Iowa City, Iowa, USA

Max Sussman BSc, PhD, CBiol, FIBiol, FRCPath
Professor Emeritus of Bacteriology, Department of Microbiology, The Medical School,
Newcastle upon Tyne, UK

Contents of Volume 3
Bacterial infections

Contents of Volumes 1, 2, 4 and 5

VOLUME 2: SYSTEMATIC BACTERIOLOGY

VOLUME 4: MEDICAL MYCOLOGY

PART I: BACKGROUND AND BASIC INFORMATION

PART II: THERAPEUTIC AGENTS AND VACCINES

PART III: SUPERFICIAL KERATINOPHILIC FUNGI

CONTRIBUTORS

Masamichi Aikawa MD, PhD
Professor, The Research Institute of Medical Sciences, Tokai University, Boseidai, Isehara, Kanagawa, Japan

Libero Ajello PhD
Adjunct Professor, Department of Ophthalmology, Emory University Eye Center, Atlanta, Georgia, USA

RP Allaker BSc, PhD
Lecturer in Oral Microbiology, Department of Oral Microbiology, St Bartholomew's and the Royal London School of Medicine and Dentistry, London, UK

Stephen D Allen MA, MD
Director, Division of Clinical Microbiology, Director of Laboratories, Department of Pathology and Laboratory Medicine, Indiana University School of Medicine, and Director, Disease Control Laboratories, Indiana State Department of Health, Indianapolis, Indiana, USA

Martin Altwegg PhD
Professor of Medical Microbiology, Head of Molecular Diagnostics Unit, Department of Medical Microbiology, University of Zurich, Zurich, Switzerland

Daniel Amsterdam PhD
Professor of Microbiology and Pathology, Associate Professor of Medicine, Director of Clinical Microbiology and Immunology, Director, Department of Laboratory Medicine, Erie County Medical Center, University of Buffalo Medical School, Buffalo, New York, USA

Larry J Anderson MD
Chief, Respiratory and Enteric Viruses Branch, Centers for Disease Control and Prevention, Atlanta, Georgia, USA

Roy M Anderson BSc, PhD, FRS
Director, Wellcome Trust Centre for the Epidemiology of Infectious Disease; Linacre Professor and Head, Department of Zoology, University of Oxford, Oxford, UK

Jørn Andreassen PhD
Assistant Professor, Department of Population Biology, Zoological Institute, University of Copenhagen, Copenhagen, Denmark

Masanori Aoki MS
Professor of Physics, School of Health Sciences, Faculty of Medicine, Kanazawa University, Kanazawa, Ishikawa, Japan

Sarath N Arseculeratne MB BS, DipBact, DPhil
Professor of Microbiology, Faculty of Medicine, University of Peradeniya, Sri Lanka

RW Ashford PhD, DSc
Professor of Medical Zoology, The Liverpool School of Tropical Medicine, Liverpool, UK

Hazel M Aucken MA, PhD
Clinical Microbiologist, Laboratory of Hospital Infection, Central Public Health Laboratory, Colindale, London, UK

L Andrew Ball D Phil
Professor of Microbiology, Department of Microbiology, University of Alabama at Birmingham, Birmingham, Alabama, USA

Albert Balows AB, MS, PhD, ABMM
Professor Emeritus, Emory University School of Medicine and Georgia State University; Former Director at The Center for Infectious Diseases, Centers for Disease Control and Prevention, Atlanta, Georgia, USA

Jangu E Banatvala MA, MD, FRCP, FRCPath, DCH, DPH
Professor of Clinical Virology, Department of Virology, United Medical and Dental Schools of Guy's and St Thomas's, St Thomas's Hospital, London, UK

PA Bates BA, PhD
Lecturer in Medical Parasitology, The Liverpool School of Tropical Medicine, Liverpool, UK

Derrick Baxby BSc, PhD, FRCPath, FRSA
Senior Lecturer in Medical Microbiology, Department
of Medical Microbiology and Genitourinary Medicine,
Liverpool University, Liverpool, UK

Norman T Begg MBCLB, DTM&H, FFPHH
Consultant Epidemiologist, Public Health Laboratory
Service Communicable Diseases Surveillance Centre,
London, UK

William J Bellini PhD
Chief, Measles Virus Section, Respiratory and
Enterovirus Branch, Centers for Disease Control and
Prevention, Atlanta, Georgia, USA

PM Bennett BSc, PhD
Reader in Bacteriology, Department of Pathology and
Microbiology, School of Medical Sciences, University of
Bristol, Bristol, UK

Ruth L Berkelman MD
Deputy Director, National Center for Infectious
Diseases, Centers for Disease Control and Prevention,
Atlanta, Georgia, USA

Jennifer M Best PhD, FRCPath
Reader in Virology, Department of Virology, United
Medical and Dental Schools of Guy's and St Thomas's,
St Thomas's Hospital, London, UK

Jochen Bockemühl MD, PhD
Head, Division of Bacteriology, Institute of Hygiene,
Hamburg, Germany

SP Borriello BSc, PhD, FRCPath
Director, Central Public Health Laboratory, Colindale,
London, UK

Edward J Bottone PhD
Director, Consultative Microbiology, Division of
Infectious Diseases, Department of Medicine, Mount
Sinai Hospital, Mount Sinai School of Medicine, New
York, New York, USA

George HW Bowden PhD
Professor, Department of Oral Biology, Faculty of
Dentistry, University of Manitoba, Winnipeg, Manitoba,
Canada

Janet M Bradbury BSc, MSc, PhD
Reader, Department of Veterinary Pathology, University
of Liverpool, Leahurst, Neston, South Wirral, UK

William J Britt MD
Professor, Department of Pediatrics, University of
Alabama at Birmingham, Birmingham, Alabama, USA

B Kay Buchanan PhD
Microbiology and Immunology Director, Microbiology
Laboratory, Sarasota Memorial Hospital, Sarasota,
Florida, USA

Donald E Burgess PhD
Associate Professor, Veterinary Molecular Biology
Laboratory, College of Agriculture, Agricultural
Experiment Station, Montana State University,
Bozeman, Montana, USA

James P Burnie MD, PhD, MSc, MA, MRCP,
FRCPath
Head of Department, Department of Medical
Microbiology, Manchester Royal Infirmary, Manchester,
UK

Colin K Campbell BSc, MSc, PhD
Clinical Scientist, Mycology Reference Laboratory,
Bristol, UK

Richard Campbell BSc, MSc, PhD
Senior Lecturer, School of Biological Sciences, Bristol,
UK

Michael Cappello MD
Assistant Professor, Pediatric Infectious Diseases,
Laboratory of Epidemiology and Public Health, Yale
University School of Medicine, New Haven,
Connecticut, USA

Keith AV Cartwright MA, BM, FRCPath
Group Director, Public Health Laboratory Service,
South West, Gloucester Royal Hospital, Gloucester, UK

Pascal Cassinotti PhD
Deputy Head, Molecular Biology Division, Institute for
Clinical Microbiology and Immunology, St Gallen,
Switzerland

E Owen Caul FIBMS, PhD, FRCPath
Deputy Director, Head of Virology, Regional Virus
Laboratory, Public Health Laboratory, Bristol, UK

Glenn H Chambliss BSc, MSc, PhD
Professor and Chair, Department of Bacteriology,
Madison, Wisconsin, USA

Francis W Chandler DVM, PhD
Professor of Pathology, Department of Pathology,
Medical College of Georgia, Augusta, Georgia, USA

Ken Charlton DVM, PhD
Formerly Research Scientist, Animal Diseases Research
Institute, Nepean, Ontario, Canada

T Cheasty BSc
Head, *E. coli* and *Shigella* Reference Unit, Laboratory of
Enteric Pathogens, Central Public Health Laboratory,
Colindale, London, UK

Ian L Chrystie TD, PhD
Lecturer, Department of Virology, United Medical and
Dental Hospitals of Guy's and St Thomas's, St
Thomas's Hospital, London, UK

Ian N Clarke BSc, PhD
Senior Lecturer in Microbiology, Molecular
Microbiology, University Medical School, Southampton
General Hospital, Southampton, UK

Jill E Clarridge PhD, ABMM
Chief, Microbiology Section, Veterans Administration
Medical Center; Associate Professor, Baylor College of
Medicine, Houston, Texas, USA

Timothy J Cleary PhD
Director of Clinical Microbiology, Department of
Pathology, University of Miami, Jackson Memorial
Hospital, Miami, Florida, USA

J Barklie Clements BSc, PhD, FRSE
Professor of Virology, Department of Virology, Institute
of Virology, University of Glasgow, Glasgow, UK

Leslie Collier MD, DSc, FRCP, FRCPath
Professor Emeritus of Virology, The London Hospital
Medical College, London; formerly Director, Vaccines
and Sera Laboratories, The Lister Institute of
Preventive Medicine, Elstree, Hertfordshire, UK

Michael J Corbel PhD, DSc, MRCPath, CBiol,
FIBiol
Head, Division of Bacteriology, National Institute for
Biological Standards and Control, Potters Bar,
Hertfordshire, UK

CS Cox BSc, PhD
Research Leader, DERA, Chemical and Biological
Defence, Porton Down, Salisbury, Wiltshire, UK

Francis EG Cox PhD, DSc
Professor of Parasite Immunology, School of Life, Basic
Medical and Health Sciences, King's College London,
London, UK

Gary M Cox MD
Assistant Professor of Medicine, Duke University
Medical Center, Durham, North Carolina, USA

Nancy J Cox PhD
Chief, Influenza Branch, Division of Viral and
Rickettsial Disease, Centers for Disease Control and
Prevention, Atlanta, Georgia, USA

Marie B Coyle PhD
Professor of Laboratory Medicine and Microbiology,
Department of Laboratory Medicine, Harbor View
Medical Center, University of Washington, Seattle,
Washington, USA

Dorothy H Crawford PhD, MD, MRCPath, DSc
Professor of Microbiology, Department of Medical
Microbiology, University of Edinburgh, Medical School,
Edinburgh, UK

DWT Crompton MA, PhD, ScD, FRSE
John Graham Kerr Professor of Zoology, Division of
Environmental and Evolutionary Biology, Institute of
Biomedical and Life Sciences, University of Glasgow,
Glasgow, UK

William L Current BS, MS, PhD
Senior Research Scientist, Infectious Diseases Research,
Lilly Research Laboratories, Eli Lilly and Company,
Indianapolis, Indiana, USA

A Curry BSc, PhD
Top Grade Clinical Scientist, Public Health Laboratory,
Withington Hospital, Manchester, UK

Melanie T Cushion PhD
Associate Professor of Medicine, Division of Infectious
Diseases, Department of Internal Medicine, University
of Cincinnati College of Medicine, Cincinnati, Ohio,
USA

William Cushley BSc, PhD
Senior Lecturer, Division of Biochemistry and
Molecular Biology, Institute of Biomedical and Life
Sciences, University of Glasgow, Glasgow, UK

David AB Dance MB ChB, MSc, FRCPath,
DTM&H
Director/Consultant Microbiologist, Public Health
Laboratory Service, Derriford Hospital, Plymouth, UK

Gregory A Dasch BA, PhD
Senior Microbiologist, Viral and Rickettsial Diseases
Program, Infectious Diseases Department, Naval
Medical Research Institute, Bethesda, Maryland, USA

AJ Davison MA, PhD
Senior Scientist, MRC Virology Unit, Institute of
Virology, Glasgow, UK

Martin Day BSc, PhD
Reader in Microbial Genetics, School of Pure and
Applied Biology, University College Wales, Cardiff, UK

DD Despommier BS, MS, PhD
Professor of Public Health and Microbiology, Division
of Environmental Health Sciences, Faculty of Medicine,
School of Public Health, Columbia University, New
York, New York, USA

Ulrich Desselberger MD, FRCPath, FRCP
Director, Clinical Microbiology and Public Health
Laboratory, Addenbrooke's Hospital, Cambridge, UK

Arthur F DiSalvo MD
Director, Nevada State Health Laboratory, Reno,
Nevada, USA

Edouard Drouhet MD
Professor of Mycology, Pasteur Institute, Mycology Unit,
Pasteur Institute, Paris, France

JP Dubey MVSC, PhD
Senior Scientist/Microbiologist, Parasite Biology and
Epidemiology Laboratory, US Department of
Agriculture, Beltsville, Maryland, USA

Brian I Duerden BSc, MD, FRCPath
Professor and Head, Department of Medical
Microbiology, University of Wales College of Medicine,
Cardiff; Deputy Director, Public Health Laboratory
Service, London, UK

Lee M Dunster PhD
Co-ordinator, Viral Haemorrhagic Fever/Arbovirus
Surveillance, Kenya Medical Research Institute, Virus
Research Centre, Nairobi, Kenya

Daniel Elad DVM, PhD
Head, General Bacteriologic and Mycologic Diagnostics
Division, Kimron Veterinary Institute, Beit Dagan, Israel

David B Elkins MSPH, PhD
Senior Research Fellow, Australian Centre for
International and Tropical Medicine and Nutrition,
Queensland Institute of Medical Research, Brisbane,
Queensland, Australia

David H Ellis BSc, MSc, PhD
Associate Professor, Department of Microbiology and
Immunology, University of Adelaide and Head,
Mycology Unit, Women's and Children's Hospital,
North Adelaide, Australia

Gisela Enders MD
Professor Dr, Institut für Virologie und Epidemiologie,
Stuttgart, Germany

Sir MA Epstein CBE, MA, MD, PhD, DSc, FRCPath,
FRS
Professor, Nuffield Department of Clinical Medicine,
University of Oxford, John Radcliffe Hospital, Oxford,
UK

Martha Espinosa Cantellano MD, DSc
Associate Professor, Department of Experimental
Pathology, Center for Research and Advanced Studies,
Mexico City, Mexico

SJ Eykyn FRCP, FRCS, FRCPath
Reader (Hon Consultant) in Clinical Microbiology,
Division of Infection, United Medical and Dental
School of Guy's and St Thomas's, St Thomas's Hospital,
London, UK

Richard R Facklam PhD
Chief, Streptococcus Laboratory, Centers for Disease
Control and Prevention, Atlanta, Georgia, USA

S Faine MD, DPhil, FRCPA, FASM
Emeritus Professor, Department of Microbiology,
Monash University, Melbourne; Armadale, Victoria,
Australia

Heinz Feldmann MD
Assistant Professor, Institut für Virologie, Philipps
University Marburg, Marburg, Germany

Hugh J Field ScD, FRCPath
Lecturer in Virology, Centre for Veterinary Science,
University of Cambridge, Cambridge, UK

Roger G Finch FRCP, FRCPath, FFPM
Professor of Infectious Diseases, Department of
Microbiology and Infectious Diseases, Nottingham City
Hospital, University of Nottingham, Nottingham, UK

Sydney M Finegold MD
Professor of Medicine; Professor of Microbiology and
Immunology, UCLA School of Medicine; Staff
Physician, Infectious Diseases Section, Veteran Affairs
Medical Center, Los Angeles, California, USA

Michelle Nett Fiordalisi PhD
Fellow, William W McLendon Clinical Immunology
Laboratory, University of North Carolina Hospitals,
Chapel Hill, North Carolina, USA

Ana Flisser BS, PhD
Director, National Institute for Epidemiological
Diagnosis and Reference, Ministry of Health, Carpio,
Mexico City, Mexico

James D Folds PhD
Professor, Pathology and Laboratory Medicine;
Director, McLendon Clinical Laboratories, University of
North Carolina Hospitals, Chapel Hill, North Carolina,
USA

Thomas M Folks BA, MS, PhD
Chief, HIV/Retrovirus Diseases Branch, DASTLR,
Centers for Disease Control and Prevention, Atlanta,
Georgia, USA

Edward AC Follett BSc, PhD, FRCPath
Adviser in Microbiology, Scottish National Blood
Transfusion Service, Regional Virus Laboratory, Ruchill
Hospital, Glasgow, UK

Jocelyn RL Forsyth MB ChB, Dip Bact, MD,
FRCPA
Senior Associate, Department of Microbiology, The
University of Melbourne, Parkville, Victoria, Australia

Hisashi Fujioka PhD
Assistant Professor of Pathology, Institute of Pathology,
Case Western Reserve University, Cleveland, Ohio, USA

Guido Funke MD, FAMH
Consultant in Medical Microbiology, Department of
Medical Microbiology, University of Zurich, Zurich,
Switzerland

Kenneth L Gage PhD
Plague Section Chief, Bacterial Zoonoses Branch,
Division of Vector-Borne Infectious Diseases, Centers
for Disease Control and Prevention, Fort Collins,
Colorado, USA

N Spence Galbraith CBE, MB, FRCP, FFPHM,
DPH
Formerly Director, Public Health Laboratory Service,
Communicable Disease Surveillance Centre, Colindale,
London, UK

Lynne S Garcia MS, F(AAM)
Manager, UCLA Brentwood Facility Laboratory,
Pathology and Laboratory Medicine, University of
California at Los Angeles Medical Center, Los Angeles,
California, USA

Nigel J Gay MA, MSc
Mathematical Modeller, Immunisation Division, Public
Health Laboratory Service, Communicable Disease
Surveillance Centre, London, UK

Edwin E Geldreich AB, MS
Microbiology Consultant in Drinking Water, Cincinnati,
Ohio, USA

Caroline Attardo Genco PhD
Associate Professor, Department of Microbiology and
Immunology, Morehouse School of Medicine, Atlanta,
Georgia, USA

Wolfram H Gerlich PhD
Professor, Institute of Medical Virology, Giessen,
Germany

Saheer E Gharbia BSc, PhD
Research Fellow (Hon), National Collection of Type
Cultures, Public Health Laboratory Service, Colindale,
London, UK

David I Gibson PhD, DSc
Head, Parasitic Worms Division, Department of
Zoology, The Natural History Museum, London, UK

RJ Gilbert MPharm, PhD, DipBact, FRCPath
Director, Food Hygiene Laboratory, Central Public
Health Laboratory, London, UK

Herbert M Gilles MSc, MD, DSc, DMedSc, FRCP,
FFPHM
Emeritus Professor, Liverpool School of Tropical
Medicine, Liverpool, UK

Youri Glupczynski MD, PhD
Head, Department of Clinical Microbiology, Centre
Hospitalier Universitaire André Vésale, Montigny-le-
Tilleul, Belgium

Robert C Good BA, MS, PhD
Guest Researcher, TB/Mycobacteriology Branch,
Division of AIDS, STD and TB Laboratory Research,
Centers for Disease Control and Prevention, Atlanta,
Georgia, USA

Michael Goodfellow PhD, DSc, CBiol, FIBiol
Professor of Microbial Systematics, Department of
Microbiology, The Medical School, Newcastle upon
Tyne, UK

Norman L Goodman PhD
Professor and Director of Clinical Microbiology
Laboratory, Department of Pathology, College of
Medicine, University of Kentucky, Lexington, Kentucky,
USA

Michael C Goodnough PhD
Assistant Scientist, Department of Food Microbiology
and Toxicology, University of Wisconsin, Madison,
Wisconsin, USA

Alexander WC von Graevenitz MD
Professor of Medical Microbiology; Director,
Department of Medical Microbiology, Department of
Medical Microbiology, Zurich University, Zurich,
Switzerland

JM Grange MD, MSc
Reader in Clinical Microbiology, Imperial College
School of Medicine, National Heart and Lung Institute,
London, UK

John R Graybill MD
Chief, Infectious Diseases Division, Audie Murphy
Veterans, Administration Hospital; and University of
Texas Health Science Center, San Antonio, Texas, USA

David Greenwood PhD, DSc, FRCPath
Professor of Antimicrobial Science, Division of
Microbiology and Infectious Diseases, Department of
Clinical Laboratory Sciences, University Hospital,
Queen's Medical Centre, Nottingham, UK

Duane J Gubler ScD, MS
Director, Division of Vector-Borne Infectious Diseases,
Centers for Disease Control and Prevention, Fort
Collins, Colorado, USA

Eveline Guého PhD
Researcher at INSERM, Unité de Mycologie, Institut
Pasteur, Paris, France

Jacques Guillot DVM, PhD
Assistant Professor of Parasitology-Mycology, Unité de
Parasitologie-Mycologie, URA-INRA Immunopathologie
Cellulaire et Moleculaire, Ecole National Vétérinaire
d'Alfort, Maisons-Alfort, France

Stephen C Hadler MD
Director, Epidemiology and Surveillance Division,
National Immunization Program, Centers for Disease
Control and Prevention, Atlanta, Georgia, USA

Thomas L Hale PhD
Department Chief, Department of Enteric Infections,
Walter Reed Army Institute of Research, Washington
DC, USA

Pekka E Halonen MD
Emeritus Professor of Virology, Department of Virology,
University of Turku; MediCity, Turku, Finland

JM Hardie BDS, PhD, DipBact, FRCPath
Professor of Oral Microbiology, Department of Oral
Microbiology, St Bartholomew's and the Royal London
School of Medicine and Dentistry, London, UK

Melissa R Haswell-Elkins BA, MSc, PhD
Senior Research Fellow, Indigenous Health
Programme, Australian Centre for International and
Tropical Health and Nutrition, University of
Queensland, Royal Brisbane Hospital, Brisbane,
Queensland, Australia

Charles L Hatheway PhD
Chief, Botulism Laboratory, Centers for Disease Control
and Prevention, Atlanta, Georgia, USA

Harald zur Hausen MD, DSc
Managing Director, Deutsches Krebsforschungszentrum,
Heidelberg, Germany

Sir David L Hawksworth CBE, DSc, FDhc, CBiol,
FIBiol, FLS
President, International Union of Biological Sciences;
Visiting Professor, Universities of Kent, London and
Reading; Director, International Mycological Institute,
Egham, Surrey, UK

Roderick J Hay DM, FRCP, FRCPath
Mary Dunhill Professor of Cutaneous Medicine, St
John's Institute of Dermatology, United Medical and
Dental Schools of Guy's and St Thomas's, Guy's
Hospital, London, UK

John C Hierholzer PhD
Former Supervisory Research Microbiologist, Centers for Disease Control and Prevention, Atlanta, Georgia, USA

Tor Hofstad MD, PhD
Professor of Medical Microbiology, Department of Microbiology and Immunology, The Gade Institute, University of Bergen, Bergen, Norway

John J Holland PhD
Professor Emeritus, Biology Department, University of California at San Diego, La Jolla, California, USA

Barry Holmes PhD, DSc, FIBiol
Clinical Scientist, National Collection of Type Cultures, Central Public Health Laboratory, Colindale, London, UK

Stanley C Holt PhD
Professor of Microbiology, Department of Microbiology, University of Texas Health Science Center at San Antonio, San Antonio, Texas, USA

Marcel Hommel MD, PhD
Alfred Jones and Warrington Yorke Professor of Tropical Medicine, Liverpool School of Tropical Medicine, Liverpool, UK

GS de Hoog PhD
Professor of Mycology, Centraalbureau voor Schimmelcultures, Baarn, The Netherlands

Douglas B Hornick MD
Associate Professor of Pulmonary and Critical Care Medicine, Department of Medicine, University of Iowa School of Medicine, Iowa City, Iowa, USA

Peter J Hotez MD, PhD
Associate Professor, Department of Pediatrics and Epidemiology, Yale University School of Medicine, New Haven, Connecticut, USA

TGB Howe MD, PhD
Senior Lecturer in Bacteriology, Department of Pathology and Microbiology, School of Medical Sciences, University of Bristol, Bristol, UK

TJ Humphrey BSc, PhD, MRCPath
Professor; Head of Public Health Laboratory Service Food Microbiology Research Unit, Heavitree, Exeter, Devon, UK

Hilary Humphreys MD, FRCPI, FRCPath
Consultant Microbiologist, Federated Dublin Voluntary Hospitals, Dublin, Ireland

Charles J Hunter MD
Fellow, Department of Pathology, Division of Infectious Diseases, University of Virginia Health Science Center, Charlottesville, Virginia, USA

Thomas J Inzana PhD
Professor of Microbiology, Department of Biomedical Sciences and Pathobiology, Virginia-Maryland Regional College of Veterinary Medicine, Blacksburg, Virginia, USA

J Michael Janda BSc, MS, PhD
Chief, Enterics and Special Pathogens Section, Microbial Diseases Laboratory, California Department of Health Services, Berkeley, California, USA

AE Jephcott MA, MD, FRCPath, DipBact
Director, Public Health Laboratory, Bristol, UK

Robert C Jerris PhD
Assistant Professor, Department of Pathology and Laboratory Medicine, Emory University School of Medicine, Atlanta, Georgia, USA

David T John MSPH, PhD
Professor of Microbiology/Parasitology; Associate Dean for Basic Sciences, Department of Biochemistry and Microbiology, Oklahoma State University, College of Osteopathic Medicine, Tulsa, Oklahoma, USA

Elizabeth M Johnson BSc, PhD
Clinical Scientist, Mycology Reference Laboratory, Bristol, UK

Eric A Johnson ScD
Professor of Food Microbiology and Toxicology, Food Research Institute, College of Agricultrual and Life Sciences, University of Wisconsin, Madison, Wisconsin, USA

Russell C Johnson PhD
Professor of Microbiology, Department of Microbiology, University of Minnesota, Minneapolis, Minnesota, USA

Dorothy Jones BSc, MSc, PhD, DipBact
Honorary Fellow, Department of Microbiology and Immunology, University of Leicester, Leicester, UK

J Zoe Jordens BSc, PhD
Clinical Scientist/Honorary Senior Lecturer, Haemophilus Reference Laboratory, Oxford Public Health Laboratory and Nuffield Department of Pathology & Bacteriology, John Radcliffe Hospital, Headington, Oxford, UK

Stephen L Josephson PhD
Director, Microbiology/Virology, APC 1136, Rhode Island Hospital, Providence, Rhode Island, USA

Kimberly L Kane BSc, PhD
Postdoctoral Fellow, Clinical Microbiology–Immunology Laboratories, University of North Carolina Hospitals, Chapel Hill, North Carolina, USA

Michael Kann MD
Research Fellow, Institute of Medical Virology, Justus-Liebig-Universität Giessen, Giessen, Germany

SHE Kaufmann PhD
Professor and Head of Immunology, Department of Immunology, University of Ulm, Ulm, Germany

Yoshihiro Kawaoka PhD
Professor, Department of Pathobiological Science, School of Veterinary Medicine, University of Wisconsin-Madison, Madison, Wisconsin, USA

Masako Kawasaki PhD
Instructor, Department of Dermatology, Kanazawa Medical University, Uchinada, Ishikawa, Japan

Rima F Khabbaz MD
Associate Director for Medical Science, Division of Viral and Rickettsial Diseases, National Center for Infectious Diseases, Centers for Disease Control and Prevention, Atlanta, Georgia, USA

Michael P Kiley BS, MS, PhD
Senior Scientific Adviser, Federal Laboratories for Health Canada and Agriculture and Agri-Food Canada, Winnipeg, Manitoba, Canada

Mogens Kilian DMD, DSc
Professor of Microbiology, Head, Department of Medical Microbiology and Immunology, University of Aarhus, Aarhus, Denmark

Hans-Dieter Klenk MD
Professor of Virology, Head, Department of Hygiene and Medical Microbiology, Institute for Virology, Philipps-University Marburg, Marburg, Germany

Wesley E Kloos PhD
Professor of Genetics and Microbiology, Department of Genetics, North Carolina State University, Raleigh, North Carolina, USA

Somei Kojima MD, PhD
Professor of Parasitology, Department of Parasitology, University of Tokyo, Minato-ku, Tokyo, Japan

Paul E Kolenbrander PhD
Research Microbiologist, National Institute of Dental Research, National Institutes of Health, Bethesda, Maryland, USA

Myriam S Künzi PhD
Postdoctoral Fellow, John Hopkins Oncology Center, Baltimore, Maryland, USA

Ralph Lainson OBE, FRS, AFTWAS, DSc
Professor (Honoris Causa), Federal University of Pará, ex Director, The Wellcome Belém Leishmaniasis Unit, Departamento de Parasitologia, Instituto Evandro Chagas, Belém, Pará, Brazil

Paul R Lambden BSc, PhD
Senior Research Fellow, Molecular Microbiology, University Medical School, Southampton General Hospital, Southampton, UK

Sandra A Larsen MS, PhD
Guest Researcher, Bacterial STD Branch, Division of AIDS, Sexually Transmitted Diseases and Tuberculosis Laboratory Research, National Center for Infectious Diseases, Centers for Disease Control and Prevention, Atlanta, Georgia, USA

Edward R Leadbetter PhD
Professor of Microbiology, Department of Molecular and Cell Biology, University of Connecticut, Storrs, Connecticut, USA

James W LeDuc PhD
Associate Director, Global Health, National Center for Infectious Diseases, Centers for Disease Control and Prevention, Atlanta, Georgia, USA

Paul F Lehmann PhD
Professor of Microbiology and Immunology, Microbiology Department, Medical College of Ohio, Toledo, Ohio, USA

Stanley M Lemon MD
Professor of Microbiology and Immunology and Internal Medicine, Chairman, Department of Microbiology and Immunology, University of Texas Medical Branch at Galveston, Galveston, Texas, USA

Lony Chong-Leong Lim PhD
Fellow, William W McLendon Clinical Immunology Laboratory, University of North Carolina Hospitals, Chapel Hill, North Carolina, USA

Graham Lloyd BSc, MSc, PhD
Head of Diagnosis, Centre for Applied Microbiology and Research, Porton Down, Salisbury, Wiltshire, UK

Alberto T Londero MD
Emeritus Professor, Department of Microbiology, Session Medical Mycology, School of Medicine, Federal University of Santa Maria, Santa Maria, RS, Brazil

Francisco J López-Antuñano MD, MPH
Consultant, Instituto Nacional de Salud, Morelos, Mexico

Mario Lozano Chiu PhD
Postdoctoral Fellow, University of Texas Medical School, Houston, Texas, USA

David M MacLaren MA, MD, FRCP, FRCPath
Emeritus Professor of Medical Bacteriology, Moidart House, Bodicote, Banbury, Oxford, UK

Alastair P MacMillan BVSc, MSc, MRCVS
Head, FAO/WHO Collaborating Centre for Reference and Research on Brucellosis, Central Veterinary Laboratory, Addlestone, Surrey, UK

CR Madeley MD, FRCPath
Consultant Virologist, Public Health Laboratory Service, Institute of Pathology, Newcastle General Hospital, Newcastle upon Tyne, UK

John T Magee PhD, MSc, FIMLS
Top Grade Scientific Officer, Department of Medical Microbiology and Public Health Laboratory, University of Wales College of Medicine, Cardiff, UK

Brian WJ Mahy PhD, ScD
Director, Division of Viral and Rickettsial Diseases, Centers for Disease Control and Prevention, Atlanta, Georgia, USA; formerly Director, The Animal Virus Research Institute, Pirbright, Surrey, UK

Scott A Martin BS, MS, PhD
Professor, Department of Animal and Dairy Science, College of Agriculture, Livestock and Poultry, University of Georgia, Athens, Georgia, USA

William J Martin PhD
Director, Scientific Resources Program, National Center for Infectious Diseases, Centers for Disease Control and Prevention, Atlanta, Georgia, USA

Adolfo Martínez-Palomo MD, DSc
Director General, Centro de Investigación y de Estudios Avanzados, Mexico City, Mexico

Tadahiko Matsumoto MD, DMSc
Director, Department of Dermatology, Toshiba Hospital, Higashi-oi, Shinagawa-ku, Tokyo, Japan

Ruth Matthews MD, PhD, MSc, FRCPath
Reader in Medical Microbiology, Department of Medical Microbiology, Manchester Royal Infirmary, Manchester, UK

Joseph E McDade PhD
Associate Director for Laboratory Science, National Center for Infectious Diseases, Centers for Disease Control and Prevention, Atlanta, Georgia, USA

Michael R McGinnis PhD
Director, Medical Mycology Research Center, Associate Director, University of Texas at Galveston-WHO Collaborating Center for Tropical Diseases, and Professor, Department of Pathology, University of Texas Medical Branch at Galveston, Galveston, Texas, USA

Jim McLauchlin PhD
Clinical Scientist, Central Public Health Laboratory, Colindale, London, UK

Heinz Mehlhorn PhD
Professor of Parasitologie, Institut für Zoomorphologie, Zellbiologie und Parasitologie, Heinrich-Heine-Universität, Düsseldorf, Germany

A Leonel Mendoza MS, PhD
Assistant Professor, Department of Microbiology, Medical Technology Program, Michigan State University, East Lansing, Michigan, USA

Volker ter Meulen MD
Chairman, Institute for Virology and Immunobiology, University of Würzburg, Würzburg, Germany

Gillian Midgley BSc, PhD
Lecturer in Medical Mycology, Department of Medical Mycology, St John's Institute of Dermatology, United Medical and Dental School of Guy's and St Thomas's, St Thomas's Hospital, London, UK

Michael A Miles MSc, PhD, DSc
Professor of Medical Parasitology and Head, Applied Molecular Biology Unit, Department of Medical Parasitology, London School of Hygiene and Tropical Medicine, London, UK

J Michael Miller PhD, ABMM
Chief, Diagnostic Microbiology Section, Hospital Infections Program, National Center for Infectious Diseases, Centers for Disease Control and Prevention, Atlanta, Georgia, USA

P Minor BA, PhD
Head, Division of Virology, National Institute for Biological Standard and Control, Potters Bar, Hertfordshire, UK

AC Minson BSc, PhD
Professor of Virology, Virology Division, Department of Pathology, University of Cambridge, Cambridge, UK

DH Molyneux MA, PhD, DSc
Director, Professor of Tropical Health Sciences, Liverpool School of Tropical Medicine, Liverpool, UK

Arnold S Monto MD
Professor of Epidemiology, School of Public Health, University of Michigan, Ann Arbor, Michigan, USA

Stephen A Morse MSPH, PhD
Associate Director for Science, Division of AIDS, STD and Tuberculosis Laboratory Research, Centers for Disease Control and Prevention, Atlanta, Georgia, USA

RP Mortlock BS, PhD
Professor of Microbiology, Section of Microbiology, Cornell University, Ithaca, New York, USA

Ralph Muller DSc, PhD, BSc, FIBiol
Formerly Director, International Institute of Parasitology, St Albans, Hertfordshire, UK

David A Murdoch MA, MBBS, MSc, MD, MRCPath
Honorary Clinical Research Fellow, Department of Microbiology, Southmead Health Services NHS Trust, Westbury-on-Trym, Bristol, UK

Frederick A Murphy DVM, PhD
Professor, School of Veterinary Medicine, University of California, Davis, California, USA

PR Murray PhD
Professor, Division of Laboratory Medicine, Departments of Pathology and Medicine, Washington University School of Medicine, St Louis, Missouri, USA

David Mutimer MBBS
Senior Lecturer, Birmingham University Department of Medicine; Honorary Consultant Physician, Liver and Hepatobiliary Unit, Queen Elizabeth Hospital, Edgbaston, Birmingham, UK

Irving I Nachamkin PhD
Professor of Pathology and Laboratory Medicine, Department of Pathology and Laboratory Medicine, University of Pennsylvania School of Medicine, Philadelphia, Pennsylvania, USA

Francis E Nano PhD
Associate Professor, Department of Biochemistry and Microbiology, University of Victoria, Victoria, British Columbia, Canada

AA Nash BSc, MSc, PhD
Professor, Department of Veterinary Pathology, University of Edinburgh, Edinburgh, UK

Neal Nathanson MD
Professor and Chair Emeritus, Department of
Microbiology, University of Pennsylvania Medical
Center, Philadelphia, Pennsylvania, USA

James C Neil BSc, PhD
Professor of Virology and Molecular Oncology,
Department of Veterinary Pathology, University of
Glasgow, Glasgow, UK

WC Noble DSc, FRCPath
Professor of Microbiology, Department of Microbial
Diseases, St John's Institute of Dermatology, United
Medical and Dental Schools of Guy's and St Thomas's,
St Thomas's Hospital, London, UK

Steven J Norris PhD
Professor of Pathology and Laboratory Medicine,
Microbiology and Molecular Genetics, Department of
Pathology, University of Texas Health Science Center,
Houston, Texas, USA

David C Old PhD, DSc, FIBiol, FRCPath
Reader in Medical Microbiology, Department of
Medical Microbiology, Ninewells Hospital and Medical
School, Dundee, UK

Arvind A Padhye PhD
Chief, Fungus Reference Laboratory, Emerging
Bacterial and Mycotic Diseases Branch, Division of
Bacterial and Mycotic Diseases, Centers for Disease
Control and Prevention, Atlanta, Georgia, USA

Norberto J Palleroni PhD
Professor of Microbiology, Center for Agricultural
Molecular Biology, Cooke College, Rutgers University,
New Brunswick, New Jersey, USA

Stephen R Palmer MA, MB, BChir, FFPHM
Professor & Director, Welsh Combined Centres for
Public Health, University of Wales College of Medicine;
Head, Communicable Disease Surveillance Centre
Welsh Unit, Cardiff, UK

Demosthenes Pappagianis PhD, MD
Professor of Medical Biology and Immunology,
Department of Medical Microbiology and Immunology,
University of California, Davis, California, USA

M Thomas Parker MD, FRCPath, DipBact
Formerly Director, Cross-Infection Reference
Laboratory, Central Public Health Laboratory,
Colindale, London, UK

D Parratt MD, FRCPath
Senior Lecturer, Department of Medical Microbiology,
Ninewells Hospital, Dundee, UK

Roger Parton BSc, PhD
Senior Lecturer, Division of Infection and Immunity,
Institute of Biomedical and Life Sciences, University of
Glasgow, Glasgow, UK

Thomas F Patterson MD
Associate Professor of Medicine, Division of Infectious
Diseases, Department of Medicine, University of Texas
Health Science Center, San Antonio, Texas, USA

Charles W Penn BSc, PhD
Reader in Microbiology, School of Biological Sciences,
University of Birmingham, Edgbaston, Birmingham, UK

T Hugh Pennington MB, BS, PhD, FRCPath, FRSE
Professor of Bacteriology, Department of Medical
Microbiology, University of Aberdeen, Aberdeen, UK

John R Perfect MD
Professor of Medicine, Duke University Medical Center,
Durham, North Carolina, USA

William A Petri Jnr MD, PhD
Professor, Department of Infectious Diseases, University
of Virginia Health Sciences Center, Charlottesville,
Virginia, USA

Paula M Pitha BS, MS, PhD
Professor of Oncology, Oncology Center and
Department of Molecular Biology and Genetics,
Baltimore, Maryland, USA

Tyrone L Pitt MPhil, PhD
Deputy Director, Laboratory of Hospital Infection,
Central Public Health Laboratory, Colindale, London,
UK

Tanja Popovic MD, PhD
Principal Investigator, Diphtheria Research Project,
Childhood and Respiratory Diseases Branch, Division of
Bacterial and Mycotic Diseases, National Center for
Infectious Diseases, Centers for Disease Control and
Prevention, Atlanta, Georgia, USA

R Scott Pore PhD
Professor of Microbiology and Immunology,
Department of Microbiology and Immunology, West
Virginia University School of Medicine, Morgantown,
West Virginia, USA

Roger Pradinaud MD
Directeur, Service de Dermato-Vénéreo-Leprologie,
Centre Hospitalier de Cayenne, Guyane Française

Craig R Pringle BSc, PhD
Professor of Biological Sciences, Biological Sciences
Department, University of Warwick, Coventry,
Warwickshire, UK

Stanley B Prusiner AB, MD
Professor of Neurology, Biochemistry and Biophysics,
Department of Neurology, University of California, San
Francisco, California, USA

Thomas J Quan PhD, MPH
Microbiologist, Imu-Tek Animal Health Inc, Fort
Collins, Colorado, USA

CP Quinn BSc, PhD
Head, Biotherapy Unit, Centre for Applied
Microbiology and Research, Porton Down, Salisbury,
Wiltshire, UK

Sharath K Rai PhD
Postdoctoral Fellow, Department of Molecular
Immunology, Bristol Myers Squibb PRI, Seattle,
Washington, USA

Anita Rampling MA, PhD, MB ChB, FRCPath
Director, Public Health Laboratory, Department of
Pathology, West Dorset Hospital, Dorchester, UK

Robert C Read MD, MRCP
Senior Clinical Lecturer in Infectious Diseases,
Department of Medical Microbiology, University of
Sheffield Medical School, Sheffield, UK

Stephen C Redd MD
Chief, Measles Elimination Activity, Epidemiology and
Surveillance Division, Centers for Disease Control and
Prevention, Atlanta, Georgia, USA

Sanjay G Revankar MD
Infectious Diseases Fellow, Department of Medicine,
Division of Infectious Diseases, University of Texas
Health Science Center, San Antonio, Texas, USA

John H Rex MD
Associate Professor, University of Texas Medical School,
Houston, Texas, USA

Malcolm D Richardson BSc, PhD, CBiol, MIBiol,
FRCPath
Director, Regional Mycology Reference Laboratory,
Department of Dermatology, Glasgow, UK

Geoffrey L Ridgway MD, BSc, MRCP, FRCPath
Consultant Microbiologist, Department of Clinical
Microbiology, University College London Hospitals;
Honorary Senior Lecturer, University College Hospital,
London, UK

Glenn D Roberts PhD
Director, Clinical Mycology and Mycobacteriology
Laboratories; Professor of Microbiology and Laboratory
Medicine, Mayo Medical School, Division of Clinical
Microbiology, Mayo Clinic, Rochester, Minnesota, USA

Betty H Robertson PhD
Chief, Virology Section, Hepatitis Branch, Division of
Viral and Rickettsial Diseases, Centers for Disease
Control and Prevention, Hepatitis Branch, Atlanta,
Georgia, USA

Frank G Rodgers PhD
Professor of Microbiology; Editor, Journal of Clinical
Microbiology, Department of Microbiology, Rudman
Hall, University of New Hampshire, Durham, New
Hampshire, USA

John T Roehrig PhD
Chief, Arbovirus Diseases Branch, Division of Vector-
Borne Infectious Diseases, National Center for
Infectious Diseases, Centers for Disease Control and
Prevention, Fort Collins, Colorado, USA

MJ Rosovitz BSc
Research Assistant, Department of Bacteriology,
University of Wisconsin-Madison, Madison, Wisconsin,
USA

Paul A Rota PhD
Research Microbiologist, Measles Virus Section, Centers
for Disease Control and Prevention, Atlanta, Georgia,
USA

Andrew H Rudolph MD
Clinical Professor of Dermatology, Dermatology
Department, Baylor College of Medicine, Houston
Texas, USA

Kathryn L Ruoff PhD
Assistant Professor of Pathology, Harvard Medical
School; Assistant Director, Microbiology Laboratories,
Massachusetts General Hospital, Boston, Massachusetts,
USA

A Denver Russell BPharm, PhD, DSc, FRCPath,
FRPharmS
Professor, Welsh School of Pharmacy, University of
Wales at Cardiff, Cardiff, UK

WC Russell BSc, PhD, FRSE
Emeritus Research Professor, School of Biological and
Medical Sciences, University of St Andrews, St Andrews,
Fife, UK

Maria S Salvato PhD
Assistant Professor, Department of Pathology and
Laboratory Medicine, Services Memorial Institute,
University of Wisconsin Medical School, Madison,
Wisconsin, USA

Anthony Sanchez PhD
Special Pathogens Branch, Division of Viral and
Rickettsial Diseases, National Center for Infectious
Diseases, Centers for Disease Control and Prevention,
Atlanta, Georgia, USA

Klaus P Schaal MD
Director, Professor of Medical Microbiology, Institute
for Medical Microbiology and Immunology, University
of Bonn, Bonn, Germany

Julius Schachter PhD
Professor of Laboratory Medicine, World Health
Organization Collaborating Centre for References and
Research on Chlamydia, Chlamydia Research
Laboratory, Department of Laboratory Medicine, San
Francisco General Hospital, San Francisco, California,
USA

Wiley A Schell MSc
Research Associate, Department of Medicine, Duke
University Medical Center, Durham, North Carolina,
USA

Walter F Schlech III MD
Professor of Medicine, Faculty of Medicine, Dalhousie
University, QE II HSC, Halifax, Nova Scotia, Canada

L Schlesinger MD
Associate Professor of Medicine, Department of
Medicine, Division of Infectious Diseases, University of
Iowa, Iowa City, Iowa, USA

Connie S Schmaljohn PhD
Chief, Department of Molecular Virology, US Army
Medical Research Institute of Infectious Diseases, Fort
Detrick, Maryland, USA

Gabriel A Schmunis MD, PhD
Coordinator, Communicable Diseases Program, Pan American Health Organization, Washington, DC, USA

Sibylle Schneider-Schaulies PhD
Lecturer, Institut für Virologie und Immunbiologie, Universität Würzburg, Würzburg, Germany

John Richard Seed PhD
Professor, Department of Epidemiology, School of Public Health, University of North Carolina, Chapel Hill, North Carolina, USA

Esther Segal PhD
Professor of Microbiology/Mycology, Department of Human Microbiology, Sackler School of Medicine, Tel Aviv University, Ramat Aviv, Tel Aviv, Israel

Bernard W Senior BSc, PhD, FRCPath
Lecturer in Medical Microbiology, Department of Medical Microbiology, Dundee University Medical School, Ninewells Hospital and Medical School, Dundee, UK

Haroun N Shah BSc, PhD, FRCPath
Head, Identification Services Unit, National Collection of Type Cultures, Central Public Health Laboratory, Colindale, London, UK

Jeffrey J Shaw PhD, DSc
Professor, Departamento de Parasitologia, Instituto de Ciências Biomédicas, Universidade de São Paulo, São Paulo, Brazil

Thomas M Shinnick PhD
Chief, Tuberculosis/Mycobacteriology Branch, Centers for Disease Control and Prevention, Atlanta, Georgia, USA

Stuart G Siddell BSc, PhD
Professor of Virology, Institute of Virology, University of Würzburg, Würzburg, Germany

Gunter O Siegl PhD
Professor and Head, Institute for Clinical Microbiology and Immunology, St Gallen, Switzerland

Lynne Sigler MSc
Curator and Associate Professor, University of Alberta Microfungus Collection and Herbarium, Devonian Botanic Garden, Edmonton, Alberta, Canada

RB Sim BSc, DPhil
MRC Scientific Staff, MRC Immunochemistry Unit, Department of Biochemistry, University of Oxford, Oxford, UK

Peter Simmonds BM, PhD, MRCPath
Senior Lecturer, Department of Medical Microbiology, University of Edinburgh Medical School, Edinburgh, UK

Anthony Simmons MA, MB, BChir, PhD, FRCPath
Senior Medical Specialist, Infectious Diseases Laboratories, Institute of Medical and Veterinary Science, Adelaide, Australia

Martin B Skirrow MB, ChB, PhD, FRCPath, DTM&H
Consultant Medical Microbiologist, Public Health Laboratory, Gloucestershire Royal Hospital, Gloucester, UK

Mary PE Slack MA, MB, FRCPath
Lecturer (Honorary Consultant) in Bacteriology, Haemophilus Reference Laboratory, Oxford Public Health Laboratory and Nuffield Department of Pathology and Bacteriology, John Radcliffe Hospital, Oxford, UK

Henry R Smith MA, PhD
Deputy Director, Laboratory of Enteric Pathogens, Central Public Health Laboratory, Colindale, London, UK

Eric J Snijder PhD
Assistant Professor, Department of Virology, Institute of Medical Microbiology, Leiden University, Leiden, The Netherlands

Phyllis H Sparling DVM, MS
Liaison, Centers for Disease Control and Prevention, Atlanta, Georgia, USA

David CE Speller MA, BM, BCh, FRCP, FRCPath
Emeritus Professor of Clinical Microbiology, University of Bristol, Bristol, UK

Carol A Spiegel PhD
Associate Professor, Department of Pathology and Laboratory Medicine, University of Wisconsin, Madison, Wisconsin, USA

Andrew Spielman ScD
Professor of Tropical Public Health, Department of Tropical Public Health, Harvard School of Public Health, Boston, Massachusetts, USA

Bret M Steiner PhD
Chief, Treponemal Pathogenesis, Division of Sexually Transmitted Diseases, Centers for Disease Control and Prevention, Atlanta, Georgia, USA

Scott J Stewart BS
Formerly of National Institute of Allergies and Infectious Diseases; 344 Roaring Lion Road, Hamilton, Montana, USA

Max Sussman BSc, PhD, CBiol, FIBiol, FRCPath
Emeritus Professor of Bacteriology, Department of Microbiology, The Medical School, Newcastle upon Tyne, UK

Roland W Sutter MD, MPH, TM
Deputy Chief for Technical Affairs, Polio Eradication Activity, National Immunization Program, Centers for Disease Control and Prevention, Atlanta, Georgia, USA

Bala Swaminathan PhD
Chief, Foodborne and Diarrhoeal Diseases Laboratory 333 Section, Foodborne and Diarrhoeal Diseases Branch, Centers for Disease Control and Prevention, Atlanta, Georgia, USA

Robert V Tauxe MD, MPH
Chief, Foodborne and Diarrhoeal Diseases Branch,
Division of Bacterial and Mycotic Diseases, Centers for
Disease Control and Prevention, Atlanta, Georgia, USA

David J Taylor MA, VetMB, PhD, MRCVS
Reader in Veterinary Microbiology, Department of
Veterinary Pathology, University of Glasgow, School of
Veterinary Medicine, Bearsden, Glasgow, UK

John M Taylor PhD
Senior Member, Fox Chase Cancer Center,
Philadelphia, Pennsylvania, USA

David Taylor-Robinson MD, MRCP, FRCPath
Emeritus Professor of Microbiology and Genitourinary
Medicine, Department of Genitourinary Medicine, St
Mary's Hospital, London, UK

Lucia Martins Teixeira PhD
Associate Professor, Universidade Federal do Rio de
Janeiro, Instituto de Microbiologia, Rio de Janeiro,
Brazil

Sam Rountree Telford III DSc
Lecturer in Tropical Health, Department of Tropical
Public Health, Harvard University, Boston,
Massachusetts, USA

Ram P Tewari PhD
Professor of Microbiology, Department of Medical
Microbiology and Immunology, Southern Illinois
University, Springfield, Illinois School of Medicine,
Springfield, Illinois, USA

E John Threlfall BSc, PhD
Grade C Clinical Scientist, Laboratory of Enteric
Pathogens, Central Public Health Laboratory,
Colindale, London, UK

Richard C Tilton BS, MS, PhD
Senior Vice President, Chief Scientific Director, BBI
Clinical Laboratories, New Britain, Connecticut, USA

Noel Tordo PhD
Head, Laboratoire de Lyssavirus, Institut Pasteur, Paris,
France

Anna Maria Tortorano PhD
Associate Professor of Hygiene, Laboratory of Medical
Microbiology, Institute of Hygiene and Preventive
Medicine, School of Medicine, Università degli Studi di
Milano, Milano, Italy

Kevin J Towner BSc, PhD
Consultant Clinical Scientist, Public Health Laboratory,
University Hospital, Queen's Medical Centre,
Nottingham, UK

JG Tully BS, MS, PhD
Chief, Mycoplasma Section, Laboratory of Molecular
Microbiology, National Institute of Allergy and
Infectious Diseases, National Institutes of Health,
Frederick, Maryland, USA

Peter C B Turnbull BSc, MS, PhD
Head, Anthrax Section, Centre for Applied
Microbiology and Research, Porton Down, Salisbury,
Wiltshire, UK

Kenneth L Tyler MD
Professor of Neurology, Medicine, Microbiology and
Immunology, Department of Neurology, University of
Colorado Health Sciences Center, and Chief,
Neurology Service Denver Veteran Affairs Medical
Center, Denver, Colorado, USA

Edward J Usherwood MA, PhD
Research Fellow, Department of Veterinary Pathology,
Edinburgh, UK

Maria Anna Viviani MD
Associate Professor of Hygiene, Laboratory of Medical
Microbiology, Institute of Hygiene and Preventive
Medicine, School of Medicine, Università degli Studi di
Milano, Milano, Italy

Martin I Voskuil BA
Research Scientist, Department of Bacteriology,
University of Wisconsin-Madison, Madison, Wisconsin,
USA

William G Wade BSc, PhD
Richard Dickinson Professor of Oral Microbiology,
Head of Oral Biology Unit, Department of Oral
Medicine and Pathology, United Medical and Dental
Schools of Guy's and St Thomas's, Guy's Hospital,
London, UK

Derek Wakelin BSc, PhD, DSc, FRCPath
Professor of Zoology, Department of Life Science,
University of Nottingham, Nottingham, UK

Alexander Wandeler MSc, PhD
Head of Rabies Unit, Animal Diseases Research
Institute, Nepean, Ontario, Canada

Audrey R Wanger PhD
Assistant Professor, Department of Pathology and
Laboratory Medicine, University of Texas Medical
School at Houston, Houston, Texas, USA

Bodo Wanke PhD, MD
Head of Laboratório de Micologia Médica, Laboratório
de Micologia, Hospital Evandro Chagas, Rio de Janeiro,
Brazil

ME Ward BSc, PhD
Professor of Medical Microbiology, Molecular
Microbiology, Southampton University School of
Medicine, Southampton General Hospital,
Southampton, UK

MFR Waters OBE, MB, FRCP, FRCPath
Formerly Consultant Leprologist and Physician,
Hospital for Tropical Diseases, London, UK

Emilio Weiss BS, MS, PhD
Emeritus Chair of Science, Naval Medical Research
Institute, Bethesda, Maryland, USA

Irene Weitzman PhD
Assistant Director, Clinical Microbiology Service, and
Associate Professor of Clinical Pathology in Medicine,
Columbia Presbyterian Medical Center, New York, New
York, USA

Lawrence J Wheat MD
Professor of Medicine, Infectious Disease Division,
Wishard Memorial Hospital, Indianapolis, Indiana, USA

Richard J Whitley MD
Professor of Pediatrics, Microbiology and Medicine,
Department of Pediatrics, University of Alabama at
Birmingham, Birmingham, Alabama, USA

James Whitworth MD, FRCP, DTM&H
Team Leader, MRC Programme on AIDS, Entebbe,
Uganda

Louis A Wilson BS, MSc, MD, FACS
Professor of Ophthalmology, Emory University School
of Medicine and Adjunct Professor of Microbiology,
Georgia State University, Atlanta, Georgia, USA

John A Wyke MA, VetMB, PhD, MRCVS, FRSE
Director of Research, Beatson Institute, Honorary
Professor at University of Glasgow, Beatson Institute for
Cancer Research, Glasgow, UK

Kentaro Yoshimura BVM, DVM, PhD
Professor of Parasitology, Chairman, Department of
Parasitology, Akita University School of Medicine, Akita,
Japan

Viqar Zaman MBBS, DSc, DTM&H, FRCPath
Professor, Department of Microbiology, The Aga Khan
University, Karachi, Pakistan

Stephen H Zinder BA, MS, PhD
Professor of Microbiology, Section of Microbiology,
Cornell University, Ithaca, New York, USA

EDITOR-IN-CHIEF'S PREFACE

The period since publication of the first edition in 1929 has seen various modifications in the form and content of *Topley and Wilson*, perhaps the most important of which was the change with the 7th edition to a multi-author work in four volumes. This, the 9th edition, marks three spectacular departures from past policy.

First, and most obviously, the work now covers every class of pathogen: viruses, bacteria, fungi and parasites, including the helminths. The arrangement is in order of complexity, ranging from *Virology* in Volume 1 through *Systematic Bacteriology* and *Bacterial Infections* in Volumes 2 and 3, *Medical Mycology* in Volume 4 and *Parasitology* in Volume 5. Each has its own index, and a general index to the entire work is provided in Volume 6.

This major expansion called for a change in authorship, which previously was almost entirely British. Clearly, the range of expertise now needed to cover every aspect of medical microbiology, including mycology and parasitology, can no longer be provided from any one country and we have been fortunate in recruiting leading experts from many parts of the world for this expanded edition. In all, there are 234 chapters, of which the USA has provided 45% and the UK 35%; the remainder come from 20 other countries.

The third important new feature is the appearance of an electronic version alongside the printed work, which will facilitate information retrieval, cross-referencing and, most important, a continual programme of revision and updating.

During the planning phase, surveys of known and potential readers indicated a majority demand for more detailed referencing than hitherto, and the provision of factual material rather than the more speculative and discursive treatment characteristic of the early editions. This trend has become increasingly apparent with successive editions, and there is now no justification for retaining the word 'Principles' in the title. Despite this change in emphasis, the readership

for whom the work is intended remains the same; it comprises primarily microbiologists working in research, diagnostic and public health laboratories and those teaching both undergraduates and postgraduates. Although it is first and foremost a treatise on microbiology, the comprehensive coverage of the clinical and pathological features of infection makes it also an invaluable source of reference for physicians dealing with infective disease.

The 8th edition comprised four volumes of text, of which the first covered *General Bacteriology and Immunity*, and was intended to service those dealing with the more specialized topics. This arrangement did not, however, prove satisfactory; the 9th edition is therefore designed to make the volumes more self-contained, and descriptions of the immune response as it relates respectively to viruses, bacteria and the eukaryotic parasites are provided in the appropriate volumes.

The arrangement of the *Virology* volume is similar to that in the 8th edition, except that it is divided into five rather than two parts. Accounts of the general characteristics of bacteria and of bacteria in the environment will now be found in Volume 2 (*Systematic Bacteriology*). Both this and Volume 3 (*Bacterial Infections*) can be read individually, but, as in past editions, they obviously complement each other. The quantity of information now available has meant a further increase in size of Volumes 1, 2 and 3, which now contain about 30% more material than did the whole of the 8th edition. The two new volumes, dealing respectively with *Medical Mycology* and *Parasitology*, greatly enhance the value of the work as a whole. Whether to include the helminths under the title *Microbiology and Microbial Infections* was a debatable point, which succeeded on the grounds that to omit them would impair coverage of the entire gamut of infection, and that a separate mention in the title would have made it unwieldy.

Some points of editorial policy deserve mention. As in previous editions, the emphasis throughout is on infections of humans; animal diseases are given much less prominence, usually receiving mention only when they cause zoonoses, serve as models of pathogenesis or are of economic importance. Sections likely to be of interest only to the more specialized reader are indicated by the use of a small typeface, and the location and cross-referencing of specific sections are now made easier by numbering them.

The standard of the illustrations, many of which are now in colour, is considerably higher than in previous editions; in particular, there is a wealth of excellent drawings and photographs in Volumes 4 and 5. The quality of the references has been greatly improved by providing the titles of papers and both first and last pages; and the international provenance of the contributors has resulted in broader surveys of the world literature than is usual in predominantly British or American texts.

In conclusion, I take this opportunity of saying how much I appreciate the efforts of all those concerned with bringing this large and complex work to fruition. Almost by definition, the more distinguished the author, the more he or she will have other pressing commitments, a consideration that applies to most of our contributors. Sincere thanks are due to them for their participation and for providing the huge fund of learning and expertise that is apparent throughout the edition. I gladly take this opportunity of expressing my gratitude to all my colleagues on the editorial team for the intensive and sustained effort they have devoted to bringing this large and complex publication to fruition. It would be invidious to single out individuals among the copy-editors and the staff at Arnold who have laboured so devotedly behind the scenes, but to each of them my gratitude is also due for their competent help and unfailing support during the preparation of this edition.

LC

VOLUME EDITORS' PREFACE

This volume deals with the fascinating world between the basic and systematic aspects of bacteriology on the one hand and clinical infectious diseases on the other. This broad area of study has never acquired its own name, probably because it is a compound of many independent sciences, including epidemiology, immunology and pathology, amongst others. In addition, continuing awareness of the history of infectious diseases often affords an important retrospective, particularly at a time when the prospect of emerging infections increasingly occupies our attention.

Readers familiar with recent editions of this work will note that the structure and arrangement of this volume have changed. The early chapters dealing with immunity and disease transmission were previously in the volume devoted to general microbiology and immunity. The sequence of the later chapters, which deal with infections due to individual or groups of pathogenic bacteria, has as far as possible been rearranged on a 'system' basis. The object is to bring closer together discussions of the different infections of single body systems, such as the respiratory tract and the gastrointestinal tract. The intriguing ability of some pathogens to cause disease in many body systems means that such an arrangement cannot be applied with absolute rigour. At the same time, the recruitment of a large number of new authors has occasioned new titles for a number of the chapters and the inclusion of new topics, including the emergence and resurgence of bacterial infectious diseases, oral infections, bartonellosis and cat scratch disease. For the first time a separate chapter is devoted to the non-sporing anaerobic bacteria.

Many chapters have undergone binary fission. The mycobacterioses other than tuberculosis have been given a separate chapter, and increasing knowledge about helicobacter infections has made it desirable to consider these separately from campylobacter infections. Similarly, plague and other yersinial infections are each dealt with in separate chapters; pasteurellosis and tularaemia are now separated from the chapter on melioidosis and glanders.

As in the past, animal diseases other than zoonoses are addressed briefly or not at all, unless they are in some special way important in the context of human disease.

The explosion of knowledge about bacterial infections in recent years is so great that some older knowledge has had to be omitted from this edition. Readers should therefore be reminded that previous editions of *Topley and Wilson* continue to be valuable sources of record and reference. This volume is an attempt to present the present state of knowledge about the bacteriology of infectious diseases together with pointers to future developments.

Many new authors have joined us for this edition, which is now for the first time truly international. Although this has meant a farewell to many past contributors, it has also meant a welcome to many new ones. We wish to thank all our authors, old and new, for their enthusiasm in the preparation of this volume.

MS
WJH

ABBREVIATIONS

5-BU	5-bromouracil
AAF/I, II	aggregative adherence fimbriae I, II
AB	*Adalia bipunctata* (bacterium)
ABC	ATP-binding cassette
ABS	Animal Biosafety Level
AC	adenylate cyclase
ACES	*N*-2-acetamido-2-amino-ethanesulphonic acid
ACIP	Advisory Committee on Immunization Practices
ACP	acyl carrier protein
ACT	adenylate cyclase toxin
ADA	adenosine deaminase
ADCC	antibody-dependent cellular cytotoxicity
ADH	arginine decarboxylase
ADP	adenosine diphosphate
AE	attaching and effacing (lesions)
AFA	afimbrial adhesin
AFB	acid-fast bacilli
AFIP	Armed Forces Institute of Pathology
Ag-EIA	antigen capture enzyme immunoassay
AGE	agarose gel electrophoresis
AGG	agglutinogen
AI	artificial insemination
AIDS	acquired immune deficiency syndrome
AMAN	acute motor axonal neuropathy
AMES	aminoglycoside-modifying enzymes
ANF	absolute non-fermenting
ANUG	acute necrotizing ulcerating gingivitis; acute necrotizing ulcerating gingivostomatitis
AOAC	Association of Official Analytical Chemists
AP	alkaline protease
APC	antigen-presenting cells; antigen-processing cells
APD	average pore diameter
APPCR	arbitrarily primed PCR
APS	adenosine 5′-phosphosulphate; adenyl sulphate
ARC	AIDS-related complex
ARDS	acute respiratory distress syndrome; adult respiratory distress syndrome
ASH test	antihyaluronidase test
ASK test	antistreptokinase test
ASO test	antistreptolysin O test
ASTPHLD	Association of State and Territorial Public Health Directors
ATCC	American Type Culture Collection
ATF	ambient temperature fimbriae
ATPase	adenosine 5′-triphosphatase
ATS	American Thoracic Society
BA	bacillary angiomatosis
BB	mid-borderline (leprosy)
BCG	bacille Calmette–Guérin
BCYE	buffered charcoal yeast extract
BFP	bundle-forming pilus
BG	Bordet–Gengou
BHI	brain–heart infusion
BI	bacterial index; biological indicator
BIG	botulism immune globulin
BL	borderline lepromatous (leprosy)
BLIS	bacteriocin-like inhibitory substances
BMT	bone marrow transplant
BOD	biochemical oxygen demand
BoNT	botulinum neurotoxin
BP	bacillary peliosis
BPASU	British Paediatric Association Surveillance Unit
BPI	bactericidal/permeability increasing protein
BPL	β-propiolactone
BSA	bovine serum albumin
BSK	Barbour–Stoenner–Kelly (medium)
BT	borderline tuberculoid (leprosy)
C1-inh	C1-inhibitor
CA	chorioallantoic
CAM	cell adhesion molecule
CAMP	Christie–Atkins–Munch-Petersen (test)
cAMP	cyclic adenosine 5′-monophosphate
CAP	catabolite gene activator protein (see also CRP)
CAPD	continuous ambulatory peritoneal dialysis
CBPP	contagious bovine pleuropneumonia
CCC DNA	covalently closed circular DNA
CCDC	Consultant in Communicable Disease Control
CCFA	cycloserine-cefoxitin-egg yolk-fructose agar
CCP	critical control point
CCPP	contagious caprine pleuropneumonia
CDC	Centers for Disease Control

CDP	cytidine 5′-diphosphonate
CDSC	Communicable Disease Surveillance Centre
CE	Chief Executive
CF	complement fixation; cystic fibrosis
CFA	complete Freund's adjuvant
CFA	cycloserine–egg yolk–fructose agar
CFA/I, II	colonization factor antigen I, II
cfu	colony-forming unit
CGD	chronic granulomatous disease
CHEF	contour-clamped homogeneous electric field electrophoresis
CHO	Chinese hamster ovary
CIE	countercurrent immunoelectrophoresis
CIN	cefsulodin–Irgasan–novobiocin
CLED	cysteine lactose electrolyte-deficient
CMA	cycloserine-mannitol agar
CMBA	cycloserine-mannitol blood agar
CMC	critical micelle concentration
CMGS	cooked meat medium containing glucose and starch
CMI	cell mediated immunity
CMP-NANA	cytidine-5′-monophospho-*N*-acetylneuraminic acid
CMR	chloroform–methanol residue
CMRNG	chromosomally resistant *Neisseria gonorrhoeae*
CMV	cytomegalovirus
CNA	Columbia colistin–nalidixic acid agar
CNS	central nervous system; coagulase-negative staphylococcus
CNW	catalase-negative or weakly reacting
COPD	chronic obstructive pulmonary disease
COVER	Cover of Vaccination Evaluated Rapidly
CP	capsular polysaccharides
CPHL	Central Public Health Laboratory
CR1	complement receptor type 1
CR2	complement receptor type 2
CRA	chlorine-releasing agent
CRD	chronic respiratory disease
CRE	catabolite responsive elements
CRF	coagulase-reacting factor
CRMOX	Congo red magnesium oxalate
CRP	cAMP receptor protein or catabolite gene activator protein (see also CAP); C-reactive protein
CRS	congenital rubella syndrome
CS1, 2, etc.	coli surface associated antigen 1, 2, etc.
CSD	cat scratch disease
CSF	cerebrospinal fluid
CT	cholera toxin
CTL	cytotoxic lymphocytes
CVD	Center of Vaccine Development
CWDF	cell wall deficient forms
DAEC	diffusely adherent *Escherichia coli*
DAF	decay-accelerating factor
DAP	diaminopimelic acid
DCA	deoxycholate–citrate agar
DCCD	*N,N*′-dicyclohexylcarbodiimide
DFA-TP	direct fluorescent antibody test for *Treponema pallidum*
DFAT-TP	direct fluorescent antibody tissue test for *Treponema pallidum*
DFD	dark, firm and dry
DGI	disseminated gonococcal infection
DHEA	dehydroepiandrosterone
DHFR	dihydrofolate reductase
DIF	direct immunofluorescence

dmfs	decayed, missing and filled surfaces (deciduous teeth)
DMFS	decayed, missing and filled surfaces (permanent teeth)
dmft	decayed, missing and filled teeth (deciduous teeth)
DMFT	decayed, missing and filled teeth (permanent teeth)
DN	double-negative
DNA	deoxyribonucleic acid
DNAase	deoxyribonuclease
DNP	2,4-dinitrophenol
DNT	dermonecrotic toxin
DoH	Department of Health
DOTS	directly observed therapy, short course
Dp	electrochemical potential
DRT	decimal reduction time; D value
DS	double-staining
DSB	double-strand break
DSO	double-strand origin
DST	Diagnostic Sensitivity Test
DT	definitive phage type
DTaP	diphtheria and tetanus toxoids and acellular pertussis vaccine
DTH	delayed-type hypersensitivity
DTP	diphtheria, tetanus, pertussis
dUMP	deoxyuridine 5′-monophosphate
E-Hly	enterohaemolysin
EAE	erythema arthriticum epidemicum
EAF	EPEC adherence factor
EAggEC	enteroaggregative *Escherichia coli*
EAST	enteroaggregative *Escherichia coli* heat-stable enterotoxin
EB	ethidium bromide
EBSS	Earle's balanced salt solution
EBV	Epstein–Barr virus
ECF-A	eosinophil chemotactic factor of anaphylaxis
ECP	extracellular products
ED	Entner–Doudoroff
EDTA	ethylenediaminetetraacetic acid
EF	oedema factor
EF-2	elongation factor 2
EGF	epidermal growth factor
EGTA	ethyleneglycol-bis(β-aminoethylether)-*N,N,N′,N′*-tetraacetic acid
EHEC	enterohaemorrhagic pathovar of *Escherichia coli*
EI, EII	enzyme I, enzyme II
EIA	enzyme immunoassay
EIEC	enteroinvasive *Escherichia coli*
ELISA	enzyme-linked immunosorbent assay
EM	environmental mycobacteria
EMB	eosin–methylene blue; ethambutol
EMC	encephalomyocarditis
EMJH	Ellinghausen, McCullough, Johnson, Harris (medium)
EMP	Embden–Meyerhof–Parnas
EMRSA	epidemic methicillin-resistant *Staphylococcus aureus*
EMS	ethylmethane sulphonate
ENL	erythema nodosum leprosum
EOP	efficiency of plating
EPEC	enteropathogenic *Escherichia coli*
EPHLS	Emergency Public Health Laboratory Service
EPS	expressed prostatic secretions; extracellular polysaccharides

ERCP	endoscopic retrograde cholangiopancreatography		HEPA	high efficiency particulate air
ERIC	enterobacterial repetitive intergenic consensus		HETES	monohydroxyeicosatetraeonic acid
			Hfr	high-frequency recombination
			HFT	high-frequency transduction
ERIC-PCR	enterobacterial repetitive intergenic consensus typing		HG	hybridization group
			Hib	*Haemophilus influenzae* type b
ERL	Epidemiological Research Laboratory		HiPIP	high potential iron protein
ESM	extended spectrum macrolide		HIV	human immunodeficiency virus
ESR	erythrocyte sedimentation rate		HLA	human major histocompatibility antigen
ET	electrophoretic type; enzyme type; epidermolytic toxin; erythrogenic toxin		HLT	heat-labile toxin
			HLY	haemolysin
ETA	exfoliatin A; exotoxin A		HMP	hexose monophosphate pathway
ETB	exfoliatin B		HMWP	high molecular weight protein
ETEC-ST	*Escherichia coli* producing heat-stable enterotoxin; enterotoxigenic *Escherichia coli*		HNIG	human normal immunoglobulin
			HPLC	high performance liquid chromatography
			HRF	homologous restriction factor
ETO	ethylene oxide		HSP, hsp	heat shock protein
ETS	exotoxin S		HSV	herpes simplex virus
ETZ	electron transparent zone		HT	haemorrhagic toxin
Ext-A	exfoliative toxin A		HTE	hamster trachea epithelial
FA	fluorescent antibody		HTIG	human tetanus immunoglobulin
FAD	flavin adenine dinucleotide		HTST	high temperature, short time
FAME	fatty acid methyl ester		HUS	haemolytic–uraemic syndrome
FAS	fluorescence actin-staining		IATS	International Antigenic Typing Scheme
FBP	ferrous sulphate, sodium metabisulphite and sodium pyruvate; fructose-1,6-biphosphate		IBK	infectious bovine keratoconjunctivitis
			ICAM	intercellular adhesion molecules
			ICC	Infection Control Committee
FD	ferredoxin		ICD	Infection Control Doctor
FDC	follicular dendritic cells		ICDDR,B	International Centre for Diarrhoeal Disease, Bangladesh
FHA	filamentous haemagglutinin			
FIGE	field inversion gel electrophoresis		ICMSF	International Committee on Microbiological Specifications for Food
FIRN	fimbriation-, inositol- and rhamnose-negative			
			ICN	Infection Control Nurse
FITC	fluorescein-isothiocyanate		ICS	intercellular spread
Fla	polar flagellum		ICSB	International Committee for Systematic Bacteriology
FMN	flavin adenine mononucleotide			
FnBP	fibronectin-binding protein		ICT	Infection Control Team
FP	flavoprotein		ICTV	International Committee for Taxonomy of Viruses
FPH2, FPH$_2$	reduced flavoprotein			
FT-IR	Fourier transform infrared		idt	indeterminate (leprosy)
FTA	fluorescent treponemal antibody		IE	infective endocarditis
FTA-ABS	fluorescent treponemal antibody-absorption (test)		IF	inactivation factor
			IFA	indirect fluorescent antibodies
GBS	Guillain–Barré syndrome		IFAT	indirect fluorescent antibody test
GDP	guanidine diphosphate		IFN	interferon
GLC	gas-liquid chromatography		IG	immune globulin
GLP	glycolipoprotein		Ig	immunoglobulin
GMCSF	granulocyte-macrophage colony-stimulating factor		IHF	integration host factor
			IJSB	International Journal of Systematic Bacteriology
GMP	guanosine 5′-monophosphate			
GMS	Gomori's methenamine silver nitrate		IL	interleukin
GPAC	gram-positive anaerobic cocci		IMIG	immune globulin intramuscular injection
GPIC	guinea pig eye inoculation with *Chlamydia psittaci*		IMP	inosine 5′-monophosphate
			IMS	immunomagnetic separation
GPL	glycopeptidolipid		INH	isoniazid
GTP	guanosine 5′-triphosphate		Ipa	invasion plasmid antigen
GUM	genitourinary medicine		IPS	intracellular polysaccharides
GVHD	graft-versus-host disease		IPV	inactivated poliovirus vaccine
HACCP	hazard analysis of critical control points		IR	intercept ratio; inverted repeat
HAP	haemagglutinin/protease		IS	insertion sequence
HAV	hepatitis A virus		ISCOM	immune stimulating complexes
HBIG	hepatitis B immunoglobulin		ISG	immune serum globulin
HBT	human blood bilayer Tween		ITU	intensive therapy unit
HBV	hepatitis B virus		IUCD	intrauterine contraceptive device
HCV	hepatitis C virus		IVD	intravascular device
HDP	hexose diphosphate (pathway)		IVDU	intravenous drug user
HE	haematoxylin–eosin		IVIG	immune globulin intravenous injection
HEA	Hektoen enteric agar			

IWGMT	International Working Group on Mycobacterial Taxonomy
JH	Jarisch–Herxheimer (reaction)
KDO	2-keto-3-deoxyoctonate; 2-keto-3-deoxyoctonic acid
KDPG	2-keto-3-deoxy-6-phosphogluconate
KIA	Kligler's iron agar
KID50	50% kidney infecting dose
KP	Kanagawa phenomenon
L–J	Lowenstein–Jensen
LAB	lactic acid bacteria
LAF	laminar air flow
Laf	lateral flagellum
LAL	*Limulus* amoebocyte lysate
LAM	lipoarabinomannan
LAMP	lipid-associated membrane proteins
LAO	lysine–arginine–ornithine
LAP	leucine aminopeptidase
Laz	lipid-associated azurin
LC	large colony
LCR	ligase chain reaction
LDC	lysine decarboxylase
LF	lactoferrin; lethal factor
Lf	lines of flocculation or flocculation units
LGV	lymphogranuloma venereum
LJP	localized juvenile periodontitis
LL	lepromatous (leprosy)
LLS	lipopolysaccharide-like substance
LOH	large, opaque, hazy edge
LOS	lipo-oligosaccharide
LP	lactoperoxidase
LPS	lipopolysaccharide
LT	*Escherichia coli* heat-labile toxin; lethal toxin; leukotriene
LTA	lipoteichoic acid
LTSF	low temperature steam with formaldehyde
LTT	lymphocyte transformation test
mA₂pm	*meso*-diaminopimelic acid (see also m-Dpm)
mAb	monoclonal antibody
MAC	membrane attack complex; *Mycobacterium avium* complex; *Mycobacterium avium–intracellulare* complex
MAFF	Ministry of Agriculture, Fisheries and Food
MAI	*Mycobacterium avium-intracellulare*
MALT	mucosa-associated lymphoid tissue
MAM	*Mycoplasma arthritidis* mitogen
MAP	major antigenic protein
MASPs	MBL-associated proteases
MAT	microscopic agglutination test
MBC	minimum bactericidal concentration
MBL	mannose-binding lectin; syn. MBP
MBP	mannose- or mannan-binding protein; syn. MBL
MCA	Medicines Control Authority
MCLO	*Mycobacterium chelonae*-like organisms
MCMP	major cytoplasmic membrane protein
MCP	membrane cofactor protein; monocytic chemotactic protein
MDP	muramyl dipeptide
m-Dpm	*meso*-diaminopimelic acid (see also mA₂pm)
MDR	multidrug resistance
MDR-TB	multidrug-resistant tuberculosis
MDT	multidrug therapy
MEE	multilocus enzyme electrophoresis; syn. MLEE

MEM	minimum essential medium
MGRSA	methicillin–gentamicin resistant *Staphylococcus aureus*
MHA-TP	microhaemagglutination assay for antibodies to *Treponema pallidum*
MHC	major histocompatibility complex
MI	morphological index
MIC	minimum inhibitory concentration
MICP	major iron-containing protein
MIF	microimmunofluorescence
MIP	macrophage infectivity potentiator
MK	menaquinone
MLEE	multilocus enzyme electrophoresis; syn. MEE
MLO	*Mycoplasma*-like organisms
MLP	mitral leaflet prolapse
MLS	macrolides, lincosamides and streptogramin B
MMO	methane mono-oxygenase
MMR	mass miniature radiology; measles, mumps and rubella
MNNG	*N*-methyl-*N'*-nitro-*N*-nitrosoguanidine; syn. NTG
MOEH	Medical Officer for Environmental Health
MOH	Medical Officer of Health
MOI	multiplicity of infection
MOMP	major outer-membrane protein
MOTT	mycobacteria other than tubercle
MP	mononuclear phagocyte
MPD	maximum pore diameter
MPL	monophosphoryl lipid A
MR	mannose-resistant; methyl red
MR/K	mannose-resistant *Klebsiella*-like
MR/P	mannose-resistant *Proteus*-like
MREHA	mannose-resistant and eluting haemagglutinin
MRM	murine respiratory mycoplasmosis
MRSA	methicillin-resistant *Staphylococcus aureus*
MRSE	methicillin-resistant *Staphylococcus epidermidis*
MRSP	mapped restriction site polymorphism
MRT	milk ring test
MS	mannose-sensitive; mutans streptococci
MSCRAMMs	microbial surface components recognizing adhesive matrix molecules
MSSA	methicillin-sensitive *Staphylococcus aureus*
MUG	methylumbelliferyl-β-D-glucuronidase
MuLV	murine leukaemia virus
MW	molecular weight
NAB	nucleic acid-binding
NAD	nicotinamide adenine dinucleotide
NADase	nicotinamide adenine dinucleotidase
NaDCC	sodium dichloroisocyanuric acid
NADPH	nicotinamide adenine dinucleotide phosphate (reduced) oxidase
NANAT	nalidixic acid, novobiocin, cycloheximide and potassium tellurite
NAP	*p*-nitro-α-acetylamino-β-propiophenone
NCCLS	National Committee for Clinical Laboratory Standards
NCHI	non-capsulate *Haemophilus influenzae*
NFA	non-fimbrial adhesins
NGU	non-gonococcal urethritis
NHS	National Health Service; normal human serum
NIBSC	National Institute of Biological Standards and Control
NIH	National Institutes of Health

NITU	neonatal intensive therapy unit	**PLC**	phospholipase C
NK	natural killer	**PLD**	phospholipase D
NMO	non-mobile	**PLET**	polymyxin–lysozyme–EDTA–thallous acetate
NNIS	National Nosocomial Infection Surveillance	**PLGA**	polylactic and polyglycolic acids
NPPC	*p*-nitrophenylphosphorylcholine	**PMC**	pseudomembranous colitis
Nramp	natural-resistance-associated macrophage protein	**PMF**	*Proteus mirabilis* fimbriae
		pmf	proton-motive force
NSAID	non-steroidal anti-inflammatory drug	**PMN**	polymorphonuclear leucocyte
NTG	*N*-methyl-*N*'-nitro-*N*-nitrosoguanidine; syn. MNNG	**PMS**	pyrolysis mass spectrometry
		PNG	polymorphonuclear neutrophilic granulocyte
NTM	non-tuberculous mycobacteria		
NVS	nutritionally variant streptococci	**PNH**	paroxysmal nocturnal haemoglobinuria
O-SP	O-specific polysaccharide	**PNS**	purple non-sulphur (bacteria)
O–R	oxidation–reduction	**POL**	physician's office laboratory
OA	oleic acid–albumin	**PPD**	Purified Protein Derivative of Tuberculin
OC	Outbreak Committee	**PPE**	porcine proliferative enteropathy
ODC	ornithine decarboxylase	**PPEM**	potentially pathogenic environmental mycobacteria
OE	outer envelope		
OF	oxidation–fermentation	**ppGpp**	guanosine 5'-diphosphate 3'-diphosphate
OM	outer membrane	**PPLO**	pleuropneumonia-like organisms
OMP	outer-membrane protein	**PPNG**	penicillinase-producing *Neisseria gonorrhoeae*
ONPG	*o*-nitrophenyl-β-D-galactopyranoside		
ONS	Office for National Statistics	**pppGpp**	guanosine 5'-triphosphate 3'-diphosphate
OPCS	Office of Population Censuses and Surveys	**PPV**	proportion of population vaccinated
OPV	oral polio vaccine	**PRAS**	pre-reduced anaerobically stabilized (media)
ORF	open reading frame		
ORT	oral rehydration treatment	**PRN**	pertactin
P-EI	phosphorylated enzyme I	**PROS**	pathogen-related oral spirochaete
P–V	Panton–Valentine (leucocidin)	**PRP**	polyribosephosphate
PA	protective antigen	**PS**	purple sulphur (bacteria)
PAF	platelet-activating factor	**PS/A**	polysaccharide adhesin
PAGE	polyacrylamide gel electrophoresis	**PSE**	pale, soft exudative
PAI	*Pseudomonas aeruginosa* autoinducer	**PSI**	photosystem I
PALCAM	polymyxin–acriflavine–lithium chloride–ceftazidime–aesculin–mannitol	**PSII**	photosystem II
		PSP	paralytic shellfish poisoning
PANTA	polymyxin, amphotericin, nalidixic acid, trimethoprim and azlocillin	**PT**	pertussis toxin
		Ptd	pertussis toxoid
Pap	pili associated with pyelonephritis	**PTS**	phosphoenolpyruvate phosphotransferase system
PAP	primary atypical pneumonia		
PAS	*p*-aminosalicylic acid; periodic acid–Schiff	**Pva**	polyvinyl alcohol
PBP	penicillin-binding protein	**PVE**	prosthetic valve endocarditis
PCF	putative colonization factor	**PYG**	peptone–yeast extract–glucose
PCP	*Pneumocystis carinii* pneumonia	**PYR**	pyrrolidonyl-β-naphthylamide
PCR	polymerase chain reaction	**PZA**	pyrazinamide
PCV	proportion of cases in the vaccinated	**QAC**	quaternary ammonium compound
PDH	pyruvate dehydrogenation complex	**r-det**	resistance determinant
PE	elastase	**RAG**	recombinant activating gene
PEA	phenylethyl alcohol agar	**RAPD**	random amplified polymorphic DNA fingerprinting
PEP	phosphoenolpyruvate		
PFGE	pulse field gel electrophoresis	**RaRF**	Ra reactive factor
Pfk	phosphofructokinase	**RAS**	Ribi Adjuvant System
pfu	plaque-forming unit	**RBP**	rose bengal plate
PG	prostaglandin	**RC**	rolling circle
PGI₂	prostacyclin	**RCA**	regulation of complement activation
PGL-I	phenolic glycolipid I	**RCCS**	random cloned chromosomal sequence
PGP	polyglycerophosphate	**rDNA**	DNA coding for RNA
PGU	post-gonococcal urethritis	**REA**	restriction endonuclease analysis
PHA	passive haemagglutination assay; poly-β-hydroxyalkanoate	**REAC**	restriction endonuclease digestion of chromosome DNA
		REAP	restriction endonuclease digestion of plasmid DNA
PHB	poly-β-hydroxybutyrate		
PHLS	Public Health Laboratory Service	**rep-PCR**	repetitive element polymerase chain reaction
PHMB	polyhexamethylene biguanide		
PI	gonococcal protein; propamidine isethionate; protein I	**REP-PCR**	repetitive extragenic palindromic element typing
PID	pelvic inflammatory disease		
PK-TP	PK-*Treponema pallidum*	**rEPA**	*Pseudomonas aeruginosa* exoprotein A
Pla	plasminogen activator protease	**RFLP**	restriction fragment length polymorphism

RGM	rapidly growing mycobacteria
RH	relative humidity
RIM	Rapid Identification Method
RIT	rabbit infectivity testing
RMAT	rapid microagglutination test
RMSF	Rocky Mountain spotted fever
RNA	ribonucleic acid
RNAase	ribonuclease
RNI	reactive nitrogen intermediate
ROI	reactive oxygen intermediate
RPLA	reversed passive latex agglutination
RPP	rapid progressive periodontitis
RPR	rapid plasma reagin
rRNA	ribosomal RNA
RSS	recurrent non-typhoidal salmonella septicaemia
RST	reagin screen test
RSV	respiratory syncytial virus
RT	ribotyping
RTD	routine test dilution
RTF	Reduced Transport Fluid; resistance transfer factor
RTX	repeats in toxin
SAF	sodium acetate–acetic acid–formalin; Syntex Adjuvant Formulation
SAK	staphylokinase
SAL	sterility assurance level
SARA	sexually acquired reactive arthritis
SASP	small acid-soluble protein
SAT	standard tube-agglutination test
SBA	sheep blood agar
SC	secretory component; small colony
SCID	severe combined immunodeficiency
SCIEH	Scottish Centre for Infection and Environmental Health
SDA	strand displacement amplification
SDH	succinate dehydrogenase
SDS	sodium dodecyl sulphate
SDS-PAGE	sodium dodecyl sulphate polyacrylamide gel electrophoresis
SE	staphylococcus enterotoxin
SE-A	staphylococcus enterotoxin A
SE-C	staphylococcus enterotoxin C
SFG	spotted fever group
ShET	*Shigella* enterotoxin
SHHD	Scottish Home and Health Department
SIDS	sudden infant death syndrome
SIM	sulphide–indole–motility
SIRS	systemic inflammatory response syndrome
SLE	systemic lupus erythematosus
SLT	Shiga-like toxin; syn. VT
SMAC	sorbitol MacConkey
SMD	smooth domed (colony morphology)
SMG	'Streptococcus milleri group'
SMT	smooth transparent (colony morphology)
SNAP	synaptosomal-associated protein
SOD	small, opaque, defined border; superoxide dismutase
SPA	species-specific surface protein antigen
SPE	streptococcal pyrogenic exotoxin
SPEA	streptococcal pyrogenic exotoxin A
SPG	sucrose phosphate glutamate
SPS	sodium polyanethol sulphonate
SRS	slow-reacting substance
SRS-A	slow-reacting substance of anaphylaxis
SRSV	small, round structured virus
SS	salmonella–shigella (agar); Stainer–Scholte (medium)

SSB	single-strand break
SSSS	staphylococcal scalded skin syndrome
SSU	small subunit
ST	*Escherichia coli* heat-stable toxin
STD	sexually transmitted disease
STM	signature tagged mutagenesis
STP	standard plate count
SXT	co-trimoxazole; sulphamethoxazole–trimethoprim (see also TMP–SMX)
TA	transaldolase
TAP	transporters associated with antigen processing
TBW	tracheobronchial washings
TCA	tricarboxylic acid; trichloroacetic acid
TCBS	thiosulphate–citrate–bile salts–sucrose
TCF	tracheal colonization factor
TCH	thiophen-2-carboxylic acid hydrazide
TCID	tissue culture infective dose
TCR	T cell receptor
TCT	tracheal cytotoxin
Td	diphtheria toxoid
TDE	transmissible degenerative encephalopathy
TDH	thermostable direct haemolysin
TDHT	5-thyminyl-5,6-dihydrothymine
TDM	trehalose dimycolate
TDP	thermal death point
TDT	thermal death time
TeTx	tetanus toxin
TF	transferrin
THF	termination host factor
TK	transketolase
TMP–SMX	trimethoprim–sulphamethoxazole (see also SXT)
TNase	thermonuclease
TNF	tumour necrosis factor
TOC	total organic carbon
TPGY	trypticase–peptone–glucose–yeast extract
TPHA	*Treponema pallidum* haemagglutination
TPI	*Treponema pallidum* immobilization
TPP	thiamine pyrophosphate
TRH	thermostable related toxin
TRUST	toluidine red unheated serum test
TSB	trypticase–soy broth
TSI	triple sugar iron (agar)
TSST-1	staphylococcal toxic shock toxin-1; toxic shock syndrome toxin-1
TT	tetanus toxoid; tuberculoid
TTP	thrombotic thrombocytopenic purpura
TWAR	Taiwan acute respiratory
UCA	uroepithelial cell adhesin
UCNC	unclassified catalase-negative coryneform
UHT	ultra-heat-treated
UMP	uridine 5'-monophosphate; uridylic acid
UNDP	undecaprenol phosphate
UPGMA	unweighted pair-group method with arithmetic averages
UPTC	urease-positive subgroup
USR	unheated serum reagin
UTI	urinary tract infection
VAMP	vesicle-associated membrane protein; vesicle-associated protein
VB	voided bladder urine
VD	venereal disease
VDRL	Venereal Disease Research Laboratory
VE	vaccine efficacy
VEE	Venezuelan equine encephalomyelitis
VFA	volatile fatty acid
VOMP	variable outer-membrane protein

VP	Voges–Proskauer	**VZV**	varicella zoster virus
VPI	Virginia Polytechnic Institute	**WC-BS**	whole cell B subunit
VSC	volatile sulphur compounds	**XLD**	xylose–lysine–deoxycholate
VT	verotoxin; syn. SLT	**XMP**	xanthosine 5′-monophosphate
VTEC	Vero cytotoxin-producing *Escherichia coli*; verotoxigenic *Escherichia coli*	**YPM**	*Yersinia pseudotuberculosis*-derived mitogen

BACTERIA AS PATHOGENS: HISTORICAL INTRODUCTION

M T Parker

1 **Pathogenicity and virulence**	3 **Antimicrobial agents**
2 **Immunity**	4 **The laboratory in the diagnosis and control of bacterial diseases**

The clinical and epidemiological study of communicable diseases was an essential preliminary to the recognition of microbes as pathogens. As early as the sixteenth century Fracatorius pointed out that certain clinically recognizable contagious diseases spread in different ways; though this gave him no clue to the nature of causative agents, it carried an implication of their multiplicity. Early in the nineteenth century, clinical studies of several communicable diseases led to their being recognized as specific entities. For example, investigation of the continuous fevers led Schönlein in 1839 to make a clear distinction between typhoid fever ('typhus abdominalis') and typhus fever ('typhus exanthematicus'). This cleared the ground for William Budd, an English country physician, to elucidate the epidemiology of typhoid fever by field studies performed in the 1850s, some 30 years before Eberth discovered its bacterial cause.

We have described (Volume 2, Chapter 1) the slow and at times unwilling acceptance by scientists of the mid-nineteenth century of Pasteur's evidence that fermentation was a consequence of the multiplication of micro-organisms and his belief that this provided a valid analogy for communicable diseases in animals and humans. The constant association of recognizable micro-organisms with specific diseases, evidence for which had been accumulating since the 1830s, was held to be consistent with a cause–effect relationship. This 'germ theory of disease' was finally justified in the 1880s, at least in respect of a number of bacterial diseases, after Koch had shown how to grow the organisms in pure culture outside the body and, in favourable instances, to reproduce their pathogenic effects by injecting them into animals.

1 PATHOGENICITY AND VIRULENCE

The term 'pathogenicity' came to be applied to the ability of certain sorts of bacteria to cause disease, but it was observed that individual strains in such a group might vary in this respect, i.e. in their 'virulence' (Miles 1955). Thus Davaine in 1872 had observed the enhancement of virulence on serial passage in animals and Pasteur in 1877–81 its attenuation on prolonged artificial culture. It was soon established that healthy persons had a rich surface flora of microbes. In 1886 Theodor Escherich described the organisms now known as *Escherichia coli* and *Klebsiella pneumoniae* in the faeces of normal babies. He subsequently recognized the ability of such coliform bacteria to cause urinary tract infection and considered the possibility that they might be responsible for infantile diarrhoea. Soon, members of well recognized pathogenic species, e.g. typhoid bacilli, were found in the faeces of healthy persons who appeared not to have suffered a clinical infection. Clearly the line of demarcation between pathogens and non-pathogens was not clear cut.

Some pathogens caused disease in a proportion of physically intact subjects who did not possess specific immunity (see p. 3). Others, a more numerous class, sometimes referred to as **opportunist pathogens**, did so only if the body's surface was breached by trauma or disease or its immunity system was damaged or deficient. Events of the First World War, notably widespread gunshot injury and malnourishment, stimulated interest in the inverse relationship between the pathogenicity of the infecting organism and the susceptibility of the host (see Miles 1955).

1.1 Virulence factors

The mechanisms of bacterial pathogenicity have proved to be various and to be related to the possession of a multiplicity of products and activities referred to as virulence factors.

Toxins

It was shown early (1888–90) that certain pathogens, e.g. the diphtheria and tetanus bacilli, formed extracellular toxic materials that reproduced the effects of the disease when injected into animals. Soon the number of such known exotoxins had increased greatly, and streptococci, staphylococci and clostridia were found to produce an imposing array of proteins and enzymes that damaged experimental animals in a variety of ways. Much later and with greater difficulty a number of exotoxins associated with diarrhoeal diseases were discovered. However, many demonstrably pathogenic bacteria did not produce exotoxins: these included gram-negative organisms that were toxic for animals when killed whole cultures were given by injection. In the 1930s these were found to form cell-bound toxic material, endotoxin, later shown to be a lipopolysaccharide (see Volume 2, Chapter 1). This is now recognized as the main cause of death in a wide range of infections, giving rise to fever, activation of complement by the alternative pathway, intravascular clotting and the formation of cytokines. Similar effects produced by severe infection with gram-positive bacteria are less clearly related to a particular component of the bacterial body. The question had to be addressed: how could an organism gain entry to the body, overcome the local defences and multiply sufficiently to produce enough toxic substance to damage the host? The leucocidal action of a number of bacterial exotoxins was a likely contributor; this effect was demonstrated in staphylococci in 1894 by van de Velde and subsequently shown to be caused by at least 3 of the exotoxins of *Staphylococcus aureus*. Leucocidins were later described in many other pathogens.

Non-toxic determinants of virulence

Bail, in a series of papers in 1900–04, drew attention to the presence in bacterial exudates of substances that, though not necessarily themselves toxic, aided the establishment of invasive infection; these he called aggressins. Investigations in the 1920s and 1930s, described in Volume 2 (see Volume 2, Chapter 1), identified several substances the ability of which to act as determinants of virulence could be inferred from the fact that antisera to them gave protection against infection with the corresponding organism. These included the capsular polysaccharides of pneumococci and the M proteins of *Streptococcus pyogenes*. Both inhibited phagocytosis; whereas the pneumococcal capsule formed a thick mechanical barrier and denied access of complement to the surface of the organism, the M protein formed only a thin surface layer but nevertheless prevented opsonization. It is now thought to hinder the access of complement by binding fibrinogen to the streptococcal surface.

Other pathogens have since been found to possess surface components associated with virulence, many of them polysaccharides. These included the K antigens of enterobacteria and the capsular polysaccharides of *Haemophilus influenzae* and *Neisseria meningitidis*. Actions attributed to them were various; in addition to inhibition of phagocytosis, these sometimes included antigenic mimicry of host tissue conferring immunity to defence mechanisms and resistance to the lytic action of complement. Hyaluronic acid capsules, described in streptococci in the 1930s, are of uncertain significance as virulence factors because the organisms generally form hyaluronidase at some stage of the growth cycle. This illustrates the difficulty of relating the in vitro production of supposed virulence factors to what happens in the body.

The role in pathogenesis of loose extracellular slime not aggregated around individual bacteria has been recognized more recently. Dextrans formed by oral streptococci contribute to the formation of dental plaque and so might be looked upon as determinants for dental caries and gingivitis. Slime-forming coagulase-negative staphylococci are now believed to initiate the formation of 'vegetations' on prosthetic devices. The alginate slime of mucoid strains of *Pseudomonas aeruginosa* appears to aid colonization of the respiratory tract in cystic fibrosis patients.

Adhesins

Interest has recently concentrated on structures that enable bacteria to adhere to mucous surfaces, such as those of epithelial cells of the respiratory, alimentary and urogenital tracts, as the first stage of the pathogenic process: adhesins. Fimbriae or pili, first described in the 1940s, were early associated with the adhesion of free-living organisms to surfaces. Their role in pathogenesis was established when it was shown that adhesion to epithelial cells of the gut was essential for the production and absorption of the enterotoxins of *E. coli*. This was first demonstrated by H W Smith and Linggard in 1971 with a fimbriate strain responsible for diarrhoea in piglets. Other fimbrial colonization factors have since been demonstrated in strains responsible for diarrhoea in various mammals, including humans. Receptors for them are usually present in a narrow range of hosts. Fimbrial adhesins have since been described in gonococci and meningococci. The flagella of the cholera vibrio may also be looked upon as a virulence factor, enabling the organism to penetrate the mucous layer to reach the epithelial surface and there form enterotoxin.

Other protein adhesins associated with virulence are found in the outer cell membrane, where they are closely associated with the lipopolysaccharide. This is true of strains of *Shigella* and *Shigella*-like strains of *E. coli* which invade and kill gut epithelial cells. Many of the protein adhesins, whether fimbrial or outer membrane in situation, have proved to be encoded on plasmids; indeed this property facilitated their recognition. Less is known of the role of adhesion in the pathogenicity of gram-positive bacteria, but Beachey and colleagues have produced evidence that the adhesion of *S. pyogenes* to pharyngeal epithelial cells is mediated by lipoteichoic acids attached to the cell membrane but protruding to the cell surface; fibronectin is the receptor for these.

ANTIGENIC VARIATION

Some bacteria avoid the host's immune defences by antigenic variation. It was recognized in the 1920s that recrudescences of relapsing fever were associated with reinvasion of the bloodstream by mutant borreliae after the development of an antibody response to the original strain. Gonococci have recently been shown to possess at least 2 mechanisms for altering their surface antigens and so attaining a similar end.

INTEGRATION OF THE ACTION OF VIRULENCE FACTORS

From the point of view of a micro-organism possessing it, pathogenicity is a means of enhancing transmission to fresh hosts and thus the long-term survival of the strain. The ideal virulence factor is not one that leads to the death of the host, but one that maximally enhances and prolongs infectivity. In the simplest of life cycles, a pathogen needs a variety of activities: to be able to enter the host, defeat its immunity mechanisms, multiply, break out of the host again, survive in the world outside, and restart the process; and many life cycles are much more complex than this.

These considerations explain the apparent excess of virulence factors found in many pathogens; several enzymes with apparently the same function, 2 enzymes with opposite actions, and so on. Finlay and Falkow (1989) have reviewed recently acquired information about how micro-organisms regulate their manifold activities, 'switching' them on and off in response to chemical and physical signals received from their surroundings.

For general accounts of bacterial pathogenicity, see Mims (1987) and Finlay and Falkow (1989).

2 IMMUNITY

Immunology was born of the study of how animals, by natural or artificial means, become immune to microbial infections or to the toxins of micro-organisms. For as long as there are written accounts of infective diseases it was recognized that recovery is often accompanied by acquired resistance, and there are many reports through the centuries of attempts to induce immunity by bringing about infection artificially. Variolation, i.e. prophylactic immunization against smallpox by attempting to induce a mild attack of the disease itself, though a hazardous procedure, had been widely practised from ancient times in Asia and the Middle East. The first step to a safer procedure was the substitution for smallpox material of inocula derived from the lesions of cowpox, a much milder disease, as practised, for example, in the 1770s by the Dorsetshire farmer, Benjamin Jesty. The first methodical investigation of the hypothesis that cowpox prevented smallpox was made by the Gloucester physician, Edward Jenner, whose memoir 'An enquiry into the causes and effects of the variola vaccinae' was published in 1798.

Between 1877 and 1881, Pasteur applied the principle of vaccination successfully to the prevention of chicken cholera and animal anthrax by giving injections of living cultures the virulence of which had been attenuated. In 1889, Pfeiffer in Koch's laboratory showed that the immune response to bacterial vaccines was highly specific. The year before, Roux and Yersin, associates of Pasteur, had given the first account of a bacterial exotoxin, and in 1890 Koch's pupils Behring and Kitasato showed that animals given injections of such a toxin developed immunity to it (see Table 1 in Volume 2, Chapter 1).

2.1 Cellular defences

The Russian zoologist, Elie Metchnikoff (1845–1916) (Fig. 1.1), was the first to recognize the significance of phagocytosis in resistance to microbial invasion of tissues. In his earliest experiments in 1883, he inserted rose thorns in the body cavity of starfish larvae and saw that they were soon surrounded by collections of motile cells. Then, in *Daphnia*, he observed the engulfment and destruction of fungal spores both by blood leucocytes and by fixed connective tissue cells. Next year he began experiments on vertebrates and described phagocytosis of anthrax bacilli and other organisms by leucocytes in rabbits. In a series of lec-

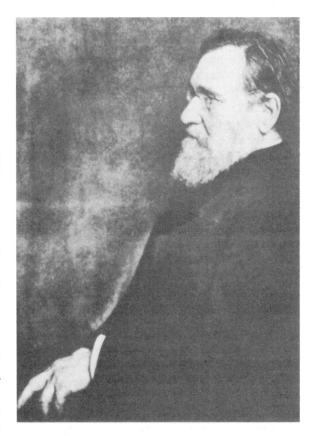

Fig. 1.1 Élie Metchnikoff. (From a photograph of 1907 by Nicola Perscheid. Courtesy of The Wellcome Trustees).

tures in 1891 Metchnikoff summarized his belief that immunity was primarily cellular. This view did not receive general acceptance, mainly because it appeared to conflict with emerging evidence for humoral immunity mechanisms (see section 2.2). However, early in the twentieth century the conflict between the cellular and humoral theories of immunity was partially resolved; the importance of phagocytosis by leucocytes and the role in it of serum factors were accepted. However, it was not until over 50 years after Metchnikoff's first publication that mechanisms of cellular immunity independent of serum factors were recognized (see p. 7).

2.2 Humoral defences

Nuttall in 1888 had shown that some species of bacteria were killed by the defibrinated blood of certain animals, and one year later Buchner found not only that cell-free serum was bactericidal but also that it ceased to be so after being heated at 50°C for 1 h. Another humoral defence was described by Behring and Kitasato in 1890: the serum of animals rendered immune to tetanus by repeated injections of toxin specifically neutralized it. In 1894 Pfeiffer and Isaeff announced that, when cholera vibrios were introduced into the peritoneal cavity of guinea pigs, they were dissolved. That the lysis of the vibrios was independent of cells was shown in 1895 by Bordet (Fig. 1.2), who defined 2 agents, both present in the serum of immunized guinea pigs, that were necessary for this effect: one was relatively heat-stable and specific for the cholera vibrio, and the other easily destroyed by heating to 55°C. The first, not always present in normal serum, appeared in large amounts in response to immunization; the other was present in any normal serum. The first sensitized the vibrios to the lytic action of the second; or, in modern terminology, the vibrios were sensitized by specific antibody present in antiserum, and lysed by complement (see section on 'Complement', below). Bordet further noticed that the antiserum clumped the vibrios before lysis occurred. This was the phenomenon of agglutination by antibody, first studied in detail by Gruber and Durham in 1896. By 1897 Kraus had established that filtrates of cultures of the plague bacillus and of the cholera vibrio formed a precipitate with antisera from an immunized animal and that the reaction was specific.

ANTIGENS AND ANTIBODIES

The heat-stable serum constituents responsible for these in vitro effects were called antibodies and the substances stimulating their formation were called antigens. By the early years of the twentieth century, reactions between antigen and antibody could be detected by tests for precipitation, agglutination, neutralization of toxins and sensitization of microbes to the action of complement.

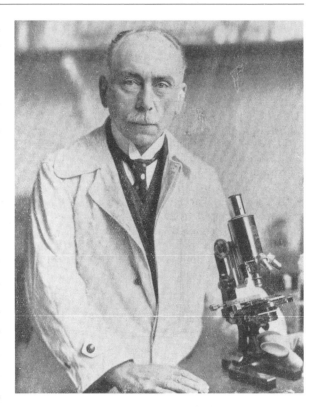

Fig. 1.2 Portrait of Jules Jean Baptiste Vincent Bordet in old age. (Courtesy of the Wellcome Institute Library, London).

COMPLEMENT

Bordet's observations in the last years of the nineteenth century had established the existence of the heat-labile component of normal serum that we now call complement, and in 1901 Bordet and Gengou set out the principles of the complement fixation test in which the disappearance of complement was used to detect the occurrence of an antigen–antibody reaction. Later it became clear that complement was not a single substance but that the term described a sequence of events that began when a serum component reacted with an antigen–antibody complex. These events, generally referred to as 'activation', formed a cascade-like series of enzymatic changes in the serum proteins; the manifold consequences of this included important beneficial effects on the host, such as the elimination of micro-organisms by lysis or opsonization, but also harmful effects, as in certain allergic reactions. In the 1950s Pillemer and his colleagues showed that many complement-like effects were independent of antibody, and that the later stages of the complement 'cascade' might be activated, through what is known as the 'alternative pathway', by many different substances, including microbial components, thus bypassing the stage of combination of antibody with antigen.

ACTIVE AND PASSIVE IMMUNIZATION

In the early decades of the twentieth century the specific antibody response was widely exploited for the treatment and prevention of bacterial diseases: by passive immunization (giving injections of human or animal serum containing the appropriate antibody) or active immunization (inducing the subject to form the antibody). In either case, success could be expected only if the antibody in question had protective activity. This consideration caused no difficulty in the prevention or treatment of diseases attributable to a single protein exotoxin, such as diphtheria and tetanus. Here the problem was how to give sufficient toxin to induce a brisk antibody response without harming the subject. Detoxification with formaldehyde ('toxoiding') was applied to tetanus toxin by Eisler and Löwenstein in 1915 and to diphtheria toxin by Glenny in 1921. Vaccines of killed whole organisms had been prepared from an early date on empirical principles in the hope that among the antibodies formed there would be at least one with protective activity. In 1897 Almroth Wright began antityphoid vaccination with heat-killed organisms and this procedure was used widely in the British Army. Its value was for a long time considered questionable, but a series of large-scale controlled trials in the 1950s and 1960s showed it to be moderately effective. A notable application of Pasteur's principle of using live vaccines of organisms of attenuated virulence was the BCG vaccine against tuberculosis, introduced by Calmette and Guérin in 1921.

Glenny and coworkers showed in 1926 that the addition of alum to diphtheria toxin enhanced antibody production. Later it was found that the addition of various irritant substances to the inoculum had a similar effect. Freund's powerful adjuvant, described in the 1940s, is an oily emulsion containing dead tubercle bacilli or mycobacterial lipid.

For a general account of the early development of immunization methods, see Parish (1965).

2.3 Hypersensitivity: delayed and anaphylactic

The introduction of microbes, or of soluble antigens such as toxins, into the animal body did not always induce increased immunity to the microbes or the toxin. Jenner in 1798 had observed that persons immunized with cowpox responded to a second inoculation of cowpox material into the skin by an exaggerated inflammatory reaction. In 1890 Koch described an analogous form of this hypersensitivity, in which guinea pigs infected with tubercle bacilli responded with an intensified inflammatory reaction to a local injection of more tubercle bacilli. A similar reaction, taking some 12–24 h to reach maximum intensity, occurred when soluble material from the tubercle bacillus, later termed tuberculin, was injected; the same amount of tuberculin was not toxic for normal animals.

Another form of hypersensitivity, first observed in 1894, occurred during immunization with certain animal products. When many doses of antigen were injected at intervals of several days, one of the later injections sometimes induced a severe and often fatal reaction. Unlike the response of the tuberculous guinea pig to tuberculin, the response of these animals occurred immediately after the injection. This paradoxical effect was studied in detail by Portier and Richet in 1902 and named anaphylaxis by them. The 2 types of hypersensitivity reaction, the one delayed in time and the other immediate, were distinguishable in another respect. Delayed hypersensitivity could not be induced in normal animals by the serum of hypersensitive animals but the immediate anaphylactic hypersensitivity was transferable in this way. This operational distinction between the 2 types of hypersensitivity reaction – passive transfer respectively by lymphoid tissue and by serum – proved to be of major importance in defining the processes of immunization at the cellular level.

2.4 The antibody response

Specificity

The outstanding feature of both immunization and hypersensitivity was the specificity of the result. In general, an antibody induced by a particular antigen reacted most strongly, and often exclusively, with the inducing antigen. Paul Ehrlich (1854–1915) (Fig. 1.3) in his 'side chain theory', advanced in 1897, postulated a chemical affinity between surface structures on the antigen and complementary groups ('receptors') on host cells; union of the 2 stimulates the cells to produce more receptors, i.e. antibody. An important element in Ehrlich's concept was the recognition that, in order to stimulate antibody production, an antigen had to be 'foreign' to the animal being immunized. For a general account of the work of Ehrlich, see Marquardt (1949).

Generally speaking, substances with antigenic properties appeared to be large molecules, such as proteins, but not all large molecules were antigenic. Purified bacterial polysaccharides, for example, though possessing antigenic specificity, did not stimulate antibody production, i.e. they were haptens (see Volume 2, Chapter 1). The first clue to the chemical nature of specificity came in 1906 from the experiments of Obermayer and Pick, who modified the surface of serum proteins by introducing nitro groups or iodine, and found that the modified antigens induced the formation of antibodies that were to a large extent specific for the nitro group or iodine. In 1914 Landsteiner showed that a wide variety of artificially introduced chemical groups would alter the specificity of antigens. From 1923 onwards, Heidelberger and Avery, in classic studies of pneumococcal type antigens, showed that their specificity was determined by differences in the composition of their capsular polysaccharides.

Nature of antibodies

Many workers from 1907 onwards found that antibody activity was associated with the serum globulins. Ultracentrifugation by Heidelberger and Pedersen in 1937 and electrophoresis by Tiselius and Kabat in 1938 showed that antibodies were in the slow-moving globulin fraction.

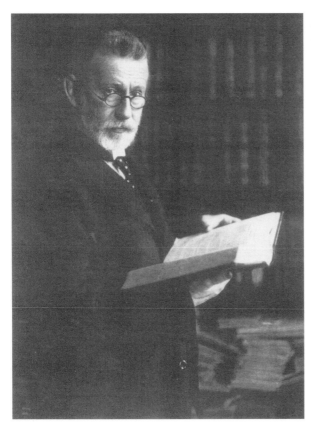

Fig. 1.3 Portrait of P Ehrlich in his study, by Alfred Krauth. (Courtesy of the Wellcome Institute Library, London).

By the 1950s antibodies had been recognized as belonging to one of the 5 classes of serum globulins described by Tiselius in 1927. Of these, immunoglobulin M is the principal component of the primary immune response and immunoglobulin G of the secondary response. Immunoglobulin E is associated with one form of hypersensitivity. Immunoglobulin A is found in 2 forms, one in serum and the other (secretory immunoglobulin A) principally on mucous surfaces of the respiratory, genital and alimentary tracts where it constitutes an important defence against entry into the body of foreign antigens.

COMBINATION OF ANTIGENS AND ANTIBODIES

The nature of this was only slowly elucidated. Ehrlich, in the 1890s, demonstrated its quantitative nature in the reaction of diphtheria toxin and antitoxin, and Ramon, in 1923, reported that optimum flocculation and neutralization of the toxin took place with a fixed proportion of antitoxin. Three years later, Dean and Webb showed that optima of this kind indicated the equivalence of antibody and antigen, but that the 2 might combine in varying proportions.

From Heidelberger's pioneer chemical analysis of specific precipitates in 1929 it became evident that molecules of both antigen and antibody were multivalent and, as Marrack first proposed, precipitates of the 2 were primarily bound in a lattice of interlinked antibody and antigen molecules.

ANTIBODY TYPES: B AND T CELLS

As early as 1898, Pfeifer and Marx suggested that antibody was formed by lymphoid tissues, but this was not clearly established until the 1940s. A major advance in the following decade was the distinction between 2 cellular systems in lymphoid tissues: bursacytes (B cells), which responded with the production ultimately of antibody, and thymocytes (T cells), which on stimulation by antigen initiated the reaction of delayed hypersensitivity and the activation of macrophages to greater microbicidal activity. Both systems of cells, when already sensitized by a particular antigen, responded vigorously to further experience of it by means of cells endowed with a specific memory for making that response. The B and T systems have proved to be more complex than is indicated above; each has subsidiary functions, including inhibitory effects that operate in the regulation of the immune response.

FORMATION OF ANTIBODIES

We have alluded to Ehrlich's view that the union of the antigen with receptors ('side chains') on the surface of cells led to the overproduction of similar receptors, which were released into body fluids as antibody. Ehrlich apparently thought that the receptors, normally concerned with attaching nutrient substances to the cell, could also attach a wide variety of different chemical substances which, if antigenic, could elicit a corresponding variety of antibodies. An opposite notion, that antibody-forming cells had a general synthetic mechanism which, in the presence of an antigen, used the antigen as a template and so produced antibody with a configuration complementary to and therefore specific for it, was proposed in 1930 by Breinl and Haurowitz. For some years this 'template' hypothesis, that antigens 'instructed' the cell about the kind of antibody it was to make, held the field. In 1955, however, Jerne proposed a mechanism which was a return to Ehrlich's notion of an already formed combining site for each of a wide variety of antigenic configurations found in nature; in Jerne's view, the preformed sites were on the serum globulin molecules. An injected antigen combined with its appropriate globulin, and the resulting complex was carried to the antibody-forming cells, which were then stimulated to produce globulins with the same configuration.

Soon after, Burnet extended the suggestion by postulating that the attachment of the required diversity of combining sites, and therefore of the cells carrying them, arose as the result of some mutations of the antibody-forming cells, and that the attachment of antigen to an appropriate site stimulated the cell to replicate, and so gave rise to a population of descendants, a clone, all of which produced antibody of the same specificity. Of the 2 rival theories of antibody formation, the **instructive** and the **selective**, the selective hypothesis as currently refined is now firmly established.

Porter's demonstration of an invariant portion of the antibody molecule and a hypervariable region that combines with antigen provided a structural basis for Jerne's postulates (Jerne 1974). With about 10^8 different regions in the lymphocytes, hypervariable by DNA recombination or somatic mutation, each capable of dealing with several antigens, it is clear that any possible molecular shape can be recognized. Six reactive groups, called idiotypes, 3 on the light and 3 on the heavy chains, presumably each stimulate antibody, the anti-idiotype, thus forming a network of antibody and anti-antibody in an equilibrium, which is disturbed in the direction of greater specific immunity by the introduction of exogenous antigen.

2.5 Cellular immunity

In 1942 Landsteiner and Chase, in experiments on delayed hypersensitivity, showed that lymphoid tissues, in addition to their role as source of antibodies, participated directly in immune reactions. Lymphocytes from an animal made hypersensitive to a particular antigen would, on transfer to a normal animal, make it hypersensitive to the same antigen. This, the first proof that a form of specific immune reactivity could be transferred passively to an animal by a cell, was a decisive advance toward the rehabilitation of Metchnikoff's thesis of the overriding importance of cells in immune reactions. In the same year, Lurie made an equally decisive advance in the same direction by showing that phagocytic macrophages from rabbits immunized against tubercle bacilli in circumstances that excluded the participation of antibody had a greater power than normal macrophages of killing the tubercle bacilli they ingested.

2.6 Monoclonal antibodies

The discovery that B cells may give rise to myelomata that are monoclonal in respect of the type of globulin they secrete opened up an entirely new field of study in the 1970s. Variants of a particular myeloma cell selected so as to produce no immunoglobulin are hybridized with lymphocytes from the spleen of an animal already stimulated with antigen and the hybridoma selected which, when grown in tissue culture or in the peritoneal cavity of an animal, will give rise to one type of antibody. Clones can be selected to yield antibody specific for a single antigenic determinant or for as much of an antigen as is desired. Monoclonal antibodies have been exploited in the making and purification of antigens and in the production of diagnostic antisera. Whether they will yield safe and potent therapeutic agents has yet to be established.

2.7 The immune response to tissues

Although it had been argued plausibly that the chief function of the immune response in the higher animals is protection against parasitic microbes, it was recognized early that it might have other equally important biological functions. Ehrlich had realized that the immune system responded only to substances 'foreign' to itself. If, however, an aberrant cell or substance arose in or was introduced into the body, the immune system might bring about its destruction or elimination. In the earlier part of the twentieth century this aspect of the immune system, as a monitor of deviations from the norm, received considerable attention, particularly in relation to cancer. In retrospect, however, this can be seen to have been fruitless because it was thought of largely in terms of humoral immunity. Landsteiner and Chase's demonstration of the carriage by lymphocytes of specific immune reactivity had far-reaching consequences in this respect. As Freund first demonstrated convincingly in 1953, the reaction of the host to 'foreign' material resembled closely that of delayed hypersensitivity.

The same kind of response occurs in tissue transplantation. Grafts are rejected by a mechanism which was shown by Medawar, first in 1958, to be another instance of the delayed hypersensitivity reaction, being immunologically specific in relation to the antigen of the grafted tissue and being mediated by lymphocytes carrying the immune reactivity.

2.8 Immune tolerance

Medawar's studies of graft rejection also brought into prominence the phenomenon of immune tolerance. He took advantage of the fact that the lymphoid tissue of an animal does not begin to mature into a system capable of immune responses until about the time of birth. When cells from a particular strain of mice, for example, were injected into fetal mice of a different genetic constitution, these mice, on reaching maturity, accepted grafts from the donor mice which they would otherwise have rejected. According to an extension of Jerne's hypothesis of antibody formation by clonal selection, any somatic mutant cell with specificity for the donor cell that arises in the maturing lymphoid tissue combines with the donor antigens present and is suppressed before it can grow into a substantial reactive clone of cells with that specificity. The recipient mouse thus remains permanently indifferent to foreign antigens introduced at this stage of its development. In the same manner, it was argued that all the mouse's own tissue substances with potentialities as antigens that have access to the maturing lymphoid system would suppress any mutant lymphoid cells with corresponding specificities. Thus the adult animal is indifferent to its own potential antigens, the state of affairs implied in Ehrlich's 'horror autotoxicus'.

The concept of immune tolerance had practical importance in relation to the task of transplanting tissues and organs from one human being to another, since the problem of making a graft acceptable was clearly seen as one of inducing, temporarily at least, an indifference to the foreign antigens of the graft.

2.9 Applications in medical microbiology

Four periods can be discerned in the application of immunology to the prevention and treatment of microbial diseases.

1   From early times until the 1880s, various attempts were made, some of them highly successful, to induce immunity to microbial diseases by bringing about a modified attack of the disease itself or of a related but milder infection. This ceased to be the only available means of inducing specific immunity with the observation in 1886 that injections of killed bacterial cultures had a similar effect. Nevertheless, new roles for live vaccines have continued to be found.

2   In the period 1890–1935 the main objectives of intervention were to administer specific antibodies or to induce the body to form them (p. 4 and 5). The most striking successes were with diseases caused by a bacterial exotoxin. From the 1890s on, killed vaccines of whole organisms were widely used on empirical grounds but without clearly defined immunological objectives. Critical assessment of them was not possible until the 1950s and 1960s when large-scale controlled trials were used to measure the amount and duration of protection afforded by typhoid and whooping cough vaccines.

3   In the 1940s there was a temporary loss of interest in the body's immune mechanisms as more and more bacterial infections were found to be susceptible to chemotherapy and antibiotic treatment, but this state of affairs did not last long. Difficulties caused by resistance to the new agents, and a growing awareness of the increased susceptibility to microbial diseases of patients with inherited or acquired immunodeficiency, rekindled interest in the body's specific defence mechanisms. Advances made in the 20 years after World War II, particularly in knowledge of the differing roles of T and B lymphocytes and of tissue immunity, made it possible to pinpoint the causes of many immunodeficiency diseases and even to propose treatments for some of them.

4   The new knowledge of the immune system, at first a minority interest that appeared to concern only a few patients with rare inherited diseases, began to move centre stage with the widespread introduction of treatments in which immunosuppression was an integral part or an inevitable side effect. An important objective was to learn how to limit or modulate this so that the minimum of harm is done in achieving the objectives of the treatment. Then, in the 1980s, the AIDS epidemic presented the problem of immunodeficiency as a consequence of a viral infection that had attained world-wide distribution. In the present state of knowledge the only recourse seems to be to seek means of preventing or eliminating the initiating viral infection and palliating the effects of the microbial complications as they appear.

3   ANTIMICROBIAL AGENTS

3.1   Chemotherapy

Paul Ehrlich has justly been described as the father of chemotherapy. As early as 1879 he had conceived the idea that chemical substances differed in their affinity for living cells. This led him to search for substances that would interfere with the metabolism of parasites at concentrations that would not damage the metabolism of host cells. He observed that methylene blue, known as a useful stain for malaria parasites, had some therapeutic action in malaria. In 1891, however, under the influence of Behring's discovery of bacterial antitoxins, he abandoned chemotherapy and devoted his energies to developing his 'side chain theory' of antibody production. In 1902 he returned to the search for chemotherapeutic agents, screening through the multitude of new organic chemicals being produced by the German dye industry. Making use of the experimental model of trypanosomiasis in rodents, he discovered the effects of trypan red and later of the organic arsenical atoxyl. Acting on the erroneous view that spirochaetes were related to trypanosomes, he then embarked on a screening of chemical relatives of atoxyl for curative action on experimental syphilis in rabbits and so discovered salvarsan, which he showed in 1910 to be effective in the treatment of human syphilis.

The next 20 years yielded a meagre harvest of therapeutically useful chemicals: hexamine and mandelic acid for infections of the urinary tract and chalmoogra oil for leprosy. Early in the twentieth century a number of inhibitory agents produced by bacteria were shown to inhibit the growth of other bacteria in vitro (see Florey et al. 1960), but attempts to obtain potent preparations of these bacteriocins that could be safely administered to patients failed. It was therefore not surprising that Fleming's brief account in 1929 of a diffusible antibacterial substance produced by a mould, *Penicillium*, attracted little immediate attention.

In the mean time, German scientists continued to test new organic chemicals for therapeutic action, and in 1935 Domagk gave a brief report that the red dye Prontosil cured experimental infections with haemolytic streptococci in laboratory animals. Next year Colebrook and Kenny demonstrated the strong therapeutic effect of Prontosil on severe puerperal streptococcal infections. Prontosil, though active therapeutically, did not inhibit streptococci in vitro, and it was soon shown that it was converted in the body into the colourless compound *p*-aminobenzene sulphonamide. This was the active agent, which inhibited streptococci by blocking the utilization of the related compound *p*-aminobenzoic acid, an essential nutrient for the organism. In 1938, Ewins and Whitby found that another sulphonamide, sulphapyridine, was a more potent agent with a broader spectrum of action on bacteria (see Foster 1970). There followed a rapid exploitation of sulphonamide derivatives, but in 1942 outbreaks of infection with sulphonamide-resistant streptococci were already being reported; by the later years of World War II the widespread prevalence of resistant strains in military camps was compromising the use of sulphonamides.

3.2 Antibiotics

THE PENICILLINS

While Fleming's agent from *Penicillium* was temporarily forgotten, Dubos in New York began a systematic search among soil organisms for agents that inhibited pyogenic cocci, and in 1939 he discovered tyrothricin, a mixture of antibiotics formed by a *Bacillus*. At about the same time, work on Fleming's agent, subsequently to be called penicillin, was resumed by Florey's team in Oxford, and in 1940 Chain and his colleagues succeeded in making a stable preparation of it. By 1943 it was being produced on an industrial scale and the antibiotic era had begun.

Within 2 years staphylococci highly resistant to penicillin had become prevalent in many hospitals in which the antibiotic was being used lavishly. Mary Barber and her colleagues in London showed that this was not because resistant mutants arose in patients being treated with penicillin; patients and staff were being colonized by already resistant staphylococci which had a selective advantage in persons whose sensitive flora was inhibited by exposure to the antibiotic. These resistant strains formed a penicillin-destroying enzyme, penicillinase. It was later established that penicillinase-forming staphylococci had been isolated and placed in a culture collection several years before Chain had made his first preparations of the antibiotic. Thus penicillinase production was a resistance mechanism awaiting a new man-made destiny.

In the late 1950s the penicillin molecule was modified to yield an antibiotic (methicillin) resistant to the action of staphylococcal penicillinase. Soon after it came into use in Britain staphylococci resistant to it were detected. This type of resistance was non-enzymic but it was found almost exclusively in strains that formed large amounts of penicillinase. It proved to be a broad spectrum tolerance for β-lactam antibiotics that was fully expressed only at temperatures well below 37°C. In the 1960s a number of methicillin-resistant staphylococci were isolated in Poland at a time when no methicillin had been imported into the country. These facts suggest that 'methicillin resistance' in staphylococci may be a supernumerary mechanism for survival in the presence of β-lactam antibiotics in general, useful to an organism establishing itself on a skin surface before it had had the opportunity to secrete much penicillinase. If so, excessive use of all β-lactam antibiotics in the 1980s may have helped to select methicillin-resistant staphylococci.

Resistance to penicillins, either enzymic or non-enzymic, is now widespread in many bacterial groups. A notable exception is *S. pyogenes*, which has continued to be highly sensitive to penicillins despite over half a century of heavy exposure to them.

OTHER ANTIBIOTICS

In 1944 streptomycin was introduced and soon afterwards several other unrelated antibiotics: chloramphenicol, the tetracyclines and the macrolides, all with rather broad spectra of activity on bacteria. This greatly extended the range of diseases that were treatable, and the range was further increased by the chemical manipulation of naturally occurring antibiotics. However, over the years, resistance has appeared to virtually every widely used antibiotic, and strains resistant to one or more antibiotics have appeared in most important pathogens. In a few situations, as in the prolonged treatment of tuberculosis with streptomycin and other agents, resistant mutants appeared often in the infecting strain during the course of treatment. With most other organisms, however, including nearly all those responsible for septic and diarrhoeal diseases, resistance was not seen until the agent had been in use for some time, even a number of years. When first encountered, the resistant organisms belonged to a single identifiable strain which then became widely disseminated in the population; later resistance appeared in other strains.

MULTIPLE-ANTIBIOTIC RESISTANCE

Very soon it became apparent that resistances to unrelated agents were tending to become aggregated in a minority of members of a particular bacterial species, and that these 'multiresistant' strains were establishing themselves endemically in hospital populations. The 'hospital staphylococci' of the 1950s and 1960s were nearly all profuse formers of penicillinase and had separate genetic determinants for several resistances, usually on plasmids. So it seemed that, at this time, the association of these resistances was ecological rather than genetic and was attributed to the selective advantage conferred by multiresistance to an organism liable to encounter a variety of antibiotics in a short time.

A different situation was revealed in outbreaks of drug-resistant bacillary dysentery in the general population of Japan; in 1963 Watanabe and coworkers reported that the resistance of the causative shigellae to several agents was encoded on a single plasmid that was transferable by cell-to-cell contact in the presence of a resistance transfer factor. Similar systems of resistance transfer were soon found in a wide range of gram-negative bacteria. These often mediated the transfer of resistance determinants between members of different species or even genera, and various mechanisms were identified for the recombination of genes and their movement from plasmid to chromosome and back again. The outcome of this genetic mobility was to increase the diversity of resistances in both potential pathogens and commensals. However, whatever the means of transmission of resistance determinants between bacteria, the frequency of resistant bacteria in a human and animal population appeared to be determined mainly by the selective advantage resistance conferred to the organism when the antibiotic was present and transmission of infection between members of the population could take place easily.

By the 1960s it was generally realized that the growing problems of resistance to antimicrobial agents were in the main attributable to the combined effects of selection of resistant organisms and their subsequent spread to fresh hosts. These processes were repeatedly demonstrated in studies of septic infections in hospital patients and later also in relation to diarrhoeal diseases in the general population. Similar situations were found in herds of animals maintained to provide food for man; excessive exposure to antibiotics given prophylactically as a substitute for hygienic rearing or to stimulate growth resulted in a formidable accumulation of multiresistant organisms in poultry, pigs and cattle.

Limiting the spread of antibiotic-resistant bacteria in hospitals now seems, in the broadest terms, to be a matter of restraint in the use of antimicrobial agents and improving hospital hygiene, both objectives easier to state than to implement. Only in the special case of domiciliary treatment of tuberculosis can increasing resistance be attributed to inadequate or uncompleted treatment schedules.

4 THE LABORATORY IN THE DIAGNOSIS AND CONTROL OF BACTERIAL DISEASES

4.1 The beginnings

Bacteriology applied to medicine began in the workrooms of Pasteur and Koch, where they and their pupils established the basic techniques of cultivating bacteria and obtaining pure cultures of them (see Volume 2, Chapter 1). When Koch moved to Berlin in 1880 to join the Prussian Government's preventive medicine organization, the Kaiserliches Gesundheitsamt, one of his first tasks was to put the action of chemical disinfectants on a firm scientific basis. But soon, while Koch transferred his attention to tuberculosis, his pupils, notably Behring, were exploiting the humoral response to bacteria and by 1890 had demonstrated the action of diphtheria and tetanus antitoxins. Controversy about the curative efficacy of diphtheria antitoxin led the Government to set up in 1896 near Berlin an institute for testing the potency of antisera under the directorship of Paul Ehrlich. In 1897 he published precise standards to be adhered to by makers of diphtheria antitoxin, based on a reference dried antiserum. Park, in extensive studies in New York between 1896 and 1900, showed that the passive immunization of contacts with diphtheria antitoxin was a valuable preventive measure. Agglutination tests for serum antibodies as a means of confirming the diagnosis of typhoid fever were described in 1895 by Durham and by Gruber, and their findings were confirmed by Widal in the next year. The complement fixation test for syphilis described by Wassermann and coworkers in 1906 was at first thought to be a means of detecting antibody to the causative treponeme. This proved not to be the case, though paradoxically the test was a fairly reliable means of confirming the diagnosis of syphilis. Its importance was to be greatly enhanced 4 years later when syphilis became the first bacterial disease to be treatable by a chemotherapeutic agent. In the early years of the twentieth century, too, Robert Koch organized a large collaborative study in southwest Germany which established the role of the typhoid carrier in the genesis of epidemics of enteric fever. Thus, by this time, the main lines of development of public health and clinical bacteriology had been laid down.

4.2 Detecting pathogenic bacteria

Koch had little difficulty in establishing the bacterial aetiology in a number of diseases in which the causative organism was present in pure culture in the blood or an internal organ, or even in cholera, in which a morphologically recognizable organism was a prominent member of the gut flora. In many diseases in which the site of the lesion was at or near the body surface, it was very difficult to decide which of the many organisms present was the pathogen. This is well illustrated by the lengths to which Eberth and Gaffky had to go in 1880–81 to detect the typhoid bacillus in the intestine and mesenteric glands of patients with enteric fever (see Foster 1970, pp. 75–7). Once it was possible to grow bacteria on solid media, colonial form was sometimes of help, but not much in this case. In 1889, Theobald Smith began to accumulate biochemical markers for the typhoid bacillus, noting its anaerogenic attack on glucose, and others soon followed. In 1889, Conradi and Drigalski described the first combined selective indicator medium on which the typhoid bacillus formed non-lactose fermenting colonies recognizable by their colour; many other organisms were inhibited. In 1942, Pollock and colleagues adopted from soil bacteriologists the principle of enrichment in a liquid medium which encourages the growth of the pathogens, in this case salmonellae, but not of many other bowel organisms. Plating on a selective medium, sometimes preceded by enrichment, was widely used for the isolation of many other sorts of pathogen. Selective agents included dyes and heavy metals, and latterly also antibiotics and other antibacterial agents. The initial stage in the identification of a pathogen was colonial recognition, aided by changes brought about in or around the colony that indicated one or more of the organism's phenotypic characters. After checking the morphology of the organisms in the indicated colony, rapid preliminary tests, such as slide agglutination, could be used to establish a provisional identification. Then, subculture to a non-selective medium was made to secure a pure culture before applying more leisurely confirmation tests.

In the early decades of the twentieth century, diagnostic bacteriology was a labour-intensive 'cottage industry' requiring considerable skill and experience. Media had to be prepared at frequent intervals from primary ingredients such as fresh meat and other animal products; media tended to vary in performance from laboratory to laboratory and also over time. Unexpected difficulties, such as heavy-metal contamination of distilled water from copper stills, might lead to inhibition of growth from small inocula. Media in containers with cotton-wool plugs had a short shelf-life. This situation changed dramatically in the 1930s when bacteriologists adopted the screw-capped bottle as the standard container for media and McCartney set up a central organization to supply bulk media for the laboratories of London's municipal hospitals. Soon, dehydrated bulk media, including a number that had been difficult to prepare consistently, became available commercially.

Further industrialization of diagnostic bacteriology occurred in the 1960s with the 'kit revolution'. Plastic strips of media-containing cupules containing a variety of substrates greatly reduced the labour of routine identification. The results of computer-assisted taxonomic studies made it possible to give confidence limits for identifications provided by patterns of positive and negative test results. Despite the manifest advantages of the newer identification methods, there were potential dangers from their overenthusiastic application of technological 'deskilling' and corner-cutting, notably by omitting time-consuming procedures such as regular microscopic examination of isolates and checks for their purity.

GROWTH REQUIREMENTS OF PATHOGENS

By the 1940s efficient anaerobic jars were appearing in routine laboratories and the less fastidious anaerobes were receiving attention. The specific nutritional and gaseous requirements of certain pathogens, e.g. haemophili, brucellae, were known. It was often difficult to distinguish between an apparent requirement for a 'rich' medium containing fresh animal products and the need to neutralize toxic constituents of the medium. Satisfaction of the need for certain lipids made it possible to grow tubercle bacilli and leptospires in otherwise quite simple liquid media.

By the 1960s, improved knowledge of growth requirements led to overconfidence among bacteriologists, who tended to equate failure to cultivate a causative bacterium with absence of a bacterial cause. This view was shaken by later events. Intensive studies by enterobacteriologists had failed to reveal one of the most common causes of acute diarrhoea, a micro-aerophilic curved gram-negative bacillus now called *Campylobacter jejuni*. The key observation, by Butzler and colleagues in 1973, was that these organisms could be separated from other intestinal organisms by their ability to pass through a 0.65 μm Millipore filter; if their gaseous requirements were met they would grow freely on ordinary laboratory media. Ten years later, Warren and Marshall in Australia disposed of the widely held view that the human stomach contents are essentially sterile. They identified another curved micro-aerophilic organism, *Helicobacter pylori*, as the cause of chronic gastritis, probably of peptic ulceration, and perhaps of gastric carcinoma. An even more remarkable situation came to light in 1977 when a common-source outbreak of pneumonia occurred in Philadelphia; McDade and his colleagues succeeded with difficulty in showing that the cause was a gram-negative bacillus now placed in the genus *Legionella*. Though normally an inhabitant of water supplies, this organism appears to satisfy its very fastidious growth requirements by parasitizing free-living amoebae. The tick-borne disease erythema chronica migrans was first recognized clinically in 1909 and is now known to be a widespread zoonotic disease of man. Its cause, a borrelia with complex growth requirements, was first cultivated in 1986. It seems unlikely that bacteriologists have yet reached the end of the road opened up by Koch.

It would be premature to attempt an assessment of recent advances in molecular genetics, such as the polymerase chain reaction, on the practice of diagnostic bacteriology.

4.3 Detecting 'marker' organisms

We may use the presence of an identifiable non-pathogen as a 'marker' for a pathogen that is difficult to detect or found only intermittently. The presence of *E. coli* in drinking water is the best example of this. Largely as a result of the work of Alexander Houston at the beginning of the twentieth century, it came to be accepted that this indicated a chance that enteric pathogens from the same source as the *E. coli* might survive in the water. The justification for this is that *E. coli* is constantly present in human excreta and that it and the enteric bacilli disappear from natural waters at about the same rate.

Methods of determining the 'most probable number' of coliform bacilli from the examination of a number of tubes containing measured volumes of water were placed on a firm statistical base by Greenwood and Yule in 1917. Tubes that yielded coliform bacilli were submitted to more specific tests for *E. coli*. Tests for *E. coli* to establish the safety of milk and other foodstuffs lack the intellectual legitimacy of the water tests.

4.4 Quantitative culture

Estimating the number of potential pathogens in samples collected from patients plays a limited part in clinical bacteriology. The one situation in which it is of vital importance is in the recognition of urinary tract infection. Samples of urine are liable to become contaminated in the course of collection with bacteria similar to those that commonly cause infection. These multiply rapidly in urine at ambient temperature. Uncertainty about the interpretation of urine cultures was partially resolved by the conclusion of Kass and his colleagues in 1956 that a count of 100 000 organisms per ml or more on a sample of urine, collected with specified precautions against contamination and cultured promptly, was 'significant' of infection. It should be emphasized that what set this limit was the ability of a competent nurse to collect a sample containing less that 100 000 organisms per ml from an uninfected patient; it is freely conceded that occasional urinary tract infections, notably with *Staphylococcus saprophyticus*, may give lower urine counts.

4.5 Typing

Members of a bacterial species, traditionally characterized by a general conformity of phenotypic characters (see Volume 2, Chapter 1) may be subdivided by differences in one class of characters: serotyping, bacteriophage typing, bacteriocin typing. John Smith of Aberdeen, in 1931 and 1933, was the first person to use a typing method to obtain evidence of the probable source and route of spread of a pathogen; he serotyped by slide agglutination isolates of *S. pyogenes* from patients with puerperal pyrexia and their attendants. Similar studies by Allison and Brown of hospital-acquired secondary infection in patients with scarlet fever followed in 1937. In 1936 Craigie and colleagues began developing a method of typing typhoid bacilli on the basis of susceptibility to lysis by a series of adaptations of a bacteriophage active only on strains possessing the Vi antigen. Felix subsequently developed the method further into a system for world-wide surveillance. Later, other typing systems based on susceptibility to arbitrarily selected and unadapted phages were developed for other salmonellae. A similar phage-typing system for *S. aureus*, described by Wilson and Atkinson in 1945 and standardized by Williams and Rippon in 1952, has been widely applied to studying the acquisition of staphylococcal infection by hospital patients. Typing systems based on a variety of other sorts of character have since been described.

The use of typing methods has been of great value in studies of the transmission of infection, particularly in hospitals, but their application has from time to time been marred by failure to understand that, though membership of different types provides good evidence for a lack of epidemiological relationship between isolates, membership of the same type never affords certainty of such a relationship. Indeed, if a type is common, membership of it by 2 strains will often be fortuitous. As early as 1956, Anderson and Williams expressed the view that the main value of typing was to exclude irrelevant isolates, so that the others belonging to the same type as the index strain could be investigated for relations to it in time and place of isolation.

4.6 Serological evidence of infection

In 1907 Dreyer followed up the earlier observations of Durham, Gruber and Widal by showing how to measure the amount of antityphoid antibody in the serum of enteric fever patients: suspensions of typhoid bacilli were mixed with progressive dilutions of serum in tubes and the end point or titre of agglutination determined. After the distinction between H and O agglutination had been made by Weil and Felix in 1917 it was possible to begin relating the antigenic structure of the various enteric bacilli to the antibodies they elicited and to distinguish antibody formed in the current illness from that attributable to earlier infection or vaccination. However, it was often necessary to examine paired sera collected at an interval to decide this issue. In the 1930s Felix showed that agglutinins against the surface Vi antigen of the typhoid bacillus provided a means of identifying chronic typhoid carriers.

The importance of agglutination tests in the diagnosis of enteric fever declined after 1945 as methods of isolating salmonellae improved and it was realized that effective antibiotic treatment inhibited the specific antibody response. Tests for Vi antibody continued to be of use in predicting the future infectivity of symptomless excreters of typhoid bacilli.

In the antibiotic era there has been a general decline in the importance of serodiagnostic tests. Their use now tends to be confined to the recognition of certain chronic bacterial diseases, such as brucellosis, and of other infections coming late to diagnosis. Serological tests for syphilis retain their importance but the Wassermann and Kahn-type tests of the early twentieth century have largely been superseded by tests for specific antitreponemal antibodies.

4.7 Skin reactions

The tuberculin skin test of Koch (p. 5) was soon recognized as a hypersensitivity reaction indicating previous experience of the mycobacterium. In 1913, Schick described a skin test that was interpretable in the contrary sense: a positive reaction indicating susceptibility to diphtheria toxin and a negative reaction immunity to it attributable to circulating antitoxin. The original use of the test to detect persons already immune to diphtheria lost importance when active immunization ceased to be a hazardous procedure.

The so-called Dick test of 1921, a skin reaction to the injection of a filtrate of *S. pyogenes*, was introduced as a means of detecting susceptibility to the erythrogenic toxin and therefore to scarlet fever. This interpretation was called into question by Kim and Watson in 1970, who revived the view expressed by Dochez and Stevens in 1927 that a positive reaction was an allergic response to past experience of the streptococcus. The virtual disappearance of severe scarlet fever from Europe and North America makes it unlikely that this controversy will be resolved.

4.8 The control of antibiotic treatment

When sulphonamides were first used it was on clinical indications of their probable therapeutic effect. Testing bacteria for their in vitro susceptibility to antimicrobial agents first became common after the introduction of penicillin, and early methods were derived from those used by Florey's Oxford team to measure the strength of antibiotic preparations. First, a standard inoculum of a test organism (the 'Oxford staphylococcus') was added to serial dilutions of antibiotic and the mixture incubated; the end point of the test was the smallest amount of antibiotic that prevented the appearance of turbidity. The process could be reversed to test other organisms for their susceptibility to the antibiotic, which was reported as the minimum inhibitory concentration (MIC) of the antibiotic for the organism (in μg ml^{-1}).

However, the MIC was not accepted universally as a guide to optimal dosage. In some circumstances, it was argued, the preferred goal should be total destruction of the bacteria, and the minimum bactericidal concentration was more relevant to this. It was also observed that, in the case of penicillinase-forming staphylococci the MIC of penicillin varied widely with the size of the inoculum and was of little value as a guide to dosage.

In any event, the demand for antibiotic susceptibility tests became so great that bacteriologists soon opted for a less labour-intensive procedure than the tube-dilution MIC method. Heatley, a member of Florey's Oxford team, had placed antibiotic-containing solutions in porcelain cylinders sealed to the surface of agar plates that had previously been seeded with a standard inoculum. After incubation, the size of the zone of inhibition of growth around the cylinder, caused by the diffusion of antibiotic, provided a measure of antibiotic activity, or, in parallel tests on the test organism and the Oxford staphylococcus, an indication of their relative susceptibility to the antibiotic. Alternatively, the antibiotic was placed in a hole punched in the agar medium or applied on a paper disk or in a tablet.

Agar diffusion tests are now usually performed with antibiotic impregnated paper disks, by one of several approved methods. Whichever method is used, the purpose is to detect organisms with significantly greater resistance to the antibiotic than a standard sensitive organism; either the standard organism is tested in parallel with the culture under examination or results obtained previously in tests of the standard organism under identical conditions provide data for comparison. The test conditions for the respective methods are so specified that organisms can be allocated to categories: 'sensitive' and 'resistant', or 'sensitive', 'intermediate' and 'resistant', according to the diameter and character of the inhibition zone, and that this will predict the action of the agent in an infected patient. It may sometimes be legitimate to equate zone sizes approximately to MIC values, but not if the organism can destroy the agent enzymatically.

Resistance mechanisms can be looked upon either (1) as aids to the survival of an organism in the presence of an antibacterial agent or (2) as a means of preventing clinical cure by the agent. In the interpretation of disk diffusion tests there are potential confusions of objective between (1) separating distinct populations of sensitive and resistant organisms and (2) identifying organisms with 'clinically significant' resistance.

REFERENCES

Finlay BB, Falkow S, 1989, Common themes in microbial pathogenicity, *Microbiol Rev*, **33**: 210–30.

Florey HW, Chain E et al., 1960, *Antibiotics*, Oxford University Press, London.

Foster WD, 1970, *A History of Medical Microbiology and Immunology*, Heinemann, London.

Jerne NK, 1974, Towards a network theory of the immune system, *Ann Inst Pasteur Immunol (Paris)*, **125C**: 373–89.

Marquardt M, 1949, *Paul Ehrlich*, Heinemann, London.

Miles AA, 1955, The meaning of pathogenicity, *Mechanisms of Microbial Pathogenicity*, 3rd Symp Soc Gen Microbiol, eds Howie JW O'Hea AJ, 1–16.

Mims CA, 1987, *The Pathogenesis of Infectious Diseases*, 3rd edn, Academic Press, London.

Parish HJ, 1965, *A History of Immunization*, Livingstone, Edinburgh.

NON-SPECIFIC RESISTANCE TO INFECTION

D M MacLaren

1 INTRODUCTION

Humans share their environment with countless microbial species, many of which have adopted, or are able to adopt, a parasitic mode of life. Within days of birth the human infant begins to be colonized by a rich and diverse commensal flora the composition and numbers of which, although showing fluctuations under the influence of hygiene, hormones and diet, remain broadly constant throughout life. This colonization is not a state of mutual indifference but can best be described as one of uneasy neutrality. Whatever benefits it confers on its host (see p. 16), the commensal flora poses 2 threats. Many of its members possess in varying degrees potential pathogenicity and constantly cross the mucosal boundaries at random into the inner tissues where they are rapidly removed. This removal is non-specific in that the phagocytic cells involved are not programmed to remove particular invaders and their ability to do so is not improved on subsequent contact. By contrast, specific immunity is directed against particular pathogens and elimination is enhanced by earlier contact. The second threat is colonization of other than the usual sites, e.g. the small intestine where colonization disrupts host physiology and leads to malabsorption. For these reasons the commensal flora must be kept within circumscribed bounds. In addition, the human host has to contend with encounters with pathogenic microorganisms against which acquired immunity has not yet been developed. Humans have acquired many non-specific mechanisms of resistance (Table 2.1). Before discussing the ways and means of non-specific resistance, some general factors that have a bearing on resistance to infection are reviewed.

Table 2.1 Factors that contribute to non-specific resistance to infection

Genetic factors
Nutrition
Commensal flora
Physical barriers
Natural antibodies
Iron limitation
Acute phase proteins
Phagocytic cells

2 GENERAL FACTORS

2.1 Genetics

Genetic inheritance probably plays a role in most infections, although in the individual it seems overshadowed by other aspects and its influence is not easily discerned. Nevertheless, infection has been a powerful selective force throughout the ages. Resistance to falciparum malaria shown by those with the sickle-cell trait is a clear example of this selection; this unfavourable sickle gene pool has been maintained in malarious regions (Hill 1992).

2.2 Nutrition

Malnutrition, which usually means deficiencies in protein, carbohydrate, vitamins and essential trace elements such as zinc, has a deleterious effect on the immune system. In the developing world malnutrition primarily affects the young, whereas in the developed world it is the elderly or those suffering from underlying debilitating disease who are affected. Malnutrition impairs cell mediated immunity and, more importantly for non-specific immunity, results in reduced concentrations of complement components. T cells are reduced in number, especially CD4 cells, whereas B cells are relatively spared so that antibody levels remain largely normal (Chandra 1993).

2.3 Age

Age influences the efficiency of host defences and at both extremes of life the immune system functions less well. The neonate shows a constellation of subnormal immunological parameters: neutrophils that function less well and a marrow reserve that is much less than in the adult. Moreover, specific antibody derived from the mother may be just adequate; prematurity results in even lower levels. Complement is also suboptimal (Berger 1990). In old age the immune system shows the senescence seen in other organs; cellular immunity is most affected (Saltzman and Peterson 1987).

2.4 Stress

Whether psychological or physical, stress adversely affects the immune response (Peterson et al. 1991, Cohen, Tyrrell and Smith 1991).

3 FIRST LINES OF DEFENCE

3.1 Physical barriers

These form an important line of defence. For example, the skin is impenetrable to most organisms and its outer dry layers, its low pH and the presence of fatty acids make it an inhospitable environment for bacteria other than adapted species (Jenkinson 1992). The continual shedding of skin squames with adherent bacteria reduces the microbial load. Should the integrity of the skin be compromised by disease, such as eczema, then it is commonly secondarily infected. The mucous membranes form a less formidable barrier, but are lined with mucus to which bacteria and viruses adhere. Mucus with entrapped bacteria is swept away by the cilia of the ciliated respiratory mucosa or the villi in the intestine. The flushing effect of bodily secretions reduces the microbial flora and, for example, the stream of relatively acid urine keeps the urinary tract free of micro-organisms as does the copious flow of secretions in the small intestine. Any slowing of the urinary flow increases the chance of ascending infection; diseases that interfere with intestinal motility, such as scleroderma, promote colonization of the small intestine and consequent malabsorption. Saliva teeming with oral bacteria flows to the back of the throat and is swallowed; gastric acidity destroys most swallowed bacteria.

3.2 Chemical factors

The barrier defences of skin and mucous membranes are reinforced by the presence of antibacterial substances. Lysozyme, an enzyme that degrades bacterial peptidoglycan, is present in most secretions. Saliva contains antibacterial H_2O_2. This peroxide, produced largely by commensal oral streptococci and other catalase-negative bacteria, in the presence of salivary peroxidase, oxidizes thiocyanate to give the bactericidal hypothiocyanite (Thomas and Aune 1978). The low pH of the stomach and vagina is inimical to most bacteria; cholera infection occurs more readily in association with achlorhydria (Nalin et al. 1978). The use of inhibitors of gastric acid production to prevent stress ulcers in seriously ill patients has the drawback that the stomach becomes colonized by gram-negative bacteria that form a source for pharyngeal colonization and possible aspiration pneumonia, especially in patients receiving assisted respiration (Driks et al. 1987).

3.3 Immunoglobulins

All classes of immunoglobulins have been detected on mucous membranes, but IgA is the most important because it is present in the greatest amounts. In addition, IgA is a dimer linked by a secretory part that not only aids transport but renders it more resistant to proteolytic enzymes in secretions. IgA is not usually involved like IgG in complement-mediated killing, but impedes adherence, an essential first step in bacterial colonization.

3.4 Commensal flora

This protects the host from colonization by pathogenic bacteria by a variety of mechanisms:

1 competition for available food and tissue receptors
2 production of toxic substances, such as fatty acids, or antagonistic substances, such as bacteriocins
3 keeping the immune system primed; in germ-free animals and neonates monocytes are less likely than in 'contaminated' individuals to bear the class II histocompatibility antigens needed for the immune response and
4 stimulation of antibodies (natural antibodies) that may cross-react with pathogenic microbes (Mackowiak 1982).

4 SECOND LINES OF DEFENCE

When the first lines of defence fail, either because of congenital or acquired defects, then the way to deeper tissues is open to bacteria and the next lines of defence come into play. Ciliary dysfunction associated with respiratory infections is one example of congenital defects (Eliasson et al. 1977). There are many examples of acquired defects; in modern medicine invasive techniques to monitor and support bodily functions bypass the physical barriers so that infections with relatively avirulent bacteria are common. The increasing use of indwelling devices provides niches for bacterial colonization and infection; these foreign bodies reduce natural resistance for various reasons, e.g. local depletion of complement. Moreover, bacteria grow on these foreign bodies in a biofilm that protects them from the host's defences (Costerton, Lewandowski and Caldwell 1995). Once the micro-organism is across the mucosal barrier, the host has 3 means of defence.

4.1 Iron limitation

Free iron is essential for bacterial growth; in man most iron is localized intracellularly as ferritin, haemosiderin or haem compounds and unavailable to the micro-organism. Free iron levels are too low to support bacterial growth, because circulating iron is bound to transferrin (present in serum and lymph) and to lactoferrin (present in neutrophils and many bodily secretions such as saliva, tears, colostrum, milk and intestinal secretions). Lactoferrin and transferrin are bacteriostatic. Pathogenic bacteria have had to develop means of wresting iron from the bodily stores (Otto et al. 1994). A response to infection is a further sequestration of iron which in chronic infections may lead to anaemia.

4.2 Acute phase proteins

During acute infections, and other acute inflammatory illnesses, acute phase proteins appear in increased amounts in the blood. These are manufactured by hepatocytes under the influence of cytokines produced by the immune system and are an important non-specific resistance mechanism that has been maintained phylogenetically. This reaction may buy time for the host until the immune response becomes fully operative (Trautwein, Boker and Manns 1994). Some of these proteins and their possible roles in resistance are listed in Table 2.2.

5 PHAGOCYTIC CELLS AND MECHANISMS

Phagocytosis is the process by which invading organisms are ingested by phagocytic cells, ingestion being followed by intracellular killing. It is vital for the wellbeing of the host. Chemotherapeutic regimens that lead to granulocytopenia as a side effect have demonstrated beyond any doubt the necessity of adequate numbers of granulocytes to prevent nosocomial infections (Bodey et al. 1966).

Phagocytosis is a non-specific defence and involves a series of reactions:

1 the activation of the phagocyte
2 the guiding of the phagocyte to the bacterium
3 attachment of the bacterium to the phagocyte and its ingestion and
4 the intracellular killing of the micro-organism.

Thereafter, the processing of the microbial antigens is an integral part of acquired immunity.

Many cells are able to ingest particles, for example endothelial cells, but 3 cells may be regarded as 'professional' phagocytes; these are polymorphonuclear neutrophils, macrophages and, to a much lesser degree, eosinophils. All are myeloid cells derived from common precursor stem cells that develop along different lines.

5.1 The neutrophil leucocyte

ORIGIN AND FATE

The polymorphonuclear neutrophil is the characteristic cell of acute inflammation, be it infectious or non-infectious in origin. As its name suggests, it has a lobed nucleus and weakly staining granules. Neutrophils can be rapidly mobilized from huge reserves in the bone marrow and quickly reach inflamed sites. Essential

Table 2.2 Some acute phase proteins

Protein	Function	Role in resistance
α_1-Acid glycoprotein	Promotes platelet adherence and collagen	Improved wound healing
Complement	Lysis and opsonization	Promotes phagocytosis
α_1-Trypsin	Protease inhibitor	Controls tissue damage by leucocyte proteases
α_1-Macroglobulin	Complexes with proteases	Increased granulopoiesis and macrophage activation
C-Reactive protein	Activates complement; modulates cytokine production	Stimulates and modulates inflammation
Haptoglobin	Binds to haemoglobin	Ingestion of complex by macrophages removes iron source from bacteria
LPS-BP	Binds to endotoxin	Complex more powerful activator of macrophages
Fibrinogen	Clotting factor	Coagulation
Ceruloplasmin	Transports copper	?

properties for the efficient functioning of neutrophils are motility, deformability and a recognition system that senses gradients of chemoattractants. During development the neutrophils acquire the characteristics of mature cells, i.e. cytoplasmic granules, receptors for chemotaxis and phagocytosis, deformability and motility. Exit from the bone marrow requires active deformation and motility, the cells squeezing through the pores of the endothelial cells that line the marrow sinuses. This exit is controlled by chemical signals and in normal circumstances a large reserve of neutrophils remains in the marrow, estimated to be about 10^9 cells per kg body weight and far exceeding the total number of neutrophils in the blood.

Neutrophils are short-lived cells that circulate in the blood, possibly for only a few hours, and survive in tissues a little longer. Their fate is uncertain, but many appear to migrate into the oral cavity and gut; others may die in the tissues and be removed by macrophages. Neutrophils have little capacity for protein synthesis so that their life span is short and their turnover is great. In humans, c. 10^{11} cells are formed and destroyed each day. The marrow reserve means that when the need arises, a neutrophil leucocytosis can rapidly be achieved. About half the blood neutrophils are circulating, whereas the other half are adherent to endothelial surfaces, a phenomenon known as 'margination'. The marginated and circulating neutrophils are in a state of flux, marginated cells freeing themselves to return to the circulation and vice versa. Non-activated neutrophils adhere to endothelium loosely and transiently through selectin proteins; the blood flow causes them to roll along the endothelial surface.

Should the neutrophil in its rolling movement come upon inflammatory stimuli and activated endothelial cells, the selectin adhesin is shed and integrin adhesins are upgraded to give rise to a firmer binding. Now the neutrophils become more flattened with a greater adhering surface and blood flow shearing stress is no longer able to displace them. Activation of neutrophils is brought about by leukotriene B4, C5a or *N*-formyl peptides; inflammatory mediators also upgrade the expression of endothelial receptors (Bevilacqua 1993).

Adherence to endothelium is the first step in the exit of the cell from the blood vessel to the tissues under the influence of chemoattractants. Inherited defects in adherence, which can involve either selectin or integrin proteins, are associated with immunodeficiency; bacterial infections are severe and are characterized by the failure to form pus, tissue necrosis and periodontitis. Though leucocytosis occurs, when tested in vitro the neutrophils show poor adherence and phagocytosis (Malech and Gallin 1987). Three integrin proteins (LFA-1, Mo-1 and p150,95) are expressed constitutively and are upgraded on activation. Mo-1 (CR3) and p150,95 (CR4) also serve as receptors for the complement fragments iC3b and C3d. Counter-receptors on endothelium are ICAM (intercellular adhesion molecules) 1 and 2. The latter is expressed constitutively whereas the former is upgraded when the endothelium is stimulated, e.g. by interleukin-1 (IL-1) or tumour necrosis factor (TNF); steroids inhibit endothelial selectin and the upgrading of ICAM-1, which accounts for some of their anti-inflammatory activity (Cronstein et al. 1992). Knowledge of adherence proteins may have practical applications because monoclonal antibodies directed against these adherence antigens can modulate the neutrophil response.

The neutrophil is a 2-edged weapon and, for example, in bacterial meningitis, the great influx of neutrophils into the CSF may have harmful consequences for the host because they are unable to phagocytose virulent bacteria in a fluid milieu in the absence of complement and antibody. Frustrated in their purpose, they discharge their highly reactive oxygen radicals, enzymes and toxic substances to the detriment of the host. Modulation of the neutrophil response may be a beneficial strategy (Tuomanen et al. 1989).

Before activation the neutrophil is often primed by mediators at concentrations too low to activate the leucocyte; these include endotoxin, chemotactic factors, cytokines and certain lipids. After priming, the leucocyte shows greater responsiveness for c. 20 min. This enhanced responsiveness is more marked to another activator than to a second dose of the same primer, which suggests possible desensitization. Priming has some cell specificity, i.e. bacterial mediators prime neutrophils whereas parasitic mediators prime eosinophils (Bass et al. 1987).

CHEMOTAXIS

Once the neutrophils are marginated on endothelium, chemotactic factors stimulate them to cross the endothelial barrier and move towards the site of inflammation. Neutrophil migration follows a carefully co-ordinated sequence of events: first migration is mediated by C5a, leukotriene B4 and IFN-γ; a second wave involves IL-8 and IL-6; and a third wave involves stimulation by IL-1 ,TNF-α and granulocyte stimulating factor (Kuhns et al. 1992). Crossing takes place through the junctions between the endothelial cells. Then the leucocytes must be able to traverse the basement membrane to reach the extravascular tissues. On flat surfaces they display amoeboid motion. Typically, the moving cell has a polarized shape with a ruffled, hyaline anterior veil (lamellipodium) that is rich in actin and myosin, but without organelles. Behind this the cell body is tapered and contains the nucleus and organelles. Sometimes a tail (uropod) with retractile fibres is seen. In 3-dimensional matrices, such as collagenous tissue, the matrix may serve as a 'climbing frame' so that the need for adherence is less strict. Moreover, in such 3-dimensional situations the leucocytes may show great variation in shape as they advance.

The speed at which leucocytes move can also be influenced. Chemokinesis refers to acceleration of movement that occurs when the neutrophil meets a constant concentration of chemoattractant. This process is complementary to chemotaxis and ensures a rapid accumulation of neutrophils at the site of infection.

Leucocyte movement through the tissues can be random or directed (chemotaxis). The latter is a response to a chemical gradient, the leucocyte being drawn to the source of the chemoattractant where the concentration is greatest. During this response, and even before movement begins, the cells are oriented so that the lamellipodium faces the source of the chemoattractant. Receptors previously distributed at random around the cell are now concentrated at the front of the cell (Snyderman and Goetzl 1981). Obviously the leucocyte must possess a sensory detector system to register differences in concentrations. It has been estimated that a neutrophil can detect a difference of concentration of 1% across its own length. This sensor must be linked to the motor apparatus of the cell by transduction mechanisms.

5.2 Chemotactic factors

Many factors have been shown to act as chemoattractants for neutrophils and other leucocytes. Some classes are shown in Table 2.3.

C5A

This is the major chemoattractant generated by complement activation (see Chapter 4) and neutrophils possess specific receptors for it. The importance of C5a as a chemoattractant in bacterial infections rests on the fact that it is generated when complement is activated at the surface of micro-organisms and diffusion results in a gradient that leucocytes can detect. This then leads them directly to the pathogenic micro-organism, even if it does not itself produce chemoattractants; for example, chemotaxis towards *Staphylococcus aureus* largely depends on this complement mechanism (Russell et al. 1976). Patients deficient in C5a suffer from serious pyogenic infections.

FORMYL METHIONYL PEPTIDES

The prokaryotic cell, in contrast to the eukaryotic cell, begins synthesis of protein from formyl methionyl peptides; the mammalian host will recognize these as foreign. One synthesized peptide is formyl-Met-Leu-Phe, which is a potent stimulus for neutrophil chemotaxis and is often used as a standard in chemotaxis experiments in vitro. Neutrophils possess receptors for these peptides (Schiffman and Gallin 1979).

LEUKOTRIENE B4

This is a lipoxygenase-derived product of arachidonic acid that is released by neutrophils and other cells by various stimuli. It is chemotactic for neutrophils and eosinophils The release from inflammatory cells of a chemoattractant amplifies the inflow of neutrophils.

LYMPHOKINES

The more general term **cytokine** is preferable to lymphokine, because cells other than lymphocytes produce these substances. They function as chemotactic factors. Cytokines recruit inflammatory cells to the site of infection by their effects on the adhesion molecules of both leucocytes and endothelium. IL-8 is a classical example of a neutrophil chemoattractant.

CYTOTAXINS

Cytotaxins are bacterial factors that are **directly** chemotactic. Much of the early work on cytotaxins failed to distinguish direct chemotaxis from chemotaxis after complement activation. Endotoxin has been regarded as a bacterial chemoattractant, but it is a powerful activator of complement. Filtrates of *Escherichia coli* are chemotactic, presumably by virtue of peptides. Filtrates of gram-positive species seem chemotactic, but may contain enzymes that degrade complement to yield chemotactic fragments. The picture is confused because *Bacteroides fragilis* seems to impair in vitro chemotaxis induced by *E. coli* (Namavar

Table 2.3 Some factors that serve as chemoattractants for leucocytes

Origin	Factor
Activated complement	C5a
Cells	
Lymphocytes	Lymphokine
Basophils	Eosinophil chemoattractant
Macrophages	Various
Neutrophils	Various
Tumour cells	Macrophage chemoattractant
Damaged tissue	Denatured protein and other products
Micro-organisms	
Bacteria	Formyl peptides
Viruses	No direct chemoattractants; chemotaxis via complement or new antigens on infected cells
Parasites	Eosinophil chemoattractants
Immune reactions	Immune complexes cause neutrophils to release neutrophil chemoattractants

et al. 1987) and different components of *S. aureus* inhibit or stimulate chemotaxis (Weksler and Hill 1969).

Apart from peptides and possibly some lipid compounds, the evidence for pure bacterial chemoattractants is confusing. Chemotaxis in viral diseases is less well understood; indeed, some viruses also inhibit leucocyte locomotion (Rabson et al. 1977). The accumulation of leucocytes in viral lesions is evidence for chemotaxis; possible mechanisms are the products of cell death or complement mediated reactions to viral antigens on the infected cell surface, or new antigens produced in response to viral infection (Snyderman, Wohlenberg and Notkins 1972).

5.3 Phagocytosis

Two steps, **attachment** and **ingestion**, are involved in phagocytosis. Attachment requires recognition of the particle at the membrane of the leucocyte; metabolic inhibitors do not affect attachment but they do inhibit ingestion which is an energy-dependent process. Phagocytosis can be classified as non-immune or immune. Non-immune phagocytosis includes ingestion of particles such as latex or carbon particles or avirulent bacteria. In the case of the latter it has been proposed that the hydrophobicity of the cell wall leads to a non-specific attachment (van Oss and Gillman 1972). Phagocytosis may, however, be mediated by proteins of neutrophil or bacterial walls that recognize sugars in the other, so-called lectinophagocytosis (Ofek and Sharon 1988). Nevertheless, the hydrophobicity of the bacterial cell wall is important for ingestion because bacteria of greater pathogenicity have evolved a hydrophilic surface, for example a capsule, that resists non-immune phagocytosis, but is susceptible to immune phagocytosis in which antibody and complement are involved. Antisera that promote phagocytosis seem to do so by making the bacterial surface hydrophobic.

Neutrophils and macrophages have surface receptors for the Fc region of IgG and for the components of complement activation C3b and iC3b. During the immunological reaction the micro-organism becomes coated with C3b and IgG antibody; the Fc portion remains free. This process was termed 'opsonization' from the Greek word for culinary seasoning. The bound IgG and C3b interact with receptors on the phagocyte and thereafter the process of ingestion is set in train. Receptors for IgG (FcgRI–III), but not for other immunoglobulins, and for C3b and iC3b are found on neutrophils (Lay and Nussenzweig 1968, Messner and Jelinek 1970). FcgII and FcgIII are low affinity receptors, whereas FcgI is a high affinity receptor expressed only after activation. The complement receptors exist as intracellular pools that can be mobilized rapidly (Berger et al. 1984). Downregulation of reactions due to receptors occurs by a reduction in the number of receptors, e.g. the normal respiratory burst is followed by downregulation of neutrophil receptors. The balance between upgrading and downgrading of receptors is presumably designed to modulate the neutrophil reaction and limit possible tissue damage (Gaither et al. 1987). In humans the main opsonizing antibodies are IgG1 and IgG3. Most pyogenic micro-organisms are eliminated by opsonic phagocytosis.

Ingestion results from the sequential binding of particle ligands to their receptors on the phagocyte. This causes polymerization of actin filaments under the point of attachment and leads to the cytoplasmic membrane flowing around the particle until it is enclosed in a phagosome (Griffin et al. 1975). The first steps of ingestion trigger a sequence of events in the leucocyte, i.e. a burst of oxidative metabolism; after fusing with the phagosome, the granules discharge their contents into it.

The neutrophil contains 2 principal types of granule, azurophil and specific granules. The specific granules fuse first, followed by the azurophil granules. Should the granules fuse with the phagosome before it has closed, their contents leak out into the surroundings. Discharge to the surroundings also occurs if the granules fuse with the cell membrane instead of the phagosome membrane. This latter event tends to happen if the phagocyte encounters particles it cannot ingest, for example those that are too large or too hydrophilic; the phenomenon has been termed 'frustrated phagocytosis'.

INTRACELLULAR KILLING

The penultimate step in the elimination of invading bacteria is their intracellular killing, and the final step in the drama is the processing of their antigens by the immune system. Although the 2 killing processes (oxidative and non-oxidative) work in concert, it is convenient for the sake of clarity to discuss them separately.

Oxidative killing

Some of the neutrophil's most potent weapons are reactive oxygen intermediates (ROI), in particular hydroxyl radicals, superoxide anions, and H_2O_2. Nevertheless, there is some disagreement over which ROI are the principal killing agents; the extreme lability and reactivity of the ROI complicate the unravelling of the problem. Catalase-positive bacteria are usually readily killed, either because of an excess of peroxide or other ROI or because non-oxidative reactions are lethal (Cohen 1994). The importance of this oxygen pathway for bacterial killing is illustrated by chronic granulomatous disease (CGD) in which a defect in one of several components results in failure to produce superoxide ions. Sufferers usually die in childhood from chronic or recurrent infections. The respiratory burst that leads to formation of superoxide anions is based on the nicotinamide adenine dinucleotide phosphate (reduced) oxidase (NADPH) system of the neutrophil. This system reacts more vigorously in 'primed' neutrophils. The most common cause of CGD is a defect in the *b* cytochrome that oxidizes NADPH to yield superoxide anion. Although careful in vitro studies with all variables identical (except for O_2 concentration) have shown that under anaerobic conditions neutrophils can kill bacteria as effectively as in aerobic conditions (Vel et al. 1984), the clinical picture of CGD leaves no doubt about the crucial importance of the oxidative mechanism in practice.

Non-oxygen-dependent mechanisms

These mechanisms depend on antimicrobial proteins and phagosomal acidity. The azurophilic granules contain a wide range of antimicrobial proteins and enzymes; they are primarily involved in microbial killing and digestion. The specific granules aid the respiratory burst and contain factors involved in inflammation. A third class of granules, tertiary granules, has been described, but their role in neutrophil function is unclear (Table 2.4). Degranulation and fusion of lysosome and phagosome are under the control of a transduction signal. A review of the most important antimicrobial proteins follows.

Defensins that are also found in intestinal cells (Selsted et al. 1992) make up about 50% of the protein of neutrophils and they are active against bacteria, fungi and viruses. Their mode of killing is not fully understood. Defensins are found in the haemolymph of insects and probably represent an ancient mode of host defence (Hoffmann and Hetru 1992).

Cathepsin G is a serine protease that binds to penicillin-binding proteins and, like penicillin, interferes with peptidoglycan synthesis (Cohen 1994). **Azuricidin** is a serine protease that kills bacteria at a low pH (5.5). **Bactericidal/permeability increasing protein** (BPI) has been widely studied. It binds to lipopolysaccharide and, as the name suggests, it increases the permeability of bacteria. It may find a place in the treatment of septic shock by modifying endotoxin. BPI reversibly inhibits the metabolism of sensitive bacteria (Cohen 1994). **Lactoferrin** may kill some bacteria (Ellison and Giehl 1991), but its main function is to deprive micro-organisms of essential iron. It is believed to play other roles, e.g. modulation of complement activity (Kijlstra and Jeurissen 1982) and production of hydroxyl radicals, and it alters cell membrane during degranulation (Boxer et al. 1982). **Acidification** can lead directly to the death of some

bacteria, but most are not killed by the pH of 6.0 found in the phagosome. The low pH enhances the activity of some antimicrobial systems, e.g. the formation of OCl^- by the action of myeloperoxidase and its lethal effect is optimal at low pH. Acidification of the phagosome is brought about by several processes, including the outpouring of acid hydrolases, the metabolism of ingested micro-organisms and active transport of hydrogen ions (Cohen 1994).

Interaction between oxidative and non-oxidative processes

The granule proteins play a role in oxidative metabolism, especially lactoferrin and myeloperoxidase. In the presence of a halide, myeloperoxidase converts H_2O_2 to OCl^- ions that can form long-acting chloramines; they can also react with superoxide to yield hydroxyl radicals. This pathway seems of only limited importance because deficiencies in myeloperoxidase do not lead to frequent infections. In the presence of iron, superoxide can react with H_2O_2 to form hydroxyl radicals more rapidly than do OCl^- ions and superoxide. Lactoferrin can regulate this reaction by sequestrating iron. Hydroxyl radicals are very destructive and this regulation may be of great importance.

5.4 Eosinophils

These resemble neutrophils in structure. They arise from bone marrow stem cells but they develop separately; IL-5 is the cytokine most involved in increasing the eosinophil count. If the neutrophil is the cell classically associated with acute inflammation, the eosinophil is associated with the reaction of acute hypersensitivity, certain skin disorders and with defence against parasitic infections. During maturation the eosinophil develops 3 types of granules: primary granules; secondary granules that contain major basic protein, cationic protein, a neurotoxin and peroxidase; and small granules that contain acid phosphatase and arylsulphatase. The eosinophil has receptors for IgA, IgG, IgE, cytokines and complement and can phagocytose, but it does so less effectively than the

Table 2.4 Some contents of neutrophil granules[a]

Azurophil	Specific	Tertiary
Acid hydrolases	Lactoferrin	Gelatinase
Cationic proteins	Lysozyme	
Defensins	Vitamin B12 binding protein	
Lysozyme	Monocyte chemotactic factor	
Myeloperoxidase	Complement receptors	
Bactericidal permeability increasing factor	Cytochrome *b*	
Acid and neutral proteases	Membrane-bound parts of the NADPH system	
Cathepsin	C3, C5 proteases	
Elastase		
β-Glucuronidase		
Arylsulphatase		

[a]Azurophil granules are mainly involved in bacterial killing and digestion, specific granules with inflammation; the function of tertiary granules is uncertain.

neutrophil. The eosinophil is able to produce superoxide and H_2O_2. It is more inclined to discharge its lethal products externally and effect extracellular killing. This reflects its antiparasite function, since parasites are too large to be ingested. Experimental studies have shown eosinophils to latch on to *Schistosoma mansoni* and to kill the parasite by discharging the granule contents (Densen et al. 1978). Less is known about the diapedesis of eosinophils and the modulation of their receptors, but they are probably regulated in an analogous manner to that of neutrophils. Eosinophils may modulate the reaction of acute hypersensitivity. They have been shown to possess substances able to inactivate the products of basophil stimulation that are involved in acute hypersensitivity: for example, eosinophil histaminase inactivates histamine produced by basophils; arylsulphatase and phospholipase can inactivate leukotrienes and platelet-activating factor (PAF). Moreover, the eosinophil can downregulate the further production of these and other mediators by basophils (Butterworth and David 1981).

6 MONONUCLEAR PHAGOCYTES

The mononuclear phagocyte is an intriguing and fascinating cell that has enjoyed a variety of names: in blood a monocyte, in tissue a histiocyte, in bone an osteoclast and in the liver a Kupffer cell. In the past the mononuclear macrophages were regarded as 'fixed' or 'free', the former being an integral part of the structure of the relevant organ. This classification is too rigid and does not accord with evidence that 'fixed' Kupffer cells can increase in number in response to a macrophage stimulator. A more widely used classification is to regard macrophages as 'resident' or 'elicited'. The elicited macrophages are those recruited by some inflammatory stimulus from the blood monocytes. The peritoneal cavity illustrates this; studies of the mouse have shown that there are resident macrophages whose biological level of activity (e.g. motility, bactericidal activity) is low, but which in concert with lymph flow are able to eliminate small bacterial inocula. Infection of the peritoneal cavity that overpowers the resident macrophages leads to a neutrophil response followed by a macrophage reaction. Analysis by monoclonal antibodies of the macrophages now present shows they are mostly elicited, i.e. they are less differentiated but more actively phagocytic than resident cells. The accepted view is that the resident and the elicited macrophages are both derived from blood monocytes.

The long-lived macrophage is a much more versatile cell than the short-lived neutrophil. Along with natural killer (NK) cells, it belongs phylogenetically to a primitive defence system. Its phagocytosis of bacteria resembles that of amoebae. It has, however, evolved to play a wider role in regulating the whole immune response. When fully developed, the monocytes leave the marrow and circulate in the blood, in far smaller numbers than the neutrophil, until they settle in the tissues where they develop in a variety of ways and are sufficiently distinctive to have been given different names. Included among the macrophages are the Langerhans cells of the skin, the interdigitating cells in lymphatic tissue and antigen-presenting cells.

The elicited macrophages are, like the neutrophils, actively phagocytic and bactericidal; they are classically summoned to deal with intracellular pathogens or chronic infections. The elicited macrophages also release cytokines such as IL-1 and TNF-α that influence lymphocyte behaviour. Different subpopulations of macrophages can be identified by detecting surface antigens with monoclonal antibodies, e.g. resident versus elicited (Verweij et al. 1991) and the presence of major histocompatibility antigens (MHC) can be detected. Resident macrophages are mostly MHC-II negative, whereas macrophages elicited by such stimuli as mycobacterial antigen show many class II-positive cells. Class II-positive cells that bear antigen interact with helper T lymphocytes and this interaction is vital for T cell-dependent immune response.

6.1 Functions of macrophages

Macrophages are 'scavenger' cells that remove particles or damaged cells from the body. The Kupffer cells and the macrophages lining the splenic sinusoids are ideally placed to filter particulate matter from the blood. Aged erythrocytes are removed in the spleen; enhanced removal of abnormal red cells is seen in haemolytic anaemias. Pulmonary macrophages efficiently remove particles that have evaded the physical barriers and reached the alveoli. Other macrophage cells function as antigen-presenting cells.

Macrophages are recruited in much the same way as neutrophils but the process is slower because there is no huge marrow reserve of macrophages. Macrophages respond to the same stimuli as neutrophils. Little is known about defects in monocyte chemotaxis, but animal and human studies have suggested that tumours can produce factors that impair monocyte locomotion (Wilkinson 1992).

Activation of macrophages is characterized by changes in their morphology (a larger membrane surface, the cell is more spread out and pinocytosis is prominent) and their biochemistry (increased synthesis of proteolytic enzymes, complement factors, plasminogen activator and leukotrienes). Superoxide production is increased and phagocytosis via C3b receptors is greater.

Macrophages can kill many bacteria, but others can survive within the macrophage. These include *Mycobacterium tuberculosis*, *Listeria monocytogenes*, *Salmonella typhi*, *Legionella pneumophila* and a number of protozoa, including *Toxoplasma gondii*. Killing of these microorganisms requires macrophage activation (see section 6.2 and Chapter 5). The non-activated macrophage can thus function as a Trojan horse by transporting micro-organisms through the body and protecting them from serum antibodies.

6.2 Macrophage activation

The importance of macrophage activation was shown with tubercle bacilli. Macrophages isolated at the start of a mycobacterial infection were unable to kill the mycobacteria, whereas macrophages isolated several weeks after the onset of the infection could do so. This enhanced killing was dependent on cell mediated immunity; transfer of this immunity could be effected by transfer of T cells from the infected animal but not by serum. Activity is not specific to the micro-organism; macrophages activated by the development of cell mediated immunity to one microbe show increased killing of other intracellular micro-organisms. Activated macrophages resemble inflammatory macrophages, i.e. they show the same heightened biochemical reactions. They do, however, produce more H_2O_2 than inflammatory macrophages. They secrete more cytokines such as IL-1 and TNF-α that have wide-reaching effects, i.e. they function as pyrogens. TNF-α is the factor responsible not only for killing tumour cells but also for the cachexia associated with malignancy and some infections, e.g. trypanosomiasis that seems out of proportion to the underlying disease.

The concept of macrophage activation has been widened to include antitumour activation; the immunological pathways for this may not be identical to those for activation against micro-organisms.

Macrophages are prominent in chronic inflammatory states, be they infectious or non-infectious, e.g. foreign-body granuloma. A distinction can be drawn between low grade inflammatory granulomas, e.g. foreign-body, and more active infectious granulomas. In the former the macrophages are relatively inactive whereas in the latter there is constant renewal of macrophages and lymphocyes. The lymphocytes secrete lymphokines that include macrophage-activating factors, the major one being interferon-α, and a co-ordinated immune response results in which the activated macrophages in turn release factors that stimulate T and B lymphocytes. Macrophages recruit more macrophages by virtue of their cytokines.

6.3 Macrophages and antigen presentation

Macrophages of MHC class II, bearing antigens, are needed for an immune response to thymus-dependent antigens. In culture these 'antigen-presenting' macrophages interact physically with T lymphocytes that form rosettes around them. Several types of 'antigen-presenting' cells have been described; some have phagocytic and degradative capabilities and would seem to be true macrophages, whereas others do not appear to be able to phagocytose and may be a different class of cell. The dendritic cells described in the spleen are smaller than macrophages, are not phagocytic, have no complement receptors, but they do possess class II antigen. The Langerhans cells of the skin may be similar, but they do possess complement receptors. Other macrophage-like cells are the 'veiled' cells seen in lymph nodes after contact sensitization. Dendritic cells are often seen after antigen stimulation and, being surrounded by lymphocytes, are involved in the immune response. Whether they are true macrophages is debatable.

7 CONCLUSION

The study of immunology has made great strides since the days when Shaw, in his play *The Doctor's Dilemma*, gently mocked Almroth Wright's immunological concepts. Advances in oncology have rendered many patients temporarily neutropenic during therapy and the vital role of the phagocyte in preventing infection has been all too dramatically demonstrated. The macrophage displays a versatility undreamed of when it was first shown to be the cell of chronic inflammation. Our knowledge of the immune system reveals a complex interacting series of reactions which provide humans with a highly organized defence against infection. Our knowledge remains incomplete; the range of cytokines with similar functions suggests some redundancy, but it is more likely that subtle differences in function will be described.

The non-specific immune system has a dark side and in many diseases the reactions are excessive or misguided so that more harm than good is done. Advances in our ability to modulate non-specific immunity without losing the benefits of resistance to infection may yield improved results in some infections and in non-infectious inflammatory states.

REFERENCES

Bass DA, Gerard C et al., 1987, Priming of the respiratory burst of neutrophils by diacylglycerol. Independence from activation or translocation of protein kinase C, *J Biol Chem*, **262:** 6643–9.

Berger M, 1990, Complement deficiency and neutrophil dysfunction as risk factors for bacterial infection in newborns and the role of granulocyte transfusion in therapy, *Rev Infect Dis*, **2 (Suppl. 4):** S401–9.

Berger M, O'Shea J et al., 1984, Human neutrophils increase expression of C3bi as well as C3b receptors, *J Clin Invest*, **74:** 1566–71.

Bevilacqua MP, 1993, Endothelial-leukocyte adhesion molecules, *Annu Rev Immunol*, **11:** 767–804.

Bodey GP, Buckley M et al., 1966, Quantitative relationships between circulating leukocytes and infection in patients with acute leukemia, *Ann Intern Med*, **64:** 328–40.

Boxer LA, Coates TD et al., 1982, Lactoferrin deficiency associated with altered granulocytic function, *N Engl J Med*, **307:** 404–10.

Butterworth AE, David JR, 1981, Eosinophil function, *N Engl J Med*, **304:** 154–6.

Chandra RK, 1993, Nutrition and immunity, *Clinical Aspects of Immunology*, 5th edn, Blackwell Scientific, London, 1325–8.

Cohen MS, 1994, Molecular events in the activation of human neutrophils for microbial killing, *Clin Infect Dis*, **18 (Suppl. 2):** 170–9.

Cohen S, Tyrrell DAJ, Smith A, 1991, Psychological stress and susceptibility to the common cold, *N Engl J Med*, **325:** 606–12.

Costerton JW, Lewandowski Z, Caldwell DE, 1995, Microbial biofilms, *Annu Rev Microbiol*, **49:** 711–45.

Cronstein BN, Kimmel SC et al., 1992, A mechanism for the anti-inflammatory effects of corticosteroids: the glucocorticoid receptor regulates leucocyte adhesion to endothelial cells and expression of endothelial-leucocyte adhesion molecule 1 and intercellular adhesion molecule1, *Proc Natl Acad Sci USA*, **89:** 9991–5.

Densen P, Mahmoud AAF et al., 1978, Demonstration of eosinophil degranulation on the surface of opsonized schistosomules by phase-contrast cinemicrography, *Infect Immun*, **22:** 282–5.

Driks MR, Craven DE et al., 1987, Nosocomial pneumonia in intubated patients given sucralfate as compared with antacids or histamine type 2 blockers, *N Engl J Med*, **317:** 1376–82.

Eliasson R, Mossberg B et al., 1977, The immotile cilia syndrome, *N Engl J Med*, **297:** 1–6.

Ellison RT III, Giehl TJ, 1991, Killing of Gram-negative bacteria by lactoferrin and lysozyme, *J Clin Invest*, **88:** 1080–91.

Gaither TA, Medley SR et al., 1987, Studies of phagocytosis in chronic granulomatous disease, *Inflammation*, **11:** 211–27.

Griffin Jr FM, Griffin SA et al., 1975, Studies on the mechanism of phagocytosis. I. Requirements for circumferential attachment of particle-bound ligands to specific receptors on macrophage plasma membrane, *J Exp Med*, **142:** 1263–82.

Hill AV, 1992, Malaria resistance genes: a natural selection, *Trans R Soc Trop Med Hyg*, **86:** 225–6.

Hoffman JA, Hetru C, 1992, Insect defensins: inducible antibacterial peptides, *Immunol Today*, **13:** 411–15.

Jenkinson DMC, 1992, The basis of the skin microflora ecosystem, *The Skin Microflora and Microbial Skin Disease*, Cambridge University Press, Cambridge, 1–32.

Kijlstra A, Jeurissen SH, 1982, Modulation of classical C3 convertase of complement by tear lactoferrin, *Immunology*, **47:** 263–70.

Kuhns DB, DeCarlo E et al., 1992, Dynamics of the cellular and humoral components of the inflammatory response elicited in skin blisters, *J Clin Invest*, **89:** 1734–40.

Lay WH, Nussenzweig V, 1968, Receptors for complement of leucocytes, *J Exp Med*, **128:** 991–1009.

Mackowiak PA, 1982, The normal microbial flora, *N Engl J Med*, **307:** 83–93.

Malech HL, Gallin JL, 1987, Neutrophils in human disease, *N Engl J Med*, **317:** 687–94.

Messner RP, Jelinek J, 1970, Receptors for gamma G globulin on human neutrophils, *J Clin Invest*, **49:** 2165–71.

Nalin DR, Levine RJ et al., 1978, Cholera, non-vibrio cholera and stomach acid, *Lancet*, **2:** 856–9.

Namavar F, Verweij-Van Vught AMJJ et al., 1987, Effect of *Bacteroides fragilis* cellular components on chemotactic activity of polymorphonuclear leukocytes towards *Escherichia coli*, *J Med Microbiol*, **24:** 119–24.

Ofek I, Sharon N, 1988, Lectinophagocytosis: a molecular mechanism of recognition between cell surface sugars and lectins in the phagocytosis of bacteria, *Infect Immun*, **56:** 538–47.

van Oss CJ, Gillman CJ, 1972, Phagocytosis as a surface phenomenon. 1. Contact angles and phagocytosis of non-opsonized bacteria, *J Reticuloendothel Soc*, **12:** 283–92.

Otto B, Sparrius M et al., 1994, Utilization of haem from the hapto-haemoglobin complex by *Bacteroides fragilis*, *Microb Pathog*, **17:** 137–47.

Peterson PK, Chao CC et al., 1991, Stress and pathogenesis of infectious disease, *Rev Infect Dis*, **13:** 710–20.

Rabson AR ,Whiting DA et al., 1977, Depressed neutrophil motility in patients with recurrent herpes simplex infections: in vitro restoration with levamisole, *J Infect Dis*, **135:** 113–16.

Russell RJ, Wilkinson PC et al., 1976, Effects of staphylococcal products on locomotion and chemotaxis of human blood neutrophils and monocytes, *J Med Microbiol*, **9:** 433–9.

Saltzman RL, Peterson PK, 1987, Immunodeficiency of the elderly, *Rev Infect Dis*, **9:** 1127–39.

Schiffman E, Gallin JI, 1979, Biochemistry of phagocyte chemotaxis, *Curr Top Cell Regul*, **15:** 203–61.

Selsted ME, Miller SI et al., 1992, Enteric defensins: antibiotic peptide components of intestinal host defense, *J Cell Biol*, **118:** 929–36.

Snyderman R, Goeztl EJ, 1981, Molecular and cellular mechanisms of leukocyte chemotaxis, *Science*, **213:** 830–7.

Snyderman R, Wohlenberg C, Notkins AL, 1972, Inflammation and viral infection: chemotactic activity resulting from the interaction of antiviral antibody and complement with cells infected with herpes simplex virus, *J Infect Dis*, **126:** 207–9.

Thomas EL, Aune TM, 1978, Lactoperoxidase, peroxide, thiocyanate antimicrobial system. Correlation of sulfhydryl oxidation with antimicrobial action, *Infect Immun*, **20:** 456–63.

Trautwein C, Boker K, Manns MP, 1994, Hepatocyte and immune system: acute phase reaction as a contribution to early defense mechanisms, *Gut*, **35:** 1163–6.

Tuomanen EI, Saukkonen K et al., 1989, Reduction of inflammation, tissue damage, and mortality in bacterial meningitis in rabbits treated with monoclonal antibodies against adhesion-promoting receptors of leucocytes *J Exp Med*, **170:** 959–69.

Vel WAC, Namavar F et al., 1984, Killing capacity of human polymorphonuclear leukocytes in aerobic and anaerobic conditions, *J Med Microbiol*, **18:** 173–80.

Verweij WR, Namavar F et al., 1991, Early events after intraabdominal infection with *Bacteroides fragilis* and *Escherichia coli*, *J Med Microbiol*, **35:** 18–22.

Weksler BB, Hill MJ, 1969, Inhibition of leukocyte migration by a staphylococcal factor, *J Bacteriol*, **98:** 1030–5.

Wilkinson PC, 1992, Macrophage/monocyte chemotaxis, *Encyclopedia of Immunology*, vol. ii, Academic Press, London, 1028–9.

IMMUNOGLOBULINS

W Cushley

Antibody (Ab) molecules are the functional products of the humoral arm of the mammalian immune system. They are glycoprotein molecules found mainly in the γ fraction of serum and are members of the immunoglobulin (Ig) family of serum proteins. Although Ig molecules exist as 5 classes, each with distinctive structural and functional properties, all Ig molecules conform to a common unit structural theme, the 4-chain model, which provides a molecular explanation for their immunological activities. Ab molecules are synthesized by B lymphocytes.

The humoral response is one arm of the specific, adaptive immune response and is characterized by the diversity of individual specific Abs which it can produce, immunological memory, and production of Abs of the most appropriate type to combat particular pathogens. The humoral response interacts with the cellular immune response, in the sense that T lymphocytes profoundly influence the nature of the humoral response and the humoral response also interfaces with components of the non-specific immune system. Thus, the non-specific immune system, which shows no specificity or immunological memory, possesses potent cytotoxic power in the form of phagocytic cells and the components of the complement cascade. The humoral response has essentially no toxic capacity in its own right, but uses Ab specifically to recruit the cytotoxic power of the non-specific system and focus it at the target of interest.

The humoral immune response displays characteristic features. After initial challenge with antigen, levels of antibody of the IgM class rise over some 4–7 days; this is the primary humoral response. If antigenic challenge persists, Abs of other classes, notably IgG, are produced; this is the secondary response. Subsequent challenge with the same antigen elicits a response that is more rapid than the primary response

and generates greater quantities of specific Ab of greater quality (i.e. different class and higher affinity) than those found in the primary response. The capacity to respond to rechallenge by a given antigen is long lived and resides in memory B cells. The secondary response encompasses antibody responses whose major components are of the IgA, IgD, IgE or IgG classes.

This chapter explores the biochemical, cellular and genetic basis of antibody function.

2   IMMUNOGLOBULIN STRUCTURE

2.1   The 4-chain model

The 4-chain model describes the overall structure of IgG molecules (Porter 1962) and this structural theme is common to all 5 Ig classes. The general features of the 4-chain model are illustrated in Fig. 3.1, using human IgG1 as example. Ab molecules are composed of 2 identical heavy chains, disulphide-bonded to 2 identical light chains in such a way that the N-terminus of each heavy and light chain is juxtaposed in 3-dimensional terms to generate the Ab combining site. Interchain disulphide bonds not only link the heavy and light chains but also link the 2 heavy chains together. The IgG molecule is bivalent with respect to antigen binding (Edelman and Poulik 1961, Porter 1962).

Controlled proteolysis of IgG molecules has provided insights into structure–function relationships by investigation of the distinct fragments of Ig molecules generated (see Fig. 3.1). Papain cleaves the intact IgG molecule to release 3 fragments of approximately equal molecular weight. Two of these fragments, derived from the N-terminus of the molecule, are

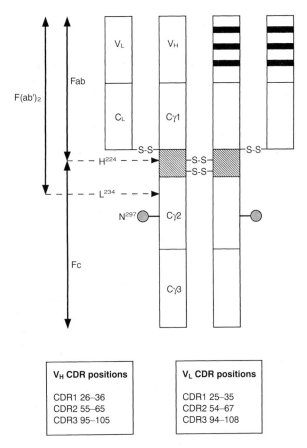

VH CDR positions

CDR1 26–36
CDR2 55–65
CDR3 95–105

VL CDR positions

CDR1 25–35
CDR2 54–67
CDR3 94–108

Fig. 3.1 Four-chain model of IgG1. The 4-chain structure of human IgG1 is illustrated, giving approximate positions of individual domains and of interchain, but not intrachain, disulphide bonds. The filled regions denote complementarity determining regions and the positions of the heavy and light chain CDRs are noted in the panels at the foot of the figure; the shaded area represents the hinge region of the molecule and the stippled circle denotes the position of the major carbohydrate group. The left hand side of the figure shows the sites of cleavage (dashed arrows) of the molecule by papain (2 × Fab + 1 × Fc) or pepsin (1 × F(ab')₂) and the fragments produced (solid double-headed arrows). Proteolytic cleavage occurs on the C-terminal side of the indicated residues and the one letter amino acid code is employed (H, histidine; L, leucine; N, asparagine). The numbering system is based on the EU IgG1 myeloma protein (Kabat et al. 1977).

identical and, because they retain antigen binding capacity, are referred to as Fab fragments (**f**ragment **a**ntigen **b**inding). Fab fragments are monovalent with respect to antigen binding and, as such, are unable to form immunoprecipitates in solution or in semi-solid media. The remaining product of papain digestion, the Fc (**f**ragment **c**rystalline) piece, is derived from the C-terminus of the intact IgG molecule and has no antigen binding capacity. It is, however, of considerable importance in the expression of antibody effector functions.

Pepsin digestion of intact IgG yields quite different proteolysis products. A large fragment of MW c. 100 kDa is the main product, the remaining material usually being small peptides. The 100 kDa fragment is

derived from the N-terminus of the intact IgG, has antigen binding capacity and is bivalent (i.e. possesses 2 equivalent antigen combining sites). This is the F(ab')₂ fragment.

2.2 Primary structure

Primary protein structure is the linear arrangement of amino acids in the polypeptide chain. Initial sequencing studies of Ig molecules were performed using Bence Jones proteins which are monomeric or dimeric light chains derived from the urine of patients with multiple myeloma (Edelman and Gally 1962). Primary sequence analysis of Bence Jones light chains revealed that they were divisible into 2 distinct regions of approximately equal size. Thus, from the amino acid 1 (the N-terminal residue) to amino acid 107, the sequence of one Bence Jones protein was different from that of any other Bence Jones protein with which it was compared, whereas the sequences from residues 108–214 were essentially identical for all Bence Jones proteins. These observations led to the division of light chains into variable (V) and constant (C) regions on the basis of the variability of amino acid sequence within the protein (Milstein 1966).

A similar structural division can be made for heavy chains. As described for the light chains, the N-terminal regions of the heavy chains possess considerable variability from one chain to another, but the C-terminal regions are relatively constant. In the case of the heavy chains, however, the variable region extends from residue 1 to residue 113, and the constant region from residue 114 to the C-terminus, which may be some 400 amino acid residues distant in the primary sequence. Furthermore, when the sequences of heavy chain C regions are analysed, it is clear that there are areas of significant homology of primary sequence along the length of the C region. The sequence can be subdivided into units of homology of approximately 100–110 amino acids. The functional importance of these domains will be discussed below in the context of tertiary structure (see section 2.3, p. 27).

The V regions of both heavy (VH) and light (VL) chains have numerous amino acid substitutions when individual polypeptide chains are compared. However, plots of variability of amino acid versus position in the primary sequence reveal that the distribution of amino acid substitutions is not random and that the variability is clustered in small regions of the primary structure. These areas of the V region are the hypervariable regions and they provide a molecular explanation for antibody specificity. Thus, the VL and VH regions of an individual antibody molecule are unique and the recognition of antigen by that Ab is similarly distinctive. Since the hypervariable regions govern the specificity of the Ab molecule, they are sometimes referred to as complementarily determining regions (CDRs).

Both heavy and light chains possess 3 CDRs. The heavy chain CDRs are located at positions 26–36, 55–65 and 95–105 in the primary sequence; the light chain CDRs are positioned at residues 25–35, 54–67 and 94–108 (Kabat et al. 1987). The above numbering is based on the EU myeloma protein (Edelman et al. 1969). The 3-dimensional arrangement of framework regions and CDRs is such that the CDRs are located very close together in a pocket at the N-terminus of the Ab and thereby give rise to the Ag binding site. Outside the hypervariable regions, or CDRs, the primary sequence of the V region is largely conserved between molecules. These conserved regions are crucial in the maintenance of the higher structure of the V_H and V_L regions and are therefore termed framework regions.

2.3   Secondary and tertiary structures

Secondary structure is the relationship between amino acids located some distance apart in the primary structure, whose interactions give rise to periodic structural motifs in the folded protein molecule (e.g. α-helix or β-pleated sheet structures). Ig molecules contain no α-helical structures but are rich in β-pleated sheets. Tertiary structure also describes the spatial relationship of amino acids which are distant in the primary sequence and, for the purposes of this discussion, refers to those cysteine residues in the primary sequence which form intrachain disulphide bridges, giving rise to individual domains within the Ig molecule.

The 'Ig-like fold' or domain is a characteristic higher structural motif of Ig structure. The primary structural data indicate that the sequences of Ig chains are divisible into homology units of approximately 110 amino acids in length. Within each of these units lies a single disulphide bridge, enclosing 65–75 residues in the V regions, and 52–59 residues in the C region domains. Clearly, the location of the cysteine residues is critical in domain formation; this is reflected not only in the conservation of this amino acid at defined positions in the polypeptide chain but also by the conservation of primary sequences surrounding the cysteine groups participating in intrachain disulphide bond formation.

The domain structure produced by disulphide bond formation is rich in β-sheet structure, with each domain in both the V and the C regions of the Ig molecule containing 2 β sheets. In each β sheet, the polypeptide structure may be considered as layers of overlapping sequence lying parallel to the long axis of the domain, one layer containing 3 strands of polypeptide and the other 4 strands. The polarity of adjacent, individual strands is antiparallel and the 2 layers are joined by the single disulphide bond. Multiple hydrophobic amino acid side chain groups protrude into the space between the layers.

The Ig-like domain, rich in β-pleated sheet structure, is found in many proteins which participate in the specific immune response, including class I and II major histocompatibility complex (MHC) molecules, the T cell antigen–receptor complex and the receptor for polymeric IgA (which eventually functions as secretory component).

2.4   Quaternary structure

Quaternary structure reflects the interaction between distinct polypeptide subunits of a multi-domain protein. In Ig molecules the interaction between particular domains is well defined and correlates well with biological activity. Thus, V_H and V_L domains interact to yield the correct conformation for generation of the antigen binding site. C_L and C_H1 domains also interact. In the C region, like domains interact. Thus, Cγ2 interacts with Cγ2 and Cγ3 with Cγ3. However, the interaction does not always involve direct contact between the faces of the 2 participating domains. In IgG molecules the Cγ2 domains are separated from each other by the large oligosaccharide unit located in this domain, whereas Cγ3 domains interact via contacts between faces of the 2 domains.

The forces which stabilize domain–domain interactions are non-covalent in character and involve weak intermolecular physical forces (i.e. hydrophobic interactions, salt bridges, hydrogen bonding). Although the physical forces which mediate domain interaction are identical for V and C domains, the faces of the protein that interact are distinct. Thus, V domains interact via those layers of the domain containing 3 strands of peptide sequence, whereas the C domains interact via the layers containing 4 strands of polypeptide.

2.5   Other structural features

The hinge region of IgG molecules is of critical importance to their function; located between the Cγ1 and Cγ2 domains, it is rich in proline and cysteine residues. The size of the hinge region varies from one IgG subclass to another, and is 10–20 residues in length in all subclasses except IgG3 where it is 60 residues long. This area of the Ig molecule has considerable segmental flexibility, which is important in the expression of the effector functions of IgG molecules. For example, the greater the segmental flexibility of given immunoglobulin isotype, the more likely it is that complement can be effectively fixed (Oi et al. 1984). The positioning of the hinge region is such that it allows the Fab arms of the IgG to adopt a wide range of orientations with respect to each other, and this feature also explains the characteristic 'Y' shape of IgG molecules visualized in antigen binding experiments in the electron microscope (Valentine and Green 1967).

The hinge region is the location of the inter-heavy chain disulphide bonds in the IgG molecule, the exact number of which varies between IgG subclasses. Thus, IgG1 and IgG4 have 2 interchain disulphide bridges, IgG2 has 4 bonds, and IgG3 possesses 15 interchain disulphide links. The region is also exposed to the solvent, with the consequence that proteolytic enzymes may attack it and generate fragments as described earlier in this chapter.

Ig molecules contain varying amounts of carbohydrate. In most instances the glycans are attached to asparagine residues (so-called N-linked oligosaccharides), but carbohydrate is also found linked to the hydroxyl groups of serine or threonine residues (O-linked sugars) in human IgD molecules and in the hinge region of human IgA molecules. In IgG molecules the principal site of glycosylation is asparagine-297, and the N-linked oligosaccharide is usually a biantennary complex structure, although the precise oligosaccharide structure can vary enormously between individual IgG molecules. The presence of certain types of carbohydrate structure has been correlated with particular autoimmune disease states (Parekh et al. 1985), but the role of the N-linked glycans themselves in disease pathogenesis is unclear. The other Ig isotypes are multiply glycosylated (Winkelhake 1978).

3   IMMUNOGLOBULIN CLASSES

Ig molecules exist as 5 classes, or isotypes, in man, each of which has characteristic structural features and particular immunological activities. The serological marker that defines Ig class or subclass is the isotype; the terms 'isotype' and 'class' (and 'subclass') are used interchangeably. All isotypes have a 4-chain unit as their fundamental structural feature and each class is named for the heavy chain of the molecule. Thus, IgG is named for the γ (gamma) heavy chain, IgM for the μ (mu) chain, and IgA for the α (alpha) chain. The principal molecular properties of the 5 human Ig classes are detailed in Table 3.1.

3.1   IgM

IgM is a pentameric structure comprising 5 identical 4-chain units; that is, it has 10 identical binding sites. The μ heavy chain has 5 domains, V_H plus 4 C regions ($C\mu1$, $C\mu2$, $C\mu3$ and $C\mu4$), and lacks a hinge region. The pentameric structure is stabilized by disulphide bonding between adjacent $C\mu3$ domains, and by the presence of the J (joining) chain. A single J chain is disulphide-bonded close to the C-terminus of the IgM pentamer (Chapuis and Koshland 1974). The critical cysteine residue (Cys-575) is part of an 18 amino acid C-terminal peptide extension located immediately following the $C\mu4$ domain, and this residue forms disulphide bonds either with J chain or with cysteines located in an identical position in other μ chains of the pentameric complex.

IgM is the principal component of the primary humoral response. Because of its large size (970 kDa, 19S), it is located mainly in the bloodstream. It is decavalent, leading to highly avid binding of antigens (thereby overcoming the potentially low affinity of the Ab–Ag interaction), and is efficient in both opsonization and complement fixation.

3.2   IgG

IgG is the main class of immunoglobulin in serum. As will be obvious from the detailed discussion of the 4-chain model, it exists as a molecule of MW 146–160 kDa (7S) in serum and is an abundant component of the secondary humoral immune response. This class of Ig is found not only in the bloodstream itself but also in extravascular spaces. It is also transported across the placental membrane and is therefore responsible for passive immunity in the fetus and neonate.

There are 4 major subclasses of the IgG isotype in man, each distinguished by minor variations in amino acid sequence in the C region and by the number and location of disulphide bridges. The structural variations have consequences for biological activity. Thus, the IgG1 and IgG3 isotypes are efficient in fixation of complement, whereas IgG2 and IgG4 subclasses are incapable of activating this effector function. Similarly, only IgG1 and IgG3 are capable of interacting with the Fc receptors on macrophages and therefore of acting as efficient opsonins.

3.3   IgA

IgA is found in 2 forms in the body, in serum where it occurs as a monomer (160 kDa, 7S), and on secretory surfaces where it exists as a dimeric molecule (385 kDa, 11S). The dimeric form is known as secretory IgA (sIgA) and is found in association with J chain and with secretory component; the latter is involved in transport of the IgA to the secretory surfaces. Secretory component is non-covalently associated with the IgA molecules in the sIgA complex. The α chain has 3 C domains and, like μ chains, possesses an 18 amino acid C-terminal sequence allowing disulphide bonding to the J chain. A small hinge region is also present. There are 2 subclasses of IgA, IgA1 and IgA2, distinguished by their distribution and by arrangement of disulphide bonds. IgA1 is the predominant form of IgA found in serum, whereas IgA1 and IgA2 isotypes are present in roughly equal proportions in sIgA; both the α1, and α2 heavy chains can interact with J chain and secretory component.

IgA is a component of the secondary humoral response. The principal antigens that elicit an IgA response are micro-organisms in the gut (e.g. antigens introduced by foodstuffs) or in the airways. IgA cannot cross the placenta and so has no role in passive immunity in the fetus. However, sIgA can be passed to the neonate during lactation and is therefore of significant protective value because the IgA transferred by the mother will reflect immune responses to pathogens present in the environment throughout the period of breast-feeding.

3.4   IgE

IgE (MW 184 kDa, 8S), sometimes referred to as reaginic antibody, is present in very small amounts in normal individuals, but levels are increased in patients with allergic conditions (e.g. hay fever). The ε (epsilon) chain has 4 C domains, and its Fc structure is specialized for interaction with high affinity receptors for the Fc piece of IgE present on mast cells and basophils. Cross-linking of IgE bound to such Fc receptors leads to degranulation of the cell, with sub-

Table 3.1 Molecular properties of immunoglobulins

	IgM	IgG1	IgG2	IgG3	IgG4	IgA1	IgA2	sIgA	IgD	IgE
Heavy chain	μ	γ_1	γ_2	γ_3	γ_4	α_1	α_2	α_1/α_2	δ	ϵ
MW (kDa)	65	51	51	60	51	56	52	52 or 56	70	72.5
Assembled form	$(\mu_2 L_2)_5$ J[a]	$\gamma_2 L_2$[b]	$\gamma_2 L_2$	$\gamma_2 L_2$	$\gamma_2 L_2$	$\alpha_2 L_2$	$\alpha_2 L_2$	$(\alpha_2 L_2)_2$ J SC[c]	$\delta_2 L_2$	$\epsilon_2 L_2$
MW (kDa)	970	146	146	160	146	160	160	385	188	184
Sedimentation coefficient	19S	7S	7S	7S	7S	7S	7S	11S	7S	8S
Valency for Ag	10	2	2	2	2	2	2	4	2	2
Serum concentration (mg ml^{-1})	1.5	9	3	1	0.5	3	0.5	0.05	0.03	0.000 05

[a]MW of J chain is 15 kDa.
[b]Written as $\gamma_2 L_2$ for convenience; formal structural formula is $(\gamma_1)_2 L_2$.
[c]MW of secretory component (SC) is 70 kDa.

sequent release of histamine and other pharmacological mediators (Ishizaka, Tomioka and Ishizaka 1971), triggering a series of physiological reactions that can result in anaphylaxis. Thus, IgE is a mediator of type I hypersensitivity reactions. IgE may have evolved originally to combat parasitic infestations (e.g. by helminths) and the development of anaphylactic responses was an unfortunate by-product. IgE does not fix complement via the classical pathway but may activate the alternative pathway. It is found in roughly equal proportions in the bloodstream and extravascular space.

3.5 IgD

IgD is present in very low concentrations in the serum and its exact functional role is unknown. The δ heavy chain has 3 C domains. IgD is most frequently found on the cell membrane of B lymphocytes, where its main function appears to be that of a cell membrane receptor for antigen.

3.6 Other immunoglobulin components

Light chains are found in 2 forms, kappa (κ) and lambda (λ), and any single antibody molecule contains only one type of light chain. The proportion of κ:λ in the human is 2:1, but this ratio varies considerably between species. The κ and λ proteins are products of independent genes located on different chromosomes.

J chain is a glycoprotein of MW 15 kDa associated with polymeric Igs (i.e. IgM or IgA) which serves to stabilize the structure of the polymerized immunoglobulins (Chapuis and Koshland 1974).

Secretory component is a glycoprotein of MW 70 kDa found almost exclusively in sIgA, although association of secretory component with IgM, to yield secretory IgM, has been described in patients with IgA deficiency (Thompson 1970). The association of secretory component with IgM molecules is a reflection of the initial identity of secretory component as the receptor for polymeric immunoglobulin on the apical surface of epithelial cells. After binding the polymeric Ig, the receptor molecule transports the Ig across the cell (a process called transcytosis) to the basolateral surface membrane where the receptor is cleaved; a portion of the cleaved receptor remains in non-covalent association with the IgA; it is this protein which is designated as secretory component. Thus, secretory component, an important component of the sIgA molecule, is not a biosynthetic product of B lymphocytes.

3.7 Immunoglobulin metabolism

Immunoglobulins are being constantly synthesized, secreted into the circulation and catabolized (Table 3.2). Once secreted into the extracellular environment, each Ig isotype has a characteristic metabolic half-life, IgG molecules tending to be the longest-lived species, and IgE molecules being most rapidly cleared from the circulation (Table 3.2). The rate of synthesis of IgG molecules in humans is 33 mg kg^{-1} per day, i.e. more than 2 g per day for a 70 kg man. IgG molecules are relatively long lived in the circulation, with a half-life of approximately 21 days; IgG3 has a half-life of 7 days. The fractional catabolic rate of IgG molecules, or the percentage turned over per day, is of the order of 17% (7% for IgG3). During an active immune response, the amount of specific antibody synthesized in terms of µg of protein is quite small and represents only a minor fraction of the total IgG present in the serum; thus, initiation of a vigorous humoral immune response does not make a large impact on the total serum concentration of immunoglobulin. The catabolism of immunoglobulin is regulated by the Fc region and involves both protein and oligosaccharide components (Winkelhake 1978).

3.8 Membrane immunoglobulin

B lymphocytes express a receptor form of Ab, membrane Ig (mIg), on their cell surfaces. As required by the clonal selection hypothesis, the receptor Ab is identical in essentially all respects to the Ab which will be secreted by the B cell upon contact with Ag; the sole difference is the presence of a hydrophobic sequence at the C-terminus of the heavy chain which allows stable insertion into the plasma membrane. The mIg forms part of the B cell antigen–receptor complex and is found associated with other proteins at the cell membrane. It should be noted that the mIg molecule is always found as a single 4-chain unit; thus, primary B cells synthesizing IgM express a single 4-chain mIgM unit at their cell surface but, once activated by Ag, secrete a polymeric IgM containing 5 4-chain IgM units. The mIg associated proteins are transmembrane proteins of 34 kDa (Ig-α) and 37 kDa (Ig-β) which have functions in efficient transport of the mIg molecule to the cell surface and in linking the B cell antigen–receptor complex to the intracellular signalling machinery of the B lymphocyte. The Ig-α and Ig-β proteins form a disulphide-bonded complex with each other and associate non-covalently with the mIg molecule (Reth 1992). The mechanisms of intracellular signalling triggered by the B cell antigen–receptor complex are extremely complex and involve recruitment of soluble protein tyrosine kinases, activation of inositol lipid hydrolysis and calcium mobilization (reviewed by Cushley and Harnett 1993). The biological response of the B cell to binding of Ag to the B cell antigen–receptor complex depends upon the state of differentiation of the B lymphocyte (see section 5.1, p. 32).

4 BIOLOGICAL EFFECTOR FUNCTIONS OF IMMUNOGLOBULINS

4.1 Range of effector functions

Antibody molecules by themselves are not directly

Table 3.2 Metabolism of immunoglobulins

	IgM	IgG1	IgG2	IgG3	IgG4	IgA1	IgA2	IgD	IgE
Serum concentration (μg ml^{-1})	1500	9000	3000	1000	500	3000	500	30	0.05
Distribution (%)[a]	80	45	45	45	45	42	42	75	50
Synthetic rate (mg kg^{-1} day^{-1})	3.3	33	33	33	33	24	24	0.4	0.002
Fractional catabolic rate (%)[b]	8.8	7	7	17	7	25	25	37	71
Half-life (days)	10	21	20	7	20	6	6	3	2

[a]Distribution is expressed as the percentage of intravascular immunoglobulin.
[b]Fractional catabolic rate is expressed as the percentage of the intravascular pool catabolized per day.

cytotoxic towards invading pathogens. In most cases, the humoral immune system depends on the recruitment of other cytotoxic systems which can eliminate invading organisms, once specifically directed to the target by Ab. Consequently, antibody molecules participate in a wide variety of effector functions (Table 3.3). These activities are triggered following binding of specific antigen and can involve a wide range of serum proteins, lymphocytes and non-specific inflammatory cells. Thus, the complement cascade is readily activated by immune complexes which contain antibodies of particular subclasses. The Fc portion of immunoglobulins can be bound by specific receptors on the plasma membranes of a wide range of cells; this interaction has consequences for the phagocytosis of target organisms, or for direction of antibody-dependent cellular cytotoxicity (ADCC) for the destruction of cellular targets. Studies with fragments of Ig molecules and with monoclonal antibodies to specific domains of the IgG molecule have demonstrated convincingly that the expression of effector functions is mediated by the Fc portion of the immunoglobulin molecule.

4.2 Neutralization

Neutralization is not strictly an effector function since it is a direct consequence of the binding of Ab to an Ag and does not require the Fc region; it is, however, an important means by which Abs protect the host against disease. Many pathogens mediate their effects by elaborating toxic agents which bind to specific receptors on target tissues to induce a biological response or, in the case of viruses and intracellular bacteria, utilize cell surface structures to gain entry to

cells where replication can occur. In such circumstances, a protective Ab is one which specifically interferes with the interaction of the toxin or pathogen with a cell surface receptor. In an immune response to a single agent, a large array of antibodies are produced which can bind at distinct sites (called epitopes or determinants) on the foreign protein or pathogen. Taking a toxin as an example, if an Ab binds to the toxin at an epitope which is required by the toxin for interaction with a cell surface receptor, then the Ab sterically hinders the binding of toxin to the cell surface receptor and is said to neutralize the biological activity of the toxin; thus, the toxin cannot bind to the receptor and so no pathology develops. The same applies to neutralizing Abs specific for viruses: if Ab blocks the interaction of a virus with a receptor then the virus cannot enter a cell and consequently no replication occurs and no overt disease develops. A goal of vaccine strategies is therefore to induce the production of neutralizing antibodies in the immunized host.

4.3 Complement fixation

The classical pathway of complement activation is readily triggered by immune complex formation, although not all isotypes are capable of participating in this reaction (Table 3.3). Thus, IgM is a potent activator of complement but IgA is unable to activate the classical pathway. It should be noted, however, that aggregated IgA molecules, and possibly IgE molecules, may activate the alternative pathway of complement fixation. The capacity to activate the complement cascade depends upon the ability to interact with the C1q

Table 3.3 Effector functions of immunoglobulins

	IgM	IgG1	IgG2	IgG3	IgG4	IgA1	IgA2	sIgA	IgD	IgE
Complement fixation	+++	++	+	+++	−	+[a]	−	−	−	−
Placental transfer	−	−	+	−	+	−	−	−	−	−
Binding to										
Mononuclear cells	−	+	−	+	−	−	−	−	−	−
Polymorphonuclear cells	−	+	−	+	−	−	−	−	−	−
Basophils and mast cells	−	−	−	−	−	−	−	−	−	+++
T and B lymphocytes	+	++	−	++	−	+	+	−	−	+

[a]Activation of the alternative pathway.
+, ++, +++, degrees of efficacy (+, poor; +++, good).
−, no reports of activity.

component and, in the case of IgG molecules, upon the segmental flexibility of the molecule.

The point of interaction between IgG and C1q has been mapped to 3 residues, glutamate-318, lysine-320 and lysine-322 in the 3-strand face of the Cγ2 domain (Duncan and Winter 1988). The carbohydrate group of IgG, located on asparagine-297, influences the effectiveness of complement fixation since absence of the oligosaccharide leads to a decrease in activation of the classical pathway, an effect which may be explained by a 3-fold increase in the dissociation constant for the interaction between IgG and C1q when non-glycosylated IgG molecules are employed (Leatherbarrow et al. 1985).

4.4   Fc receptor interactions

Receptors specific for the Fc portion of immunoglobulin molecules are found on a wide variety of cells, including B and T lymphocytes, macrophages and monocyte and polymorphonuclear cells (reviewed by Burton 1985). The presence of Fc receptors (FcRs) on macrophage and polymorphonuclear cells has implications for the successful eradication of bacterial infections. Thus, the humoral response to an invading bacterium will result in opsonization (coating) of the cell wall by antibody molecules; some damage will result from complement fixation. In addition, the FcR of a phagocytic cell will bind to antibody molecules (IgG1 and IgG3 isotypes) and phagocytosis is promoted. A bonus in this situation is that many cells also possess receptors for complement components which are themselves opsonins; complement fixation by antibody therefore results in potentiation of phagocytosis. A variation of this process occurs when larger cellular targets are coated by antibody. The polymorphonuclear cells become bound to the target, via FcR mediated binding to immune complexes, and mediate lysis of the cells to which they have been directed by the antibody.

The capacity of IgG to interact with the high affinity monocyte FcR is a particular property of the Cγ2 domain of the molecule (Burton 1985, Woof et al. 1986) and leucine-235 in the Cγ2 domain is critical in the interaction (Duncan et al. 1988). As with the IgG–C1q interaction, the carbohydrate groups seem to be necessary for optimal receptor–ligand interaction, as absence of oligosaccharides severely reduces binding of IgG to FcR; the precise molecular role of the oligosaccharides is not well understood.

High affinity IgE receptors are found on mast cell and basophil membranes (Hulett and Hogarth 1994), and the Cε3 and Cε4 domains appear to be critical for receptor–ligand interaction. IgE also binds to a low affinity receptor, denoted CD23, found on the surface of lymphocytes and other haematopoietic cells. CD23 is believed to have a role in the regulation of IgE production by B lymphocytes (Bonnefoy et al. 1995).

5   CELLULAR AND GENETIC BASIS OF ANTIBODY PRODUCTION

5.1   B lymphocytes in the humoral response

B lymphocytes are the cellular seat of synthesis of Ab molecules. In humans, B cells are derived from pluripotent haematopoietic stem cells via a multi-step differentiation programme initiated in the bone marrow. A range of B lymphocyte precursors are detectable in the bone marrow and the purpose of differentiation at this stage is to provide the B cells with a single receptor for Ag (i.e. via somatic recombination of Ig genes as discussed below). Once a B cell expresses an Ag receptor and emerges into the periphery, the fate of that cell is inextricably linked to contact with Ag. An immature B cell (which expresses only mIgM) will be driven into apoptosis (programmed cell death) by contact with Ag, whereas a mature B cell (expressing both mIgM and mIgD) will be clonally expanded by Ag binding to give rise to many IgM secreting cells and also to memory B cells. Resting memory B cells are also driven to synthesize Ab by contact with Ag.

Analysis of the immune response to an Ag reveals that the initial (or primary) response consists largely of IgM antibodies of low affinity, whereas the secondary (or memory) response comprises Ab of other isotypes and of much higher affinity. The development of B cells with higher affinity for Ag is a manifestation of immunological memory. Upon activation by Ag, a mature B cell will secrete IgM Abs, which will bind Ag and form immune complexes, and will be driven to proliferate. The proliferating cells give rise to germinal centres in lymphoid organs, such as the spleen and tonsil, which contain a large number of proliferating B cells, called centroblasts, derived from one or a very few primary B cells. The centroblasts form the part of the germinal centre known as the dark zone (due to its histological appearence) and lose expression of mIgM (and mIgD); at this point, the Ig genes of the centroblast are subject to hypermutation in the V regions and to isotype switch for the C region genes. These processes give rise to non-proliferating cells, centrocytes, which express mIg of a different isotype (e.g. mIgG), with V regions that are subtly different from those of the initial primary B cell from which they were derived; individual receptors may be of lower or higher affinity for Ag. IgM immune complexes sequestered on the surface of follicular dendritic cells in the light zone of the germinal centre provide the means of selection of high affinity memory B cells. Centrocytes are programmed to die by apoptosis and will only survive if the hypermutated receptor which the cell expresses can bind Ag on the follicular dendritic cell; since Ag is present in small and limiting amounts, centrocytes with the higher affinity receptors will be favoured for survival (Liu et al. 1989). Those cells which are rescued by their ability to bind Ag (and which receive other survival signals) form the cohort of memory B cells for the initial Ag.

The processing of B cells in germinal centres therefore provides a cellular explanation for the observation of increased affinity of Abs in the secondary immune response to an Ag.

5.2 Theories of antibody production

The primary structural analysis of Ig molecules indicates that the humoral immune system is capable of recognizing a vast array of antigens in a specific manner. Two schools of thought emerged to account for this diversity: instruction of the immune system by each Ag or selection of pre-existing Ab by Ag. Evidence to support the selective theory was provided by studies of denatured and reduced Fab fragments of purified antiribonuclease Ab (Haber 1964). Reactivity to ribonuclease was always recovered after renaturation in the absence of ribonuclease, indicating that antigen (Ag) did not 'instruct' the antibody to recognize it. Thus, the information for antibody specificity must be contained in the primary structure of the immunoglobulin.

The clonal selection theory (Burnet 1959) was developed to provide a framework to explain the synthesis of antibody molecules by B lymphocytes; all B lymphocytes, whether those responding to antigen for the first time or daughter memory cells undergoing activation in response to rechallenge, obey the rules of this theory. The principal tenets of this theory are:

1 The capacity to respond to a given antigen exists prior to antigen exposure.
2 Each B lymphocyte possesses a single receptor specificity for antigen.
3 The binding specificity of the receptor is identical to that of the antibody which the cell will secrete in response to antigen binding.
4 Specific antigen is the sole signal for clonal expansion.
5 The antibody produced by a cell is subject to allelic exclusion (i.e. only one set of antibody-determining genes is activated).

The mechanisms of somatic recombination involved in the formation of active genes and in the generation of antibody diversity have been elucidated and the data are entirely consistent with the above tenets (Schatz, Oettinger and Schissel 1992).

5.3 Immunoglobulin genes and antibody diversity

The pioneering experiments of Tonegawa and his colleagues demonstrated that the genetic elements encoding V and C regions of the polypeptide are located some distance from each other in the DNA of non-B cells, but are fused together in Ab-synthesizing B cells (Hozumi and Tonegawa 1976). Indeed, in the case of the genetic material encoding V region sequences, multiple separate elements were shown to be involved. Thus, for κ chains, there are multiple V genes (250–300) and 4 functional J 'mini-genes'. V and J genes are separated by a great distance in germ-line DNA but, in a B cell, one V element is found joined to a single J element, giving a continuous unit of VJ information; that is, V and J elements undergo somatic recombination. A simple arithmetic calculation reveals that between 1000 and 1200 different VJ units can be formed by somatic recombination at the κ locus. A similar rearrangement of V and J information is observed at the λ locus (Fig. 3.2). At the heavy chain locus, there is an additional mini-gene family located between the V and J genes, called the D (diversity) genes. Two somatic recombination events are therefore required at the heavy chain locus to give a complete and active V gene: one D and one J element are recombined to give a DJ unit, followed by fusion of a single V gene to give a continuous VDJ gene. Somatic recombination is independent of antigen, thus conforming to the rules of the clonal selection theory.

The recombination process is controlled by highly conserved nucleotide sequences flanking the genes to be rearranged, and is mediated by the recombinase activating gene (RAG) products. The recombination process is not exact, and shifts in the frame of recombination can increase diversity and, in the case of fusion to the D genes, the enzyme terminal deoxyribonucleotidyl transferase can add nucleotides (usually G) to 3′ hydroxyl groups in a non-template directed manner; these are referred to as N regions. The joining of any V gene to any J gene (or DJ for heavy chains) results in deletion of all intervening DNA. Gene rearrangement proceeds in a specific order, heavy chains rearranging first, followed by κ genes; finally, and only if the κ genes do not rearrange successfully, the λ genes undergo somatic recombination. Successful recombination on one of the 2 chromosomes bearing a given Ig gene prevents rearrangement on the other chromosome, thus suggesting an explanation for allelic exclusion.

The active Ig gene is transcribed into a primary nuclear RNA (nRNA) transcript which contains not only the coding elements (exons) for V and C regions but also all the non-coding sequences (introns). Introns are found between the recombined VJ or VDJ unit and its appropriate C gene and, in the case of heavy chains only, between the exons which encode the individual domains of the heavy chain polypeptide. Introns are removed by RNA splicing to yield an mRNA molecule in which all the V and C information is continuous. This is translated to yield the functional Ig polypeptide.

Clonal selection requires the receptor Ig to have the same structure as the Ab which the B cell will later secrete. B cells simultaneously synthesize discrete mRNAs which programme the synthesis of the structurally distinct receptor and secretory forms of their heavy chain polypeptide (Singer, Singer and Williamson 1980). This is again accomplished by RNA splicing, in this case by selective use of 2 small exons, located at the 3′ end of the C gene for each heavy chain isotype, which encode hydrophobic sequences allowing stable insertion into the plasma membrane; these are the M (membrane) exons (Alt et al. 1980).

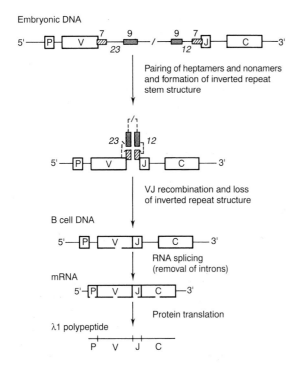

Embryonic DNA

Fig. 3.2 Generation of a functional λ_1 immunoglobulin light chain gene. The organization of coding (exons) and non-coding (introns) sequences in embryonic and B cell DNA are illustrated. The exons, depicted as open boxes, encode the leader peptide (P), the variable region gene (V), the joining mini-gene (J), and the constant region coding sequence (C). Introns are shown as thin solid lines. A pair of conserved sequences located at the 3' end of the V gene and the 5' end of the J gene serve to guide the recombination process. The first of these is a heptanucleotide motif of sequence CACTGTG (hatched box), and the other is a nonanucleotide (filled box) of sequence GGTTTTTGT. Within a single strand of DNA, the elements located at the 5' end of the J gene are precisely complementary to those at the 3' end of the V gene, thus promoting base pairing within the DNA strand to generate the inverted repeat stem structure shown in the figure. Note that, for recombination to occur, the conserved elements must be separated by spacers of different lengths (12 and 23 bases) as this generates the recognition structure for the RAG products important in somatic recombination. Once brought into close proximity, there is scission of the DNA to release intervening DNA and ligation of the termini of the V and J genes to form a contiguous VJ unit. Following transcription, the primary nuclear RNA transcript undergoes processing to remove the intronic sequences to generate a messenger RNA in which all the coding sequences are continuous and which programmes the synthesis of a functional λ_1 polypeptide.

Heavy and light chain mRNA molecules are synthesized on distinct membrane-bound polyribosomes and, in common with all secretory and membrane proteins, the nascent chains are guided across the endoplasmic reticulum membrane by a hydrophobic sequence, the signal peptide, which is proteolytically removed during transit across the membrane. Glycosylation of the nascent chain occurs cotranslationally and assembly of 4-chain units occurs in the lumen of the endoplasmic reticulum; in the case of IgM and IgA molecules, polymerization and addition of J chains are

late events, probably occurring immediately before the final secretory event. Ig synthesis proceeds in different B cells at distinct rates which reflect the state of differentiation of the B cell. Thus, a small resting B cell synthesizes 10^6 Ig molecules per day, mostly for use as receptor Ig, whereas a plasma cell can produce up to 2000 Ig molecules per second, essentially all of which is of the secretory form.

Immunological memory in the humoral response is reflected in the production of higher affinity Abs of non-IgM isotypes (e.g. IgG). Increased affinity is a function of somatic hypermutation of V region sequences and selection of antigen mediated selection of high affinity clones in germinal centres, whereas isotype switching at the level of the DNA results from movement of the VDJ gene from its original position just 5' to the Cμ gene to a new position immediately 5' to, for example, the Cγ gene. All intervening DNA is deleted during this rearrangement process, called switch recombination, but the molecular signals are different from those controlling VDJ and VJ recombination events (Harriman et al. 1993). The exception is the simultaneous production of mIgM and mIgD by mature B cells; the synthesis of the δ heavy chain does not involve switch recombination. It is the result of the RNA splicing of a long transcript that contains VDJ, all the Cμ information and the Cδ gene (Blattner and Tucker 1984).

6 ANTIBODIES IN HEALTH AND DISEASE

6.1 Protective value of the humoral response

Antibody molecules play an important role in protection against a wide variety of invading organisms. The value of the humoral response in protection of the host is best illustrated in individuals whose humoral immune function is impaired. The severest form of congenital immunodeficiency is severe combined immunodeficiency (SCID), in which there is an almost complete lack of a functional immune system. The prognosis for such patients is very poor. SCID occurs in several forms including an X-linked defect in a cytokine receptor component (Russell et al. 1994) and an autosomal abnormality in nucleotide metabolism (adenine deaminase deficiency). An example of a more B cell selective immunodeficiency is the X-linked Bruton's agammaglobulinaemia, a condition in which the capacity to mount antibody responses is absent (Sideras and Edvard Smith 1995). The defect in this instance can be traced to a mutation in a tyrosine kinase activity (*btk*, or Bruton's tyrosine kinase) which is found only in B cells and is necessary for the early development of B cells. The consequence of the deficiency is that patients tend to suffer from a wide variety of recurrent bacterial infections, although the T cell component of the immune response is normal in such patients and the ability to resist viral and fungal infections is relatively unimpaired. Similarly, defects caused by mutation in, or deletion of, particular C region genes can predispose the individual to a tight range of diseases; for example, ataxia telangiectasia patients frequently have a specific deficiency in IgA production and suffer repeated sinopulmonary infections, thus illustrating the value of sIgA in protecting secretory surfaces. By contrast, patients suffering from DiGeorge's syndrome, an autosomal recessive disease characterized by the absence of a thymus, possess no cellular immunological functions and are consequently extremely susceptible to viral and fungal infections. Such patients have a comparatively normal primary humoral response and can readily eradicate bacterial infection. Thus, the humoral immune response plays a critical role in defence against both primary and secondary bacterial infections, whereas the cellular immune system affords protection against primary viral infections.

6.2 Immunological damage mediated by antibody

The ability of antibodies to eliminate pathogens depends upon their ability to recruit the potent cytotoxic power of the non-specific immune system. However, there are instances in which the damaging effects of phagocytic cells, complement or other mediators is directed towards self tissues, resulting in tissue damage and loss of function. This is manifest as allergy or autoimmune disease. As noted earlier, allergies can arise due to induction of IgE synthesis, but IgG antibodies also cause significant damage if undesirable specificities are present. Thus, penicillin is a small β-lactam ring-containing antibiotic which, due to its small size, is generally non-immunogenic (i.e. it is unable to provoke an antibody response). However, in some individuals the penicillin binds to platelets and, in this form, it is highly immunogenic. On a first treatment with the drug, IgM antibodies are produced and immunological memory established; although there is damage to platelets by the primary response, this is generally not severe. On taking penicillin on a second or subsequent occasion, IgG antibodies of high affinity are elicited which bind to the drug associated with the platelet membrane. The formation of the immune complex is the signal for delivery of lethal complement mediated damage to the platelets and to their uptake by phagocytes.

Penicillin allergy is an example of accidental damage to self tissues. In other cases, B lymphocytes bearing receptor specificity for self components are not removed during development and antibodies to self tissues, autoantibodies, are produced. In some instances, for example in Hashimoto's thyroiditis, the antibodies focus complement and phagocytic activity directly at a particular target tissue, leading to loss of function, whereas in other syndromes the effect of the antibody is more indirect; thus, antibodies to intrinsic factor block uptake of vitamin B12 from the gut, resulting in pernicious anaemia. In certain autoimmune disease states, the pathology is related to the formation of immune complexes of autoantibody and autoantigen and accumulation of these complexes in particular tissues. Thus, in rheumatoid arthritis, anti-IgG antibodies form immune complexes with IgG and these deposit in the joints. The non-specific immune system responds to the presence of an immune complex by complement activation leading to local tissue damage, inflammation, pain and loss of function. A similar situation develops in systemic lupus erythematosis in which anti-DNA antibodies complex with DNA and precipitate in the kidney, resulting in damage to basement membrane. In each case, the non-specific immune system is targeted to the self tissue by autoantibody. The value of tolerance to self tissues is therefore evident.

6.3 Immunotechnology: monoclonal antibodies

The specificity of antibodies makes them excellent tools for use in diagnostics and therapy. The critical advance that revolutionized the technological application of antibodies was the development of monoclonal antibodies (mAbs). In short, this technology allows the establishment of an immortal cell line which secretes a single antibody of defined specificity. In practical terms, the procedure exploits the enormous specificity present in a sample of normal lymphocytes and the capacity for infinite growth found in B cell tumours. Thus, a sample of normal lymphocytes from an immunized host are fused to tumour cells in the test tube to make a hybrid cell. The normal lymphocytes are programmed to die rapidly, so any which do not fuse to the tumour cells simply die out over a few days. The tumour cells used in the fusion are chosen on the basis of a minor defect in nucleotide metabolism which means that addition of certain nucleotide analogues to the cultures will selectively cause death of the tumour cells. The normal lymphocytes have intact nucleotide metabolism and, when fused to a tumour cell, gain the immortal properties of the tumour and contribute both their antibody specificity and their normal nucleotide metabolism; it is this combination which allows only the hybrid cells to survive in the presence of the selecting drug. The hybrids, called hybridomas, can be cloned at limiting dilution and screened for the desired mAb specificity. Once a suitable clone is identified it can be grown in large cultures and gram quantities of homogenous antibody produced.

mAbs have found many applications in medicine. Perhaps the most obvious example of an immunodiagnostic product is the readily available pregnancy testing kit, which employs mAbs to human chorionic gonadotrophin and yields a definitive result in less than 5 min. mAbs specific for a range of cell surface markers find use in haematology laboratories in the diagnosis of leukaemia and other disorders and in routine clinical biochemistry laboratories for accurate quantitation of blood proteins and hormones. Immunotherapeutics using antibodies envisages infusion of mAbs, either alone or coupled to radionuclides or potent biological toxins, as means to eliminate tumour cells. Although the use of mAbs in this way has not yet met with universal success, there are isolated instances of remission of certain tumours, which offers significant promise for the future of immunotherapeutics.

REFERENCES

Alt FW, Bothwell ALM et al., 1980, Synthesis of secreted and membrane-bound immunoglobulin μ-chains is directed by mRNAs that differ at their 3′ ends, *Cell*, **20**: 293–301.

Blattner FR, Tucker PW, 1984, The molecular biology of immunoglobulin D, *Nature (London)*, **307**: 417–22.

Bonnefoy JY, Gauchat JF et al., 1995, Regulation of IgE synthesis by CD23/CD21 interaction, *Int Arch Allergy Immunol*, **107**: 40–2.

Burnet FM, 1959, *The Clonal Selection Theory of Immunity*, Vanderbilt Press, New York.

Burton DR, 1985, Immunoglobulin G; functional sites, *Mol Immunol*, **22**: 161–206.

Chapuis RM, Koshland ME, 1974, Mechanisms of IgM polymerization, *Proc Natl Acad Sci USA*, **71**: 657–61.

Cushley W, Harnett MM, 1993, Cellular signalling mechanisms in B lymphocytes, *Biochem J*, **292**: 313–32.

Duncan AR, Winter G, 1988, The binding site for C1q on IgG, *Nature (London)*, **332**: 738–40.

Duncan AR, Woof JM et al., 1988, Localisation of the binding site for the human high-affinity Fc receptor on IgG, *Nature (London)*, **332**: 563–4.

Edelman GM, Gally JA, 1962, The nature of Bence Jones proteins. Chemical similarities to polypeptide chains of myeloma globulins and normal γ-globulins, *J Exp Med*, **116**: 207–27.

Edelman GM, Poulik MD, 1961, Studies on structural units of the γ-globulins, *J Exp Med*, **113**: 861–84.

Edelman GM, Cunningham BA et al., 1969, The covalent structure of an entire gamma G immunoglobulin molecule, *Proc Natl Acad Sci USA*, **63**: 78–85.

Haber E, 1964, Recovery of antigenic specificity after denaturation and complete reduction of disulfides in a papain fragment of antibody, *Proc Natl Acad Sci USA*, **52**: 1099–106.

Harriman W, Volk H et al., 1993, Immunoglobulin class switch recombination, *Annu Rev Immunol*, **11**: 361–84.

Hozumi N, Tonegawa S, 1976, Evidence for somatic rearrangement of immunoglobulin genes coding for variable and constant regions, *Proc Natl Acad Sci USA*, **73**: 3628–32.

Hulett MD, Hogarth MP, 1994, Molecular basis of Fc receptor function, *Adv Immunol*, **57**: 1–127.

Ishizaka T, Tomioka H, Ishizaka K, 1971, Degranulation of human basophil leukocytes by anti-γE antibody, *J Immunol*, **106**: 705–10.

Kabat EA, Wu TT et al., 1987, *Sequences of Proteins of Immunological Interest*, 4th edn, US Department of Health and Human Services, Public Health Service, NIH, Bethesda, MD.

Leatherbarrow RJ, Rademacher TW et al., 1985, Effector functions of a monoclonal aglycosylated mouse IgG2a: binding and activation of complement component C1 and interaction with human monocyte Fc receptor, *Mol Immunol*, **22**: 407–15.

Liu YJ, Joshua DE et al., 1989, Nature of antigen-driven selection in germinal centres, *Nature (London)*, **342**: 929–31.

Milstein C, 1966, Variations in amino-acid sequence near the disulphide bridges of Bence Jones proteins, *Nature (London)*, **209**: 370–3.

Oi VT, Vuang TM et al., 1984, Correlation between segmental flexibility and effector fuctions of antibodies, *Nature (London)*, **307**: 136–40.

Parekh RB, Dwek RA et al., 1985, Association of rheumatoid arthritis and primary osteoarthritis with changes in the glycosylation patterns of total serum IgG, *Nature (London)*, **316**: 452–5.

Porter RR, 1962, Structure of γ-globulins, *Symposium on Basic Problems in Neoplastic Disease*, eds Gelhorn A, Hirschberg E, Columbia University Press, New York, 177.

Reth M, 1992, Antigen receptors on B lymphocytes, *Annu Rev Immunol*, **10**: 97–121.

Russell SM, Johnston JA et al., 1994, Interaction of IL-2Rβ and γc chains with Jak1 and Jak3: implications for XSCID and XCID, *Science*, **266**: 1042–4.

Schatz DG, Oettinger MA, Schissel MS, 1992, V(D)J recombination: molecular biology and regulation, *Annu Rev Immunol*, **10**: 359–83.

Sideras P, Edvard Smith CI, 1995, Molecular and cellular aspects of X-linked agammaglobulinemia, *Adv Immunol*, **59**: 135–223.

Singer PA, Singer HH, Williamson AR, 1980, Different species of messenger RNA encode receptor and secretory IgM mu chains differing at their carboxy termini, *Nature (London)*, **285**: 294–300.

Thompson RA, 1970, Secretory piece linked to IgM in individuals deficient in IgA, *Nature (London)*, **226**: 946–8.

Valentine RC, Green NM, 1967, Electron microscopy of an antibody–hapten complex, *J Mol Biol*, **27**: 615–17.

Winkelhake JL, 1978, Immunoglobulin structure and effector functions, *Immunochemistry*, **15**: 695–714.

Woof JM, Partridge LJ et al., 1986, Localisation of the monocyte binding region on human immunoglobulin G, *Mol Immunol*, **23**: 319–30.

C h a p t e r   4

COMPLEMENT

R B Sim

1   INTRODUCTION

The complement system is an important component of immune defence against infection. It is part of the innate (non-adaptive) immune system, and can respond to challenges by micro-organisms before an adaptive immune response has developed. Hereditary deficiencies of complement proteins are rare, but individuals who lack part of the complement system are generally at increased risk of recurrent infection. Complement promotes and regulates the phagocytosis or lysis of foreign cells, particles or macromolecules and the breakdown products of host tissue.

The human complement system is composed of more than 30 proteins, both soluble (in blood plasma and other body fluids) and membrane-bound (on blood cells and other tissues), that interact with each other when the system is activated by various stimuli. The properties of the major soluble proteins are summarized in Table 4.1. The cell surface proteins act as receptors for fragments of soluble complement proteins or as regulatory proteins that control the activities of soluble complement proteins, and protect from attack by complement the cells on which they are situated.

In addition to its role in innate immunity, complement interacts with the adaptive immune system in several ways. These include recognition and activation of complement by antibody–antigen complexes, roles in the regulation of B lymphocyte activity, and participation in the localization of some antigens to antigen-presenting cells.

Various proteins of the complement system detect 'targets' (Fig. 4.1) and bind to them, usually by mechanisms that involve the recognition of charge distribution patterns or of carbohydrate on the surface of the target. Recognition and activation occurs by 2 major routes, named the classical and alternative path-

ways. The binding of complement proteins to targets results in activation of the complement system and formation, on the target, of unstable complex proteases, the C3 convertases. The C3 convertases (designated C4b2a or C3bBb, see Fig. 4.1) of the 2 complement pathways are each made up of 2 protein components. One component (C4b or C3b) is covalently bound to the surface of the complement activator and the other (C2a or Bb) is a serine protease that is able to cleave and activate C3, the most abundant complement component. The major fragment of activated C3, C3b, binds covalently to complement-activating surfaces, such as cells, viruses and immune complexes. When large amounts of C3b or its proteolytic breakdown product iC3b have been deposited on activating surfaces, phagocytosis of the coated substance is greatly enhanced. This occurs partly through the interaction of the surface-bound C3 fragments with C3 receptors located on phagocytic cells. If the complement activator has a lipid bilayer, lysis can also occur through interaction with the membrane of components C5, C6, C7, C8 and C9, which bind together to form the membrane attack complex (MAC) (Law and Reid 1996, Sim 1993, Sim and Malhotra 1994).

The complement system in humans is very well characterized at the biochemical level. The primary sequences of almost all the proteins of the system are known, and information about their secondary and tertiary structure is being obtained. The activities of the proteins in vitro is generally known in considerable detail, but many uncertainties remain about their activities in vivo (for reviews see Law and Reid 1996, Sim 1993). The major and well established activities in vivo are opsonization/phagocytosis and cell lysis, and roles in the control of vascular permeability and neutrophil chemotaxis. Other activities that contribute to the regulation of lymphocyte function are being explored (Fearon and Carter 1995, Gustavsson,

Table 4.1   Properties of the soluble complement proteins

Protein	MW (kDa)	Serum concentration (mg l^{-1})	No. of polypeptide chains	Homology group or homologues
C1q	465	80–100	18	MBL, SPA
C1r	85	35–50	1, cleaved to 2 on activation	Serine protease
C1s	85	35–50	1, cleaved to 2 on activation	Serine protease
C4	195	300–450	3	C3, C5, α2m
C2	110	15–25	1, cleaved to 2 on activation	Abnormal serine protease homologous to factor B
C3	185	1000–1350	2	C4, C5, α2m
C5	185	60–90	2	C3, C4, α2m
C6	120	60–90	1	Homologous to C7, C9, C8 α and β chains
C7	115	50–80	1	Homologous to C6, C9, C8 α and β chains
C8	160	60–100	3	α and β chains homologous to C6, C7, C9
C9	75	50–80	1	Homologous to C6, C7, C8 α and β chains
Factor B	90	180–250	1, cleaved to 2 on activation	Abnormal serine protease homologous to C2
Factor D	25	2	1	Serine protease
Properdin	220	20–30	Oligomeric, usually tetramer of 56 kDa subunit	Thrombospondin
Factor H	155	100–150	1	Member of RCA family, with CR1, CR2, MCP, DAF
Factor I	88	30–40	2	Serine protease
C4bp	540	200–400	7 × 70 kDa plus 1 × 50 kDa	Member of RCA family, with CR1, CR2, MCP, DAF
C1-Inh	110	150–300	1	Serpin

α2m, α2 macroglobulin; DAF, decay-accelerating factor; MBL, mannose-binding lectin; MCP, membrane cofactor protein; RCA, regulation of complement activation; SPA, surfactant protein A.

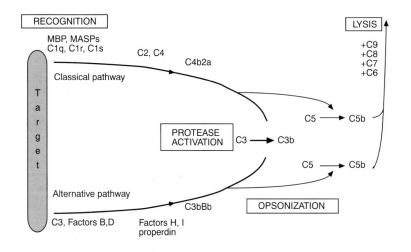

Fig. 4.1   The complement system. A simplified flow diagram of complement activation, showing the stages of recognition, protease activation, opsonization and cell lysis.

Kinoshita and Heyman 1995). A complement system similar to the human system occurs in all mammals that have been examined and variants of the system occur in all other vertebrate classes. In invertebrates, a few proteins similar to vertebrate complement proteins have been described and these may represent stages in the development of the activities of the mammalian complement system (Dodds and Day 1993).

Since the system is involved in the removal of materials from the circulation and tissues, it also has the potential to opsonize or lyse host cells. In addition to the beneficial effects of complement, undesirable complement-mediated tissue damage may occur in many situations. These include mechanical injury, viral infection, tissue damage initiated by autoantibodies, and rheumatoid arthritis. Diminished complement activity that arises through consumption of complement or from genetic defects is associated with susceptibility to infection and inadequate removal of immune complexes from the circulation, which may lead to damage of small blood vessels, particularly of the skin and kidneys.

2 THE CLASSICAL PATHWAY: ACTIVATION AND COMPONENTS

The classical pathway of complement consists of the glycoproteins C1q, C1r, C1s, and C2–C9 (Figs 4.1 and 4.2). One molecule of C1q, 2 of C1r, and 2 of C1s associate in the presence of Ca^{2+} ions to form a large protein complex called C1. C1q is the molecule that interacts with most potential targets; it provides specificity in activation of this pathway. Classical pathway activation has mostly been studied with immune complexes that contain IgG or IgM antibodies as the activator. Many other substances also activate the classical pathway, without a requirement for antibody (Taylor 1993, Sim and Malhotra 1994). These include:

1 nucleic acid and chromatin
2 cytoplasmic intermediate filaments (vimentin-type)
3 mitochondrial membranes possibly via cardiolipin or via mitochondrial proteins
4 some viruses, e.g. murine leukaemia virus (MuLV)
5 gram-positive bacteria, e.g. some pneumococci, streptococci, via capsular polysaccharide
6 gram-negative bacteria via the lipid A component of the lipopolysaccharide of the cell wall.

The initial step for classical pathway activation is the binding of C1q to the activator. C1q has a complex quaternary structure often described as a 'bunch of tulips' (see Fig. 4.3). Each molecule has 6 globular head regions and each of these contains 3 non-identical domains that can bind immunoglobulin or other targets. Each of the 3 domain types may have a different binding specificity, but it has not yet been possible to investigate this experimentally. The head regions are connected by a collagen triple helix to a central core. Activation of complement requires multiple interactions between a single molecule of C1q and the activator and, therefore, the activator is usually of high molecular weight and has a repetitive structure, such as exposed lipid A on bacterial surfaces or multiple antibody molecules bound to a particulate antigen. On binding of 2 or more C1q globular heads to the target, a conformational change occurs in C1q which is transmitted to the serine protease proenzymes C1r and C1s, which are bound to the collagenous region of C1q. This allows autoactivation of C1r, which then activates C1s. Activated C1s cleaves C4, the larger fragment of which, C4b (Fig. 4.2), has

an exposed thiol ester that is able to react non-specifically with any available nucleophiles (Fig. 4.4). These nucleophiles may be hydroxyl groups, for example on sugars, that form an ester bond to the carbonyl of the thiol ester, or amino groups located on a variety of surfaces, which form an amide bond. A proportion, usually less than 10%, of the C4b formed ends up covalently bound to the complement activator. The remainder reacts with water and diffuses away from the site of complement activation. C2 binds to the surface-bound C4b and, if it is appropriately positioned close to activated C1s, it is cleaved to form a complex, C4b2a (Fig. 4.2).

The C4b2a complex is the classical pathway C3 convertase enzyme, which is able to cleave and activate C3, a homologue of C4. Activation of C3 is similar to that of C4; activated C3b, as with C4b, contains an exposed thiol ester group through which C3b binds covalently to the surface of the complement activator. As with C4b, covalent binding of C3b is non-specific and requires only surface –OH or $-NH_2$ groups on the target (Fig. 4.4). Specificity of binding of C3b, or C4b, is conferred not by the covalent binding reaction, but by the fact that C3 and C4 are activated by enzymes already localized on the target surface. Activated C3b and C4b cannot diffuse far from the site of activation, because they are rapidly hydrolysed and inactivated. The specificity of C3b and C4b binding is, therefore, determined by the binding of C1q onto a target surface. When C4b2a activates some C3 molecules, one of the C3b product molecules can bind covalently to C4b to form a C4b2a3b complex. The C4b + C3b in this complex bind and orient C5 for cleavage by the C2a protease. C5b is homologous to C3b and C4b but has no thiol ester. C5b initiates assembly of the MAC. The freshly activated C5b binds C6, and a large complex that consists of C5b, C6, C7, C8 and C9 is built up. During assembly, the MAC associates with lipid bilayer membranes and may cause lysis and death of the target cell. If the complement activator does not contain a lipid bilayer, the MAC has no suitable target and is inactivated by soluble control proteins, including S protein (vitronectin) or SP-40,40 (clusterin). Attack on host cells by the MAC is inhibited mainly by the cell surface regulatory protein, CD59, which binds to the MAC and alters its mode of interaction with the membrane.

Molecules other than C1q can also participate in the activation of the classical pathway (Sim and Malhotra 1994, Holmskov et al. 1994, Malhotra et al. 1994, 1995). The protein, mannose-binding lectin (MBL), is able to substitute for C1q (Fig. 4.1). MBL is also sometimes called Ra reactive factor (RaRF), because it was characterized by binding to the Ra chemotype of *Salmonella*. Another name for MBL is mannose- or mannan-binding protein (MBP), but the abbreviation MBL is preferred to avoid confusion with 'major basic protein' or 'myelin basic protein'. Purified MBL activates C1r and C1s after interaction with mannose-rich structures on yeasts, bacteria and viruses. It does not bind to normal IgG, but it activates complement on interaction with the carbohydrate

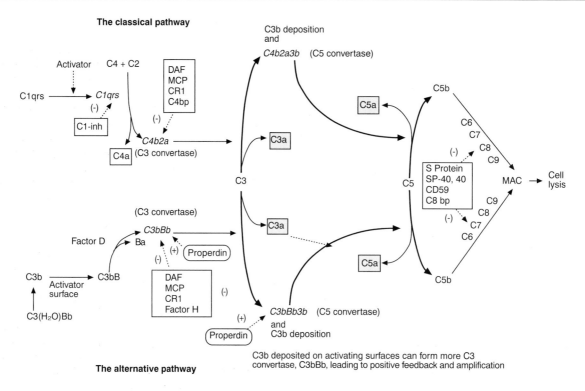

Fig. 4.2   The classical and alternative pathways of complement activation. The routes of activation of both pathways are shown, together with regulatory proteins (boxed). For the classical pathway, MBL and MASPs, shown in Fig. 4.1, may act similarly to C1q, C1r and C1s.

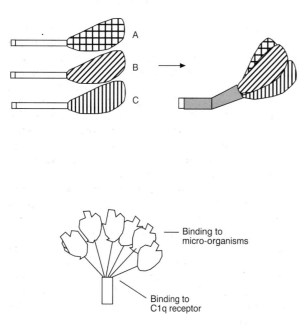

Fig. 4.3   The structure of C1q. C1q is made up of 3 types of polypeptide chains, A, B and C. The collagenous regions of these intertwine to form a collagen triple helix and a globular 'head' made up of 3 lobes: one from an A chain, one from B and one from C. Six such subunits associate covalently and non-covalently to form a 'bunch of tulips' structure. MBL is built up in the same way, and has the same shape. For MBL, however, all the polypeptide chains are identical, and each lobe of the globular head is a C-type lectin domain.

groups of a glycosylation variant of IgG, termed IgG-G0, or agalactosyl IgG, which is present at elevated levels in rheumatoid arthritis (Malhotra et al. 1995). The structure of MBL resembles that of C1q, in that it has collagenous segments and up to 6 globular heads (see Fig. 4.3). In MBL, each globular head is made up of 3 identical C-type lectin domains, which interact with carbohydrates in a calcium ion-dependent manner. Whether MBL activates C1r and C1s in vivo, or whether it is associated with other proteases that are structurally similar to C1r and C1s, and termed MBL-associated proteases (MASPs), is a matter of controversy (Holmskov et al. 1994, Malhotra et al. 1994, Vorup-Jensen et al. 1996). The 2 MASPs (MASP-1 and MASP-2) are not yet fully characterized in terms of function, but they are likely to act like C1r plus C1s, becoming activated and cleaving C2 and C4. They may be able to activate C3 directly at a low rate. MBL and MASPs are much less abundant in the circulation than are C1q, C1r and C1s, and as a result their quantitative role in complement activation is at present difficult to assess. In infants, MBL deficiency is associated with severe recurrent bacterial infections (Turner 1994, Garred et al. 1995). This deficiency was first characterized by an assay that showed severely defective opsonization of yeast (*Saccharomyces cerevisiae*) in vivo.

The acute phase protein C-reactive protein (CRP) forms complexes with charged species, including the phosphate-containing pneumococcal C-polysaccharide. Complexed CRP then interacts with C1q, and this interaction also activates the classical pathway (Jiang, Siegel and Gewurz 1991, Sim and Malhotra 1994).

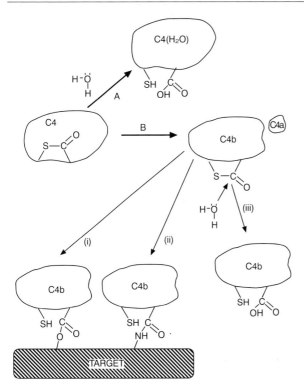

Fig. 4.4 The covalent binding reaction of C3 and C4. C4 is shown; C3 behaves very similarly. When C4 is activated by a convertase (B) it is cleaved to form C4a and C4b. The thiol ester in C4b becomes exposed to the environment, where it rapidly reacts with surface hydroxyl or amine groups to form ester (i) or amide (ii) bonds. Most of the C4b formed, however, reacts with water (iii) and so does not become bound to the surface of a complement activator. In the circulation, the thiol ester of unactivated C3 (or C4) can be attacked at a very slow rate, by low molecular weight nucleophiles, such as water or ammonia (A), to form, for example, C3 (H_2O) which has some of the properties of C3b.

The classical pathway is therefore activated by a wide range of stimuli. C1q and CRP are principally involved in recognizing charge clusters, including charged carbohydrates, such as C-polysaccharide and lipid A. In contrast, MBL recognizes neutral sugars.

Several plasma glycoproteins are involved in the regulation of activation of the classical pathway, as are a number of membrane-associated molecules that act as regulators, receptors for fragments of activated complement, or both (Law and Reid 1996). These are discussed later (see section 4, p. 42).

3 THE ALTERNATIVE PATHWAY

The proteins of the alternative pathway are factor D, factor B, C3 and C5–C9. Components C5–C9 are common to both pathways and C3 has a central role in both pathways (see Figs 4.1 and 4.2). The regulatory proteins factor H, factor I and properdin have major roles in controlling activation of the alternative pathway. Activation of the alternative pathway, like that of the classical pathway, can be both antibody-dependent and antibody-independent (Sim 1993, Taylor 1993,

Sim and Malhotra 1994). Antibody-dependent activation takes place via IgG, IgA and, rarely, IgE immune complexes. Antibody-independent activation can be effected by a whole spectrum of substances located on the surfaces of bacteria, fungi, viruses, multicellular parasites and tumour cells.

The mechanism by which targets are recognized by the alternative pathway is less well understood than for the classical pathway. In the classical pathway the 'recognition' molecule is almost always C1q (or MBL). In the alternative pathway, however, several proteins are involved simultaneously in recognition; it is thought that perturbations in the interaction between C3b deposited on the activating surface and regulatory molecules determine whether complement is activated or not.

The most obvious similarity between the alternative and classical pathways is the C3 convertase enzyme (see Figs 4.1 and 4.2). The C3 convertase of the alternative pathway is C3bBb, which is very similar to the classical pathway C3 convertase, C4b2a. Thus, C4b is a homologue of C3b, and C2 is a homologue of factor B. Factor D is a serine protease that cleaves factor B into fragments Ba and Bb when factor B is bound to C3b. In this way factor D has a role similar to the classical pathway C1s, which cleaves C2 when this is bound to C4b. The alternative pathway does not, however, have proteins similar to C1q or C1r. A paradoxical situation arises in which C3b, the product of C3 cleavage, is required in order to assemble the enzyme responsible for C3 cleavage. How do the first molecules of C3b arise?

Fearon and Austen (1975) showed that C3 that had not been proteolytically activated was able to generate C3b in the presence of factor D and factor B. It is now generally accepted that C3 in the circulation undergoes conversion, at a slow rate, to a form that behaves like C3b, but is not cleaved. This may be due to normal thermal unfolding, which results in the exposure of the reactive thiol ester group in C3 to the solvent. Small nucleophiles such as H_2O or ammonia gain access to the internal thiol ester and cleave it (see Fig. 4.4). In solution in the presence of factor B and factor D, this 'C3b-like' molecule, sometimes referred to as C3(H_2O) or C3u or C3i, is able to form a C3 convertase (C3(H_2O)Bb), and this is able to cleave and activate C3 (Fig. 4.2). The C3b so formed, if in the vicinity of a surface, is able to bind covalently via its exposed thiol ester and generate another C3 convertase (Fig. 4.2). In this way an amplification loop can be formed whereby, once C3b is deposited on a surface, very many bound and activated C3b molecules are formed.

In vivo the classical pathway is also present and the amplification of C3b deposition, via the alternative pathway, also occurs if the classical pathway C3 convertase (C4b2a) is the source of the initial C3b molecule. Multiple C3b molecules are deposited in clusters on the complement activator. This cluster formation is important in mediating multiple interactions with C3 receptors on phagocytic cells.

Whether a substance is an activator or non-activator

of the alternative pathway depends on the survival of the first C3b deposited on the surface. Once formed, C3b can be proteolysed very rapidly to a form called iC3b. This reaction is mediated by the regulatory protease factor I, which attacks C3b only when C3b has formed a complex with another regulatory protein, factor H. It is thought that the C3b on an activator is in a 'protected' site so that the control proteins, which normally convert it to iC3b, are unable to do so, leaving it able to generate more C3b via formation of a C3bBb complex. Factor H has an apparent affinity for C3b bound to non-activators 8–10 times greater than that for C3b bound to activators (Horstmann, Pangburn and Muller-Eberhard 1985, Meri and Pangburn 1990). It has been suggested that sites located on factor H interact both with C3b and with sialylated oligosaccharides or other polyanions commonly found on the surface of non-activators. When factor H interacts with a surface via both sites, that is with C3b and a feature of the surface, the apparent affinity of factor H for the bound C3b is increased. This leads to formation of a C3b–H complex, in which the C3b is attacked by factor I and cleaved to iC3b. Although the mechanism for this is not yet clearly understood, in practical terms factor H has been shown to have an important role in distinguishing between activator and non-activator surfaces (Horstmann, Pangburn and Muller-Eberhard 1985, Meri and Pangburn 1990).

There is constant turnover of C3, with C3b formation by the hydrolysis mechanism and formation of $C3(H_2O)Bb$ as discussed above. A small proportion of the C3b formed binds randomly to any available surface. Thus, some C3b will be deposited on all host cells, as well as on exogenous material. The deposited C3b will nearly always be destroyed rapidly, so that amplification of C3b fixation does not occur. On suitable surfaces, however, which provide a 'protected environment' for C3b, C3bBb will form, and the alternative pathway will be activated. This constant random fixation of C3b is a type of surveillance mechanism, in which all materials in contact with blood are tested for their capacity to activate complement. Host cells have surface regulatory proteins, including complement receptor type 1 (CR1), decay-accelerating factor (DAF) and membrane cofactor protein (MCP), which behave like factor H, and so inhibit formation of C3bBb, or promote cleavage of the C3b to iC3b (see section 4.2). This prevents opsonization of the host cell surface.

The C5 convertase of the alternative pathway is formed by the binding of an activated C3b molecule to surface bound C3bBb. As with the classical pathway C5 convertase, it is proposed that a second C3b molecule binds to C3b in a C3bBb complex. C5 recognizes and binds to both C3b molecules and is thus presented to the catalytic unit of the enzyme complex, Bb. Once the C5 convertase is assembled, the late stages of complement activation, involving assembly of the MAC, proceed as described for the classical pathway.

4 REGULATION OF COMPLEMENT ACTIVATION

As might be expected for a pathway in which a high degree of amplification occurs, regulation is exerted by way of a large number of control proteins that operate at various stages of the pathway. This is necessary to prevent damage to host tissues and also depletion of C3 and the subsequent depletion of the late complement components. Control proteins influence 3 main stages of complement activation:

1 direct inhibition of serine proteases
2 decay and destruction of convertases
3 control of the membrane attack complex.

4.1 Inhibition of serine proteases

All the proteases of the complement system are serine proteases, and all have a very high degree of specificity, i.e. they are not known to cleave any proteins other than their complement system substrates. Many serine proteases in blood have relatively specific natural inhibitors that belong to the 'serpin' family, which includes α_1-antitrypsin and α_2-antiplasmin, amongst others. Of the complement proteases, only C1r and C1s, and possibly both MASPs, are controlled by a serpin, named C1-inhibitor (C1-inh). C1-inh forms a covalent complex with the activated proteases C1r and C1s, thereby blocking the active site of each. This reaction causes C1r and C1s to dissociate from the C1q–activator complex, to leave the collagenous region of C1q available to interact with C1q receptor (Holmskov et al. 1994, Malhotra et al. 1994). Hereditary or acquired lack of C1-inh causes angio-oedema. The other serine proteases of the complement system do not appear to have any natural inhibitor. For factor D and factor I, which circulate in active rather than proenzymic form, activity is controlled by the fact that their substrates are only transiently present. Thus, factor I attacks C3b or C4b only when they are bound to a 'factor I-cofactor' protein, namely factor H, CR1 or MCP (see section 4.2), whereas factor D cleaves factor B only when it is in the form of a C3bB complex. Factor D is identical to the adipocyte protease adipsin and may have other roles outside the complement system. C2 and factor B circulate as proenzymes and are activated by C1s and factor D, respectively. They are, however, active against their natural protein substrates, C3 and C5, only when the C2a fragment is bound to C4b, or when Bb is bound to C3b. For the cleavage of C5, there is the further requirement that the trimolecular complexes C4b2a3b or $C3b_2Bb$ are assembled. As noted in section 4.2, the convertase enzymes are unstable and C2a or Bb dissociate from C4b or C3b with half-lives of less than 5 min.

4.2 Control of convertases

The C3 and C5 convertases are controlled in 3 ways (Fig. 4.5). First, the enzymatic subcomponents, C2a and Bb, dissociate from C4b or C3b, and do not rebind. Second, a group of regulatory proteins bind to the C4b2a or C3bBb complexes and accelerate their dissociation. Proteins with decay-accelerating activity include the soluble proteins factor H and C4b-binding protein (C4bp), and the membrane proteins complement receptor type 1 (CR1) and decay-accelerating factor (DAF). Third, once C2a or Bb have dissociated, the remaining C4b or C3b is inactivated by the protease, factor I.

The action of factor I requires the presence of one of several protein cofactors that bind to the substrate, C4b and/or C3b. C3b or C4b complexed to one of these cofactors is the substrate for factor I. The factor I-cofactor proteins are factor H, C4bp, CR1 and membrane cofactor protein (MCP). In decay-acceleration and factor I-cofactor activities, factor H acts only on C3b, and C4bp only on C4b. The other proteins interact with both classical and alternative pathways. C4bp and factor H are present at high concentration in plasma and they control fluid-phase, as well as surface-associated activation of C3 and C5. DAF and MCP are widely distributed on human tissues and have an important role in preventing amplification of C3b fixation to host tissues. CR1 has a more restricted tissue distribution, on erythrocytes, most leucocytes, tissue macrophage, and human kidney, and functions both as a C3b receptor and as a surface-bound regulatory protein.

Another regulatory protein acts only on the alternative pathway convertases, and acts as a positive, rather than a negative control. Properdin, sometimes called factor P, binds to C3bBb or C3b$_2$Bb and stabilizes the complex, providing a moderate increase in stability.

The regulatory proteins factor H, C4bp, MCP, DAF and CR1 are closely related homologous proteins, made up of small, independently folding domains, each 60 amino acids long (summarized in Sim et al. 1993). For example, factor H contains 20 such domains, whereas MCP and DAF each have 4. These proteins, together with complement receptor type 2

(CR2) are all encoded in the same region of the human genome, on the long arm of chromosome 1. This region is referred to as the RCA (regulation of complement activation) gene cluster.

4.3 Control of the membrane attack complex (MAC)

Assembly and regulation of the MAC is under the control of several soluble and membrane-bound proteins. Two soluble proteins, S protein (vitronectin) and SP-40,40 (also called clusterin) inhibit the insertion of the MAC into lipid bilayers, ensuring that lytic complexes cannot diffuse far from the site of complement activation. This limits possible damage to bystander cells. Membrane-bound regulatory proteins also act at this stage of the pathway; they protect the cells on which they are located from damage by complement. The more important of these is a widely distributed 20 kDa protein CD59 (also called HRF-20 or protectin), which binds the C5b–8 complex in such a way that C9 cannot bind, and in this way insertion of C9 into the bilayer is prevented. Another membrane-associated MAC regulator is a 70 kDa species, homologous restriction factor (HRF), which is less well characterized than CD59.

The importance of the membrane-bound MAC inhibitors is illustrated by paroxysmal nocturnal haemoglobinuria (PNH), a condition in which spontaneous lysis of erythrocytes takes place. In this condition, affected erythrocytes lack phosphatidyl–inositol-linked membrane proteins, including HRF and CD59. DAF is also absent from these cells, but comparison with rare cases of specific DAF deficiency indicates that absence of DAF alone is not associated with clinically significant haemolysis (Reid et al. 1991).

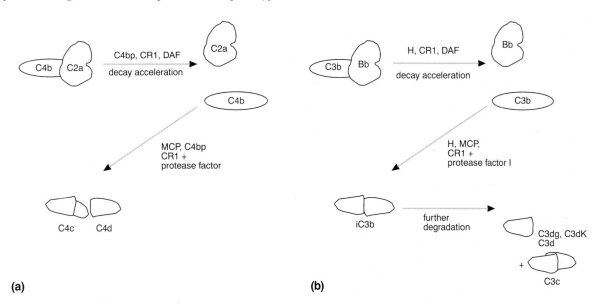

(a) **(b)**

Fig. 4.5 Control of convertases. The actions of control proteins are shown that regulate (a) C4b2a and (b) C3bBb.

Table 4.2 Receptors for C3 fragments

Receptor	Ligand	Characteristics
CR1 (CD35)	C3b	Polymorphic in size: 210 kDa to >300 kDa; main variant made up of 30 CCP domains; elongated, string-like structure, >80 nm long. Found on erythrocytes and most leucocytes, tissue macrophage and kidney. Major role in transport and phagocytosis of C3b-bearing immune complexes
CR2 (CD21)	(C3b) iC3b C3d, EBV	140 kDa; made up of 15 or 16 CCP domains; elongated structure, as CR1. Distribution limited to B and some T lymphocytes, follicular dendritic cells. Major role is regulation of B cell activities. Also a receptor for EBV
CR3 (CD11b, 18)	iC3b	Member of integrin family: 2 non-covalently-linked polypeptides, 165 and 90 kDa; multidomain structure. Found on phagocytic cells. Major role in phagocytosis. Has binding sites for other, non-complement, ligands
'CR4' (CD11c, 18) (p150, 95)	iC3b	Homologous to CR3: role as an iC3b receptor not well established. Distribution similar to CR3, and may have similar role. Also binds to other non-complement ligands
'CR5'	C3d/C3dg	Uncharacterized at the molecular level; defined as a binding activity for soluble (oligomeric) C3d on polymorphs

EBV, Epstein–Barr virus.

5 COMPLEMENT RECEPTORS

In addition to the membrane-bound regulatory proteins of the complement system, there are several receptors for complement proteins or their activation fragments. These receptors are involved in a wide range of biological activities. A number of these, particularly the receptors for C3 fragments, complement receptor types 1, 2, 3 and 4 (named CR1–4), are well characterized at the biochemical level, but others are identified only by their binding function. The properties of complement receptors have been reviewed by Sim and Walport (1987) and Brown (1995).

5.1 Receptors for C3 fragments

When C3 is activated, it is cleaved into 2 fragments, C3b (178 kDa) and C3a (9 kDa). C3b, which may be surface bound or free in solution (see Fig. 4.3), is further rapidly cleaved to iC3b (see Fig. 4.5). The latter is broken down slowly into 2 fragments, C3d and C3c. In the case of surface-bound C3b, the C3d remains on the surface; C3c diffuses away and does not seem to have any further biological role. There are several receptors that bind to C3 fragments. Their properties and possible roles are summarized in Table 4.2. The C3 receptors have major roles in immune complex clearance, phagocytosis, and regulation of lymphocytes.

5.2 Receptors for other complement proteins and fragments

Other receptors of major interest in the complement system are the receptors through which the small anaphylatoxins C4a, C3a and C5a exert their effects. These small fragments, cleaved from C3, C4 and C5 during complement activation, have effects on a wide range of cells, but their major effect is to increase vascular permeability. C5a is also a chemotactic factor. More than one receptor type may exist for these peptides, and to date the chemotaxis receptor for C5a (Boulay et al. 1991, Gerard and Gerard 1991) and a leukocyte receptor for C3a (Crass et al. 1996; Ames et al. 1996) have been characterized.

A C1q receptor (also called the collectin receptor) has been isolated and partially characterized. It also serves as a receptor for MBL and for a small family of proteins, the collectins, which are related in structure to C1q and MBL (Malhotra et al. 1990, 1992). This receptor may be involved principally in phagocytosis of C1q-bearing particles, or collectin-coated particles. Further receptors for factor H, fragments of factor B and various other complement fragments have been reported, but their biological significance is uncertain.

REFERENCES

Ames RS, Li Y et al., 1996, Molecular cloning and characterization of the human anaphylotoxin C3a receptor, *J Biol Chem,* **271:** 20231–4.

Boulay F, Tardif M et al., 1991, Expression cloning of a receptor for C5a anaphylotoxin on differentiated HL60 cells, *Biochemistry,* **30:** 2993–9.

Brown EJ, 1995, Phagocytosis, *Bioessays,* **17:** 109–17.

Crass T, Raffetseder U et al., 1996, Expression cloning of the human C3a receptor (C3aR) from U-937 cells, *Eur J Immunol,* **26:** 1944–50.

Dodds AW, Day AJ, 1993, The phylogeny and evolution of the complement system, *Complement in Health and Disease,* 2nd edn, eds Whaley K, Loos M, Weiler JM, Kluwer Academic Publishers, Dordrecht, Netherlands, 39–88.

Fearon DT, Austen KF, 1975, Initiation of C3 cleavage in the alternate complement pathway, *J Immunol*, **115:** 1357–61.

Fearon DT, Carter RH, 1995, The CD19/CR2/TARA-1 complex of B lymphocytes, *Ann Rev Immunol*, **13:** 127–49.

Garred P, Madsen HO et al., 1995, Increased frequency of homozygosity of abnormal mannan-binding protein alleles in patients with suspected immunodeficiency, *Lancet*, **346:** 941–3.

Gerard NP, Gerard C, 1991, The chemotactic receptor for human C5a anaphylotoxin, *Nature (London)*, **349:** 614–17.

Gustavsson S, Kinoshita T, Heyman B, 1995, Antibodies to murine complement receptor 1 and 2 can inhibit the antibody response in vivo without inhibiting T-helper cell induction, *J Immunol*, **154:** 6524–8.

Holmskov U, Malhotra R et al., 1994, Collectins: collagenous C-type lectins of the innate immune defense system, *Immunol Today*, **15:** 67–74.

Horstmann RD, Pangburn MK, Muller-Eberhard HJ, 1985, Species specificity of recognition by the alternate pathway of complement, *J Immunol*, **134:** 1101–4.

Jiang H, Siegel JN, Gewurz H, 1991, Bonding and activation by C-reactive protein via the collagen-like region of C1q and inhibition of these reactions by monoclonal antibodies to C-reactive protein and C1q, *J Immunol*, **146:** 2324–30.

Law SKA, Reid KBM, 1996, *Complement*, 2nd edn, IRL Press, Oxford.

Malhotra R, Thiel S et al., 1990, Human leukocyte C1q receptor binds other soluble proteins with collagen domains, *J Exp Med*, **172:** 955–9.

Malhotra R, Haurum J et al., 1992, Interaction of C1q receptor with lung surfactant protein A, *Eur J Immunol*, **22:** 1437–45.

Malhotra R, Lu J et al., 1994, Collectins, collectin receptors and the lectin pathway of complement activation, *Clin Exp Immunol*, **97, Suppl. 2:** 4–9.

Malhotra R, Wormald MR et al., 1995, Glycosylation changes of IgG associated with rheumatoid arthritis can activate complement via the mannose-binding protein, *Nature Med*, **1:** 237–43.

Meri S, Pangburn M, 1990, Discrimination between activators and nonactivators of the alternative pathway of complement: regulation via a sialic acid/polyanion binding site on factor H, *Proc Natl Acad Sci USA*, **87:** 3982–6.

Reid ME, Mallinson G et al., 1991, Biochemical studies on red blood cells from a patient with the Inab phenotype (decay accelerating factor deficiency), *Blood*, **78:** 3291–7.

Sim RB (ed.), 1993, *Activators and Inhibitors of Complement*, Kluwer Academic Publishers, Dordrecht, Netherlands.

Sim RB, Kölble K et al., 1993, Genetics of deficiencies of the soluble regulatory proteins of the complement system, *Int Rev Immunol*, **10:** 65–86.

Sim RB, Malhotra R, 1994, Interaction of carbohydrate with lectins and complement, *Biochem Soc Trans*, **22:** 106–11.

Sim RB, Walport MJ, 1987, C3 receptors, *Complement in Health and Disease*, ed. Whaley K, MTP Press, Lancaster, 125–61.

Taylor PW, 1993, Non-immunoglobulin activators of the complement system, *Activators and Inhibitors of Complement*, ed. Sim RB, Kluwer Academic Publishers, Dordrecht, Netherlands, 37–68.

Turner MW, 1994, Mannose-binding protein, *Biochem Soc Trans*, **22:** 88–94.

Vorup-Jensen T, Stover C et al., 1996, Cloning of cDNA encoding a human MASP-like protein (MASP-2), *Mol Immunol*, **33, Suppl. 1:** 81.

Chapter 5

CELL MEDIATED IMMUNITY AND INTRACELLULAR BACTERIAL INFECTIONS

S H E Kaufmann

1 INTRODUCTION

The immune system has evolved to protect the mammalian host from infectious disease but it did not develop independently of microbial pathogens; rather, they have co-evolved. Each strategy of microbial parasites to achieve their major goal of exploiting a suitable biotope for multiplication has been countered by an appropriate host response. Conversely, the pathogen responsible for each infectious disease has found a means to overcome, at least partially, host defence. In principle, the survival strategies of intracellular bacteria within the host are based on mechanisms that promote entry into and survival within host cells. These pathogens are hidden from attack by antibodies, complement and other factors. They have not, however, succeeded in concealing themselves completely from the immune system, because specialized host cells have evolved that present to T lymphocytes the surface antigens of intracellular parasites and so stimulate them. These T cells mobilize potent effector mechanisms capable of controlling intracellular pathogens. Occasionally the immune response achieves total eradication and sometimes it only restricts microbial growth and thus limits the detriment to the host.

Living intracellularly often means dependence on host cells, but many intracellular bacteria strikingly avoid causing harm to their host. Conversely, infection and disease are often markedly separated in time. Thus, intracellular bacteria that persist at their cellular site may later cause disease, when the sensitive balance between pathogen and immune response is tipped in favour of the infectious agent. Unfortunately, the immune response not only protects the host; as clinical disease unfolds, immunopathology develops. This chapter describes the general mechanisms of cell mediated immunity responsible for protection against and for pathogenesis of intracellular bacterial infections.

2 TWO TYPES OF INTRACELLULAR BACTERIA

The term 'intracellular bacteria' describes microbial pathogens that have an obligatory or facultative intracellular lifestyle (Moulder 1985). Major intracellular bacteria of both groups are listed in Table 5.1. Facultative intracellular bacteria reside mainly in mononuclear phagocytes (MPs) but certain other host cells may also become infected. Because MPs are major effectors of antimicrobial defence, living in these cells requires successful evasion of intracellular killing mechanisms. Obligate intracellular bacteria are more frequently found in host cells other than the MPs, such as epithelial and endothelial cells. These pathogens have further adapted to their intracellular habitat by losing the ability to live an extracellular lifestyle. Pathogenic rickettsiae, for example, depend on the availability of host coenzymes, such as coenzyme A, nicotinamide adenine dinucleotide (NAD) and adenosine triphosphate (ATP), which they require for their own energy production. Intracellular bacteria are found in various genera and they cause a wide variety of diseases. The general hallmarks of intracellu-

Table 5.1   Major intracellular bacteria

Pathogen	Disease	Preferred target cell	Preferred location in host cell	References
Facultative intracellular				
Mycobacterium tuberculosis M. bovis	Tuberculosis	Macrophages	Phagosome, cytosol (?)	Bloom 1994
Mycobacterium leprae	Leprosy	Macrophages, Schwann cells, numerous other host cells	Phagolysosome	Hastings 1994
Salmonella typhi/S. paratyphi	Typhoid fever	Macrophages	Phagosome	Finlay and Falkow 1989
Brucella sp.	Brucellosis	Macrophages	Phagolysosome	Smith and Ficht 1990, Baldwin, Jiang and Fernandes 1993
Legionella pneumophila	Legionnaire's disease	Macrophages	Phagosome	Barbaree, Breimann and Dufour 1993
Listeria monocytogenes	Listeriosis	Macrophages, hepatocytes	Cytosol	Kaufmann 1988b, Portnoy et al. 1992
Francisella tularensis	Tularaemia	Macrophages	Phagosome	Sandström 1994
Obligate intracellular				
Rickettsia rickettsii	Rocky Mountain spotted fever	Endothelial cells, smooth muscle cell	Cytosol	Mandell, Douglas and Bennett 1990
Rickettsia prowazekii	Endemic typhus	Endothelial cells	Cytosol	Mandell, Douglas and Bennett 1990
Rickettsia typhi	Typhus	Endothelial cells	Cytosol	Mandell, Douglas and Bennett 1990
Rickettsia tsutsugamushi	Scrub typhus	Endothelial cells	Cytosol	Mandell, Douglas and Bennett 1990
Coxiella burnetii	Q fever	Macrophages, lung parenchyma cells	Phagolysosome	Baca and Paretsky 1993
Chlamydia trachomatis	Urogenital infection, conjuctivitis, trachoma, lymphogranuloma venerum (different serovars)	Epithelial cells	Phagosome	Beatty, Morrison and Byrne 1994, Brunham and Peeling 1994
Chlamydia psittaci	Psittacosis	Macrophages, lung parenchyma cells	Phagosome	Beatty, Morrison and Byrne 1994
Chlamydia pneumoniae	Pneumonia	Lung parenchyma cells	Phagosome	Beatty, Morrison and Byrne 1994

Table 5.2 Essential and conditional features of intracellular bacterial infections

Essential
Intracellular habitat
T cell mediated protection
Delayed-type hypersensitivity
Granulomatous tissue reaction

Conditional
Labile balance between persistent infection and protective immune response
Dissociation of infection from disease
Chronic disease
Low intrinsic toxicity
Immunologically mediated pathology

lar bacterial infections are depicted in Table 5.2. Some of these features are shared by all and others by only some infections.

3 PROFESSIONAL PHAGOCYTES

Professional phagocytes include MPs and polymorphonuclear neutrophilic granulocytes (PNGs). These are the principal effector cells of antibacterial immunity and they are distinct in this respect from all other host cells, the non-professional phagocytes (Rabinovitch 1995). PNGs are found preferentially in the vascular bed from where they are rapidly attracted to sites where bacteria lodge and where they bring about an acute inflammatory response. These cells are short-lived and express aggressive host defence mechanisms (Haslett, Savill and Meagher 1989). Hence, they are central to the acute inflammatory response and required for the initial control of a bacterial infection. Phagocytosis by PNGs is lethal for all extracellular and most intracellular bacteria. Moreover, at the site of bacterial replication PNGs cause local tissue damage. These 2 mechanisms may co-operate in early host defence. In the murine listeriosis model, hepatocytes that harbour listeriae are lysed by PNGs at the beginning of infection and then the released bacteria

are killed by the same effector cells (Weiss 1989, Conlan and North 1993). Once intracellular bacteria have established themselves within host cells, they are less accessible to PNGs which increasingly lose their impact as the infection becomes chronic.

MPs comprise various tissue macrophages and blood monocytes (Adams and Hamilton 1984, Gordon et al. 1995). Tissue macrophages are long-lived cells which, in their resting state, express moderate antibacterial capacity. Once activated by T cell cytokines, in particular interferon-γ (IFN-γ), they disclose potent antimicrobial capacities and become the central effector cells in chronic intracellular bacterial infections (Table 5.3). Only a few intracellular bacteria, such as *Mycobacterium tuberculosis*, can resist activated macrophages by interfering with macrophage activation and by counteracting their effector functions (Table 5.3). The description below emphasizes the antibacterial mechanisms of MPs. Where appropriate, reference is made to PNGs and non-professional phagocytes. However, MPs are a highly heterogeneous group that express different functional capacities which are not always taken into account in the following description; rather it emphasizes the full antibacterial potential of MPs.

3.1 Phagocytosis and invasion

The term phagocytosis describes the internalization of particles, such as bacteria, by host cells (Rabinovitch 1995). Phagocytosis is a central event in the encounter between an intracellular parasite and its host. Phagocytosis is necessary to establish infection and for pathogen eradication. The process is initiated by interaction with receptor ligands, including broadly reactive receptors, such as mannose receptors that react with sugar ligands present on various micro-organisms, and more specific receptors, such as Fc receptors and complement receptors respectively with specificity for IgG or complement breakdown products (Brown 1991, Ravetch and Kinet 1991, Stahl 1992). Receptor ligand interactions induce invagination of the MP plasma membrane and so bring about phagosome formation. In the early phagosome, bacteria reside in

Table 5.3 Major antibacterial capacities of activated macrophages and microbial evasion mechanisms

Macrophage effector capacity	Microbial evasion mechanism
Defensins	Evasion into cytosol
Phagosome acidification	Phagosome neutralization
Phagosome–lysosome fusion	Inhibition of phagosome–lysosome fusion
Lysosomal enzymes	Resistance against enzymes
Intraphagolysosomal killing	Evasion into cytosol
	Robust cell wall
Reactive oxygen intermediates (ROI)	CR-mediated uptake, ROI detoxifiers, ROI scavengers
Reactive nitrogen intermediates (RNI)	Unknown (ROI and ROI detoxifiers may interfere with RNI)
Iron starvation	Microbial iron scavengers, e.g. siderophores
Tryptophan starvation	Unknown

a virtually external milieu which then undergoes step-wise changes; after a brief period of alkalization, the phagosome becomes acidic. Toxic products, such as reactive nitrogen and oxygen intermediates, are introduced into the phagosome and kill many bacteria. The phagosome then fuses with the lysosomes to make phagosomal bacteria accessible to degradative lysosomal enzymes.

As is indicated by their designation, professional phagocytes are particularly equipped for microbial uptake and killing. In contrast, non-professional phagocytes are poor to non-phagocytic, unless phagocytosis is induced by a microbial pathogen. This process is generally called invasion. Although microbial invasion is initiated by the pathogen, it is generally a function of the host cell. Invasion is induced by specific bacterial invasins that bind to host cell receptors, such as integrins or growth factor receptors, which then initiate phagocytosis (Isberg 1991, Bliska, Galán and Falkow 1993). The capacity to invade host cells is not restricted to intracellular bacteria. For various bacteria, invasion of mucosal epithelial cells is the first step of entry into the host (Goldberg and Sansonetti 1993). Examples are the facultative intracellular bacteria *Salmonella typhi*, *S. paratyphi* and *Listeria monocytogenes*, the obligate intracellular bacterium *Chlamydia trachomatis* and the extracellular bacterium *Shigella*. This type of invasion need not, however, result in stable intracellular residence, because most bacteria traverse epithelial cells only to be spread to other tissue sites.

3.2 Intracellular residence

The intracellular habitat imposes advantages and disadvantages on bacteria. Since many pathogens persist in the host for long periods of time, a fragile balance develops between microbial survival and host defence. Three different situations can be distinguished:

1 PNGs provide the most aggressive though relatively short-lived intracellular milieu for bacteria. Thus, these host cells represent a poor intracellular habitat and primarily serve host defence functions. PNGs are rapidly attracted to the site of microbial implantation, where they restrict microbial growth at the outset of infection. This is particularly important with acute infections. A major contribution of PNGs to protection against persistent intracellular infection is less compelling.
2 Non-professional phagocytes serve primarily as a protective habitat for intracellular bacteria. Although some antimicrobial mechanisms (e.g. tryptophan or iron starvation) can be activated in these cells, their overall contribution to antibacterial defence is limited.
3 MPs are the central target cells for intracellular bacteria. They serve a dual function by supplying a habitat for many intracellular bacteria in their resting state and by acting as major defenders when they have been activated.

Various non-professional phagocytes provide a habitat for obligate intracellular bacteria and for certain facultative intracellular bacteria. The pathogenic rickettsiae and chlamydiae, respectively, preferentially localize in endothelial and epithelial cells (Mandell, Douglas and Bennet 1990, Beatty, Morrison and Byrne 1994). Hepatocytes and Schwann cells, respectively, serve as the major habitat for *L. monocytogenes* and for *Mycobacterium leprae* (Portnoy et al. 1992, Hastings 1994). MPs serve as the principal host for all facultative and some obligate intracellular bacteria. Successful macrophage activation, therefore, represents the paradigm shift in protection against many intracellular bacteria; failure of this step has dramatic consequences. For the host, insufficient macrophage activation results in disseminated, often fatal disease, whereas for the pathogen, insufficient resistance to activated macrophages causes death and eradication before clinical disease can be established. Full macrophage activation opposed by highly resistant bacteria results in a sensitive balance between host and pathogen, which leads to disease only when immunity is compromised.

3.3 Phagosome alkalization and defensins

Phagocytosis results in a rapid rise in pH within the phagosome, which provides the alkaline milieu necessary for a group of low molecular weight peptides to express their antimicrobial activities (Lehrer 1993, Boman 1995). Antibacterial peptides that contain 6 cysteine residues, the defensins, are abundant in human PNGs and in epithelial cells of the gastrointestinal tract. MPs from some species also possess high concentrations of defensins. Although these and other basic antibacterial peptides are toxic for various bacteria, including certain intracellular bacteria such as *S. typhimurium*, *L. monocytogenes*, *Legionella pneumophila* and *M. tuberculosis*, their contribution to protection against intracellular bacteria remains to be established, particularly because they are rare to absent in human macrophages. Their great abundance in gastrointestinal and oropharyngeal epithelia, however, suggests an important role for these peptides in local defence at the port of entry for many pathogens.

3.4 Phagosome acidification and phagolysosome fusion

The initially alkaline pH soon falls to become acidic and this acidic milieu is itself inhibitory to bacterial growth. It can be partially neutralized by bacterial cations, such as NH_4^+, which are produced intraphagosomally by *M. tuberculosis* (Gordon, D'Arcy Hart and Young 1980, Russell 1995). The low pH is optimal for the lysosomal enzymes that are discharged into the phagosome as a result of phagosome–lysosome fusion (Bainton 1981). Lysosomes contain various hydrolases that digest and degrade proteins, lipids, carbohydrates and nucleic acids. These lysosomal enzymes facilitate microbial killing by toxic effector molecules and, more importantly, degrade killed bacteria. In principle, attack by lysosomal enzymes can be counteracted in 2 ways. Some bacteria, including *S. typhimur-*

ium, *L. pneumophila* and *Chlamydia* spp., inhibit phagosome–lysosome fusion (Finlay and Falkow 1989, Barbaree, Breimann and Dufour 1993, McClarty 1994). Other intracellular bacteria, such as *M. leprae* and *Brucella* spp., resist attack by lysosomal enzymes within the fused phagolysosome (Baldwin, Jiang and Fernandes 1993, Hastings 1994). *M. tuberculosis* seems to exploit both alternatives (Bloom 1994). This highly resistant pathogen not only interferes with phagosome–lysosome fusion by means of NH_4^+ production, but also resists lysosomal enzymes because of its very robust waxy cell wall.

3.5 Production of toxic effector molecules

The reactive nitrogen and oxygen intermediates (RNI and ROI) are central to bacterial killing. The so-called oxidative burst, which results in ROI production, is stimulated in both PNGs and MPs (Elsbach and Weiss 1983, Adams and Hamilton 1984). Major inducers of ROI are IFN-γ and IgG through their respective receptors, IFN-γR and FcR (Ravetch and Kinet 1991, Farrar and Schreiber 1993). A series of enzymatic and non-enzymatic reactions results in the conversion of molecular oxygen to ROI, O_2^-, H_2O_2, OH^-, $^1O_2$ and OH^+ radicals. Human PNGs and blood monocytes possess myeloperoxidase which induces halogenation of microbial proteins (Elsbach and Weiss 1983, Adams and Hamilton 1984). The damage caused by oxidation and halogenation is lethal for many bacteria. Nevertheless, intracellular bacteria frequently survive attack by ROI, because they have developed various evasion mechanisms (Kaufmann and Reddehase 1989). These include the complement receptors CR1 and CR3 that facilitate uptake of bacteria, such as *L. pneumophila*, *M. leprae* and *M. tuberculosis*, without stimulating a respiratory burst. Numerous intracellular bacteria, including *L. monocytogenes*, *S. typhimurium*, *L. pneumophila* and *Coxiella burnetii*, produce detoxifying enzymes, such as superoxide dismutase and catalase, which inactivate O_2^- and H_2O_2, respectively. Finally, microbial components, such as the acid phosphatase of *Coxiella burnetii* and the phenolic glycolipid of *M. leprae*, scavenge ROI.

The high concentrations of RNI necessary to kill bacteria are produced by murine MPs and PNGs, whereas high level RNI production by human MPs remains controversial (Denis 1994, Nathan and Xie 1994). Rapid and potent RNI production depends on the inducible NO synthase (i-NOS), which is most strongly induced by IFN-γ. This enzyme is central to the transformation of L-arginine to L-citrulline that leads to •NO release, which has been identified as the principal effector of antibacterial resistance against numerous intracellular bacteria in mice. Specific mechanisms of evasion from RNI attack by intracellular bacteria are unknown, but maximum RNI production can be partially affected in various ways.

3.6 Iron and tryptophan starvation

Limiting the availability of essential molecules is a powerful means of controlling intracellular bacterial growth, provided the host cell itself is not affected by such deprivation. The effects of iron and tryptophan starvation are the best studied examples of this phenomenon. Iron is necessary for bacterial growth and for antibacterial defence (Payne 1993). A great part of intracellular iron is bound to special proteins, particularly ferritin, which is its principal storage molecule, and some intracellular iron is complexed to sulphur and haem proteins. Professional phagocytes also contain lactoferrin which binds iron with high efficiency. Hence, release of lactoferrin into the phagosome limits iron availability and so contributes to controlling the growth of certain intracellular bacteria, such as *L. pneumophila* (Barbaree, Breimann and Dufour 1993). Most of the iron in the extracellular space is bound to transferrin and lactoferrin. The supply of intracellular iron is, therefore, controlled by the density of surface-expressed transferrin receptors. Bacteria mobilize iron by releasing it from host iron binding proteins, or by means of specialized iron-binding proteins, the siderophores (Payne 1993), or by a combination of both.

The best studied example of essential amino acid deprivation is growth inhibition of *Chlamydia psittaci* and *C. trachomatis* by tryptophan deprivation (McClarty 1994). Degradation of tryptophan to kynurenine by indole-amine-2,3-deoxygenase restricts growth of these pathogens not only in macrophages but also in epithelial cells.

3.7 Escape into the cytosol

In order to avoid self-damage, antibacterial effector mechanisms are focused on the phagosome. Therefore, escape from the endosome into the cytosol represents a general means of intracellular survival that is used by intracellular bacteria such as *L. monocytogenes*, *M. leprae* and *Rickettsia* spp. (Portnoy et al. 1992, Hastings 1994, Winkler 1995). In the case of *L. monocytogenes* the SH-activated cytolysin, listeriolysin, has been identified as being essential and several phospholipases have been identified as supportive, for phagosome escape (Portnoy et al. 1992). Macrophage activation by IFN-γ counteracts the passage of *Listeria* into the cytosol and so renders the organisms susceptible to endosomal killing.

4 T LYMPHOCYTES AS SPECIFIC MEDIATORS OF PROTECTION AGAINST INTRACELLULAR BACTERIA

4.1 T lymphocytes

Lymphocytes are the mediators of specific immunity. There are 2 distinct lymphocyte populations: B cells and T cells. Both express unique receptors responsible for antigen recognition and are members of the immunoglobulin supergene family. B cells express surface Ig, the direct interaction of which with free antigen leads to antibody secretion. Accordingly, B cells mediate humoral immune responses. The antigen receptor of T lymphocytes, termed the T cell receptor (TCR), remains cell bound and does not directly recognize antigen (Germain 1994). Rather, it 'sees' foreign antigen presented by surface molecules that are encoded by genes of the major histocompatibility complex (MHC). T cells are, therefore, responsible for cell mediated immune responses. The TCR is a disulphide-linked heterodimer composed either of an α and a β chain or of a γ and a δ chain (Haas, Pereira and Tonegawa 1993). In mouse and man, more than 90% of mature T cells express TCRα/β and a minor T cell population (less than 10%) expresses TCRγ/δ. A given T cell clone possesses a unique TCR that is responsible for its exquisite antigen specificity (Davis and Chien 1995). The capacity to respond to the myriad of microbial antigens is counteracted by the equally wide diversity of the T cell system. At the genetic level, this diversity is achieved principally by rearrangements of the TCR chain genes. A series of negative and positive selection events in the thymus is responsible for reactivity against the wide diversity of foreign antigens and for deletion or inactivation of self-reactive T cell clones (Jameson, Hogquist and Bevan 1995). The TCR itself fails to transduce activation signals as a result of antigen recognition. This task is performed by the CD3 complex which is closely associated with the TCR (Chan, Desai and Weiss 1994). Both TCR and CD3 are required for antigen-specific T cell activation. Accordingly, these 2 molecules are essential markers of mature T cells.

T lymphocytes express other surface molecules in addition to the TCR–CD3 complex. Some of these molecules characterize distinct T cell populations with specialized biological functions. The most important of these markers are the CD4 and CD8 co-receptors on mature T cells that are expressed in a mutually exclusive way and respectively interact with conserved regions of the MHC class II or MHC class I molecule (Janeway 1992). A minor population of TCRα/β cells and the majority of TCRγ/δ cells lack both CD4 and CD8 and hence are termed double-negative (DN). Interactions of the CD4 or CD8 molecule with MHC class II or MHC class I gene products are central to thymic T cell development and to antigen-induced activation of mature T cells. Accordingly, CD4 or CD8 T cells are termed MHC class II or MHC class I restricted. Double-negative T cells do not obey stringent MHC restriction and often act independently of conventional MHC products. However, stimulation of these cells also requires antigen presentation on the surface of host cells usually by so-called non-classical MHC class Ib products such as CD1 (Shawar et al. 1994, Beckman and Brenner 1995).

The CD4 and CD8 TCRα/β lymphocytes not only encompass the vast majority of all mature T cells but are also of utmost importance for cell mediated immunity, including acquired resistance against intra-

cellular microbes. The following discussion will, therefore, focus primarily on these 2 T cell subsets. Nevertheless, double-negative TCRα/β and TCRγ/δ lymphocytes appear to contribute to antibacterial defence and so cannot be completely neglected (Kaufmann 1995).

CD4 T cells are generally helper T cells, that is they produce a variety of cytokines that activate immune cells and certain other host cells, such as epithelial and endothelial cells (Janeway 1992). In addition, CD4 T cells also express cytolytic activities. These CD4 T lymphocytes are central mediators of acquired resistance against intracellular bacteria (Kaufmann 1993a). CD8 T cells are preferentially cytolytic T lymphocytes (CTL) and specifically lyse target cells by direct cell contact (Janeway 1992); they also produce cytokines. The role of CD8 T cells in protection against intracellular bacteria is increasingly recognized. In summary, the functional activity spectra of CD4 and CD8 T cells show a remarkable overlap. Accordingly, activation requirements and antigen restriction rather than distinct biological functions underlie the different roles of CD4 and CD8 T cells in immunity to intracellular pathogens.

4.2 The MHC as antigen presentation molecule to T cells

The MHC encodes surface molecules that are responsible for the presentation of foreign peptides to T lymphocytes (Germain 1994). The MHC class II molecule is composed of 2 non-covalently linked glycoproteins of similar size: the α and the β chain (Cardell et al. 1994). The polymorphic domains of both chains form a pocket, the so-called peptide binding groove that accommodates an antigenic peptide 13 or more amino acids in length, which is presented to CD4 T lymphocytes. The MHC class I molecule is composed of a heavy or α chain which is non-covalently linked to a small non-MHC-encoded molecule, the β_2-microglobulin (Raulet 1994). The 2 polymorphic domains of the heavy chain form the peptide binding groove which presents foreign peptides 8–10 amino acids in length to CD8 T cells.

The MHC genes are highly polymorphic and so differ between individuals. Moreover, the MHC encompasses numerous genes that are expressed in different combinations. Therefore, only few individuals share the same MHC phenotype. On the one hand, MHC polymorphism is responsible for rejection of tissue transplants by unrelated individuals and on the other, restriction of antigen-specific T cell activation by the surface-expressed self-MHC molecules is essential for antigen-controlled T cell activation. The extensive polymorphism of the MHC genes accommodates a wide variety of different peptides. Because of their peptide selectivity, MHC molecules from different individuals bind distinct peptides from a single protein. As a consequence, the fine peptide specificity of T cells from different individuals for a given protein can vary remarkably. This represents a major limitation for the design of peptide-based vaccines against infectious agents (Kaufmann 1993a).

4.3 The impact of intracellular antigen localization and MHC processing on activation of CD4 and CD8 T cells

Infection with intracellular pathogens is regarded as a major driving force in the evolution of CD4 and CD8 T cells. There is a division of labour between the 2 T cell populations; CD4 T cells are responsible for intracellular bacteria and CD8 T cells for viruses. MHC class I molecules are present on virtually all host cells and, therefore, almost any cell can present antigens through MHC class I molecules to CD8 T cells. Constitutive MHC class II expression is largely restricted to immune cells, such as B cells, MPs and dendritic cells. Hence, presentation of antigens through MHC class II molecules to CD4 T cells is restricted to these so-called antigen-presenting cells (APC). Bacteria are engulfed by professional phagocytes, such as PNGs and MPs. Since the latter also expresses MHC class II, they are particularly suited for presenting microbial antigens. Most intracellular bacteria in the phagosome are degraded by lysosomal enzymes and the resulting peptides are attached to MHC class II molecules that shuttle between endosome and cell surface (Harding et al. 1995). Presentation of bacterial peptides by MHC class II gene products then stimulates CD4 T cells that activate the antibacterial capacities in macrophages.

In contrast to bacteria, viral pathogens are replicated by host cells. Accordingly, synthesis of viral proteins follows that of host cells. Viral proteins are present in the cytosol compartment where they are degraded in specialized organelles, in particular the so-called proteosomes. The resulting peptides are transported into the endoplasmic reticulum by specific transporters associated with antigen processing (TAP), where they are introduced to the MHC class I molecules (Germain 1994, Benham, Tulp and Neefjes 1995). If necessary, further trimming of the peptides takes place and complexes of MHC class I plus peptides 8–10 amino acids in length are transported to and presented on the cell surface to activate CD8 T cells.

Although the notion of differential presentation of viral and bacterial antigens in the context of MHC class I or MHC class II molecules, respectively, has been instrumental in understanding T cell responses, it has more recently been realized that there are major exceptions to this rule (Fig. 5.1). Importantly, antigens from intracellular bacteria have access to the MHC class I pathway and, consequently, CD8 T cells contribute to immunity against this group of pathogens (Kaufmann 1988a, 1993a, Harding et al. 1995). First, a group of bacterial pathogens, such as *L. monocytogenes* and rickettsiae, are capable of evasion by entering the cytosol. Localization of these pathogens in the cytosol promotes introduction of the antigen into the MHC class I pathway. Second, even antigens from the many intracellular bacteria that remain in the endosome can find their way into the MHC class I pathway. This occurs either by a so far unknown transport mechanism from the endosome into the cytosol or by extrusion of endosomal peptides to facilitate their extracellular association with surface-expressed MHC class I molecules. Correspondingly, protective immunity against all intracellular bacteria depends on both CD4 and CD8 T cells. There are probably quantitative differences in this dependency, so that protection against bacteria, such as *L. monocytogenes*, which escape into the cytosol, is primarily CD8 T cell dependent and resistance against phagosomal bacteria, such as *M. bovis* BCG, is primarily CD4 T cell dependent.

4.4 The impact of protein display on antigenicity for T cells

Since the majority of intracellular bacteria survive within resting MPs, their somatic proteins are not accessible to degradation and MHC processing (Fig. 5.1). Such bacteria are, however, metabolically active and secrete proteins that undergo antigen processing. Hence, soon after infection, secreted antigens are the major source of T cell antigens. After MP activation, an appreciable proportion of bacteria are killed and somatic proteins become available for antigen processing. At later stages of infection, therefore, somatic antigens gain increasing importance. The more intracellular bacteria resist macrophage killing, the more secreted antigens will be dominant over somatic antigen. Dormant pathogens with minimal metabolic activity are a poor source of any kind of antigen and the importance of antigen display for rational design of subunit vaccines is increasingly recognized (Hess et al. 1994). Because vaccination should activate protective T cells immediately after microbial invasion, secreted antigens will in future represent attractive candidates for vaccines against intracellular bacteria.

4.5 Unconventional γ/δ T cells and α/β T cells in antibacterial immunity

Although the major burden of antibacterial protection rests on the CD4 and CD8 T lymphocytes that express TCRα/β, an additional contribution to immunity against intracellular bacteria by less common T cell subsets appears likely.

γ/δ T CELLS

These appear to have a particular bias for intracellular bacteria, most prominently mycobacteria (Kaufmann 1993a). Peripheral blood γ/δ T lymphocytes from normal individuals are strikingly expanded by in vitro stimulation with mycobacterial and other bacterial components and such responsive γ/δ T cells express the Vγ9Vδ2 chain combination. Moreover, during reactional stages in leprosy lesions and in tuberculous lymphadenitis, an increased accumulation of γ/δ T cells has been described. The stimulatory ligands are

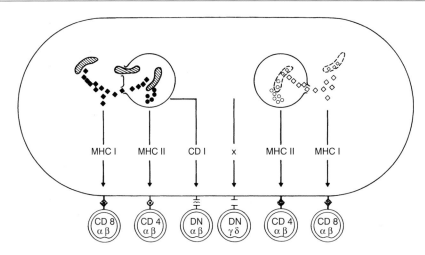

Fig. 5.1   The impact of bacterial localization and antigen display on the type of activated T lymphocyte. *Left panel*: Bacteria that survive in host cells display their antigens in secreted form and somatic antigens are not at this stage available. Secreted antigens from bacteria that remain in the endosomal compartment are preferentially introduced into the MHC II pathway to stimulate CD4 T cells. Recent evidence suggests that antigen from endosomal bacteria can be transported into the MHC I pathway in the cytosol. Some intracellular bacteria can evade into the cytosol where the MHC I pathway can be charged with secreted antigens. *Middle panel*: Recent evidence suggests that non-protein bacterial antigens are presented by molecules of the CD1 complex to double-negative (DN) α/β T cells and by other surface molecules to γ/δ T cells. Some CD8 T cells also recognize bacterial ligands presented by non-classical MHC Ib molecules. Very little is known about these pathways. *Right panel*: As a result of macrophage activation at least some intracellular bacteria are killed and in this way somatic antigens become accessible to MHC processing. As discussed above, endosomal antigens are processed through MHC II to stimulate CD4 T cells, while cytosolic antigens are processed through MHC I to stimulate CD8 T cells.

phosphorylated alkyl derivatives or carbohydrates (Kaufmann 1995). Recent findings in the mouse model have directly demonstrated a prominent role for γ/δ T cells in protection against intracellular bacteria (Kaufmann 1993a). Since γ/δ T lymphocytes precede α/β T cells at the site of replication of *Listeria*, it can be assumed that γ/δ T cells form a link between innate immunity by NK cells and specific acquired immunity due to α/β T lymphocytes.

DOUBLE-NEGATIVE α/β T CELLS

Double-negative α/β T cells have been identified that are stimulated by mycolic acid or lipoarabinomannan from mycobacteria (Kaufmann 1995). Although the biological functions of these cells remain to be established, it is tempting to speculate that they also contribute to antibacterial immunity.

CD8 T CELLS WITH SPECIFICITY FOR *N*-FORMYL PEPTIDES

In mice, T cells have been described that express the conventional phenotype, CD8+ CD4 - TCRα/β, which responds to *N*-formyl peptides (Shawar et al. 1994), which are the signal sequence for protein export in bacteria. *N*-Formyl peptides are virtually absent from mammalian cells, being present only in mitochondria. T lymphocytes with this specificity have been identified as potent mediators of protection against infection with *L. monocytogenes*.

Finally, it appears that a number of unconventional T cells that recognize unusual ligands participate in optimum protection against intracellular bacteria. Common to these T cells is their restriction by the so-called non-classical MHC-Ib and the CD1 molecules

(Fig. 5.1) (Shawar et al. 1994, Kaufmann 1995). CD1 and most non-classical MHC Ib molecules are surface expressed in association with β₂-microglobulin, but they are far less polymorphic than classical MHC class I molecules (Shawar et al. 1994). In addition, these T cells are focused on less diverse ligands, some of which are present in various microbes but absent from host cells. These recent observations have a profound impact on our understanding of immunity, in general, and rational vaccine design against bacterial pathogens, in particular. First, they demonstrate that the antigen repertoire of T cells is not restricted to peptides but also encompasses lipids and carbohydrates. Second, specificity for ligands abundant in pathogenic bacteria, but absent from host cells, does away with the need for self versus non-self discrimination and, conversely, the danger of autoimmune reactions. It suggests that T cells of this type evolved directly to counteract bacterial pathogens. Third, the low polymorphism of the restricting elements, together with the conservation of microbial antigens, indicates that the same antigenic entities stimulate these rare T cells in various individuals of an outbred population.

5   NATURAL KILLER CELLS

Natural killer (NK) cells are important cellular components of the innate host immune response (Bancroft 1993, Scott and Trinchieri 1995, Yokoyama 1995). Originally these cells were identified by their ability to kill susceptible tumour cells in the absence of nominal antigens and they were therefore considered to be important for tumour surveillance. Since then it has been realized that NK cells also play a major role in anti-infectious defence. NK cells are a distinct lymphocyte population that lacks the TCR–CD3 complex and surface Ig, respectively of T and B cells but the cells express various unique markers. At present, CD16 (a special Fc receptor) and CD56 (NKH-1) represent the best characterized markers of human NK cells. Recent work suggests that this potent effector cell type is controlled by both inhibitory and stimulatory signals. In the mouse Ly49 and in man CD94 are expressed by NK cells and transmit an inhibitory signal as long as they interact with a conserved region of MHC class I on target cells. Tumour cells that express a reduced density of MHC class I molecules on their surface are, therefore, more susceptible to NK cell lysis than normal host cells. In rats and mice the stimulatory signal is transmitted by a receptor called NKR-P1 with specificity for carbohydrates on susceptible tumour cells or microbial pathogens. In human NK cells CD69 may perform similar functions. NK cells also lyse autologous targets infected with intracellular bacteria by direct cell contact. Since NK cells express special Fc receptors (CD16), they are also able to lyse antibody-coated target cells. This process is generally termed antibody-dependent cellular cytotoxicity (ADCC). Moreover, circumstantial evidence has been presented for direct growth inhibition of certain bacteria and fungi by NK cells. Significantly, NK cells are potent IFN-γ producers and in this way they contribute to early resistance against intracellular bacteria (Bancroft 1993). NK cells are activated by cytokines from macrophages infected with intracellular bacteria. The relevance of NK cells to antibacterial resistance is best shown by studies of experimental infection in SCID and RAG mice that respectively lack functional T and B lymphocytes. At first these mice are highly resistant to listeriosis, because they have IFN-γ-producing NK cells (Bancroft 1993), but the pathogens are not completely eradicated and ultimately these immunodeficient mice succumb to infection.

6 CYTOKINES

Cytokines are soluble glycoproteins that are produced by and act on various immune and non-immune cells (Paul and Seder 1994). Cytokines serve as transmitters between various leucocyte populations and they also promote interactions with other host cells, such as endothelial and epithelial cells. To emphasize interactions between different leucocytes, the term interleukin (IL) was coined for these numerous cytokines (see Fig. 5.2). T lymphocytes and MPs are major cellular sources of cytokines which, respectively, are termed lymphokines or monokines. CD4 T cells are the most potent producers of lymphokines, but all other T cell populations have also been shown to produce cytokines. A single cell can secrete several cytokines and many cytokines have pleiotropic activity and act on a variety of host cells. Different cytokines may express similar functions, a redundancy that compensates for certain cytokine deficiencies. Cytokines can

act on the producing cell (autocrine action), on cells in the vicinity (paracrine action), or on cells at a greater distance (endocrine action).

Cytokines are central during all phases of intracellular bacterial infections. Soon after infection the so-called proinflammatory cytokines and the chemokines induce leucocyte migration to and cause early inflammation at the site of bacterial replication. Later, cytokines are responsible for the development of granulomatous tissue responses. Other cytokines are responsible for T cell differentiation into distinct effector cells and for the maturation of MPs. The well known activation of antibacterial capacities in macrophages by T cells is mediated by cytokines. In most cases, different cytokines act in a synergistic or an antagonistic manner. It is, therefore, often the cytokine milieu rather than a single cytokine that defines the outcome of the particular response. In the following account, cytokines of major relevance to immunity

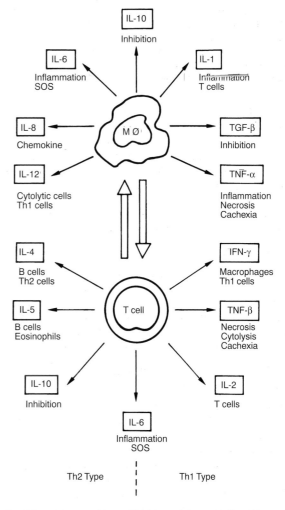

Fig. 5.2 Major cytokines. This figure shows the cytokines of major relevance to immunity against intracellular bacteria. Monocyte or T cell derived cytokines are often termed monokines or lymphokines, respectively. Cytokines of Th1 type are central to protective immunity against intracellular bacteria, while cytokines of Th2 type are important for protection against helminths and in allergic responses.

against intracellular bacteria are briefly described (Fig. 5.2).

6.1 Monokines

The monokines IL-1, IL-6 and TNF-α are important proinflammatory cytokines (Dinarello 1992, Vassalli 1992, Akira, Taga and Kishimoto 1993). When produced in sufficiently high concentrations to enter the vascular system, endocrine effects prevail. These 3 monokines cause acute phase responses by inducing the release from hepatocytes of various plasma proteins that signal SOS. IL-1 and TNF-α act as endogenous pyrogens that stimulate hypothalamic cells to cause fever. TNF-α is also known as cachectin, because it is responsible for cachexia, the characteristic signs of wasting, for example in tuberculosis. At lower concentrations these three cytokines induce local inflammation by an auto- or paracrine activation mode of action at the site of bacterial growth. TNF-α and IL-1 activate PNGs and endothelial cells in which they induce the secretion of cytokines, such as IL-6 and chemokines (see p. 59). TNF-α and IL-1 cause leucocyte migration by stimulating leucocyte adhesion to endothelial cells (Bevilacqua 1993, Imhof and Dunon 1995). Finally, together with IFN-γ, TNF-α stimulates macrophage activation (see p. 59) and it is a major inducer of granuloma formation, the typical tissue response to intracellular bacteria. IL-8 and a number of similar cytokines of low molecular weight, such as RANTES (**r**egulated upon **a**ctivation, **n**ormal **T** cell **e**xpressed and **s**ecreted) and MCP-1 (monocyte chemotactic protein 1), further promote leucocyte attraction to the site at which microbes lodge (Baggiolini, Dewald and Moser 1994). For these chemotactic cytokines, the term chemokines has been coined. The combined action of proinflammatory cytokines and chemokines is ultimately responsible for the inflammatory response that controls and contains microbial growth at an early stage of infection.

IL-12 is produced primarily by activated B lymphocytes and MPs (Trinchieri 1995) and various bacterial components are potent inducers of IL-12 secretion. Early IL-12 production by macrophages infected with intracellular bacteria is a crucial step in the development of a protective T cell response. IL-12 is also a potent stimulant of 2 central biological functions in antibacterial immunity, namely IFN-γ production and target cell lysis. These activities are induced in both T cells and NK cells. IL-12 is therefore crucial to both innate and acquired resistance.

Transforming growth factor β (TGF-β) and IL-10 are best characterized as immune inhibitors, although they also activate various immune functions (Mosmann 1994, Wahl 1994). In intracellular bacterial infections, the immune inhibitory functions of these 2 cytokines prevail. In response to bacterial infection, TGF-β is induced in T cells and macrophages. This interferes with inflammatory cytokines and chemokines and so appears to be involved in the termination of inflammatory responses. Yet, this pleiotropic cytokine also stimulates functions relevant to antibacterial immunity. Thus, it induces angiogenesis and collagen synthesis and promotes IgA production by mucosal B cells. IL-10 is produced by activated T cells, B cells and macrophages. It interferes with the protective immune response against intracellular bacteria by counteracting IFN-γ and IL-12 effects. Although some inhibition by IL-10 of T cell differentiation into IFN-γ-secreting helper T cells has been described, more pronounced effects are evident at the stage of macrophage activation by IFN-γ. Moreover, IL-10 induces IgG secretion in B cells and so contributes to humoral immune responses.

6.2 Lymphokines

IL-2 is an important T cell growth and differentiation factor and so is central to various aspects of cell mediated immunity (Taniguchi and Minami 1993).

IFN-γ is the principal cytokine of protective immunity against intracellular bacteria (Farrar and Schreiber 1993) and acts on macrophages in which it stimulates various antimicrobial functions, including ROI and RNI production. Although IFN-γ also participates in humoral immunity by inducing secretion of IgG2a and IgG3, it is primarily a B cell antagonist. This is primarily due to its potent inhibition of IL-4- and IL-5-secreting T cells (see p. 57). IFN-γ production further contributes to antibacterial resistance by stimulating NK cells, PNGs and leucocyte migration. IFN-γ is produced not only by T cells, but also by NK cells; it is therefore available during the innate and the acquired immune responses.

T cells produce a homologue of TNF-α, termed TNF-β or lymphotoxin (Vassalli 1992, Tracey and Cerami 1993). Although both cytokines share numerous biological activities, TNF-β effects are normally restricted to paracrine and autocrine functions because T cells secrete much lower concentrations of TNF-β as compared with the TNF-α produced by activated macrophages.

IL-4 and IL-5 are potent B cell stimulators (Paul and Seder 1994, Takatsu, Takaki and Hitoshi 1994) and though both are typical T cell products, they are also produced by other cells, primarily mast cells and basophils. IL-4 induces B cell maturation and is also responsible for IgE secretion, whereas IL-5, together with TGF-β, is central to IgA secretion. In addition, IL-5 directly stimulates eosinophils. Hence, IL-4 and IL-5 are essential for humoral immunity and are central to allergic reactions and resistance against helminths. IL-4 also stimulates leucocyte adhesion to endothelial cells and, therefore, sustains inflammatory responses. IL-4 is a strong antagonist of IFN-γ, thus interfering with acquired resistance against intracellular bacteria. It interferes with the development of IFN-γ-producing cells, with IFN-γ synthesis and with IFN-γ stimulation of macrophages. Hence, IL-4 strongly counteracts acquired resistance against intracellular bacteria.

7 TH1 AND TH2 CELLS

The plethora of cytokines produced by CD4 helper T cells imposes the central control function in immunity on this population. The enormous diversity of biological activities regulated by CD4 T cells, some of them counterproductive, makes this task impossible for a single cell type. Accordingly, there is further division within the CD4 T cell population. According to their cytokine profiles, so-called Th1 and Th2 cells, both derived from a Th0 precursor cell, can be distinguished (Fig. 5.3) (Sher and Coffman 1992, Romagnani 1994). The Th1 cells preferentially secrete IFN-γ and IL-2 which respectively activate macrophages and cytotoxic lymphocytes (CTL). They are, therefore, central to cell mediated immunity against viruses, bacteria, fungi and protozoa. IFN-γ produced by Th1 cells also induces secretion of IgG2a and IgG3 isotypes with complement activating and opsonizing capacities that contribute to antimicrobial immunity. In contrast, Th2 cells preferentially produce IL-4, IL-5 and IL-10. IL-4 is also the central cytokine in B cell activation and IL-4, IL-5 and IL-10 stimulate IgG1, IgA, or IgG4, respectively. Hence, Th2 cytokines are essential for humoral immunity. IL-4 also induces IgE production which, in turn, activates basophils and mast cells and IL-5 directly activates eosinophils. Thus, Th2 cells are principal mediators of resistance against helminths and allergic responses. Other cytokines are produced by both Th types. Because of the global importance of microbial infections and the increasing incidence of allergic problems in industrialized nations, Th1 cells are often viewed as helpful and Th2 cells as detrimental. However, this bias neglects the world-wide health problems caused by helminths and the profound contribution of Th2 cells to humoral immunity against microbial infections (Locksley 1994).

Differentiation of Th1 and Th2 cells is controlled at 2 major stages. Soon after antigen encounter, cells of the innate immune system produce cytokines that promote preferential differentiation of either Th type. Rapid production of IL-12 and IFN-γ, respectively, by macrophages or NK cells at the outset of infection with bacterial pathogens ensures preferential Th1 cell development (Trinchieri 1995). By contrast, early IL-4 production promotes Th2 cell development with further support by IL-10 from macrophages. The cellular source of IL-4 is as yet ill-defined and probably includes basophils, mast cells and an unusual CD4+ NK1.1+ T cell population in the mouse (Paul and Seder 1994). At the stage of an established immune response, Th1 and Th2 cells counter-regulate each other with IFN-γ from Th1 cells and IL-4 from Th2 cells interfering with the other Th subset (Romagnani 1994).

In most cases, Th1 and Th2 cells are not activated exclusively in response to a given antigenic stimulus, but rather there are quantitative differences (see Fig. 5.3). In experimental leishmaniasis, activation of protective Th1 cells preponderates in resistant mouse strains, whereas in susceptible strains, disease-exacer-

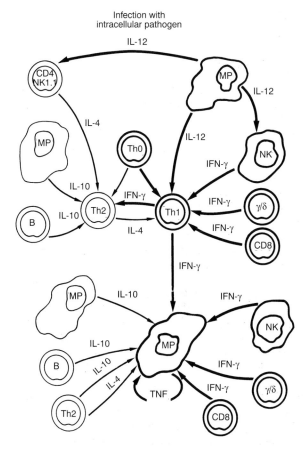

Fig. 5.3 The Th1 Th2 cytokine network in antibacterial immunity. The protective immune response against intracellular bacteria is dominated by Th1 cells (bold arrows). Potent stimulation of IL-12 and IFN-γ by cells of the innate immune system promotes preferential development of Th1-type immune responses. Th2-type cytokines are only weakly stimulated by infections with intracellular bacteria (faint arrows). Nevertheless, some Th2-type cytokines are produced and may help to terminate the immune response before it harms the host. In certain infections (leishmaniasis, leprosy) overactivation of Th2 cells may interfere with the protective immune response.

bating Th2 cell responses are preferentially stimulated (Reiner and Locksley 1995). A similar situation seems to exist in leprosy with dominant Th1 cytokines in tuberculoid leprosy and high Th2 cytokine levels in lepromatous leprosy (Bloom, Modlin and Salgame 1992). Thus, in these infections Th1 cells can be viewed as beneficial and Th2 cells as detrimental. In general, however, Th1 cells act as inducers, and Th2 cells as terminators, of cell mediated immunity against intracellular pathogens. Hence, both T cell subsets seem to be necessary for the successful combat of microbial invaders without enduring damage to the host. This can only be achieved by the activation of Th1 and Th2 cells in a highly co-ordinated and sequential manner.

8 CYTOLYTIC MECHANISMS

Cytolytic mechanisms are an essential part of the immune response against intracellular bacteria and they participate in both protection and pathogenesis (Kaufmann 1993b); cytolytic host cell destruction can be specific or non-specific. Although MHC class I restricted CD8 T lymphocytes are the principal mediators of specific cytolysis, MHC class II restricted CD4 T cells and double-negative γ/δ T cells also express specific cytolytic activity. Target cell lysis may be brought about by 2 independent mechanisms. First, CTL store specialized cytolytic molecules – perforins and granzymzes – in granules (Berke 1994, Podack 1995) and these cytolysins are secreted as the result of target cell recognition by way of the TCR–CD3 complex. The perforins polymerize in the extracellular space to yield complexes that form pores in the target cell membrane. These complexes structurally and functionally resemble the membrane attack complex of the complement system. Pore formation allows the influx of ions and water from the extracellular into the intracellular milieu, with resulting osmotic swelling and ultimately target cell lysis. Moreover, high concentrations of granzymes enter the target cells and damage intracellular proteins. This process is best compared with active killing, whereas the second mechanism is induced by CTL in the target cells and resembles suicide. Interactions between the Fas antigen on the target cell and the Fas ligand on CTL induces apoptosis (Nagata 1994), a fragmentation of DNA with subsequent disruption of the nucleus. The Fas antigen is related to the tumour necrosis factor (TNF) receptor family and the Fas ligand resembles membrane-bound TNF. NK cells have a killer potential similar to that of CTL (Berke 1994).

The pathological sequelae of target cell lysis are obvious; they cause tissue damage but it appears likely that target cell lysis also contributes to protection. Intracellular bacteria that persist in non-professional phagocytes or in deactivated tissue macrophages are shielded from more proficient phagocytes, such as the blood monocytes. Liberation of bacteria by lysis of incapacitated host cells may be a necessary preliminary step in their elimination (Kaufmann 1988a).

A second type of host cell injury is caused by PNGs and, to a lesser extent, by MPs (Weiss 1989, Conlan and North 1993). Liberation of proteolytic enzymes, such as elastase and collagenase, and the toxic effector molecules ROI and RNI, from the lysosomal compartment causes extensive tissue damage. The release of hypochlorous acid by PNG inactivates extracellular proteinase inhibitors which, as a result, cannot interfere with the extracellular activities of lysosomal proteases. In addition, PNGs rapidly die at the site of inflammation and as a consequence of this autolysis lysosomal enzymes are released, further contributing to tissue injury. Tissue macrophages also secrete proteolytic enzymes, but not hypochlorous acid. Since MPs are long-lived, uncontrolled liberation of lysosomal proteases as a result of autolysis rarely occurs. Thus, MPs are less harmful and tend rather to cause circumscribed lesions.

9   DELAYED-TYPE HYPERSENSITIVITY (DTH)

Administration of soluble proteins from an intracellular bacterium causes a skin reaction in individuals who have been infected with the same agent (Hahn and Kaufmann 1981). This DTH response is indicative for specific immunity and so provides a helpful diagnostic tool but it does not distinguish between asymptomatic infection and clinical disease. Moreover, DTH is an immunological phenomenon that may persist for a time after successful eradication of the pathogen. Therefore, DTH cannot determine whether the organism persists in the host or not. The tuberculin test is widely used for diagnosis of infection with *M. tuberculosis*. The DTH reaction is mediated by MHC class II restricted CD4 T cells which, at the site of antigen administration, induce an inflammatory response characterized by mononuclear phagocytes. Chemokines and IFN-γ seem to be the principal mediators of this reaction, with some contribution by TNF. Although DTH is often regarded as indicative of protective immunity, this assumption has recently been questioned. Soluble proteins are used to elicit DTH responses which primarily stimulate MHC class II restricted CD4 T cells. By contrast, effective protection against intracellular bacteria encompasses MHC class I restricted CD8 T cells and probably unconventional double-negative T cells, which are not or are only poorly activated by soluble proteins. A positive DTH response, therefore, does not reflect the complete T cell armamentarium of antibacterial protection.

10   COURSE OF INFECTION

Soon after host invasion, intracellular bacteria find their preferred cellular niche. Some pathogens remain at the site of entry, such as *C. trachomatis*, which multiplies in the epithelium. Other pathogens (e.g. *M. tuberculosis*, which, after being inhaled, multiplies in resident macrophages in the lung parenchyma) find their niche in the close vicinity of the site of entry. Yet other pathogens (e.g. *L. monocytogenes*, which lodges in hepatocytes and Kupffer cells in the liver) find their biotope at distant sites. Since the courses of infection vary significantly, the major hallmarks will be highlighted below by describing 5 different examples of infection (Fig. 5.4).

EXPERIMENTAL *L. MONOCYTOGENES* INFECTION

This is an acute type of infectious disease that is completely eradicated within 2 weeks (Kaufmann 1988b) because bacterial multiplication causes secretion of proinflammatory cytokines and chemokines in infected cells. These cytokines, in turn, induce phagocyte migration to the site of bacterial growth (Fig. 5.5) and PNGs strikingly reduce the initial course of infection (Conlan and North 1993), whereas in other intracellular bacterial infections the acute inflammatory response may vary in strength and in its capacity to

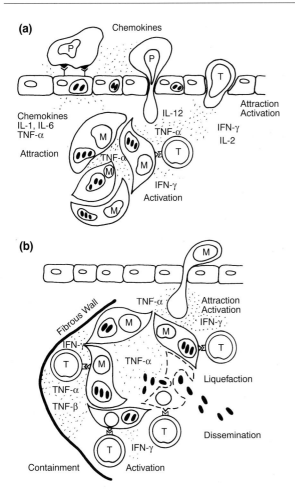

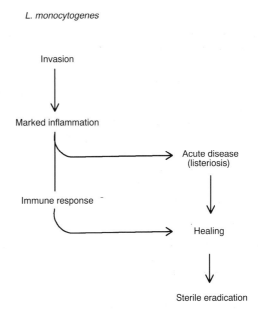

Fig. 5.5 Principal mechanisms in *L. monocytogenes* infection.

Fig. 5.4 Major steps of granuloma formation. (a) At the site of bacterial implantation, proinflammatory cytokines and chemokines are produced that induce migration of professional phagocytes. Although the majority of bacteria may be killed by these inflammatory phagocytes, some persist within macrophages. Macrophage activation is achieved by specific T lymphocytes which enter the stage later. TNF-α from infected macrophages and T cell cytokines, including IFN-γ, induce granuloma formation. (b) *Left section*: Within the granuloma, often encapsulated by a fibrous wall, T cells and macrophages achieve bacterial containment. Although the bacteria may not be completely eradicated, dissemination is prevented. *Right section*: Rupture of the granuloma occurs when the equilibrium between bacterial persistence and host immune response in the granuloma is altered. The cells are destructed and bacteria disseminated over the body. Active disease unfolds. M, macrophage; P, phagocyte; T, T cell; IFN-γ, interferon-γ; IL-1, interleukin-1; IL-2, interleukin-2; IL-6, interleukin-6; IL-12, interleukin-12, TNF-α, tumour necrosis factor α; TGF-β, transforming growth factor β.

limit microbial replication. For example, slow-growing *M. tuberculosis* and *M. leprae* that cause chronic diseases are less vulnerable to this early PNG attack.

Macrophages infected with intracellular bacteria also produce high levels of IL-12 and TNF-α that activate IFN-γ-secreting NK cells (Bancroft 1993, Trinchieri 1995). These NK cells produce the first wave of IFN-γ, which activates macrophages, thus sustaining the initial reduction of listeriae. The next wave of IFN-γ is provided by γ/δ T lymphocytes which are the first

T cells to arrive at the inflammatory lesion (Haas, Pereira and Tonegawa 1993). Subsequently, specific α/β T cells are activated. In listeriosis CD8 T cells are the major mediators of acquired resistance (Kaufmann 1988a). High concentrations of IL-12 and IFN-γ and minute levels of IL-4, produced at the outset of infection, promote the development of CD4 T cells of Th1 type and of CD8 CTL.

The inflammatory lesion at the site of listerial infection is succeeded by a granulomatous lesion. The granuloma is the characteristic tissue response of cell mediated immunity against intracellular bacteria (Fig. 5.5). Although T cells are essential for granuloma formation, this is initiated by TNF-α from infected macrophages. *L. monocytogenes* is highly susceptible to host defence and is, therefore, eliminated before a full granuloma has developed. Accordingly, lesions remain immature and only have a marginal influence on antilisterial protection.

EPIDEMIC TYPHUS

This is an acute, often fatal infectious disease (Fig. 5.6) due to *Rickettsia prowazekii*, an obligate intracellular pathogen that can survive in the resting, but not in the activated macrophage (Mandell, Douglas and Bennett 1990). Vascular endothelial cells, therefore, represent the major niche of persistent survival. The resulting endothelial injury may have fatal consequences for highly oxygen-dependent tissues, such as central nervous system and heart muscle. In approximately half of diseased individuals, cell mediated immunity achieves complete cure. However, even in the convalescent individual, the pathogen is often not entirely eradicated. The organisms persist asymptomatically and, several years later, they may be reactivated to cause the milder Brill–Zinsser disease.

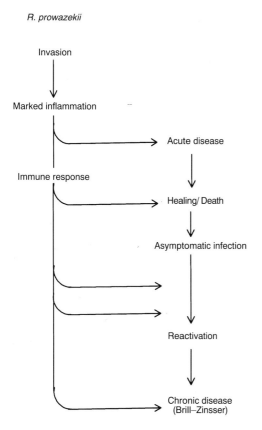

Fig. 5.6 Principal mechanisms in *R. prowazekii* infection.

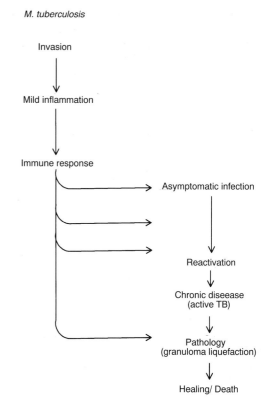

Fig. 5.7 Principal mechanisms in *M. tuberculosis* infection.

TUBERCULOSIS

This is the paradigm of chronic infectious diseases caused by intracellular bacteria (Fig. 5.7). Tuberculosis is typically a disease of the lung, although any organ may be affected (Bloom 1994). On the one hand, the pathogen is highly resistant to macrophage killing; on the other, it has low intrinsic toxicity. *M. tuberculosis* may, therefore, persist in the host for years without causing clinical symptoms. The balanced encounter between persisting pathogen and host immune mechanisms is focused on the granulomatous lesion (Fig. 5.7), where the bacteria are contained and prevented from spreading to other tissue sites. Macrophages in the granuloma differentiate into multinucleated giant cells that harbour dormant tubercle bacilli (Dannenberg 1991). Interactions between different macrophage populations and T cell subsets markedly constrain bacteria within the granuloma but do not succeed in eradicating them. The granulomatous lesion is walled off by a fibrous wall, further improving containment and TNF is essential for the formation and encapsulation of the granuloma (Vassalli 1992). Later the sensitive balance between tubercle bacilli and host defence may be altered, so that disease results and reactivation of dormant infection is a major cause of adult tuberculosis. Expanding lesions cause injury to the tissue and this may become worse, if the lesions liquefy. Bacteria then grow to large numbers in the cellular detritus and are dissemi-

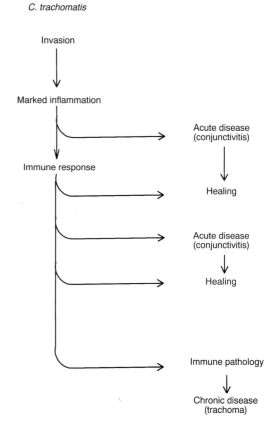

Fig. 5.8 Principal mechanisms in *C. trachomatis* infection.

nated to distant tissue sites. At this stage, high levels of TNF-α are produced so that its endocrine effects cause the well known wasting syndromes of tuberculosis (Tracey and Cerami 1993). In this case pathology is caused, at least in part, by an immune response out of balance.

EYE INFECTION WITH *C. TRACHOMATIS*

C. trachomatis causes inclusion conjunctivitis and trachoma that can be controlled by the immune system (Beatty, Morrison and Byrne 1994) (Fig. 5.8). However, repeated immune challenge, either in response to reinfection or against persisting bacteria, ultimately causes scars that lead to blindness. Thus, immunity is the principal mediator of pathology in this disease (Brunham and Peeling 1994).

LEPROSY

Leprosy is a disease of broad spectrum, in which the polar lepromatous form is more malignant than the tuberculoid form (Hastings 1994) (Fig. 5.9). Although disease is generally focused on the skin and peripheral nerves, any tissue may be affected. In the tuberculoid form, the encounter between pathogen and protective immunity is concentrated in granulomatous lesions that resemble those of tuberculosis. The T cells in tuberculoid lesions produce IL-2, IFN-γ and TNF-β and are thus of Th1 type. Damage of peripheral nerves by immune mechanisms results in anaesthesia, which is the cause of secondary infections and mechanical injury. Autoaggressive immune mechanisms are most obvious in reversal reactions that frequently occur during chemotherapy. In lepromatous leprosy the abundant *M. leprae* and the predominance of foamy macrophages with reduced numbers of T cells within lesions suggest immunosuppression. In fact, the few lymphocytes present in lepromatous lesions express the unusual phenotype CD8$^+$ CD28$^-$ and the Th2-type

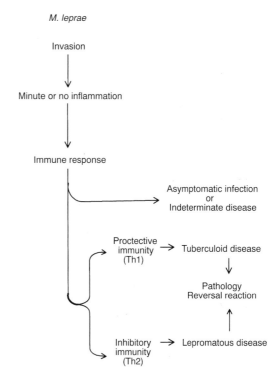

Fig. 5.9 Principal mechanisms of *M. leprae* infection.

cytokines IL-4, IL-5 and IL-10 predominate over the Th1 cytokines IL-2, IFN-γ and TNF-β (Bloom, Modlin and Salgame 1992). This strongly suggests the emergence of CD8 T cells of Th2 type that are responsible for immunosuppression. Although the determining factors are unknown, it is obvious that in leprosy the balance between Th1 and Th2 cytokines respectively is decisive for protection or the exacerbation of disease.

REFERENCES

Adams DO, Hamilton TA, 1984, The cell biology of macrophage activation, *Annu Rev Immunol*, **2:** 283–318.

Akira S, Taga T, Kishimoto T, 1993, Interleukin-6 in biology and medicine, *Adv Immunol*, **54:** 1–78.

Baca OG, Paretsky D, 1993, Q-fever and *Coxiella burnetii*: a model for host–parasite interactions, *Microbiol Rev*, **47:** 127–49.

Baggiolini M, Dewald B, Moser B, 1994, Interleukin-8 and related chemotactic cytokines – CXC and CC chemokines, *Adv Immunol*, **55:** 97–179.

Bainton DF, 1981, The discovery of lysosomes, *J Cell Biol*, **91:** 66S–76S.

Baldwin CL, Jiang X, Fernandes DM, 1993, Macrophage control of *Brucella abortus*: influence of cytokines and iron, *Trends Microbiol*, **1:** 99–104.

Bancroft GJ, 1993, The role of natural killer cells in innate resistance to infection, *Curr Opin Immunol*, **5:** 503–10.

Barbaree JM, Breimann RF, Dufour AP, 1993, Legionella. *Current Status and Emerging Perspectives*, ASM, Washington DC.

Beatty WL, Morrison RP, Byrne GI, 1994, Persistent chlamydiae: from cell culture to a paradigm for chlamydial pathogenesis, *Microbiol Rev*, **58:** 686–99.

Beckman EM, Brenner MB, 1995, MHC class I-like, class II-like and CD1 molecules: distinct roles in immunity, *Immunol Today*, **16:** 349–52.

Benham A, Tulp A, Neefjes J, 1995, Synthesis and assembly of MHC–peptide complexes, *Immunol Today*, **16:** 359–62.

Berke G, 1994, The binding and lysis of target cells by cytotoxic lymphocytes: molecular and cellular aspects, *Annu Rev Immunol*, **12:** 735–73.

Bevilacqua MP, 1993, Endothelial-leukocyte adhesion molecules, *Annu Rev Immunol*, **11:** 767–804.

Bliska JB, Galán JE, Falkow S, 1993, Signal transduction in the mammalian cell curing bacterial attachment and entry, *Cell*, **73:** 903–20.

Bloom BR, 1994, *Tuberculosis. Pathogenesis, Protection, and Control*, ASM, Washington DC.

Bloom BR, Modlin RL, Salgame P, 1992, Stigma variations: observations on suppressor T cells and leprosy, *Annu Rev Immunol*, **10:** 453–88.

Boman HG, 1995, Peptide antibiotics and their role in innate immunity, *Annu Rev Immunol*, **13:** 61–92.

Brown EJ, 1991, Complement receptors and phagocytosis, *Curr Opin Immunol*, **3:** 76–83.

Brunham RC, Peeling RW, 1994, *Chlamydia trachomatis* antigens: role in immunity and pathogenesis, *Infect Agents Dis*, **3:** 218–33.

Cardell S, Merkenschlager M et al., 1994, The immune system of mice lacking conventional MHC class II molecules, *Adv Immunol*, **55:** 423–40.

Chan AC, Desai DM, Weiss A, 1994, The role of protein tyrosine kinases and protein tyrosine phosphatases in T cell antigen receptor signal transduction, *Annu Rev Immunol*, **12:** 555–92.

Conlan W, North R, 1993, Neutrophil-mediated lysis of infected hepatocytes, *ASM News*, **59:** 563–7.

Dannenberg AM Jr, 1991, Delayed-type hypersensitivity and cell-mediated immunity in the pathogenesis of tuberculosis, *Immunol Today*, **12:** 228–33.

Davis MM, Chien Y-H, 1995, Issues concerning the nature of antigen recognition by αβ and γδ T-cell receptors, *Immunol Today*, **16:** 316–18.

Denis M, 1994, Human monocytes/macrophages: NO or no NO?, *J Leukoc Biol*, **55:** 682–4.

Dinarello CA, 1992, Role of interleukin-1 in infectious diseases, *Immunol Rev*, **127:** 119–46.

Elsbach P, Weiss J, 1983, A reevaluation of the roles of the O_2-dependent and O_2-independent microbicidal systems of phagocytes, *Rev Infect Dis*, **5:** 843–53.

Farrar MA, Schreiber RD, 1993, The molecular cell biology of interferon-γ and its receptor, *Annu Rev Immunol*, **11:** 571–612.

Finlay BB, Falkow S, 1989, Salmonella as an intracellular parasite, *Mol Microbiol*, **3:** 1833–41.

Germain RN, 1994, MHC-dependent antigen processing and peptide presentation: providing ligands for T lymphocyte activation, *Cell*, **76:** 287–99.

Goldberg MB, Sansonetti PJ, 1993, *Shigella* subversion of the cellular cytoskeleton: a strategy for epithelial colonization, *Infect Immun*, **61:** 4941–6.

Gordon AH, D'Arcy Hart P, Young MR, 1980, Ammonia inhibits phagosome–lysosome fusion in macrophages, *Nature (London)*, **286:** 79–80.

Gordon S, Clarke S et al., 1995, Molecular immunobiology of macrophages: recent progress, *Curr Opin Immunol*, **7:** 24–33.

Haas W, Pereira P, Tonegawa S, 1993, γ/δ T-cells, *Annu Rev Immunol*, **11:** 637–85.

Hahn H, Kaufmann SHE, 1981, The role of cell mediated immunity in bacterial infections, *Rev Infect Dis*, **3:** 1221–50.

Harding CV, Song R et al., 1995, Processing of bacterial antigens for presentation to class I and II MHC-restricted T lymphocytes, *Infect Agents Dis*, **4:** 1–12.

Haslett C, Savill JS, Meagher L, 1989, The neutrophil, *Curr Opin Immunol*, **2:** 10–18.

Hastings RC, 1994, *Leprosy*, 2nd edn, Churchill Livingstone, Edinburgh, London, Melbourne.

Hess J, Szalay G et al., 1994, Vaccination strategies using viable carrier systems against intracellular pathogens, *Behring Inst Mitt*, **95:** 67–79.

Imhof BA, Dunon D, 1995, Leukocyte migration and adhesion, *Adv Immunol*, **58:** 345–416.

Isberg RR, 1991, Discrimination between intracellular uptake and surface adhesion of bacterial pathogens, *Science*, **252:** 934–8.

Jameson SC, Hogquist KA, Bevan MJ, 1995, Positive selection of thymocytes, *Annu Rev Immunol*, **13:** 93–126.

Janeway CA, 1992, The T cell receptor as a multicomponent signalling machine: CD4/CD8 coreceptors and CD45 in T cell activation, *Annu Rev Immunol*, **10:** 645–74.

Kaufmann SHE, 1988a, CD8+ T lymphocytes in intracellular microbial infections, *Immunol Today*, **9:** 168–74.

Kaufmann SHE, 1988b, Listeriosis: new findings – current concern, *Microb Pathog*, **5:** 225–31.

Kaufmann SHE, 1993a, Immunity to intracellular bacteria, *Annu Rev Immunol*, **11:** 129–63.

Kaufmann SHE, 1993b, Immunity to intracellular bacteria, *Fun-*

damental Immunology, ed. Paul WE, Raven Press, New York, 1251.

Kaufmann SHE, 1995, Immunity to intracellular microbial pathogens, *Immunol Today*, **16:** 338–42.

Kaufmann SHE, Reddehase MJ, 1989, Infection of phagocytic cells, *Curr Opin Immunol*, **2:** 43–9.

Lehrer RI, 1993, Defensins: antimicrobial and cytotoxic peptides of mammalian cells, *Annu Rev Immunol*, **11:** 105–28.

Locksley RM, 1994, Th2 cells: help for helminths, *J Exp Med*, **179:** 1405.

McClarty G, 1994, Chlamydiae and the biochemistry of intracellular parasitism, *Trends Microbiol*, **2:** 157–64.

Mandell GL, Douglas RG, Bennett JE, eds, 1990, Section D: Rickettsiosis, *Principles and Practice of Infectious Diseases*, Churchill Livingstone, New York.

Mosmann TR, 1994, Properties and functions of interleukin-10, *Adv Immunol*, **56:** 1–26.

Moulder JW, 1985, Comparative biology of intracellular parasitism, *Microbiol Rev*, **49:** 298–337.

Nagata S, 1994, Fas and Fas ligand: a death factor and its receptor, *Adv Immunol*, **57:** 129–44.

Nathan C, Xie Q-W, 1994, Nitric oxide synthases: roles, tolls, and controls, *Cell*, **78:** 915–18.

Paul WE, Seder RA, 1994, Lymphocyte responses and cytokines, *Cell*, **76:** 241–51.

Payne SM, 1993, Iron acquisition in microbial pathogenesis, *Trends Microbiol*, **1:** 66–9.

Podack ER, 1995, Execution and suicide: cytotoxic lymphocytes enforce Draconian laws through separate molecular pathways, *Curr Opin Immunol*, **7:** 11–16.

Portnoy DA, Chakraborty T et al., 1992, Molecular determinants of *Listeria monocytogenes* pathogenesis, *Infect Immun*, **60:** 1263–7.

Rabinovitch M, 1995, Professional and non-professional phagocytes: an introduction, *Trends Cell Biol*, **5:** 85–8.

Raulet DH, 1994, MHC class I-deficient mice, *Adv Immunol*, **55:** 381–421.

Ravetch JV, Kinet J-P, 1991, Fc receptors, *Annu Rev Immunol*, **9:** 457–92.

Reiner SL, Locksley RM, 1995, The regulation of immunity to *Leishmania major*, *Annu Rev Immunol*, **13:** 151–77.

Romagnani S, 1994, Lymphokine production by human T cells in disease states, *Annu Rev Immunol*, **12:** 227–57.

Russell DG, 1995, Mycobacterium and leishmania: stowaways in the endosomal network, *Trends Cell Biol*, **5:** 125–8.

Sandström G, 1994, The tularaemia vaccine, *J Chem Tech Biotechnol*, **59:** 315–20.

Scott P, Trinchieri G, 1995, The role of natural killer cells in host–parasite interactions, *Curr Opin Immunol*, **7:** 34–40.

Shawar SM, Vyas JM et al., 1994, Antigen presentation by major histocompatibility complex class I-b molecules, *Annu Rev Immunol*, **12:** 839–80.

Sher A, Coffman RL, 1992, Regulation of immunity to parasites by T cells and T cell-derived cytokines, *Annu Rev Immunol*, **10:** 385–410.

Smith LD, Ficht TA, 1990, Pathogenesis of *Brucella*, *Crit Rev Microbiol*, **17:** 209–30.

Stahl PD, 1992, The mannose receptor and other macrophage lectins, *Curr Opin Immunol*, **4:** 49–52.

Takatsu K, Takaki S, Hitoshi Y, 1994, Interleukin-5 and its receptor system: implications in the immune system and inflammation, *Adv Immunol*, **57:** 145–90.

Taniguchi T, Minami Y, 1993, The IL-2/IL-2 receptor system: a current overview, *Cell*, **73:** 5–8.

Tracey KJ, Cerami A, 1993, Tumor necrosis factor, other cytokines and disease, *Annu Rev Cell Biol*, **9:** 317–43.

Trinchieri G, 1995, Interleukin-12: a proinflammatory cytokine with immunoregulatory functions that bridge innate resistance and antigen-specific adaptive immunity, *Annu Rev Immunol*, **13:** 251–76.

Vassalli P, 1992, The pathophysiology of tumor necrosis factors, *Annu Rev Immunol*, **10:** 411–52.

Wahl SM, 1994, Transforming growth factor ß: the good, the bad, and the ugly, *J Exp Med*, **180:** 1587–90.

Weiss SJ, 1989, Tissue destruction by neutrophils, *N Engl J Med*, **320:** 365–76.

Winkler HH, 1995, *Rickettsia prowazekii*, ribosomes and slow growth, *Trends Microbiol*, **3:** 196–8.

Yokoyama WM, 1995, Natural killer cell receptors, *Curr Opin Immunol*, **7:** 110–20.

Chapter 6

THE IMMUNOLOGICAL BASIS OF TISSUE DAMAGE

D Parratt

| 1 Introduction | 3 Superantigens |
| 2 Hypersensitivity | 4 Cytokines and nitric oxide |

1 INTRODUCTION

The immunological basis of tissue damage in infection is an evolving topic. There is little doubt that immunological mechanisms, particularly hypersensitivities, have an important role in causing damage in infections and the literature on this topic is reviewed below. However, there are now further aspects to be considered. The cause of tissue damage has extended beyond the mechanisms of hypersensitivity to include the actions of cytokines, superantigens and the reactions which generate nitric oxide. All of these are potentially capable of causing damage. What is not clear is how and when such damage occurs.

The difficulty is that the totality of events in any infection is poorly understood. There is no field theory that will predict the progress of infection in an individual. It is possible to describe the events that occur in an infection, particularly the damaging events, but it is not possible to predict (or define) when these events will occur. This is a significant problem for the practising clinician who is faced with the difficulty of predicting the outcome of 2 infinitely variable parameters. One of these is the growth of the micro-organism and the other is the effect of the immune response.

This chapter will describe the **possible** effects of such an interaction in respect of damage caused by immune responses. It is not feasible, however, to predict when these damaging effects might occur. The review will begin with hypersensitivity and consider later the other aspects of immune mediated damage.

2 HYPERSENSITIVITY

Hypersensitivity is an abnormal immune response that produces damage, either histopathological or physiological, in the host. Early bacteriologists were well acquainted with some forms of bacterially induced hypersensitivity, which they termed 'anaphylaxis' or 'anaphylactic shock', and which they distinguished from 'toxic' phenomena by the specificity of the response and its reproducibility in the same host after months or years. These hypersensitivities could be transferred between animals by serum; the anaphylaxis that resulted could be local with an inflammatory reaction at the injection site or generalized with shock, respiratory distress due to bronchospasm and urticaria. Analogous reactions were observed in man, often with antigens of non-bacterial origin, such as therapeutic horse serum.

Hypersensitivities are of different types, with varying mechanisms, and have been classified by Gell and Coombs (1963). This classification (Table 6.1) describes the main clinical events that occur with each type of hypersitivity reaction. Patients do not always present in classic fashion and several types of hypersensitivity may be seen in the same patient at a given time. However, difficulties such as these are common in medicine and do not negate the use of a classification that is generally helpful.

2.1 Antibody mediated hypersensitivity

Of the 4 types of hypersensitivity, 3 are mediated by antibody (types I, II and III). The term 'immediate' is sometimes used for all of these to distinguish them from type IV or 'delayed' hypersensitivity. However, the term 'immediate' is best restricted to type I, anaphylactic hypersensitivity.

Table 6.1   Classification of hypersensitivity states (see Gell and Coombs 1963)

Type	Description	Clinical conditions
1	Anaphylactic; immediate; IgE mediated	Dermatitis; eczema; asthma; hay fever; generalized anaphylaxis
2	Cytotoxic	Transfusion reactions; some 'autoimmune diseases' (e.g. Goodpasture's syndrome); acquired haemolytic anaemias
3	Immune complex mediated; Arthus; serum sickness	Drug-induced serum sickness; acute glomerulonephritis
4	Delayed; T cell mediated; cell mediated hypersensitivity	Contact dermatitis; 'granulomatous' lesions of tuberculosis and leprosy; drug reactions

TYPE I HYPERSENSITIVITY

Anaphylactic or **immediate** type I hypersensitivity is mediated by IgE antibody and is due to the powerful effects of histamine and other vasoactive amines. The hypersensitivity may be local or generalized, depending upon the amount of vasoactive amines released, the site of their release and the route of entry of the stimulating antigen. Generally, small amounts of antigen administered to mucous membranes or skin will induce local anaphylaxis, whereas larger amounts of antigen administered systemically may cause generalized anaphylaxis. Early work on this type of hypersensitivity and the discovery and definition of IgE are reviewed by Bennich and Johannsson (1971).

IgE antibody production

All healthy individuals produce IgE antibody specific for most antigens they encounter. The IgE is in addition to the IgM, IgG and IgA antibodies with which we are more familiar; generally the quantity produced is very small. In a variety of pathological states, IgE production is not controlled and when large amounts are present, a type I hypersensitivity may occur.

IgE antibodies bind to mast cells and basophils which exist in large numbers in the submucosal and mucosal layers of the respiratory tract, gut wall and skin. These cells have a high affinity for the Fc fragment of the IgE molecule so that the IgE molecules are bound with the Fab regions exposed and ready to bind antigen (Kay 1981). In this way, mast cells and basophils become 'primed' to react. It is thought that mast cells acquire their IgE in regional lymph nodes before migrating to the tissues.

A second and subsequent exposure to antigen may invoke the hypersensitivity reaction by triggering the mast cells to release histamine and other vasoactive amines.

The derivation of IgE responses is still not clear. Experimental studies in mice and man have shown that the cells involved are from subsets of CD4+ Th (helper) cells. These have been designated Th2 cells and they secrete IL-4 (interleukin-4), IL-5 but not interferon-γ (IFN-γ). Secretion of IL-4 causes increased IgE synthesis by B cells, a response that is suppressed by secretion of IFN-γ which can come from

several different cells including Th1 cells. The developing concept is that certain antigens, termed allergens, preferentially stimulate Th2 cells to secrete IL-4 and increase IgE antibody formation (Maggi and Romagnani 1994). It is not clear whether this action is due to the molecular structure of the antigen or to the type of antigen-processing cell (APC) which presents the antigen to the other immune-active cells, or to both these factors. The concept does, however, provide an explanation for the regular stimulation of IgE by antigens from helminths in allergic and non-allergic alike. It suggests that these have a molecular structure or handling characteristics which the immune system would interpret in the form of a Th2 response which would lead to high IgE antibody levels (Leung 1994).

By contrast, the genetic background of allergic individuals is critical in furthering the IgE response against allergens and it is believed that the cytokine environment in these persons is responsible for the generation of the abnormal Th2 cell response (Leung 1994).

Mast cells, long associated with allergic responses, have recently been shown to produce IL-4 and to provide a T cell-independent mechanism for the enhancement of IgE production (Howarth et al. 1994). Thus, Th2 cells are triggered by allergen on antigen-presenting cells bearing IgE and these release IL-4 which enhances the IgE response. Mast cells respond to the subsequent antigen IgE antibody interaction and release IL-4 which enhances the effect and this establishes an amplification loop (Leung 1994). Allergic or atopic individuals may be more efficient than others at amplifying the IgE response to antigens and this may result in their allergic disease.

The importance of this recent work is that abnormal IgE antibody responses may be modified by cytokine administration. The propensity towards an abnormal IgE response is countered by IFN-γ (Maggi and Romagnani 1994). It would seem logical that abnormal production of IgE could, therefore, be suppressed by treatment with IFN-γ. There is some evidence that this is the case in animal models (Lack et al. 1992) and that the abnormal response could be converted to a protective response. In this respect, IFN-α and IL-12 may also be important by changing the response from Th2 (IgE-producing) to Th1 (IgE non-producing) (Maggi and Romagnani 1994).

For the microbiologist, the challenge is to determine whether micro-organisms have antigens which can stimulate IgE production by activating the above mechanisms. Helminths are clearly important as a source of these antigens but many other micro-organisms may be as important, but remain unrecognized.

Mechanisms of type I hypersensitivity

When antigen attaches to IgE antibody bound by mast cells, cross-linking of the antibody molecules may occur. There may be as many as 130 000 high-affinity binding sites on each mast cell (Coleman and Godfrey 1981) and cross-linking stimulates phospholipid metabolism, opening channels in the cell membrane, leading to calcium influx (Church et al. 1982). An energy-dependent disorganization of the intracellular granules occurs, with eventual release of the granule contents into the extracellular fluids. The substances released from the granules are histamine, glycosidases, proteases, chemotactic factors and heparin. In addition, the changes occurring in phospholipid metabolism make arachidonic acid available and this substance acts as a substrate for the production of further active compounds. Activity on arachidonic acid through the cyclo-oxygenase pathway leads to the formation of prostaglandin D_2 (PGD_2), whereas activity through the lipoxygenase pathway produces monohydroxyeicosatetraeonic acid (HETES) and the leukotrienes, which are important mediators of inflammation. The leukotriene LTB4 is a chemotaxin for eosinophils, mononuclear cells and neutrophils; leukotrienes LTC4, LTD4 and LTE4 collectively form 'slow-reacting substance of anaphylaxis' (SRS-A), which is one of the mediators belonging to a group of slow-reacting substances (SRS). SRS-A may be synthesized by mast cells after activation but its components can also be produced by eosinophils and macrophages. The recruitment of this help by other cells follows the initial release of the preformed mediators in the mast cell granules. In a similar way, prostaglandin E_2 (PGE_2) is generated by smooth muscle, thromboxane A2 by platelets and PGI_2 (prostacyclin) by vascular epithelium, after initial release of mast cell contents. Further influx of neutrophils, eosinophils and macrophages takes place as a result of the release of the HETES and leukotrienes from mast cells, which increases and prolongs the inflammatory response (for review, see Holgate and Kay 1984).

The effect of the mediator release is varied and due to the activities shown in Table 6.2. Vascular dilatation and increased vessel permeability are notable events that lead to local oedema and, when sufficiently severe, to a fall in blood pressure, the latter being a particular problem when histamine and other active substances are released systemically and when the degree of sensitization of mast cells is high. The effects of mediator release on smooth muscle are also notable in the lung, where peripheral airway resistance, producing asthma, occurs. In addition, at any site where mediators are released, inflammatory cells will be attracted, notably eosinophils, neutrophils and mononuclear cells; these, together with the early release of destructive enzymes from mast cells, cause tissue destruction and inflammation. The accompanying induced oedema and platelet aggregation cause further disruption of blood flow in the area and inflammation increases. A further increase in damage may occur as a result of cytokine release stimulated by the activated neutrophils. These events begin within 30 min of antigen challenge in suitably sensitized persons and may persist for many hours, particularly when the inflammatory changes are severe.

The clinical manifestations of type I hypersensitivities vary according to the degree of sensitization and the site at which antigen challenge, and therefore mast cell degranulation, occurs. In the lung, asthma is the clinical manifestation, in the skin it is urticaria and in the systemic circulation it is generalized anaphylaxis, characterized by a profound fall in blood pressure.

Type I hypersensitivity and infection

Type I hypersensitivity probably plays a part in many infections although firm evidence has been difficult to obtain. The microbiologist is most likely to encounter this hypersensitivity with parasitic and fungal infections and with drug reactions to antibiotics.

IgE antibody responses are frequent in helminth infections which suggests that this type of reaction is probably important in defence against the parasite. Some investigators have explored this possibility, notably in schistosomiasis. The major antigens of schistosomula preferentially induce specific IgE antibody, which, acting with macrophages, eosinophils and platelets, induces antibody-dependent cellular cytotoxicity (ADCC). The specific IgE antibody is protective but its involvement with cells is essential (Capron and Dessaint 1985). As indicated earlier, regulation of the IgE response involves complex interactions of cytokines which stimulate a Th2 type of response rather than a Th1 response, although parasitic antigens may stimulate the former type of response regardless of the genetic make-up of the host (reviewed by Leung 1994).

Elevated IgE antibodies exist in most helminth and many protozoal infections. For example, in schistosomiasis most patients infected with *Schistosoma haematobium* or *Schistosoma mansoni* have raised amounts of IgE antibody to worm and egg antigens of the parasites. The total IgE level is also raised, although with treatment it decreases more rapidly than the titre of specific IgE. The detection of specific IgE can be used diagnostically and epidemiologically and titres correlate well with immediate skin test reactivity to worm and egg antigens (see Maddison 1986 for review). The serum titres of total and specific IgE are raised in up to 100% of patients with *Echinococcus granulosus* infections. It has been known for many years that rupture of a cyst in this infection induces anaphylaxis, and it is now believed that the reaction is largely IgE mediated (Schantz and Gottstein 1986). It should be noted that the cyst fluid can induce anaphylaxis, albeit of lesser degree, in sheep that have not been sensitized to the parasite and have no IgE antibody.

Table 6.2   Mediators of tissue inflamation in type I hypersensitivity

Histamine	Found in mast cells, basophils, platelets. Action via H1 receptor leads to increased vascular permeability, contracts smooth muscle, increases goblet cell secretion of mucus. Action via H2 receptors leads to increased gastric secretion and decreased mediator release from mast cells and basophils.
	Chemotactic for eosinophils.
LTC4	Produce slow contraction of smooth muscle, leading
LTD4	to vasoconstriction and peripheral airway resistance.
LTE4	Increase vascular permeability.
	LTC4 stimulates goblet cell secretion of mucus. LTB4 is chemotactic for eosinophils, neutrophils and mononuclear cells.
	All detected by same monoclonal antibody (de Weck 1992) and comprise the substance previously known as SRS-A (slow-reacting substance of anaphylaxis).
Eosinophil chemotactic factor of anaphylaxis (ECF-A)	Released from mast cells and basophils. Selectively chemotactic for eosinophils.
Platelet activating factor (PAF)	Induces platelet aggregation and secretion. May amplify anaphylactic reactions.
Prostaglandins	Wide tissue distribution. Released during anaphylaxis. PGD_2, PGE_2, cause vasodilatation. PGD_2, $PGF_{2\alpha}$, cause airway constriction. Some intermediates of prostaglandin synthesis are important mediators of platelet aggregation and smooth muscle contraction.
HETES	Synthesized by activated mast cells. Stimulates mucus secretion. Chemotaxin for eosinophils, neutrophils and mononuclear cells.
Enzymes	Mast cells secrete proteolytic and glycosidase enzymes which damage neighbouring cells.

This apparent conflict may be explained by the finding that vasoactive amine release from mast cells is possible by a direct stimulating mechanism independent of IgE antibody (de Weck 1992). The effects of a type I hypersensitivity are therefore seen without the involvement of IgE. Whilst these effects have been reported for simple molecules such as drugs, it seems possible that antigens from organisms such as worms might have the same effect.

Increased levels of specific IgE antibody have been described in toxocariasis (Glickman, Schantz and Grieve 1986), filariasis (Ambroise-Thomas and Peyron 1986) and onchocerciasis (Mackenzie, Burgess and Sisley 1986).

However useful IgE antibody responses may be in infections, tissue damage can occur, as with all hypersensitivities. The extent and range of tissue damage is not well understood in most of the infections discussed above, although hydatid disease provides an exception. The destruction of ocular tissues in toxocariasis and ascariasis infection has also been well described (Rockey et al. 1981).

Aspergillus spp. are important causes of type I reactions and of asthma in susceptible individuals. This may occur as a result of inhalation of *Aspergillus* spores without infection, or as an effect of pulmonary asper-

gillosis, when the organism is growing in a cavity or infarcted area of the lung. Other fungi such as *Cladosporium* spp. and *Penicillium* spp. can induce asthma, although this is not associated with true infection. Dermatophyte fungi, particularly *Trichophyton*, have been shown to induce specific IgE antibody and immediate skin reactions and some workers believe that a type I hypersensitivity is responsible for the intense itching that characterizes these infections (Platts-Mills et al. 1987). A similar hypothesis has been put forward to explain the chronic irritation in atopic dermatitis. In this case IgE antibody specific for *Staphylococcus aureus* has been demonstrated in approximately 30% of patients; it is suggested that colonization or infection of abraded skin by the organism triggers histamine release and adds to the local irritation (Motala et al. 1986).

Type I hypersensitivities are not frequently described in virus infections although they may be important, particularly in respiratory infections. Specific IgE antibodies are elevated in the sera of children infected with respiratory syncytial virus (RSV) and correlate with the severity of wheezing and bronchiolitis. After treatment, the IgE levels decrease (Bui et al. 1987). The same report indicates that RSV-infected children have elevated titres of IgG, although these antibodies are not thought to induce symptoms. The role of IgG4 in type I hypersensitivity is uncertain, although it has been regarded as a mediator of passive cutaneous anaphylaxis (Parish 1970) and is therefore a possible inducer of type I hypersensitivity.

Other important type I hypersensitivities are those induced by antibiotics, most of which can produce type I hypersensitivity although it is uncommon. For example, with penicillin G the maximum reported rate is 0.04% of treated patients. The penicilloyl derivative of the drug is thought to be the important hapten and, because it can be induced by other antibiotics of the penicillin family, this type of hypersensitivity is cross-reactive. A true anaphylactic response to a penicillin means that the use of other penicillins is contraindicated thereafter. The mortality from these rare reactions is approximately 10% (see Kucers and Bennett 1987). The more common hypersensitivities to antibiotics, such as serum sickness (type III), are due to other mechanisms (see section on 'Mechanisms of type III hypersensitivity', p. 70).

TYPE II HYPERSENSITIVITY

Antibody mediated cytotoxic damage is the principal feature of type II hypersensitivity. The antigen forms part of the membrane of the cell under attack, or alternatively is firmly bound to the membrane (e.g. haptens, drugs). The binding of antibodies is followed by activation of the complement pathways (see Chapter 4). The effect is to produce damage to the cell wall which becomes 'leaky', loses high molecular weight products and takes up water, ultimately lysing. Immune haemolysis of transfused blood by preformed antibodies to red cell antigens and 'autoimmune' haemolytic anaemia are obvious examples of type II reactions in clinical practice.

Immunoglobulin class and type II hypersensitivity

The most important property of antibody for participation in this type of hypersensitivity is the ability to activate complement. In man, most IgM antibodies and IgG antibodies of the IgG1 and IgG3 subclass types are able to activate complement. The demonstration of these antibodies on the surface of host cells by immunofluorescence provides a basis for recognizing this hypersensitivity, although where red blood cells are the target the Coombs test (passive haemagglutination) may be useful.

Mechanisms of type II hypersensitivity

In theory, any host cell is susceptible to attack by type II hypersensitivity. It only requires the development of an antibody specific for a cell surface antigen, followed by the attachment of that antibody and activation of complement to lyse the cell. In practice, this event occurs only in rare 'autoimmune' diseases such as idiopathic haemolytic anaemia when a change in red cell surface antigens predisposes to the immune attack. This change may be induced by infection or by the attachment to the surface of the cell of haptens which, when combined with cellular proteins, create 'new' antigens which stimulate antibody. Antibiotics

are examples (Weitzman, Stossel and Desmond 1978). It is probable that in many infections cell surface antigens are changed by virus-encoded antigen expression or are modified by the attachment of haptens or antigens (Oldstone 1987). The secreted substances of bacteria, fungi and other parasites may attach to host cells, 'targeting' them for attack by the formation of antibody.

Type II hypersensitivity and infection

Although it is likely that a number of infections will, in time, be shown to exert their pathogenic effect by this hypersensitivity mechanism, it has been difficult to prove this in many infections. As described above, the concept is that organisms either change host cell antigens or produce products that attach to host cell membranes.

Another idea is that the antigens of the organism molecularly mimic host antigens and may, on occasion, induce an antibody response that is directed against host cells. The concept of molecular mimicry has been reviewed by Oldstone (1987). Examples cited include: the cross-reaction of the neutralizing domain of coxsackie B4 virus with heart muscle, which may explain the involvement of this virus in myocarditis; the reaction between part of the α-gliadin molecule and the E1B-coded polypeptides of adenovirus-12 and evidence of the involvement of this virus in coeliac disease; and the established cross-reaction between *Klebsiella pneumoniae* nitrogenase and HLA-B27 sequences in patients with ankylosing spondylitis or Reiter's syndrome. Oldstone (1987) correctly indicated that the propensity to develop disease following infection with the relevant organisms is variable and unpredictable, even though the known cross-reactivities are present. The effect of environmental factors on the outcome is currently immeasurable in most situations. A further useful example of the effect of type II hypersensitivity in a bacterial infection occurs with *Helicobacter pylori*, now acknowledged to be the major cause of peptic ulcer disease and gastritis. This organism has been shown to induce cross-reactive antibodies which are specific for gastric antigens (Negrini et al. 1991); the resulting damage to the gastric mucosa is thought to be due to the cross-reactive autoimmune reaction that results. It may be that other diseases such as myasthenia gravis, Guillain–Barré syndrome and type I diabetes, which have been associated with virus infections, have similar mechanisms (Oldstone 1987).

Type II hypersensitivity may also be important in the treatment of many infections because of its involvement in the destruction of neutrophils, 'sensitized' by the adduction of antibiotic molecules to the surface of the cells (Weitzman, Stossel and Desmond 1978).

It is clear that the investigation of type II hypersensitivity in infection will be difficult. The introduction to this chapter indicated that the interaction between host and parasite was infinitely variable and that the task of interpreting the interaction is bound to be difficult. The examples of type II hypersensitivity quoted above demonstrate this problem well.

TYPE III HYPERSENSITIVITY

Type III hypersensitivity is caused by immune complexes which activate complement (see Chapter 4) and stimulate an inflammatory reaction. This may occur in localized tissues, in which case it is termed an Arthus reaction, or in the systemic circulation. The Arthus reaction in skin is characterized by oedema, hyperaemia, erythema which may proceed to necrosis, and susceptibility to this reaction can be passively transferred by the injection of serum.

It is now clear that the formation of antigen–antibody complexes in serum, with subsequent deposition of the complexes in tissues is the key event in type III hypersensitivity. The complexes will cause damage to the tissues only if complement is activated; the complement activation is primarily determined by the ratio of antigen to antibody within the complexes. Briefly, complexes with a large excess of either antigen or antibody will not activate the classical pathway of complement. Complexes that are formed at equivalence, when the number of antibody-binding sites equals exactly the number of antigenic determinants, are the best complement activators. Complexes with a slight excess of antigen or antibody, although less efficient than equivalence complexes, nevertheless activate complement well. There is a difference in the half-life of these complement-activating complexes which is short for equivalence and slight antibody excess complexes and prolonged for those with modest antigen excess (Cochrane and Koffler 1973).

Immunoglobulin class and type III hypersensitivity

The isotype of immunoglobulin involved in type III hypersensitivity is probably important. At present, it is difficult to determine which isotype is important because of problems in the measurement of any of the antibodies that form complexes and initiate damage. Early work concentrated on 'precipitins', usually IgG antibodies, but the inherent problems of this approach were demonstrated when it was shown that type III reactions could occur even when precipitin tests were negative (Parratt et al. 1982). A different approach has been to quantitate immune complexes rather than the antibody that may be a component of the complex. Many such methods have been described and have been reviewed by Espinoza (1983). IgM-, IgG-, IgA- and IgE-containing complexes have been regularly detected in many diseases, including infections. It has been assumed that complexes containing IgG or IgM will activate complement and cause damage, although some investigators have discounted the importance of IgM complexes in type III hypersensitivity (Levinsky 1981). An alternative view is that IgA- and IgE-containing complexes, which probably only activate the alternative pathway of complement, may be important causes of tissue damage in nephritis and asthma (Maire et al. 1983, Nawata et al. 1984). It is unfortunate that, due to the difficulties of measuring and analysing immune complexes in any infection, our understanding of the relevance of different immunoglobulin isotypes in complexes has advanced little in the last few years.

Mechanisms of type III hypersensitivity

Activation of complement in the tissues releases chemotactic factors and mediators of inflammation. The reaction, initially occurring in the vascular endothelium, causes an influx of polymorphonuclear leucocytes (Cochrane and Koffler 1973), causing damage to the vessel wall. Leakage of the vessel contents causes enlargement of the lesion in the surrounding tissues. As a general rule the severity of the tissue inflammation, which heals by fibrosis with loss of function, is related to the degree of complement activation; this is determined by the amount of immune complex deposited in the tissue, which in turn depends both on the quantity of complex generated and on the amount removed by normal processes of elimination.

The quantity of immune complex generated is directly determined by the amounts of antibody and antigen that interact. Type III hypersensitivity can never occur in the absence of an antibody response to the challenge antigen. However, as indicated above, it is believed that the ratio of antigen to antibody is important in producing damaging complement-fixing immune complexes. The interaction of antibody with antigen might produce complexes that do not activate complement and are incapable of causing damage. Therefore the absolute amount of available antibody is not important. It is the amount of antibody that combines with antigen at the critical, damaging, ratios that determines the severity of the hypersensitivity. It is quite possible for a patient with high titres of antibody to be injected with small amounts of antigen without untoward effects. The converse of this, antigen overloading, is also seen in patients with infectious mononucleosis who have been taking ampicillin. Such patients have antibody to ampicillin by virtue of their infection and develop a severe rash (McKenzie, Parratt and White 1976). On continuing the administration of the ampicillin (antigen) the rash disappears.

A similar phenomenon has been observed in mice, in which glomerular deposits of complexes in the kidney have been removed by the injection of a large excess of antigen (Mannik and Striker 1980). In these instances it is presumably the change to antigen excess complexes that do not activate complement which halts the inflammatory reaction. In clinical practice, therefore, the recurrence of a type III hypersensitivity is unpredictable even in the same patient, because it is rarely possible to determine the quantities of interactive antigen and antibody.

Removal of immune complexes by host mechanisms further complicates the picture. IgG-containing immune complexes bind to Fc receptors on neutrophils, monocytes, tissue macrophages and Kupffer cells, and in so doing stimulate their own uptake by these cells. Platelets also have receptors for immune complexes although it is not clear whether there is subsequent removal of the bound complexes. Human erythrocytes have receptors for C3b, a breakdown product of complement that is incorporated in complement-activating complexes, and it is thought that immune complexes can be removed from circulation by attachment to these cells. Such an effect has been demonstrated in monkeys (Cornacoff, Herbert and Smead 1983). Complement also assists in the removal of immune complexes, probably by activating the C3b receptors, and it has been shown that patients with deficiencies of the complement system have a higher than usual incidence of immune complex hypersensitivity (Tomino et al. 1984). This may seem paradoxical but can be understood if it is postulated that complement activation of complexes is beneficial only until the removal mechanisms are saturated and high levels of complexes accumulate in the blood and tissues. Complement activation then becomes an instrument of damage.

The outcome of antigen–antibody interaction in terms of immune complex hypersensitivity is therefore highly, if not infinitely, variable. When hypersensitivity occurs clinically it is either confined to a local site such as skin or lung where the reaction resembles the originally described Arthus lesion or, more commonly, the reaction is generalized because of the presence of large amounts of circulating immune complexes, which are filtered out in important organs and tissues. The kidney, muscles, joints and skin are particularly affected and the prototype of this disorder is 'serum sickness'. The classic form of serum sickness is now rarely seen because of the rarity of administration of foreign proteins, although it can occur with drugs and in autoimmune diseases such as systemic lupus erythematosus (SLE). In SLE the immune complex hypersensitivity may become chronic over many months or years, leading to severe damage to tissue and organs.

Type III hypersensitivity may occur in any response to a soluble antigen in which antibody is produced by the host. The resultant disease may be acute or chronic, generalized or localized, and all such variants have been well documented in infections.

Type III hypersensitivity and infection

Raised serum levels of immune complexes have been demonstrated in many kinds of infections. Examples of bacterial infections are endocarditis, meningococcal and gonococcal infections, infected shunts in children, leprosy and syphilis. Viral infections such as dengue haemorrhagic fever, cytomegalovirus infections, hepatitis B, infectious mononucleosis and subacute sclerosing panencephalitis are represented, as are the parasitic infections malaria, trypanosomiasis, schistosomiasis, filariasis and toxoplasmosis (see Villarreal et al. 1983). This list is not exhaustive but serves to demonstrate that immune complex formation is common in many infections. This is not surprising because immune complexes will always form when antibody coexists with the antigen which has stimulated it. In many infections antibody produced against the responsible micro-organism is ineffective in eradicating the organism, which continues to multiply and release more antigen. Further stimulation of antibody follows and a cycle of damage results from the steady increase in immune complex levels. However, hypersensitivity does not always result. If the organism is

eliminated by some other defence mechanism, formation of complexes ceases. Furthermore, as indicated above, the ratio of antigen to antibody in the complexes is important and an individual may escape the formation of complexes that inflict damage in the tissues. It is therefore necessary to distinguish between immune complex formation and immune complex hypersensitivity in infections. For example, in infective endocarditis, high levels of circulating immune complexes correlate well with glomerular injury (Hooper et al. 1983) and the presence of complexes in CSF accords with cerebral disease in African trypanosomiasis (Lambert, Berney and Kazyumba 1981). By contrast, there is no simple relationship between circulating immune complexes and glomerular damage in schistosomiasis (Bout et al. 1977).

Glomerular injury is one of the most common manifestations of postinfection type III hypersensitivity. The classic disease is post-streptococcal glomerulonephritis in which it is believed that complexes of streptococcal antigen and its respective antibody are deposited on the glomerular membranes with subsequent complement activation, inflammation and fibrosis. Hypersensitivity is suggested by the latent period between streptococcal infection and the onset of glomerulonephritis, decreased serum complement levels, deposits of immunoglobulin and complement in the glomeruli and the absence of viable streptococci in the lesions. Some investigators have reported the demonstration of streptococcal antigens in renal biopsy specimens (Michael et al. 1966, Lange et al. 1976), although others have failed to confirm these findings. Other hypotheses to account for the glomerular damage have been proposed, including the concept that streptococcal infection sensitizes the host to glomerular basement membrane antigens, thus triggering a type II hypersensitivity. The tenor of this argument, well reviewed by Villarreal et al. (1983), is that there is something different about the strains of streptococci causing glomerulonephritis that distinguishes them from other group A streptococci and from other species of bacteria. However, Villarreal et al. (1983) also reported that microbial antigens of many other species can be demonstrated in glomerular deposits. The referenced list they provide includes *S. aureus*, *Pseudomonas aeruginosa*, *Salmonella typhi*, *Treponema pallidum*, various streptococci (including *Streptococcus pneumoniae*), *Mycobacterium*, *Klebsiella* and *Yersinia* spp. *Candida albicans* and *Coccidioides immitis* are also documented together with 9 viruses (hepatitis B, measles, Epstein–Barr virus, varicella zoster virus, coxsackie B, cytomegalovirus, mumps, ECHO viruses and oncornaviruses). Parasites are included in the list, some of which have been discussed above. That so many micro-organisms have been incriminated suggests that cross-antigenicity is very unlikely and that type III hypersensitivity is a more plausible explanation. Type III hypersensitivity is liable to occur whenever antigen and antibody coexist in the circulation. This is likely to happen in most infections; complexes thus formed will have their most dramatic effect in the kidney which, because of its high blood flow and filtering action, retains the damaging complexes. It is probable that immune complex events occur very commonly in many infections and that thorough investigation may reveal the cause of their induction and the degree of damage which results. The crucial test is the demonstration of microbial antigens in the immune complexes. This can be achieved in tissue sections (e.g. in a renal biopsy by immunofluorescence) but is more difficult with circulating immune complexes. In the latter case one of the techniques used most frequently is to isolate the complexes from serum, disrupt them and separate the antigen for some form of immunological identification. An early example of this approach was the analysis of serum complexes in human schistosomiasis (Bout et al. 1977). More recently, similar studies have been carried out in HIV-infected humans and it has been shown that diagnosis is improved by measurement of antigen derived from dissociated immune complexes (Nielson et al. 1995). The methods used to dissociate the complexes are cumbersome but represent the first steps towards antigen-specific immune complex assay. Similar studies have shown the diagnostic value of this type of approach in pneumococcal pneumonia (Mellancamp et al. 1987), Lyme disease (Schutzer et al. 1990), human infection with *S. haematobinum* (Manca et al. 1988) and in animal models of *Coxiella burnetii* infection infection (Bo-Hai and Shu-Rong 1987). As the amount of damage caused to tissues is related directly to the amount of immune complexes generated, the development of such antigen-specific immune complex assays and their refinement should allow a more detailed analysis of immune complex damage in the future.

2.2   Cell mediated hypersensitivity

TYPE IV HYPERSENSITIVITY

The tissue-damaging events in this form of hypersensitivity are mediated by T lymphocytes, not by antibody. The process is also referred to as 'cell mediated' or 'delayed' hypersensitivity. The use of the term 'delayed' reflects the very different time scale of this type of response if compared with immediate hypersensitivity, mediated by antibodies. After primary exposure to antigen, a period of 7–10 days or longer elapses before the production of the sensitized T lymphocytes, which migrate to the site of antigen deposition. Secondary responses take 24–72 h to appear, again because of the time taken for proliferation of the relevant T cells and for their migration into the affected tissues. For many bacterial and viral infections the presence of multiple antigenic determinants will stimulate both antibody production and the proliferation of specific T cells. Examples of immunological responses that involve both major mechanisms are discussed later in this section. The tuberculin skin test is the best known example of an evoked delayed hypersensitivity reaction but the complex antigenic structure of *Mycobacterium tuberculosis* and of tuberculin or Purified Protein Derivative (PPD) must be recognized as inducing responses that are not 'pure' T cell. The

historical aspects of this reaction were reviewed in the last edition of this book.

The role of T lymphocytes in type IV hypersensitivity

Recent work on this topic has centred on the activities of T lymphocytes in the lesions of leprosy caused by *Mycobacterium leprae*. This is a useful model to consider and has been reviewed by Sieling and Modlin (1994).

In the 'tuberculoid' variant of this disease in which cell mediated immunity is most pronounced and granuloma formation is most evident, CD4 T cells predominate over CD8 T cells in a ratio of almost 2:1. In the absence of cell mediated immunity (i.e. in lepromatous leprosy) this ratio is reversed in favour of CD8 cells. The CD4 cells found in the granulomata are mainly memory cells and the CD8 cells are cytotoxic. The distribution of the cells, histologically, is interesting. CD4+ memory cells are located in the centre of the granuloma with macrophages, whereas the CD8+ cells are in the periphery of the lesion. There is also a predominance of Langerhans cells, CD1+ and antigen-presenting in character, at the periphery. However, of functional importance is the presence of increased levels of cytokines in the T cells of the granuloma. These cytokines include IL-2, IFN-γ, IL-1β and TNF-α. In addition, cells that contain serine esterase or RNA are frequently found, suggesting T cytotoxic activity in the lesion.

The presence of T cells producing IL-2 and IFN-γ in the granulomatous lesions of tuberculoid leprosy suggests the presence of a Th1-type immune response, which activates macrophages, which in turn kill the intracellular pathogens. The element of hypersensitivity here is one of degree. Provided the response leads to limited tissue destruction and effective killing of the pathogen, immunity results. When the Th1 response is so vigorous as to result in macrophage destruction of normal tissue, albeit in the vicinity of abnormal infected tissue, a hypersensitivity results. There are as yet no clear data to define the control mechanisms used in this type of response. However, it has been shown that the T cells that infiltrate the lesions in tuberculoid leprosy have TCR receptors which are predominantly Vβ6, and that some Vβ receptors (i.e. 1–6.4 subfamilies) are more commonly associated with lesion formation than others (i.e. 6.5–6.7 subfamilies). It may be that the type of T cell, defined according to Vβ family, will influence the outcome in respect of hypersensitivity versus immunity.

The inflammatory response in the lesion is clearly due to the combined effects of T cells and macrophages. T cells can be directly cytotoxic independently of antibody and complement. In this cytotoxic action cell contact, Mg^{2+} and phospholipase or trypsin-like enzymes are probably all essential to achieve the destructive effect on target cells (Henney 1980). Cell membrane changes caused by the enzymes lead to loss of potassium from the cell and a failure to regulate sodium ions, leading to cell death.

Examples of cell mediated hypersensitivity in other infections are reviewed below.

Type IV hypersensitivity and infection

Tuberculosis is a good example of cell mediated hypersensitivity in infection. There is a spectrum of infection similar to that of leprosy, described above (Lenzini, Rottoli and Rottoli 1977). Patients with granuloma formation, strong and classic Mantoux reactivity and lymphocyte responsiveness in vitro are termed 'reactive' and correspond to those with tuberculoid leprosy. Such patients respond well to treatment whereas those at the 'unreactive' end of the spectrum, with poorly responsive T lymphocytes, do not respond well to therapy and may have disseminated disease. In other models, animal experiments have indicated that bacterial strain differences influence the T cell response of mice to *Salmonella typhimurium* (Killar and Eisenstein 1986). Some mice develop effective and protective T cell immunity without evidence of hypersensitivity (i.e. negative skin reactivity to antigen) whereas other strains regularly produce a T cell mediated hypersensitivity reaction. The dose of antigen administered is also important; Ptak and colleagues (1980) showed that the route or mechanism by which the antigen is processed often influences the outcome. In this study, in which a hapten was used to investigate contact sensitivity in mice, it was established that delayed hypersensitivity can be observed in 2 forms. The first is an 'evanescent' reaction in skin, which declines rapidly and can be induced by altering the mode of antigen presentation by using material that has undergone phagocytosis. The second, more delayed, type of response, with cellular infiltration, occurs when the hapten is presented by Langerhans cells. Intravenous injection of haptenated epidermal cells is also effective. In human tuberculosis there is the same division of skin reactivity into early and late reactions (Lenzini, Rottoli and Rottoli 1977), the latter being characterized by cellular infiltration, induration and central necrosis, a classic delayed hypersensitivity reaction. By contrast, the early reactions comprise chiefly erythema and oedema, and it could be speculated that this form of response is due to the lymphocyte factors which release 5-HT from eosinophils and basophils (Kops et al. 1986).

The mechanisms that determine whether an individual will respond with a hypersensitivity and be susceptible to damage are poorly understood; they are clearly important and it is no longer sufficient to consider cell mediated immunity (a beneficial state) and cell mediated (type IV) hypersensitivity to be one and the same thing. The distinction is even more important when one considers the central role of T cell mediated responses in infection.

3 SUPERANTIGENS

It has become clear that some micro-organisms can exert a pathogenic effect, and thus cause damage, by releasing substances (often toxins) which induce vigorous stimulation of immune cells. One of the mechanisms by which this occurs is the release of so-called superantigens, which stimulate subsets of T cells and bring about the release of cytokines which initiate cell and tissue damage. This is not a 'classical' hypersensitivity reaction as defined above, but, nevertheless, is a plausible cause of host-implemented self-destruction. The topic has been reviewed by Zumia (1992). The concept of superantigenicity relies on the finding that T lymphocytes specifically recognize foreign antigens when these are associated with or presented by MHC class I or class II molecules on antigen-producing cells and that this specificity is due to TCRs (T cell receptors), which are in contact with the MHC–antigen complex. TCRs are made up from 2 chains, α and β, or γ and δ, and conventional antigen recognition requires either the recognition of α and β or γ and δ receptors. The 2 chains produce a structural groove into which the antigen 'fits'.

Superantigens bypass this mechanism by binding to MHC class II molecules outside the antigen groove in such a way that they can stimulate T cells which are expressing relevant TCR Vβ gene products. In this way, they may cause the activation of between 5 and 25% of T cells. Most activation appears to be of cells bearing members of the Vβ gene products (approximately 24) although activation of cells with γ/δ TCR has been demonstrated. Of particular interest is the fact that superantigens may cause unresponsiveness on the part of T cells (anergy) as well as overstimulation of these cells.

Some superantigens have been found to be endogenous proteins but many are exogenous and derived from micro-organisms.

3.1 Micro-organisms as a source of superantigens

The classic examples are the toxins of *S. aureus* and *Streptococcus pyogenes*. In the case of *S. aureus*, 3 groups of toxins have been shown to have superantigen effects. Thus the enterotoxin SE-A has been shown to be the most potent T cell mitogen yet discovered. In addition, the exfoliative toxin ExT-A and the toxic shock syndrome toxin (TSST-1) both have considerable superantigen activity. The erythrogenic toxins (ET) of group A β-haemolytic streptococci (A, B and C antigenic variants) have superantigen properties (Müller-Alouf et al. 1994), as does a fragment of the M protein molecule of this organism (Zumia 1992). Apart from these 'classical' toxins, it has been shown that a soluble product from *Mycoplasma arthritidis* has superantigen activity (Mehindate et al. 1994). Zumia (1992) postulates similar activities for the exotoxin A of *P. aeruginosa*, antigens from malarial parasites, and HIV-1 encoded superantigens. TSST-1 has been postulated as the cause of Kawasaki syndrome (Leung et al. 1993), a disease with no known aetiology at present.

3.2 The clinical relevance of superantigens

It is not clear at present what role superantigens play in disease. Certainly, *S. aureus* and *S. pyogenes* are associated with fulminant shock syndromes where the action of toxins is likely to be central to their activity. In other instances, these organisms produce infections that are not fulminant. This paradox may be partly explained by the fact that superantigens have a variable activity, either stimulating or suppressing T cells in different circumstances (Zumia 1992). The explanation may be simpler, as described by Takei, Arora and Walker (1993), who showed that antibody to the staphylococcal toxin superantigens could neutralize the superantigen effects of the toxin. Taken together, these findings demonstrate the unpredictability of any host parasite effects in the individual patient, a matter referred to in the introduction to this chapter (see section 1, p. 65).

The mechanism by which superantigens do induce fulminant shock is of interest. Bacterially induced shock is the result of cytokine release. In a comparative study (Müller-Alouf et al. 1994), it was shown that the erythrogenic toxins of *S. pyogenes* (ETA and ETC), known to be superantigens, stimulated IL-8 and TNF-α from peripheral blood mononuclear cells. By contrast, lipopolysaccharide (LPS) from gram-negative bacteria, also a shock-inducing substance, stimulated the release of IL-1α, IL-1β, IL-6 and TNF-α only from monocytes but not T cells. The release of cytokines clearly followed different pathways but had a common expression in the activation of TNF-α.

4   Cytokines and nitric oxide

It is becoming clear that some cytokines, the chemical 'messengers' that bring about communication between cells of the immune system, are capable of causing tissue damage (Bellanti, Kadlec and Escobar-Gutiérrez 1994). In particular, levels of TNF-α, IL-1, IL-6 and IL-8 are often increased in infectious diseases. According to Bellanti, Kadlec and Escobar-Gutiérrez (1994), the levels of some of these cytokines, such as IL-1, can be elevated from 10 to 20 times normal values, and the mechanisms of the shock syndrome induced by IL-1 are related to the capacity of this cytokine to stimulate production of platelet aggregating factor (PAF), prostaglandins and nitric oxide. These induce shock, which may be irreversible and may lead to death. Paradoxically, IL-1 has been shown to be beneficial in animals by protecting them from bacterial and fungal infections (Dinarello and Wolff 1993). A partial explanation of such a paradox may be provided by the recognition that the release of minute amounts of stimulating material from micro-organisms (e.g. LPS) may be more important than large amounts of the same (Rabinovici, Fuerstein and Neville 1994). These investigators argue that the collision or interaction between LPS and PAF, another cytokine, is more important than the actual amounts of LPS released. They cite the importance of studies (Dubois, Bissonnette and Rola-Pleszczynski 1989), which indicate a synergistic interaction between LPS and PAF. Clearly, there is much to be learned about the dynamic aspects of the stimulation of these cytokines. As indicated

above, another cytokine, IL-8, is found in increased amounts in infections. Further work on the role of this cytokine in bacterial infections has been reviewed by Kunkel, Lukacs and Strieter (1994). These investigators have indicated that the development of adult respiratory distress syndrome (ARDS), which is now assumed to be a cytokine mediated response to bacterial onslaught, is significantly associated with the appearance of IL-8 in the lungs, and that this cytokine, which may induce damage, is generated from alveolar macrophages. IL-8 is chemotactic for neutrophils and its generation is not caused directly by stimulation of alveolar macrophages by endotoxin (LPS) from gram-negative bacteria. It appears that endotoxin stimulates other cytokines, such as IL-1 and TNF, which in turn 'recruit' the help of macrophages; these cells respond by releasing IL-8. Kunkel, Lukacs and Strieter (1994) describe the involvement of this cytokine in other infections besides those leading to ARDS and indicate that measurement of the cytokine may be useful for predicting the prognosis in serious infection.

Indeed, it is clear from the evidence to date that a thorough understanding of the cytokine interactions in infections is required in order both to predict outcome and to manipulate these pathways with appropriate therapy. The missing link at present is information about parasite behaviour that causes cytokine activation. For example, some patients with gram-negative bacteraemia quickly become shocked and develop major organ failure and ARDS whereas others with identical infections do not. Presumably the **severity** of the infection has something to do with this difference and this is a factor which is not quantifiable at present.

4.1   Nitric oxide

Nitric oxide production by cells may be an extremely important factor in the outcome of host–parasite interaction. There is evidence that the production of this substance will aid the killing of organisms (Virta, Karp and Vuorinen 1994) and that it increases the resistance of the host to infections such as mucosal candidosis (Vazgueztorres et al. 1995). However, it is clear from other investigations that nitric oxide production may cause host tissue damage. Rodriguez-Del Valle et al. (1994) investigated the effect of endotoxin (LPS) on hepatocytes and showed that excessive nitric oxide was produced by these cells and that this increased production was associated with inhibition of proliferation, protein synthesis and the appearance of degraded cytoplasmic DNA which they regarded as indicative of damage to injured hepatocytes. In another study, Wizemann and Laskin (1994) showed that lipopolysaccharide produced an excess of nitric oxide in damaged lung macrophages although this was more marked in alveolar macrophages than in the interstitial variety. Although the exact role of this substance in inflammatory responses to infection is unclear, it must remain an important area for future work. It has even been suggested that nitric oxide may have immunoregulatory functions (Yamamoto, Friedman and Klein 1994).

REFERENCES

Ambroise-Thomas P, Peyron F, 1986, Filariasis, *Immunodiagnosis of Parasitic Diseases*, vol. 1, eds Walls KW, Schantz PM, Academic Press, London, 233–48.

Bellanti JA, Kadlec JV, Escobar-Gutiérrez A, 1994, Cytokines and the immune response, *Pediatr Clin North Am*, **41:** 597–621.

Bennich H, Johansson SGO, 1971, Structure and function of human immunoglobulin E, *Adv Immunol*, **13:** 1–55.

Bo-Hai W, Shu-Rong Y, 1987, Antigen specific circulating immune complexes in *Coxiella burnetii* infected guinea pigs, *Exp Mol Pathol*, **47:** 175–84.

Bout D, Santoro F et al., 1977, Circulating immune complexes in schistosomiasis, *Immunology*, **33:** 17–22.

Bui RH, Molinaro GA et al., 1987, Virus specific IgE and IgG$_4$ antibodies in serum of children infected with respiratory syncytial virus, *Pediatrics*, **110:** 87–92.

Capron A, Dessaint JP, 1985, Effector and regulatory mechanisms in immunity to schistosomes: a heuristic view, *Annu Rev Immunol*, **3:** 455–76.

Church MK, Pao GJK, Holgate ST, 1982, Characterization of histamine secretion from mechanically dispersed human lung mast cells: effects of anti-IgE, calcium ionophore A23187, compound 48/50 and basic polypeptides, *J Immunol*, **129:** 2116–21.

Cochrane CG, Koffler D, 1973, Immune complex disease in experimental animals and man, *Adv Immunol*, **16:** 185–264.

Coleman J, Godfrey RC, 1981, The number and affinity of IgE receptors on dispersed human lung mast cells, *Immunology*, **44:** 859–63.

Cornacoff JB, Herbert LA, Smead WL, 1983, Private erythrocyte-immune complex clearing mechanism, *J Clin Invest*, **71:** 236–44.

Dinarello CA, Wolff SM, 1993, The role of interleukin-1 in disease, *N Engl J Med*, **328:** 106–13.

Dubois C, Bissonnette E, Rola-Pleszczynski M, 1989, Platelet activating factor (PAF) enhances tumor necrosis factor production by alveolar macrophages: prevention by PAF receptor antagonists and lipoxygenase inhibitors, *J Immunol*, **143:** 964–70.

Espinoza LR, 1983, Assays for circulating immune complexes, *Circulating Immune Complexes: their Clinical Significance*, eds Espinoza LR, Osterland CK, Futura, New York, 27.

Gell PGH, Coombs RRA (eds), 1963, *Clinical Aspects of Immunology*, 2nd edn, Blackwell Scientific, Oxford, 761.

Glickman LT, Schantz PM, Grieve RB, 1986, Toxocariasis, *Immunodiagnosis of Parasitic Diseases*, vol. 1, eds Walls KW, Schantz PM, Academic Press, London, 201–55.

Henney CS, 1980, The mechanism of T cell mediated lysis, *Immunol Today*, **1:** 36–41.

Holgate ST, Kay AB, 1984, Mast cells and the lung, *Hosp Update*, **10:** 151–61.

Hooper DC, Bayer AS et al., 1983, Circulating immune complexes in prosthetic valve endocarditis, *Arch Intern Med*, **143:** 2081–4.

Howarth PH, Bradding P et al., 1994, Cytokines and airway inflammation, *Ann NY Acad Sci*, **725:** 69–82.

Kay AB, 1981, *The Inflammatory Process*, eds Venge P, Lindblom J, Almqvist and Wiksell International, Stockholm, 293.

Killar LM, Eisenstein TK, 1986, Delayed type hypersensitivity and immunity to *Salmonella typhimurium*, *Infect Immun*, **52:** 504–8.

Kops SK, Ratzlaff RE et al., 1986, Interaction of antigen-specific T cell factors with unique 'receptors' on the surface of mast cells: demonstration in vitro by an indirect resetting technique, *J Immunol*, **136:** 4515–24.

Kucers A, Bennett NMcK, 1987, *The Use of Antibiotics*, 4th edn, Heinemann Medical, London, 33.

Kunkel SL, Lukacs NW, Strieter RM, 1994, The role of interleukin-8 in the infectious process, *Ann NY Acad Sci*, **730:** 134–43.

Lack G, Renz H et al., 1992, Nebulized interferon-gamma (IFN-gamma) decreases IgE production in a murine model of airways sensitization, *J Allergy Clin Immunol*, **89:** Abstr. 382.

Lambert PH, Berney M, Kazyumba G, 1981, Immune complexes in serum and in cerebrospinal fluid in African trypanosomiasis, *J Clin Invest*, **67:** 77–85.

Lange K, Ahmed U et al., 1976, A hitherto unknown streptococcal antigen and its probable relation to acute post-streptococcal glomerulonephritis, *Clin Nephrol*, **5:** 207–15.

Lenzini P, Rottoli P, Rottoli L, 1977, The spectrum of human tuberculosis, *Clin Exp Immunol*, **27:** 230–7.

Leung DYM, 1994, Mechanisms of the human allergic response: clinical implications, *Clin Immunol*, **41:** 727–43.

Leung DYM, Meissner HC et al., 1993, Toxic shock syndrome toxin-secreting *Staphylococcus aureus* in Kawasaki syndrome, *Lancet*, **2:** 1385–8.

Levinsky RJ, 1981, The measurement of immune complexes, *Immunol Today*, **2:** 94–7.

Mackenzie CD, Burgess PJ, Sisley BM, 1986, Onchocerciasis, *Immunodiagnosis of Parasitic Diseases*, vol. 1, eds Walls KW, Schantz PM, Academic Press, London, 255–83.

McKenzie H, Parratt D, White RG, 1976, IgM and IgG antibody levels to ampicillin in patients with infectious mononucleosis, *Clin Exp Immunol*, **26:** 214–21.

Maddison SE, 1986, Schistosomiasis, *Immunodiagnosis of Parasitic Diseases*, vol. 1, eds Walls KW, Schantz PM, Academic Press, London, 1–28.

Maggi E, Romagnani S, 1994, Role of T cells and T cell-derived cytokines in the pathogenesis of allergic diseases, *Ann NY Acad Sci*, **725:** 2–12.

Maire MA, Barnet M et al., 1983, Identification of components of IC purified from human sera, *Clin Exp Immunol*, **51:** 215–24.

Manca F, Cauda R et al., 1988, Detection of parasite related antigens associated with conglutinin binding immune complexes in patients with *Schistosoma haematobium*, *Trans R Soc Trop Med Hyg*, **82:** 254–7.

Mannik M, Striker GE, 1980, Removal of glomerular deposits of immune complexes in mice by administration of excess antigen, *Lab Invest*, **42:** 438–89.

Mehindate K, Al-Daccak R et al., 1994, Modulation of *Mycoplasma arthritidis*-derived superantigen-induced cytokine gene expression by dexamethasone and interleukin-4, *Infect Immun*, **62:** 4716–21.

Mellencamp MA, Preheim LC et al., 1987, Isolation and characterization of circulating immune complexes from patients with pneumococcal pneumonia, *Infect Immun*, **55:** 1737–42.

Michael AF, Drummond KM et al., 1966, Acute post-streptococcal glomerulonephritis; immune deposit disease, *J Clin Invest*, **45:** 237–48.

Motala C, Potter PC et al., 1986, Anti-*Staphylococcus aureus* – specific IgE in atopic dermatitis, *Allergy Clin Immunol*, **78:** 583–9.

Müller-Alouf H, Alouf JE et al., 1994, Comparative study of cytokine release by human peripheral blood mononuclear cells stimulated with *Streptococcus pyogenes* superantigenic erythrogenic toxins, heat-killed streptococci and lipopolysaccharide, *Infect Immun*, **62:** 4915–21.

Nawata Y, Koike T et al., 1984, Anti-IgE autoantibody in patients with bronchial asthma, *Clin Exp Immunol*, **58:** 348–56.

Negrini R, Lisato L et al., 1991, *Helicobacter pylori* infection induces antibodies cross-reacting with human gastric mucosa, *Gastroenterology*, **101:** 437–55.

Nielsen K, Santos E et al., 1995, Immune complex-dissociated p24 antigenaemia in the diagnosis of human immunodeficiency virus infection in vertically infected Brazilian children, *Pediatr Infect Dis J*, **14:** 67.

Oldstone MBA, 1987, Molecular mimicry and autoimmune disease cell, *Cell*, **50:** 819–20.

Parish WE, 1970, Short-term anaphylactic IgG antibodies in human sera, *Lancet*, **2:** 591–2.

Parratt D, McKenzie H et al., 1982, *Radioimmunoassay of Antibody*, John Wiley, Chichester, 105.

Platts-Mills TAE, Fiocco GP et al., 1987, Serum IgE antibodies to *Trichophyton* in patients with urticaria, angioedema, asthma and rhinitis: development of a radioallergosorbent test, *Allergy Clin Immunol*, **79**: 40–5.

Ptak W, Rozycka D et al., 1980, Role of antigen presenting cells in the development and persistence of contact hypersensitivity, *J Exp Med*, **151**: 362–75.

Rabinovici R, Fuerstein G, Neville LF, 1994, Cytokine gene and peptide regulation in lung microvascular injury: new insights on the development of adult respiratory distress syndrome, *Ann NY Acad Sci*, **725**: 346–53.

Rockey JH, Donnelly JJ et al., 1981, Immunopathology of ascarid infection of the eye, *Arch Ophthalmol*, **99**: 1831–40.

Rodriguez-Del Valle M, Hwang SM et al., 1994, Role of nitric oxide in hepatic injury following acute endotoxaemia, *Ann NY Acad Sci*, **730**: 329–31.

Schantz PM, Gottstein B, 1986, Echinococcosis (hydatidosis), *Immunodiagnosis of Parasitic Diseases*, vol. 1, eds Walls KW, Schantz PM, Academic Press, London, 84.

Schutzer SE, Coyle PK et al., 1990, Sequestration of antibody to *Borrelia burgdorferi* in seronegative Lyme disease, *Lancet*, **1**: 312–15.

Sieling PA, Modlin RL, 1994, Regulation of cytokine patterns in leprosy, *Ann NY Acad Sci*, **730**: 42–51.

Takei S, Arora YK, Walker SM, 1993, Intravenous immunoglobulin contains specific antibodies inhibitory to activation of T cells by staphylococcal toxin superantigens, *J Clin Invest*, **91**: 602–7.

Tomino Y, Sakai H et al., 1984, Solubilization of intraglomerular deposits of IgG immune complexes by human sera or gamma-globulin in patients with lupus nephritis, *Clin Exp Immunol*, **58**: 42–8.

Vasqueztorres A, Carson JJ et al., 1995, Nitric oxide enhances resistance of SCID mice to mucosal candidosis, *J Infect Dis*, **172**: 192–7.

Villarreal J, Canseco M et al., 1983, Post-streptococcal glomerulonethritis. The role of immune complexes, *Circulating Immune Complexes: their Clinical Significance*, eds Espinoza LR, Osterland CK, Futura, New York, 191–218.

Virta M, Karp M, Vuorinen P, 1994, Nitric oxide donor-mediated killing of bioluminescent *Escherichia coli*, *Antimicrob Agents Chemother*, **38**: 2775–9.

de Weck AL, 1992, Perspectives in allergy diagnosis, *Int Arch Allergy Immunol*, **99**: 252–6.

Weitzman SA, Stossel TP, Desmond M, 1978, Drug-induced immunological neutropenia, *Lancet*, **1**: 1068–71.

Wizemann TM, Laskin DL, 1994, Effects of acute endotoxemia on production of cytokines and nitric oxide by pulmonary alveolar and interstitial macrophages, *Ann NY Acad Sci*, **730**: 336–7.

Yamamoto Y, Friedman H, Klein TW, 1994, Nitric oxide has an immunoregulatory role other than antimicrobial activity in *Legionella pneumophila* infected macrophages, *Ann NY Acad Sci*, **730**: 342–4.

Zumia A, 1992, Superantigens, T cells and microbes, *Clin Infect Dis*, **15**: 313–20.

Chapter 7

Infections associated with immunodeficiency and immunosuppression

D Amsterdam

1 Compromised host defences	3 Infections in specific host groups
2 Principal opportunistic pathogens and clinical infections	4 The management of immunodeficient hosts
	5 Future considerations

Immunodeficiency and immunosuppression are outcomes of the processes that compromise the host defence mechanisms such that the individual is at increased risk for infection due to an opportunistic or more common pathogen(s). The immunological abnormality or dysfunction is associated with specific host defence mechanisms that are either modified or absent. These host defence processes may be acquired or in some cases are primary immunodeficiencies that are genetically determined or linked disorders in which the immune system is the sole or major system affected by the genetic defect. The factors that predispose to infection are:

1 granulocytopenia related to underlying immunological malignancies, cancer chemotherapy, alcohol, and specific bacterial and viral infections
2 cellular immune dysfunction due to congenital disorders, diseases such as Hodgkin's disease and AIDS, and resultants of immunosuppressive regimens administered to leukaemic patients or organ transplant recipients
3 humoral immune dysfunction due to agammaglobulinaemia, diseases such as multiple myeloma and chronic lymphocytic leukaemia, and splenectomized individuals
4 exposure to foreign bodies associated with invasive procedures such as venepuncture, endoscopy, surgery, placement of central venous catheters, grafts, shunts, and artificial joints
5 obstructive conditions associated with tumours and other medical conditions that block the natural drainage of secretions and vital organs leading to obstruction, abscess formation and infection and

6 central nervous system dysfunction which is associated with degrees of aspiration and result in the potential for pneumonia in any situation in which there is a partial or complete loss of the gag reflex.

The spectrum of host factors that predispose to infection, the clinical syndrome and the most common pathogens associated with these infections are outlined in Table 7.1.

1 Compromised host defences

1.1 Granulocytopenia and defects in phagocytic defences

The most thoroughly investigated and extremely common immune defect is granulocytopenia, a condition frequently associated with acute leukaemia, aplastic anaemia and intensive myelosuppressive chemotherapy or other drug reactions. The incidence of infection associated with this condition begins to rise as the granulocyte count falls below 500 cells ml^{-1} with a very substantial rise when the count approaches zero. Most severe infections in nearly all cases of bacteraemia occur when the count is <100 cells ml^{-1} of whole blood (de Jongh et al. 1986). As the absolute number of circulating granulocytes diminishes, the greater the risk for serious bacterial and fungal infections appears. In acute leukaemic patients, the risk becomes most pronounced when the absolute granulocyte count drops below 100 cells ml^{-1} of whole blood. Other associated risks include the extent of granulocytopenia and the rate of granulocyte decline.

Table 7.1   Immunodeficiencies, associated host clinical syndromes and infectious agents

Immunodeficiency	Clinical syndrome	Infectious agents
Granulocytopenia	Bacteraemia, sepsis, pneumonia, UTI, sinusitis	Gram-negative bacilli: *Escherichia coli* and other enterics; *Salmonella* spp.; *Pseudomonas* spp.; *Legionella* Gram-positive cocci and bacilli: *Staphylococcus aureus*; *Staphylococcus epidermidis* (and other coagulase-negative spp.); *Streptococcus pneumoniae*; *Streptococcus pyogenes*; *Enterococcus* spp.; Anaerobes: *Bacteroides* spp.; *Clostridium* spp.; and *Fusobacterium* spp. Fungi: *Candida* spp.; *Aspergillus* spp.
Cellular immune disorders	Pneumonia, enteritis, proctitis, retinitis, stomatitis disseminated disease (mycobacteria), invasive candidiasis	*Legionella pneumophila*; *Listeria monocytogenes*; *Mycobacterium* spp.; *Nocardia* spp.; *Salmonella* spp.; *Coccidioides immitis*; *Cryptococcus neoformans*; *Histoplasma capsulatum*; *Pneumocytis carinii*; EBV, CMV, HSV, VZ; *Cryptosporidium*, *Toxoplasma gondii*, *Strongyloides stercoralis*
Humoral immune disorders	Bacteraemia, sepsis, meningitis, pneumonia	*Streptococcus pneumoniae*; *Haemophilus influenzae*
Foreign bodies (vascular access devices)	Bacteraemia, exit site and tunnel infections	*Staphylococcus aureus*, *Staphylococcus epidermidis*, JK corynebacteria

UTI, urinary tract infection.

Clearly, granulocytopenia predisposes to infection; however, the occurrence of infection and the setting of granulocytopenia are dependent on the presence or absence of other associated predisposing factors that act in concert with the absence of granulocytes. When cancer chemotherapy damages mucosal membranes the most frequent sites of infection in granulocytopenic patients are the peridontium, oropharynx, lung, distal oesophagus, perineal area and skin. It is generally accepted that the organism that causes infection has colonized the area that becomes diseased. Organisms considered of low pathogenic index can, in the presence of a damaged mucosal barrier, ciliary dysfunction, obstruction, etc., and associated with the absence or diminution of normal numbers of granulocyte, invade. Thus, pneumonias are usually associated with organisms that have colonized the patient's oronasopharynx and perianal lesions are caused by one or more of the organisms colonizing the lower intestinal tract (Schimpff et al. 1972). The combination and association of anatomical barrier damage and absence of granulocytes facilitates the rapid progression to bloodstream invasion, sepsis and death. If patients have been hospitalized prior to the development of infection, they are likely to be colonized with a different assortment of bacteria and fungi that are likely to have antimicrobial resistance patterns indicative of the institutional setting in which they were acquired. The hospital-acquired micro-organisms tend to be more resistant to the usual array of antimicrobial agents utilized and vary widely from hospital to hospital. Thus, the organisms colonizing patients may well be organisms that have been acquired subsequent to admission to the hospital and are not truly part of the patients' normal endogenous flora. More than 50% of infections occurring during neutropenia are due to these hospital-acquired pathogens and thus may prove to be more virulent and more resistant to commonly used antibiotics (see Chapter 13).

The majority (over 85%) of bacterial infections in this group of patients are due to 6 organisms: the gram-negative bacilli, *Escherichia coli*, *Klebsiella pneumoniae* and *Pseudomonas aeruginosa* and 3 gram-positive cocci, *Staphylococcus epidermidis*, α-haemolytic *Streptococcus* species and *Staphylococcus aureus* (EORTC 1987). In comparison, more than 85% of fungal infections are associated with 2 genera as follows: *Aspergillus flavus*, *Aspergillus fumigatus*, *Candida albicans* and *Candida tropicalis* (Walsh et al. 1991).

1.2 Cellular immune dysfunction

The inability of monocytes and macrophages to kill intracellular pathogens effectively is referred to as the immune defect associated with cellular immune dysfunction. This is a very broad generalization, but useful as a means of subclassifying the compromised host with regard to factors that predispose to infection. In certain disease conditions, e.g. AIDS and Hodgkin's disease, there is an integral dysfunction of cellular immunity associated with the disease whereas patients with renal transplants or those who suffer from acute lymphocytic leukaemia or patients with bone marrow transplantation demonstrate substantial dysfunction of cellular immunity as a result of the immunosuppressive regimens formulated to heal them (Schimpff and Klastersky 1993).

Various opportunistic pathogens that can produce infection in the compromised setting of defective cellular immunity are listed in Table 7.1. In the general population, clinical infections caused by most of these micro-organisms are infrequent except for tuberculosis, childhood varicella and recurrent herpes labialis. It should be noted that the micro-organisms noted in Table 7.1 associated with patients with cellular immunodeficiency do not occur in all patient groups with the same frequency.

1.3 Humoral immune dysfunction

Multiple myeloma, splenectomy and other conditions associated with hypogammaglobulinaemia, such as chronic lymphocytic leukaemia, result in humoral immune dysfunction and pose a significant risk for the development of infections caused by encapsulated pyogenic bacteria. The most frequent of these infections are due to *Streptococcus pneumoniae* and *Haemophilus influenzae*. Humoral immune dysfunction can be described as the host defence's defect that results from the impairment of specific antibody binding to respective antigens. This antigen–antibody binding plays an important role in opsonizing micro-organisms for phagocytosis and for neutralizing toxins. Individuals with agammaglobulinaemia have a fairly predictable spectrum of infections as they do not have in their serum opsonizing antibodies to the common encapsulated pyogenic bacteria. This condition impairs the activity of all phagocytic cells including granulocytes, monocytes and macrophages. Multiple myeloma is the prototype malignancy for demonstrating infections associated with humoral immunodeficiency (Jacobson and Zolla-Prazner 1986). Infections in this condition relate to the specific opsonizing antibody needed to defend against infection caused by the offending encapsulated pathogen. As a result, some patients will not have infections with *S. pneumoniae*, whereas others will have multiple recurrent episodes of pneumococcal infection caused by the same or different serotypes.

The spleen has 2 major anti-infective roles: clearing the bloodstream of bacteria through its mononuclear phagocytic function and production of antibody.

Although the liver is efficient at removing opsonized bacteria, the spleen is capable of sequestering particles and is more efficient in removing non-opsonized bacteria. Infections that arise after splenectomy, whether it be due to trauma, staging in Hodgkin's disease or autosplenectomy, are usually due to *S. pneumoniae* and occasionally *H. influenzae* or *Neisseria meningitidis*.

1.4 Foreign and obstructive events

It makes little difference in patient outcome as to the manner in which the host is compromised. When integumentary and mucosal barriers to infections provided by the intact skin, alimentary tract, mucosa and respiratory mucosa, which make up the host primary defence mechanism against organism invasion, are inoperative the host is open to infection. The individual with multiple trauma and the patient with leukaemia undergoing chemotherapy are examples that characterize both the surgical and medical patient in whom alteration to anatomical barriers is an important predisposing factor to infection. Increasingly common in the past 20 years is the use of peripheral and central indwelling vascular catheters, surgically implanted prosthetic devices, vascular grafts and impregnated shunts and pacing devices. These devices have become an important component for the treatment of patients through administering blood products, chemotherapy and parenteral hyperalimentation, repairing obstructed veins and arteries, replacing various joints and valves, and pacing arrhythmic heart beats; as foreign bodies, however, they serve as the sites that compromise host defences.

Micro-organisms gain access to the breakdown in mucosal barriers or they may attach directly to the foreign body inserted in the patient and thus gain access to the bloodstream, causing clinical disease. Treatment can prove difficult and frequently requires prolonged intensive antimicrobial therapy. Ultimately the infected device itself may have to be removed as the seeding nidus of infection.

The agent responsible for infection that is likely to occur in the patient with an indwelling catheter or implanted medical device depends to a large extent on the underlying disease and its associated immunodeficiency. However, there is an association for certain types of infection. In cancer and AIDS patients, indwelling central venous catheters are most likely to become infected with gram-positive organisms, usually the coagulase-negative staphylococci. These infections are treatable with parenteral antimicrobial therapy such as vancomycin or teicoplanin and do not necessarily require removal of the infected catheter. Infections with gram-negative bacteria and the *Candida* genus more often require catheter removal as well as aggressive systemic antimicrobial therapy.

1.5 Tumours and other medical conditions

Malignant processes generally lead to some degree of impaired host defences. Depending upon the nature of the malignancy, any of the major host defence mechanisms may become impaired. Associated with the primary immunodeficiency that is linked to a specific malignant condition, tumours may also obstruct vital organ function. In these situations the infecting micro-organisms are usually the ones that have colonized the site near the tumour. The normal flora found at the site of the tumours are likely to be affected by the hospitalization of the patient, previous antibiotic therapy and other medical and surgical interventions.

2 PRINCIPAL OPPORTUNISTIC PATHOGENS AND CLINICAL INFECTIONS

2.1 Gram-positive bacteria

The ubiquitous *S. aureus* and *S. epidermidis* have distinctive propensities for invading skin and adjacent tissue at cutaneous puncture sites and at the sites of indwelling intravenous catheters. Within 48–72 h staphylococci are demonstrable on these foreign bodies. The frequency of clinical infection is directly related to the duration that catheters remain in place. During the last decade the use of long-term central access devices, such as the central venous catheters (Hickman) and long-term subcutaneous implantable ports (Port-a-Cath), have become a frequent occurrence, particularly in leukaemic patients. Infections associated with these devices are relatively common and occur as either exit site infections of the surrounding skin structures or as intravascular infections which may develop subsequently as a bacteraemia. In the evaluation of patients with unexplained fever of unknown origin it is necessary to consider the role of these central access devices in causing bacteraemia and blood should be cultured. Additionally, until specific agents are isolated and antimicrobial susceptibility studies done, empirical therapy should be directed against the more likely agents such as *Staphylococcus*, and the JK corynebacteria.

S. pneumoniae infection occurs at a higher frequency in patients with humoral immune deficiencies, particularly those who have had a splenectomy. Patients with multiple myeloma who are incapable of producing adequate antibody response to *Streptococcus* are also at risk and, for as yet unexplained reasons, are more likely to develop pneumococcal pneumonia than bacteraemia or meningitis. With the increasing frequency of penicillin-resistant *S. pneumoniae* it is important that susceptibilities with antimicrobial tube dilution studies be done to determine clearly the resistant nature of the diplococcus (Klugman 1990).

Staphylococci and streptococci are recoverable on nutrient agar medium containing 5% blood (usually sheep cells). Microscopic morphology, coagulase clumping, optochin susceptibility and catalase reactivity assist in their identification.

LISTERIA MONOCYTOGENES

L. monocytogenes is widely distributed in nature; however, it seldom causes serious disease in healthy persons other than the fetus or newborn. In adults it gives rise to meningitis and septicaemia in individuals debilitated by old age, alcoholism, diabetes and especially in immunosuppressed hosts. Individuals are usually exposed by the food-borne route.

The 2 forms of the disease that are best recognized are septicaemia often progressing to meningitis or meningeal involvement, and cerebritis often progressing to brain abscess which is particularly seen in severely immunodepressed patients. Other manifestations include arthritis, endocarditis and eye and skin involvement (Salata et al. 1986). The role of *L. monocytogenes* in central nervous system infections in cancer patients was reviewed by Chernik and colleagues (1977) who found that the organism was the most frequent cause of meningitis, accounting for approximately one-third of all bacterial infections in their study. Patients with lymphoma or leukaemia were especially susceptible.

Listeriosis is a common opportunistic infection in renal transplant recipients and in individuals receiving prolonged immunosuppressive drug therapy. Infrequent reports of clusters of cases in transplant units raise the possibility of horizontal transmission of infection. However, it is frequently difficult to identify the source or mechanism of spread of these infections (Gantz et al. 1975). It is uncommon for *Listeria* to be associated with infection in AIDS patients although the marked cellular immunodeficiency of AIDS patients would seem to dispose them. An explanation for this event is the possibility that the frequent antimicrobial coverage given to these individuals may provide protection from *Listeria* infection (Mascola et al. 1988).

The immunological response to *Listeria* infection has been studied in experimental animals. It has been established that the principal host defence is cell mediated. In order to stimulate a T lymphocyte response, bacterial growth within macrophages is required (Berche, Gaillard and Sansonetti 1987). Production of bacterial haemolysin has also been a factor in promoting cellular responses (Portnoy 1988). As is common with other intracellular pathogens, specific T cell lysis of infected macrophages is dependent on recognition of Ia antigens in mice and the equivalent histocompatibility proteins in man (Kauffmann et al. 1987).

The gram-positive pleomorphic organism can be detected microscopically in gram-stained preparations of the spinal fluid or other clinical material. Microscopically, organisms appear diphtheroid-like, exhibit typical tumbling motility and are readily recovered from blood and spinal fluid using a blood agar basal medium containing 5–10% red blood cells.

2.2 Gram-negative bacteria

Granulocytopenia is the major risk factor associated with aerobic gram-negative infection. Septicaemia is the most common clinical manifestation and in approximately one-third of this patient population no other source of infection can be documented. The clinical presentation for this type of infection ranges from a low grade fever to overt septic shock.

The most common pathogen identified in these patients is *E. coli*. When the absolute granulocyte count dips below 500 ml^{-1} of blood, the risk of *Pseudomonas aeruginosa* bacteraemia rises markedly. *P. aeruginosa* is able to invade the endothelial cell lining of major blood vessels which may serve as foci of infection. Mortality rate of the infections is higher than that associated with other gram-negative organisms. One of the complications of gram-negative septicaemia is the resultant dissemination to other sites, particularly the lung. When this occurs, mortality rates are generally twice as high as those for bacteraemia alone. Initially patients present with clinical signs of pneumonia, which may be minimal, and normal chest radiology. A lack of granulocytes reduces the initial inflammatory response and makes clinical diagnosis complex.

LEGIONELLA SPECIES

Several species of *Legionella* have been established as human pathogens and include predominantly *Legionella pneumophila* and *Legionella micdadei*. *L. pneumophila* was first isolated from patients with pneumonia who attended the 1976 American Legion Convention in Philadelphia, but was identified as a human pathogen as early as 1947 (Fraser et al. 1977). Various risk factors and underlying conditions have been identified and predispose individuals to infection. These include: male gender, middle age and older, cigarette smoking, corticosteroid therapy, organ transplantation with immunosuppression, diabetes and chronic obstructive pulmonary disease. Additional risk factors that have been identified based upon data from the Centers for Disease Control (CDC) include lung cancer, haematological malignancies and AIDS (Marston, Lipman and Breiman 1994).

Clinical disease associated with *Legionella* infections may take the form of acute pneumonia with a high fatality rate, fever or extrapulmonary infections which include cellulitis and fasciitis.

Legionella is a fastidious, weakly gram-negative micro-organism that is found intracellularly and extracellularly. It does not grow on commonly used laboratory media which renders clinical diagnosis difficult. More than 30 species of *Legionella* have been isolated and up to 50 serogroups have been identified. *L. pneumophila* is the most common cause of Legionnaires' disease and there are 6 serotypes of this organism. *L. pneumophila* is found in aquatic habitats including chlorinated potable water systems and the delivery system of large residential communities. The organism gains access to the lung via inhalation of aerosolized droplets. Once in the lung, *L. pneumophila* is phago-cytosed by alveolar macrophages, but is not killed. Within the macrophage reproduction continues until the cell ruptures and bacteria are released. The bacteria in turn are phagocytosed and the cell cycle continues (Nguyen et al. 1991, Yu 1991, 1995).

Patients with Legionnaires' disease present with initial manifestations that are non-specific: malaise, weakness and lethargy. Fever is present in almost all patients and rapidly rises. Cough, also present in almost all patients, is initially non-productive but later produces purulent sputum. Gastrointestinal symptoms are common and include abdominal discomfort and non-bloody diarrhoea. Clinically there is frequently bilateral pneumonia affecting several lobes of the lung; nodular lesions or abscesses can develop during the course of illness. However, there are no characteristic chest x-ray findings; both cavitary and non-cavitary lesions have been reported (Kirby et al. 1980, Nguyen et al. 1991, Edelstein 1993, Yu 1995).

The diagnosis of *L. pneumophila* infection can only be established by laboratory methods. A sputum cultured on buffered charcoal yeast extract agar supplemented with antimicrobial agents to avoid overgrowth of other micro-organisms appears to be the most sensitive medium (Edelstein 1993). A frequently used rapid method for detection of *Legionella* is direct fluorescent antibody staining. Other approaches include a DNA probe of respiratory secretions, indirect fluorescence antibody testing of blood and respiratory secretions and detection of urinary antigen by enzyme immunoassay (EIA) (Edelstein 1993, Yu 1995).

The treatment of choice for *L. pneumophila* pneumonia has been erythromycin over a time course of 14–21 days (Roig, Carreres and Domingo 1993). The newer macrolides, azithromycin and clarithromycin, may be superior to erythromycin because of enhanced in vitro activity, improved pharmacokinetics and fewer side effects. Alternative treatments include erythromycin plus rifampicin, co-trimoxazole, doxycycline and minocycline, all with documented in vitro and in vivo activity against *L. pneumophila* (Roig, Carreres and Domingo 1993). Roig, Carreres and Domingo (1993) have indicated that the fluoroquinolones (ciprofloxacin and ofloxacin) may be more appropriate for transplant recipients in order to avoid potential interactions between macrolides and immunosuppressive drugs. However, clinical data supporting the activity of quinolones are pending.

2.3 Acid-fast bacteria

MYCOBACTERIA

Tuberculosis is the leading cause of infectious death in the world. It has been estimated that one-third of the world's population, approximately 1.7 billion people, have latent TB infection (Sudre, ten Dam and Kochi 1992, Raviglione, Snider and Kochi 1995). According to the World Health Organization, almost 3.8 million cases of TB were reported in 1990. Nearly one-half the reported cases occur in South East Asia and sub-Saharan Africa, the countries of the Western

Pacific rim accounting for another third of cases (DeCock et al. 1989). The HIV epidemic has played a significant role in the resurgence of TB. The largest increase in new cases of active TB has occurred in the age group 25–44 years and a lower, but substantial, increase in incidence has been associated with those younger than 15 years. Immigrants and refugee populations have accounted for almost one-third of TB cases (Centers for Disease Control and Prevention 1995). Between 25 and 50% of AIDS patients in Africa, India, Thailand and some Latin American countries develop clinical TB. HIV infection enhances the risk of reactivation of latent TB infection and a primary progressive TB following initial infection. As a secondary consequence, this results in an increase in transmission from the larger reservoir of individuals who are actively infected.

Utilizing molecular epidemiological techniques, investigators have shown that more cases of TB are due to recent infection than was previously thought (Alland et al. 1994, Small et al. 1994). By using the technique of restriction fragment length polymorphisms (RFLPs) these researchers determined the DNA fingerprints of isolates and found that nearly 40% of the TB cases were due to recent infection.

Although several abnormalities in the immune response to *Mycobacterium tuberculosis* have been described in people with HIV infection, the loss of CD4+ T cells is the most important predictor of the risk of developing TB. In individuals with latent TB infection and high CD4+ T cell counts (i.e. >600) the risk of reactivation is low. However, as the CD4+ T cell count drops the risk of primary disease increases (Daley et al. 1992) (Fig. 7.1).

The stage of HIV disease and the associated immune status influence the clinical presentation of TB. Typically, patients with higher CD4+ T cell counts tend to have more typical presentations with a higher incidence of cavitary disease and fewer extrapulmonary complications. Atypical presentations are more usual in later stages of HIV, with bacteraemias and diffuse infiltrates.

Multidrug-resistant tuberculosis (MDR-TB), defined as *M. tuberculosis* resistant to at least isoniazid and rifampicin, is an increasing world-wide problem. The prevalence of MDR-TB is greater in Asia, Africa and Latin America than in North America and Europe

(Narain, Raviglione and Koch 1992). In some countries there is concern that MDR-TB strains may replace drug-susceptible TB as the main cause of disease.

In the USA, MDR-TB occurs in 2 types of patients: individuals with inadequately treated TB and those exposed to MDR-TB infected individuals prior to their diagnosis in outbreak settings. This latter group comprises largely immunosuppressed patients infected with HIV (Centers for Disease Control 1992).

The *Mycobacterium avium–intracellulare* complex (MAC) is now the most common opportunistic bacterial infection in patients with AIDS in developed countries (Horsburgh 1991, Chaisson et al. 1992, Jacobson 1992). These organisms are ubiquitous in nature and have been isolated from soil, water, animals and food. There is little information about transmission and horizontal or animal-to-person transmission is thought to be unlikely. It is unclear which environmental factors play a role in infection with MAC. Although water, soil, dust and food have all been suspected, recent studies have identified specific exposures associated with infection. These include contact with soil from indoor potted plants (Yajko et al. 1995) and ingestion of hard cheeses (Horsburgh et al. 1994). Daily showering was associated with a decreased risk of MAC infection and other water exposure, such as drinking water, swimming, sitting in hot tubs, was not associated with a greater risk of infection (Horsburgh et al. 1994). von Reyn and associates (1994) have recently shown that clinical isolates were genetically similar to MAC of a hospital water supply.

The diagnosis of MAC requires isolation and identification of the organism. The standard method for diagnosing disseminated MAC is blood culture (Kiehn et al. 1985). MAC diagnosis can also be made by culture of any normally sterile site, especially bone marrow, lymph node, or liver. As with other mycobacteria, MAC is slow-growing and requires 2–6 weeks for colony formation on solid agar. Blood culture is the preferred and most reliable method, yielding 98% sensitivity in one study (Hawkins et al. 1986). The identification of the organism can be confirmed with the use of a DNA probe.

The increasing awareness associated with the HIV epidemic has placed other mycobacteria species in the forefront and these have been recorded with greater frequency in AIDS patients (Wolinsky 1992, Straus et

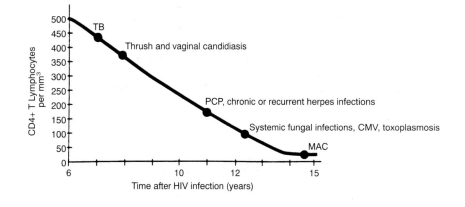

Fig. 7.1 Opportunistic infections associated with progressive immunodeficiency as determined by CD4+ lymphocyte count in AIDS. (Reprinted from Dobkin 1995, with permission).

al. 1994, Stracher and Sepkowitz 1995). These myco-bacteria, the clinical features of infections that they present and the typical treatment regimens are included in Table 7.2.

The role of *M. tuberculosis* infections in patients with underlying malignancy was recognized more than 60 years ago (Parker et al. 1932). The association was marked in cases of Hodgkin's lymphoma and to a lesser extent in leukaemia and in other cancers.

It has been shown (Kaplan, Armstrong and Rosen 1974) that significant mortality is attributable to tuberculosis in patients with malignant diseases. In those patients receiving steroids and chemotherapy, infections were most severe and tended to be dissemi-nated. When the rate of mycobacterial infection was compared in cancer patients and the normal popu-lation, it was found that a 3-fold higher incidence of infection was found in cancer patients (Feld, Brodey and Groschel 1976). When the aetiological agent was of the non-tuberculous mycobacterial species, in 30 such cases, 12 were due to *Mycobacterium kansasii* and 7 to *Mycobacterium fortuitum*. In all of these disseminated infections none was of miliary nature. In the study in which the patient groups included those with haema-tological malignancies and renal transplant recipients who were receiving steroid therapy, *M. kansasii*, *M. for-tuitum* and MAC were the predominant pathogenic species (Wolinsky 1979). In cancer patients *M. fortui-tum* infections have been associated with the use of intravenous catheters (Hoy et al. 1987).

NOCARDIA ASTEROIDES

Nocardia asteroides is an acid-fast staining micro-organ-ism whose morphological shape has led to confusion with mycobacteria in stained smears. However, nocar-diosis is a very different disease with a different clinical presentation consisting of abscess formation targeted

in the lung as the organ initially infected. The organ-ism spreads haematogenously and results in abscess formation in the brain and less frequently in skin, soft tissues and other internal organs. The typical patient infected with *Nocardia* is receiving long-term mainten-ance immunosuppressive therapy. Of the 3 nocardial species known to be pathogenic for man – *N. asteroides*, *N. farcinica* and *N. brasiliensis* – *N. asteroides* is the most frequently recovered (Beaman et al. 1976). *Nocardia* spp. are distributed in soil and decaying vegetable matter; humans acquire the organism usually by inha-lation, although direct inoculation of the skin as a result of trauma can occasionally occur. The occur-rence of clusters of cases of *Nocardia* infection suggests common source acquisition and this has been described in renal transplant units where dust-borne transmission as a result of building construction has been suggested (Houang et al. 1980, Stevens et al. 1981). Person-to-person transmission has not been demonstrated.

Neutrophils mount the initial host response in the early stages of *Nocardia* infection. The neutrophils themselves may contain the offending organism; how-ever, they are not the definitive defence mechanism as they kill nocardiae poorly. Probably the more important mechanism operative during the later stages of infection is through activated macrophages and immune T cells (Filice and Niewoehner 1987). The outcome of this interaction depends not only on the status of the host cells but on the virulence of the nocardial strain. Experimental studies using a murine model indicate that some isolates of *Nocardia* are able to survive the normal bactericidal activity of macro-phages by direct inhibition of phagosome–lysosome solidification (Davis-Scibienski and Beaman 1980).

Since an early 1960s study of clinical cases of nocar-diosis (Murray et al. 1961) the number of cases has

Table 7.2 Atypical mycobacteria, clinical features and treatment in patients with HIV

Mycobacterium	**Clinical features**	**Treatment**
M. bovis	Identical to TB	INH + RIF + EMB + STM
M. fortuitum–chelonei complex	Pulmonary disease, soft tissue abscesses, cutaneous lesions	Surgical excision + CEFOX + AMIK
M. genavense	MAC-like disease, anaemia organomegaly, diffuse disseminated infection	CLARITH + EMB + RIF
M. gordonae	Pulmonary disease, systemic symptoms, cutaneous lesions	INH + RIF + EMB + CLOF
M. haemophilum	Cutaneous lesions, arthritis systemic symptoms	CLARITH + CIPRO + RIF ± AMIK
M. kansasii	TB-like disease (pulmonary and extrapulmonary)	INH + RIF + EMB ± STM
M. malmoense	Pulmonary disease, systemic symptoms, mediastinal adenopathy	INH + RIF + EMB
M. xenopi	Pulmonary disease, hepatic infections	INH + EMB + RIF or STM

AMIK, amikacin; EMB, ethambutol; CIPRO, ciprofloxacin; CLARITH, clarithromycin; CLOF, clofazimine; INH, isoniazid; MAC, *Mycobacterium avium* complex; RIF, rifampicin; STM, streptomycin.
Adapted from Stracher and Sepkowitz 1995.

risen sharply. This probably is a reflection of the increasing population of immunocompromised patients. In one large series, most patients with nocardiosis had serious underlying disease (Williams, Krick and Remington 1976). Infrequently, *Nocardia* infection has been the presenting feature of a congenital immunodeficiency–chronic granulomatous disease (Jonsson et al. 1986). Patients at risk for nocardiosis include those with Hodgkin's lymphoma, pulmonary alveolar proteinosis, chronic malnutrition, renal and heart transplantation, and conditions requiring prolonged steroid administration (Arduino et al. 1993). More recently AIDS has been a contributing factor. On occasion, individuals are dually infected with *M. tuberculosis* or other non-tuberculous mycobacteria and these infections involve the lung. The majority of infections involve the lung; in the more serious cases, single or multiple pulmonary abscesses appear. In about 25% of cases there is dissemination to extrapulmonary sites, especially to the brain; a typical lesion presents as a non-capsulated abscess. Other sites favoured by the *Nocardia* are the skin, liver, kidneys, joints and eyes.

The laboratory diagnosis of *Nocardia* infection is difficult. In about one-third of cases sputum cultures are positive and more invasive methods are required for sampling the lung. Blood cultures are of some value in disseminated disease as they are only occasionally positive. The diagnosis of brain abscess will usually require brain biopsy because the organism is infrequently found in the cerebrospinal fluid.

Nocardia spp., specifically *asteroides*, are susceptible to a range of antimicrobial agents that include the sulphonamides, tetracycline and the macrolides.

Additional information about the nocardiae and other actinomyces can be found in Volume 2 (see Volume 2, Chapter 20).

2.4 Fungi

YEASTS

Candida species are common, offending fungal pathogens associated with granulocytopenia and cellular immunodeficiencies. In granulocytopenic patients, these infections tend to be life threatening. Factors predisposing to serious fungal infections include: prolonged, broad spectrum antimicrobial therapy, indwelling intravascular catheters, extended length of hospital stay, corticosteroid therapy, and hyperalimentation – all factors common in the severely ill cancer patient. Morbidity and mortality rates for *Candida* infection in cancer patients have increased. Although *C. albicans* is the major pathogen of this group, there is a noticeable increase in infections due to other *Candida* species including *Candida tropicalis*, *Candida glabrata* and *Candida parapsilosis* (Horn et al. 1985).

These yeasts, especially *C. albicans*, commonly colonize mucosal surfaces throughout the body. As a result they are part of the commensal flora of the oropharyanx, gastrointestinal and female lower genital tract. During heavy immunosuppressive and antibody therapy, it is not unusual to find laboratory cultures overgrown with these organisms. The major problem is to determine if this is sufficient evidence to document clinical infection. Documenting invasive disease as a result of the isolation of these organisms from superficial sites is tentative and should be interpreted with caution. Factors that predispose patients to mucosal or skin invasion and result in access to the circulation and organ systems include prolonged periods of neutropenia, indwelling catheters, surgical operations, parenteral nutrition, underlying disease (e.g. diabetes mellitus) and intravenous drug abuse. Infections with opportunistic viruses of the herpes group can predispose tissue invasion at these sites.

The principal host defence against *Candida* infection is the phagocytic cell. Intracellular killing of *C. albicans* has been demonstrated in neutrophils and is mediated by the myeloperoxidase system.

The diagnosis of invasive candidiasis is difficult because of the poor sensitivity of laboratory detection methods. Blood cultures are positive in no more than half of cases with disseminated disease. Antigenic detection of circulating *Candida* antigen has not proved fruitful but is a laboratory approach to the determination of invasive disease (Fung, Dunta and Tilton 1986).

The primary therapeutic regimen for treatment of *Candida* infections is amphotericin B, although fluconazole has proved to be an agent with ancillary killing power.

CRYPTOCOCCUS NEOFORMANS

Both immunosuppressed patients and individuals without known immunodeficiency contract cryptococcal infections after exposure to the air-borne basidiospores of *Cryptococcus neoformans*. In non-compromised patients, cryptococcal infection usually manifests itself as a mild, self-limited pulmonary disease and only less commonly does symptomatic pulmonary disease or manifestations of dissemination to chronic meningitis result. Immunosuppressed patients, however, tend to develop more acute or disseminated forms in the clinical guise of acute meningitis or meningoencephalitis or possibly as a diffuse pneumonia. Dissemination of *Cryptococcus* occurs by the faecal droppings of pigeons, which harbour the organism. Subsequent inhalation of viable fungus by humans results in development of symptomatic or asymptomatic pulmonary infection. Because of their high body temperature, pigeons harbouring the organism in their intestinal tract are seemingly immune from disease and thus do not develop invasive disease. These same pigeons are considered to be the reservoir for infection of humans. Haematogenous spread from the lungs leads to metastatic disease in a variety of organ systems. However, there is a propensity for infection of the central nervous system. The most common clinical manifestations of disseminated cryptococcal disease is that of a relatively slowly evolving meningitis in patients with underlying lymphoma or AIDS. The older picture is that of association with malignant lymphoma, especially Hodgkin's disease.

Defects in T cell dependent cellular immunity are

strongly linked to infection with *C. neoformans*. Patients who contract cryptococcosis have lowered reactivity to skin tests with cryptococcin and depressed in vitro synthesis of leucocyte migration inhibition factor on stimulation with *C. neoformans* (Schimpff and Bennett 1975).

The determinant for virulence of the organism is the polysaccharide capsule. The capsule seemingly confers resistance to ingestion by phagocytic cells. The first line of host defence is the resident alveolar macrophage which has a limited capacity to phagocytose and kill the organism (Diamond, Root and Bennett 1972). Neutrophils have a greater capacity to kill by antibody and the activation of both complement pathways. Perhaps the most important host defence against this organism is the delayed-type hypersensitivity response that results in activation of macrophages by T lymphocytes. The principal trigger for this is thought to be a mannoprotein which is a constituent of the capsular antigen (Murphy et al. 1988).

The incidence of cryptococcosis varies widely and is related to the underlying disease. In AIDS patients it has been estimated to occur at a rate of 6–10% in American patients (Zuger et al. 1986) whereas in the UK the rate has been anywhere from 3.2% to 13% (Eng et al. 1986). The incidence of cryptococcosis undoubtedly differs with patient selection.

A frequent clinical presentation of cryptococcosis is meningitis, although this is presumed to be a result of haematogenous spread from an initial focus in the lung. In one series, cryptococcal meningitis ranked second in frequency among the infectious agents causing neurological disease in AIDS patients (Levy and Bredesen 1988).

The yeast can be detected in about 50% of cases by visualization of the capsule in an India ink stain preparation of the cerebrospinal fluid deposit. The organism can be cultured from clinical specimens, especially CSF, but culture is frequently of low diagnostic sensitivity. Cryptococcal antigen can be detected in the spinal fluid by means of a latex agglutination test with a commercial reagent. This improved sensitivity is over 90% and is very specific. Antigens can also be detected in serum and in other body fluids. A low cell count in the CSF with a high antigen titre usually is predictive of poor outcome. Antigen titres in both serum and CSF are frequently extremely high and may range from 1 to 10 000 and higher.

The standard therapy for acute cryptococcal meningitis is intravenous amphotericin B. The combination of amphotericin B and 5-flucytosine can augment success in treatment and is reported to be superior to the newer triazole, fluconazole (Diamond 1995).

ASPERGILLUS SPECIES

Of the approximately 200 or more species of this group of septate filamentous fungi belonging to the Ascomycetes, only a few species are consistently isolated from clinical material. These include *Aspergillus fumigatus*, *Aspergillus flavus*, *Aspergillus niger*, *Aspergillus nidulans*, *Aspergillus terreus* and *Aspergillus glaucus*.

Aspergilli naturally reside in soil and can readily be recovered from air. Spore counts are subject to seasonal variation, the highest numbers being found during the winter months. Infection is acquired by inhalation of spores which due to their small size gain access to the terminal bronchi and alveoli. It is assumed that fungal cell components including aflatoxin, mannans and catalase impede host defences. Additionally, diffusible substances from the spores of *A. fumigatus* inhibit the microbicidal action of phagocytic cells in vitro (Robertson et al. 1987).

The most frequently encountered species, *A. fumigatus*, has been implicated in 3 forms of pulmonary disease: aspergilloma following saprophytic colonization of an old lung cavity or abscess; allergic lung disease manifesting as asthma, extrinsic alveolitis, or allergic bronchopulmonary aspergillosis; and invasive aspergillosis which may disseminate to extrapulmonary organs and is the form most typically seen in immunocompromised hosts.

Host defence mechanisms are mediated by alveolar macrophages that inhibit germination of the spores. This effect appears to be non-specific as it can take place in neutropenic as well as in athymic hosts (Fromtling and Shadomy 1986). Yet, neutrophils play a critical role in preventing the organism from establishing an invasive infection. The damaging effects of human neutrophils on aspergillosis hyphae have been demonstrated by Diamond and Clark (1982). In experimental studies determining the effects of cortisone treatment on cellular defences it was observed that macrophages failed to arrest fungal growth and germination. In these cortisone-treated animals many went on to develop invasive pneumonia (Merkow et al. 1968).

Neutropenia complicating the treatment of haematological malignancy is a major risk factor for the development of invasive aspergillosis (Young et al. 1970). Patients' susceptibility steadily increases with the duration of neutropenia (Gerson et al. 1984). Recipients of bone marrow transplants in whom there is failure of engraftment of the donor marrow are particularly at risk (Pirsch and Maki 1986). Those individuals receiving solid organ transplants have been recognized at risk, largely as a consequence of steroid immunosuppression.

Mortality rates from aspergillosis infection in immunosuppressed patients is high. This is attributable to the lack of a reliable method for the early detection of pulmonary infection (Repentigny and Reiss 1984) and the poor activity of available antifungal regimens. Prevention of aspergillosis infection is provided by the use of filtered air in transplant units to prevent spores from gaining access and has proved to be effective in reducing the incidence of aspergillosis (Sherertz et al. 1987, Barnes and Rogers 1989). The only drug with a record of therapeutic success against this fungus is amphotercin B (Fisher et al. 1981).

PNEUMOCYSTIS CARINII

There still appears to be some controversy over whether to classify *P. carinii* as a protozoon or a fungus. At least in this volume it appears that the classification is as a fungus (see Volume 4, Chapter 34 and Volume 5, Chapter 22). *P. carinii* is able to cause pneumonia and, rarely, other organ system infections in the host with compromised cell mediated immunity. *P. carinii* infects individuals early in life but infection rarely causes disease in the immunocompetent host. Immunosuppression permits the organism to replicate and cause clinical disease.

P. carinii pneumonia (PCP) is the most common AIDS-defining opportunistic infection in the USA. In 1991 PCP comprised about 46% of newly diagnosed AIDS cases. The vast majority of cases (80%) of PCP are initiated when the CD4+ T cell count falls below 200 ml^{-1} (Bernard et al. 1992, Centers for Disease Control and Prevention 1992, Walzer 1995) (see Fig. 7.1).

Extrapulmonary disease occurs in a limited number (c. 3%) of AIDS patients, especially those who have not been maintained prophylactically on pentamidine. The most commonly affected extrapulmonary sites are the lymph nodes, spleen, liver and bone marrow (Northfelt, Clement and Safrin 1990).

P. carinii has not been cultured from infected human tissue. Histological identification, however, is rapid by use of specific staining techniques. Several morphological forms corresponding to life cycle states can be observed in appropriately stained material. The most common form is the cyst, approximately 5–8 μm in diameter. Cysts are spherical, crescentic or disc-like with a thick (100 μm) wall that is clearly stained black by Gomori's methenamine silver (GMS) nitrate, or stained violet purple by toluidine blue. Pear-shaped or amoeboid intracystic bodies or sporozoites reside within cysts. The smaller (1–5 μm) trophozoites are more numerous than the better visualized cysts. These extra cystic forms can be identified using Giemsa or other stains. The direct fluorescent antibody technique can detect both cysts and trophozoite forms and increases the sensitivity of detection of PCP in infected individuals. A definitive diagnosis is established by identifying the organism in sputum obtained preferably by sputum induction or lung tissue, bronchoalveolar lavage or transbronchial lung biopsy (Walzer 1995).

The mortality for HIV-infected patients with untreated PCP is nearly 100%. Oral and parenteral trimethoprim–sulphamethoxazole (TMP–SMX) and parenteral pentamidine (Conte et al. 1990) have been effective in a majority of cases (Centers for Disease Control and Prevention 1992). Clinical improvement in patients with PCP and AIDS is slower than that observed in individuals with other types of immunosuppression.

2.5 Protozoa and metazoa

CRYPTOSPORIDIUM

This coccidial organism may be acquired from animals but it may also be transmitted from person to person. In immunocompetent individuals it is responsible for self-limited diarrhoeal episodes with abdominal cramps and bloating and occasional cases of malabsorption. Full recovery within 2–3 weeks is usual. The parasite is confined to the intestinal tract and both large and small bowel are affected. The pathogenesis of the disease is not clearly understood.

The increased severity of cryptosporidiosis in patients with impaired cellular or humoral immunity was addressed in early reports (Meisel et al. 1976) and has since been confirmed (Soave and Armstrong 1986), especially in AIDS. Predisposing disorders are congenital immunodeficiencies including selective IgA deficiency, AIDS and various forms of active immunosuppression. Clinically there is a greatly increased pool of stool output, with weight loss and malabsorption which occurs as part of a protracted illness. Occasional cases of extraintestinal disease – of the lung or biliary tract – have been described. Diagnosis of *Cryptosporidium* is usually made by demonstrating the oocysts in smears prepared from concentrated stool samples and stained by a modified acid-fast method. Immunofluorescent detection of oocyst by means of a monoclonal IgM is warranted in several situations as the sensitivity of the immunoassay is greater than that of microscopic observation. Chemotherapy is not highly effective but there are reports that symptoms are ameliorated by the administration of opiates and spiramycin (Portnoy et al. 1984).

MICROSPORIDIUM

The microsporidia are small unicellular parasites that are considered eukaryotes. These obligate, intracellular, spore-forming protozoan organisms have a wide host range that includes most invertebrates and all classes of vertebrates. Five microsporidial genera are recognized but the majority of infections in HIV persons are attributed to *Enterocytozoon bieneusi* (Weber and Bryan 1994).

In humans, microsporidia have a predilection to infect individuals with impaired cell mediated immunity. The source of human infection is unknown. Person-to-person transmission has not been demonstrated and the pathology of human microsporidial infection is not understood. Infection with this parasite activates antibody production; however, antibodies alone do not yield protection. A competent cellular immune response has been shown experimentally to suppress microsporidial multiplication (Shadduck 1989). The parasite may invade cells of the muscles, liver, kidney, intestine, cornea and nervous system (Shadduck 1989). In both latent and active infections it can be demonstrated in the stool and urine. Although serological assays have been used to demonstrate latent infections, these tests are not feasible for diagnosis of human infection. Currently diagnosis depends on the morphological demonstration of the organism, preferably by electron microscopic examination.

There is limited experience with therapy for these infections. The compound albendazole has potential utility for infections with *Encephalitozoon* species. However, therapy for *E. bieneusi* has been limited. Metronidazole is considered a prospect for therapy.

GIARDIA LAMBLIA

This fragmented protozoon is a frequently encountered cause of acute chronic diarrhoea which in the later form of the infection may be accompanied by malabsorption. It is world wide in distribution, but most infections in otherwise healthy persons are asymptomatic. In patients with humoral immunodeficiency, notably hypogammaglobulinaemia, giardiasis causes particularly severe symptoms that include vomiting, diarrhoea, malabsorption and weight loss (Ament et al. 1977). Achlorhydria and pancreatic dysfunction are thought to increase the risk of giardiasis.

Cysts of *Giardia* spp. are observed in the stool of some 30% of chronically infected patients. When giardiasis is strongly suspected repeated examinations of faecal concentrate should be made for cysts or biopsy material for trophozoites. A monoclonal antibody that results in increased sensitivity is now available for detection of *Giardia*. Initial treatment of this organism is with metronidazole or tinidazole.

TOXOPLASMA GONDII

This coccidian organism is an obligate intracellular parasite. In immunodeficient patients this parasite may result from a current acquisition of the organism or from reactivation of a latent infection. A characteristic feature is disseminated disease affecting the heart, lungs, liver or kidneys, with a particular predilection for the central nervous system. Underlying diseases that predispose to toxoplasmosis are usually those that cause a deficiency of cell mediated immunity (Ruskin and Remington 1976).

T. gondii is the most common cause of latent CNS infection in individuals with AIDS (Luft and Remington 1992, Porter and Sande 1992). Seroepidemiological studies indicate that this organism affects approximately one-third of the general population of the USA. Reactivation of a pre-existent latent infection frequently occurs when the CD4+ T cell count is less than 100 ml^{-1}. *T. gondii* can infect a variety of tissues and toxoplasmic encephalitis is the most common clinical infection. Pulmonary toxoplasmosis is less common than toxoplasmic encephalitis, but it is an important clinical concern in people with AIDS. *T. gondii* is an obligate, intracellular protozoon with a complex life cycle of tachyzoites (formerly termed trophozoites), tissue cysts and oocytes. The infection is transmitted to carnivores, including humans, by ingestion of raw or undercooked meat or by inhalation of oocytes in faeces of recently infected cats. Transmission can also occur transplacentally from an infected mother to the fetus.

The diagnosis of systemic toxoplasmosis may be made by demonstrating parasitaemia, or more often by means of serological tests for specific IgM and IgG antibodies in the serum.

Toxoplasmosis of the central nervous system can be confirmed only by brain biopsy. Radiologically, CT scan with the use of contrast is the recommended study (Luft and Remington 1992). Diagnostic CT scans will demonstrate the pattern of enhancement (ring or nodular) in more than 90% of patients who have toxoplasmosis encephalitis.

Treatment may involve a combination of pyrimethamine and sulphadiazine The empirical use of these agents when toxoplasmosis is suspected has yielded good clinical outcomes equivalent to treating cases confirmed by brain biopsy. The relapse rate associated with discontinuing treatment may be as high as 100% in AIDS patients. For these individuals, lifelong maintenance therapy is necessary (Beamen, Luft and Remington 1992).

LEISHMANIA DONOVANI

This organism causes widespread infection in many tropical and subtropical countries (Bryceson 1987). It is transmitted to man by the sand fly. Most infections in man are subclinical; however, a proportion even in supposedly normal individuals takes a form of visceral leishmaniasis or kala azar, a potentially fatal chronic disease characterized by splenomegaly with fever and weight loss. Visceral leishmaniasis may appear in association with immunodeficiency. Fernandez-Guerrero and colleagues (1987) described 10 such patients who had a renal transplant, suffered from leukaemia or systemic lupus erythematosus (SLE) or were HIV-positive.

The diagnosis of *L. donovani* is made by demonstrating amastigotes in Giemsa-stain smears of bone marrow or splenic aspirates. Treatment is available via a pentavalent antimony compound, sodium stibogluconate.

BABESIA DIVERGENS

The tick-borne intraerythrocytic babesiae are protozoa found in many species of mammals. Two of them are known to cause disease in man. *Babesia microti*, a parasite of rodents transmitted by ixodid ticks, causes a febrile disease in otherwise healthy persons exposed to ticks in northern USA. The other predominant species, *Babesia divergens*, is a parasite of cattle, also transmitted by the same group of ticks; it causes sporadic human infections in several European countries, but only in persons who have previously suffered splenectomy (Ruebush 1987). The parasite can be seen in blood films stained by Giesma's or a similar methodology; however, they may be mistaken for malaria parasites. Chemotherapy has not generally been shown to be effective. Prompt blood transfusion, renal dialysis and even exchange transfusion may be required.

STRONGYLOIDES STERCORALIS

Infection with this worm is widespread in the tropics and subtropics. Individuals who have lived in an endemic area may have a latent infection that can persist for many years. Under conditions which are favourable to the parasite, notably impairment of cellular immunity (Scowden, Schaffner and Stone 1978), the organism may go through a number of successive generations in the same host. This process of multiplication may lead to an overwhelming infection with intestinal and pulmonary complications that manifest as nausea, vomiting, diarrhoea, cough and haemoptysis. Infection may be complicated by the appearance of septicaemia, meningitis and shock due to secondary infection by gram-negative aerobic bacteria. In the temperate zones, severe strongyloides infection is often associated with the administration of steroids (Longworth and Weller 1986). Other conditions that predispose to infections with this nematode include haematological malignancy, chronic renal failure, malnutrition, alcoholism and AIDS.

The diagnosis of this nematode may be made by detecting the filariform larvae in the faeces; in heavy infestations they can also be observed in the sputum. Thiabendazole is the treatment of choice.

2.6   Viruses

Viruses that have pathogenic potential for immunocompetent members of the population result in infections of increased severity in immunodeficient hosts. Respiratory syncytial virus (RSV) is an example of a virus that usually causes diseases only in infants, but is responsible for pneumonia in immunodeficient adults and children. Similarly, measles and influenza viruses can initiate pneumonia and encephalitis in immunodeficient subjects (Pullan et al. 1976).

Viral infections may occur as primary infection or reactivation of latent disease. Related to the extent of impairment of cell mediated immunity of the host, viral infections may present a wide spectrum of symptoms ranging from asymptomatic shedding of the virus to fulminant disease. Most notably, members of the herpes group have a propensity to reactivate infection. The herpes viruses are frequent and troublesome opportunistic pathogens and are responsible for a wide range of clinical disease. Important sequelae of virus infections include: virus-induced immunosuppression (Rouse and Horohov 1986) causing bacterial or fungal superinfection; malignancy, as associated with Epstein–Barr virus (EBV)-induced lymphoma in organ-transplant recipients; and autoimmune phenomena.

Several drugs are now available for treating viral infections. Aciclovir is effective in controlling infection due to herpes simplex virus (HSV) and varicella zoster virus (VZV) and ganciclovir and foscarnet have been shown to be effective against cytomegalovirus (CMV) retinitis (AIDS Clinical Trials Group 1992).

Viral infections frequently encountered in immunodeficient patients are presented in Table 7.3. Additional information can be found in Volume 1 (see Volume 1, Chapter 42) and in other chapters in Volume 1 devoted to specific viral infections.

3   INFECTIONS IN SPECIFIC HOST GROUPS

3.1   Primary (congenital) immunodeficiencies

Although these diseases are individually uncommon,

they are now increasingly recognized; new syndromes are being described as clinicians have become aware of their existence and more sophisticated immunological and screening tests have become available. The principal congenital immunodeficient disorders and their associated infectious complications are shown in Table 7.4. They have recently been reviewed by Christenson and Hill (1994) and previously by Fischer (1992). These disorders occur with a frequency of about 1:10 000. The most frequently encountered, common variable immunodeficiency and X-linked agammaglobulinaemia, are manifested primarily or exclusively as defects in B cell humoral immunity; less frequent are those forms of primary immunodeficiency in which cellular immunity is impaired. Given the central role that T cells play in cellular immunity (particularly CD4 T cells), profound deficits in T cell function will result in secondary deficits in B cell function and humoral immunity.

Disorders of this group most commonly manifest as:

1   an increased severity or frequency of infection with pathogenic microbes and
2   opportunistic infection with micro-organisms of low virulence.

The appearance of severe infection with an opportunistic micro-organism such as *P. carinii* within the early months of life in an infant who is not receiving any immunosuppressive medication is sufficient evidence to warrant a detailed immunological investigation. Additionally, recurrent pulmonary, cutaneous or bloodstream infections associated with organisms such as *S. aureus* or an encapsulated strain of pneumococcus, meningococcus or *H. influenzae* should initiate a prompt search for an underlying immunodeficiency.

3.2   Secondary immunodeficiencies

Patients with underlying malignancy often suffer, as a complication of their disease, defects in immune response frequently affecting T cell function. The development of an opportunistic infection may be the first evidence of this defect. Associations include tuberculosis with lymphoma and legionellosis with childhood leukaemia. In patients with advanced malignancy, T cell responses are particularly depressed but malnutrition probably has an important supplementary role in this situation. In patients with extensive bone marrow replacement due to leukaemia, infections arise as a result of quantitative deficiencies of phagocytic cells. This function of humoral immunity is a hallmark of multiple myeloma.

Common variable hypogammaglobulinaemia is generally regarded as an acquired disorder since the disease usually appears in children or young adults. However, the finding of immunological abnormalities in relatives (Douglas, Goldberg and Fudenberg 1970) suggests that some forms may be inherited (see Table 7.4). The isolation of retroviruses has been reported in several patients with hypogammaglobulinaemia (Webster et al. 1986) and poses the possibility that this is a virus-induced immunodeficiency. Low levels of cir-

Table 7.3 Features of viral infections in immunosuppressed hosts

Virus	Principal patient groups affected	Major clinical manifestations	Principal diagnostic methods	Treatment
Herpes viruses				
Herpes simplex	Leukaemia BMT Organ transplant	Mucositis, oesophagitis hepatitis, pneumonia, encephalitis	Culture	Aciclovir
Cytomegalovirus	Organ transplant BMT	Pneumonia, hepatitis, colitis	Antigen detection, culture, biopsy	Ganciclovir, phosphonoformate, foscarnet
Epstein–Barr virus	BMT Renal transplant	Hepatitis, lymphoproliferative syndrome	Serology	–
Varicella zoster virus	BMT Organ transplant	Pneumonia, encephalitis	Serology	Aciclovir
Polyomaviruses				
BK	Renal transplant BMT	Haemorrhagic cystitis	Electron microscopy, serology, biopsy	–
JC	Leukaemia Lymphoma Renal transplant	Multifocal leucoencephalopathy		
Adenoviruses	BMT Organ transplant	Pneumonia, encephalitis, myocarditis, colitis	Culture	–
Enteroviruses	BMT Organ transplant	Enteritis, pneumonia	Culture	
Measles	Leukaemia	Pneumonia, encephalitis	Culture, biopsy	–
Respiratory syncytial virus	BMT Organ transplant	Pneumonia	Antigen, detection culture	Ribavirin
Hepatitis B virus	Liver transplant Heart transplant	Chronic hepatitis	Serology	Interferon-α2b
Hepatitis C virus	BMT Organ transplant	Chronic hepatitis	EIA	Interferon-α2b

culating IgG, sometimes accompanied by IgM or IgA deficiency, are the main feature of this disorder, with predisposition to respiratory infection with encapsulated bacteria, and gastrointestinal infections such as giardiasis. In some cases there is an accompanying T cell deficiency which may account for the development of lymphoreticular malignancies. Long-term treatment with gammaglobulin appears to be the only available support of therapy for this condition and reduces the incidence of intermittent infections.

3.3 Acquired immunodeficiency syndrome (AIDS)

The aetiological agent of AIDS is a retrovirus designated human immunodeficiency virus type 1 (HIV-1). The CD4+ T lymphocyte is the primary target for HIV infection because of the affinity of the virus for the CD surface marker. The CD4+ T lymphocyte co-ordinates a number of important immunological functions and a loss of these functions results in regressive

Table 7.4 Primary (congenital) immunodeficiency disorders and associated infections

Combined T and B cell defects	
Severe combined immunodeficiency (SCID), e.g Swiss-type agammaglobulinaemia; Nezelof's syndrome; reticular dysgenesis	Bacterial, viral, and *Pneumocystis* pneumonias; 'BCGosis'; cutaneous and systemic yeast infections; chronic diarrhoea; failure to thrive from birth
Wiskott–Aldrich syndrome	Sinusitis, otitis media, pneumonia due to *Haemophilus influenzae* and *Streptococcus pneumoniae*; gastroenteritis; eczema; thrombocytopenia
Ataxia telangiectasia	Recurrent sinus and chest infections due to pneumococcus, *H. influenzae*, *Staphylococcus aureus*
Pure T cell defects	
DiGeorge syndrome	*Pneumocystis* pneumonia; cutaneous and systemic yeast infections; diarrhoea; failure to thrive; cardiac anomalies; parathyroid hormone deficiency
Chronic mucocutaneous candidiasis	Skin and mucosal *Candida* infection
B cell defects	
Sex-linked hypogammaglobulinaemia, with deficiencies of IgG, IgM, IgA	Otitis media, sinusitis, pneumonia, septicaemia due to *S. pneumoniae*, *H. influenzae*, *S. aureus*, meningococcus; chronic enterovirus infection
IgM deficiency	Pneumococcal, *H. influenzae*, *E. coli* septicaemia and meningitis
IgA deficiency	Otitis media, sinopulmonary infections; diarrhoea due to *Giardia* and *Cryptosporidium* spp.
Common variable hypogammaglobulinaemia	Pneumococcal, *H. influenzae*, *S. aureus* sinusitis, pneumonia, septicaemia; chronic diarrhoea; chronic hepatitis
Complement–component defects	
C2 + alternative pathway	Pneumococcal, *H. influenzae*, meningococcal sepsis
C3, C5	Sinusitis, pneumonia, septicaemia due to *S. pneumoniae*, *H. influenzae*, *E. coli*, *Streptococcus pyogenes*
C6, C7, C8	Meningococcal septicaemia, meningitis
Phagocyte defects	
Microbicidal	
Chronic granulomatous disease (see Chapter 4)	Recurrent abscesses, pneumonia, due to *S. aureus*, *E. coli*, *Klebsiella*, *Serratia*, *Salmonella*, *Candida* and *Aspergillus* spp.
Chediak–Higashi syndrome	*S. aureus* and *Candida* infections, including abscesses
NK cell deficiency	Herpes group viruses
Chemotactic	
'Lazy' leucocyte syndrome	Gingivitis, recurrent otitis media, rhinitis
+ hyperimmunoglobulin E (some cases referred to as Job syndrome, see Chapter 4)	Otitis media, chest infection, septicaemia, eczema due to *S. aureus* and *Candida*
Neutropenia	
Infantile agranulocytosis (also familial and cyclic neutropenia)	*E. coli* and other 'gram-negative' sepsis

impairment of the immune response. Studies of the natural history of HIV infection have documented a wide spectrum of disease manifestations, ranging from asymptomatic infection to life-threatening conditions characterized by severe immunodeficiency, serious opportunistic infections and cancers. Although immunoglobulin levels may be normal or even elevated, there is accompanying evidence of humoral dysfunction and also of functional abnormalities of polymorphs.

AIDS represents the end of a spectrum of disease resulting from progression of infection with HIV which is typically symptomless in the initial stages, followed by generalized lymphadenopathy or AIDS-related complex (ARC). As part of the prodrome of AIDS, patients may suffer from continued fever, diarrhoea, weight loss and malaise. At this time, infections often arise which have been shown to be in strong association with the lowering of the CD4+ T lymphocytes. As can be seen in Fig. 7.1, the earliest infections are associated with oral candidiasis and localized herpes infections. Subsequently, the first manifestation of HIV infection may be *Pneumocystis* pneumonia which is the initial element in the large majority of cases. A wide range of infections with other organisms (bacteria, fungi, viruses and protozoa) also occurs (see Table 7.5). The incidence of opportunistic infection as the CD4+ T lymphocyte count falls below 200 μl^{-1} is depicted in Fig. 7.2. Mixed or multiple infections are characteristic of AIDS, especially in the later stages.

Symptomatic disease that does not meet the case definition of AIDS as defined by the Centers for Disease Control (CDC) is frequently referred to as ARC, a non-specific appellation for the combination of any 2 clinical symptoms with 2 laboratory test abnormalities that are not attributable to an identifiable, unrelated illness in an HIV-infected person. Pneumonia with or without bacteriological diagnosis is probably the leading cause of HIV-related morbidity and death (Centers for Disease Control 1992).

The World Health Organization recommends that an alternative definition be used for case reporting in countries where extensive laboratory investigation of infection and immunity may not be readily obtainable. This modified definition is based upon clinical presentation alone, and is manifest as a combination of at least one major and 2 minor signs in the absence of known reason for immunosuppression. Major signs include weight loss of 10% or more and diarrhoea or fever that persists for 1 month or longer. Minor signs include persistent cough, general pruritic dermatitis, recurrent zoster or progressive or disseminated herpes, oropharyngeal candidiasis and generalized lymphadenopathy.

Throughout the world, pulmonary TB is the hallmark infection in persons with HIV (Raviglione, Narain and Kochi 1992). The addition of pulmonary TB to the list of AIDS infections indicates disease is based upon the strong epidemiological link between HIV infection and the development of TB (Centers for Disease Control 1992).

Gastrointestinal infections may be caused by CMV, *Cryptosporidium*, *Entamoeba histolytica*, MAC and a disease array of microbial pathogens (see Table 7.5).

Toxoplasmosis is the most frequent of the various causes of mass lesions in the central nervous system. In some series its incidence is thought to be as high as 40%. Treatment for cerebral toxoplasmosis (pyrimethamine plus sulphadiazine or clindamycin) is frequently given on the basis of findings of computerized tomographic scanning (CT) and the presence of a distinct radiological pattern (ring form) is typical confirmation of the presence of toxoplasmosis. Because of the high rate of relapse once treatment is terminated, long-term prophylaxis is usually recommended.

3.4 Malignant diseases

The objective of cancer therapy is to produce a remission of the underlying disease and thus to achieve long-term cure. The chemotherapy and other treatments used may be expected to cause profound immunosuppression and, together with other factors that inhibit host defences, are responsible for the high rate of infection that cancer patients experience. Over the last decade, individuals with underlying malignant diseases have succumbed less frequently to overwhelming bacterial sepsis, which used to be the primary cause of death during the most intensive stages of treatment. However, other opportunistic micro-organisms have assumed increasing importance. The risk of developing a major episode of infection, such as bacteraemia and subsequently septicaemia, in the course of hospital treatment is related closely to the underlying malignancy. In patients with solid tumours of the CNS, head and neck, skin or lung the risk of infection is low whereas it is considerable in cases of acute leukaemia (Bodey et al. 1986).

Neutropenia, defined as less than 0.5×10^6 neutrophils per ml is a key factor predisposing to opportunistic infection during the treatment of haematological malignancy. Septic complications are observed more frequently during periods of marked neutropenia (Bodey et al. 1966, Storring et al. 1977). At one time, *E. coli* and other members of the resident intestinal microbiota were the predominant causes of septicaemia and related complications (Bodey et al. 1986). Breaches of the bowel mucosa occurring as a consequence of drug or radiation toxicity probably provided the main portal of entry for these organisms; the urinary tract was considered as another access route. *P. aeruginosa* is responsible for many of the more serious infections in neutropenic patients. Infections with this organism were often complicated by septic shock and pneumonia, which explains the 30–50% mortality rates that have been reported (Bodey, Jadeja and Elting 1985).

There has been a gradual shift in the spectrum of micro-organisms causing septicaemia; as new pathogens become part of the nosocomial microflora of institutions they will be recovered from residents with increasing frequency (see Chapter 13). Gram-positive bacteria can now be expected to be the most frequent agents recovered from blood cultures in neutropenic leukaemic patients. The high prevalence of coagulase-negative staphylococci (see Chapter 13 and Volume 2, Chapter 27), particularly *S. epidermidis*, has been associated with the widespread use of long-term indwelling venous catheters (Hickman et al. 1979, Darbyshire, Weightman and Speller 1985). *S. aureus* continues to be an important pathogen in this setting although the portal of entry of this organism is unknown in 70% of cases (Espersen et al. 1987). Espersen and colleagues (1987) reported on a series of patients with haematological malignancy or agranulocytosis, in which *S. aureus* accounted for 7% of the episodes of septicaemia. The mortality rate was 3-fold higher than that of leukaemia.

Anaerobes (non-sporing, gram-negative) cause perirectal and other abscesses in neutropenic hosts (Glenn et al. 1988). In addition some species of *Clostridium* are responsible for lower bowel disease and septicaemia. *Clostridium septicum* has been implicated in the pathogenesis of neutropenic enterocolitis (King et al. 1984) and this may be complicated by septicaemia. *Clostridium tertium* is considered a cause of less serious

Table 7.5 Micro-organisms and disease syndromes in HIV-infected persons[a]

Micro-organism	Syndrome
Gram-positive bacteria	
Staphylococcus aureus	Impetigo, sinusitis, cellulitis, SSS[b] septic bursitis, pneumonia, bacteraemia, osteomyelitis
Streptococcus pneumoniae	Pneumonia (lobar), septic arthritis, bacteraemia, sinusitis, mastoiditis, meningitis, endocarditis
Streptococcus	Fasciitis, soft-tissue infection, meningitis
Listeria monocytogenes	Meningitis, hepatitis, bacteraemia, disseminated infection
Corynebacterium diphtheriae	Cutaneous infection
Corynebacterium jeikeium	Skin nodules, bacteraemia, disseminated infection
Clostridium difficile	Pseudomembranous enterocolitis, bacteraemia
Gram-negative bacteria	
Aeromonas hydrophilia	Proctocolitis
Bordetella	Pertussis, pneumonia, sinusitis, bronchitis
Campylobacter spp.	Bacteraemia, enteritis, enterocolitis, endocarditis, disseminated infection, osteomyelitis
Bactonella (Rochalimaea)	Bacillary angiomatosis, hepatosplenic infection, bacteraemic endocarditis, encephalitis, lymphadenitis
Haemophilis influenzae	Bronchitis, pneumonia, sinusitis, otitis/mastoiditis
Kingella denitrificans	Granulomatous disease
Klebsiella rhinoscleromatis	Oropharyngeal infection
Legionella pneumophila	Pneumonia, sinusitis
Methylobacterium (Protomonas extorquens)	Bacteraemia
Neisseria meningitidis	Disseminated infection, meningitis
Pseudomonas spp.	Sinusitis, ostomyelitis, bacteraemia, pneumonia, indwelling catheter infection
Salmonella spp.	Bacteraemia, enteritis, endocarditis, cholecystitis, septic arthritis, osteomyelitis pneumonia, disseminated infection
Shigella flexneri	Enteritis, bacteraemia, disseminated infection
Actinomycetes	
Nocardia spp.	Pneumonia, brain abscess, liver abscess
Rhodococcus equi	Pneumonia, pleural effusion, bacteraemia, disseminated infection
Actinomyces israelii	Cervicofacial infections, oesophagitis
Spirochaetes	
Treponema pallidum	Syphilis (all forms), cutaneous infection, diarrhoea, proctitis
Fungi	
Yeasts	
Candida spp.	Candidaemia, mucositis, disseminated/cutaneous infection, pyarthrosi endocarditis, endopthalmitis, hepatosplenic infection, brain abscess
Cryptococcus spp.	Pulmonary infection, meningitis, fungaemia, joint infection, primary cutaneous infection, pericarditis, mycocarditis, prostatitis, retinochorditis, pleural effusion, bone marrow infection, lymphadenitis
Trichosporon beigelii	Cutaneous infection, fungaemia, disseminated infection
Torulopsis glabrata	Osteomyelitis, mucositis, fungaemia
Saccharomyces cerevisiae	Pneumonia, fungaemia
Rhodotorula rubra	Fungaemia (catheter related)
Sporobolomyces salmonicolor	Pulmonary infection, fungaemia
Other fungi (including but not limited to)	
Alternaria spp.	Cutaneous infection, brain abscess, pneumonia, disseminated infection, fungaemia, hepatobiliary infection, oesophagitis, endocarditis, sinusi meningitis, pulmonary infection, pharyngeal infection
Fusarium spp.	
Penicillium spp.	
Aspergillus spp.	
Rhizopus spp.	
Prototheca wickerhamii	
Pneumocystis carinii	

Table 7.5 Continued

Micro-organism	Syndrome
Viruses (see Volume 1, Chapters 38 and 42)	
DNA viruses	Retinitis, disseminated infection, oesophagitis, encephalitis, hepatitis, cystitis, dermatitis, enterocolitis, CNS and Burkitt's lymphoma (EBV), pneumonitis, Kaposi's sarcoma, persistent anaemia, RBC aplasia (HPV-B19), progressive multifocal leucoencephalopathy (JO papovavirus)
RNA viruses	Chronic hepatitis C infection, encephalitis, pneumonia, exacerbation of respiratory problems, gastroenteritis, increased severity of illness and mortality
Protozoa	
Acantamoeba spp.	Granulomatous amoebic encephalitis, skin ulcers, granulomatous sinus
Babesia spp.	Babesiosis (fever and bloodstream infection)
Cryptosporidium parvum	Chronic diarrhoea, cholangitis, pneumonia
Cyclospora cayetanensis	Chronic diarrhoea
Encephalitozoan hellem	Keratoconjunctivitis, disseminated microsporidiosis
Enterocytozoon bieneusi	Chronic diarrhoea, cholangitis, pneumonia
Isospora belli	Chronic diarrhoea
Leishmania spp.	Visceral leishmaniasis
Septata intestinalis	Chronic diarrhoea, cholangitis, disseminated microsporidiosis
Toxoplasma gondii	Encephalitis, myocarditis, pneumonitis, hepatitis, disseminated disease
Trypanosoma cruzi	Meningoencephalitis, myocarditis
Stronglycoides stercoralis	Pulmonary infection
Arthropods	
Sarcoptes scabei	Severe crusted scabies

[a]Adapted from Kaplan et al. 1995; 156 citations that reference 111 genera and species.
[b]Scalded skin syndrome.

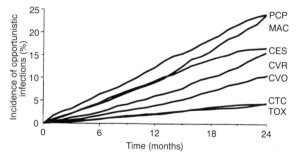

Fig. 7.2 Kaplan–Meier estimates of months from first observed CD4+ lymphocyte count of $<20\,\mu l^{-1}$ to incident diagnosis of selected opportunistic infection. PCP, *Pneumocystis carinii*; MAC, disseminated infection with *Mycobacterium avium* complex; CES, *Candida* oesophagitis; CVR, cytomegalovirus retinitis; CVO, cytomegalovirus disease other than retinitis; CTC, cryptococcosis; and TOX, toxoplasmosis. (Reprinted from Kaplan et al. 1995, with permission).

infections, although it is observably less resistant to antimicrobial agents than other members of the clostridia group (Speirs, Warren and Rampling 1988).

When neutropenia is prolonged (i.e. more than 3 weeks) it is thought to be the major factor accounting for the increased incidence of serious fungal infections in leukaemic patients (Gerson et al. 1984).

Among the other contributory factors is selective pressure on the host's resident microflora as a result of repeated regimens of parenteral antimicrobial agents (Barnes and Rodgers 1987). Fungal infections are the leading cause of problems associated with patients undergoing leukaemia chemotherapy (Bodey 1988) and *C. albicans* is the most frequently encountered fungal pathogen in these patients. There has been an increase both in other species of *Candida* (notably *C. tropicalis* and *C. kreusii* in some institutions) and in *A. fumigatus* infections. There have been other reports of infection associated with relatively infrequently encountered fungal agents such as *Fusarium* species and *Trichosporon*. Mortality rates due to these mycoses are higher than for systemic bacterial infections.

A frequent and painful complication of acute immunosuppression is mucositis, usually associated with herpes simplex virus (HSV) infection. Viral shedding can be detected in oropharyngeal cultures in the majority of patients with latent infection. The higher incidence of HSV mucositis in leukaemic rather than in other groups of patients is a reflection of the more intensive immunosuppression associated with leukaemia chemotherapy (Greenberg et al. 1987). Oesophagitis, viraemia and encephalitis are occasional complications of HSV infection. Reactivation of varicella zoster virus (VZV) usually occurs later in the course of treatment for malignancy and it may reflect as many as 10% of adult patients with leukaemia or lymphoma. A high rate of dissemination may be expected in patients with relapsed disease (Rusthoven et al. 1988).

In children, the late complications of leukaemia chemotherapy have been studied by Ninane and Chessells (1981). In their study population, among children who had completed their course of induction treatment, nearly half required subsequent readmission for treatment of infectious diseases. The majority of these infections were of the respiratory tract and the primary agents were bacteria, CMV and *P. carinii*. The highest mortality rates were in cases of measles and septicaemia.

3.5   Organ transplant recipients

Patients who are about to receive an organ transplant for failure of one of their organs are more susceptible to infection than otherwise healthy individuals. In addition to a complete history and physical examination, the susceptibility of the patient to infectious diseases should be determined. Infections to which the patient may have been previously exposed may now be dormant and this information should be discovered prior to transplantation. Examples include a history of exposure to tuberculosis as determined by Purified Protein Derivative (PPD) skin tests, hepatitis infections (B, C and δ), recurrent herpetic lesions, varicella and exposure to bacterial and fungal infections. The geographical location of the recipient's residence in areas endemic for certain aetiological agents (e.g. *Histoplasma capsulatum, Coccidioides immitis* and *Strongyloides stercoralis*) should be considered and evaluated. In addition, human infection with human immunodeficiency virus may be a contraindication to transplantation.

In the non-transplant population certain underlying conditions prove to be a risk for infection and these include diabetics, individuals with osteomyelitis infections, and patients with a history of dental problems. Each of these conditions will be exacerbated by the use of corticosteroids and immunosuppressive agents in the course following transplantation. It is not uncommon for a potential recipient of liver, heart or lung transplants to be hospitalized for prolonged periods awaiting a suitable donor organ. It is in this time frame within the hospital setting that potential recipients can become colonized and infected with nosocomial micro-organisms present in the hospital. In these patients, a pretransplantation antimicrobial prophylaxis regimen should be considered to cover the resident microflora in the hospital or cultured as colonizers from the patient. In potential liver transplant recipients most of the infections occur early in the post-transplant period and are due to gram-negative aerobic micro-organisms and fungi that colonize the gastrointestinal tract. In an attempt to decrease these infections, most transplantation centres have instituted selective bowel decontami-

nation which involves the use of non-absorbable oral antimicrobial agents in combination, such as polymixin E, tobramycin and the antifungal agent fluconazole, or the quinolone norfloxacin and nystatin. The period for initiation of these medications is dependent upon the transplant centre; they may be initiated prior to and through 5 days following transplantation. Infection rates in the small bowel decontamination treated groups range from 6% to 11% compared with 50–53% in non-treated patients (Smith et al. 1993).

Transplant recipients who are hepatitis B surface antigen (HBsAg) negative prior to transplantation are at greater risk than the normal population for exposure to hepatitis B virus (HBV) and these patients should receive recombinant HBV vaccine prior to transplantation. Administration of recombinant HBV vaccine is recommended in this group of patients although one study suggests that the response rate for developing hepatitis B surface antibody is approximately 29% (Berner et al. 1993).

EVALUATION OF THE TRANSPLANT DONOR

Like the recipient, the organ donor must undergo extensive evaluation for the presence of infection. Obviously the transmission of infection from infected organs can be considered a direct inoculation of potential agents and is contraindicated. A list of recommended tests for determining infections that are potentially transmitted by organ donation are outlined in Table 7.6 (Gottesdiener 1989). Regulatory groups in various countries usually mandate a list of agents to be tested. In the USA, the United Network for Organ Sharing (UNOS) and the American Red Cross recommends HIV, HTLV, CMV, hepatitis B and C, tuberculosis, bacteria, fungi and syphilis. Others are ruled out according to risk factors of the individual and areas of endemicity.

INFECTIONS IN GENERAL

More than 80% of transplant recipients experience one episode of clinical infection postoperatively (Tolkoff-Rubin and Rubin 1988). Each transplanted solid organ and immunosuppression regimen confers certain risk factors that predispose allograft recipients to infection. Some of these have been mentioned above (e.g. diabetes mellitus, prior hepatitis B and C infection, leucopenia, splenectomy, uraemia, the use of cadaveric donor organs and repeated treatment of persistent or recurrent rejection). The use of immunomodulating agents to suppress the body's defence mechanisms to accept the transplanted organ is a dual-edged approach that protects the transplanted donor organ from the body's immune defences but at the same time exposes the recipient to increased potential for infection.

Transplant recipients are at risk for the usual infections seen in immunocompetent hosts just as they are at risk for opportunistic infections. These infections derive from the transplanted allograft, technical complications of surgical manipulation, reactivation of latent infection and environmental exposure to new microbes in the environment where transplantation

Table 7.6 Screening transplant donors for infectious agents

Infection	Test[a]	Positive test comment
Human immunodeficiency virus (HIV-1/2)	HIV-1/2[b] (EIA)[c]	Contraindicates organ use
HTLV-1 (human T lymphocytic virus type I)	HTLV-1 (EIA)	Contraindicates organ use
Epstein–Barr virus (EBV)	EBV-VCA[d]	Poses increased risk for recipient
Cytomegalovirus (CMV)	CMV-Ab	Poses increased risk for recipient
Hepatitis B	HBsAg (EIA)	Recipient at risk unless HBsAg-positive
Hepatitis C	Anti-HCV (EIA)	Potential risk for HCV
Syphilis	Reaginic test[e]	Treat recipient after transplant
Bacteria	Culture of perfusate	Possible transmission of infection
Tuberculosis	PPD	Possible transmission of infection
Fungi	Culture	Possible transmission of infection
Malaria[f]	Microscopic examination of thick smear	Possible transmission to recipient
Schistosomiasis[f]	Schistosoma antibody	Possible transmission to recipient
Toxoplasmosis	Toxoplasma antibody	Possible transmission to recipient; heart transplants at greatest risk
Trypanosomiasis[f]	Trypanosoma antibody	Possible transmission to recipient

[a]For most of the viral agents, molecular based (PCR) assays are available which are more sensitive but less specific in the general donor population.
[b]The HIV-1p24 antigen can be used to shorten the window period for development and detection of an antibody.
[c]Enzyme immunoassay.
[d]Viral capsid antigen.
[e]Positive screen is confirmed.
[f]Donors from endemic areas.

was rendered. The infectious agents vary in a predictable pattern depending upon the organ transplanted, the immunosuppressive regimen and the duration of the postoperative course. When considering infections and contributing micro-organisms associated with transplants it is wise to consider that the organ transplant recipients are at risk for increased susceptibility of infection associated with the transplanted organ during the first months following transplantation. Thus, renal transplant recipients are at risk for developing pyleonephritis, liver transplant recipients develop cholangitis, heart transplant recipients develop endocarditis, and lung transplant recipients tend to develop bronchitis and pneumonia. These infections are related to the altered anatomy, the condition of the host, and the acceptability of the foreign tissue to infection.

More than 15 years ago, Rubin and coworkers (1981) elucidated time posts that indicate the course of bacterial, fungal, viral or other infections that occur after transplantation. For this schema, the authors used kidney transplantation, but in general their guide seems to be true for most solid organ transplants. The time pattern for these agents to appear is indicated in Table 7.7. Infections occurring within the first month after transplantation are probably a result of transplanting an infectious agent during surgery. The period from 1 to 6 months after transplantation is the frame for opportunistic infections that result from the high initial levels of immunosuppression required to prevent acute rejection (Peterson et al.

1981, Rubin 1991). During the 6 months to 1 year interval, there is a return to routine bacterial infections and the development of slower growing chronic fungal and mycobacterial infections as the recipient receives a lower dosage of immunosuppressive agents.

BONE MARROW TRANSPLANTS (BMT)

The patient who receives an allogeneic bone marrow transplant is subject to a wide array of microbial infections as outlined in Fig. 7.3 (Schimpff and Klastersky 1993). In terms of frequency of infection there are 3 time posts as can be seen in the figure. In the first 20 days following transplantation there is a very high rate of reactivation of HSV. In the 3 weeks immediately following transplantation, there is a period of aplasia with consequent high risk for gram-negative and gram-positive bacteraemia followed by increasing risk for invasive infections associated with *Candida* and *Aspergillus*. This is probably a result of prior antibiotic therapy which shifts the local flora. As the marrow engrafts and neutropenia resolves, acute graft-versus-host disease (GVHD) begins, initially burdening the predisposition to *Aspergillus* and later, about day 40, leading to a high incidence of CMV interstitial pneumonia during the phase of intense cellular immune dysfunction. As acute GVHD diminishes and becomes chronic GVHD, it is likely that herpes zoster infections appear, often with dissemination and death unless treated with high dose aciclovir. In part associated with the chronic GVHD, these patients in later stages may have serious episodes of pneumococcal bacteraemia which can

Table 7.7 Patterns of infectious complications in transplant recipients

Transplant	Immunosuppression	Months after transplantation		
		0–1	**2–6**	**7–12+**
Bone marrow	CSP-A Cyclophosphamide Total body irradiation HDMP (G) Azathioprine (G)	Herpes mucositis Candida stomatitis Septicaemia	CMV pneumonia Candidaemia Aspergillosis *Pneumocystis* pneumonia	Pneumococcal pneumonia, septicaemia Varicella zoster
Kidney	CSP-A HDMP (R)	Herpes mucositis Wound, urinary tract infection; device-related infection	CMV pneumonia *Listeria* meningitis Aspergillosis Cryptococcosis Nocardiosis	CMV retinitis
Liver	CSP-A Hydrocortisone Prednisolone ATG (R) HDMP (R)	Herpes mucositis Abdominal and liver abscess Wound infection Cholangitis Pneumonia Septicaemia Candidaemia	CMV pneumonia Aspergillosis *Pneumocystis* pneumonia Toxoplasmosis	Varicella zoster
Heart	CSP-A HDMP (R) ATG (R)	Herpes mucositis Wound infection (sternal, mediastinal) Bacterial pneumonia Septicaemia	CMV pneumonia Candidaemia Aspergillosis Urinary tract infection Varicella zoster Toxoplasmosis *Pneumocystis* pneumonia Nocardia	

CSP-A, cyclosporine A; HDMP, high dose methylprednisolone; ATG, anti-T lymphocyte globulin; R, use in rejection episodes; G, use in graft-versus-host disease; CMV, cytomegalovirus.

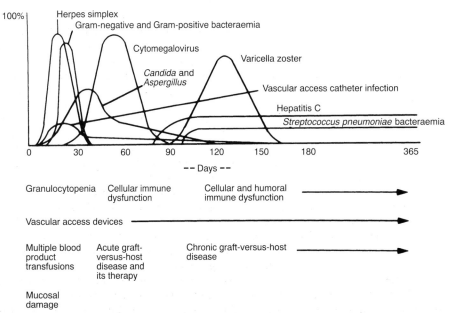

Fig. 7.3 Infection in allogeneic bone marrow transplantation. (Reprinted from Schimpff and Klastersky 1993, with permission).

begin at approximately day 100. At this time, hepatitis C, if not ruled out as part of the pretransplant screen, may become apparent. The hepatitis C virus is frequently transfused with platelets in the first 3 weeks and develops at this time as an acute hepatitis syndrome.

It should be noted that at any time after insertion, the vascular access devices may become associated with exit site infection, tunnel infection or catheter-related bacteraemia. This is true for BMT and other solid organ transplants.

KIDNEY TRANSPLANTATION

The early experience emphasized the frequency of morbidity due to opportunistic bacteria and viruses (Myerowitz, Medeiros and O'Brien 1972) but the current 95% survival rate for this procedure demonstrates experience in controlling potential infections. As with all transplant procedures some infections arise from the surgical placement of the donor kidney, others are consequences of drug-induced and associated immunosuppression (Tolkoff-Rubin and Rubin 1992).

During the perioperative period and the succeeding few weeks, the principal complications are wound, urinary tract and intravascular device-related infections which may be complicated by an episode of bacteraemia and septicaemia. The rate for these infections varies, depending upon the series, from 2 to 50%; good surgical technique and patient management play an important role in reducing the risk. The major causative organisms are *E. coli*, other coliform bacteria, *P. aeruginosa*, *S. faecalis*, *S. aureus* and coagulase-negative staphylococci. Perioperative antibiotic prophylaxis has proved to be effective in reducing rates of sepsis in the initial week following transplantation but has little influence on the total number of infections observed in the first month (Cohen, Rees and Williams 1988). Indwelling urinary catheters pose a particular risk for kidney transplant recipients. The reported incidence of urinary tract infections in this patient population has been as high as 83% (Rubin et al. 1981, Dunn 1990, Dunn and Najarian 1991).

The incidence of mycobacterial infections in renal transplant recipients is 0.8% compared with 0.1% in the general population (Lichtenstein and MacGregor 1983, Delaney et al. 1993). Of these infections approximately 30% are associated with the atypical mycobacteria, *M. kansasii*, *Mycobacterium chelonei* and *Mycobacterium haemophilum* (Delaney et al. 1993). *M. tuberculosis* infection is most often due to reactivation of disease. There have been reports of possible allograft transmission in patients who were PPD skin test negative prior to transplantation and nosocomial transmission in a renal transplant unit (Peters, Reiter and Bowell 1984, Jereb et al. 1993). The most common site of infection is the lung but extrapulmonary and disseminated diseases have also been seen involving skin, lymph nodes, musculoskeletal system and urinary tract.

Although fungal infections are the major cause of morbidity and mortality throughout the transplant period, their incidence in renal transplantation is at the lower end of the range (5%) as compared with 40% in liver transplant patients (Paya 1993). Eighty per cent of fungal infections occur within the first 2 months of transplantation. *Candida* and *Aspergillus* account for more than 80% of these infections. The mortality from these infections is high and ranges from 30 to 100%. The urinary tract is the most common site of fungal infection, especially with *Candida*. This can disseminate and lead to candidaemia which requires prompt antifungal therapy.

Around the 2–6 month time frame in post-transplant recovery, the principal opportunist is CMV. Most CMV infections are due to reactivation of latent virus, whereas a smaller proportion of patients who were seronegative prior to transplantation develop primary infection as a result of transmission of the virus in the donor kidney if this was not ruled out. It has become clear that reinfection from this source but with a different strain of CMV may occur in seropositive patients (Chou 1986). Primary infections are generally more severe than those due to reactivation and are likely to be exacerbated by the use of antilymphocytoglobulin for the treatment of rejection episodes. In addition, CMV is often implicated as a trigger for rejection. The clinical presentation of CMV infection ranges from mild constitutional symptoms to life-threatening pneumonia. Extrapulmonary manifestations are encephalitis, intestinal ulceration or haemorrhage. Viraemia is likely to accompany these systemic features. Retinitis accompanied by visual impairment is a later complication of chronic CMV infection.

Other viruses that are reactivated during this time frame include EBV, BK and JC polyoma viruses and adenoviruses. Reactivation of hepatitis B virus in the absence of the normal serum markers usually seen in immunocompetent individuals has also been recorded and frequently progresses to chronic hepatitis (Degos et al. 1988).

LIVER TRANSPLANTATION

Experience with liver transplantation is more recent than with kidney and the experience of the Pittsburgh (PA) Transplant Team indicates that 80% of patients who have undergone liver transplantation develop at least one episode of infection. These complications, especially septicaemia, CMV disease and invasive mycoses, contribute significantly to mortality (Kusne et al. 1988). Abdominal infections occur most frequently in liver transplant recipients and account for more than 50% of the bacterial infections (Paya et al. 1989). These infections include hepatic abscess, cholangitis and peritonitis. Abdominal infections are usually polymicrobial, involving enteric organisms such as, *E. coli*, *Enterococcus*, *Enterobacter*, *Klebsiella* and yeast. Infection with *Pseudomonas* is less common (Korvich et al. 1991). Agents associated with wound infections in this group of patients are gram-negative bacteria, anaerobic organisms and yeasts. Polymicrobial septicaemia has a frequency of 10% or greater (Keating and Wilhelm 1993). The rate at which these infections occur is closely related to the duration of the surgical procedure and is greater in patients who are undergoing second or subsequent transplant operations.

The incidence of fungal infections in liver transplantation is the highest of all the organ groups and is at the 40% level. Eighty per cent of fungal infections occur within the first 2 months following transplantation. *Candida* and *Aspergillus* account for the greatest majority, 80% of these infections. Mortality from fungal infections is extremely high and ranges from 30 to 100%. The reasons for this extreme in mortality rate include the problems encountered in recognizing early infections and the lack of effective therapy, at least against *Aspergillus*, and limited experience and data on effective antifungal prophylactic regimens. Infections with mycobacteria have also been reported (Strencek et al. 1992).

In this transplant group the majority of CMV infections appear within 2 months of transplantation. Virus shedding can be detected in about 60% of adult patients (Singh et al. 1988) usually as a result of reactivation of latent infection.

Other important opportunistic infections that appear at times over the ensuing 6 months are *P. carinii* pneumonia and toxoplasmosis. Subsequently, VZV is a significant cause of morbidity and affects 5–10% of patients.

HEART AND LUNG TRANSPLANTATION

Early infectious complications in this group relate principally to the surgical procedure and the intensive supportive care that is necessary during the time frame after transplant. Wound infections in this group are frequently due to organisms found in the pulmonary allograft. These infections may result from direct infective inoculation of the median sternotomy site. The organisms most frequently causing early sternal wound infections are *S. aureus*, *C. albicans* and *Mycoplasma hominis*. In later infections, *P. aeruginosa* has been implicated. When the lung is involved, the overall prevalence of pulmonary infection is greater than 60% (Dauber, Paradis and Dummer 1990, Mauer et al. 1992). The predisposing factors that contribute to this high prevalence include injury to the airway mucus with disruption of mucociliary clearance, airway anastomosis, impairment of the transport of mucus up the trachea, elimination of the cough reflex and interruption of lymphatic drainage (Dauber, Paradis and Dummer 1990). Pneumonia may be associated with the organisms that colonize the donors. Three-quarters of all pneumonias in heart–lung patients are attributable to gram-negative rods, principally, Enterobacteriaceae and the pseudomonads. The remainder are due to *S. aureus*, *H. influenzae* and *S. pneumoniae* (Dauber, Paradis and Dummer 1990).

Fungi have been reported to account for as many as 10% of all infections observed and may affect the lungs, heart and occasionally other organs in disseminated infection.

P. carinii infection occurs in the first 6 months following transplantation and is frequently seen in association with CMV infection. The highest incidence of PCP occurs in heart–lung transplant recipients (Dummer et al. 1986). About 1 month after transplantation CMV becomes a major opportunistic pathogen, reaching a peak incidence at about the seventh postoperative week. Disseminated infection has been observed in up to one-third of infected patients but without any difference in frequency between primary and reactivation events (Hofflin et al. 1987).

T. gondii poses a threat to all recipients of solid organs as this organism may remain dormant but can reactivate in immunosuppressed transplant recipients. Serious consequences can result when a toxoplasma-infected heart is transplanted into a seronegative recipient.

3.6   Chronically immunodeficient hosts

Long-term survivors of organ transplantation and leukaemia chemotherapy are continuously susceptible to infections by opportunistic micro-organisms during their period of immunosuppressive management. For some patients this may be a lifelong requirement.

A significant complication, particularly seen with chronic immunosuppression, is infection of the CNS. In one series of patients there were 55 documented CNS infections with a 60% mortality rate (Hooper, Pruitt and Rubin 1982). The most frequently encountered causative organisms in this group were *C. neoformans*, *L. monocytogenes* and *A. fumigatus*.

In patients with collagen-vascular diseases such as SLE and other autoimmune mediated disorders, a high dose of immunosuppressive therapy with steroids is required. Bacteria, especially gram-negative micro-organisms, are the most frequently encountered infecting organisms in this patient group and may be responsible for urinary tract, wound or chest infections occasionally complicated by septicaemia. Some of these patients who develop renal failure require dialysis and as a result are at risk for peritonitis; in the case of those undergoing haemodialysis, arterial venous shunt infection may also be extant complicated by episodes of septicaemia (Cohen et al. 1982). Opportunistic viral and fungal infections are a less common, though major cause of morbidity, especially when complicated by pneumonia.

As a result of loss of splenic function, either from hyposplenism or following splenectomy, the host loses 2 major anti-infective roles of the spleen: clearing the bloodstream of bacteria through its mononuclear–phagocyte function and the production of antibody. Functional hyposplenism occurs in haematological disorders such as sickle cell anaemia, coeliac disease and in bone marrow transplant recipients. The risk of pneumococcal pneumonia and fulminant septicaemia in splenectomized patients has been recognized for some time (Robinette and Fraumeni 1977). It is noteworthy that in patients with chronic leukaemia who undergo splenectomy, the major pathogen may be *P. aeruginosa* (Mower, Hawkins and Nelson 1986).

3.7 Other immunodeficient groups

Among other hosts at increased risk of infection because of antecedent disease or compromised circumstances are those in which the nature of the predisposing factors are less readily understood. It has been suggested that trauma, surgical intervention and extensive burns contribute to immunosuppression and that this renders patients prone to invasive bacterial diseases. It is uncertain whether these conditions are due to specific inhibition of cellular or humoral defences (Zimmerli 1985). In a trauma or burn process the early exposure and infection with bacteria into a newly inflicted wound surface permits multiplication to take place before the cellular inflammatory response has been mobilized. This event, coupled with the large area of exposed tissue, are the primary predisposing factors. Experimental studies of wound or burn infections initiated at various periods after exposure, and the success of very brief periods of perioperative chemoprophylaxis, tend to support this view.

In critically ill patients there is impairment of local non-specific host defences that predisposes to colonization of the oropharynx and the upper gastrointestinal tract by potential pathogens or opportunistic micro-organisms, notably aerobic gram-negative bacteria (Hudson 1989). This may be aggravated by treatment of the patient with H2 receptor antagonists that do not present a chemical barrier to the advance of these organisms. Recognition of these pathogenic mechanisms has led to the selective decontamination of the bowel (see section 3.5, p. 94) to prevent colonization.

Malnutrition and metabolic disease are additional secondary aspects that contribute to immunodeficiency. Clinical observations suggest that malnutrition, at least in its extreme forms, inhibits host defence mechanism. With HIV infection, protein energy malnutrition is a frequent cause of impaired cell mediated immunity (Chandra 1993) and frequently plays a role in malignant diseases. Malnutrition results in involution of the thymus and a parallel reduction in T cell dependent areas in the lymph nodes and spleen, thereby reducing the number of circulating T cells. Fatal measles virus infection is a major problem related to malnutrition; risk of progressive or severe tuberculosis and herpes virus infections is greater. The original descriptions of *Pneumocystis* pneumonia were in malnourished children. The reduction or impairment in cell mediated immunity and T lymphocyte numbers is reversible over a period of weeks to months with restoration of regular nutritional levels (Locksley and Wilson 1995).

Diabetes is an example of the interaction of metabolic disease and infection. It is associated with increased susceptibility to a number of infections but only when the diabetes is uncontrolled. It is attributable to impaired functioning of the PMNs, defective chemotaxis, phagocytic uptake and intracellular killing. Infections associated with disease in its uncontrolled state include urinary tract infections, staphylo-coccal infections, skin sepsis and perinephric abscesses. Tuberculosis, malignant otitis externa due to *P. aeruginosa* and a variety of fungal infections have also been observed (Alberti and Hockaday 1987).

The inhibition of normal phagocyte activity associated with chronic alcoholism is also associated with increased susceptibility to various bacterial infections. This is attributable to the inhibition of phagocytic activity by ethanol or acetaldehyde.

Immunodeficiency secondary to infectious processes has been observed to impair host defences. There are several examples other than of AIDS of one infection predisposing to another (Greenwood 1987). Viral infections, most notably HIV, are associated with impaired cell mediated immunity. Measles virus, each of the herpes group viruses (CMV, EBV and HHV6), influenza virus and RSV are some of the examples of viruses that impair function of the cellular immune system through the production of proteins or induction of host cells directly through downregulation of cell mediated immunity by soluble mediators. Some examples of these secondary infections are the forms of bacterial pneumonia following influenza; gastroenteritis, tuberculosis and bacterial pneumonia following measles; and labial herpes simplex following measles or meningococcal or pneumococcal infection. Infections with intraerythrocytic parasites such as *Bartonella* (see Volume 2, Chapter 63) or malaria parasites may predispose to septicaemia due to *Salmonella* or other enterobacteria. Similarly, *Salmonella* osteomyelitis associated with sickle cell crisis may be caused by monocyte blockade.

4 THE MANAGEMENT OF IMMUNODEFICIENT HOSTS

4.1 Prevention of infection

The compromised host that is immunosuppressed by virtue of a therapeutic course or extrinsic factors can become part of a carefully planned course of treatment such that prophylactic or therapeutic strategies can be implemented on the basis of expected infectious complications (see Table 7.1, p. 78). In the febrile granulocytopenic patient with underlying malignant disease, the original targets of empirical antibiotic therapy are gram-negative bacteria, particularly *P. aeruginosa*. Although gram-negative, bacillary infections such as *E. coli* and *Klebsiella* still predominate in some cancer centres, infections due to *P. aeruginosa* have declined. At the same time, some cancer treatment centres have observed a significant increase in the frequency of infections due to *Enterobacter* or to *Xanthomonas maltophila*. By contrast, infections due to the gram-positive organisms *S. aureus* and *S. epidermidis* have increased, particularly those associated with the use of indwelling intravenous catheters.

The use of broad spectrum antimicrobial agents is paramount in treating the clinically ill compromised host. The mainstay of such treatment, especially in the febrile, granulocytopenic patient, includes at least 2 bactericidal antibiotics effective against *Pseudomonas* and other aerobic bacteria. An aminoglycoside plus an antipseudomonal β-lactam antibiotic or 2 antipseudomonal β-lactams are the usual initial choices. Indwelling central venous catheters can usually be left in place unless gram-negative bacilli, *Candida*, or corynebacteria or other gram-positive organisms are recovered from blood or the line site. If lesions that represent typical or atypical viral infections are present, antiviral therapy should be initiated. Empirical antiviral therapy should not be considered unless some evidence of clinical suspicion for viral agents is present.

The role of active immunization with bacterial and viral vaccines has been especially important in children in preventing potentially lethal infectious diseases such as poliomylitis, pertussis, diphtheria and tetanus. Although killed vaccines or toxoids can be administered with safety, live vaccines should be avoided as their safety in immunodeficient patients is uncertain. An exception to this is varicella vaccine, widely used in the USA and Japan to protect susceptible children with leukaemia or other malignant diseases. A major drawback of active immunization for immunosuppressed patients is the possible inability of the host to provide an adequate immune response to the vaccination. Conversely, the use of immunostimulants in some organ transplant recipients has led to accelerated rejection of the donor organ.

Preliminary studies have been initiated on the effect of immunomodulators such as cytokines, interleukins and interferons. Other biological compounds such as granulocyte colony-stimulating factor, which prevents infection in patients with chemotherapy-induced neutropenia, and granulocyte-macrophage colony-stimulating factor (GMCSF), which accelerates the recovery of bone marrow function in neutropenic patients, appear to be effective in preventing bacterial infections. A drawback associated with these biological preparations is the difficulty in obtaining adequate yields of cells and the risk to the recipients of virus transmission which has restricted their widespread use. The use of recombinant DNA technology to synthesize these compounds is an alternative approach.

Granulocyte transfusions can provide a brief respite to clinically ill granulocytopenic patients. Use of these immunomodulating agents should be limited to controlling a known bacterial infection in those patients receiving appropriate antibiotics who fail to respond to therapy. Specific monoclonal antibody therapy and the use of cytokine therapy are being considered in control trials and are considerations for the future.

It is becoming clear that the traditional strategies for the treatment and prevention of infection that have centred on antimicrobial agents directed at the offending organism will be altered. The use of immunomodulating agents (biological response modifiers or biological therapeutics) will have (and in some cases has had) an important role as adjuvant therapy in infection. An all too common example is the development of sepsis following gram-negative infection. The release of endotoxin from the cell wall of these organisms initiates a cascade of events that includes macrophage activation and cytokine release that frequently leads to clinical sepsis and its complications and, ultimately, death of the patient. Antibiotic therapy directed at the organism alone cannot block the sequence of events that follows. Antibody directed at the core LPS or lipid A of gram-negative organisms is thought to have sufficient broad specificity that it would be useful in treating infections before the identity of the aetiological agent is known. Clinical trials with such a biological product have been initiated but the results did not clearly demonstrate the superiority of the product to license its use – at least in the USA (Greenberg et al. 1992). Additional clinical trials have been initiated.

4.2 Diagnosis and treatment of infection

Prompt recognition of the onset of infection and the identification of the aetiological agent(s) associated with it are essential if treatment is to succeed. Some indication of the likely aetiological agents that cause infection in this group of patients can be inferred from the nature of the patient's underlying disease or the type of immunosuppressive therapy employed (see section 3, p. 88). When planning the initial empirical antimicrobial treatment regimen for these patients it is often necessary to 'cover' the range of possible aetiological agents.

Heretofore laboratory diagnostic methods lacked sensitivity and speed of performance. In the clinical microbiology laboratory there has been a traditional dependence on cultural methods; however, there is a trend toward the use of non-cultural methods and the use of antigen detection, molecular methods using PCR-based assays, and non-specific markers for the early detection of infection (see Chapter 12). Generally, the fundamental approach involves cultures taken of blood and any site and body fluid suspected of being infected.

An appreciation of the rapidity and analytical sensitivity of the several diagnostic approaches practised today is outlined in Table 7.8. A typical criticism of molecular-based diagnoses is that the antimicrobial susceptibility of the offending aetiological agent cannot be determined because it has not as yet been recovered and isolated. However, it should be noted that selected genetic loci within the organism genome can be probed for those targets that can express resistance to a particular antimicrobial agent so that the laboratory could simultaneously **detect, identify** and **determine the resistance profile of** a pathogen. The table also clarifies for clinicians the conundrum of how a microscopic smear for acid-fast bacilli could be reported as negative when the culture (some 5–8 weeks later) is positive for *M. tuberculosis*.

The approach to the diagnosis and management of patients with specific clinical syndromes will vary, but 3 conditions that are typical of microbial infections in immunodeficient patients follow.

Table 7.8 Limits of diagnostic modalities; comparative rapidity (TAT)[a] and analytical sensitivity

Diagnostic modality	TAT	Analytic sensitivity (cfu)[b]
Microscopy (light)[c]	10 min	10^5–10^6
Culture	19 h	1
Immunological[d]	10–20 min	10^{4-5}
LAL[e]	~1 h	10^3
Probe, nucleic acid	2–4 h	$10^{3.5-4.5}$
PCR	~4 h	<1

[a]Turn-around time; time interval from receipt of clinical specimen to report.
[b]Colony forming units.
[c]UV light increases (lowers) the detection limit.
[d]Includes latex agglutination and coaggutination; EIA and countercurrent immunoelectrophoresis (CIE) require additional time.
[e]*Limulus* amoebocyte lysate.

FEBRILE NEUTROPENIC HOSTS

Fever almost invariably complicates the course of remission-induction therapy for leukaemia and bone marrow transplant recipients, especially when patients suffer profound bone marrow failure for several weeks. Fever is the hallmark of infection but is not specific for it. An infection can begin and progress in the absence of fever. Frequently in this patient group there are recurrent febrile episodes and on each occasion the possibility of septicaemia should be considered, especially in the presence of shock and despite the absence of any localized signs of infection. Because of the patient's inability to mount an immunological response, the typical signs of infection due to soft tissue invasion are often absent.

The prime concern is to institute prompt antibiotic prophylaxis-treatment while pursuing the laboratory diagnosis. Heavy reliance is placed upon blood culture for the detection of bacteraemia, but conventional or automated radiometric, fluorometric, or colorimetric techniques give positive results in a limited number of cases, c. 50%. Several studies of blood cultures have indicated that for patients not previously receiving antimicrobial therapy, most pyogenic organisms showed detectable growth after 3 days of incubation. If, however, the patient has received antimicrobial therapy, the growth of organisms may be suppressed for longer periods. If 3 sets of blood cultures are drawn they are adequate to diagnose bacteraemia and any more than this number is unnecessary (Washington 1975). Fungi are difficult to detect in the blood, especially *Aspergillus* species, as they may spread through the lymphatics rather than the bloodstream. When fungaemia is suspected, supplementary cultures by another blood culture method, for example the lysis–centrifugation method, should be considered. Immunological approaches for the detection of fungal antigens by latex or ELISA methods may prove to be a significant advantage.

Measuring the serum level of acute phase reactant has been examined as a tool for distinguishing bacterial from fungal or viral infection or at least infective from non-infective causes of fever. Elevated serum levels of C-reactive protein can usually distinguish bacterial from non-bacterial aetiologies; however, there is a time delay before significant elevation is reached, by which time treatment may already have been initiated.

In earlier studies of infection in neutropenic patients, the enterobacteria were the predominant pathogens. The combination of a broad spectrum penicillin with an aminoglycoside became well established as the first line of empirical therapy against this group of organisms (Gaya 1984). The increasing incidence of gram-positive bacteraemia associated with infection of indwelling vascular catheters has demonstrated the larger role of gram-positive organisms and it has become necessary to consider the use of vancomycin empirically in fevers.

Probably the most important determinant of success of treatment is bone marrow recovery. Generally, patients with prolonged profound neutropenia fare less well. The use of granulocyte transfusion and the use of specific antibacterial sera are questionable supplements to antimicrobial therapy in the treatment of gram-negative septicaemia. The use of adjuvant therapy in this group of patients continues to be explored (see section 4.1, p. 99).

FEVER WITH PULMONARY INFILTRATES

Pulmonary abnormalities may take the form of consolidation, diffuse infiltration, or nodular or excavating lesions or both (Fishman 1986). However, non-microbial disorders such as pulmonary oedema or embolism or malignant disease may present similar appearances. Occasionally extrapulmonary symptoms present with septicaemic diseases or Legionnaires' disease or cryptococcosis.

Every effort should be made to provide prompt laboratory confirmation of this impairment. Suitable respiratory specimens are difficult to obtain and some form of invasive sampling procedure such as fibreoptic bronchoscopy with bronchoalveolar lavage is often required. Antigen detection methods for CMV and *Pneumocystis* have the advantage of sensitivity and rapidity, but cultural examination should not be omitted because it is often more sensitive, serves to detect mixed infections and provides opportunities to test the susceptibility of pathogens to antimicrobial agents (see Table 7.8). Examination of specimens from extrapulmonary sources should also be considered; blood and bone marrow culture and the examination of serum and urine for fungal antigens are advisable.

CENTRAL NERVOUS SYSTEM INVOLVEMENT

Infections in this area develop as part of the disseminated disease and are well recognized in chronically immunosuppressed patients and as a feature of AIDS. Often, there is an insidious onset and the infection is not diagnosed or recognized until at an advanced stage.

The major causes of CNS infection are the established opportunistic pathogens such as *C. neoformans*, *L. monocytogenes* and *N. asteroides*, but collectively conventional pathogens are more often implicated in the immunosuppressed (Hooper, Pruitt and Rubin 1982). Infrequently, infection is due to neurotropic agents such as JC virus which is responsible for multifocal leucoencephalopathy.

Neurological and radiological investigations that include electroencephalogram and CT scan can distinguish focal from diffuse lesions in the brain and the difficulty in obtaining histological material may lead to delay in establishing diagnosis. CSF examination should include microscopy, cryptococcal antigen detection and culture for conventional as well as unusual agents of meningitis and viruses. The quantity of cells, glucose and protein levels in the CNS are good indicators of bacterial, viral, or 'aseptic' meningitis. Blood cultures and serological tests are also advised.

DIARRHOEA

Enteric pathogens are frequently the cause of diarrhoea as part of systemic infection but for individuals in the hospital for more than 3 days it is unlikely that the typical enteric pathogens (*Salmonella, Shigella, Yersinia*) should be considered as aetiology for this condition. A more likely reason is the possibility of antibiotic-associated enterocolitis and testing for toxin associated with *Clostridium difficile* is a major finding. Viral gastroenteritis due to the adenovirus, rotavirus and enteroviruses is common and often clinically severe in immunodeficient children. In addition to conventional microscopic and culture examination of faeces, it may be necessary to utilize special staining methods for *Cryptosporidium* species along with antigen detection and culture examination for viruses.

5 FUTURE CONSIDERATIONS

As we advance inexorably to the next millennium, one must pose the question of how Herculean advances in clinical medicine will further predispose patients to new and as yet undiagnosed aetiological agents. The iatrogenic manipulations of medical practitioners clearly will place patients at risk for new or emerging agents. The potential use of xenografts, artificial blood supplies and blood sterilizing and exchange equipment will produce, no doubt, other infections that compromise the host as a result of his or her underlying condition. The advances that have been made are the use of antimicrobial-impregnated vascular access devices and catheters to reduce the risk of infection associated with these devices and the use of biotherapeutics. Emerging pathogens challenge both the diagnostic laboratory and clinician with the recognition and detection of these agents; they also raise the spectre of new avenues for resistant mechanisms to be expressed against the dwindling armamentarium of effective anti-infective agents.

REFERENCES

AIDS Clinical Trials Group, 1992, Mortality in patients with the acquired immunodeficiency syndrome treated with either foscarnet or ganciclovir for cytomegalovirus retinitis, *N Engl J Med*, **326:** 213–20.

Alberti KGMM, Hockada TDR, 1987, *Oxford Textbook of Medicine*, 2nd edn, eds Weatherall DJ, Ledingham JGG, Warrell DA, Oxford University Press, Oxford, 951.

Alland D, Kalkut GE et al., 1994, Transmission of tuberculosis in New York City: an analysis by DNA fingerprinting conventional epidemiologic methods, *N Engl J Med*, **330:** 1710–16.

Ament ME, Ochs HD et al., 1977, Structure and function of the gastrointestinal tract in primary immunodeficiency syndromes, a study of 39 patients, *Medicine (Baltimore)*, **52:** 227–50.

Arduino RC, Johnson PC et al., 1993, Nocardiosis in renal transplant recipients undergoing immunosuppression with cyclosporine, *Clin Infect Dis*, **16:** 505–12.

Barnes RA, Rogers TR, 1987, An evaluation of empirical antibiotic therapy in febrile neutropenic patients, *Br J Haematol*, **66:** 137–40.

Barnes RA, Rogers TR, 1989, Control of an outbreak of nosocomial aspergillosis by laminar air-flor isolation, *J Hosp Infect*, **14:** 89–94.

Beamen MIH, Luft BJ, Remington JS, 1992, Prophylaxis for toxoplasmosis in AIDS, *Ann Intern Med*, **117:** 163–4.

Beaman BL, Burnside J et al., 1976, Nocardial infections in the United States, 1972–1974, *J Infect Dis*, **134:** 286–93.

Berche P, Gaillard J-L, Sansonetti PJ, 1987, Intracellular growth of *Listeria monocytogenes* as a prerequisite for in vivo induction of T cell-mediated immunity, *J Immunol*, **138:** 2266–71.

Bernard EM, Kent A et al., 1992, *The Medical Clinics of North America Series: Medical Management of AIDS Patients*, WB Saunders, Philadelphia, 107–19.

Berner J, Kadian M et al., 1993, Prophylactic recombinant hepatitis B vaccine in patients undergoing orthotopic liver transplantation, *Transplant Proc*, **25:** 1751–2.

Bodey GP, 1988, The emergence of fungi as major hospital pathogens, *J Hosp Infect*, **11, Suppl. A:** 411–26.

Bodey GP, Jadeja L, Elting L, 1985, *Pseudomonas* bacteremia. Retrospective analysis of 410 episodes, *Arch Intern Med*, **145:** 1621–9.

Bodey GP, Buckley M et al., 1966, Quantitative relationships between circulating leukocytes and infection in patients with acute leukemia, *Ann Intern Med*, **64:** 328–40.

Bodey GP, Elting L et al., 1986, *Escherichia coli* bacteremia in cancer patients, *Am J Med*, **81, Suppl. 1A:** 85–95.

Bryceson ADM, 1987, *Oxford Textbook of Medicine*, 2nd edn, eds Weatherall DJ, Ledingham JGG, Warrell DA, Oxford University Press, Oxford, 524.

Centers for Disease Control, 1992, National action plan to combat multidrug-resistant tuberculosis, *Morbid Mortal Weekly Rep*, **41:** 59–71.

Centers for Disease Control and Prevention, 1992, Recommendations for prophylaxis against *Pneumocystis carinii* pneumonia for adults and adolescents infected with human immunodeficiency virus, *Morbid Mortal Weekly Rep*, **RR-4:** 1–11.

Centers for Disease Control and Prevention, 1995, Tuberculosis morbidity – United States, 1994, *Morbid Mortal Weekly Rep*, **44:** 387–9, 395.

Chaisson RE, Moore RD et al., 1992, Incidence and natural history of *Mycobacterium avium* complex infections in patients with advanced HIV disease treated with zidovudine, *Am Rev Respir Dis*, **146:** 285–9.

Chandra RK, 1993, Nutrition and immunity, *Clinical Aspects of Immunology*, 5th edn, eds Lackham BJ, Peter K et al., Blackwell Scientific, London, 1325–38.

Chernik NL, Armstrong D, Posner JB, 1977, Central nervous system infections in patients with cancer, *Cancer*, **40:** 268–74.

Chou S, 1986, Acquisition of donor strains of cytomegalovirus by renal-transplant recipients, *N Engl J Med*, **314:** 1418–23.

Christenson JC, Hill HR, 1994, Infections complicating congenital immunodeficiency syndromes, *Clinical Approach to Infection in the Compromised Host*, 3rd edn, eds Rubin RH, Young LS, Plenum, New York, 521–43.

Cohen J, Rees AJ, Williams G, 1988, A prospective randomized trial of perioperative antibiotic prophylaxis in renal transplantation, *J Hosp Infect*, **11**: 357–63.

Cohen J, Pinching AJ et al., 1982, Infection and immunosuppression, *Q J Med*, **51**: 1–15.

Conte JE Jr, Chernoff D et al., 1990, Intravenous or inhaled pentamidine for treating *Pneumocystis carinii* pneumonia in AIDS. A randomized trial, *Ann Intern Med*, **113**: 203–9.

Daley CL, Small PM et al., 1992, An outbreak of tuberculosis with accelerated progression among persons infected with the human immunodeficiency virus: an analysis using restriction-length polymorphisms, *N Engl J Med*, **326**: 231–5.

Darbyshire PJ, Weightman NC, Speller DCE, 1985, Problems associated with indwelling central venous catheters, *Arch Dis Child*, **60**: 129–34.

Dauber JH, Paradis IL, Dummer JS, 1990, Infectious complications in pulmonary allograft recipients, *Clin Chest Med*, **11**: 291–308.

Davis-Scibienski C, Beaman BL, 1980, Interaction of *Nocardia asteroides* with rabbit alveolar macrophages: effect of growth phase and viability on phagosome-lyosome fusion, *Infect Immunol*, **29**: 24–9.

DeCock KM, Benoit S et al., 1989, Tuberculosis and HIV infection in sub-Saharan Africa, *JAMA*, **268**: 1581–7.

Degos F, Lugassy C et al., 1988, Hepatitis B virus and hepatitis B-related viral infection in renal transplant recipients, *Gastroenterology*, **94**: 151–6.

Delaney V, Sumrani N et al., 1993, Mycobacterial infections in renal allograft recipients, *Transplant Proc*, **25**: 2288–9.

Diamond RD, 1995, *Cryptococcus neoformans, Principles and Practice of Infectious Diseases*, 4th edn, eds Mandell GL, Bennett JE, Dolin R, Churchill Livingstone, New York, 2331–40.

Diamond RD, Clark RA, 1982, Damage to *Aspergillus fumigatus* and *Rhizopus oryzae* hyphae by oxidative and nonoxidative microbicidal products of human neutrophiles in vitro, *Infect Immun*, **38**: 487–95.

Diamond RD, Root RK, Bennett JE, 1972, Factors influencing killing of *Cryptococcus neoformans* by human leukocytes in vitro, *J Infect Dis*, **125**: 367–76.

Dobkin JF, 1995, Opportunistic infections and AIDS, *Infect Med*, **12**: 58–79.

Douglas SD, Goldberg LS, Fudenberg HH, 1970, Clinical, serologic and leukocyte function studies on patients with idiopathic 'acquired' agammaglobulinemia and their families, *Am J Med*, **48**: 48–53.

Dummer SJ, Montero GC et al., 1986, Infections in heart–lung transplant recipients, *Transplantation*, **41**: 725–9.

Dunn DL, 1990, Problems related to immunosuppression, *Crit Care Clin*, **6**: 955–77.

Dunn DL, Najarian JS, 1991, Infectious complications of transplant surgery, *Principles and Management of Surgical Infections*, eds Davis JM, Shires JG, JB Lippincott, Philadelphia, 425–63.

Edelstein PH, 1993, Legionnaires' disease, *Clin Infect Dis*, **16**: 741–9.

Eng RH, Bishburg E et al., 1986, Cryptococcal infections in patients with acquired immunodeficiency syndrome, *Am J Med*, **81**: 19–23.

EORTC, 1987, Ceftazidime combined with a short or long course of amikacin for empirical therapy of gram-negative bacteremia in cancer patients with granulocytopenia. The EORTC International Antimicrobial Therapy Cooperative Group, *N Engl J Med*, **317**: 1692–8.

Espersen F, Frimodt-Moller N et al., 1987, *Staphylococcus aureus* bacteremia in patients with hematological malignancies and/or agranulocytosis, *Acta Med Scand*, **222**: 465–70.

Feld R, Bodey GP, Groschel D, 1976, Mycobacteriosis in patients with malignant disease, *Arch Intern Med*, **136**: 67–70.

Fernandez-Guerrero ML, Aguada JM et al., 1987, Visceral leish-

maniasis in immunocompromised hosts, *Am J Med*, **83**: 1098–102.

Filice GA, Niewoehner DE, 1987, Contribution of neutrophils and cell-mediated immunity to control of *Nocardia asteroides* in murine lungs, *J Infect Dis*, **156**: 113–21.

Fischer A, 1992, Severe combined immunodeficiencies, *Immunodefic Rev*, **3**: 83–100.

Fisher B, Armstrong D et al., 1981, Invasive aspergillosis, *Am J Med*, **71**: 571–7.

Fishman JA, 1986, Diagnostic approach to pneumonia in the immunocompromised host, *Semin Respir Infect*, **1**: 133–44.

Fraser DW, Tsai TR et al., 1977, Legionnaires disease: description of an epidemic of pneumonia, *N Engl J Med*, **297**: 1189–97.

Fromtling RA, Shadomy HJ, 1986, An overview of macrophage–fungal interactions, *Mycopathologia*, **93**: 77–93.

Fung JC, Donta ST, Tilton RC, 1986, Candida detection system (CAND-TEC) to differentiate between *Candida albicans* colonization and disease, *J Clin Microbiol*, **24**: 542–7.

Gantz NM, Myeromitz RL et al., 1975, Listeriosis in immunosuppressed patients. A cluster of eight cases, *Am J Med*, **58**: 637–43.

Gaya H, 1984, Rational basis for the choice of regimens for empirical therapy of sepsis in granulocytopenic patients, *Clin Haematol*, **13**: 573–86.

Gerson SL, Talbot GH et al., 1984, Prolonged granulocytopenia: the major risk factor for invasive pulmonary aspergillosis in patients with acute leukemia, *Ann Intern Med*, **100**: 345–51.

Glenn J, Cotton D et al., 1988, Anorectal infections in patients with malignant diseases, *Rev Infect Dis*, **10**: 42–52.

Gottesdiener KM, 1989, Transplanted infections: donor-to-host transmission with the allograft, *Ann Intern Med*, **110**: 1001–16.

Greenberg MS, Friedman H et al., 1987, A comparative study of herpes simplex infection in renal transplant and leukemic patients, *J Infect Dis*, **156**: 280–7.

Greenberg RN, Wilson KM et al., 1992, Observations using anti-endotoxin antibody (E5) as adjuvant therapy in humans with suspected gram-negative sepsis, *Crit Care Med*, **20**: 730–5.

Greenwood BM, 1987, *Oxford Textbook of Medicine*, 2nd edn, eds Weatherall DJ, Ledingham JGG, Warrell DA, Oxford University Press, Oxford, 51.

Hawkins CC, Gold JW et al., 1986, *Mycobacterium avium* complex infections in patients with the acquired immunodeficiency syndrome, *Ann Intern Med*, **105**: 184–8.

Hickman RO, Buckner CD et al., 1979, A modified right atrial catheter for access to the venous system in marrow transplant recipients, *Surg Gynecol Obstet*, **148**: 871–5.

Hofflin JM, Potasman I et al., 1987, Infectious complications in heart transplant recipients receiving cyclosporine and corticosteroids, *Ann Intern Med*, **106**: 209–16.

Hooper DC, Pruitt AA, Rubin RH, 1982, Central nervous system infection in the chronically immunosuppressed, *Medicine (Baltimore)*, **61**: 166–88.

Horn R, Wong B et al., 1985, Fungemia in a cancer hospital: changing frequency, earlier onset, and results of therapy, *Rev Infect Dis*, **7**: 646–55.

Horsburgh CR Jr, 1991, *Mycobacterium avium* complex infection in the acquired immunodeficiency syndrome, *N Engl J Med*, **324**: 1332–8.

Horsburgh CR Jr, Chin DP et al., 1994, Environmental risk factors for acquisition of *Mycobacterium avium* complex in person with human immunodeficiency virus infection, *J Infect Dis*, **170**: 362–7.

Houang ET, Lovett IS et al., 1980, *Nocardia asteroides* infection – a transmissible disease, *J Hosp Infect*, **1**: 31–40.

Hoy JF, Rolston KV et al., 1987, *Mycobacterium fortuitum* bacteremia in patients with cancer and long-term catheters, *Am J Med*, **83**: 213–17.

Hudson LD, 1989, *Infection Control by Selective Decontamination*, Springer-Verlag, Berlin, 34.

Jacobson DR, Zolla-Prazner S, 1986, Immunosuppression and infection in multiple myeloma, *Semin Oncol*, **13**: 282–90.

Jacobson MA, 1992, Mycobacterial diseases: tuberculosis and *Mycobacterium avium* complex, *The Medical Management of AIDS*, 3rd edn, ed. Sandi MA, WB Saunders, Philadelphia, 284–96.

Jereb JA, Burwen DR et al., 1993, Nosocomial outbreak of tuberculosis in renal transplant unit: application of a new technique for restriction fragment length polymorphism analysis of *Mycobacterium tuberculosis* isolates, *J Infect Dis*, **168**: 1219–24.

de Jongh CA, Joshi JH et al., 1986, Antibiotic synergism and response in gram-negative bacteremia in granulocytopenic cancer patients, *Am J Med*, **80**: 96–100.

Jonsson S, Wallace RJ et al., 1986, Recurrent *Nocardia pneumonia* in an adult with chronic granulomatous disease, *Am Rev Respir Dis*, **133**: 930–2.

Kaplan JE, Masur H et al., 1995, USPHS/IFDSA guidelines for the prevention of opportunistic infections in persons infected with human immunodeficiency virus: introduction, *Clin Infect Dis*, **21, Suppl. 1**: S1–11.

Kaplan MH, Armstrong D, Rosen P, 1974, Tuberculosis complicating neoplastic disease. A review of 201 cases, *Cancer*, **33**: 850–8.

Kauffmann SH, Hug E et al., 1987, Specific lysis of *Listeria mono-cytogenes*-infected macrophages by class II-restricted L3T4 + T cells, *Eur J Immunol*, **17**: 237–46.

Keating MR, Wilhelm MR, 1993, Management of infectious complications following liver transplantation, *Curr Clin Top Infect Dis*, **13**: 226–49.

Kiehn TE, Fitzroy F et al., 1985, Infections caused by *Mycobacterium avium* complex in immunocompromised patients: diagnosis by blood culture and fecal examination, antimicrobial susceptibility tests, and morphological and seroagglutination characteristics, *J Clin Microbiol*, **21**: 168–73.

King A, Rampling A et al., 1984, Neutropenic enterocolitis due to *Clostridium septicum* infection, *J Clin Pathol*, **37**: 335–43.

Kirby BD, Snyder KM et al., 1980, Legionnaires' disease: report of 65 nosocomially acquired cases and a review of the literature, *Medicine (Baltimore)*, **59**: 188–205.

Klugman KP, 1990, Pneumococcal resistance to antibiotics, *Clin Microbiol Rev*, **3**: 171–96.

Korvich JA, Marsh WJ et al., 1991, *Pseudomonas aeruginosa* bacteremia in patients undergoing liver transplantation: an emerging problem, *Surgery*, **109**: 662–8.

Kusne S, Dummer JS et al., 1988, Infections after liver transplantation. An analysis of 101 consecutive cases, *Medicine (Baltimore)*, **67**: 132–43.

Levy RM, Bredesen DE, 1988, Central nervous system dysfunction in acquired immunodeficiency syndrome, *J Acquired Immune Defic Syndr*, **1**: 41–64.

Lichtenstein IH, MacGregor RR, 1983, Mycobacterial infections in renal transplant recipients: report of five cases and review of the literature, *Rev Infect Dis*, **5**: 216–26.

Locksley RM, Wilson CB, 1995, Cell-mediated immunity and its role in host defenses, *Principles and Practice of Infectious Disease*, 4th edn, eds Mandell GL, Bennett JE, Dolin R, Churchill Livingstone, New York, 102–49.

Longworth DL, Weller PF, 1986, *Current Clinical Topics in Infectious Diseases*, eds Remington JS, Scwartz MN, McGraw-Hill, New York, 1.

Luft BJ, Remington J, 1992, Toxoplasmic encephalitis in AIDS, *Clin Infect Dis*, **15**: 211–22.

Marston BJ, Lipman HB, Breiman RF, 1994, Surveillance for Legionnaires' disease: risk factors for morbidity and mortality, *Arch Intern Med*, **154**: 2417–22.

Mascola L, Lieb L et al., 1988, Listeriosis: an uncommon opportunistic infection in patients with acquired immunodeficiency syndrome, *Am J Med*, **84**: 162–4.

Mauer JR, Tullis ED et al., 1992, Infectious complications following isolated lung transplantation, *Chest*, **101**: 1056–9.

Meisel JL, Perera DR et al., 1976, Overwhelming watery diarrhea associated with a *Cryptosporidium* in an immunosuppressed patient, *Gastroenterology*, **70**: 1156–60.

Merkow L, Pardo M et al., 1968, Lysosomal stability during phagocytosis of *Aspergillus flavus* spores by alveolar macrophages of cortisone-treated mice, *Science*, **160**: 79–81.

Mower WR, Hawkins JA, Nelson EW, 1986, Postsplenectomy infection in patients with chronic leukemia, *Am J Surg*, **152**: 583–6.

Murphy JW, Mosley RL et al., 1988, Serological, electrophoretic, and biological properties of *Cryptococcus neoformans*, *Infect Immun*, **56**: 424–31.

Murray JF, Finegold SM et al., 1961, The changing spectrum of nocardiosis, *Am Rev Respir Dis*, **8**: 315–30.

Myerowitz RL, Medeiros AA, O'Brien TF, 1972, Bacterial infection in renal homotransplant recipients. A study of fifty-three bacteremic episodes, *Am J Med*, **53**: 308–14.

Narain JP, Raviglione MC, Koch IA, 1992, HIV-associated tuberculosis in developing countries: epidemiology and strategies for prevention, *Tuberc Lung Dis*, **73**: 311–21.

Nguyen ML, Yu VL et al., 1991, Legionella infection, *Clin Chest Med*, **12**: 257–68.

Ninane J, Chessells JM, 1981, Serious infections during continuing treatment of acute lymphoblastic leukaemia, *Arch Dis Child*, **56**: 841–4.

Northfelt DW, Clement MJ, Safrin S, 1990, Extrapulmonary pneumocystis: clinical features in human immunodeficiency virus infection, *Medicine (Baltimore)*, **69**: 392–8.

Parker F Jr, Jackson H Jr et al., 1932, Studies of diseases of lymphoid and myeloid tissues; coexistence of tuberculosis with Hodgkin's disease and other forms of malignant lymphoma, *Am J Med Sci*, **184**: 694–9.

Paya CV, 1993, Fungal infections in solid-organ transplantation, *Clin Infect Dis*, **16**: 677–88.

Paya CV, Hermans PE et al., 1989, Incidence, distribution, and outcome of episodes of infection in 100 orthotopic liver transplantations, *Mayo Clin Proc*, **64**: 555–64.

Peters TG, Reiter CG, Bowell RI, 1984, Transmission of tuberculosis by kidney transplantation, *Transplantation*, **38**: 514–15.

Peterson PK, Balfour HH et al., 1981, Fever in renal transplant recipients: causes, prognostic significance and changing patterns at the University of Minnesota Hospital, *Am J Med*, **71**: 345–51.

Pirsch JD, Maki DG, 1986, Infectious complications in adults with bone marrow transplantation and T-cell depletion of donor marrow. Increased susceptibility to fungal infections, *Ann Intern Med*, **104**: 619–31.

Porter SB, Sande MA, 1992, Toxoplasmosis of the central nervous system in the acquired immunodeficiency syndrome, *N Engl J Med*, **327**: 1643–8.

Portnoy DA, 1988, Role of hemolysin for the intracellular growth of *Listeria monocytogenes*, *J Exp Med*, **167**: 1459–71.

Portnoy D, Whiteside HE et al., 1984, Treatment of intestinal cryptosporidiosis with spiramycin, *Ann Intern Med*, **101**: 202–4.

Pullan CR, Noble TC et al., 1976, Atypical measles infections in leukaemic children on immunosuppressive treatment, *Br Med J*, **1**: 1562–5.

Raviglione MC, Narain JP, Kochi A, 1992, HIV-associated tuberculosis in developing countries: clinical features, diagnosis, and treatment, *Bull W H O*, **70**: 515–26.

Raviglione MC, Snider DE, Kochi A, 1995, Global epidemiology of tuberculosis: morbidity and mortality of a worldwide epidemic, *JAMA*, **273**: 220–6.

de Repentigny L, Reiss E, 1984, Current trends in immunodiagnosis of candidiasis and aspergillosis, *Rev Infect Dis*, **6**: 301–12.

von Reyn CF, Maslow JN et al., 1994, Persistent colonization of potable water as a source of *Mycobacterium avium* infection in AIDS, *Lancet*, **343**: 1137–41.

Robertson MD, Seaton A et al., 1987, Suppression of host defenses by *Aspergillus fumigatus*, *Thorax*, **42**: 19–25.

Robinette LD, Fraumeni Jr JF, 1977, Splenectomy and subsequent mortality in veterans of the 1939–45 war, *Lancet*, **2:** 127–9.

Roig J, Carreres A, Domingo C, 1993, Treatment of Legionnaire's disease, *Drugs*, **46:** 63–79.

Rouse BT, Horohov DW, 1986, Immunosuppression in viral infections, *Rev Infect Dis*, **8:** 850–73.

Rubin RH, 1991, Pre-emptive therapy in immunocompromised hosts, *N Engl J Med*, **324:** 1057–9.

Rubin RH, Wolfson JS et al., 1981, Infections in the renal transplant recipient, *Am J Med*, **70:** 405–11.

Ruebush TK, 1987, *Babesia, Oxford Textbook of Medicine*, 2nd edn, eds Weatherall DJ, Ledingham JGG, Warrell DA, Oxford University Press, Oxford, 5.502–5.504.

Ruskin J, Remington JS, 1976, Toxoplasmosis in the compromised host, *Ann Intern Med*, **84:** 193–9.

Rusthoven JJ, Ahlgren P et al., 1988, Varicella-zoster infection in adult cancer patients. A population study, *Arch Intern Med*, **148:** 1561–6.

Salata RA, King RE et al., 1986, *Listeria monocytogenes* cerebritis bacteremia, and cutaneous lesions complicating hairy cell leukemia, *Am J Med*, **81:** 1068–72.

Schimpff SC, Bennett JE, 1975, Abnormalities in cell-mediated immunity in patients with *Cryptococcus neoformans* infection, *J Clin Immunol*, **55:** 430–41.

Schimpff SC, Klastersky J, 1993, Infectious complications in bone marrow transplantation, *Recent Results Cancer Res*, 132.

Schimpff SC, Young VM et al., 1972, Origin of infection in acute nonlymphocytic leukemia. Significance of hospital acquisition of potential pathogens, *Ann Intern Med*, **77:** 707–14.

Scowden EB, Schaffner W, Stone WJ, 1978, Overwhelming strongyloidiasis, *Medicine (Baltimore)*, **57:** 527–44.

Shadduck JA, 1989, Human microsporidiosis and AIDS, *Rev Infect Dis*, **11:** 203–7.

Sheretz RJ, Belani A et al., 1987, Impact of air filtration on nosocomial *Aspergillus* infections, *Am J Med*, **83:** 709–18.

Singh N, Dummer JS et al., 1988, Infections with cytomegalovirus and other herpes viruses in 121 liver transplant recipients: transmission by donated organ and the effect of OKT3 antibodies, *J Infect Dis*, **158:** 124–31.

Small PM, Hopewell PC et al., 1994, The epidemiology of tuberculosis in San Francisco: a population-based study using conventional and molecular methods, *N Engl J Med*, **330:** 1703–9.

Smith S, Jackson R et al., 1993, Selective bowel decontamination in pediatric liver transplants, *Transplantation*, **55:** 1306–9.

Soave R, Armstrong D, 1986, Cryptosporidium and cryptosporidiosis, *Rev Infect Dis*, **8:** 1012–23.

Speirs G, Warren RE, Rampling A, 1988, *Clostridium tertium* septicemia in patients with neutropenia, *J Infect Dis*, **158:** 1336–40.

Stevens DA, Pier AC et al., 1981, Laboratory evaluation of an outbreak of nocardiosis in immunocompromised hosts, *Am J Med*, **71:** 928–34.

Storring RA, Jameson B et al., 1977, Oral non-absorbed antibiotics prevent infection in acute non-lymphoblastic leukaemia, *Lancet*, **2:** 837–40.

Stracher AR, Sepkowitz KA, 1995, Atypical mycobacterial infections in HIV disease, *The AIDS Reader*, **5:** 14–25.

Straus WL, Ostroff SM et al., 1994, Clinical and epidemiologic characteristics of *Mycobacterium haemophilum*, an emerging pathogen in immunocompromised patients, *Ann Intern Med*, **120:** 118–25.

Strencek M, Ferrell L et al., 1992, Mycobacterial infection after liver transplantation: a report of three cases and review of the literature, *Clin Transplant*, **6:** 55–61.

Sudre P, ten Dam G, Kochi A, 1992, Tuberculosis: a global overview of the situation today, *Bull W H O*, **70:** 149–59.

Tolkoff-Rubin NE, Rubin HR, 1988, Infections in the organ transplant recipient, *Organ Transplantation and Replacement*, ed. Cerilli JG, JB Lippincott, Philadelphia, 445–61.

Tolkoff-Rubin NE, Rubin R, 1992, Opportunistic fungal and bacterial infections in renal transplant recipient, *J Am Soc Nephrol*, **2:** S264–9.

Walsh TJ, Lee J et al., 1991, Empiric therapy with amphotericin B in febrile granulocytopenia patients, *Rev Infect Dis*, **13:** 496–503.

Walzer PD, 1995, *Pneumocystis carinii, Principles and Practice of Infectious Diseases*, 4th edn, eds Mandell GL, Bennett JE, Dolin R, Churchill Livingstone, New York, 2475–87.

Washington JA II, 1975, Blood cultures – principles and techniques, *Mayo Clin Proc*, **59:** 91–8.

Weber R, Bryan RT, 1994, Microsporidial infections in immunodeficient and immunocompetent patients, *Clin Infect Dis*, **19:** 517–21.

Webster AD, Dalgleish AG et al., 1986, Isolation of retroviruses from two patients with 'common variable' hypogammaglobulinaemia, *Lancet*, **1:** 581–3.

Williams DM, Krick JA, Remington JS, 1976, Pulmonary infection in the compromised host, *Am Rev Respir Dis*, **114:** 359–94.

Wolinsky E, 1979, Nontuberculous mycobacteria and associated diseases, *Am Rev Respir Dis*, **119:** 107–59.

Wolinsky E, 1992, Mycobacterial diseases other than tuberculosis, *Clin Infect Dis*, **15:** 1–12.

Yajko DM, Chin DP et al., 1995, *Myobacterium avium* complex in water, food, and soil samples collected from the environment of HIV-infected individuals, *J AIDS Hum Retroviruses*, **9:** 176–82.

Young RC, Bennett JE et al., 1970, Aspergillosis: the spectrum of the disease in 98 patients, *Medicine (Baltimore)*, **49:** 147–73.

Yu VL, 1991, *Legionella pneumophila* and related species, *J Infect Control*, **8, Suppl. A:** S29–35.

Yu VL, 1995, *Legionella pneumophilia* (Legionnaires' disease), *Principles and Practice of Infectious Diseases*, 4th edn, eds Mandell GL, Bennett JE, Dolin R, Churchill Livingstone, New York, 2087–97.

Zimmerli W, 1985, Impaired host defense mechanisms in intensive care unit patients, *Intensive Care Med*, **11:** 174–8.

Zuger A, Louie E et al., 1986, Cryptococcal disease in patients with acquired immunodeficiency syndrome. Diagnostic features and outcome of treatment, *Ann Intern Med*, **104:** 234–40.

Chapter 8

ACTIVE AND PASSIVE IMMUNIZATION

M N Fiordalisi, L C L Lim, K L Kane and J D Folds

In this volume, established vaccines and antisera for preventing or treating bacterial infections are discussed in detail in the relevant chapters (Table 8.1). Here, we give as background an outline of the humoral and cell mediated responses to immunization; a description of the types of vaccine licensed for use in humans; and indications of promising lines of research now being pursued on new types of immunizing agents and methods of delivery. A summary of routine immunizations recommended in the USA is provided as an Appendix. Further information on antibodies and cell mediated immunity will be found in Chapter 3. The immunoprophylaxis of viral diseases is dealt with in Volume 1, Chapter 45.

1 HISTORICAL NOTE

The concept of immunization was based on the observation that those who survived certain diseases often failed to develop the disease a second time. The practice of inoculating material from smallpox pustules for the prevention of the disease (variolation) was practised in China, India and Persia long before it was introduced into Europe (Blaxall 1930). Lady Mary Wortley Montagu (1689–1762), wife of the British Ambassador at Constantinople, saw variolation carried out by Turkish women, and is credited with its popularization in England. Edward Jenner noted that farm workers exposed to open cowpox pustules were not susceptible to the more fatal smallpox infection and suggested that previous exposure to cowpox provided protection against subsequent exposure to smallpox. In 1798, Jenner tested this hypothesis by inoculating a young boy with material from a cowpox pustule on the hand of a milkmaid. He subsequently challenged the boy with the contents of a smallpox pustule and the boy failed to develop smallpox.

Jenner's theory was advanced by the work of other scientists, including Louis Pasteur, Benjamin Waterhouse and Thomas Cimsdale, who demonstrated a causal relationship between micro-organisms and disease. Pasteur also showed that micro-organisms varied in their capacity to produce disease in a host (virulence) and proposed that the virulence of an organism could be altered to develop a strain that would be safe for use as a vaccine against the more serious natural infection. Pasteur demonstrated that during growth under suboptimal conditions or passage in an unrelated host, some micro-organisms lose their virulence, that is they become 'attenuated' but retain the capacity to stimulate protective immunity in the host (Eyquem 1986). Pasteur's concept of virulence and attenuation ultimately led to the use of vaccination as a means of preventing disease. Several of the vaccines currently in use are based on an attenuated form of the infectious organism.

Effective vaccination does not necessarily depend on exposure to an intact micro-organism. In 1888, Roux and Yersin noted that the diphtheria bacillus produced an exotoxin in liquid culture and showed that the disease could be reproduced by injection of the bacteria-free medium of a diphtheria culture (Ada 1993, Grossman 1994). Two years later, von Behring and Kitasato developed a diphtheria antitoxin and demonstrated that serum from an individual exposed to the toxin protected against exposure to the same toxin (passive immunization) (Griffiths 1984). These initial methods of immunization were refined as immunology developed during the late nineteenth

Table 8.1 Summary of licensed vaccines

Vaccine	Type	Chapter	Page	Remarks
Clostridium tetani	Formol toxoid	36	713	These 3 vaccines are adsorbed to alum and given in various combinations
Corynebacterium diphtheriae	Formol toxoid	19	352	
Bordetella pertussis	Whole cell inactivated	18	338	
Bordetella pertussis	Subunit ('acellular')	18	338	Contains various combinations of immunogens. Expensive. Recommended for booster only
Vibrio cholerae	Whole cell inactivated	26	508	See Table 26.3 for parenteral and oral vaccines available
Salmonella Typhi	Inactivated and attenuated	24	472	See Table 24.5 for efficacy of various formulations
Mycobacterium bovis (BCG)	Attenuated	21	405	
Bacillus anthracis	Culture filtrate	40	814	Live spore vaccines used in Russia and China
Yersinia pestis	Inactivated whole cell	44	899	Efficacy uncertain. Recommended only for those at high risk
Haemophilus influenzae (Hib)	Conjugated polysaccharide	17	312	
Neisseria meningitidis	Polysaccharide	17	308	Serogroups A and C. Serogroup B vaccines under development
Streptococcus pneumoniae	Polysaccharide	18	328	Contains antigens of 23 serotypes

and early twentieth centuries and have led to the use of immunization as an important public health measure.

2 OUTLINE OF THE IMMUNE RESPONSE

An appreciation of the challenges involved in the development of successful vaccines requires an understanding of the normal immune response. The basic concepts of humoral and cell mediated immunity will, therefore, be presented here briefly. It will be convenient below to use the term immunogen for substances that initiate or stimulate immune responses, whereas the term antigen will be reserved for substances that combine specifically with antibodies.

2.1 Humoral immunity

Humoral immunity is mediated by immunoglobulins directed specifically against immunogenic foreign substances. Amongst other properties, circulating antibodies have the following roles in humoral immunity:

1 binding to and neutralizing bacterial toxins
2 preventing the entry of bacteria and viruses into cells by blocking their attachment to the cells of the host and
3 binding specifically to bacteria and other particles and so facilitating their phagocytosis (opsonization).

The humoral immune response results in the development of memory B lymphocytes capable of responding to the same antigen as elicited the original response; they have a long functional life span and express immunoglobulin-like (Ig-like) receptors on their surface. These receptors, which are generated on memory B cells in the germinal centres of the lymph nodes and the spleen, are capable of interaction with specific epitopes on the antigen that elicited the response. Since memory cells have previous experience of the antigen and are present in large numbers, they give a more rapid and vigorous secondary antibody response than occurs on first exposure to the antigen.

THE PRIMARY ANTIBODY RESPONSE

Two types of lymphocyte are distinguished according to their site of origin: B lymphocytes arise in the bone marrow (originally observed in the bursa of Fabricius of chickens) and T lymphocytes develop in the thymus (Glick, Chang and Jaap 1956, Claman, Chaperon and Triplett 1966). A primary antibody response is initiated when a foreign substance is specifically recognized by a B lymphocyte. Substances capable of inducing an immune response by B lymphocytes or T lymphocytes are termed immunogens. Their recognition depends on complementarity between the binding region of the surface immunoglobulin (Ig) molecules on the B lymphocyte and an exposed region on the antigen (epitope). During a first (primary) immunogenic challenge, a specifically reacting clone of B lymphocytes proliferates: part of the expanded clone transforms into plasma cells with a limited life span and the remainder become long-lived memory cells. Some evidence suggests that the persistence of memory lymphocytes may depend on the continued presence of immunogen (Gray 1993). The plasma cells are highly specialized and secrete large amounts of immunoglobulins of 5 different classes (IgM, IgD, IgG, IgA and IgE). For a detailed description of immunoglobulins see Chapter 3.

Activation of resting B cells requires 2 signals. The first is provided by the binding of antigen to surface IgM or IgD on a resting B lymphocyte: selective activation follows, since only B cells that express Ig specific for the immunogen are triggered. The second activation signal is provided by contact with T helper lymphocytes (Th) in an antigen-restricted manner and will be discussed in more detail later (Mosier and Coppleson 1968). It takes 5–10 days for B cells to differentiate into plasma cells following antigen activation. This results in a latent period during which serum antibody is not detectable and infection may become established.

Antibodies produced during the primary response belong predominantly to the IgM class, since resting B lymphocytes express only surface IgM and IgD. IgM antibodies bind antigen with low affinity (a measure of strength and stability of interaction). During proliferation, particularly during a second or subsequent exposure to the immunogen, B lymphocytes may be stimulated by interaction with cytokines to switch from production of IgM to other classes of antibodies such as IgG (Esser and Radbruch 1990, Finkelman, Holmes and Katona 1990). IgG is often produced in small amounts during the primary antibody response, but its production usually follows a few days after that of IgM, when isotype switching occurs (Fig. 8.1). Apart from isotype switching, somatic mutation occurs in the Ig genes with the result that antibody of higher affinity is expressed on some B lymphocytes. As the amount of available immunogen decreases, B lymphocytes with high affinity surface Ig are selectively stimulated to proliferate. As a result, the affinity of the Ig produced tends to increase during the course of the response.

THE SECONDARY ANTIBODY RESPONSE

Re-exposure to the immunogen evokes a secondary immune response that differs from the primary response in 4 important ways:

1 only protein antigens induce a secondary antibody response
2 antibody is produced more rapidly, often within 1–3 days
3 it is produced to a higher concentration
4 the higher concentration is maintained for longer.

The secondary antibody response results from the stimulation by the immunogen of resting memory cells that differentiated from activated B lymphocytes during the primary response. The rapid secondary immune response is due to the pre-existing pool of specific memory B lymphocytes ready to respond to rechallenge with immunogen. These cells differentiate into antibody-secreting plasma cells in fewer generations than naive B lymphocytes.

Since memory B lymphocytes are derived from activated B lymphocytes that have undergone somatic mutation and class switching, they are activated by lower doses of antigen than naive B lymphocytes and differentiate into plasma cells that produce predominantly IgG antibodies.

2.2 Cell mediated immunity

Humoral antibody responses do not provide adequate protection against intracellular pathogens, including viruses and intracellular bacteria such as *Listeria monocytogenes* and *Salmonella* Typhi, fungi, yeasts and protozoa. For this purpose the host relies upon cell mediated immunity to contain and clear infection.

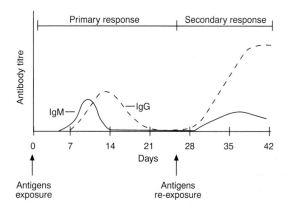

Fig. 8.1 Diagram of antibody production during the primary and secondary humoral responses.

T lymphocytes are the effectors of cell mediated immunity.

Briefly, T lymphocytes bind and respond only to protein antigens that have been processed by and presented on the surface of antigen-presenting cells (APCs) in the context of major histocompatibility (MHC) molecules (Trowsdale, Ragoussis and Campbell 1991). MHC molecules present antigen in a context that helps T lymphocytes to distinguish between self and foreign antigens. Class I MHC proteins are expressed on all nucleated cells whereas class II MHC molecules are expressed only on a subset of immune cells (primarily B cells and macrophages). T lymphocytes recognize the antigen–MHC complexes directly through the variable region domain of their T cell receptors (TCRs) (Fig. 8.2). The TCR is associated with a second protein receptor (CD4 or CD8) on the surface of the T lymphocyte, which restricts the T lymphocyte to interaction with only one MHC class: CD4 T lymphocytes recognize class II MHC molecules and CD8 T lymphocytes recognize class I MHC molecules. Resting T lymphocytes express a TCR with a unique specificity determined by the variable domain and, therefore, only a small fraction (0.1%) of T lymphocytes responds to a particular immunogen.

T lymphocytes are activated by physical interaction with APCs and by the binding of cytokines, such as IL-1 and tumour necrosis factor (TNF), released by the APCs. After activation, T lymphocytes release cytokines that stimulate their own growth and differentiation, attract other immune cells to the site of infection, and promote phagocytosis of organisms and particles by macrophages. Some T lymphocytes become cytotoxic (cytotoxic T lymphocytes, CTL), express CD8, and are capable of destroying infected cells directly, in part by the release of proteases onto the targeted cell. Other T lymphocytes, called helper T cells (Th), express CD4 and direct the immune response by secreting various combinations of cytokines. The T helper 1 (Th1) subset, which secretes IFN-γ and IL-2, promotes cell mediated immunity and the T helper 2 (Th2) subset, which secretes IL-4, IL-5, IL-6 and IL-10, induces humoral immunity. Cell mediated immunity responds to immunogen exposure and re-exposure in a manner analogous to that seen in humoral immunity. The primary cell mediated response generates antigen-specific memory T cells that mediate a more rapid and expanded secondary response upon re-exposure to antigen.

2.3 Cellular interactions of the immune response

B cell activation and T helper cells

T-independent immunogens induce antibody production during the humoral immune response without the assistance of T cells. These immunogens and are divided into 2 classes: type I antigens activate B cells in a polyclonal manner and include components of bacterial cell walls, such as lipopolysaccharide; type II immunogens require cytokines fully to induce antibody synthesis and are non-protein polymers with frequently repeating units, such as dextran and pneumococcal polysaccharide.

T-dependent antigens, on the other hand, require T lymphocytes to trigger antibody synthesis; most protein antigens are T-dependent. In order fully to activate B lymphocytes, intact T-dependent antigens must first be bound by the appropriate B lymphocyte Ig. After endocytosis, the B lymphocyte (acting as an APC) digests the antigen by proteolysis, and portions of it are then presented on the B lymphocyte surface bound to class II MHC molecules. A small subset of activated CD4 - Th lymphocytes recognize and bind to the peptide class II MHC molecules on the B lymphocyte (Fig. 8.2). This cell-to-cell contact is enhanced by accessory receptor–ligand interactions between the B and T lymphocytes. Of particular importance is the co-stimulatory effect of the binding of CD40 ligand on the Th lymphocyte to CD40 on the B lymphocyte. Although this cell–cell contact serves to stimulate both B and Th lymphocytes, it is called cognate B cell activation (Parker 1993). Activation of B lymphocytes by Th lymphocytes is further augmented by secretion by the latter of cytokines that help to direct antibody synthesis. The complex interactions of B lymphocytes and Th lymphocytes result in a highly specific, potent and tightly regulated response to protein antigens.

(a)

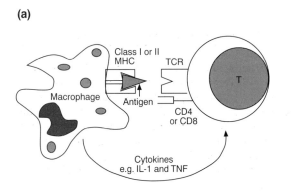

(b)

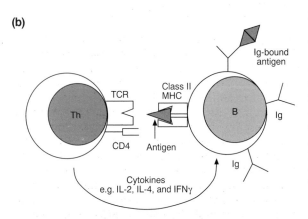

Fig. 8.2 Antigen-specific activation of (a) T lymphocytes and (b) B lymphocytes.

3 ACTIVE IMMUNIZATION

Active immunization is induced when an immuno-competent host develops an immune response as the result of exposure to an immunogen. Usually, both humoral and cell mediated responses are evoked, and the immunogen is recognized and eliminated. Active immunization can be induced by natural or artificial means. Natural active immunization occurs when a host is exposed to a pathogen, and develops immunity against re-exposure to the same pathogen. For example, the development of whooping cough after infection with *Bordetella pertussis* produces immunity to a second infection with the same serotype. By contrast, artificial active immunization involves administration of a vaccine that contains a killed or avirulent form or an immunoprotective component of a pathogen, designed to elicit protective immunity. On subsequent exposure to the infectious pathogen, it is recognized and eliminated, thereby affording protection against the disease. In the case of, for example, whooping cough, vaccination with a killed vaccine that contains a mixture of the prevalent bacterial serotypes elicits immunity to infection.

4 THE IMMUNOGENICITY OF BACTERIAL VACCINES

Antigens vary widely in the degree to which they are immunogenic; immunogenicity is determined primarily by 3 factors:

1 molecular weight
2 chemical complexity and
3 'foreignness' (Benjamin 1984).

Immunogens are macromolecules, and their immuno-genicity increases with molecular weight. Although there is no lower limit, substances smaller than 5 kDa are rarely immunogenic. Immunogenicity also tends to increase with chemical complexity, which may reflect the diversity of distinct compositional units, including amino acids, carbohydrates and prosthetic groupings. Included in this complexity are secondary or tertiary molecular structure. Thus, because of their complex secondary and tertiary structure, globular proteins are more immunogenic than polysaccharides.

An important function of the immune system is to distinguish self (host) from non-self (foreign). Therefore, the more dissimilar a molecule is from host molecules, the greater its immunogenicity. Some organisms avoid immune recognition by expressing molecules that are not antigenic because of their identity or close resemblance to host molecules, a phenomenon known as mimicry.

Molecules that express an epitope and bind antibody but are too small to activate the immune system are defined as haptens; they are antigenic but not immunogenic. Haptens fail to activate Th lymphocytes or B lymphocytes, and so they do not stimulate an antibody response. Haptens do, however, become immunogenic when coupled to a carrier molecule.

Carriers are proteins that are themselves immuno-genic, especially for T lymphocytes; immunization with hapten–carrier complexes induces antibodies against both hapten and the carrier.

Successful immunization requires a vaccine that induces an immune response that resembles as closely as possible the response to the natural infection. This can be achieved by the use of immunogens that are active during natural infections, generating B and T memory lymphocytes specific for protective antigens. These memory cells subsequently respond rapidly on re-exposure to the infection. The ideal vaccine is highly immunogenic and elicits life-long immunity. It should also be easily administered, preferably in a single dose, without adverse effects. None of the currently available vaccines possesses all these characteristics.

5 LICENSED VACCINES

Table 8.1 summarizes the main characteristics of bacterial vaccines that are licensed and commercially available in various countries. The childhood immunization schedules currently recommended in the USA are listed in the Appendix. Corresponding schedules are published by the Department of Health and other Health Departments of the UK.

5.1 Whole cell inactivated vaccines

Most bacterial vaccines are of this type. They include pertussis, cholera, typhoid and plague vaccines and are produced by killing the micro-organisms with heat or by treatment with chemicals such as formaldehyde or phenol (Plotkin 1980, Crawford et al. 1984, Provost et al. 1986, Hoke, Nisalak and Sangawhipa 1988). Although the infectivity of the pathogens is destroyed by these treatments, much of their antigenic integrity remains.

5.2 Whole cell attenuated vaccine

Although a number of viral vaccines are attenuated, the only bacterial vaccines in this category are the bacillus Calmette–Guérin (BCG) strain of *Mycobacterium bovis*, used to vaccinate against tuberculosis (Colditz et al. 1995), and a typhoid vaccine. The advantage of using viable micro-organisms is that they tend for a time to reproduce in the host, allowing for continuous stimulation of immunoresponsive cells, including T and B lymphocytes and macrophages. In the case of viral vaccines, a single dose usually evokes firm and long-lasting protective immunity. The performance of BCG in this respect is more open to doubt. The contraindications to BCG immunization include immunological defects, HIV infection and generalized septic skin conditions.

5.3   Toxoid vaccines

Highly immunogenic vaccines are made from the exotoxins produced by *Corynebacterium diphtheriae* and *Clostridium tetani*. Their toxicity is removed by treatment with formalin, and the inactivated toxin (toxoid) is used in vaccine preparations (Ramon 1923, Glenny and Pope 1926, Wassilak, Orenstein and Sutter 1994). These toxoids, nearly always adsorbed to an alum adjuvant, evoke high titres of antitoxic IgG antibodies. Diphtheria and tetanus toxoids may be combined with pertussis and other vaccines.

5.4   Acellular pertussis vaccine

An acellular form of the pertussis vaccine that contains various combinations of protective antigens is available and produces fewer side effects than whole cell vaccines (Blackwelder et al.1991, Blumberg et al. 1991; and see Chapter 18, p. 338). It is licensed for use in the USA by the Food and Drug Administration (Marwick 1996).

5.5   Polysaccharide vaccines

Examples of polysaccharide vaccines are purified capsular polysaccharides used in the pneumococcus and meningococcus vaccines. The pneumococcus vaccine consists of the polysaccharides of 23 capsular types of *Streptococcus pneumoniae* (Lee, Banks and Li 1991, Shapiro 1991) and the meningococcus vaccine is composed of capsular polysaccharide of types A, C, Y and W-135, of *Neisseria meningitidis* (Armand et al. 1982, Hankins et al. 1982). Both preparations are useful for the prevention respectively of pneumonia and meningitis in at-risk populations. Since the polysaccharides consist of repeating units, T-independent immune responses result in the production of IgM that opsonizes and eliminates *S. pneumoniae* and *N. meningitidis* (Stein 1992).

In *Haemophilus influenzae* type b (Hib) vaccine the polyribose phosphate capsular polysaccharide is conjugated to diphtheria or tetanus toxoid or an outer-membrane protein of group B *N. meningitidis*. Since this vaccine is a polysaccharide–protein conjugate it elicits a T-dependent immune response and an IgG antibody response develops to provide immunity (Deveikis, Ward and Kim 1988, Granoff, Weinberg and Shackelford 1988).

Children do not develop efficient T-independent immune responses, and the ability to raise a T-dependent response is especially important in children younger than 24 months (Stein 1992). The Hib vaccine produces protective immunity in this group of children.

5.6   Adverse reactions to bacterial vaccines

In general, bacterial vaccines do not cause systemic adverse reactions other than occasional malaise and low grade pyrexia within 24–48 h of administration. Local pain, swelling and tenderness are caused by some whole cell vaccines but resolve within a day or so.

Because whole micro-organisms are used, responses are elicited not only against protective antigens but also against non-protective antigens. The latter may cross-react with host tissues and, therefore, have the potential to elicit autoreactive immune responses. The whole cell killed pertussis vaccine has been implicated in the causation of encephalopathy in c. 1 in 100 000 of infants receiving it (see Chapter 18, p. 338) but estimates of incidence vary and the mechanism is not fully understood (Mortimer and Jones 1979, Manclark and Cowell 1984).

The alum adjuvant used in toxoid vaccines may cause local reactions, e.g. pain, tenderness and swelling. Treatment is symptomatic.

6   ADJUVANTS

A single dose of killed inactivated vaccine does not always induce optimal levels of protective immunity, and one or more booster doses are necessary to achieve effective immunity. Alum adjuvants are incorporated in some inactivated vaccine preparations to potentiate their immunogenicity. The simplest explanation of their effect is that they bind vaccine components and subsequently release them slowly to maintain continuous stimulation of immunoresponsive cells (White 1972); however, their modes of action are not fully understood and probably vary from adjuvant to adjuvant.

6.1   Aluminium salts

Alum adjuvants are made from aluminium hydroxide or phosphate salts (Glenny and Pope 1926, Aprile and Wardlaw 1966) and are the only adjuvants approved for human use.

Freund's adjuvants are not approved for human use but are widely used in experimental animals. Complete Freund's adjuvant (CFA) is a suspension of killed strain C *Mycobacterium tuberculosis* or *Mycobacterium butyricum* in mineral oil combined with an emulsifier, such as Arlacel A (Freund 1956). A different form of adjuvant is an incomplete Freund's adjuvant (IFA) that contains only mineral oil and emulsifier but no bacteria (Edelman 1980). It is a less effective adjuvant than CFA, which was at one time approved for human use but was discontinued because of serious side effects.

6.2   Adjuvants under development

Since only alum adjuvants are approved for clinical use, research is in progress to identify and develop more potent and safer adjuvants for use in humans. The following are examples of preparations under study.

MURAMYL DIPEPTIDE DERIVED ADJUVANTS

The adjuvant action of CFA is attributed to muramyl dipeptide (MDP) present in mycobacteria (Ellouz et al. 1974). When purified and used as an adjuvant, MDP has adjuvant activity similar to that of CFA, but is toxic in humans. Derivatives of MDP have been developed, including murabutide, muramyl tripeptide and threonyl-MDP (Allison and Byars 1990). The latter in a squalene–pluronic polymer emulsion or Syntex Adjuvant Formulation (SAF) is the most promising MDP derivative (Allison and Byars 1990). SAF enhances adjuvant activity with various immunogens but does not evoke adverse reactions in animals and humans.

LIPOPOLYSACCHARIDE, LIPID A AND MONOPHOSPHORYL LIPID A ADJUVANTS

Lipopolysaccharides (LPS) of gram-negative bacteria have adjuvant activity (Johnson, Gaines and Landy 1956), which resides in the lipid A moiety (Quershi and Takayama 1990). Lipid A is, however, highly toxic and a non-toxic derivative, monophosphoryl lipid A (MPL), has been derived (Rudbach et al. 1990). When used as an adjuvant, MPL has adjuvant effects similar to that of LPS, but with reduced toxicity. To enhance its activity further, MPL has been used together with trehalose dimycolate, a derivative of MDP, to form the Ribi Adjuvant System (RAS) (Masihi et al. 1986). When used in experimental animals, RAS has adjuvant activity similar to that of CFA but with reduced toxicity.

SAPONIN, QUIL A AND QS21 ADJUVANTS

Saponin, isolated from the tree bark of *Quillaja saponaria*, has potent adjuvant properties, but is highly toxic in its crude form (Dalsgaard 1974). Its purified derivative, quil A, has adjuvant properties in experimental animals but it is too toxic for human use (Dalsgaard 1978). The biochemical analysis of quil A has led to the purification of a derivative, QS21 (Kensil et al. 1991), which is a potent adjuvant when used with various vaccine preparations (Kensil, Wu and Soltysik 1995).

7 VACCINE DELIVERY SYSTEMS UNDER DEVELOPMENT

LIPOSOMES

Liposomes are prepared from lipid membrane constituents to form microparticles that can be used to deliver vaccine preparations. Most liposomes consist of multilamellar or unilamellar vesicles. When vaccines are delivered in liposomes, they are more immunogenic than when given alone (van Rooijen 1990, Pietrobon 1995). The immunogenicity of vaccines is further enhanced when they are combined with an adjuvant in liposomes (Fortin and Therien 1993). This is attributed to the slow release of the vaccine from the liposomes and the adjuvant system, and sustained stimulation of immunoresponsive cells. Liposomes can be constructed to accommodate different sizes of antigen molecules and they reduce the toxicity of adjuvants such as MDP, lipid A and quil A (Alving et al. 1992, Alving 1993, Gupta et al. 1993).

IMMUNE STIMULATING COMPLEXES

Immune stimulating complexes (ISCOMs) are made by solubilizing quil A, cholesterol compounds and vaccines, to give 'cage-like' complexes in which the vaccines are encapsulated (Morein et al. 1987). When used to deliver vaccines, ISCOMs stimulate both humoral and cell mediated immune responses (Hoglund et al. 1989). Although ISCOMs have been widely used in veterinary vaccines, they are not as yet approved for human use because of the potential side effects of quil A used in their construction.

BIODEGRADABLE POLYMER MICROSPHERES

Microspheres used as delivery systems for vaccine preparations are usually made from polymers that contain polylactic and polyglycolic acids (PLGA) (Aguado and Lambert 1992). When PLGA microspheres are used to deliver vaccine preparations, humoral and cell mediated immune responses are elicited (Eldridge et al. 1993). Although the strength of the immune responses is similar to those elicited with alum adjuvants, PLGA microspheres have the added advantages of providing a protective enclosure for the vaccines, allowing for their gradual release, and most importantly, of being safe without causing adverse effects. Vaccines enclosed in microspheres are usually protected from the effects of pH, bile salts and proteolyic enzymes, and are widely used for delivery on mucosal surfaces (Nedrud and Lamm 1991). By varying the molecular weight and ratio of lactic and glycolic acids, PLGA microspheres can be designed to deliver vaccines at different rates, from a few days or weeks to months, allowing for a sustained release that minimizes the number of vaccine doses that have to be administered (Langer 1981). Finally, PLGA microspheres should be safe for use in humans, since PLGA is used to manufacture surgical sutures that have a proven safety record.

8 VACCINES UNDER DEVELOPMENT

RECOMBINANT PROTEIN VACCINES

The advent of recombinant DNA technology has made possible the genetic manipulation of the protective protein antigens of pathogens for vaccine development. Usually, the protective antigen is identified in vitro by antibody neutralization and killing assays, and in vivo with experimental animal protection studies. The gene that encodes the protective antigen is identified and cloned into a plasmid vector, which is then introduced into a bacterial, yeast, insect or mammalian cell expression system, in which the desired recombinant protein is expressed in large quantities and then purified by biochemical methods. When administered as a vaccine, the recombinant protein is immunogenic and elicits protective immunity.

Since the gene of the protective antigen can be sequenced and manipulated, genetic methods can be used to identify the most immunogenic epitope(s) to elicit protective immunity. At present hepatitis B vaccine is the only recombinant protein vaccine preparation licensed for human use. It contains genetically engineered hepatitis B surface antigen in an alum adjuvant and confers good protection (McAleer et al. 1984, Zajac et al. 1986). Recombinant DNA technology is now widely used in vaccine research to develop subunit vaccines designed to contain only immunogenic protective antigens. There is a good chance that such preparations will eventually replace at least some of the bacterial vaccines now in use.

ANTI-IDIOTYPE ANTIBODY VACCINES

Idiotopes are the hypervariable domains of the antibody molecules (Ab1) that serve as the paratope or antigen-combining site. Therefore the idiotope of Ab1 is the 'mirror image' of the epitope or antigenic determinant that it binds. When Ab1 is used to generate anti-idiotype antibody (Ab2), the latter recognizes the Ab1 idiotope. It is the 'internal image' of the epitope that Ab1 binds. Likewise, when an anti-idiotype antibody (Ab2) is used to generate anti-anti-idiotype antibody (Ab3), the latter recognizes the Ab2 idiotope because it is the 'mirror image' of the epitope, similar to that of Ab1 (Kohler et al. 1988). Since the idiotopes of anti-idiotypic antibodies are 'internal images' of the epitope, anti-idiotype antibodies could be used in vaccine preparations as a substitute for the protective epitope(s) of pathogens. Anti-idiotypic antibodies are especially useful when the epitope(s) of the pathogen is difficult to identify or synthesize. A schematic representation of idiotypic antibody production is shown in Fig. 8.3.

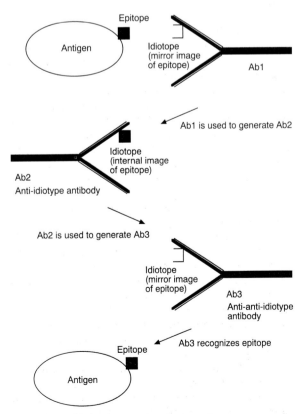

Fig. 8.3 Diagram of idiotypic antibody production.

Anti-idiotype antibody vaccines are safe and free from the adverse side effects associated with vaccine preparations that contain whole cell pathogens or their components. A major disadvantage of anti-idiotype antibodies in vaccine preparations is that their immunogenicity is weak. Experimental anti-idiotype antibody vaccines have been developed for hepatitis B (Kennedy et al. 1983), herpes simplex (Gell and Moss 1985), rabies (Reagen et al. 1983), human immunodeficiency virus (Kang et al. 1992), *S. pneumoniae* (McNamara, Ward and Kohler 1984), and *Schistosoma mansoni* (Grzych et al. 1985).

SYNTHETIC PEPTIDE-BASED VACCINES

Synthetic peptides used as vaccines are derived from the amino acid sequences of protective epitopes and determinants of pathogens that activate B and T cells (Brown 1990). By means of molecular biological approaches, oligopeptides 3–12 amino acids in length are synthesized and used as vaccines. Since the peptide design is highly specific, only immunoresponsive B or T cells that recognize the peptide are stimulated and the desired humoral or cell mediated immune response is stimulated. Antibodies to specific epitopes can be generated and specific helper and cytotoxic T cell responses can also be elicited with peptide-based vaccines.

Peptides used as vaccines are safe because they do not contain undesirable components of the pathogen. Moreover, peptides can be designed to eliminate epitopes with the potential to be autoreactive or suppressive. They can also be combined to contain various combinations of B and T cell epitopes. However, when peptides are used in vaccine preparations, they are poor immunogens and require the use of adjuvants, conjugation to carrier proteins (Clarke et al. 1987) or multiple repeating peptide units (Tam 1988) to enhance immunogenicity.

Another disadvantage of peptides as vaccines is the configuration and recognition of peptides by immunoresponsive cells (Laver et al. 1990). Peptides usually present as linear determinants and are recognized by T cells in the context of MHC molecules and B cell epitopes, but the latter also recognize conformational determinants. Thus, the generation of a B cell response against a protective conformational determinant may not be possible. Peptide-based vaccines are also limited for human use because of the polymorphism of MHC class I and II molecules in different individuals. Since the linear determinant of a peptide is highly specific and recognized only by a restricted set of MHC molecules, a 'universal peptide' must be added to peptide preparations to overcome this problem. Experimental peptide-based vaccines have been developed for use against hepatitis B (Dreesman et al. 1985), influenza (Muller, Shapiro and Arnon 1982), measles (Partidos, Stanley and Steward 1992), human immunodeficiency virus (Wang et al. 1991) and malaria (Zavala et al. 1987).

LIVE VIRAL AND BACTERIAL VECTOR VACCINES

Vector vaccine preparations are usually made up of attenuated micro-organisms that are genetically manipulated to express the protective protein antigen from another pathogen. The gene that encodes the protective antigen is inserted into the genome of the attenuated micro-organism by molecular biological techniques. The inserted gene, together with the genome of the micro-organism, is transcribed and translated and the desired protective antigen, along with other proteins of the micro-organism, is expressed. Vector vaccines elicit humoral and cell mediated immune responses to the proteins of the micro-organism and the desired protective antigen. Since an attenuated micro-organism is used as the vector, the degree to which the immune response is stimulated is consistent with that of an attenuated vaccine. Most micro-organisms used as vectors are the same as are used in attenuated vaccine preparations. Careful selection of vectors allows this approach to vaccine preparation to target protective immunity against at least 2 different pathogens. For example, the use of a attenuated varicella zoster virus vector (Lowe et al. 1987) that expresses a protective antigen against hepatitis B, evokes protective immunity against both viruses. Other viral vectors commonly used include vaccinia virus (Moss et al. 1984, Collins et al. 1990), and adenovirus (Johnson et al. 1988, Yuasa et al. 1991). Similarly, the BCG strain of *M. bovis* (Aldovini and Young 1991, Stover et al. 1991) and *Salmonella typhimurium* (Sadoff et al. 1988, Strugnell et al. 1990) are used as bacterial vectors. The major safety concerns with the use of live vector vaccines are similar to those associated with attenuated vaccines. Moreover, the use of live vectors may eliminate the need for subsequent booster vaccinations.

NUCLEIC ACID VACCINES

Nucleic acid vaccines, constructed by recombinant DNA technology, are plasmid DNA vectors that contain the gene of an immunogen (Vogel and Sarver 1995, Ertl and Xiang 1996). Plasmid vectors are administered parenterally in aqueous solution or are coated onto gold beads and given intramuscularly or subcutaneously (Williams et al. 1991, Cheng, Ziegelhoffer and Tang 1993). The plasmid vectors are taken up, usually by muscle cells, at the site of inoculation. They remain extrachromosomal within these cells, and are transcribed and translated into the desired immunogen. The proteins expressed by nucleic acid vaccination are usually processed and presented by MHC class I pathways, similarly to viral antigens, and elicit cytotoxic T cell responses. Helper T cell and antigen-specific humoral responses are also elicited (Davis, Michel and Whalen 1993, Irwin et al. 1994). In experimental animal systems, nucleic acid vaccination elicits protective immunity against challenge with several different viral pathogens (Montgomery et al. 1993, Robison, Hunt and Webster 1993, Webster et al. 1994). Clinical trials with plasmid DNA vectors con-taining various HIV genes are in progress in seropositive HIV individuals (Vogel and Sarver 1995). The major advantages of DNA in nucleic acid vaccines include its stability, and the ability to manipulate the desired gene(s) genetically into plasmid DNA vectors for large scale production and purification. The use of 'naked' DNA has, however, raised serious safety issues. Although it has been demonstrated that the plasmid vectors do not integrate into the host cell and remain extrachromosomal, the opportunity remains for integration of 'naked' DNA into host DNA and for oncogenic mutagenesis. Another safety concern involves the development of anti-DNA antibodies that may lead to the development of autoimmunity.

Nucleic acid vaccines based on mRNA also elicit humoral and cell mediated responses (Martinon et al. 1993). Since RNA does not integrate into chromosomal DNA, its use in nucleic acid vaccines appears to be safer than the use of DNA. However, RNA is more unstable than DNA and may prove impractical for use in the large scale production of nucleic acid vaccines.

9 PASSIVE IMMUNIZATION

Passive immunization is the administration of preformed antibodies produced by another individual or animal. This method of immunization provides immediate protection against a pathogen or toxin without the need for a course of immunization. The most common reason for the passive immunization of healthy immunocompetent individuals is exposure to a toxin or poison (Grossman 1994).

Passive immunization is given to neutralize diphtheria, botulinum and tetanus toxins; after known or presumed exposure to rabies, passive immunization is given to protect against the immediate threat of disease while active immunization is administered to prevent long-term incubation of the infection.

Immunocompromised or immunodeficient individuals, who cannot mount a humoral response, may also be given passive immunization. Children with hypogammaglobulinaemia, individuals with AIDS, patients receiving chemotherapy, and organ transplant recipients receiving immunosuppressive therapy cannot respond appropriately to natural infection or active immunization and, therefore, may require passive immunization and supportive immune globulin transfusions to prevent severe infection (Bussel, Fitzgerald-Pedersen and Feldman 1990, De Simone et al. 1990, Buckley and Schiff 1991, Kuroda et al. 1991). As prophylaxis such patients may be given intravenous immunoglobulin on a weekly or monthly basis in the absence of known exposure. Children with leukaemia are often given varicella zoster immunoglobulin after exposure to chickenpox. Transplant patients may be given cytomegalovirus immunoglobulin to prevent cytomegalovirus infections while on immunosuppressive therapy.

A major disadvantage of passive immunization is its brief period of effectiveness: transferred immunoglobulins have a short half-life (typically 25 days for

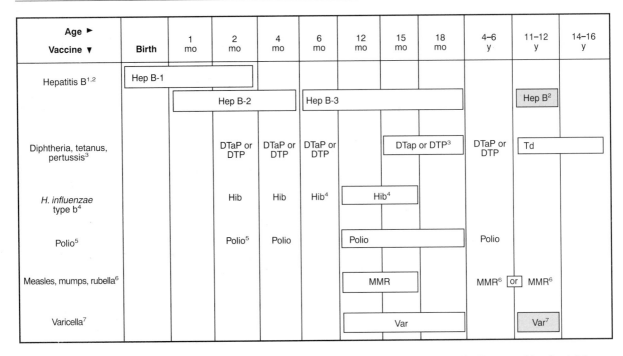

Age ▶ Vaccine ▼	Birth	1 mo	2 mo	4 mo	6 mo	12 mo	15 mo	18 mo	4–6 y	11–12 y	14–16 y
Hepatitis B[1,2]	Hep B-1		Hep B-2		Hep B-3					Hep B[2]	
Diphtheria, tetanus, pertussis[3]			DTaP or DTP	DTaP or DTP	DTaP or DTP		DTap or DTP[3]		DTaP or DTP	Td	
H. influenzae type b[4]			Hib	Hib	Hib[4]	Hib[4]					
Polio[5]			Polio[5]	Polio		Polio			Polio		
Measles, mumps, rubella[6]						MMR			MMR[6] or MMR[6]		
Varicella[7]						Var				Var[7]	

Fig. 8.4 Recommended childhood immunization schedule, USA, January to December 1997. (Approved by the Advisory Committee on Immunization Practices, the American Academy of Pediatrics and the American Academy of Family Physicians.) This schedule indicates the recommended age for routine administration of currently licensed childhood vaccines. Some combination vaccines are available and may be used whenever administration of all components of the vaccine is indicated. Providers should consult the manufacturers' package inserts for detailed recommendations. Vaccines are listed under the routinely recommended ages. Open bars indicate the range of acceptable ages for vaccination. Shaded bars indicate 'catch-up' vaccination: at 11–12 years of age, hepatitis B (Hep B) vaccine should be administered to children not previously vaccinated, and varicella virus vaccine should be administered to unvaccinated children who lack a reliable history of chickenpox.

1 Infants born to HBsAg-negative mothers should receive the first dose of vaccine at birth or by 2 months of age, and a second dose ≥ 1 month later. Infants born to HBsAg-positive mothers should receive 0.5 ml hepatitis B immunoglobulin (HBIG) within 12 h of birth, and a dose of vaccine at a separate site. The second dose is recommended at 1–2 months of age and the third at 6 months of age. For infants born to mothers whose HBsAg status is unknown at time of delivery, blood should be drawn at the time of delivery to determine the mother's HBsAg status; if it is positive, the infant should receive HBIG as soon as possible (no later than 1 wk of age). The dosage and timing of subsequent vaccine doses should be based upon the mother's HBsAg status.

2 Children and adolescents who have not been vaccinated against hepatitis B in infancy may begin the series during any childhood visit. Those who have not previously received 3 doses of hepatitis B vaccine should initiate or complete the series at the age of 11–12 years. The second dose should be administered at least 1 month after the first dose, and the third dose at least 4 months after the first dose and at least 2 months after the second dose.

3 DTaP (diphtheria and tetanus toxoids and acellular pertussis vaccine) is the preferred vaccine for all doses in the vaccination series, including completion of the series in children who have received ≥1 dose of whole-cell DTP vaccine. Whole-cell DTP is an acceptable alternative to DTaP. The fourth dose of DTaP may be administered as early as the age of 12 months, provided 6 months have elapsed since the third dose, and if the child is considered unlikely to return at the age of 15–18 months Td (tetanus and diphtheria toxoids, adsorbed, for adult use) is recommended at the age of 11–12 years if at least 5 years have elapsed since the last dose of DTP, DTaP or DT. Subsequent routine Td boosters are recommended every 10 years.

4 Three *Haemophilus influenzae* type b (Hib) conjugate vaccines are licensed for infant use. If PRP-OMP is administered at 2 and 4 months of age, a dose at 6 months is not required. After completing the primary series, any Hib conjugate vaccine may be used as a booster.

5 Two poliovirus vaccines are currently licensed in the USA; inactivated poliovirus vaccine (IPV) and oral poliovirus vaccine (OPV). The following schedules are all acceptable by the Advisory Committee on Immunization Practices, the American Academy of Pediatrics and the American Academy of Family Physicians, and parents and providers may choose among them: (1) IPV at the ages 2 and 4 months, OPV at the ages 12–18 months and 4–6 years; (2) IPV at the ages 2, 4, 12–18 months and 4–6 years; (3) OPV at the ages 2, 4, 6–18 months and 4–6 years. The Advisory Committee on Immunization Practices routinely recommends schedule 1. IPV is the only poliovirus vaccine recommended for immunocompromised persons and their household contacts.

6 The second dose of MMR is routinely recommended at 4–6 or 11–12 years of age, but may be administered at any time provided at least 1 month has elapsed since the first dose, and that both doses are administered at or after 12 months of age.

7 Susceptible children may receive Varicella vaccine (Var) during any visit after the first birthday, and unvaccinated persons who lack a reliable history of chickenpox should be vaccinated at 11–12 years of age. Susceptible persons older than 13 years should receive 2 doses, at least 1 month apart.

IgG) and passive immunization does not evoke immunological memory in the recipient. In addition, passive immunization may produce serious side effects and, therefore, its use is more limited than active immunization.

Originally, antisera used for passive immunization were produced in animals, commonly horses, immunized against the pathogen or toxin. The use of animal sera has declined because of the risk of severe adverse reactions, particularly serum sickness, and the short half-life of animal Ig (7–23 days). Individuals immunized many times with animal sera may develop severe allergic reactions including acute anaphylaxis, serum sickness and the Arthus reaction. Sera used for passive immunization are now derived from alcohol-fractionated pooled human plasma taken from donors irrespective of their natural infection or immunization history. Such pools of sera or plasma contain IgG of multiple specificities, and are likely to contain antibodies against the most common infectious diseases. This type of preparation is designated immune serum globulin (ISG; human normal immunoglobulin, HNIG, in the UK) and is used to provide protection after exposure to hepatitis A and for treating individuals with hypogammaglobulinaemia. Non-specific immunoglobulin is available as a preparation for intramuscular injection (IMIG) and as a preparation for intravenous injection (IVIG), from which high molecular weight Ig complexes capable of activating complement have been removed (Grossman 1994). A second type of human immunoglobin used for passive immunization is obtained from human subjects who have been immunized against or naturally infected with specific organisms. These preparations include tetanus, varicella zoster and rabies immunoglobulin.

APPENDIX: RECOMMENDED CHILDHOOD IMMUNIZATION SCHEDULE, USA, JANUARY TO DECEMBER 1997

This schedule appears in Volume 1, Chapter 45. It is reproduced above, as Fig. 8.4, by courtesy of Drs S C Hadler and R W Sutter.

REFERENCES

Ada GL, 1993, Vaccines, *Fundamental Immunology*, 3rd edn, ed. Paul WE, Raven Press, NY, 1309–54.

Aguado MT, Lambert PH, 1992, Controlled-release vaccines – biodegradable polylactide/polyglycolide (PL/PG) microspheres as antigen vehicles, *Immunobiology*, **184**: 113–25.

Aldovini A, Young RA, 1991, Humoral and cell-mediated responses to live recombinant BCG-HIV vaccines, *Nature (London)*, **351**: 479–82.

Allison AC, Byars NE, 1990, *New Generation Vaccines*, Marcel Dekker, New York, 129–40.

Alving CR, 1993, Lipopolysaccharide, lipid A, and liposomes containing lipid A as immunologic adjuvants, *Immunobiology*, **187**: 430–46.

Alving CR, Verma JN et al., 1992, Liposomes containing lipid A as a potent non-toxic adjuvant, *Res Immunol*, **143**: 197–8.

Aprile MA, Wardlaw AC, 1966, Aluminum compounds as adjuvants for vaccine and toxoids in man: a review, *Can J Public Health*, **57**: 343–54.

Armand J, Arminjon F et al., 1982, Tetravalent meningococcal polysaccharide vaccine groups A, C, Y, W-135: clinical and serological evaluation, *J Biol Stand*, **10**: 335–9.

Benjamin DC, 1984, The antigenic structure of proteins: a reappraisal, *Annu Rev Immunol*, **2**: 67–101.

Blackwelder WC, Storsaeter J et al., 1991, Acellular pertussis vaccines. Efficacy and evaluation of clinical case definitions, *Am J Dis Child*, **145**: 1285–9.

Blaxall FR, 1930, Smallpox, *A System of Bacteriology MRC*, **vol. 7**: HMSO, London, 84–132.

Blumberg DA, Mink CM et al., 1991, Comparison of acellular and whole-cell pertussis-component diphtheria-tetanus-pertussis vaccines in infants, *J Pediatr*, **119**: 194–204.

Brown F, 1990, The potential of peptides as vaccines, *Semin Virol*, **1**: 67–74.

Buckley R, Schiff R, 1991, The use of intravenous immune globulin in immunodeficiency diseases, *N Engl J Med*, **325**: 110.

Bussell JB, Fitzgerald-Pedersen J, Feldman C, 1990, Alteration of two doses of intravenous gammaglobulin in the maintenance treatment of patients with immune thrombocytopenic prupura, *Am J Hematol*, **33**: 184–8.

Cheng L, Ziegelhoffer PR, Tang NS, 1993, In vivo promoter activity and transgene expression in mammalian somatic tissues evaluated by using particle bombardment, *Proc Natl Acad Sci USA*, **90**: 4455–9.

Claman HN, Chaperon EA, Triplett RF, 1966, Thymus-marrow cell combinations: synergism in antibody production, *Proc Soc Exp Biol Med*, **122**: 1167–71.

Clarke BE, Newton SE et al., 1987, Improved immunogenicity of a peptide epitope after fusion to hepatitis B core protein, *Nature (London)*, **330**: 381–4.

Colditz GA, Berkley CS et al., 1995, The efficacy of bacillus Calmette–Guerin vaccination of newborns and infants in the prevention of tuberculosis: meta-analyses of the published literature, *Pediatrics*, **96**: 29–35.

Collins PL, Purcell RH et al., 1990, Evaluation in chimpanzees of vaccinia virus recombinants that express the surface glycoproteins of human respiratory syncytial virus, *Vaccine*, **8**: 164–8.

Crawford CR, Faiza AM et al., 1984, Use of zwitterionic detergent for the preparation of an influenzae virus vaccine 1. Preparation and characterization of disrupted virions, *Vaccine*, **2**: 193–8.

Dalsgaard K, 1974, Saponin adjuvants III. Isolation of a substance from *Quillaja saponaria* Molina with adjuvant activity in foot-and-mouth disease vaccines, *Arch Ges Virusforsch*, **44**: 243–54.

Dalsgaard K, 1978, A study of the isolation and characterization of the saponin quil A. Evaluation of its adjuvant activity, with a special reference to the application in the vaccination of cattle against foot-and-mouth disease, *Acta Vet Scand*, **69**: 1–40.

Davis HL, Michel ML, Whalen RG, 1993, DNA-based immunization induces continuous secretion of hepatitis B virus surface antigen and high levels of circulating antibody, *Human Mol Genet*, **2**: 1837–51.

De Simone C, Antonaci S et al., 1990, Report of the symposium on the use of intravenous gammaglobulin adults infected with the human immunodeficiency virus, *J Clin Lab Anal*, **4**: 313–17.

Deveikis A, Ward J, Kim KS, 1988, Functional activities of human antibody induced by the capsular polysaccharide or polysaccharide-conjugate vaccines against *Haemophilus influenzae* type b, *Vaccine*, **6**: 14–18.

Dreesman RM, Sparrow JT et al., 1985, Synthetic hepatitis B surface antigen peptide synthesis, *Adv Exp Med Biol*, **185**: 129–37.

Edelman R, 1980, Vaccine adjuvants, *Rev Infect Dis*, **2**: 370–83.

Eldridge JH, Staas JK et al., 1993, New advances in vaccine delivery systems, *Semin Hepatol*, **30, Suppl. 4**: 16–25.

Ellouz F, Adam A et al., 1974, Minimal structural requirements for adjuvant activity of bacterial peptidoglycan derivatives, *Biochem Biophys Res Commun*, **59**: 1317–25.

Ertl HCJ, Xiang Z, 1996, Novel vaccine approaches, *J Immunol*, **156**: 3579–82.

Esser C, Radbruch A, 1990, Immunoglobulin class switching: molecular and cellular analysis, *Annu Rev Immunol*, **8**: 717–35.

Eyquem A, 1986, One century after Louis Pasteur's victory against rabies, *Am J Reprod Immunol Microbiol*, **10**: 132–4.

Finkelman FD, Holmes J, Katona IM, 1990, Lymphokine control of in vivo immunoglobulin isotope selection, *Annu Rev Immunol*, **8**: 303–33.

Fortin A, Therien HM, 1993, Mechanism of liposome adjuvanticity: an in vivo approach, *Immunobiology*, **188**: 316–22.

Freund J, 1956, The mode of action of immunological adjuvants, *Adv Tuberc Res*, **7**: 130–48.

Gell PGH, Moss PAH, 1985, Production of cell-mediated immune responses to herpes simplex virus by immunization with anti-heteroantisera, *J Gen Virol*, **66**: 1801–4.

Glenny AT, Pope CG, 1926, The antigenic value of toxoid precipitated by potassium alum, *J Pathol Bacteriol*, **29**: 38–45.

Glick B, Chang TS, Jaap RG, 1956, The bursa of Fabricius and antibody production, *Poult Sci*, **35**: 224–31.

Granoff DM, Weinberg GA, Shackelford PG, 1988, IgG subclass response to immunization with *Haemophilus influenzae* type b polysaccharide-outer membrane protein conjugated vaccine, *Pediatr Res*, **24**: 180–5.

Gray D, 1993, Immunological memory, *Annu Rev Immunol*, **11**: 49–77.

Griffiths J, 1984, Doctor Thomas Cimsdale and smallpox in Russia, *Bristol Med Chir J*, **99**: 14–16.

Grossman M, 1994, Immunization, *Basic and Clinical Immunology*, 8th edn, eds Stites DP, Terr AI, Parslow TG, Appleton and Lange, Norwalk, CT, 717–38.

Grzych JM, Capron M et al., 1985, An idiotype vaccine against experimental schistosomiasis, *Nature (London)*, **316**: 74–6.

Gupta RK, Relyveld EH et al., 1993, Adjuvants – a balance between toxicity and adjuvanticity, *Vaccine*, **11**: 293–306.

Hankins WA, Gwaltney JM et al., 1982, Clinical and serological evaluation of a meningnococcal polysaccharide vaccine. Groups A, C, Y, and W-135, *Proc Soc Exp Biol Med*, **169**: 54–7.

Hoglund S, Dalsgaard K et al., 1989, ISCOMs and immunostimulation with viral antigens, *Subcell Biochem*, **15**: 39–68.

Hoke CH, Nisalak A, Sangawhipa N, 1988, Protection against Japanese encephalitis by inactivated vaccines, *N Engl J Med*, **319**: 608–14.

Irwin MJ, Laube LS et al., 1994, Direct injection of a recombinant retroviral vector induces human immunodeficiency virus-specific immune responses in mice and nonhuman primates, *J Virol*, **68**: 5036–44.

Johnson AG, Gaines S, Landy M, 1956, Studies on the O antigen of *Salmonella typhosa* V. Enhancement of antibody response to protein antigens by the purified lipopolysaccharide, *J Exp Med*, **103**: 225–46.

Johnson DC, Ghosh-Choudhury G et al., 1988, Abundant expression of herpes simplex virus glycoprotein gB using an adenovirus vector, *Virology*, **164**: 1–14.

Kang YC, Nara P et al., 1992, Anti-idiotypic monoclonal antibody elicits broadly neutralizing anti-gp 120 antibodies in monkeys, *Proc Natl Acad Sci USA*, **89**: 2546–50.

Kennedy RC, Adler-Storthz K et al., 1983, Immune response to hepatitis B surface antigen: enhancement by prior injection of antibodies to the idiotype, *Science*, **221**: 853–5.

Kensil CR, Wu JY, Soltysik S, 1995, Structural and immunological characterization of the vaccine adjuvant QS-21, *Vaccine Design: The Subunit and Adjuvant Approach*, eds Powell MF, Newman MJ, Plenum Publishing, New York, 525–41.

Kensil CR, Patel U et al., 1991, Separation and characterization of saponins with adjuvant activity from *Quillaja saponaria* Molina cortex, *J Immunol*, **146**: 431–7.

Kohler H, Kaveri S et al., 1988, Overview of idiotypic networks and the nature of molecular mimicry, *Methods Enzymol*, **78**: 3–35.

Kuroda Y, Takashima H et al., 1991, Treatment of HTLV-I-associated myelopathy with high-dose intravenous gammaglobulin, *J Neurol*, **238**: 309–14.

Langer R, 1981, Polymers for the sustained release of macromolecules: their use in a single-step method of immunization, *Methods Enzymol*, **73**: 57–75.

Laver WG, Air GM et al., 1990, Epitopes on protein antigens. Misconceptions and realities, *Cell*, **61**: 553–6.

Lee CJ, Banks SD, Li JP, 1991, Virulence, immunity, and vaccine related to *Streptococcus pneumoniae*, *Crit Rev Microbiol*, **18**: 89–114.

Lowe RS, Keller PM et al., 1987, Varicella-zoster virus as a live vector for the expression of foreign genes, *Proc Natl Acad Sci USA*, **84**: 3896–900.

McAleer WJ, Buynak EB et al., 1984, Human hepatitis B vaccine from recombinant yeast, *Nature (London)*, **307**: 178–80.

McNamara MK, Ward RE, Kohler H, 1984, Monoclonal idiotope vaccine against *Streptococcus pneumoniae* infection, *Science*, **226**: 1325–6.

Manclark CR, Cowell JL, 1984, Pertussis, *Bacterial Vaccines*, ed. Germanier R, Academic Press, New York, 69–106.

Martinon F, Krishnan S et al., 1993, Induction of virus-specific cytotoxic T lymphocytes in vivo by liposome-entrapped mRNA, *Eur J Immunol*, **23**: 1719–22.

Marwick C, 1996, Acellular pertussis vaccine is licensed in infants, *JAMA*, **276**: 576–8.

Masihi KN, Lange W et al., 1986, Immunobiological activities of non-toxic lipid A: enhancement of non- specific resistance in combination with trehalose dimycolate against viral infections and adjuvant effects, *Int J Immunopharmacol*, **8**: 339–45.

Montgomery DL, Shiver JW et al., 1993, Heterologous and homologous protection against influenza A by DNA vaccination: optimization of DNA vectors, *Dan Cell Biol*, **12**: 777–8.

Morein B, Lovgren K et al., 1987, The ISCOM. An immunostimulating complex, *Immunol Today*, **8**: 333–8.

Mortimer EA Jr, Jones PK, 1979, An evaluation of pertussis vaccine, *Rev Infect Dis*, **1**: 927–32.

Mosier ED, Coppleson LW, 1968, A three-cell interaction required for the induction of the primary immune response in vitro, *Proc Natl Acad Sci USA*, **61**: 542–6.

Moss B, Smith GL et al., 1984, Live recombinant vaccinia virus protects chimpanzees against hepatitis B, *Nature (London)*, **311**: 67–71.

Muller GM, Shapiro M, Arnon R, 1982, Anti-influenza response achieved by immunization with a synthetic conjugate, *Proc Natl Acad Sci USA*, **79**: 569–73.

Nedrud JG, Lamm ME, 1991, Adjuvants and the mucosal immune system, *Topics in Vaccine Adjuvant Research*, eds Spriggs DR, Koff WC, CRC, Boca Raton, FL, 51–67.

Parker DC, 1993, T cell-dependent B cell activation, *Annu Rev Immunol*, **11**: 331–60.

Partidos C, Stanley C, Steward M, 1992, The effect of orientation of epitopes on the immunogenicity of chimeric synthetic peptides representing measles virus protein sequences, *Mol Immunol*, **29**: 651–8.

Pietrobon PJF, 1995, Liposome design and vaccine development, *Vaccine Design: The Subunit and Adjuvant Approach*, eds Powell MF, Newman MJ, Plenum Publishing, New York, 347–61.

Plotkin SA, 1980, Rabies vaccine prepared in human cell cultures: progress and perspectives, *Rev Infect Dis*, **2**: 433–47.

Provost PJ, Hughes JV et al., 1986, An inactivated hepatitis A viral vaccine of cell culture origin, *J Med Virol*, **19**: 23–31.

Quershi N, Takayama K, 1990, Structure and function of lipid A, *The Bacteria. Vol. XI. Molecular Basis of Bacterial pathogenesis*, eds Iglewski BH, Clark VL, Academic Press, San Diego, 319–38.

Ramon G, 1923, Sur le pouvoir flocculant et sur les propriétés immunisantes d'une toxin diphtérique rendue anatoxique (anatoxine), *C R Acad Sci*, **177**: 1338–40.

Reagen KJ, Wunner WH et al., 1983, Anti-idiotypic antibodies induce neutralizing antibodies to rabies virus glycoprotein, *J Virol*, **48**: 660–6.

Robison HL, Hunt LA, Webster RG, 1993, Protection against a lethal influenza virus challenge by immunization with a hemagglutinin-expressing plasmid DNA, *Vaccine*, **11**: 957–60.

van Rooijen N, 1990, *Bacterial Vaccines, Advances in Biotechnological Processes*, vol. 13, Wiley-Liss, New York, 255–79.

Rudbach JA, Cantrell JL et al., 1990, Immunotherapy with bacterial endotoxin, *Endotoxin*, eds Friedman H, Klein TW et al., Plenum Publishing, New York, 665–76.

Sadoff JC, Ballou WR et al., 1988, Oral *Salmonella typhimurium* vaccine expressing circumsporozoite protein protects against malaria, *Science*, **240**: 336–8.

Shapiro ED, 1991, Pneumococcal vaccine, *Vaccines and Immunotherapy*, ed. Cryz SJ Jr, Pergamon Press, Oxford, 127–39.

Stein KE, 1992, Thymus-independent and thymus-dependent responses to polysaccharide antigens, *J Infect Dis*, **165, Suppl. 1**: S49–52.

Stover CK, de la Cruz VF et al., 1991, New use of BCG for recombinant vaccines, *Nature (London)*, **351**: 456–60.

Strugnell RA, Maskell D et al., 1990, Stable expression of foreign antigen from the chromosome of *Salmonella typhimurium* vaccine strain, *Gene*, **88**: 57–63.

Tam JP, 1988, Synthetic peptide vaccine design: synthesis and properties of a high density multiple antigenic peptide system, *Proc Natl Acad Sci USA*, **85**: 5409–13.

Trowsdale J, Ragoussis J, Campbell RD, 1991, Map of the human MHC, *Immunol Today*, **12**: 445–8.

Vogel FR, Sarver N, 1995, Nucleic acid vaccines, *Clin Microbiol Rev*, **8**: 406–10.

Wang CY, Looney DJ et al., 1991, Long-term high-titer neutralizing activity induced by octameric synthetic HIV antigen, *Science*, **254**: 285–8.

Wassilak SGF, Orenstein WA, Sutter RW, 1994, Tetanus toxoid, *Vaccines*, 2nd edn, eds Plotkin SA, Mortimer EA Jr, WB Saunders, Philadelphia, 57–90.

Webster RG, Fynan EF et al., 1994, Protection of ferrets against influenza challenge with a DNA vaccine to haemagglutinin, *Vaccine*, **12**: 1495–8.

White RG, 1972, Concepts of the mechanism of action of adjuvants, *Immunogenicity*, ed. Borek F, North Holland, Amsterdam, 112–30.

Williams RS, Johnson SA et al., 1991, Introduction of foreign genes into tissue of living mice by DNA-coated microprojectiles, *Proc Natl Acad Sci USA*, **88**: 2726–30.

Yuasa T, Kajino K et al., 1991, Preferential expression of the large hepatitis B virus surface antigen gene by an adenovirus-hepatitis B virus recombinant, *J Gen Virol*, **72**: 1927–34.

Zajac BA, West DJ et al., 1986, Overview of clinical studies with hepatitis B vaccine made by recombinant DNA, *J Infect*, **13, Suppl. A**: 39–45.

Zavala F, Tam JP et al., 1987, Synthetic peptide vaccine confers protection against murine malaria, *J Exp Med*, **166**: 1591–6.

Chapter 9

THE EPIDEMIOLOGY OF BACTERIAL INFECTIONS

S R Palmer and N S Galbraith

Epidemiology is the study of the patterns of occurrence and causes of disease in populations. It does not stand alone but is complementary to microbiology and environmental risk assessment methods of investigation. For general accounts of epidemiology see Hennekins and Buring (1987), Holland, Detels and Knox (1991) and Beaglehole, Bonita and Kjellstrom (1993). The occurrence of an episode of microbial disease is a result of the interaction of the agent, host and environmental factors that leads to the exposure of the host to sufficient numbers of the agent in the appropriate transmission mode. Successful investigation and control require that not only the microbiological, but also behavioural, genetic, environmental and social factors which influence the occurrence and presentation of the disease be taken into account. Close collaboration between epidemiologists, microbiologists and other public health workers is therefore essential. Accurate laboratory diagnosis is usually a major factor in successful control, though epidemiological methods alone may be sufficient to indicate appropriate interim control measures. For example, the modes of transmission and the risk behaviour leading to the acquired immune deficiency syndrome (AIDS) were identified by epidemiological methods 2 years before the causative agent was discovered. Advice to the public about reducing the risk of infection did not need to be revised substantially when the human immunodeficiency virus (HIV) was identified. The discovery of HIV was a major advance and allowed the development of diagnostic tools that are now used to study epidemiological characteristics of the infection, e.g. incubation period, progression rate to AIDS,

spectrum of clinical disease, period of infectivity. Increasingly, the epidemiological method is seen by microbiologists as a necessary tool in setting priorities for the use of scarce resources. Applications of epidemiology in microbiological disease include population surveillance to monitor trends in disease and infections and to detect case clusters, the investigation of sources and modes of transmission of micro-organisms, applying public health measures to control outbreaks of disease, and devising and evaluating preventive and control programmes.

1 CONCEPTS IN THE EPIDEMIOLOGY OF INFECTIOUS DISEASE

RESERVOIR OF INFECTION

This is where the infectious agent normally lives and where it may multiply or survive; it may be human (e.g. in chickenpox), animal (e.g. in brucellosis) or the inanimate environment (e.g. in tetanus).

SOURCE OF INFECTION

Infection may be derived from the patient's own microflora (endogenous), or from another human being, or an animal (zoonosis) or an environmental source (exogenous). The source of an exogenous infection may sometimes be different from its reservoir. For example, in an outbreak of listeriosis in Canada the reservoir of infection was a flock of sheep, from which manure was used as fertilizer on a cabbage field. Contaminated cabbages from the field were used to make coleslaw which become the source of infection for human subjects (Schleck et al. 1983). When the source of infection is inanimate, e.g. food, water or fomites, it is termed the **vehicle** of infection.

MODE OF TRANSMISSION

The mechanism by which an infectious agent passes from the reservoir or source of infection to the person can be classified as follows.

Food-, drink- or water-borne infection

Examples of this type of infection are typhoid and cholera. The term 'food poisoning' has in the past sometimes been restricted to incidents of acute disease in which the agent has multiplied in the food vehicle before ingestion (e.g. food-borne salmonellosis), or where it may have formed toxins (e.g. botulism).

Direct or indirect contact

This includes spread from cases or carriers, animals or the environment to other persons who are 'contacts'. Within this category possible routes include: faeces-to-hand-to-mouth spread (e.g. shigellosis); sexual transmission (e.g, gonorrhoea); skin or mucous membrane contact (e.g. wound infection, cutaneous anthrax).

Percutaneous infection

This includes: insect-borne transmission via the bite of an infected insect either directly from saliva (e.g. malaria); or indirectly from insect faeces contaminating the bite wound (e.g. typhus); transfusion of contaminated blood and inoculation of blood or blood products from needle stick injuries (e.g. hepatitis B); direct transmission through intact skin (e.g. schistosomiasis), or broken skin (e.g. leptospirosis).

Air-borne infection

Infectious organisms may be inhaled as: droplets (e.g. streptococcal pharyngitis); droplet nuclei (e.g. tuberculosis); aerosols (e.g. Legionnaires' disease); dust (e.g. ornithosis); spores (e.g. anthrax).

Transplacental infection

An example of this is rubella.

OCCURRENCE

An infection that is continuously in a population is said to be **endemic**, whereas an increase in incidence above the endemic level is described as an **epidemic**, or **pandemic** when the epidemic is world wide. Cases may be **sporadic**, that is, not known to be related to other cases or infections, or clustered in **outbreaks** which may be defined as 2 or more related cases or infections, suggesting the possibility of a common source or transmission between cases. Three commonly used measures of occurrence of disease or infection are the **incidence rate**, the rate of occurrence of new cases in a defined population (e.g. 10 cases per 100 000 persons per year); **cumulative incidence** or risk, which is the proportion of people who

get a disease during a specific period; and **prevalence**, the proportion of a defined population with the disease at a point in time (**point prevalence**) or during a defined period of time (**period prevalence**). The prevalence of a disease depends upon its incidence and duration. In chronic diseases, prevalence may be high although incidence is low, but in short-duration infectious diseases prevalence approximates to incidence.

The **attack rate** during an outbreak is a type of cumulative incidence, the proportion of the population at risk at the beginning of a time period who became ill during the period. The **secondary attack rate** is the attack rate in the contacts of primary cases due to person-to-person spread.

INCUBATION PERIOD

This is the time from infection to the onset of symptoms. For each organism there is a characteristic range within which infecting dose and portal of entry, as well as host factors such as age (Glynn and Palmer 1992) and immunosuppression, give rise to individual variability.

HOST RESPONSE

This depends upon the dose of the infecting agent and the susceptibility of the host, perhaps influenced by genotype, age, sex, other concurrent disease, immunity and 'risk factors' such as smoking for Legionnaires' disease. In an outbreak of infection there is often a spectrum of clinical response ranging from no symptoms to fulminant disease and death.

COMMUNICABILITY

The infectious agent may be passed to others over a variable time, **the period of communicability**; in some infections even from symptomless temporary or chronic **carriers** (e.g. *Salmonella* Typhi).

2 EPIDEMIOLOGICAL METHODS

2.1 Collection of observations

Investigation of the occurrence and distribution of disease requires accurate definition of the disease and its possible determinants and the measurement of their frequency in the population. A clear case definition is essential in epidemiological studies. If serological or cultural confirmation of the diagnosis is not possible, because a specific laboratory test is lacking or appropriate samples were not collected, the case definition will depend upon the clinical features as, for example, with AIDS before the discovery of HIV. During the investigation of an outbreak, laboratory confirmation of the diagnosis may be possible only in a few cases; a clinical definition will then need to be used in further studies. The specificity of the diagnosis in some patients may be doubtful; in these circumstances it is helpful to classify cases as 'definite', 'probable' and 'possible'. When case definitions are based on the presence of symptoms these must be precisely defined, e.g. 'by diarrhoea we mean at least ≥ 3 loose or watery stools in a 24 h period', so that all respondents understand the questions in the same way and the comparability of different studies can be assessed.

Routine sources of data on infectious diseases are described in a later section (see section 3.1, p. 129). In detailed epidemiological enquiries, however, other sources must be used: medical records, interviews with patients, and questionnaires.

2.2 Medical records

Clinical records may contain data on symptoms, investigations performed and their results, and personal details of patients, but for epidemiological purposes clinical records are seldom sufficient. The data recorded are likely to be accurate but incomplete, since they are not collected in a standard way from each patient. Scrutiny of these records may be useful in confirming the reported diagnosis and assessing whether the patient meets the case definition and laboratory records usually provide an invaluable source of microbiological data and data on age, sex and the geographical distribution of cases. However, to obtain detailed accurate clinical information, interviews with patients are usually required. For example, in a survey of hydatid disease, a review of clinical records yielded data on the patients' age, sex and home address, and on the results of clinical investigations and pathological tests. However, data on past history of residence, occupation and exposure to dogs were seldom recorded; this could be obtained only by questioning the patients (Palmer and Biffin 1987).

2.3 Epidemiological interviews and questionnaires

To ensure accurate and comparable records of all persons included in the enquiry and to facilitate analysis, the data should be collected on a carefully designed standard form or questionnaire. Whenever possible the questionnaire should be tested on a few cases and changes made as necessary before use in the main study. Administration of the questionnaire will often be by direct face-to-face interview by a single investigator or group of investigators trained to administer the questionnaire. Interview by telephone may be useful in obtaining data quickly. When numbers are large and the enquiry is straightforward, a self-administered postal questionnaire is cheaper and quicker to administer, but the response rate and accuracy of the data may be less than those obtained by interview.

When designing questionnaires it is important to take into account the limitations of people's recall of events. For example, in one study, food consumption recalled by people 2–3 days after a luncheon was compared with that observed at the time and recorded on video tape (Decker et al. 1986). Only 4 of 32 patients made no errors in reporting. The sensitivity of the food-history questionnaire was 87.6% and its specificity 96.1%. Thirteen per cent of the respondents reported eating one or both of 2 food items that were

on the questionnaire but not served at the luncheon. Such errors in recall can be reduced by providing background details of events, by design of good questionnaires and by making use of other sources to check data, such as diaries, menus, discussion with relatives, etc. Random errors in recall are unlikely to give rise to false associations between illness and, for example, an item of food, but they will reduce the power of the study to identify the true vehicle of infection. For some types of data, such as history of immunization, recall by patients or parents is of very limited value; studies of vaccine efficacy usually require validation of vaccine history from medical records.

2.4 Descriptive analysis

Variables measured may be:

1 fixed or discrete (e.g. sex, occupation, nationality) or
2 continuous (e.g. age, white blood cell count).

Analysis of the distribution will usually be by calculation of proportions of people who fall within certain categories or rates of occurrence of disease within subgroups of the population. Analysis of continuous variables is more complex because values obtained from a population will form a continuous distribution, usually approximating to a normal or skewed normal distribution (Fig. 9.1). This distribution may be summarized by the mean, median, mode and the standard deviation; these measures are commonly used to compare continuous variables in different populations.

The data should first be analysed within the 3 classical epidemiological parameters of time, place and person, taking into account interactions of these variables.

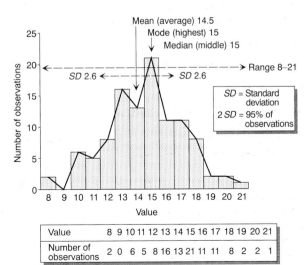

Fig. 9.1 Frequency distribution and measures of continuous variable.

TIME

The epidemic curve is the most useful and immediate means of assessing the type of outbreak (Fig. 9.2). In point-source outbreaks in which all cases are exposed at a given time, onset of symptoms of all primary cases will cluster within the range of the incubation period. For example, in the winter term of 1982, 2 campylobacter outbreaks were reported in boarding schools in the south of England. In the first of these (Fig. 9.2a), 102 of 780 boys were admitted to the sanatorium with gastrointestinal illness, 46 of them on one day; this explosive outbreak was probably due to post-pasteurization contamination of the milk supply on one particular day. The other outbreak occurred in a school supplied with unpasteurized milk and was due to a continuing or recurring source of contamination. In this case the epidemic curve extended over several incubation periods (Fig. 9.2b); 35 of 370 boys were admitted to the sanatorium over the first weeks of the term. In some outbreaks, a point-source of infection may be followed by person-to-person spread as in an outbreak of *Salmonella* Typhimurium, phage-type 10, infection affecting 66 students and one member of staff in a university hall of residence in Bristol in March 1980 (Palmer et al. 1981). The main wave of the outbreak was due to the consumption of contaminated meat pie but subsequent cases were due to person-to-person spread, prolonging the decline in the epidemic curve (Fig. 9.2c). In outbreaks propagated from person to person the occurrence of cases will be spread over several incubation periods with peaks at intervals of the incubation period. For example, an outbreak of measles affecting 151 persons in a circumscribed rural community in Oxfordshire between February and June 1981 (Fig 9.2d) showed a smooth epidemic curve but with distinct peaks at 1, 2, 3 and 4 incubation-period intervals after the case (Knightley and Mayon-White 1982). In larger community outbreaks of diseases spread from person to person, the epidemic curve is usually smoother and the peaks at the generation time of the new cases less obvious.

The onset of disease and the epidemic curve should be studied in relation to other events in the environment of the patients; this may draw attention to possible sources of the infection. For example, investigation of a hospital outbreak of Legionnaires' disease in 1983 revealed that a few weeks earlier the domestic hot-water temperatures in the building had been reduced from c. 55°C at outlets to c. 45°C, a temperature at which legionellae flourish. Subsequent investigations confirmed that the domestic water supply in the hospital was the source of infection (Palmer et al. 1986).

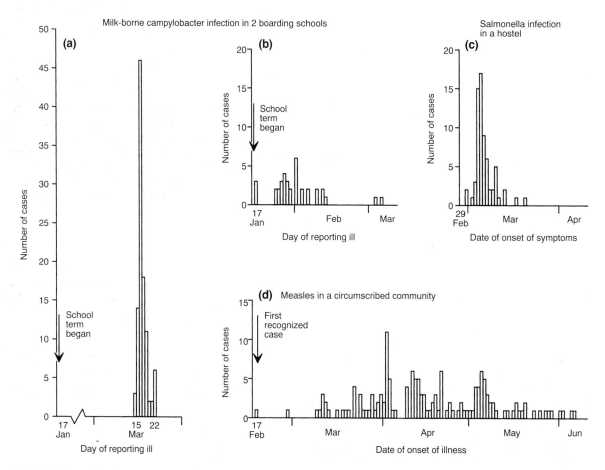

Fig. 9.2 The epidemic curve. (Reproduced from Galbraith NS, 1985, *Oxford Textbook of Public Health*, eds Holland WW, Detels R, Knox G, Vol. 4, Chapter 1, Oxford University Press, by permission of the Oxford University Press).

PLACE

The geographical distribution of disease may provide evidence of its source or method of spread. For example, the crucial factor in the recognition of Lyme disease and the role of tick bites in transmission of *Borrelia burgdorferi* was geographical clustering of presumed childhood rheumatoid arthritis in Old Lyme, Connecticut (Steere, Broderick and Malawista 1978). Investigation revealed that the incidence of illness was higher in communities on the east than on the west side of the Connecticut River, and field studies showed that *Ixodes* ticks were particularly abundant in the former area. Case clustering in a particular place of work or neighbourhood may indicate the existence of a point-source of infection or of person-to-person spread. In outbreaks of hospital-acquired infection, movement of patients between wards may hide clusters; it is therefore necessary to identify and plot the location of the patients at the time of likely exposure.

PERSON

This includes analysis by age, sex, occupation and any other relevant characters which preliminary enquiries indicate may be relevant (e.g. food histories, history of travel, leisure activities and medical or nursing care). For example, food-borne outbreaks of infection due to milk, ice cream and confectionery characteristically affect children rather than adults. A sudden increase in isolations of *Salmonella* Ealing mainly affecting infants led to the recognition and early control of a nationwide outbreak of salmonellosis due to infant-formula dried milk (Rowe et al. 1987). In contrast, in an outbreak of *Salmonella* Oranienburg infection in Norway in 1981 and 1982, 83% of 121 cases were aged 25 years or more, suggesting a food vehicle restricted to adults. This proved to be home-cured meats, the organism originating from contaminated black pepper used as one of the ingredients (Gustavsen and Breen 1984). In another outbreak, of *Salmonella* Cubana infection in hospital patients, the predominance of patients with gastrointestinal dysfunction led to identification of carmine dye, used in investigations, as the vehicle of infection (Lang et al. 1967).

2.5 Epidemiological surveys and analytical studies

Descriptive analysis may suggest hypotheses about the source or mode of transmission of an infection, but is not always a sufficient base for introducing control measures. Analytical epidemiology refers to the use of epidemiological techniques to answer specific questions or to test specific hypotheses. The epidemiological approach is complementary to the microbiological. For example, when microbiological investigations reveal legionellae in a hospital cooling tower this does not in itself identify the source of infection because legionellae commonly colonize water systems without causing disease. Epidemiological evidence is necessary to demonstrate an association between exposure to contaminated water and disease (Bartlett, Macrae and Macfarlane 1986).

EXPERIMENTAL AND INTERVENTION STUDIES

Studies of the efficacy of treatments and vaccines are usually undertaken by randomized controlled trials (Cockburn 1955). Random allocation of people to treatment and non-treatment groups is used to overcome bias that can arise if treated and untreated groups differ in underlying factors; for example, if the groups differed in susceptibility to disease, this might produce a favourable result wrongly attributed to the treatment. Treated and untreated groups are then followed to determine the outcome, and incidence rates are compared. With the exception of vaccine trials, most measures of infectious-disease control have not been subject to randomized controlled trials.

Figure 9.3 shows an epidemiological study design for an experimental study.

PREVALENCE AND INCIDENCE STUDIES

In prevalence or cross-sectional studies (Fig. 9.4) the aim is to measure the proportion of a population with disease or other variable at a point in time. Prevalence studies are often used in descriptive epidemiology, for example, in the surveillance of HIV infection in which the proportions of different risk groups who are HIV-antibody positive are calculated at different times to monitor the spread of infection in the population. Crucial to the success of such studies is the representativeness of the sample of the population studied. Studies of AIDS and HIV infection are hampered by inability to identify the population of homosexuals and drug abusers from which to select a representative sample. Patients attending clinics for sexually transmitted diseases (STD) probably represent the extreme end of the spectrum of sexual activity and are likely to have the highest prevalence of HIV infection. On the other hand, high risk patients may attend private medical facilities so that STD clinic populations cannot be considered necessarily representative even of highly sexually active homosexuals, although they may

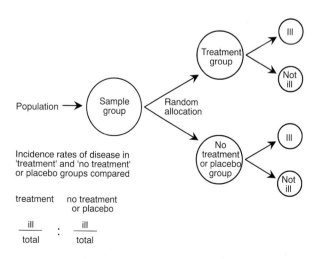

Fig. 9.3 Epidemiological study design – experimental study.

provide a suitable population for monitoring trends in infection.

The methodology of prevalence studies requires the definition of a population and the study sample. The list of names of the population (e.g. electoral register, school register, general practice age-and-sex register), is referred to as the 'sampling frame'; if a sample is to be taken this should be selected either by random, systematic, stratified or cluster sampling (Abramson 1984), so that findings are representative of the practice population. Information on the presence of disease or symptoms is collected by questionnaire or proforma, together with other data on personal characteristics or potential risk factors. The proportions of persons with various characteristics or exposures are then compared to identify high risk groups or exposures associated with high prevalence.

Incidence, longitudinal or follow-up studies measure the rate of occurrence of disease; for these purposes, observations on the population must be made at more than one point in time. Incidence studies may be used descriptively, for example, in following the age incidence of measles to monitor the impact of measles vaccination in a community, in describing the natural history and fatality rates from HIV infection by following cohorts of infected people over several years, or in monitoring cross-infection rates in hospitals. However, they are often also used to test specific hypotheses.

ANALYTICAL COHORT STUDIES

The analytical cohort study is an application of the incidence study; it attempts to investigate causes of disease by using a natural experiment in which a proportion of a population is exposed and a proportion unexposed. It differs from the true experiment in that exposure is not controlled and may not be random; caution is therefore needed when interpreting the data. If the at-risk population is large, a random sample can be investigated and the results extrapolated to the total population.

Cohort studies may be prospective, when the disease occurs after the study has begun and the characteristics of the population have been identified. For example, in a study to identify risk factors for HIV infection, a serological survey of homosexual men was carried out and seronegative men were enrolled in the study. Baseline data on sexual activity were recorded, and 6 months later the sera of the same men were again tested and seroconversion rates were calculated for groups with a particular sexual behaviour. Seroconversion rates were significantly higher in men practising receptive anal intercourse (Kingsley et al. 1987) than in those who practised other forms of sexual activity. In a study in the USA of the influence of socio-economic factors on the incidence and outcome of cytomegalovirus infection in pregnancy, 2 cohorts of women were selected by enrolling those attending a private clinic and those attending a state health department clinic. Seroconversion rates were significantly higher in the lower socioeconomic group (Stagno et al. 1986). Retrospective or historical cohort studies are possible when the population has been defined and identified previously for other purposes. In investigations of food-poisoning outbreaks that have taken place in institutions or after attendance at receptions it is usually possible to identify retrospectively all those exposed and to relate the attack rates to food consumed (food-specific attack rates).

Several possible types of bias may lead to misinterpretation of results of analytical studies (Palmer and Swan 1991) and should be considered at the design stage. One potential problem is that of misclassification of cases and non-cases. For example, in the outbreak already described, of *Salmonella* Typhimurium in 1981 in a university hostel, it was not possible to detect the vehicle of infection by comparing food-specific attack rates if a case definition based upon the presence of gastrointestinal symptoms was used. Faeces samples were obtained from the whole cohort and only when symptomless excreters had been excluded from the well group did a significant difference in food-specific attack rates emerge. To help overcome this problem it is usual to ask all the individuals in the cohort about symptoms over the appropriate time period, so that those who may have been unrecognized cases can be excluded from the analysis or reclassified as cases. The feasibility of serotesting, swabbing or otherwise testing controls to exclude symptomless infected persons should always be considered.

Another important possible bias may arise from 'loss to follow-up'. The loss of cases or controls from the study because of refusal to be interviewed or failure to trace patients can seriously bias results since exposures in non-responders may differ from those of responders. A poor response rate may invalidate the results of a study.

CASE-CONTROL STUDIES

The essential difference between a case-control study (Fig. 9.5) and a cohort study is that the former begins with the identification of people with and without the

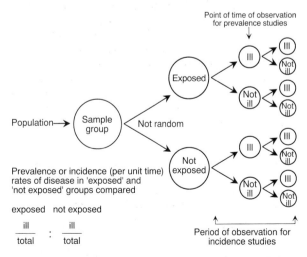

Fig. 9.4 Epidemiological study design – prevalence and incidence studies.

infection and then attempts retrospectively to identify factors associated with disease. In cohort studies, on the other hand, groups of people are identified other than by the presence of disease, and then information on disease occurrence in this group is sought. When the population affected cannot be accurately determined or cases are few, case-control studies are appropriate. Their use should be confined to the testing of specific hypotheses. For example, in the outbreak of *Salmonella* Ealing infection in infants, the hypothesis that the vehicle of infection was infant-formula dried milk was tested by a case-control study that showed a strong association between illness and consumption of one particular brand. Subsequently, *Salmonella* Ealing was cultured from the milk powder and from the factory where it was produced (Rowe et al. 1987). Case-control studies are relatively quick and cheap to perform but their design and analysis can be complex (Schlesselman 1982) and special attention must be paid to potential sources of bias (Kopec and Esdaile 1990).

Cases and controls should be representative of the infected and uninfected population, respectively, from which they came and should have had equal opportunity for exposure to the suspected source. Possible bias in the detection of cases may occur if, for example, only patients admitted to hospital are studied; those who have died of fulminant disease or have only mild illnesses may as a result be excluded. Variables significantly associated with disease in a biased sample may merely reflect the factors that caused the bias, for example, admission to hospital. 'Sampling frames' commonly used to select controls include electoral registers, hospital admissions lists, general practitioner age–sex registers, hotel and reception guest lists, family members of cases, neighbours of cases, acquaintances nominated by cases, and persons investigated by the laboratory but who were negative for the disease in question. When only a few cases are identified the statistical power of the study can be increased by increasing the number of controls per case up to 5 before the efficiency of the study falls.

Interpretation of differences in the proportions of cases and controls with a particular variable must take into account the possible effect of confounding factors. A confounding factor is one that is not the source of infection but is associated both with the cases and independently with the suspected source. The association with the occurrence of disease may lead to a misinterpretation of the source of the infection. When confounding factors can be reasonably predicted they may be excluded by selecting controls that are matched to cases for exposure to those factors. For example, in the first recognized outbreak of haemorrhagic colitis in the USA in 1982, interviews with cases suggested that food eaten at one fast-food restaurant chain were associated with illness. Since exposure to the particular restaurant chain depended upon the location of the restaurants, and probably also on age, controls were matched with cases for neighbourhood of residence and age. A significant association between illness and the restaurant chain was found and subsequently frozen hamburger meat from one restaurant yielded the causative organism *Escherichia coli* O:157 H:7 (Riley et al. 1983). Full details of possible sources of bias in case-control studies are given by Sackett (1979).

The major drawback of case-control studies is that accurate and complete data may not be available retrospectively. Medical records are notoriously incomplete and the recall of patients may be faulty. The latter problem is lessened in acute incidents, because there is usually little delay between the event and the interview. A particular problem is that of 'rumination bias'; because of their illness, sufferers will have gone over in their minds possible exposures and recall may be biased by their own preconceptions or by speculation in the press or other 'media'. Cases may also have been interviewed on many occasions; as well as promoting a more detailed recall, this may introduce bias from suggestions made by interviewers.

STATISTICAL ANALYSIS

In both cohort and case-control studies the basic analysis is made by a comparison of proportions. The data can be presented in a contingency table (Table 9.1).

In cohort studies the ratio $a/(a+b)$ is the attack rate in the exposed. The ratio $[a/(a+b)]:[c/(c+d)]$ is the ratio of the attack rates in the exposed and the unexposed and is called the **relative risk**. The size of the relative risk is an indication of the causative role of the factor concerned. In case-control studies there are usually no denominators from which risks can be estimated and it is necessary to work with the 'odds' of infection or exposure. The odds of a case having been

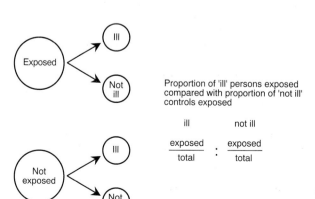

Proportion of 'ill' persons exposed compared with proportion of 'not ill' controls exposed

$$\frac{\text{exposed}}{\text{total}} : \frac{\text{exposed}}{\text{total}}$$

Fig. 9.5 Epidemiological study design – case-control study.

Table 9.1 Contingency table for cohort and case-control studies

	Case	Not case	Total
Exposed	a	b	$a + b$
Not exposed	c	d	$c + d$
Total	$a + c$	$b + d$	$a + b + c + d$

exposed are a/c and the odds of a control having been exposed are b/d. The odds ratio, ad/bc, or cross-product ratio, is a very useful measure of association. It approximates to the relative risk when the disease is rare. If there is no association between exposure and infection the odds ratio will be unity.

In both the cohort and case-control studies dose response effects can be examined if data on different levels of exposure are collected. If the relative risk or odds ratio increases with increasing exposure, the strength of the evidence to determine causality is greatly enhanced. Dose response may be the only way of showing an association between exposure and disease if the exposure is universal (e.g. water consumption).

In analytical studies it is desirable that the relative risk and the odds ratios are presented, together with confidence intervals, rather than depending solely on p values. The p value is the probability of obtaining a difference between the proportion of cases and non-cases who are exposed which is as large or larger than that observed in the study if there is no association between disease and exposure. The p value depends not only on the size of the effect but also on the sample size. A study may fail to show an odds ratio or relative risk significantly greater than unity even when a real difference exists because the study size is too small (type II error). Analysis of data sets usually begins by looking at exposure variables one at a time (univariate analysis). Associations between variables and the outcome measures may be causal or they may be due to shared associations with another variable, such as age or sex, known as a confounding variable. The latter can be investigated by stratified analysis in which associations between exposure and disease are examined within subcategories of the confounding variable. The Mantel–Haenszel method is frequently used and logistic regression modelling methods are increasingly used. When matched studies are performed the matching should be preserved in analysis and McNemar's test and the exact binominal probability should be calculated in place of χ^2 and Fisher's exact test. For further discussion of statistical methods see Breslow and Day (1980, 1987) and Altman (1991).

3 EPIDEMIOLOGICAL SURVEILLANCE

In this chapter epidemiological or population surveillance describes the measurement and reporting of infection in a geographically defined population that may be local, national or international, or may be a particular group at special risk of infections such as hospital in-patients or personnel in certain industries in which there are particular infectious disease hazards. It has been defined as the ongoing systematic collection, analysis and interpretation of outcome-specific data, closely integrated with the timely dissemination of these data to those responsible for preventing and controlling disease (Thacker and Berkelman 1988).

One of the earliest recorded surveillance programmes was developed in the City of London in the sixteenth and seventeenth centuries to detect the appearance of plague, so that the City administration could decide when to close the theatres of the City to limit the assembly of large crowds of people, and the Royal Court could be advised if and when it was desirable to leave London to escape the disease. The parish clerks of the City were responsible for data collection; each parish appointed 2 lay searchers to ascertain burials of plague victims, which were then recorded by the clerks along with other burials in the parish burial registers. These data were summated each week by the parish clerks in returns to the Warden of the Hall of Parish Clerks, who then prepared a statistical tabulation of burials by parish. This was published in a weekly bulletin, the 'Bill of Mortality', together with information on the total plague burials compared with the previous week and the number of parishes affected by plague and the number free of the disease (Wilson 1927). The long-term trends in burials in London derived from these Bills of Mortality were studied in 1662 by John Graunt, a City draper, who assessed the validity of the data and demonstrated a higher mortality in towns than in the country by comparing London with Romsey in Hampshire, and drew attention to the high mortality in young children. Greenwood (1948) regarded John Graunt and William Petty, with whom Graunt worked, as the founders of present-day medical statistics.

Thacker and Berkelman (1988) wrote of the USA that: the 'basic elements of surveillance were present in Rhode Island in 1741 when the colony passed an act requiring tavern keepers to report contagious diseases among their patrons. Two years later, the colony passed a law requiring the reporting of small pox, yellow fever and cholera.' Systematic reporting of disease began in the USA in 1874 in Massachusetts, when the State Board of Health introduced voluntary weekly reporting of disease by physicians using a standard postcard.

In the UK, the need for more accurate and complete mortality data led to the introduction of medical certification of death and the civil registration of births, marriages and deaths in 1836. The General Register Office for England and Wales was established in London, later known as the Office of Population Censuses and Surveys (OPCS) (Nissel 1987) and in 1996 it became part of the Office for National Statistics (ONS). Similar national register offices exist in the other countries of the UK. William Farr, the first Compiler of Abstracts (medical statistician) at the General Register Office, during his 41 years in office, initiated the present international classification of causes of death and developed further the surveillance of communicable disease, establishing a method of influenza surveillance that remains in use today. Dr John Simon, the first Medical Officer to the Local Government Board (Chief Medical Officer), said of William Farr: 'Eminently he was the man to bring into statistical relief, and to make intelligible to the common mind, whatever broad lessons were latent in the life-and-death registers of that great counting house...' (the General Register Office). This provision of readily comprehensible information to those who need it for prompt action remains a crucial component of surveillance.

Surveillance has now assumed even greater importance because of the increased threat of national and international spread of infections arising from the escalating speed, distance and volume of human travel and the expanding national and international distribution of foodstuffs and other materials which may carry pathogenic organisms (Dorolle 1968). For example, surveillance may be the only means of detecting outbreaks when the victims have travelled during the incubation period from the place of exposure to many different destinations, or when the vehicle of infection is widely distributed geographically and sometimes also in time. In the face of this threat, national and international surveillance of communicable disease was revived and developed beginning in the 1950s (Langmuir 1963, Raska 1966). More recently, it has been appreciated that increasing human social, technical, environmental and population change is likely to promote the evolution of new pathogens and facilitate the return of old diseases, now termed 'emerging and re-emerging infections', and that this requires increased surveillance on a global scale to ensure rapid detection, investigation and control (Lederberg, Shope and Oaks 1992, Murphy 1994).

The 6 main objectives of epidemiological surveillance for communicable disease are:

1 early detection of changes in disease pattern to enable rapid investigation and application of appropriate control measures
2 monitoring long-term trends in disease and infection, including serological surveillance, to assess the need for intervention and to predict future trends
3 determining the prevalent infections in a population so that clinicians may be alerted
4 collation of data about newly recognized or rare diseases at national or international level so that their epidemiology can be described and a basis for research is provided
5 evaluation of disease-control measures and preventive programmes
6 planning and costing of health services for the prevention and control of communicable disease.

The method of surveillance remains similar to that of plague surveillance in the seventeenth century, namely:

1 the systematic collection of data
2 analysis of these data to produce statistics
3 interpretation of the statistics to provide information
4 timely distribution of this information in a readily assimilable form to all those who require it so that action can be taken
5 continuing surveillance to evaluate the action.

The main principles of successful surveillance are simplicity, timeliness, accuracy and regular analysis and reporting to those who provide data and to those who are responsible for control action. Surveillance is, by definition, an ongoing activity and can be sustained only when the burden placed on the data provider is light. Surveillance data should be limited to the minimum required to meet its specified objectives. Reporting methods should be simple and streamlined. Successful systems have been developed using modern information technology such as the Minitel system in France (Valleron and Garnerin 1993). Electronic data collection should be linked to electronic systems for dissemination of high quality surveillance information. For accuracy, surveillance data ideally require clear case definitions as have been developed by the Centers for Disease Control in the USA (Wharton et al. 1990).

Guidelines for the evaluation of surveillance systems have been proposed (Klaucke et al. 1988). These include the following features:

1 a description of the public health importance of the health event including incidence and prevalence, severity of disease as measured by mortality rates and case fatality rates, and preventability
2 a description of the system including the objectives, the population under surveillance, case definitions, a flow chart of data collection, details of data transfer, data analysis and dissemination of information
3 a measure of the usefulness of the surveillance system including decisions and actions taken as a result of the information generated
4 evaluation of key attributes of the system including: simplicity, flexibility, acceptability, sensitivity, predictive value positive, respresentativeness and timeliness
5 costs of the system.

3.1 Data-collection systems

Surveillance data may be sought actively or acquired passively by making use of routinely generated data. Most active data-collecting systems are based on carefully designed standard case definitions. For example, the surveillance of certain rare childhood disorders, including Reye's syndrome, in the UK is maintained by the British Paediatric Association Surveillance Unit (BPASU), by monthly mailing of paediatricians to detect cases, followed by subsequent detailed clinical and epidemiological enquiry. These data are then assessed to ensure that all cases meet the standard case definitions before being analysed to describe the epidemiology of the diseases (Hall and Glickman 1988). A unit, similar to the BPASU, was created in 1994 for the active surveillance of neurological disease, the British Neurological Surveillance Unit. A clinical reporting system, set up in 1982 for surveillance of the AIDS epidemic, relies partly on the passive reporting of clinical cases, deaths and laboratory data for the detection of cases and partly on the active collection of data when these were incomplete. The cases are then scrutinized to ensure that they meet the internationally agreed case definition so that the changing epidemiology of the syndrome can be accurately described (PHLS AIDS Centre 1991).

Passive data-collection systems are based upon clinical or microbiological diagnoses which often do not have precise definitions and despite the absence of case definitions, these are invaluable for detecting episodes or cases for further study. For example, in all countries in the UK, cases of typhoid and paratyphoid fevers are detected nationally by statutory notifications, laboratory reports and referral of cultures of the organisms for identification to the Food and Enteric Reference Division of the Central Public Health Laboratory (CPHL); these 3 data sources are then linked. Further active enquiries are made by questionnaire to find out the country where the infection was acquired and possible sources of infection, so that preventive action may be taken. Similarly, cases of Legionnaires' disease are detected by laboratory and incident reports and subsequent active enquiries made, nationally and internationally, to discover cases associated with a common environmental source of infection, so that control measures can be quickly applied.

The main routine data-collecting systems by which information is collected passively in England and Wales and their uses in the surveillance of some specific communicable diseases are shown in Table 9.2. Similar systems are used in other parts of the UK.

Mortality data

Mortality data on communicable diseases have limited use because they do not usually cause death. However, they can be made available quickly, are usually accurate and probably nearly complete. They have been used in the surveillance of influenza since the epidemic of 1847, now in combination with morbidity data from general practitioners and laboratory reports (Tillett and Spencer 1982), and in the surveillance of the acquired immune deficiency syndrome (AIDS) (McCormick 1994). The death entry is a public document and this may sometimes deter the doctor from entering the correct diagnosis on the death certificate, for example in deaths due to syphilis or AIDS, although the doctor may subsequently provide further information about a death in confidence, after the death entry has been completed.

Statutory notification

Notification of infectious disease was first introduced in Huddersfied in 1876 by local act of Parliament; other local authorities followed and in 1899 it became mandatory throughout England and Wales. Weekly summaries of these data began in 1910 and were first published in 1922. The current list of notifiable infectious diseases in England and Wales is shown in Table 9.3. The Public Health (Control of Disease) Act 1984, Section 11, states 'if a registered medical practitioner becomes aware, or suspects, that a patient whom he is attending ... is suffering from a notifiable disease'

he/she shall notify forthwith the proper officer of the local authority (usually the Consultant in Communicable Disease Control, CCDC). The CCDC in turn sends each week a return of the number of notifications to the OPCS received in the preceding 7 days (except leprosy which is reported in strict confidence to the Communicable Disease Surveillance Centre, CDSC). Weekly summaries of these data were previously published in the *OPCS Monitor*, but this ceased publication at the end of 1994 and the data have since been available electronically on the Public Health Laboratory Service (PHLS) computer network, EPINET, and from September 1995 have been published in the weekly *Communicable Disease Report* (*CDR*) (Communicable Disease Surveillance Centre 1995). The data are later corrected and published quarterly and annually by the ONS. Similar systems operate in Scotland and Northern Ireland (Ashley, Cole and Kilbane 1991). The chief advantages of these data are that they are available quickly, they relate to defined populations so that rates by age and sex can be calculated and they provide an invaluable means of monitoring trends for diseases that are not often confirmed in the laboratory, for example whooping cough and mumps. The defects of the data are that the clinical diagnosis may not always be correct; the diagnosis may vary between clinicians especially because there are no case definitions (except for ophthalmia neonatorum and food poisoning); under-notification frequently occurs and may vary from place to place and at different times. These deficiencies can be partially overcome by training notifying clinicians and by regular feedback of local and national information, but it appears that neither the legal obligation to notify nor the payment of a fee promotes more complete notification (McCormick 1993).

In the USA, systems for the notification of selected diseases such as cholera, smallpox, plague and yellow fever began to be introduced in 1878. By 1903 notification to local authorities for selected diseases was required in all states. In 1925 all states joined a national morbidity reporting system which was taken on after 1948 by the National Office of Vital Statistics which continued to produce weekly morbidity statistics. These reports have been developed as the *Morbidity and Mortality Weekly Report*, which since 1961 has been the responsibility of the Centers for Disease Control (CDC) in Atlanta. Currently, notifiable diseases are reported by states to CDC through the National Notifiable Diseases Surveillance System using the National Electronic Telecommunications System for Surveillance (Centers for Disease Control 1991).

Laboratory reporting of microbiological data

The routine voluntary reporting of laboratory-diagnosed infections forms the core of communicable-disease surveillance in England and Wales and also in Scotland, where a somewhat similar reporting system operates. This reporting system was originally developed by the PHLS in the 1940s and 1950s (Grant and Eke 1993) and comprises confidential reporting

Table 9.2 The main routine data-collecting systems used in communicable disease surveillance in England and Wales

Disease	Data-collecting system				
	Death registration	Statutory notification	Laboratory reports	RCGP reports	GUM clinic reports
Anthrax		++	+		
Brucellosis			++		
Chickenpox	+		+	++	
Herpes zoster	+		+	++	
Cholera		+	++		
Diphtheria		++	++		
Food poisoning	+	++	++	+	
Gonorrhoea			+		++
Hepatitis A	+	++	++	+	
Hepatitis B	+	+	++		+
HIV infection (AIDS)	+		++		+
Hydatid disease	+		++		
Influenza	++		++	++	
Infectious mononucleosis			+	++	
Legionnaires' disease			++		
Leptospirosis	+	+	++		
Malaria	+	+	++		
Measles	+	++	++	++	
Meningitis	+	++	++	+	
Mumps		++	+	++	
Ornithosis			++		
Pneumonia	+		+	+	
Poliomyelitis		++	++		
Rubella	+	++	++	++	
Shigellosis		++	++		
Syphilis	+		+		++
Tetanus	++	++	++		
Tuberculosis	+	++	++		
Typhoid and paratyphoid		+	++		

RCGP, Royal College of General Practitioners; GUM, genitourinary medicine.

by medical microbiologists to the Directors of CDSC and Scottish Centre for Infection and Environmental Health (SCIEH), each week on specially designed forms, of specified infections diagnosed in their laboratories. At CDSC data are analysed within a week of receipt to produce tables and line lists which are used in compiling narrative reports for publication in the CDR. Statistics derived from these data are also available on-line to staff in CDSC, and to CCDCs and medical microbiologists through the PHLS computer network, EPINET (Palmer and Henry 1992). Reporting by manual means has begun to be replaced by electronic reporting systems (Grant and Eke 1993) and by the end of 1995 about 50% of the approximately 250 000 laboratory reports received in that year were transmitted electronically. The main benefits of laboratory reports are that they are very precise, in that they are based on laboratory-diagnosed infections and the fine typing of the infecting organisms; they often include clinical and epidemiological details; and they allow for free-text comment. Furthermore, the reporting system is flexible, so that any important, unusual or new infections can be reported, even though they were not necessarily included in the orig-

inal reporting instructions. However, the reports have some drawbacks: they are limited to infections in which there is a suitable laboratory test; infections which are easily diagnosed clinically tend to be poorly covered; and the reports are not population based, that is the data do not usually have a population denominator, so that incidence rates cannot be calculated. Moreover, as with all routine morbidity reporting systems, the data are incomplete, not all laboratories report and the completeness of the reports received may vary between laboratories and over time, so that trends are sometimes difficult to interpret.

GENERAL PRACTICE REPORTING OF CLINICAL DATA

Morbidity data from general practice were studied first in 1955, following which 4 national morbidity studies have taken place, the last in 1991–92 (McCormick, Fleming and Charlton 1995). Continuously collected clinical data from general practice, which is more useful in communicable-disease surveillance, first became available in 1966 when the Royal College of General Practitioners (RCGP) set up a reporting system based on first consultations in a limited number of volunteer

Table 9.3   Statutorily notifiable diseases in England and Wales

Under the Public Health (Control of Disease) Act 1984	
Cholera	Relapsing fever
Food poisoning	Smallpox
Plague	Typhus

Under the Public Health (Infectious Diseases) Regulations 1988	
Acute encephalitis	Ophthalmia neonatorum
Acute poliomyelitis	Paratyphoid fever
Anthrax	Rabies
Diphtheria	Rubella
Dysentery (amoebic and bacillary)	Scarlet fever
Leprosy	Tetanus
Leptospirosis	Tuberculosis
Malaria	Typhoid fever
Measles	Viral haemorrhagic fever
Meningitis	Viral hepatitis
Meningococcal septicaemia (without meningitis)	Whooping cough
Mumps	Yellow fever

Notes 'Viral haemorrhagic fever' means Argentine haemorrhagic fever (Junin), Bolivian haemorrhagic fever (Machupo), Chikungunya fever, Congo/Crimean haemorrhagic fever, dengue fever, Ebola virus disease, haemorrhagic fever with renal syndrome (Hantaan), Kyasanur forest disease, Lassa fever, Marburg disease, Omsk haemorrhagic fever and Rift Valley disease.
There are minor differences in notifiable diseases in Scotland and Northern Ireland (see Ashley, Cole and Kilbane 1991).
Some diseases are notifiable locally, for example, psittacosis in Cambridge.
AIDS is not statutorily notifiable, but clinicians report cases voluntarily, in strict confidence, to the directors of the CDSC in England and Wales and of the SCIEH in Scotland. Advice about reporting is available from these centres and from genitourinary medicine physicians.

practices (Fleming and Crombie 1985). In 1996 there were 367 participating general practitioners in 93 practices serving a population of about 700 000 people; data from 40 of the practices were recorded manually and sent by post, and from the other 53 the data were entered into computer and transferred electronically to the RCGP Research Unit in Birmingham, where they were analysed each week and statistics produced. These weekly analyses are sent to the ONS, the CDSC, the Department of Health (DoH) and other organizations concerned with national surveillance, and were published in the weekly *OPCS Monitor* until 1994. They are published annually by the RCGP Research Unit in the annual reports of the unit. Analogous general practitioner reporting schemes operate in Wales (Palmer and Smith 1991) and some other parts of the UK. These general practitioner reporting systems act primarily as early warning systems providing data rapidly within 10 days of reporting and have the advantages that the data are related to defined practice populations and are unique for some common diseases which are not notifiable and for which laboratory tests are not usually performed, such as chickenpox, herpes zoster and infectious mononucleosis (see Table 9.2). In the RCGP system guidelines to diagnosis are provided and in the Welsh system a set of standard case definitions, but the precise definition of an infection is less important than the speedy recognition of an emerging outbreak which may require prompt investigation. However, there are some deficiencies: reporting may not always be complete; the population covered may not be representative geographically or demographically of the whole country and is too small for the surveillance of less common diseases.

In Europe a network of sentinel sites (Eurosentinel) was established in 1988 and funded by the European Union. In 1992 there were 16 sentinel systems in 9 countries collaborating (Van Casteran and Leurquin 1992).

REPORTS OF SEXUALLY TRANSMITTED DISEASES

Legislation in the nineteenth and early twentieth centuries required the registration, regular examination and, if necessary, detention of prostitutes, and compulsory admission to hospital for other sufferers from venereal disease (VD) was recommended. However, when a national VD service came into being in 1916, these legal powers were discontinued and a free confidential service for diagnosis and treatment was established at VD clinics, now genitourinary medicine (GUM) clinics. At the same time, a system of quarterly clinic returns began, providing the number of new episodes of specified infections by gender and for some diseases in age groups, which, with variations and additions, has continued ever since. Sexually transmitted diseases, including AIDS, have not been made statutorily notifiable in the UK because of fears that a legal obligation to report individual patient data might lead to some individuals concealing their infections, consequently hindering the control of these infections. The clinic returns are analysed by the UK departments of health and are collated by CDSC and SCIEH; periodic reviews of trends are published, the most recent for the decade 1981–90 (Catchpole 1992). The clinic returns provide data that are probably accurate, being based on specialist clinical diagnosis, often supported by laboratory tests, are unlikely to vary between clinics and over time, and provide a unique set of data extending over nearly three-quarters of a century for some infections. However, the reports record episodes of infection rather than patients, are incomplete because they do not include patients treated outside GUM clinics, and the proportion of patients treated outside the clinics is unknown and may vary by diagnosis, between clinics and over time.

HOSPITAL DATA

Data from a 10% sample of hospital discharges and deaths were available from 1955 to 1985, but had limited use in communicable-disease surveillance because the data did not become available until about 2 years after collection (Ashley, Cole and Kilbane 1991). In 1995, these data were replaced by Hospital Episode Statistics which are currently being assessed for their possible value in communicable-disease surveillance. Paget (1897) in his book *Wasted Records of Disease*, referring to hospital records, commented: 'At present these records of disease are rarely utilized for public purposes, and they represent in their present circumstances little more than so much waste of time, material, and intelligence.' A century later, a satisfactory method of capturing these data for the surveillance of communicable diseases and other acute diseases has still to be found.

ROUTINE SEROLOGICAL SURVEILLANCE

In 1990 a serological study to measure the spread of human immunodeficiency virus (HIV) infection in the population was begun; it has continued since and become a routine surveillance system. Samples from sera collected for clinical purposes are unlinked from personal identifiers but remain linked to epidemiological information; sera remaining unused are then tested for HIV infection. This Unlinked Anonymous HIV Prevalence Monitoring Programme demonstrated an initial decline in prevalence rates of infection in homosexual men and injecting drug users in the mid-1980s, but, more recently, a rise amongst pregnant women in London (Report 1995).

OTHER ROUTINE DATA-COLLECTING SYSTEMS

Work-absence data have been used in the surveillance of influenza, but surveillance is now based principally on mortality data, laboratory reports and general practitioner reports. CCDCs report voluntarily to the CDSC outbreaks occurring in their districts and are required to report serious outbreaks; these reports are usually of food-borne diseases, notably salmonellosis, and provide supplementary data for surveillance of these diseases. Each week, members of the Medical Officers of Schools Association voluntarily report, to the CDSC, illness in around 10 000 children in 35–40 boarding schools in England and Wales, providing data on outbreaks of infectious disease, which are particularly valuable in influenza surveillance.

3.2 Action consequent on surveillance

The routine data-collecting systems used for communicable-disease surveillance are managed by several different organizations and it is the responsibility of the CDSC in England and Wales and the SCIEH in Scotland to analyse and collate these data and interpret them to provide a comprehensive view of communicable disease. A flow diagram showing the production of the weekly *CDR*, the CDSC information bulletin, is shown in Fig. 9.6.

Changes in numbers of reports were hitherto usually discovered by examining the data in either numerical or graphical form, but statistical and computer techniques are now often used to assist in the detection of significant variations from previously recorded experience (Tillett and Spencer 1982, Farrington and Beale 1993). Such variations may indicate changes in the incidence of disease but they may also result from changing interest of disease, altered diagnostic techniques or reporting methods, or fluctuations in the number of microbiologists, laboratories, clinicians, practices or clinics participating in the reporting system. It is usual, therefore, to compare the data from all the relevant data-collecting systems to validate the observed trends. Often, especially if there is a rapid increase in reports, field investigation is necessary to substantiate an increase and determine its cause.

Routine, regular and systematic dissemination of information to the providers of the data and to disease-control authorities is essential for successful surveillance (Langmuir 1963). In England and Wales this is maintained through the weekly *CDR* and the monthly *CDR* review and in Scotland the *SCIEH Weekly Report*, which are available without charge to professional staff concerned with the control of communicable disease. These bulletins contain narrative reports of newly identified or suspected outbreaks of disease, reviews of prevalent communicable diseases and related topics as well as numerical data on certain organisms, notifiable diseases and general practitioner reports. More extensive reviews are published in quar-

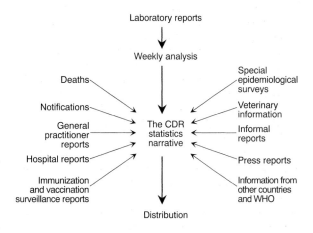

Fig. 9.6 Weekly Communicable Disease Report: information flow.

terly reviews, annual reports and in the medical press. Sometimes when an acute episode of infection is identified, more rapid transmission of information electronically, by phone or facsimile is required.

The uses of epidemiological surveillance may be illustrated by examples that refer to its main objectives.

EARLY DETECTION FOR RAPID CONTROL

In January 1988 there was an increase in laboratory reports of an unusual organism, *Salmonella typhimurium* definitive type 124. During the month the organism was identified in cultures from 63 patients, but there had been fewer than this number of reports in the whole of the previous year. A rapid descriptive epidemiological study of 15 patients suggested that wrapped salami sticks, a widely available meat product, might be the vehicle of infection. This hypothesis was tested by a case-control study which showed a statistically significant association between infection and eating the salami sticks. The organism was later isolated from salami sticks sampled from a shop associated with one of the cases. The product was withdrawn from the market and a public warning issued within 7 days of the identification of the outbreak (Cowden et al. 1989). Many similar examples of the early detection of outbreaks and their rapid control have been published in the *CDR* and other medical journals.

ASSESSING THE NEED FOR INTERVENTION

Notifications of viral hepatitis (infectious jaundice until 1988) declined throughout the 1970s particularly in the age group 5–14 years. Since there had been no change in laboratory reports of acute hepatitis B, it was concluded that there had been a fall in the incidence of hepatitis A infection. This was supported by a similar decline in laboratory reports of *Shigella sonnei*, another infection spread mainly by the faecal–oral route in children. However, notifications rose again in the early 1980s to reach a peak in 1982, a rise that was mirrored by a smaller increase in laboratory reports of hepatitis A based on serological tests, which first

became available in 1979 (Fig. 9.7). Although most of the increase was in children, there were rises in adults, particularly in the first quarter of 1981 and the first half of 1982, which corresponded in time to reports of outbreaks of hepatitis A due to shellfish, reported mostly in southeast England. As a result of these surveillance findings, a case-control study of notified viral hepatitis was conducted in 19 local authority districts, all but one of them close to the Thames estuary. This showed a statistically significant association between illness and the consumption of shellfish, particularly cockles (O'Mahony et al. 1983). An investigation of shellfish production followed, with subsequent intervention by hygienic improvements in the cleansing and cooking of shellfish (Millard, Appleton and Parry 1987). Continuing surveillance demonstrated a general decline in notifications and laboratory reports of hepatitis A.

A rise in laboratory reports of hepatitis B then followed in 1984, associated in time with increased notifications of drug addicts to the Home Office and several reports of outbreaks of hepatitis B in injecting drug users. Intervention included the augmentation of health education about drug misuse and extension of hepatitis B vaccination, but the part these measures played in the subsequent decline in laboratory reports is unclear because of the impact of the AIDS epidemic on the spread of hepatitis B infection.

A second rise in notifications began in 1988 and continued until 1992 and was more closely mirrored by laboratory reports of hepatitis A than in the previous 10 years, probably because easily applied salivary tests for anti-HAV IgM had by this time become available. There were other differences between the 2 rises; notifications in the 1988–92 rise were higher in the north than in the south, predominantly in children under 15 years and shellfish-associated outbreaks were less common than in the earlier rise. As a consequence of these findings a large case-control study was undertaken in 201 local authorities in England in 1990–91, with about 1500 cases and nearly the same number of controls. This showed a highly significant

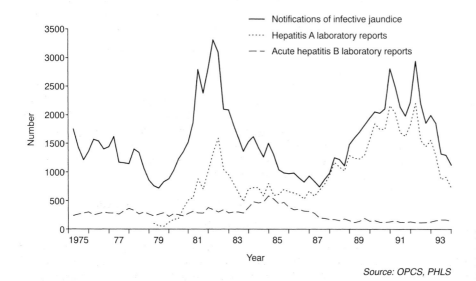

Fig. 9.7 Viral hepatitis. Quarterly notifications and laboratory reports, England and Wales 1975–93.

Source: OPCS, PHLS

association with household contact with a known case, which may lead to an evaluation of vaccination as well as the use of normal human immune globulin in these circumstances. A significant association was also shown with eating shellfish in the north and west of England; the absence of an association in the south and east was probably due to the processing equipment installed after the previous outbreaks. An association with travel abroad was also demonstrated, supporting the recommendation for vaccination of frequent travellers to areas where hepatitis A is endemic (Maguire et al. 1995).

Determining prevalent infections as an aid to clinical care

Trends in the incidence of respiratory pathogens were monitored by laboratory reports. These showed a regular 4 year cycle of outbreaks of *Mycoplasma pneumoniae* infection, annual winter peaks of respiratory syncytial virus and summer peaks of parainfluenza type 3 virus infection but a less regular pattern of infection due to parainfluenza types 1 and 2, adenoviruses and coxsackie A viruses. Detection of these changes enables clinicians to be alerted early, assisting them in prompt diagnosis and the selection of appropriate therapy. Another example of the value of surveillance data for clinical use was laboratory reports of antibiotic-resistant strains of *Neisseria gonorrhoeae* leading to changes in the clinical management of the disease (Jephcott 1992).

Important developments in communicable disease may be brought to the attention of clinicians when required, by Chief Medical Officer letters, by reports of specialist associations, and by the medical press. The increasing use of electronic communication may give clinicians access to communicable disease information by Internet in the future.

Detecting new or rare diseases for study

The surveillance of Reye's syndrome began in 1981. This showed that the annual incidence varied between 0.3 and 0.6 per 100 000 in the British Isles with the highest rate in Northern Ireland. No clear seasonal peaks were seen but 59% of patients had an onset of disease in autumn or winter. The median age was 14 years and the sex distribution equal. The national collection of data on cases that met the standard case definition enabled an analytical study to be made of risk factors in the disease. This suggested an association with the use of aspirin, similar to that seen previously in the USA, and led to the withdrawal of paediatric aspirin preparations and cessation of the general use of aspirin in childhood in 1986. The surveillance scheme continued and demonstrated a decline in the number of cases in subsequent years despite more active data collection (Newton and Hall 1993).

Evaluation of preventive programmes

Surveillance of whooping cough was at first based on notifications that started in 1939. These showed a substantial decline in the 1950s after the introduction of routine immunization in childhood, from an average of nearly 140 000 per year during 1950–59 to fewer than 25 000 per year during 1960–69. In the 1960s, 2 further sources of routine data were used, laboratory reports of *Bordetella pertussis* and general practitioner reports of whooping cough from the Birmingham Research unit of the RCGP; all 3 indices declined demonstrating the efficacy of immunization. However, in 1974 the publication of a report about possible neurological complications of immunization against whooping cough was followed by public controversy about vaccine safety. At the same time, by an unfortunate coincidence, the post of Medical Officer of Health (MOH) with the responsibility for immunization programmes was abolished in the 1974 National Health Service (NHS) reorganization. Immunization acceptance rates fell dramatically; by 1978 only 30% of children under 2 years of age had been immunized and large outbreaks followed in 1978 and 1982 (Fig. 9.8). These outbreaks coincided with an increase in *M. pneumoniae* infections, which gave rise to suggestions that this organism and other respiratory pathogens might have been the cause of the outbreaks, but continuing surveillance of whooping cough showed an increase in all 3 indices, indicating that the outbreaks were indeed due to *B. pertussis*. Another large outbreak was expected in 1986; a rise in the 3 indices in 1985 suggested that this was imminent, but it failed to develop due to a rise in immunization acceptance to nearly 70%. This was supported by a regional analysis of the data, which showed a notification rate of 462 per 100 000 in regions with acceptance rates of 50–59% compared with 333 per 100 000 in those with acceptance rates of 70% or more. The rise in immunization acceptance rates followed publication of the conclusion that the association of neurological disease with immunization was not causal and coincided with the appointment of immunization co-ordinators in NHS districts, replacing the function of the former MOH. The next 4 year outbreak of whooping cough in 1990 was much smaller than previous outbreaks and by 1994, when immunization uptake rates had reached 93%, the expected outbreak did not occur. Surveillance had shown that whooping cough was at last controlled in England and Wales.

Planning and costing of health services

Surveillance data on AIDS and HIV infection have been used to make future projections of the likely numbers of cases of AIDS and severe HIV disease for planning purposes (Report 1996) and employing surveillance data on salmonellosis. Sockett (1995) assessed the costs of the disease and estimated the cost-benefits of preventive measures.

3.3 Surveillance of immunization programmes

The development of large-scale, strictly controlled field trials of vaccines in the early 1950s (Cockburn 1955) provided a reliable means of establishing the

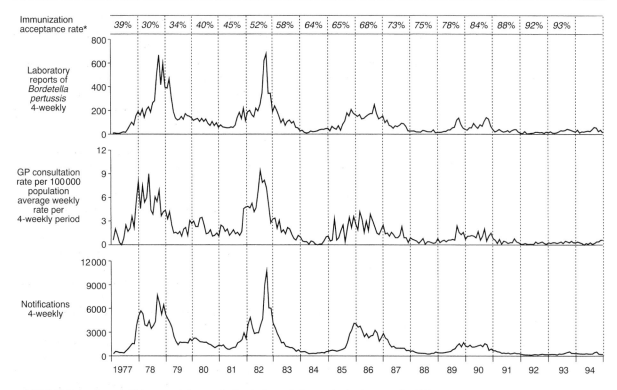

Fig. 9.8 Whooping cough, England and Wales 1977–94.

efficacy and safety of vaccines in the field and of ensuring that laboratory measures of antigenicity correlated with protection against infection in vaccinated subjects. For example, the earlier failure to appreciate these requirements resulted in the widespread use of alcoholized typhoid vaccine in the 1940s, which was thought to give better protection than phenolized vaccine because it was shown in mice to preserve the Vi antigen, then considered responsible for immunity. However, in subsequent controlled field trials it was shown to give little, if any, protection (Yugoslav Typhoid Commission 1962). Conversely, painstaking whooping cough vaccine trials in the 1950s demonstrated the correlation of the mouse protection test with protection against pertussis in children (Medical Research Council 1956), which has been used to test the potency of whole cell whooping cough vaccines ever since.

More recently it was appreciated that after licensing and general release of a vaccine, ensuing surveillance was also necessary, not only to demonstrate the influence of the immunization programmes on disease incidence but also to identify subsequent possible changes in vaccine efficacy under field conditions, to reveal groups of susceptible subjects and to detect unsuspected, rare or new vaccine reactions that would not become apparent in the smaller population immunized in the initial vaccine trials (Begg and Miller 1990). The main objects of surveillance of immunization programmes are, therefore, the continual measurement of efficacy, safety and uptake of vac-

cines, and also the assessment of disease-control measures other than immunization used in the prevention of the relevant diseases. The methods used are the same as for epidemiological surveillance, but they require additional data-collecting systems and different analyses.

Vaccine efficacy

Potency testing

Vaccines manufacturers are required by the Medicines Act 1976 to submit to the Medicines Control Authority (MCA) a detailed application for licensing of all new vaccines. These applications include information about the quality assurance laboratory tests that they will subsequently carry out on all batches of vaccines that they produce before they are released, to ensure they meet agreed standards of efficacy and safety and conform with World Health Organization (WHO) and European Union standards. The National Institute of Biological Standards and Control (NIBSC), acting on behalf of MCA, receives samples of all batches before release and verifies that they meet the required standards. The MCA and NIBSC also visit the manufacturers at least annually to inspect the vaccine production units and review their production and quality assurance procedures. After the batches of vaccine are released by the MCA, samples taken from the field are in certain circumstances retested by NIBSC, for example, in the event of vaccine-associated disease or when there is a need to investigate the handling and storage of vaccines. In warm climates special measures are required to ensure the stability of vaccines, particularly live virus vaccines, because of their sensitivity to environmental conditions, and cold-chain monitors (temperature-sensitive colour cards) are usually included in vaccine packs to monitor these circumstances. These are now coming into use in temperate areas to ensure careful attention to vaccine handling and storage.

Causative organisms

Changes in the antigenic structure and prevalence of different serotypes of the causative organisms of the diseases in the immunization programmes need to be continually studied to detect changes which might render the vaccines less effective. For example, because of continual small antigenic changes in the influenza A virus (antigenic drift) and occasional larger changes (antigenic shift), viral isolates from all parts of the world are collected and studied in WHO centres, so that the most appropriate strains may be selected for vaccine production (Pereira 1979). The efficacy of whooping cough vaccine appeared to decrease in the 1960s and was found to be due to a change in the prevalent serotypes of *B. pertussis* (Preston 1965); it was subsequently corrected by the inclusion of the new serotypes in the vaccine.

Serological studies

After licensing and general release of a vaccine, serological studies provide valuable information about immunity in selected individuals who have been immunized routinely and the duration of immunity in samples of immunized people. Samples of sera derived from the whole population (serological surveillance) can be used to determine immunity in different age groups so that the appropriate ages for immunization can be selected (Morgan-Capner et al. 1988) and changes in population immunity detected. For example, serological surveillance in England and Wales between 1986 and 1991 showed that the proportion of school-aged children who were susceptible to measles was increasing following the introduction of measles, mumps and rubella (MMR) vaccination in 1988 and, using mathematical models, a major epidemic was predicted in the mid-1990s (Ramsay et al. 1994). A national vaccination programme for school-aged children ensued in November 1994 and an epidemic was averted.

Epidemiological studies

Vaccine efficacy (VE) can be calculated from the following equation (where ARu = attack rate in the unvaccinated and ARV = attack rate in the vaccinated):

$$VE = \frac{(ARu - ARv)}{ARu} \times 100$$

The epidemiological techniques for measuring vaccine efficacy in the field were reviewed by Orenstein et al. (1985). There are 5 main methods:

1   Screening. If a vaccine has a 90% efficacy, an attack rate of over 10% in vaccinated subjects indicates the need for investigation.
2   Outbreak investigation. The assumption which must be satisfied in the above equation is that both vaccinated and unvaccinated subjects have had equal exposure to infection, an assumption which is likely to be satisfied in outbreaks in confined populations when the attack rate is high (e.g. in institutional outbreaks of measles where case ascertainment will also probably be complete and immunization records easily available). The method can also be applied in community-wide outbreaks in a defined population or in samples of that population.
3   Secondary attack rates in households. This method has been used to determine the efficacy of whooping cough vaccine, because here again the contacts of the index cases in households are likely to have an equal exposure to infection. By adding together the data from several households sufficient numbers become available for analysis.
4   Routine data-collecting systems. These can be used to estimate vaccine efficacy if the data can be linked with immunization histories. The proportion of cases in the vaccinated (PCV) is related to VE and the proportion of the population vaccinated (PPV). Using a variation of the formula:

$$PCV = \frac{PPV - (PPV \times VE)}{1 - (PPV \times VE)}$$

Orenstein et al. (1985) showed that by means of this formula it was possible to estimate vaccine efficacy when the attack rates in vaccinated and in unvaccinated individuals were not known (Fig. 9.9).
5   Case-control studies. Clarkson and Fine (1987) developed case-control methods to determine vaccine efficacy by comparing the immunization status of notified cases with that of children on the child-health computer file, which is available in most parts of the UK.

VACCINE SAFETY

No vaccine can be considered entirely safe (Wilson 1967). Common local or systemic reactions are likely to be identified in large-scale clinical trials before the introduction of vaccines into general use and at this time will be assessed and any necessary action taken to reduce their frequency and severity. Data on vaccine reactions are collected passively and actively in the UK. The principal passive data-collecting system entails medical practitioners reporting reactions and suspected reactions following immunization to the Committee on the Safety of Medicines, using specially designed yellow cards which are available in every edition of the *British National Formulary*. These reports are reviewed regularly by the Joint Committee on Vaccination and Immunization. Other sources of data are complaints to vaccine manufacturers and informal

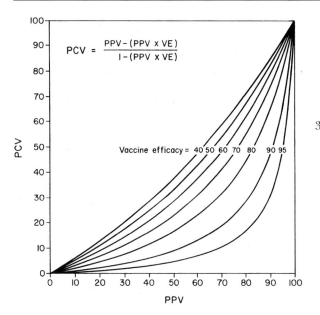

$$PCV = \frac{PPV - (PPV \times VE)}{1 - (PPV \times VE)}$$

Vaccine efficacy = 40 50 60 70 80 90 95

Fig. 9.9 The relationship between the percentage of cases vaccinated (PCV) and the percentage of the population vaccinated (PPV) for 7 different percentage values of vaccine efficiency (VE). (From Orenstein et al. (1985), reprinted by permission of the World Health Organization).

reports to NIBSC, CDSC and the National Poisons Centres. Unfortunately, none of these passive data collecting systems normally involves the doctors responsible for immunization, the immunization co-ordinators, and consequently they are liable to remain unaware of adverse reactions taking place locally in their immunization programmes. Active data collection has been used in the surveillance of polio vaccination since its inception in the 1950s and after the introduction of oral polio vaccine (OPV) in 1962, it provided valuable evidence of the safety of OPV, enabling the programme to continue despite reports of suspected vaccine-induced disease (Galbraith 1964). More recently active surveillance has been used in special studies of bacille Calmette–Guérin (BCG), measles and MMR vaccines (Begg and Miller 1990).

The detection of rare events associated with immunization poses difficulties, but the investigation of these events to determine whether or not they were caused by immunization presents even greater problems. There are 4 methods of investigation that may suggest a causal relationship between immunization and the event:

1   Case clusters. When clusters of disease or reactions are detected in apparent association with immunization, field investigation may discover the cause and lead to prevention of a recurrence. For example, an epidemiological inquiry into a cluster of severe local reactions to BCG vaccine in one health district in 1982 identified faulty vaccination technique of one inadequately trained doctor as the cause. Subsequently, a new on-going training scheme for staff in the BCG vaccination programme was implemented.

2   Pathological investigations. These may detect the

agent of a live vaccine in the lesion which has followed immunization, for example, osteomyelitis following BCG vaccination may be shown to contain the vaccine bacillus, and the cerebrospinal fluid in meningoencephalitis after mumps vaccination may be shown to contain vaccine virus (Maguire, Begg and Handford 1991).

3   Case-control studies. The comparison of the vaccine histories of cases experiencing vaccine reactions with those of a control group, matched for age and sex, may reveal a temporal association between vaccination and the reaction, but this association may not be causal. For example, a strict case-control study showed an association between whooping cough immunization and serious acute neurological illness (Miller et al. 1981), but after several years of further studies and continuing debate, sometimes acerbic, it was concluded that this association was not causal (Griffith 1989). Cohort studies, comparing disease in a vaccinated group with that in an unvaccinated group, are not suitable for studying rare vaccine reactions because the incidence in the study population is likely to be too low to find significant differences between the 2 groups.

4   Case series analysis. Farrington, Nash and Miller (1996) have described a method for estimating the incidence of clinical events after vaccination compared with a control period, based upon data from the cases alone, which may be used for monitoring vaccine safety when a vaccine is in widespread use. This method has the great advantage of reducing the need to follow up large population cohorts or of selecting and investigating control groups.

VACCINE UPTAKE

Vaccine uptake in the UK is measured by 4 main methods:

1   Vaccine usage gives a coarse measure of vaccine uptake. Despite being inaccurate because vaccine wastage and incomplete courses are not taken into account, the method enables major changes to be recognized quickly, which can then be investigated in the field.

2   Annual reports from health authorities to the departments of health in the UK of the numbers of children completing primary courses of immunization and given reinforcing doses in the previous year. Although these data are published quickly, in the middle of the following year, a drawback is that they refer to children whose immunization began up to 3 years earlier. The denominators used to calculate uptake rates are now district resident populations, but prior to 1988 the number of live births in the district was used for this purpose, which gave unreliable rates because they did not allow for the movement of children from one district to another.

3   The Cover of Vaccination Evaluated Rapidly (COVER) programme. Using the computerized child-health register, quarterly cohorts of children

are studied just after reaching the age of immunization to determine the numbers immunized. Quarterly uptake rates are calculated using the resident populations of the health authorities and the results made available quickly to immunization co-ordinators (Begg, Gill and White 1989).

4 In the WHO Expanded Programme of Immunization, cluster sampling has been used to randomly select groups of children whose immunization histories are then recorded and used as an estimate of the vaccine uptake of the area sampled. Repeated sampling over time can reveal trends in uptake (Henderson and Sundaresan 1982).

ASSESSMENT OF DISEASE CONTROL MEASURES

In some vaccine-preventable diseases the benefits of vaccination may diminish as the disease is controlled or the vaccination programme may cease to be cost-effective or the disease may be prevented by other means which may change as the programme progresses. For example, routine vaccination against smallpox in childhood was discontinued in the UK in 1971 because the benefits no longer outweighed the risks (Dick 1971). Routine BCG vaccination of all schoolchildren aged 11–13 years probably ceased to be cost-effective in the 1970s (Stilwell 1976) and a study of the consequences of discontinuing this programme indicated that if the routine vaccination was stopped there would be a slowing in the rate of decline of tuberculosis in young people for about 15 years, but the decline would then accelerate again. A national policy decision is awaited soon; however, in the meantime several health authorities have already ceased routine BCG vaccination (Watson 1995). Typhoid immunization programmes may be valuable in countries with defective sewage disposal and poor water supplies, but as water-borne sewage systems are developed and chlorinated water supplies introduced immunization may no longer be appropriate.

INFORMATION

The regular provision of readily assimilable information is an essential component of the surveillance of immunization programmes, just as it is of disease surveillance. In England and Wales, information on efficacy and safety is published in reports in the *CDR* and elsewhere in the medical press. Some of these are produced regularly, such as the annual reports on rubella and congenital rubella (Miller et al. 1994); others are produced as new circumstances develop, for example, the publication on meningoencephalitis associated with MMR vaccine (Maguire, Begg and Handford 1991), or in reports on surveillance of particular diseases such as poliomyelitis (Joce, Wood and Brown 1992). Information on vaccine uptake is published for the whole of the UK, derived both from the reports to the departments of health and from the COVER programme, in regular quarterly reports in the *CDR* and annually by the DoH (White et al. 1995). However, there is not yet an annual review bringing together all aspects of the surveillance of immunization programmes in the UK.

4 THE INVESTIGATION OF OUTBREAKS

In the past the detection of outbreaks of disease relied mainly on the appearance of groups of cases associated in time or place. With the advent of epidemiological surveillance it became possible to search actively for less apparent outbreaks and other variations in disease pattern, recently aided by the use of computer programs (Farrington and Beale 1993). The investigation of outbreaks, or indeed a single case, requires a systematic approach (Goodman, Buchler and Koplan 1990) to achieve rapid and effective disease control. This can also be assisted by computer programs, for example, 'Epi-Info' produced by the Centers for Disease Control, Atlanta, now widely used throughout the world. The epidemiological methods used for this purpose were pioneered by John Snow in his famous study of cholera near Golden Square, London in 1854 (Snow 1855) and remain in use today. They may be considered under 6 main headings:

1 preliminary enquiry
2 management
3 identification of cases and collection and analysis of data
4 control
5 communication
6 further epidemiological and laboratory studies (Palmer and Swan 1991).

It is not always appropriate to follow this sequence of action; the order will depend upon the particular circumstances of an outbreak and often several of the steps are taken at the same time. There is a useful list of sources of information available in the UK for communicable disease control, designed particularly for CCDCs (Morgan, O'Mahony and Stanwell-Smith 1992).

4.1 Preliminary enquiry

The objects of the preliminary enquiry are:

1 to confirm that there is in reality an outbreak
2 to verify the provisional diagnosis of the disease
3 to agree a case definition for epidemiological investigation
4 to formulate tentative hypotheses of the source and spread of the infection and
5 to initiate immediate control measures if required.

CONFIRMING THE OUTBREAK

An increase in the reported number of cases of a disease may not necessarily be caused by an outbreak but could be due to changes in recognition or reporting. For example, the increase may be related to improved ascertainment of cases following the introduction of new or more sensitive diagnostic procedures, to the need to detect as many cases as possible because of the availability of a new specific treatment, or to more extensive investigation of a disease because of special interests of new clinicians or microbiologists.

Reporting may increase because of changes in the population size or structure, or as a consequence of improved data handling procedures such as computerization, or as a result of false positive laboratory or other tests, or because of the misinterpretation of the original data (Shears 1996).

CONFIRMING THE DIAGNOSIS

The clinical diagnosis can usually be established by a study of the case histories of a few affected persons. Laboratory tests are essential to confirm this in most infections, but epidemiological investigations should begin as soon as possible and not normally be delayed until the laboratory results become available.

CASE DEFINITION

A clear case definition should be agreed at this stage and applied consistently throughout the investigation by all investigators; this is of particular importance in a previously unrecognized disease or one in which there are no satisfactory confirmatory laboratory tests.

TENTATIVE HYPOTHESIS

The preliminary enquiry should include detailed interviews with a few of the affected persons, so that obvious common features may be identified quickly; for example, the association with a specific food, or contact with a particular person or place. Hypotheses can then be developed of the sources and mode of spread of the infection and a questionnaire designed to test these hypotheses in subsequent analytical studies (see section 2.3, p. 123).

IMMEDIATE CONTROL

It may be possible in some circumstances to take immediate control measures based on the tentative hypothesis before this can be confirmed, so that further cases may be prevented. For example, in serious infections that spread from person to person, such as diphtheria, hepatitis B or poliomyelitis, as soon as the diagnosis is suspected it is necessary to identify individuals who may have been the source of infection so that they are isolated if appropriate, and to identify those who may have been exposed to infection so that they can be traced and given protection by vaccines or chemotherapy. If a common vehicle or source of infection is suspected, appropriate action should be taken to interrupt the spread and control the source.

4.2   Management of an incident

If the preliminary enquiry confirms that the outbreak is indeed real, an early decision should be made on the management of the investigation. Small outbreaks will usually be managed by the CCDC with the appropriate and usually essential assistance of a consultant microbiologist and an environmental health officer. In hospitals an outbreak will usually be managed by the Control of Infection Officer assisted by the Infection Control Nurse (Hospital Infection Working Group 1995). The CCDC is obliged by the Public

Health (Infectious Diseases) Regulations 1988 to inform the Chief Medical Officer for England, or for Wales as appropriate, and the CDSC of 'any serious outbreak of any disease' and of cases of disease subject to the International Health Regulations (meaning here cholera, plague, smallpox and yellow fever). He/she should also report to CDSC any case of leprosy, malaria or rabies contracted in Great Britain, and viral haemorrhagic fever. In serious incidents, that is, large outbreaks, severe diseases, geographically widespread outbreaks and those of public interest, an outbreak control team should be formed. This should include, in addition to the CCDC, a PHLS consultant microbiologist, a CDSC consultant epidemiologist, and a consultant physician in infection. Other agencies may also be involved, for example in suspected water-borne disease these may include the local water companies, river authorities, veterinary services and the Department of the Environment (Report of the Group of Experts 1990). The control team will require an administrator or non-medical epidemiologist to manage an 'incident room' where information on the outbreak should be collated and made available to those who require it. The control team should define the responsibilities of its members and allocate to one person the task of spokesperson for the press and other news media, often through the local authority, health authority or DoH press officers. The control team should meet frequently until the acute incident is over when its tasks may be devolved to the local authorities, health authorities and the CDSC.

4.3   Identification of cases, collection and analysis of data

The cases first reported in an outbreak usually comprise only a small proportion of the total and may not be a representative sample. Investigation of these cases alone may be misleading for 3 main reasons:

1 in diseases spread from person to person, such as diphtheria, missed cases or carriers may be responsible for spreading the infection
2 in point-source outbreaks, such as those of Legionnaires' disease or food-borne diseases, the presenting cases may have come to light because of a chance association with a place or potential vehicle of infection
3 without knowing the population from which the cases have come the denominator of 'persons at risk' is not available to calculate attack rates and so determine whether or not a particular exposure was associated with an increased incidence of the disease.

Identification of the exposed population will enable thorough case finding to be accomplished, for example, by scrutinizing school or hotel registers, lists of institutional residents, pay-rolls and other occupational records, nominal rolls of travellers and lists of persons attending functions associated with the disease. If such studies are not possible, as is often the case in community outbreaks, case finding may be undertaken by reviewing routine mortality and morbidity data used for communicable disease surveillance, by individual household enquiry, and by special appeal to medical and lay persons through the press and other news media.

The aim of the enquiry will be to collect data from those affected and those at risk but not affected, by careful questionnaire (see section 2.3, p. 123). The data routinely sought from cases include name, date of birth, gender, occupation, recent travel, immunization history, date of onset of symptoms, description of the illness and the names and addresses of the medical attendants. Other details will depend on the nature of the infection and possible modes of spread. The case data will then be analysed by time, place and person to determine the mode of spread, source of infection and persons who may have been exposed (see section 2.4, p. 123). The date or time of onset of symptoms of cases should be plotted on a graph so that the type of epidemic curve can be recognized, and on a map to reveal the geographical distribution of the cases. Cases that do not conform to the time or geographical distribution may sometimes provide valuable evidence of the source of infection. For example, in John Snow's classic study of the outbreak of cholera near Golden Square, Soho, in 1854, a widow died of the disease in West Hampstead, several miles from Soho and provided the most conclusive evidence of the source of infection because she had previously resided in Broad Street and had delivered to her daily a large bottle of water from her favourite supply, the Broad Street pump (Snow 1855). Comparisons of attack rates by age, gender, location, food history, and other appropriate parameters may provide evidence of the source and spread of infection which may then be confirmed by analytical epidemiological studies already described.

4.4 Control

Control measures may be directed towards the source of infection, the mode of transmission or people at risk, or a combination of these.

CONTROL OF THE SOURCE

The source may be human, animal or environmental.

Human source

Infections derived from a human source can be controlled by the physical isolation of cases and carriers and, if necessary, treatment until they are free from infection, provided that the cases and carriers are easily identified and carrier rates are low. For example, it is possible to control diphtheria and typhoid fever in this way because cases can be recognized clinically and confirmed by laboratory tests and because carrier rates are low and carriers can readily be detected microbiologically. In contrast, meningococcal infection is not susceptible to control by isolation because pharyngeal carrier rates in excess of 20% in the population are common during outbreaks and it is usually impractical to detect and isolate all the carriers. The method of physical isolation used depends upon the mode of spread and severity of the disease; for example, negative-pressure plastic isolators are used in Britain for the African viral haemorrhagic fevers, room isolation for diphtheria, and special precautions in the disposal of secretions and excretions (isolation by 'barrier nursing') in typhoid fever. Isolation of human sources of infection can also be accomplished in some diseases by 'ring immunization', that is, by encircling the case or carrier with a barrier of immune persons which blocks the spread of infection to susceptible people outside the 'ring'. This method was first used in Leicester in the nineteenth century and later throughout the UK for smallpox control; when modified and accompanied by meticulous surveillance world wide it helped to achieve the eradication of the disease (Fenner et al. 1988). It has also been applied in the control of poliomyelitis by mass immunization and in measles by immunization of contacts in school and institutional outbreaks.

Animal source

When animals are the source of an infection, it is sometimes possible to control an outbreak by eradication of that source, for example, in ornithosis by slaughtering the birds and disinfecting the cages and premises. Rabies may be controlled by the destruction of rabid animals and of wild or stray animals that may harbour the virus, and by the muzzling of domestic dogs. Outbreaks of food-borne zoonoses are usually controlled by removing the vehicle of infection: eradication plays a major part in the long-term control of these zoonoses, for example, bovine tuberculosis and brucellosis.

Environmental source

The source of Legionnaires' disease and primary amoebic meningoencephalitis, both recognized in the 1970s, is water in the environment. Outbreaks of Legionnaires' disease were usually associated with water-cooling systems of air-conditioning plants, water-distribution systems in large buildings, or whirlpool spas. Primary amoebic meningoencephalitis was usually contracted from warm unchlorinated natural water sources, such as warm springs, sometimes used to supply swimming pools. Both these infections may be controlled by appropriate cleansing and disinfection. Other pathogens, mainly gram-negative bacteria, may contaminate the inanimate environment of man; for example, salmonellae are found on work surfaces, utensils and equipment in kitchens and coliform organisms and pseudomonads on surfaces and equipment in hospitals. Control measures include appropriate cleansing, disinfection or sterilization of these environmental sources.

CONTROL OF SPREAD

Food- and water-borne infections can be curtailed by withdrawal from sale of the contaminated product or treatment of the product to render it safe, for example, the recall of a contaminated meat product (Cowden et al. 1989), and the pasteurization of a contaminated milk supply.

Direct contact infections may be reduced by avoiding contact, for example, in cutaneous anthrax by not handling potentially contaminated animal products such as unsterilized bone meal.

Indirect contact infections, for example, staphylococcal infections in hospitals, may be reduced by strict aseptic techniques and meticulous hand washing, accompanied in the case of wound infection by the use of 'no touch' dressing techniques.

Faecal–oral spread, such as in bacillary dysentery and hepatitis A infection, may also be restricted by scrupulous attention to hand washing and by the careful and frequent disinfection of surfaces in lavatories and toilet areas.

Percutaneous spread by insects, such as in malaria, typhus and yellow fever, may be controlled by vector destruction, protective clothing and insect repellents. Infections spread by percutaneous inoculation, such as hepatitis B and HIV, may be prevented by measures to avoid accidental inoculation and the contamination of broken skin by infected blood or tissue fluids.

Air-borne spread may be limited by ventilation in buildings and in special circumstances the physical isolation of highly susceptible subjects.

CONTROL OF PERSONS AT RISK

It is sometimes possible to control disease by active or passive immunization or by chemoprophylaxis in persons exposed to risk. For example, active immunization against measles within 72 h of exposure may prevent the disease. Human immunoglobulins are commonly given for passive protection, for example, rabies immunoglobulin in addition to active immunization as part of post-exposure prophylaxis given as soon as possible after exposure, hepatitis B immunoglobulin in post-exposure prophylaxis after accidental inoculation injury and for infants of carrier mothers, and zoster immunoglobulin in the newborn and immunodeficient patients after exposure to chickenpox. Chemoprophylaxis is offered to close contacts of cases of meningococcal meningitis, such as household contacts and children in the same class at school, and long-term chemoprophylaxis against pneumococcal infection is given to patients after splenectomy.

4.5   Communication

Accurate and timely information about an outbreak is of major importance, especially if the outbreak is of national interest and is receiving wide publicity. To achieve this, it is helpful for the CCDC to maintain a check list of authorities and individuals to be informed (Morgan, O'Mahony and Stanwell-Smith 1992). These would normally include the local consultant physician in infection, microbiologist, chief environmental health officer and director of public health, but depending upon the type of outbreak might also include the local divisional veterinary officer, employment medical adviser, education officer and clinicians in hospital and general practice, and similar persons in neighbouring areas. In a major incident, national authorities including the PHLS and its CDSC, the

DoH, the Ministry of Agriculture, Fisheries and Food (MAFF), the Health and Safety Executive and others may be involved. An initial written report should normally be completed within 24–48 h after the preliminary enquiry and circulated to all the authorities and individuals concerned; a final report suitable for publication should be produced at the end of the investigation and interim reports may be necessary if the investigation is complex or prolonged. In a major incident it may also be necessary for frequent bulletins of updated information to be issued by the spokesperson of the 'outbreak control team' from the 'incident room'.

4.6   Further epidemiological and microbiological studies

Analytical studies (see section 2.5, p. 124) may be necessary to confirm the association of disease with a particular vehicle or source of infection. Often case-control studies are undertaken early in an enquiry because they can be accomplished quickly and cheaply, but more time-consuming cohort studies may be required to determine the relative risk so that the most cost-effective long-term control measures can be implemented.

An outbreak may suggest a previously unknown source or vehicle of infection and microbiological surveys may be needed to discover the extent, frequency and mode of transmission so that long-term control measures can be designed and implemented. For example, the discovery that bulk egg products were a vehicle of infection of paratyphoid B and other salmonella infections led to extensive studies of the bacteriology of these products and to improved hygienic methods of production and pasteurization. The identification of Legionnaires' disease and its association with cooling towers of air-conditioning systems and with piped water systems in large buildings led to studies of the growth of legionellae in these systems and subsequently to improvements in design and maintenance to prevent colonization and growth of the organism.

5   THE UK COMMUNICABLE DISEASE CONTROL SERVICES

Local public health services for the investigation, control and prevention of disease were developed in the nineteenth century in the wake of the devastating cholera epidemics of 1831–32 and 1849–50. The famous report of the Poor Law Commissioners, 'On an inquiry into the sanitary condition of the Labouring Population of Great Britain', published in 1842, advocated 'that for the promotion of the means necessary to prevent disease it would be good economy to appoint a district medical officer'. This proposal was first taken up by the City of Liverpool with the appointment of Dr William Henry Duncan as 'Officer of Health' in 1847 and soon after in 1848 by the City of London when Dr John Simon was appointed Medical Officer of Health (MOH). Further appointments followed the Public Health Act 1848, which assigned to local authorities legal responsibility for public health and empowered them to appoint a MOH to carry out their new duties, an appointment which became mandatory in 1872 (Lewis 1991).

The ensuing improvements in hygiene and sanitation, rising standards of living, better nutrition and immunization programmes played an important part in bringing about a dramatic decline in infectious disease. In the middle of the nineteenth century, one death in 3 was attributed to infectious diseases, about one-third due to tuberculosis and one-fifth to scarlet fever and diphtheria; by the turn of the century infectious diseases accounted for one in 5 deaths and by the 1960s they were no longer a major cause of death (Nissel 1987). Morbidity also declined; by 1970, diphtheria, tetanus, whooping cough and poliomyelitis were controlled by immunization, smallpox eradication was nearing completion, bovine tuberculosis was virtually eliminated and many other infections, such as streptococcal disease, meningococcal meningitis and septicaemia, and tuberculosis had become treatable with new specific antimicrobial drugs. The outlook for patients suffering from infectious diseases changed so radically that infection was no longer perceived as a hazard to health and the traditional role of the MOH in the investigation, control and prevention of infectious disease began to seem superfluous.

It is understandable, therefore, that when this post was discontinued under the National Health Service Reorganisation Act 1973, infection control was overlooked. MOHs were transferred to the NHS in the new role of 'community physician' and most of them were absorbed into the management structure of the new NHS. Complacency about infection, however, was soon dispelled by the appearance of Lassa fever and other new African viral haemorrhagic fevers, which caused particular concern in the 1970s because of evidence of air-borne spread in an African hospital outbreak and consequently fears of community spread by the air-borne route in Britain (Galbraith et al. 1978); it seemed as though a new scourge had arrived, replacing the age old one of smallpox as soon as it was eradicated. New arrangements for the control of infectious disease were then made in haste in October 1973, when local authorities were asked to designate a community physician of the local health authority to carry out their functions of infectious disease control (Department of Health and Social Security 1973). This appointment was termed the Medical Officer for Environmental Health (MOEH) in England and Wales and in Scotland the Community Medicine Specialist (Infectious Diseases and Environmental Health). The MOEH, unlike the MOH, was not a statutory appointment; most of the duties were advisory and there was no clear accountability to either the health authority or the local authority. Furthermore, some of the former responsibilities of the MOH were not included in the new post; for example, that of managing immunization programmes lapsed and was not replaced until 1985 when district immunization

co-ordinators were first appointed (Begg and Nicoll 1994). The inadequacies and the anomalous situation of the MOEH soon became evident and eventually led to abolition of the post and the creation of a new NHS appointment in health authorities in England and Wales (Report 1988), which became known as the Consultant in Communicable Disease Control (CCDC).

The CCDC is accountable to the health authority for the control of communicable diseases, including the control of infection in hospitals. It is usual for the incumbent to be appointed to the geographically corresponding local authority(ies) for their statutory functions in the control of infectious disease and also for medical aspects of the control of non-infectious environmental hazards. Medical microbiologists as well as public health physicians were recruited to these new posts and specialist training programmes devised to meet the needs of each specialty (Reports of a Working Group 1994).

5.1 The Public Health Laboratory Service (PHLS)

The Emergency Public Health Laboratory Service (EPHLS) was set up in 1939, at the outbreak of the Second World War, to improve the microbiological and epidemiological capability of local authorities in dealing with outbreaks of infectious disease expected to occur during wartime. In the event, there were no major epidemics, but the EPHLS proved invaluable in supporting MOHs in the investigation and control of communicable disease, for example, in diphtheria control and in tracing the source of multiple outbreaks of salmonellosis associated with imported spray-dried egg (Williams 1985). As a result, the Service was included as a permanent part of the public health organization of England and Wales in the National Health Service Act 1946, dropping the word 'Emergency' from its title to become the Public Health Laboratory Service (PHLS). Reference laboratories were brought together at Colindale in north London to form the Central Public Health Laboratory (CPHL), which included an epidemiological unit, the Epidemiological Research Laboratory (ERL), initially formed to undertake field trials of whooping cough vaccines. At the same time, the primary diagnostic public health laboratories (area and regional laboratories) began to be transferred to hospital sites, where they were amalgamated with the hospital microbiological laboratories and their work extended to encompass both public health and hospital microbiology. The Service was at first administered by the Medical Research Council, but in 1961 was transferred to a newly created PHLS Board and the Headquarters Office was later moved from central London to Colindale. In 1996, there were 49 public health laboratories in 10 regional groups, undertaking both public health and hospital microbiology, and on a new site at Colindale, there were the CPHL with research and reference laboratories, the Communicable Disease Surveillance Centre (CDSC), established in 1977, as well as the Headquarters Office of the Service.

Since its commencement, the Service has monitored laboratory-diagnosed infections in the population, including hospital-acquired infections, a function extended by the first Director of the ERL to include data from hospital as well as public health laboratories, so assembling a national database of laboratory diagnosed infections. The Service has provided reference services, supported local and health authorities in the investigation and control of infectious disease and undertaken a wide range of research (Williams 1985).

5.2   The Communicable Disease Surveillance Centre (CDSC)

Government responsibility for the prevention of disease rests with the Secretary of State for Health and the Secretaries of State for Northern Ireland, Scotland and Wales. Sections of the DoH, the Northern Ireland and Welsh Offices, and the Scottish Home and Health Department (SHHD), carry this responsibility for communicable disease, although the day-to-day activities for the national surveillance of communicable disease and the investigation and control of these diseases in England and Wales were transferred to the CDSC in 1977 and 1978.

The CDSC co-ordinates, advises and assists CCDCs and has a duty to offer assistance when this appears appropriate and to respond promptly to requests for assistance. The CDSC is not only the national centre for the surveillance and control of communicable disease in England and Wales, but also the epidemiological unit of the PHLS with other responsibilities, including the surveillance of immunization programmes and epidemiological research, functions of the former ERL with which it amalgamated in 1985, as well as teaching and training in the epidemiology of communicable diseases. A unit of the CDSC was established for Wales in 1983, situated in Cardiff, and posts of 'regional epidemiologist' were created in several English NHS regions, but a formal regional epidemiological service, with epidemiologists in all 8 English NHS regions did not come into being until 1996.

5.3   Arrangments in Scotland

An informal network of laboratories exists and there is a national epidemiological centre, the Scottish Centre for Infection and Environmental Health (SCIEH), which is administered by the Common Service Agency of the Scottish Home and Health Department (SHHD). It performs similar functions to and works in close association with the CDSC.

6   COMMUNICABLE DISEASE SURVEILLANCE AND CONTROL IN THE USA

Primary responsibility for communicable disease surveillance and control rests with local authorities with powers delegated from the states. The federally funded Centers for Disease Control and Prevention (CDC) grew out of the Public Health Service's Office of Malaria Control, formed in 1942 in Atlanta. In 1951, Langmuir developed at CDC the Epidemiologic Intelligence Service which has an international reputation for field investigations and training of epidemiologists who may be deployed anywhere to assist in field outbreak investigation and control. In addition, CDC carries out national surveillance of infectious diseases, with weekly production of the *Morbidity and Mortality Weekly Reports* (*MMWR*).

7   COMMUNICABLE DISEASE SURVEILLANCE AND CONTROL IN EUROPE

A review of infectious disease surveillance systems in Europe, exhibiting a variety of different organizational models, has been published by Salmon and Bartlett (1995). Collaborative international surveillance has been successful for AIDS, legionella and salmonella infection. In addition, increasing co-operation between states has allowed the development of a European CDC training programme.

REFERENCES

Abramson JH, 1984, *Survey Methods in Community Medicine*, 3rd edn, Churchill Livingstone, Edinburgh.

Altman DG, 1991, *Practical Statistics for Medical Research*, Chapman and Hall, London.

Ashley JSA, Cole SK, Kilbane MPJ, 1991, Health information resources: United Kingdom – health and social factors, *Oxford Textbook of Public Health*, vol. 2, eds Holland WW, Detels R, Knox G, Oxford University Press, Oxford, 30–53.

Bartlett CLR, Macrae AD, Macfarlane JT, 1986, *Legionella Infections*, Edward Arnold, London, 20.

Beaglehole R, Bonita R, Kjellstrom T, 1993, *Basic Epidemiology*, WHO, Geneva.

Begg NT, Gill ON, White JM, 1989, COVER (Cover of Vaccination Evaluated Rapidly): description of the England Wales scheme, *Public Health*, **103:** 81–9.

Begg N, Miller E, 1990, Role of epidemiology in vaccine policy, *Vaccine*, **8:** 180–9.

Begg N, Nicoll A, 1994, Immunisation, *Br Med J*, **309:** 1073–5.

Breslow NE, Day NE, 1980, *Statistical Methods in Cancer Research, Volume 1, The Analysis of Case-control Studies*, WHO International Agency for Research on Cancer, Lyon.

Breslow NE, Day NE, 1987, *Statistical Methods in Cancer Research, Volume 2, The Design and Analysis of Cohort Studies*, WHO International Agency for Research on Cancer, Lyon.

Catchpole MA, 1992, Sexually transmitted diseases in England and Wales: 1981–1990, *Commun Dis Rep*, **1:** R1–7.

Centers for Disease Control, 1991, National electronic telecommunications system for surveillance – United States, *Morbid Mortal Weekly Rep*, **40:** 502–3.

Clarkson JA, Fine PEM, 1987, An assessment of methods for routine local monitoring of vaccine efficacy, with particular reference to measles and pertussis, *Epidemiol Infect*, **99:** 485–99.

Cockburn WC, 1955, Large-scale field trials of active immunizing agents, *Bull W H O*, **13:** 395–407.

Communicable Disease Surveillance Centre, 1995, Notifications of infectious diseases: a new feature in the CDR Weekly, *Commun Dis Rep*, **5:** 185.

Cowden JM, O'Mahony M et al., 1989, A national outbreak of *Salmonella typhimurium* DT 124 caused by contaminated salami sticks, *Epidemiol Infect*, **103:** 219–25.

Decker MD, Booth AL et al., 1986, Validity of food consumption histories in a foodborne outbreak investigation, *Am J Epidemiol*, **124:** 859–63.

Dick G, 1971, Routine smallpox vaccination, *Br Med J*, **2:** 163–6.

Department of Health and Social Security, 1973, *Reorganisation of Local Government, Reorganisation of National Health Service. Transitional Arrangements and Organisation and Development of Services. Control of Notifiable Diseases and Food Poisoning*, HRC(73)34, Circular 58/73, DHSS, London.

Dorolle P, 1968, Old plagues in the jet age. International aspects of present and future control of communicable disease, *Br Med J*, **2:** 789–92.

Farrington CP, Beale AD, 1993, Computer-aided detection of temporal clusters of organisms reported to the Communicable Disease Surveillance Centre, *Commun Dis Rep*, **3:** R78–82.

Farrington CP, Nash J, Miller E, 1996, Case series analysis of adverse reactions to vaccines: a comparative evaluation, *Am J Epidemiol*, **143:** 1165–73.

Fenner F, Henderson DA et al., 1988, *Smallpox and its Eradication*, WHO, Geneva.

Fleming DM, Crombie DL, 1985, The incidence of common infectious diseases: the weekly returns service of the Royal College of General Practitioners, *Health Trends*, **17:** 13–16.

Galbraith NS, 1964, Poliomyelitis surveillance in England and Wales 1962, *Proceedings of the Ninth Symposium of the European Association against Poliomyelitis and Allied Diseases, Stockholm, 1963*, 92–106.

Galbraith NS, Berrie JRH et al., 1978, Public health aspects of viral haemorrhagic fevers in Britain, *J R Soc Health*, **98:** 152–61.

Glynn JR, Palmer SR, 1992, Incubation period, severity of disease, and infecting dose: evidence from a *Salmonella* outbreak, *Am J Epidemiol*, **136:** 1369–77.

Goodman RA, Buchler JW, Koplan JP, 1990, The epidemiologic held investigation: science and judgment in public health practice, *Am J Epidemiol*, **132:** 9–16.

Grant AD, Eke B, 1993, Application of information technology to the laboratory reporting of communicable disease in England and Wales, *Commun Dis Rep*, **3:** R75–8.

Greenwood M, 1948, *Medical Statistics from Graunt to Farr*, Cambridge University Press, Cambridge.

Griffith AH, 1989, Permanent brain damage and pertussis vaccination: is the end of the saga in sight?, *Vaccine*, **7:** 199–210.

Gustavsen S, Breen O, 1984, Investigation of an outbreak of *Salmonella oranienburg* infections in Norway, caused by contaminated black pepper, *Am J Epidemiol*, **119:** 806–12.

Hall SM, Glickman M, 1988, British Paediatric Association. The British Paediatric Surveillance Unit, *Arch Dis Child*, **63:** 344–6.

Henderson RH, Sundaresan T, 1982, Cluster sampling to assess immunization coverage: a review of experience with a simplified sampling method, *Bull W H O*, **60:** 253–60.

Hennekins CH, Buring JE, 1987, *Epidemiology in Medicine*, Little, Brown and Company, Boston/Toronto.

Holland WW, Detels R, Knox G (eds), 1991, *Oxford Textbook of Public Health, Volume 2, Methods of Public Health*, 2nd edn, Oxford Medical Publishers, Oxford.

Hospital Infection Working Group, 1995, *Hospital Infection Control. Guidance on the Control of Infection in Hospitals*, DOH and PHLS, London.

Jephcott AE, 1992, The work of the Gonococcus Reference Unit, *PHLS Microbiol Dig*, **9:** 155–9.

Joce R, Wood D et al., 1992, Paralytic poliomyelitis in England and Wales 1985–91, *Br Med J*, **305:** 79–82.

Kingsley LA, Detels R et al., 1987, Risk factors for seroconversion to human immunodeficiency virus among male homosexuals. Results from a Multi-center AIDS Cohort Study, *Lancet*, **1:** 345–9.

Klaucke DN, Buehler JW et al., 1988, Guidelines for evaluating surveillance systems, *Morbid Mortal Weekly Rep*, **37, SS-5:** 1–18.

Knightley MJ, Mayon-White RT, 1982, Measles epidemic in a circumscribed community, *J R Coll Gen Pract*, **32:** 675–80.

Kopec JA, Esdaile JM, 1990, Bias in case-control studies. A review, *J Epidemiol Community Health*, **44:** 179–86.

Lang DJ, Kunz J et al., 1967, Carmine as a source of nosocomial salmonellosis, *N Engl J Med*, **276:** 829–32.

Langmuir AD, 1963, The surveillance of communicable disease of national importance, *N Engl J Med*, **268:** 182–92.

Lederberg J, Shope RE, Oaks SC, 1992, *Emerging Infections. Microbial Threats to Health in the United States*, National Academic Press, Washington, DC.

Lewis J, 1991, The origins and development of public health in the UK, *Oxford Textbook of Public Health*, eds Holland WW, Detels R, Knox G, Oxford University Press, Oxford, **1:** 23–34.

McCormick A, 1993, The notification of infectious diseases in England and Wales, *Commun Dis Rep*, **3:** R19–25.

McCormick A, 1994, The impact of human immunodeficiency virus on the population of England and Wales, *Population Trends*, **76:** 1–7.

McCormick A, Fleming D, Charlton J, 1995, *Morbidity Statistics from General Practice: Fourth National Study 1991–1992*, Series MB5, No.3, HMSO, London.

Maguire HC, Begg NT, Handford SG, 1991, Meningoencephalitis associated with MMR vaccine, *Commun Dis Rep*, **1:** R60–1.

Maguire HC, Handford S et al., 1995, A collaborative case control study of sporadic hepatitis A in England, *Commun Dis Rep*, **5:** R33–40.

Medical Research Council, 1956, Vaccination against whooping cough. Relation between protection in children and results of laboratory tests, *Br Med J*, **2:** 454–62.

Millard J, Appleton H, Parry JV, 1987, Studies on heat inactivation of hepatitis A virus with special reference to shellfish, *Epidemiol Infect*, **98:** 397–414.

Miller DL, Ross EM et al., 1981, Pertussis immunization and serious acute neurological illness in children, *Br Med J*, **282:** 1595–9.

Miller E, Tookey P et al., 1994, Rubella surveillance to June 1994: third report from the PHLS and the National Congenital Surveillance Programme, *Commun Dis Rep*, **4:** R146–52.

Morgan D, O'Mahony M, Stanwell-Smith RE, 1992, From the briefcase to the bookshelf: information sources for communicable disease control, *Commun Dis Rep*, **2:** R91–5.

Morgan-Capner P, Wright J et al., 1988, Surveillance of antibody to measles, mumps and rubella by age, *Br Med J*, **297:** 770–2.

Murphy FA, 1994, New, emerging, and reemerging infectious diseases, *Adv Virus Res*, **43:** 1–52.

Newton L, Hall SM, 1993, Reye's syndrome in the British Isles: report for 1990/91 and the first decade of surveillance, *Commun Dis Rep*, **3:** R11–16.

Nissel M, 1987, *People Count. A History of the General Register Office*, HMSO, London.

O'Mahony MC, Gooch CD et al., 1983, Epidemic hepatitis A from cockles, *Lancet*, **1:** 518–20.

Orenstein WA, Bernier RH et al., 1985, Field evaluation of vaccine efficacy, *Bull W H O*, **63:** 1055–68.

Paget CE, 1897, *Wasted Records of Disease*, Edward Arnold, London, 78–9.

Palmer SR, Biffin A, 1987, The changing incidence of human hydatid disease in England and Wales, *Epidemiol Infect*, **99:** 693–700.

Palmer SR, Henry R, 1992, Epinet in Wales: PHLS Cadwyn Cymru. Development of a public health information system, *PHLS Microbiol Dig*, **9 (3):** 107–9.

Palmer SR, Smith RMM, 1991, GP surveillance of infections in Wales, *Commun Dis Rep*, **3:** R25–8.

Palmer SR, Swan AV, 1991, The epidemiological approach to infection control, *Rev Med Microbiol*, **2:** 187–93.

Palmer SR, Jephcott AE et al., 1981, Person-to-person spread of *Salmonella typhimurium* phage type 10 after a common-source outbreak, *Lancet*, **1:** 881–4.

Palmer SR, Zamiri I et al., 1986, Legionnaire's disease cluster and reduction in hospital hot water temperatures, *Br Med J (Clin Res Ed)*, **292:** 1494–5.

Pereira MS, 1979, Global surveillance of influenza, *Br Med Bull*, **35:** 9–14.

PHLS AIDS Centre, 1991, The surveillance of HIV-1 infection and AIDS in England and Wales, *CDR (Lond Engl Rev)*, **1:** R51–R6.

Preston NW, 1965, Effectiveness of pertussis vaccines, *Br Med J*, **2:** 11–13.

Ramsay M, Gay N et al., 1994, The epidemiology of measles in England and Wales: rationale for the 1994 national vaccination campaign, *Commun Dis Rep*, **4:** R141–6.

Raska K, 1966, National and international surveillance of communicable diseases, *WHO Chron*, **20:** 315–21.

Report, 1988, *Public Health in England. The Report of the Committee of Inquiry into the Future Development of the Public Health Function*, CMD 289, HMSO, London.

Report, 1995, *Unlinked Anonymous HIV Prevalence Monitoring Programme: England and Wales. Data to the End of 1994*, Department of Health, London.

Report, 1996, The incidence and prevalence of AIDS and prevalence of other severe HIV disease in England and Wales for 1995 to 1999: projections using data to the end of 1994, *Commun Dis Rep*, **6:** R1–24.

Report of the Group of Experts, 1990, *Cryptosporidium in Water Supplies*, HMSO, London, 45–56.

Reports of a Working Group, 1994, Training of consultants in communicable disease control, *Commun Dis Rep*, **4:** R37–49.

Riley W, Remis RS et al., 1983, Hemorrhagic colitis associated with a rare *Escherichia coli* serotype, *N Engl J Med*, **308:** 681–5.

Rowe B, Begg NT et al., 1987, *Salmonella ealing* infections associated with consumption of infant dried milk, *Lancet*, **2:** 900–3.

Sackett DL, 1979, Bias in analytic research, *J Chronic Dis*, **32:** 51–68.

Salmon RL, Bartlett CLR, 1995, European surveillance systems, *Rev Med Microbiol*, **6:** 267–76.

Schesselman JJ, 1982, *Case-control Studies*, Oxford University Press, New York/Oxford.

Schleck WF III, Lavigne PM et al., 1983, Epidemic listerosis – evidence for transmission by food, *N Engl J Med*, **308:** 203–6.

Shears P, 1996, Pseudo-outbreaks, *Lancet*, **347:** 138.

Snow J, 1855, *On the Mode of Communication of Cholera*, Churchill, London.

Sockett PN, 1995, The epidemiology and costs of diseases of public health significance, in relation to meat and meat products, *J Food Safety*, **15:** 91–112.

Stagno S, Pass RF et al., 1986, Primary cytomegalovirus infection in pregnancy, incidence, transmission to fetus and clinical outcome, *JAMA*, **256:** 1904–8.

Steere AC, Broderick TF, Malawista SE, 1978, Erythema chronicum migraines and lyme arthritis: epidemiologic evidence for a tick vector, *Am J Epidemiol*, **1980:** 312–21.

Stilwell JA, 1976, Benefits and costs of the schools' BCG vaccination programme, *Br Med J*, **1:** 1002–4.

Thacker SB, Berkelmann RL, 1988, Public health surveillance in the United States, *Epidemiol Rev*, **10:** 164–90.

Tillett HE, Spencer I, 1982, Influenza surveillance in England and Wales using routine statistics, *J Hyg Camb*, **88:** 83–94.

Valleron AJ, Garnerin P, 1993, Computerised surveillance of communicable diseases in France, *Commun Dis Rep CDR Rev*, **3:** R82–7.

Van Casteran V, Leurquin P, 1992, Eurosentinel: development of an international sentinel network of general practitioners, *Methods Inform Med*, **31:** 147–52.

Watson JM, 1995, BCG – mass or selective vaccination?, *J Hosp Infect*, **30, Suppl.:** 508–13.

Wharton M, Chorba TL et al., 1990, Case definitions for public health surveillance, *Morbid Mortal Weekly Rep*, **39:** RR-13.

White JM, Rush M et al., 1995, COVER/Korner 95-1 (April to June 1995) vaccination coverage statistics for children up to 2 years old in the United Kingdom, *Commun Dis Rep*, **5:** R186–7.

Williams REO, 1985, Microbiology for the public health, *The Evolution of the Public Health Laboratory Service 1939–1980*, Public Health Laboratory Service, London.

Wilson FP, 1927, *The Plague in Shakespeare's London*, Clarendon Press, London.

Wilson GS, 1967, *The Hazards of Immunization*, Athlone Press, London.

Yugoslav Typhoid Commission, 1962, A controlled field trial of the effectiveness of phenol and alcohol typhoid vaccines, *Bull W H O*, **26:** 357–69.

THEORY OF INFECTIOUS DISEASE TRANSMISSION AND HERD IMMUNITY

N T Begg and N J Gay

1 INTRODUCTION

Successful control of an infectious disease requires an understanding of the agent responsible for the disease, its interaction with the host it infects and the environment. Though this may appear obvious, history is littered with failed attempts to control infectious diseases through ignorance of basic factors such as the mode of transmission, natural reservoirs of infection and the role of carriers. Thus, in the early nineteenth century cholera was thought to be an airborne disease. At that time efforts at control were based on remedies to ward off contaminated atmosphere ('miasma'). It was not until 1854 that John Snow, an English epidemiologist, showed that cholera was a water-borne infection. His discovery was based on the simple observation that during a cholera epidemic attack rates were highest among people who obtained their drinking water from one particular pump (Fig. 10.1). Snow's remedy – to remove the handle of the pump and thereby stop the outbreak – revolutionized the control of cholera and presaged a series of public health measures aimed at improving the safety of drinking water. Unfortunately, ignorance about cholera control persists to the present day. When the seventh cholera pandemic reached Latin America in 1991, the response of most countries was to introduce a requirement that all visitors be vaccinated. Though cholera vaccine may provide some protection against disease to individuals, it does not prevent excretion of *Vibrio cholerae* by cases (Finkelstein 1984). Vaccination with existing vaccines therefore has no value as a public health measure for the control of infection.

In recent years knowledge about disease trans-

mission and herd immunity has had a very marked impact on the practice of immunization. Several characteristics of an infection determine the readiness with which it may be controlled by immunization. These include the infectivity of the agent, the length of the incubation period, the duration of naturally acquired and vaccine-induced immunity and the presence or absence of subclinical infection and non-human hosts (Allwright 1988). Mathematical modelling techniques that incorporate these factors can be used to predict the outcome of alternative vaccine strategies, under varying assumptions about vaccine efficacy and coverage. This type of information has been crucial in the design of successful immunization programmes against diseases such as smallpox, poliomyelitis and measles.

In this chapter the basic theory of infectious disease transmission and herd immunity will be described and the way in which the application of theory contributes to the control of communicable disease in man will be considered.

2 HISTORICAL PERSPECTIVE

The theory of infectious disease transmission has its origins in the first decade of the twentieth century. After the discovery of germ theory in the nineteenth century, attempts were made to understand the cycles in the incidence of many infectious diseases. In particular, explanations were sought for the regularity with which epidemics of diseases such as measles occurred and why these epidemics peaked and died out before all susceptible persons had been infected. In 1906, Hamer proposed a model in which he considered the

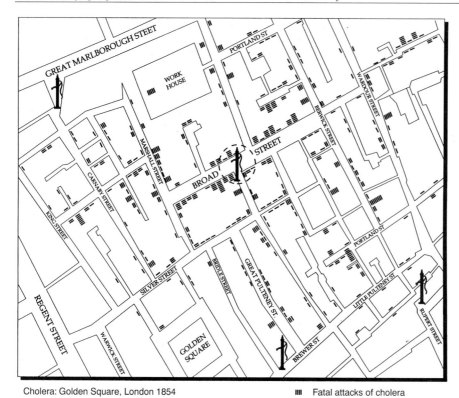

Cholera: Golden Square, London 1854   ▥ Fatal attacks of cholera

Fig. 10.1 Distribution of cholera deaths, Golden Square, 1854.

cases to occur in discrete, 2 week generations. The number of cases of disease in one generation was assumed to be a constant multiple of the number of cases in the previous generation and of the number of susceptible individuals. On this simple assumption, he was able to explain the epidemic nature of measles. The regular cycles were due to the reduction in the number of susceptibles during an epidemic, followed by a gradual reaccumulation as more children were born. His argument was not, however, widely accepted at the time. An alternative, empirically derived theory, due to Brownlee (1907, 1909), was based on Farr's (1840) observations of the shape of epidemic curves. According to this theory, the infectivity of the agent was reduced by a constant factor with each successive generation of cases in the course of an epidemic; the decay of an epidemic was due to this attenuation of infectivity rather than lack of susceptible persons. An account of Brownlee's work is given by Fine (1979). Contemporary with this debate was the proposal by Ross (1909, 1911) of a model of malaria transmission along lines similar to those of Hamer's theory of measles. Ross and Hamer were well aware that their models represented a considerable simplification of the heterogeneity of real populations, but they realized that they had captured the fundamental mechanisms that underlie the observed patterns of disease incidence.

It was against this background that Topley and Wilson commenced their classical series of experimental studies of the spread of infection among mice. Carefully controlled conditions in mouse populations were ideal for testing the competing theories. At the beginning of this research Topley (1919a, 1919b, 1919c),

in his Goulstonian Lectures to the Royal College of Physicians of London, set out the main problems to be investigated. It is clear that he was influenced by Brownlee's ideas but he did not dismiss Hamer's theory: 'Though reasons have been given for believing that the outstanding feature in the subsidence of an epidemic is a loss of infectivity by the bacterial virus, yet the resistance of the host cannot be a negligible factor. It will operate by decreasing the concentration of susceptible individuals, and hence the chances of successful transference.'

After 5 years of experimentation, Topley and Wilson (1923) were led to the conclusion that 'the question of immunity as an attribute of a herd should be studied as a separate problem, closely related to, but in many ways distinct from, the problem of the immunity of an individual host'. Theirs was the first published reference of the term 'herd immunity'. Its use indicates that the focus of the research was moving away from the properties of the infective agent towards properties of the herd or population. The most fundamental result that had been established was that the addition of a number of susceptible mice to a population in which a bacterial parasite was at equilibrium produced an outbreak of disease (Topley 1923). This was confirmed experimentally by Webster (1946) in the USA. Similar observations in a human population were made by Dudley (1926) on the incidence of diphtheria in a boarding school. Outbreaks recurred when the admission of sufficient susceptible new boys had removed the herd immunity. As the experimental evidence mounted, Hamer's theory became accepted; no evidence was obtained to support Brownlee's theory of varying infectivity. A full account of the mouse experiments is given in the final report (Greenwood et al. 1936).

Further theoretical progress was made during this period by Kermack and McKendrick (1927) who proved the existence of an epidemic threshold, i.e. that an epidemic would occur if and only if the proportion susceptible exceeded a given level. Soper (1929) provided a clear statement of Hamer's model and its continuous time equivalent. He showed that the continuous model produced damped oscillations around the equilibrium solution and derived the period of small oscillations. Soper also noted the similarity with laws for chemical reactions and for this reason the model acquired the tag 'mass action'. The inability of this model to yield the undamped epidemic cycles observed for measles was seen as a major flaw, until Bartlett (1956) showed that this problem could be overcome by a stochastic formulation of the Hamer–Soper model. His numerical simulations generated recurrent epidemics with no tendency to the equilibrium. Bartlett noted that the size of the population affected the pattern of epidemics; larger towns had more regular cycles, whereas 'fade out' of infection often occurred in simulations with a small population. This led him to derive a critical community size above which fade out was unlikely (Bartlett 1957), a result that accorded well with observations. Bailey provided the first comprehensive account of 'the mathematical theory of epidemics' in which these developments were discussed (Bailey 1957). This included methods for estimating parameters, such as latent and infectious periods, from epidemiological data.

In the USA, meanwhile, Reed and Frost were developing a model which has become the basis for the study of outbreaks in small populations. This included a non-linear term to discount the effect of 2 or more infectious individuals contacting the same susceptible person (Frost 1976). The first study to include heterogeneity in contacts between members of a population was that of Fox et al. (1971) who explored the effects of superimposing family and other structures on a Reed–Frost model. Their stochastic simulations led them to emphasize the important role that small pockets of susceptible individuals can play in sustaining transmission.

The concept of the basic reproduction number (R_0) was introduced into infectious disease epidemiology by Macdonald (1957) in the context of his studies of malaria. R_0 has become a central feature of the theory of infectious diseases since Dietz (1975) and Hethcote (1983) first used it in the study of directly transmitted infections. It provides a simple method for comparing diseases and the difficulty of eliminating them. Dietz (1975) showed how, in a simple homogeneous model, R_0 can be estimated from the average age at infection. Diekmann et al. (1990) provided a rigorous mathematical framework for the definition of R_0 in models of disease transmission in heterogeneous populations. These include the models with age-dependent transmission rates developed by Anderson and May (1984, 1985a, 1985b) and others (Hethcote 1983, Schenzle 1984) that have been used to investigate the dynamics of a wide range of infections and to explore the effects of different vaccination programmes (Anderson and May 1985a, 1990, Anderson and Grenfell 1986, Anderson, Crombie and Grenfell 1987, Halloran et al. 1994, Babad et al. 1995). Such work has become increasingly influential on vaccination policy decisions.

Much attention has recently focused on the epidemiology of HIV and AIDS. Models for sexually transmitted diseases may require many population subgroups with widely differing sexual activity levels, and the long incubation period for AIDS and the changes in infectivity present further complications. Developments across the entire spectrum of modelling approaches have been reviewed by Mollison, Isham and Grenfell (1994) who also highlighted areas in which further research is necessary.

3 BASIC PRINCIPLES

3.1 Infection in the individual

The several stages in an episode of infectious disease are presented in Fig. 10.2. The process begins when a susceptible individual is exposed to an infectious case. If transmission of the infectious organism takes place and it begins to multiply in the tissues of the exposed individual, that individual can be considered to have been infected. However, not all exposures result in transmission, and of these only a small proportion progress to clinical disease. At this early stage the individual is not yet infectious, a stage known as the latent period of infection.

The next stage marks the end of latency and the beginning of the period of infectivity, when the infected individual begins to shed the organism from the respiratory or gastrointestinal tract or in body fluids such as blood or urine. At this point the individual is infectious, that is he is able to transmit the organism to others.

Throughout the latent period and the early stages of the period of infectivity, the individual does not have symptoms. The onset of the first symptom heralds the end of the incubation period, which is defined as the interval between the initial exposure and the onset of symptoms. In some patients, symptoms appear at the same time as infectivity, but it is more usual for the latter to precede symptoms by a few days.

The next stage is reached when the individual is no longer infectious. Normally this occurs while symptoms are present, although in some cases, particularly in immunosuppressed individuals, shedding can continue after symptoms have resolved. When shedding becomes persistent, the individual has become a carrier. Knowledge of carrier states is particularly important for understanding the dynamics of disease transmission. Some patients, as for example in typhoid fever, may be asymptomatic carriers for years (Kaye et al. 1967).

In some infections the symptoms resolve and the patient is no longer infectious but the organism

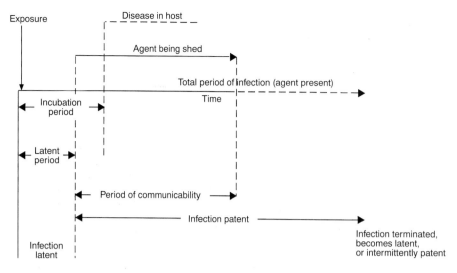

Fig. 10.2 Stages of infection.

remains dormant; the infection has re-entered the latent period. The disease may subsequently reactivate, sometimes years later, with shedding of the organism; varicella and malaria are examples of infections that commonly become latent.

The duration of the latent and infectious periods are important parameters of mathematical models. Classic epidemiological studies that observed the interval between primary and secondary cases within households made it possible to estimate these parameters for measles and other infections (Hope Simpson 1948, Bailey 1956a, 1956b).

DEVELOPMENT OF IMMUNITY

The immunological basis for the development of immunity to bacterial infections is considered in Chapter 5. From the perspective of infectious disease transmission theory, a number of key components must be considered.

Some infections, for example gonorrhoea, do not result in natural immunity. For infections that do stimulate an immune response, the duration of immunity affects the rate at which susceptibles accumulate in a population. Generally speaking, naturally acquired immunity is longer lasting than vaccine-induced immunity; in some infections immunity may be life-long.

It is particularly important to distinguish between immunity against infection and immunity against disease. For example, live oral polio vaccine (DPV) protects against both infection and disease whereas the inactivated vaccine (IPV) protects predominantly against disease. This difference has significant implications for control programmes – control of a polio epidemic can be achieved much more rapidly, and with lower vaccine coverage with live vaccine than with inactivated vaccine.

Finally, in infections where transmission is common among young children, the influence of maternal antibody is a highly significant factor. For example, the incidence of meningococcal disease in infants bears an inverse relationship to the decline in maternal antibody (Fig. 10.3). The peak incidence is at 6 months of

age and coincides with the nadir in maternal antibody. After 6 months, naturally acquired immunity begins to develop and the disease incidence declines. The significance for control measures is that vaccines intended for use in a mass immunization programme need to be effective during the window of susceptibility in early life.

3.2 Infection in the population

The course of infection in the individual has a strong influence on the pattern of disease in a population. Diseases that confer permanent immunity after a short infection, such as measles and rubella, occur naturally in a cycle of regularly recurring epidemics. Diseases for which individuals become susceptible to reinfection on recovery (e.g. gonorrhoea), or some infected individuals become long-term carriers (e.g. hepatitis B), tend to occur at a more steady rate.

Factors specific to each population, including demographic factors and behavioural patterns, also affect the incidence of the disease. These determine whether, and at what level, an infection can remain endemic in a particular population. Many infections have widely differing levels of endemic infection in developed and developing countries. Hepatitis B is commonly acquired in childhood in sub-Saharan Africa, but in developed countries it is largely confined to adults in particular risk groups. Hepatitis A, and other infections transmitted by the faecal–oral route, are acquired at a younger age in countries where sanitation is poor (see section 5.1, p. 161). The difference is less striking for infections such as measles and rubella, but these, too, are acquired at a younger age in less developed countries. The contrasting epidemiology of infections in different populations may necessitate entirely different approaches to disease control.

BASIC REPRODUCTION NUMBER

The basic reproduction number R_0 for an infection in a population summarizes the effect of many of these factors in a single parameter. R_0 is variously termed

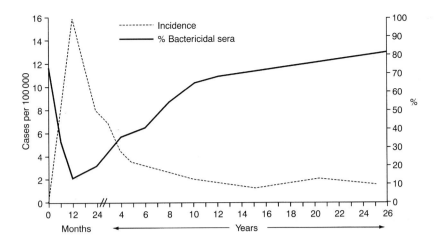

Fig. 10.3 Relationship between age-specific incidence of meningococcal infection and immunity (after Goldschneider, Gotschlich and Artenstein 1969).

the basic reproductive or reproduction rate, ratio or number by different authors. It is defined as the number of secondary infections that would be produced in a completely susceptible population by a typical infectious individual (Anderson and May 1991, Dietz 1993). Thus R_0 depends on both the properties of the infective organism and the social and demographic characteristics of the population. It may vary between infections, but also for the same infection in different populations. R_0 can be interpreted as the average number of contacts made by an individual during the infectious period, where a contact is defined as any encounter in which an infectious individual would transmit infection to a susceptible individual. This definition is clearly disease specific.

EFFECTIVE REPRODUCTION NUMBER

In most real situations not all individuals in the population are susceptible to infection; some are immune either as a result of previous infection or through vaccination. Contacts of an infectious person with immune individuals do not result in new infections but will be 'wasted'. The effective reproduction number R is defined as the number of secondary infections produced by a typical infectious individual (Anderson and May 1991). Clearly, R depends on R_0 and the susceptibility of the population. For a simple homogeneous model, in which contact between any 2 individuals is assumed to be equally likely, $R = R_0 x$, where x denotes the proportion of the population who are susceptible.

Persistence thresholds

An infection can establish itself in a population only if $R_0 > 1$. Any such infection has an endemic equilibrium state at which $R = 1$, where a typical infectious individual produces one secondary infection. At this equilibrium state only one of the R_0 contacts made by an infective individual is with a susceptible individual. In the simple model, the proportion of the population who are susceptible is $1/R_0$. The equilibrium at $R = 1$ is a threshold; if $R > 1$ the number of infections increases and if $R < 1$ the number of infections decreases. Many infections show this threshold behaviour in their natural epidemic cycles. During these

cycles R oscillates around 1 as the proportion susceptible oscillates around the equilibrium value.

The $R = 1$ threshold is the key to designing vaccination programmes. If a vaccination programme aims to eliminate a disease, it must maintain $R < 1$, so that the number of infections decreases with each successive generation of cases. In order to achieve elimination, the proportion of the population that is susceptible must be maintained below the threshold. The necessary level of immunity can in the long term be achieved by immunizing at birth a proportion p of the population, where $p = 1 - 1/R_0$, so that only a proportion $1 - p = 1/R_0$ of newborns remains susceptible. Diseases with a high R_0 are therefore more difficult to eliminate than those with low R_0. For example, a disease with $R_0 = 20$ requires $p = 95\%$, whereas one with $R_0 = 4$ requires $p = 75\%$.

HERD IMMUNITY

The arguments above suggest that it is possible to eliminate an infection without immunizing every member of the population. It is this concept of indirect protection of susceptible individuals to which the term 'herd immunity' has been attached, although many authors have been deliberately vague in any definition. Fox et al. (1971) discussed a dictionary definition of herd immunity as 'the resistance of a group to attack by a disease to which a large proportion of the members are immune, thus lessening the likelihood of a patient with a disease coming into contact with a susceptible individual'. Fine (1993) pointed out the ambiguity of this definition; it fails to distinguish between total protection, when the immunity of the herd is above the threshold and the disease cannot persist, and partial protection, when the presence of some immune individuals lessens the risk to a susceptible individual. The threshold concept is the more appealing and it leads to a definition of a population as having herd immunity when $R < 1$. An equivalent statement of this definition is 'a population is said to have herd immunity to an infection if a typical primary infection produces less than one secondary infection'. Such a concise definition has the advantage of clarifying a sometimes vague concept; either a population has herd immunity, or it does not.

The amount by which the population falls above or below the herd immunity threshold is quantified by the effective reproduction number R.

Although the concept of herd immunity has been defined, it is still necessary to clarify what is meant by a 'typical' infective. In a simple homogeneous model all individuals in the population are assumed to have the same number of contacts; every infective is typical. In more complex models that incorporate heterogeneity in the contact process, the typical infective is defined as some suitably weighted average of all infectives. The typical infective is determined through a defined mathematical framework as the fastest growing stable distribution of infectives (Diekmann et al. 1990). The definition of a population with herd immunity, if $R<1$, is applicable to these more complex models. The factors determining the effective reproduction number are the number of contacts made by infectives and the levels of susceptibility. The immunity of the herd does not depend necessarily on the immunity of individuals. For example, a population in which an infection has an $R_0<1$ has herd immunity to that infection even if no individuals are immune.

Estimation of R_0

Dietz (1993) has reviewed the various methods that have been used to estimate the basic reproduction number for infectious diseases. Many require data on the endemic state of the disease before the introduction of any control measures. Perhaps the simplest of these methods is that of Anderson and May (1991):

$$R_0 = N/B(A - m)$$

where N is the population size, B the annual number of births, A the average age at infection and m the average duration of protection from infection provided by maternally derived antibodies. For stable populations this expression reduces to $R_0 = L/(A - m)$, where L is the life expectancy. A brief heuristic justification of this formula is possible for populations where virtually all individuals are infected during their lifetime. $A - m$ is the average duration of susceptibility so that the proportion susceptible $x = (A - m)/L$, and at equilibrium $R_0 = 1/x$. In deriving these simple formulae it is assumed that the risk of infection for a susceptible individual, often called the 'force of infection', is independent of age. The complications introduced by an age-dependent force of infection, that preclude the derivation of an explicit formula for R_0, are discussed below.

3.3 Mathematical modelling

The essential requirement of a mathematical model is that it accounts for the mechanism that underlies the process it is intended to describe. The key to models of infectious diseases is an understanding of the interactions between infectious and susceptible individuals that result in the transmission of infection. These should be described by a set of clearly stated assumptions, which can then be expressed as mathematical

equations that relate the variables and parameters of the model. The model is simply the means of evaluating the consequences of a set of assumptions.

When formulating a model, a compromise must be reached between simplicity and overcomplication. Simple models, which may have explicit solutions, clearly demonstrate the effect of each parameter but may grossly oversimplify the complexities of the transmission process. More complicated models provide greater flexibility, but each additional refinement introduces further parameters that increase the task of parameter estimation and make it more difficult to discern the effect of any individual parameter. In general, simple models are most useful for investigating qualitative effects, whereas more detailed models are necessary for quantitative predictions.

When the results of any modelling exercise are interpreted it is essential to bear in mind the assumptions on which the model is based. No model can fully describe all the complexities of the transmission of a disease in a population. They can, however, greatly enhance the understanding of the processes that underlie disease transmission, and play an important role in the design of control programmes.

The examples in this chapter exemplified by measles will concentrate on infections for which humans are the only host, that have short latent and infectious periods that confer permanent immunity (exemplified by measles). A flow diagram illustrates the basic structure of a model for such an infection showing the compartments that may be included (Fig. 10.4). For models of other infections, such as those that do not confer immunity or that have a carrier state, this structure must be adapted accordingly. Models with different structures, suitable for a wide range of infectious diseases, have been presented and discussed by Anderson and May (1991).

Dynamic behaviour

Numerical simulations of infectious disease transmission proceed in discrete time steps to describe the changes over time in the number of individuals in each of the compartments of the model. The values at each time step are calculated from the values at the previous time step, starting from some specified initial values. This procedure is essentially the same for all models, but complex models may have more compartments or further stratification by age, sex, etc.

The rates at which transitions between compartments occur are determined by the assumptions and parameters of the model. For example, the rate at which individuals move from the latent to the infectious compartment is governed by the latent period, and the rate of movement from infectious to immune by the infectious period. The crux of all models of disease transmission is the rate at which susceptibles are infected, the force of infection, and how this is assumed to depend on the number of infectious individuals.

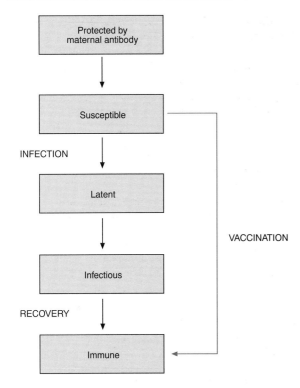

Fig. 10.4 Flow chart showing the compartmental structure of mathematical models.

The mass action assumption

The force of infection, λ, is the rate at which susceptible persons acquire infection. The probability that a given susceptible individual will acquire infection in a short period δt is $\lambda \delta t$. For a directly transmitted infection, the force of infection at any time depends on the infectives present in the population at that time. The simplest assumption is that the force of infection is directly proportional to the total number of infectives. The rate at which new infections occur in the population is then proportional to the product of the number of susceptibles and the number of infectives. This model is known as the mass action model because of its similarity to the model for chemical reactions.

Discrete time model of Hamer

The simplest version of a mass action model is that originally used by Hamer (1906) to describe measles epidemics in London. He considered infections as occurring in discrete generations and denoted the number of susceptibles and infectives in the nth generation by S_n and I_n, respectively. The number of susceptibles and cases in the following generation were calculated from the difference equations:

$$I_{n+1} = (1/m) I_n S_n$$

$$S_{n+1} = S_n - I_{n+1} + b$$

Thus the number of new infections is assumed to be proportional to the number of susceptibles and the number of infections – the 'mass action' assumption.

All infections from the previous generation are removed by recovery or death. The number of susceptibles is decreased by the number of new infections and increased by the influx of b susceptibles during each time step; it is assumed that there is no mortality of susceptibles.

The only parameters of the model are the time between generations, the number of susceptibles added during each time step and the critical number of susceptibles, m. The critical number of susceptibles m can be written in terms of the basic reproduction number R_0 and the population size N as $m = N/R_0$. The mass action assumption then has the interpretation that each of the I_n cases makes R_0 contacts, of whom a proportion S_n/N are susceptible; leading to $I_{n+1} = R_0 I_n S_n/N$ cases in the next generation. Hamer used a generation time of 2 weeks, the sum of the latent and infectious periods for measles, and the values $b = 4400$ (there were approximately 2500 births per week but 300 of these babies died before losing protection from maternal antibodies at 6 months of age) and $m = 150\,000$ (determined empirically).

The model produces a series of undamped regularly recurring epidemics, the magnitude and period of which depend on the parameters and initial conditions. Hamer used initial values of $I_0 = 12\,800$, $S_0 = 150\,000$ to produce a cycle with a period of 18 months (i.e. 39 periods of 2 weeks) (Fig. 10.5). He noted that the number of susceptibles was fairly stable during the course of an epidemic cycle, oscillating by just 20% around the equilibrium number of 150 000. If the number of susceptibles exceeds this threshold, there are more infections in the next generation, i.e. $I_{n+1} > I_n$ if $S_n > m$; if the number of susceptibles is below the threshold, the number of infections decreases. The effective reproduction number at the nth generation is S_n/m and oscillates around 1 during the epidemic cycle.

Continuous time model

The continuous time equivalent of Hamer's model produces damped epidemic cycles (Soper 1929). The period of these cycles, T, can be calculated analytically (Soper 1929) and expressed in terms of the average age at infection, A, and the combined length of the latent and infectious periods D, where

$$T = 2\pi\sqrt{AD}$$

Use of this formula to predict the interepidemic period corresponds well with observed values for many infections (Anderson and May 1991).

Reed–Frost model

The Reed–Frost model is preferred to the mass action model for outbreaks in small populations. Again we consider cases as occurring in discrete generations and let p be the probability of contact between any 2 individuals in each time step. The probability of a susceptible being infected is modelled as the probability of meeting at least one infective, which is $1 - (1 - p)^{I_n}$. In this formulation the number of new infec-

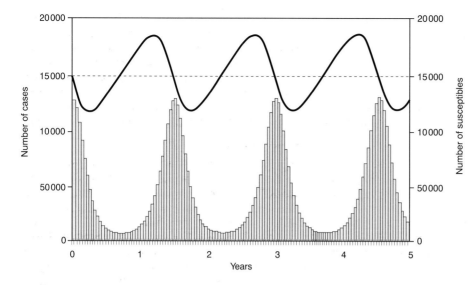

Fig. 10.5 Number of cases and susceptible individuals predicted by Hamer's discrete time model for measles in London.

tives is not proportional to the number of infectives in the previous generation, because the model accounts for the possibility that a susceptible may be contacted by more than one infectious individual.

HETEROGENEITY

The models considered so far have been homogeneous models in which all susceptibles in the population experience the same force of infection. This is undoubtedly a gross simplification of most real situations. For infections such as measles, mumps and rubella, the force of infection is highly age-dependent because of the heterogeneity in contact patterns (Farrington 1990, Grenfell and Anderson 1985, Anderson and May 1985a); in schools, children have most contact with other children of the same age. Changes in transmission rate as schools open and close can account for the seasonality of measles (Fine and Clarkson 1982a, Schenzle 1984). For sexually transmitted diseases, the degree of mixing between different subgroups of the population may be crucial in determining the spread of infection. For other infections, spatial factors, such as population density, may play a role or there may be genetic differences in susceptibility (Anderson and May 1984). Heterogeneity in the application of control measures, such as vaccination, may introduce further problems, e.g. pockets of susceptibility from unvaccinated communities or clustering of vaccination failures. The simple homogeneous model can be generalized in order to investigate these effects (Anderson and May 1991).

DETERMINISTIC AND STOCHASTIC MODELS

The transmission of an infection between individuals in a population depends on a number of chance events. In a large population with many such events the observed behaviour will be close to that expected from the averaging of random effects. Deterministic models examine the expected behaviour of a system and running a deterministic simulation under the same conditions gives the same result every time. This makes them easy to work with.

The major weakness of deterministic models is their behaviour in a situation with a small number of susceptibles or infectives, in which individual random events may affect the outcome. This may arise from an outbreak in a small population, such as a school, or from a very low level of infection in a large population, perhaps as the result of a successful vaccination programme. Stochastic models, which use randomly generated numbers to determine the outcomes of individual events, are better suited to such situations. Stochastic simulations are usually repeated many times to generate a range of results, so that the probability of an outbreak of a particular size or duration can be inferred.

The difference between deterministic and stochastic formulations is illustrated by the case of the introduction of a single infective into a population in which there is no infection. If $R > 1$, a deterministic model will always generate the same outbreak, whereas with a stochastic model one possibility is that no secondary transmission occurs and this may even be the most likely outcome. Alternatively, if $R < 1$, no significant spread occurs in a deterministic model, whereas a stochastic model has a finite probability of generating a large outbreak.

A combination of stochastic and deterministic approaches may be required at different stages of the same problem. The investigation of the effects of introducing a mass vaccination programme is an appropriate application for a deterministic model. If the programme were implemented successfully to eliminate endemic infection, stochastic modelling could be used to yield the distribution of the size of outbreaks expected from any imported infections.

3.4 Strategies for disease control

The strategy adopted to control an infectious disease will depend on many factors, including the aim of the programme, the availability of resources and the epidemiology of the disease. This section outlines the possible aims, describes the strategies available and discusses when they are appropriate.

AIM OF A CONTROL PROGRAMME

Programmes for disease control must have a clearly defined aim. The programme can be designed to meet this aim and its success in achieving it can be assessed. The 3 levels of control are containment, elimination and eradication (Allwright 1988).

Containment

Containment is the most modest control option; infection remains endemic in the population, but morbidity from the disease is reduced to an 'acceptable' level. An example of a containment aim was the WHO measles target for 1995 – a 90% reduction in measles cases and a 95% reduction in measles deaths from the levels before vaccine was introduced.

Elimination

Elimination of an infectious disease from a population requires that there is no endemic transmission of infection within the population and that an imported infection produces no more than an isolated outbreak. This is achieved through the herd immunity of the population; the effective reproduction number must be maintained below one.

Eradication

Eradication of an infectious disease requires the destruction of the pathogen that causes it. It allows the cessation of all control measures, yielding huge savings for future generations. Smallpox is the only disease that has so far been eradicated; the last case of wild smallpox infection occurred in 1977. A WHO programme to eradicate poliomyelitis is in progress; elimination from the Americas has been achieved and significant advances have been made in all other regions (World Health Organization 1995).

ROUTINE VACCINATION

Routine vaccination is the most common method for administering vaccine to a population; children are vaccinated when they reach a target age. Such a programme requires maintenance of a suitable infrastructure to ensure a regular supply of vaccine, etc. If the vaccine provides protection against infection, and not just against disease, the introduction of a vaccination programme will affect the circulation of infection. The dynamic interaction between susceptible and infectious individuals in the population can lead to counter-intuitive results.

Age at infection

A vaccination programme that leads to reduced circulation of infection will cause the average age of infection to rise (Fig. 10.6). Unprotected individuals experience a reduced force of infection and so remain susceptible for longer and thus are older when they eventually become infected. The change in the age distribution of cases is even more marked if transmission rates are higher in older age groups.

The increase in age at infection is beneficial if disease is most severe at a young age, e.g. pertussis and measles in developing countries, but it can lead to an increase in morbidity if disease severity increases with age. For diseases such as poliomyelitis and rubella (see section 4.3, p. 158) vaccination programmes must achieve high coverage so that the reduction in circulation outweighs the problem of increasing age at infection.

Honeymoon periods

The 'honeymoon period' is the name given to the period of low incidence that is frequently observed after introduction of a routine vaccination programme, but which is inevitably followed by a resurgence of infection if vaccination coverage or efficacy is not sufficiently high (McLean and Anderson 1988, Chen et al. 1994, McLean 1995). When the vaccine is first introduced, many of those above the age of vaccination will be immune through natural infection; vaccination reduces the proportion susceptible to well below the threshold. However, the resulting low force of infection allows unprotected individuals, who are not vaccinated or in whom vaccination fails to induce immunity, to accumulate. Once the threshold is exceeded, a post-honeymoon epidemic can occur (Fig. 10.7). If the vaccination programme is maintained the infection will settle into a new epidemic cycle with an epidemic period longer than before vaccination.

VACCINATION CAMPAIGNS

Vaccination campaigns aim to vaccinate all children in a target age range within a short period of time, often one day, week or month. Campaigns may be used to supplement routine programmes, either as a one-off or as a method of giving a second dose, or as an alternative to these. They are often favoured in countries that do not have the infrastructure to maintain a high coverage through routine vaccination programmes.

The advantage of a suitably targeted campaign is that it removes most of the susceptible individuals from the population, thus reducing the reproduction number R well below the $R = 1$ threshold. This has a dramatic effect on transmission which may be interrupted within a few generations if sufficient coverage is achieved. The follow-up programme must maintain herd immunity, either by routine immunization or by periodic campaigns. If the latter approach is chosen, the interval between follow-up campaigns should be determined so as to maintain $R<1$; a campaign is necessary whenever the herd immunity threshold is about to be exceeded. Serological surveillance data make it possible to target a campaign for maximum effect.

This basic strategy is behind the attempt by WHO to eradicate poliomyelitis, and attempts by PAHO to eliminate measles from the Americas (de Quadros et al. 1996). The elimination of measles by mass campaigns was pioneered in the Gambia in 1968–1970, based on modelling simulations by Macdonald (Thacker and Millar 1991), and revived in Cuba

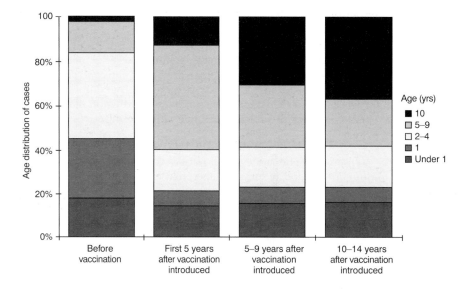

Fig. 10.6 Modelled change in the age distribution of infection following the introduction of vaccination. Simulation of measles in a developing country before and after the introduction of a routine vaccination programme that immunizes 80% of children at age 9–12 months. Parameter values: basic reproduction number $R_0 = 20$; life expectancy $L = 50$ years; latent period 1 week; infectious period 1 week; duration of protection by maternal antibody $m = 6$ months.

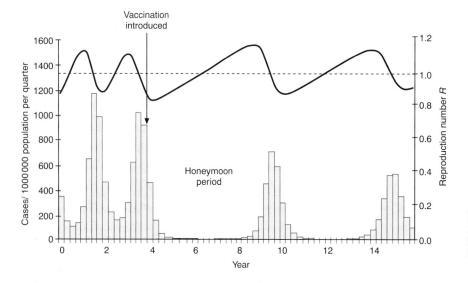

Fig. 10.7 Modelled number of cases of infection following the introduction of vaccination (for details see Fig. 10.6).

(Sabin 1991). Elimination of measles from the Americas may pave the way for eventual eradication.

OUTBREAK CONTROL

Outbreak control may be used to complement or even replace mass vaccination programmes when disease incidence is low. It is, however, only suitable for infections where outbreaks can be identified at an early stage, so that control measures can be taken before widespread transmission occurs. This requires that cases can be diagnosed rapidly and accurately, preferably clinically, and that asymptomatic infections are uncommon. Low transmissibility of infection and a long latent period are also advantageous because they cause outbreaks to develop slowly, permitting time for interventions.

Aggressive outbreak control was an integral part of the smallpox eradication strategy; smallpox satisfies all the above criteria. However, attempts in the USA to control outbreaks of measles through targeted vaccination proved largely unsuccessful (Davis et al.

1987). Infections for which vaccine is currently used to control community outbreaks include hepatitis A and meningococcal infection, neither of which is ideally suited to such an approach because of the high proportion of subclinical infections (hepatitis A) and the relative lack of vaccine efficacy (menigococcal disease), but the low incidence of disease in the population does not justify the expense of mass vaccination.

QUARANTINE AND ISOLATION

A quarantine strategy may be used to prevent the introduction of an infection into a population from which it is absent. It is appropriate only if the population is isolated from the potential source of infection. No attempt is made to create herd immunity in the population and so failure of the quarantine measures can lead to a sizeable outbreak. Quarantine policies should therefore be backed up by outbreak control procedures. Quarantine measures were used extensively in North America in the nineteenth century to prevent the introduction of infections such as cholera, smallpox and typhus by ships from Europe. They are still used to exclude rabies from the UK.

Isolation of infectious individuals is another method of preventing spread of infection through an unprotected population. Such a policy can be successful only if infectives are identified before they transmit infection. The isolation of HIV positive individuals in sanatoria is a major and controversial part of the strategy in Cuba for the prevention of AIDS.

4 HERD IMMUNITY AND VACCINATION PROGRAMMES

Most communicable diseases have a regular cyclical pattern (Noah 1989) but some infections are less predictable. Epidemics of meningococcal disease occurred during both World Wars, in the early 1970s, and again since the mid-1980s. Influenza epidemics are even less predictable and are associated with major antigenic shift. In general, the epidemic cycles of viral infections are more regular than those of bacterial diseases.

Introduction of a vaccine that protects against transmission of infection disrupts the natural epidemic cycle of a disease. Models that simulate the transmission of infection within a population may be used to predict the effects of vaccination programmes on the incidence of disease. The predictability of epidemics has been greatly enhanced in recent years by serological surveillance, where the proportion susceptible to an infection by age is determined by large cross-sectional antibody prevalence studies. In the UK, routine serological surveillance for measles, mumps and rubella antibody was established in 1986, before the introduction of combined measles, mumps, rubella vaccine (Morgan-Capner et al. 1988). The application of mathematical models to serological surveillance data has recently made possible the anticipation of a measles epidemic in the UK, which was then averted by a national immunization campaign (see section 4.4, p. 160).

4.1 Diphtheria

The symptoms of diphtheria are caused by the production of an exotoxin which is produced by the infecting organism, *Corynebacterium diphtheriae* (see Chapter 19 and Volume 2, Chapter 25). Naturally acquired antitoxic immunity provides protection that is usually life-long. The traditional method for measuring diphtheria immunity – the Schick test – is no longer available and has been superseded by the assessment of neutralizing antitoxin in serum. A concentration of 0.1 units of antitoxin per ml or more indicates long-term immunity. In the prevaccination era, most babies were born with maternally derived passive immunity and infection was relatively uncommon in the first year of life. Attack rates were highest in the group aged 1–5 years and by early adulthood most individuals were immune to diphtheria (Fig. 10.8).

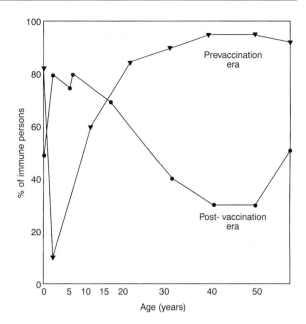

Fig. 10.8 Diphtheria immunity by age in the pre- and post-vaccine eras.

Close contact is required for transmission of diphtheria and therefore epidemics occurred particularly under conditions of crowding and poor hygiene. The importance of closeness and duration of contact in determining the spread of disease was first described by Dudley in 1926. Children sleeping in the same school dormitory were at greater risk than those in casual contact during working hours (Dudley 1926). In temperate countries the disease was commonest in the colder winter months whereas in tropical countries transmission occurred all the year round. In tropical countries the principal source of infection is from cutaneous diphtheria lesions whereas in temperate countries pharyngeal diphtheria is more common.

Routine immunization with diphtheria toxoid, which protects against the effects of the toxin, was introduced in the 1940s. Immunization very rapidly reduced the disease incidence in temperate countries and by the 1960s diphtheria had virtually been eliminated. As a result, the pattern of immunity in the population has changed completely. Because the organism no longer circulates in the community, adults born since the introduction of immunization rely solely on vaccine-induced immunity, which is generally lower than naturally acquired immunity. Immunization is commenced at 2 months of age so that young infants very rapidly acquire vaccine-induced immunity, which is boosted by further immunizations given at school entry and, since 1993, on leaving school. However, older adults, in whom the last dose of vaccine was given many years ago, have waning immunity and in Britain up to a third of older adults may now be susceptible to diphtheria (Maple et al. 1995). Fortunately, this immunity gap does not appear to have led to significant outbreaks despite the fact that cases of toxigenic diphtheria continue to be imported from developing countries (Begg and Balraj

1995). In the former USSR, diphtheria has re-emerged in recent years. This is only partly explained by waning immunity in adults. Other factors include mass population movements and lower vaccine coverage in young children.

Since vaccine-induced immunity protects against the toxic effects of the disease, it might be expected that diphtheria immunization would not reduce circulation of the organism. Nevertheless, isolation of a toxigenic strain of *C. diphtheriae* is now very rare and it appears that vaccine interrupts transmission in addition to preventing disease. This is probably related to the fact that transmission of *C. diphtheriae* by clinical cases is much more efficient than that by subclinical carriers.

The level of diphtheria immunity in the population required to achieve herd immunity is not known precisely, but is generally considered to be between 70 and 90% (Simonsen and Kjeldsen 1987).

4.2 Pertussis

Immunity to pertussis is complicated and many components of *Bordetella pertussis* appear to have a role (see Chapter 18 and Volume 2, Chapter 38). At present the serological correlates of immunity are not known and thus population immunity data are of little value in mathematical modelling.

In Britain, pertussis epidemics occurred at intervals of 4 years before the introduction of routine immunization in the 1950s (Fig. 10.9). There were more than 100 000 reported cases per year and about 1 per 1000 patients died from the disease. The mortality rate and the risk of complications from pertussis depend greatly on age. Most deaths occur in young children under the age of 6 months. After this age the severity of the disease declines progressively and in adults it may be a relatively mild, self-limiting illness. Because the risk of severe disease is greatest in the first few months of life, it is important that pertussis vaccines are given as early as possible. For this reason, an accelerated schedule of immunization, at 2, 3 and 4 months of age, was introduced in the UK in 1992.

Pertussis vaccines were introduced in the 1950s. Coverage was initially high (over 80%) and the magnitude of epidemics decreased considerably. Only 2000 cases were recorded in 1972. In the mid-1970s, however, doubts were cast over the safety of the vaccine and vaccine coverage dropped from 80% to 30%; this led to a resurgence in epidemics, the size of which had not been seen for over 20 years. Subsequently, vaccine coverage has improved and the epidemics have again decreased in size. In 1995 only 1873 cases were notified, the lowest annual figure ever recorded.

The interesting feature throughout this period is that despite the introduction of vaccination with great fluctuations in coverage, there has been little change in the length of the interepidemic cycle. This led to the suggestion that pertussis vaccine may have no effect on carriage but that it simply protects against disease (Fine and Clarkson 1982b). However, a decrease in the incidence of pertussis in children too young to be vaccinated points to some reduction in transmission (Miller, White and Fairley 1994). A recent study that used an age-structured model to simulate the transmission of pertussis in England and Wales suggested that both these observations are consistent with a vaccine efficacy against transmission of approximately 80% (Miller and Gay 1996). In this scenario, the recent improvements in coverage to more than 95% would lead to a discernible lengthening of the epidemic period and an increasing proportion of infections would occur in adults. Increasing evidence suggests that adults with clinically inapparent or mild infection may act as important reservoirs of infection.

The question of whether vaccine protects against the transmission of infection has important implications for the control of pertussis. If the current vaccines do not protect against transmission, elimination of the infection would be impossible. It remains to be seen whether the recently developed subunit vaccines for which there is preliminary evidence suggesting that they affect transmission, will in fact prove to do so. Field trials of efficacy have recently established the efficacy of acellular pertussis vaccines in infants from 2 months of age.

4.3 Rubella: the prevention of congenital rubella syndrome

Most cases of rubella present as a mild illness with rash. Infection in pregnancy, however, can cause congenital rubella syndrome (CRS), which results in severe malformation of the fetus, including cataracts, deafness and heart defects (Gregg 1941, Miller, Cradock-Watson and Pollock 1982) (see Volume 1, Chapter 28). The purpose of a rubella vaccination programme is to reduce the number cases of CRS by preventing infections in pregnant women. Various strategies have been used to achieve this goal since the vaccine became available in 1970. To make informed policy decisions possible, the risks and benefits of each vaccination programme can be evaluated with mathematical models (Anderson and Grenfell 1986).

Before vaccination was introduced in developed countries, rubella epidemics occurred every 4–5 years

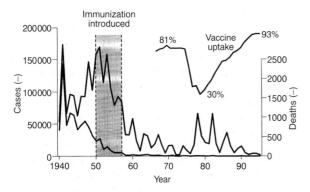

Fig. 10.9 Whooping cough notifications: cases and deaths, England and Wales 1940–95. (Prepared by CDSC; source OPCS).

and the average age of infection was approximately 10 years. About 85% of the population experienced the disease by the age of 16 years, leaving 15% who remained susceptible to infection as adults; a significant number of infections in pregnancy and consequent cases of CRS resulted. In developing countries, rubella is acquired at a much younger age; almost everyone is infected in childhood and cases of CRS are uncommon. However, rubella vaccination may become necessary if social and environmental changes lead to a reduction in transmission rates.

POLICY OPTIONS

The number of rubella infections in pregnancy depends on the number of susceptible pregnant women and the risk of infection in pregnancy. Vaccination programmes were designed to reduce the number of infections in pregnancy by reducing one of these contributing factors. The 2 main options of universal and selective vaccination are respectively often termed the US and UK policies after the countries in which they were originally used.

The universal policy

The universal policy was designed to eliminate CRS by the elimination of rubella, which was to be achieved by a high vaccine coverage of all children at a young age. Susceptible pregnant women would be protected from infection by the herd immunity of the population.

The selective policy

The selective policy was designed to reduce the incidence of CRS by reducing the level of susceptibility among pregnant women, by vaccinating only girls at the age of 10–14 years. This would allow the virus to remain endemic, so that many girls would be infected and acquire immunity before they were vaccinated. Vaccination would serve to reduce the number of susceptible girls. Further reductions could be achieved by screening pregnant women and vaccinating those found to be susceptible.

RISKS AND BENEFITS

A universal policy offers the greater benefit of the elimination of CRS but also entails more risk. If vaccination coverage is low, the number of infections in pregnancy may actually be increased by the vaccination programme. Vaccination reduces the force of infection acting on the unvaccinated population, causing them to remain susceptible longer until they acquire infection at an older age. The number of susceptible pregnant women may increase. If the increase in susceptibility among pregnant women outweighs the reduction in the force of infection, more cases of CRS will occur.

By contrast, a selective policy can only eliminate CRS with 100% coverage; the risk to susceptible pregnant women is not reduced by the vaccination programme. However, the policy does not carry the risk of increasing the incidence of CRS; the reduction in the incidence of CRS is the same as the coverage achieved.

Anderson and Grenfell (1986) used an age-structured model to calculate the number of cases of CRS expected at different levels of coverage for each of the 2 policies at the long-term steady state (Fig. 10.10). Under the universal policy, there was an increase in the number of cases of CRS for coverages less than 60%, but rubella and CRS were eliminated for coverage greater than 80–85%. If coverage exceeded 75%, the universal policy prevented more cases of CRS than a selective policy with the same coverage. Short-term dynamic simulations produced similar results.

Policy implications

The USA introduced a universal rubella vaccination programme in 1969. Following a decline in the number of infections through the 1970s and 1980s to very low levels, there was a resurgence of rubella in 1989–91 (Lindegren et al. 1991, Centers for Disease Control 1994). Many cases were in unvaccinated young adults, including pregnant women (56 cases of CRS were reported in 1990–91) or in children from communities who refused vaccination. Since these outbreaks the incidence of rubella has returned to low levels. The USA aims to eliminate indigenous rubella and CRS by 1996, maintaining herd immunity through high vaccination coverage.

The UK introduced a selective vaccination programme in 1970, and achieved 80–85% coverage at a time when the coverage of measles vaccination was less than 60%. Although this resulted in a considerable reduction in the number of infections in pregnancy, their continuing occurrence prompted a switch to a universal policy in 1988. A vaccination campaign amongst children 5–16 years of age in 1994 removed many susceptibles from these cohorts, but in 1995 10–15% of males aged 18–30 remained susceptible to rubella. This led to a resurgence of rubella in 1996, which included many outbreaks in universities and military barracks. The legacy of the selective vaccination programme is that less than 2% of women are susceptible to rubella, thus limiting the number of infections in pregnancy (Miller et al. 1997).

In São Paulo State, Brazil, a universal rubella vaccination programme was introduced in 1992, following a modelling study to explore strategy options. This is an exemplary approach to vaccination programme design. At the start of the programme, in which vaccine is given to children at 15 months of age, a one-off vaccination campaign was carried out among older children to prevent the resurgent epidemics experienced in the USA. The upper age limit of the campaign was set as 10 years, because models suggested that little benefit was to be gained by including older children, though the estimated seroprevalence in this age group was only 70–80% (Massad et al. 1994). The transmission rates of the model were based on an age-specific force of infection estimated from a serological survey that included only 54 samples from persons aged 10 years or more (de Azevedo Neto et al. 1994). The experience of the next 10–15 years will determine whether the decision not to include chil-

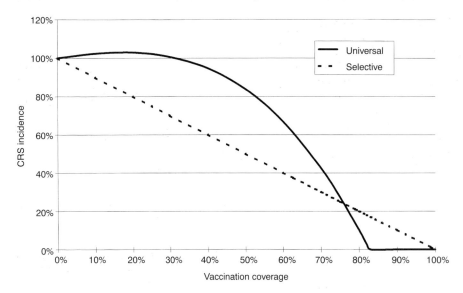

Fig. 10.10 Predicted equilibrium incidence of congenital rubella syndrome (relative to its incidence in the absence of vaccination) by vaccine coverage for selective and universal rubella vaccination programmes (after Anderson and Grenfell 1986).

dren aged 11–15 years in the campaign will show that modelling saved unnecessary expenditure, or that too much faith was placed in the predictions of insufficiently robust models.

4.4   Measles: vaccination strategy in England and Wales

Measles is the most infectious of the vaccine-preventable diseases and causes significant morbidity and mortality if it is not controlled by vaccination (see Volume 1, Chapter 23). In this section we review the history of measles vaccination in England and Wales, in particular the role of models in the planning of the national vaccination campaign conducted in 1994.

BACKGROUND

Before measles vaccination was introduced in England and Wales epidemics occurred in alternate years, causing an average of 100 deaths per year. Almost everyone experienced measles infection as a young child; 55% of notified cases were in those under 5 years, 42% in those aged 5–9 years and only 3% were in persons aged over 10 years. Vaccination was introduced in 1968, but uptake was initially low with only 50% of children being vaccinated up to 1980. Coverage then increased steadily, reaching 80% by 1988. Over this period measles notifications and deaths showed a downward trend, but coverage was sufficiently low for the virus to remain endemic. Children who were not vaccinated became infected, resulting in continuing morbidity and mortality.

In 1988 combined measles, mumps and rubella vaccine (MMR) replaced single antigen measles vaccine and coverage increased to 93% within 2 years. This, together with an MMR catch-up programme targeted at preschool children, resulted in a marked reduction in measles incidence in all age groups. Unvaccinated children, therefore, had little opportunity to acquire immunity through infection, and they remained susceptible. The ageing of cohorts with higher levels of

susceptibility caused an increase in the proportion of school children who were susceptible to measles, detected by serologiocal surveillance (Fig. 10.11).

The shift of measles susceptibility was also reflected by a change in the age distribution of measles infections. A study with laboratory salivary diagnosis demonstrated that notifications, based on clinical diagnosis, were unreliable, especially in young children (Brown and Ramsay 1994). Most infections were occurring in those aged 10 years or more and outbreaks in secondary schools were becoming more common (Calvert and Cutts 1994, Morse et al. 1994, Ramsay et al. 1994).

MODELLING

Two separate approaches were used to predict the incidence of measles. Both models summarize their results using the reproduction number *R*. If *R*<1 the population has herd immunity and resurgence of disease cannot occur.

The first study used models to interpret the serological surveillance data, to examine whether the

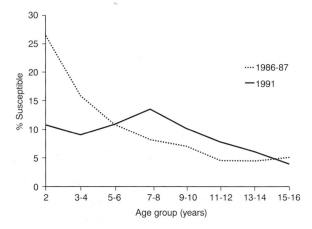

Fig. 10.11 Serological surveillance data: proportion of samples negative for measles IgG antibody by age, England 1986–87 and 1991.

increase in susceptibility would be sufficient to exceed the threshold at $R = 1$ (Gay et al. 1995). The model divided the population into 5 age groups. The reproduction number was determined by the level of susceptibility in each age group and the transmission rates within and between age groups. This calculation is the age stratified equivalent of $R = R_0 x$. The level of susceptibility expected in each year in each age group was projected from the serological data, assuming that no infection occurred. Transmission rates were derived from age-specific notification data from the prevaccination period (Fig. 10.12). Because of the difficulty in obtaining a precise estimate for the transmission rate within the 10–14 year age group a range of values was used. (These values were a multiple α of the transmission rate within the 5–9 year age group, with α ranging from 1 to 2.). The model predicted that as the most susceptible cohorts moved into the age group with the highest transmission rates (10–14 years) the reproduction number, R, would exceed 1. This would occur sometime before 1998, depending on the transmission rate assumed for the 10–14 year age group (Fig. 10.13). The scenario that best reflected the observed changes in the age distribution of cases suggested that this would occur sooner rather than later. This provided the potential for a resurgence of measles in 1995–96 involving more than 100 000 cases with most occurring in persons aged 10 years or more. Because of the increased severity with age, such a resurgence would result in a disproportionately high level of morbidity and mortality.

The second study simulated measles transmission in England and Wales with a dynamic model fed with vaccination coverage statistics (Babad et al. 1995). The model provided a good reflection of historical data. The study concluded that a single-dose vaccination policy would not be sufficient to eliminate measles and investigated the options for supplementary vaccination measures. A vaccination campaign covering all children aged 5–16 years would reduce R well below the threshold. The introduction of a second routine vaccine dose at the age of 4 years immediately after the campaign would maintain the herd immunity of the population.

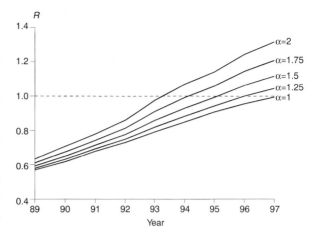

Fig. 10.13 Calculated value of the reproduction number for measles in England for a range of values of the age-specific transmission rates (Gay et al. 1995).

EFFECT OF THE CAMPAIGN

A national campaign to immunize children aged 5–16 with a combined measles and rubella vaccine was carried out in 1994 (Miller 1994). All children were offered vaccine, irrespective of their previous history of vaccination or disease and a 92% coverage was achieved. The incidence of measles dropped dramatically after the campaign and the few cases that occurred were in a pattern consistent with limited spread from imported infections (Gay et al. 1997). The introduction of a second dose into the routine vaccination schedule at school entry should sustain the herd immunity achieved. Continued surveillance is essential to monitor the effect of the programme. Salivary investigation of all suspected cases makes it possible to identify outbreaks and serological surveillance monitors the maintenance of herd immunity.

5 ENVIRONMENTAL AND SOCIAL EFFECTS AND POPULATION IMMUNITY

Changes in environmental and social conditions may affect the population in a number of ways. Poor hygiene facilitates spread of infections by the faecal–oral route, such as dysentery, whereas crowded accommodation facilitates the spread of air-borne infections, such as tuberculosis and meningococcal disease. Temperature and other environmental conditions affect the survival of infectious disease agents. Social conditions such as sexual behaviour and patterns of occupation influence the likelihood of exposure to specific infectious agents.

5.1 Control of disease by hygiene

In countries where hygiene is poor, enteric infections spread easily. For example, hepatitis A (see Volume 1, Chapter 34) is endemic in many developing countries where basic hygiene measures such as hand washing and safe sewage disposal are lacking. Most children

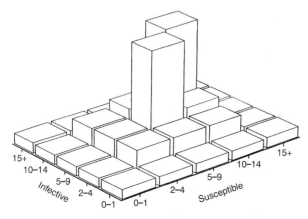

Fig. 10.12 Age-specific transmission rates for measles in England and Wales (with $\alpha = 1$) (Gay et al. 1995).

become infected in the first few years of life. In this young age group, a large proportion of infections are subclinical and icteric cases are relatively uncommon. Where hygiene is good, infection in young children is relatively uncommon and most reach adulthood without immunity to hepatitis A (Fig. 10.14). In these countries, most infections occur in adults, in whom symptomatic infection is very common. Two main patterns of disease are observed – slowly evolving community outbreaks lasting for months or even years in which infection is transmitted from person to person, and explosive point source outbreaks that arise from a contaminated food or water source (Tang et al. 1991). In countries in transition between high and low states of endemicity there is often a rapid reduction in the incidence of infection (Lim and Yeoh 1992, Yap and Guan 1993, Perez-Trallero et al. 1994). Models suggest that this may be followed by a substantial resurgence of endemic disease (Gay 1996).

Hepatitis A vaccines have recently become available and are of value in protecting those likely to be most at risk, such as travellers to highly endemic areas. Largely on the grounds of cost, no country has yet implemented hepatitis A for routine use, but vaccines against hepatitis A that can be incorporated into other vaccines are being developed. In countries with good hygiene the basic reproduction number for hepatitis A is relatively low; it is approximately 2 in England and Wales (Gay et al. 1994), and herd immunity could be achieved with modest vaccination coverage. Mass vaccination programmes may, however, be most appropriate for countries in the transitional phase.

Poliomyelitis is another example of a disease that is affected by changes in hygiene. During the early part of this century, when hygiene was poor in Britain, polio circulated widely among preschool children. In this age group paralysis was relatively uncommon and the number of paralytic cases was therefore small. During the 1940s and 1950s, as hygiene improved and the

circulation of wild virus diminished, the average age of infection rose. This led to epidemics of paralytic disease in older children and young adults (Fig. 10.15). Poliomyelitis vaccines became available in the 1950s and rapidly reduced the incidence of the disease. Global eradication of polio is now planned by the World Health Organization. Its eradication is feasible, because there is no known non-human reservoir of the disease and the virus does not survive long in potential environmental sources such as sewage. Live oral vaccine is able to interrupt transmission and also to prevent disease, and it is relatively cheap and easily delivered.

5.2 Sexually transmitted diseases

Sexually transmitted diseases are the best examples of infections whose incidence is affected by behaviour. The incidence of a disease is affected not only by the mean rate of partner acquisition but particularly by the degree of heterogeneity in behaviour within a population. The importance of core groups in the transmission of infection is well documented (Yorke, Hethcote and Nold 1978, Jacques et al. 1988). Changes in the behaviour of the core groups can have a dramatic effect on the incidence of infection.

The studies of gonorrhoea (see Chapter 33) by Yorke, Hethcote and Nold (1978) and Hethcote and Yorke (1984) were the first detailed investigations of the transmission dynamics of a sexually transmitted disease. They described how changes in behaviour affect the level of endemic disease. In recent years, interest in the AIDS epidemic has produced explosive growth in the literature. However, the complexity of the interactions between subgroups of the population and the problem of collecting suitable data from which parameters can be estimated make modelling particularly difficult. Population-based surveys (Johnson et al. 1992) can provide a basis for initial parameter estimates but transmission models remain most useful for assessing the relative contribution of various factors to future trends in the incidence of AIDS, rather than for making quantitative predictions (Williams and Anderson 1994).

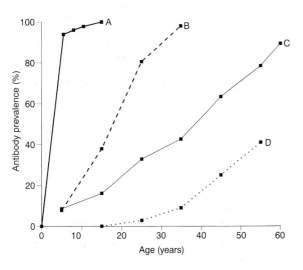

Fig. 10.14 Prevalence of antibody to hepatitis A in several countries: A, Cameroon, 1989 (Stroffolini et al. 1991); B, Spain, 1986 (Perez-Trallero et al. 1994); C, England, 1987 (Gay et al. 1994); D, Sweden, 1977 (Iwarson et al. 1978).

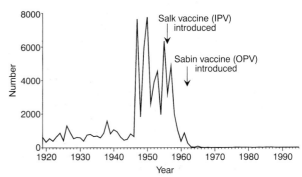

Fig. 10.15 Poliomyelitis notifications, England and Wales 1919–95. (Prepared by CDSC).

5.3 Vector control

Malaria (see Volume 5, Chapter 20) was the first infection in which population dynamics were extensively studied. Transmission of malaria depends on several factors, but the most important relate to the anopheline mosquito vector. The calculation of the basic reproduction number and eradication threshold are different in vector borne and directly communicable infections. The contact parameter is a function of the density, survival rate and feeding behaviours of the vector populations. The estimates of the basic reproduction number for malaria range between 5 and 100. These reflect considerable variations in the epidemiology of malaria, which is observed even within relatively small geographical areas. Macdonald (1957) developed a formula for the likelihood of infection based on the proportion of anopheline mosquitoes with sporozoites in their salivary glands. Malaria transmission in Macdonald's model was proportional to the density of the vector, the number of times each day that the mosquito bites a human, and the probability of that mosquito surviving for one day. Macdonald's model has been refined in recent years, but it illustrates some important points relevant to the control of malaria. Vector longevity is the most important factor in determining transmission and therefore focuses control measures on the adult mosquito. Control programmes are most likely to be effective where vector longevity is short and the basic reproduction number is low. This was the situation in Europe where the reproduction level was low in many areas and the vector was found mainly within houses where it could be attacked with insecticides. There is also considerable variation between different species of anopheline mosquitoes in their ability to transmit malaria (the vectorial capacity). Each vector has its own behaviour patterns and breeding grounds. Malaria is often seasonal, coinciding with the rainy season, which provides water for mosquito breeding, and the increased humidity that favours mosquito survival.

Several malaria vaccines are currently under development and these may have individual as well as population actions. They are being designed to act at various stages of the infection cycle; some of the candidate vaccines may protect only against transmission and not against disease.

6 GENETIC FACTORS IN POPULATION IMMUNITY

Studies of herd immunity must clearly take into account genetic differences in resistance. Much of the work in this area was done on mice by Webster and others in the 1920s (Webster 1946). They were able to show genetic effects in resistance to infection which emerged as a result of inbreeding and other genetic manipulations, but the extent to which this work can be extrapolated to man is not clear. Observations in human populations are beset by confounding factors. There is no doubt that some populations are more susceptible to certain infectious diseases than others. Of particular note are sex differences in disease rates for many childhood infectious diseases. For example, mumps is more common among boys than among girls. The incidence of meningococcal disease and other infections caused by bacteria with polysaccharide capsules varies enormously in different parts of the world. Certain populations, for example Aboriginal Australians, have very high rates of disease and respond poorly to polysaccharide vaccines (Pearce et al. 1995).

REFERENCES

Allwright SPA, 1988, Introduction, *Elimination or Reduction of Diseases? Opportunities for Health Service Action in Europe*, eds Silman AJ, Allwright SPA, Oxford Medical Publications, Oxford, 5–7.

Anderson RM, Crombie JA, Grenfell BT, 1987, The epidemiology of mumps in the United Kingdom: a preliminary study of virus transmission, herd immunity and the potential impact of immunisation, *Epidemiol Infect*, **99:** 65–84.

Anderson RM, Grenfell BT, 1986, Quantitative investigations of different rubella vaccination policies for the control of congenital rubella syndrome (CRS) in the United Kingdom, *J Hyg Camb*, **96:** 305–33.

Anderson RM, May RM, 1984, Spatial, temporal and genetic heterogeneity in host populations and the design of vaccination programmes, *IMA J Math Appl Med Biol*, **1:** 233–66.

Anderson RM, May RM, 1985a, Age-related changes in the rate of disease transmission: implications for the design of vaccination programmes, *J Hyg Camb*, **94:** 365–435.

Anderson RM, May RM, 1985b, Vaccination and herd immunity to infectious diseases, *Nature (London)*, **318:** 323–9.

Anderson RM, May RM, 1990, Immunisation and herd immunity, *Lancet*, **335:** 641–5.

Anderson RM, May RM, 1991, *Infectious Diseases of Humans: Dynamics and Control*, 2nd edn, Oxford University Press, Oxford.

de Azevedo Neto RS, Silveira AS et al., 1994, Rubella seroepidemiology in a non-immunized population of Sao Paulo State, Brazil, *Epidemiol Infect*, **113:** 161–73.

Babad HR, Nokes DJ et al., 1995, Predicting the impact of measles vaccination in England and Wales: model validation and analysis of policy options, *Epidemiol Infect*, **114:** 319–41.

Bailey NTJ, 1956a, On estimating the latent and infectious period of measles. I. Families with two susceptibles only, *Biometrika*, **43:** 15–22.

Bailey NTJ, 1956b, On estimating the latent and infectious periods of measles. II. Families with three or more susceptibles, *Biometrika*, **43:** 322–31.

Bailey NTJ, 1957, *The Mathematical Theory of Epidemics*, Griffin, London.

Bartlett MS, 1956, *Proceedings of the Third Berkeley Symposium on Mathematical Statistics and Probability*, University of California Press, Berkeley, 81–109.

Bartlett MS, 1957, Measles periodicity and community size, *J R Stat Soc A*, **120:** 48–60.

Begg N, Balraj V, 1995, Diphtheria: are we ready for it?, *Arch Dis Child*, **73:** 568–72.

Brown DW, Ramsay ME, 1994, Salivary diagnosis of measles: a study of notified cases in the United Kingdom, 1991–3, *Br Med J*, **308:** 1015–17.

Brownlee J, 1907, Statistical studies in immunity. The theory of an epidemic, *Proc R Soc Edinb*, **26:** 484–521.

Brownlee J, 1909, Certain considerations of the causation and course of epidemics, *Proc R Soc Med (Epidemiol Sect)*, **2**: 243–58.

Calvert N, Cutts FT, 1994, Measles among secondary school children in West Cumbria: implications for vaccine policy, *Commun Dis Rep*, **4**: R70–3.

Centers for Disease Control, 1994, Rubella and congenital rubella syndrome – United States, January 1, 1991–May 7, 1994, *Morbid Mortal Weekly Rep*, **43**: 391–401.

Chen RT, Weierbach R et al., 1994, A 'post-honeymoon period' measles outbreak in Muyinga sector, Burundi, *Int J Epidemiol*, **23**: 185–93.

Davis RM, Whitman ED et al., 1987, A persistent outbreak of measles despite appropriate prevention and control measures, *Am J Epidemiol*, **126**: 438–49.

Diekmann O, Heesterbeek JAP, Metz JAJ, 1990, On the definition and the computation of the basic reproduction ratio R0 in models for infectious diseases in heterogeneous populations, *J Math Biol*, **28**: 365–82.

Dietz K, 1975, *Mathematical Models for the Spread of Infectious Diseases*, Society for Industrial and Applied Mathematics, Philadelphia, PA, 104–21.

Dietz K, 1993, The estimation of the basic reproduction number for infectious diseases, *Stat Methods Med Res*, **2**: 23–41.

Dudley SF, 1926, *The Spread of Droplet Infection in Semi-isolated Communities*, Medical Research Council special report series, No 111, HMSO, London.

Farr W, 1840, *Progress of Epidemics*, Second Report of the Registrar General of England and Wales, London, 16–20.

Farrington CP, 1990, Modelling forces of infection for measles, mumps and rubella, *Stat Med*, **9**: 953–67.

Fine PEM, 1979, John Brownlee and the measurement of infectiousness: an historical study in epidemic theory, *J R Stat Soc A*, **142**: 347–62.

Fine PEM, 1993, Herd immunity: history, theory, practice, *Epidemiol Rev*, **15**: 265–302.

Fine PEM, Clarkson JA, 1982a, Measles in England and Wales – I: an analysis of factors underlying seasonal patterns, *Int J Epidemiol*, **11**: 5–14.

Fine PEM, Clarkson JA, 1982b, The recurrence of whooping cough: possible implications for assessment of vaccine efficacy, *Lancet*, **1**: 666–9.

Finkelstein RA, 1984, *Bacterial Vaccines*, Academic Press, Orlando, FL, 107.

Fox JP, Elveback L et al., 1971, Herd immunity: basic concept and relevance to public health immunization practices, *Am J Epidemiol*, **94**: 179–89.

Frost WH, 1976, Some conceptions of epidemics in general, *Am J Epidemiol*, **103**: 141–51.

Gay NJ, 1996, A model of long term decline in disease transmissibility: implications for the incidence of hepatitis A, *Int J Epidemiol*, **25**: 854–61.

Gay NJ, Morgan-Capner P et al., 1994, Age-specific antibody prevalence to hepatitis A: implications for disease control, *Epidemiol Infect*, **113**: 113–20.

Gay NJ, Hesketh LM et al., 1995, Interpretation of serological surveillance data for measles using mathematical models: implications for vaccine strategy, *Epidemiol Infect*, **115**: 139–56.

Gay NJ, Ramsay M et al., 1997, The epidemiology of measles in England and Wales since the 1994 vaccination campaign, *Commun Dis Rep*, **7**: R17–21.

Goldschneider I, Gotschlich EC, Artenstein MS, 1969, Human immunity to the meningococcus. II. Development of natural immunity, *J Exp Med*, **129**: 1327–48.

Greenwood M, Bradford Hill A et al., 1936, *Experimental Epidemiology*, Medical Research Council special report series, No. 209, HMSO, London.

Gregg NM, 1941, Congenital cataract following German measles in the mother, *Trans Ophthalmol Soc Aust*, **3**: 35.

Grenfell BT, Anderson RM, 1985, The estimation of age related rates of infection from case notifications and serological data, *J Hyg Camb*, **95**: 419–36.

Halloran ME, Cochi SL et al., 1994, Theoretical epidemiologic and morbidity effects of routine varicella immunization of preschool children in the United States, *Am J Epidemiol*, **140**: 81–104.

Hamer WH, 1906, The Milroy Lectures on epidemic disease in England – the evidence of variability and of persistency of type, *Lancet*, **1**: 733–9.

Hethcote HW, 1983, Measles and rubella in the United States, *Am J Epidemiol*, **117**: 2–13.

Hethcote HW, Yorke JA, 1984, Gonorrhea: transmission dynamics and control, *Lect Notes Biomath*, **56**: 1–105.

Hope Simpson RE, 1948, The period of transmission in certain epidemic diseases, *Lancet*, **2**: 755–60.

Iwarson S, Frosner GG et al., 1978, The changed epidemiology of hepatitis A infection in Scandinavia, *Scand J Infect Dis*, **10**: 155–6.

Jacques JA, Simon CP et al., 1988, Modelling and analysing HIV transmission: the effect of contact patterns, *Math Biosci*, **92**: 119–99.

Johnson AM, Wadsworth J et al., 1992, Sexual lifestyles and HIV risk, *Nature (London)*, **360**: 410–12.

Kaye D, Merseilis DG et al., 1967, Treatment of chronic enteric carriers of *Salmonella typhosa* with ampicillin, *Ann NY Acad Sci*, **145**: 429–35.

Kermack WO, McKendrick AG, 1927, Contributions to the mathematical theory of epidemics, part 1, *Proc R Soc Edinb*, **115**: 700–21.

Lim WL, Yeoh EK, 1992, Hepatitis A vaccination, *Lancet*, **339**: 304.

Lindegren ML, Fehrs LJ et al., 1991, Update: rubella and congenital rubella syndrome, 1980–1990, *Epidemiol Rev*, **13**, 341–8.

Macdonald G, 1957, *The Epidemiology and Control of Malaria*, Oxford University Press, London.

McLean AR, 1995, After the honeymoon in measles control, *Lancet*, **345**: 272.

McLean AR, Anderson RM, 1988, Measles in developing countries. Part II. The predicted impact of mass vaccination, *Epidemiol Infect*, **100**: 419–22.

Maple PA, Efstratiou A et al., 1995, Diphtheria immunity in UK blood donors, *Lancet*, **345**: 963–5.

Massad E, Burattini MN et al., 1994, A model-based design of a vaccination strategy against rubella in a non-immunized community of Sao Paulo State, Brazil, *Epidemiol Infect*, **112**: 579–94.

Miller E, 1994, The new measles campaign, *Br Med J*, **309**: 1102–3.

Miller E, Cradock-Watson JE, Pollock TM, 1982, Consequences of confirmed maternal rubella at successive stages of pregnancy, *Lancet*, **2**: 781–4.

Miller E, Gay NJ, 1996, Epidemiological determinants of pertussis, *Dev Biol Stand*, **89**: 15–23.

Miller E, White JM, Fairley CK, 1994, Pertussis vaccination, *Lancet*, **344**: 1575–6.

Miller E, Waight P et al., 1997, The epidemiology of rubella in England and Wales before and after the 1994 measles and rubella vaccination campaign, *Commun Dis Rep*, **7**: 1226–32.

Mollison D, Isham V, Grenfell BT, 1994, Epidemics: models and data, *J R Stat Soc A*, **157**: 115–49.

Morgan-Capner P, Wright J et al., 1988, Surveillance of antibody to measles, mumps and rubella by age, *Br Med J*, **297**: 770–2.

Morse D, O'Shea M et al., 1994, Outbreak of measles in a teenage school population: need to immunise susceptible adolescents, *Epidemiol Infect*, **113**: 355–65.

Noah ND, 1989, Cyclical patterns and predictability in infection, *Epidemiol Infect*, **102**: 175–90.

Pearce MC, Slendan JW et al., 1995, Control of Group C meningococcal disease in Australian Aboriginal children by mass rifampicin chemoprophylaxis and vaccination, *Lancet*, **346**: 20–3.

Perez-Trallero E, Cilla G et al., 1994, Falling incidence and prevalence of hepatitis A in northern Spain, *Scand J Infect Dis*, **26**: 133–6.

de Quadros CA, Olivé JM et al., 1996, Measles elimination in the Americas: evolving strategies, *JAMA*, **275**: 224–9.

Ramsay ME, Gay NJ et al., 1994, The epidemiology of measles in England and Wales: rationale for the 1994 national vaccination campaign, *Commun Dis Rep*, **4**: R141–6.

Ross R, 1909, *Report on the Prevention of Malaria in Mauritius*, J and A Churchill, London.

Ross R, 1911, *The Prevention of Malaria*, 2nd edn, Murray, London.

Sabin AB, 1991, Measles, killer of millions in developing countries: strategy for rapid elimination and continuing control, *Eur J Epidemiol*, **7**: 1–22.

Schenzle D, 1984, An age-structured model of pre- and post-vaccination measles transmission, *IMA J Math Appl Med Biol*, **1**: 169–91.

Simonsen O, Kjeldsen K, 1987, Susceptibility to diphtheria in populations vaccinated before and after the elimination of indigenous diphtheria in Denmark, *Acta Pathol Microbiol Immunol Scand*, **95**: 225–31.

Soper HE, 1929, The interpretation of periodicity in disease prevalence, *J R Stat Soc*, **92**: 34–73.

Stroffolini T, Chiaramonte M et al., 1991, A high degree of exposure to hepatitis A infection in urban children in Cameroon, *Microbiologica*, **14**: 199–203.

Tang YW, Wang JX et al., 1991, A serologically confirmed, case-control study of a large outbreak of hepatitis A in China

associated with consumption of clams, *Epidemiol Infect*, **107**: 651–7.

Thacker SB, Millar JD, 1991, Mathematical modeling and attempts to eliminate measles: a tribute to the late Professor George Macdonald, *Am J Epidemiol*, **133**: 517–25.

Topley WWC, 1919a, The Goulstonian Lectures on the spread of bacterial infection, *Lancet*, **2**: 1–5.

Topley WWC, 1919b, The Goulstonian Lectures on the spread of bacterial infection, *Lancet*, **2**: 45–9.

Topley WWC, 1919c, The Goulstonian Lectures on the spread of bacterial infection, *Lancet*, **2**: 91–6.

Topley WWC, 1923, The spread of bacterial infection: some general considerations, *J Hyg Camb*, **21**: 226–36.

Topley WWC, Wilson GS, 1923, The spread of bacterial infection. The problem of herd immunity, *J Hyg Camb*, **21**: 243–9.

Webster LT, 1946, Experimental epidemiology, *Medicine (Baltimore)*, **25**: 77–109.

Williams JR, Anderson RM, 1994, Mathematical models of the transmission dynamics of human immunodeficiency virus in England and Wales: mixing between different risk groups, *J R Stat Soc A*, **157**: 69–87.

World Health Organization, 1995, *Report of the First Meeting of the Global Commission for the Certification of the Eradication of Poliomyelitis*, World Health Organization, Geneva, 1–31.

Yap I, Guan R, 1993, Hepatitis A sero-epidemiology in Singapore: a changing pattern, *Trans R Soc Trop Med Hyg*, **87**: 22–3.

Yorke JA, Hethcote HW, Nold A, 1978, Dynamics and control of the transmission of gonorrhea, *Sex Transm Dis*, **5**: 51–6.

Chapter   1 1

THE EMERGENCE AND RESURGENCE OF BACTERIAL INFECTIOUS DISEASES

R L Berkelman

1 **Demographic changes**	6 **Microbial adaptation and change**
2 **International travel and commerce**	7 **Breakdown of public health infrastructure**
3 **Societal changes**	8 **Infectious origins of chronic diseases**
4 **Changes in technology**	9 **Summary**
5 **Land use patterns and ecological change**	

In recent years, the world has witnessed an emergence and resurgence of infectious diseases. Despite predictions earlier in this century to the contrary, infectious diseases remain the leading cause of death world wide and the potential threats posed by infectious diseases are increasing (Lederberg 1988, Institute of Medicine 1992, Krause 1992). The factors contributing to the emergence of infectious diseases are multiple and complex (Morse 1995). They include demographic changes, changing life-styles and unprecedented population growth; political instability; global travel and commerce; development of new technologies; ecological changes; microbial adaptation and natural variation or mutation of micro-organisms; and deterioration of national and international infrastructures for the control of infectious agents. These factors may contribute to the emergence of a wide array of micro-organisms including bacteria, viruses, parasites and fungi.

As broadly defined by the 1992 US Institute of Medicine report, *Emerging Infections: Microbial Threats to Health in the United States*, emerging infections are those whose incidence in humans has increased within the past 2 decades or whose incidence threatens to increase in the near future. These include the emergence of new agents, the re-emergence of agents that previously had declined in incidence, and the development of antimicrobial resistance. The term also includes the recognition that an established disease has a previously unknown infectious origin.

1   DEMOGRAPHIC CHANGES

Increasing population density and urban poverty in many areas of the world are major factors favouring the emergence and re-emergence of diseases such as tuberculosis, shigellosis and cholera. The population of the world currently exceeds 5 billion and by the year 2050 is expected to grow to between 7.8 and 12.5 billion (Fig. 11.1) (Rousch 1994).

Along with the population surge, the geographical distribution of the world's population is shifting. Since 1950, an increasing percentage of persons are living in Asia and Africa. It is predicted that Africa's percentage of the world's population will continue to increase, from 12% in 1990 to 23% by the year 2050 (Rousch 1994). In turn, the percentage of the world's population living in Europe or North America is

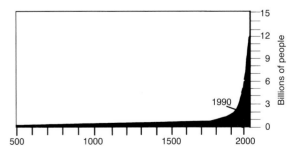

Fig. 11.1   World population through 1990, with projections by United Nations demographers of high and low scenarios. (Abstracted with permission from Rousch W, 1994, Population: the view from Cairo, *Science*, **265**: 1164–7. Copyright 1994 American Association for the Advancement of Science).

declining. There is also a dramatic trend towards urbanization. By the year 2000, the United Nations projects that there will be 21 cities of 10 million population or more, and all but 4 will be in developing countries. Overcrowding and development of slum areas are growing factors in a complex set of interactions that contribute to disease emergence.

2   INTERNATIONAL TRAVEL AND COMMERCE

The dramatic increases in international travel and commerce are also playing a significant role in the emergence of infectious diseases. The current volume of global traffic, together with the speed at which destinations can be reached, is unprecedented. In the early 1990s, more than 500 million international trips on commercial airplane flights were recorded (World Tourism Organization, unpublished data) and carried persons with drug-resistant tuberculosis, cholera and other diseases (Fig. 11.2). Occasionally, the transport vehicles are themselves the sites of dissemination of disease, as with Legionnaires' disease on cruise ships (Centers for Disease Control and Prevention [CDC] 1994c) or food-borne illnesses or tuberculosis on airlines (Driver et al. 1994, Hedberg, MacDonald and Osterholm 1994).

There are many examples of human movement resulting in geographical dispersion of a pathogen; recent advances in molecular epidemiology have been instrumental in documenting the course of a number of pathogens. In the 1970s, a group of closely related strains of serogroup B *Neisseria meningitidis* were first identified in Europe. The strains were identified by multilocus enzyme electrophoresis as members of a distinctive group of closely related clones (the ET-5 complex). The ET-5 complex was recovered in Europe

for the first time in 1974 and the closeness of the clones suggests a relatively recent origin of this group. The circulation of this strain has resulted in epidemic disease, lasting more than a decade in Norway (Caugant et al. 1986). The strains were subsequently found in Cuba and several South American countries (e.g. Brazil, Argentina, Chile) in the 1980s. The appearance of ET-5 in Miami in 1981 was associated with the large influx of Cuban immigrants that occurred in the early 1980s. More recently, highly genetically related *N. meningitidis* serogroup B strains of the ET-5 clones have been isolated in the Pacific Northwest; these strains closely match isolates from Chile (Reeves et al. 1995).

In the early 1990s, an estimated 20 million persons were refugees, a group that may be at higher risk of many infectious diseases (Wilson 1995). Drug-resistant tuberculosis has been common among refugees entering developed countries from developing ones and has contributed to the resurgence of tuberculosis witnessed in some developed countries.

Acute disasters, such as earthquakes or displacement of persons through civil strife, may have an impact on food and water supplies and often require temporary living quarters, which frequently resemble slums. Following civil strife in Rwanda in 1994, an estimated 50 000 Rwandan refugees died within the first month as cholera and *Shigella dysenteriae* type 1 swept through the camps in Zaire (Goma Epidemiology Group 1995).

Global commerce has also been an important factor in transporting pathogens. Importation of turtles, iguanas and other reptiles carrying *Salmonella* (CDC 1995b), the carriage of *Vibrio cholerae* in the ballast water of ships, and shipment of fresh fruits and vegetables contaminated with *Shigella* or enterotoxigenic *Escherichia coli* from one geographical area to another (Hedberg, MacDonald and Osterholm 1994) have resulted in outbreaks of disease geographically distant from the source of the pathogen (Wilson 1995).

Although most fruits and vegetables used to be locally grown and consumed, the increasing trend towards global commerce has led to expanded importation of fresh fruits and vegetables from developing countries into more developed ones, and workers within developed countries today are often low-paid migrant workers (Hedberg, MacDonald and Osterholm 1994). These factors increase the potential for products to be contaminated in the field, during packing, or during distribution to retail markets and have contributed to the changes in the epidemiology of food-borne diseases, which has witnessed an increasingly wider array of pathogens including bacteria, parasites and viruses.

Travel, migration and commerce allow global mixing of microbial species. Disease emergence may occur if circumstances in the new environment are propitious, allowing survival and proliferation of an introduced microbial pathogen.

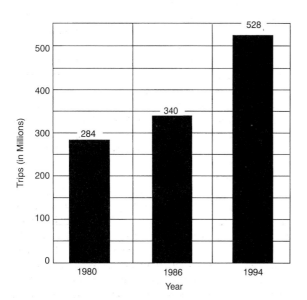

Fig. 11.2   Growth in annual numbers of international airline passengers, 1980–1994, based on data from the World Tourism Organization.

3 SOCIETAL CHANGES

Changes in individual and collective behaviour can affect the risk of exposure to infectious agents. For example, as the association was made between cardio-vascular disease risk and consumption of selected foods such as beef, people changed their dietary habits, including the consumption of different food items. In the USA and many other developed countries, the per capita consumption of whole milk and beef has declined, and consumption of cheese, poultry, and fresh fruits and vegetables has increased (Hedberg, MacDonald and Osterholm 1994). The variety of food has also changed; compared to 50 years ago, a markedly increased number of items are stocked in the average grocery store in developed countries. The place of consumption has also changed; the number of fast-food restaurants has increased, as have such features as salad bars to accompany the changing dietary preferences.

The proliferation of fast-food restaurants with uniform methods of preparation and frequent use of single sources of food has further expanded the opportunities for a large number of persons to be exposed to contaminated food. In an outbreak of haemolytic–uraemic syndrome (HUS) and haemorrhagic colitis in western USA caused by hamburger contaminated with *E. coli* O157:H7 (Bell et al. 1994), scores of restaurants affiliated with a single fast-food chain were implicated.

In some economies, there has been an expanding participation of women in the workforce and a rising proportion of single-parent families, accompanied by growth in the use of child care services. In the USA, 90% of families with preschool children use full- or part-time child day-care services (Thacker et al. 1992). Because children are frequently in close or direct physical contact and have poor personal hygiene, pathogens may be more readily transferred from one child to another in these facilities. Use of child care centres has been associated with an increased risk of transmission of many enteric and respiratory pathogens.

Outbreaks of diarrhoeal illness in child care centres have resulted from many enteric pathogens including *Shigella*, *Salmonella*, *Campylobacter* and *E. coli* O157:H7 (Thacker et al. 1992). Children attending day-care centres are at a 1.6–3.4 times greater risk of a diarrhoeal illness compared with children who receive care at home. The risk is greatest for those not yet toilet trained (Thacker et al. 1992). Secondary spread to household and community contacts may also occur.

The incidence of respiratory illnesses, including those caused by *Streptococcus pneumoniae* and group A *Streptococcus*, is also elevated for children attending child care centres. Accumulating evidence suggests that day-care attendees are at greater risk for acute otitis media, which often follows upper respiratory infections, than children cared for at home. Increased use of child care centres may account partially for the marked increase in visits to physicians for otitis media documented in the USA between 1975 and 1990, from approximately 10 million visits to over 24 million visits per year (Schappert 1992). Outbreaks of tuberculosis in family day-care homes have also been reported.

Changes in sexual behaviour have also affected changes in disease patterns (Wasserheit 1994). The rates of sexually transmitted diseases are closely associated with changes in the number of sexual partners, use of drugs and adequacy of health care services. Recent increases in reported rates of chlamydial infection in the USA are related not only to improvement in surveillance but also to increases in sexual activity of very young women. High rates of oral contraceptive use may foster rapid transmission of chlamydial infection.

4 CHANGES IN TECHNOLOGY

Changes in technology have also resulted in the emergence of newly recognized pathogens. New methods of food production have led to new niches for pathogens. Mass production, with its increased complexity of operations, can greatly magnify the public health significance of microbial contamination. A pathogen present in some of the raw material may contaminate a large batch of final product. For example, there have been dramatic changes in how hamburger meat is produced in the USA. Today, a single hamburger patty typically includes meat from many cattle, and cattle from many different farms (Boyce, Swerdlow and Griffin 1995). Over a quarter million hamburgers contaminated with *E. coli* O157:H7 were recalled in a single outbreak (Bell et al. 1994, Berkelman 1994). Contaminated cheese from one plant distributed to 4 other processors, which subsequently shredded it and thereby contaminated cheeses from other sources, led to a widespread outbreak of salmonellosis (Hedberg et al. 1992).

Medical and technological advances in the medical care of patients have resulted in benefits to many patients, but many of these advances have also been accompanied by an increased risk of infections. The escalation in the use of chemotherapy, radiation and other immunosuppressive therapy has increased the frequency of opportunistic infections. Bacteraemias and fungaemias associated with intravascular devices have increased dramatically. Renal dialysis units expose susceptible patients and personnel to complex equipment that frequently is difficult to decontaminate (Favero, Alter and Bland 1992). Surgery is performed on patients who are already highly susceptible to infections.

Special attention must be given to the risk of transmission of infection through transfusion of blood or blood products. In the USA, there has been an increase in the number of episodes of sepsis caused by *Yersinia enterocolitica*; prolonged storage of the packed red blood cell units have resulted in high bacterial and endotoxin concentrations in the transfused unit (Tipple et al. 1990, CDC 1991). In addition, there have been more reports of infections with staphylococcal species resulting in sepsis or death associated with contaminated platelets; most of these units had pooled units with long storage times (Zaza et al. 1994).

The use of organ transplants has also grown dramatically in many countries in the past decade. Organ transplants pose special risks; the organ may harbour a pathogen, and the transplantation procedure is accompanied by immunosuppressive therapy (Hibberd and Rubin 1992). The number of opportunistic bacterial, fungal and other infections has also risen as a result of the emergence of human immunodeficiency virus (HIV). This increase is expected to continue as the HIV epidemic affects larger numbers of persons.

Legionnaires' disease has emerged in developed countries as a result of technological change. Cooling towers, air conditioners, whirlpool spas, respiratory therapy equipment, and ultrasonic mist machines have all provided new opportunities for the *Legionella* bacterium to become aerosolized and infect humans (CDC 1994b).

Technology related to tampon development and use has been associated with the emergence of menstrual-associated toxic shock syndrome. This illness is due to in vivo production of a unique toxin, toxic shock syndrome toxin-1, by *Staphylococcus aureus*, and the epidemic of toxic shock syndrome witnessed in 1980 was associated with the introduction and marketing of hyperabsorbable tampons. The molecular basis for increased toxin production in the presence of tampon fibres has been debated (Kass 1987).

5 LAND USE PATTERNS AND ECOLOGICAL CHANGE

Ecological changes have contributed to the emergence of tick-borne diseases in many areas of the world. Lyme disease, caused by transmission of *Borrelia burgdorferi* through tick bites, has become the most common vector-borne disease in the USA and reported cases of disease continue to increase. The disease is also well recognized across Europe and northern Asia; cases have also been reported from other continents (Berglund et al. 1995). Sites of intense transmission of *B. burgdorferi* often represent newly reforested areas that had recently been farmed. The suburban encroachment on the newly reforested areas, along with increased recreational use of forested areas, has also increased the exposure of humans to ticks.

Since 1986, 2 tick-borne diseases caused by *Ehrlichia* spp. have been recognized in the USA (Dumler and Bakken 1995). *Ehrlichia chaffeensis* causes human monocytic ehrlichiosis, a syndrome characterized by fever, headache and laboratory findings such as leucopenia and thrombocytopenia. A species closely related to *Ehrlichia equi* causes a similar syndrome known as human granulocytic ehrlichiosis. Persons affected in the USA have spent time in tick-infested areas where *Ixodes scapularis* is common. Infected *I. scapularis* have been identified by polymerase chain reaction assays.

Alterations in the aquatic environment may result in changes in the occurrence of water-borne diseases. The seasonality of cholera has been related to coastal algae blooms (Epstein et al. 1994). Other changes in

human ecology, such as urbanization and the development of periurban slums, may also contribute to an increased risk of diseases such as cholera (Levine and Levine 1994).

6 MICROBIAL ADAPTATION AND CHANGE

New pathogens may emerge as a result of a mutation's causing enhanced virulence. Such a mutation may explain the emergence of Brazilian purpuric fever in 1984, caused by *Haemophilus aegyptius*; it was the first time this agent had been shown to cause invasive disease (CDC 1985, Brazilian Purpuric Fever Study Group 1987). Since its recognition in Brazil, this virulent pathogen has been found in Australia; other parts of the world may be at risk for epidemics.

In 1993, the clonal spread of a novel non-O1 serotype of *V. cholerae* was documented (Ramamurthy et al. 1993); *V. cholerae* O139 was first detected in southern Asia and quickly replaced *V. cholerae* O1 strains in many affected areas. Previous natural infection or receipt of cholera vaccine was found to afford little or no protective benefit. The strains hybridized with DNA probes specific for the cholera toxin gene, but did not hybridize with the DNA probe specific for the heat-stable enterotoxin of *V. cholerae* non-O1.

The development of resistance to antimicrobial agents is also a powerful example of bacteria's capacity to adapt. Almost all major bacterial pathogens acquire antibiotic-resistance genes (Tomasz 1994) and the problem has been amplified by the increased use of antibiotics world wide.

The introduction of penicillin in the 1940s was soon followed by the detection of resistant bacteria. Bacterial resistance has grown with the addition of large numbers of antibiotics with distinct mechanisms of action. These antibiotics have increasingly had a wider antibacterial spectrum. Antibiotics have been introduced not only for therapeutic use in persons but also in large scale in animal feed. Endtz et al. (1991) demonstrated the rise in prevalence of *Campylobacter* strains that were resistant to ciprofloxacin in both poultry products and in human stools in the Netherlands. Extensive use of fluoroquinolones in the poultry industry between 1982 and 1989 is likely to have resulted in the resistance observed.

Once genes for resistance have been acquired, the progeny of these bacteria with their resistance genes tend to spread with great rapidity within the species. Production of β-lactamase by staphylococci was rare before the introduction of penicillin; by 1960, *S. aureus* strains carrying the β-lactamase gene spread world wide (Shlaes, Binczewski and Rice 1993). More than 90% of all isolates of *S. aureus* now carry the β-lactamase gene, in both the USA and Europe, and methicillin resistance has increased rapidly in the 1980s. Strains with and without genes for resistance demonstrate similar virulence in terms of toxin production. Methicillin resistance is mediated most frequently by the production of a novel penicillin-binding protein.

The incidence of infections with vancomycin-resistant enterococci has also increased; more than 10% of isolates tested by CDC from patients in intensive care units are resistant to vancomycin (Hospital Infection Control Practices Advisory Committee 1995). At least 3 structurally different genes and gene products are likely to be involved in this resistance (Shlaes, Binczewski and Rice 1993). Vancomycin resistance, emerging amidst the increasing incidence of high-level resistance to penicillins and aminoglycosides, has limited treatment options. Vancomycin use is a risk factor for colonization and infection with vancomycin-resistant enterococci and may also increase the possibility of the emergence of vancomycin-resistant *S. aureus*. Noble, Virani and Cree (1992) demonstrated conjugative transfer of high-level vancomycin resistance from *Enterococcus faecalis* to *S. aureus* in the laboratory and concern exists that resistance may be transferred to wild-type *S. aureus*. Spread of resistant strains within hospitals may be limited by aggressive infection control measures and prudent vancomycin use.

Drug-resistant *S. pneumoniae* were first documented in Australia and South Africa in the 1960s and 1970s; reports of similar isolation were made with increasing frequency from other parts of the world in the 1980s. By 1992, more than 16% of pneumococcal isolates submitted to CDC were resistant to at least one drug class, paralleling documentation of increased use of broader spectrum antimicrobial drugs (Breiman et al. 1994, McCaig and Hughes 1995). The rapid emergence of drug-resistant strains is complicating the management of pneumococcal infections and demonstrates the need for more judicious use of antimicrobial agents (Reichler et al. 1992, Hofman et al. 1995).

Penicillinase-producing *Neisseria gonorrhoeae* was first recognized in 1976. By the 1990s, 32% of *N. gonorrhoeae* isolates were resistant to penicillin or tetracycline, and resistance to fluoroquinolones was recognized (CDC 1993). *N. gonorrhoeae* also demonstrates the increasingly diverse array of mechanisms of resistance, including both plasmid- and chromosomally mediated resistance to the penicillins and tetracyclines.

Antibacterial resistance is also a problem for the developing world. In central and southern Africa, isolates of *S. dysenteriae* 1 have been demonstrated to be resistant to all readily accessible oral antibiotics, including ampicillin, chloramphenicol, nalidixic acid, tetracycline and trimethoprim–sulphamethoxazole (Ries et al. 1994, Tuttle et al. 1995). The need to monitor, regularly and frequently, the prevailing antimicrobial resistance patterns in different geographical areas has been repeatedly demonstrated. Preventive measures may be more successful than therapy for control of many epidemics.

7 BREAKDOWN OF PUBLIC HEALTH INFRASTRUCTURE

Complacency has also resulted in the re-emergence of pathogens previously controlled. Basic tenets of public health, such as close monitoring of disease in a population accompanied by a rapid response for diseases such as shigellosis and salmonellosis, and control programmes for diseases such as tuberculosis and diphtheria, have been neglected in many areas of the world as public health attention towards the control of all but a few selected conditions declined in the 1970s and 1980s (Berkelman et al. 1994). In addition, the emergence of new pathogens such as *E. coli* O157:H7 has been inadequately addressed.

Cases of tuberculosis in the USA increased 18% from 1985 through 1991; yet, by 1992, most public health laboratories had not incorporated the more rapid radiometric methods for routine culture or drug susceptibility testing of mycobacteria. The erosion of public health services together with the mistaken perception of tuberculosis as a disease of declining public health significance resulted in decreased funding for many laboratories in the USA and resulted in the delay in implementation of newer, more rapid diagnostic technologies for tuberculosis (Bloom and Murray 1992, Dowdle 1993, Huebner, Good and Tokars 1993) as well as a decline in resources for control programmes.

In 1994, reports of widespread transmission of pneumonic plague within India resulted in estimated economic losses to India of over $1 billion dollars (Campbell and Hughes 1995). Intense investigation revealed that most reported cases of plague were incorrectly diagnosed and that no transmission of pneumonic plague was identified in any major city but Surat. Effective surveillance coupled with laboratory expertise in plague might have averted some of the economic loss.

The epidemic levels of cholera reached in South America in the early 1990s, after almost a century of absence of the disease from the continent, were attributed, in part, to breakdowns in public health measures (Institute of Medicine 1992). Contaminated municipal water supplies contributed to the spread of the epidemic after the pathogen was introduced along the coastal waters of Peru (Blake 1993). As both the population and the percentage of the population in poverty grow in South America, the potential for spread of diarrhoeal illnesses increases.

In the early 1990s, Russia and many of the newly independent states experienced a dramatic resurgence of diphtheria (CDC 1995a) (Fig. 11.3). Inadequate immunization of the population, crowding and low socioeconomic conditions, and high mobility of the infected individuals may have contributed to this outbreak, which has resulted in thousands of deaths.

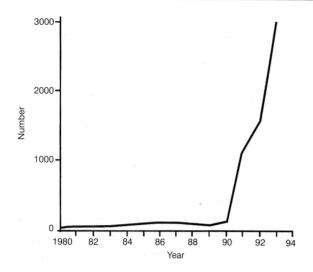

Fig. 11.3 Diphtheria cases in the Ukraine, 1980–1994, based on World Health Organization estimates.

8 INFECTIOUS ORIGINS OF CHRONIC DISEASES

A number of diseases or conditions, previously considered to be non-infectious, have recently been recognized to have an infectious aetiology. *Helicobacter pylori* was first isolated from humans in 1982 and is now known to play a central role in the development of diffuse gastritis and duodenal ulceration (Marshall 1989). More than 90% of patients with duodenal ulceration are infected with *H. pylori* and treatment with antimicrobial therapy heals duodenal ulcers; additionally, lower recurrence rates are associated with eradication of *H. pylori*. Presence of *H. pylori*, as determined by serological studies, is also associated with a 3–6-fold higher risk of gastric cancer (Fuchs and Mayer 1995); gastric cancer is the second most common cause of cancer-related deaths in the world. Evidence has been accumulating that *Chlamydia pneumoniae* may have an aetiological role in the development of atherosclerosis (Saikku et al. 1992).

Guillain–Barré syndrome, a leading cause of acute paralysis, has been associated with infection with *Campylobacter jejuni*; in a study conducted in England and Wales, 26% of 96 patients with Guillain–Barré syndrome had evidence of infection with *C. jejuni* (Rees et al. 1995). Peripheral nerves may share epitopes with *C. jejuni*. Other syndromes that are ill-defined and often considered to be immune mediated may soon also be discovered to have infectious micro-organisms playing a central role in aetiology, possibly through molecular mimicry (Bolton 1995).

In addition, techniques to identify organisms that do not rely on cultivation have been developed. To identify the bacillus causing Whipple's disease, the bacterial 16S ribosomal RNA sequence from infected tissue was amplified and its phylogenetic relations have been described (Relman et al. 1992).

9 SUMMARY

Following the 1992 publication of the US Institute of Medicine report on emerging infections, CDC released a prevention strategy to address emerging infectious disease threats for the USA (CDC 1994a). In 1994, the World Health Organization defined goals to guide implementation of a global effort on emerging infectious diseases (World Health Organization 1994); in 1995, the World Health Assembly passed a resolution calling for attention to the problem of new and re-emerging infections. An international partnership is needed to develop an effective global disease and response network (National Science and Technology Council 1995). The need to increase laboratory expertise in basic diagnostics, to develop inexpensive and easy diagnostic tests for field use, and to have available the diagnostic reagents, drugs, and vaccines needed has been emphasized. As the speed with which the world changes continues to accelerate, the challenges confronting us by the re-emergence of old pathogens or the recognition of new ones will likewise be heightened.

REFERENCES

Bell BP, Goldoft M et al., 1994, A multistate outbreak of *Escherichia coli* O157:H7 associated bloody diarrhea and hemolytic uremic syndrome from hamburgers: the Washington experience, *JAMA*, **272:** 1349–53.

Berglund J, Eitrem R et al., 1995, An epidemiologic study of Lyme disease in southern Sweden, *N Engl J Med*, **333:** 1319–24.

Berkelman RL, 1994, Emerging infectious diseases in the United States, 1993, *J Infect Dis*, **170:** 272–7.

Berkelman RL, Bryan RT et al., 1994, Infectious disease surveillance: a crumbling foundation, *Science*, **264:** 368–70.

Blake PA, 1993, Epidemiology of cholera in the Americas, *Gastroenterol Clin North Am*, **22:** 639–60.

Bloom BR, Murray CJL, 1992, Tuberculosis: commentary on a reemergent killer, *Science*, **257:** 1055–64.

Bolton CF, 1995, The changing concepts of Guillain–Barré syndrome (editorial), *N Engl J Med*, **333:** 1415–17.

Boyce TG, Swerdlow DL, Griffin PM, 1995, *Escherichia coli* O157:H7 and the hemolytic–uremic syndrome, *N Engl J Med*, **333:** 364–8.

Brazilian Purpuric Fever Study Group, 1987, *Haemophilus aegyptius* bacteraemia in Brazilian purpuric fever, *Lancet*, **2:** 761–3.

Breiman RF, Butler JC et al., 1994, Emergence of drug-resistant pneumococcal infections in the United States, *JAMA*, **271:** 1831–5.

Campbell GL, Hughes JM, 1995, Plague in India: a new warning from an old nemesis, *Ann Intern Med*, **122:** 151–3.

Caugant DA, Frøhom LO et al., 1986, Intercontinental spread of a genetically distinctive complex of clones of *Neisseria meningitidis* causing epidemic disease, *Proc Natl Acad Sci USA*, **83:** 4927–31.

Centers for Disease Control, 1985, Preliminary report: epidemic fatal purpuric fever among children – Brazil, *Morbid Mortal Weekly Rep*, **34:** 217–19.

Centers for Disease Control, 1991, Update: *Yersinia enterocolitica* bacteremia and endotoxin shock associated with red blood cell transfusions – United States, 1991, *Morbid Mortal Weekly Rep*, **40:** 176–8.

Centers for Disease Control and Prevention, 1993, Sentinel surveillance for antimicrobial resistance in *Neisseria gonorrhoeae* – United States, 1988–1991, *Morbid Mortal Weekly Rep*, **42 (SS-3):** 29–39.

Centers for Disease Control and Prevention, 1994a, Addressing emerging infectious disease threats: a prevention strategy for the United States, US Department of Health and Human Services, Public Health Service, Atlanta, Georgia, 1–46.

Centers for Disease Control and Prevention, 1994b, Legionnaires' disease associated with cooling towers – Massachusetts, Michigan, and Rhode Island, 1993, *Morbid Mortal Weekly Rep*, **43:** 491–3 and 99.

Centers for Disease Control and Prevention, 1994c, Update: outbreak of Legionnaires' disease associated with a cruise ship, 1994, *Morbid Mortal Weekly Rep*, **43:** 574–5.

Centers for Disease Control and Prevention, 1995a, Diphtheria epidemic – New Independent States of the former Soviet Union, 1990–1994, *Morbid Mortal Weekly Rep*, **44:** 177–80.

Centers for Disease Control and Prevention, 1995b, Reptile-associated salmonellosis – selected states, 1994–1995, *Morbid Mortal Weekly Rep*, **44:** 347–50.

Dowdle WR, 1993, The future of the public health laboratory, *Annu Rev Public Health*, **14:** 649–64.

Driver CR, Valway SE et al., 1994, Transmission of *Mycobacterium tuberculosis* associated with air travel, *JAMA*, **272:** 1031–5.

Dumler JS, Bakken JS, 1995, Ehrlichial diseases of humans: emerging tick-borne infections, *Clin Infect Dis*, **20:** 1102–10.

Endtz HP, Ruijs GJ et al., 1991, Quinolone resistance in campylobacter isolated from man and poultry following the introduction of fluoroquinolones in veterinary medicine, *J Antimicrob Chemother*, **27:** 199–208.

Epstein PR, Ford TE et al., 1994, Marine ecosystem health: implications for public health, *Disease in Evolution*, 1st edn, eds Wilson ME, Levins R, Spielman A, The New York Academy of Sciences, New York, 13–23.

Favero MS, Alter MJ, Bland LA, 1992, Dialysis-associated infections and their control, *Hospital Infections*, 3rd edn, eds Bennett JV, Brachman PS, Little, Brown and Company, Boston/Toronto/London, 375–403.

Fuchs CS, Mayer RJ, 1995, Gastric carcinoma, *N Engl J Med*, **333:** 32–41.

Goma Epidemiology Group, 1995, Public health impact of Rwandan refugee crisis: what happened in Goma, Zaire, in July, 1994? *Lancet*, **345:** 339–44.

Hedberg CW, Korlath JA et al., 1992, A multistate outbreak of *Salmonella javianna* and *Salmonella oranienburg* infections due to consumption of contaminated cheese, *JAMA*, **268:** 3203–7.

Hedberg CW, MacDonald KL, Osterholm MT, 1994, Changing epidemiology of food-borne disease: a Minnesota perspective, *Clin Infect Dis*, **18:** 671–82.

Hibberd PL, Rubin RH, 1992, Infection in transplant recipients, *Hospital Infections*, 3rd edn, eds Bennett JV, Brachman JS, Little, Brown and Company, Boston/Toronto/London, 899–921.

Hofmann J, Cetron MS et al., 1995, The prevalence of drug-resistant *Streptococcus pneumoniae* in Atlanta, *N Engl J Med*, **333:** 481–6.

Hospital Infection Control Practices Advisory Committee (HICPAC), 1995, Recommendations for preventing the spread of vancomycin resistance, *Infect Control Hosp Epidemiol*, **16:** 105–13.

Huebner RE, Good RC, Tokars JI, 1993, Current practices in mycobacteriology: results of a survey of state public health laboratories, *J Clin Microbiol*, **31:** 771–5.

Institute of Medicine, 1992, *Emerging Infections: Microbial Threats to Health in the United States*, National Academy Press, Washington, DC, 1–294.

Kass EH, 1987, On the pathogenesis of toxic shock syndrome, *Rev Infect Dis*, **9, Suppl. 5:** S482–9.

Krause RM, 1992, The origin of plagues: old and new, *Science*, **257:** 1073–8.

Lederberg J, 1988, Medical science, infectious disease, and the unity of humankind, *JAMA*, **260:** 684–5.

Levine MM, Levine OS, 1994, Changes in human ecology and behavior in relation to the emergence of diarrheal diseases, including cholera, *Proc Natl Acad Sci USA*, **91:** 2390–4.

McCaig LF, Hughes JM, 1995, Trends in antimicrobial drug prescribing among office-based physicians in the United States, *JAMA*, **273:** 214–19.

Marshall BJ, 1989, History of the discovery of *C. pylori*, Campylobacter pylori *in Gastritis and Peptic Ulcer Disease*, 1st edn, ed. Blaser MJ, Igaku Shoin Medical Publishers, New York, 7–23.

Morse SS, 1995, Factors in the emergence of infectious diseases, *Emerg Infect Dis*, **1:** 7–15.

National Science and Technology Council (NSTC), 1995, *Report of the NSTC Committee on International Science, Engineering, and Technology (CISET) Working Group on Emerging and Re-emerging Infectious Diseases*, Executive Office of the President of the United States, Washington, DC, 1–55.

Noble WC, Virani Z, Cree RGA, 1992, Co-transfer of vancomycin and other resistance genes from *Enterococcus faecalis* NCTC 12201 to *Staphylococcus aureus*, *FEMS Microbiol Lett*, **93:** 195–8.

Ramamurthy T, Garg S et al., 1993, Emergence of novel strain of *Vibrio cholerae* with epidemic potential in southern and eastern India (corresp.), *Lancet*, **341:** 703–4.

Rees JH, Soudain SE et al., 1995, *Campylobacter jejuni* infection and Guillian–Barré syndrome, *N Engl J Med*, **333:** 1374–417.

Reeves MW, Perkins BA et al., 1995, Epidemic-associated *Neisseria meningitidis* detected by multilocus enzyme electrophoresis, *Emerg Infect Dis*, **1:** 53–4.

Reichler MR, Allphin AA et al., 1992, The spread of multiply resistant *Streptococcus pneumoniae* at a day care center in Ohio, *J Infect Dis*, **166:** 1346–53.

Relman DA, Schmidt TM et al., 1992, Identification of the uncultured bacillus of Whipple's disease, *N Engl J Med*, **327:** 293–301.

Ries AA, Wells JG et al., 1994, Epidemic *Shigella dysenteriae* type 1 in Burundi: panresistance and implications for prevention, *J Infect Dis*, **169:** 1035–41.

Rousch W, 1994, Population: the view from Cairo, *Science*, **265:** 1164–7.

Saikku P, Leinonen M et al., 1992, Chronic *Chlamydia pneumoniae* infection as a risk factor for coronary heart disease in the Helsinki heart study, *Ann Intern Med*, **116:** 273–8.

Schappert SM, 1992, *Office Visits for Otitis Media: United States, 1975–90*, Advance data from vital and health statistics, no. 214, National Center for Health Statistics, Hyattsville, MD.

Shlaes DM, Binczewski B, Rice LB, 1993, Emerging antimicrobial resistance and the immunocompromised host, *Clin Infect Dis*, **17, Suppl. 2:** S527–36.

Thacker SB, Addiss DG et al., 1992, Infectious diseases and injuries in child day care: opportunities for healthier children, *JAMA*, **268:** 1720–6.

Tipple MA, Bland LA et al., 1990, Sepsis associated with transfusion of red cells contaminated with *Yersinia enterocolitica*, *Transfusion*, **30:** 207–13.

Tomasz A, 1994, Multiple-antibiotic-resistant pathogenic bacteria: a report on the Rockefeller University Workshop, *N Engl J Med*, **330:** 1247–51.

Tuttle J, Ries AA et al., 1995, Antimicrobial-resistant epidemic *Shigella dysenteriae* type 1 in Zambia: modes of transmission, *J Infect Dis*, **171:** 371–5.

Wasserheit JN, 1994, Effect of changes in human ecology and behavior on patterns of sexually transmitted diseases, including human immunodeficiency virus infection, *Proc Natl Acad Sci USA*, **91:** 2430–5.

Wilson ME, 1995, Travel and the emergence of infectious diseases, *Emerg Infect Dis*, **1:** 39–46.

World Health Organization, 1994, Emerging infectious diseases, *Wkly Epidemiol Rec*, **69:** 234–6.

Zaza S, Tokars JI et al., 1994, Bacterial contamination of platelets at a university hospital: increased identification due to intensified surveillance, *Infect Control Hosp Epidemiol*, **15:** 82–7.

C h a p t e r   1 2

THE LABORATORY DIAGNOSIS OF BACTERIAL DISEASES

J M Miller

1 The role of the laboratory	4 Test methods
2 The testing process	5 Antimicrobial sensitivity tests
3 The management of specimens	6 Quality assurance

1 THE ROLE OF THE LABORATORY

The microbiology section of the laboratory plays a critical role in establishing the diagnosis of infectious disease. However, the technical approach is often very different from that of every other section of the laboratory. In diagnostic microbiology, interpretative judgement by skilled microbiologists remains the primary means of arriving at a result that is accurate and clinically relevant. In order to interpret results properly, the microbiologist must have a good knowledge of host–parasite relationships and know how to relate results to the diagnostic needs of the clinician. Indeed, many microbiologists believe that skilled personnel are more important than advanced technology in making accurate identifications and in affording microbiology laboratories their reputation for diagnosing infectious disease. Health care providers should insist on having competent specialists to provide the most cost-effective, clinically relevant microbiology results available for the care of their patients (D'Amato and Isenberg 1991, D'Amato 1995, Baron, Francis and Peddecord 1996, Editorial 1996a).

The microbiology laboratory provides analytical information that supports the diagnosis of the patient's illness and subsequent therapeutic intervention, and analytical and demographic data to support the infection control needs of the health care facility or community (McGowan and Metchock 1996). Public health laboratories use the same type of data to facilitate interventions within populations rather than on individual patients. This chapter is devoted to an overview of the appropriate use of the microbiology laboratory for the diagnosis of bacterial diseases. Further details of identification tests on bacteria and of bacterial immunoserology are given in Volume 2, Chapters 4 and 18, respectively, and in the chapters devoted to specific micro-organisms.

2 THE TESTING PROCESS

Historically, the microbiology laboratory served only as the site for analysis of specimens. It can, however, make a broader contribution to a successful outcome for the patient by also contributing to specimen selection, collection, transport and storage, and to the post-analytical steps of reporting and interpretation.

Early in the identification process, specimens are evaluated by a variety of methods including gross examination and one or more stains to determine if they represent a true disease process or whether they contain large numbers of commensal flora that might compromise accurate interpretation of results. On the basis of the information provided on the requisition, the laboratory selects the most appropriate approach for confirming a suspected diagnosis. This may include direct antigen testing by latex agglutination or enzyme immunoassay (EIA), which may be manual or automated; phenotypic analysis of bacterial isolates using a variety of biochemical or enzymatic methods, which also may be manual or automated; or newer molecular genetic techniques such as DNA probes, the polymerase chain reaction (PCR), ligase chain reaction (LCR), and related methods. For bacterial isolates and some fungi, the laboratory must use standard procedures, such as those published in the USA by the National Committee for Clinical Laboratory Standards (NCCLS 1997a, 1997b) or its international counterparts, for susceptibility testing of appropriate isolates to assist in evaluating or initiating a therapeutic regimen.

3 THE MANAGEMENT OF SPECIMENS

Several authors discuss the management of specimens, e.g. Miller and Wentworth (1985), Baron, Peterson and Finegold (1994), Miller and Holmes (1995), Miller (1996). Their selection, collection and transport to the laboratory are all of critical importance.

3.1 The requisition

Requisitions (request forms) for microbiology analysis should contain as much information as possible to assist the microbiologist in interpreting the results of culture. A patient's travel history, epidemiological associations, significant past medical history, and current therapy are usually helpful in interpretation and should be included on the requisition. A clear indication should be given of any special risk of infection, e.g. with hepatitis B or human immunodeficiency virus (HIV) associated with handling the specimen.

Because of the complexity and importance of specimen management, it is recommended that laboratories, physicians' offices, and nurses' stations in hospitals have a manual on hand to assist in this process (Miller 1996).

3.2 Transport to the laboratory

Each specimen should be transported in a package appropriate for the type of organism suspected. Transport media for bacteria will not be adequate if a viral aetiology is suspected (see Volume 1, Chapter 44). *Chlamydia* require special attention to specimen collection and transport, as do anaerobic bacteria. Because many of these agents are highly fastidious, improper packaging and transport may cause them to die before arrival in the laboratory or may so reduce their numbers as to compromise the ability of the laboratory to recover them. Clearly, if bacteria are allowed to multiply or die before the specimen arrives in the laboratory, it is no longer representative of the disease process.

Once in the laboratory, the suitability of the specimen must be evaluated by the microbiologist. Biosafety is of prime importance in handling specimens, particularly blood or body fluids. One must consider all transport containers contaminated to some degree and it is recommended that all specimens be handled with gloved hands and that the containers be manipulated and media inoculated within the confines of a biosafety cabinet if one is available.

3.3 Commensal flora

One common problem with specimen analysis by culture is the presence of commensal or normal flora that may mask the true aetiological agent or make its isola-

tion more difficult. Of particular difficulty are specimens from sites listed in Table 12.1. Some body sites have more resident flora than others. Often, a gram stain can help to determine the suitability of the specimen for processing since the presence of epithelial cells usually signals the presence of contaminating flora. If for any reason the results might be inaccurate, incomplete, or misleading, the laboratory must note this on the report and suggest that they be interpreted with caution.

4 TEST METHODS

There are 4 primary issues to consider in determining whether a test method, product, or system should be selected for use in the laboratory (Sewell and Schifman 1995). First and foremost is the value of the test for patient care. Is there a clinical need for it, or is value gained by using the test? The second is an evaluation of the performance of the method and comparison of its performance to those of other techniques. The evaluation protocol should include, where appropriate, measures of precision, linearity, accuracy, sensitivity, specificity, predictive values, and reference ranges for the local population. Sensitivity represents the frequency of a positive test in patients with the disease (true positives among all positive patients) and specificity represents the frequency of a negative test in individuals without the disease (true negatives among all negative patients). These 2 values are independent of the prevalence of the disease in the population. The positive predictive value of a test is the probability that a positive test indicates that the patient has the disease (true positives among all positive tests) and the negative predictive value is the probability that a negative test rules out disease (true negatives among all negative tests) (Table 12.2). These values are affected by the prevalence of disease in the population tested. Third, an evaluation of the actual cost of providing the test should be undertaken. This is influenced by the cost of reagents, instruments, technologists' time, the amount or extent of quality control required with each test, the number of tests per run, and the requirements to confirm a positive result. Fourth, it is important to determine the degree of expertise required of microbiologists to perform the test with maximum accuracy. Special collection and transport devices may involve additional costs. Indirect costs may also be included if required by local accounting policy.

4.1 Phenotypic identification

The phenotypic identification of bacteria in the laboratory is accomplished through several basic steps. However, simply isolating one or more organisms from a specimen may not have clinical significance, making interpretation of results a complex issue, particularly if both potential pathogens and commensal flora are found together in the same specimen. If the specimen submitted for culture has been compro-

Table 12.1 Sites of infection and common sources of contamination[a]

Site of infection	Source of contamination
Middle ear	External ear canal
Lower respiratory tract	Oropharynx
Nasal sinus	Nasopharynx
Endometrium	Vagina
Superficial wounds/subcutaneous infections	Skin and mucous membranes
Fistulae	Gastrointestinal tract
Bladder	Urethra and external genitalia

[a]Adapted from Bartlett (1985).

Table 12.2 Predictive value of positive and negative test results

Sensitivity	$= \dfrac{\text{Number who had the infection and gave a positive result}}{\text{Total number infected}} \times 100\%$
Specificity	$= \dfrac{\text{Number who did not have the infection and gave a negative result}}{\text{Total number not infected}} \times 100\%$
Predictive value of a positive result	$= \dfrac{\text{Number who had the infection and gave a positive result}}{\text{Total number who gave a positive result}} \times 100\%$
Predictive value of a negative result	$= \dfrac{\text{Number who did not have the infection and gave a negative result}}{\text{Total number who gave a negative result}} \times 100\%$

mised in any way, as described earlier, the results may be misleading and foster misdiagnosis and inappropriate therapy.

From the specimen source, the microbiologist determines which growth media are selected and under what conditions they will be incubated. For instance, many enriched media and those containing blood are incubated at 35–37°C in an atmosphere of 5% carbon dioxide in anticipation of detecting fastidious isolates. Non-enriched media and media designed for isolating members of the Enterobacteriaceae should not, however, be placed into a carbon dioxide environment.

The selection of the appropriate media for culture is critical to successful isolation and characterization of bacterial pathogens. Whether commercially purchased or prepared 'in-house', the microbiologist must be assured that the media will support the growth of the pathogens most likely to be found in the submitted specimen. Examples of specific media selections are available (Baron, Peterson and Finegold 1994). For instance, urine specimens should be cultured on media that will support the growth of both gram-positive and gram-negative organisms. The gram-positive organisms may include some fastidious species and the medium for them should therefore be enriched with blood or an equivalent product. Gram-negative bacteria in urine probably originate from intestinal sources and the media chosen should inhibit the growth of gram-positive organisms and facilitate the growth of gram-negative bacteria. Therefore, 2 media would probably be selected for urine culture. When, as in the case of faeces, the normal flora is so profuse as to make recognition of a pathogen unlikely even on selective medium, primary culture is preceded by enrichment culture.

Surgical or deep wound specimens may contain both aerobic and anaerobic bacteria and media must be selected to accommodate the growth of virtually all groups of bacteria. Since strictly anaerobic bacteria may not survive even brief periods of exposure to oxygen, the laboratory should provide both an oxygen-free transport system for specimen collection and media specifically designed to support the growth of fastidious anaerobic bacteria. Several media are likely to be necessary including blood agar; an agar specific for gram-negative rods; a chocolate agar for more fastidious isolates; 2 anaerobic agar plates, one designed for fastidious anaerobes and another selective for gram-negative species of anaerobes; and perhaps a broth medium to enrich or enhance the growth of anaerobes.

Because of the generation times of most bacteria, inoculated plates must be held at their incubation temperature of 35–37°C for a full 18–24 h before examination. For adequate growth, fastidious organisms and anaerobes may require incubation for 48 h. For this reason, media inoculated with specimens from most body sites should be held for 48–72 h before reporting a negative result. Whereas *Escherichia coli* may require less than 18 h to develop readable colonies, organisms such as *Neisseria gonorrhoeae* and many anaerobic species may need 48 h or more before adequate growth has been achieved. *Mycobacterium tuberculosis* requires 4–6 weeks under ideal conditions before adequate growth on solid media is obtained.

The microbiologist observes culture plates for characteristic colonial morphology, odours, pigments, or medium interactions to gain clues to the identity of the organism or to the next step in its identification. The next steps will probably be a gram stain, a specific stain or microscopic observation (Table 12.3), selection of isolated colonies for transfer to fresh media to obtain a pure culture, a spot test as described below, or inoculation of a substrate utilization system for identification of the organism. In many cases, an assessment of the colonial morphology, evaluation of the specimen type and information about the patient may lead to a final report indicating that no further testing is needed.

4.2   Blood cultures

The diagnosis of bacteraemia by blood culture is an important aspect of the work of a medical microbiology laboratory and is considered in detail in Chapter 16, section 2.

4.3   Rapid tests

The use of spot tests for bacterial identification provides a rapid means of reporting that is surprisingly accurate. In some cases, microbiologists can supply presumptive identification of an organism within 30 min of discovering the isolate.

Generally, results from this type of test are available immediately since little or no incubation is required. Such rapid tests include spot indole with Kovac's reagent (Arnold and Weaver 1948) or with para-dimethylaminocinnamaldehyde (Miller and Wright 1982), oxidase test (Clark et al. 1984), rapid urease test (Qadri et al. 1984), various disc tests including β-lactamase disks and L-pyrrolidonyl-β-naphthylamide (PYR), coagulase test (with commercial latex formulations) for staphylococci, and the catalase test. These spot tests, along with the gram stain results, can assist in the rapid identification of many aetiological agents. For example, a flat, dry lactose-fermenting (pink) colony on MacConkey agar that is also spot indole-positive and oxidase-negative can be reported presumptively as *E. coli*. These organisms may comprise over half the isolates from positive urine cultures. Organisms that swarm on 5% sheep blood agar, exhibit a characteristic odour, and are oxidase-negative can be presumptively identified as *Proteus* spp. With further testing by spot indole, the positive isolates may be presumptively reported as *Proteus vulgaris* and the negative ones as *Proteus mirabilis*. *Proteus penneri* is also indole-negative but is less likely to be encountered. With the rapid results available from spot tests, along with the known antimicrobial susceptibility profile of the local hospital isolates, empirical therapy can be initiated or adjusted before routine susceptibility test results are available. The organisms

for which spot testing can be used, however, are limited to those few whose characteristics are so unique as to set them apart from all others. The majority of species isolated from clinical specimens cannot be identified by spot tests. Most laboratories must select one of the commercially available substrate utilization systems (see section 4.4), and its utility must be determined at the local level by a rational, scientific approach (Miller 1991).

4.4   Substrate utilization systems

Rapid biochemical identification by automated identification systems can often be accomplished within 2–6 h of incubation, but this process cannot begin until at least 18–24 h after the specimen arrives in the laboratory. The first 18–24 h is necessary for initial processing. Isolates are selected from this first incubation to be used as inocula for instrument- or system-based identification and susceptibility testing. The utility of the available automated systems has been evaluated (Stager and Davis 1992) and the role of non-automated commercially available substrate utilization systems summarized (Miller and Holmes 1995). The accuracy of all these systems varies, depending largely on the organism under test. Most microbiologists feel confident reporting a genus and species identification if the system indicates that the likelihood of accuracy (usually listed as a percentage) is high enough. For example, for members of the Enterobacteriaceae family, one would expect and confidently report results based on a likelihood of 95% or greater. For the more fastidious, slower growing gram-negative non-Enterobacteriaceae and for anaerobic bacteria, the microbiologist might accept a likelihood of 85% or greater. There are no universal guidelines or standards of accuracy for accepting and reporting identification results. However, an alternative test method must be available should the likelihood percentage fall below the values set by the individual laboratory. Indeed, one must not blindly accept results from any identification system if the observations made by the microbiologist suggest that an alternative identification may be the correct one. Phenotypic characters and susceptibility profiles must confirm the reported results. If both the standard and alternative test methods provide unacceptable responses, the organism should be submitted to an outside reference laboratory for identification.

Most of the available commercial substrate utilization systems are based on one of the following mechanisms: pH-based reaction (most 18–24 h systems), enzyme profiles (many 4 h systems), carbon source utilization that measures metabolic activity, volatile or non-volatile acid detection, or visual detection of growth.

Some commercial systems do not require growth of the organisms in order to arrive at a genus and species identification. Systems that detect the presence of preformed enzymes are available and accurate after an incubation period of only 4 h. Enzyme detection methods are available for most groups of bacteria,

Table 12.3 Microscopic examination methods[a]

Microscopic method	Application	Principle	Time required (min)	Advantage	Disadvantage
Wet mount	Stool, vaginal discharge, urine sediment	Detects motility, parasite morphology, fungal elements	1	Rapid and specific	Limited contrast and resolution. Experienced microscopist required
Methylene blue	Stool for WBCs	WBCs in stool stain blue; their presence suggests invasive process	1	Rapid recognition of WBCs	Stool must be examined immediately or cells distort or disintegrate
Gram stain	Differential bacterial stain; also used to evaluate adequacy of specimen for culture	Gram-positive bacteria and yeast stain blue; gram-negative bacteria stain red	3–4	Rapid; assists in organism classification; helps correlate stain to culture results	Skill in stain procedure required; background material may confuse; older cultures may stain unpredictably
Acid-fast stains	Detects *Mycobacterium* spp., *Nocardia* spp. and some parasites	Mycolic acids in cell wall resist decolorization by acid alcohol, causing retention of red dye	15 (depends on method used)	Acid-fast character specific for mycobacteria, *Nocardia*, *Cryptosporidium*, *Sarcocystis* and *Isospora belli*. Good diagnostic test	Low numbers of organisms makes reading difficult. Stained tissues may mask presence of organisms
Auramine–rhodamine	Detection of mycobacteria and other acid-fast organisms	Non-specific fluorochromes bind to mycolic acids. Cells fluoresce orange-yellow with UV light	30	Allows rapid screening at low magnification. May be more sensitive than acid-fast stain. Can do AFB stain on same slide	Single organism or low number may be hard to confirm
Acridine orange	Detects bacteria in blood, buffy coats; detects fungi and yeasts	Fluorochrome stains nucleic acids. Bacterial DNAs fluoresce orange; mammalian DNA fluoresces green	3	Rapid and sensitive for screening body fluids. Thickness of smear not a factor. Can gram stain same slide	Cellular specimens with abundance of DNA may be difficult to interpret
Antibody-conjugated stain	Detection of specific organisms in clinical material and confirmation from culture	Monoclonal antibodies labelled with fluorescent dye detects antigens in stained smears	60	Useful for *Bordetella*, *Legionella*, *Pneumocystis* and for viruses	Adequate clinical material must be submitted

[a]Adapted from Chapin (1995).

including both gram-positive and gram-negative organisms.

4.5   Conventional biochemical tests

Reference laboratories to which unidentified or difficult-to-identify organisms are sent may employ a conventional biochemical test approach to identification using up to 50 or more substrates in test tubes. This historical approach is the basis on which the biochemical definitions of organisms are generated and described in classic reference texts such as *Bergey's Manual of Systematic Bacteriology* (Krieg 1984). Until the newer molecular identification methods, such as 16S rRNA technology or specific molecular probes, can be shown to be at least equivalent in accuracy to those originally described, the conventional approach will still be necessary to resolve problems in identification. A final report can usually be produced after an incubation period of 7 days in the conventional biochemical test array. Generation of reports on fastidious isolates and anaerobic species may take longer. By definition, a genus and species identification from a standard conventional set of biochemical tests would represent a 100% accurate response. This would be the response (the 'gold standard') to which alternative test methods would be compared.

4.6   Immunoassays

Some alternative phenotypic methods are available for diagnostic testing of specimens. There are several immunoassay formats including enzyme immunoassays (EIA) and radioimmunoassays (RIA). The advantages of EIA versus RIA mainly include ease or convenience of use, better stability of EIA reagents, and the environmental and personal concerns about the radiological safety of RIA reagents. Both approaches offer tests that are highly sensitive and specific for a wide variety of microbial antigens and antibodies. Most solid-phase EIAs used for diagnostic purposes employ either a plastic microtitre plate or beads with antigen or antibody adsorbed onto the solid phase. In some formats, an antibody is attached to the solid phase to capture the antigen used in the final assay for the antibody to a specific aetiological agent. In most clinical applications, chromogenic substrates are used as a final test indicator, although fluorogenic, radioactive and luminescent ones are also available.

EIAs using enzyme-labelled antigen are also available for the detection of IgG and IgM antibodies to many, if not most, of the common infectious diseases. These are especially useful when the laboratory is unable to culture for a specific pathogen. Sensitivities may vary from 60 to 95%, however, and the literature should be consulted to determine the capability of a test and the experience of other users dealing with similar patients.

4.7   Immunofluorescence tests

Fluorescent antibody (FA) techniques for both antigen and antibody detection have been available for many years (see also Volume 2, Chapter 18). Their value depends on the quality of both the conjugate and the microscope used for reading the results. Antigens are usually detected by a direct FA procedure in which a specimen such as sputum, nasal washings, cells from lesions, or exudates are placed onto a glass slide, processed, and incubated with a fluorescein-labelled antibody (direct test) or with specific antibody followed by a fluorescein-labelled antiglobulin (indirect test). Detection of antibodies by FA is available for a number of bacterial, viral and parasitic infections.

Monoclonal antibodies are now increasingly used for immunofluorescence tests because they are highly specific and of constant quality. In order to increase sensitivity while retaining specificity, individual monoclonal antibodies can be combined. The disadvantages of immunofluorescence include the cost of the equipment, the need for skilled observers and the subjective nature of the end point. Since dead organisms can be detected by immunofluorescence, the method may be of value when patients have been treated with antimicrobial drugs before the specimen was taken.

4.8   Chromatography

Chromatography methods including gas-liquid chromatography (GLC), thin layer chromatography (TLC), and high performance liquid chromatography (HPLC) can be useful in classifying clinically significant organisms (Onderdonk and Sasser 1995). As their names imply, gas and liquid chromatography respectively use a gas and a liquid as the mobile phase. A method using gas as a mobile phase and a liquid as the stationary phase is termed GLC, whereas TLC uses a liquid mobile phase and a solid stationary phase. HPLC is a form of liquid-solid chromatography that forces the liquid phase over the solid phase under pressure.

GLC has long been a standard to assist in the definitive diagnosis of anaerobic bacterial infection, whereas TLC is less frequently used in clinical applications. Many GLC systems (chromatographs) use a packed-column method at temperatures ranging from 135 to 150°C, a thermal conductivity detector, and helium as a carrier gas (mobile phase). Flame ionization detectors are also available that require different gases for operation. The high temperature in the injector port volatilizes the fatty acids that are forced along the column at different rates depending upon their size. Since anaerobic bacteria cannot oxidize nutrients to carbon dioxide and water, they produce intermediate products of short-chain fatty acids, organic acids and alcohols that are relatively distinctive for specific groups of anaerobic bacteria. These end products of metabolism, when used in conjunction with other laboratory tests, are particularly helpful for difficult-to-identify anaerobic gram-positive bacilli. For instance, *Propionibacterium* spp. usually produce large amounts of propionic acid detectable by GLC analysis, whereas *Actinomyces* spp. produce succinic, acetic, and, for some species, lactic acid. With the advent of newer methods of identification such as commercial systems for detecting preformed enzymes, many diagnostic laboratories no longer use GLC routinely to complete the identification of anaerobes since the chromatograph instruments add significantly to test costs.

HPLC does not depend upon heated columns. This process uses a solvent as a mobile phase travelling under pressure over a solid phase housed within a metal or glass column. Detection of analytes is done by a variety of detectors. As with GLC, libraries of data generated from the HPLC profiles of specific organisms can be stored in a computer and subsequent analyses compared rapidly to the existing library to arrive at an identification.

4.9 Diagnostic kits

Kits are easy to use, provide rapid results, and utilize computer-assisted or numerical profile-assisted interpretation. The use of kits in the microbiology laboratory is not limited to biochemical identification. Packaged systems are available for direct antigen detection (e.g. tests for group A streptococcus from throat swabs or for common bacterial causes of meningitis from cerebrospinal fluid specimens), for toxin detection (e.g tests for toxin A, B or both, of *Clostridium difficile* from faecal specimens), for detection of *Giardia*-specific antigens from faecal specimens, and many other micro-organisms or their products. Indeed, some molecular diagnostic methods are now available in 'kit' form. DNA probes for *M. tuberculosis* and *Mycobacterium avium-intracellulare* and DNA probes for *N. gonorrhoeae* and *Chlamydia* are available commercially for use by clinical laboratories.

Although such kits may offer convenience and the luxury of testing for agents that may otherwise require lengthy incubation periods, the clinician and the microbiologist must also recognize their limitations. Establishing any laboratory test without first assessing its effectiveness and accuracy is unwise (Easmon 1990). Tests must be introduced after having been compared either to an existing procedure (keeping in mind that the new procedure may be more accurate than the existing one) or to a reference standard. At a minimum, a review of the literature would be in order to assist in establishing the sensitivity, specificity and predictive values of the results for the patient population for which the test or kit is to be used. All test results must be taken in the context of clinical data and evaluated carefully in order to facilitate an accurate diagnosis or to serve as a guide for antimicrobial therapy.

4.10 Tests for toxins

Toxins of micro-organisms, particularly bacteria, are responsible for a number of conditions ranging from less serious to life-threatening illness. Endotoxins are produced primarily by gram-negative bacteria and are a lipopolysaccharide component of the bacterial cell wall. They produce fever and can lead to circulatory collapse and some tissue damage in patients. Exotoxins of both gram-positive and gram-negative bacteria are produced in the cytoplasm of the cell and then released. Each exotoxin usually produces a characteristic effect on the patient.

The detection of a bacterial toxin may have advantages over identifying the organism responsible for an infection. This is the case in the diagnosis of botulism in which the toxin may be detectable by intraperitoneal injection into mice of the serum of untreated patients. The test is rapid and specific, because the signs of botulism in the mouse are characteristic and neutralized by polyvalent antiserum against the toxin. In the investigation of antibiotic-associated diarrhoea (see Chapter 35), cytotoxin (toxin B) can be demonstrated in extracts of faeces by its cytopathic effect on cultured cells, which are specifically neutralized by antiserum. This has the advantage over isolating *C. difficile* from the faeces in that transient carriage can be distinguished from colonization with resulting disease.

In the investigation of outbreaks of food poisoning, the detection of toxins such as staphylococcal enterotoxins (see Volume 2, Chapter 27) and botulinum toxin (see Chapter 37) in food may be useful for establishing which of several foods was responsible for illness. In the case of *Clostridium botulinum* food poisoning it may also provide guidance for serotherapy.

Detection of toxin production may be difficult for most laboratories unless a kit system is available such as that used for the detection of toxin produced by *C. difficile*, *Staphylococcus aureus*, or *E. coli* O157:H7. In many cases, the isolate must be submitted to an appropriate reference laboratory that has the capability of performing tests such as the toxin neutralization test. These neutralization procedures may be done in vitro or in vivo using laboratory animals, as is done with *Clostridium perfringens* toxins. A precipitin test, the Elek plate, is used to detect the toxin of *Corynebacterium diphtheriae* but this test should be done in a reference laboratory since the incidence of diphtheria is low in most areas and the test poses numerous technical problems because of the variability of reagents.

The *Limulus* assay is a highly sensitive procedure that can detect as little as 10–20 pg of endotoxin per millilitre. This test uses a lysate of blood cells from the horseshoe crab, *Limulus polyphemus*, which form a gel in the presence of lipopolysaccharide; it may be used to detect contamination of intravenous solutions prior to administration.

4.11 Molecular diagnostics

Futurists in the field of infectious disease diagnosis may speculate with some confidence that conventional culture methods will become outmoded within our lifetime. Indeed, current technology has been introduced that will allow the genetic detection and identification of some microbes without the need for culture (Wolcott 1992, van Belkum 1994, Bottger 1996). For the present, the costs of genetic identification tests and the expertise required to perform some of them exceed those of routine culture methods. Conversely, the time required for a final report may be significantly reduced by molecular techniques, and this may be of benefit to the patient. The molecular methods also have a clear role in infection control (Miller 1993, van Belkum 1994). The benefits notwithstanding, the sensitivity and specificity of these molecular methods are not 100%, as might be expected. Therefore, the replacement of conventional microbiology methods with molecular diagnostics will probably not be readily accepted by all clinicians and microbiologists until the issues of cost, special expertise and sensitivity and specificity are resolved.

DNA probes have clearly had an impact on the laboratory identification of some pathogens. Probe technology is currently available both for the direct detection of micro-organisms in clinical specimens and for confirmation of the identification of isolates taken from culture media. Table 12.4 provides a partial list of the ever-increasing number of DNA probes available for use (Podzorski and Persing 1995). Probes are short, single-stranded sequences of nucleotides designed to bind to specific regions of a target sequence of nucleotides on the chromosome of the organism to be detected. The greater the degree of homology between the nucleotides of the probe and the target, the more stable the bond. If the probe is bound tightly to its target, it will not be washed away in processing and its presence will be detected by some type of tag or label. Probe sizes may range from 10 to 10 000 base pairs but average from 14 to 40 base pairs (as a comparison, the chromosome is about 4.2 $\times 10^6$ base pairs in size). Probes have been designed to detect genera, species, and even strains within a species. The targets are often found within cellular DNA but can also be found in RNA.

Another molecular approach is to amplify the amount of target DNA to a detectable level. A partial list of nucleic acid amplification techniques available to recognize microbial pathogens includes:

1 polymerase chain reaction – developed in 1983; current applications include modifications such as nested PCR, multiplex PCR, and PCR amplification of RNA
2 self-sustained sequence replication (3SR) – developed in 1989
3 strand displacement amplification (SDA) – developed in 1991
4 Q-β replicase – developed in 1988
5 ligase chain reaction (LCR) – developed in 1989.

Other methods are emerging as are modifications of existing ones. PCR is based on the unique properties of DNA that allow its denaturation into single-stranded DNA (ssDNA) at 94°C for 15–60 s, hybridization of primers at 52°C for 15–120 s, and polymerase strand synthesis at 72°C for 15–180 s. This thermal cycle is repeated for 25–35 cycles, yielding up to 1 000 000 copies of the target DNA which can be detected by electrophoretic means. This process is automated and requires thermal cyclers and strict aseptic conditions. Any DNA, wanted or unwanted, can be amplified. In fact, the PCR process is so sensitive to external DNA contamination, that procedures are best accomplished in separate, dedicated rooms of the laboratory to minimize the chance of any microbe from the environment or from the microbiologist finding its way into the reaction vessels of the procedure. Nested PCR uses 2 sets of amplification primers, one set within the other. Multiplex PCR is accomplished when 2 or more target DNA sequences are amplified simultaneously. PCR amplification for RNA is usually reserved for the detection of RNA viruses.

3SR is used to amplify an RNA target. Because 3SR is isothermal, it is somewhat simpler to accomplish than those processes that require thermal cycling and its reaction kinetics are very rapid. Three enymes are used in the process: a reverse transcriptase that forms ssDNA from the RNA target, RNAase H that degrades the initial RNA of the hybrids, leaving DNA for the reaction, and a DNA-dependent RNA polymerase that uses the DNA as a template to replace the RNA used to continue the cycle.

SDA is also an isothermal amplification method but is based on the displacement of one probe when DNA polymerase is used to extend a second probe. The displaced probe then becomes the target for another set of probes and double-stranded DNA re-enters the cycle. In this process, the restriction site in the DNA is nicked, not cleaved, so that polymerization displaces the first probe. Q-β replicase, though not being pursued commercially, is an amplification method that uses the replicase from the Q-β bacteriophage. This is an RNA-directed RNA polymerase that assembles RNA from an RNA template. The amplification of RNA serves as a reporter system, and is not amplified simply to increase the amount of the target sequence. Colorimetric detection is simple because of the amount of RNA produced.

In the ligase chain reaction, the entire target sequence must be known and this target sequence is amplified. The critical part of this reaction is the joining of a thermostable enzyme with 2 oligonucleotides that are directly adjacent to each other. The reaction is isothermal but cyclic where denaturation, annealing and ligation occur. Ligated pairs then become the templates for the next cycle. As few as 10 nucleic acid targets can be detected with this method. An excellent and well illustrated review of these and other molecular genetic processes is available (Wolcott 1992).

Microchip technology presents a prospect of particular interest that could transform diagnostic bacteriology (Editorial 1996b). Oligonucleotides can be fixed to silica chips by light-directed synthetic methods (photolithography) to yield microchips potentially bearing very large numbers of oligonucleotides. The chips are then hybridized with the material under test; if the target nucleic acid is labelled with a fluorescent

Table 12.4 Micro-organisms identified by DNA probe technology[a]

Probes for direct detection of organisms	Probes for culture confirmation
Bacteria	Bacteria
Chlamydia trachomatis	*Campylobacter* spp.
Streptococcus pyogenes	*Enterococcus* spp.
Legionella pneumophila	Group A and B *Streptococcus*
Gardnerella vaginalis	*Haemophilus influenzae*
Mycobacterium tuberculosis	*Neisseria gonorrhoeae*
	Streptococcus pneumoniae
	Staphylococcus aureus
	Listeria monocytogenes
	Mycobacterium (6 species)
Protozoa	Protozoa
Trichomonas vaginalis	Not routinely cultured
Fungi	Fungi
Candida spp.	*Blastomyces dermatitidis*
	Coccidioides immitis
	Cryptococcus neoformans
	Histoplasma capsulatum
Viruses	Viruses
Human papillomavirus	Human papillomavirus

[a]This list is likely to change constantly. Many more probes for other organisms are presented in the literature but may not be available for commercial or widespread use.
Adapted from Podzorski and Persing (1995).

grouping, the signal can be detected by scanning confocal microscopy. The method is very fast (c. 30 min).

Whether a laboratory elects to employ conventional, automated, or molecular approaches to diagnosis, or a combination of methods, is a local decision. There are no recommended guidelines for selecting any one procedure. However, the primary consideration for any test is its benefit to the patient. One or more selected tests will probably identify the pathogen and provide useful data about its susceptibility to antimicrobial agents, for example, whether treatment could be changed from a relatively toxic broad spectrum antibiotic to a more specifically directed agent that might be less expensive and could allow the patient to receive therapy on an out-patient basis.

Tests and protocols can be carefully evaluated and selected that are cost-effective and achieve a result that is both accurate and clinically useful (Thomas 1994, Boyce et al. 1995, Cavagnolo 1995, Cover and Blaser 1995, Morris et al. 1995, 1996, Perkins, Mirrett and Reller 1995, Bird et al. 1996, Jarvis, Cookson and Robles 1996).

5 ANTIMICROBIAL SUSCEPTIBILITY TESTS

Although it is not within the scope of this chapter to detail the many protocols available for testing susceptibility to antimicrobial agents, this activity is clearly an important function of the microbiology laboratory; a detailed description of test methods can be found in Volume 2, Chapter 9, section 7.1. Procedures and interpretative criteria are also available from the National Committee for Clinical Laboratory Standards

(NCCLS 1997a, 1997b) in the USA and from counterparts throughout the world. Because the results of susceptibility tests can have a major impact on the success of treatment, it is imperative that the laboratory follows precisely the protocols outlined for each organism. For example, standardized methods that are less complex than those required for accurate testing of *N. gonorrhoeae*, *Haemophilus influenzae* and *Streptococcus pneumoniae* can be used for rapidly growing Enterobacteriaceae and the staphylococci. The simplest and least costly method is the disc diffusion test. Although zones of inhibition must be carefully measured and interpreted as 'susceptible', 'intermediate', or 'resistant', many studies have provided minimum inhibitory concentration (MIC) values equivalent to specific zone sizes. Most rapidly growing and non-fastidious organisms can be tested with standardized disc diffusion methods. Specifically, if the NCCLS disc diffusion procedure, or the related procedure published by the World Health Organization (Report 1995), is used one must perform strict quality control, use Mueller–Hinton agar, carefully adjust the inoculum, incubate at a specified temperature, and measure zone sizes after growth for 18–24 h. If these steps are not followed, the test results cannot be interpreted reliably.

Most organisms, including fastidious ones, can be tested with an agar or broth dilution MIC method. MIC tests can be manipulated to some degree to accommodate special nutritional or atmospheric requirements of an isolate whereas the disc diffusion procedure cannot. After the incubation period, a quantitative value, the MIC, can be given to each antibiotic–microbe combination tested. In many cases, the MIC value is more valuable in directing therapy than a simple sensitive (S), intermediate (I), resistant (R), result since the physician can determine the potential success or failure of therapy based on the MIC value and the amount of drug achievable in the infected body site. A newer method of susceptibility testing using a ceramic strip impregnated with an antibiotic gradient has also proved very useful for a broad range of eugonic and fastidious bacteria. This method, which is similar to disc diffusion in format, allows one to read an MIC value directly off the impregnated strip where the zone of inhibition intersects the test strip. This is currently the most expensive of the methods described if several drugs are tested. It is not unusual to find laboratories selectively incorporating all 3 susceptibility methods into the daily routine (Woods and Washington 1995).

A matter of great concern is the increasing prevalence of pathogens highly resistant to individual antimicrobial agents. It is clear that such resistance is related to the use of antimicrobial agents in community and hospital practice, and probably also in animal husbandry. Hospitals should, therefore, have a clear policy on the use of these agents, particularly those to be kept in reserve for treating infections resistant to first-line antimicrobial agents (see Chapter 13, section 8 and Volume 2, Chapter 9, sections 7 and 8).

6 QUALITY ASSURANCE

Inappropriate, incorrect or even excessive information can be misleading and facilitate an incorrect diagnosis and inappropriate therapy. A quality assurance programme encompasses the policies and procedures that actively promote good practice. Quality assurance includes the administrative and professional policies that provide the basis for an efficient service and addresses the issues of personnel, equipment, instrumentation, laboratory safety and technical procedures. Quality control involves methods that validate and document the accuracy of the technical procedures that are a part of the quality assurance programme. Microbiologists must rely on the accurate performance of the media, reagents and stains used in the laboratory. Although the analytical component is only a part of the total laboratory testing process, its role in patient care is clear and its accuracy must be ensured by continual monitoring.

The corner stone of quality control is careful record keeping of virtually every test and decision made on each specimen. Details of quality assurance and quality control in the microbiology laboratory are available in several publications (Miller and Wentworth 1985, Murray et al. 1995). These documents describe the necessity for both internal (procedural validations) and external (proficiency testing) quality control programmes.

REFERENCES

Arnold WM Jr, Weaver RH, 1948, Quick microtechniques for the identification of cultures, *J Lab Clin Med*, **33:** 1334–7.

Baron EJ, Francis D, Peddecord KM, 1996, Infectious disease physicians rate microbiology services and practices, *J Clin Microbiol*, **34:** 496–500.

Baron EJ, Peterson LR, Finegold SM, 1994, *Bailey and Scott's Diagnostic Microbiology*, 9th edn, Mosby, St Louis, MO, 53–64.

Bartlett RC, 1985, Quality control in clinical microbiology, *Manual of Clinical Microbiology*, 4th edn, eds Lennette EH, Balows A et al., American Society for Microbiology, Washington, DC.

van Belkum A, 1994, DNA fingerprinting of medically important microorganisms by use of PCR, *Clin Microbiol Rev*, **7:** 174–84.

Bird BR, Denniston MM et al., 1996, Changing practices in mycobacteriology: a follow-up survey of state and territorial public health laboratories, *J Clin Microbiol*, **34:** 554–9.

Bottger EC, 1996, Approaches for identification of microorganisms, *ASM News*, **62:** 248–50.

Boyce TG, Pemberton AG et al., 1995, Screening for *Escherichia coli* O157:H7 – a nationwide survey of clinical laboratories, *J Clin Microbiol*, **33:** 3275–7.

Cavagnolo R, 1995, Evaluation of incubation times for urine cultures, *J Clin Microbiol*, **33:** 1954–6.

Chapin K, 1995, Clinical microscopy, *Manual of Clinical Microbiology*, 6th edn, eds Murray PR, Baron EJ et al., American Society for Microbiology, Washington, DC, 33–51.

Clark WA, Hollis DG et al., 1984, *Identification of unusual pathogenic gram-negative aerobic and facultatively anaerobic bacteria*, US department of Health and Human Services, PHS, Washington, DC, 20.

Cover TL, Blaser MJ, 1995, *Helicobacter pylori*: a bacterial cause of gastritis, peptic ulcer disease and gastric cancer, *ASM News*, **61:** 21–5.

D'Amato RF, 1995, Can clinical microbiologists be fiscally responsible and not compromise patient care?, *Clin Microbiol Updates*, **2:** 1–3.

D'Amato RF, Isenberg HD, 1991, Practical and fiscally responsible application of clinical microbiology to patient care, *ASM News*, **57:** 22–6.

Easmon CSF, 1990, Laboratory diagnosis of bacterial disease, *Topley & Wilson's Principles of Bacteriology, Virology and Immunity*, vol. 3, 8th edn, eds Parker MT, Collier LH, B C Decker Inc., Philadelphia, PA, 1–9.

Editorial, 1996a, ABMM diplomate-directed labs score higher quality rating, *ASM News*, **62:** 174–5.

Editorial, 1996b, To affinity...and beyond, *Nature Genet*, **14:** 367–70.

Jarvis WJ, Cookson ST, Robles MB, 1996, Prevention of nosocomial bloodstream infections: a national and international priority, *Infect Contr Hosp Epidemiol*, **17:** 272–5.

Krieg NR (ed.), 1984, *Bergey's Manual of Systematic Bacteriology*, vol. 1, Williams & Wilkins, Baltimore, MD.

McGowan JE, Metchock BG, 1996, Basic microbiologic support for hospital epidemiology, *Infect Control Hosp Epidemiol*, **17:** 298–302.

Miller JM, 1991, Evaluating biochemical identification systems, *J Clin Microbiol*, **29:** 1559–61.

Miller JM, 1993, Molecular technology for hospital epidemiology, *Diagn Microbiol Infect Dis*, **16:** 153–7.

Miller JM, 1996, *A Guide to Specimen Management in Clinical Microbiology*, American Society for Microbiology, Washington, DC.

Miller JM, Holmes HT, 1995, Specimen collection, transport and storage, *Manual of Clinical Microbiology*, 6th edn, eds Murray PR, Baron EJ et al., American Society for Microbiology, Washington, DC, 19–32.

Miller JM, Wentworth BB, 1985, *Methods for Quality Control in*

Diagnostic Microbiology, American Public Health Association, Washington, DC.

Miller JM, Wright JW, 1982, Spot indole test: evaluation of four reagents, *J Clin Microbiol*, **15:** 589–92.

Morris AJ, Wilson SJ et al., 1995, Clinical impact of bacteria and fungi recovered only from broth cultures, *J Clin Microbiol*, **33:** 161–5.

Morris AJ, Smith LK et al., 1996, Cost and time savings following introduction of rejection criteria for clinical specimens, *J Clin Microbiol*, **34:** 355–7.

Murray PR, Baron EJ et al. (eds), 1995, *Manual of Clinical Microbiology*, 6th edn, American society for Microbiology, Washington, DC.

NCCLS, 1997a, *M7–A4. Methods for Dilution Antimicrobial Susceptibility Tests for Bacteria that Grow Aerobically*, 4th edn, National Committee for Clinical Laboratory Standards, Wayne, PA.

NCCLS, 1997b, *M2–A6. Performance Standards for Antimicrobial Disk Susceptibility Tests*, 6th edn, National Committee for Clinical Laboratory Standards, Wayne, PA.

Onderdonk AB, Sasser M, 1995, Gas-liquid and high performance liquid chromatographic methods for the identification of microorganisms, *Manual of Clinical Microbiology*, 6th edn, eds Murray PR, Baron EJ et al., American Society for Microbiology, Washington, DC, 123–9.

Perkins MD, Mirrett S, Reller LB, 1995, Rapid bacterial antigen detection is not clinically useful, *J Clin Microbiol*, **33:** 1486–91.

Podzorski RP, Persing DH, 1995, Molecular detection and identification of microorganisms, *Manual of Clinical Microbiology*, 6th edn, eds Murray PR, Baron EJ et al., American Society for Microbiology, Washington, DC, 131.

Qadri SMH, Skubairi S et al., 1984, Simple spot test for rapid detection of urease activity, *J Clin Microbiol*, **20:** 1198–9.

Report, 1995, *The Use of Essential Drugs*, 6th report. WHO Tech Rep Ser, World Health Organization, Geneva, 77–89.

Sewell DL, Schifman RB, 1995, Quality assurance: quality improvement, quality control and test validation, *Manual of Clinical Microbiology*, 6th edn, eds Murray PR, Baron EJ et al., American Society for Microbiology, Washington, DC, 55–66.

Stager CE, Davis JR, 1992, Automated systems for identification of microorganisms, *Clin Microbiol Rev*, **5:** 303–27.

Thomas JG, 1994, Survey results of routine CSF antigen detection: nothing to be proud of, *Clin Microbiol Newslett*, **16:** 187–90.

Wolcott MJ, 1992, Advances in nucleic acid-based detection methods, *Clin Microbiol Rev*, **5:** 370–86.

Woods GL, Washington JA, 1995, Antibacterial susceptibility tests: dilution and disk diffusion methods, *Manual of Clinical Microbiology*, 6th edn, eds Murray PR, Baron EJ et al., American Society for Microbiology, Washington, DC, 1336.

HOSPITAL-ACQUIRED INFECTION

David C E Speller and Hilary Humphreys

1 INTRODUCTION

Of the infections dealt with in this volume very many may be acquired in hospital, but these hospital infections have special features. Hospitals bring together uniquely vulnerable hosts and subject them to particular risks of infection from animate and inanimate sources. Apart from being the cause of morbidity and mortality, infection limits the effectiveness and adds greatly to the cost of medical treatment.

The term hospital-acquired infection (syn. nosocomial infection) is applied to any infection causing illness that was not present or in its incubation period when the subject entered hospital or received treatment in an out-patient or accident and emergency department. It includes not only incidents in which a single micro-organism spreads from person to person ('cross-infection') or from a common source in the hospital but also single and apparently unconnected infections. **Sporadic** and **endemic** hospital-acquired infections may be less striking than **epidemic** ('outbreaks') but they predominate numerically and their control or reduction present the greater challenge.

Some hospital-acquired infections do not differ from infections with the same micro-organism in the general population, but many are profoundly affected by the patient's underlying illnesses or by medical or surgical treatments to which they are subjected while in hospital. The source of the infecting organism may be **exogenous**, from another patient or a member of the hospital staff, or from the inanimate environment in the hospital; or it may be **endogenous**, from the patient's own flora, which at the time of infection may include organisms brought into hospital at admission and others acquired subsequently. In either case, the infecting organisms may spontaneously invade the tissues of the patient or be introduced into them by surgical operation, instrumental manipulation or nursing procedure. The concentration of patients with particular illnesses and undergoing similar treatments in specialist hospital units often creates unique niches for hospital pathogens. Hospital-acquired infection may also affect discharged in-patients, out-patients and staff, and an episode of hospital infection may be initiated by the admission of an infected patient from the general population. Hospital infection may spill over into the community, necessitating investigation and control in both populations. In all considerations of hospital-acquired infection, the **source**, the **mode of infection** and **host susceptibility** must all be kept in mind.

2 OCCURRENCE, CONSEQUENCES AND COST OF HOSPITAL-ACQUIRED INFECTION

Information about the extent of hospital infection in general may be obtained from **incidence** or **prevalence** studies (Chapter 9). The relationship between the results of these 2 types of survey is complex (Freeman and Hutchison 1980). Most investigations are limited to particular sites of infection, such as surgical wounds, or to individual hospital services, such as intensive care. However, in the USA it has been estimated that more than 2 million, and perhaps as many as 4 million, patients are infected in hospital each year. Study of a random sample of patients from 6449 acute care hospitals gave an incidence of 5.7 infections per 100 admissions (Haley et al. 1985a, 1985b). Ongoing nationwide surveillance of nosocomial infection in the USA is reported in terms of specific infection sites (National Nosocomial Infections Surveillance (NNIS) System 1995).

In Great Britain and Ireland, a cross-sectional prevalence survey (Emmerson et al. 1996) suggested an overall nosocomial infection prevalence rate of 9.0%, with significantly higher prevalence in teaching (11.2%) than in non-teaching (8.4%) hospitals. A previous survey (Meers et al. 1981) found a similar overall prevalence (9.2%) but Emmerson et al. (1996) point out differences in the study methods and medical practice in the 2 periods. For example, earlier patient discharge in the more recent survey implied that many surgical wound infections would be detected after discharge from hospital and therefore not included (Bailey et al. 1992, Weigelt, Dryer and Haley 1992, Byrne et al. 1994, Emmerson 1995). Nationwide prevalence surveys in Spain (EPINE 1992, 1995) have shown an overall nosocomial infection rate of 8.5% in 1990, falling to 7.2% in 1994. A similar investigation in Norway found a prevalence of 6.3%, which was a fall in comparison with previous years (Aavitsland, Stormark and Lystad 1992). A prevalence survey in Hong Kong (Kam and Mak 1993) found 8.6% of patients to have a hospital-acquired infection. Caution is needed when comparing these and similar figures, as there may be differences in the spectrum of patients, in medical practice and in definitions of infection. Indeed, there were important differences between the individual hospitals in all these investigations. A similar body site distribution of infections was seen in the studies, with 4 sites predominating: urinary tract, respiratory tract, surgical wound and skin (Fig. 13.1). Improvements in prevalence figures are often due mainly to control of urinary tract infection.

A prevalence of hospital infection between 6% and 9% has frequently been observed in recent years and it has been questioned whether the 'irreducible minimum' of hospital-acquired infections has been reached (Ayliffe 1986). This stability may indicate some success, in that an increase in the infection rate might have been expected because modern methods of treatment create more opportunities for infection and highly susceptible patients are surviving in greater numbers. Nevertheless, an examination of many aspects of current hospital practice suggests that the incidence of infection could be reduced.

Most types of hospital infection cause appreciable morbidity and may lead to residual disability and even death, although a significant worsening of outcome may be difficult to demonstrate statistically except in very large samples of patients (Freeman, Rosner and McGowan 1979). Some impression of the impact of hospital infection can be gained from the large prevalence and incidence studies, as can an estimate of the increased cost of care. Martone et al. (1992) suggested that, in the USA, a hospital-acquired infection results in an average of 4.0 extra days of stay. The average extra charges (1992) were $2100, giving an estimated annual national cost of more than $4.5 billion. It was estimated that more than 19 000 deaths were due directly to hospital infection and that this was contributory to a further 58 000 deaths. Similar figures are not available in Europe. In a 1988 case-control study it was established that hospital infection in surgical patients added an average of 8.2 days to hospital stay with added costs of £1041 (Coello et al. 1993). Antibiotic resistance in the infecting organism adds to costs and reduces the effectiveness of treatment (Holmberg, Solomon and Blake 1987). The control of hospital-acquired infection has been characterized as one of the most cost-effective of health care interventions (Haley et al. 1985b, Chaudhuri 1993, Wenzel 1995).

3 HISTORY OF KNOWLEDGE OF HOSPITAL-ACQUIRED INFECTION

A chapter devoted to hospital-acquired infection appeared for the first time in the seventh edition of this book, reflecting the growth of interest in hospital epidemiology and infection control, but the subject is not new. The need to isolate patients with obviously infectious diseases has been recognized since ancient times and the spread of infection that might ensue from the introduction of such patients into hospitals has been known for centuries. However, segregation of fever hospitals from general hospitals dates only from the early nineteenth century and the usefulness of this measure was not demonstrated statistically until

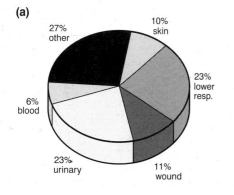

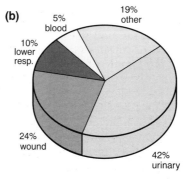

Fig. 13.1 Occurrence of hospital-acquired infection by site: (a) UK, prevalence survey (Emmerson et al. 1996); (b) USA, incidence survey (Haley et al. 1985b).

much later. Hospital-acquired infection and the consequent mortality probably reached their peak in the nineteenth century. The following brief account includes only the salient references, but the more recent papers referred to (e.g. Cruickshank 1944, Williams 1956) supply more detail.

3.1   The nineteenth century

Urban overpopulation and hospital overcrowding made hospitals places of dread for the poor; there was uncontrolled puerperal sepsis, and surgical sepsis caused death in most cases of compound fracture admitted to hospital. Cross-infection in children's hospitals was associated with mortality rates of 25–40%. The now well known work of Semmelweiss (1861) on puerperal sepsis was largely disregarded at the time. He observed its association with medical staff and students who attended patients and also performed autopsies. Semmelweiss deduced that the disease was spread by 'morbid matter' on their hands derived from cadavers or other affected patients. A dramatic reduction in infection rates was achieved by the introduction of hand-washing with chlorinated lime.

At the same time, and to greater immediate effect, Florence Nightingale, after her experience of hospital sepsis at Scutari and her reform of the army medical services, turned her attention to British hospitals. In a much quoted remark in her book *Notes on Hospitals* (Nightingale 1863) she states:

'It may seem a strange principle to enunciate as the very first requirement in a Hospital that it should do the sick no harm ... the actual mortality in hospitals, especially in those of large crowded cities, is very much higher than any calculation founded on the mortality of the same class of diseases among patients treated *out of* hospital ....'

Florence Nightingale established important principles of nursing, hospital design and hygiene, while remaining sceptical of the germ theory of disease. Further evidence was provided by the survey of the sequelae of amputation by Simpson (1869) which established that sepsis, gangrene and pyaemia were very much more common in large urban hospitals than in rural practice.

At about this time Lister (1867a, 1867b) introduced his 'antiseptic surgery', with extensive use of carbolic acid to pack wounds, especially of compound fractures, sterilize instruments and sutures, decontaminate his hands, and as an air spray. He observed a considerable improvement in the results of treatment of compound fractures and of surgical operations. Lister came to appreciate that the air spray did not add greatly to the effectiveness of the other measures, and that what he was introducing was a barrier between the patients' tissues and infection. 'Antiseptic surgery' was later replaced by von Bergman's 'asepsis' (Schimmelbusch 1894) and by the end of the century, with the introduction of surgical gloves in the USA (see Halsted 1913), the measures in use in a modern operating theatre had to a large extent been introduced.

During these years, when many fundamental discoveries in bacteriology were being made, other principles of hospital infection control were established. Flügge (1897, 1899) showed the importance of droplet and aerial spread of tuberculosis and, with Hutinel (1894) and others, established basic isolation systems for diphtheria and other infectious diseases in children's and fever hospitals.

3.2   The early twentieth century

The discovery of pathogenic bacteria provided a new basis for the study of hospital infection, and the importance of *Streptococcus pyogenes* was demonstrated during this period, in burn (Cruickshank 1935) and postoperative (Okell and Elliott 1936) infections. Cubicle and barrier nursing was introduced widely (Crookshank 1910) and was shown to be effective in preventing the spread of childhood fevers, except chickenpox and measles.

Aseptic surgery was for a time deemed adequate to keep wound infection to a low level, but this complacency was shattered by the experience of the 2 World Wars, when large open wounds readily became infected in the base hospitals (Cruickshank 1944). The local application of mild antiseptics to the wounds proved ineffective (Cruickshank 1944, Williams 1956). The arrival of penicillin in the later years of World War II gave considerable benefit (Fraser 1984).

Though Dukes (1929) recognized the importance of the indwelling catheter as a means of introducing infection into the bladder, this was forgotten. The idea was revived much later with the introduction of closed drainage systems (Gillespie 1956, Kunin and McCormack 1966).

3.3   The antibiotic era

The introduction of penicillin banished from hospitals the terrible cases of chronic sepsis, mainly caused by *Staphylococcus aureus* (Fletcher 1984). Nevertheless, the era of antibiotics ushered in for the first time a period in which staphylococcal, rather than streptococcal, infection dominated the scene (Williams 1956). Penicillin-resistant, and later multiply-resistant, *S. aureus* strains (Clarke, Dalgleish and Gillespie 1952) which had additional properties of transmissibility and virulence, caused serious wound, burn and other sepsis. Interest in air-borne and dust-borne spread, as well as transmission on the hands of attendants, revived. From this period date many of the established methods of infection control: the supply of clean air for operating theatres, procedures for wound dressings and the provision of isolation units, for example (Williams et al. 1960). So does the present general system for hospital-infection control: the appointment in the UK of medical control of infection officers (hospital epidemiologists), infection control nurses (nurse practitioners) and control of infection committees (Colebrook 1955, Subcommittee of the Central Health Services Council 1959, Gardner et al. 1962). Similar arrangements were established in the USA, where the first nurse practitioner in the discipline was appointed in 1963 (Osterman 1981).

3.4   More recent developments

For a period the importance of multiply-resistant *S. aureus* appeared to fade (Ayliffe, Lilly and Lowbury 1979) and interest shifted to gram-negative bacilli: antibiotic-resistant enterobacteria, such as *Klebsiella* and later *Serratia* spp., which caused large outbreaks of colonization, with some clinical infections. Infection by *Pseudomonas aeruginosa* came into prominence with the increasing number of patients rendered susceptible by illness or treatment. The infecting bacteria appeared to be favoured by the antibiotics in current use in the hospitals. More recently, possibly as a result of the introduction of new antibiotics, and the extensive use of indwelling medical devices, gram-positive cocci have again become the predominant causes of infection. *S. aureus* strains resistant to even more antibiotics ('methicillin-resistant *S. aureus*', see section 7.1, p. 207) have been as difficult to control as those encountered in the 1950s and multiply-resistant strains of *Staphylococcus epidermidis* have been the commonest pathogens in some units. *Enterococcus* spp. resistant to all current antibiotics including vancomycin (see section 7.2, p. 208) have presented problems in specialized units. Outbreaks of colitis caused by *Clostridium difficile* (see section 7.3, p. 208) have followed the use of broad spectrum antibiotics, such as cephalosporins. The increase in tuberculosis in immunosuppressed patients (see section 7.6, p. 209) and the occurrence of multiply-resistant strains have revived the need for isolation facilities and procedures to prevent air-borne spread of infection to patients and staff. On the other hand, the rediscovery of the principles of effective antibiotic prophylaxis in surgery has done much to prevent endogenous wound infection, for example, in colonic surgery.

The spread of viruses from patients admitted to hospital to other already sick patients remains an uncontrolled problem, particularly with respiratory syncytial virus (RSV) and other respiratory viruses in children's hospitals. Spread of viral gastrointestinal infection has been a major problem (see section 7.8, p. 211). The larger numbers of immunosuppressed patients has been associated with an increasing incidence and variety of fungal infection (see section 7.9, p. 214).

Methods of controlling hospital infection established earlier have been questioned. The UK Medical Research Council (Medical Research Council, Subcommittee of the Committee on Hospital Infection 1968) conducted an enquiry into the measures used in operating theatres. In the USA efforts to establish the cost-effectiveness of infection control measures culminated in the SENIC study (see section 9.3, p. 217) which demonstrated cost savings by the employment of effective numbers of infection control staff and the institution of preventive measures. Methods of surveillance have been further refined and computerization of records has assisted in this process. It has been important to focus the system of surveillance and control of hospital infection on areas of most effective cost benefit. The need to integrate infection control in the hospital with the wider community has been re-emphasized.

4 MODE OF SPREAD OF INFECTION IN HOSPITALS

4.1 Air-borne spread

With the tradition of the spread of disease by effluvium or miasma it is not surprising that air-borne spread of infection, for example of tuberculosis, was demonstrated early in the scientific era of bacteriology (Flügge 1897, 1899). Interest in this route went into eclipse in the early years of this century (Williams 1956) to be revived in the later 1930s and the 1940s. The contribution of the air-borne route to much common hospital infection remains the subject of controversy. Clearly, the effectiveness of this route depends on the source; on the number of micro-organisms present and the degree of dispersal, whether in droplets, in droplet nuclei or on skin scales; on survival and retention of pathogenicity by the micro-organisms in the air or environment (or their death, impairment or dilution there); on the size of the infecting dose; and on the local or general susceptibility of the

persons exposed to infection. Air-borne spread of infection has been reviewed in detail by Ayliffe and Lowbury (1982) (see also Volume 2, Chapter 14).

Bacteria can be counted in air by the slit sampler, which draws in air and impacts the particles on to a moving culture plate. Settle plates, which are agar plates exposed on horizontal surfaces for measured periods of time, capture a limited range of the particles from the air and are not quantitative. Small hand-held samplers (e.g. centrifugal samplers) are now available. They are easier and less disturbing to use in a busy operating theatre than the slit sampler, and are adapted to making counts during operations and in different areas near the operation itself. Some, however, extract only some of the particles and give results that are not as accurate as, or comparable with, those obtained with the slit sampler (Whyte 1981). Outside the operating theatre, the provision of good quality air for severely neutropenic patients in the absence of high efficiency particulate air (HEPA) filters, especially in the context of preventing aspergillus infection, is the other major indication for occasional air sampling. The absence of agreed standards, however, makes interpretation of air sampling outside the operating theatre difficult (Humphreys 1993).

TUBERCULOSIS

Clinical experience and experiments with guinea pigs indicate that air-borne spread of tuberculosis can occur by the transfer of very few micro-organisms. Patients differ greatly in their ability to transmit tuberculosis (Riley et al. 1962) and the susceptibility of the recipient is also very significant. Only patients with smear-positive pulmonary tuberculosis are regarded as constituting an infection risk and requiring single room isolation. Infectivity declines rapidly after effective treatment is initiated so that only 2 weeks of isolation during treatment is recommended (but see section 7.6, p. 209). Multidrug-resistant (MDR) tuberculosis in HIV patients during recent years has been associated with nosocomial spread to patients and health care workers and emphasizes the need for early identification of positive patients and patient isolation (Beck-Sagué et al. 1992).

PNEUMOCOCCAL INFECTION

Much infection by *Streptococcus pneumoniae* is endogenous and it has not been customary to isolate patients with pneumococcal pneumonia. The appearance of penicillin-resistant and multi-resistant strains has been associated with significant mortality (Pallares et al. 1995). The ready transmission of these emerging organisms has demonstrated the need to contain such infections (Gould, Magee and Ingham 1987), but clusters of cases also occur with some more sensitive strains, which appear to have the ability to cause lobar pneumonia in the relatively healthy (Davies et al. 1984). When the disease has been convincingly diagnosed by a gram stain of sputum, it may therefore be advisable to isolate patients with pneumococcal pneumonia for the first 24 h of treatment. Protection of vulnerable patients with the currently available polyvalent vaccine becomes more important as resistance increases (Austrian 1994).

MENINGOCOCCAL INFECTION

Meningococcal infection acquired in hospital is uncommon, but isolation for the first 48 h of treatment is advised. Among staff, only those who have had particularly close contact with the patient, as in mouth-to-mouth resuscitation, need be offered prophylactic antibiotics.

OTHER BACTERIAL INFECTIONS

The evidence for spread by air of *S. aureus* and *S. pyogenes* is contradictory (see Chapters 14 and 15). These bacteria are carried by many normal people (Williams et al. 1960); streptococci are readily shed from the upper respiratory tract, by coughing, sneezing and singing (Lidwell 1974), as are staphylococci on skin squames during physical activity. There is considerable variation in the degree of shedding. *S. aureus* is carried particularly in the perineum and nares and males tend to shed more staphylococci than females. Infected lesions on patients provide rich sources of these bacteria and release into the air is brought about by movement of secondarily contaminated articles, such as bedclothes, protective clothing, bed curtains and dressings, and of dust. The numbers in the air can be reduced by disinfection with ultraviolet light or chemicals, by such simple measures as damp, rather than dry, dusting or cleaning, and by control of air circulating between infected and susceptible persons. These measures are not, however, always effective in reducing infection rates. Striking results are most common when the prevailing infection rate is very high, as where dressings are handled, or where there is a large exposure of undefended tissue, as in burns. The important experiments in burned patients by Lowbury et al. (1970) suggested that infection by gram-negative bacilli, e.g. *P. aeruginosa*, was almost entirely by contact, infection by *S. pyogenes* by air and staphylococcal infection by both routes. Measures to control ventilation have on occasion resulted in a decline in the rate of nasal acquisition of organisms by patients. Several workers have found it impossible to control the spread of resistant strains of staphylococci by contact barriers alone but have achieved success with the use of a separate isolation unit or decontamination of the environment (Pearman et al. 1985). It may be that for these strains the selection pressure of antibiotics administered to the recipient is of importance in allowing colonization from very small inocula. These are situations in which air control is likely to yield good results.

Gram-negative bacilli tend to die when desiccated and infection by the aerial route is confined mainly to spread by nebulized spray (see p. 193).

VIRAL INFECTION

Smallpox was notorious as being readily transmitted by very few infective particles by the air-borne route. The most common viral infections transmitted by air in hospital are chickenpox, measles, influenza and RSV. Availability of immunofluorescence techniques for the rapid diagnosis of RSV renders isolation or 'cohort nursing' (placing patients with similar infections in the same ward or area) shortly after admission to hospital an increasing possibility and it is recommended (Editorial 1992). It seems that transmission of other childhood exanthems requires closer contact. Small round structured viruses (SRSVs) are an increasing cause of nosocomial diarrhoea and vomiting. Large inocula are present in vomitus and the air-borne inhalation route as well as the faecal route is now recognized as important means of transmission (Caul 1994).

FUNGAL INFECTION

Dispersal by spores is a feature of most filamentous fungi, but only *Aspergillus* spp. have been shown to be a significant cause of air-borne infection; this may occur after cardiac surgery or in immunosuppressed patients (see Chapter 7). Outbreaks have been associated with building work in hospitals (Opal et al. 1986) or inexpert filter changing in operating theatre ventilation systems. Other fungi occasionally cause clusters of infections by aerial spread, e.g. phycomycetes (del Palacio Hernanz et al. 1983). Exceptionally, other fungi that cause cardiac valve infection are thought to have arrived via air. Effectively filtered air should be supplied to certain classes of susceptible patients (Rhame et al. 1984). *Cryptococcus neoformans* is frequently found in pigeon droppings around hospitals but there is no convincing evidence of air-borne spread from this source to susceptible patients.

INFECTION IN THE OPERATING THEATRE

The pathogenesis of postoperative infection is complex but most infections arise from the patient's own flora and the remainder are acquired mainly from staff in the operating theatre (Ayliffe 1991). At one time 'aseptic surgery' appeared to offer all that was needed to minimize postoperative infection. In the 1940s, partly stimulated by cases of clostridial infection thought to be due to dust, interest was revived in the possibility that improved ventilation of operating theatres and other measures designed to limit air-borne infection would reduce it further. This was reflected in the principles of modern systems of operating theatre ventilation and the design of modern operating areas, including plenum ventilation to ensure flow of air from the theatre to the outside rather than the reverse (Humphreys 1993). Satisfactory operating theatre clothing, small operating teams with the minimum of movement and restriction of the patient's blankets, dressings, etc. to anterooms are other important factors in minimizing postoperative infection, because all these measures reduce the air count of bacteria in the theatre. Even so, any human activity raises the counts in a conventionally ventilated theatre, but these bursts should be quickly suppressed by effective ventilation.

The bacteria found in the air of a properly ventilated operating theatre are rarely pathogens in the usual sense; for example, they rarely include *S. aureus* or *S. pyogenes*. Indeed, it is difficult to find proof that reducing the air counts by conventional ventilation systems is beneficial in preventing surgical wound infection, although there have been instances in which the introduction of the systems described above have apparently resulted in a fall from an undesirably high incidence of wound infection (Blowers et al. 1955, Shooter et al. 1956).

It was an early suggestion that in surgical operations on healthy tissues with good defences a small degree of contamination with air-borne bacteria is unlikely to result in infection, but that less healthy tissues and areas such as the meninges may not be able to deal with such contamination (Cairns 1939). In the very specialized field of orthopaedic surgery, the incidence of infection has fallen with increased expertise, and it is now clear that the spectrum of infecting agents includes *S. epidermidis* and propionibacteria, such as are found in significant numbers in the air of a conventional operating theatre. Charnley and Eftekhar (1969) and others found very low rates of clinical infection when ultra-clean air was provided, but increased operative skill and the prophylactic use of antibiotics may have played a part in this. A multi-centre trial (Lidwell et al. 1982) compared conventional theatre conditions, provision of ultra-clean air, exhaust-ventilated clothing and, incidentally, use of prophylactic antibiotics, in 8055 operations (6781 hip replacements; 1274 knee replacements). The results (Fig. 13.2) showed a cumulative benefit for the 3 measures and indicated that antibiotic prophylaxis alone would achieve more than the expensive provision of ultra-clean air alone. A close relation was found between the air counts of bacteria and the risk of infection, and between staphylococci isolated in infected joints and those found in the patient or operating team at the time of operation. The benefit of very low air counts has not yet been proven for other types of surgery, but it would probably apply to the insertion of other prostheses, such as artificial heart valves and cerebrospinal fluid shunts.

4.2 Infection associated with water

LEGIONNAIRES' DISEASE

The Legionellaceae are widespread in water (see Volume 2, Chapter 49), including potable water supplies and many cases of Legionnaires' disease occur sporadically in the community. In one study in the UK they accounted for 15% of pneumonia cases (Macfarlane et al. 1982) but in other studies they were much less common. Hospitals are not spared the occurrence of legionellae in their water supplies (Tobin, Swann and Bartlett 1981) and have suffered a series of outbreaks (Bartlett, Macrae and Macfarlane 1986) mainly of infection with *Legionella pneumophila* (particularly serotype 1) but also with *Legionella micdadei*, *Legionella bozemanii* and *Legionella longbeachae*.

The factors that favour hospital-acquired Legionnaires' disease are as follows. Hospital patients include a number of individuals with an impaired immune system who are more likely to become clinically infected

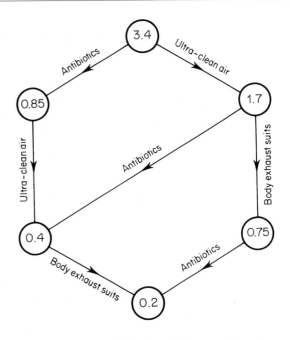

Fig. 13.2 Reduction of infection in joint prostheses by various measures (% rate of infection). (Reproduced, with permission, from Lidwell OM, 1986, *Clin Orthop Rel Res*, **211**: 91).

with legionellae and who have a higher mortality than otherwise healthy subjects. Hospital-acquired infection occurs in patients rather than in staff who may nevertheless have circulating antibodies, which suggests exposure. Water in medical equipment that delivers a nebulized spray may become contaminated (Arnow et al. 1982). Hospitals are large buildings with extended hot-water systems; it has been customary to run these at lower than usual temperatures, for economy and for the safety of patients; peak demand may lead to a further fall in temperature. Legionellae can tolerate temperatures to 55°C and can grow at 35–45°C and thus are adept at surviving and flourishing in the water systems of buildings (Latham et al. 1992). There have been many examples of the association of cases in hospital with hot-water systems, particularly with those supplying showers (Tobin et al. 1980) or run at a low temperature (Meenhorst et al. 1985). Ancillary systems used only intermittently may discharge water that has stagnated, allowing growth of legionellae in sludge or biofilm, perhaps assisted by substances from plumbing materials (Bartlett, Macrae and Macfarlane 1986). Cases associated with release of stagnant water into the general system have been described (Fisher-Hoch, Smith and Colbourne 1982). Hospital ventilation systems often have air-cooling towers in which potentially contaminated water flows over pipes through which air is circulated. Faults in such a system may allow direct access of the water to the air, or drift from the tower may contaminate the air at a later stage. Outbreaks caused by contaminated cooling towers can be explosive, occurring over a short period of time, whereas those due to domestic water systems may be more insidious and may only be revealed after active surveillance.

The source of infection of patients in hospital is thus environmental water; person-to-person spread is unknown. As legionellae are ubiquitous in water systems, regular monitoring is of little value in hospitals that have had no previous problems, but this is more problematical in hospitals where documented cases or outbreaks of nosocomial infection have occurred (Fallon 1994). Prevention depends on the good design, installation and maintenance of hot-water and ventilation systems and of the use wherever possible of air-cooled condensers rather than water-cooling towers; on keeping domestic hot water at high temperatures (>60°C for storage and >50°C at the point of delivery) unless patients are thereby exposed to risk of scalding, as for example, in mental-handicap departments; on flushing those parts of the hot-water system that are subject to stagnation; on chlorination and biocide treatment of water; and on the use of sterile water in nebulizers, etc. A recent outbreak was terminated by a series of measures including the use of copper and silver ions introduced into the water system as disinfectants (Colville et al. 1993). Preventive measures, which should involve clinicians, microbiologists and engineers, must be accompanied by good surveillance for the occurrence of Legionnaires' disease with adequate diagnostic facilities, and by contingency plans to be brought into action when possible hospital-acquired infections occur (Joint Health and Safety Executive and Department of Health Working Party on Legionellosis 1992). For further information about Legionnaires' disease see Chapter 18.

OTHER BACTERIA IN WATER AND IN DAMP AREAS IN THE HOSPITAL

Other gram-negative bacteria may be present in hospital water supplies, and their multiplication is encouraged by warmth and the other factors enumerated above. They may then act as opportunist pathogens in hospital patients. *Aeromonas hydrophila*, for example, causes pneumonia and sepsis in immunologically impaired patients. Picard and Goullet (1987) found *A. hydrophila* in maximal numbers in hospital water in hot weather, with counts running parallel to the total colony count. Risks of infection exist whenever aqueous fluids or damp objects in or on which gram-negative bacteria have had an opportunity to multiply, and have not subsequently been destroyed, come into intimate contact with susceptible patients. Examples include dental water-cooling systems, cooling cycles in autoclaves, pressure-monitoring systems on arterial lines, unsterilized lotions and irrigation solutions.

Pseudomonas spp. are to be found in mains water supplies and may multiply in any moist area; they have simple growth requirements and often show considerable resistance to antibiotics and may even survive in disinfectants, such as those prepared for multiple use. *P. aeruginosa* is ubiquitous in wet hospital sites; it has been found in food and water, ice machines (also implicated recently with infections due to *Stenotrophomonas maltophilia* in neutropenic patients in the UK), pharmacy preparations, plaster of Paris, mouthwash, dental water units, nebulizers, whirlpools and other hot baths, mattresses, sinks, taps, potted plants, flowers, flower vases, and so on. In some instances, particularly when the organisms have been introduced into the gastrointestinal or respiratory tract or the patients were particularly susceptible, colonization and later infection have been shown to have arisen from such sources. In other instances, however, the strains carried by the patients were different from those found only at inanimate sites in the wards. The patients' strains contaminated the immediate surroundings of the carrier-patients and the hands of members of the staff and were occasionally transferred to other patients (Levin et al. 1984, Allen et al. 1987). A more recent potential hazard that has been highlighted is pseudomonas infection following birth in water baths.

Burkholderia (*Pseudomonas*) *cepacia*, and other bacteria such as *Burkholderia* (*P.*) *pickettii*, possess the attributes that make them suitable for the role of hospital opportunists. Under certain conditions *B. cepacia* grows in distilled water and in the presence of aqueous chlorhexidine and quaternary ammonium compounds and may cause infections in neonates (Kahyaoglu, Nolan and Kumar 1995). It has frequently been isolated from badly formulated, unsterilized supplies of these antiseptics, and even from povidone-iodine. Infection from a contaminated disinfectant or other fluid is generally associated with application to an open wound (Bassett, Stokes and Thomas 1970), intravenous injection (Phillips et al. 1971), or urethral catheterization (Speller, Stephens and Viant 1971). *B. cepacia* is increasingly recognized as an important pathogen in patients with cystic fibrosis. In this group of patients the most important source is respiratory secretions with subsequent patient-to-patient spread and consequently patient segregation is advisable (Pankhurst and Philpott-Howard 1996).

4.3 Infection acquired from food

As in the general population, gastrointestinal pathogens may be transmitted by foods served to patients. Hospital food can also be a source of antibiotic-resistant bacteria, which may colonize the gut and later cause infection in susceptible patients. Of 1280 outbreaks of infectious intestinal disease reported to the Communicable Disease Surveillance Centre during the period 1992–94 (Djuretic et al. 1996), 189 occurred in hospitals. Salmonella infections were particularly associated with poultry or eggs, and *Clostridium perfringens* infections with meat. Outbreaks of salmonella infection in hospitals are important because they may cause serious effects in the very young, the elderly and in patients with impaired immunity (Taylor et al. 1982) and may disrupt the working of the hospital (Kumarasinghe et al. 1982). The catering faults most often responsible are failures of catering staff to follow good practice: incomplete defrosting of frozen meats and poultry, insufficient cooking of large amounts of food, use of raw or insufficiently cooked egg products, inadequate chilling and storage, and contact between food to be consumed without further cooking and raw poultry. Effective processing of all foods, including poultry and eggs, and safe preparation, storage and distribution of food, are important in hospitals, where particularly susceptible patients are exposed to risk (Wilkinson 1988). The system of centralized preparation of food that is immediately chilled to safe storage temperatures and later regenerated in a standard system after distribution ('cook-chill' or variations on this theme) allows, and demands, careful control and monitoring of bacterial content (Wilkinson 1988, Wilkinson, Dart and Hadlington 1991, Shanaghy, Murphy and Kennedy 1993).

Most outbreaks of salmonellosis in hospital are not food-borne but are caused by person-to-person spread or contaminated fomites. In the 3 year survey by Djuretic et al. (1996), only 19 of 189 hospital episodes were mainly food-borne, whereas 156 were mainly person to person; in 7 both routes were equally involved and in 7 the mode of spread was unknown. Similar figures have been reported in the USA (Baine et al. 1973). In a prospective investigation during a period of 2 years, food-borne spread probably accounted for only 11% of hospital outbreaks, although these tended to be the larger incidents (Palmer and Rowe 1983). Careful epidemiological investigation is required to determine the mode of spread and to define the population for further study (Palmer and Rowe 1983).

Hospital food is well known to be a source of often antibiotic-resistant gram-negative bacilli that colonize patients: *P. aeruginosa*, *Escherichia coli*, *Klebsiella* spp. and others (Shooter et al. 1969, Cooke et al. 1970, 1980, Casewell and Phillips 1978). It is possible for dietary components, equipment and preparation areas to become contaminated with nosocomial bacteria, particularly in facilities for the preparation of individualized diets, including enteral feeds (Casewell 1982). Colonization of the bowel is an important source of infection of other sites, for example of bacteraemia in granulocytopenic patients, who may benefit from a diet of low microbial content, with avoidance of foods likely to contain pathogenic or antibiotic-resistant bacteria (Schimpff 1993).

4.4   Infection by contact

FROM STAFF

Micro-organisms on the hands of staff may be **resident** (persistent over time and not readily removed by hand-washing) or **transient** (recently acquired from another source). It is generally accepted that the hands of staff are an important vehicle and that hand-washing makes a significant contribution to the control of hospital-acquired infection (Reybrouck 1983, Larson 1988). The relevant micro-organisms can readily be demonstrated on the hands of staff and may easily be transferred to the skin of others by brief contact (Marples and Towers 1979). Introduction of hand-washing has been accompanied by reduction of the infection rate in many studies, from that of Semmelweiss (1861) to more recent investigations of infection by gram-negative bacilli, e.g. Casewell and

Phillips (1977). The literature of more than 100 years was reviewed by Larson (1988) who concluded that the evidence strongly supported a causal connection between hand-washing and control. The effect has been observed in a variety of settings under many different hygienic circumstances (Larson 1988).

The most important micro-organisms spread by hand contact are *S. aureus* and gram-negative bacilli such as *Klebsiella* and *Serratia* spp. Carriage on the hands has been suggested as important in the transmission of antibiotic-resistant enterococci (Rhinehart et al. 1990) and of *C. difficile* (Kim et al. 1981, McFarland et al. 1989) but this has not been a consistent finding. In addition, the route has been described for many other hospital-spread pathogens, including *Candida albicans* (Burnie 1986) and even respiratory pathogens: *Corynebacterium diphtheriae* (in the past) and viruses, such as RSV and rhinoviruses (Pancic, Carpentier and Came 1980). With *S. aureus* attention has been focused on long-term carriage (Williams et al. 1960); gram-negative bacilli also have been demonstrated to persist for long periods on the hands of some persons (Casewell and Phillips 1977, Adams and Marrie 1982). Transient carriage resulting from recent contact with an infected or colonized patient may often be more important. Casewell and Desai (1983) demonstrated that strains of gram-negative bacilli, particularly of *Klebsiella* and *Serratia*, that had caused outbreaks in which infection was apparently spread by staff from patient to patient, survived longer on the hands of volunteers than did strains capable of causing outbreaks only from a point source in food or the environment. The ability of glycopeptide-resistant enterococci to survive for 1 h on fingers has also been shown (Noskin et al. 1995).

The preparations available for hand decontamination and the methods for assessing them have been reviewed (Ayliffe 1980, Reybrouck 1986). Hand hygiene may be designed for the removal of transient flora (Price 1938), which may be achieved by a simple wash with soap or detergent, or even better by an aqueous preparation of an antiseptic with a detergent. Sometimes a residual disinfectant action is needed, with or without reduction of the resident flora, as in the preoperative preparation of a surgeon's hands, or in high-dependency units in the hospital. Iodophors, the bisguanide chlorhexidine, and trichlorohydroxyphenol and related compounds may all be used and all have some residual activity (Ayliffe 1980). Alcoholic preparations, or alcohols alone, are more rapid in action than aqueous preparations and are more effective (Lowbury, Lilly and Ayliffe 1974). Their drying action on the skin can be prevented by the addition of glycerol or other emollients. A minimum of skin flora cannot be reduced further by these processes (Lilly, Lowbury and Wilkins 1979). Methods should be adopted that are suitable for the particular purpose and that avoid damage to the skin and development of resistant flora on repeated use (Ayliffe 1980, Reybrouck 1986). One clinical trial (Doebbeling et al. 1992) compared different hand-washing methods in consecutive periods in intensive care units. A reduction in nosocomial infection was directly demonstrated when chlorhexidine (rather than soap or alcohol) was used; the effect may have been partly due to better compliance by staff. Poor compliance with the prescribed measures is frequently observed and may vary with the professional group, the handwashing system prescribed and its ready availability (Albert and Condie 1981, Doebbeling et al. 1992, Gould 1994, Wurtz, Moye and Jovanovic 1994).

The clothing of personnel can be shown to become contaminated with potential pathogens, such as *S. aureus* and, less frequently, gram-negative bacilli, particularly after the handling of heavily colonized patients (Babb, Davies and Ayliffe 1983). The significance of this in the spread of infection is unknown.

FROM THE PATIENT'S ENVIRONMENT

The immediate environment readily becomes contaminated with the bacteria carried by a patient. It has sometimes been difficult to prove that organisms from environmental surfaces cause infection (Maki et al. 1982), partly because the virulence of the bacteria may become impaired. Nevertheless, if heavily contaminated (Sanderson and Rawal 1987), such surfaces must be regarded as a potential source of air-borne organisms and also of infection by direct contact with another patient or via the hands of staff. This has been shown, for example, with methicillin-resistant *S. aureus* and with *Acinetobacter* spp. Particularly in the case of bacteria carried in the bowel, which can survive in the environment for long periods, contamination of the environment or equipment may be responsible for the clustering of cases, as with *C. difficile* (Cartmill et al. 1994) and *Enterococcus* spp. (Karanfil, Murphy and Josephson 1992).

FROM EQUIPMENT

Infection from surgical instruments is now extremely rare, but other items of equipment, even if they do not penetrate the tissue, may convey infection from one patient to another. Some of these escaped attention because the risks associated with them appeared to be low or had not been perceived. Others are pieces of equipment that are difficult to clean and disinfect adequately, or are expensive and in short supply.

Many items that come into contact with patients usually do not need to be supplied sterile, but patients with impaired immunity may be susceptible to opportunist organisms present on or in these. For example, patients with debilitating illnesses may develop superficial and subcutaneous phycomycosis in macerated areas under adhesive plaster contaminated with *Rhizopus* spp. (Gartenberg et al. 1978). Premature babies have become infected by *Rhizopus* spp. from unsterile wooden tongue depressors, used as limb splints (Mitchell et al. 1996).

Bedpans and urinals have been blamed for the spread of enteric bacteria, such as *C. difficile* and antibiotic-resistant gram-negative bacilli (Curie et al. 1978). The bacterial load may be high if the washing process is not efficient, and bedpan washer-disinfectors often do not maintain an adequate temperature for the intended time. The practice of decontaminating urinals in tanks of phenolic disinfectant is often ineffective because of inaccurate dilution of the disinfectant, or its inactivation by organic matter, or by the survival of bacteria in biofilm on surfaces (Curie et al. 1978). Special decontamination measures may be necessary for particularly resistant pathogens, e.g. *C. difficile* and *Cryptosporidium* spp. Rectal thermometers have been believed to be responsible for the spread of salmonellae (Im, Chow and Chau 1981) and enterococci (Livornese, Dial and Samel 1992); all thermometers should be decontaminated after use (Nystrom 1980).

Many fibreoptic endoscopes for gastrointestinal and bronchial use are difficult to disinfect because they do not withstand heating; also their complex channels are difficult to clean. Numerous species have been transmitted by such endoscopes (Spach, Silverstein and Stamm 1993). Among the commonest have been *Salmonella* spp. and *P. aeruginosa* in the gastrointestinal tract and *Mycobacterium tuberculosis* and other mycobacteria in the respiratory system. Endoscopes are readily contaminated with *Helicobacter pylori* and transmission by endoscopy has been demonstrated (Langenberg et al. 1990). Thus, transmission may result in colonization or infection locally. In the impaired patient infection of other sites and bacteraemia may result (Schimpff 1993); bacteraemia is particularly likely to follow biliary endoscopy (Struelens et al. 1993). Hepatitis B has rarely been transmitted on endoscopes although they readily become contaminated with the virus (see Ridgway 1985). Spread of human immunodeficiency virus via endoscopes has not been reported. Such accidents can be avoided by a thorough regimen of cleaning and disinfection with a suitable chemical agent, which may be carried out manually or by special apparatus (Fraser et al. 1993, Bradley and Babb 1995) if sufficient endoscopes can be provided (Anon 1988, Fantry, Zheng and James 1993, Babb and Bradley 1995).

4.5 Infection by inoculation

Since the universal introduction of single-use disposable needles and other devices and satisfactory procedures for the sterilization of surgical instruments, with a wide safety margin, transmission of infection by this route in the developed world has been infrequent. Few agents can resist the standard sterilization processes. The prions or 'slow viruses' responsible for transmissible spongiform encephalopathies (e.g. Creutzfeldt–Jakob disease), previously associated with neurosurgery, are highly resistant to most sterilization procedures and therefore instruments used on patients with these conditions should either be disposed of or subjected to prolonged autoclaving at high temperature (Advisory Committee on Dangerous Pathogens 1994). However, there remain infections (1) transmitted by blood transfusion or tissue donation, (2) resulting from accidental injury from contaminated sharp instruments, (3) from contaminated blood, and (4) from other contaminated infusion fluids.

Infection transmitted by blood transfusion and tissue donation

Infectious agents may from time to time be transmitted to patients by donors of blood, blood products or tissue. The risk of transmission of the 3 most important agents, hepatitis B and C viruses and human immunodeficiency virus (HIV), has been reduced to a low level by a combination of donor selection, screening of donations for antigen or antibody, and heat treatment of blood products, but not before countless cases of 'serum hepatitis' had occurred and a considerable proportion of haemophilia sufferers received factor VIII infected with HIV (Editorial 1984b). Efforts should also be made to exclude other, less common, blood-transmitted infections such as other forms of hepatitis, including δ agent and possibly hepatitis G in the future, cytomegalovirus, Epstein–Barr virus, parvovirus, HTLV-1, brucellosis, syphilis, salmonellosis, malaria, trypanosomiasis, toxoplasmosis, babesiosis and filariasis (see Mollison, Engelfriet and Contreras 1987). Acquisition of transmissible spongiform encephalopathies is not considered likely to follow blood transfusion. A recent epidemiological survey of Creutzfeldt–Jakob disease in the UK revealed that only 16 of 202 cases had a history of blood transfusion and this was not significantly different from controls (Esmonde et al. 1993). Further efforts to exclude infections less common than those already currently screened for in the blood supply must be balanced against the considerable cost of such screening and the impact this might have on blood donation.

Tissue donations have been responsible for the transmission of cytomegalovirus, HIV (L'Age-Stehr et al. 1985) and rabies (Helmick, Tauxe and Vernon 1987) and may also transmit hepatitis B and hepatitis C. Creutzfeldt–Jakob disease may be acquired during surgical procedures that involve tissue transfer and when this occurs, the incubation period is a matter of months rather than years (Hart 1995).

Infection from accidental inoculation

In the past tuberculosis of the skin ('prosector's wart') was a common consequence of inoculation and is once again a potential risk from HIV patients heavily infected with *M. tuberculosis* (Kramer et al. 1993). In the pre-antibiotic era, infection by a needlestick injury with *S. pyogenes* might result in septicaemia and death, as observed by Semmelweiss in his colleague, Kolletschka. Such events remain a hazard, though a much reduced one (Hawkey, Pedler and Southall 1980). The main risks of such injuries, however, are infection with hepatitis B and C viruses, and HIV.

Hepatitis B and C and HIV infection in hospitals

Hepatitis B and C viruses, and HIV are the pathogens most likely to be transmitted from blood and tissue fluids. Bodily secretions from infected patients contain much lower concentrations of virus, or none at all. The risk of transmission to staff is greatest for those with the highest exposure to blood and to injuries with sharp instruments, but a history of a definite incident is not always given by hospital staff members who develop hepatitis B. The risk of acquiring hepatitis B from an infectious carrier in an inoculation incident is significant, especially if the patient is e antigen positive (HBeAg). An investigation following the identification of a HBeAg-positive cardiac surgeon revealed that 13% of susceptible patients contracted hepatitis B despite good infection control practice (Harpaz et al. 1996).

It is clear that the risk of transmission of HIV to staff is very small; of 1036 subjects included in several series, with adequate epidemiological and serological investigation of percutaneous or mucous-membrane exposure to blood or tissue fluid from known HIV positive patients, only 3 (0.3%) showed seroconversion (Centers for Disease Control 1987). More recently, only 4 of 1103 health care workers with percutaneous exposure to HIV infected blood seroconverted and in one case this occurred following post-exposure zidovudine (Tokars et al. 1993). The risk of a patient acquiring HIV from an infected health care worker has been the subject of much debate, some of it ill-informed, but has raised the issue of screening health care workers for HIV. A retrospective study of more than 6400 patients of an infected Florida dentist revealed 28 with HIV infection, of whom 24 had behavioural risk factors. Analysis of the viral gene sequences from the dentist and his patients excluded a possible link with the 24 with behavioural risk factors, but not with the remaining 4 (Jaffe et al. 1994). A survey of 22 171 patients of 51 infected health care workers conducted by the Centers for Disease Control, Atlanta, USA failed to reveal evidence of transmission from health care worker to patient (Robert et al. 1995). A cost-benefit analysis of screening surgeons for HIV as a strategy to minimize transmission to patients did not support this approach as cost-effective (Owens et al. 1995). In the UK, recommendations on the investigation of patients who have been cared for by a member of staff who is subsequently identified as HIV-positive, are available (Expert Advisory Group on AIDS 1993).

Hepatitis C (see Volume 1, Chapter 35), recognized in the last decade as the major cause of non-A non-B hepatitis following blood transfusion, is encountered world wide with especially high prevalence in Japan and the southern part of the USA, and may persist in 80% of infected patients (van der Poel, Cuypers and Reesink 1994). Some patient groups have a higher seroprevalence; 3.3% of Dutch haemophilia patients were positive compared with 0.03% of blood donors (Schneeberger, Vos and van Dijk 1993). Acquisition associated with particular occupations is also described; oral surgeons had a higher incidence (9.3%) than dentists (0.97%) or unselected blood donors (0.14%) in one study (Klein et al. 1991). The risk of seroconversion following a needlestick incident is not as clear as that with hepatitis B but in one study it was reported as 23% (Kiyosawa et al. 1991), which is intermediate between HIV and hepatitis B. At present the risk of a hepatitis C-positive health care worker transmitting infection to patients is also not certain. An investigation of an incident involving a hepatitis C-positive cardiac surgeon revealed that 6 of 222 patients followed up contracted postoperative hepatitis; in 5 patients the viral gene sequences were similar to those of the surgeon (Esteban et al. 1996).

Active hepatitis B immunization can be given to those at greatest risk (Mulley, Silverstein and Dienstag 1982) and this and hepatitis B immune globulin may be used as post-exposure prophylaxis (Grady et al. 1978). Other measures are clearly to be directed against the risk of inoculation of blood. With the recognition in the last decade of new agents (e.g. hepatitis C) transmissible by blood and the likelihood of others to follow, control measures have more and more emphasized good practice when handling blood, blood products and other fluids such as cerebrospinal fluid, irrespective of patient source (Expert Advisory Group on AIDS 1990). These are referred to as universal precautions and include greater awareness of the risks by staff, staff covering cuts or abrasions, careful disposal of sharps and clinical waste, and the use of gloves and gowns when in contact with body fluids (Expert Advisory Group on AIDS 1990, Board of Science and Education 1996). Additional precautions may be taken with known infected patients, or those suspected of being infected (e.g. intravenous drug abusers) but the adoption of universal precautions at all times minimizes the risks to staff and patients when a patient is not known or considered to be in an at-risk group. Recent guidelines issued in the UK to minimize acquisition of hepatitis B and HIV during surgery, which would also largely apply to hepatitis C, emphasize good practice at all times, e.g. avoidance of passing sharps by hand, with additional precautions such as double gloving when operating on positive patients or those in at-risk groups (Joint Working Party of the Hospital Infection Society and the Surgical Infection Study Group 1992). Continuing education on basic techniques to avoid inoculation risk incidents is important; taking sharps boxes for the disposal of needles to the patient's bedside reduced the number of recapped needles (a practice likely to place the health care worker at risk of a needlestick incident) from 33% to 18% (Makofsky and Cone 1993).

Testing for hepatitis B surface antigen (HBsAg) has been used to define more closely the patients who present an 'inoculation risk' and identification of HBeAg and antibody (HBeAb) to define the degree of infectivity. Screening of patients for hepatitis C is not usually indicated as an infection control measure. Testing for HIV with consent is not recommended at present, partly because of the implications of detecting seropositivity in a symptomless patient and partly because of the lack of a sufficiently sensitive and specific antigen test to identify infected patients before antibody appears. Testing for hepatitis B, C

and HIV is essential before tissue donation and recommended in certain other defined situations.

Containment measures for identified patients should concentrate on the risks associated with invasive procedures and bleeding, and especially with surgical operations and obstetric deliveries. Single-room isolation is required only for certain patients, e.g. those with mental disturbance, uncontrolled bleeding, or dual infection with HIV and another disease, such as tuberculosis. In deciding whether a patient requires single-room isolation, consideration should also be given to the psychological effects this may have. The standard decontamination measures for crockery, bedpans, etc. are adequate. For invasive procedures, limiting the number of staff present, providing adequate protective clothing, including precautions against splash on mucous membranes, limiting and containing blood loss as far as possible, care with sharp instruments, and adequate decontamination of instruments are the principles to apply. Detailed recommendations for the care of HBsAg or HIV risk patients have been formulated (Speller et al. 1990).

INFECTION FROM CONTAMINATED BLOOD

Extrinsic contamination of donor blood with small numbers of bacteria is not uncommon and serious consequences of this are rare. Occasionally stored blood may contain large numbers of bacteria (Braude, Carey and Siemienski 1955), often psychrotrophs, and septicaemia and shock may occur in the recipient (McEntegart 1956). The range of possible organisms and the risks associated with erythrocytes, whole blood and platelets together with advice on how to investigate outbreaks and prevent such occurrences have been well reviewed (Wagner, Friedman and Dodd 1994).

INFECTION FROM CONTAMINATED INFUSION FLUIDS

Major outbreaks of serious infection and endotoxic shock have been caused by heavily colonized infusion fluids other than blood. Some accidents were due to failure of sterilization during commercial manufacture (Meers et al. 1973), and others to the introduction of micro-organisms from cooling water in sterilizers (Phillips, Eykyn and Laker 1972) or from contaminated closures which release their bacteria into the infusion fluid during manipulation in the ward. Infusion fluid in reservoirs or administration sets can become colonized during use, from cracks in containers or during manipulations and additions (Duma, Warner and Dalton 1971). Indeed, a significant proportion of containers becomes contaminated with small numbers of bacteria (Maki, Goldmann and Rhame 1973). Fluids for total parenteral nutrition, such as protein hydrolysate with or without dextrose, readily support the growth of micro-organisms, particularly of *Klebsiella* and *Enterobacter* spp. and the like, and of *Candida* spp. Disseminated fungal infection has been particularly associated with total parenteral nutrition, but not all episodes have resulted from contamination of fluid in the reservoir or administration set (Goldmann and Maki 1973). The risk can be reduced by care with all manipulations or by having all additions to intravenous fluids made by skilled staff working in controlled environmental conditions. Containers and administration sets should be changed every 48 h; more frequent changing is unnecessary (Buxton et al. 1979). The use of bacterial filters, i.e. in administration sets, has done little to reduce infection (Collin et al. 1973). This may indicate that infection related to the intravascular cannula is more common than colonization of fluid in the rest of the system.

5 HOSPITAL INFECTIONS AT VARIOUS BODY SITES

5.1 Surgical wounds and other soft tissue sites

Infection of surgical wounds is important numerically and as a cause of morbidity and prolonged hospital stay. In a prevalence survey (Emmerson et al. 1996) it accounted for 12.3% of hospital-acquired infections. In the USA incidence study, surgical wound infection accounted for 24% of nosocomial infection. In some surveys the definition of wound infection was based on a simple, easily observed character such as the presence of pus in the wound and this has the advantages of minimizing observer variability. A more complex definition, making use of several other signs of inflammation (e.g. erythema), can be used with an elaborate scoring system (Wilson AP 1995). This may increase the likelihood that significant differences will be observed in comparative trials. The definition should be based on clinical observation; it may be useful to culture all infected wounds for microbiological surveillance purposes, but the presence of pathogenic bacteria in itself does not imply infection. The recorded incidence of infection will also depend on the length of postoperative stay and the degree of follow-up after discharge from hospital (Bailey et al. 1992, Weigelt, Dryer and Hayley 1992, Byrne et al. 1994, Emmerson 1995).

Several investigations have been made, in sufficiently large numbers of patients, of the factors predisposing to surgical wound infection, to determine where improvements in practice should be directed (e.g. Cruse and Foord 1973). Regression analysis has been employed to separate variables. Surgical procedures may be crudely divided as follows: 'clean', when no inflammation is encountered and no colonized body system is entered; 'clean contaminated', when a colonized system, e.g. gastrointestinal or respiratory, is entered, but there is no significant spillage; 'contaminated', when inflammation, but not pus, is encountered or spillage from a viscus occurs; and 'dirty', when a perforated viscus or pus is encountered. The incidence of infection should be less than 5% for clean operations; some surgical teams may record a rate of less than 1% (Cruse and Foord 1973). On the other hand, operations on the left colon or

rectum may be followed by wound infection in more than 30% of patients if antibiotic prophylaxis is not given. Refinements of this classification system have been suggested; it may be more useful to consider individual types of operation separately. For example, caesarean section, though included in 'clean' surgery, may have a high infection rate (Beattie et al. 1994, Henderson and Love 1995).

In general investigations, the factors most consistently associated with an increased incidence of postoperative infection are age over 60 years, long preoperative stay in hospital, long duration of operation, pre-existing infection at the site of the wound, and bacteria in the wound at the end of the operation. Underlying disease, such as diabetes, immunosuppression or irradiation and, in some studies, malnutrition and administration of adrenocorticosteroids, are also important. In preoperative preparation, shaving of hair from the site, rather than treatment with depilatories or clipping, has been associated with a much greater frequency of infection (Seropian and Reynolds 1971), but other aspects of skin preparation appeared not to exert a consistent effect. Factors of significance in some studies but not in others are male sex, emergency operations, and the use of surgical drains. It is generally agreed that good surgical technique is most important, but it is difficult to single out particular surgical practices. The use of diathermy was associated with increased infection in one series (Cruse and Foord 1973).

Overall, *S. aureus* is the dominant species in surgical wound infection, followed by the enterobacteria (Meers et al. 1981). The microbiological findings vary with the site and type of operation and also with the adequacy of culture methods, which often underestimate the role of anaerobic bacteria, such as *Bacteroides* spp. These, with other gut bacteria, often in mixed growth, are typical of infections after a colonized viscus is entered (Dunn and Simmons 1984). *S. aureus* may occur in all types of wound and is the typical cause of the less frequent wound infection in 'clean' surgery. Most infection of surgical wounds occurs at the time of operation. Evidence from animal experiments (Burke 1961) and studies of the effectiveness of antibiotic prophylaxis (e.g. Stone et al. 1976) suggest that there is a short period after bacterial contamination during which infection is initiated. In the great majority of cases, the origin of the bacteria appears to be the patient's own body flora. Much less often it is from a member of the operating team, but in many instances the origin is obscure. Occasionally a cluster of infections can be related to an organism present in a septic lesion or at a carrier site in a member of the operating team, but this is uncommon. The route by which a patient becomes infected is often not clear. The air-borne route is important in the implantation of prostheses, and in rare episodes in general surgery, which were linked with an identifiable source among the theatre staff, the circumstances strongly suggested the air as the vehicle. More usual routes are direct spread from incised organs, and intraoperative contamination of instruments and of surgeons' gloves and clothing. Contamination from apparatus such as that providing an extracorporeal circulation has occasionally been described.

STERNAL WOUNDS

Infection of the sternal wound after a cardiac operation, though difficult to recognize clinically in the early stages, may later be associated with mediastinitis, osteomyelitis, septicaemia and colonization of prosthetic material, and thus with significant morbidity and mortality. Prevention may be a major role for the prophylactic antibiotics that are used almost universally in cardiac surgery (Farrington 1986). Among factors that have been cited as predisposing to this type of postoperative infection are long and double procedures, excessive trauma to the sternum, postoperative haematoma formation and reopening of the wound (Sarr, Gott and Townsend 1984), as well as the features already described as predisposing to surgical wound infection in general.

Infection occurs at the time of operation from the many sources outlined above; it is probable that a relatively small inoculum is needed in the inevitably damaged tissue. As might be expected, *S. aureus*, coagulase-negative staphylococci and other skin bacteria predominate, followed by Enterobacteriaceae and *P. aeruginosa*. It has been reported that the incidence of infection is greater in coronary artery bypass surgery when leg veins are used, and that the infecting organisms, particularly gram-negative bacilli, may be transferred from the leg; infection of the leg wound itself is also common (Wells, Newsom and Rowlands 1983, Farrington et al. 1985).

BURNS

Burns provide a suitable site for bacterial multiplication; when this has taken place, the burn is a richer and more persistent source of infection than the surgical wound because a larger area of tissue is exposed for a longer time. The clinical consequences of infection in burns may be very serious; a large proportion of the mortality in burned patients who have survived the initial trauma and shock has been due to infection. Multiple-antibiotic resistance in the infecting agents has for many years presented difficulties in the treatment of burned patients.

S. aureus and *P. aeruginosa* are the commonest isolates in most burns units, followed by various enterobacteria and other gram-negative bacilli, such as *Acinetobacter* spp. *S. pyogenes*, once a cause of serious trouble in burns units (Cruickshank 1935), now colonizes comparatively few patients (Lawrence 1985). Nevertheless, *S. pyogenes* is important both in episodes of acute infection and in causing the death of skin grafts. As in other hospital areas, the emergence of resistant gram-positive bacteria, including multi-resistant enterococci and *S. aureus*, has been seen in burns units (Phillips, Heggers and Robson 1992, Donati et al. 1993).

As in many other sites, colonization without invasion is far commoner than invasive infection, but the frequency and clinical severity of septicaemic infections caused by most of the potential pathogens, particularly by *P. aeruginosa*, encourage regular monitoring by the culture of swabs from burns. A greater understanding of the relationship between the bacteria present and the host tissues can be obtained by examining punch biopsies (Pruitt and McManus 1992). Septicaemia may follow surgical intervention; this may be prevented by systemic antibiotic prophylaxis, as is applied in most burns units (Papini et al. 1995).

Bacteria reach burns mainly by indirect contact; airborne infection has been demonstrated on occasions (p. 191) and is more important for *S. aureus* than for gram-negative bacilli. Occasionally mattresses, baths and hydrotherapy pools have been incriminated (Ayliffe and Lilly 1985, Tredget et al. 1992). In some studies, standard infection control measures, including controlled ventilation, have not been shown greatly to influence the colonization of burns by bacteria, including antibiotic-resistant strains (Ayliffe and Lawrence 1985), although it has been suggested that single-room isolation reduces the problem of infection by gram-negative bacilli (Pruitt and McManus 1992, McManus et al. 1994). It is clear that improvements in the surgical management of burns, including judicious use of excision and timely closure, and the use of topical chemotherapy with agents such as silver sulphadiazine, have considerably reduced infection in many units.

Infection associated with extensive skin disease and major plastic surgery presents problems that are to some extent similar to those with burns.

THE EYE

The cornea is considered sterile but the conjunctiva is colonized by a number of different bacterial genera, predominantly coagulase-negative staphylococci, *Corynebacterium* spp. and *Propionibacterium* spp. (Willcox and Stapleton 1996). Resident flora and other physiological factors, e.g. immunoglobulins in tears, prevent colonization by more pathogenic bacteria. The use of contact lenses is associated with colonization by *S. aureus* and gram-negative bacilli. Postoperative infections of the eye are uncommon but may result in considerable disability and are difficult to treat. An aetiological diagnosis is usually possible only if material for culture is obtained from within the eye. Preoperative monitoring of the eye flora is not usually indicated unless there are clinical signs of infection on the surface of the eye. It may, however, be useful to examine swabs from the skin round the eye and from the anterior nares for *S. aureus*, particularly if the patient has a skin disease, so that extra care can be taken with skin preparation if *S. aureus* is grown.

Endophthalmitis is an infection of the intraocular structures and sclera and usually occurs following intraocular surgery or penetrating trauma, or as part of a generalized infection, such as systemic candidiasis. Infection after cataract surgery has declined in recent years and is now less than 0.1% (Das and Symonds 1996). Gram-positive bacteria predominate; a survey of 64 centres in France identified *S. epidermidis* as the most important pathogen (Fisch et al. 1991). A similar finding was reported in a UK study (Hassan, MacGowan and Cook 1992). The somewhat surprising emergence of *S. epidermidis*, traditionally associated with the immunocompromised host and with foreign body related infection, may represent improved diagnostic techniques. Various fungi cause occasional infections, presumably by the air-borne route. Many donor corneas yield microbial growth but few patients develop infection with organisms similar to those found on the cornea. The importance of making a microbiological diagnosis should not be underestimated as management is difficult, partly because antimicrobial agents penetrate poorly into the anterior and vitreous chambers of the eye.

Keratoconjunctivitis is usually community-acquired and is most commonly caused by *S. aureus* but *P. aeruginosa* may be associated with corneal ulceration in hospital and *Haemophilus influenzae* with infection in children (Limberg 1991). Epidemics caused by adenovirus type 8 are essentially an infection of hospitals and clinics, possibly spread by instruments such as tonometers, but also by the hands of staff, and otherwise only by close, person-to-person, family or other contact. Scrupulous hand-washing, decontamination of equipment – by chemical means if it is heat-sensitive – and use of individual containers for ophthalmic preparations, will terminate an outbreak (Barnard et al. 1973). Other adenoviruses may also be transmitted in this way (Tullo and Higgins 1980). Hospital-acquired bacterial conjunctivitis is common only in neonatal units, where minor conjuctival infection with *S. aureus* is more common than neonatal ophthalmitis due to *Chlamydia trachomatis* or *Neisseria gonorrhoeae* acquired from the birth canal.

THE PERITONEUM

Peritonitis is one of the classical associations of surgery: a breach in the bowel wall is followed by invasion of the peritoneum by a mixture of enteric bacteria, possibly acting synergistically. Advances in the classification and pathogenesis of sepsis, including peritonitis (Bone 1991), have raised the possibility of new therapeutic strategies. Patients who require intensive care have a mortality of 63%; amongst the poor prognostic features are advancing age, the presence of septic shock, failure to clear the source of sepsis and an upper gastrointestinal source (McLauchlan et al. 1995).

With the development of peritoneal dialysis for renal failure, and particularly of continuous ambulatory peritoneal dialysis (CAPD) for its chronic management, a very different form of peritonitis has become common. Short-term peritoneal dialysis, in patients unsuitable for haemodialysis, is often complicated by peritoneal infection caused by gram-negative bacilli. CAPD peritonitis has a different spectrum of aetiological agents and coagulase-negative staphylococci, particularly *S. epidermidis*, account for about half the cases (Spencer 1988, von Graevenitz and Amsterdam 1992). Factors important in the pathogenesis of such infections include the size of the bacterial inoculum, adaptation of bacteria to the local micro-environment, especially adherence to plastics, and diminished phagocytic activity in peritoneal fluid (von Graevenitz and Amsterdam 1992). Many factors have been invoked to explain the success of *S. epidermidis* as a pathogen in CAPD and there is increasing interest in

bacterial phenotypic variation in peritoneal dialysis fluid. Differences in iron regulating proteins, cell wall and cytoplasmic membrane protein profiles have been demonstrated when strains are grown in peritoneal dialysis fluid rather than in nutrient broth (Wilcox et al. 1991). Other gram-positive cocci and other skin bacteria, enterobacteria and the Pseudomonadaceae account for most other cases; anaerobic bacteria and fungi are less common. Special cultural methods may be needed to reveal the presence of intracellular organisms or organisms that for other reasons are difficult to grow. The major cause of infection is a lapse in technique by the patient or attendants in changing the containers of dialysis fluid. Patient motivation is therefore important in minimizing infection. A number of specific measures, including good surgical technique at the time of catheter insertion and the use of occlusive dressings (Ludlam et al. 1989), have been advocated to reduce infections, especially those due to *S. aureus*, which are difficult to treat. The infecting organisms may reach the peritoneum from the abdominal skin, with or without overt 'tunnel' infection. Other sources are the bowel – mixed infection with multiple enterobacteria or anaerobes, which suggests perforation (Editorial 1982) – the bloodstream and the female genital tract. Episodes of infection may be treated with antibiotics without removal of the catheter (Working Party of the British Society for Antimicrobial Chemotherapy 1987), but repeated infection in association with tunnel infection and certain pathogens, such as *S. aureus*, *P. aeruginosa* and fungi, make success less likely.

PREVENTION OF POSTOPERATIVE WOUND INFECTION

The measures taken in the operating suite to prevent postoperative wound infection have been classified into the following categories (Medical Research Council Subcommittee of the Committee on Hospital Infection 1968):

1 established
2 provisionally established
3 rational methods
4 rituals.

Since then some time-honoured practices have been discarded. Nevertheless, there is still a lack of firm evidence to justify a number of the 'rational' measures that are taken to protect the patient. This chapter gives only an outline that applies to operations generally and not to special situations such as orthopaedic implants. Many measures can be deduced from the risk factors already outlined. Thus, an operation carried out expeditiously with meticulous technique will have a reduced risk of infection.

In elective surgery, patients may be investigated preoperatively at assessment clinics, to avoid a long period in hospital before the operation. Underlying disease and existing infections should, as far as possible, be controlled. Nasal carriage of *S. aureus* is associated with postoperative infection but eradication has not yet been shown to reduce the risk (Wenzel and Perl

1995). Preoperative monitoring for pathogens such as *S. aureus* or *S. pyogenes* is commonly carried out before high-risk operations, such as those on the heart, but its usefulness has not been established (Ridgway, Wilson and Kelsey 1990). The value of total-body antiseptic treatment, as with chlorhexidine detergent, is also controversial (Lynch et al. 1992). Antiseptic skin preparation in the operating theatre, with alcoholic solutions of chlorhexidine or an iodophor, applied with some friction, is very effective (Davies et al. 1978). There is no evidence that longer applications are beneficial, except perhaps when clostridial spores must be removed (Lowbury, Lilly and Bull 1964). The use of specially impermeable material, whether woven or adhesive plastic, or of disinfectant-impregnated material, for the drapes around the operative field, is not supported by firm evidence (Lewis, Leaper and Speller 1984). Hair should, whenever possible, be clipped or removed by depilatory methods rather than by shaving.

A full discussion of the prophylactic use of antibiotics to prevent surgical wound infection is beyond the scope of this chapter (Leaper 1994, Sheridan, Tompkins and Burke 1994). The usefulness of very short perioperative courses of aptly chosen antibiotics has been decisively established for operations with a high incidence of endogenous infection. Examples are colonic surgery, upper gastrointestinal surgery in conditions of bacterial overgrowth, some operations on the biliary system, and vaginal hysterectomy. Prophylactic antibiotics are also justified for operations with a lower incidence of infection when the consequences would be very serious as, for example, for the insertion of orthopaedic and other implants, cardiac surgery and dental procedures in those at risk of endocarditis; the value of such prophylaxis has been established only for joint replacement surgery (Lidwell et al. 1982). Prophylaxis with cephalosporins, which is associated with a very low complication rate, is beneficial for patients undergoing other categories of 'clean' operations. The degree to which this extension of prophylaxis should be encouraged is under debate (Page et al. 1993, Lewis et al. 1995).

The measures customarily taken to establish a safe environment in the operating theatre have been reviewed by Hambraeus and Laurell (1980), and the principles of theatre suite design by Humphreys (1993). Briefly, ventilation is provided with clean filtered air sufficient in volume to suppress as far as possible the air-borne particles produced by human movement, in particular in the region of the operative field. This is far less important in other areas, such as near the floor. The effectiveness of conventional ventilation systems is readily upset by unsatisfactory building design or by undisciplined human activity. Transfer of bacteria from the operating team to the wound is somewhat reduced by the exclusion of staff with clinical infection and by the wearing of clean, frequently changed clothes and an operation gown. However, if the latter is made of conventional fabrics its effectiveness as a barrier to skin micro-organisms is small. Masks to filter or deflect upper respiratory particles

and caps to reduce contamination from the hair should be worn by the immediate surgical team (Dineen and Drusin 1973). Hand-washing with chlorhexidine or iodophor solutions before donning gloves should be careful and thorough but not necessarily prolonged (Larson 1984). Gloves are very commonly perforated during operations, and this may be associated with an increased risk of infection for the patient (e.g. Cruse and Foord 1973) and of blood-borne infection for the surgeon (p. 197) (Palmer and Rickett 1992).

Effective sterilization of surgical instruments, with a large margin of safety (Russell, Hugo and Ayliffe 1992), is now universal, but it was not always so (Howie 1988). Heat-sensitive equipment may give rise to difficulties and the need for a rapid turnover may force the use of less stringent decontamination methods, even for instruments that penetrate tissue.

5.2 The urinary tract

Most hospital-acquired infections of the urinary tract are associated with urethral catheterization. The circumstances under which this is practised are discussed in Chapter 32. Even the single passage of a catheter is associated with a definite, though usually low, infection risk (Kunin 1987). With an indwelling catheter eventual colonization of the bladder is almost inevitable, but it may be considerably delayed by the system of closed drainage, first introduced by Dukes (1929) and developed by Gillespie and others (Gillespie 1956, Miller et al. 1958). The closed system is not interrupted for the taking of urine specimens, and irrigation after operation can be provided without opening the system (Miller et al. 1958).

In spite of closed drainage, bladder colonization nevertheless occurs; it may reach about 10% of patients per day (Kunin and McCormack 1966). The route of infection is not via the lumen of the catheter but between the catheter and the urethral wall. Early infection is by local commensals, such as *E. coli*, coagulase-negative staphylococci and enterococci. Later, more resistant hospital-associated gram-negative bacilli such as *Klebsiella*, *Proteus*, *Serratia*, *Pseudomonas* and *Providencia* spp. may invade, particularly under the selective influence of antibiotics. Restriction of catheterization to cases of absolute necessity, avoidance of prolonged catheterization where possible, and the use of catheters with the narrowest lumen and made of newer improved materials all reduce the risks of infection (Falkiner 1993). Careful passage of the catheter by skilled staff under conditions of strict asepsis and scrupulous catheter care thereafter are also important (Falkiner 1993). Much attention has been given to the use of disinfectants in preventing infection (Stickler and Chawla 1987). Chlorhexidine may usefully be included in the local anaesthetic applied to the urethra, or used as an initial 'flush' after the catheter has been passed. Chlorhexidine irrigations reduce the colonization rate (Kirk et al. 1979) but the prolonged application of chlorhexidine may damage the bladder mucosa. Little evidence supports the use of disinfectants in established infection (Davies et al. 1987) or in the long-term protection of indwelling catheters (Stickler and Chawla 1987). Periurethral disinfection, beyond simple toilet, has not been shown to be beneficial (Burke et al. 1983), nor has the inclusion of disinfectants in the catheter-drainage bag (Gillespie et al. 1983). They may, however, prevent the spread of resistant strains of bacteria (Noy, Smith and Watterson 1982), presumably via the hands of those who empty the drainage bags; such spread is better avoided by an improved nursing regimen. The bacteria that cause urinary tract infection are variably sensitive to the antiseptics that can be used in contact with tissues (Hammond, Morgan and Russell 1987), especially when the bacteria are present in biofilm on the surface of the bladder (Stickler, Clayton and Chawla 1987). It has been suggested but not proved that extensive use of chlorhexidine may account for the spread of relatively resistant gram-negative bacilli in certain hospital departments (Dance et al. 1987).

The presence of bladder bacteriuria is benign and symptomless in many patients, but its subtle long-term effects have not been studied, and upper tract infection may itself be silent. There is no doubt that urinary infection prolongs hospital stay and worsens the prognosis (Jepsen et al. 1982). The prevalence of hospital-acquired urinary infection was lower in a recent study in the UK and Ireland when compared with 1980 (Emmerson et al. 1996) and this may reflect improved practice and catheter care. A proportion of patients develop pyelonephritis and other complications, such as epididymo-orchitis. Urinary tract infection is one of the commonest causes of bacteraemia in hospital (see p. 205); it frequently follows urethral procedures (catheter passing, catheter removal, cystoscopy, transurethral prostatectomy) in patients with colonized urine and may lead to septicaemia and even death. Thus, perioperative bacteraemia was demonstrated by Murphy et al. (1984) in 60% of patients with infected urine undergoing urethral operations and, in similar patients in the same hospital, Cafferkey et al. (1982) recorded 6% of clinical septicaemia arising in these circumstances. Of 31 patients with postoperative septicaemia investigated by Cafferkey et al. (1980), 8 suffered severe shock and 4 died.

The risk of septicaemia may be avoided by the preoperative or perioperative administration of suitable antibiotics to patients with colonized urine, especially those due to undergo urological procedures such as prostatectomy and bladder resection (Amin 1992). There may also be a case for the administration of antibiotics to patients with sterile urine who have had indwelling catheters for some time, because damage to the urethra may encourage significant passage of bacteria into the bloodstream. In a study of prophylactic ciprofloxacin in carefully selected patients undergoing vaginal repairs there was a reduction in symptomatic and asymptomatic bacteriuria compared with controls (van der Wall et al. 1992) but the long-term implications in terms of cost and the emergence of resistance should be carefully considered before this can be recommended for routine use. Antibiotic

prophylaxis has no place in other situations and treatment of urinary infection in the catheterized should be limited to dealing with clinical illness (Gillespie 1986).

Alternatives to bladder catheterization that may be feasible are suprapubic catheterization, which has in some studies been accompanied by less bladder infection than urethral catheterization, and intermittent catheterization, including self-catheterization, which may be successful in patients with neurogenic bladder disorders (Pearman 1984). When catheterization appears necessary to achieve dryness in incontinent patients, external, condom drainage may be used, or effective incontinence pads may be substituted with success (Nordqvist et al. 1984), with other measures to encourage regular micturition.

5.3 The respiratory tract

Infections of the respiratory tract represent a significant proportion of all hospital-acquired infections. In the recent prevalence study, respiratory tract infection accounted for approximately 25% of hospital infection and was as common as that of the urinary tract (Emmerson et al. 1996). Mortality is between 25 and 35%, but depends on the patient population, the diagnostic approach and whether the mortality rate is crude or takes into account other factors that contribute to a fatal outcome.

A firm diagnosis of pneumonia is not easy to make and it is even more difficult to establish its microbial aetiology. Sputum may be contaminated with bacteria from the upper respiratory tract and cultures may give misleading results. The use of bronchoscopic or alternative non-bronchoscopic approaches in the intensive care unit to obtain representative samples from the lower respiratory tract with quantitation of the organisms isolated is increasingly emphasized (Baselski and Wunderink 1994). The results from brush and lavage specimens correlate with histology even in patients on antimicrobial therapy (Chastre et al. 1995). Bronchoscopy may not, however, always be possible and it requires experience. Non-bronchoscopic lavage, with a catheter inserted through an endotracheal or tracheostomy tube, combined with semi-quantitation, can relatively easily be incorporated into routine practice (Humphreys et al. 1996).

The aetiology of pneumonia varies according to the patient population, diagnostic approaches used, local practices and procedures, and geographical location. Gram-negative bacilli, especially *P. aeruginosa*, and *S. aureus* account for the majority of cases (Dal Nogare 1994) but *S. pneumoniae* may be responsible for up to 20% of nosocomial pneumonia (Berk and Verghese 1989). Resistant enterobacteria, e.g. *Klebsiella*, *Serratia* and *Enterobacter* spp., *P. aeruginosa*, *Acinetobacter* spp. and methicillin-resistant *S. aureus* (MRSA) pose particular difficulties, especially in high dependency areas of hospitals, because of fewer treatment options and the propensity of some of these organisms to spread. For a more general account of the aetiology of pneumonia see Chapter 18.

The general conditions that predispose to pneumonia are similar to those for wound infection: obesity, advanced age and some underlying diseases. The most important factors, however, are respiratory intubation and tracheostomy. Tracheal intubation removes an important barrier to invasion of the lower respiratory tract, and even brief intubation allows oropharyngeal bacteria to pass into the trachea (Nair, Jani and Sanderson 1986). High gastric pH, often induced deliberately to prevent stress ulcers in patients in intensive therapy, encourages overgrowth of potential pathogens that may then pass into the respiratory tract of the intubated patient. It has been suggested that fibronectin is a barrier to colonization by *P. aeruginosa* and that it is breached by the increased protease content of saliva during illness (Woods et al. 1981). Molecular approaches to understanding the pathogenesis of pneumonia reveal a complex interaction between host factors, such as cytokine release, phagocytosis and lymphocyte activation, and virulence determinants of the pathogen, including lipopolysaccharide and bacterial enzymes, such as elastase. For patients in the ICU this is further complicated by other conditions such as the adult respiratory distress syndrome (Meduri and Estes 1995).

Sporadic cases and outbreaks of pneumonia may be associated with contamination of respiratory equipment, such as anaesthetic machines, ventilators, humidifiers, nebulizers, resuscitation equipment and suction catheters (Hovig 1981). Better design of equipment, improved decontamination methods and the use of filters should lessen the importance of these sources. The importance of maintaining respiratory equipment in good order has become better recognized after outbreaks with highly resistant bacteria such as *Acinetobacter* spp. (Vandenbrouke-Grauls et al. 1988, Getchell-White, Donowitz and Gröschel 1989). The causative bacteria may also be spread by indirect hand contact, and from there colonize the oropharynx before causing infection. Antibiotic administration encourages colonization by more resistant gram-negative bacilli.

The above account indicates some of the appropriate preventive measures. These include hand-washing, early removal of nasogastric and endotracheal tubes, maintenance of gastric acidity and elevating the head of the bed to 30° (Dal Nogare 1994). This conventional approach to prevention, with an assessment of which practices have been validated, has been expanded upon elsewhere (Tablan et al. 1994). Nebulized antibiotics for prophylaxis may at first give satisfactory results but later lead to problems with resistant bacteria (Feeley et al. 1975). Selective decontamination of the digestive tract, incorporating the use of topical antimicrobial agents to preserve colonization resistance and the protective effect of normal flora (van der Waaij et al. 1990), has been advocated to reduce ICU-acquired infection, including pneumonia (van Saene, Stoutenbeek and Stoller 1994). The results have, however, been conflicting and have led some to advise against its routine introduction as a preventive measure (Hamer and Barza 1993, Hurley 1995).

Though legionellosis (see section on 'Legionnaires' disease', p. 192) is predominantly community-acquired, nosocomial cases accounted for 15% of cases in England and Wales between 1980 and 1992 (Joseph et al. 1994). Hospital-acquired infection should prompt a search for its source and for active preventive measures, including chemical disinfection, control of circulating water temperature and surveillance (Hoge and Breiman 1991, Joseph et al. 1994). In young children, RSV and at times other viruses, such as enteroviruses, are significant causes of hospital-acquired respiratory infection. Without special precautions, nosocomial acquisition of RSV can be high, and a combination of cohort nursing and the use of gloves and plastic aprons significantly reduces spread (Madge et al. 1992).

5.4 Infection associated with indwelling medical devices

The increasing practice of inserting devices, usually made of various plastics, into the body of patients, and the selection pressure of antibiotics, have shifted the spectrum of significant micro-organisms commonly encountered in diagnostic laboratories.

Almost every type of indwelling device may become colonized. The predominant bacteria are coagulase-negative staphylococci, particularly *S. epidermidis.* Other colonizing organisms are *S. aureus* and other skin organisms such as corynebacteria, including *Corynebacterium jeikeium* (see Volume 2, Chapter 25), propionibacteria, streptococci, many of low-grade pathogenicity, various gram-negative aerobic bacilli, yeasts and filamentous fungi. *S. epidermidis* strains associated with such infections appear to produce greater quantities of extracellular slime than do strains from other sources. The slime binds the bacteria to the polymer surface and interferes with the body's response to infection (Gristina et al. 1993, Jansen and Peters 1993). Some corynebacteria also produce slime (Bayston, Compton and Richards 1994).

The choice of plastic, its modification or the coating of its surface may influence the likelihood of colonization (Sheth et al. 1983, An and Friedman 1996) but no currently available implantable polymers totally resist the adherence of *S. epidermidis.* The incorporation into plastics of antimicrobial substances (antibiotics, disinfectants or metal salts) is promising in experimental systems (Bach et al. 1994, Raad et al. 1995, 1996, An and Friedman 1996). A novel experimental approach to prevent colonization is the production of a small electric current in an intravascular cannula (Liu et al. 1993).

INTRAVASCULAR CANNULAE

Plastic cannulae allow infusions to be given via the same vessel for much longer than do steel needles, but they are also associated with bacterial colonization and resulting infection (Maki, Goldman and Rhame 1973). At first it was recommended that the site of infusion should be changed frequently, but with better materials, better cannula design and careful placement, cannulae such as the Hickman and Broviac catheters may now be left in situ for long periods, albeit with a low but significant infection rate (Darbyshire, Weightman and Speller 1985).

The colonization of intravascular cannulae may remain silent or be associated with a simple fever. However, if it is due to more pathogenic organisms, especially *S. aureus*, it may result in septicaemia or disseminated infection. Even with *S. epidermidis*, metastatic infection, particularly of other prosthetic material, endocarditis or even immune-complex nephritis, such as that associated with cerebrospinal fluid shunts, may occur. The rate of colonization of intravascular cannulae is very variable, depending on the site of cannulation, the fluid infused, the plastic used in the cannula, the design of the cannula and the care to achieve asepsis at insertion. Investigations up to 1973 have been reviewed (Maki et al. 1973). The use of lower limb veins is associated with an increased incidence of infection, as is umbilical cannulation in babies. Solutions for total parenteral nutrition readily support microbial growth and, alone or in admixture with circulating plasma near the cannula, they encourage colonization and a high risk of catheter-related septicaemia (see p. 197). The use of the same line for infusion of blood products and clear fluids, or its use for pressure monitoring and the taking of blood specimens, also increases the colonization rate.

The cuff of the implanted Hickman or Broviac catheter may prevent infection from tracking between catheter and tissues. The importance for cannula colonization of a side port closely related to the cannula is the subject of controversy. Reports of side port colonization are common, but there seems to be no significant difference in the rate of catheter-associated bacteraemia between cannulae with and without side ports (Cheesbrough, Finch and Macfarlane 1984). Careful adherence to instructions for the setting up and care of the infusion reduces the rate of colonization and subsequent infection. The source of colonizing organisms is usually the skin of the patient. Several studies have shown a correlation between micro-organisms on the skin and those recovered from the catheter after removal (e.g. Fuchs 1971). For this reason, careful antiseptic preparation of the skin before cannula insertion, toilet of the area, careful choice of dressings to prevent skin maceration, and the application of antibiotic or antiseptic preparations to the entry site are recommended (e.g. Hill and Casewell 1991). Convincing evidence of the effectiveness of antiseptics is, however, lacking and antibiotic preparations may on occasion encourage the proliferation of *Candida* spp. (Norden 1969). In some circumstances, as with Hickman and Broviac catheters with their cuff and protective tunnel, and other central lines, but also at times with simple peripheral cannulae, contamination of the connections of the cannula with the administration set and other reservoirs appears to be of importance (Sitges-Serra et al. 1983, Cheesbrough, Finch and Macfarlane 1984, Weight-

man et al. 1988). Care with manipulation of the apparatus may be important in cannula colonization, as it is in contamination of fluid in the rest of the system. Occasionally, cannulae are infected by the haematogenous route (Maki et al. 1973). Preventive measures and their success, depends on the postulated entry route for micro-organisms (Weightman et al. 1988, Parras et al. 1994). The route of infection may determine the preponderant site of colonization, whether the micro-organisms are on the outside of the cannula or in the lumen, and thus the best means of culturing the cannula tip after its removal. The technique devised by Maki, Weise and Sarafin (1977) for peripheral cannulae may not be as suitable for central lines. Catheter colonization may be detected in lines already being used for the taking of blood, by comparing the microbial count of a specimen of blood taken through the cannula with one from a distant vein; a simple pour-plate method will suffice (Weightman et al. 1988). It has been stated that colonized cannulae should be removed (Eykyn 1984, Jansen and Peters 1993) but in the case of Hickman and Broviac catheters, antibiotics, such as vancomycin for *S. epidermidis* (Elliott 1988), may eradicate the bacteria or suppress them sufficiently to prevent recurrence of the clinical problem (Weightman et al. 1988).

INTRAVASCULAR GRAFTS

A similar spectrum of micro-organisms is seen in infected cardiac valve prostheses and patches of polymers, and grafts in vessels (Liekweg and Greenfield 1977). This may be influenced by the antibiotic prophylaxis in use, because this may alter the flora of patients and hospital staff (Archer and Armstrong 1983).

Endocarditis on prosthetic valves may be caused by micro-organisms implanted at the time of operation or soon afterwards (Marples et al. 1978) when many intravascular lines are in situ and the graft has not yet become endothelialized. It may follow sternal-wound infection (Braimbridge and Eykyn 1987) or it may arise later from haematogenous seeding, as happens with diseased natural valves. This latter gives a microbial spectrum close to that seen in infections of natural valves (Heimberger and Duma 1989). Though the incidence of early prosthetic valve endocarditis is now less than 1%, the mortality is high. Perioperative infection may manifest after a delay and the various types of endocarditis cannot be separated by an arbitrary time after the operation (Braimbridge and Eykyn 1987, Freeman 1995). An incidence in the first year of 1.4–3.0% has been calculated (Karchmer 1991). Reliance should be placed on general measures to prevent perioperative infection and on antibiotic prophylaxis at critical times when bacteraemia is likely (Karchmer 1991).

JOINT PROSTHESES

Infection of total joint replacements is a very serious and costly complication (Strachan 1993, An and Friedman 1996). As techniques have improved, the incidence has fallen from c. 12% to less than 2% for hip replacements and from c. 15% to less than 4% for knee replacements. The effects of ultra-clean air and of prophylactic antibiotics on the incidence of infection have been discussed above (p. 192). In addition to the use of systemic antibiotics, incorporation of antibiotics in the bone cement is now standard practice for revision operations and is used by some in primary operations. Gentamicin may be used or a heat-stable antibiotic can be chosen to correspond to known infecting strains (Strachan 1993). The spectrum of infecting bacteria (An and Friedman 1996) is dominated by *S. aureus* and coagulase-negative staphylococci, with smaller numbers of enterobacteria and other gram-negative bacilli. The prognosis of infections with gram-negative organisms is worse after reoperation than infections with gram-positive organisms (Buchholz et al. 1981). Fungal infection is rare. Some recent series have shown increased numbers of streptococci (especially of enterococci) and of anaerobic cocci. Infection of a joint prosthesis almost always requires its removal, with replacement as a one- or 2-stage procedure, under local and general antibiotic cover. Occasionally, with a low-grade pathogen sensitive to oral antibiotics infecting a stable joint, medical treatment may succeed, but this form of management should rarely be undertaken as it is beset with complications.

Cerebrospinal fluid shunts

In ventriculoatrial or ventriculoperitoneal shunts, infection may give rise to systemic illness from bacteraemia, to ventriculitis or to shunt blockage. *S. epidermidis* is by far the most common infecting agent (Ersahin, Mutluer and Guzelbag 1994). As in the case of cannula infections, there may be a long lag between colonization and clinical illness. Most infecting organisms are probably implanted in the tissues at the time of operation (Pople, Bayston and Hayward 1992) but other routes may occasionally be followed (Price 1984, Ronan, Hogg and Klug 1995). These infections are managed by a combination of surgical management, including shunt removal, and chemotherapy (Bayston 1985, Walters 1992). There is no consensus about the benefits of prophylactic antibiotic use in shunt insertion (Brown 1993) but a meta-analysis suggests a statistically significant advantage (Haines and Walters 1994).

5.5 **Bacteraemia**

Although bacteraemia is not the most common hospital-acquired infection, or the most significant in adding to costs, it is of greatest importance as a cause of serious illness and death. Extensive studies in the USA have reported hospital-acquired bacteraemia in 0.2–0.4% of hospital admissions; these account for about half the total bacteraemias observed. Much higher rates have been reported for tertiary referral centres than for general hospitals (Bryan et al. 1986).

The micro-organisms that cause hospital-acquired bacteraemia and the circumstances in which they do this are fully discussed in Chapter 16. Briefly, the infecting organism may arise from a focus of infection in another system (secondary bacteraemia) or no source may be identified clinically or after additional investigations such as ultrasound (primary bacteraemia). The organisms isolated and their resistance to antibiotics to a large extent reflect those prevailing in the hospital. In a study conducted in a UK tertiary referral centre, *E. coli* was the commonest cause and accounted for 27% of cases, followed by other enterobacteria and *S. aureus* (11%); polymicrobial bacteraemia was responsible for 7% of cases (Ispahani, Pearson and Greenwood 1987). Between 1980 and 1992, the crude bacteraemia rate in a US centre increased from 6.7 to 18.4 per 1000 patient discharges and a considerable proportion of this increase was due to gram-positive cocci (Pittet and Wenzel 1995). An increasing proportion of bloodstream infections due to coagulase-negative staphylococci, enterococci and *Candida* has been documented in recent years. This may reflect the changing hospital patient population and the increasing use of invasive devices. Central venous lines and blood transfusion were independent risk factors for hospital-acquired bacteraemia in Australia (Duggan et al. 1993). Coagulase-negative staphylococci are especially important in the paediatric age group (see p. 207) and were responsible for 43% of bacteraemia in Great Ormond Street Hospital, London (Holzel and de Saxe 1992). They were the third most common bloodstream pathogen after group B streptococci and *S. aureus* in a Swedish neonatal unit (Faxelius and Ringertz 1987).

The increasing proportion of bacteraemia due to gram-positive bacteria is seen in immunocompromised patients who may require an in situ intravascular device for a long period and for whom repeated courses of broad spectrum antimicrobial agents are often necessary. Viridans streptococcal bacteraemia in neutropenic patients is associated with chemotherapy-induced mucositis as shown by the finding that blood and oral isolates were indistinguishable by ribotyping (Richard et al. 1995). Enterococcal bacteraemia, especially that due to *Enterococcus faecium*, is closely linked with the presence of cancer, neutropenia, renal failure, steroids and recent antibiotics (Noskin, Peterson and Warren 1995). The risk factors for candidaemia are similar but include recent abdominal surgery (Nielsen, Stenderup and Bruun 1991). On the other hand, the incidence of bacteraemia due to *Bacteroides* spp. has declined in many places since the introduction of effective prophylaxis for operations on the large gut (Young 1982).

Clusters of cases may reflect a hospital outbreak of infection. Thus, 9 cases of gram-negative bacteraemia involving different organisms and occurring after open heart surgery were traced to an aqueous disinfectant, used to clean pressure-monitoring equipment that was assembled before surgery and left open and uncovered overnight in the operating theatre (Rudnick et al. 1996). Care must be taken to exclude pseudobacteraemia, due to the contamination of blood culture media or their additives, contaminated skin disinfectants, specimen containers or blood-gas analysers or, in the laboratory, from contaminated apparatus or carriers among the staff (Maki 1980).

Mortality rates depend largely on the age and underlying illnesses of the patients, whether there is a removable or remediable focus of infection, and on the microbial cause. Thus infection with enterobacteria has a worse prognosis than infection with coagulase-negative staphylococci. Polymicrobial bacteraemia also has a poor prognosis. Candidaemia is associated with a mortality of 76% (Nielsen, Stenderup and Bruun 1991), which reflects the severity of underlying disease in such patients. In the intensive care patient with severe sepsis and shock, bacteraemia is associated with a poor outcome but the category of organisms appears to be less important (Brun-Buisson et al. 1995). Recent efforts to develop and use monoclonal antibodies directed against the gram-negative bacterial cell wall or cytokine mediators such as tumour necrosis factor (TNF) in these patients, have been disappointing. A multicentre study in 15 centres revealed that blocking TNF activity with high doses of a competitive inhibitor led to a higher mortality compared with placebo (Fisher et al. 1996). Further work on the pathogenesis of severe sepsis and bacteraemia will be necessary before useful and safe immunomodulatory agents can routinely be used in management.

For bacteraemia resulting from the contamination of intravenous fluids or additives to these, see section on 'Infection from contaminated infusion fluids' (p. 197).

6 HOSPITAL INFECTION AT THE EXTREMES OF LIFE

6.1 Geriatric and long-stay facilities

Hospital infection and infection control in aged patients have been somewhat neglected, but their importance is undeniable. Patients older than 65 years account for a disproportionate number of hospital-acquired infections (Smith 1988). The relative frequency of infection at different sites depends, for example, on whether simple colonization of the bladder or of an ulcer is included, but the 3 most frequently infected systems are the respiratory tract, the urinary tract and the skin. The last is more common in long-stay units (Darnowski, Gordon and Simor 1991, Jackson et al. 1992) than in acute geriatric units (Hussain et al. 1996).

Particular difficulties may be the declining defences and multiple underlying chronic diseases in the patients and, in some long-stay hospitals, a lack of facilities, including isolation facilities, low staffing levels and a comparative lack of access to medical assessment. Patients may be ambulant and have poor hygienic practices, and there may be close contact among patients. This may result in the spread of infections, such as adenovirus conjunctivitis, ringworm, scabies, etc., not seen in acute units. Chronic infections, such as tuberculosis, may spread insidiously. Carriage of MRSA may cause more severe problems when patients are transferred to surgical units or other services with vulnerable patients than in the geriatric unit itself (Combined Working Party of the British Society for Antimicrobial Chemotherapy and the Hospital Infection Society 1995). Infections in nursing homes have been reviewed by Nicolle, Strausbaugh and Garibaldi (1996).

Long-term indwelling urethral catheters are common in the elderly. Most surveys have shown a high prevalence of bacteriuria due to a number of different species. The most common are of *Proteus* or *Providencia* spp. rather than *E. coli* (Standfast et al. 1984, Lee et al. 1992). The clinical significance of most of this bacteriuria may be doubted (Jewes et al. 1988).

Nosocomial pneumonia in the elderly resembles, in aetiology and in risk factors such as tracheal intubation, that in younger age groups, but it is associated with malnutrition and neuromuscular disease and has a particularly poor prognosis (Craven et al. 1992, Hanson, Weber and Rutala 1992, Woodhead 1994). Infection by respiratory viruses, including influenza A, is common and may cause serious illness and death.

The grave consequences of salmonella infection in aged patients have been reported frequently (e.g. Committee of Inquiry 1986). Clusters of cases of diarrhoeal disease are common; when an aetiological agent is identified it is frequently a Norwalk-like virus (Stevenson et al. 1994, Augustin et al. 1995) but rotavirus outbreaks have also been reported (Holzel and Cubitt 1982).

6.2 Neonatal units

Intrauterine and perinatal infections of maternal origin, such as rubella, listeriosis, group B streptococci infection, candidiasis and infection by HIV will not be considered here. However, many of these agents may, occasionally, be spread among babies via staff or equipment.

Unlike well-baby nurseries, the prevalence of infection may exceed 20% in neonatal intensive therapy units, and on this there may be superimposed outbreaks of infection by particularly virulent and usually antibiotic-resistant strains. The babies in these units, particularly when premature, have undeveloped defences and lack a normal flora. Ill babies require much handling by staff, and it is therefore difficult to prevent the spread by contact of infection from one to another.

Infection with *S. aureus* was the main concern in the 1950s. Babies in nurseries for the newborn were regularly colonized and some developed septic skin lesions of varying severity that sometimes progressed to fatal generalized infections. The causative staphylococci showed considerable differences in virulence. The problem was ameliorated by standard infection control measures, early discharge of healthy babies from hospital and prophylactic use of topical hexachlorophane (Alder et al. 1980). Withdrawal of hexachlorophane after overdosing had been shown to give rise to neurological damage was followed by a recrudescence of staphylococcal infections (De Souza et al.

1975, Allen, Ridgway and Parsons 1994). The neonatal unit has often been a focus of infection by MRSA (Reboli, John and Levkoff 1989, Tam and Yeung 1988). In neonatal intensive therapy units there may occasionally be outbreaks of infection by enterobacteria such as *Klebsiella, Serratia* spp. and *P. aeruginosa*, sometimes resistant to many antimicrobial agents and with ability to spread rapidly and cause serious illness (Davies and Bullock 1981, Lewis et al. 1983, Coovadia et al. 1992). Colonization by such bacteria without infection is very common. Routine monitoring of carriage sites contributes little to preventing illness (Jolley 1993) but may help in formulating a rational policy for antibiotic prescribing. Surveillance is better directed towards identifying strains with the potential to spread widely and cause serious illness (Goldmann 1988).

In recent years *S. epidermidis* or other coagulase-negative staphylococci have been the most frequent cause of infection in many neonatal units (Thompson et al. 1992, Nataro and Corcoran 1994). Such infections are generally more benign than those due to gram-negative aerobic bacilli. The reason for their current prevalence is unknown, but may partly reside in their resistance to commonly used antibiotics and the increased use of intravascular cannulae and respiratory apparatus. Some strains spread within a unit, but there is no evidence of the emergence of particularly virulent or transmissible strains of coagulase-negative staphylococci. Indeed, several different strains may simultaneously infect a single patient (Simpson et al. 1986, Kacica et al. 1994).

Necrotizing enterocolitis has increased in incidence in recent years and has features, such as clustering of cases, that suggest an infective aetiology; at times tightening of infection control procedures appeared to abort an outbreak (Willoughby and Pickering 1994). However, attempts to demonstrate a specific microbial cause have been unsuccessful (de Louvois 1986, Gupta et al. 1994).

Outbreaks of virus infection in neonatal units can be serious and difficult to control. Enteroviruses such as echovirus 11 (Nagington et al. 1978), adenovirus 7 (Finn et al. 1988) or adenovirus 8 (Piedra et al. 1992), rotaviruses (Holzel and Cubitt 1982) and RSV (Hall et al. 1979) may be responsible. *Candida* spp. may on occasion cause cross-infection in neonatal units (Finkelstein et al. 1993, Reagan et al. 1995).

7 THE ROLE OF INDIVIDUAL PATHOGENS

7.1 *Staphylococcus aureus*

This organism has probably always been an important cause of hospital-acquired infection but it was first seriously investigated in the early years of the antibiotic era (see Williams et al. 1960). Certain strains that could be identified by phage typing (see Volume 2, Chapter 27) and were resistant to penicillin, and often also to other antibiotics, became prevalent in hospi-

tals. Some of these multi-resistant strains were exceptionally virulent, able to cause severe infections in otherwise healthy persons and to colonize widely. These so-called 'epidemic strains' caused many outbreaks of skin sepsis, most notably in the postnatal period, and were the main cause of postoperative wound infection in the 1950s (Shanson 1981).

During the 1960s, hospital-acquired infection by multi-resistant strains became progressively less common (Ayliffe, Lilly and Lowbury 1979). MRSA strains (see Chapter 14 and Volume 2, Chapter 27) were recognized at this time but they seldom spread widely. In the late 1970s, however, strains that were methicillin-resistant and often also resistant to aminoglycosides became prevalent in many parts of the world and have subsequently spread widely in hospitals. Patients particularly affected are those in hospital for prolonged periods, elderly or debilitated patients, those with wounds or burns, and those who have had recent treatment with antibiotics (Brumfitt and Hamilton-Miller 1989). Clinical and laboratory evidence suggests that MRSA are not less virulent than sensitive isolates (French et al. 1990) and in severely ill patients under intensive care, mortality from pneumonia may be high (Rello et al. 1994). The financial impact of MRSA is increasingly recognized (Casewell 1995); the additional measures necessary to control an outbreak with a new epidemic strain that involved over 400 patients in England amounted to £400 000 (Cox et al. 1995).

Control of epidemic MRSA strains in hospital can be difficult and failure to eradicate them has led some hospitals to accept their presence (King and Harvey 1985). Measures recommended to control spread (Combined Working Party of the Hospital Infection Society and the British Society for Antimicrobial Chemotherapy 1990) may not take account of the practical difficulties that follow when MRSA becomes endemic in a clinical facility. These include difficulties in identifying the index case, and the impact of ward closures and severe disruption of clinical services (Barrett, Teare and Sage 1993). However, incisive measures taken early may be successful, especially when combined with effective surveillance in high dependency areas (Hartstein et al. 1995). Control measures include early detection of strains carried by patients and staff and sampling of lesions from carriage sites by selective methods, including enrichment cultures (Combined Working Party of the Hospital Infection Society and the British Society for Antimicrobial Chemotherapy 1990, Ayliffe 1996). Recognition of epidemic strains may be assisted by noting the origin of the patient, the clinical illness, the type of infected lesion, the antibiotic-sensitivity pattern, and phage type. Collecting this information and the use of a simple computerized database can provide useful information on local epidemiology (Rossney, Pomeroy and Keane 1994). The complexity of strains isolated and the presence of phage non-typable strains means that a combination of phenotypic and genotypic typing methods (see section 9.2, p. 216) is now often required to determine source and spread (Tenover et al. 1994).

Colonized or infected patients should be treated in isolation, preferably in a single room or designated isolation facility, with precautions against both contact and aerial spread. Contaminated environmental surfaces may be a source for continuation of an outbreak. When large numbers of patients are involved, cohort nursing in separate areas of the hospital may be necessary; but control may be impossible without a dedicated isolation unit (Pearman et al. 1985). Mupirocin seems particularly effective in eliminating carriage (Casewell and Hill 1986) but resistance to this agent has emerged and is related to prolonged or repeated use in MRSA patients and patients with chronic skin disease (Cookson 1990). Carriage may be unresponsive to a variety of antiseptics and increasing numbers of carriers are found in non-acute units and in the community.

7.2 *Enterococcus* spp.

Recent interest in *Enterococcus* spp. as hospital pathogens has focused on unusually antibiotic-resistant strains of *Enterococcus faecium* and *Enterococcus faecalis*. Resistance may be multiple and include high-level resistance to penicillins and to aminoglycosides, such as gentamicin, which are important in providing synergistic bactericidal combinations with penicillins. They may also be resistant to glycopeptides such as vancomycin, which had been regarded as universally active against gram-positive bacteria that may infect humans, apart from intrinsically resistant genera of minor importance such as *Pediococcus*, *Leuconostoc* and *Lactobacillus* (Woodford et al. 1995).

Resistance to vancomycin in enterococci was first reported in a cluster of hospital-acquired infections in the UK (George et al. 1989) and such strains are increasingly found in oncology, renal, transplant and intensive care units (Hospital Infection Control Practices Advisory Committee 1995). The epidemiology of resistant enterococci is not entirely clear; treatment, particularly with cephalosporins and glycopeptides, may encourage colonization with enterocccci, which may then spread from patient to patient by indirect contact, via staff and environment, and thus cause persistent problems.

For epidemiological purposes, enterococci may be typed by ribotyping, but pulsed field gel electrophoresis is more discriminating. The strains are heterogeneous but the evidence suggests that particular epidemiological types spread between hospitals (Chadwick, Chadwick and Oppenheim 1996, Morrison, Woodford and Cookson 1996). Guidelines for the prevention of spread have been issued in the USA (Hospital Infection Control Practices Advisory Committee 1995) and discussed in the UK (Chadwick, Chadwick and Oppenheim 1996). These guidelines are similar to those for the control of MRSA (see above).

7.3 *Clostridium difficile*

C. difficile has emerged during the last decade as a significant hospital-acquired pathogen. It was recognized in the late 1970s as the main cause of antibiotic-associated diarrhoea, which may be associated with pseudomembraneous colitis (PMC) (Chapter 35). The number of laboratory reports of *C. difficile* infection sent to the UK Communicable Disease Surveillance Centre increased 10-fold between 1982 and 1991 (Joint DH/PHLS Working Group 1994). *C. difficile* may be part of the normal bowel flora, especially in the elderly, and may also be recovered from the hospital environment. Antibiotics, especially broad spectrum agents, disrupt the normal bowel flora and render patients susceptible to colonization. *C. difficile* rarely if ever affects health care personnel and spread from patient to staff is unusual.

The increasing numbers of elderly and debilitated patients admitted to hospitals, the misuse of antimicrobial agents and changes in health care, including greater diagnostic and therapeutic interventions, have all probably contributed to the increased colonization with *C. difficile*. Whilst most cases are sporadic, clusters or outbreaks also occur. In the UK, a large outbreak involving 175 patients occurred in 3 hospitals in Manchester in 1992. Most of the patients were over 60 years old and infection was believed to have contributed to 17 deaths (Cartmill et al. 1994). In smaller outbreaks or clusters, epidemiological evidence usually suggests a traceable chain of person-to-person spread between wards or hospitals (Nolan et al. 1987). Apart from significant morbidity and mortality in an already vulnerable population, management and control of this condition have significant financial implications. In a case-control study it was calculated that 94% of the additional costs associated with *C. difficile* infection were due to increased duration of hospital stay and the total cost was in excess of £4000 per case (Wilcox et al. 1996).

Even before the advent of newer typing techniques, clinical and epidemiological evidence suggested that patient-to-patient spread occurred by the faecal–oral route and that precautions were necessary to prevent spread. More than 20% of patients may carry *C. difficile* at some stage during hospitalization, especially if they share a room with a positive patient, and environmental and patient isolates are often indistinguishable (McFarland et al. 1989, Samore et al. 1996). Control measures should be aimed at minimizing the risk of antibiotic-associated diarrhoea by good antimicrobial prescribing, scrupulous hand-washing, the isolation or cohorting of affected patients, treatment of persistently symptomatic patients, careful disposal of contaminated laundry and, finally, environmental disinfection/decontamination (Joint DH/PHLS Working Group 1994, Gerding et al. 1995). Further research is necessary to assess the role of asymptomatic carriers in spread, especially amongst the elderly, to determine whether particular strains are more likely to cause symptoms or spread more rapidly, to clarify whether environmental disinfection with, for example hypochlorite, significantly reduces spread as compared with simple cleaning, and to improve understanding of how and when spread of *C. difficile* occurs between patients in hospital.

7.4 Enterobacteriaceae

E. coli is one of the most frequently encountered bacteria in hospital-acquired infection (Jarvis and Martone 1992). It causes urinary tract infection (Chapter 32), intra-abdominal and gut-related wound infection and bacteraemia (Chapter 16), but infection is almost always endogenous and sporadic; even resistant strains appear seldom to spread between hospital patients (Hart 1982). However, cross-infection by strains with the potential to cause enteric infection, including verocytotoxin-producing *E. coli* strains, is common in hospitals and other health care facilities (Carter, Borczyk and Carlson 1987, Kohli et al. 1994).

Other Enterobacteriaceae are more important in the spread of non-enteric infection in hospitals. This is due to antibiotic resistance, transmissibility and virulence, which interact in hospital units that accumulate patients with similar medical problems who undergo similar procedures and receive similar antibiotics. For example, *Klebsiella* spp. have come into prominence in outbreaks caused by multi-resistant strains that produce extended spectrum β-lactamases (see Volume 2, Chapter 42) (Johnson et al. 1992, Meyer et al. 1993, Quinn 1994). Ease of transmission from patient to patient, resulting in large-scale epidemics and inter-ward spread rather than small clusters of infections or common-source outbreaks, may be related to better survival on hands (Casewell and Desai 1983) or on inanimate surfaces (Hart, Gibson and Buckles 1981), but other factors must be involved (Fryklund, Tullus and Burman 1995). The characteristics of hospital infection by members of the various enterobacterial genera are outlined in Table 13.1. Infection by *Salmonella* spp. has been mentioned under infection transmitted by food (p. 193).

7.5 *Pseudomonas aeruginosa*

P. aeruginosa has been recognized as a pathogen of hospital patients only in the modern era of intensive treatment and antibiotic administration. Its ability to grow in moist conditions with simple nutrients and its comparative resistance to antibiotics and disinfectants have allowed it to become established, often in very large numbers, in fluids and wet places in the hospital and to colonize the mucous membranes and skin of patients. Respiratory infection in intensive therapy units, and infection of burns, in neonates, in abdominal surgery and after trauma, are among the most characteristic presentations, but cases may be encountered in any acute hospital unit.

Strains of *P. aeruginosa* can be distinguished by serotyping, pyocine typing, phage typing (see Volume 2, Chapter 47) and by genotypic methods. Strains may differ markedly in virulence and some epidemics are caused by particularly virulent strains or by exposure of a sensitive body site, such as the eye, to heavily contaminated fluids or apparatus. Mostly, however, infections are endemic or sporadic, and colonization is more common than clinical disease. Indeed, in some hospital units clinical infection may be rare, though colonization may be almost universal. It may, therefore, be difficult to interpret the significance of the isolation of *P. aeruginosa* from patients' specimens (Davies and Bullock 1981).

Normal subjects may carry *P. aeruginosa* in their bowel. The apparent prevalence depends on the sensitivity of isolation methods (Shooter et al. 1966) and antibiotic treatment encourages such carriage. The importance of strains at inanimate sites in the hospital varies but their spread to patients has been reported (e.g. Doring et al. 1993). Strains found at such sites are, however, often different from those found in the patients (Kropec et al. 1993). Clearly, there is much greater likelihood of infection when the patient comes into close contact with the infected source or object, such as contaminated medicaments, inhalants or splashing from sinks. It is, therefore, essential that medicaments and aqueous disinfectants intended for application to patients are supplied sterile and preferably in single-use portions. Patient-to-patient spread may occur when there is a breakdown in infection control measures, such as failure to disinfect urinals and bedpans and failure of hand hygiene (Lowbury et al. 1970). In these situations rectal and other colonization usually precedes infection.

P. aeruginosa is the most common persistent pathogen in chest infection in cystic fibrosis, but the degree to which cross-colonization occurs in hospital units appears to differ widely.

7.6 *Mycobacterium* spp.

In the past tuberculosis was a serious occupational risk for health care staff. This is no longer the case in most clinical situations where tuberculin testing and immunization, supplemented by selective chest x-ray, are available for staff in contact with patients and those handling pathological material (Joint Tuberculosis Committee of the British Thoracic Society 1994). Nosocomial acquisition of tuberculosis by patients in the developed world is also uncommon. Risk factors for transmission to patients and staff include delayed diagnosis, drug-resistant strains and lapses in administrative, engineering and infection control practices (Menzies et al. 1995). Multidrug-resistant tuberculosis in HIV patients is of increasing concern as presenting a risk to staff and other patients. Previous admission to hospital, failure to isolate positive patients in a single room and the absence of positive pressure ventilation are associated with spread (Pearson et al. 1992).

The risk of infection depends on the infectivity of the primary source, the duration and proximity of the exposure, and the susceptibility of the recipient (George et al. 1986). Infectivity depends on the amount of cough and the concentration of bacteria in the sputum. Thus, '3-smear-negative', culture-positive patients with pulmonary tuberculosis and patients with

Table 13.1   Enterobacteriaceae of importance in hospital infection

Genus[a]	Source and mode of infection	Circumstances of infection	Antibiotic characteristics of hospital strains	References
Escherichia (*E. coli*)	Endogenous; cross-infection uncommon (except enteric infection)	Common (especially urinary, bloodstream)	Ampicillin R common	Volume 2, Chapter 39 (enteric infection Chapter 27); Olesen et al. 1995
Citrobacter (*C. freundii, C. diversus*)	Infrequent, endogenous infection	Bloodstream, etc.	Often multi-R including cephalosporins	Volume 2, Chapter 39; Thurm and Gericke 1994
Klebsiella (*K. pneumoniae, K. oxytoca*)	Endogenous, but cross-infection common, with faecal carriage; transmission via hands	Bloodstream, urinary (especially catheterized), respiratory; ICUs especially neonatal, urological units	Ampicillin R; frequently aminoglycoside R; increasingly R to newer cephalosporins	Volume 2, Chapter 39; Johnson et al. 1992, Meyer et al. 1993, Quinn 1994
Serratia (non-pigmented *S. marcescens*)	Cross-infection common, also environmental sources implicated; skin, throat carriage, but faecal carriage less common; hand spread	Urinary, respiratory; ICUs, especially neonatal	R to ampicillin, early cephalosporins; frequently R to aminoglycosides and newer cephalosporins; emergent R during treatment; characteristic polymyxin R	Volume 2, Chapter 39; Lewis et al. 1983, Coria-Jimenez and Ortiz-Torres 1994, Luzzaro et al. 1995
Enterobacter (*E. cloacae, E. aerogenes*)	Endogenous and hospital infection from common source, e.g. medicaments, food, apparatus; hand spread less common; throat and faecal carriage	Respiratory, urinary, bloodstream; ICUs especially neonatal, burns units	Ampicillin R; frequently R to cephalosporins; emergent R during treatment	Volume 2, Chapter 39; Gaston 1988, Weischer and Kolmos 1992
Proteus (*P. mirabilis, P. vulgaris,* also *Morganella*)	Endogenous and small clusters; faecal carriage	Urinary, bloodstream; ICUs, urological units	Variable (see Volume 2, Chapter 43)ˈ	Volume 2, Chapter 43; Williams et al. 1983, Watanakunakorn and Perni 1994
Providencia (*P. stuartii*)	Endogenous; slow transmission among patients; faecal carriage	Urinary, occasionally other sites; geriatric, paraplegia units; mixed infection with *Proteus* spp. common	Aminoglycoside R common	Volume 2, Chapter 43; Hawkey 1984, Woods and Watanakunakorn 1996

R, resistance or resistant; ICUs, intensive care units.
[a]Only more important species are listed. For *Salmonella* see Chapter 28.

non-pulmonary tuberculosis are usually regarded as non-infective. Sputum infectivity declines rapidly during chemotherapy, including that with rifampicin, with a 99% decline in viability after 2 weeks, but scanty bacteria may survive for much longer (Jindani et al. 1980). Isolation for 2 weeks in a well ventilated side ward, without recirculation of the air to other parts of the hospital, is recommended while patients are infectious (Joint Tuberculosis Committee of the British Thoracic Society 1994). Susceptible individuals are the young and those whose immunity is depressed by disease or treatment. Care should be exercised in the handling of fomites from sputum-positive patients and in protecting highly susceptible patients from exposure (George 1988). This may entail prolonged isolation of smear-positive patients and the segregation of smear-negative or non-pulmonary cases of tuberculosis. Contact tracing should be undertaken after incidents in which staff or patients were exposed to infection (Joint Tuberculosis Committee of the British Thoracic Society 1994). Control measures can halt the transmission of multidrug-resistant strains (Wenger et al. 1995). The use by health care staff of HEPA respirators is expensive, inconvenient and is not believed to be cost-effective (Adal et al. 1994).

Hospital infection, including keratitis and systemic disease, caused by opportunist mycobacteria, such as *Mycobacterium chelonei*, *Mycobacterium gordonae* and *Mycobacterium fortuitum*, has been observed (Watt 1995). Contributory factors are the ability of these mycobacteria to survive and multiply in moist environments, inadequate decontamination procedures, and poor hygienic precautions in renal dialysis, bronchoscopy, hydrotherapy and cardiac surgery units (George 1988). Contamination of specimens by the use of tap water to rinse disinfected bronchoscopes has led to 'pseudo-outbreaks' (Nye et al. 1990). The extent to which cross-infection is responsible for the *Mycobacterium avium* complex infections seen in patients with AIDS (Chapter 7) is unknown. The *M. avium* complex may be recovered from standing water and food sources (Horsburgh 1991) and clusters of cases may therefore reflect acquisition from a common source rather than person-to-person spread.

7.7 Other bacteria

The main features of hospital infection by other bacterial species are given in Table 13.2.

7.8 Viruses

The prevalence of nosocomial viral infection is probably underestimated. Most surveys of hospital-acquired infection concentrate on bacteria and the subclinical nature of many viral illnesses together with limited diagnostic facilities partly explains why viruses do not figure prominently. Viral infections are, however, important in neonatal and paediatric patients and in immunosuppressed patients. In paediatrics, rotavirus may be the commonest individual pathogen encountered.

Community-acquired infection by respiratory syncytial virus is almost universal in children in the early years of life. In hospital this is a particular danger to premature neonates and children with cardiorespiratory abnormalities. Staff and adult patients may be reinfected, with minor respiratory symptoms, but severe disease may occur in the immunodeficient adult. The virus spreads by respiratory secretions entering the eye or nose, with or without an intervening period on surfaces or fomites. The risks of infection may be reduced by a combination of cohort nursing and the wearing of gowns and gloves (Snydman et al. 1988, Madge et al. 1992). Such a proactive approach is made possible by the availability of rapid antigen detection facilities (Editorial 1992). Similar principles apply to control of the childhood exanthemata, when infected patients are admitted to hospital (Breuer and Jeffries 1990). Staff working with pregnant women should be immune to rubella. Apart from classical influenza, influenza virus A can cause a variety of syndromes in hospital patients, including a particularly dangerous form of pneumonia in the elderly. Selective immunization of patients can be helpful and a case can be made for the routine immunization of some health workers (Heimberger et al. 1995).

Viral gastroenteritis is common in neonatal and paediatric units, in general wards and in long-stay accommodation for the elderly (Holzel and Cubitt 1982). Rotavirus is the most frequent causative agent in children. In the elderly, outbreaks of diarrhoea caused by SRSV, such as Norwalk, and other agents, can affect large numbers of patients. Spread occurs via the faecal–oral and probably also via the air-borne routes. Prevention of spread may be achieved by early diagnosis, for example by electron microscopy, and strict precautions that include wearing of aprons and gloves, strict hand-washing routines, availability of separate toilet facilities and restriction on the movement of symptomatic patients and staff caring for them, as well as good communications between hospitals to minimize inadvertent spread (Caul 1994, Rao 1995).

Enterovirus infections, though usually subclinical, are also common in hospitals (Dowsett 1988). Besides hepatitis A, coxsackie A and B and echoviruses may cause generalized febrile infections and meningitis, particularly in the newborn, generalized illness with bowel symptoms in immunodeficient persons, and minor infections in staff. Spread may occur by the oral and respiratory routes and by hands, fomites and such shared facilities as hydrotherapy pools. The same groups of patients are particularly susceptible to the herpes group of viruses. Cytomegalovirus, as well as being transmitted in utero and at birth from mother to baby, may be conveyed in donations of blood or tissue, and infections in the immunosuppressed often result from reactivation. Varicella-zoster may be conveyed by the vesicular exudate or respiratory secretions of patients with chickenpox and, less frequently, zoster. Both diseases necessitate barrier precautions and patients must be segregated from susceptible persons, who may, when appropriate, be protected with immune globulin. This will also protect

Table 13.2   Other bacteria[a] associated with hospital infection

Bacteria	Source and mode of spread	Circumstances of infection	Antibiotic characteristics of hospital strains	References
Gram-positive bacteria				
Coagulase-negative staphylococci	Endogenous; 'hospital' strains by contact, air	Implants; intravascular cannulae; sternal wounds; neonates (see pp. 199, 203, 206)	Variable; often multi-R especially to isoxazolylpenicillins, aminoglycosides; usually S to vancomycin, rifampicin	Chapter 14; Stillman, Wenzel and Donowitz 1987, Patrick et al. 1992
Streptococcus				
S. pyogenes (streptococcus Lancefield group A)	Endogenous; uncommon hospital spread from cases and throat, nose, skin, rectal carriers; contact, air	Wounds, burns, skin lesions; parturient women	Invariably S to benzylpenicillin; variable to erythromycin, tetracycline	Chapter 15; Garrod 1979, Easmon 1984
S. agalactiae (streptococcus Lancefield group B)	Endogenous (faeces, vagina); occasionally contact in neonatal units	Usually congenital in neonates; postpartum infection; skin and soft tissue lesions	Consistently benzylpenpenicillin S	Chapter 15; Easmon 1984, Zangwill et al. 1992
S. pneumoniae	Endogenous; occasionally air spread of more virulent or antibiotic-resistant strains	Pneumonia, etc., in respiratory or general impairment; children	Hospital clusters showing penicillin R or intermediate R and multi-R	Chapter 18; Millar et al. 1994
Other streptococci: viridans or indifferent; *S. anginosus* (syn. *milleri*); β-haemolytic streptococci groups C and G	Endogenous; rarely contact spread	Abdominal surgery; implants; neutropenic patients	May be relatively R to β-lactams	Chapter 15 and Volume 2, Chapter 28, Editorial 1984a, 1985
Corynebacteria (especially *C. jeikeium*)	Endogenous; skin colonization may precede infection	Implants; cannulae; immune impairment; antibiotic treatment	Multiple R; vancomycin S	Chapter 19 and Volume 2, Chapter 25, McGowan 1988
Clostridium				
C. perfringens, etc.	Usually endogenous (faeces); indirect contact spread of enteritic strains	Abdominal surgery; amputations; diabetics: elderly (enteritic)	Benzylpenicillin S	Chapter 35; Lowbury and Lilly 1958, Borriello and Barclay 1986
C. tetani	In the past, environmental and operative materials; now possibly endogenous	Very rare postoperative infection	Benzylpenicillin S	Chapter 36; Parker and Mandal 1984

Table 13.2   Continued

Bacteria	Source and mode of spread	Circumstances of infection	Antibiotic characteristics of hospital strains	References
Bacillus spp.	Environmental; may resist sterilization processes	Opportunistic; soft tissue and occasional systemic infection	Often R to β-lactams	Volume 2, Chapter 31; Weber and Rutala 1988
Rhodococcus equi	Unknown, possibly by air from soil, etc.	Pneumonia, etc. in immunocompromised, e.g. HIV infection		Volume 2, Chapter 25; Verville et al. 1994
Nocardia asteroides	Inanimate environment; possibly air-borne spread from cases	Respiratory tract infection; immunosuppression		Chapters 39 and Volume 2, Chapter 20; Houang et al. 1980, Javaly, Horowitz and Wormser 1992
Gram-negative bacteria				
Pseudomonas spp. and similar 'environmental' gram-negative bacilli	Water; damp areas; liquid medicaments; moist equipment; faecal carriage; direct and indirect contact (hands)	Colonization more frequent than infection. Chronic disease; renal failure; immune impairment; major surgery; burns; broad spectrum antibiotic treatment; neonates; implants; cannulae; catheters; respiratory equipment	Often multi-R	Volume 2, Chapters 46 and 47
Burkholderia (*Pseudomonas*) *cepacia*	Unsterilized aqueous solutions, e.g. disinfectants; nebulisers; patient-to-patient infection, probably air-borne	Various from solutions; late infection in cystic fibrosis	Often R to all classes	Volume 2, Chapter 47; Pankhurst and Philpott-Howard 1996
Stenotrophomonas (*Xanthomonas*) **maltophilia**	Multiple epidemiological types; source and spread not clear	Bacteraemia; device-related infections; broad spectrum antibiotics, including penems	Multi-R; characteristic R to penems	Vartivarian et al. 1994, Laing et al. 1995, Gerner-Smidt et al. 1995, Spencer 1995
Acinetobacter spp. (*A. baumannii*, *A. calcoaceticus*)	Endogenous; also indirect contact staff and equipment	Bacteraemia; respiratory infection; ICUs; broad spectrum antibiotics	Increasingly multi-R	Bergogne-Berezin 1995, Mulin et al. 1995, Seifert, Strate and Pulverer 1995
Achromobacter xylosoxidans		Uncommon bacteraemia, respiratory infection	Aminoglycoside R and trimethoprim S typical	Schoch and Cunha 1988, Legrand and Anaissie 1992

Table 13.2 Continued

Bacteria	Source and mode of spread	Circumstances of infection	Antibiotic characteristics of hospital strains	References
Flavobacterium spp.		*F. meningosepticum* associated with infantile meningitis; others as *Pseudomonas* spp.	Often S to some antibiotics usually thought of as 'anti-gram-positive'	Ratner 1984
Aeromonas spp.		Bacteraemia; soft tissue infection; outbreaks and invasive infection uncommon. Toxigenic strains may be enteritic		Mellersh, Norman and Smith 1984, Murphy et al. 1995
Capnocytophaga spp.	Endogenous; usually from oropharynx	Bacteraemia; immunosuppression, neutropenia	Aminoglycoside and trimethoprim R, β-lactam S typical	Volume 2, Chapter 58; Hawkey et al. 1984, Kristensen et al. 1995

S, sensitivity; R, resistance.
[a]Other than anaerobic gram-negative bacilli (Chapter 38), *Legionella* spp. (p. 192 and Chapter 18 and Volume 2, Chapter 49), *S. aureus* (p. 207 and Chapter 14), *Enterococcus* spp. (p. 208 and Volume 2, Chapter 29), *C. difficile* (p. 208 and Chapter 35), *Mycobacterium* spp. (p. 209 and Chapter 22) and *P. aeruginosa* (p. 209 and Volume 2, Chapter 47).

health care staff, of whom approximately 15% may not be immune. A register of staff immunity may be useful, especially in clinical areas where varicella infection may be more common such as paediatric wards (Breuer and Jeffries 1990). Herpetic whitlows occasionally develop in staff not protected from exposure to the respiratory secretions of patients.

Viral haemorrhagic fevers such as Lassa, Marburg and Ebola, have been responsible for infections of hospital staff and patients in tropical countries where equipment and staffing are inadequate and medical practice poor (Fisher-Hoch et al. 1995). In developed countries, a high index of suspicion and early transfer to a specialist unit are essential to reduce the chances of spread within hospital. Blood-borne infection by inoculation presents the greatest risk. Strict isolation in a secure unit should be imposed if viral haemorrhagic fever is suspected (Department of Health and Social Security and Welsh Office 1986).

For other blood-borne viruses (hepatitis B and C and HIV) see p. 196.

The control and prevention of viral infection amongst hospital staff is best managed by occupational health departments, by staff screening, immunization and education programmes, preferably working in tandem with infection control personnel.

7.9 Fungi and protozoa

Fungal infection continues to increase in hospitals (Pfaller and Wenzel 1992), as more effective and broader spectrum antibacterial agents and immunosuppressive regimens are deployed and increase the number of patients at risk (see Chapter 7). The commonest significant fungal isolate is *Candida albicans*, a bowel commensal that in most cases gives rise to endogenous infection. Members of other species, such as *Candida tropicalis*, *Candida parapsilosis*, *Candida krusei* and *Candida glabrata*, are becoming more common. Their source is particularly associated with the skin, and therefore with intravascular cannulae. Less common fungi such as *Fusarium* and *Trichosporon beigelii* are emerging causes of infection in cancer and bone marrow transplant recipients (Pfaller and Wenzel 1992). Clusters of infections with the same strain of *Candida*, with evidence of colonization of the hands of staff may occur under selective pressure from broad spectrum antibiotics (Burnie et al. 1985). Typing of *C. albicans* for epidemiological purposes is difficult. Phenotypic typing such as biotyping may be useful but DNA-based approaches are likely to be increasingly used. *Aspergillus* infection is related to the air-borne spread of spores, particularly when these reach high concentrations, as during building repairs near patients with neutropenia (Rogers and Barnes 1988; see p. 191) and occasionally other vulnerable groups such as ICU patients (Humphreys et al. 1991). Molecular typing techniques allow the comparison of isolates from patients and the environment (Leenders et al. 1996). Clusters of infections due to non-*A. fumigatus* may indicate an environmental source (Loudon et al. 1996). Strategies for the prevention of aspergillus infection include pre-emptive antifungal therapy; isolation of especially vulnerable patients in laminar flow ventilated facilities has been recommended.

There is no good evidence for the hospital spread

of *Cryptococcus neoformans*. Phycomycetes may be transmitted to susceptible patients by dressings (Gartenberg et al. 1978; see p. 195) or by air (del Palacio Hernanz et al. 1983). Dermatophytes occasionally spread in geriatric units by close contact, or on clothing or apparatus (Peachey and English 1974).

The epidemiology of *Pneumocystis carinii* is obscure. Dormant infection has been said to be ubiquitous and reactivated by immune suppression, as may be infection by *Toxoplasma gondii*. On the other hand, airborne spread of *P. carinii* can be shown in animals and there have been suggestions of clusters of linked cases (Rhame et al. 1984, Haron et al. 1988).

Cryptosporidium, a coccidian protozoon, is an important cause of debilitating diarrhoea in the immunosuppressed, such as AIDS patients (Goodgame 1996). The oocysts are comparatively resistant to disinfection and may survive well in the inanimate environment. There is evidence of case-to-case spread and of transmission to staff and to other patients, in hospitals (Martino et al. 1988), presumably by the faecal–oral route. A nosocomial outbreak in Denmark was linked to a ward ice machine (Ravn et al. 1991).

Scabies can be very disruptive in chronic institutions or hospital wards for the elderly (Holness, DeKoven and Nethercott 1992). Infestation in patients with underlying skin disease or Norwegian scabies (extensive hyperkeratotic lesions) are especially contagious (Moberg, Löwhagen and Hersle 1984). Early and reliable diagnosis, effective treatment, for example with permethrin, applied extensively to the body, and decontamination of bed linen and fomites are important to limit spread.

8 ANTIBIOTIC USE AND ANTIBIOTIC RESISTANCE IN HOSPITALS

Antibiotic treatment and hospital infection control are intimately entwined. The use of antibiotics, although not the only influence, has altered the prevailing pathogens in hospital infection; *S. pyogenes* was almost banished and, later, resistant gram-negative bacilli replaced *S. aureus*. Then gram-positive bacteria *S. aureus*, coagulase-negative staphylococci, enterococci, certain corynebacteria and *C. difficile* re-emerged. The emergence of resistant gram-negative bacteria, such as *Klebsiella* spp. with extended spectrum β-lactamases, *Stenotrophomonas maltophilia* and *Acinetobacter baumannii*, has occupied much attention recently. Changes in hospital practice may favour particular pathogens irrespective of their susceptibility to antibiotics. An example is the association of coagulase-negative staphylococci of varied antibiotic sensitivity with prostheses and cannulae. The availability of antibiotics has allowed the development of modern medical treatment, for example major surgery and the use of immunosupression, associated with new infection risks and a new range of pathogens.

Antibiotic resistance may increase the impact of hospital infection that would otherwise be of small importance and may necessitate a change to less satisfactory and more expensive antibiotics. It also appears to worsen the prognosis of infection (Hart 1982, Holmberg, Solomon and Blake 1987, French et al. 1990). On occasion it may exclude the possibility of using antibiotics to remove the source of infection in an outbreak. Hospital infection control measures, such as isolation, are extremely important in preventing the spread of resistant bacteria.

The development of multiple resistance in hospital pathogens, without the prospect of new antibiotics to deal with them, is alarming. There have been reports of infection by strains resistant to all established antibiotics (Murray 1991, Tomasz 1994), accounts of untoward failures of treatment (Armstrong et al. 1995) and trends towards resistance to agents favoured for treatment and prophylaxis, such as the late generation cephalosporins and the fluoroquinolones (Burwen, Banerjee and Gaynes 1994, Jones et al. 1994, Goldstein and Acar 1995). It has been suggested that the end of the antibiotic era may be near, or that the safety of some forms of hospital treatment may be severely compromised (Kunin 1993, Tomasz 1994). Much evidence suggests that particular resistance problems in hospital-acquired infection have resulted from the routine, unthoughtful, or 'blanket' use of antibiotics in courses that are too long. Restraint, enlightened prescribing and control of antibiotic use in hospitals may prevent a worsening of the problem (Gould 1988, Report 1995, Editorial 1996, Tenover and McGowan 1996).

9 INVESTIGATION AND SURVEILLANCE OF INFECTION

9.1 Investigation of outbreaks

An outbreak is defined as 2 or more cases of symptomatic infection or of symptomatic infection and colonization, suspected on clinical or laboratory evidence. An outbreak may be obvious, such as a number of cases of acute diarrhoea occurring in a ward over a few hours, or it may not be apparent for some time, such as deep staphylococcal infection after hip replacement in several patients over a period of months.

Outbreaks may be detected by simple laboratory surveillance with informal sources of clinical intelligence but more subtle occurrences may be detected only by a more formal investigation. This should at the same time follow the epidemiological and the microbiological approaches. A first essential is definition of a case in clinical or microbiological terms. Outbreaks defined by an increase in the infection rate at a single body site may have a multiple bacterial aetiology and the question arises whether there is in fact an outbreak. There may simply have been heightened awareness of infective episodes, a series of unlinked but significant clinical events, unrelated cases of infection by similar micro-organisms or a 'pseudo-outbreak' due to specimen contamination (McGowan and Metchock 1996).

The spread of infection may be:

1 from a point-source at one time
2 from a point-source with continued exposure
3 by person-to-person spread
4 from infected persons with secondary contamination of the environment or
5 by a mixture of these.

Outbreaks should be defined epidemiologically in terms of time, place and persons involved, and an epidemic curve should be plotted where the outbreak is relatively large (Palmer 1989). The shape of this curve and the microbiological cause may yield information for follow-up.

Small outbreaks purely of hospital concern may be dealt with by the Infection Control Team or equivalent (see section 10, p. 218) in association with clinical staff and local managers. More serious outbreaks and those with community implications require the involvement of those responsible for infection control in the community, i.e. local public health authorities and public health laboratories (see Chapter 9). When a major incident is found or suspected that is of potential seriousness for patients, or involves many patients or more than one hospital, or is liable to cause public concern, a formal action group or outbreak committee should be established (Hospital Infection Working Group of the Department of Health and Public Health Laboratory Service 1995). The responsibilities of such a group are to investigate and control the outbreak; to ensure that affected patients are adequately cared for and that there are sufficient staff and supplies in ward and laboratory; to disseminate information to patients, staff, relatives and the general public; to record the episode, prepare a report and to consider future prevention (Hospital Infection Working Group of the Department of Health and Public Health Laboratory Service 1995).

Depending on the nature of the outbreak (e.g. nosocomial legionellosis) or its extent (e.g. a large number of cases of hospital-acquired food poisoning), national bodies with specialized epidemiological skills such as the Communicable Disease Surveillance Centre (UK) or Centers for Disease Control (USA) may need to be involved. Larger outbreaks, particularly those arising from a single source, whether or not microbiological indicators are available, may require formal epidemiological studies, particularly case-control studies (Rothman 1986; see also Chapter 9). The descriptive epidemiology may have produced hypotheses to be tested. This approach may be more satisfactory than use of extended case-control studies to investigate a variety of possible factors. However, case-control studies provide a powerful means to study some types of hospital outbreak and may give more rapid answers than microbiological methods, particularly if microbiological diagnosis of the particular infection is difficult or slow, e.g. legionellosis and some forms of viral gastroenteritis. Particularly in point-source outbreaks, 'cohort' studies (Rothman 1986) may be possible. In such studies, 2 or more groups that differ in exposure to a postulated source of infection may be compared for incidence of the infection. An example is the identification of the responsible food consumed in a food-borne outbreak. Such approaches are less useful in many hospital outbreaks that are due to person-to-person spread.

The increasing numbers of compromised hospital patients, the greater awareness of the hospital environment as a source and means of transmission of infection, and the emergence of more resistant microbes may require the use of considerable laboratory support to identify or confirm the extent of the outbreak and to confirm that preventive measures have been effective. The successful control of an outbreak requires good clinical investigation and in some instances up-to-date typing techniques such as ribotyping, polymerase chain reaction based techniques, etc. (Emori and Gaynes 1993, Wendt and Wenzel 1996).

9.2 Epidemiological typing

Epidemiological typing, characterization of isolates to intraspecies level, is useful (Parker 1978, Pitt 1994) to define the extent of an outbreak and to elucidate the sources and spread of infection and the effectiveness of prevention. Established typing methods, that permit stable and discriminatory subdivisions, are available for some common hospital pathogens, such as *S. aureus* (Volume 2, Chapter 27). However, the continued appearance of new strains that are not typable by the existing systems, and the progress of newly significant species, diminish the value of classically established methods. This is a stimulus for the development of new methods, preferably those of more general applicability. The need is for simple, reproducible and discriminatory methods; fine discrimination can sometimes be attained by applying 2 or more typing methods sequentially. The aim is to define with reasonable confidence the strain responsible for an incident of infection by distinguishing all epidemiologically irrelevant isolates (Anderson and Williams 1956).

Well established phenotypic methods of typing include serotyping, phage typing (including 'reverse' phage typing; de Saxe and Notley 1978) and bacteriocin typing (see Volume 2, Chapter 8). Methods in common use for more local studies include biotyping and comparison of antibiotic-sensitivity patterns, which is often the first clue to a common-source outbreak, but it is an unreliable epidemiological tool. Other methods that have proved to be of value for typing particular organisms include morphotyping of *C. albicans* (Brown-Thomsen 1968), the Dienes phenomenon for swarming strains of *Proteus* spp. (see Volume 2, Chapter 43) and resistotyping (Elek and Higney 1970).

Analysis of DNA and other cellular constituents may provide a means of discriminating between strains that are similar by conventional typing methods, and makes possible the 'fingerprinting' of diverse species for which standard methods have not been established. The ease with which such methods can be applied has sometimes encouraged their use without proper critical evaluation of their suitability (Pitt 1994, Struelens et al. 1996). Electrophoretic analysis of cellular proteins (total cellular proteins, outer-membrane proteins, or essential enzymes) has been applied to several species, with discrimination by pattern recognition or automated mathematical analysis. Electrophoretic demonstration of plasmids, with or without treatment by restriction endonucleases, has been widely used (Mayer 1988). Chromosomal analysis is more difficult because of the larger size of the genome and the many fragments produced by endonuclease action. Nucleic acid probes can be applied to endonuclease digests (Bingen, Denamur and Elion 1994). The polymerase chain reaction can be used in a variety of ways to characterize the genome of micro-organisms (Van Belkum 1994).

The various epidemiological typing and 'finger-printing' methods have been reviewed, and criteria for their use and evaluation proposed, by a Study Group of the European Society for Clinical Microbiology and Infectious Diseases (Struelens et al. 1996).

9.3 Surveillance

Surveillance is the systematic observation and recording of disease. It is an active process and implies the analysis and dissemination of data so that direct or indirect action can subsequently be taken to improve patient care. Unlike the investigation of an outbreak or epidemic, surveillance is ongoing and the results can be used as an indicator of the quality of care, e.g. surgical wound infection rates (Glenister 1993). In his summary of the Proceedings of the First International Conference on Nosocomial Infections, Williams (1971) stated: 'Quite clearly, the first message from this conference is the need for surveillance. It is essential that hospital staff know what is going on in the hospital.' It is important to analyse surveillance activities critically to determine their usefulness in control, rather than to undertake them for their own sake, or with a false idea of their usefulness. The increasing availability of computer databases makes the analysis of data easier but more traditional and time-consuming methods such as a card recording system can be used equally well. In Britain, laboratory-based surveillance, with a variable degree of clinical reporting of infection, especially of organisms such as MRSA, has been the norm. In the USA, partly because of accreditation requirements and the fear of litigation, much staff time is devoted to the continuous gathering of data (Casewell 1980, Wenzel 1986). Justification for the latter approach comes from the Study of the Efficacy of Nosocomial Infection Control (SENIC) (Haley et al. 1985b). This large and expensive investigation determined the infection rates in 1970 and 1976, by a validated retrospective case-paper review, in a large sample of patients from 338 US hospitals. The rates were compared with the very variable infection control activities of the hospitals, expressed in terms of 2 indices, surveillance and control. The

conclusion was that optimal measures would prevent 32% of hospital-acquired infections of the urinary tract, the lower respiratory tract, surgical wounds and the bloodstream.

It should be recognized that comparisons of data collected, for example, in different institutions, are of limited value (Haley 1988). Even the most basic of surveillance activities, the detection of cases of hospital-acquired infection, is difficult and expensive, and many systems give results far below the actual rate. Furthermore, differences in case definitions between centres make reliable comparisons difficult. A comparison of different approaches, with a 'standard' of prospective identification, by an infection control physician who examined patients and records is shown in Table 13.3 (Freeman and McGowan 1981). Physician self-reporting is the least reliable method of recording infections. In the UK, Glenister (1993) assessed a number of different methods and compared these with a reference method. A laboratory-based telephone method took 3.1 h for every 100 beds but was only 51% sensitive in detecting hospital-acquired infection whereas a laboratory-based ward liaison method was 76% sensitive but more time-consuming.

The dissemination of the results of surveillance is crucial if a beneficial effect on patient care in the form of improved practices and reduced hospital-acquired infection rates are to result. Wound infection rates should be reported to individual surgeons (Cruse et al. 1980). The prevalence of all types of nosocomial infection fell from 10.5% to 5.6% over a period of 3 years following surveillance in the form of repeat prevalence surveys accompanied by improvements in infection control policies (French et al. 1989).

It is not always feasible to conduct unit or hospital-wide surveillance. Consequently, targeted or selective surveillance is recommended (Hospital Infection Working Group of the Department of Health and Pub-

Table 13.3 Hospital-acquired infection: sensitivity of methods of case finding

Method	Sensitivity
Physician self-report forms	0.14–0.34
Fever	0.47
Antibiotic use	0.48
Fever plus antibiotic use	0.59
Microbiology reports	0.33–0.65
Selected chart review with 'Kardex' clues	0.85
Total chart review	0.90
SENIC pilot project	
Prospective data collection	0.52–0.90
Retrospective chart review	0.66–0.80
Standard method	1.00

SENIC, Study on the Efficiency of Nosocomial Infection Control.
Standard method, clinical detection of infection by a trained physician, who examined all the patients and reviewed all the data in respect of them, is given a sensitivity of 1.00 by definition.
Modified from Freeman J, McGowan JE, 1981, *Rev Infect Dis*, **3**: 658 (© The University of Chicago) with permission.

lic Health Laboratory Service 1995). Targeted surveillance concentrates on areas where infection is particularly important and where it has a major impact on patient morbidity and mortality, e.g. intensive care and oncology units. Selective surveillance addresses problem areas or units or specialties with potential problems, outside the occurrence of a clearly defined epidemic, where infection rates might be higher than expected, or following the opening of a new specialist unit or facility. As the duration of hospital stay becomes shorter, it is important not to underestimate hospital infection presenting in the community after discharge (see p. 188). With the availability of newer typing techniques (see above), it may become easier to trace the spread of organisms that cause nosocomial infection so that preventive strategies to reduce cross-infection may be based on clearer scientific evidence.

10 ORGANIZATION OF HOSPITAL INFECTION CONTROL

Systems for the management of infection control in hospitals developed in parallel in Great Britain and in the USA, and essentially similar systems have been adopted in other European countries and in other parts of the world (Hambraeus 1995).

In the UK, the staff who provide infection control expertise in hospitals have been reviewed and guidance has been issued (Hospital Infection Working Group of the Department of Health and Public Health Laboratory Service 1995). Executive action in infection control, though a responsibility of the Chief Executive (CE) of the unit, is the function of an Infection Control Team (ICT), which must maintain close liaison with the CE, or appointed deputy, and other managers. In its simplest form the ICT consists of an Infection Control Doctor (ICD) and an Infection Control Nurse (ICN) (Gardner et al. 1962). The ICD is the Control of Infection Officer (Colebrook 1955, Subcommittee of the Central Health Services Council 1959) and the leader of the team, and may be formally appointed with responsibility to the medical consultants' committee or to the CE, and may report directly to the Health Authority. The ICT may be augmented by the active participation of medical microbiologists, infectious-disease physicians, scientists, medical laboratory scientific officers and others, and should be supported by an Infection Control Committee (ICC) (Hospital Infection Working Group of the Department of Health and Public Health Laboratory Service 1995).

The ICD has a wide-ranging role in the Health District and is the specialist adviser on hospital infection to the Authority and to managers and planners. The ICD is expected to develop an infection control programme, policies and procedures and to ensure that all staff are educated in infection control and that suitable audit is carried out. The ICD has the primary responsibility for surveillance and the investigation of outbreaks and advises about infectious disease in hospital staff and its prevention, including immunization policy. The ICD is the leader of the ICT and works closely with and supports the ICN. The ICD is usually the Chairman of the ICC, a role that is usually filled by a medical microbiologist. In the USA the equivalent is the Infection Control Epidemiologist.

The ICN is responsible for infection control matters to the ICD and undertakes similar activities either with the ICD or independently under his or her general guidance. The ICN may provide clinical surveillance, day by day and in outbreaks, and has particular responsibility for the application of policies and procedures and for the training of staff. The ICN often has close links with various ancillary departments, such as the pharmacy, domestic services, laundry, etc. The counterpart of the ICN in the USA is the Infection Control Practitioner (Goldmann 1986).

The ICC, which includes the augmented ICT, together with representatives of clinical departments and service departments, is not to be confused with the Outbreak Committee (OC, p. 216) but is usually the body for discussing, monitoring and approving the activities of the ICT listed above and lends it authority. It produces an action plan for infection control; it also produces general policies, encourages education, and reviews the implementation of the measures.

It is important that the hospital ICT should have strong links with the community. This connection has been responsible for preventing many outbreaks of infection both in hospitals and outside. The Consultant for Communicable Disease Control (CCDC) has a general responsibility for infection control in the whole district and provides the main communication channel for the hospital ICT on such matters. In major outbreaks with implications wider than the hospital unit both the ICD and the CCDC will be actively involved. In outbreaks of typical nosocomial infection mainly restricted to hospital patients the ICD will lead the OC, with information to the CCDC.

The present arrangements for infection control in England and Wales were reviewed by Howard (1988) for the Hospital Infection Society and of the 207 Health Districts and London postgraduate hospitals approached, 93% responded. They were responsible for 95% of 'acute' hospital beds and 85% of other beds. Their replies identified 264 ICDs, of whom 82% were medical microbiologists; ICCs had been established in 92% of Districts; 205 ICNs were in post and 93% of these worked closely with a medical microbiologist who was usually the ICD.

Thus the ICT, however constituted, has responsibility for the investigation of untoward occurrences and, even more importantly, for establishing microbiologically safe conditions in the hospital, for the provision of necessary supplies, and for ensuring safe practices in the day-to-day care of patients. Written statements of policies and procedures must be provided; the ICC and ICT must oversee the implementation of these and the education of staff in their use and interpretation. For detailed recommendations the reader is referred to reviews (Bennett and Brachman 1992, Wenzel 1993, Philpott-Howard and Casewell 1994, Wilson J 1995). Individual procedures may be required for special units, e.g. neonatal, paediatric, obstetric, intensive therapy, dialysis, transplantation and oncology.

Matters to be dealt with, in many cases in liaison with other groups of staff, are listed in Table 13.4.

Table 13.4 General subjects for which infection control policies may be required

Provision of safe air supply (to operating theatres and accommodation for immunosuppressed patients)
Safe provision of water and food
Cleaning and general hygiene
Pest control
Waste disposal
Laundry
Decontamination (cleaning, disinfection, sterilization) of all equipment and materials
Ward procedures, including dressings and minor invasive procedures, urinary catheterization
Disposal of excreta
Venepuncture and vascular cannulation
Operating theatre procedures
Antibiotic use, including prophylaxis
Isolation of patients and 'barrier nursing', to prevent spread of infection ('source isolation') or to protect susceptibles ('protective isolation')
Notification of infective disease and other liaison with community officers
Laboratory and pharmacy procedures
Staff health, immunization and carriage of pathogenic micro-organisms

In spite of the uniformity of approach to infection control in Europe, practices are diverse, as was revealed during a survey of infection in intensive care units (Vincent et al. 1995). In the USA and in Europe there is an increasing movement towards providing and unifying standards in hospital infection control against which practice can be judged and audit can be carried out (Infection Control Standards Working Party 1993, Cookson 1995, Jepsen 1995, McGowan 1995). It has been suggested that these should be 'outcome' rather than 'process' oriented (McGowan 1995). Although the methods available for measuring health benefit are limited, improving the health of the population by reducing the morbidity, mortality and use of resources incurred by hospital-acquired infection must remain the aim of all the systems outlined above.

REFERENCES

Aavitsland P, Stormark M, Lystad A, 1992, Hospital-acquired infections in Norway. A national prevalence survey in 1991, *Scand J Infect Dis*, **24:** 477–83.

Adal KA, Anglim AM et al., 1994, The use of high-efficiency particulate air-filter respirators to protect hospital workers from tuberculosis, *N Engl J Med*, **331:** 169–73.

Adams BG, Marrie TJ, 1982, Hand carriage of gram-negative rods may not be transient, *J Hyg*, **89:** 33–46.

Advisory Committee on Dangerous Pathogens, 1994, *Precautions for Work with Human and Animal Transmissible Spongiform Encephalopathy*, HMSO, London.

Albert RK, Condie F, 1981, Hand-washing patterns in medical intensive-care units, *N Engl J Med*, **304:** 1465–6.

Alder VG, Burman D et al., 1980, Comparison of hexachlorophane and chlorhexidine powders in neonatal infection, *Arch Dis Child*, **55:** 277–80.

Allen KD, Ridgway EJ, Parsons LA, 1994, Hexachlorophane powder and neonatal staphylococcal infection, *J Hosp Infect*, **27:** 29–33.

Allen KD, Bartzokas CA et al., 1987, Acquisition of endemic *Pseudomonas aeruginosa* in an intensive therapy unit, *J Hosp Infect*, **10:** 156–64.

Amin M, 1992, Antibacterial prophylaxis in urology: a review, *Am J Med*, **92, Suppl. 4A:** 114S–17S.

An YH, Friedman RJ, 1996, Prevention of sepsis in total joint arthroplasty, *J Hosp Infect*, **33:** 93–108.

Anderson ES, Williams REO, 1956, Bacteriophage typing of enteric pathogens and staphylococci and its use in epidemiology, *J Clin Pathol*, **9:** 94–127.

Anon, 1988, Cleaning and disinfection of equipment for gastro-intestinal flexible endoscopy: interim recommendations of a Working Party of the British Society of Gastroenterology, *Gut*, **29:** 1134–51.

Archer GL, Armstrong BC, 1983, Alteration of staphylococcal flora in cardiac surgery patients receiving antibiotic prophylaxis, *J Infect Dis*, **147:** 642–9.

Armstrong D, Neu H et al., 1995, The prospects of treatment failure in the chemotherapy of infectious disease in the 1990s, *Microb Drug Resist*, **1:** 1–4.

Arnow PM, Chou T et al., 1982, Nosocomial Legionnaires' disease caused by aerosolized tap water from respiratory devices, *J Infect Dis*, **146:** 460–7.

Augustin AK, Simor AE et al., 1995, Outbreaks of gastroenteritis due to Norwalk-like virus in two long-term care facilities, *Can J Infect Control*, **10:** 111–13.

Austrian R, 1994, Confronting drug-resistant pneumococci, *Ann Intern Med*, **121:** 807–9.

Ayliffe GAJ, 1980, The effect of antibacterial agents on the flora of the skin, *J Hosp Infect*, **1:** 111–24.

Ayliffe GAJ, 1986, Nosocomial infection – the irreducible minimum, *Infect Control*, **7, Suppl.:** 92–5.

Ayliffe GAJ, 1991, Role of the environment of the operation suite in surgical wound infection, *Rev Infect Dis*, **13, Suppl. 10:** S800–4.

Ayliffe GAJ, 1996, *Recommendations for the Control of Methicillin-resistant* Staphylococcus aureus *(MRSA)*, World Health Organization, Geneva.

Ayliffe GAJ, Lawrence JC (eds), 1985, *Infection in Burns*, *J Hosp Infect*, **6, Suppl. B:** 1–66.

Ayliffe GAJ, Lilly HA, 1985, Cross infection and its prevention. In *Infection in Burns*, eds Ayliffe GAJ, Lawrence JC, *J Hosp Infect*, **6, Suppl. B:** 47–57.

Ayliffe GAJ, Lilly HA, Lowbury EJL, 1979, Decline of the hospital staphylococcus? Incidence of multiresistant *Staph. aureus* in three Birmingham hospitals, *Lancet*, **1:** 538–41.

Ayliffe GAJ, Lowbury EJL, 1982, Airborne infection in hospital, *J Hosp Infect*, **3:** 217–40.

Babb JR, Bradley CR, 1995, Endoscope decontamination: where do we go from here?, *J Hosp Infect*, **30, Suppl.**: 543–51.

Babb JR, Davies JG, Ayliffe GAJ, 1983, Contamination of protective clothing and nurses' uniforms in an isolation ward, *J Hosp Infect*, **4**: 149–57.

Bach A, Bohrer H et al., 1994, Prevention of bacterial colonization of intravenous catheters by antiseptic impregnation of polyurethane polymers, *J Antimicrob Chemother*, **33**: 969–78.

Bailey IS, Karran SE et al., 1992, Community surveillance of complications after hernia surgery, *Br Med J*, **304**: 469–71.

Baine WB, Gangarosa EJ et al., 1973, Institutional salmonellosis, *J Infect Dis*, **128**: 357–60.

Barnard DL, Hart JC et al., 1973, Outbreak in Britain of conjunctivitis caused by adenovirus type 8, and its epidemiology and control, *Br Med J*, **2**: 165–9.

Barrett SP, Teare EL, Sage R, 1993, Methicillin resistant *Staphylococcus aureus* in three adjacent Health Districts of south-east England 1986–91, *J Hosp Infect*, **24**: 313–25.

Bartlett CLR, Macrae AD, Macfarlane JT, 1986, Legionella *Infections*, Arnold, London, 92, 100.

Baselski VS, Wunderink RG, 1994, Bronchoscopic diagnosis of pneumonia, *Clin Microbiol Rev*, **7**: 533–58.

Bassett DCJ, Stokes KJ, Thomas WRG, 1970, Wound infection with *Pseudomonas multivorans*, *Lancet*, **1**: 1188–91.

Bayston R, 1985, Hydrocephalus shunt infections and their treatment, *J Antimicrob Chemother*, **15**: 259–61.

Bayston R, Compton C, Richards C, 1994, Production of extracellular slime by coryneforms colonizing hydrocephalus shunts, *J Clin Microbiol*, **32**: 1705–9.

Beattie PG, Rings TR et al., 1994, Risk factors for wound infection following caesarean section, *Aust NZ J Obstet Gynaecol*, **34**: 398–402.

Beck-Sagué C, Dooley SW et al., 1992, Hospital outbreak of multidrug-resistant *Mycobacterium tuberculosis* infections. Factors in transmission to staff and HIV-infected patients, *JAMA*, **268**: 1280–6.

van Belkum A, 1994, DNA fingerprinting of medically important microorganisms by the use of PCR, *Clin Microbiol Rev*, **7**: 174–84.

Bennett JV, Brachman PS, 1992, *Hospital Infections*, 3rd edn, Little Brown, Boston.

Bergogne-Berezin E, 1995, The increasing significance of outbreaks of *Acinetobacter* spp: the need for control and new agents, *J Hosp Infect*, **30, Suppl.**: 441–52.

Berk SL, Verghese A, 1989, Emerging pathogens in nosocomial pneumonia, *Eur J Clin Microbiol Infect Dis*, **8**: 11–14.

Bingen E, Denamur E, Elion J, 1994, Use of ribotyping in epidemiological surveillance of nosocomial outbreaks, *Clin Microbiol Rev*, **7**: 311–27.

Blowers R, Mason GA et al., 1955, Control of wound infection in a thoracic surgery unit, *Lancet*, **2**: 786–94.

Board of Science and Education, 1996, *A Guide to Hepatitis C*, British Medical Association, London.

Bone RC, 1991, The pathogensis of sepsis, *Ann Intern Med*, **115**: 457–69.

Borriello SP, Barclay FE, 1986, An in-vitro model of colonisation resistance to *Clostridium difficile* infection, *J Med Microbiol*, **21**: 299–309.

Bradley CR, Babb JR, 1995, Endoscope decontamination: automated vs manual, *J Hosp Infect*, **30 Suppl.**: 537–42.

Braimbridge MWV, Eykyn SJ, 1987, Prosthetic valve endocarditis, *J Antimicrob Chemother*, **20, Suppl. A**: 173–80.

Braude AI, Carey FJ, Siemienski J, 1955, Studies of bacterial transfusion reactions from refrigerated blood: the properties of cold-growing bacteria, *J Clin Invest*, **34**: 311–25.

Breuer J, Jeffries DJ, 1990, Control of viral infections in hospitals, *J Hosp Infect*, **16**: 191–221.

Brown EM, 1993, Antimicrobial prophylaxis in neurosurgery, *J Antimicrob Chemother*, **31, Suppl. B**: 49–63.

Brown-Thomsen J, 1968, Variability in *Candida albicans* (Robin)

Berkhout studies on morphology and biochemical activity, *Hereditas*, **60**: 355–98.

Brumfitt W, Hamilton-Miller J, 1989, Methicillin-resistant *Staphylococcus aureus*, *N Engl J Med*, **320**: 1188–96.

Brun-Buisson C, Doyon F et al., 1995, Incidence, risk factors, and outcome of severe sepsis and septic shock in adults, *JAMA*, **274**: 968–74.

Bryan CS, Hornung CA et al., 1986, Endemic bacteremia in Columbia, South Carolina, *Am J Epidemiol*, **123**: 113–27.

Buchholz HW, Elson RA et al., 1981, Management of deep infection of total hip replacement, *J Bone Joint Surg [Br]*, **63**: 342–53.

Burke JF, 1961, The effective period of preventive antibiotic action in experimental incisions and dermal lesions, *Surgery*, **50**: 161–8.

Burke JP, Jacobson JA et al., 1983, Evaluation of daily neonatal care with poly-antibiotic ointment in prevention of urinary catheter-associated bacteriuria, *J Urol*, **129**: 331–4.

Burnie JP, 1986, *Candida* and hands, *J Hosp Infect*, **8**: 1–4.

Burnie JP, Odds FC et al., 1985, Outbreak of systemic *Candida albicans* in intensive care unit caused by cross-infection, *Br Med J*, **290**: 746–8.

Burwen DR, Banerjee SN, Gaynes RP, 1994, Ceftazidime resistance among selected nosocomial gram-negative bacilli in the United States. National Nosocommial Infections Surveillance System, *J Infect Dis*, **170**: 1622–5.

Buxton AE, Highsmith AK et al., 1979, Contamination of intravenous infusion fluid: effects of changing administration sets, *Ann Intern Med*, **90**: 764–8.

Byrne DJ, Lynch W et al., 1994, Wound infection rates: the importance of definition and post-discharge wound surveillance, *J Hosp Infect*, **26**: 37–43.

Cafferkey MT, Conneely B et al., 1980, Post-operative urinary infection and septicaemia in urology, *J Hosp Infect*, **1**: 315–20.

Cafferkey MT, Falkiner FR et al., 1982, Antibiotics for the prevention of septicaemia in urology, *J Antimicrob Chemother*, **9**: 471–7.

Cairns H, 1939, Bacterial infection during intracranial operations, *Lancet*, **1**: 1193–8.

Carter AO, Borczyk AA, Carlson JAK, 1987, A severe outbreak of *Escherichia coli* O157:H7-associated hemorrhagic colitis in a nursing home, *N Engl J Med*, **317**: 1496–500.

Cartmill TDI, Panigrahi H et al., 1994, Management and control of a large outbreak of diarrhoea due to *Clostridium difficile*, *J Hosp Infect*, **27**: 1–15.

Casewell MW, 1980, Surveillance of infection in hospitals, *J Hosp Infect*, **1**: 293–7.

Casewell MW, 1982, Bacteriological hazards of contaminated enteral feeds, *Hosp Infect*, **3**: 329–31.

Casewell MW, 1995, New threats to the control of methicillin-resistant *Staphylococcus aureus*, *J Hosp Infect*, **30, Suppl.**: 465–71.

Casewell MW, Desai N, 1983, Survival of multiply-resistant *Klebsiella aerogenes* and other Gram negative bacilli on finger-tips, *J Hosp Infect*, **4**: 350–60.

Casewell MW, Hill RLR, 1986, The carrier state: methicillin-resistant *Staphylococcus aureus*, *J Antimicrob Chemother*, **18, Suppl. A**: 1–12.

Casewell M, Phillips I, 1977, Hands as a route of transmission for *Klebsiella* species, *Br Med J*, **2**: 1315–17.

Casewell MW, Phillips I, 1978, Food as a source of *Klebsiella* species for colonisation and infection of intensive care patients, *J Clin Pathol*, **31**: 845–9.

Caul EO, 1994, Small round structured viruses: airborne transmission and hospital control, *Lancet*, **1**: 1240–2.

Centers for Disease Control, 1987, Recommendations for prevention of HIV in health care settings, *Morbid Mortal Weekly Rep*, **36, Suppl. 2S**: 3S–18S.

Chadwick PR, Chadwick CD, Oppenheim BA, 1996, Report of a meeting on the epidemiology and control of glycopeptide-resistance enterococci, *Hosp Infect*, **33**: 83–92.

Charnley J, Eftekhar N, 1969, Postoperative infection in total prosthetic hip replacement arthroplasty of the hip joint. With special reference to the bacterial content of the air of the operating room, *Br J Surg*, **56**: 641–9.

Chastre J, Fagon J-Y et al., 1995, Evaluation of bronchoscopic techniques for the diagnosis of nosocomial pneumonia, *Am J Respir Crit Care Med*, **152**: 231–40.

Chaudhuri AK, 1993, Infection control in hospitals: has its quality-enhancing and cost-effective role been appreciated?, *J Hosp Infect*, **25**: 1–6.

Cheesbrough JS, Finch RG, Macfarlane JT, 1984, The implications of intravenous cannulae incorporating a valved injection side port, *J Hyg*, **93**: 497–504.

Clarke SKR, Dalgleish PG, Gillespie WA, 1952, Hospital cross-infections with staphylococci resistant to several antibiotics, *Lancet*, **1**: 1132–4.

Coello R, Glenister H et al., 1993, The cost of infection in surgical patients: a case-control study, *J Hosp Infect*, **25**: 239–50.

Colebrook L, 1955, Infection acquired in hospital, *Lancet*, **2**: 885–91.

Collin J, Tweedle DEF et al., 1973, Effect of a Millipore filter on complications of intravenous infusions: a prospective clinical trial, *Br Med J*, **4**: 456–8.

Colville A, Crowley J et al., 1993, Outbreak of Legionnaires' disease at University Hospital, Nottingham. Epidemiology, microbiology and control, *Epidemiol Infect*, **110**: 105–16.

Combined Working Party of the British Society for Antimicrobial Chemotherapy and the Hospital Infection Society, 1995, Guidelines on the control of methicillin-resistant *Staphylococcus aureus* in the community, *J Hosp Infect*, **31**: 1–12.

Combined Working Party of the Hospital Infection Society and the British Society for Antimicrobial Chemotherapy, 1990, Revised guidelines for the control of epidemic methicillin-resistant *Staphylococcus aureus*, *J Hosp Infect*, **16**: 351–77.

Committee of Inquiry, 1986, *Report of the Committee of Inquiry into an Outbreak of Food Poisoning at the Stanley Royd Hospital, Wakefield*, HMSO, London.

Cooke EM, Kumar PJ et al., 1970, Hospital food as a possible source of *Escherichia coli* in patients, *Lancet*, **1**: 436–7.

Cooke EM, Sazegar T et al., 1980, *Klebsiella* species in hospital food and kitchens: a source of organisms in the bowel of patients, *J Hyg*, **84**: 97–101.

Cookson BD, 1990, Mupirocin resistance in staphylococci, *J Antimicrob Chemother*, **25**: 497–503.

Cookson BD, 1995, Progress with establishing and implementing standards for infection control in the UK, *J Hosp Infect*, **30, Suppl.**: 69–75.

Coovadia YM, Johnson AP et al., 1992, Multiresistant *Klebsiella pneumoniae* in a neonatal nursery: the importance of maintenance of infection control policies and procedures in the prevention of outbreaks, *J Hosp Infect*, **22**: 197–205.

Coria-Jimencz R, Ortiz-Torres C, 1994, Aminoglycoside resistance patterns of *Serratia marcescens* strains of clinical origin, *Epidemiol Infect*, **112**: 125–31.

Cox RA, Conquest C et al., 1995, A major outbreak of methicillin-resistant *Staphylococcus aureus* caused by a new phage-type (EMRSA-16), *J Hosp Infect*, **29**: 87–106.

Craven DE, Steger KA et al., 1992, Nosocomial pneumonia: epidemiology and infection control, *Intensive Care Med*, **18, Suppl. 1**: S3–9.

Crookshank FG, 1910, Control of scarlet fever, *Lancet*, **1**: 477–80.

Cruickshank R, 1935, The bacterial infection of burns, *J Pathol Bacteriol*, **41**: 367–9.

Cruickshank R, 1944, Hospital infection: a historical review, *Br Med Bull*, **2**: 272–6.

Cruse PJE, Foord R, 1973, A five-year prospective study of 23,649 surgical wounds, *Arch Surg*, **107**: 206–10.

Cruse PJE, Foord R et al., 1980, The epidemiology of wound infection. A 10-year prospective study of 62,939 wounds, *Surg Clin North Am*, **60**: 27–40.

Curie K, Speller DCE et al., 1978, A hospital epidemic caused by gentamicin-resistant *Klebsiella aerogenes*, *J Hyg*, **80**: 115–23.

Dal Nogare AR, 1994, Nosocomial pneumonia in the medical and surgical patient. Risk factors and primary management, *Med Clin North Am*, **78**: 1081–90.

Dance DAB, Pearson AD et al., 1987, A hospital outbreak caused by a chlorhexidine and antibiotic-resistant *Proteus mirabilis*, *J Hosp Infect*, **10**: 10–16.

Darbyshire PJ, Weightman NC, Speller DCE, 1985, Problems associated with indwelling central venous catheters, *Arch Dis Child*, **60**: 129–34.

Darnowski S, Gordon M, Simor A, 1991, Two years of infection surveillance in a geriatric long-term care facility, *Am J Infect Control*, **19**: 185–90.

Das I, Symonds JM, 1996, Endophthalmitis, *Rev Med Microbiol*, **7**: 133–42.

Davies AJ, Bullock DW, 1981, *Pseudomonas aeruginosa* in two special care baby units – patterns of colonization and infection, *J Hosp Infect*, **2**: 241–7.

Davies AJ, Hawkey PM et al., 1984, Pneumococcal cross-infection in hospital, *Br Med J (Clin Res Ed)*, **288**: 1195.

Davies AJ, Desai HN et al., 1987, Does instillation of chlorhexidine into the bladder of catheterized geriatric patients help reduce bacteriuria?, *J Hosp Infect*, **9**: 72–5.

Davies J, Babb JR et al., 1978, Disinfection of the skin of the abdomen, *Br J Surg*, **65**: 855–8.

De Souza SW, Lewis DM et al., 1975, Hexachlorophane dusting powder for newborn infants, *Lancet*, **1**: 860–1.

Department of Health and Social Security and Welsh Office, 1986, *The Control of Viral Haemorrhagic Fevers*, HMSO, London.

Dineen P, Drusin L, 1973, Epidemics of postoperative infection associated with hair carriers, *Lancet*, **2**: 1157–9.

Djuretic T, Wall PG et al., 1996, General outbreaks of infectious intestinal disease in England and Wales 1992 to 1994, *CDR Rev*, **6**: R57–63.

Doebbeling BN, Stanley GL et al., 1992, Comparative efficacy of alternative hand-washing agents in reducing nosocomial infections in intensive care units, *N Engl J Med*, **327**: 88–93.

Donati L, Scamazzo F et al., 1993, Infection and antibiotic therapy in 4000 burned patients treated in Milan, Italy, between 1976 and 1988, *Burns*, **19**: 345–8.

Doring G, Horz M et al., 1993, Molecular epidemiology of *Pseudomonas aeruginosa* in an intensive care unit, *Epidemiol Infect*, **110**: 427–36.

Dowsett EG, 1988, Human enteroviral infections, *J Hosp Infect*, **11**: 103–15.

Duggan J, O'Connell D et al., 1993, Causes of hospital-acquired septicaemia – a case control study, *Q J Med*, **86**: 479–83.

Dukes C, 1929, Urinary infections after excision of the rectum: their cause and prevention, *Proc R Soc Med*, **22**: 259–69.

Duma RJ, Warner JF, Dalton HP, 1971, Septicemia from intravenous infusion, *N Engl J Med*, **284**: 257–60.

Dunn DL, Simmons RL, 1984, The role of anaerobic bacteria in intra-abdominal infections, *Rev Infect Dis*, **6, Suppl. 1**: 5139–46.

Easmon CSF, 1984, What is the role of beta-haemolytic streptococcal infection in obstetrics? Discussion paper, *J R Soc Med*, **77**: 302–8.

Editorial, 1982, Ambulatory peritonitis, *Lancet*, **1**: 1104–5.

Editorial, 1984a, Group G streptococci, *Lancet*, **1**: 144.

Editorial, 1984b, Blood transfusion, haemophilia and AIDS, *Lancet*, **2**: 1433–5.

Editorial, 1985, *Streptococcus milleri*, pathogen in various guises, *Lancet*, **2**: 1403–4.

Editorial, 1992, Nosocomial infection with respiratory syncytial virus, *Lancet*, **340**: 1071–2.

Editorial, 1996, Thoughtful drug use can overcome antibiotic resistance, *ASM News*, **62**: 12–13.

Elek SD, Higney L, 1970, Resistogram typing, a new epidemiological tool: application to *Escherichia coli*, *J Med Microbiol*, **3**: 103–10.

Elliott TSJ, 1988, Plastic devices: new fields for old microbes, *Lancet*, **1**: 365–6.

Emmerson AM, 1995, The impact of surveys on hospital infection, *J Hosp Infect*, **30, Suppl.**: 421–40.

Emmerson AM, Enstone JE et al., 1996, The Second National Prevalence Survey of Infection in Hospitals – overview of the results, *J Hosp Infect*, **32**: 175–90.

Emori TG, Gaynes RP, 1993, An overview of nosocomial infections, including the role of the microbiology laboratory, *Clin Microbiol Rev*, **6**: 428–42.

EPINE (Working Group), 1992, Prevalence of hospital-acquired infections in Spain, *J Hosp Infect*, **20**: 1–13.

EPINE (Groupo de Trabajo EPINE), 1995, *Prevalencia de las Infecciones Nosocomiales en los Hospitales Españoles*, Sociedad Española de Hygiene y Medicina Preventiva Hospitalanas y Grupo de Trabajo EPINCAT Grafimed Publicidad, Barcelona.

Ersahin Y, Mutluer S, Guzelbag E, 1994, Cerebrospinal fluid shunt infections, *J Neurosurg Sci*, **38**: 161–5.

Esmonde TFG, Will RG et al., 1993, Creutzfeldt–Jakob disease and blood transfusion, *Lancet*, **341**: 205–7.

Esteban JI, Gomez J et al., 1996, Transmission of hepatitis C virus by a cardiac surgeon, *N Engl J Med*, **334**: 555–60.

Expert Advisory Group on AIDS, 1990, Guidance for Clinical Health Care Workers: Protection against Infection with HIV and Hepatitis Viruses, UK Health Departments, HMSO, London.

Expert Advisory Group on AIDS, 1993, AIDS-HIV Infected Health Care Workers: Practical Guidance on Notifying Patients, UK Health Departments, HMSO, London.

Eykyn SJ, 1984, Infection and intravenous catheters, *J Antimicrob Chemother*, **14**: 203–5.

Falkiner FR, 1993, The insertion and management of indwelling urethral catheters – minimizing the risk of infection, *J Hosp Infect*, **25**: 79–90.

Fallon RJ, 1994, How to prevent an outbreak of legionnaires' disease, *J Hosp Infect*, **27**: 247–56.

Fantry GT, Zheng QX, James SP, 1995, Conventional cleaning and disinfection techniques eliminate the risk of endoscopic transmission of *Helicobacter pylori*, *Am J Gastroenterol*, **90**: 227–32.

Farrington M, 1986, The prevention of wound infection after coronary artery bypass surgery, *J Antimicrob Chemother*, **18**: 656–9.

Farrington M, Webster M et al., 1985, Study of cardiothoracic wound infection at St Thomas's Hospital, *Br J Surg*, **72**: 759–62.

Faxelius G, Ringertz S, 1987, Neonatal septicemia in Stockholm, *Eur J Clin Microbiol*, **6**: 262–5.

Feeley TW, Du Moulin GC et al., 1975, Aerosol polymyxin and pneumonia in seriously ill patients, *N Engl J Med*, **293**: 471–5.

Finkelstein R, Reinhertz G et al., 1993, Outbreak of *Candida tropicalis* fungemia in a neonatal intensive care unit, *Infect Control Hosp Epidemiol*, **14**: 587–90.

Finn A, Anday E, Talbot GH, 1988, An epidemic of adenovirus 7a infection in a neonatal nursery: course, morbidity and management, *Infect Control Hosp Epidemiol*, **9**: 398–404.

Fisch A, Salvanet A et al., 1991, Epidemiology of infective endophthalmitis in France, *Lancet*, **338**: 1373–6.

Fisher CJ, Agosti JM et al., 1996, Treatment of septic shock with the tumor necrosis factor receptor: Fc fusion protein, *N Engl J Med*, **334**: 1697–701.

Fisher-Hoch SP, Smith MG, Colbourne JS, 1982, *Legionella pneumophila* in hospital hot water cylinders, *Lancet*, **1**: 1073.

Fisher-Hoch SP, Tomori O et al., 1995, Review of cases of nosocomial Lassa fever in Nigeria: the high price of poor medical practice, *Br Med J*, **311**: 857–9.

Fletcher C, 1984, First clinical use of penicillin, *Br Med J*, **289**: 1721–3.

Flügge C, 1897, Ueber Luftinfektion, *Z Hyg Infektionskr*, **25**: 179–224.

Flügge C, 1899, Die Verbreitung der Phthise durch staubförmiges Sputum und durch beim Husten verspritzte Tröpfchen, *Z Hyg Infektionskr*, **30**: 107–24.

Fraser I, 1984, Penicillin: early clinical trials, *Br Med J*, **289**: 1723–5.

Fraser VJ, Zuckerman G et al., 1993, A prospective randomized trial comparing manual and automated endoscope disinfection methods, *Infect Control Hosp Epidemiol*, **14**: 383–9.

Freeman J, Hutchison GB, 1980, Prevalence, incidence and duration, *Am J Epidemiol*, **112**: 707–23.

Freeman J, McGowan JE, 1981, Methodologic issues in hospital epidemiology. 1. Rates, case-finding and interpretation, *Rev Infect Dis*, **3**: 658–67.

Freeman J, Rosner BA, McGowan JE, 1979, Adverse effects of nosocomial infections, *J Infect Dis*, **140**: 732–40.

Freeman R, 1995, Prevention of prosthetic valve endocarditis, *J Hosp Infect*, **30, Suppl.**: 44–53.

French GL, Cheng AFB et al., 1989, Repeated prevalence surveys for monitoring effectiveness of hospital infection control, *Lancet*, **2**: 1021–3.

French GL, Cheng AFB et al., 1990, Hong Kong strains of methicillin-resistant and methicillin-sensitive *Staphylococcus aureus* have similar virulence, *J Hosp Infect*, **15**: 117–25.

Fryklund B, Tullus K, Burman LG, 1995, Survival on skin and surfaces of epidemic and non-epidemic strains of enterobacteria from neonatal special care units, *J Hosp Infect*, **29**: 201–8.

Fuchs PC, 1971, Indwelling intravenous polyethylene catheters. Factors influencing the risk of microbial colonization and sepsis, *JAMA*, **216**: 1447–50.

Gardner AMN, Stamp M et al., 1962, The Infection Control Sister. A new member of the Control of Infection Team in general hospitals, *Lancet*, **2**: 710–11.

Garrod LP, 1979, The eclipse of the haemolytic streptococcus, *Br Med J*, **1**: 1607–8.

Gartenberg G, Bottone EJ et al., 1978, Hospital-acquired mucormycosis (*Rhizopus rhizopodiformis*) of skin and subcutaneous tissue: epidemiology, mycology and treatment, *N Engl J Med*, **299**: 1115–18.

Gaston MA, 1988, *Enterobacter*: an emerging nosocomial pathogen, *J Hosp Infect*, **11**: 197–208.

George RH, 1988, The prevention and control of mycobacterial infections in hospitals, *J Hosp Infect*, **11, Suppl. A**: 386–92.

George RH, Gully PR et al., 1986, An outbreak of tuberculosis in a children's hospital, *J Hosp Infect*, **8**: 129–42.

George RC, Uttley AHC et al., 1989, High-level vancomycin-resistant enterococci causing hospital infection, *Epidemiol Infect*, **103**: 173–81.

Gerding DN, Johnson S et al., 1995, *Clostridium difficile*-associated diarrhea and colitis, *Infect Control Hosp Epidemiol*, **16**: 459–77.

Gerner-Smidt P, Bruun B et al., 1995, Diversity of nosocomial *Xanthomonas maltophilia* (*Stenotrophomonas maltophilia*) as determined by ribotyping, *Eur J Clin Microbiol Infect Dis*, **14**: 137–40.

Getchell-White SI, Donowitz LG, Gröschel DHM, 1989, The inanimate environment of an intensive care unit as a potential source of nosocomial bacteria: evidence for long survival of *Acinetobacter calcoaceticus*, *Infect Control Hosp Epidemiol*, **10**: 402–7.

Gillespie WA, 1956, Infection in urological patients, *Proc R Soc Med*, **49**: 1045–7.

Gillespie WA, 1986, Antibiotics in catheterized patients, *J Antimicrob Chemother*, **18**: 149–51.

Gillespie WA, Simpson RA et al., 1983, Does the addition of disinfectant to urinary drainage bags prevent infection in catheterized patients?, *Lancet*, **1**: 1037–9.

Glenister HM, 1993, How do we collect data for surveillance of wound infection?, *J Hosp Infect*, **24**: 283–9.

Goldmann DA, 1986, Nosocomial infection control in the United States of America, *J Hosp Infect*, **8**: 116–28.

Goldmann DA, 1988, The bacterial flora of neonates in intensive care – monitoring and manipulation, *J Hosp Infect*, **11, Suppl. A**: 340–51.

Goldmann DA, Maki DG, 1973, Infection control in total parenteral nutrition, *JAMA*, **223**: 1360–4.

Goldstein FW, Acar JF, 1995, Epidemiology of quinolone resistance: Europe and North and South America, *Drugs*, **49, Suppl. 2:** 36–42.

Goodgame RW, 1996, Understanding intestinal spore-forming protozoa: cryptosporidia, microsporidia, *Isospora*, and *Cyclospora*, *Ann Intern Med*, **124:** 429–41.

Gould D, 1994, Nurses' hand decontamination practice: results of a local study, *J Hosp Infect*, **28:** 15–30.

Gould FK, Magee JG, Ingham HR, 1987, A hospital outbreak of antibiotic-resistant *Streptococcus pneumoniae*, *J Infect*, **15:** 77–9.

Gould IM, 1988, Control of antibiotic use in the United Kingdom, *J Antimicrob Chemother*, **22:** 395–7.

Grady GF, Lee VA et al., 1978, Hepatitis B immune globulin for accidental exposures among medical personnel: final report of a multicenter controlled trial, *J Infect Dis*, **138:** 625–38.

von Graevenitz A, Amsterdam D, 1992, Microbiological aspects of peritonitis associated with continuous ambulatory peritoneal dialysis, *Clin Microbiol Rev*, **5:** 36–48.

Gristina AG, Giridhar G et al., 1993, Cell biology and molecular mechanisms of artificial device infections, *Int J Artif Organs*, **16:** 755–63.

Gupta S, Morris JG et al., 1994, Endemic necrotizing enterocolitis: lack of association with a specific infectious agent, *Pediatr Infect Dis J*, **13:** 728–34.

Haines SJ, Walters BC, 1994, Antibiotic prophylaxis for cerebrospinal fluid shunts: a metanalysis, *Neurosurgery*, **34:** 87–92.

Haley RW, 1988, The vicissitudes of prospective multihospital surveillance studies: the Israeli Study of Surgical Infections 1988, *Infect Control Hosp Epidemiol*, **9:** 228–31.

Haley RW, Culver DH et al., 1985a, The nationwide infection route. A new need for vital statistics, *Am J Epidemiol*, **121:** 159–67.

Haley RW, Culver DH et al., 1985b, The efficiency of infection surveillance and control programs in preventing nosocomial infections in US hospitals, *Am J Epidemiol*, **121:** 182–205.

Hall CB, Kopelman AE et al., 1979, Neonatal respiratory syncytial virus infection, *N Engl J Med*, **300:** 393–6.

Halsted WS, 1913, Ligature and suture materials the employment of fine silk in preference to catgut and the advantages of transfixion of tissues and vessels in control of hemorrhage, also an account of the introduction of gloves, gutta-percha tissue and silver foil, *JAMA*, **60:** 1119–26.

Hambraeus A, 1995, Establishing an infection control structure, *J Hosp Infect*, **30, Suppl.:** 232–40.

Hambraeus A, Laurell G, 1980, Protection of the patient in the operating suite, *J Hosp Infect*, **1:** 15–30.

Hamer DH, Barza M, 1993, Prevention of hospital acquired pneumonia in critically ill patients, *Antimicrob Agents Chemother*, **37:** 931–8.

Hammond SA, Morgan JR, Russell AD, 1987, Comparative susceptibility of hospital isolates of gram-negative bacteria to antiseptics and disinfectants, *J Hosp Infect*, **9:** 255–64.

Hanson LC, Weber DJ, Rutala WA, 1992, Risk factors for nosocomial pneumonia in the elderly, *Am J Med*, **92:** 161–6.

Haron E, Bodey GP et al., 1988, Has the incidence of *Pneumocystis carinii* pneumonia in cancer patients increased with the AIDS epidemic?, *Lancet*, **2:** 904–5.

Harpaz R, von Seidlein L et al., 1996, Transmission of hepatitis B virus to multiple patients from a surgeon without evidence of inadequate infection control, *N Engl J Med*, **334:** 549–54.

Hart CA, 1982, Nosocomial gentamicin- and multiply-resistant enterobacteria at one hospital. Factors associated with carriage, *J Hosp Infect*, **3:** 165–72.

Hart CA, 1995, Transmissible spongiform encephalopathies, *J Med Microbiol*, **42:** 153–5.

Hart CA, Gibson MF, Buckles AM, 1981, Variation in skin and environmental survival of hospital gentamicin-resistant enterobacteria, *J Hyg*, **87:** 277–85.

Hartstein AI, Denny MA et al., 1995, Control of methicillin-resistant *Staphylococcus aureus* in a hospital intensive care unit, *Infect Control Hosp Epidemiol*, **16:** 405–11.

Hassan IJ, MacGowan AP, Cook SD, 1992, Endophthalmitis at the Bristol Eye Hospital: an 11-year review of 47 patients, *J Hosp Infect*, **22:** 271–8.

Hawkey PM, Malnick H et al., 1984, *Capnocytophaga ochracea* infection: two cases and a review of the literature, *J Clin Pathol*, **37:** 1059–65.

Hawkey PM, Pedler SJ, Southall PJ, 1980, *Streptococcus pyogenes*: a forgotten occupational hazard in the mortuary, *Br Med J*, **281:** 1058.

Heimberger T, Chang H-G et al., 1995, Knowledge and attitudes of healthcare workers about influenza: why are they not getting vaccinated?, *Infect Control Hosp Epidemiol*, **16:** 412–14.

Heimberger TS, Duma RJ, 1989, Infection of prosthetic heart valves and cardiac pacemakers, *Infect Dis Clin North Am*, **3:** 221–45.

Helmick CG, Tauxe RV, Vernon AA, 1987, Is there a risk to contacts of patients with rabies?, *Rev Infect Dis*, **9:** 511–18.

Henderson E, Love EJ, 1995, Incidence of hospital-acquired infections associated with caesarean section, *J Hosp Infect*, **29:** 245–55.

Hill RL, Casewell MW, 1991, Reduction in the colonization of central venous cannulae by mupirocin, *J Hosp Infect*, **19, Suppl. B:** 47–57.

Hoge CW, Breiman RF, 1991, Advances in the epidemiology and control of *Legionella* infections, *Epidemiol Rev*, **13:** 329–41.

Holmberg SD, Solomon SL, Blake PA, 1987, Health and economic impacts of antimicrobial resistance, *Rev Infect Dis*, **9:** 1065–78.

Holness D, DeKoven JG, Nethercott JR, 1992, Scabies in chronic health care institutions, *Arch Dermatol*, **128:** 1257–60.

Holzel H, de Saxe M, 1992, Septicaemia in paediatric intensive-care patients at the Hospital for Sick Children, Great Ormond Street, *J Hosp Infect*, **22:** 185–95.

Holzel HS, Cubitt WD, 1982, Enteric viruses in hospital-acquired infection, *J Hosp Infect*, **3:** 101–4.

Horsburgh CR, 1991, *Mycobacterium avium* complex infection in the acquired immunodeficiency syndrome, *N Engl J Med*, **324:** 1332–8.

Hospital Infection Control Practices Advisory Committee (HICPAC), 1995, Recommendations for preventing the spread of vancomycin resistance, *Infect Control Hosp Epidemiol*, **16:** 105–13.

Hospital Infection Working Group of the Department of Health and Public Health Laboratory Service, 1995, *Hospital Infection Control. Guidance on the Control of Infection in Hospitals*, Department of Health, London.

Houang T, Lovett IS et al., 1980, *Nocardia asteroides* infection – a transmissible disease, *J Hosp Infect*, **1:** 31–40.

Hovig B, 1981, Lower respiratory tract infections associated with respiratory therapy and anaesthesia equipment, *J Hosp Infect*, **2:** 301–15.

Howard AJ, 1988, Infection control organization in hospitals in England and Wales 1986. Report of a survey undertaken by a Hospital Infection Society Working Party, *J Hosp Infect*, **11:** 183–91.

Howie J, 1988, Upgrading surgeons' autoclaves – a personal recollection, *J Infect*, **16:** 231–4.

Humphreys H, 1993, Infection control and the design of a new operating theatre suite, *J Hosp Infect*, **23:** 61–70.

Humphreys H, Johnson EM et al., 1991, An outbreak of aspergillosis in a general ITU, *J Hosp Infect*, **18:** 167–77.

Humphreys H, Winter R et al., 1996, Comparison of bronchoalveolar lavage and catheter lavage to confirm ventilator-associated lower respiratory tract infection, *J Med Microbiol*, **45:** 226–31.

Hurley JC, 1995, Prophylaxis with enteral antibiotics in ventilated patients: selective decontamination or selective cross-infection?, *Antimicrob Agents Chemother*, **39:** 941–7.

Hussain M, Oppenheim BA et al., 1996, Prospective survey of the incidence, risk factors and outcome of hospital-acquired infections in the elderly, *J Hosp Infect*, **32:** 117–26.

Hutinel V, 1894, La dipthérie aux enfants-assistés de Paris; sa suppression; étude de prophylaxie, *Rev Mens Mal Enfants*, **12:** 515–30.

Im SWK, Chow K, Chau PY, 1981, Rectal thermometer mediated cross-infection with *Salmonella wandsworth* in a paediatric ward, *J Hosp Infect*, **2:** 171–4.

Infection Control Standards Working Party, 1993, *Standards in Infection Control in Hospitals*, Central Public Health Laboratory, London.

Ispahani P, Pearson NJ, Greenwood D, 1987, An analysis of community and hospital acquired bacteraemia in a large teaching hospital in the United Kingdom, *Q J Med*, **241:** 427–40.

Jackson M, Flerer J et al., 1992, Intensive surveillance for infections in a three-year study of nursing home patients, *Am J Epidemiol*, **135:** 685–96.

Jaffe HW, McCurdy JM et al., 1994, Lack of HIV transmission in the practice of a dentist with AIDS, *Ann Intern Med*, 855–9.

Jansen B, Peters G, 1993, Foreign body associated infection, *J Antimicrob Chemother*, **32, Suppl. A:** 69–75.

Jarvis WR, Martone WJ, 1992, Predominant pathogens in hospital infections, *J Antimicrob Chemother*, **29, Suppl. A:** 19–24.

Javaly K, Horowitz HW, Wormser GP, 1992, Nocardiosis in patients with human immunodeficiency virus infection. Report of 2 cases and review of the literature, *Medicine (Baltimore)*, **71:** 128–38.

Jepsen OB, 1995, Towards European Union standards in hospital infection control, *J Hosp Infect*, **30, Suppl.:** 64–8.

Jepsen OB, Larsen SO et al., 1982, Urinary tract infection and bacteraemia in hospitalized medical patients – a European multicentre prevalence survey on nosocomial infection, *J Hosp Infect*, **3:** 241–52.

Jewes LA, Gillespie WA et al., 1988, Bacteriuria and bacteraemia in patients with long-term indwelling catheters – a domiciliary study, *J Med Microbiol*, **26:** 61–5.

Jindani A, Aber VR et al., 1980, The early bactericidal activity of drugs in patients with pulmonary tuberculosis, *Am Rev Respir Dis*, **121:** 939–49.

Johnson AP, Weinbren MJ et al., 1992, Outbreak of infection in two UK hospitals caused by a strain of *Klebsiella pneumoniae* resistant to cefotaxime and ceftazidime, *J Hosp Infect*, **20:** 97–103.

Joint DH/PHLS Working Group, 1994, *The Prevention and Management of* Clostridium difficile *Infection*, Department of Health and Public Health Laboratory Service, London.

Joint Health and Safety Executive and Department of Health Working Party on Legionellosis, 1992, *The Prevention and Control of Legionellosis: review and forward look*, NHS Management Executive HSG(92)45, London.

Joint Tuberculosis Committee of the British Thoracic Society, 1994, Control and prevention of tuberculosis in the United Kingdom: Code of Practice 1994, *Thorax*, **49:** 1193–200.

Joint Working Party of the Hospital Infection Society and the Surgical Infection Study Group, 1992, Risks to surgeons and patients from HIV and hepatitis: guidelines on precautions and management of exposure to blood or body fluids, *Br Med J*, **305:** 1337–43.

Jolley AE, 1993, The value of surveillance cultures on neonatal intensive care units, *J Hosp Infect*, **25:** 153–9.

Jones RN, Kehrberg EN et al., 1994, Prevalence of important pathogens and antimicrobiol activity of parenteral drugs at numerous medical centers in the United States, I. Study on the threat of emerging resistance: real or perceived, *Diagn Microbiol Infect Dis*, **19:** 203–15.

Joseph CA, Watson JM et al., 1994, Nosocomial Legionnaires' disease in England and Wales, 1980–92, *Epidemiol Infect*, **112:** 329–45.

Kacica MA, Morgan MJ et al., 1994, Relatedness of coagulase-negative staphylococci causing bacteremia in low-birthweight infants, *Infect Control Hosp Epidemiol*, **15:** 658–62.

Kahyaoglu O, Nolan B, Kumar A, 1995, *Burkholderia cepacia* sepsis in neonates, *Pediatr Infect Dis J*, **14:** 815–16.

Kam KM, Mak WP, 1993, Territory-wide survey of hospital infection in Hong-Kong, *J Hosp Infect*, **23:** 143–51.

Karanfil LV, Murphy M, Josephson A, 1992, A cluster of vancomycin-resistant *Enterococcus faecium* in an intensive care unit, *Infect Control Hosp Epidemiol*, **13:** 195–200.

Karchmer AW, 1991, Prosthetic valve endocarditis: a continuing challenge for infection control, *J Hosp Infect*, **18, Suppl. A:** 355–6.

Kim KH, Fekety R et al., 1981, Isolation of *Clostridium difficile* from the environment and contacts of patients with antibiotic associated colitis, *J Infect Dis*, **143:** 42–50.

King K, Harvey K, 1985, MRSA revisited, *Med J Aust*, **142:** 88–9.

Kirk D, Dunn M et al., 1979, Hibitane bladder irrigation in the prevention of catheter-associated urinary infection, *Br J Urol*, **51:** 528–31.

Kiyosawa K, Sodeyama T et al., 1991, Hepatitis C in hospital employees with needlestick injuries, *Ann Intern Med*, **115:** 367–9.

Klein RS, Freeman K et al., 1991, Occupational risk for hepatitis C virus infection among New York City dentists, *Lancet*, **338:** 1539–42.

Kohli HS, Chaudhuri AKR et al., 1994, A severe outbreak of E. *coli* O157 in two psychogeriatic wards, *J Public Health Med*, **16:** 11–15.

Kramer F, Sasse SA et al., 1993, Primary cutaneous tuberculosis after a needlestick injury from a patient with AIDS and undiagnosed tuberculosis, *Ann Intern Med*, **119:** 594–5.

Kristensen B, Schonheyder HC et al., 1995, *Capnocytophaga* (*Capnocytophaga ochracea* group) bacteremia in hematological patients with profound granulocytopenia, *Scand J Infect Dis*, **27:** 153–5.

Kropec A, Huebner J et al., 1993, Exogenous or endogenous reservoirs of nosocomial *Pseudomonas aeruginosa* and *Staphylococcus aureus* infection in a surgical intensive care unit, *Intensive Care Med*, **19:** 161–5.

Kumarasinghe G, Hamilton WJ et al., 1982, An outbreak of *Salmonella muenchen* infection in a specialist paediatric hospital, *J Hosp Infect*, **3:** 341–4.

Kunin CM, 1987, *Detection, Prevention and Management of Urinary Tract Infection*, 4th edn, Lea & Febiger, Philadelphia.

Kunin CM, 1993, Resistance to antimicrobial drugs – a worldwide calamity, *Ann Intern Med*, **118:** 557–61.

Kunin CM, McCormack RC, 1966, Prevention of catheter-induced urinary-tract infection by sterile closed drainage, *N Engl J Med*, **274:** 1156–61.

L'Age-Stehr J, Schwarz A et al., 1985, HTLV-III infection in kidney transplant recipients, *Lancet*, **2:** 1361–2.

Laing FP, Ramotar K et al., 1995, Molecular epidemiology of *Xanthomonas maltophilia* colonization and infection in the hospital environment, *J Clin Microbiol*, **33:** 513–18.

Langenberg W, Ramos EA et al., 1990, Patient-to-patient transmission of *Campylobacter pylori* infection by fiberoptic gastroduodenoscopy and biopsy, *J Infect Dis*, **161:** 507–11.

Larson E, 1984, Current handwashing issues, *Infect Control*, **5:** 15–17.

Larson E, 1988, A causal link between handwashing and mode of infection. Examination of the evidence, *Infect Control*, **9:** 28–36.

Latham RH, Schaffner W et al., 1992, Nosocomial Legionnaires' disease, *Curr Sci*, 512–17.

Lawrence JC, 1985, The bacteriology of burns, *J Hosp Infect*, **6, Suppl. B:** 3–17.

Leaper DJ, 1994, Prophylactic and therapeutic role of antibiotics in wound care, *Am J Surg*, **167:** 15S–20S.

Lee YL, Thrupp LD et al., 1992, Nosocomial infection and antibiotic utilization in geriatric patients: a pilot prospective surveillance program in skilled nursing facilities, *Gerontology*, **38:** 223–32.

Leenders A, van Belkum A et al., 1996, Molecular epidemiology of apparent outbreak of invasive aspergillosis in a hematology ward, *J Clin Microbiol*, **34:** 345–51.

Legrand C, Anaissie E, 1992, Bacteremia due to *Achromobacter xylosoxidans* in patients with cancer, *Clin Infect Dis*, **14:** 479–84.

Levin MH, Olson B et al., 1984, *Pseudomonas* in the sinks in an intensive care unit: relation to patients, *J Clin Pathol*, **37:** 424–7.

Lewis DA, Leaper DJ, Speller DCE, 1984, Prevention of bacterial colonization of wounds at operation: comparison of iodine-impregnated ('Ioban') drapes with conventional methods, *J Hosp Infect*, **5:** 431–7.

Lewis DA, Hawkey PM et al., 1983, Infection with netilmicin resistant *Serratia marcescens* in a special care baby unit, *Br Med J*, **287:** 1701–5.

Lewis RT, Weigand FM et al., 1995, Should antibiotic prophylaxis be used routinely in clean surgical procedures: a tentative yes, *Surgery*, **742–6, 746–7.**

Lidwell OM, 1974, Aerial dispersal of micro-organisms from the human respiratory tract, *The Normal Microbial Flora of Man*, eds Skinner A, Carr J, Academic Press, London, 135–54.

Lidwell OM, Lowbury EJL et al., 1982, Effect of ultraclean air in operating rooms on deep sepsis in the joint after total hips or knee replacement: a randomised study, *Br Med J*, **285:** 10–14.

Liekweg WG, Greenfield LJ, 1977, Vascular prosthetic infections: collected experience and results of treatment, *Surgery*, **81:** 335–42.

Lilly HA, Lowbury EJ, Wilkins MD, 1979, Limits to progressive reduction of resistant skin bacteria by disinfection, *J Clin Pathol*, **32:** 382–5.

Limberg MB, 1991, A review of bacterial keratitis and bacterial conjunctivitis, *Am J Ophthalmol*, **112:** 2S–9S.

Lister J, 1867a, On a new method of treating compound fracture, abscess, etc., with observations on the conditions of suppuration, *Lancet*, **1:** 326–9, 357–9, 387–9.

Lister J, 1867b, On a new method of treating compound fracture, abscess, etc., *Lancet*, **2:** 95–6.

Liu WK, Tebbs SE et al., 1993, The effects of electric current on bacteria colonising intravenous catheters, *J Infect*, **27:** 261–9.

Livornese LL, Dial S, Samel C, 1992, Hospital-acquired infection with vancomycin-resistant *Enterococcus faecium* transmitted by electronic thermometers, *Ann Intern Med*, **117:** 112–16.

Loudon KW, Coke AP et al., 1996, Kitchens as a source of *Aspergillus niger* infection, *J Hosp Infect*, **32:** 191–8.

de Louvois J, 1986, Necrotising enterocolitis, *J Hosp Infect*, **7:** 4–12.

Lowbury EJL, Lilly HA, 1958, The sources of hospital infection of wounds with *Clostridium welchii*, *J Hyg*, **56:** 169–82.

Lowbury EJL, Lilly HA, Ayliffe GAJ, 1974, Preoperative disinfection of surgeons' hands: use of alcoholic solutions and effects of gloves on skin, *Br Med J*, **4:** 369–72.

Lowbury EJL, Lilly HA, Bull JP, 1964, Methods for disinfection of hands and operation sites, *Br Med J*, **2:** 531–6.

Lowbury EJL, Thom BT et al., 1970, Sources of infection with *Pseudomonas aeruginosa* in patients with tracheostomy, *J Med Microbiol*, **3:** 39–56.

Ludlam HA, Young AE et al., 1989, The prevention of infection with *Staphylococcus aureus* in continuous ambulatory peritoneal dialysis, *J Hosp Infect*, **14:** 293–301.

Luzzaro F, Pagani L et al., 1995, Extended spectrum beta-lactamases conferring resistance to monobactams and oxyimino-cephalosporins in clinical isolates of *Serratia marcescens*, *J Chemother*, **7:** 175–8.

Lynch W, Davey PG et al., 1992, Cost-effectiveness analysis of the use of chlorhexidine detergent in preoperative whole-body disinfection in wound infection prophylaxis, *J Hosp Infect*, **21:** 179–91.

McEntegart MG, 1956, Dangerous contaminants in stored blood, *Lancet*, **2:** 909–11.

McFarland LV, Mulligan ME et al., 1989, Nosocomial acquisition of *Clostridium difficile* infection, *N Engl J Med*, **320:** 204–9.

Macfarlane JT, Finch RG et al., 1982, Hospital study of adult community acquired pneumonia, *Lancet*, **2:** 255–8.

McGowan JE, 1988, JK coryneforms: a continuing problem for hospital infection control, *J Hosp Infect*, **11, Suppl. A:** 358–66.

McGowan JE, 1995, Success, failures and costs of implementing standards in the USA – lessons for infection control, *J Hosp Infect*, **30, Suppl.:** 76–87.

McGowan JE, Metchock BG, 1996, Basic microbiologic support for hospital epidemiology, *Infect Control Hosp Epidemiol*, **17:** 298–302.

McLauchlan GJ, Anderson ID et al., 1995, Outcome of patients with abdominal sepsis treated in an intensive care unit, *Br J Surg*, **82:** 524–9.

McManus AT, Mason AD et al., 1994, A decade of reduced gram-negative infections and mortality associated with improved isolation of burned patients, *Arch Surg*, **129:** 1306–9.

Madge P, Paton JY et al., 1992, Prospective controlled study of four infection-control procedures to prevent nosocomial infection with respiratory syncytial virus, *Lancet*, **340:** 1079–83.

Maki DG, 1980, Through a glass darkly. Nosocomial pseudo-epidemics and pseudobacteremia, *Arch Intern Med*, **140:** 26–8.

Maki DG, Goldman DA, Rhame FS, 1973, Infection control in intravenous therapy, *Ann Intern Med*, **79:** 867–87.

Maki DG, Weise CE, Sarafin HW, 1977, A semiquantitative culture method for identifying intravenous-catheter-related infection, *N Engl J Med*, **296:** 1305–9.

Maki DG, Alvarado CJ et al., 1982, Relation of the inanimate hospital environment to endemic nosocomial infection, *N Engl J Med*, **307:** 1562–6.

Makofsky D, Cone JE, 1993, Installing needle disposal boxes closer to the bedside reduces needle-recapping rates in hospital units, *Infect Control Hosp Epidemiol*, **14:** 140–4.

Marples RR, Towers AG, 1979, A laboratory method for the investigation of contact transfer of microorganisms, *J Hyg*, **82:** 237–48.

Marples RR, Hone R et al., 1978, Investigation of coagulase-negative staphylococci from infection in surgical patients, *Zentralbl Bakteriol Parasitenkd Infektionskr Hyg Abt 1 Orig*, **241:** 140–56.

Martino P, Gentile G et al., 1988, Hospital-acquired cryptosporidiosis in a bone marrow transplantation unit, *J Infect Dis*, **158:** 647–8.

Martone WJ, Jarvis WR et al., 1992, Incidence and nature of endemic and epidemic nosocomial infections, *Hospital Infections*, eds Bennett JV, Brachman PS, Little Brown, Boston, 577–96.

Mayer LW, 1988, Use of plasmid profiles in epidemiologic surveillance of disease outbreaks and in tracing the transmission of antibiotic resistance, *Clin Microbiol Rev*, **1:** 228–43.

Medical Research Council, Subcommittee of the Committee on Hospital Infection, 1968, Aseptic methods in the operating suite, *Lancet*, **1:** 705–9, 763–8, 831–9.

Meduri GU, Estes RJ, 1995, The pathogenesis of ventilator-associated pneumonia: II. The lower respiratory tract, *Intensive Care Med*, **21:** 452–61.

Meenhorst PL, Reingold AL et al., 1985, Water-related nosocomial pneumonia caused by *Legionella pneumophila* serogroups 1 and 10, *J Infect Dis*, **152:** 356–64.

Meers PD, Calder MW et al., 1973, Intravenous infusion of contaminated dextrose solution: the Devonport incident, *Lancet*, **2:** 1189–92.

Meers PD, Ayliffe GAJ et al., 1981, Report on the National Survey of Infection in Hospitals, 1980, *J Hosp Infect*, **2, Suppl. 1:** 1–39.

Mellersh AR, Norman P, Smith GH, 1984, *Aeromonas hydrophila*: an outbreak of hospital infection, *J Hosp Infect*, **5:** 425–30.

Menzies D, Fanning A et al., 1995, Tuberculosis among health care workers, *N Engl J Med*, **332:** 92–9.

Meyer KS, Urban C et al., 1993, Nosocomial outbreak of klebsiella infection resistant to late generation cephalosporins, *Ann Intern Med*, **119:** 353–8.

Millar MR, Brown NM et al., 1994, Outbreak of infection with penicillin-resistant *Streptococcus pneumoniae* in a hospital for the elderly, *J Hosp Infect*, **27:** 99–104.

Miller A, Gillespie WA et al., 1958, Postoperative infection in urology, *Lancet*, **2**: 608–12.

Mitchell SJ, Gray J et al., 1996, Nosocomial infection with *Rhizopus microsporus* in preterm infants: association with wooden tongue depressors, *Lancet*, **348**: 441–3.

Moberg SA, Löwhagen GE, Hersle KS, 1984, An epidemic of scabies with unusual features and treatment resistance in a nursing home, *J Am Acad Dermatol*, **11**: 242–4.

Mollison PL, Engelfriet CP, Contreras M, 1987, *Blood Transfusion in Clinical Medicine*, 8th edn, Blackwell, Oxford, 764.

Morrison D, Woodford N, Cookson BD, 1996, Epidemic vancomycin-resistant *Enterococcus faecium* in the UK, *Clin Microbiol Infect*, **1**: 146–7.

Mulin B, Talon D et al., 1995, Risks for nosocomial colonization with multiresistant *Acinetobacter baumanii*, *Eur J Clin Microbiol Infect Dis*, **14**: 569–76.

Mulley AG, Silverstein MD, Dienstag JL, 1982, Indication for use of hepatitis B vaccine, based on cost effectiveness analysis, *N Engl J Med*, **307**: 644–52.

Murphy DM, Stassen L et al., 1984, Bacteraemia during prostatectomy and other transurethral operations: influence of timing of antibiotic administration, *J Clin Pathol*, **37**: 673–6.

Murphy OM, Gray J, Pedler SJ, 1995, Non-enteric aeromonas infections in hospitalized patients, *J Hosp Infect*, **31**: 55–60.

Murray BE, 1991, New aspects of antimicrobial resistance and the resulting therapeutic dilemmas, *J Infect Dis*, **163**: 1185–94.

Nagington J, Wreghitt TG et al., 1978, Fatal echovirus 11 infections in outbreak in special-care baby unit, *Lancet*, **2**: 725–8.

Nair P, Jani K, Sanderson PJ, 1986, Transfer of oropharyngeal bacteria into the trachea during endotracheal intubation, *J Hosp Infect*, **8**: 96–103.

Nataro JP, Corcoran L, 1994, Prospective analysis of coagulase-negative staphylococcal infection in hospitalized infants, *J Pediatr*, **125**: 798–804.

National Nosocomial Infections Surveillance (NNIS) System, 1995, National Nosocomial Infections Surveillance (NNIS) Semiannual report, May 1995, *Am J Infect Control*, **23**: 377–85.

Nicolle LE, Strausbaugh LJ, Garibaldi RA, 1996, Infections and antibiotic resistance in nursing homes, *Clin Microbiol Rev*, **9**: 1–17.

Nielsen H, Stenderup J, Bruun B, 1991, Fungemia in a university hospital 1984–1988, *Scand J Infect Dis*, **23**: 275–82.

Nightingale F, 1863, *Notes on Hospitals*, Longman, London.

Nolan NPM, Kelly CP et al., 1987, An epidemic of pseudomembranous colitis: importance of person to person spread, *Gut*, **28**: 1467–73.

Norden CW, 1969, Application of antibiotic ointment to the site of venous catheterization – a controlled trial, *J Hosp Infect*, **120**: 611–15.

Nordqvist P, Ekelund P et al., 1984, Catheter-free geriatric care. Routines and consequences for clinical infection, care and economy, *J Hosp Infect*, **5**: 298–304.

Noskin GA, Peterson LR, Warren JR, 1995, *Enterococcus faecium* and *Enterococcus faecalis* bacteremia: acquisition and outcome, *Clin Infect Dis*, **20**: 296–301.

Noskin GA, Stosor V et al., 1995, Recovery of vancomycin-resistant enterococci on fingertips and environmental surfaces, *Infect Control Hosp Epidemiol*, **16**: 577–81.

Noy MF, Smith CA, Watterson LL, 1982, The use of chlorhexidine in catheter bags, *J Hosp Infect*, **1**: 365–7.

Nye K, Chadha DK et al., 1990, *Mycobacterium chelonei* isolation from broncho-alveolar lavage fluid and its practical implications, *J Hosp Infect*, **16**: 257–61.

Nystrom B, 1980, The disinfection of thermometers in hospitals, *J Hosp Infect*, **1**: 345–8.

Okell SC, Elliott SD, 1936, Cross-infection with haemolytic streptococci in otorhinological wards, *Lancet*, **2**: 836–42.

Olesen B, Kolmos HJ et al., 1995, Bacteraemia due to *Escherichia coli* in a Danish university hospital, 1986–1990, *Scand J Infect Dis*, **27**: 253–7.

Opal SM, Asp AA et al., 1986, Efficacy of infection control measures during a nosocomial outbreak of disseminated aspergillosis associated with hospital construction, *J Infect Dis*, **153**: 634–7.

Osterman CA, 1981, The infection control practitioner, *CRC Handbook of Hospital Acquired Infections*, ed. Wenzel RP, CRC Press, FL, 19–32.

Owens DK, Harris RA et al., 1995, Screening surgeons for HIV infection, *Ann Intern Med*, **122**: 641–52.

Page CP, Bohnen JH et al., 1993, Antimicrobial prophylaxis for surgical wounds. Guidelines for clinical care, *Arch Surg*, **128**: 79–88.

del Palacio Hernanz A, Fereres J et al., 1983, Nosocomial infection by *Rhizomucor pusillus* in a clinical haematology unit, *J Hosp Infect*, **4**: 45–9.

Pallares R, Linares J et al., 1995, Resistance to penicillin and cephalosporin and mortality from severe pneumococcal pneumonia in Barcelona, Spain, *N Engl J Med*, **333**: 474–80.

Palmer JD, Rickett IW, 1992, The mechanisms and risks of surgical glove perforation, *J Hosp Infect*, **22**: 279–86.

Palmer SR, 1989, Epidemiology in search of infectious diseases: methods in outbreak investigation, *J Epidemiol Community Health*, **43**: 311–14.

Palmer SR, Rowe B, 1983, Investigation of outbreaks of salmonella in hospitals, *Br Med J*, **287**: 891–3.

Pancic F, Carpentier DC, Came PE, 1980, Role of infectious secretions in the transmission of rhinovirus, *J Clin Microbiol*, **12**: 467–71.

Pankhurst CL, Philpott-Howard J, 1996, The environmental risk factors associated with medical and dental equipment in the transmission of *Burkholderia* (*Pseudomonas*) *cepacia* in cystic fibrosis patients, *J Hosp Infect*, **32**: 249–55.

Papini RP, Wilson AP et al., 1995, Wound management in burn centres in the United Kingdom, *Br J Surg*, **82**: 505–9.

Parker L, Mandal BK, 1984, Postoperative tetanus, *Lancet*, **2**: 407.

Parker MT, 1978, *Hospital-acquired Infections: Guidelines to Laboratory Methods*, WHO Regional Publications European Series No. 4, WHO, Copenhagen.

Parras F, Ena J et al., 1994, Impact of an educational program for the prevention of colonization of intravascular catheters, *Infect Control Hosp Epidemiol*, **15**: 239–42.

Patrick CH, John JF et al., 1992, Relatedness of strains of methicillin-resistant coagulase-negative staphylococcus colonizing hospital personnel and producing bacteremias in a neonatal intensive care unit, *Pediatr Infect Dis J*, **11**: 935–40.

Peachey RDG, English MP, 1974, Outbreak of *Trichophyton rubrum* infection in a geriatric hospital, *Br J Dermatol*, **91**: 389–97.

Pearman JW, 1984, Infection hazards in patients with neuropathic bladder dysfunction, *J Hosp Infect*, **5**: 355–8.

Pearman JW, Christiansen KJ et al., 1985, Control of methicillin-resistant *Staphylococcus aureus* (MRSA) in an Australian metropolitan teaching hospital complex, *Med J Aust*, **142**: 103–8.

Pearson ML, Jereb JA et al., 1992, Nosocomial transmission of multidrug-resistant *Mycobacterium tuberculosis*, *Ann Intern Med*, **117**: 191–6.

Pfaller M, Wenzel R, 1992, Impact of the changing epidemiology of fungal infections in the 1990s, *Eur J Clin Microbiol Infect Dis*, **11**: 287–91.

Phillips I, Eykyn S, Laker M, 1972, Outbreak of hospital infection caused by contaminated autoclaved fluids, *Lancet*, **1**: 1258–60.

Phillips I, Eykyn S et al., 1971, *Pseudomonas cepacia* (*multivorans*) septicaemia in an intensive-care unit, *Lancet*, **1**: 375–7.

Phillips LG, Heggers JP, Robson MC, 1992, Burn and trauma units as sources of methicillin-resistant *Staphylococcus aureus*, *J Burn Care Rehabil*, **13**: 293–7.

Philpott-Howard J, Casewell M, 1994, *Hospital Infection Control Policies and Practical Procedures*, WB Saunders, London.

Picard B, Goullet P, 1987, Seasonal prevalence of nosocomial *Aeromonas hydrophila* infection related to aeromonas in hospital water, *J Hosp Infect*, **10**: 152–5.

Piedra PA, Kasel JA et al., 1992, Description of an adenovirus type 8 outbreak in hospitalized neonates born prematurely, *Pediatr Infect Dis J*, **11:** 460–5.

Pitt TL., 1994, Bacterial typing systems: the way ahead, *J Med Microbiol*, **40:** 1–2.

Pittet D, Wenzel RP, 1995, Nosocomial bloodstream infections, *Arch Intern Med*, **155:** 1177–84.

van der Poel CL, Cuypers HT, Reesink HW, 1994, Hepatitis C virus six years on, *Lancet*, **344:** 1475–9.

Pople IK, Bayston R, Hayward RD, 1992, Infection of cerebrospinal fluid shunts in infants: a study of etiological factors, *J Neurosurg*, **77:** 29–36.

Price EH, 1984, *Staphylococcus epidermidis* in cerebrospinal fluid shunts, *J Hosp Infect*, **5:** 7–17.

Price PB, 1938, The bacteriology of normal skin: a new quantitative test applied to a study of the bacterial flora and the disinfectant action of mechanical cleaning, *J Infect Dis*, **63:** 301–18.

Pruitt BA, McManus AJ, 1992, The changing epidemiology of infection in burn patients, *Can J Surg*, **16:** 56–67.

Quinn JP, 1994, Clinical significance of extended-spectrum β-lactamases, *Eur Clin Microbiol Infect Dis*, **13, Suppl. 1:** S39–42.

Raad I, Darouiche R et al., 1995, Antibiotics and prevention of microbial colonization of catheters, *Antimicrob Agents Chemother*, **39:** 2397–400.

Raad I, Hachem R et al., 1996, Silver-iontophoretic catheter: a prototype of a long-term antiinfective vascular access device, *J Infect Dis*, **173:** 495–8.

Rao GG, 1995, Control of outbreaks of viral diarrhoea in hospitals – a practical approach, *J Hosp Infect*, **30:** 1–6.

Ratner H, 1984, *Flavobacterium meningosepticum*, *Infect Control*, **5:** 237–9.

Ravn P, Lundgren JD et al., 1991, Nosocomial outbreak of cryptosporidiosis in AIDS patients, *Br Med J*, **302:** 277–80.

Reagan DR, Pfaller MA et al., 1995, Evidence of nosocomial spread of *Candida albicans* causing bloodstream infection in a neonatal intensive care unit, *Diagn Microbiol Infect Dis*, **21:** 191–4.

Reboli AC, John JF, Levkoff AH, 1989, Epidemic methicillin-gentamicin-resistant *Staphylococcus aureus* in a neonatal intensive care unit, *Am J Dis Child*, **143:** 34–9.

Rello J, Torres A et al., 1994, Ventilator-associated pneumonia by *Staphylococcus aureus*: comparison of methicillin-resistant and methicillin-sensitive episodes, *Am J Respir Crit Care Med*, **150:** 1545–9.

Report, 1995, Report of the ASM Task Force on Antibiotic Resistance, *Antimicrob Agents Chemother*, **Suppl.:** 1–23.

Reybrouck G, 1983, Role of the hands in the spread of nosocomial infection, *J Hosp Infect*, **4:** 103–10.

Reybrouck G, 1986, Handwashing and hand disinfection, *J Hosp Infect*, **8:** 5–23.

Rhame FS, Streifel AJ et al., 1984, Extrinsic risk factors for pneumonia in the patient at high risk of infection, *Am J Med*, **76, Suppl. 5A:** 42–52.

Rhinehart E, Smith N, et al., 1990, Rapid dissemination of beta-lactamase-producing aminoglycoside-resistant *Enterococcus faecalis* among patients and staff on an infant-toddler surgical ward, *N Engl J Med*, **323:** 1814–18.

Richard P, Del Valle GA et al., 1995, Viridans streptococcal bacteraemia in patients with neutropenia, *Lancet*, **345:** 1607–9.

Ridgway EJ, Wilson AP, Kelsey MC, 1990, Preoperative screening cultures in the identification of staphylococci causing wound and valvular infections in cardiac surgery, *J Hosp Infect*, **15:** 55–63.

Ridgway GL, 1985, Decontamination of fibreoptic endoscopes, *J Hosp Infect*, **6:** 363–8.

Riley RL, Mills CC et al., 1962, Infectiousness of air from a tuberculosis ward, *Am Rev Respir Dis*, **85:** 511–25.

Robert LM, Chamberland ME et al., 1995, Investigations of patients of health care workers infected with HIV, *Ann Intern Med*, **122:** 653–7.

Rogers TR, Barnes RA, 1988, Prevention of airborne fungal

infection in immunocompromised patients, *J Hosp Infect*, **11, Suppl. A:** 15–20.

Ronan A, Hogg GG, Klug GL, 1995, Cerebrospinal fluid shunt infection in children, *Pediatr Infect Dis J*, **14:** 782–6.

Rossney AS, Pomeroy HM, Keane CT, 1994, *Staphylococcus aureus* phage typing, antimicrobial susceptibilty patterns and patient data correlated using a personal computer: advantages for monitoring the epidemiology of MRSA, *J Hosp Infect*, **26:** 219–34.

Rothman KJ, 1986, *Modern Epidemiology*, Little Brown, Boston, 57, 62 and 237.

Rudnick JR, Beck-Sagué CM et al., 1996, Gram-negative bacteremia in open-heart-surgery patients traced to probable tap-water contamination of pressure-monitoring equipment, *Infect Control Hosp Epidemiol*, **17:** 281–5.

Russell AD, Hugo WB, Ayliffe GAJ (eds), 1992, *Principles and Practice of Disinfection, Preservation and Sterilisation*, Blackwell, Oxford.

van Saene HKF, Stoutenbeek CC, Stoller JK, 1992, Selective decontamination of the digestive tract in the intensive care unit: current status and future prospects, *Crit Care Med*, **20:** 691–703.

Samore MH, Venkataraman L et al., 1996, Clinical and molecular epidemiology of sporadic and clustered cases of nosocomial *Clostridium difficile* diarrhea, *Am J Med*, **100:** 32–40.

Sanderson PJ, Rawal P, 1987, Contamination of the environment of spinal cord injured patients by organisms causing urinary-tract infection, *J Hosp Infect*, **10:** 173–8.

Sarr MG, Gott VL, Townsend TR, 1984, Mediastinal infection after cardiac surgery, *Ann Thorac Surg*, **38:** 415–23.

de Saxe MJ, Notley CM, 1978, Experiences with the typing of coagulase-negative staphylococci and micrococci, *Zentralbl Bakteriol [Orig A]*, **241:** 46–59.

Schimmelbusch C, 1894, *The Aseptic Treatment of Wounds*, trans. Rake AT, Lewis, London.

Schimpff SC, 1993, Gram-negative bacteremia, *Support Care Cancer*, **1:** 5–18.

Schneeberger PM, Vos J, van Dijk WC, 1993, Prevalence of antibodies to hepatitis C virus in a Dutch group of haemodialysis patients related to risk factors, *J Hosp Infect*, **25:** 265–70.

Schoch PE, Cunha BA, 1988, Nosocomial *Achromobacter xylosoxidans* infections, *Infect Control Hosp Epidemiol*, **9:** 84–7.

Seifert H, Strate A, Pulverer G, 1995, Nosocomial bacteremia due to *Acinetobacter baumannii*. Clinical features, epidemiology and predictors of mortality, *Medicine (Baltimore)*, **74:** 340–9.

Semmelweiss IF, 1861, *The Aetiology, the Concept and the Prophylaxis of Childbed Fever*, trans. Murphy FP, Classics of Medicine Library, Birmingham.

Seropian R, Reynolds BM, 1971, Wound infections after preoperative depilatory versus razor preparation, *Am J Surg*, **121:** 251–4.

Shanaghy N, Murphy F, Kennedy K, 1993, Improvements in the microbiological quality of food samples from a hospital cook-chill system since the introduction of HACCP, *J Hosp Infect*, **23:** 305–14.

Shanson DC, 1981, Antibiotic-resistant *Staphylococcus aureus*, *J Hosp Infect*, **2:** 11–36.

Sheridan RL, Tompkins RG, Burke JF, 1994, Prophylactic antibiotics and their role in the prevention of surgical wound infection, *Adv Surg*, **27:** 43–65.

Sheth NK, Franson TR et al., 1983, Colonization of bacteria on polyvinylchloride and Teflon intravascular catheters in hospitalized patients, *J Clin Microbiol*, **18:** 1061–3.

Shooter RA, Taylor GW et al., 1956, Post-operative wound infection, *Surg Gynecol Obstet*, **103:** 257–62.

Shooter RA, Walker KA et al., 1966, Faecal carriage of *Pseudomonas aeruginosa* in hospital patients. Possible spread from patient to patient, *Lancet*, **2:** 1331–4.

Shooter RA, Gaya H et al., 1969, Food and medicaments as possible sources of hospital strains of *Pseudomonas aeruginosa*, *Lancet*, **1:** 1227–9.

Simpson JY, 1869, Our existing system of hospitalization and its effects. Part III. Provincial hospitals of Great Britain, etc. Chapter XII Some comparisons etc., between the limb amputations in country practice and in the practice of large and metropolitan hospitals, *Edinburgh Med J*, **15**: 523.

Simpson RA, Spencer AF et al., 1986, Colonization by gentamicin-resistant *Staphylococcus epidermidis* in a special care baby unit, *J Hosp Infect*, **7**: 108–20.

Sitges-Serra A, Jaurrieta E et al., 1983, Bacteria in total parenteral nutrition catheters: where do they come from?, *Lancet*, **1**: 531.

Smith PW, 1988, Nosocomial infections in the elderly, *Infect Dis Clin North Am*, **3**: 763–77.

Snydman DR, Greer C et al., 1988, Prevention of nosocomial transmission of respiratory syncytial virus in a newborn nursery, *Infect Control Hosp Epidemiol*, **9**: 105–8.

Spach DH, Silverstein FE, Stamm WE, 1993, Transmission of infection by gastrointestinal endoscopy and bronchoscopy, *Ann Intern Med*, **118**: 117–28.

Speller DCE, Stephens ME, Viant AC, 1971, Hospital infection by *Pseudomonas cepacia*, *Lancet*, **1**: 798–9.

Speller DC, Shanson DC et al., 1990, Acquired immune deficiency syndrome: recommendations of a Working Party of the Hospital Infection Society, *J Hosp Infect*, **15**: 7–34.

Spencer RC, 1988, Infection in continuous ambulatory peritoneal dialysis, *J Med Microbiol*, **27**: 1–9.

Spencer RC, 1995, The emergence of epidemic, multiple antibiotic-resistant *Stenotrophomonas* (*Xanthomonas*) *maltophilia* and *Burkholderia* (*Pseudomonas*) *cepacia*, *J Hosp Infect*, **30, Suppl.**: 453–64.

Standfast SJ, Michelsen PB et al., 1984, A prevalence survey of infections in a combined acute and long-term care hospital, *Infect Control*, **5**: 177–84.

Stevenson P, McCann R et al., 1994, A hospital outbreak due to Norwalk virus, *J Hosp Infect*, **26**: 261–72.

Stickler DJ, Chawla JC, 1987, The role of antibiotics in the management of patients with long-term indwelling bladder catheters, *J Hosp Infect*, **10**: 219–28.

Stickler DJ, Clayton CL, Chawla JC, 1987, The resistance of urinary tract pathogens to chlorhexidine bladder washouts, *J Hosp Infect*, **10**: 28–39.

Stillman RI, Wenzel RP, Donowitz LC, 1987, Emergence of coagulase negative staphylococci as major nosocomial bloodstream pathogens, *Infect Control*, **8**: 108–12.

Stone HH, Hooper CA et al., 1976, Antibiotic prophylaxis in gastric biliary and colonic surgery, *Ann Surg*, **184**: 443–52.

Strachan CJL, 1993, Antibiotic prophylaxis in peripheral vascular and orthopaedic prosthetic surgery, *J Antimicrob Chemother*, **31, Suppl. B**: 65–78.

Struelens MJ, Rost F et al., 1993, *Pseudomonas aeruginosa* and Enterobacteriaceae bacteremia after biliary endoscopy: an outbreak investigation using DNA macrorestriction analysis, *Am J Med*, **95**: 489–98.

Struelens MJ and the Study Group on Epidemiological Markers (ESGEM) of the European Society for Clinical Microbiology and Infectious Diseases (ESCMID), 1996, Consensus guidelines for appropriate use and evaluation of microbial epidemiologic typing systems, *Clin Microbiol Infect*, **2**: 2–11.

Subcommittee of the Central Health Services Council, 1959, *Staphylococcal Infection in Hospital*, HMSO, London.

Tablan OC, Anderson LJ et al., 1994, Guidelines for prevention of nosocomial pneumonia. Part I. Issues on prevention of noscomial pneumonia – 1994, *Am J Infect Control*, **22**: 247–92.

Tam AY, Yeung CY, 1988, The changing pattern of severe neonatal staphylococcal infection: a 10-year study, *Aust Paediatr J*, **24**: 275–9.

Taylor DN, Bied JM et al., 1982, *Salmonella dublin* infections in the United States, 1979–1980, *J Infect Dis*, **146**: 322–7.

Tenover FC, McGowan JE, 1996, Reasons for the emergence of antibiotic resistance, *Am J Med Sci*, **311**: 9–16.

Tenover FC, Arbeit R et al., 1994, Comparison of traditional and molecular methods of typing isolates of *Staphylococcus aureus*, *J Clin Microbiol*, **32**: 407–15.

Thompson PJ, Greenough A et al., 1992, Nosocomial bacterial infections in very low birth weight infants, *Eur J Pediatr*, **151**: 451–4.

Thurm V, Gericke B, 1994, Identification of infant food as a vehicle in a nosocomial outbreak of *Citrobacter freundii*: epidemiological subtyping by allozyme, whole-cell protein and antibiotic resistance, *J Appl Bacteriol*, **76**: 553–8.

Tobin JO'H, Swann RA, Bartlett CLR, 1981, Isolation of *Legionella pneumophila* from water systems: methods and preliminary results, *Br Med J*, **282**: 515–17.

Tobin JO'H, Beare J et al., 1980, Legionnaires' disease in a transplant unit: isolation of the causative agent from shower baths, *Lancet*, **2**: 118–21.

Tokars JI, Marcus R et al., 1993, Surveillance of HIV infection and zidovudine use among health care workers after occupational exposure to HIV-infected blood, *Ann Intern Med*, **118**: 913–19.

Tomasz A, 1994, Rockefeller University Workshop special report. Multiple antibiotic-resistant pathogenic bacteria, *N Engl J Med*, **330**: 1247–51.

Tredget EE, Shankowsky HA et al., 1992, Epidemiology of infections with *Pseudomonas aeruginosa* in burn patients: the role of hydrotherapy, *Clin Infect Dis*, **15**: 941–9.

Tullo AB, Higgins PG, 1980, An outbreak of adenovirus type 4 conjunctivitis, *Br J Ophthalmol*, **64**: 489–93.

Vandenbrouke-Grauls CMJE, Kerver AJH et al., 1988, Endemic *Acinetobacter anitratus* in a surgical intensive care unit: mechanical ventilators as reservoir, *Eur J Clin Microbiol Infect Dis*, **7**: 485–9.

Vartivarian SE, Papadakis KA et al., 1994, Mucocutaneous and soft tissue infections caused by *Xanthomonas maltophilia*. A new spectrum, *Ann Intern Med*, **121**: 969–73.

Verville TD, Huycke MM et al., 1994, *Rhodococcus equi* infection of humans. 12 cases and a review of the literature, *Medicine (Baltimore)*, **73**: 119–32.

Vincent JL, Bihari DJ et al., 1995, The prevalence of nosocomial infection in intensive care units in Europe. Results of the European Prevalence of Infection in Intensive Care (EPIC) Study. EPIC International Advisory Committee, *JAMA*, **274**: 639–44.

van der Waaij D, Manson WL et al., 1990, Clinical use of selective decontamination: the concept, *Intensive Care Med*, **16**: S212–15.

Wagner SJ, Friedman LI, Dodd RY, 1994, Transfusion-associated bacterial sepsis, *Clin Microbiol Rev*, **7**: 290–302.

van der Wall E, Verkooyen RP et al., 1992, Prophylactic ciprofloxacin for catheter-associated urinary-tract infection, *Lancet*, **339**: 946–51.

Walters BC, 1992, Cerebrospinal fluid shunt infection, *Neurosurg Clin North Am*, **3**: 387–401.

Watanakunakorn C, Perni SC, 1994, *Proteus mirabilis* bacteremia: a review of 176 cases during 1980–1992, *Scand J Infect Dis*, **26**: 361–7.

Watt B, 1995, Lesser known mycobacteria, *J Clin Pathol*, **48**: 701–5.

Weber DJ, Rutala WA, 1988, *Bacillus* species, *Infect Control Hosp Epidemiol*, **9**: 368–73.

Weigelt JA, Dryer D, Haley RW, 1992, The necessity and efficiency of wound surveillance after discharge, *Arch Surg*, **127**: 77–81.

Weightman NC, Simpson EM et al., 1988, Bacteraemia related and indwelling central venous catheters: prevention, diagnosis and treatment, *Eur J Clin Microbiol Infect Dis*, **7**: 125–9.

Weischer M, Kolmos HJ, 1992, Retrospective 6-year study of enterobacter bacteraemia in a Danish university hospital, *J Hosp Infect*, **20**: 15–24.

Wells FC, Newsom SWB, Rowlands C, 1983, Wound infection in cardiothoracic surgery, *Lancet*, **1**: 1209–10.

Wendt C, Wenzel RP, 1996, Value of the hospital epidemiologist, *Clin Microbiol Infect*, **1:** 154–9.

Wenger PN, Otten J et al., 1995, Control of nosocomial transmission of multidrug-resistant *Mycobacterium tuberculosis* among healthcare workers and HIV-infected patients, *Lancet*, **345:** 235–40.

Wenzel RP, 1986, Old wine in new bottles, *Infect Control*, **7:** 485–6.

Wenzel RP, 1993, *Prevention and Control of Nosocomial Infections*, Williams & Wilkins, Baltimore.

Wenzel RP, 1995, The Lowbury Lecture. The economics of nosocomial infections, *J Hosp Infect*, **31:** 79–87.

Wenzel RP, Perl TM, 1995, The significance of nasal carriage of *Staphylococcus aureus* and the incidence of wound infection, *J Hosp Infect*, **31:** 13–24.

Whyte W, 1981, The Casella Slit Sampler or the Biotest Centrifugal Sampler – which is more efficient?, *J Hosp Infect*, **2:** 297–9.

Wilcox MH, Williams P et al., 1991, Variation in the expression of cell envelope proteins of coagulase-negative staphylococci cultered under iron-restricted conditions in human peritoneal dialysate, *J Gen Microbiol*, **137:** 2561–70.

Wilcox MH, Cunniffe JG et al., 1996, Financial burden of hospital-acquired *Clostridium difficile* infection, *J Hosp Infect*, **34:** 23–30.

Wilkinson PJ, 1988, Food hygiene in hospitals, *J Hosp Infect*, **11, Suppl. A:** 77–81.

Wilkinson PJ, Dart SP, Hadlington CJ, 1991, Cook-chill, cook-freeze, cook-hold sous vide: risks for hospital patients, *J Hosp Infect*, **19:** 225–30.

Willcox MDP, Stapleton F, 1996, Ocular bacteriology, *Rev Med Microbiol*, **7:** 123–31.

Williams EW, Hawkey PM et al., 1983, Serious nosocomial infection caused by *Morganella morganii* and *Proteus mirabilis* in a cardiac surgery unit, *J Clin Microbiol*, **18:** 5–9.

Williams REO, 1956, The progress of ideas on hospital infection, *Bull Hyg*, **31:** 965–79.

Williams REO, 1971, Summary of Conference, *Proceedings of the International Conference on Nosocomial Infections*, eds Brachman PS, Eickhoff TC, American Hospital Association, Chicago, 318.

Williams REO, Blowers R et al., 1960, *Hospital Infection. Causes and Prevention*, Lloyd-Luke London, 30.

Willoughby RE, Pickering LK, 1994, Necrotizing enterocolitis and infection, *Clin Perinatol*, **21:** 307–15.

Wilson AP, 1995, Surveillance of wound infection, *J Hosp Infect*, **29:** 81–6.

Wilson J, 1995, *Infection Control in Clinical Practice*, Baillière Tindall, London.

Woodford N, Johnson AP et al., 1995, Current perspectives on glycopeptide resistance, *Clin Microbiol Rev*, **5:** 585–615.

Woodhead M, 1994, Pneumonia in the elderly, *J Antimicrob Chemother*, **34, Suppl. A:** 85–92.

Woods DE, Straus DC et al., 1981, Role of salivary protease activity in adherence of gram-negative bacilli to mammalian buccal epithelial cells in vivo, *J Clin Invest*, **68:** 1435–40.

Woods TD, Watanakunakorn C, 1996, Bacteremia due to *Providencia stuartii*: review of 49 episodes, *South Med J*, **89:** 221–4.

Working Party of the British Society for Antimicrobial Chemotherapy, 1987, Diagnosis and management of peritonitis in continuous ambulatory peritoneal dialysis, *Lancet*, **1:** 845–9.

Wurtz R, Moye G, Jovanovic B, 1994, Handwashing machines, handwashing compliance, and potential for cross-contamination, *Am J Infect Control*, **22:** 228–30.

Young SEJ, 1982, Bactaeraemia 1975–1980: a survey of cases reported to the PHLS Communicable Disease Surveillance Centre, *J Hosp Infect*, **5:** 19–26.

Zangwill KM, Schuchat A et al., 1992, Group B streptococcal disease in the United States, 1990: report from a multistate active surveillance system, *Morbid Mortal Weekly Rep CDC Surveill Summ*, **41:** 25–32.

Chapter 14

STAPHYLOCOCCAL DISEASES

W C Noble

1 INTRODUCTION

The staphylococci are normal inhabitants of the body surface of man and other animals (see Volume 2, Chapter 27); their ability to cause disease appears to be a secondary feature. Many staphylococci have some ability to multiply in tissue but are kept in check by natural defence mechanisms. Nevertheless, staphylococcal disease is common because the conditions that permit the organism to gain access to the tissues are numerous and occur frequently.

The most important pathogen in the genus is *Staphylococcus aureus* which, in general, causes 2 forms of disease:

1 **Acute inflammation** that usually begins at or near the site of entry of the organisms to the tissue. In most instances it is relatively mild and localized but at times spreads widely by direct extension and occasionally leads to generalized infection. Examples are boils, furuncles and surgical wound infection.

2 **Acute toxaemia** that results from the absorption of extracellular products formed by staphylococci multiplying at a lesion site, a carrier site, or outside the body. Examples include exfoliation of the skin caused by epidermolytic toxins, staphylococcal diarrhoea usually accompanied by vomiting caused by multiplication of the organisms in food (staphylococcal food poisoning) or in the gut (staphylococcal postantibiotic diarrhoea) or toxic shock syndrome, a generalized toxaemia associated with growth of staphylococci at carrier sites or in tissues.

Some examples of infection due to *S. aureus* are listed in Table 14.1.

The ability of *S. aureus* to gain access to the tissues appears to be determined as much by host factors as by the characteristics of the infecting strain. The

Table 14.1 Examples of infection with *Staphylococcus aureus*

Primary infection
Superficial infection
folliculitis
furunculosis
impetigo
Deep infection
abscess
wound infection
pneumonia
osteomyelitis
septicaemia
Secondary infection
eczema
decubitus ulcers
Toxin mediated disease
food poisoning
toxic shock syndrome
scalded skin syndrome

organism may enter by penetrating apparently unbroken skin or through a break in the skin due to accidental trauma or surgical intervention or through a mucous membrane damaged by viral infection or other pathological process, or even through a normally sterile cavity such as the bladder. One of the main determinants for staphylococcal infection is a local or general lowering of host resistance, though individual strains of *S. aureus* differ in their ability to invade and establish infection.

Outside hospital many staphylococcal infections are self-infections and appear to be sporadic, though some, such as impetigo, are epidemic. Staphylococcal infection may be a communicable disease and this is most evident in hospitals and semi-closed communities where populations of particularly susceptible individuals may be infected by single strains.

Since the extensive introduction of foreign bodies such as catheters and prostheses in surgery, the coagulase-negative staphylococci have become much more important as agents of infection. Although they rarely cause localized inflammation in the absence of foreign bodies, deep infections such as peritonitis, endocarditis and chronic septicaemia are well documented in patients receiving peritoneal dialysis, prosthetic heart valves, joint prostheses or long-term intravenous catheters.

The pathogenesis of infection in animals other than humans is less well understood though much has been learned in recent years. The study of natural infection in animals has sometimes illuminated disease in humans.

2 STAPHYLOCOCCUS AUREUS

2.1 Carriage

Although it is common to assume that *S. aureus* is the only coagulase-positive staphylococcus encountered in humans, a small number of normal individuals carry *Staphylococcus intermedius* in the anterior nares (Harvey, Marples and Noble 1994). This animal pathogen coagulates plasma in the tube coagulase test but is negative for clumping factor and is rarely positive with commercial kit tests that rely on clumping factor and protein A. In the past it has probably been described as 'atypical' *S. aureus*.

In persons without skin disease, resident carriage of *S. aureus* on unspecialized skin sites is rare, though assiduous examination with sensitive culture techniques will reveal small numbers of cells in about 50% of the population. In normal individuals, carriage in the anterior nares is found in 20–40% of the population and in the axillae, groin (perineum) and toe-webs of about 10%, 20% and 5% respectively (Noble, Valkenburg and Wolters 1967, Polakoff et al. 1967). All rates are subject to considerable variation; successive monthly random samples each of about 240 individuals from a normal population yielded rates of 29%, 37%, 24%, 36%, 25% and 23% (Noble, Valkenburg and Wolters 1967), making it difficult to determine whether particular populations such as those with AIDS (Ganesh et al. 1989, Amir et al. 1995) or diabetes (Boyco et al. 1989) have significantly different carrier rates (Table 14.2). There is a family propensity to carry *S. aureus* in the nose and this may be related to the HLA-Dr tissue type (Kinsman, McKenna and Noble 1983). Patients with skin disease such as atopic dermatitis have nose and skin carriage rates that may be in excess of 80% (Bibel, Greenberg and Cook 1977, Hauser et al. 1985).

2.2 Infections of skin and soft tissues

LOCALIZED INFECTION

S. aureus is responsible for about 70% of all soft tissue infections in humans but the proportion due to specific organisms is very site specific; for example, half of all axillary abscesses contain *S. aureus* but only 8% of vulvovaginal abscesses do so (Meislin et al. 1977). Folliculitis is a mild form of infection but may cause problems at particular sites, for example, the eye (styes). The characteristic staphylococcal lesion is the boil (furuncle), a subepidermal collection of pus, often around the root of a hair follicle. It has been estimated that about 5–9% of the population have one or more minor skin infections a year, most of which are boils (Gould and Cruickshank 1957, Kay 1962). About one-third of the patients have 2 or more lesions in succession and over 10% have recurrent infections over years or months (Roodyn 1960, Steele 1980, Hedstrom 1981). Infections occur more frequently in the first 40 years of life with peaks in those of 1–10 years and 30–40 years (Kay 1962). In about 65% of cases the infecting strain is the same as that carried in the nose, especially where the lesion is of the head or neck. The proportion contributed by perineal carriage is not known. In industrial injuries to the hand local contamination is more important than nasal carriage (Williams and Miles 1949).

In the 1950s, sepsis of the skin was more common among close family contacts of persons recently discharged from hospital, and especially babies born in hospital, than in the rest of the community (Ravenholt, Wright and Mulhearn 1957, Hurst and Grossman 1960, Galbraith 1960) but this was not the experience in later studies (Oliver et al. 1964). This may in part be due to the decline in the prevalence of staphylococci of types 52/52A/80/81 in the later years.

The host factors associated with the development of boils or furuncles are numerous, including pressure, minor trauma and some immunological deficiencies. Boils on the neck are often ascribed to wearing tight collars and this is accentuated in hot, humid climates where wearing western-style suits predisposes to local infections to a greater degree than wearing a local form of dress (Selwyn, Verma and Vaishnav 1967). Minor trauma in industry (Williams and Miles 1949), or occupation (Decker et al. 1986), experimental occlusion of skin (Singh, Marples and Kligman 1971) or tight contaminated surgical stitches (Elek and Conen 1957) also increase the probability of infection. Sports injuries may also increase the risk of infection (Sosin et al. 1989). Patients with chronic furunculosis are frequently reported to have a defect of cell mediated immunity (Yocum et al. 1976, Blum and Fish 1977, Rebora et al. 1978).

LOCALIZED INFECTION IN ANIMALS

Most species of domestic animal suffer localized infections similar to those in humans; for commercial reasons much attention is paid to mastitis in cattle, sheep, goats and rabbits (reviewed by Lloyd 1993). In most cases infection is due to animal biotypes of *S. aureus* but some infections, especially in dogs, are due to *S. intermedius*, formerly described as *S. aureus* biotypes E and F. Most infections follow some form of trauma; pyoderma in dogs is associated with scratching and flea allergy, furunculosis in horses occurs most

Table 14.2 Nasal carrier rates of *Staphylococcus aureus* in various populations

Population	N	Percentage nasal carriers
Normals, Netherlands		
Mean rate	1418	29 ± 7 *SD*
range	c. 240	23–35
HIV-negative, UK	56	27
HIV-positive, UK	47	45
HIV-negative, Kenya	290	17
HIV-positive, Kenya	264	27
Non-diabetics, USA	363	21
Diabetics (non-insulin-requiring), USA	188	27

Based on Noble, Valkenburg and Wolters 1967, Boyko et al. 1989, Ganesh et al. 1989, Amir et al. 1995.

commonly in the area covered by the saddle and girths.

2.3 Exfoliative diseases

These are characterized by separation of the superficial layers of the skin by sideways pressure or the formation of bullae (blisters) as a result of the action of epidermolytic toxins. Early reports (Parker, Tomlinson and Williams 1955) indicated that most of the *S. aureus* responsible were of phage group II and lysed only by phage 71; they were egg yoke opacity negative and most produced a bacteriocin, later shown to be encoded on a plasmid that also bears the gene for epidermolytic toxin B. Later reports (da Azavedo and Arbuthnott 1981) showed that about a quarter of strains did not belong to phage group II and belonged to a large range of phage types.

Impetigo presents in 2 basic forms; simple or crusted lesions are formed when vesicles develop, burst and discharge copious amount of serous fluid. This forms the characteristic 'honey coloured stuck-on crusts'. In bullous impetigo the lesions appear as blisters (bullae) which rupture to reveal an erythematous base and are named variously according to their severity, extent and distribution: including bullous impetigo and pemphigus neonatorum (a misnomer). Staphylococcal impetigo is chiefly a disease of children but may occur in adults living under conditions of poor hygiene; staphylococci are readily recovered from the initial lesions. In the European literature the term impetigo has generally implied a staphylococcal infection, whereas in North America it was more often used for streptococcal disease. There are indications that staphylococci have more often been involved in North America in recent years (Demidovitch et al. 1990). Streptococcal and mixed infections are also found. Impetigo may be epidemic in schools and closed communities (Mobacken et al. 1975, Kaplan et al. 1986, Dancer et al. 1990b).

Bullous impetigo forms the mild end of a spectrum of disease, the extreme of which, scalded skin syndrome, is seen in neonates and young children and is chiefly reported in its epidemic form (Curran and Al Salihi 1980, Dancer et al. 1988, Richardson et al. 1990,

Dave et al. 1994). It is rare in immunocompetent adults (Opal, Johnson-Winegar and Cross 1988) but seen occasionally in those with immunosuppression or renal incompetence (Peterson et al. 1977, Goldberg et al. 1989). In adult patients with AIDS an extensive, atypical bullous impetigo may be seen (Duvic 1987). Scalded skin syndrome was first described by Ritter von Rittershain in 1878 – hence the term 'Ritter's disease' – and later by Lyell (1979) as the scalded skin syndrome; the early literature frequently described this disease as 'toxic epidermal necrolysis', a term now reserved for a drug-induced splitting of the skin seen most frequently in adults. The staphylococcal and drug-induced diseases are differentiated by the level and manner in which the skin splits (Amon and Dimond 1975, Manzella et al. 1980). The onset is abrupt, with generalized erythema closely resembling that of scarlet fever; within 1–2 days the skin becomes wrinkled and peels off on light stroking (Nikolsky's sign). Large flaccid bullae appear and extensive areas of skin may be exfoliated; there may be acute toxaemia followed by death. The causative organisms are not found in the unopened bullae but may be secondary invaders of the damaged skin. The epidermolytic toxins ETA and ETB are serine proteases (Bailey and Smith 1990, Dancer et al. 1990a) that cause the skin to split at the stratum granulosum (de Dobbeleer and Achten 1975, Elias, Fritsch and Epstein 1977); the toxins act at sites distant from the infected lesion which may be facial impetigo or an umbilical stump.

Melish and Glasgow (1971) reported scarlatiniform rashes in 11 young children. These were distinguished from scarlet fever chiefly by the absence of an enanthem and by the presence of a transient Nikolsky's sign in 9 cases. This suggests that exfoliative toxins may cause the rash, but there are reports of a more specific staphylococcal scarlet fever due to the action of the pyrogenic exotoxins (Schlievert 1981, Rahman and Rammelkamp 1982). Scarlatiniform rashes are also seen in toxic shock syndrome accompanied by extensive exfoliation at a late stage but epidermolytic toxins are not involved in toxic shock syndrome.

EXFOLIATIVE DISEASE IN ANIMALS

Although newborn mice and the adult hairless mouse (hrhr) are also susceptible to epidermolytic toxins and form an excellent animal model of the disease, most animals are not susceptible (Fritsch, Kaaserer and Elias 1979). There remain occasional reports of a scalded skin syndrome-like reaction in dogs (Love and Davis 1980) infected with *S. intermedius* and toxins similar to ETA and ETB have been reported from *Staphylococcus hyicus* recovered from pigs (Amtsberg 1979). Most recently a new epidermolytic toxin, termed ETC, has been reported from *S. aureus* skin infection of a horse; ETC acts on the skin of mice and day-old chicks, whereas ETA and ETB of human origin act only on the mouse and the epidermolytic toxin from *S. hyicus* only on chicks (Sato et al. 1994).

2.4 Secondary infection

Lesions of atopic dermatitis and adjacent normal skin in adults are almost universally colonized at high density by *S. aureus* (Leyden, Marples and Kligman 1974, Ogawa et al. 1994) though this is less frequent in children (David and Cambridge 1986, Hoeger et al. 1992). At bacterial densities over about 10^5 cm^{-2} the lesions may appear clinically infected and require antibiotic therapy; there is current speculation that infection involves the superantigen activity of the enterotoxins and toxic shock syndrome toxin (McFadden, Noble and Camp 1993), perhaps by formation of IgE antibody resulting in histamine release from basophils (Leung et al. 1993). Other non-infective skin lesions such as psoriasis may also become colonized but to a much lesser extent than in atopic dermatitis. Secondary infection of viral lesions such as chickenpox and of scabies also occurs regularly but usually without serious consequences.

2.5 Sepsis in wounds and burns

S. aureus is the most common cause of sepsis in minor trauma and remains responsible for about one-third to one-half of all surgical wound infection. The frequency of infection depends on the type of operation, the age of the patient, the length of incision and other parameters (Lidwell 1961, Abussaud and Meqdem 1986). Burn wounds often carry *S. aureus* but it does not usually cause delay in healing or rejection of a graft.

2.6 Infections of the urinary tract

Cystitis and pyelonephritis due to *S. aureus* rarely occur outside hospital but may follow catheterization or operations on the bladder or prostate. They form only a small proportion of hospital-acquired urinary tract infection but may have serious consequences; up to 15% may be complicated by bacteraemia (Demuth, Gerding and Crossley 1979). Haematogenous spread to the kidneys may also occur.

2.7 Staphylococcal pneumonia

S. aureus may invade the lungs from the bloodstream, giving rise to abscesses; more often it causes a primary pneumonia. This occurs in 3 classes of patients:

1 young infants
2 healthy young adults secondary to influenza
3 adults suffering from serious diseases.

Infection of infants tends to occur in the premature or sickly and in the past was frequently due to strains with particular epidemic potential. Currently fewer such patients are seen than formerly though the infection still leads to a rapidly progressive disease with significant mortality (Knight and Carman 1992). Post-influenzal pneumonia is the main cause of death in young adults following influenza A infection. The onset of the staphylococcal disease is rapid, sputum is watery, profuse and evenly blood-tinged. Death may occur in 1–2 days. Massive numbers of staphylococci are found in the lungs, a result of the damage to tissue which occurs as a result of viral infection. Staphylococcal pneumonia is rare in young adults in the absence of influenza, except in those who are HIV-positive where 6% of episodes of pulmonary infection were due to *S. aureus* and had a mortality rate of 38% (Levine, White and Fels 1990). Isolation of *S. aureus* may be a poor guide to the frequency of staphylococcal pneumonia in debilitated hospital patients. Only 3% of isolations from sputum on admission to hospital and 17% of apparent acquisitions were clinically significant. However, patients with head injuries more often had *S. aureus* in the respiratory tract (19% of 91) compared with other patients (1.8% of 549) receiving ventilation and about half (8 of 17) of the head injury patients had pneumonia (Inglis et al. 1993). Coma is a significant factor in the development of hospital-acquired pneumonia (Rello et al. 1990).

Staphylococcal lung infection is common in patients with cystic fibrosis but is probably of less significance than infection with *Pseudomonas aeruginosa* (Hudson, Wielinski and Regelmann 1993). Staphylococci in cystic fibrosis patients have no distinctive properties (Branger et al. 1994) and are replaced by pseudomonas as the disease progresses.

2.8 Osteomyelitis

In its acute form this is frequently caused by *S. aureus* and is usually accompanied by bacteraemia. Recent data indicate a decline in the importance of *S. aureus*, at least in children, and a shift in the most prevalent site from the long bones to the vertebral column (Espersen et al. 1991, Craigen, Watters and Hackett 1992).

2.9 Generalized infection

S. aureus may spread from a localized lesion through the tissue planes or along the lymphatics to the regional lymph nodes, but it often causes a more serious disease when it spreads by the bloodstream.

Occasionally this may follow a local trivial lesion in an apparently healthy person. Indeed, the fact that staphylococcal osteomyelitis seldom follows a recognized local lesion but may be precipitated by mild injury to the bone suggests that transient staphylococcal bacteraemia is quite common. Abscesses of the kidney (renal carbuncle) also result from the deposition of staphylococci from the blood; they develop in the renal cortex, do not communicate with the renal collecting system and tend to spread to the adjacent perinephric tissue. Nowadays they are less common than formerly except in association with intravenous drug abuse.

STAPHYLOCOCCAL SEPTICAEMIA, PYAEMIA AND ENDOCARDITIS

Acute septicaemia may occur in association with local suppuration, such as wound sepsis, pneumonia or osteomyelitis, or it may occur spontaneously. Septicaemia often develops in patients who are predisposed to it by a serious underlying disease such as neoplasia, liver disease, diabetes, rheumatoid arthritis, or certain extensive skin diseases or by septic complications of procedures for their relief, notably surgical operations and intravenous cannulation (Lautenschlager, Herzog and Zimmerli 1993, Espersen et al. 1994). The special liability of patients with severe rheumatoid arthritis to suffer from staphylococcal septicaemia, often with pyoarthritis, is only partly attributable to treatment with steroids. Parenteral drug abusers with endocarditis due to S. aureus are especially likely to develop rheumatoid factor (24%) compared with 7% of control non-infected drug abusers (Sheagren et al. 1976). The foot is a frequent source of infection in patients with rheumatoid disease (Morris and Eade 1978).

Endocarditis develops in many cases of septicaemia. According to Nolan and Beaty (1976), endocarditis occurs rather infrequently in cases of septicaemia in which there is an identifiable primary staphylococcal infection. When the primary focus is one that can easily be removed, for example, an infected cannula site, the septicaemia usually responds to a short course of antimicrobial therapy. Septicaemia without an obvious primary source is more commonly associated with endocarditis and with the subsequent development of pyaemic abscesses elsewhere in the body (Nolan and Beaty 1976) and is much more difficult to eradicate. Surgical intervention in congenital heart disease has changed the natural history of endocarditis in children with a decrease in S. aureus infections (Awadallah et al. 1991). S. aureus is one of the important causes of endocarditis associated with intravenous drug abuse (Tuazon, Cardella and Sheagren 1975, Robbins et al. 1986). Fulminating attacks of staphylococcal septicaemia may be associated with thrombocytopenia, disseminated intravascular coagulation, glomerulonephritis and occasionally symmetrical peripheral gangrene (Murray, Tuazon and Sheagren 1977), which may be attributed to activation of the alternative complement pathway (O'Connor, Wiseman and Fierer 1978).

Meningitis due to S. aureus may result from haematogenous spread, especially in older patients with underlying disease, but is more frequently associated with trauma and foreign body infection (Jensen et al. 1993).

S. aureus is often present in considerable numbers in the urine of patients with staphylococcal septicaemia even in the absence of renal abscess (Lee, Crossley and Gerding 1978).

Tropical pyomyositis is a generalized staphylococcal disease that affects apparently healthy young people; large abscesses (frequently multiple) develop in voluntary muscles. The disease is more common in tropical than in temperate climates and has been especially common in Central Africa and New Guinea (Shepherd 1983). Infection does not appear to follow skin sepsis, but various predisposing factors have been described including intravenous drug abuse, diabetes and other staphylococcal sepsis (Jimenez-Mejias et al. 1992, Belsky Teates and Hartman 1994). The source of the staphylococci is not known but a preponderance of phage group II strains suggests a degree of epidemic spread.

Septicaemic infection in animals is exemplified by tick pyaemia in lambs and exudative epidermitis in pigs. Infected lambs may die from septicaemia a few days after birth; those that escape suffer chronic abscesses of the joints and liver. The disease occurs only in geographical areas in which sheep are infected with the tick *Ixodes ricinus*, causing a profound neutropenia (tick-borne fever); experimentally it has been shown that the tick acts as a vector for the introduction of S. aureus which are normally present on the lamb's skin (Webster and Mitchell 1989). In pigs less than 8 weeks old severe cases of exudative epidermitis (greasy pig disease) due to S. hyicus begin as a facial dermatitis which progresses to the mouth, lips and coronets; systemic infection is followed by death in 3–8 days (Lloyd 1993).

2.10 Staphylococcal toxic shock syndrome

Under this name Todd and colleagues (1978) described a characteristic syndrome of high fever, headache, confusion, conjunctival reddening, subcutaneous oedema, vomiting and diarrhoea, and profound hypotensive shock in children and adults. In the more severe cases, acute renal failure, disseminated intravascular coagulation, peripheral gangrene, and even death occurred. All the patients had a scarlatiniform rash; fine desquamation of the hands and feet often occurred during convalescence. Patients examined bacteriologically yielded S. aureus from one or more sites.

In 1979, cases of a similar illness in young women began to be reported with increasing frequency in the USA. A striking association was shown with the use of highly absorbent intravaginal tampons during menstruation, especially when these were used continuously and changed infrequently (Davis et al. 1980, Shands et al. 1980). Two or more attacks, each associated with menstruation and the use of tampons, were reported in a number of women. Patients with toxic shock syndrome lack pre-existing antibodies to the toxin; not all patients develop antibody after an initial illness, accounting for recurrences (Davis et al. 1980, Vergeront et al. 1983). The low incidence of toxic shock syndrome in very young children may be attributable to maternal antibody (Jacobson et al. 1987). The conditions under which toxin is formed in tampons are not wholly established. Apart from extended use, the density of the packing material (related to the absorbency), which increases the surface area and controls the air content, appears to encourage greater growth of staphylococci and more toxin production (Reiser, Hinzman and Bergdoll 1987) though toxin is not produced under strictly anaerobic conditions (Tierno and Hanna 1989). It has been suggested that the polyacrylate component of high absorbency tampons may absorb magnesium and permit production of the toxin. The results of studies on Mg^{2+} on toxin production are conflicting but may be summarized as follows: in vitro low levels of Mg^{2+} (2–5 mg ml^{-1}) result in increased production but higher levels (c. 15 mg ml^{-1}) suppress toxin production; low levels of Zn^{2+} and Fe^{2+} enhance the effect of Mg^{2+} on production (Reeves 1989). However, not all workers agree with these findings; this may be due in part to the diverse in vitro models that have been employed.

In 1979–80 the incidence of toxic shock syndrome in Wisconsin was 6 per 10 000 menstruating women (Davis et al. 1980) but it appears to have been less common outside North America (de Saxe et al. 1982). Withdrawal from sale of the super absorbent tampons substantially reduced the incidence of this disease and currently only about 50–70% of toxic shock syndrome cases are associated with tampons (Reingold 1991, Schuchat and Broome 1991, Marples and Wieneke 1993). Non-menstrual cases may follow wound infection, as in the original description by Todd et al. (1978) or from apparently trivial local lesions.

Schlievert, Schoettle and Watson (1979) reported a toxin, pyrogenic exotoxin C, which enhanced the effect of enterobacterial endotoxin by 50 000-fold (Schlievert 1981). Bergdoll et al. (1981) reported, as enterotoxin F, a toxin with the general properties of an enterotoxin; its presence was detected immunologically from 94% of *S. aureus* strains from the vagina of patients with toxic shock syndrome but from only 10% of *S. aureus* from other sources. Antibody titres showed the reverse distribution. Enterotoxin F and pyrogenic exotoxin C are now accepted as identical and are referred to as toxic shock syndrome toxin-1 (TSST-1) (Bonventre et al. 1983). The presence of a temperate phage probably determines production of the toxin, accounting for the description of menstrual isolates as 'clonal' (Kreiswirth et al. 1989). The majority of TSST-1 producing strains are phage group I, lysed particularly by phage 29. Toxic shock syndrome associated with enterotoxin B in the absence of TSST-1 has been reported (DiTomaso and Warner 1994, Renaud et al. 1994). Given the role of TSST-1 and the enterotoxins as superantigens, this may not be surprising. A variant of toxic shock syndrome, described as recalcitrant, ery-

thematous and desquamating, has been described in patients with AIDS (Cone et al. 1992) associated with the production of TSST-1 and enterotoxins A and B. The presence of enterotoxin C in the kidneys of about one-third of cases of sudden infant death syndrome has been reported (Malam et al. 1992) though other enterotoxins and TSST-1 are not seen. As superantigens, TSST-1 and the enterotoxins are able to activate T cells non-specifically, resulting in the massive release of cytokines including interleukins 1 and 2 and tumour necrosis factor.

Strains of *S. aureus* recovered from animals also produce TSST-1 but the associated pathology has been little explored. Thus 28.6% of bovine mammary isolates of *S. aureus* produced one or more of the enterotoxins or TSST-1 (Kenny et al. 1993). In goats about 25% of strains produced TSST-1 and over 40% of animals had antibody to TSST-1 in serum or milk, indicating production of the toxin in vivo (Valle et al. 1991). Comparable figures for strains of human origin are that about 60% of phage group I strains produce TSST-1 and about 10% of other phage groups, a mean of about 30% (Ejlertsen et al. 1994).

DIARRHOEA AND VOMITING

It has been known for many years that diarrhoea and vomiting follow ingestion of food contaminated with preformed staphylococcal enterotoxins. The symptoms occur within 30 min to 6 h of ingestion with a peak at about 2 h; enterotoxin A is most frequently implicated (Richards et al. 1993, Wieneke, Roberts and Gilbert 1993).

During the period 1950–65 there were cases of acute staphylococcal diarrhoea in which the organisms were multiplying in the gut. Soon after the introduction of the tetracyclines there were reports of severe choleriform diarrhoea in patients undergoing treatment with one of these antibiotics. Severe dehydration and death often followed. The normal coliform gut flora had been replaced by an overgrowth of *S. aureus* resistant to tetracycline. Prompt treatment with an antibiotic to which the staphylococci were sensitive resulted in speedy amelioration of the symptoms. Similar diarrhoea attacks were reported to follow the use of other antibiotics. In the early 1960s many cases were associated with preoperative preparation of the bowel by the use of neomycin. With more sophisticated decontamination regimens this problem has almost disappeared. Many episodes were associated with the staphylococcal strains then endemic in the wards. Most of these were phage group III and produced enterotoxin B, though enterotoxin A was also formed (Dack 1956).

In retrospect it seems improbable that all cases of post-antibiotic diarrhoea during the 1950–65 period were caused by *S. aureus*. Later discoveries revealed that a cytotoxin is secreted by *Clostridium difficile* that can cause necrosis of the bowel tissue and enterocolitis related to antibiotic therapy (see Chapter 35), suggest that other microbial species may well have been involved.

3 PATHOGENESIS OF THE LOCAL INFLAMMATORY LESION

Remarkably little has been added to our knowledge of the pathogenesis of local lesions and it remains probable that a cocktail of enzymes, toxins or a combination of both is responsible for the observed lesion. The intradermal or subcutaneous injection of *S. aureus* into human subjects does not result in the appearance of a local lesion unless the infecting dose is very large. Much smaller inocula suffice in man, mice and guinea pigs, but not rabbits, if a foreign body is used to introduce the staphylococci; in rabbits a burn or other form of skin injury has a similar effect. A consideration of the diverse experiments performed indicates that a staphylococcal lesion in skin or soft tissue is likely to be found under the following local conditions:

1 vasoconstriction
2 necrosis
3 acute inflammation due to another organism
4 a hypersensitivity reaction
5 the presence of a foreign body.

Anti-inflammation agents, including the endotoxin of gram-negative bacilli (Conti, Cluff and Scheder 1961) and some, but not all, corticosteroids (Agarwal 1967b), enhance the severity of the lesion.

Comparison of the lesions in mice formed by introducing *S. aureus* subcutaneously either in fluid medium or on a cotton dust plug (Noble 1965) showed that the effect of a foreign body was to slow down the rate of exudation of fluid and migration of leucocytes into the lesions (Agarwal 1967a), permitting the staphylococci to multiply. In humans, acute inflammation also results from placing small numbers of *S. aureus* on the skin after the outer epidermal layers have been removed by repeated skin stripping with adhesive tape (Singh, Marples and Kligman 1971). The conditions necessary for a severe lesion are that:

1 the area is kept moist
2 serum exudes from the surface
3 leucocytes do not migrate into the exudate until the lesion is established
4 few competing organisms are present.

Extensive spreading cellulitis appears regularly if a few hundred cocci are applied soon after the skin is stripped. If the inoculation is delayed by 24 h the lesion is less severe and more localized; if delayed for 48 h it is minimal or absent. Protection of the staphylococci from the cellular defences of the body and delay in mobilizing them for only a short time thus appear to be important determinants of wound infection.

Little is known about how *S. aureus* penetrates the apparently unbroken skin to cause a boil. The anatomy of the lesion suggests that it often begins in a hair follicle. Experimental infections appear to require much larger numbers of organisms than are found on normal human skin. Serendipitous observations made during studies on gene transfer on skin have revealed that the minor trauma caused by pulling out hairs during removal of adhesive tape results in folliculitis, whereas the simple presence of large numbers of staphylococci does not.

The fact that almost all *S. aureus* strains that cause boils form a lipase active on Tween 80 and opacity in egg yolk broth suggests that the ability to attack certain skin lipids is a determinant for the formation of boils. This hypothesis has been tested by taking Tween-negative variants of boil producing strains, prepared by lysogenic conversion, and comparing with the wild-type the ability of these organisms to cause lesions when instilled into the hair follicles of pigs (Jessen and Bülow 1967). Lipase-negative variants failed to cause boils in this model whereas the lipase-positive strains resulted in localized boil-like infection. This is unlikely to be the only determinant for boil production, however, since Tween-positive phage group III strains, which cause postoperative wound infection, rarely cause boils. Suppression of skin surface lipid during aggressive therapy of acne vulgaris by isotretinoin results in up to half the treated patients developing lesions due to *S. aureus* (Leyden and Jones 1987, Williams et al. 1992). However, such treatments alter the general skin structure and also reduce the potentially competing flora. Removing skin lipid (and also skin flora) with ethanol as well as creating a high surface humidity favours local multiplication of staphylococci (Foster and Hutt 1960, Singh, Marples and Kligman 1971). This may lead to a lesion that is papulovesicular rather than a boil; the staphylococci are confined to the superficial layers of the epidermis; and necrosis, oedema and haemorrhages appear in the underlying tissue. According to Singh, Marples and Kligman (1971) this is a toxic dermatitis due to staphylococcal extracellular products. Similar lesions form spontaneously under occlusive dressings on the skin of carriers of neomycin-resistant *S. aureus* if they are treated with neomycin (Marples and Kligman 1969).

ADHERENCE

It is self-evident that bacteria that cannot adhere to tissue will rapidly be removed by desquamation, blood flow, etc., and are therefore much less liable to cause infection. Much interest has been generated in the ability of *S. aureus* to adhere to extracellular matrix proteins, especially fibronectin, and specific fibronectin-binding proteins have been explored (Proctor 1987, Wadström 1987). Fibronectin binding to *S. aureus* does not encourage phagocytosis, playing little part in opsonization (Verbrugh et al. 1981). Deposition of fibronectin on catheters, sutures and other implants facilitates the adherence of staphylococci and permits growth and expression of pathogenesis. A glycocalyx forms round adherent micro-organisms and protects them against phagocytosis and perhaps from the action of antibiotics. Mayberry-Carson et al. (1983) observed glycocalyx formation on catheters in an osteomyelitis model. Fibronectin and protein A are important in adherence of *S. aureus* to human mesothelial cell monolayers (Glancey et al. 1993, Poston et al. 1993). Collagen binding proteins have been shown to play a part in experimental septic arthritis; mutant *S. aureus* that lack a collagen binding gene were much less likely to cause infection in mice (Patti et al. 1994), whereas *S. aureus* strains from human patients with septic arthritis possess the ability to adhere to cartilage (Switalski et al. 1993).

PHAGOCYTOSIS

Various serum factors (opsonins) are necessary for the phagocytosis of staphylococci. Most human sera contain antibacterial (opsonic) antibodies, the action of which is enhanced by complement. In addition, complement is activated by staphylococci through the alternative pathway and primary opsonic activity independent of the presence of specific antibody. However, opsonization by the antibody-dependent classical pathway is rapid and efficient in contrast to the alternative pathway (Quie et al. 1981). After phagocytosis in the presence of serum, there is an initial rapid fall in the number of viable *S. aureus* though a small number survive; under similar conditions, coagulase-negative staphylococci are usually completely destroyed.

The increased susceptibility to *S. aureus* infections of patients with various abnormalities of the phagocytic system indicates that this cellular element of the early inflammatory response may be of primary importance in the development of septic lesions. This has been reviewed by Quie and colleagues (Quie, Hill and Davies 1974, Quie et al. 1981). Absence of antibody and abnormalities of the complement cascade leading to poor opsonization, are causes of increased susceptibility to staphylococcal infection. Various miscellaneous causes are described but in late stage infections phagocytic cells express reduced chemotaxis and phagocytosis compared with healthy controls (Ellis et al. 1988, Pos et al. 1992). By contrast, human pulmonary alveolar macrophages from HIV-positive patients without pneumonia were more actively phagocytic than those from healthy controls. In HIV-positive patients with pneumonia, usually due to *Pneumocystis carinii*, phagocytic function is, however, much reduced (Musher et al. 1990). Before the advent of AIDS the most striking effects on phagocytosis were seen in diseases resulting from deficiencies in the response of leucocytes to chemotactic stimulation or in their bactericidal function.

Job's syndrome is a rare disease in which recurrent, severe 'cold' staphylococcal abscesses and chronic eczema are associated with a very high serum IgE concentration associated with a deficit of anti-*S. aureus* serum IgA (Dreskin, Goldsmith and Gallin 1985). The leucocytes of these patients exhibit a profoundly depressed leucotactic response. A variant of this syndrome was seen in a patient with end stage renal disease, chronic eczema and high IgE levels who suffered more than 15 episodes of peritonitis while receiving continuous ambulatory peritoneal dialysis (CAPD) (Khan and Bank 1994). Formation of fibrin in the dialysate by *S. aureus* may account for the interference with phagocytosis (Davies et al. 1990). Depression of leucotaxis has also been reported in juvenile rheumatoid arthritis and in diabetes mellitus (Quie, Hill and Davies 1974).

In **chronic granulomatous disease** phagocytosis is normal but does not lead to the usual oxidative burst of metabolic activity that results in the intracellular accumulation of H_2O_2 that is necessary for the bactericidal action of the myeloperoxidase. As a result, patients suffer from repeated chronic, septic infections, notably of the cervical glands and lungs, caused by catalase-positive bacteria including staphylococci.

The importance of a capsule in resistance to phagocytosis has been re-evaluated in recent years. Capsular types 5 and 8, the most common in bloodstream isolates of *S. aureus*, are described as microcapsular and the cocci are readily phagocytosed and killed in normal serum containing complement. This does not hold true for encapsulated type 1 strains (Xu, Arbeit and Lee 1992). In experimental infections in mice (Lee et al. 1987) an exopolysaccharide capsule rendered the strain more able to cause disease. Vaccination with capsular material has been proposed for the prevention or reduction of staphylococcal infections (Foster 1991).

Bacteriostasis by serum

Coagulase-positive staphylococci have a much greater ability than coagulase-negative staphylococci to grow in normal serum. Serum in which coagulase-positive staphylococci have grown will, however, support the growth of the coagulase-negative cocci. The importance of this for pathogenesis is unclear. Strains of *S. aureus* and sera both differ in the degree to which inhibition occurs.

CELLULAR VIRULENCE FACTORS

Some staphylococcal strains form substances that delay the mobilization of local defence mechanisms. The bacterial cell wall has aggressive activity, so that the addition of dead organisms to living ones favours the production of a lesion (Fisher 1963, Gow et al. 1963); this effect is attributable to heat- and acid-resistant material in the cell wall. Noble (1965) showed that strains of *S. aureus* differed in their ability to cause a necropurulent lesion when mixed with cotton dust and injected subcutaneously in mice. Aggressive action in this model was due to an ability to delay the inflammatory response (Agarwal 1967b). In further experiments Hill (1968) obtained similar lesions by injecting a small amount of cell wall material from an 'aggressive' strain with a subinfecting dose of viable cocci. The cell wall material appeared to be peptidoglycan complexed with protein; such residues from 'aggressive' but not from 'non-aggressive' *S. aureus* strains inhibited the production of oedema around the cotton plug and the migration of leucocytes (Weksler and Hill 1969). Active immunization of mice with the aggressin gave protection against infection by this experimental route (Hill 1969). The problems inherent in dissecting pathogenicity or virulence in staphylococci can be seen from the fact that peptidoglycan induces histamine release from human basophils in vitro (Espersen and Jarlov 1984); it will also activate complement and induce chemotaxis, that is, peptidoglycan alone provokes an inflammatory response.

Capsulate strains of *S. aureus* have a poor ability to cause local lesions in the subcutaneous cotton dust test (Easmon 1980) when compared with strains that possess the cell wall aggressin; the reverse is, however, true for intraperitoneal infection. It has been suggested that protein A may act as an aggressin by forming complexes with γ-globulin and cause a local hypersensitivity reaction (Gustafson et al. 1968). When injected intradermally in humans, protein A provokes an apparent immediate and delayed-type hypersensitivity response (White and Noble 1985) which is more difficult to reproduce in mice except by injection of the footpads (Kinsman, White and Noble 1981). Nevertheless, protein A deficient mutants derived by allele replacement are slightly less virulent for mice than the parent strain (Patel and Nowlan 1987). Hale and Smith (1945) considered that the production of free coagulase protects staphylococci from phagocytosis by the deposition of fibrin around the cocci. However, no difference in virulence was seen between coagulase-positive staphylococci and negative variants produced by site-specific mutation in an experimental endocarditis model (Baddour et al. 1994). Repeated passage of *S. aureus* in rabbits greatly enhances its virulence for rabbits by the intrathoracic route. This is associated with an increase in the resistance of the organisms to intracellular killing by rabbit polymorphonuclear leucocytes, to the bactericidal substances released by lysed leucocytes, and to the bactericidal action of rabbit serum, but not to inhibition of phagocytosis (Adlam et al. 1970).

THE ROLE OF EXTRACELLULAR TOXINS

It would be reasonable to think that damage to tissues by the extracellular toxins of *S. aureus* may contribute to the production of septic lesions, but few of these substances appear to be formed by all the strains that cause disease in their respective natural hosts. On at least 2 occasions (Kellaway, MacCallum and Terbutt 1928, Olin and Lithander 1948), the injection into human patients of medicaments in which *S. aureus* had multiplied led within a few hours to vomiting, high fever, cyanosis, convulsions and, in a number of cases, death. Staphylococcal α-toxin may have caused these effects but this could not definitely be established at the time (Wilson 1967) and these incidents need to be reassessed in the light of superantigen activity. The α-toxin may contribute to the necrosis and perhaps to the delayed mobilization of leucocytes in the natural local staphylococcal lesion since α-toxin negative mutants derived by allele replacement are significantly less virulent in experimental subcutaneous infections of mice (Patel and Nowlan 1987) than is the parent strain. This confirms the observations of Agarwal (1967b) on challenge by the subcutaneous cotton dust model that antibody to α-toxin reduces infection, though in neither this study, nor that of Goshi, Cluff and Johnson (1961) on burns in rabbits was it certain that anti-α-toxin was the only antibody

formed. Immunization of rabbits with purified toxin leads to a more rapid infiltration of staphylococcal lesions with leucocytes, to the inhibition of necrosis and of multiplication of the organisms (Goshi et al. 1963) but in both rabbit and humans it leads to dermal hypersensitivity which is proportional to the anti-α-toxin titre (Goshi, Cluff and Norman 1963, Smith et al. 1963). Such immunization does not protect lactating mice against mastitis after intramammary infusion of *S. aureus* but it prevents the lethal haemorrhagic form of the disease caused by certain highly virulent strains (Adlam et al. 1977). Extracellular staphylococcal products may enhance the chemotactic activity of leucocytes (Russell et al. 1976); the most striking effect on polymorphonuclear cells was observed when staphylococci or their products had first been incubated with plasma, but monocytes exhibited a direct chemotactic effect. Although high doses of α-toxin damage polymorphs, small doses enhance their ability to take up and kill staphylococci (Gemmell et al. 1982).

Animal strains of staphylococci of known pathogenicity less frequently produce α-toxin but many produce β-toxin though no definite part in pathogenesis can be ascribed to this latter toxin (Adlam et al. 1977). Staphylokinase might conceivably aid the dissemination of staphylococci by causing dislodgement of infected clots in veins, but it is rarely formed by the β-toxin producing strains.

HYPERSENSITIVITY

Early experiments with whole cells or culture filtrates of *S. aureus* to 'immunize' rabbits resulted in an increase in susceptibility to subcutaneous infection and to the appearance of a delayed-type hypersensitivity. Easmon and Glynn (1975) found that after repeated infections caused by the injection of *S. aureus* on cotton dust plugs, mice showed a T lymphocyte mediated delayed hypersensitivity to staphylococcal cell walls. The mice were hypersensitive to the peptidoglycan but not to the teichoic acid or to protein A of *S. aureus* and not to the cell wall constituents of other species of staphylococci (Easmon and Glynn 1978). The sera of hypersensitive mice protected uninfected mice against the dermonecrotic effect of subsequent challenge by the subcutaneous route. However, the transfer of spleen cells increased susceptibility and the appearance of severe dermonecrotic lesions. When both serum and spleen cells were transferred, the effect was similar to that of serum alone, that is, the harmful effects of delayed hypersensitivity were expressed only in the absence of a humoral response (Easmon and Glynn 1975). In subsequent studies (Easmon and Glynn 1977, 1979) evidence was obtained for a humoral factor in infected mice that suppressed the delayed hypersensitivity response, but its effects were overridden by repeated infections. This suggested (Easmon 1980) that cell mediated hypersensitivity was likely to influence the severity of natural disease only when staphylococci or their cellular constituents persisted in the tissues, as when a patient has a defect in the mechanism of phagocytosis or intracellular killing of staphylococci. It must be remembered, however, that the serum antibody response to staphylococcal products in humans is often remarkably poor.

3.1 Sources and routes of infections

The majority of staphylococcal infections arise from endogenous sources. This is true not only of sporadic infections, minor wound sepsis and post-influenzal pneumonia in the community, but also of a considerable proportion of surgical wound infections and neonatal sepsis. Sometimes, however, staphylococci from another carrier or a contaminated object will reach, and cause infection in, a patient. Air-borne transmission may also occur. Carriage of *S. aureus* can be considered in the light of self-infection or as a source for cross-infection.

CARRIAGE

The carriage of *S. aureus* was first described by Hallman (1937) and has since been studied intensively (see Williams 1963). At any time about 35% of normal adults carry *S. aureus* in the anterior nares. Populations of primitive peoples are reported with lower carrier rates (7–25%, see Rountree 1967) usually associated with high carrier rates of Enterobacteriaceae. However, successive monthly random samples of about 240 individuals from a normal European population yielded variable nasal carrier rates, making it difficult to assess the significance of different rates usually measured in a small population (Noble, Valkenburg and Wolters 1967). About 65% of anterior nasal carriers also carry on the turbinates and posterior nasal space (Noble et al. 1964) and seeding from this site may account for apparent intermittent carriage in the anterior nares. High carrier rates are recorded for infants: by the age of 2 weeks rates of 60–70% of those born at home and 80–100% of those born in hospital. The rate declines to 20% by the end of infancy and rises again to reach the adult level by about 5–8 years. In elderly persons it declines to 20–25%.

Repeated sampling of the same population yields cumulative nasal carrier rates of 60–90%; 20–35% of persons are persistent carriers, 30–70% are intermittent carriers and 10–40% are never carriers (Williams 1963). Persistent carriers usually harbour the same strain for months or years, indicating a marked stability in the nasal flora. Those who acquired a 'hospital staphylococcus' in the nose while an in-patient, were frequently readmitted carrying their original domestic strain (Noble et al. 1964). Application of lysostaphin to the anterior nares, which removes *S. aureus* but has little effect on other nasal micro-organisms, showed that natural recolonization with *S. aureus* occurs more slowly than when antibiotics that tend to eliminate other species, as well as the staphylococcus, were used. The success of the antibiotic mupirocin (SmithKline Beecham) in ridding the nose of hospital-acquired *S. aureus* (Hill, Duckworth and Casewell 1988) may result

partly from the fact that the coryneform flora of the nose is not eliminated by this antibiotic.

Information on throat carriage of *S. aureus* is discrepant, with reported rates varying from 4 to 64% (Williams 1963). A random sample survey of a normal population showed winter carriage rates of about 15% but in spring these dropped to about 3%, suggesting that the discrepant rates may be seasonally related (Noble, Valkenburg and Wolters 1967).

Faecal carriage rates in infants generally reflect nasal carriage; in normal adults faecal carrier rates are about 20% at a single examination and only small numbers of cells are found. This probably also reflects nasal carriage.

Skin carrier rates reported by various authors vary widely; this is most probably because in most instances the number of colony-forming units on normal skin is small and the proportion of persons detected as carriers therefore reflects the total area of skin sampled and the efficiency of culture techniques. Most *S. aureus* on normal skin are transients and can be removed by washing; they chiefly represent 'contamination' from resident carrier sites such as the nose or perineum. Nevertheless, a small proportion of normal persons and most patients with certain skin diseases, such as atopic dermatitis (atopic eczema), may be densely colonized (Noble 1992). By far the most common site of 'independent' skin carriage is the perineum where 10–20% of normal persons, half of whom are not nasal carriers, yield large numbers of *S. aureus* (Polakoff et al. 1967, Dancer and Noble 1991). Resident carriage also occurs normally in the axillae and toewebs in about 5% of the population.

Patients with chronic skin disease, especially the eczemas, are almost universally heavily colonized by *S. aureus*. Patients with other skin diseases are less prone to colonization unless large amounts of steroid have been used in therapy (Noble and Savin 1968).

AIR-BORNE DISSEMINATION

Few staphylococci are disseminated directly into the air from the respiratory tract; much larger numbers reach the environment from the body surface carried on air-borne desquamated skin scales (Davies and Noble 1963). Some individuals disperse organisms very efficiently in this way; some, but not all, are heavy nasal carriers (Solberg 1965, Noble et al. 1976) and may contribute to environmental contamination in hospital wards (Noble 1962). Profuse dispersal is more common in males than females and is related to dispersal from skin areas below the waist (Bethune et al. 1965, Noble et al. 1976). Much dispersal results from friction of clothing removing scales from the skin surface but some dispersal takes place even from those who are naked.

The equivalent particle diameter of air-borne particles carrying *S. aureus* is about 12 μm with a range of 4–24 μm (Noble, Lidwell and Kingston 1963). These particles remain suspended on air currents for long periods of time allowing wide dispersal and are able to pass through ordinary cotton fabrics, including surgical gowns (Whyte, Vesley and Hodgson 1976). A number of outbreaks of surgical sepsis acquired in the operating room have been traced to dispersers (Ayliffe and Collins 1967, Shanson and McSwiggan 1980, Tanner et al. 1980). Nevertheless, only about 10% of air-borne staphylococci survive the first 24 h, about half dying during the initial desiccation process; the infectivity of these dried organisms is not known.

DISSEMINATION BY CONTACT

Less is known about the transmission of staphylococci by contact than by the air-borne route, because suitable methods of studying it quantitatively have not been developed and evaluated. The undoubted reduction in wound sepsis rate which followed the introduction of 'no touch' dressing techniques (see Williams 1971) and clear accounts of the role of hands in contaminating wounds (Wu and Shen 1993, Wu and Liu 1994) indicate the importance of this route of infection.

Nasal carriers of *S. aureus* frequently contaminate their fingers with their nasal strain (Noble, Valkenburg and Wolters 1967, Doebbeling 1994) and suppression of nasal carriage with the antibiotic mupirocin has been shown to result in a reduction in hand carriage (Reagen et al. 1991).

ACQUISITION AT CARRIER SITES

The neonatal period

Newborn babies are very susceptible to colonization with *S. aureus*, which is the usual consequence of their first exposure to the organism; clinical sepsis seldom develops without prior colonization. Many studies on colonization or infection of infants with *S. aureus* were carried out during the 1950s and early 1960s when *S. aureus* of phage type 80/81 was pandemic. During that period babies tended to acquire their staphylococci from other babies rather than from their mother or nurses. Mothers and babies were in hospital for longer periods than is now common. Colonization of the nose, umbilical stump, or both rapidly approached 100% but if the stump was treated with hexachlorophane the nasal carrier rate was reduced (Gezon et al. 1964). When the use of hexachlorophane ceased in the early 1970s carrier rates rose (Hargiss and Larson 1978) but the introduction of chlorhexidine treatment reversed this trend (Bygdeman et al. 1984). All are agreed that colonization predisposes to infection.

Staphylococci may be spread in nurseries by the air-borne or contact route. Rammelkamp and his colleagues (Wolinsky et al. 1960, Mortimer et al. 1962, 1966) compared the rate of colonization from an index source in the same room when they were attended to:

1 with unwashed hands
2 with effectively washed hands
3 with gloved hands and
4 without direct manual contact with the source of infection.

Briefly, contact with unwashed hands caused 5 times as many acquisitions as air-borne infection but if the hands were carefully washed or gloved the 2 routes of acquisition were about equal.

LATER ACQUISITIONS

Patients admitted to hospital acquired staphylococci in the nose roughly in proportion to the duration of stay in hospital and to the amount of air-borne staphylococci to which they are exposed (Noble et al. 1964, Lidwell et al. 1966, 1970, 1971), suggesting that the inhalation of air-borne particles bearing staphylococci is the most important route. However, patients admitted to dermatology wards also acquired *S. aureus* on the chest and perineum, though at slightly lower rates than in the nose (Wilson, White and Noble 1971). Patients with eczema acquired *S. aureus* on the chest more often than did those with psoriasis, but nasal and perineal acquisition occurred at the same rate in each group of patients. Application of topical antibiotics was more likely to lead to nasal and chest acquisition than were systemic antibiotics but any antibiotic therapy was more likely to lead to acquisition than was absence of antibiotic therapy. This agrees generally with the many studies of nasal acquisition and the role of antibiotic therapy.

3.2 The characters of 'hospital' strains

The strains that established themselves in hospitals in the 1950s and 1960s were in general resistant to antibiotics in common use at the time. There is little evidence that, as a class, they differed from less resistant strains found outside hospital either in pathogenicity or communicability; they certainly showed considerable variability amongst themselves in these respects. The same arguments can be advanced in respect of the methicillin-resistant *S. aureus* (MRSA) that are currently epidemic within sections of hospitals such as intensive care units.

ANTIBIOTIC RESISTANCE

Penicillinase-forming strains of *S. aureus* existed in small numbers before penicillin was used therapeutically. The rapid increase in their prevalence in hospitals in the mid-1940s was a consequence of their spread by cross-infection. Soon afterwards, resistances to antibiotics other than penicillin, which in most instances had not been detected before the corresponding antibiotic had been taken into use, appeared in a minority of penicillinase producers. These strains, generally termed 'multiple antibiotic resistant', became widespread in hospitals in their turn. The spectrum of resistance in individual strains became progressively wider and encompassed, in the vast majority, penicillinase production plus resistance to any combination of antibiotics then in use. This situation has not, in essence, changed; modern hospital strains remain penicillinase producers and are resistant to a number of currently used antibiotics. Antibiotic resistance in strains encountered outside hospital reflects the resistance of hospital strains but usually at a lower prevalence. In a study of 500 normal women attending routine antenatal out-patient clinics,

Dancer and Noble (1991) found 76% of staphylococci were penicillinase producers, 13% were resistant to tetracycline, 4% to erythromycin, 1.2% to neomycin and 0.6% to gentamicin. Three isolates (1.75%) were resistant to methicillin.

The genetic determinants for resistance to various antimicrobial agents comprise a series of plasmid or chromosomally borne genes, some of which appear distinct and others of which are shared, especially with the enterococci. The acquisition and accumulation of genes by 'hospital' staphylococci can generally be explained on ecological rather than genetic grounds.

When a new antibiotic comes into use, resistance to it sometimes appears promptly but in several instances has not appeared until some years have elapsed. For example, the appearance of resistance to gentamicin was delayed for about 10 years after its introduction but in 1976 several clearly distinguishable strains appeared almost simultaneously (for references see Shanson 1981). At the time of writing naturally vancomycin-resistant strains of *S. aureus* have not appeared despite the introduction of vancomycin almost 40 years ago, though it has not until recently been used extensively. By contrast, strains resistant to mupirocin appeared within 2 years of the antibiotic becoming available; in this case resistance was due to an exogenous gene acquired by *S. aureus* at least 20 years before the drug was available (Dyke et al. 1991). Resistance to ciprofloxacin, which is due to a point mutation in the DNA gyrase gene, rose to 5.3% of *S. aureus* in New York City hospitals within 6 months of the introduction of the antibiotic (Schaefler 1989). The initial mutation to resistance or the acquisition of a pre-existing gene from elsewhere is a rare event but once resistance occurs it will be selected by the use of that antibiotic. In general then, selection and cross-infection were, and remain, the main factors responsible for building up and maintaining populations of resistant staphylococci and the hospital environment is a fertile place for this to occur.

TYPING OF *S. AUREUS* STRAINS

The epidemiology of *S. aureus* infections, especially in hospitals and other closed communities, has traditionally been followed by phage typing and complementary techniques such as plasmid profiling (Richardson, Noble and Marples 1992). Phage typing has remained a valuable tool except in the case of MRSA where it may offer poor discrimination. Molecular methods involving the polymerase chain reaction (Gürtler and Barrie 1995) or restriction endonuclease fragment analysis with a 'rare cutting' enzyme such as *Sma*I and separating the generated fragments by pulsed field gel electrophoresis (Bannerman et al. 1995) have proved more successful. The latter technique has been proposed to replace phage typing.

Phage typing patterns have been used since 1947 to characterize *S. aureus* strains prevalent in hospitals. Whilst invaluable for relatively short-term studies, it later became apparent that such patterns may give misleading results when used to study the course of long continual endemic prevalence of particular strains. Changes in typing pattern may occur as a result of the acquisition or loss of a prophage and this concealed the continued prevalence of an epidemic strain (Asheshov and Rippon 1959, Rosendal and Bülow 1971). The relationship between phage typing pattern and antibiotic resistance has been reviewed by Parker (1983).

S. aureus phage types can be placed into a number of phage groups and there are interesting correlations between these phage groups and the diseases with which they are associated (Table 14.3). The patterns of lysis within a group may be determined by the lysogenic status of the individual strain but the groups may be determined by restriction/modification systems. It is known that groups II and V are restriction groups (Asheshov, Coe and Porthouse 1977, Stobberingh and Winkler 1977). Strains of phage group I are commonly associated with boils and those lysed by phage 29 are frequently associated with the production of TSST-1. Phage group II strains are frequently implicated in impetigo and scalded skin syndrome whereas phage group III or I and III are often multiresistant strains associated with hospital infection and with enterotoxin A production. These correlations are not, however, absolute. There is no particular distribution of phage types among nasal carriers in the normal population; Dancer and Noble (1991) found 15% of 184 strains types as phage group I, 14% as group II, 20% as group III, 34% were non-typable and the remaining 17% were mixed phage groups.

PATHOGENICITY AND TRANSMISSIBILITY

The behaviour of individual staphylococcal strains in hospitals provides evidence that they differ not only in the frequency with which they cause infection but also in the nature of the resulting lesion. Moreover, some spread more easily than others, but this is not always attributable to a wider spectrum of resistance to antibiotics.

The concept of 'epidemic' strains was first proposed in the pre-antibiotic era in connection with neonatal sepsis; this was perhaps because attention was drawn to outbreaks of exfoliative skin lesions in newborns. In 1952 a single strain rapidly spread throughout Australia and later this phage type 80/81 strain was recovered world wide. By 1970, however, this and related strains had almost disappeared from the UK (Parker et al. 1974). Later hospital epidemic strains were chiefly from phage group III and were multiresistant. It was evident from studies in this period that some strains may spread from patient to patient, detected chiefly as nasal carriage, without causing infection (Barber et al. 1953, Shooter et al. 1958), whereas others might become widespread in the air yet fail to colonize new patients (Noble 1962).

By 1975, only some 20% of infections in London hospitals were caused by multiresistant strains of *S. aureus* and strains resistant only to penicillin were responsible for one-half (Parker 1983) but generally only small outbreaks were seen. The only identifiable 'new' strains to assume importance in the 1970s were phage group V strains lysed by phages 94 and 96

Table 14.3 Correlation between *Staphylococcus aureus* phage group and disease

Phage group	Phages*	Diseases
I	29, 52, 52A, 79, 80	Furuncles Toxic shock syndrome (especially phage 29)
II	3A, 3C, 55, 71	Impetigo Scalded skin syndrome Tropical pyomyositis
III	6, 42E, 47, 53, 54, 75, 77, 83, 84, 85	Surgical wound infection (especially multiresistant strains) Food poisoning

*Phages of International set only.

(Marraro and Mitchell 1975, Asheshov, Coe and Porthouse 1977), which were resistant to few antibiotics. By 1980 strains resistant to gentamicin and methicillin were becoming more widespread and serious local outbreaks of infection were reported from Australia, the USA, Ireland and Britain (Crossley, Landesman and Zeske 1979, Graham et al. 1980, Price, Brain and Dickson 1980, Shanson and McSwiggan 1980, King et al. 1981, Cafferkey et al. 1983, Cooke et al. 1986, Marples and Cooke 1988). Some of these outbreaks were extensive and long continued with evidence of interhospital spread.

Current preoccupations are with MRSA. An epidemic strain (EMRSA) was identified which caused particular problems in London and south east England (Marples, Richardson and de Saxe 1986). Originally this epidemic strain typed readily with phages 84 and 85 but changes have occurred in this pattern and successive waves of EMRSA have been identified (Table 14.4), each new strain apparently displacing the previous strains (Mackintosh et al. 1991).

Similar patterns have been seen elsewhere (Linnemann et al. 1991). Various attempts have been made to find characteristics that might explain the ability of E(MRSA) to spread or cause disease. In vitro adherence of MRSA and methicillin-sensitive strains (MSSA) to nasal epithelial cells has been shown not to differ (Ward 1992) whilst there are profound differences within MRSA in adherence to extracellular matrix proteins (Cree et al. 1994) and in resistance to desiccation and the action of free fatty acids (Farrington et al. 1992). Bacteraemias caused by MRSA and MSSA cannot be separated with regard to symptoms or apparent virulence (Lewis and Saravolatz 1985). If epidemic and non-epidemic MRSA are considered, however, a combination of protein A production, α-toxin and capsular type will predict epidemicity with a specificity of 75% (van Wamel et al. 1995).

Over the past 50 years it has proved virtually impossible to predict the behaviour of 'hospital' staphylococci. The impact of effective antibiotic control and infection control of the hospital staphylococcus is debatable. This situation is likely to continue.

Table 14.4 Some characteristics of EMRSA from the UK

Strains	Phage type*	Resistance pattern								Selected others	Urease
		Te	Mn	Em	Da	Km	Gm	Sm	Nm		
1	85/88A/932	R	R	R	R	(R)	(R)	R	–		++
2	80/85/90/932	(R)	–	R	–	–	–	–	–		–
3	75/83A/932	–	–	R	–	R	R	R	R		–
4	85/90/932	R	R	R	–	–	–	R	–		+
5	77/84	R	R	–	–	R	R	R	–	Rif Bc	++
6	90/932	R	R	R	–	R	–	R	R		–
7	85	R	R	R	–	–	–	R	–		+
8	83A/83C/932	R	R	–	–	–	–	R	–		++
9	77/84/932	R	R	R	–	R	R	R	–	Cm	++
10	77/83A/29/75/85	R	R	R	–	R	R	–	–	Cm	–
11	84	R	R	R	R	R	R	R	R	Bc	++
12	75/83A/83C/932	R	R	R	–	R	–	R	R	Fc	++
13	29/83C/932	R	R	–	R	R	R	R	R	Fc Bc	++
14	29+/6/47/54/90/932	R	R	–	–	R	–	R	R	Fc	–

Based on Kerr et al. 1990.
*Underlining indicates phages lysing only at 100 × routine test dilution.
All strains were resistant to penicillin and methicillin: R, resistant; Tc, tetracycline; Mn, minocycline; Em, erythromycin; Da, dalacin; Km, kanamycin; Gm, gentamicin; Sm, streptomycin; Nm, neomycin; Rif, rifampicin; Bc, bacitracin; Cm, chloramphenicol; Fc, fusidic acid.

INFECTION OF WOUNDS

Outside hospital the patient is probably the chief source of his infection. For surgical wound infection the position is more complex and probably varies between hospitals and at various times in the same hospital. Estimates of self-infection and cross-infection vary widely. Williams and his colleagues (1959) reported wound sepsis rates of 7.1% in nasal carriers and 2% in non-carriers. Other workers have not found this relationship (Moore and Gardner 1963) and it may be that at times operating room infection is more common. Nevertheless, the increased likelihood of infection in nasal carriers has been echoed in many studies of infection of dialysis patients, both haemodialysis (Kirmani et al. 1978) and peritoneal dialysis (Sesso et al. 1989). Thus, Rebel and colleagues (1975) found that in a single dialysis unit, 10 nasal carriers suffered 15 colonizations and 5 infections of the haemodialysis shunt site whereas 22 non-carriers suffered 8 colonizations and 4 infections. Davies et al. (1989) reported that nasal carriage increased the risk of exit site infection in peritoneal dialysis by 6-fold. Much of this may be attributable to contact transfer from the nose to the sensitive site via the hands. This and similar routes of transfer may account for much hospital infection, since acquisition of a 'hospital' staphylococcus in the nose would lead to transfer to a wound by the same nose–hand–wound route.

In HIV-positive patients the prevalence of nasal carriage of *S. aureus* increased with the severity of the underlying disease and was judged to be a risk factor in the development of septicaemia in those with AIDS (Weinke et al. 1992).

Exogenous infection in the operating room may originate from the surgeon or an assistant who touches or contaminates the wound or instruments (Shooter et al. 1957, Penikett, Knox and Liddell 1958). On occasion a disperser of staphylococci present in the operating room, but not in contact with the patient, such as a porter or technician may also contribute to operating room infection (Ayliffe and Collins 1967, Tanner et al. 1980). Operating room clothing has been designed in an attempt to reduce dispersal of organisms (Mitchell, Evans and Kerr 1978, Dankert, Zijlstra and Lubberding 1979) but it has been difficult to assess the efficacy of special clothing or of increased operating room ventilation in the reduction of surgical sepsis due to the other routes by which organisms may be spread (Lidwell 1976).

3.3 Diagnosis

Standard microbiological methods continue to be satisfactory for diagnosing most cases of sepsis caused by *S. aureus*. However, when the organism is seen or cultured from a site that is not normally sterile, care must be taken with interpretation. *S. aureus* grows well on standard nutrient or blood agar. Differentiation from coagulase-negative cocci can be made by the tube coagulase test. The use of latex particles coated with plasma to detect protein A or clumping factor is satisfactory but some of the available commercial test kits may perform poorly with methicillin-resistant strains (MRSA) that lack cell bound protein A (Mathieu and Picard 1991).

The detection of *S. aureus* antigens in blood and body fluids has not been used extensively for rapid diagnosis. The non-specific binding of protein A to IgG may lead to difficulties and a variety of heat-labile materials in serum can interfere with immunoassays for staphylococcal antigen (Tabbarah et al. 1979). High levels of antibody to *S. aureus* tend to form immune complexes with available staphylococcal antigen (Wheat et al. 1979). Despite these problems, staphylococcal antigens (teichoic acid and peptidoglycan) have been detected in severe staphylococcal sepsis (Ribner, Keusch and Robbins 1975, Jackson et al. 1978, Wergerland et al. 1989) but are also found in normal individuals. Antibody to staphylococcal protein A can be detected in the sera of patients with bacteraemia or endocarditis but the tests are not sufficiently specific for diagnostic purposes (Greenberg et al. 1990).

Serological methods play no part in the diagnosis of most localized staphylococcal infections. They have been used for the detection of certain chronic or subacute deep-seated infections such as endocarditis and osteomyelitis. Taylor et al. (1975) recommended a combination of antibody tests for both α- and γ-toxin as being effective for diagnosis of staphylococcal bone disease. Titres of antibody to staphylococcal nuclease may be raised in some cases of osteomyelitis in which anti-α and anti-γ titres are not increased (Taylor, Fincham and Cook 1976). A major complication of all serological tests is that nasal carriage may result in high antibody titres; for example, male nasal carriers of TSST-1 producing strains may have moderate to high antibody levels in the absence of staphylococcal disease (Ritz et al. 1984).

3.4 Treatment

Whether or not to give specific treatment for a particular staphylococcal infection, and the choice of antimicrobial therapy and other measures such as surgical treatment, are matters for clinical judgement. Antibiotics alone will not cure closed septic lesions, such as abscesses, without surgical drainage; indeed, for small superficial lesions adequate surgical drainage alone may be sufficient. By contrast, prompt effective chemotherapy is necessary for severe staphylococcal sepsis such as osteomyelitis, endocarditis and septicaemia, extensive exfoliative disease, pneumonia and the toxic shock syndrome.

One of the main problems is the duration of chemotherapy needed in a case of staphylococcal bacteraemia, given the risk of endocarditis or metastatic complications. A short course of treatment is reasonable for those in whom bacteraemia is associated with a clear focus of infection, where there is no evidence of a defect in the host defences, cardiac valvular damage, or of developing metastatic lesions and where the organism is fully sensitive to the drugs chosen and the clinical response is prompt. Patients who do not satisfy these criteria probably need treatment for 4 weeks.

The choice of antimicrobial agents should be based on in vitro sensitivity tests. Few strains of *S. aureus*, whether from the community or hospital environment, are now sensitive to penicillin. The penicillinase-stable penicillins, for example, flucloxacillin and oxacillin, are still the mainstay of antistaphylococcal chemotherapy. In serious infections they may be combined with an aminoglycoside or fusidic acid. Combination of a penicillin plus clavulanic acid is also effective in skin and soft tissue infections. First and second generation cephalosporins are also effective but third generation cephalosporins should be avoided because they are less active against staphylococci. Clindamycin is useful in cases of osteomyelitis. Patients allergic to penicillins may be given erythromycin, vancomycin, or first generation cephalosporins. Mupirocin is useful for skin infections.

Infections with methicillin-resistant staphylococci cannot be treated with penicillins or cephalosporins. Such strains usually show multi-antibiotic resistance but currently remain sensitive to vancomycin and teichoplanin. Rifampicin, fusidic acid and ciprofloxacin may also be of value.

3.5 Prevention

Most of the measures we take to prevent staphylococcal infections in hospital form part of a general programme for the prevention of septic infections. Briefly, the main objectives are:

1 to prevent the access of *S. aureus* to susceptible sites from which it can invade the tissues
2 to lessen the chance that organisms that do reach the tissues can cause sepsis and
3 to reduce as far as possible the number of sources of *S. aureus* in the immediate neighbourhood of the patient.

Eliminating the predisposing factors discussed earlier in this chapter (see section 3, p. 237) may be most helpful. There is no doubt that careful surgical technique lessens the risk of infection. The prophylactic use of antibiotics may be a useful means of preventing the multiplication of organisms implanted into wounds. However, this must be carried out according to strictly defined protocols if the disadvantages, such as selection of resistant variants, are not to outweigh the advantages. The frequency of carriage of *S. aureus* by normal persons makes it impracticable, save under exceptional circumstances, to ensure that a patient will not be exposed to the organism.

It is seldom possible to insist that members of the hospital staff should be non-carriers, except for those few engaged in special tasks. General attempts to abolish nasal carriage, in patients or staff, by mass chemoprophylaxis have not proved very effective and have frequently created problems of antibiotic resistance (Williams et al. 1966). However, the removal and treatment, preferably outside hospital, of individual members of staff who have been the source of infections,

is justified. Although the topical application of creams containing gentamicin, neomycin or vancomycin usually frees the nose of staphylococci, the preferred antibiotic is mupirocin which has proved to be very effective in reducing nasal carriage. It has proved particularly valuable for treating hospital staff who have become carriers of methicillin-resistant *S. aureus* (Casewell and Hill 1986, Frank et al. 1989, Doebbeling et al. 1993). Use of this antibiotic to suppress nasal carriage has been reported to be effective in reducing infection in patients with jugular cannulae (Hill et al. 1990) and haemodialysis (Boelaert et al. 1991), doubtless because of reduced contamination of the hands (Reagan et al. 1991).

Reduction of hand contamination and suppression of staphylococcal growth, especially on the skin of newborns, was formerly accomplished with hexachlorophane. This was applied regularly as a powder, detergent washing fluid or cream and was most effective (for references see Williams et al. 1966). Evidence of its toxicity led to a great reduction in its use with concomitant increase in staphylococcal infection among newborns (Dixon et al. 1973, Kaslow et al. 1973, Scopes, Eykyn and Phillips 1974). For a review of the hazards of hexachlorophane to newborn infants, of the circumstances in which it may be used safely and for alternatives to it, see Editorial (1982). Chlorhexidine has been recommended for routine cord care in newborns, and is effective in suppressing colonization (Bygdeman et al. 1984, Seeberg et al. 1984), and for routine preoperative and general hand disinfection (Kjolen and Andersen 1992).

The value of bacterial interference as a means of preventing colonization with epidemic virulent strains of *S. aureus* was well established during the years when *S. aureus* phage type 80/81 was pandemic. Shinefield and colleagues (1963) showed that instillation of large inocula of a strain of *S. aureus* '502A' into the anterior nares of newborns protected them from colonization by the pandemic strain and subsequent sepsis. However, strain 502A is itself capable of causing infection, though this is usually minor, and the process was generally discontinued when the type 80/81 strains were no longer pandemic. The process of deliberate nasal colonization as a preventive method has been used more recently in patients with chronic furunculosis where it has limited value (Hedstrom 1981). More success with interference, though not with strain 502A, has been achieved in animal studies where it can protect against infections with *S. hyicus* (Allaker et al. 1990). The potential for this procedure remains.

In recent years the prevention of infection caused by MRSA has been a particular concern. Guidelines covering all aspects of hospital care and microbiological methodology have been produced for control of infections caused by these staphylococci (Report 1986).

3.6 Active immunization

Toxic filtrates of *S. aureus* may be rendered innocuous by treatment with formalin. A course of injection with toxoid results in a high concentration of anti-α-toxin in the blood, in animals and humans. There is little convincing evidence, however, that it influences the course of chronic or recurrent infections. Staphylococcus toxoid also contains variable amounts of Panton–Valentine (P–V) leucocidin and several workers have reported a prophylactic effect that they attribute to the formation of antileucocidin (Bänffer and Franklin 1967). The potential for vaccines against *S. aureus* based on components of cell surface polysaccharides and proteins has been reviewed by Foster (1991).

4 CARRIAGE OF THE COAGULASE-NEGATIVE STAPHYLOCOCCI

Many of the coagulase-negative staphylococci can be recovered from human or animal skin where they form a major part of the normal, resident population (Noble 1992). There are some differences between the flora recovered from apparently similar populations in various parts of the world and also in the distribution of the staphylococcal species on the individual human body. For example, *Staphylococcus epidermidis* is the most common species on the face and thorax whereas *Staphylococcus hominis* is the most common on the arms and legs. The significance of this for pathology has not been established.

4.1 Infections due to coagulase-negative staphylococci and micrococci

Coagulase-negative staphylococci are frequently recovered from swabs of wounds and other skin lesions, but it is difficult to determine the significance of this because of their universal colonization of the skin. They have been assigned a pathogenic role in minor pustules of the skin (Lotem et al. 1988) and since some, at least, produce potential pathogenicity factors, this cannot be wholly discounted. However, the role of some organisms in other types of infection, especially those associated with catheterization or the insertion of prostheses, is well established. The predominant species in all such infections is *S. epidermidis* (Table 14.5).

URINARY TRACT INFECTION

Mild infections, usually caused by *S. epidermidis*, but less frequently by *Staphylococcus haemolyticus* or *Staphylococcus warneri*, may follow operations on or instrumental manipulation of the lower urinary tract (Larsen and Burke 1986, Leighton and Little 1986). Occasional infections, not associated with catheters and due to *S. epidermidis*, have also been described, especially in children (Hall and Snitzer 1994).

A distinct species, *Staphylococcus saprophyticus*, causes spontaneous acute urinary tract infection in previously healthy individuals, chiefly, though not exclusively, in women aged 16–25 years (Hovelius, Colleen and Mardh 1984, Pead, Maskell and Morris 1985). The

symptoms resemble urinary tract infection by *Escherichia coli*; many of the patients show evidence of pyelonephritis, but the disease is usually self-limiting. The cocci most probably enter the urinary tract by the ascending route. Indistinguishable organisms are found on the skin of the arms and legs of a small percentage of normal males and females (Kloos and Musselwhite 1975), but occur in high numbers on the feet of females aged 16–25 years, but not males, in the absence of urinary tract infection (Reuther and Noble 1993). Food and the animals from which it is derived, have also been suggested as potential sources of *S. saprophyticus* (Hedman et al. 1990, 1993).

It is probable that many species of staphylococci are introduced into the urinary tract mechanically or by physiological means. *S. saprophyticus* adheres to urinary tract epithelium more readily than, for example, *S. epidermidis* (Colleen et al. 1979, Fujita et al. 1992); isolates from urinary tract infections show a high capacity to adhere to laminin (Paulsson, Ljungh and Wadström 1992). *S. saprophyticus* possesses a powerful urease, which is a significant pathogenicity factor, at least in experimental studies (Gatermann, John and Marre 1989). Other potential pathogenicity factors include a sheep red cell haemagglutinin (Hovelius and Mardh 1979). Host factors that may play a part in colonization that precedes disease include previous urinary tract infection, a recent menstrual period, recent intercourse and recent or concurrent vaginal candidiasis; there is also a seasonal variation (Rupp, Soper and Archer 1992) with a summer and autumn peak.

SYSTEMIC INFECTIONS

The presence of coagulase-negative staphylococci as a major part of the skin flora has always made interpretation of their role in systemic infection difficult. Although occasional closed abscesses are reported from which only coagulase-negative staphylococci can be recovered (Surani, Chandna and Weinstein 1993, Waghorn 1994), the majority of infections are associated with a catheter or prosthesis; an exception is native valve endocarditis.

A proportion of coagulase-negative staphylococci possess enzymes, toxins, or both, that are more commonly associated with *S. aureus*. Gemmel (1983) reported that α-, β- and δ-lysin production is common in coagulase-negative staphylococci from infective processes; Lambe and colleagues (1990) extended this observation to include the species *Staphylococcus lugdunensis* and *Staphylococcus schleiferi*, finding them to be equivalent to *S. epidermidis* in an experimental foreign body infection. They reported that all species produced exoenzymes, α- and δ-lysins, as potential pathogenicity factors, but remarked that production did not always correlate with abscess production. A feature that has engaged much attention is the production of a glycocalyx (slime) by strains of coagulase-negative staphylococci. Slime is produced when the organisms are growing on a solid surface such as a plastic catheter (Christensen et al. 1982), allowing the formation of surface microcolonies. Slime protects the staphylococci against host defences such as phagocytosis and

Table 14.5 Percentage distribution of coagulase-negative staphylococci in clinical material

Country Source	Germany General	Greece General	Norway General	UK CAPD	USA Central venous catheters
S. capitis	1.5	0.8	0.8	1.5	0
S. epidermidis	61	63	73.8	78	62
S. haemolyticus	10	3.3	5.3	7.4	6
S. hominis	19	8.3	6.9	6.4	15
S. saprophyticus	1.5	8.3	6.1	1.2	0
S. simulans	1.8	1.7	2.2	0	0
S. warneri	4.5	1.7	4.6	5	6
Others	0.3	12.5	0.8	0	0
N	336	120	131	405	34

Based on Papapetropoulos et al. 1981, Iwantscheff et al. 1985, Haslett et al. 1988, Spencer 1988, Refsahl and Andersen 1992.

against the action of antibiotics (Peters et al. 1987). Slime is implicated in the adherence of staphylococci to catheters (Davenport et al. 1986, Diaz Mitona et al. 1987, Baddour et al. 1988), but others have reported that there is no correlation with disease (Alexander and Rimland 1987, Souto, Ferreiros and Criado 1991). In an in vivo study of infection, in an infant mouse weight gain retardation model, Gunn (1989) found that slime production was most common in strains of *S. lugdunensis* though this species was almost the least virulent by the test method.

Study of the adherence of coagulase-negative staphylococci to surfaces is made complex by the presence of slime, but adherence to individual extracellular matrix proteins is a valuable tool (Paulsson, Ljungh and Wadström 1992). In a study of strains from patients with endocarditis, Cree, Phillips and Noble (1995) reported that strains from native valve endocarditis were more likely to adhere to laminin and to tissue culture cells than strains from prosthetic valves. Slime production was similar at about 45% in both groups.

Coagulase-negative staphylococci are the principal pathogens in 3 important types of disease: peritonitis in patients undergoing chronic ambulatory peritoneal dialysis (CAPD), endocarditis, especially that associated with prosthetic valves, and ventricular shunt infections. They are also regularly recovered from infections of prosthetic joints.

PERITONITIS

Coagulase-negative staphylococci account for about 40% of all cases of peritonitis in patients undergoing CAPD with *S. epidermidis* the most common, followed by *S. haemolyticus*. The organisms frequently originate from the skin that surrounds the abdominal exit site of the peritoneal catheter or from the hands of the patient or a nurse whilst changing bags of dialysis fluid. Although evidently part of the normal flora of the skin, the infecting organisms may in fact be recently acquired members of the skin flora (Ludlam et al. 1989). In some centres, however, organisms that originate from the patient's skin are in a minority.

Nevertheless, poor catheter technique or maintenance is the main cause of infection (Eisenberg et al. 1987, Beard-Pegler et al. 1989).

In experiments it is important to consider the conditions encountered in nature, since growth of organisms and the activity of some, but not all, antibiotics differs in used dialysis fluid from that in nutrient broths (Verbrugh et al. 1984). An important factor in the establishment of peritonitis is the low level of host defences in the peritoneal cavity. There is a small resident population of macrophages that is diluted in the large volumes of dialysis fluid. Experimentally, 10^6 phagocytes per ml are required to obtain a bacteriostatic effect (Verbrugh et al. 1984). Similarly, in the uninfected peritoneal cavity amounts of immunoglobulin and complement are low (Easmon and Clark 1987). Small numbers of staphylococci can survive within peritoneal macrophages protected from antibiotics and this may contribute to persistent and recurrent infection (Buggy, Schaberg and Schwarz 1984, Brown et al. 1991). Antibody to coagulase-negative staphylococci develops soon after insertion of the catheter but appears not to be protective (Dryden et al. 1993).

ENDOCARDITIS

This may occur in 2 quite distinct circumstances:

1. spontaneously in persons with previously damaged heart valves, though there may be no history of this (Baltimore 1992) and
2. after an open operation on the heart (Quinn, Cox and Drake 1966).

In the first, endocarditis is often of the subacute form, the blood culture may be intermittently positive and the staphylococcus may be sensitive to antibiotics except penicillin and can be eradicated by intensive treatment. Coagulase-negative staphylococci are among the less common causes of infection in patients with chronically damaged heart valves or intravenous drug abusers in whom they cause about 5% of infections (Whitener et al. 1993) though the rate may be increasing slowly (Etienne and Eykyn 1990). Postcardiotomy endocarditis is usually of the acute form, the blood culture is in most cases uniformly positive, the staphylococcus is usually resistant to penicillin and several other antibiotics, and the prognosis may be poor. Coagulase-negative staphylococci are the most frequently isolated pathogens in prosthetic valve endocarditis (Whitener et al. 1993) and may present months after surgery. The operations on the heart after which endocarditis develops are usually those in which a valve has been replaced by a rigid prosthesis. The most consistent lesion in fatal cases develops immediately adjacent to the site of attachment of the prosthesis; microabscesses may form and extend into the surrounding tissue; vegetations on the prosthetic valve are a less constant feature (Arnett and Roberts 1977).

The causative organism in native and prosthetic valve endocarditis is usually described as *S. epidermidis* and this species causes about 60–80% of infections, but other species are also involved (Cree, Phillips and Noble 1995). Most native valve infections are community-acquired and most prosthetic valve infections are hospital-acquired with corresponding differences between the staphylococci responsible not only in antibiotic resistance patterns but also in the ability to adhere to plastics, tissue culture cells or extracellular matrix proteins (Cree, Phillips and Noble 1995). There are occasional reports of cross-infection in hospital-acquired prosthetic valve endocarditis (Blouse et al. 1978, Marples et al. 1978). Infection is most probably acquired from operating room staff, perhaps via instruments.

Amongst the individual species, other than *S. epidermidis*, recovered from endocarditis there has been a preponderance of reports on *S. lugdunensis* with suggestions that infections with this species are more severe than is usual for the coagulase-negative staphylococci (Shuttleworth and Colby 1992, Schonheyder et al. 1993, Vandenesch et al. 1993).

VENTRICULAR SHUNT INFECTIONS

Ventricular shunt infections develop in children after the insertion of a valve to drain off cerebrospinal fluid (CSF) in cases of hydrocephalus, usually, but not always, into the cardiac atrium. These infections were amongst the earliest catheter-associated coagulase-negative infections to be recognized (Callaghan, Cohen and Stewart 1961, Holt 1969) and may be characterized by splenomegaly and anaemia. Coagulase-negative staphylococci are responsible for about two-thirds of all infections of these shunts; the organism is usually present in the blood and less often in the CSF (Pople, Bayston and Hayward 1992). The disease differs from postcardiotomy infections in that the vegetation is regularly present on the prosthesis and the heart valves are unaffected even when the tip of the atrial catheter is in contact with it. Most infections occur within 8 weeks of insertion of the shunt and are difficult to eradicate unless the infected prosthesis is removed (Younger et al. 1987).

OTHER PROSTHESIS INFECTIONS

Coagulase-negative staphylococci occur chiefly in late infections, for example, more than 6 months after insertion of joint prostheses, where they may account for one-third of all infections; highly resistant strains may complicate therapy of these infections (James et al. 1994). Coagulase-negative staphylococci are also responsible for half the infections of prosthetic vascular grafts (Edmiston, Schmitt and Seabrook 1989, O'Brien and Collin 1992).

4.2 Typing coagulase-negative staphylococci

In contrast to *S. aureus*, phage typing the coagulase-negative species has not proved to be as valuable a tool. Up to 75% of *S. epidermidis* can be phage typed with certain phages provided that the strains have been heat shocked. Plasmid profiling, restriction endonuclease typing and other molecular techniques are also valuable and many studies of the epidemiology of coagulase-negative staphylococci have resorted to using a combination of 3 or more methods (Richardson, Noble and Marples 1992).

5 INFECTION DUE TO *MICROCOCCUS* AND *STOMATOCOCCUS*

Some infections formerly assigned to genera other than *Staphylococcus* must now be subsumed within the staphylococci; an example is endocarditis due to *S. saccharolyticus*, an anaerobic species formerly assigned to *Peptococcus* (Westblom et al. 1990). However, a small number of bloodstream infections have been reported due to *Micrococcus* spp. (Old and McNeill 1979, Marples and Richardson 1980, Magee et al. 1990); foot infection (pitted keratolysis) has also been reported as due to *Micrococcus sedentarius* (Nordstrom et al. 1987). The former *Micrococcus mucilaginosus* has been transferred to the genus *Stomatococcus* and has been reported from endocarditis and peritonitis (Rubin, Lyon and Murcia 1978, Lanzerdorfer, Zaruba and von Graevenitz 1988, Weinblatt, Sahdev and Berman 1990).

REFERENCES

Abussaud MJ, Meqdem MM, 1986, A study of some factors associated with wound infection, *J Hosp Infect*, **8:** 300–4.

Adlam C, Pearce JH, Smith H, 1970, The interaction of staphylococci grown in vivo and in vitro with polymorphonuclear leucocytes, *J Med Microbiol*, **3:** 157–63.

Adlam C, Ward PD et al., 1977, Effect of immunization with highly purified alpha- and beta-toxins on staphylococcal mastitis in rabbits, *Infect Immun*, **17:** 259–66.

Agarwal DS, 1967a, Subcutaneous staphylococcal infection in mice. 1. The role of cotton-dust in enhancing infection, *Br J Exp Pathol*, **48:** 436–49.

Agarwal DS, 1967b, Subcutaneous staphylococcal infection in mice. 3. Effect of active and passive immunization and anti-inflammatory drugs, *Br J Exp Pathol*, **48:** 483–500.

Alexander W, Rimland D, 1987, Lack of correlation of slime production with pathogenicity in continuous ambulatory peritoneal dialysis caused by coagulase negative staphylococci, *Diagn Microbiol Infect Dis*, **8:** 215–20.

Allaker RP, Lloyd DH et al., 1990, Interaction of *Staphylococcus hyicus* with inhibitor-producing bacteria on the skin of gnotobiotic piglets, *Microb Ecol Health Dis*, **3:** 19–24.

Amir M, Paul J et al., 1995, Nasopharyngeal carriage of *Staphylococcus aureus* and carriage of tetracycline-resistant strains associated with HIV-seropositivity, *Eur J Clin Microbiol Infect Dis*, **14:** 34–40.

Amon RB, Dimond RL, 1975, Toxic epidermal necrolysis. Rapid differentiation between staphylococcal and drug induced disease, *Arch Dermatol*, **111:** 1433–7.

Amtsberg G, 1979, Demonstration of exfoliatin-producing substances in cultures of *Staphylococcus hyicus* of pigs and *Staphylococcus epidermidis* type 2 of cattle, *Zentralbl Veterinärmed*, **B26:** 257–72.

Arnett EN, Roberts WC, 1977, Clinicopathology of prosthetic valve endocarditis, *Infections of Prosthetic Heart Valves and Vascular Grafts*, ed. Duma RJ, University Park Press, Baltimore, 17–41.

Asheshov EH, Coe AW, Porthouse A, 1977, Properties of strains of *Staphylococcus aureus* in the 94, 96 complex, *J Med Microbiol*, **10:** 171–8.

Asheshov EH, Rippon JE, 1959, Changes in typing pattern of phage-type 80 staphylococci, *J Gen Microbiol*, **20:** 634–43.

Awadallah SM, Kavey RE et al., 1991, The changing pattern of infective endocarditis in children, *Am J Cardiol*, **68:** 90–4.

Ayliffe GAJ, Collins BJ, 1967, Wound infections acquired from a disperser of an unusual strain of *Staphylococcus aureus*, *J Clin Pathol*, **20:** 195–8.

da Azavedo J, Arbuthnott JP, 1981, Prevalence of epidermolytic toxin in clinical isolates of *Staphylococcus aureus*, *J Med Microbiol*, **14:** 341–4.

Baddour LM, Smalley DL et al., 1988, Proposed virulence factors among coagulase negative staphylococci isolated from two healthy populations, *Can J Microbiol*, **34:** 901–5.

Baddour LM, Tayidi MM et al., 1994, Virulence of coagulase-deficient mutants of *Staphylococcus aureus* in experimental endocarditis, *J Med Microbiol*, **41:** 259–63.

Bailey CJ, Smith TP, 1990, The reactive serine residue of epidermolytic toxin A, *Biochem J*, **269:** 535–7.

Baltimore RS, 1992, Infective endocarditis in children, *Pediatr Infect Dis J*, **11:** 907–12.

Bänffer JRJ, Franken JF, 1967, Immunization with leucocidin toxoid against staphylococcal infection, *Pathol Microbiol*, **30:** 166–74.

Bannerman TL, Hancock GA et al., 1995, Pulsed-field gel electrophoresis as a replacement for bacteriophage typing of *Staphylococcus aureus*, *J Clin Microbiol*, **33:** 551–5.

Barber M, Wilson BDR et al., 1953, Spread of *Staphylococcus aureus* in a maternity department in the absence of severe sepsis, *J Obstet Gynecol*, **60:** 476–82.

Beard-Pegler MA, Gabelish CL et al., 1989, Prevalence of perito-

nitis associated coagulase-negative staphylococci on the skin of continuous ambulatory peritoneal dialysis patients, *Epidemiol Infect*, **102:** 365–78.

Belsky DS, Teates CD, Hartman ML, 1994, Case report: diabetes mellitus as a predisposing factor in the development of pyomyositis, *Am J Med Sci*, **308:** 251–4.

Bergdoll MS, Crass BA et al., 1981, A new staphylococcal enterotoxin, enterotoxin F, associated with toxic-shock-syndrome *Staphylococcus aureus* isolates, *Lancet*, **1:** 1017–21.

Bethune DW, Blowers R et al., 1965, Dispersal of *Staphylococcus aureus* by patients and surgical staff, *Lancet*, **1:** 480–3.

Bibel DJ, Greenberg JH, Cook JL, 1977, *Staphylococcus aureus* and the microbial ecology of atopic dermatitis, *Can J Microbiol*, **23:** 1062–8.

Blouse LE, Lathrop GA et al., 1978, Epidemiologic features and phage types associated with nosocomial infections caused by *Staphylococcus epidermidis*, *Zentrabl Bakteriol Parasitenkd Infektionskr Hyg Abt 1*, **A241:** 119–35.

Blum R, Fish LA, 1977, Recurrent severe staphylococcal infections, eczematoid rash, extreme elevation of IgE, eosinophilia, and divergent chemotactic responses in two generations, *J Pediatr*, **90:** 607–9.

Boelaert JR, de Baere YA et al., 1991, The use of mupirocin ointment to prevent *Staphylococcus aureus* bacteraemias in haemodialysis patients: an analysis of cost effectiveness, *J Hosp Infect*, **19, Suppl. B:** 41–6.

Bonventre PF, Weckbach L et al., 1983, Production of staphylococcal enterotoxin F and pyrogenic exotoxin C by *Staphylococcus aureus* isolates from toxic shock syndrome associated sources, *Infect Immun*, **40:** 1023–9.

Boyco EJ, Lipsky BA et al., 1989, NIDDM and prevalence of nasal *Staphylococcus aureus* colonization, *Diabetes Care*, **12:** 189–92.

Branger C, Fournier JM et al., 1994, Epidemiology of *Staphylococcus aureus* in patients with cystic fibrosis, *Epidemiol Infect*, **112:** 489–500.

Brown AL, Stephenson JR et al., 1991, Recurrent CAPD peritonitis caused by coagulase-negative staphylococci: re-infection or relapse determined by clinical criteria and typing methods, *J Hosp Infect*, **18:** 109–22.

Buggy BP, Schaberg DR, Swartz RD, 1984, Intraleukocytic sequestration as a cause of persistent *Staphylococcus aureus* peritonitis in continuous ambulatory peritoneal dialysis, *Am J Med*, **76:** 1035–40.

Bygdeman S, Hambraeus A et al., 1984, Influence of ethanol with and without chlorhexidine on the bacterial colonization of the umbilicus of newborn infants, *Infect Control*, **5:** 275–8.

Cafferkey MT, Hone R et al., 1983, Gentamicin and methicillin-resistant *Staphylococcus aureus* in Dublin hospitals: clinical and laboratory studies, *J Med Microbiol*, **16:** 117–27.

Callaghan RP, Cohen SJ, Stewart GT, 1961, Septicaemia due to colonization of Spitz Holter valves by staphylococci, *Br Med J*, **1:** 860–2.

Casewell MW, Hill RLR, 1986, Elimination of nasal carriage of *Staphylococcus aureus* with mupirocin ('pseudomonic acid') – a controlled trial, *J Antimicrob Chemother*, **17:** 365–72.

Christensen GD, Simpson WA et al., 1982, Adherence of slime producing strains of *Staphylococcus epidermidis* to smooth surfaces, *Infect Immun*, **37:** 318–26.

Colleen S, Hovelius B et al., 1979, Surface properties of *Staphylococcus saprophyticus* and *Staphylococcus epidermidis* as studied by adherence tests and two-polymer, aqueous phase systems, *Acta Pathol Microbiol Scand*, **B87:** 321–8.

Cone LA, Woodward DR et al., 1992, A recalcitrant, erythematous, desquamating disorder associated with toxin-producing staphylococci in patients with AIDS, *J Infect Dis*, **165:** 638–43.

Conti CR, Cluff LE, Scheder EP, 1961, Studies on the pathogenesis of staphylococcal infection. IV. The effect of bacterial endotoxin, *J Exp Med*, **113:** 845–59.

Cooke EM, Casewell MW et al., 1986, Methicillin-resistant *Sta-*

phylococcus aureus in the UK and Ireland. A questionnaire survey, *J Hosp Infect*, **8**: 143–8.

Craigen MA, Watters J, Hackett JS, 1992, The changing epidemiology of osteomyelitis in children, *J Bone Joint Surg [Br]*, **74**: 541–5.

Cree RGA, Aleljung P et al., 1994, Cell surface hydrophobicity and adherence to extra-cellular matrix proteins in two collections of methicillin-resistant *Staphylococcus aureus*, *Epidemiol Infect*, **112**: 307–14.

Cree RGA, Phillips I, Noble WC, 1995, Adherence characteristics of coagulase-negative staphylococci isolated from patients with infective endocarditis, *J Med Microbiol*, **43**: 161–8.

Crossley K, Landesman B, Zaske D, 1979, An outbreak of infections caused by strains of *Staphylococcus aureus* resistant to methicillin and aminoglycosides. II. Epidemiological studies, *J Infect Dis*, **139**: 280–7.

Curran JP, Al Salihi FL, 1980, Neonatal staphylococcal scalded skin syndrome: massive outbreak due to an unusual phage type, *Pediatrics*, **66**: 285–90.

Dack GM, 1956, The role of enterotoxin of *Micrococcus pyogenes* var *aureus* in the etiology of pseudomembranous enterocolitis, *Am J Surg*, **92**: 765–9.

Dancer SJ, Noble WC, 1991, Nasal, axillary, and perineal carriage of *Staphylococcus aureus* among women: identification of strains producing epidermolytic toxins, *J Clin Pathol*, **44**: 681–4.

Dancer SJ, Simmons NA et al., 1988, Outbreak of staphylococcal scalded skin syndrome among neonates, *J Infect*, **16**: 87–103.

Dancer SJ, Garratt R et al., 1990a, The epidermolytic toxins are serine proteases, *FEBS Lett*, **268**: 129–32.

Dancer SJ, Poston SM et al., 1990b, An outbreak of pemphigus neonatorum, *J Infect*, **20**: 73–82.

Dankert J, Zijlstra JB, Lubberding H, 1979, A garment for use in the operating theatre: the effect upon bacterial shedding, *J Hyg Camb*, **82**: 7–14.

Dave J, Reith S et al., 1994, A double outbreak of exfoliative toxin-producing strains of *Staphylococcus aureus* in a maternity hospital, *Epidemiol Infect*, **112**: 104–14.

Davenport DS, Massanari RM et al., 1986, Usefulness of test for slime production as a marker for clinically significant infections with coagulase-negative staphylococci, *J Infect Dis*, **153**: 332–9.

David TJ, Cambridge GC, 1986, Bacterial infection and atopic eczema, *Arch Dis Childh*, **61**: 20–3.

Davies RR, Noble WC, 1963, Dispersal of staphylococci on desquamated skin, *Lancet*, **1**: 1111.

Davies SJ, Ogg CS et al., 1989, *Staphylococcus aureus* nasal carriage, exit-site infection and catheter loss in patients treated with continuous ambulatory peritoneal dialysis (CAPD), *Periton Dial Bull*, **9**: 61–4.

Davies SJ, Yewdall VM et al., 1990, Peritoneal defence mechanisms and *Staphylococcus aureus* in patients treated with continuous ambulatory peritoneal dialysis, *Periton Dial Int*, **10**: 135–40.

Davis JP, Chesney PJ et al., 1980, Toxic-shock syndrome: epidemiologic features, recurrence, risk factors, and prevention, *N Engl J Med*, **303**: 1429–35.

Decker MD, Lybarger JA et al., 1986, An outbreak of staphylococcal skin infection among river rafting guides, *Am J Epidemiol*, **124**: 969–76.

Demidovitch CW, Witler RR et al., 1990, Impetigo: current etiology and comparison of penicillin, erythromycin and cephalexin therapies, *Am J Dis Child*, **144**: 1313–15.

Demuth PJ, Gerding DN, Crossley K, 1979, *Staphylococcus aureus* bacteriuria, *Arch Intern Med*, **139**: 78–80.

Diaz-Mitoma D, Harding GKM et al., 1987, Clinical significance of a test for slime production in ventriculoperitoneal shunt infections caused by coagulase-negative staphylococci, *J Infect Dis*, **156**: 555–60.

DiTomaso A, Warner EA, 1994, Case report: toxic shock syndrome arising from cellulitis, *Am J Med Sci*, **308**: 110–11.

Dixon RE, Kaslow RA et al., 1973, Staphylococcal disease outbreaks in hospital nurseries in the United States – December 1971 through March 1972, *Pediatrics*, **51**: 413–17.

de Dobbeleer G, Achten G, 1975, Staphylococcal scalded skin syndrome. An ultrastructural study, *J Cutan Pathol*, **2**: 91–6.

Doebbeling BN, 1994, Nasal and hand carriage of *Staphylococcus aureus* in health care workers, *J Chemother*, **6, Suppl. 2**: 11–17.

Doebbeling BN, Breneman DL et al., 1993, Elimination of *Staphylococcus aureus*, nasal carriage in health care workers. Analysis of six clinical trials with calcium mupirocin ointment, *Clin Infect Dis*, **17**: 466–74.

Dreskin SC, Goldsmith PK, Gallin JI, 1985, Immunoglobulins in the hyperimmunoglobulin E and recurrent infection (Job's) syndrome. Deficiency of anti-*Staphylococcus aureus* immunoglobulin A, *J Clin Invest*, **75**: 26–34.

Dryden MS, Talsania H et al., 1993, Serological response to coagulase-negative staphylococci in patients with peritonitis on continuous ambulatory peritoneal dialysis, *Eur J Clin Microbiol Infect Dis*, **12**: 87–92.

Duvic M, 1987, Staphylococcal infection and pruritis in AIDS related complex, *Arch Dermatol*, **123**: 1599.

Dyke KGH, Curnock SP et al., 1991, Cloning of the gene conferring resistance to mupirocin in *Staphylococcus aureus*, *FEMS Microbiol Lett*, **61**: 195–8.

Easmon CSF, 1980, Experimental staphylococcal infection in mice, *J Med Microbiol*, **13**: 495–506.

Easmon CSF, Clark LA, 1987, Opsonization of *Staphylococcus epidermidis*, *Zentralbl Bakteriol Mikrobiol Hyg Abt 1*, **Suppl. 16**: 169–76.

Easmon CSF, Glynn AA, 1975, Cell mediated immune responses in *Staphylococcus aureus* infections in mice, *Immunology*, **29**: 75–85.

Easmon CSF, Glynn AA, 1977, Effect of cyclophosphamide on delayed hypersensitivity to *Staphylococcus aureus* in mice, *Immunology*, **33**: 767–76.

Easmon CSF, Glynn AA, 1978, Role of *Staphylococcus aureus* cell wall antigens in the stimulation of delayed hypersensitivity after staphylococcal infection, *Infect Immun*, **19**: 341–2.

Easmon CSF, Glynn AA, 1979, The cellular control of delayed hypersensitivity to *Staphylococcus aureus* in mice, *Immunology*, **38**: 103–8.

Editorial, 1982, Hexachlorophene today, *Lancet*, **1**: 87–8.

Edmiston CE Jr, Schmitt DD, Seabrook GR, 1989, Coagulase-negative staphylococcal infections in vascular surgery: epidemiology and pathogenesis, *Infect Control Hosp Epidemiol*, **10**: 111–17.

Eisenberg ES, Ambalu M et al., 1987, Colonization of skin and development of peritonitis due to coagulase-negative staphylococci in patients undergoing peritoneal dialysis, *J Infect Dis*, **156**: 478–82.

Ejlertsen T, Jensen A et al., 1994, Epidemiology of toxic shock syndrome toxin-1 production in *Staphylococcus aureus* strains isolated in Denmark between 1959 and 1990, *Scand J Infect Dis*, **26**: 599–604.

Elek SD, Conen PE, 1957, The virulence of *Staphylococcus pyogenes* for man. A study of the problem of wound infection, *Br J Exp Pathol*, **38**: 573–86.

Elias PM, Fritsch P, Epstein EH, 1977, Staphylococcal scalded skin syndrome. Clinical features, pathogenesis, and recent microbiological and biochemical developments, *Arch Dermatol*, **113**: 207–19.

Ellis M, Gupta S et al., 1988, Impaired neutrophil function in patients with AIDS or AIDS-related complex: a comprehensive evaluation, *J Infect Dis*, **158**: 1268–76.

Espersen F, Jarlov JO, 1984, *Staphylococcus aureus* peptidoglycan induces histamine release from basophil human leukocytes in vitro, *Infect Immun*, **46**: 710–14.

Espersen F, Frimodt-Moller N et al., 1991, Changing pattern of bone and joint infections due to *Staphylococcus aureus*: study of cases of bacteraemia in Denmark, 1959–1988, *Rev Infect Dis*, **13**: 347–58.

Espersen F, Rosdahl VT et al., 1994, Epidemiology of *Staphylococcus aureus* bacteraemia in Denmark, *J Chemother*, **6:** 219–25.

Etienne J, Eykyn S, 1990, Increase in native valve endocarditis caused by coagulase-negative staphylococci: an Anglo-French clinical and microbiological study, *Br Heart J*, **64:** 381–4.

Farrington M, Brenwald N et al., 1992, Resistance to desiccation and skin fatty acids in outbreak strains of methicillin-resistant *Staphylococcus aureus*, *J Med Microbiol*, **36:** 56–60.

Fisher S, 1963, Experimental staphylococcal infection of the subcutaneous tissue of the mouse. II. Promotion of the infection with staphylococcal cells and products, *J Infect Dis*, **113:** 213–18.

Foster TJ, 1991, Potential for vaccination against infections caused by *Staphylococcus aureus*, *Vaccine*, **9:** 221–7.

Foster WD, Hutt MSR, 1960, Experimental staphylococcal infections in man, *Lancet*, **2:** 1373–6.

Frank U, Lenz W et al., 1989, Nasal carriage of *Staphylococcus aureus* treated with topical mupirocin (pseudomonic acid) in a children's hospital, *J Hosp Infect*, **13:** 117–20.

Fritsch PO, Kaaserer G, Elias PM, 1979, Action of staphylococcal epidermolysin: further observations on its species specificity, *Arch Dermatol Res*, **264:** 287–91.

Fujita K, Yokata T et al., 1992, In vitro adherence of *Staphylococcus saprophyticus*, *Staphylococcus epidermidis*, *Staphylococcus haemolyticus*, and *Staphylococcus aureus* to human ureter, *Urol Res*, **20:** 399–402.

Galbraith NS, 1960, Staphylococcal infections in general practice, *Proc R Soc Med*, **53:** 253–5.

Ganesh R, Castle D et al., 1989, Staphylococcal carriage and HIV infection, *Lancet*, **2:** 558.

Gatermann S, John J, Marre R, 1989, *Staphylococcus saprophyticus* urease: characterization and contribution to uropathogenicity in unobstructed urinary tract infection of rats, *Infect Immun*, **57:** 110–16.

Gemmel CG, 1983, Extra-cellular toxins and enzymes of coagulase-negative staphylococci, *Staphylococci and Staphylococcal Infection*, vol. 2, eds Easmon CSF, Adlam C, Academic Press, London, 809–27.

Gemmell CG, Peterson PK et al., 1982, Effect of staphylococcal alpha-toxin on phagocytosis of staphylococci by human polymorphonuclear leukocytes, *Infect Immun*, **38:** 975–80.

Gezon HM, Thompson DJ et al., 1964, Hexachlorophene bathing in early infancy, *N Engl J Med*, **270:** 379–86.

Glancey G, Cameron JS et al., 1993, Adherence of *Staphylococcus aureus* to cultures of human peritoneal mesothelial cells, *Nephrol Dial Transplant*, **8:** 157–62.

Goldberg NS, Ahmed T et al., 1989, Staphylococcal scalded skin syndrome mimicking acute graft-versus-host disease in a bone marrow transplant recipient, *Arch Dermatol*, **125:** 85–7.

Goshi K, Cluff LE, Johnson JE, 1961, Studies on the pathogenesis of staphylococcal infection. III. The effect of tissue necrosis and antitoxic immunity, *J Exp Med*, **113:** 259–70.

Goshi K, Cluff LE, Norman PS, 1963, Studies on the pathogenesis of staphylococcal infection. VI. Mechanism of immunity conferred by anti-alpha hemolysin, *Bull Johns Hopkins Hosp*, **112:** 31–47.

Goshi K, Smith EW et al., 1963, Studies on the pathogenesis of staphylococcal infection. VII. Characterization of the dermal reaction to purified alpha hemolysin in normal and immune animals, *Bull Johns Hopkin Hosp*, **113:** 183–201.

Gould JC, Cruickshank JD, 1957, Staphylococcal infection in general practice, *Lancet*, **2:** 1157–61.

Gow TL, Sweeney FJ et al., 1963, Abscess-forming factor(s) produced by *Staphylococcus aureus*. I. Collodian bag implantation technique, *J Bacteriol*, **86:** 611–18.

Graham DR, Correa-Villasenor A et al., 1980, Epidemic neonatal gentamicin-methicillin-resistant *Staphylococcus aureus* infection associated with nonspecific topical use of gentamicin, *J Pediatr*, **97:** 972–8.

Greenberg DP, Bayer AS et al., 1990, Antibody responses to protein A in patients with *Staphylococcus aureus* bacteremia and endocarditis, *J Clin Microbiol*, **28:** 458–62.

Gunn BA, 1989, Comparative virulence of human isolates of coagulase-negative staphylococci tested in an infant mouse weight retardation model, *J Clin Microbiol*, **27:** 507–11.

Gürtler V, Barrie HD, 1995, Typing of *Staphylococcus aureus* strains by PCR-amplification of variable-length 16S–23S rDNA spacer regions: characterization of spacer sequences, *Microbiology*, **141:** 1255–65.

Gustafson GT, Stalenheim G et al., 1968, 'Protein A' from *Staphylococcus aureus*. IV. Production of anaphylaxis-like cutaneous and systemic reactions in non-immunized guinea-pigs, *J Immunol*, **100:** 530–4.

Hale JH, Smith W, 1945, The influence of coagulase on the phagocytosis of staphylococci, *Br J Exp Pathol*, **26:** 209–16.

Hall DE, Snitzer JA III, 1994, *Staphylococcus epidermidis* as a cause of urinary tract infections in children, *J Pediatr*, **124:** 437–8.

Hallman FA, 1937, Pathogenic staphylococci from anterior nares: incidence and differentiation, *Proc Soc Exp Biol Med*, **36:** 789–94.

Hargiss C, Larson E, 1978, The epidemiology of *Staphylococcus aureus* in a newborn nursery from 1970 through 1976, *Pediatrics*, **61:** 348–53.

Harvey RG, Marples RR, Noble WC, 1994, Nasal carriage of *Staphylococcus intermedius* in humans in contact with dogs, *Microb Ecol Health Dis*, **7:** 225–7.

Haslett TM, Isenberg HD et al., 1988, Microbiology of indwelling central intravascular catheters, *J Clin Microbiol*, **26:** 696–701.

Hauser C, Wuethrich B et al., 1985, *Staphylococcus aureus* skin colonization in atopic dermatitis patients, *Dermatologica*, **170:** 35–9.

Hedman P, Ringertz O et al., 1990, *Staphylococcus saprophyticus* found to be a common food contaminant, *J Infect*, **21:** 11–19.

Hedman P, Ringertz O et al., 1993, The origin of *Staphylococcus saprophyticus* from cattle and pigs, *Scand J Infect Dis*, **25:** 57–60.

Hedstrom SA, 1981, Recurrent staphylococcal furunculosis. Bacteriological findings and epidemiology in 100 cases, *Scand J Infect Dis*, **13:** 115–19.

Hill MJ, 1968, A staphylococcal aggressin, *J Med Microbiol*, **1:** 33–43.

Hill MJ, 1969, Protection of mice against infection by *Staphylococcus aureus*, *J Med Microbiol*, **2:** 1–7.

Hill RLR, Duckworth GJ, Casewell MW, 1988, Elimination of nasal carriage of methicillin-resistant *Staphylococcus aureus* with mupirocin during a hospital outbreak, *J Antimicrob Chemother*, **22:** 377–84.

Hill RLR, Fisher AP et al., 1990, Mupirocin for the reduction of colonization of internal jugular cannulae – a randomized controlled trial, *J Hosp Infect*, **15:** 311–21.

Hoeger PH, Lenz W et al., 1992, Staphylococcal skin colonization in children with atopic dermatitis: prevalence, persistence, and transmission of toxigenic and non-toxigenic strains, *J Infect Dis*, **165:** 1064–8.

Holt RJ, 1969, Studies on staphylococci from colonized ventriculo-atrial shunts, *J Clin Pathol*, **22:** 745–6.

Hovelius B, Colleen S, Mardh PA, 1984, Urinary tract infections in men caused by *Staphylococcus saprophyticus*, *Scand J Infect Dis*, **16:** 37–41.

Hovelius B, Mardh PA, 1979, Haemagglutination by *Staphylococcus saprophyticus* and other staphylococcal species, *Acta Pathol Microbiol Scand*, **B87:** 45–50.

Hudson VL, Wielinski CL, Regelmann WE, 1993, Prognostic implications of initial pharyngeal bacterial flora in patients with cystic fibrosis diagnosed before the age of two years, *J Pediatr*, **122:** 854–60.

Hurst V, Grossman M, 1960, The hospital nursery as a source of staphylococcal disease among families of newborn infants, *N Engl J Med*, **262:** 951–6.

Inglis TJ, Sproat LJ et al., 1993, Staphylococcal pneumonia in ventilated patients: a twelve-month review of cases in an intensive care unit, *J Hosp Infect*, **25:** 207–10.

Iwantscheff A, Kühnen E, Brandis H, 1985, Species distribution of coagulase-negative staphylococci isolated from clinical sources, *Zentralbl Bakteriol Mikrobiol Parasitenkd Infektionskr Hyg*, **A260:** 41–50.

Jackson LJ, Sottile MI et al., 1978, Correlation of antistaphylococcal antibody titers with severity of staphylococcal disease, *Am J Med*, **64:** 629–33.

Jacobson JA, Kasworm EM et al., 1987, Low incidence of toxic shock syndrome in children with staphylococcal infection, *Am J Med Sci*, **294:** 403–7.

James PJ, Butcher IA et al., 1994, Methicillin-resistant *Staphylococcus epidermidis* in infection of hip arthroplasties, *J Bone Joint Surg [Br]*, **76:** 725–7.

Jensen AG, Espersen F et al., 1993, *Staphylococcus aureus* meningitis. A review of 104 nationwide, consecutive cases, *Arch Intern Med*, **153:** 1902–8.

Jessen O, Bülow P, 1967, Changes in pathogenicity of *Staphylococcus aureus* by lysogenic conversion influencing lipase production, as evidenced by experimental skin infection in pigs, *Acta Pathol Microbiol Scand Suppl*, **187:** 48–9.

Jimenez-Mejias ME, Lozano de Leon F et al., 1992, Pyomyositis caused by *Staphylococcus aureus*, *Med Clin (Barc)*, **99:** 201–5.

Kaplan MH, Chmel H et al., 1986, Importance of exfoliatin toxin A production by *Staphylococcus aureus* strains isolated from clustered epidemics of neonatal pustulosis, *J Clin Microbiol*, **23:** 83–91.

Kaslow RA, Dixon RE et al., 1973, Staphylococcal disease related to hospital nursery bathing practices – a nationwide epidemiologic investigation, *Pediatrics*, **51:** 418–29.

Kay CR, 1962, Sepsis in the home, *Br Med J*, **1:** 1048–52.

Kellaway CH, MacCallum P, Terbutt AH, 1928, *Report of the Commission to the Government of the Commonwealth of Australia*, Melbourne, Australia.

Kenny K, Reiser RF et al., 1993, Production of enterotoxins and toxic shock syndrome by bovine mammary isolates of *Staphylococcus aureus*, *J Clin Microbiol*, **31:** 706–7.

Kerr S, Kerr GE et al., 1990, A survey of methicillin-resistant *Staphylococcus aureus* affecting patients in England and Wales, *J Hosp Infect*, **16:** 35–48.

Khan GA, Bank N, 1994, An adult patient with hyperimmunoglobulinemia E (Job's) syndrome, end-stage renal disease and repeated episodes of peritonitis, *Clin Nephrol*, **41:** 233–6.

King K, Brady LM, Harkness JL, 1981, Gentamicin-resistant staphylococci, *Lancet*, **2:** 698–9.

Kinsman OS, McKenna R, Noble WC, 1983, Association between histocompatibility antigens (HLA) and nasal carriage of *Staphylococcus aureus*, *J Med Microbiol*, **16:** 215–20.

Kinsman OS, White MI, Noble WC, 1981, Inflammatory reactions to staphylococcal protein A in mice, *Br J Exp Pathol*, **62:** 142–5.

Kirmani N, Tuazon CU et al., 1978, *Staphylococcus aureus* carriage rate of patients receiving long term haemodialysis, *Arch Intern Med*, **138:** 1657–9.

Kjolon H, Anderson BM, 1992, Handwashing and disinfection of heavily contaminated hands – effective or ineffective?, *J Hosp Infect*, **21:** 61–71.

Kloos WE, Musselwhite MS, 1975, Distribution and persistence of *Staphylococcus* and *Micrococcus* species and other aerobic bacteria on human skin, *Appl Microbiol*, **30:** 381–95.

Knight GJ, Carman PG, 1992, Primary staphylococcal pneumonia in childhood: a review of 69 cases, *J Paediatr Child Health*, **28:** 447–50.

Kreiswirth BN, Projan SJ et al., 1989, Toxic shock syndrome toxin is encoded by a variable genetic element, *Rev Infect Dis*, **11, Suppl. 1:** S83–8.

Lambe DW Jr, Ferguson KP et al., 1990, Pathogenicity of *Staphylococcus lugdunensis*, *Staphylococcus schleiferi* and three other coagulase-negative staphylococci in a mouse model and possible virulence factors, *Can J Microbiol*, **36:** 455–63.

Lanzendorfer H, Zaruba K, von Graevenitz A, 1988, *Stomatococcus mucilaginosus* as an agent of CAPD peritonitis, *Zentralbl Bakteriol Mikrobiol Hyg [A]*, **270:** 326–8.

Larsen RA, Burke JP, 1986, The epidemiology and risk factors for nosocomial catheter-associated bacteriuria caused by coagulase-negative staphylococci, *Infect Control*, **7:** 212–15.

Lautenschlager S, Herzog C, Zimmerli W, 1993, Course and outcome of bacteremia due to *Staphylococcus aureus*: evaluation of different clinical case definitions, *Clin Infect Dis*, **16:** 567–73.

Lee BK, Crossley K, Gerding DN, 1978, The association between *Staphylococcus aureus* bacteremia and bacteriuria, *Am J Med*, **65:** 303–6.

Lee JC, Betley MJ et al., 1987, Virulence studies, in mice, of transposon-induced mutants of *Staphylococcus aureus* differing in capsule size, *J Infect Dis*, **156:** 741–50.

Leighton PM, Little JA, 1986, Identification of coagulase-negative staphylococci isolated from urinary tract infections, *Am J Clin Pathol*, **85:** 92–5.

Leung DY, Harbeck R et al., 1993, Presence of IgE antibodies to staphylococcal exotoxins on the skin of patients with atopic dermatitis. Evidence for a new group of allergens, *J Clin Invest*, **93:** 1374–80.

Levine SJ, White DA, Fels AO, 1990, The incidence and significance of *Staphylococcus aureus* in respiratory cultures from patients infected with the human immunodeficiency virus, *Am Rev Respir Dis*, **141:** 89–93.

Lewis E, Saravolatz LD, 1985, Comparison of methicillin-resistant and methicillin-sensitive *Staphylococcus aureus* bacteremia, *Am J Infect Control*, **13:** 109–14.

Leyden JJ, Jones WD, 1987, *Staphylococcus aureus* infection as a complication of isotretinoin prescription, *Arch Dermatol*, **123:** 606–8.

Leyden JJ, Marples RR, Kligman AM, 1974, *Staphylococcus aureus* in the lesions of atopic dermatitis, *Br J Dermatol*, **90:** 525–30.

Lidwell OM, 1961, Sepsis in surgical wounds. Multiple regression analysis applied to records of post-operative wound sepsis, *J Hyg Camb*, **59:** 259–70.

Lidwell OM, 1976, Clean air, less infection, *Hosp Engng*, **30:** 9–17.

Lidwell OM, Polakoff S et al., 1966, Staphylococcal infection in thoracic surgery: experience in a subdivided ward, *J Hyg Camb*, **64:** 321–37.

Lidwell OM, Polakoff S et al., 1970, Nasal acquisition of *Staphylococcus aureus* in a subdivided and mechanically ventilated ward: endemic prevalence of a single staphylococcal strain, *J Hyg Camb*, **68:** 417–33.

Lidwell OM, Davies J et al., 1971, Nasal acquisition of *Staphylococcus aureus* in partly divided wards, *J Hyg Camb*, **69:** 113–23.

Linnemann CC Jr, Moore P et al., 1991, Reemergence of epidemic methicillin-resistant *Staphylococcus aureus* in a general hospital associated with changing staphylococcal strains, *Am J Med*, **91:** 238S–44S.

Lloyd DH, 1993, Bacterial and fungal skin disease in animals, *The Skin Microflora and Microbial Skin Disease*, ed. Noble WC, Cambridge University Press, Cambridge, 264–90.

Lotem M, Ingber A et al., 1988, Skin infection provoked by coagulase-negative staphylococci resembling Gram-negative folliculitis, *Cutis*, **42:** 443–4.

Love DN, Davis PC, 1980, Isolation of *Staphylococcus aureus* from a condition in greyhounds histologically resembling 'staphylococcal scalded skin syndrome' of man, *J Small Anim Pract*, **21:** 351–7.

Ludlam HA, Noble WC et al., 1989, The epidemiology of peritonitis caused by coagulase-negative staphylococci in continuous ambulatory peritoneal dialysis, *J Med Microbiol*, **30:** 167–74.

Lyell A, 1979, Toxic epidermal necrolysis (the scalded skin syndrome): a reappraisal, *Br J Dermatol*, **100:** 69–86.

McFadden JP, Noble WC, Camp RDR, 1993, Superantigenic exotoxin-producing potential of staphylococci isolated from atopic eczematous skin, *Br J Dermatol*, **128:** 631–2.

Mackintosh CA, Marples RR et al., 1991, Surveillance of methicillin-resistant *Staphylococcus aureus* in England and Wales, 1986–1990, *J Hosp Infect*, **18:** 279–92.

Magee JT, Burnett IA et al., 1990, *Micrococcus* and *Stomatococcus* spp. from human infections, *J Hosp Infect*, **16**: 67–73.

Malam JE, Carrick GF et al., 1992, Staphylococcal toxins and sudden infant death syndrome, *J Clin Pathol*, **45**: 716–21.

Manzella JP, Hall CB et al., 1980, Toxic epidermal necrolysis in childhood: differentiation from staphylococcal scalded skin syndrome, *Pediatrics*, **66**: 291–4.

Marples RR, Cooke EM, 1988, Current problems with methicillin-resistant *Staphylococcus aureus*, *J Hosp Infect*, **11**: 381–92.

Marples RR, Kligman AM, 1969, Pyoderma due to resistant *Staphylococcus aureus* following topical application of neomycin, *J Invest Dermatol*, **53**: 11–13.

Marples RR, Richardson JF, 1980, Micrococcus in the blood, *J Med Microbiol*, **13**: 355–62.

Marples RR, Richardson JF, de Saxe MJ, 1986, Bacteriological characters of strains of *Staphylococcus aureus* submitted to a reference laboratory related to methicillin resistance, *J Hyg Camb*, **96**: 217–23.

Marples RR, Wieneke AA, 1993, Enterotoxins and toxic shock syndrome toxin-1 in non-enteric staphylococcal disease, *Epidemiol Infect*, **110**: 477–88.

Marples RR, Hone R et al., 1978, Investigation of coagulase-negative staphylococci from infections in surgical patients, *Zentrabl Bakteriol Parasitenkd Infektionskr Hyg*, **A241**: 140–56.

Marraro RV, Mitchell JL, 1975, Experiences and observations with the typing of *Staphylococcus aureus* phage 94, *J Clin Microbiol*, **12**: 180–4.

Mathieu D, Picard V, 1991, Comparative evaluation of five agglutination techniques and a new miniaturized system for rapid identification of methicillin-resistant strains of *Staphylococcus aureus*, *Int J Med Microbiol*, **276**: 46–53.

Mayberry-Carson KJ, Tober-Meyer B et al., 1983, Bacterial adherence and glycocalyx formation in osteomyelitis experimentally induced with *Staphylococcus aureus*, *Infect Immun*, **43**: 825–33.

Meislin HW, Lerner SA et al., 1977, Cutaneous abscesses. Anaerobic and aerobic bacteriology and outpatient management, *Ann Intern Med*, **87**: 145–9.

Melish ME, Glasgow LA, 1971, Staphylococcal scalded skin syndrome: the expanded clinical syndrome, *J Pediatr*, **78**: 958–67.

Mitchell NJ, Evans DS, Kerr A, 1978, Reduction of skin bacteria in theatre air with comfortable, non-woven disposable clothing for operating-theatre staff, *Br Med J*, **1**: 696–8.

Mobacken H, Holst R et al., 1975, Epidemiological aspects of impetigo contagiosa in western Sweden, *Scand J Infect Dis*, **7**: 39–44.

Moore B, Gardner AMN, 1963, A study of post-operative wound infection in a provincial general hospital, *J Hyg Camb*, **61**: 95–113.

Morris IM, Eade AW, 1978, Pyogenic arthritis and rheumatoid disease: the importance of the infected foot, *Rheumatol Rehabil*, **17**: 222–6.

Mortimer EA Jr, Lipsitz PJ et al., 1962, Transmission of staphylococci between newborns, *Am J Dis Child*, **104**: 289–95.

Mortimer EA Jr, Wolinsky E et al., 1966, Role of airborne transmission in staphylococcal infections, *Br Med J*, **1**: 319–22.

Murray HW, Tuazon CV, Sheagren JN, 1977, Staphylococcal septicemia and disseminated intravascular coagulation. *Staphylococcus aureus* endocarditis mimicking meningococcemia, *Arch Intern Med*, **137**: 844–7.

Musher DM, Watson DA et al., 1990, The effect of HIV infection on phagocytosis and killing of *Staphylococcus aureus* by human pulmonary alveolar macrophages, *Am J Med Sci*, **299**: 158–63.

Noble WC, 1962, The dispersal of staphylococci in hospital wards, *J Clin Pathol*, **15**: 552–8.

Noble WC, 1965, The production of subcutaneous staphylococcal skin lesions in mice, *Br J Exp Pathol*, **46**: 254–62.

Noble WC, 1992, Staphylococci on the skin, *The Skin Microflora and Microbial Skin Disease*, ed. Noble WC, Cambridge University Press, Cambridge, 135–52.

Noble WC, Lidwell OM, Kingston D, 1963, The size distribution of airborne particles carrying microorganisms, *J Hyg Camb*, **61**: 385–91.

Noble WC, Savin JA, 1968, Carriage of *Staphylococcus aureus* in psoriasis, *Br Med J*, **1**: 417–19.

Noble WC, Valkenburg HA, Wolters CHL, 1967, Carriage of *Staphylococcus aureus* in random samples of a normal population, *J Hyg Camb*, **65**: 567–73.

Noble WC, Williams REO et al., 1964, Some aspects of nasal carriage of staphylococci, *J Clin Pathol*, **17**: 79–83.

Noble WC, Habbema JDF et al., 1976, Quantitative studies on the dispersal of skin bacteria into the air, *J Med Microbiol*, **9**: 53–61.

Nolan CM, Beaty HN, 1976, *Staphylococcus aureus* bacteremia. Current clinical patterns, *Am J Med*, **60**: 495–500.

Nordstrom KM, McGinley KJ et al., 1987, Pitted keratolysis: the role of *Micrococcus sedentarius*, *Arch Dermatol*, **123**: 1320–5.

O'Brien T, Collin J, 1992, Prosthetic vascular graft infection, *Br J Surg*, **79**: 1262–7.

O'Connor DT, Weisman MH, Fierer J, 1978, Activation of the alternate complement pathway in *Staphylococcus aureus* infective endocarditis and its relationship to thrombocytopenia, coagulation abnormalities, and acute glomerulonephritis, *Clin Exp Immunol*, **34**: 179–87.

Ogawa T, Katsuoka K et al., 1994, Comparative study of the staphylococcal flora of the skin surface of atopic dermatitis patients and healthy subjects, *J Dermatol*, **21**: 453–60.

Old DC, McNeill GP, 1979, Endocarditis due to *Micrococcus sedentarius incertae sedis*, *J Clin Pathol*, **32**: 951–2.

Olin G, Lithander A, 1948, Toxin-forming staphylococci, as a cause of deaths on the injection of infected bacteriological preparations, *Acta Pathol Microbiol Scand*, **25**: 152–60.

Oliver VL, Sargent CA et al., 1964, The spread of sepsis contracted in hospital to the family, *Am J Hyg*, **79**: 302–9.

Opal SM, Johnson-Winegar AD, Cross AS, 1988, Staphylococcal scalded skin syndrome in two immunocompetent adults caused by exfoliatin B-producing *Staphylococcus aureus*, *J Clin Microbiol*, **26**: 1283–6.

Papapetropopoulos M, Pappas A et al., 1981, Distribution of coagulase-negative staphylococci in human infections, *J Hosp Infect*, **2**: 145–53.

Parker MT, 1983, The significance of phage-typing patterns in *Staphylococcus aureus*, *Staphylococci and Staphylococcal Infections*, vol. 1, eds Easmon CSF, Adlam C, Academic Press, London, 33–62.

Parker MT, Tomlinson AJH, Williams REO, 1955, Impetigo contagiosa. The association of certain types of *Staphylococcus aureus* and of *Streptococcus pyogenes* with superficial skin lesions, *J Hyg Camb*, **53**: 458–73.

Parker MT, Asheshov EH et al., 1974, Epidemic staphylococcal infections in hospitals, *Ann NY Acad Sci*, **236**: 466–84.

Patel A, Nowlan P, 1987, Virulence of protein-A deficient and alpha-toxin-deficient mutants of *Staphylococcus aureus* isolated by allele replacement, *Infect Immun*, **55**: 3103–10.

Patti JM, Bremell T et al., 1994, The *Staphylococcus aureus* collagen adhesin is a virulence determinant in experimental septic arthritis, *Infect Immun*, **62**: 152–61.

Paulsson M, Ljungh A, Wadström T, 1992, Rapid identification of fibronectin, vitronectin, laminin, and collagen cell surface binding proteins on coagulase-negative staphylococci by particle agglutination assays, *J Clin Microbiol*, **30**: 2006–12.

Pead L, Maskell R, Morris J, 1985, *Staphylococcus saprophyticus* as a urinary pathogen: a six year prospective survey, *Br Med J Clin Res Ed*, **291**: 1157–9.

Penikett EJK, Knox R, Liddell J, 1958, An outbreak of post-operative sepsis, *Br Med J*, **1**: 812–14.

Peters G, Schumacher-Perdrau F et al., 1987, Biology of *Staphylococcus epidermidis* extracellular slime, *Zentralbl Bakteriol Mikrobiol Hyg Abt 1*, **Suppl. 16**: 15–32.

Peterson PK, Laverdiere M et al., 1977, Abnormal neutrophil chemotaxis and T-lymphocyte function in staphylococcal scalded skin syndrome in an adult patient, *Infection*, **5**: 128–31.

Polakoff S, Richards IDG et al., 1967, Nasal and skin carriage of *Staphylococcus aureus* by patients undergoing surgical operation, *J Hyg Camb*, **65**: 559–66.

Pople IK, Bayston R, Hayward RD, 1992, Infection of cerebrospinal fluid shunts in infants: a study of etiologic factors, *J Neurosurg*, **77**: 29–36.

Pos O, Stevenhagen A et al., 1992, Impaired phagocytosis of *Staphylococcus aureus* by granulocytes and monocytes of AIDS patients, *Clin Exp Immunol*, **88**: 23–8.

Poston SM, Glancey GR et al., 1993, Co-elimination of *mec* and *spa* genes in *Staphylococcus aureus* and the effect of *agr* and protein A production on bacterial adherence to cell monolayers, *J Med Microbiol*, **39**: 422–8.

Price EH, Brain A, Dickson JAS, 1980, An outbreak of infection with a gentamicin and methicillin-resistant *Staphylococcus aureus* in a neonatal unit, *J Hosp Infect*, **1**: 221–8.

Proctor RA, 1987, The staphylococcal fibronectin receptor: evidence for its importance in invasive infections, *Rev Infect Dis*, **9, Suppl. 4**: S335–40.

Quie PG, Hill HR, Davies AT, 1974, Defective phagocytosis of staphylococci, *Ann NY Acad Sci*, **236**: 233–43.

Quie PG, Verhoef J et al., 1981, Host determinants of staphylococcal infections, *The Staphylococci*, eds MacDonald A, Smith G, Aberdeen University Press, Aberdeen, 83–93.

Quinn EL, Cox F, Drake EH, 1966, Staphylococcic endocarditis, *JAMA*, **196**: 815–18.

Rahman AN, Rammelkamp CH, 1982, Scarlet fever, toxic-shock syndrome and the staphylococcus, *Am J Med Sci*, **284**: 36–9.

Ravenholt RT, Wright P, Mulhern M, 1957, Epidemiology and prevention of nursery-derived staphylococcal disease, *N Engl J Med*, **257**: 789–95.

Reagan DR, Doebbeling BN et al., 1991, Elimination of coincidental *Staphylococcus aureus* nasal and hand carriage with intranasal application of mupirocin calcium ointment, *Ann Intern Med*, **114**: 101–6.

Rebel MH, van Furth R et al., 1975, The flora of renal haemodialysis shunt sites, *J Clin Pathol*, **28**: 29–32.

Rebora A, Nunzi E et al., 1978, Buckley's syndrome, *Br J Dermatol*, **99**: 569–72.

Reeves MW, 1989, Effect of trace metals on the synthesis of toxic shock syndrome toxin-1, *Rev Infect Dis*, **11, Suppl. 1**: S145–9.

Refsahl K, Andersen BM, 1992, Clinically significant coagulase-negative staphylococci identification and resistance patterns, *J Hosp Infect*, **22**: 19–31.

Reingold AL, 1991, Toxic shock syndrome: an update, *Am J Obstet Gynecol*, **165**: 1236–9.

Reiser RF, Hinzman SJ, Bergdoll MS, 1987, Production of toxic shock syndrome toxin-1 by *Staphylococcus aureus* restricted to endogenous air in tampons, *J Clin Microbiol*, **25**: 1450–2.

Rello J, Quintana E et al., 1990, Risk factors for *Staphylococcus aureus* nosocomial pneumonia in critically ill patients, *Am Rev Respir Dis*, **142**: 1320–4.

Renaud F, Bornstein N et al., 1994, Clonal study of enterotoxin-B producing strains of *Staphylococcus aureus*, *Epidemiol Infect*, **112**: 501–11.

Report, 1990, Revised Guidelines for the control of epidemic methicillin-resistant *Staphylococcus aureus*. Report of a combined working party of the Hospital Infection Society and British Society for Antimicrobial Chemotherapy, *J Hosp Infect*, **7**: 193–201.

Reuther JWA, Noble WC, 1993, An ecological niche for *Staphylococcus saprophyticus*, *Microb Ecol Health Dis*, **16**: 351–77.

Ribner B, Keusch GT, Robbins JB, 1975, *Staphylococcus aureus* antigen in cerebrospinal fluid crossreactive with *Haemophilus influenzae* type b antiserum, *Ann Intern Med*, **83**: 370–1.

Richards MS, Rittman M et al., 1993, Investigation of a staphylococcal food poisoning outbreak in a centralized school lunch program, *Public Health Rep*, **108**: 765–71.

Richardson JF, Noble WC, Marples MR, 1992, Species identification and epidemiological typing of the staphylococci, *Identification Methods in Applied and Environmental Microbiology*, Blackwell Scientific Publications, Oxford, 193–219.

Richardson JF, Quoraishi AHM et al., 1990, Beta-lactamase negative, methicillin-resistant *Staphylococcus aureus* in a newborn nursery: report of an outbreak and laboratory investigation, *J Hosp Infect*, **16**: 109–21.

Ritz HL, Kirkland JJ et al., 1984, Association of high levels of serum antibody to staphylococcal toxic shock antigen with nasal carriage of toxic shock antigen-producing strains of *Staphylococcus aureus*, *Infect Immun*, **43**: 954–8.

Robbins MJ, Frater RW et al., 1986, Influence of vegetation size on clinical outcome of right-sided infective endocarditis, *Am J Med*, **80**: 165–71.

Roodyn L, 1960, Recurrent staphylococcal infections and duration of the carrier state, *J Hyg Camb*, **58**: 11–19.

Rosendal K, Bülow P, 1971, A subdivision of *Staphylococcus aureus* belonging to the 83A, 84, 85, 6557, 592 complex with special reference to antibiotic resistance, *Acta Pathol Microbiol Scand*, **B79**: 377–84.

Rountree PM, Beard MA et al., 1967, Further studies on the nasal flora of people of Papua-New Guinea, *Med J Aust*, **1**: 967–9.

Rubin SJ, Lyons RW, Murcia AJ, 1978, Endocarditis associated with cardiac catheterization due to a Gram-positive coccus designated *Micrococcus mucilaginosus incertae sedis*, *J Clin Microbiol*, **7**: 545–9.

Rupp ME, Soper DE, Archer GL, 1992, Colonization of the female genital tract with *Staphylococcus saprophyticus*, *J Clin Microbiol*, **30**: 2975–9.

Russell RJ, Wilkinson PC et al., 1976, Effects of staphylococcal products on locomotion and chemotaxis of human blood neutrophils and monocytes, *J Med Microbiol*, **8**: 433–7.

Sato H, Matsumori Y et al., 1994, A new type of staphylococcal exfoliative toxin from a *Staphylococcus aureus* strain isolated from a horse with phlegmon, *Infect Immun*, **62**: 3780–5.

de Saxe MJ, Wieneke A et al., 1982, Toxic shock syndrome in Britain, *Br Med J*, **284**: 1641–2.

Schaefler A, 1989, Methicillin resistant strains of *Staphylococcus aureus* resistant to quinolones, *J Clin Microbiol*, **27**: 335–6.

Schlievert PM, 1981, Staphylococcal scarlet fever: role of pyrogenic exotoxins, *Infect Immun*, **31**: 732–6.

Schlievert PM, Schoettle DJ, Watson DW, 1979, Purification and physicochemical and biological characterization of a staphylococcal pyrogenic exotoxin, *Infect Immun*, **23**: 609–17.

Schonheyder HC, Hansen VK et al., 1993, *Staphylococcus lugdunensis*: an important cause of endocarditis. A case report, *APMIS*, **101**: 802–4.

Schuchat A, Broome CV, 1991, Toxic shock syndrome and tampons, *Epidemiol Rev*, **13**: 99–112.

Scopes JW, Eykyn S, Phillips I, 1974, Staphylococcal infection of the newborn, *Lancet*, **2**: 1392.

Seeberg S, Brinkhoff B et al., 1984, Prevention and control of neonatal pyoderma with chlorhexidine, *Acta Paediatr Scand*, **73**: 498–504.

Selwyn S, Verma BS, Vaishnav VP, 1967, Factors in the bacterial colonization and infection of the human skin, *Indian J Med Res*, **55**: 652–6.

Sesso R, Draibe S et al., 1989, *Staphylococcus aureus* skin carriage and development of peritonitis in patients on continuous ambulatory peritoneal dialysis, *Clin Nephrol*, **31**: 264–8.

Shands KN, Schmid GP et al., 1980, Toxic-shock syndrome in menstruating women: association with tampon use and *Staphylococcus aureus* and clinical features in 52 cases, *N Engl J Med*, **303**: 1436–42.

Shanson DC, 1981, Antibiotic resistant *Staphylococcus aureus*, *J Hosp Infect*, **2**: 11–36.

Shanson DC, McSwiggan DA, 1980, Operating theatre acquired infection with a gentamicin-resistant strain of *Staphylococcus aureus*: outbreaks in two hospitals attributable to one surgeon, *J Hosp Infect*, **1**: 171–2.

Sheagren JN, Tuazon CU et al., 1976, Rheumatoid factor in acute bacterial endocarditis, *Arthritis Rheum*, **19**: 887–90.

Shepherd JJ, 1983, Tropical myositis: is it an entity and what is its cause?, *Lancet*, **2**: 1240–2.

Shinefield HR, Ribble JC et al., 1963, Bacterial interference: its effect on nursery acquired infection with *Staphylococcus aureus*. I. Preliminary observations on artificial colonization of newborns, *Am J Dis Child*, **105**: 646–54.

Shooter RA, Griffiths JD et al., 1957, Outbreak of staphylococcal infection in a surgical ward, *Br Med J*, **1**: 433–6.

Shooter RA, Smith MA et al., 1958, Spread of staphylococci in a surgical ward, *Br Med J*, **1**: 607–13.

Shuttleworth R, Colby WD, 1992, *Staphylococcus lugdunensis* endocarditis, *J Clin Microbiol*, **30**: 1948–52.

Singh G, Marples RR, Kligman AM, 1971, Experimental *Staphylococcus aureus* infection in humans, *J Invest Dermatol*, **57**: 149–52.

Smith EW, Goshi K et al., 1963, Studies on the pathogenesis of staphylococcal infection. VIII. The human cutaneous reaction to injection of alpha hemolysin, *Bull Johns Hopkins Hosp*, **113**: 247–60.

Solberg CO, 1965, A study of carriers of *Staphylococcus aureus*, *Acta Med Scand*, **178, Suppl. I**: 1–96.

Sosin DM, Gunn RA et al., 1989, An outbreak of furunculosis among high school athletes, *Am J Sports Med*, **17**: 828–32.

Souto MJ, Ferreiros CM, Criado MT, 1991, Failure of phenotypic characteristics to distinguish between carrier and invasive isolates of *Staphylococcus epidermidis*, *J Hosp Infect*, **17**: 107–15.

Spencer RC, 1988, Infections in continuous ambulatory peritoneal dialysis, *J Med Microbiol*, **27**: 1–9.

Steele RW, 1980, Recurrent staphylococcal infection in families, *Arch Dermatol*, **116**: 189–90.

Stobberingh EE, Winkler KC, 1977, Restriction-deficient mutants of *Staphylococcus aureus*, *J Gen Microbiol*, **99**: 359–67.

Surani S, Chaudna H, Weinstein RA, 1993, Breast abscess: coagulase-negative staphylococcus as sole pathogen, *Clin Infect Dis*, **17**: 701–4.

Switalski LM, Patti JM et al., 1993, A collagen receptor on *Staphylococcus aureus* strains isolated from patients with septic arthritis mediates adherence to cartilage, *Mol Microbiol*, **7**: 99–107.

Tabbarah ZA, Kohler RB et al., 1979, Inhibitory effect of heat-labile serum factors on detection of staphylococcal, pseudomonas, and hepatitis B surface antigens by solid-phase radioimmunoassay, *J Infect Dis*, **140**: 822–5.

Tanner EI, Bullin J et al., 1980, An outbreak of post-operative sepsis due to a staphylococcal disperser, *J Hyg Camb*, **85**: 219–25.

Taylor AG, Fincham WJ, Cook J, 1976, Staphylococcal antibodies in osteomyelitis: the use of anti-staphylococcal nuclease levels in diagnosis, *Zentralbl Bakteriol Parasitenkd Infektionskr Hyg Abt 1*, **Suppl. 5**: 911–16.

Taylor AG, Cook J et al., 1975, Serological tests in the differentiation of staphylococcal and tuberculous bone disease, *J Clin Pathol*, **28**: 284–8.

Tierno PM Jr, Hanna B, 1989, Ecology of toxic shock syndrome: amplification of toxic shock toxin-1 by materials of medical interest, *Rev Infect Dis*, **11, Suppl. 1**: S182–6.

Todd J, Fishaut M et al., 1978, Toxic-shock syndrome associated with phage-group-I staphylococci, *Lancet*, **2**: 1116–18.

Tuazon CU, Cardella TA, Sheagren JN, 1975, Staphylococcal endocarditis in drug users. Clinical and microbiologic aspects, *Arch Intern Med*, **135**: 1555–61.

Valle J, Vadillo S et al., 1991, Toxic shock syndrome toxin (TSST-1) production by staphylococci isolated from goats and presence of specific antibodies to TSST-1 in serum and milk, *Appl Environ Microbiol*, **57**: 889–91.

Vandenesch F, Etienne F et al., 1993, Endocarditis due to *Staphylococcus lugdunensis*: report of 11 cases and review, *Clin Infect Dis*, **17**: 871–6.

Verbrugh HA, Peterson PK et al., 1981, Human fibronectin binding to staphylococcal surface protein and its relative inefficiency in promoting phagocytosis by human polymorphonuclear leukocytes, monocytes, and alveolar macrophages, *Infect Immun*, **1981**: 811–19.

Verbrugh HA, Keane WF et al., 1984, Bacterial growth and killing in chronic ambulatory peritoneal dialysis, *J Clin Microbiol*, **20**: 199–203.

Vergeront JM, Stolz SJ et al., 1983, Prevalence of serum antibody to staphylococcal enterotoxin F among Wisconsin residents: implications for toxic-shock syndrome, *J Infect Dis*, **148**: 692–8.

Wadström T, 1987, Molecular aspects on pathogenesis of wound and foreign body infections due to staphylococci, *Zentralbl Bakteriol Mikrobiol Hyg [A]*, **266**: 191–211.

Waghorn DJ, 1994, *Staphylococcus lugdunensis* as a cause of breast abscess, *Clin Infect Dis*, **19**: 814–15.

van Wamel WJB, Fluit AC et al., 1995, Phenotypic characterization of epidemic versus sporadic strains of methicillin-resistant *Staphylococcus aureus*, *J Clin Pathol*, **33**: 1769–74.

Ward TT, 1992, Comparison of in vitro adherence of methicillin-sensitive and methicillin-resistant *Staphylococcus aureus* to human nasal epithelial cells, *J Infect Dis*, **166**: 400–4.

Webster KA, Mitchell GB, 1989, Experimental production of tick pyaemia, *Vet Parasitol*, **34**: 129–33.

Weijmer MC, Neering H, Welten C, 1990, Preliminary report: furunculosis and hypoferraemia, *Lancet*, **336**: 464–6.

Weinblatt ME, Sahdev I, Berman M, 1990, *Stomatococcus mucilaginosus* infections in children with leukemia, *Pediatr Infect Dis J*, **9**: 678–9.

Weinke T, Schiller R et al., 1992, Association between *Staphylococcus aureus* nasopharyngeal colonization and septicemia in patients infected with the human immunodeficiency virus, *Eur J Clin Microbiol Infect Dis*, **11**: 985–9.

Weksler BB, Hill MJ, 1969, Inhibition of leukocyte migration by a staphylococcal factor, *J Bacteriol*, **98**: 1030–5.

Wergeland HI, Haaheim LR et al., 1989, Antibodies to staphylococcal peptidoglycan and its peptide epitopes, teichoic acid, and lipoteichoic acid in sera from blood donors and patients with staphylococcal infections, *J Clin Microbiol*, **27**: 1286–91.

Westblom TU, Gorse GJ et al., 1990, Anaerobic endocarditis caused by *Staphylococcus saccharolyticus*, *J Clin Microbiol*, **28**: 2818–19.

Wheat LJ, Kohler RB et al., 1979, Circulating staphylococcal antigen in humans and immune rabbits with endocarditis due to *Staphylococcus aureus*: inhibition of detection by preexisting antibodies, *J Infect Dis*, **140**: 54–61.

White MI, Noble WC, 1985, The cutaneous reaction to staphylococcal protein A in normal subjects and patients with atopic dermatitis or psoriasis, *Br J Dermatol*, **113**: 179–83.

Whitener C, Caputo GM et al., 1993, Endocarditis due to coagulase-negative staphylococci: microbiologic, epidemiologic, and clinical considerations, *Infect Dis Clin North Am*, **7**: 81–96.

Whyte W, Vesley D, Hodgson R, 1976, Bacterial dispersion in relation to operating room clothing, *J Hyg Camb*, **76**: 367–78.

Wieneke AA, Roberts D, Gilbert RJ, 1993, Staphylococcal food poisoning in the United Kingdom 1969–90, *Epidemiol Infect*, **110**: 519–31.

Williams REO, 1963, Healthy carriage of *Staphylococcus aureus*: its prevalence and importance, *Bacteriol Rev*, **27**: 56–71.

Williams REO, 1971, Changing perspectives in hospital infection, *Proceedings of the International Conference on Nosocomial Infections*, eds Brachman PS, Eickhoff TC, American Hospitals Association, Chicago, 1–10.

Williams REO, Miles AA, 1949, *Infection and Sepsis in Industrial Wounds of the Hand*, Medical Research Council Special Report Series, No. 262, Medican Research Council, London, 1–87.

Williams REO, Jevons MP et al., 1959, Nasal staphylococci and sepsis in surgical patients, *Br Med J*, **2**: 658–62.

Williams REO, Blowers R et al., 1966, *Hospital Infection: Causes and Prevention*, 2nd edn, Lloyd-Luke, London.

Williams RE, Doherty VR et al., 1992, *Staphylococcus aureus* and intranasal mupirocin in patients receiving isotretinoin for acne, *Br J Dermatol*, **126:** 362–6.

Wilson GS, 1967, *The Hazards of Immunization*, Athlone Press, London, 75–88.

Wilson PE, White PM, Noble WC, 1971, Infections in a hospital for patients with diseases of the skin, *J Hyg Camb*, **69:** 125–32.

Wolinsky E, Lipsitz PJ et al., 1960, Acquisition of staphylococci by newborns. Direct versus indirect transmission, *Lancet*, **2:** 620–2.

Wu SX, Liu YX, 1994, Molecular epidemiologic study of burn wound infection caused by *Staphylococcus aureus* in children, *Chin Med J*, **107:** 570–3.

Wu S, Shen L, 1993, Plasmid analysis and phage typing in the study of staphylococcal colonization and disease in newborn infants, *Chin Med Sci J*, **8:** 157–61.

Xu S, Arbeit RD, Lee JC, 1992, Phagocytic killing of encapsulated and microencapsulated *Staphylococcus aureus* by human polymorphonuclear leukocytes, *Infect Immun*, **60:** 1358–62.

Yocum MW, Strong DM et al., 1976, Selective immunoglobulin M (IgM) deficiency in two immunodeficient adults with recurrent staphylococcal pyoderma, *Am J Med*, **60:** 486–94.

Younger JJ, Christensen GD et al., 1987, Coagulase negative staphylococci isolated from cerebrospinal fluid shunts: importance of slime production, species identification, and shunt removal to clinical outcome, *J Infect Dis*, **156:** 548–54.

Chapter 15

STREPTOCOCCAL DISEASES

K L Ruoff

1 INTRODUCTION

An association between streptococci and various infections was first noted in the late nineteenth century. Chain-forming cocci were described by Billroth, Pasteur and Rosenbach, who in 1884 originated the name *Streptococcus pyogenes*. In 1919 Brown described the varying haemolytic reactions of streptococci, allowing for differentiation of these organisms. Strains capable of lysing red blood cells (β-haemolytic streptococci) were the focus of most twentieth century streptococcal research and are the organisms examined in this chapter. Beginning in the late 1920s, Lancefield developed a serological system for subdividing the β-haemolytic streptococci into groups based on polysaccharide antigens and into types within a given group on the basis of protein antigens (M and T proteins). Lancefield's system greatly facilitated studies of the aetiology and epidemiology of streptococcal diseases.

The 'pyogenic' streptococci of Lancefield's serological group A (*S. pyogenes*) were eventually linked to a host of serious infections as well as to diseases that occurred as sequelae to pyogenic infection (acute rheumatic fever, acute glomerulonephritis). During the twentieth century the incidence of serious disease due to *S. pyogenes* began declining in certain areas even before the antibiotic era. This trend toward seemingly less virulent strains continued until the 1980s, when we began to see a reappearance of highly virulent streptococci capable of causing severe pyogenic infections, sometimes accompanied by a toxic shock-like syndrome, and 'rheumatogenic' strains associated with outbreaks of rheumatic fever (Denny

1994). During the last half of the twentieth century β-haemolytic streptococci of other serological groups (B, C, G) have also been recognized as agents of serious infection. Information on the habitats and diseases caused by these streptococci in humans is summarized in Table 15.1.

2 DISEASES CAUSED BY *STREPTOCOCCUS PYOGENES* (GROUP A STREPTOCOCCI)

2.1 Pharyngitis and infections of the respiratory tract

Streptococcal pharyngitis is characterized by pain, redness and swelling of the posterior pharynx, accompanied by greyish white tonsillar exudate, tenderness of the anterior cervical lymph nodes, fever and general malaise. *S. pyogenes* may also cause less severe forms of pharyngitis without constitutional symptoms. While streptococcal pharyngitis can affect any age group, it is a common infection of school-aged children, usually spread from person to person via respiratory or saliva droplets.

Although pharyngitis caused by *S. pyogenes* is normally self-limiting, its possible suppurative complications include infections of the upper and lower respiratory tracts, such as peritonsillar and retropharyngeal abscess, acute sinusitis, acute otitis media, cervical lymphadenitis and pneumonia. Many of these complications are caused by spread of streptococci from the throat, but the majority of *S. pyogenes* pneu-

Table 15.1 β-Haemolytic streptococci causing infections in humans

Streptococcus	Lancefield group	Sites of colonization	Diseases
S. pyogenes	A	Throat Nose Skin Rectum	Pharyngitis Respiratory infection Rheumatic fever Glomerulonephritis Skin and soft tissue infection
S. agalactiae	B	Genital tract Gastrointestinal tract Throat Skin	Neonatal infection Urogenital infection Endocarditis Skin and soft tissue infection
Group C and G (large colony-forming strains)[a]	C or G	Throat Gastrointestinal tract Genital tract Skin	Pharyngitis Respiratory infection Glomerulonephritis Endocarditis Skin and soft tissue infection
Small colony-forming 'S. milleri' group strains	A, C, F, G	Oral cavity Respiratory tract Gastrointestinal tract	Oral infections Abscess or purulent infection

[a]Group C strains are traditionally differentiated into the species *S. equi, S. equisimilis, S. zooepidemicus* and *S. dysgalactiae.*

monias are associated with chronic repiratory disease or are preceded by viral respiratory infections rather than streptococcal pharyngitis (Bisno 1995a).

Streptococcal M protein plays a central role in the pathogenesis by virtue of its antiphagocytic properties. Fibrinogen binds to streptococci expressing M protein and blocks complement deposition on the bacterial cell surface (Chhatwal, Dutra and Blobel 1985). M protein also binds factor H, a complement control protein. The net effect is inhibition of opsonization by the alternative complement pathway. M protein is a major virulence factor; streptococcal strains lacking this protein are avirulent and host antibody to a given M protein type confers protective immunity. M protein types are determined by regions of the molecule that display variation in amino acid sequence. These regions are oriented towards the outer surface of the cell, while the conserved regions of the filamentous M protein molecule are anchored in the cell membrane. Over 100 immunologically distinct M protein types have been discerned, allowing for strain typing of group A streptococci (Robinson and Kehoe 1992). Additional antiphagocytic factors possessed by *S. pyogenes* include its hyaluronic acid capsule and a C5a peptidase which inactivates C5a, a chemotactic factor generated in the complement cascade (Whitnack 1993).

Colonization of mucosal surfaces by group A streptococci is a prerequisite for infection and is mediated by bacterial cell surface fibrils composed of lipoteichoic acid and M protein. Complexes between the glycerolphosphate backbone of lipoteichoic acid and M protein are thought to allow for orientation of the lipid moieties of lipoteichoic acid towards the surface of the bacterial cell. The lipid portion of the lipoteichoic acid molecules can then interact with hydrophobic regions of fibronectin coating host cells, facilitating adherence of the bacteria (Beachey and Courtney 1987). Studies with M protein-positive and negative isogenic strains have suggested, however, that M proteins do not play a direct role in adherence (Robinson and Kehoe 1992). A streptococcal fibronectin-binding protein (protein F) has also been identified (Hanski and Caparon 1992) and the studies of Natanson and coworkers (1995) have demonstrated a correlation between the presence of this protein and M type, suggesting a relationship between fibronectin-binding ability and virulence.

Hasty and coworkers (1992) reviewed mechanisms of streptococcal adhesion and noted that the use of different target substrata in in vitro studies of adherence generated different conclusions concerning the streptococcal molecules involved in this phenomenon. These included lipoteichoic acid, fibronectin-binding protein, M protein, vitronectin-binding protein and the C carbohydrate (group-specific antigen). These authors advocated a 2-step adhesion model for *S. pyogenes* in which the initial step is somewhat non-specific, consisting of a weak hydrophobic interaction mediated by a hydrophobic moiety such as lipoteichoic acid. Once this initial weak adherence occurs, additional specific streptococcal adhesins (M protein, fibronectin-binding protein, etc.) can react with receptors on the target cells. Possession of different specific secondary adhesins could explain the observation that streptococcal isolates from pharyngitis bind better in in vitro assays to buccal cells while streptococci isolated from cutaneous infections bind more effectively to skin cells.

Some group A streptococci produce an α-lipoproteinase capable of opacifying horse serum. Production of this serum opacity factor is associated with strains producing one of the 2 major classes of M protein (Fischetti 1989). Pharyngeal infection with serum opacity factor-positive isolates is characterized by reduced immune response to streptococcal M protein (Bisno 1995a).

The haemolysins produced by *S. pyogenes* are capable of lysing many kinds of cells in addition to erythrocytes. Two distinct haemolysins, streptolysins O and S, have been identified. Streptolysin O is oxygen-labile and antigenic whereas host antibodies to the oxygen-stable streptolysin S have not been detected. Subsurface growth of *S. pyogenes* strains in blood-containing media displays stronger haemolysis than surface growth due to the functioning of both haemolysins in the absence of oxygen.

Group A streptococci manufacture other products that are assumed to contribute to pathogenicity. Factors that could facilitate the spread of infection through tissue include hyaluronidase (capable of destroying the hyaluronic acid in the ground substance of host tissues), DNAases and streptokinase, which facilitates the destruction of clots. NADase is another extracellular streptococcal enzyme that could contribute to virulence. A number of these streptococcal products are antigenic and host response to them can be used to assess previous streptococcal infection (see section 8, p. 267). IgG Fc receptors may also contribute to pathogenicity (Lebrun et al. 1982).

Streptococcal pyrogenic exotoxins, also referred to as erythrogenic toxins, are important virulence factors in streptococcal infections and are discussed in sections 2.2 and 2.4, pp. 259 and 262.

EPIDEMIOLOGY OF PHARYNGITIS AND RESPIRATORY INFECTIONS

Group A streptococci are usually transmitted from person to person, via respiratory or saliva droplets, although epidemics of streptococcal pharyngitis caused by contaminated food or drink have also been documented. Widespread pasteurization has greatly reduced reports of infection by contaminated milk. Contamination of food with infected respiratory secretions are thought to be the most common cause of foodborne streptococcal infection, but skin infections of those handling food may also be the ultimate source of contamination (Farley et al. 1993b). Streptococci present on clothing, bedding or in dust do not seem to contribute to the spread of pharyngitis. Crowded conditions occurring in schools, military barracks and in indoor environments in cold weather favour the spread of streptococci.

Antibiotic treatment rapidly reduces the streptococcal burden in the nares and throat whereas untreated patients may harbour a slowly decreasing number of streptococci for weeks after the resolution of acute infection. Carriage rates in healthy children are usually higher than those in adults and have been estimated at 15–20%, varying with the locale and the season. In a survey of group A streptococci collected in the United States during 1988–1990, M serotypes 1, 2, 4 and 12 were the most commonly isolated strains from uncomplicated pharyngitis (Johnson, Stevens and Kaplan 1992).

2.2 Scarlet fever

Scarlet fever occurs when pharyngitis or other types of streptococcal infection is caused by a pyrogenic (erythrogenic) toxin-producing strain. The genetic information specifying production of scarlet fever toxin is provided to the streptococcal strain by a lysogenic bacteriophage (Zabriskie 1964). While the clinical course of the infection is similar to that caused by non-toxigenic strains, infection with toxin-producing *S. pyogenes* is distinguished by development of a red rash that usually starts on the upper chest and then spreads to other body areas. If antitoxin is injected intradermally, blanching of the rash is observed (Schultz–Charlton reaction). Immunity to the toxin in previously infected patients can be demonstrated by the development of erythema surrounding the site of intracutaneous injection of the toxin (the Dick test). Neither of the aforementioned methods is in current clinical use (Bisno 1995a). Severe forms of scarlet fever (malignant scarlet fever, toxic scarlet fever) may be life threatening and are characterized by invasive extension of infection from the pharynx, extremely high fever, bacteraemia and shock (Stevens 1992).

EPIDEMIOLOGY OF SCARLET FEVER

The occurrence of scarlet fever cases should logically parallel the dissemination of pharyngitis-associated, toxin-producing *S. pyogenes* strains. Dramatic rises and falls in the incidence of this disease have been documented. The number of severe cases of scarlet fever in England and Wales peaked in the late nineteenth century, but by 1900 the mean annual death rate from scarlet fever among children less than 15 years of age had dropped to less than 500 from a high of close to 2500 approximately 30 years previously (Kass 1971). This occurred, of course, without the benefit of antibiotic treatment to control streptococcal pharyngitis. Musser and colleagues (1993b) analysed strains isolated from temporally and geographically separated epidemics of scarlet fever, using multilocus enzyme electrophoresis and comparative sequencing of the streptococcal pyrogenic exotoxin A (the scarlet fever toxin) gene. Their observations led them to suggest that epidemics of scarlet fever are associated with an increased incidence of streptococcal clones displaying allelic variation in their scarlet fever toxin genes. This genetic variety may enhance the ability of a strain to overcome herd immunity against heterologous toxin allelic variants. Streptococcal pyrogenic toxins are discussed in more detail in section 2.4 (p. 262).

2.3 Acute rheumatic fever and acute glomerulonephritis

While the pathogenesis of the non-suppurative sequelae of streptococcal infection is still not completely understood, the deleterious effects of these diseases on the health and wellbeing of their sufferers have been well documented. In the late nineteenth century Walter Butler Cheadle, a London paediatrician, defined rheumatic fever as a disease entity, in spite of its varied manifestations. By the 1930s the association between *S. pyogenes* and rheumatic fever had been established by Collis in the UK and Coburn in the USA. Rheumatic fever persisted as an important disease through the first half of the twentieth century and then seemed to recede in developed countries and temperate climates (in the United States and western Europe). Its incidence during the second half of the twentieth century seemed to increase, however, in developing countries in tropical areas (Stollerman 1990). The widespread use of penicillin for the control of group A pharyngitis was thought to be responsible for dramatically diminishing the incidence of acute rheumatic fever in the United States, but a trend towards decreasing incidence of the disease was seen even before the antibiotic era. Despite the widespread availability of antibiotics, an increase in the incidence of rheumatic fever was noted in the 1980s in the USA (Massell et al. 1988).

Acute rheumatic fever and acute glomerulonephritis occur as non-suppurative sequelae of infection by *S. pyogenes*. Rheumatic fever may follow streptococcal pharyngitis but not cutaneous infection, whereas glomerulonephritis is preceded by either skin or throat infection. Attack rates of acute rheumatic fever among sufferers of streptococcal pharyngitis have been documented to range from less than 0.5% to 3% (Wannamaker 1979). The concept of 'rheumatogenic' and 'nephritogenic' strains of streptococci is supported by the association of different M serotypes with rheumatic fever, glomerulonephritis following pharyngitis and glomerulonephritis following cutaneous infection. Rheumatogenic strains usually lack the ability to produce serum opacity factor and often produce copious capsular material that leads to the formation of colonies with a mucoid appearance. In spite of evidence supporting the existence of *S. pyogenes* strains with enhanced propensity to cause either rheumatic fever or glomerulonephritis, no bacterial virulence factor has been shown to be solely responsible for these diseases.

Rheumatic fever is an acute self-limiting illness characterized by inflammatory lesions of the heart, joints, subcutaneous tissues and central nervous system. Pathological findings include Aschoff's nodules, which when observed in cardiac tissue display a rosette of giant multinuclear and large mononuclear cells surrounding a central area of necrosis. Damage to heart valves may occur as a result of acute rheumatic fever

and this damage may persist or progress, leading to cardiac failure years after the initial attack. Since the clinical symptoms of rheumatic fever are diverse and can mimic those of other diseases, diagnosis is based on clinical symptoms and documentation of antecedent (within 1–5 weeks prior to the onset of rheumatic fever) pharyngeal infection by *S. pyogenes*. Serological tests are often employed to document previous streptococcal infection (see section 8, p. 267). The clinical criteria for the diagnosis of rheumatic fever were summarized by Jones and updated by the American Heart Association (Denny 1994). These modified 'Jones criteria' appear in Table 15.2 and encompass the major and minor manifestations of acute rheumatic fever and acceptable methods for documenting preceding streptococcal infection (Bisno 1995b).

Theories to explain the pathogenesis of rheumatic fever have focused on tissue damage caused by streptococcal products (i.e. streptolysins), or antigen–antibody complexes (as in serum sickness). A more recently embraced theory of rheumatic fever pathogenesis incorporates the concepts of molecular mimicry and autoimmunity. Various streptococcal cellular components have been shown to mimic the structure of molecules found in human tissue; antibodies directed against streptococcal products are thought to cross-react with host tissue, producing autoimmune damage. Similarities in structure and subsequent serological cross-reactivity of streptococcal cell constituents (M protein, membrane antigens, group carbohydrate) with human heart, skin, joint and brain tissues has been demonstrated. Patients exhibiting rheumatic fever are found to harbour antibodies that cross-react with both streptococcal products and human tissue components.

Although cross-reacting host antibodies could explain some of the pathogenesis of rheumatic fever, other factors relating to the host's immune system and genetic predisposition towards the development of rheumatic fever appear to play a role in this disease. Acute rheumatic fever is usually a relatively rare complication of streptococcal pharyngitis, often occurs in more than one member of a family and tends to recur in a given individual. Studies aimed at establishing a link between certain major histocompatibility complex (MHC) antigens and a predisposition for rheumatic fever have been either inconclusive or only suggestive of an association. However, certain B cell alloantigens have been found to be more prevalent in rheumatic

Table 15.2 Updated (1992) Jones criteria for diagnosis of acute rheumatic fever

Manifestations		Documentation of previous group A infection
Major	**Minor**	
Carditis	Arthralgia	Positive culture or streptococcal antigen test
Polyarthritis	Fever	
Chorea	Elevated erythrocyte sedimentation rate	Serological tests: elevated or rising titres of streptococcal antibodies
Erythema marginatum	Elevated C-reactive protein	
Subcutaneous nodules	Prolonged P–R interval	

Adapted from Denny 1994.

fever patients than in the general population, lending support to the concept of a genetic predisposition to the disease (Froude et al. 1989).

Acute glomerulonephritis may follow either pharyngitis or cutaneous streptococcal infection. Clinical symptoms include pallor, oedema, hypertension and hypoalbuminaemia. Urinalysis reveals elevated levels of protein, leucocytes and red blood cells; the urine may have a 'rusty' or 'smoky' appearance. The severity of acute glomerulonephritis can range from subclinical to extremely serious, resulting in renal failure (Whitnack 1993).

As with rheumatic fever, the pathogenesis of acute glomerulonephritis is incompletely understood. Renal biopsy specimens from glomerulonephritis patients reveal 'humps' on the epithelial side of the glomerular basement membrane. These deposits are composed of IgG and complement and are thought to represent immune complex deposits that cause an inflammatory response. The principle of molecular mimicry is again illustrated by cross-reaction with human glomeruli of antibodies raised against streptococcal membrane fractions. Common antigenic determinants have also been noted in renal glomeruli and streptococcal M protein (Froude 1989).

During the initial stages of acute glomerulonephritis a protein named endostreptosin can be detected beneath the glomerular basement membrane. This antigen reacts with antibodies produced by patients with glomerulonephritis (Lange et al. 1976). Nephritogenic streptococci harbour protein antigens that may be identical to the endostreptosin found in glomeruli (Johnson and Zabriskie 1986, Yoshizawa et al. 1992).

EPIDEMIOLOGY OF ACUTE RHEUMATIC FEVER AND ACUTE GLOMERULONEPHRITIS

Since the development of acute rheumatic fever and acute glomerulonephritis is directly linked to antecedent streptococcal infection, the epidemiology of most cases of these diseases is similar to that of streptococcal pharyngitis. The variables in the development of rheumatic fever and glomerulonephritis are, as mentioned above, the 'rheumatogenicity' or 'nephritogenicity' of the streptococcal strain and an apparent predisposition of the host to suffer these sequelae. Acute rheumatic fever is most common in school-aged children and also occurs typically in people living in crowded situations (military barracks, areas of poverty). The incidence of rheumatic fever during the second half of the twentieth century decreased dramatically in the USA and western Europe (especially during the 1960s and 1970s) but showed no signs of declining in certain developing areas of the world (parts of Africa, South America, the Middle East and India). Surveys performed in the 1970s indicated incidences of rheumatic heart disease in schoolchildren ranging from 1.2 to 21 per 1000 in severely affected areas compared to an incidence of 0.1 per 1000 in the USA.

A resurgence of rheumatic fever occurred in the USA in the mid-1980s. Clusters of disease were noted among schoolchildren and in military camps. One notable feature of the civilian outbreaks was their occurrence in middle class families as opposed to families living in overcrowded, poverty-stricken conditions. Outbreak-associated *S. pyogenes* strains were found to belong to M types that had previously been associated with acute rheumatic fever (1, 3, 5, 6, 18). There was a notable association of highly encapsulated, mucoid M type 18 strains and rheumatic fever cases (Stollerman 1990).

Acute glomerulonephritis displays a relatively high attack rate of 10–15% of individuals infected with a nephritogenic strain. Unlike rheumatic fever, recurrences are rare, but the occurrence of multiple cases within families is common. Although there are some common characteristics of acute glomerulonephritis preceded by either pharyngeal or cutaneous streptococcal infection, some of the epidemiological aspects of this disease are linked to the type of streptococcal infection that preceded it. Wannamaker (1970) noted that pharyngitis-associated glomerulonephritis was more likely to affect early school-aged children in the winter and spring months. The latent period preceding illness was 10 days and the incidence among male children was twice that observed in female children. Acute glomerulonephritis associated with skin infections (pyoderma) was more frequent in preschool-aged children, displayed a longer latent period (3 weeks), was more common in the late summer and early autumn and was more frequent in warmer climates. Equal numbers of male and female children were affected. Different serotypes of group A streptococci are responsible for pharyngitis-associated and cutaneous infection-associated glomerulonephritis. Although the incidence of rheumatic fever seemed to increase in the USA during the 1980s, a decline in acute glomerulonephritis cases severe enough to warrant hospital admission was reported in at least one location in the USA (Roy and Stapleton 1990) and in Singapore (Yap, Chia and Murugasu 1990).

Much valuable data on the epidemiology, treatment and prevention of streptococcal pharyngitis and its non-suppurative sequelae were gathered from a 'captive audience' composed of members of the US military during the 1940s and 1950s. Lowell Rantz (1958) called attention to the magnitude of the rheumatic fever problem during World War II in certain military installations in the USA, noting an incidence of 49.9 cases per 1000 at Fort Warren in Wyoming. Data assembled by the Streptococcal Disease Laboratory, established in 1949 at Warren Air Force Base, document a rheumatic fever attack rate of 3–4 per 1000 during the first 3 years of operation of the laboratory. Studies conducted by the Streptococcal Disease Laboratory demonstrated that rheumatic fever could be prevented by penicillin treatment of streptococcal pharyngitis within 9 days of the onset of infection and that a 10 day course of treatment was more effective than treatment lasting 5 days. The staff of the Streptococcal Disease Laboratory at Warren Air Force Base included Rammelkamp (the Laboratory Director), Wannamaker, Denny, Dingle, Brink, Houser, Hahn, Stetson and Kasper, some of the foremost streptococcal researchers of their day. Their other accomplishments included the evaluation of antibiotics other than penicillin for the treatment of streptococcal pharyngitis; studies on the effects of anti-inflammatory agents on the course of rheumatic fever; the demonstration that close contact, but not fomites, enhanced streptococcal spread; the demonstration of enhanced infectiousness of epidemic strains of *S. pyogenes*; research suggesting that streptococcal immunity was due to anti-M protein antibodies; and the demonstration of nephritogenicity in type 12 strains of *S. pyogenes* (Denny 1994).

2.4 Skin and soft tissue infections caused by *S. pyogenes*

Streptococcal infections of the skin and soft tissues can range from mild and self-limiting to life threatening. The specific infections considered here include impetigo (pyoderma), erysipelas, cellulitis and necrotizing fasciitis. While some streptococcal skin infections are thought to be primary infections, initiated by streptococci colonizing intact skin, others are considered secondary infections of traumatized skin, including surgical wounds and burns. Surgical wound infections are infrequently caused by *S. pyogenes*, but such infections can be extremely serious and are usually associated with transmission via a streptococcal carrier. Health care personnel cultured during outbreaks of surgical wound infections have been found to carry group A streptococci in the upper respiratory tract, rectum and vagina and one report documents carriage and subsequent dissemination from psoriatic lesions on the scalp of an operating room technician (Mastro et al. 1990).

Impetigo

Streptococcal impetigo is characterized by superficial skin lesions, usually less than 2.5 cm (1 inch) in diameter, that resolve spontaneously within 1–2 weeks of the initial appearance. The lesion evolves from a papule to a small vesicle surrounded by a zone of erythema. The vesicles turn into pustules that eventually develop a thick crust. In streptococcal ecthyma, a more severe form of impetigo, the lesions are ulcerated, often with raised oedematous edges. The lesions of staphylococcal impetigo are distinguished from those of streptococcal disease in that they begin as large vesicles or bullae that develop a thin crust after rupture.

Ferrieri and colleagues (1972) studied patients with streptococcal impetigo at the Red Lake Indian Reservation in the USA. They found that streptococci can produce lesions within 10 days of colonization of the skin. Lesions are thought to arise when colonizing organisms are introduced into broken skin via minor trauma or insect bites. These authors also demonstrated transfer of streptococci colonizing the skin to the nose and throat, within 14 and 20 days, respectively, of initial skin colonization. While impetigo occurred regularly during the summer months in the population studied, acute glomerulonephritis outbreaks occurred only when nephritogenic strains were prevalent as agents of impetigo (Ferrieri et al. 1970).

Epidemiology of impetigo

Although impetigo is often associated with warm, humid climates, it also occurs in northern areas, typically in the summer season. Preschool-aged children, prison inmates, residents of mental institutions and workers who handle raw meat have been among the groups in whom streptococcal impetigo has been documented. Poor hygiene seems to be a predisposing factor. Transmission of impetigo is not completely understood. Direct contact or transfer of streptococci via environmental agents or insect vectors are possible mechanisms of transmission.

Impetigo is associated with restricted M types of *S. pyogenes*, different from those that normally colonize the pharynx. Although pharyngitis-associated M types are rarely isolated from streptococcal skin infection, strains that normally cause impetigo can frequently be found as throat colonizers. These strains rarely cause symptoms of pharyngitis and can account for the majority of throat-colonizing strains in areas where streptococcal skin infection is common (Anthony et al. 1976). Skin-colonizing *S. pyogenes* strains display great variety in their M types and some strains have been observed to lose detectable M protein after repeated subculture on artificial media. Consequently, T protein antigens have been used to type these organisms. The T typing system has, however, proven inadequate, since strains may produce antigens that react with more than one T typing antiserum and these T reaction patterns are not specific for a given M type (Johnson and Kaplan 1993).

Erysipelas

Group A streptococci can cause an acute, spreading inflammation of the skin, often on the face, known as erysipelas. Erysipelas most often occurs in adults and infants and is seen more frequently in the winter months in temperate climates. The inflammatory lesion is erythematous, swollen, limited by a well demarcated edge and may be accompanied by clinical symptoms of fever and chills. Erysipelas may be preceded by streptococcal infection of the upper respiratory tract or infection of broken skin, but in many cases the aetiology is unknown. Lesions usually resolve spontaneously within a few days to 2 weeks, but repeated attacks in the same patient, often on the same area of the skin, are not uncommon.

Isolation of streptococci from erysipelas lesions is difficult and it has been hypothesized that this condition may be caused by a toxin, or by hypersensitivity to some streptococcal component. Norrby and colleagues (1992) studied group A strains isolated from cases of erysipelas and found a predominance of serotype T1M1. They noted only low-level production of erythrogenic toxin A, but high-level production of erythrogenic toxins B and C in the majority of strains (see 'Severe streptococcal infection accompanied by toxic shock syndrome', p. 263, for more information on these toxins). These workers also observed a higher frequency of polymorphism in the *emm* gene (responsible for M protein) among erysipelas strains than among a group of isolates from cases of bacteraemia.

CELLULITIS

Streptococcal cellulitis can occur when organisms gain access to broken skin; it is characterized by pain, swelling and redness of the skin. These localized symptoms may be accompanied by fever, chills, lymphangitis and bacteraemia. In contrast to erysipelas lesions, streptococcal cellulitis lesions are neither raised nor clearly demarcated. Injecting drug users and those with impaired lymphatic drainage in the extremities are predisposed to the development of this infection (Bisno 1995a).

NECROTIZING FASCIITIS

Necrotizing fasciitis is the term used currently to describe the invasive soft tissue infection originally referred to by Meleney as 'streptococcal gangrene' (Meleney 1924). This infection may be caused by bacteria other than group A streptococci (e.g. clostridia, staphylococci), by mixtures of different bacteria, or by *S. pyogenes* alone. Infection is initiated after trauma that may be minor or even inapparent. During the first 24 h after introduction of the streptococci into the subcutaneous tissues mild erythema may be the only symptom, but more often swelling and tenderness develop and spread outward from the initial lesion. Within 24–48 h the erythema darkens to a purplish then blue hue and bullae appear. By the fourth or fifth day the affected area becomes gangrenous and within 7–10 days after infection the edges of the lesion become sharply demarcated and the skin breaks down to expose severe necrosis of the subcutaneous tissues. The infection is accompanied by constitutional symptoms of fever and prostration. Metastatic abscesses may also develop (Stevens 1992). In severe, rapidly progressing forms of this infection treatment must be initiated early in the infection and usually involves extensive surgical debridement of infected tissue in order to prevent a fatal outcome.

SEVERE STREPTOCOCCAL INFECTION ACCOMPANIED BY TOXIC SHOCK SYNDROME

In the late 1980s rheumatic fever was joined by severe invasive streptococcal infection, usually in soft tissues, as a resurgent disease. Although both these entities were well known in the early twentieth century, their frequencies had decreased until the occurrence of recent cases. Invasive soft tissue infection accompanied by a toxic shock-like syndrome has been described in North America, Europe and Australia (Cone et al. 1987, Stevens et al. 1989, Chomarat 1990, Cherchi et al. 1992, Stevens 1992, Demers et al. 1993, Donaldson et al. 1993). These infections have occurred typically in otherwise healthy adults, although cases have also been reported in children (Belani et al. 1991, Jackson, Burry and Olson 1991).

Infections accompanied by streptococcal toxic shock syndrome often begin with skin wounds or minor non-penetrating traumas evidenced by bruising or haematoma. The site of infection becomes intensely painful, usually within 24–72 h of the initial trauma; common additional symptoms include fever, tachycardia and hypotension. Soft tissue infection can proceed to necrotizing fasciitis or myositis, requiring extensive surgical debridement. Shock, renal failure and acute respiratory distress syndrome (ARDS) are complications of severe invasive infections caused by *S. pyogenes*. In spite of appropriate and timely treatment, approximately 30% of severe group A streptococcal infections accompanied by toxic shock have been fatal (Stevens 1992).

Attempts at understanding the virulence factors of *S. pyogenes* strains capable of these rapid and devastating infections have focused on streptococcal pyrogenic exotoxins (SPEs), of which 3 immunologically distinct types (SPEA, SPEB, SPEC) have been identified. These toxins are responsible for the rash of scarlet fever, are pyrogenic and can contribute to the production of shock by virtue of their ability to induce the synthesis of cytokines. According to current hypotheses, SPEA may act as a 'superantigen' as do staphylococcal toxic shock syndrome toxin 1 and staphylococcal enterotoxins. Superantigens can interact directly (without processing) with regions of class II MHC molecules on antigen-presenting cells and with the Vβ chain of T cell receptors. Each superantigen recognizes 1–5 Vβs and all T cells with one of these Vβ regions, regardless of antigenic specificity, will be stimulated by the superantigen. The resulting massive cytokine release can account for the symptoms of toxic shock (Schlievert 1993).

Stevens (1992) hypothesized that the pathogenesis of streptococcal toxic shock syndrome was dependent not only on bacterial virulence, but also on host factors. In his model, streptococci with M protein type 1 or 3 (common among streptococcal toxic shock isolates) are more invasive (mechanism unknown) than other strains. If such a virulent strain encounters a host who lacks specific protective anti-M protein antibodies, an invasive infection will ensue. If the infecting strain also produces an SPE to which the host has no antibodies, full blown infection accompanied by toxic shock will occur. Toxic shock syndrome has been associated with SPEA or SPEB, but not SPEC. Host antibodies to M protein will abort infection, whereas antibodies to the SPE only would allow for invasive infection with less devastating consequences, proving fatal only to neonates, the elderly, or the compromised patient. Support for this hypothesis is suggested by the data of Holm and coworkers (1992) who found that lower levels of acute antibody to SPEB correlated with fatal infection due to SPEB-producing strains, whereas less severe outcomes were noted in patients with higher antibody titres.

In epidemiological studies that have attempted to explain the recent increase in severe toxic shock-associated infections, it was noted that in the USA an increase in the frequency of streptococcal isolates with M protein types 1, 3 or 18 occurred during the period spanning 1972–1988 (Schwartz, Facklam and Breiman 1990). These 3 serotypes were more frequently isolated from patients with serious invasive infections in a group of strains collected during 1988–1990 (Johnson, Stevens and Kaplan 1992). Within a collection of 34 strains of M type 1 or 3 isolated from toxic shock cases, Hauser and colleagues (1991) found that whereas only 53% of strains produced SPEA under in vitro conditions, 85% contained the gene encoding the SPEA toxin, compared with a published value of presence of the SPEA gene in 15% of a sample of unselected *S. pyogenes* isolates. All strains in the study of Hauser and coworkers contained the gene for SPEB (production of toxin was demonstrated in 59%) and only 21% of the isolates contained the gene encoding SPEC. Musser and colleagues (1993a) used molecular methods to characterize isolates from severe disease in the 1920s and 1930s as well as recently isolated strains. Their data suggested that variations can occur in clone-virulence factor (SPEA) allele combinations and this variation may contribute to fluctuations in the incidence of severe streptococcal disease.

2.5 Other invasive streptococcal infections

PUERPERAL FEVER

Puerperal fever, or infection of the endometrium and surrounding structures, was a serious, life-threatening complication of childbirth or abortion before the antibiotic era. Streptococci commonly invade tissue, lymphatics and the bloodstream in this classic infection. Semmelweis, in the 1860s, correctly thought that puerperal fever could be transmitted by the midwife or doctor. Alternatively, *S. pyogenes* strains colonizing the patient's respiratory tract could also serve as the ultimate source of infection. Puerperal sepsis characterized by toxic shock syndrome has been noted (Silver and Heddleston 1992).

MYOSITIS

Streptococcal infection of muscle (myositis) is rarely reported and may occur alone or in the presence of necrotizing fasciitis. Adams et al. (1985) noted that only 21 cases of streptococcal myositis had been reported during the first 85 years of the twentieth century. Streptococcal myositis is reported to occur spontaneously, or to be preceded by minor trauma or muscle strain. Clinically, patients present with pain, swelling and erythema. Since antibiotics alone are insufficient for treatment, extensive surgical debridement is the recommended method of treatment for this infection (Stevens 1992).

BACTERAEMIA

Group A streptococci rarely gain entrance into the bloodstream from infections of the pharynx, although this site is the source for bacteraemia in the small proportion of scarlet fever patients who become septic. Cutaneous infections, including cellulitis and erysipelas, are more likely to provide a focus for bacteraemia. Formerly streptococcal bacteraemias were commonly seen in young children and elderly patients with predisposing factors such as burns, varicella, malignancy, diabetes, peripheral vascular disease and

immunosuppression. Currently these infections are associated with intravenous drug use, or with severe soft tissue infection by particularly invasive strains of *S. pyogenes* (Stevens 1992). Endocarditis due to group A streptococci has become an infrequent infection since the advent of antibiotics.

3 INFECTIONS IN HUMANS CAUSED BY *STREPTOCOCCUS AGALACTIAE* (GROUP B STREPTOCOCCI)

β-Haemolytic streptococci with Lancefield's group B antigen were recognized as pathogens in cattle during the nineteenth century, but it was not until the 1930s that these organisms were identified as agents of human disease (Fry 1938). Cases of infection caused by group B streptococci were reported only infrequently until the 1960s, when attention was called to the participation of these organisms in postpartum and neonatal infection (Eickhoff et al. 1964). The apparent increase of group B infection during the ensuing decades may have been due to enhanced awareness and more accurate identification of these streptococci by clinical laboratories. Another possible factor is an increase in the number of immature neonates who might not have survived in the past. Hussain and colleagues (1995) reported that paediatric patients older than 3 months of age (past the period for classical neonatal disease) accounted for 13% of 143 paediatric patients with group B infection during a 7.5 year period at one US hospital. Two-thirds of these non-neonatal paediatric patients had an underlying condition that would predispose them to infection. Group B streptococci are currently also recognized as agents of infection in adults, many of whom are predisposed to infection.

3.1 Neonatal infections

Infections of newborns by group B streptococci are classified either as early onset (occurring within the first few days of life) or late onset (beginning within 1 week to 3 months of age). Pre-term infants and neonates whose mothers exhibited obstetrical complications are typical of early onset group B infection victims. Neonates exhibit lethargy, poor feeding, fever and respiratory symptoms. Early onset disease is characterized by bacteraemia with no obvious focus, pneumonia and meningitis. Late onset disease is not correlated with maternal obstetrical complications or less than full term infants. As in early onset disease, babies exhibit lethargy, poor feeding and fever. Bacteraemia, meningitis and bone and joint infections are characteristic of late onset infection, which often has a more favourable outcome than early onset disease. A rapidly progressing, fulminant form of late onset disease is also seen and is associated with the development of neurological sequelae (Edwards and Baker 1995). Risk factors for development of neonatal group B streptococcal infection include maternal colonization, maternal infection and prolonged rupture of membranes. Heavy maternal colonization is correlated with development of disease as opposed to asymptomatic colonization of neonates, who are thought to acquire group B streptococci during birth via their respiratory or alimentary tracts or skin. In cases of maternal infection, the infant may already be ill at birth. Ascending infection may initiate premature rupture of membranes, a predisposing factor for group B infection.

Group B streptococcal capsules have been examined as virulence factors. The polysaccharide capsular material and protein antigens form the basis of a serotyping scheme, delineating types Ia, Ib/c (formerly Ib), Ia/c (formerly Ic), II, III, IV, V and VI. Provisional serotypes have also been proposed (Wessels and Kasper 1993). Serotype III has been most often associated with neonatal disease (Henrichsen et al. 1984, Jelinková and Motlová 1985). Wessels and coworkers (1989) constructed a mutant type III strain that produced a capsule identical to the wild type except for the presence of sialic acid. This mutant strain showed reduced virulence in a neonatal rat model of group B infection, lending credence to the theory that sialylation of bacterial surface molecules enhances infectivity by inhibiting activation of the alternative pathway of complement. Since this pathway helps to defend non-immune hosts against bacterial infection, sialylated capsules may enhance infection in premature neonates with low levels of maternal antibody. These infants have been shown to be at increased risk for infection by serotype III group B streptococci (Baker and Kasper 1976). Higher (>2 μg ml^{-1}) levels of type III antibody are correlated with enhanced opsonophagocytic killing of group B streptococci via the alternative complement pathway (Ferrieri 1990). Other factors influencing the susceptibility of neonates to infection by group B streptococci may be lowered amounts of complement components or a reduced capability for phagocytosis by the leucocytes of neonates (Wessels and Kasper 1993).

3.2 Infections in adults

In addition to causing postpartum infection, group B streptococci have become recognized as pathogens in non-pregnant adults. In a retrospective study in the Atlanta, Georgia area, Schwartz and colleagues (1991) reported an annual incidence of 2.4 cases per 100 000 during 1982–83. A prospective study during 1989–90 in the same population noted an annual incidence of 4.4 per 100 000, suggesting an increasing frequency of group B streptococcal disease (Farley et al. 1993a). Mortality rates in these 2 studies and one other by Gallagher and Watanakunakorn (1985) ranged from 21 to 70%.

Group B streptococci cause a variety of infections in adults, including bacteraemia, skin and soft tissue infection, bone infection, urosepsis, pneumonia, endocarditis and meningitis. In the bacteraemia cases studied, the ultimate focus of the infection could not always be discovered (Gallagher and Watanakunakorn

1985). Adults with group B streptococcal infection are usually older (published mean ages are approximately 60 years or more) and the risk of infection seems to increase with advancing age. Other predisposing factors are diabetes mellitus, cancer and HIV infection. Schwartz and coworkers (1991) noted that the risk of group B streptococcal infection was increased 10.5-fold in patients with diabetes mellitus and 16.4-fold in those with malignancies. A recent report by Schlievert, Gocke and Deringer (1993) described a case of toxic shock-like syndrome associated with group B streptococcal infection in a previously healthy young adult. The authors isolated a novel pyrogenic exotoxin from the patient's isolate and from 3 other group B strains isolated from toxic shock cases.

3.3 Epidemiology of group B streptococcal infections

Transmission of group B streptococci from mother to child can occur during birth in the case of vaginal colonization, or before birth in the setting of maternal infection. Colonization of newborns may occur without infection; organisms can be isolated from neonatal skin and mucous membranes. Vertical transmission from mother to baby is well described in early onset neonatal disease and, whereas the mother may be the ultimate source of streptococci in late onset illness, horizontal transmission can also occur. Nosocomial spread of streptococci from baby to baby via health care workers has been demonstrated to occur in nurseries (Noya et al. 1987).

Studies of carriage of group B streptococci suggest that the presence of these organisms in the vagina may be intermittent, leading to the hypothesis that the normal habitat of group B streptococci is the intestine. Group B streptococci can be isolated from faeces and the contents of the small intestine (Anthony et al. 1983), but the rectum and anorectal areas appear to be the major sites of colonization (Islam and Thomas 1980, Easmon et al. 1981). In pregnant women anorectal specimens are more likely to be positive than those obtained from the urethra or vagina (Ross and Cumming 1982). Vaginal carriage rates have been found to be higher in the earlier part of the menstrual cycle, in teenagers compared to older women, in sexually active women and in women with a history of 3 or fewer pregnancies. Virgins and certain ethnic groups, notably Mexican-American women, have displayed decreased rates of vaginal carriage (Baker et al. 1977, Anthony et al. 1981). The number of specimens cultured and culture methods (selective or non-selective) also influence the recovery of group B streptococci from genital specimens and thus the determination of carriage rates. Published carriage rate values have ranged from approximately 5 to 25% in surveys of pregnant women (Baker and Barrett 1973, Reid 1975, Finch, French and Phillips 1976).

In addition to serotype III, types Ia, Ib and II are the most common types isolated from infected neonates (Wessels and Kasper 1993). Studies employing multi-locus enzyme electrophoresis have suggested that disease-causing serotype III isolates are genetically related and constitute a clone that may be responsible for much of the observed group B streptococcal infection (Musser et al. 1989). Using the same techniques, Helmig and coworkers (1993) also demonstrated relatedness of disease-associated strains, but observed greater genetic variety among non-disease-producing isolates colonizing healthy pregnant women. Thus, widely disseminated virulent clones of group B streptococci may play a key role in neonatal disease.

4 INFECTIONS IN HUMANS CAUSED BY GROUP C AND G STREPTOCOCCI

β-Haemolytic streptococci producing Lancefield's group C or G antigen can be differentiated into 2 categories on the basis of colony size and other characteristics. Large colony formers are classic pyogenic streptococci and will be considered in this section, whereas small colony-forming strains belong to the 'Streptococcus milleri' group of species and are discussed in section 5. Large colony-forming group C and G streptococcal strains are closely related genetically, and a proposal to include them in a single species, regardless of heterogeneity of Lancefield antigens, has been forwarded (Farrow and Collins 1984). In traditional classification schemes strains of these streptococci with the group C antigen were separated into the species *Streptococcus equi* (a pathogen of horses), *Streptococcus equisimilis*, *Streptocccus zooepidemicus* and *Streptococcus dysgalactiae* on the basis of carbohydrate fermentation patterns.

Group C and G β-haemolytic streptococci have been isolated as commensals from the pharynx (Forrer and Ellner 1979), the intestine (Barnham 1983), the skin (Gaunt and Seal 1987) and the female genital tract (Christensen et al. 1974). The large colony-forming strains resemble *S. pyogenes* in terms of their virulence factors and pathogenic potential. M-like proteins have been identified in both group C and G strains (Efstratiou et al. 1989, Campo, Schultz and Bisno 1995). In the case of group G strains, the M protein has been shown to inhibit phagocytosis and to be homologous to the class I M proteins of *S. pyogenes* (Schnitzler et al. 1995). Group C and G strains may also produce virulence-associated extracellular products like haemolysins, hyaluronidase and streptokinase (Efstratiou et al. 1989).

Large colony-forming group C and G streptococci can cause pharyngitis that is similar in its clinical manifestations to infection produced by *S. pyogenes* (McCue 1982, Efstratiou 1989, Turner et al. 1990). Although no cases of rheumatic fever following infection with group C or G strains have been documented, acute glomerulonephritis may occur after pharyngeal infection or other types of infection with these streptococci (Duca et al. 1969, Stryker, Fraser and Facklam 1982, Barnham, Thornton and Lange 1983, Cohen et al. 1987, Gann et al. 1987, Manian et al. 1992). In addition to pharyngitis, group C and G large colony-

forming β-haemolytic streptococci are well documented as agents of a variety of serious infections. These include bacteraemia (Bradley et al. 1991), endocarditis, skin and soft tissue infections, pneumonia, septic arthritis, puerperal sepsis and meningitis (Mohr et al. 1979, Stamm and Cobbs 1980, Gaunt and Seal 1987, Arditi et al. 1989, Barnham et al. 1989, Salata et al. 1989, Ortel, Kalliano and Gallis 1990).

5 INFECTIONS CAUSED BY SMALL COLONY-FORMING β-HAEMOLYTIC STREPTOCOCCI

Small colony-forming β-haemolytic streptococcal strains (the 'minute haemolytic streptococci' described by Long and Bliss in 1934) may evidence Lancefield group A, C, F or G antigens, or be non-groupable in the Lancefield system. These organisms are genetically different from large colony-forming pyogenic group A, C and G streptococci and are included in the species comprising the 'S. milleri' group. According to the currently accepted classification of these organisms, which may have variable haemolytic reactions, β-haemolytic strains are found principally in the species *Streptococcus anginosus* and *Streptococcus constellatus* (Whiley et al. 1990). Chapter 20 of this volume should be consulted for additional information on this group of organisms. The small colony-forming β-haemolytic streptococci constitute part of the normal flora of the pharynx and upper respiratory tract and can also be isolated from faeces (Smith and Sherman 1938).

Small colony-forming β-haemolytic strains have been recognized as participants in serious infections in a variety of body sites. Mucosal trauma or disease is thought to be a major predisposing factor encouraging infection of normally sterile tissues by these organisms. Possible pathogenic factors of small colony-forming β-haemolytic streptococci include fibronectin-binding ability and production of hydrolytic enzymes (Ruoff and Ferraro 1987, Unsworth 1989, Willcox and Knox 1990). These organisms have been isolated from purulent infections of the oral cavity, upper respiratory tract, central nervous system, gastrointesinal and genitourinary tracts, abdominal cavity, skin, soft tissues and bone (Ball and Parker 1979, Gossling 1988, Ruoff 1988, Whitworth 1990, Whiley et al. 1992).

6 INFECTIONS IN HUMANS CAUSED BY OTHER β-HAEMOLYTIC STREPTOCOCCI

Streptococcus suis serotype 2 is a pathogen of swine, but may also cause disease in humans. This streptococcal species is often β-haemolytic on horse blood agar, but α-haemolytic on sheep blood agar and produces Lancefield's group R, S or T carbohydrate antigen (Kilpper-Bälz and Schleifer 1987). Human infections with this organism are seen in meat handlers and may include presentations of septicaemia or meningitis (Arends and Zanen 1988). *Streptococcus porcinus*, another swine pathogen, is a β-haemolytic streptococcus with Lancefield's E, P, U or V antigen. This organism has been recovered infrequently from human clinical cultures (Facklam et al. 1995), as have β-haemolytic group L streptococci, which are normally pathogens of animals (Barnham 1987).

7 INFECTIONS CAUSED BY VIRIDANS STREPTOCOCCI

Organisms known as viridans streptococci are common inhabitants of the oral cavity, upper respiratory passages, intestine and female genital tract. They differ from 'pyogenic' streptococci in that they lack the overt virulence factors that have been well characterized in the latter group. Viridans streptococci have traditionally been described as α-haemolytic, although non-haemolytic and even β-haemolytic strains are included in this ill-defined streptococcal division. Viridans species or species groups include *Streptococcus mutans*, *Streptococcus salivarius*, *Streptococcus sanguis*, *Streptococcus mitis*, *Streptococcus bovis* and 'Streptococcus milleri'. β-Haemolytic organisms classified as 'Streptococcus milleri' are mentioned in section 5 of this chapter (p. 266).

In spite of the absence of characteristics normally associated with virulence, viridans streptococci can participate in a variety of infections. As with other low-virulence opportunistic pathogens, infections caused by viridans streptococci usually occur in compromised or predisposed hosts in normally sterile tissues to which the streptococci have gained access. Colonization and subsequent infection has been linked to the ability of viridans streptococci to adhere to host tissue. This behaviour is thought to be mediated by association of bacterial lipoteichoic acid with host tissue fibronectin (Hogg and Manning 1988). Extracellular polysaccharides such as dextran have also been implicated as virulence factors, since dextran production seems to correlate with virulence in endocarditis (Pelletier, Coyle and Petersdorf 1978).

Within its natural habitat of the oral cavity, *S. mutans* is responsible for the most prevalent infectious disease of humans, dental caries. Although many theories on the aetiology of dental caries have been advanced, the association of *S. mutans* with caries has been well established since the 1960s. Carious lesions are favoured by high levels of dietary sucrose which provide a substrate for acid production by *S. mutans* and other bacteria inhabiting dental plaque. Although efforts to prevent this almost universal bacterial disease have included hygenic regimens, antibacterial agents and immunization, it still remains a widespread problem.

Viridans streptococci that become introduced into the bloodstream by trauma to oral mucosal surfaces usually produce only transient and insignificant bacteraemias. In some cases, however, these bacteria may colonize heart tissue and cause subacute bacterial endocarditis. Individuals with damaged cardiac valvular endothelium or cardiac abnormalities that produce altered blood flow patterns within the heart are often at risk of developing this infecton. Colonization of heart tissue is thought to be mediated by the adherence of streptococci to platelet and fibrin vegetations that form at the site of damage to the cardiac endothelium. Fibronectin, also present in these non-bacterial thrombotic vegetations, may facilitate bacterial adherence (Scheld et al. 1985). Once colonization occurs, streptococcal dextran presumably provides a stratum for growth and possible protection of the streptococci from the action of antibiotics (Dall et al. 1987). Endocarditis caused by viridans streptococci is subacute and usually characterized by fever, cardiac murmurs and constitutional symptoms such as malaise and weight loss. Continuous bacteraemia, revealed by multiple positive blood cultures, is also characteristic. Antibiotic therapy is usually successful in treating this infection.

Viridans streptococci are also infrequently recovered from other infections such as meningitis and pneumonia. Recent studies have implicated these organisms as emerging agents of bacteraemia and septicaemia in patients undergoing anti-cancer treatments (Sotiropoulos et al. 1989, Kern, Kurrle and Schmeiser 1990, Awda et al. 1992). Association of a shock syndrome with viridans streptococcal septicaemia in this patient population has also been noted (Elting, Bodey and Keefe 1992).

8 HOST RESPONSE TO STREPTOCOCCAL INFECTIONS

The measurement of humoral responses to streptococcal infection is of value in the diagnosis of the non-suppurative sequelae acute rheumatic fever and acute glomerulonephritis. By the time these diseases appear, suppurative infection has resolved and streptococcal culture is often negative. Demonstration of elevated antibody levels to various streptococcal products will, however, support the probability of antecedent infection and aid in establishing a diagnosis of rheumatic fever or post-streptococcal glomerulonephritis. In general, anti-streptococcal antibody levels rise above normal limits within 2–3 weeks of the acute infection. Table 15.3 summarizes characteristics of 3 of the major tests for streptococcal antibodies. In addition to the ASO, anti-DNAase B and anti-A-CHO tests, antibodies to the following streptococcal products or components can also be assayed: streptokinase (ASK test), hyaluronidase (ASH test), NADase (anti-NADase test), M protein (type-specific antibody test).

The test for antistreptolysin O, developed by Todd, will detect about 85% of rheumatic fever cases; antibody to this streptococcal haemolysin will not be detected in all patients with antecedent pharyngitis and is not a reliable indicator of previous skin infection with group A streptococci. Consequently, more than one test for anti-streptococcal antibodies is desirable when the ASO results are normal but previous streptococcal infection is suspected. A commercially

Table 15.3 Principal streptococcal antibody tests

Test	Antigen	Method
ASO	Streptolysin O	Antistreptolysin O antibodies in patient serum inhibit streptolysin O-mediated red blood cell lysis in reaction mixture. End point is last serum dilution that shows no haemolysis. Titres may be expressed in Todd units or international units depending on how streptolysin O was standardized
Anti-DNAase B	DNAase B	Anti-DNAase B antibodies in patient serum inhibit DNAase B from hydrolysing a DNA–methyl green coloured conjugate. End point is last serum dilution with an arbitrary (2+ to 4+) degree of colour
Anti-A-CHO	Group A carbohydrate	ELISA assay measuring amount of antibody in patient serum binding to purified group A carbohydrate

available agglutination test employs erythrocytes coated with streptolysin O, DNAase B, streptokinase, hyaluronidase and adenine dinucleotide glycohydrolase in an effort to detect elevated antibodies to one or more of these streptococcal products. Antistreptolysin O and other anti-streptococcal antibodies may also be produced in response to infection with large colony-forming group C and G streptococci (Efstratiou et al. 1989). Additional information on the performance and use of anti-streptococcal antibody tests can be found in Ayoub and Harden (1992) and in the 8th edition of this book.

9 LABORATORY CONSIDERATIONS

9.1 Specimens

Suitable specimens for the detection of streptococci include infected tissues, sputum, blood and other body fluids. Swabs containing purulent material are also suitable for submission to the laboratory. Throat swabs should be obtained by swabbing the tonsils, avoiding the tongue and uvula. Any visible exudate should be collected on the swab. Most β-haemolytic streptococci survive desiccation and special transport conditions are usually not required. This applies especially to throat specimens that are to be screened only for *S. pyogenes*. In specimens thought to contain other pathogens that may be more fragile than streptococci, rapid transport to the laboratory or use of a transport medium is advisable. Throat swabs to be cultured only for group A streptococci may be stored in tubes containing silica gel if an extended interval will elapse between collection and planting. A filter paper transport system for the detection of *S. pyogenes* in throat specimens has also been described (Facklam and Washington 1991).

9.2 Culture methods

Complex media enriched with blood are recommended for the recovery of streptococci. These media not only encourage the growth of streptococci, but also allow detection of haemolytic reactions which aid in the identification process. Haemolytic reactions may vary with different types of animal blood and the basal medium employed. The β-haemolytic streptococci discussed in this chapter should reliably produce β-haemolysis on media supplemented with either horse or sheep blood. While *S. pyogenes*, group B streptococci and large colony-forming group C and G streptococci grow well in ambient atmospheres at 35°C, some small colony-forming β-haemolytic strains may require an atmosphere containing an elevated (5%) CO_2 concentration. This requirement can be met with a CO_2 incubator or a candle jar. All streptococci grow well in anaerobic atmospheres and haemolysis may be enhanced due to the functioning of the oxygen labile streptolysin O. As 'aerotolerant anaerobes' growth of these organisms is not inhibited by the presence of oxygen.

Sheep blood agar is useful for the culture of throat swabs because it contains inadequate amounts of NAD to support the growth of the NAD-requiring commensal *Haemophilus haemolyticus*. If present on the throat culture plate, the β-haemolytic colonies of this normal flora constituent would have to be investigated as possible β-haemolytic streptococcal colonies, complicating the workup of the culture. Material from throat swabs is transferred to the agar surface and then streaked to produce isolated colonies. The practice of making numerous stabs into the agar with the inoculating loop serves to deposit bacteria beneath the surface of the agar where the oxygen concentration may be low enough to enable the functioning of streptolysin O. This results in enhanced haemolysis in the area of the stab and facilitates detection of group A streptococci in the mixture of throat flora. Procedures that employ overnight incubation of swabs in broth for enrichment of streptococci and a pour-streak method facilitating detection of haemolytic reactions in subsurface colonies have also been described (Facklam and Washington 1991). Since the pharyngeal streptococcal load is much greater in infection than in carriage states, semiquantitative evaluation of group A streptococci may be desirable, but variation in sampling can also influence the numbers of streptococci recovered by culture.

Numerous selective media formulations and incubation conditions have been employed to inhibit normal throat flora and enhance recovery of group A streptococci from throat specimens. Media additions include antibiotics such as trimethoprim–sulphamethoxazole and incubation conditions have varied from ambient atmospheres to elevated CO_2 concentrations to anaerobic conditions. Different studies have reached different conclusions on the most effective way to recover group A streptococci, but Kellog (1990), in a review of this matter, concluded that 90–95% of group A strains will be recovered from symptomatic patients using any of the following protocols: anaerobically incubated (48 h) sheep blood agar; sheep blood incubated in an ambient atmosphere for 48 h (a sterile cover glass may be placed over the inoculation area to reduce oxygen tension and enhance haemolysis); trimethoprim–sulphamethoxazole-supplemented sheep blood agar incubated in an atmosphere containing 5–10% CO_2 for 48 h; or anaerobically incubated (48 h) trimethoprim–sulphamethoxazole-supplemented sheep blood agar.

Efforts to identify expectant mothers at risk of delivering infants infected with group B streptococci have led to the formulation of special culture media and methods for recovery of these organisms. Selective enrichment media consisting of Todd–Hewitt broth supplemented with colistin and nalidixic acid (Jones et al. 1983), gentamicin and nalidixic acid (Persson and Forsgren 1987), or trimethoprim and sulphamethoxazole (Altaie and Dryja 1994) have been described.

9.3 Antigen detection methods

Detection of the Lancefield antigens of streptococci present in a specimen allows for direct and rapid diagnosis of infection without culture of streptococci on laboratory media. This method has been applied to the detection of *S. pyogenes* in throat swab specimens and numerous commercially available products have been evaluated in comparison to the 'gold standard' of detection, culture. Antigen detection methods for group A streptococci involve an antigen extraction step; this is usually accomplished by immersing material from the throat swab in a solution of enzymes (pronase) or nitrous acid. After extraction of Lancefield antigen from organisms present in the specimen, various techniques are applied for antigen detection. These have included agglutination (Gerber 1986), enzyme immunoassay (Hoffman 1990, Drulak et al. 1991), liposome immunoassay (Gerber, Randolph and DeMeo 1990) and optical immunoassay (Harbeck et al. 1993). Extensive evaluations of antigen detection methods for group A streptococci on throat swabs have concluded that these methods are rapid and specific. They are, however, lacking in sensitivity when compared to culture. This occurs notably in cases where small numbers of streptococci are present in the specimen. It has been concluded that results of these screening tests can be accepted with confidence only when positive for group A streptococci. Specimens producing negative antigen detection results should be cultured to confirm the absence of *S. pyogenes* (Gerber 1986).

Since colonization of the female genital tract with group B streptococci is sporadic throughout pregnancy, antepartum or intrapartum detection of these organisms with a rapid test would be desirable. Although heavy vaginal colonization by group B streptococci is correlated with the risk of neonatal infection, lightly colonized mothers may also give birth to infected infants. Thus, a reliable test should be able to detect all levels of colonization. Cultural methods, especially those involving an enrichment step, are able to do this (Lim, Morales and Walsh 1987), but antigen detection methods appear to be lacking in sensitivity. This has been demonstrated in recent evaluations of latex agglutination assays (Green et al. 1993) and enzyme immunoassays (Granato and Petosa 1991, Wust, Hebisch and Peters 1993). Antigen detection methods for group B streptococci may also be used for the examination of infected body fluids, such as cerebrospinal fluid.

Fluorescent antibody (FA) staining may also be employed as a rapid and sensitive technique for direct detection of group A and B streptococci. The technically demanding nature of FA techniques has made them less attractive since the advent of commercially available, simple to use agglutination reagents. Detailed information on FA methods can be found in other sources (Facklam 1980).

9.4 Serological methods

The streptococcal antibody tests described in section 8 of this chapter (p. 267) are useful in establishing previous streptococcal infection in cases of suspected rheumatic fever or glomerulonephritis. It is difficult to demonstrate a rising antibody titre by the time the patient presents with symptoms of non-suppurative sequelae; therefore, sera are evaluated for titres that are elevated above the 'upper limit of normal', a value that is variable in populations of different ages, in different locations and with different frequencies of streptococcal infection. Table 15.4 displays upper limits of normal values collected by Wannamaker and Ayoub (1960) for various streptococcal tests. In order to exclude a diagnosis of rheumatic fever or glomerulonephritis, negative results in 2 or 3 serological tests are considered as conclusive.

9.5 Other methods

The gram stain has been used as a rapid method for diagnosing colonization of expectant mothers with group B streptococci. There is an inherent lack of specificity in this technique due to the normal presence of other streptococcal species in the female genital tract. Variable sensitivity has been noted in evaluations of this technique (Holls, Thomas and Troyer 1987, Sandy, Blumenfeld and Iams 1988).

Table 15.4 Normal limits of streptococcal antibody titres

Antibody	Upper limits of normal[a]		Lower limits for rheumatic fever[b]
	5–12 years	young adults	
Antistreptolysin O	333	200	250
Antihyaluronidase	110	80	300
Anti-DNAase B		80	320
Anti-NADase		130	175

Adapted from Wannamaker and Ayoub 1960, and the 8th edition of this text.
[a]Titres of 80% of the population studied are less than or equal to these values.
[b]Titres of 80% of the population studied are greater than or equal to these values.

Nucleic acid probe methods for the rapid detection of both group A and B streptococci are now available (Davis and Fuller 1991, Heiter and Borbeau 1993). The usefulness and cost-effectiveness of these methods compared to existing protocols has yet to be fully evaluated.

10 TREATMENT

β-Haemolytic streptococci continue to be susceptible to penicillin, which remains the drug of choice for the treatment of most infections caused by these organisms. The streptococci are similarly susceptible to other cell wall active agents like cephalosporins and vancomycin. Minimum inhibitory concentrations (MICs) for penicillin range from 0.006 to 0.25 µg ml^{-1}. The uniform susceptibility of β-haemolytic streptococci to cell wall active agents makes routine susceptibility testing of these organisms unnecessary. Group B streptococcal strains are often able to withstand higher penicillin concentrations than streptococci of other serogroups and consequently serious infections (e.g. meningitis) caused by these strains are often treated with a synergistic bactericidal combination of penicillin and gentamicin (Sahm 1994). High-level resistance to gentamicin and other aminoglycosides, which obviates the synergistic effect observed when these antimicrobials are combined with cell wall active agents, has been described in group B streptococci but seems so far to be uncommon (Buu-Hoï, LeBouguenac and Horaud 1990). The frequency of resistance of group A β-haemolytic streptococci to erythromycin, often used as a treatment alternative for penicillin-allergic patients, is variable and has been found to be quite high in some geographical areas (Spencer et al. 1989, Seppälä et al. 1992, Coonan and Kaplan 1994).

Various hypotheses have been advanced to explain the observation of occasional penicillin treatment failures, often in cases of pharyngitis. One theory holds that a large enough number of β-lactamase-producing normal throat flora organisms could prevent streptococcal eradication by destroying penicillin. A second hypothesis, based on in vitro results, invokes the concept of antibiotic tolerance. The growth of tolerant bacteria is inhibited by relatively low concentrations of an antibiotic, but extremely high concentrations (≥ 32 times the MIC) are required to kill the organisms. Tolerance is demonstrated in the laboratory by determination of and comparison between the MIC and the minimum bactericidal concentration (MBC) of an antimicrobial agent for a given bacterial strain. The phenomenon of tolerance has been documented in group A streptococci (Krasinski et al. 1986, Dagan 1987), but it should be remembered that variations in technique can influence the results of these determinations and it is not known if the same phenomenon is operational under in vivo conditions.

11 PREVENTION

Although streptococcal pharyngitis may resolve spontaneously, antibiotic therapy aimed at eradicating *S. pyogenes* from the pharynx will prevent the development of rheumatic fever, even if initiated as late as 9 days after the onset of pharyngitis. Prolonged administration of penicillin or other antimicrobial agents, rather than a single high dose, is most effective. Such treatment will also prevent the suppurative sequelae of pharyngeal infection (Bisno 1995a). The spread of streptococcal pharyngitis and its subsequent sequelae can be controlled with antibiotic prophylaxis of the population at risk. This principle was established and well documented during military epidemics of World War II and is still used as an effective method for the control of streptococcal disease in military populations today (Thomas et al. 1988).

Cases of group B streptococcal neonatal disease can be diminished by preventing the vertical transmission of streptococci from mother to infant. Intrapartum administration of intravenous ampicillin has been shown to reduce significantly group B streptococcal colonization of neonates born to colonized mothers (Boyer and Gotoff 1986, Lim et al. 1986). The development of a vaccine is a second strategy being investigated in the effort to reduce group B neonatal disease. The immunization of pregnant women with type III capsular polysaccharide results in the formation of IgG, which can cross the placenta. With maternal immunization, infant antibody levels are sufficiently high (greater than 2 µg ml^{-1}) to cause enhancement of bactericidal opsonization and phagocytosis via the alternative complement pathway, as occurs in infants with these levels of natural immunity. Antibodies in infants persist throughout the first 2–3 months of life and consequently could be beneficial in the prevention of late onset disease (Baker et al. 1988). Since polysaccharides show variable immunogenic activity, efforts have been directed at developing protein conjugates of capsular polysaccharide types that commonly cause neonatal infection, the goal being a multivalent conjugate vaccine that could prevent the majority of cases of group B streptococcal neonatal disease (Wessels and Kasper 1993).

12 STREPTOCOCCAL DISEASES IN ANIMALS

Domestic animals suffer infections caused by a variety of β-haemolytic streptococci with the notable exception of group A strains. Although occasional infections of monkeys by group A streptococci have been documented, most serious diseases of domesticated animals are caused by β-haemolytic strains belonging to group B, C, G and other serogroups.

12.1 Infections in cattle

Mastitis is a common disease in cattle and was caused principally by *S. agalactiae* (group B) before the widespread availability of antibiotics. The group B strains causing mastitis are distinct from those infecting humans and can spread rapidly through dairy herds. Intramammary instillation of penicillin and decontamination of structures housing cows will usually stop the spread of infection. Streptococci belonging to Lancefield group C (*S. dysgalactiae* and *S. zooepidemicus*) and G are infrequently isolated as agents of bovine mastitis, while the non-β-haemolytic *Streptococcus uberis* has become a more common agent of this disease in recent years. As with group B streptococci, group G bovine isolates appear to form a population that is distinct from that in humans (Clark et al. 1984). β-Haemolytic group L strains have also been isolated from infections in cattle (Barnham 1987).

12.2 Infection in horses

S. equi, a β-haemolytic species with the group C antigen, is an important agent of disease in horses. It can cause regional or generalized suppurative lymphadenitis, a condition known as 'strangles', often following acute infection of the pharynx or nasopharynx. Effective vaccines are available to protect against this disease, which is especially devastating to young horses. Infection by the group C species *S. zooepidemicus* usually occurs in tissues that have been damaged by trauma or by previous viral infection in the case of the respiratory tract.

12.3 Infections in swine

β-Haemolytic streptococci are normal inhabitants of the respiratory and genital tracts of pigs, but some of these organisms are also important agents of disease. *S. suis* strains may produce Lancefield group R, S, T or RS antigens or be non-groupable (Kilpper-Bälz and Schleifer 1987). Although these streptococci can share antigens with Lancefield group D organisms, they are unrelated to the latter group. Over 20 capsular serotypes of *S. suis* have been described; serotype 2 is recognized as the most prevalent isolate from cases of pneumonia, meningitis and arthritis (Gottshalk et al. 1989). β-Haemolytic streptococci with Lancefield group E, P and U antigens, classified as *S. porcinus* (Collin et al. 1984), group L strains (Barnham 1987) and group C strains identified as *S. equisimilis* have also been described as pathogens in pigs.

12.4 Infections in sheep

Group C streptococci classified as *S. dysgalactiae* have been documented as agents of septicaemia and pneumonia in lambs. β-Haemolytic group L strains have also been isolated as agents of ovine disease (Barnham 1987).

12.5 Infections in dogs

A survey of 254 β-haemolytic streptococcal strains isolated from canine infections revealed a preponderance of group G strains, along with isolates of groups C, E and one of group A (Biberstein, Brown and Smith 1980). The group G species *Streptococcus canis* was established to include canine strains and also isolates of bovine origin. *S. canis* can be differentiated from human group G strains by physiological characteristics (Devriese et al. 1986). Group L streptococci have also been isolated as agents of infection in dogs (Barnham 1987).

REFERENCES

Adams EM, Gundmundsson S et al., 1985, Streptococcal myositis, *Arch Intern Med*, **145:** 1020–3.

Altaie SS, Dryja D, 1994, Detection of group B *Streptococcus*. Comparison of solid and liquid culture media with and without selective antibiotics, *Diagn Microbiol Infect Dis*, **18:** 141–4.

Anthony BF, Kaplan EL et al., 1976, The dynamics of streptococcal infections in a defined population of children: serotypes associated with skin and respiratory infections, *Am J Epidemiol*, **104:** 652–66.

Anthony BF, Eisenstadt R et al., 1981, Genital and intestinal carriage of group B streptococci during pregnancy, *J Infect Dis*, **143:** 761–6.

Anthony BF, Carter JA et al., 1983, Isolation of group B streptococci from the proximal small intestine of adults, *J Infect Dis*, **147:** 776.

Arditi M, Shulman ST et al., 1989, Group C β-hemolytic streptococcal infections in children: nine pediatric cases and review, *Rev Infect Dis*, **11:** 34–45.

Arends JP, Zanen HC, 1988, Meningitis caused by *Streptococcus suis* in humans, *Rev Infect Dis*, **10:** 131–7.

Awada A, van der Auwera P et al., 1992, Streptococcal and enterococcal bacteremia in patients with cancer, *Clin Infect Dis*, **15:** 33–48.

Ayoub EM, Harden E, 1992, Immune response to streptococcal antigens: diagnostic methods, *Manual of Clinical Immunology*, 4th edn, eds Rose NR, DeMacario EC et al., American Society for Microbiology, Washington DC, 427–34.

Baker CJ, Barrett FF, 1973, Transmission of group B streptococci among parturient women and their neonates, *J Pediatr*, **83:** 919–25.

Baker CJ, Kasper DL, Correlation of maternal antibody deficiency with susceptibility to neonatal group B streptococcal infection, 1976, *N Engl J Med*, **294:** 753–6.

Baker CJ, Goroff DK et al., 1977, Vaginal colonization with group B *Streptococcus*: a study in college women, *J Infect Dis*, **135:** 392–7.

Baker CJ, Rench MA et al., 1988, Immunization of pregnant women with a polysaccharide vaccine of group B streptococcus, *N Engl J Med*, **319**: 1180–5.

Ball LC, Parker MT, 1979, The cultural and biochemical characters of *Streptococcus milleri* strains isolated from human sources, *J Hyg Camb*, **82**: 63–78.

Barnham M, 1983, The gut as a source of the haemolytic streptococci causing infection in surgery of the intestinal and biliary tracts, *J Infect*, **6**: 129–39.

Barnham M, 1987, Group L beta-haemolytic streptococcal infection in meat handlers: another streptococcal zoonosis?, *Epidemiol Infect*, **99**: 257–64.

Barnham M, Thornton TJ, Lange K, 1983, Nephritis caused by *Streptococcus zooepidemicus* (Lancefield group C), *Lancet*, **1**: 945–8.

Barnham M, Kerby J et al., 1989, Group C streptococci in human infection: a study of 308 isolates with clinical correlations, *Epidemiol Infect*, **102**: 379–90.

Beachey EH, Courtney HS, 1987, Bacteria adherence: the attachment of group A streptococci to mucosal surfaces, *Rev Infect Dis*, **9, supplement 5**: S475–81.

Belani K, Schlievert P et al., 1991, Association of exotoxin-producing group A streptococci and severe disease in children, *Pediatr Infect Dis J*, **10**: 351–4.

Biberstein EL, Brown C, Smith T, 1980, Serogroups and biotypes among beta-hemolytic streptococci of canine origin, *J Clin Microbiol*, **11**: 558–61.

Bisno AL, 1995a, *Streptococcus pyogenes*, *Principles and Practice of Infectious Diseases*, 4th edn, eds Mandell GL, Bennett JE, Dolin R, Churchill Livingstone, New York, 1786–99.

Bisno AL, 1995b, Nonsuppurative poststreptococcal sequelae: rheumatic fever and glomerulonephritis, *Principles and Practice of Infectious Diseases*, 4th edn, eds Mandell GL, Bennett JE, Dolin R, Churchill Livingstone, New York, 1799–810.

Boyer KM, Gotoff SP, 1986, Prevention of early-onset neonatal group B streptococcal disease with selective intrapartum chemoprophylaxis, *N Engl J Med*, **314**: 1665–9.

Bradley SF, Gordon JJ et al., 1991, Group C streptococcal bacteremia: analysis of 88 cases, *Rev Infect Dis*, **13**: 270–80.

Buu-Hoï A, LeBouguenec C, Horaud T, 1990, High-level chromosomal gentamicin resistance in *Streptococcus agalactiae* (group B), *Antimicrob Agents Chemother*, **34**: 985–8.

Campo RE, Schultz DR, Bisno AL, 1995, M proteins of group G streptococci: mechanisms of resistance to phagocytosis, *J Infect Dis*, **171**: 601–6.

Cherchi GB, Kaplan EL et al., 1992, First reported case of *Streptococcus pyogenes* infection with toxic shock-like syndrome in Italy, *Eur J Clin Microbiol Infect Dis*, **11**: 836–8.

Chhatwal GS, Dutra IS, Blobel H, 1985, Fibrinogen binding inhibits the fixation of the third component of human complement on surface of groups A, B, C, and G streptococci, *Microbiol Immunol*, **29**: 973–80.

Chomarat M, Chapuis C et al., 1990, Two cases of severe infection with beta-haemolytic group A streptococci associated with a toxic shock-like syndrome, *Eur J Clin Microbiol Infect Dis*, **9**: 901–3.

Christensen KK, Christensen P et al., 1974, Frequencies of streptococci of groups A, B, C, D and G in urethra and cervix swab specimens from patients with suspected gonococcal infection, *Acta Pathol Microbiol Scand*, **B82**: 470–4.

Clark RB, Berrafati JF et al., 1984, Biotyping and exoenzyme profiling as an aid in the differentiation of human from bovine group G streptococci, *J Clin Microbiol*, **20**: 706–10.

Cohen D, Ferne M et al., 1987, Food-borne outbreak of group G streptococcal sore throat in an Israeli military base, *Epidemiol Infect*, **99**: 249–55.

Cone LA, Woodard DR et al., 1987, Clinical and bacteriologic observations of a toxic shock-like syndrome due to *Streptococcus pyogenes*, *N Engl J Med*, **317**: 146–9.

Coonan KM, Kaplan EL, 1994, *In vitro* susceptibility of recent North American group A streptococcal isolates to eleven oral antibiotics, *Pediatr Infect Dis J*, **13**: 630–5.

Dagan R, Ferne M et al., 1987, An epidemic of penicillin-tolerant group A streptoccal pharyngitis in children living in a closed community: mass treatment with erythromycin, *J Infect Dis*, **156**: 514–16.

Dall L, Barnes WG et al., 1987, Enzymatic modification of glycocalyx in the treatment of experimental endocarditis due to viridans streptococci, *J Infect Dis*, **156**: 736–40.

Davis TE, Fuller DD, 1991, Direct identification of bacterial isolates in blood cultures by using a DNA probe, *J Clin Microbiol*, **29**: 2192–6.

Demers B, Simor AE et al., 1993, Severe invasive group A streptococcal infections in Ontario, Canada: 1987–1991, *Clin Infect Dis*, **16**: 792–800.

Denny FW, 1994, A 45-year perspective on the streptococcus and rheumatic fever: the Edward H. Kass lecture in infectious disease history, *Clin Infect Dis*, **19**: 1110–22.

Donaldson PMW, Naylor B et al., 1993, Rapidly fatal necrotising fasciitis caused by *Streptococcus pyogenes*, *J Clin Pathol*, **46**: 617–20.

Devriese LA, Hommez J et al., 1986, *Streptococcus canis* sp. nov.: a species of group G streptococci from animals, *Int J Syst Bacteriol*, **36**: 422–5.

Drulak M, Bartholomew W et al., 1991, Evaluation of the modified Visuwell Strep-A enzyme immunoassay for detection of group-A *Streptococcus* from throat swabs, *Diagn Microbiol Infect Dis*, **14**: 281–5.

Duca E, Teodorovici GR et al., 1969, A new nephritogenic streptococcus, *J Hyg Lond*, **67**: 691–8.

Easmon CSF, Tanna A et al., 1981, Group B streptococci– gastrointestinal organisms?, *J Clin Pathol*, **34**: 921–3.

Edwards MS, Baker CJ, 1995, *Streptococcus agalactiae* (group B *Streptococcus*), *Principles and Practice of Infectious Diseases*, 4th edn, eds Mandell GL, Bennett JE, Dolin R, Churchill Livingstone, New York, 1835–45.

Efstratiou A, Teare EL et al., 1989, The presence of M proteins in outbreak strains of *Streptococcus equisimilis* T-type 204, *J Infect*, **19**: 105–11.

Eickhoff TC, Klein JO et al., 1964, Neonatal sepsis and other infections due to group B beta-hemolytic streptococci, *N Engl J Med*, **271**: 1221–8.

Elting LS, Bodey GP, Keefe BH, 1992, Septicemia and shock syndrome due to viridans streptococci: a case-control study of predisposing factors, *Clin Infect Dis*, **14**: 1201–7.

Facklam RR, 1980, Streptococci and aerococci, *Manual of Clinical Microbiology*, 3rd edn, eds Lennette EH, Balows A et al., American Society for Microbiology, Washington DC, 88–110.

Facklam RR, Washington JA II, 1991, *Streptococcus* and related catalase-negative gram-positive cocci, *Manual of Clinical Microbiology*, 5th edn, eds Balows A, Hausler WJ et al., American Society for Microbiology, Washington DC, 238–57.

Facklam R, Elliott J et al., 1995, Identification of *Streptococcus porcinus* from human sources, *J Clin Microbiol*, **33**: 385–8.

Farley MM, Harvey RC et al., 1993a, A population-based assessment of invasive disease due to group B streptococcus in nonpregnant adults, *N Engl J Med*, **328**: 1807–11.

Farley TA, Wilson SA et al., 1993b, Direct inoculation of food as the cause of an outbreak of group A streptococcal pharyngitis, *J Infect Dis*, **167**: 1232–5.

Farrow JAE, Collins MD, 1984, Taxonomic studies on streptococci of serological groups C, G, and L and possibly related taxa, *Syst Appl Microbiol*, **5**: 483–93.

Ferrieri P, 1990, Neonatal susceptibility and immunity to major bacterial pathogens, *Rev Infect Dis*, **12**: S394–400.

Ferrieri P, Dajani AS et al., 1970, Appearance of nephritis associated with type 57 streptococcal impetigo in North America, *N Engl J Med*, **283**: 832–6.

Ferrieri P, Dajani AS et al., 1972, Natural history of impetigo. I. Site sequence of acquisition and familial patterns of spread of cutaneous streptococci, *J Clin Invest*, **51**: 2851–62.

Finch FG, French GL, Phillips I, 1976, Group B streptococci in the female genital tract, *Br Med J*, **1**: 1245–7.

Fischetti VA, 1989, Streptococcal M protein: molecular design and biological behavior, *Clin Microbiol Rev*, **2**: 285–314.

Forrer OB, Ellner PD, 1979, Distribution of hemolytic streptococci in respiratory specimens, *J Clin Microbiol*, **10**: 69–71.

Froude J, Gibofsky A et al., 1989, Cross-reactivity between streptococcus and human tissue: a model of molecular mimicry and autoimmunity, *Curr Top Microbiol Immunol*, **145**: 5–26.

Fry RM, 1938, Fatal infections by haemolytic streptococcus group B, *Lancet*, **1**: 199–201.

Gallagher PG, Watanakunakorn C, 1985, Group B streptococcal bacteremia in a community teaching hospital, *Am J Med*, **78**: 795–800.

Gann JW, Gray BM et al., 1987, Acute glomerulonephritis following group G streptococcal infection, *J Infect Dis*, **156**: 411–12.

Gaunt PN, Seal DV, 1987, Group G streptococcal infections, *J Infect*, **15**: 5–20.

Gerber MA, 1986, Diagnosis of group A beta-hemolytic streptococcal pharyngitis, use of antigen detection tests, *Diagn Microbiol Infect Dis*, **4**: 5S–15S.

Gerber MA, Randolph MF, DeMeo KK, 1990, Liposome immunoassay for rapid identification of group A streptococci directly from throat swabs, *J Clin Microbiol*, **28**: 1463–4.

Gossling J, 1988, Occurrence and pathogenicity of the *Streptococcus milleri* group, *Rev Infect Dis*, **10**: 257–85.

Gottschalk M, Higgins R et al., 1989, Description of 14 new capsular types of *Streptococcus suis*, *J Clin Microbiol*, **27**: 2633–6.

Granato PA, Petosa MT, 1991, Evaluation of a rapid screening test for detecting group B streptococci in pregnant women, *J Clin Microbiol*, **29**: 1536–8.

Green MA, Dashefsky B et al., 1993, Comparison of two antigen assays for rapid intrapartum detection of vaginal group B streptococcal colonization, *J Clin Microbiol*, **31**: 78–82.

Hanski E, Caparon M, 1992, Protein F, a fibronectin-binding protein, is an adhesin of group A streptococci, *Proc Natl Acad Sci USA*, **89**: 6172–6.

Harbeck RJ, Teague J et al., 1993, Novel, rapid optical immunoassay technique for detection of group A streptococci from pharyngeal specimens: comparison with standard culture methods, *J Clin Microbiol*, **31**: 839–44.

Hasty DL, Ofek I et al., 1992, Multiple adhesins of streptococci, *Infect Immun*, **60**: 2147–52.

Hauser AR, Stevens DL et al., 1991, Molecular analysis of pyrogenic exotoxins from *Streptococcus pyogenes* isolates associated with toxic shock-like syndrome, *J Clin Microbiol*, **29**: 1562–7.

Heiter BJ, Bourbeau PP, 1993, Comparison of the Gen-Probe group A streptococcus direct test with culture and a rapid streptococcal antigen detection assay for diagnosis of streptococcal pharyngitis, *J Clin Microbiol*, **31**: 2070–3.

Helmig R, Uldbjerg N et al., 1993, Clonal analysis of *Streptococcus agalactiae* isolated from infants with neonatal sepsis or meningitis and their mothers and from healthy pregnant women, *J Infect Dis*, **168**: 904–9.

Henrichsen J, Ferrieri P et al., 1984, Nomenclature of antigens of group B streptococci, *Int J Syst Bacteriol*, **34**: 500.

Hoffman S, 1990, Detection of group A streptococcal antigen from throat swabs with five diagnostic kits in general practice, *Diagn Microbiol Infect Dis*, **13**: 209–15.

Hogg SD, Manning JE, 1988, Inhibition of adhesion of viridans streptococci to fibronectin-coated hydroxyapatite beads by lipoteichoic acid, *J Appl Bacteriol*, **65**: 483–9.

Holls WM, Thomas J, Troyer V, 1987, Cervical Gram stain for rapid detection of colonization with β-streptococcus, *Obstet Gynecol*, **69**: 354–7.

Holm SE, Norrby A et al., 1992, Aspects of pathogenesis of serious group A streptococcal infections in Sweden, *J Infect Dis*, **166**: 31–7.

Hussain SM, Luedtke GS et al., 1995, Invasive group B streptococcal disease in children beyond early infancy, *Pediatr Infect Dis J*, **14**: 278–81.

Islam AKMS, Thomas E, 1980, Faecal carriage of group B streptococci, *J Clin Pathol* , **33**: 1006–8.

Jackson MA, Burry VF, Olson LC, 1991, Multisystem group A β-hemolytic streptococcal disease in children, *Rev Infect Dis*, **13**: 783–8.

Jelinková J, Motlová J, 1985, Worldwide distribution of two new serotypes of group B streptococci: type IV and provisional type V, *J Clin Microbiol*, **21**: 361–2.

Johnson DR, Kaplan EL, 1993, A review of the correlation of T-agglutination patterns and M-protein typing and opacity factor production in the identification of group A streptococci, *J Med Microbiol*, **38**: 311–15.

Johnson DR, Stevens DL, Kaplan EL, 1992, Epidemiologic analysis of group A streptococcal serotypes associated with severe systemic infections, rheumatic fever, or uncomplicated pharyngitis, *J Infect Dis*, **166**: 374–82.

Johnson KH, Zabriskie JB, 1986, Purification and partial characterization of the nephritis strain-associated protein from *Streptococcus pyogenes*, group A, *J Exp Med*, **163**: 697–712.

Jones DE, Friedl EM et al., 1983, Rapid identification of pregnant women heavily colonized with group B streptococci, *J Clin Microbiol*, **18**: 558–60.

Kass EH, 1971, Infectious diseases and social change, *J Infect Dis*, **123**: 110–14.

Kellog J, 1990, Suitability of throat culture procedures for detection of group A streptococci and as reference standards for evaluation of streptococcal antigen detection kits, *J Clin Microbiol*, **28**: 165–9.

Kern W, Kurrle E, Schmeiser T, 1990, Streptococcal bacteremia in adult patients with leukemia undergoing aggressive chemotherapy. A review of 55 cases, *Infection*, **18**: 138–45.

Kilpper-Bälz R, Schleifer KH, 1987, *Streptococcus suis* sp. nov., nom. rev., *Int J Syst Bacteriol*, **37**: 160–2.

Krasinski K, Hanna B et al., 1986, Penicillin tolerant group A streptococci, *Diagn Microbiol Infect Dis*, **4**: 291–7.

Lange K, Ahmed U et al., 1976, A hitherto unknown streptococcal antigen and its probable relation to acute poststreptococcal glomerulonephritis, *Clin Nephrol*, **5**: 207–15.

Lebrun L, Pillot J et al., 1982, Detection of human Fc (γ) receptors on streptococci by indirect immunofluorescence staining: a survey of streptococci freshly isolated from patients, *J Clin Microbiol*, **16**: 200–1.

Lim DV, Morales WJ, Walsh AF, 1987, Lim group B strep broth and coagglutination for rapid identification of group B streptococci in preterm pregnant women, *J Clin Microbiol*, **25**: 452–3.

Lim DV, Morales WJ et al., 1986, Reduction of morbidity and mortality rates for neonatal group B streptococcal disease through early diagnosis and chemoprophylaxis, *J Clin Microbiol*, **23**: 489–92.

Long PH, Bliss EA, 1934, Studies upon minute hemolytic streptococci. I. The isolation and cultural characteristics of minute beta hemolytic streptococci, *J Exp Med*, **60**: 619–31.

McCue JD, 1982, Group G streptococcal pharyngitis: analysis of an outbreak at a college, *JAMA*, **248**: 1333–6.

Manian FA, Chor P et al., 1992, Acute glomerulonephritis and encephalomyelitis following group G streptococcal bacteremia, *Clin Infect Dis*, **14**: 784–6.

Massell BF, Chute CG et al., 1988, Penicillin and the marked decrease in morbidity and mortality from rheumatic fever in the United States, *N Engl J Med*, **318**: 280–6.

Mastro TD, Farley TA et al., 1990, An outbreak of surgical-wound infections due to group A streptococcus carried on the scalp, *N Engl J Med*, **323**: 968–72.

Meleny FL, 1924, Hemolytic streptococcus gangrene, *Arch Surg*, **9**: 317–64.

Mohr DN, Feist DJ et al., 1979, Infections due to group C streptococci in man, *Am J Med*, **66**: 450–6.

Musser JM, Mattingly SJ et al., 1989, Identification of a high-virulence clone of type III *Streptococcus agalactiae* (group B

Streptococcus) causing invasive neonatal disease, *Proc Natl Acad Sci USA*, **86**: 4731–5.

Musser JM, Kapur V et al., 1993a, Geographic and temporal distribution and molecular characterization of two highly pathogenic clones of *Streptococcus pyogenes* expressing allelic variants of pyrogenic exotoxin A (scarlet fever toxin), *J Infect Dis*, **167**: 337–46.

Musser JM, Nelson K et al., 1993b, Temporal variation in bacterial disease frequency: molecular population genetic analysis of scarlet fever epidemics in Ottawa and in Eastern Germany, *J Infect Dis*, **167**: 759–62.

Natanson S, Sela S et al., 1995, Distribution of fibronectin-binding proteins among group A streptococci of different M types, *J Infect Dis*, **171**: 871–8.

Norrby A, Eriksson B et al., 1992, Virulence properties of erysipelas-associated group A streptococci, *Eur J Clin Microbiol Infect Dis*, **11**: 1136–43.

Noya FJD, Rench MA et al., 1987, Unusual occurrence of an epidemic of type Ib/c group B streptococcal sepsis in a neonatal intensive care unit, *J Infect Dis*, **155**: 1135–44.

Ortel TL, Kallianos J, Gallis HA, 1990, Group C streptococcal arthritis: case report and review, *Rev Infect Dis*, **12**: 829–37.

Pelletier LL Jr, Coyle M, Petersdorf R, 1978, Dextran production as a possible virulence factor in streptococcal endocarditis, *Proc Soc Exp Biol Med*, **158**: 415–20.

Persson K M-S, Forsgren A, 1987, Evaluation of culture methods for isolation of group B streptococci, *Diagn Microbiol Infect Dis*, **6**: 175–7.

Rantz LA, 1958, Hemolytic streptococcal infections, *Preventive Medicine in World War II. Vol. 4. Communicable Diseases transmitted chiefly through Respiratory and Alimentary Tracts*, Office of the Surgeon General, Washington DC, 229–57.

Reid TMS, 1975, Emergence of group B streptococci in obstetric and perinatal infections, *Br Med J*, **2**: 533–5.

Robinson JH, Kehoe MA, 1992, Group A streptococcal M proteins: virulence factors and protective antigens, *Immunol Today*, **13**: 362–7.

Ross PW, Cumming CG, 1982, Group B streptococci in women attending a sexually transmitted diseases clinic, *J Infect*, **4**: 161–6.

Roy S III, Stapleton FB, 1990, Changing perspectives in children hospitalized with poststreptococcal acute glomerulonephritis, *Pediatr Nephrol*, **4**: 585–8.

Ruoff KL, 1988, *Streptococcus anginosus* ('*Streptococcus milleri*'): the unrecognized pathogen, *Clin Microbiol Rev*, **1**: 102–8.

Ruoff KL, Ferraro MJ, 1987, Hydrolytic enzymes of '*Streptococcus milleri*', *J Clin Microbiol*, **25**: 1645–7.

Sahm DF, 1994, Streptococci and staphylococci: laboratory considerations for in vitro susceptibility testing, *Clin Microbiol Newslett*, **16**: 9–14.

Salata RA, Lerner PI et al., 1989, Infections due to Lancefield group C streptococci, *Medicine (Baltimore)*, **68**: 225–39.

Sandy EA, Blumenfeld ML, Iams JD, 1988, Gram stain in the rapid determination of maternal colonization with group B β-streptococcus, *Obstet Gynecol*, **71**: 796–8.

Scheld WM, Strunk RW et al., 1985, Microbial adhesion to fibronectin *in vitro* correlates with production of endocarditis in rabbits (42205), *Proc Soc Exp Biol Med*, **180**: 474–82.

Schlievert PM, 1993, Role of superantigens in human disease, *J Infect Dis*, **167**: 997–1002.

Schlievert PM, Gocke JE, Deringer JR, 1993, Group B streptococcal toxic shock-like syndrome: report of a case and purification of an associated pyrogenic toxin, *Clin Infect Dis*, **17**: 26–31.

Schnitzler N, Podbielski A et al., 1995, M or M-like protein gene polymorphisms in human group G streptococci, *J Clin Microbiol*, **33**: 356–63.

Schwartz B, Facklam RR, Breiman RF, 1990, Changing epidemiology of group A streptococcal infection in the USA, *Lancet*, **336**: 1167–71.

Schwartz B, Schuchat A et al., 1991, Invasive group B streptococcal disease in adults, *JAMA*, **266**: 1112–14.

Seppälä J, Nissinen A, et al., 1992, Resistance to erythromycin in group A streptococci, *N Engl J Med*, **326**: 292–7.

Silver RM, Heddleston LN, 1992, Life-threatening puerperal infection due to group A streptococci, *Obstet Gynecol*, **79**: 894–6.

Smith FR, Sherman JM, 1938, The hemolytic streptococci of human feces, *J Infect Dis*, **62**: 786–9.

Sotiropoulos SV, Jackson MA et al., 1989, Alpha-streptococcal septicemia in leukemic children treated with continuous or large dosage intermittent cytosine arabinoside, *Pediatr Infect Dis J*, **8**: 755–8.

Stamm AM, Cobbs CG, 1980, Group C streptococcal pneumonia: report of a fatal case and review of the literature, *Rev Infect Dis*, **2**: 889–98.

Spencer RC, Wheat PF et al., 1989, Erythromycin resistance in streptococci, *Lancet*, **1**: 168.

Stevens DL, 1992, Invasive group A streptococcus infections, *Clin Infect Dis*, **14**: 2–13.

Stevens DL, Tanner MH et al., 1989, Severe group A streptococcal infections associated with a toxic shock-like syndrome and scarlet fever toxin A, *N Engl J Med*, **321**: 1–7.

Stollerman GH, 1990, Rheumatogenic group A streptococci and the return of rheumatic fever, *Ann Intern Med*, **35**: 1–26.

Stryker WS, Fraser DW, Facklam RR, 1982, Foodborne outbreak of group G streptococcal pharyngitis, *Am J Epidemiol*, **116**: 533–40.

Thomas RJ, Conwill DE et al., 1988, Penicillin prophylaxis for streptococcal infections in United States Navy and Marine Corps recruit camps, 1951–1985, *Rev Infect Dis*, **10**: 125–30.

Turner JC, Hayden GF et al., 1990, Association of group C β-hemolytic streptococci with endemic pharyngitis among college students, *JAMA*, **264**: 2644–7.

Unsworth PF, 1989, Hyaluronidase production in *Streptococcus milleri* in relation to infection, *J Clin Pathol*, **42**: 506–10.

Wannamaker LW, 1970, Differences between streptococcal infections of the throat and of the skin, *N Engl J Med*, **282**: 23–31.

Wannamaker LW, 1979, Changes and changing concepts in the biology of group A streptococci and in the epidemiology of streptococcal infections, *Rev Infect Dis*, **1**: 967–73.

Wannamaker LW, Ayoub EM, 1960, Antibody titers in acute rheumatic fever, *Circulation*, **21**: 598–614.

Wessels MR, Kasper DL, 1993, The changing spectrum of group B streptococcal disease, *N Engl J Med*, **328**: 1843–4.

Wessels MR, Rubens CE et al., 1989, Definition of a bacterial virulence factor: sialylation of the group B streptococcal capsule, *Proc Natl Acad Sci USA*, **86**: 8983–7.

Whiley RA, Fraser H et al., 1990, Phenotypic differentiation of *Streptococcus intermedius*, *Streptococcus constellatus*, and *Streptococcus anginosus* strains within the '*Streptococcus milleri* group', *J Clin Microbiol*, **28**: 1497–501.

Whiley RA, Beighton D et al., 1992, *Streptococcus intermedius*, *Streptococcus constellatus*, and *Streptococcus anginosus* (the *Streptococcus milleri* group): association with different body sites and clinical infections, *J Clin Microbiol*, **30**: 243–4.

Whitnack E, 1993, Streptococci, *Mechanisms of Microbial Disease*, 2nd edn, eds Schaecter M, Medoff G, Eisenstein BI, Williams & Wilkins, Baltimore, 198–212.

Whitworth JM, 1990, Lancefield group F and related streptococci, *J Med Microbiol*, **33**: 135–51.

Willcox MDP, Knox KW, 1990, Surface-associated properties of *Streptococcus milleri* group strains and their potential relation to pathogenesis, *J Med Microbiol*, **31**: 259–70.

Wust J, Hebisch G, Peters K, 1993, Evaluation of two enzyme immunoassays for rapid detection of group B streptococci in pregnant women, *Eur J Clin Microbiol Infect Dis*, **12**: 124–7.

Yap HK, Chia KS, Murugasu B, 1990, Acute glomeruloneptritis – changing patterns in Singapore children, *Pediatr Nephrol*, **4**: 482–4.

Yoshizawa N, Oshima S et al., 1992, Role of a streptococcal antigen in the pathogenesis of acute poststreptococcal glomerulonephritis, *J Immunol*, **148**: 3110–16.

Zabriskie J, 1964, The role of temperate bacteriophage in the production of erythrogheic toxin by group A streptococci, *J Exp Med*, **119**: 761–7.

Chapter 16

BACTERAEMIA, SEPTICAEMIA AND ENDOCARDITIS

S J Eykyn

1 INTRODUCTION

Bacteria may enter the bloodstream, giving rise to **bacteraemia**, from an existing focus of infection, from a site with commensal flora, or by direct inoculation of contaminated material into the vascular system. These organisms are often cleared from the blood within minutes so that the bacteraemia is silent and transient, but if the immune system is overwhelmed or evaded, organisms persist in the blood, resulting in the symptoms and signs of **septicaemia**. The differentiation of septicaemia from bacteraemia, whilst theoretically attractive, is not a practical proposition. Although **septicaemia** (literally sepsis of the blood) implies a more serious clinical condition than **bacteraemia** (literally bacteria in the blood), in practice many clinicians and microbiologists use the terms interchangeably, confusing their students and others. The definitions are further complicated by the clinical description of a 'septicaemic' or 'septic' patient who clearly has a severe infection but from whose blood the laboratory staff fails to culture any bacteria. The 'sepsis syndrome' is increasingly used to describe patients severely ill from infection who may or may not have positive blood cultures, particularly in intensive therapy units (ITU), and this term has much to commend it. Traditionally the term **bacteraemia** referred to the transitory presence of bacteria in the blood of a patient in the absence of symptoms; the origin of the bacteria was usually from a site of commensal colonization. The term **septicaemia** meant the presence of bacteria in the blood with clinical signs and symptoms of infection. Their origin was from a focus of infection from which they entered the circulation. The distinction between bacteraemia and septicaemia is now largely ignored in the medical literature and, for the purposes of this chapter, the term bacteraemia will be

used. If the vascular endothelium is already damaged, most often in the heart, or the organism causing the bacteraemia has the necessary virulence factors, intravascular infection, usually **endocarditis**, may occur. Lastly, as a sequel to a persistent bacteraemia, metastatic (haematogenous) infection may arise at any site, although some bacterial species have a predilection (or tropism) for specific sites. Common sites to be seeded in this way are bones (especially the vertebrae in adults), joints and heart valves (usually previously normal). The condition of **pyaemia** (literally pus in the bloodstream), referring to bacteraemia with metastatic infection, is now rarely used and has a somewhat archaic connotation. The complex relationships between the sources and consequences of bacterial invasion of the bloodstream are outlined in Fig. 16.1.

The **clinical** condition of septicaemia is difficult to define precisely. The symptoms are characteristically

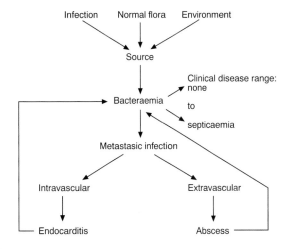

Fig. 16.1 The origins of bacteraemia and septicaemia.

non-specific, ranging from fever and malaise to over-whelming illness with profound toxaemia and rigors. Septicaemic patients are almost always febrile, some-times markedly so, although a minority, including some of the most gravely ill, may have a subnormal temperature. Patients with severe community-acquired bacteraemia caused by virulent pathogens may initially complain of muscle aches (myalgia) and gastrointes-tinal symptoms in addition to chills and fevers. A pro-portion of patients with clinical evidence of septi-caemia will develop circulatory collapse and hypotension. The main cause of this state of shock is loss of fluid from the circulation as plasma leaks through damaged capillary walls. Similar changes in the lungs lead to the respiratory distress syndrome with pulmonary oedema and hypoxia. Septicaemic patients usually have an initial leucocytosis; in over-whelming infection there may be leucopenia but with left shift and toxic granulation in the neutrophils. There may also be a consumptive coagulopathy, with a low platelet count and disordered clotting. Inadequate perfusion results in multi-organ failure with anuria, metabolic acidosis and jaundice. Without adequate support cardiac failure then occurs from hypoxia and acidosis. Patients may die from septicaemia, but their underlying condition at the time they acquired the infection is also an important predictor of a fatal out-come.

2 LABORATORY DIAGNOSIS

2.1 Blood culture

The rapid and reliable detection of bacteraemia by culturing the blood is one of the most important func-tions of a clinical microbiology laboratory. Whilst the demonstration of endotoxin in the blood of a patient infected with gram-negative organisms has been shown to be a good predictor of the development of the clinical syndrome of septicaemia (van Deventer et al. 1988), this is not routinely available. Although the basic objective of all blood culture methods, namely to recover small numbers of bacteria from the blood, is similar, actual blood culture practices vary and are almost idiosyncratic to each laboratory. Whatever sys-tem is used, it essentially comprises the aseptic collec-tion of blood from the patient, culture of this in a liquid medium, a means of detecting the presence of bacteria growing in the medium, and a final phase of subculture on a solid medium for identification and sensitivity testing.

TIMING OF COLLECTION OF BLOOD CULTURES

Bacteraemia can be continuous, intermittent or transi-ent and to obtain the maximum yield of organisms, blood should be collected at an appropriate time. With most bacteraemias the number of organisms in the blood varies with the temperature of the patient. The optimal time for blood culture is 1 h before the temperature rises with the next best time just as the

temperature starts to rise (Shanson 1989). Whenever possible blood for culture should be taken before anti-biotics are given. This will usually be when a patient has a high or persistent fever or complains of sweats or chills. Specific guidelines concerning preferred tim-ing of blood cultures are quite impractical and are not recommended.

PREPARATION OF THE SKIN BEFORE VENEPUNCTURE FOR BLOOD CULTURE

Before blood is withdrawn for culture, but after the vein has been located and palpated, the patient's skin must be cleaned and disinfected to minimize the risk of contamination with skin flora. Such contamination can be a major source of confusion in the interpret-ation of blood cultures. Stokes et al. (1993) recom-mend cleaning the skin with an isopropyl alcohol wipe and allowing it to dry thoroughly before vene-puncture; they also emphasize that the hands of the operator should be thoroughly washed and dried before the procedure. Some institutions recommend that the operator wear surgical gloves.

COLLECTION OF BLOOD FOR CULTURE

Blood is always collected with a sterile needle and syr-inge or with a proprietary sterile system of needle and evacuated tube or bottle of blood culture medium, for example, the Vacutainer System (Becton Dickinson). Indwelling intravascular catheters should not be used as the sole route for obtaining blood for culture because they become colonized with organisms that do not necessarily invade the bloodstream. However, blood from this source, even via different lumens of the catheter, is often used in conjunction with periph-eral venous samples to assess whether or not blood-stream invasion has occurred or whether there is only bacterial colonization of the catheter, particularly in febrile neutropenic patients.

CONTAMINATION OF BLOOD CULTURES; PSEUDOBACTERAEMIA

Contamination of some blood cultures is inevitable. Washington's survey (1992) found that only 15 (22%) of 67 participating international medical centres reported a contamination rate of less than 2%; an additional 24 (35%) reported rates of 2–5% and rates above 8% were not uncommon. Anecdotally at St Tho-mas' Hospital, there tends to be an increase in con-taminants when the new house staff arrive. In addition to contamination with normal skin flora, blood cul-ture systems can be contaminated from sources out-side the patient's bloodstream, creating what is known as **pseudobacteraemia**. This was first reported in 1968, but the term was not used extensively until much later when it replaced the entities of pseudosepticaemia and pseudosepsis. Pseudobacteraemia is under-reported; it can be very difficult to recognize and in some cases has taken months to identify and led to much clinical confusion. Most reports of pseudo-bacteraemia involve organisms that are unusual patho-gens, predominantly gram-negative bacteria such as coliforms and pseudomonads. Most of these are resistant to many antibiotics and antiseptics and readily survive in the environment. In their review of pseudobacteraemia, Jumaa and Chattopadhyay (1994) give a useful summary both of the bacteria isolated in reported episodes and of the sources of contamination. The latter include contaminated skin antiseptics, thrombin vials, blood gas analysers and penicillinase. A commonly encountered source of pseudobacteraemia is the initial inoculation of an aliquot of the blood drawn for culture into some other test bottle whose surface or contents (such as anticoagulant) is already contaminated. Examples include ESR bottles and blood gas machines. Such a practice is to be deprecated. Blood culture bottles must always be inoculated first. Pseudobacteraemia is largely preventable and the laboratory should keep a close check on blood culture results so that unusual organisms or patterns of isolation can be speedily reviewed.

NUMBER OF SETS OF BLOOD CULTURES

Washington's survey (1992) noted that clinical laboratories in the USA were more likely than those in Europe or Asia to recommend collection of more than one blood culture set per septic episode. The value of more than a single blood culture has been clearly established and the guidelines published by Aronson and Bor (1987) recommend obtaining 2 separate sets of blood cultures if the probability of septicaemia (i.e. bacteraemia) is high and the anticipated pathogen is not an organism regarded as normal skin flora. Additional blood cultures are recommended if the patient has received antibiotics or if the anticipated pathogen is an organism commonly regarded as a contaminant, for example, a coagulase-negative staphylococcus. In practice, it is clinicians, rather than microbiologists, who usually determine how many cultures are taken. In the UK at least, the majority of 'septic' patients have one set of blood cultures and those with suspected endocarditis have several.

VOLUME OF BLOOD FOR CULTURE

Since the number of bacteria in the blood in bacteraemia may be small, often about 1–2 ml^{-1}, sometimes less, it is not surprising that the volume of blood per culture is a major determinant of the bacterial yield, regardless of the blood culture system used. Most European laboratories and some in the USA in Washington's survey (1992) cultured 10 ml of blood though recommendations vary.

BLOOD CULTURE SYSTEMS; REQUIREMENT FOR BOTH AEROBIC AND ANAEROBIC BOTTLES

There are many possible methods for culturing bacteria from blood, both manual and semi-automated. Washington's survey (1992) showed that many different systems were used in clinical laboratories, probably reflecting market availability. It also showed that broth-based systems were frequently used in conjunction with other systems, particularly the lysis centrifugation method (Dupont Isolator System). This is a rapidly changing field with automated systems such as Bactec (Becton Dickinson) and Vital (bioMérieux) increasingly used; such systems detect, by different means, the carbon dioxide produced as the organisms metabolize the substrate in the medium. Further modifications to these systems are expected and thus a more detailed description of current systems will not be given here. Most laboratories with a heavy workload will require such systems, despite their capital cost, as they are efficient and labour saving. Conventional methods are nevertheless still used and have the advantage of flexibility and a larger volume of blood. Convention has always dictated, and with good reason, that both aerobic and anaerobic culture bottles should always be used, since few media are optimal for both strict aerobes and strict anaerobes. However, there has been a recent trend in some laboratories, in the USA at least, to limit the use of anaerobic blood cultures to patients undergoing colorectal or gynaecological surgery and trauma services, and to set up 2 aerobic bottles or systems on other patients. The incidence of anaerobic bacteraemia has markedly decreased in many medical centres; it accounted for only 1.5% of cases of clinically significant bacteraemia and fungaemia in the study reported by Roberts, Gaere and Coldman (1991). The decision to omit anaerobic cultures, or to limit them to selected cases, must be based on local information and needs. The advent of AIDS and the realization that disseminated mycobacterial infections, particularly *Mycobacterium avium-intracellulare* (MAI), was common in such patients led to the development of a specific mycobacterial blood culture bottle. Such cultures are indicated only in patients susceptible to this type of infection.

REMOVAL OF ANTIMICROBIAL AGENTS FROM THE BLOOD

Blood cultures are sometimes indicated when patients are already on systemic antibiotics and in such cases neutralization or inactivation of the antimicrobial is required. Simple dilution will contribute to this, but β-lactamases of the appropriate type can be added to remove some penicillins and cephalosporins; however, this addition is associated with an increased risk of contamination. If β-lactamase is used it should be tested simultaneously for sterility. Liquoid (sodium polyanethol sulphonate 0.05%), which is sometimes included in aerobic blood culture media, is antagonistic to some aminoglycosides and some media, including thiol broth, are antagonistic to other antibiotics. Devices that contain cation resin for the removal of antibiotics have given variable results and they are expensive.

DETECTION OF GROWTH AND LENGTH OF INCUBATION

The earlier bacteria are detected in blood cultures, the sooner the laboratory can provide the clinician with helpful information. This usually means the reporting of a gram-stained smear result, though with diphasic media and the Isolator more detailed initial information may be possible. With conventional broth blood cultures, turbidity or haemolysis initiates a gram stain and subcultures are performed at 24 and 48 h and usually at 1 week. Automated systems flag up growth, either, as with the newer systems, by continuous monitoring, or when the bottles are monitored, usually twice a day. Whilst the information that a gram-negative bacillus has been detected in the aerobic bottle may be useful clinically, information about gram-positive cocci in clumps is of no help at all; on the balance of probabilities they are much more likely to be coagulase-negative staphylococci (and hence probably contaminants) than *Staphylococcus aureus* and there is no quick reliable method of knowing which. What clinicians want is the identity of the organism and its antimicrobial susceptibility pattern. This takes longer, though in some instances direct tests on the blood culture bottle contents to detect bacterial antigens, such as Pneumotex for pneumococci or direct Lancefield groups for streptococci or enterococci, can provide a rapid identification. Weak or non-specific reactions may lead to confusion. The clinical microbiologist wants, on the one hand, to provide information about positive blood cultures as soon as possible but, on the other hand, is only too aware of the clinical frustrations of what is viewed as incomplete information. Furthermore, a verbal report of 'gram-positive cocci in clumps, probably staphylococci' is all too often (mis)interpreted as 'presumptive *S. aureus*'. With conventional systems a terminal subculture is performed before the broths are discarded at 5–7 days and most (though not all) of the organisms causing bacteraemia would be recovered within this time. Terminal subcultures are seldom done on bottles with negative readings in automated systems; this assumes that all microbes can be detected by the system, which is not always so. Certain fastidious organisms, particularly those that occasionally cause endocarditis such as *Haemophilus* spp., *Actinobacillus actinomycetemcomitans* and *Cardiobacterium hominis*, can take longer than a week to grow, but extended incubation must be specifically requested in suspected endocarditis as it is not cost-effective to prolong routinely the incubation time for all blood cultures.

3 BACTERAEMIA

3.1 Frequency

It is conventional to express the incidence of bacteraemia as the number of episodes per 1000 patient admissions. Inevitably medical centres vary in their definitions of a bacteraemic episode and in their evaluation of blood cultures yielding coagulase-negative staphylococci; the number and mix of hospital admissions also varies. It is therefore hardly surprising that the reported rates of bacteraemia are variable; in Washington's survey (1992) these varied from 2 to 100, approximately one-third of the reporting centres exceeding 20 cases per 1000 admissions. In this study the rates among US hospitals that included clinical evaluation for defining a septic episode were similar

(11, 13 and 17, respectively) and fell within the range of those reported in the UK (5–18 per 1000 admissions). There is little doubt that the incidence has increased over the past 3 decades; in St Thomas' Hospital, over the 25 year period 1970–94, it has increased from 3.8 to 8.8 episodes per 1000 admissions in a series of over 6000 prospectively documented episodes.

3.2 Causative organisms

In Washington's survey (1992) the rank order of the 10 most frequent organisms causing bacteraemia varied, both nationally and internationally. *Escherichia coli* was the most frequent isolate in European and Asian medical centres but in none of the participating USA centres. In most centres coagulase-negative staphylococci were more common than *S. aureus*. Enterococci were more common in the USA than elsewhere. MAI was among the 10 most frequently encountered organisms in 2 USA centres. Inevitably the list of bacteraemic isolates will vary according to the type of hospital and the patients it admits. Information about the frequency of isolation of particular organisms from all cases of bacteraemia is thus really of only limited interest. For a detailed examination of the pathogenesis and epidemiology of these infections, and consideration of their treatment with antimicrobial agents, it is necessary to distinguish infections acquired in the community from those that arise in hospital or result from infected devices (usually intravascular) inserted in hospital that might best be classified as hospital (or device)-associated infections. The last decade has seen a sizeable increase in people with long-term intravenous access who either administer their drugs at home, or who attend hospital, usually as out-patients. Such patients include, amongst others, oncology patients and patients dialysing via intravenous lines. The pathogens in all these patients are fundamentally different from those seen in patients with true community-acquired infections. Unfortunately not all papers on bacteraemia recognize this and consider bacteraemia as a homogeneous entity. Hospital-acquired infections, often referred to as nosocomial infections, are largely iatrogenic (see 'Hospital acquired bacteraemia', p. 284). Although some studies have analysed community- and hospital-acquired bacteraemias separately, for example, the Nottingham study (Ispahani, Pearson and Greenwood 1987) and the Colorado study (Weinstein et al. 1983), there seem to be no published studies that analyse these data from one centre over a long time; such data are available for St Thomas' Hospital and will be referred to as the STH study. Table 16.1 lists the commonest organisms isolated from episodes of community-acquired bacteraemia in St Thomas' Hospital during the 1970s, 1980s and the first half of the 1990s. Table 16.2 provides similar information for episodes of hospital-acquired bacteraemia. Since the data were all collected prospectively, they are likely to be more accurate than a retrospective analysis.

Table 16.1   Organisms isolated in community-acquired bacteraemia at St Thomas' Hospital 1970–95

	1970–79 (665 episodes) (%)	1980–89 (1088 episodes) (%)	1990–95 (977 episodes) (%)
Gram-positive organisms			
Streptococcus pneumoniae	25.3	19.1	14.0
Staphylococcus aureus	10.8	8.8	7.6
CN staphylococci	0.1	0.8	1.0
Oral streptococci	6.3	6.0	4.1
Streptococcus milleri group	2.2	2.4	0.8
Streptococcus pyogenes	2.0	2.0	3.2
Group B streptococci	1.5	1.5	2.7
Group G streptococci	0.8	1.4	1.3
Group C streptococci	0.1	0.2	0.2
Enterococcus spp.	1.7	1.1	3.0
Streptococcus bovis	1.0	1.1	1.0
Listeria monocytogenes	0.7	1.0	0.3
	(52.5)	(45.4)	(39.2)
Gram-negative organisms			
Escherichia coli	22.2	27.1	26.1
Klebsiella spp.	3.2	3.4	4.1
Proteus spp.	2.0	3.9	2.2
Pseudomonas aeruginosa	1.5	1.3	2.4
Enterobacter spp.	0.4	0.3	1.0
Citrobacter spp.	0.4	0.5	0.3
Salmonella spp.	3.4	2.3	3.0
Shigella spp.	0.1	0.1	–
Campylobacter spp.	0.1	0.2	0.7
Haemophilus spp.	3.0	4.5	2.7
Neisseria meningitidis	4.0	1.9	2.4
Neisseria gonorrhoeae	1.5	0.2	0.2
	(41.8)	(45.7)	(45.1)
Anaerobes	3.6	6.1	3.7
Yeasts	–	–	0.8
Mycobacterium spp.	–	0.1	6.9
Others	2.5	2.7	4.3

CN, coagulase-negative.

COMMUNITY-ACQUIRED BACTERAEMIA

The proportion of bacteraemias acquired in the community in a particular medical centre depends on its type and the patients that it admits. In the USA, two-thirds of bacteraemias were community-acquired at a community hospital (Schekler 1977), whereas only a third were community-acquired in the Colorado study. In the UK, nearly 60% of episodes in the Nottingham study were community-acquired, whereas in the STH study the figure was only just over 40%; this proportion has not altered over 25 years. Community-acquired bacteraemia frequently occurs in previously healthy people and, perhaps paradoxically, is often more severe than hospital-acquired bacteraemia and more often than not is caused by organisms sensitive to many antibiotics. Many cases occur in association with demonstrable infection at a local site from which the organisms enter the bloodstream, as in pneumococcal pneumonia or a coliform urinary or biliary tract infection. In other community-acquired bacteraemias,

the bacteria enter the blood from some (usually undetected) site and subsequently produce metastatic (haematogenous) infection, as in staphylococcal osteomyelitis. Still other bacteraemias are generalized septicaemic illnesses *ab initio*, such as enteric fever, brucellosis and meningococcaemia. These latter infections may (but frequently do not) result in localized metastatic infection.

The organisms responsible for community-acquired bacteraemia most often come from the patient's own commensal flora, for example *S. aureus*, *E. coli* and *Streptococcus pneumoniae*, though it is not always clear why they become invasive. Pathogens may also be acquired from other people, animals or environmental sources. Often the organisms isolated from the blood will also be present at a local site of infection. The bacteria most frequently isolated in community-acquired bacteraemias are *E. coli*, *S. pneumoniae* and *S. aureus*. This pattern has been the same for 25 years, although as Table 16.1 shows, *S. pneumoniae* accounts

Table 16.2 Organisms isolated in hospital-acquired bacteraemias at St Thomas' Hospital 1970–95

	1970–79 (866 episodes) (%)	1980–89 (1409 episodes) (%)	1990–95 (1285 episodes) (%)
Gram-positive organisms			
Staphylococcus aureus (MRSA)	21.0 (0)	19.0 (0.5)	17.5 (1.1)
CN staphylococci	2.4	10.9	15.7
Streptococcus pneumoniae	3.4	1.4	2.6
Streptococcus pyogenes	1.8	0.4	0.7
Group B streptococci	1.5	1.0	0.7
Group G streptococci	0.3	0.4	0.7
Group C streptoccoci	0.5	0.1	0.2
Oral streptococci	0.8	1.7	1.2
Streptococcus milleri group	0.6	1.0	0.7
Enterococcus spp.	3.1	5.9	7.7
Streptococcus bovis	0.3	0.2	0.1
	(35.7)	(42.0)	(47.8)
Gram-negative organisms			
Escherichia coli	20.1	19.2	12.0
Klebsiella spp.	10.1	8.7	6.0
Proteus spp.	6.1	5.4	3.7
Pseudomonas aeruginosa	9.0	7.7	9.7
Enterobacter spp.	2.4	2.7	4.8
Serratia spp.	0.5	1.1	1.1
Acinetobacter spp.	0.8	0.4	1.0
Citrobacter spp.	0.7	1.0	1.4
Pseudomonas spp.	2.0	0.2	0.3
	(51.7)	(46.4)	(40.0)
Anaerobes	7.2	4.4	3.6
Yeasts	1.4	1.7	2.4
Others	4.0	5.5	6.2

CN, coagulase-negative; MRSA, methicillin-resistant *Staphylococcus aureus*.

for fewer episodes in the 1990s (14%) than it did in the 1970s (25.3%) as does *S. aureus* (7.6% versus 10.8%). By contrast, the proportion accounted for by *E. coli* has remained the same, or even marginally increased (22.2% versus 26.1%). The commonest 3 pathogens have accounted for a decreasing proportion of episodes at STH over 25 years: 58% in the 1970s, 55% in the 1980s and 48% in the 1990s. This difference is at least in part explained by the increasing incidence of mycobacterial bacteraemia, usually, but not exclusively, MAI, which in the 1990s reached 6.9%. This incidence is linked to the number of HIV-positive patients who attend the hospital. The 3 commonest organisms will be considered in more detail.

Escherichia coli The commonest cause of community-acquired bacteraemia, and in Europe of all bacteraemia, is *E. coli*; it accounted for 26.1% of community-acquired episodes in the 1990s at STH, for 28% in the Nottingham study and for 22% in the Colorado study. About 60% of these episodes result from urinary tract infections and a urinary focus is even more likely in women (72.7% episodes at STH) than men (39.3%). Bacteraemic urinary tract infections have a variety of clinical presentations ranging from the classical symptoms of acute pyelonephritis (usually in young women) to rather non-specific illness, often without symptoms referable to the urinary tract, in elderly or diabetic patients, again predominantly female. In elderly men community-acquired bacteraemic urinary tract infections usually occur in association with retention of urine or other obstructive pathology. The second most common focus of infection for community-acquired *E. coli* bacteraemia is the biliary tract, usually associated with cholelithiasis and occasionally local malignancy. These infections accounted for about 15% of episodes at STH. Other foci include the gastrointestinal tract and vertebral osteomyelitis.

E. coli, whatever its focus of infection, originates from the patient's colonic flora. The commonest serogroups of *E. coli* in order of frequency are O6, O2, O4, O1, O18 and O75 but many others are found (Gransden, Eykyn and Phillips 1990b). Whether the predominance of certain O serogroups in urinary tract infections reflects their uropathogenicity or their prevalence in the colonic flora is uncertain. In any event, outbreaks of infection caused by particular strains of *E. coli* have rarely been recognized either in the community or in hospitals. However, in 1986–87, a community-based epidemic of infection with a multiresistant *E. coli* O15 occurred in south-east London.

This was mainly manifest as urinary tract infection, which in many cases was severe and accompanied by bacteraemia. The infecting epidemic strain was resistant to ampicillin, amoxycillin, trimethoprim, sulphonamide, tetracycline and chloramphenicol (Phillips et al. 1988). In STH, some 45% of strains of *E. coli* isolated from the bloodstream in community-acquired infections are currently resistant to ampicillin and amoxycillin and 20% to trimethoprim.

Streptococcus pneumoniae Pneumococci are second only to *E. coli* as a cause of community-acquired bacteraemia; they accounted for 13% of episodes in the Nottingham study and 16% in the Colorado study. In STH they now account for only 14% of episodes compared with 25.3% in the 1970s. All 3 studies confirm that the majority of cases of pneumococcal bacteraemia (and indeed of all pneumococcal infection) are acquired in the community. Most cases are associated with respiratory tract infection, usually pneumonia. Meningeal infection occurs in a small number of cases of community-acquired pneumococcaemia, 7.7% in the STH study; this figure was lower than that in 2 earlier reports from the UK (Young 1982, Gruer, McKendrick and Geddes 1984) and lower than the 17% found by Kuikka et al. (1992) in Finland. Patients with pneumococcaemic meningitis often also have pneumonia. Foci of infection other than the respiratory tract or the meninges are rare.

In some patients with pneumococcaemia, no focus of infection is found. Such cases include, at one end of the spectrum, the overwhelming bacteraemia (usually fatal) that occasionally occurs in patients who have had a splenectomy for disease or trauma, or who are functionally asplenic from sickle cell disease, and, at the other end of the spectrum, cases of 'occult pneumococcaemia', a condition seen in young children, usually under 2 years, who present with what is thought to be a viral respiratory infection, sometimes with a febrile convulsion, and are later found to have pneumococci in a blood culture. Pneumococcaemia without focal disease was first described by Belsey in 1967, and has subsequently been referred to as occult bacteraemia which seems an appropriate term. Occult pneumococcaemia appears to be more frequent, or probably more frequently recognized, in the USA and Finland than in the UK where reports of the condition are rare and few paediatricians are aware of it. This may reflect different paediatric practice: UK general practitioners would be most unlikely to do a blood culture on a febrile child and only those children referred to hospital would thus have a blood culture. The nationwide study from Finland of all invasive pneumococcal infections in children from 1985 to 1989 detected 310 cases of occult pneumococcaemia in a total of 452 episodes (69%) (Eskola et al. 1992). This study also reported the serogroups of the pneumococci and found that type 14 was the commonest cause of occult bacteraemia in young children and our own small study (22 cases seen at STH since 1970) also had a preponderance of type 14. This type was the commonest type seen in pneumococcaemia

(other than occult) at all ages in the 500 cases seen at STH; types 3, 8 and 1 were the next most common in adults, but types 1 and 3 were rarely seen in children. Although pneumococcaemia can occur in previously healthy people, it is now more commonly seen in those with underlying disorders such as bronchopulmonary disease or, increasingly, alcoholism and HIV infection.

Staphylococcus aureus Community-acquired bacteraemia due to *S. aureus* occurs with moderate frequency; the incidence was 11.4% in the Nottingham study and 12.2% in the Colorado study. In STH, it was 7.6% in the 1990s, a slight decrease from that found in the 1980s (8.8%) and the 1970s (10.8%). Community-acquired methicillin-resistant *S. aureus* (MRSA) bacteraemia has not been detected at STH and is rarely seen in the UK. Sometimes community-acquired *S. aureus* bacteraemia arises from a local tissue infection that is obvious to the clinician, and in such cases, which are uncommon, the bacteraemia is 'secondary' to the local infection. In other cases there is no obvious local site of infection or only a trivial site (which may be detected retrospectively) yet the patient is unwell, sometimes with marked systemic disturbance. In such cases the staphylococcus has gained access to the blood via the skin lesion (or simply from the skin) and the resultant bacteraemia has been called 'primary'. This designation is confusing as it implies that the staphylococci have appeared in the blood *de novo*. The staphylococci in the blood then localize at a particular site and the commonest sites are bone, joint and heart valves with others such as the respiratory tract and perinephric abscess much less common. Bone or joint infections accounted for 36% of cases of community-acquired *S. aureus* bacteraemia seen at STH.

The pattern of haematogenous staphylococcal osteomyelitis has changed over the past 30 years: acute ostetomyelitis of the long bones, which used to be seen in young children, usually boys, has become much less common, whereas the incidence of haematogenous vertebral osteomyelitis has dramatically increased and is most common in the elderly (Espersen et al. 1991). In STH, the percentage of episodes of staphylococcal bacteraemia associated with vertebral osteomyelitis was only 1.2% in the 1970s, but 5.6% in the 1980s and 13.3% in the 1990s. In staphylococcal vertebral osteomyelitis, the isolation of *S. aureus* from blood cultures is frequently the first indication that the patient's neckache or backache has an infective aetiology. Staphylococcal septic arthritis is less common than osteomyelitis. It can occur in previously healthy people but is even more likely in patients with pre-existing joint pathology, such as rheumatoid arthritis; in such patients more than one joint may be affected and the diagnosis can be very difficult because the symptoms are usually attributed to the underlying disease. The relevance of *S. aureus* in the blood culture may not be appreciated. Second only to bone or joint as the focus of infection in community-acquired staphylococcaemia is endocarditis (21% in the STH series) and this is considered in detail in section 4 (p. 287). Other foci of infection are much less common.

Other organisms These are uncommon individually, but some may cause particularly severe infections. Remarkably in STH in the 1990s, *Mycobacterium* spp., mostly MAI, acccounted for almost as many episodes of community-acquired bacteraemia as *S. aureus* (6.9% versus 7.6%). Any hospital microbiology laboratory that serves a large HIV-positive population will be aware of the need to set up mycobacterial cultures in these patients. Amongst other gram-positive aerobes we detected a small increase in *Streptococcus pyogenes* bacteraemia in the 1990s and there has been a well documented increase in severe *S. pyogenes* infections in many countries since the mid-1980s. Many of these severe infections are caused by M1 and M3 strains and occur in previously healthy people. Various other streptococci, mostly of the 'viridans' type, also cause community-acquired bacteraemia and many of these patients will have infective endocarditis. There was an increase in *Listeria monocytogenes* bacteraemia during the 1980s, much of which resulted from contaminated pâté and unpasteurized cheese. Even then, listeriosis, despite intense publicity, remained a rare infection and its incidence has now decreased. Gram-negative bacteraemias include infections with various salmonellas, occasional coliforms other than *E. coli*, a decreasing number of cases of *Haemophilus* spp. (the result of Hib vaccination) and *Neisseria meningitidis*, which occasionally causes a devastating septicaemic illness, usually in children and young adolescents. It should be noted that in many cases of meningococcal meningitis, bacteraemia is not detected. Anaerobes account for only a small proportion of episodes (3.7% in STH in the 1990s).

It is thus evident that whereas many community-acquired bacteraemias are caused by microbes that are also common causes of hospital-acquired infections (e.g. *E. coli* and *S. aureus*), others, such as *S. pneumoniae*, are seldom acquired in hospital and yet others, such as *N. meningitidis*, are never acquired in hospital.

HOSPITAL-ACQUIRED BACTERAEMIA

As might be expected, the incidence of hospital-acquired bacteraemia varies according to the type of institution studied and is highest in tertiary care centres such as teaching hospitals and others with large numbers of 'complicated' patients. Technological advances and, in particular, invasive procedures, have brought a concomitant increase in hospital-acquired bacteraemia. Whereas in the 1970s, more episodes were caused by gram-negative aerobes than gram-positive organisms, in the subsequent years the situation has changed and gram-positive bacteria, mainly staphylococci, are now more common. This increase has mainly involved the coagulase-negative staphylococci whose incidence in STH has risen from 2.4% in the 1970s to 15.7% in the 1990s, whereas the incidence of *S. aureus* has decreased from 21% in the 1970s to 17.5% in the 1990s. There has also been a steady increase in enterococcal infections. The commonest organisms will be considered in more detail.

Gram-positive aerobes

Coagulase-negative staphylococci There has been a dramatic increase in coagulase-negative staphylococcal bacteraemia in hospital practice over the past decade and in some hospitals they are the commonest bacteria isolated. They also remain the commonest contaminants isolated from blood cultures; in some cases it is difficult to determine their clinical relevance. Most episodes of coagulase-negative staphylococcal bacteraemia occur in patients on adult ITUs, in premature babies on neonatal units and in haematological (usually neutropenic) and oncological patients (many of whom are at home whilst receiving chemotherapy with Hickman lines in situ); almost all are associated with intravascular lines. Respiratory colonization with coagulase-negative staphylococci is also common in premature babies on neonatal units and this may result in respiratory infection and associated bacteraemia. Since these babies usually also have intravenous lines, they, rather than the respiratory tract, probably pre-empt the bacteraemia. There has been a tendency in the past to refer (without further investigation) to coagulase-negative staphylococci as *S. epidermidis* (*sensu lato*) but speciation, which can now be readily performed in routine laboratories, shows that although *S. epidermidis* (*sensu stricto*) is indeed the commonest species of coagulase-negative staphylococcus, it accounted for 75% of the cases at STH, other species are also seen, and at STH *S. haemolyticus* was the commonest of these (12.3%). Hospital-acquired coagulase-negative staphylococci are frequently multiresistant and methicillin-resistant.

Staphylococcus aureus In the STH series, *S. aureus* was, with *E. coli*, the commonest isolate in hospital-acquired bacteraemia in the 1970s (21.0% and 20.1%, respectively) and 1980s (19.0% and 19.2%, respectively). In the 1990s the incidence of *E. coli* fell (12.0%) and *S. aureus* was the most common isolate (17.5%), though it was only marginally more common than the coagulase-negative staphylococci. It accounted for fewer episodes (about 10%) in the Nottingham and Colorado studies. Such differences may be explained by the numbers of patients on haemodialysis, a notorious cause of *S. aureus* infections. In contrast to community-acquired staphylococcaemia, hospital-acquired infections are nearly always secondary to infection at a local site, by far the commonest of which is a vascular access site. A small but significant proportion of patients with intravascular lines subsequently develop endocarditis. The other main site of infection in hospital-acquired *S. aureus* bacteraemia is a surgical wound. Such infections usually occur after 'clean' surgical operations and include sternal wound sepsis after cardiothoracic surgery as well as abdominal wound infections after caesarean section (and not always emergency sections) and hysterectomy.

Enterococcus spp. In parallel with the large increase in coagulase-negative staphylococcal bacteraemia, there has been an increase in enterococcal bacteraemia. In STH enterococci accounted for 7.7% of episodes in the 1990s, but some hospitals, usually those with specialized renal and liver units, have seen an even greater increase. As with the coagulase-negative staphylococci, many of the enterococcal bacteraemias are associated with intravascular lines and sometimes both microbes are isolated from such infections. These enterococci include not only *Enterococcus faecalis* and *Enterococcus faecium*, but also occasionally other species. Strains can be vancomycin-resistant, ampicillin and amoxycillin-resistant, resistant to high-level gentamicin and sometimes resistant to all. The use of large quantities of cephalosporins and ciprofloxacin as well as vancomycin itself may well encourage selection of such strains.

Gram-negative organisms

Escherichia coli The commonest gram-negative organism isolated from hospital-acquired bacteraemia remains *E. coli* although its incidence is decreasing. In about half (52% in STH series) the episodes of *E. coli* bacteraemia the organism originated in the urinary tract; in about half (46% in STH series) these, urethral manipulation, such as a change of catheter or a bladder washout, or instrumentation, such as cystoscopy or urethral dilatation, were involved. In such cases the urine is almost always already infected and it is the manipulation that causes the bacteraemia. Other foci of infection include the biliary tract (9.3%) where, again, manipulation such as endoscopic retrograde cholangiopancreatography (ERCP) or stenting can be the triggering factor, and the gastrointestinal tract (13.2%). Many gram-negative aerobic bacilli cause infection of intravascular lines yet, curiously, *E. coli*, the commonest gram-negative bacillus isolated from the blood, very seldom causes these infections. In the STH series, only 8 of 712 (1.1%) episodes of hospital-acquired bacteraemia from intravascular lines were caused by *E. coli*. Although multiresistant strains are seen, most *E. coli* acquired in hospital have similar antibiotic sensitivity patterns to strains acquired in the community. The predominant serogroups are also similar to those seen in community-acquired bacteraemia but a wider variety of serogroups were encountered. All these organisms originate in the patient's bowel flora.

Other gram-negative bacilli These organisms are individually much less common than *E. coli*. Many species cause bacteraemia in hospital patients; the commonest are the pseudomonads, mostly *Pseudomonas aeruginosa* (9.7% of all hospital-acquired bacteraemias in STH in the 1990s), *Klebsiella* spp. (6.0%), *Enterobacter* spp. (4.8%) and *Proteus* spp. (3.7%). The incidence of *Enterobacter* spp., *Serratia* spp., *Acinetobacter* spp. and *Citrobacter* spp. has increased over the past decade and is probably linked to increased prescribing of cephalosporins. Over all, enterobacteria other than *E. coli* account for about 20% of hospital-acquired bacteraemia (21.1% in STH in the 1990s; 19.9% in the Nottingham study and 19.4% in the Colorado study). In common with *E. coli*, the greater proportion of other enterobacterial bacteraemias also arise from the urinary tract (35.3% in STH series) but a significant proportion (18.2% in STH series) are associated with infected intravascular lines. *P. aeruginosa*, in common with the enterobacteria, is also frequently associated with urinary tract infection, but this incidence (24.1% in the STH series) was less than for enterobacteria; the incidence of infected intravascular lines was similar. *Pseudomonas* spp. bacteraemias (and this includes those genera that were previously classified as *Pseudomonas* spp. such as *Comamonas*, *Stenotrophomonas*, *Burkholderia* and *Shewanella*) are most frequently associated with infected intravascular lines.

Other organisms Anaerobic bacteraemia has decreased in incidence; in the STH series, it was highest in the 1970s (7.2%), fell to 4.4% in the 1980s, and was 3.6% in the 1990s. This decrease is almost certainly the result of the widespread use of effective anti-anaerobic prophylaxis for dirty and contaminated surgery. Yeast bacteraemia has increased; it almost always results from infected intravascular lines and is most often seen in patients on the ITU. Such patients have always received, or often are still receiving, broad spectrum antibiotics. Although most isolates are *Candida albicans*, an increasing number of other species are encountered, some of which, for example *Candida glabrata*, are resistant to fluconazole which is one of the most widely used systemic antifungal agents. Cross-infection with these yeasts has also been a problem in some ITUs.

3.3 Outcome

Although it is possible to quote an 'overall' mortality rate for bacteraemic patients, or mortality rates according to the infecting organism, such data are, with few exceptions, of limited value. The outcome of bacteraemic infection depends on both the virulence of the pathogen and the underlying condition of the patient at the onset of the bacteraemia. It is unusual for a patient to die directly and solely as a result of bacteraemia, that is from sepsis, but when this does occur the infection is much more likely to be community-acquired than hospital-acquired. The more recent published series of bacteraemia have analysed mortality rates according to whether the death was or was not directly related to the bacteraemia (Weinstein et al. 1983, Ispahani, Pearson and Greenwood 1987). Older series, which tended to concentrate on gram-negative bacteraemia, analysed mortality rates according to the underlying condition of the patient: McCabe and Jackson (1962) categorized their patients' underlying disease as 'rapidly fatal', 'ultimately fatal' or 'non-fatal'. DuPont and Spink (1969) divided their patients into those with a good prognosis, those with a poor prognosis who were not expected to recover from their primary disease during their hospital admission, and an intermediate group. In their study of 860 patients with bacteraemia due to gram-negative aerobic bacilli, the mortality rate for patients with a good prognosis was 23%, for those with an intermediate prognosis it was 62% and for those with a poor prognosis it was 88%. The much larger series from STH (Eykyn, Grandsen and Phillips 1990,

Gransden, Eykyn and Phillips 1990a) which has been in operation continuously from 1970, categorizes patients with bacteraemia (at the time of the positive blood culture) according to the the the same criteria as Dupont and Spink (1969); the mortality rates for patients with community- and hospital-acquired bacteraemia for this period are shown in Table 16.3, analysed according to underlying prognosis and whether or not death was directly attributable to the bacteraemia. In the STH series, the overall mortality for patients with a good prognosis was 4.1% and it was higher for community-acquired infections (5.2%) than for those acquired in hospital (1.8%). This difference can be explained by the innate virulence of some of the pathogens acquired in the community. For patients with an intermediate prognosis the overall mortality was 15.1% and again it was higher for community-acquired infections (18.4% versus 13.1%). The patients with a poor prognosis had the highest overall mortality (62.5%), slightly higher for the community-acquired infections (68.9% versus 60.2%). In the STH study and the Nottingham and Colorado studies, deaths were also assessed as to whether they were directly related to the bacteraemia (i.e. to sepsis *per se*) or to other factors in addition to the bacteraemia. The overall mortality rate at STH was 20.6%, but that directly related to bacteraemia was only 5.8%. Somewhat higher figures were reported from the Nottingham study in which the total death rate was 28.8% and that related to bacteraemia was 19.5%. In the Colorado study, patients who developed bacteraemia in hospital were more likely to die as a result of infection than those with community-acquired infection (24% versus 13%) and deaths that were not directly related to bacteraemia were more than 6 times as common in hospital-acquired infections as in those acquired in the community (17% versus 2.5%) but the patients' underlying prognosis was not differentiated. The figures from the STH study are rather different; here the total mortality was similar for hospital- and community-acquired infections (22.1% versus 18.7%) but the mortality directly related to infection was 3 times higher in community-acquired infections than in those acquired in hospital (9.4% versus 3.1%). The mortality related to underlying disease plus bacteraemia was higher (14.8%) and this was twice as high

in hospital-acquired infections as in those acquired in the community (19.0% versus 9.3%).

It is clear from the data shown that patients with a good prognosis at the time they become bacteraemic seldom die of infection and when they do, the infection is much more likely to have been acquired in the community than in the hospital. Fatal community-acquired bacteraemia is caused by virulent pathogens such as *N. meningitidis*, *S. pyogenes* and *S. aureus*. There has been a decrease in fatal community-acquired bacteraemia in healthy people since the STH records began in 1970; whereas in the 1970s, 18 (3.9%) of 302 patients died of their infection, in the 1990s, 9 (2.3%) of 290 did. This decrease undoubtedly relates to advances in ITU management; it is nothing to do with antibiotics. Deaths directly related to hospital-acquired bacteraemia in patients with a good prognosis have always been very uncommon but there were no cases at STH in the 1990s.

Septic shock

Septic shock, sometimes known as bacteriogenic shock, has a high mortality rate, perhaps 40–60%; it is characterized by the 'sepsis syndrome' plus hypotension that is not explained by hypovolaemia or cardiac causes. Although a patient with septic shock has clinical evidence of infection, there may or may not be a bacteraemia and 30–60% of patients with septic shock have negative blood cultures. The confusion with the terms bacteraemia and septicaemia has already been discussed (p. 277); throughout this chapter bacteraemia has been used to signify a positive blood culture from a patient with clinical evidence of infection. The term septicaemia now seems to have been largely discarded and the 'sepsis syndrome' introduced to identify patients with a generalized systemic response (i.e. evidence of infection plus tachycardia, tachypnoea and hyper- or hypothermia) plus evidence of organ dysfunction. Septic shock refers to a subset of patients with the sepsis syndrome who also have hypotension not explained by hypovolaemia or cardiac causes. This terminology is further complicated by the entity known as the 'systemic inflammatory response syndrome' (SIRS), a rather broad description that encompasses non-infective conditions such as pancreatitis and burns that can mimic bacterial sepsis.

Table 16.3 Mortality for patients with bacteraemia St Thomas' Hospital 1970–95

	All patients			Good prognosis			Intermediate prognosis			Poor prognosis		
	Total	Died (%)	DB (%)	Total	Died (%)	DB (%)	Total	Died (%)	DB (%)	Total	Died (%)	DB (%)
All	6294	1298 (20.6)	368 (5.8)	1562	64 (4.1)	57 (3.6)	3635	548 (15.1)	222 (6.1)	1097	686 (62.5)	89 (8.1)
C-A	2731	511 (18.7)	258 (9.4)	1067	55 (5.2)	49 (4.6)	1368	252 (18.4)	148 (10.8)	296	204 (68.9)	61 (20.6)
H-A	3563	787 (22.1)	110 (3.1)	495	9 (1.8)	8 (1.6)	2267	296 (13.1)	74 (3.3)	801	482 (60.2)	28 (3.5)

C-A, community-acquired; H-A, hospital-acquired; DB, died of infection (bacteraemia).

What is clear is that once shock and organ failure occur in a septic patient, the mortality is very high despite intensive care.

The pathogenesis of septic shock involves both microbial virulence and host factors. For many years it was thought that shock was caused by gram-negative bacteria and it was often referred to as 'gram-negative shock' or 'endotoxic shock'. In fact, septic shock is as likely to be caused by gram-positive bacteria as gram-negative and may be polymicrobial. Bacteria produce a variety of extracellular and cell wall constituents which stimulate the immune system to produce inflammatory mediators that bring about septic shock. The subject is well reviewed by Sriskandan and Cohen (1995). In shock caused by gram-negative organisms, bacterial endotoxin or lipopolysaccharide (LPS) binds to a number of different carrier molecules and the resultant complex then interacts via cell surface molecules with host monocytes and endothelial cells. Superantigenic bacterial toxins such as staphylococcal toxic shock toxin-1 (TSST-1) and streptococcal pyrogenic exotoxin A (SPEA) cause profound hypotension, inflammation and organ failure in animal models and the strains of *S. aureus* and *S. pyogenes* that express these toxins cause the staphylococcal and streptococcal toxic shock syndrome in man. These toxins trigger T lymphocyte activation and proliferation with release of cytokines. Other extracellular products of bacteria such as pore-forming exotoxins are able to disrupt immune cell membrane integrity. The host immune system is stimulated by infection and, in an attempt to combat this, produces numerous proinflammatory mediators which assist the target cells in eradicating the pathogen. Modulating and anti-inflammatory mediators are released simultaneously and if the balance is inappropriate the host may suffer harmful consequences. Thus, host factors produced in response to infection can produce deleterious effects and contribute to the pathogenesis of septic shock. Attempts have been made to treat patients with septic shock with monoclonal antibodies against LPS and tumour necrosis factor (TNF) but these have not been shown to be beneficial.

3.4 Antibiotic susceptibility of isolates and approaches to treatment of bacteraemia

Most reported studies on bacteraemia give little or no information concerning the antibiotic susceptibility of the causative microbes. In the STH study (Phillips et al. 1990) multiresistant bacteria were uncommon and when they did occur it was almost exclusively in hospital-acquired infections. Most of these resistant organisms were enterobacteria other than *E. coli*, and they were isolated from patients who were receiving (or had recently received) β-lactam antibiotics. Multiresistant gram-positive bacteria include both *S. aureus* and coagulase-negative staphylococci, but in most UK hospitals the latter are more common. The antibiotic sensitivity of the causative microbe will rarely be known early enough to provide definitive guidance on the **initial** treatment of a bacteraemic patient; this must be based on the prediction of the likely pathogen and its usual sensitivity to antibiotics. The microbiologist should always be able to provide information about the antibiotic sensitivity patterns of common microbes. Few could object to broad spectrum combinations for initial treatment of a septic patient but they can seldom be justified as definitive therapy. There will often be important clues to the identity of the pathogen when the blood culture is taken. In many patients with community-acquired bacteraemia a local site of infection such as the urinary tract or (less often) the respiratory tract can be sampled directly at the time of the blood culture and the likely pathogen defined, or the clinical history and signs will indicate the site of infection as with biliary tract, respiratory tract or gastrointestinal tract infections and the probable pathogen can be predicted. In hospital-acquired bacteraemia, too, there are also often useful clues to the site of infection such as postoperative wounds or intravascular access sites. Sometimes in bacteraemia associated with urinary catheterization or instrumentation, a recent specimen of urine may already have been cultured before the patient became bacteraemic. However, occasionally there are no obvious clues and then the nature of the pathogen is less easily predicted.

Once a significant pathogen has been isolated from the blood and its antibiotic sensitivity known, definitive treatment should be given and this should rarely require more than 2 antibiotics, and usually one. The in vitro testing of combinations of antibiotics for synergy has little place in a routine laboratory and there is scant evidence that such synergy results in more appropriate treatment of bacteraemic patients except in enterococcal endocarditis. The results of such tests are seldom available in time to influence the choice of antibiotics and their results are not always reproducible. Nor is there any evidence that estimation of the serum bactericidal titre against the causative pathogen is of any value in the management of infection.

4 INFECTIVE ENDOCARDITIS

In infective endocarditis (IE) there is infection, almost always bacterial, of the endocardium, generally of a heart valve or valves, but sometimes on septal defects or other congenital abnormalities. The advent of intracardiac prostheses over 30 years ago brought the realization that these, too, or strictly the tissues into which they are sewn, can also become infected. The terminology used to describe what has universally come to be known as **infective endocarditis** has changed. The old term 'bacterial endocarditis' excludes fungal and other non-bacterial causes of the disease and is generally best avoided, as is the traditional classification of the disease as 'acute', 'subacute' (still referred to by many doctors as 'SBE' and used indiscriminately for any case of endocarditis) and 'chronic' endocarditis; this classification is largely of historical interest because it related to the usual course of untreated disease. The acute form was a fulminating infection, usually caused by *S. aureus, S. pneumoniae, S. pyogenes* or *N. gonorrhoeae*, and it resulted in the death of the patient in less than 6 weeks, sometimes in days. These infections occurred in patients without a previous cardiac abnormality. The subacute form of the disease resulted in death after 6 weeks to 3 months, and the chronic form after 3 months or more. The indolent forms of the disease were usually caused by 'viridans' streptococci and occurred in patients with damaged heart valves. Although the general concept of acute and subacute endocarditis can sometimes be helpful, it is important to realize that many organisms do not fit neatly into one or other category, that an increasing number of patients with subacute disease do not have known heart disease, and that patients with an acute clinical presentation may have valvular disease. Furthermore, endocarditis caused by 'viridans' streptococci can present acutely, usually because the diagnosis has been delayed or missed. Whilst a classification based on the nature of the causative pathogen is frequently used, even this is not ideal as other factors are also important. In this chapter the following classification will be used: **native valve endocarditis**, **prosthetic valve endocarditis** and **endocarditis in intravenous drug users (IVDU)**. Most cases of IE are acquired in the community but there is now an increasing number of cases of **hospital-acquired (nosocomial) endocarditis** and this can affect both native and prosthetic valves. It usually results from surgery or other invasive procedures. Table 16.4 gives details of organisms isolated from patients with IE seen at STH from 1970 to 1995 according to these categories. Although most cases of IE are caused by a fairly limited number of pathogens, heart valves, and in particular prosthetic valves, can become infected with just about any microbe or fungus; the bigger the series the greater will be the variety encountered.

Although many patients have definite IE on clinical, pathological, echocardiographic and other grounds, in others it is much less clear, yet they still may be treated for the disease. Attempts have been made to produce hard diagnostic criteria. von Reyn et al. (1981) introduced the categories of 'definite', 'probable' and 'possible' IE but their 'definite' category relied on direct evidence from histology or microbiology at surgery or autopsy. Echocardiography was not widely available then. Their 'definite' catgory was too restrictive. Over a decade later Durack et al. (1994) proposed new criteria of 'definite' and 'possible' IE based on a much more comprehensive assessment that included clinical and echocardiographic findings and these have gained widespread acceptance.

4.1 Incidence of infective endocarditis

Infective endocarditis is an uncommon disease. Scheld and Sande (1995), in a review of 10 large American series, quote a frequency of about one case per 1000 hospital admissions with a range of 0.16–5.4 cases per 1000 admissions. In the STH study (1970–95) IE was diagnosed in about 5% of episodes of bacteraemia. There has been no prospective national study of IE in the UK since that conducted in 1981–82 (Bayliss et al. 1983b) which reported 544 episodes in the 2 year period. It has been estimated that there are about 1000 cases of IE per annum in the UK, that is 20 cases per million population (Young 1987); thus, there is likely to have been a considerable shortfall in the reporting of cases in the prospective study. A more recent prospective survey from the North East Thames Region (population 3.375 million), in which every effort was made to contact all physicians and hospitals, gave an annual incidence of 22 cases per million (Skehan, Murray and Mills 1988). In Europe, a recent prospective national study from the Netherlands (population 14.5 million) detected 438 cases in 2 years, giving an

Table 16.4 Distribution of infecting organisms in community- and hospital-acquired native and prosthetic valve endocarditis St Thomas' Hospital 1970–95

Organism	Native valve endocarditis (320)			Prosthetic valve endocarditis (72)		
	Community-acquired (277)	Hospital-acquired (43)	Total	Community-acquired (40)	Hospital-acquired (32)	Total
Oral (viridans)						
Not speciated	9	0	9	4	0	4
S. oralis/S. mitis	45	0	45	8	1	9
S. sanguis/S. gordonii	44 (1 IVDU)	0	44	6	0	6
S. mutans	13	0	13	0	0	0
S. salivarius	6	0	6	1	0	1
S. morbillorum (now reclassified to *Gemella*)	0	0	0	1	0	1
S. acidominimus	1 Σ118	0	1	0 Σ20	0	0
Other streptococci						
'S. milleri group'	8 (1 IVDU)	0	8	0	0	0
S. bovis	17	0	17	0	0	0

Table 16.4   Continued

Organism	Native valve endocarditis (320)			Prosthetic valve endocarditis (72)		
	Community-acquired (277)	Hospital-acquired (43)	Total	Community-acquired (40)	Hospital-acquired (32)	Total
Streptococcus pneumoniae	9	1	10	0	0	0
Group B streptococci	11	1	12	0	0	0
Group G streptococcus	1 Σ12	0	1	0	0	0
Enterococci						
E. faecalis	16	0	16	1	0	1
E. durans	1	0	1	0	0	0
E. avium	1 Σ18	0	1	0	0	0
Staphylococci						
S. aureus	59 (17 IVDU)	26 (IVDU)	85	3	13	16
Coagulase-negative staphs						
S. epidermidis	9	7	16	0	3	3
S. hominis	3	0	3	0	0	0
S. capitis	0	1	1	1	0	1
S. simulans	1	0	1	0	0	0
S. lugdunensis	1	0	1	1	1	2
S. caprae	1	0	1	0	0	0
Unclassifiable CN staphs	0	1	1	0	0	0
Micrococcus sedentarius	0 Σ15	0 Σ9	0 Σ24	0	1	1
Others						
Corynebacterium spp.	1	1	2	1	5	6
Lactobacillus rhamnosus	1	0	1	0	0	0
Listeria monocytogenes	0	0	0	1	0	1
Erysipelothrix rhusiopathiae	0	0	0	1	0	1
Rhodococcus sp.	0	0	0	1	0	1
Haemophilus parainfluenzae	2	0	2	2	0	2
Haemophilus aphrophilus	2	0	2	0	0	0
Haemophilus sp.	1	0	1	0	0	0
Cardiobacterium hominis	1	0	1	0	0	0
Campylobacter fetus	0	0	0	1	0	1
Actinobacillus actinomycetemcomitans	0	0	0	3	0	3
Brucella melitensis	0	0	0	1	0	1
Escherichia coli	3 (1 IVDU)	0	3	1	0	1
Proteus mirabilis	0	1	1	0	0	0
Actinetobacter spp.	0	1	1	0	1	1
Pseudomonas aeruginosa	0	0	0	0	1	1
Pseudomonas picketii	0	0	0	0	3	3
Coxiella burnetii	6	0	6	2	0	2
Chlamydia psittaci	2	0	2	0	0	0
Bartonella sp.	1	0	1	0	0	0
Fungi						
Candida albicans	0	2	2	0	2	2
Candida sp.	0	0	0	0	1	1
Aspergillus sp.	0	1	1	0	0	0
Histoplasma capsulatum	1	0 Σ21	1	0 Σ14	0	0

CN, coagulase-negative; IVDU, intravenous drug user; Σ, totals.

annual incidence of 15 cases per million person-years. When this incidence was adjusted for age and sex the incidence was 19 per million person-years (van der Meer et al. 1992a). There is a well recognized increased incidence of IE with age, and over all the infection is more common in males than females. A study from 3 French regions detected 386 cases in a year, giving an annual incidence of 23 cases per million (Delahaye et al. 1992).

The population at risk for IE has changed, at least

in affluent countries, in the post-antibiotic era; rheumatic heart disease has largely disappeared whereas degenerative heart disease has increased as have, in certain areas, the number of IVDUs. There is also an increasing number of patients with prosthetic heart valves.

4.2 Native valve infective endocarditis: community-acquired

IE may develop on a native heart valve that was previously normal or one that is abnormal as a result of congenital malformation or acquired disease. Congenital abnormalities that predispose to IE include bicuspid aortic valves, mitral leaflet prolapse (MLP) (with a murmur) and, less often, septal defects. Patients with bicuspid aortic valves and those with MLP, and their doctors, may be unaware of the abnormality until IE occurs. The predominant cause of acquired valvular abnormality was formerly rheumatic heart disease, but increasingly now it is degenerative heart disease secondary to atherosclerosis which is frequently undetected until IE develops. Fifty years ago native valve IE was mainly a disease of young people: in Cates and Christie's study (1951) of 442 cases of 'subacute bacterial endocarditis' seen between 1945 and 1948, 62% of patients were aged between 15 and 35 years. Since then native valve IE has become a disease of the middle-aged and elderly.

Streptococcal and enterococcal endocarditis

Two-thirds of cases of community-acquired native valve IE are caused by streptococci or enterococci: 214 of 326 (65.6%) in the Dutch series and 182 of 277 (65.7%) in the STH series. However, streptococcal and enterococcal IE cannot be considered as a homogeneous entity since both the pathogenesis of the infection and the disease itself differ according to the species responsible. The largest group are the oral streptococci which are usually referred to as the 'viridans' streptococci because most produce α-haemolysis (greening) on blood agar; these will be considered first.

Oral ('viridans') streptococci

For many years these streptococci were known as '*Streptococcus viridans*' and this inaccurate though convenient designation is still used by some clinicians. This bacterial grouping includes a number of different species, some of which have undergone recent taxonomic changes as a result of the application of chemotaxonomic and molecular techniques in microbial systematics. These taxonomic changes are well reviewed by Hardie and Whiley (1994), but it seems that further reclassification of some species is inevitable. The oral streptococci include *S. oralis* (previously *S. mitior*), *S. sanguis* (some strains previously included in this species have now been reclassified as *S. gordonii*), *S. mitis*, *S. mutans* and *S. salivarius* as well as some others. In Parker and Ball's study (1976) of streptococci associated with systemic disease,

the oral streptococci so defined accounted for about two-thirds of the 317 streptococci isolated from the blood in IE, presumably mostly native valve disease though not specified. In the Dutch study (van der Meer et al. 1991), 125 of the 190 (66%) cases of native valve streptococcal IE were caused by the oral streptococci listed above and the figures for STH were virtually identical (108 of 164, 65.9%). The predominant species of oral streptococci are *S. oralis* and *S. sanguis*. Many of the oral streptococci seldom cause bacteraemic infection other than IE; this is particularly true of *S. mutans*, which does not cause infection elsewhere in the body. Thus, the presence of these organisms in blood cultures, particularly in more than one set, should raise the possibility of IE as this diagnosis may not always be obvious clinically. A recent report of the identification of 47 strains of oral streptococci from cases of IE found that 31.9% were *S. sanguis*, 29.8% *S. oralis* and 12.7% *S. gordonii*. Other species were much less common (Douglas et al. 1993).

Although bacteraemia is an essential component of the pathogenesis of streptococcal IE, the valvular endothelium must first be changed by blood turbulence or other factors which result in the deposition of platelets and fibrin; this has been called non-bacterial thrombotic endocarditis. Streptococci reaching the site via the bloodstream then adhere to and colonize the site, producing vegetations. The transient bacteraemia has been generally assumed to result from dentistry, particularly dental extractions, in the 3 months before the onset of symptoms. Such a history is only obtained in a minority of cases, although many, perhaps most, have dental sepsis or caries. Most studies have relied on retrospective analyses of patients' notes which do not always include information on their dental health. Patients with poor oral hygiene undoubtedly suffer repeated bacteraemia with oral streptococci whilst chewing or brushing their teeth; these procedures may induce bacteraemia in people with good oral hygiene. Cates and Christie (1951) in their study of 'subacute bacterial endocarditis' 40 years ago found that only 12.3% of their 187 cases of 'viridans' streptococcal IE had had a tooth extraction less than 3 months before the onset of symptoms, whereas 34.8% had dental sepsis or caries. More than 30 years later, Bayliss et al. (1983a) reported a similar incidence of 13.7% of cases occurring within 3 months of a dental procedure. Our findings at STH were similar and 18% of our patients with IE were edentulous. Even if there is no overt dental focus it can still be assumed that the oral streptococci have originated in the mouth. Transient bacteraemia with oral streptococci may also follow procedures such as tonsillectomy or adenoidectomy and (rarely) bronchoscopy or gastroscopy, but there is no evidence that these procedures result in IE. Although oral streptococci account for only one-third of bacteraemias after dental trauma (Rogosa et al. 1960), they cause virtually all the cases of IE that follow these procedures.

The different species of oral streptococci differ in their habitat and in their propensity to cause IE. *S. salivarius*, for example, is found mainly on the mucosa of the tongue and is an infrequent cause of IE. The rest of the oral streptococci are found mainly on dental surfaces. Of these, *S. mutans* and *S. sanguis* produce dextran that contributes to the formation of dental plaque, which accounts for the close adherence of bacteria to the tooth surface. Dextran production may be a virulence factor in the pathogenesis of IE, but since not all species of streptococci that cause IE are dextran producers (including most strains of *S. oralis*, one of the commonest of the oral streptococci to cause IE), other factors must also be involved. Platelet aggregation is also important in the development of vegetations and certain oral streptococci, particularly *S. sanguis*, have been shown to aggregate platelets.

The *Streptococcus milleri* group

There are currently 3 recognized species that are conveniently referred to as the *S. milleri* group, *S. anginosus*, *S. constellatus* and *S. intermedius*. There are significant differences in the distribution of these species in man (Hardie and Whiley 1994). Although such speciation within the *S. milleri* group is now possible, many authors still refer to these strains as *S. milleri*; indeed, in the past they were often misidentified as anaerobic streptococci since on initial isolation they tend to prefer anaerobic conditions. In any event, organisms of the *S. milleri* group seldom cause native valve IE. The Dutch study (van der Meer et al. 1991) is the only published series with data on species within the group. In a total of 326 cases of native valve IE they reported 12 cases of *S. intermedius* and 3 of *S. constellatus* (interestingly no *S. anginosus*), giving an overall incidence for the *S. milleri* group of 4.6%. This is similar to the 2–5% incidence in the 5 reports quoted by Douglas et al. (1993) although they included prosthetic infections as well as native. The incidence of IE at STH in native valve disease was 2.9% of 277 cases, but speciation of the responsible streptococci was available in only 2 cases (one *S. intermedius*, one *S. constellatus*). Unlike the 'viridans' streptococci, the *S. milleri* group are commonly isolated from septic lesions at a variety of sites, including abscesses of internal organs such as the liver and brain, either in pure culture or more commonly in polymicrobial infections with anaerobes. However, *S. milleri* group IE does not occur in association with such septic conditions; it seems to be an entirely separate entity. There are indications that IE caused by these organisms tends to be a more acute and severe infection that that usually associated with the 'viridans' streptococci.

Streptococcus bovis

S. bovis was as common as *S. sanguis* and *S. mitior* (*oralis*) as a cause of streptococcal IE (valves not specified) in Parker and Ball's (1976) series in which it was responsible for 15.8% of 317 cases and for nearly a quarter of the cases in patients over 55 years. In the Dutch study it caused 7.7% of 326 cases of native valve IE, a similar figure to STH where 6.1% of 277 cases of native valve IE were caused by *S. bovis*. The disease it produces is similar to that caused by 'viridans' strep-

tococci. In the past the organism was often misidentified as *Enterococcus* (previously *Streptococcus*) *faecalis* since the 2 species are biochemically quite similar. The advent of streptococcal identification kits such as the API 20 Strep (bioMérieux) and the Rapid ID 32 Strep (bioMérieux), which are commonly used in many laboratories, has made accurate speciation of *S. bovis* much easier. Two biotypes of *S. bovis* are described, of which biotype I (dextran-producing, mannitol-fermenting) is the more common in IE. They are conveniently considered together.

S. bovis is a bowel organism and is seldom found in the mouth. In 1977, Klein et al. reported 2 patients with *S. bovis* endocarditis and adenocarcinoma of the colon. Since then others have noted an association between *S. bovis* bacteraemia and not only colonic cancer but also polyposis and other gastrointestinal disorders. In their study of 90 cases of *S. bovis* bacteraemia during 1951–80, Hønberg and Gutschik (1987) identified 15 patients (17%) with gastrointestinal cancer and concluded that there was a high frequency of neoplasms in patients with a history of *S. bovis* bacteraemia, particularly in those with IE, even several years after the episode of bacteraemia. Leport et al. (1987), in a study of 77 cases of group D streptococcal endocarditis, found a significantly higher frequency of colonic polyps and neoplasms in patients with *S. bovis* endocarditis than in those with enterococcal endocarditis and they emphasized the need for colonoscopy in any patient with *S. bovis* endocarditis.

Streptococcus pneumoniae

In the pre-antibiotic era, *S. pneumoniae* accounted for about 10% of cases of IE (Scheld and Sande 1995) but it is now rarely seen. Only 5 cases (1.5%) of native valve pneumococcal endocarditis were reported in the Dutch series and at STH there were 9 cases (3.2%), more than half of which were postmortem diagnoses. The pneumococcus causes an acute fulminating infection, generally on a previously normal valve. Pneumococcal IE tends to occur in alcoholics and these patients usually have concomitant pneumonia and meningitis. The pneumococcus clearly originated in the patient's respiratory tract.

Pyogenic streptococci

β-Haemolytic pyogenic streptococci of Lancefield groups A, B, C and G occasionally cause endocarditis, usually attacking normal valves. The group B streptococci (*S. agalactiae*) are by far the most common and their incidence has recently increased. At STH they accounted for 4% of cases of native valve endocarditis and for a similar number in the Dutch series (2.8%). Although group B streptococci have a well recognized though unexplained predilection for diabetics, most cases of IE do not occur in diabetic patients. They are aggressive pathogens and, as in staphylococcal IE (see 'Staphylococcal endocarditis', other sites of infection are often found; these include septic arthritis, vertebral osteomyelitis, meningitis and endophthalmitis. Group G streptococci are more commonly seen than either group A or C; there were 5 cases in the Dutch series (1.5%) but only one at STH (0.4%). Like the group B strains, the other pyogenic streptococci also cause acute destructive disease.

Enterococci

Enterococci, still known by many clinicians as *Streptococcus faecalis*, account for about 7% of cases of native valve IE; in the Dutch series they acounted for 7.4% of 326 cases and at STH for 6.5% of 277 cases. Most cases are caused by *Enterococcus faecalis* (20 of 24 in the Dutch series, 16 of 18 at STH) but there are occasional cases of other species such as *E. faecium*, *E. durans* and *E. avium*. Although uncommon, enterococcal endocarditis is more difficult to treat than streptococcal endocarditis because enterococci are intrinsically more resistant to antibiotics than streptococci; the recent emergence of high-level gentamicin resistance and vancomycin resistance in enterococci has rendered IE with such strains virtually untreatable with antibiotics alone. Some 40% of patients with enterococcal IE have no previous history of heart disease or murmurs (Scheld and Sande 1995); it is thus presumed that enterococci can attack normal heart valves but this remains unproven. Enterococcal endocarditis is most commonly seen in elderly men, many of whom have had genitourinary infection, urinary tract or other manipulation or trauma in the preceding 3 months. Enterococci are normal inhabitants of the gastrointestinal tract; they are also occasionally found in the urethra and they may cause urinary tract infection, particularly after instrumentation. Enterococcal bacteraemia has been reported after colonoscopy, proctoscopy, sigmoidoscopy and barium enema. Enterococcal endocarditis has only very rarely followed such procedures although they are frequently performed.

STAPHYLOCOCCAL ENDOCARDITIS

Staphylococci now account for nearly 30% of community-acquired native valve IE (26.7% at STH) and they are also an important cause of hospital-acquired IE (see section 4.3, p. 293). Most of these staphylococci are *S. aureus*, but an increasing proportion are now coagulase-negative staphylococci.

Staphylococcus aureus

Some 80% of the staphylococci isolated from cases of community-acquired native valve IE are *S. aureus*. This organism attacks normal or abnormal valves, producing severe fulminating infection; valvular destruction with abscess formation may occur within days. The infection arises from a bacteraemia which itself arises from a trivial septic lesion or, usually, with no detectable local lesion. The disease begins with quite nonspecific 'flu-like symptoms, often with gastrointestinal upset and meningism. The cerebrospinal fluid usually contains polymorphs but is generally sterile on culture. Heart murmurs are seldom present initially unless there was a previous cardiac abormality. The physician is thus confronted with a toxic ill patient with *S. aureus* in the blood without localizing signs except possibly for meningitis but the cerebrospinal

fluid proves sterile. In about a quarter of cases the urine will contain both pus cells and staphylococci, the result of microabscesses in the kidney, and this can lead to further diagnostic confusion. This, the classical presentation of staphylococcal endocarditis, was accurately described over a century ago by William Osler in his Gulstonian lectures on 'malignant endocarditis' (1885) but it still seems largely unknown to many clinicians. There is nothing 'subacute' about *S. aureus* endocarditis; it is a devastating infection in which diagnostic delay may result in death. Any patient who is unwell with a *S. aureus* bacteraemia but no obvious site of infection should be assumed to have IE and treated accordingly. Native valve IE with *S. aureus* may occur at any age but is more common in the middle-aged and elderly; it occurs in the previously healthy as well as in those with underlying diseases such as diabetes. *S. aureus* is also the commonest cause of IE in intravenous drug users (IVDU) (see section 4.5, p. 294).

Coagulase-negative staphylococci

Although still regarded by many as pathogens of prosthetic rather than native valves, coagulase-negative staphylococci also cause native valve infection and this has become more common, or certainly more commonly recognized, since the early 1980s (Etienne and Eykyn 1990). In the STH series, coagulase-negative staphylococci accounted for 5.4% of community-acquired native valve IE and the Dutch series reported a similar incidence (4.9%) but did not specify whether the infections were community- or hospital-acquired. The infecting species is most often *S. epidermidis* (*sensu stricto*); this species accounted for about 60% of cases in the Dutch series and at STH. However, in many reports the designation *S. epidermidis* tends to be used for any unspeciated coagulase-negative staphylococcus. Many other species have been reported to cause native valve IE, including *S. hominis*, *S. lugdunensis*, *S. simulans*, *S. warneri*, *S. capitis*, *S. caprae* and *S. sciuri*. Coagulase-negative staphylococci are normal inhabitants of the skin and different species vary in their distribution throughout the body. Thus, it seems likely that native valve coagulase-negative staphylococcal IE is an endogenous infection. Sometimes a presumptive predisposing (usually very minor) skin lesion can be detected but often there is none, a situation akin to that in IE caused by *S. aureus*. Most patients have a pre-existing cardiac abnormality. Although the clinical presentation of coagulase-negative staphylococcal IE can be similar to that caused by 'viridans' streptococci (i.e. 'subacute'), it is becoming increasingly clear that these organisms, and particularly *S. lugdunensis* (Vandenesch et al. 1993) but also other species, can be aggressive pathogens producing an infection similar to that produced by *S. aureus* and they may express similar virulence factors.

OTHER ORGANISMS

A small proportion of cases (6.1% in the Dutch series, 7.6% at STH) of community-acquired native valve IE are caused by organisms other than streptococci, enterococci or staphylococci. A wide variety of microbes is found, including some that are fastidious and slow to grow on primary isolation from blood cultures or that cannot readily be isolated on conventional culture media. They include species that have a predilection for the heart valve and rarely cause infections other than IE, as, for example, those known as the HACEK group (*Haemophilus aphrophilus*, *H. paraphrophilus*, *Actinobacillus actinomycetemcomitans*, *Cardiobacterium hominis*, *Eikenella corrodens* and *Kingella kingae*), whose isolation from blood cultures is virtually diagnostic of IE. Anaerobes that are found in large numbers in the normal mouth, in the mouth with dental caries and which are the predominant flora of the bowel, have rarely been reported to cause endocarditis. No case was seen in the Dutch series or at STH, yet according to Felner and Dowell (1970) non-streptococcal anaerobic bacteria accounted for 1.3% of cases of IE and some other authors have reported a higher incidence, especially in IVDUs and polymicrobial infections (Dorsher, Wilson and Rosenblatt 1989). All members of the HACEK group of organisms form part of the normal upper respiratory commensal flora. In the STH series, *Coxiella burnetii* (Q fever) accounted for 2.2% of community-acquired native valve IE and endocarditis is a recognized, though rare (and very late) sequel of acute *C. burnetii* infection. Most infections occur in middle-aged men with pre-existing heart disease. The reservoir of the organism in the UK is sheep and cattle but the source and mode of transmission of many human cases is unknown. In contrast to most other cases of IE, the diagnosis is usually made serologically although *C. burnetii* can be recovered on culture with special techniques. In view of this it is likely that *C. burnetii* endocarditis is underdiagnosed and some cases labelled 'culture-negative' endocarditis. Other organisms occasionally causing IE that cannot be isolated in routine laboratories include *Chlamydia* spp. and the more recently recognized *Bartonella* (lately *Rochalimaea*) spp.

4.3 Native valve endocarditis: hospital-acquired

Increasing use of intravascular devices (IVD) has brought a parallel increase in associated bacteraemia and such devices are now the commonest cause of hospital-acquired bacteraemia. Occasionally such bacteraemias result in endocarditis, sometimes on a previously normal heart valve. Endocarditis has resulted from infected peripheral venous, central venous and pulmonary artery catheters and from intracardiac pacemakers. In their review of 21 cases of endocarditis associated with central venous catheterization Tsao and Katz (1984) found that two-thirds of cases had right-sided infection, suggesting a parallel with the animal model in which catheter-induced traumatic sterile vegetations become infected after bacteraemia. In fact, although IVD-related bacteraemia may result in right-sided endocarditis, the infection is not invariably right-sided. In most but not all cases the IVD will have been in situ for some time, often many weeks. In STH, 13.4% of all cases of native valve IE

were hospital-acquired and most of these were attributable to infected IVDs. Many of these patients were undergoing haemodialysis and endocarditis has long been recognized as a complication of haemodialysis (Goodman et al. 1969, King et al. 1971). Staphylococci are the predominant microbes, usually *S. aureus*. Fungal IE can also result from infected IVDs with *Candida* spp. the most usual pathogens. The STH series included a case of *Acinetobacter* sp. endocarditis in a severely burned patient and IE has been called 'a silent source of sepsis in the burn patient' (Baskin, Rosenthal and Pruitt 1976). Endocarditis in burned patients results from infected IVDs and associated thrombophlebitis (Srivastava and MacMillan 1979). It has been suggested that burned patients are potentially more susceptible to IVD-associated endocarditis because of their hyperdynamic state and the hypercoagulability of their blood (Ehrie et al. 1978).

Hospital-acquired endocarditis can result from procedures other than IVDs and these include cardiac catheterization and genitourinary instrumentation.

4.4 Prosthetic valve endocarditis

Prosthetic valve endocarditis (PVE) is an uncommon but potentially disastrous complication of cardiac valve replacement; intracardiac prostheses are inherently more susceptible to bacterial colonization than native heart valves. The risk of an individual patient developing PVE at any particular time is difficult to determine from reported studies of PVE. As Rutledge, Kim and Applebaum (1985) pointed out, to cite a frequency of PVE of 4% as most studies do is not very valuable; it does not differentiate between times of high risk (early onset PVE <60 days postoperation) and low risk (late onset PVE >60 days postoperation) and it depends on the length and completeness of the follow-up. It is more useful to give the number of episodes of PVE per number of patient-days at risk and they reported a frequency of 5.9 episodes per 1000 patient-years. If a patient survived the early postoperative period without developing PVE then the frequency was 3.7 per 1000 patient-years. They found, using actuarial techniques, that the patient was at greatest risk of contracting PVE during the first 150 days after the operation; after this the risk stabilized and remained constant for the rest of the follow-up period (up to 20 years). Late PVE is more common because there are more patients at risk.

PVE has conventionally been considered as 'early' and 'late' with 60 days regarded as the time limit for early cases (Dismukes et al. 1973) because of differences between the microbiology and pathogenesis of infection in the 2 time periods. Early PVE results from perioperative contamination and is thus a hospital-acquired infection. Not all these 'early' infections present within 60 days of operation and this has led some investigators to suggest that the time limit for early disease should be extended to 6 months or even a year. It may be more logical to refer to cases of PVE as hospital-acquired or community-acquired and this classification has been used in the STH series since prosthetic valves can also become infected at any interval after surgery via infected IVD. Whatever classification is used, it is clear that the causative microbes of PVE acquired in hospital and the severity of disease differ from PVE acquired in the community, often many years after valve replacement. Early and late infections will be considered separately.

EARLY ONSET PVE

The incidence of early PVE has fallen since the advent of valve replacement surgery over 40 years ago but the commonest infecting organisms are still likely to be staphylococci, both coagulase-negative staphylococci (generally reported as *S. epidermidis sensu lato*) and *S. aureus*. These are skin organisms and although strains of *S. aureus* are usually acquired endogenously from the patient's own commensal flora (sometimes preoperative nasal carriage with the same phage type can be demonstrated), the pathogenesis of coagulase-negative staphylococcal infections is less readily defined and may be from theatre staff or the patient. Other skin organisms that cause early PVE are the corynebacteria, again from either staff or patient. When infection is caused by *S. aureus* there is almost always an antecedent sternal wound infection which may initially appear deceptively trivial. Other organisms are much less common but include gram-negative bacilli and fungi. Unusual sources of infection have included contamination of glutaraldehyde-fixed porcine prosthetic valves with *Mycobacterium chelonae* (Centers for Disease Control 1978), the inadvertent infusion of intravenous fluids contaminated with *Pseudomonas thomasii* (now *picketii*) (Phillips, Eykyn and Laker 1972) and, at STH, the use of an operating theatre water bath contaminated with *P. aeruginosa* to thaw fresh frozen plasma before infusion. There are undoubtedly others. The mortality of early PVE is high, particularly for that caused by *S. aureus*. Since early PVE is associated with contamination of the valve at the time of surgery or soon afterwards, it should be largely preventable by stringent antisepsis. Early and appropriate treatment of staphylococcal sternal wound infection is also very important.

LATE ONSET PVE

The pathogenesis of late PVE differs from that of early PVE and is similar to that of native valve endocarditis with bacteria from the bloodstream localizing on the prosthesis or damaged endocardium. As with community-acquired native valve IE, the commonest pathogens in late PVE are streptococci, enterococci and staphylococci, but a larger percentage of cases than in native valve disease are caused by organisms other than these (35% versus 7.6% in the STH series). It is becoming increasingly clear that virtually any organism can infect a prosthetic valve and the STH series includes cases of *Listeria monocytogenes*, *Erysipelothrix rhusiopathiae*, *Campylobacter fetus* and *Brucella melitensis*. The mortality of late PVE is less than that of early infection and not much different than for native valve infection. Patients with late PVE are likely to present to doctors earlier than many of those with native valve infection and hence to be referred to specialist departments earlier. Both these factors are relevant to outcome.

4.5 Endocarditis in intravenous drug users

Endocarditis was one of the earliest recognized medical complications of intravenous drug abuse and it is the commonest cause of bacteraemia in IVDUs. It is much more common in certain USA centres than in the UK. Over all, the predominant pathogen is *S. aureus* (including MRSA in some parts of the USA) and a much wider spectrum of organisms has been reported from the USA than that as yet encountered in the UK. These include pyogenic streptococci, pseudomonads, other gram-negative bacilli and fungi as well as polymicrobial infections. Most cases involve a previously normal tricuspid valve and result from repeated intravenous injection of foreign material and organisms. Left-sided IE is uncommon in IVDUs unless they have previous heart disease. Tricuspid endocarditis presents with the signs of systemic infection and respiratory symptoms from septic pulmonary emboli and not with the 'classical signs' of endocarditis. Such symptoms (and the chest x-ray findings) may be misdiagnosed as pneumonia by clinicians unfamiliar with right-sided IE. The presentation and clinical manifestations are similar in IVDUs whether they are HIV positive or negative. The causative organisms are usually acquired from the patient's own flora although the drug 'works' have been implicated in cases of *P. aeruginosa* infection. Most IVDUs with tricuspid endocarditis have a good prognosis but the mortality rate is markedly increased in those with very large vegetations. Recurrent attacks of IE, either with the same or different pathogens, are common in IVDUs.

4.6 'Culture-negative' endocarditis

Most reported series of IE include a variable number of cases that are designated 'culture-negative', that is they have negative blood cultures. Although the incidence is reported to vary from 2.5 to 31% (Scheld and Sande 1995), it is now thought to be much nearer the former figure and in the Dutch study it was 1.1% (van der Meer et al. 1992a); some earlier studies used poorly defined diagnostic criteria and possibly inadequate culture techniques. Unfortunately when the term 'culture-negative' IE is used it tends to imply that the condition has nothing to do with microbes and thus tends to confuse the reader. There are patients in whom a clinical diagnosis of IE is made but who have negative blood cultures; there are various explanations for this as follows.

PREVIOUS ANTIBIOTIC ADMINISTRATION

Previous administration of antibiotics will reduce the incidence of positive blood cultures, particularly in streptococcal IE. The duration of previous antibiotic therapy is also an important factor. After only 2–3 days of antibiotic treatment, blood cultures that were initially negative often then become positive, but after longer courses they may remain persistently negative. Blood cultures in patients on appropriate antibiotic treatment for IE become negative before organisms are eradicated from the vegetations. Patients with IE rarely have classical 'textbook' signs and it is only too easy for the diagnosis never to be entertained and antibiotics given on some other pretext. In such cases the antibiotics should be stopped and repeated blood cultures performed; however, if the clinical and echocardiographic evidence for IE is convincing, few clinicians will be prepared to withhold antibiotics indefinitely while the microbiological search for a pathogen is pursued. A history of recent dentistry or (and more probably) the presence of dental sepsis or caries may suggest a streptococcal aetiology in some patients.

Fastidious slow growing organisms

These are uncommon causes of IE but may take much longer to grow in blood cultures than the more usual 'viridans' streptococci or staphylococci. Examples include the HACEK group and the nutritionally variant streptococci (NVS) such as *Streptococcus adjacens* and *Streptococcus defectivus*. The HACEK group may not be detected automatically in blood culture systems such as Bactec and terminal subcultures are required. They are also only sometimes isolated from some sets (or bottles) of blood cultures rather than being consistently isolated as is usual with most cases of streptococcal IE. The NVS may be detected on a gram-stained film from the blood culture bottle but fail to grow on subculture unless provided with the necessary growth factors.

Organisms requiring special isolation techniques or serological diagnosis

Examples of these uncommon but important causes of IE include *Coxiella burnetii*, *Chlamydia psittaci* and perhaps *Chlamydia pneumoniae*, *Bartonella* (lately *Rochalimaea*) spp. and certain fungi such as *Aspergillus* spp. Although specialized culture techniques are available for some of these pathogens, most laboratories will still rely on serological diagnosis. Sometimes features in the history will prompt these investigations: exposure to psittacines (or other birds) will suggest psittacosis and intravenous lines, multiple antibiotics or drug addiction will suggest a fungal aetiology. More often the significance of the history is only appreciated retrospectively when a general serological screen has revealed the diagnosis.

A different diagnosis

This is probably quite common since physicians are rightly concerned not to miss a case of IE. In such cases the microbiologist may often be able to provide reassurance that microbes are not responsible for the patient's illness and thus pre-empt unnecessary antibiotic treatment. Once clinicians commit a patient to treatment for presumptive IE they may be reluctant to stop.

4.7 Treatment of infective endocarditis

In the pre-antibiotic era, IE was almost uniformly fatal and no-one can deny that antibiotics have dramatically reduced the mortality of the disease. However, a major further reduction followed the introduction of valve replacement surgery some 40 years ago. It is remarkable that an infected valve can safely be excised at the start of antibiotic therapy (even with positive blood cultures) if the clinical condition of the patient warrants it; indeed, delay in valve replacement may be disastrous. The mortality of IE depends on various factors, not least the causative pathogen and the valve; it is highest for *S. aureus* in early PVE and lowest for 'viridans' streptococcal native valve infection. Mortality will only be reduced by earlier diagnosis and earlier referral for specialist care. Although patients with IE may be seen initially by different types of clinician, they should always be seen by or referred to a cardiologist and, where necessary, to a cardiac surgeon as soon as possible. Antibiotic therapy is only one (albeit essential) part of the management of the disease and the principles on which it should be based are essentially similar for any case of IE, as follows.

Unless the patient is very unwell, toxic and septic, antibiotics should preferably be withheld until the blood culture results are available. Many patients with IE will have been ill for several weeks or even months, and thus a delay of a day or 2 in starting antibiotics cannot make any difference to the course of the disease. Antibiotics cannot possibly prevent emboli in such patients, an argument that is sometimes advanced for treating the patient before the blood culture results are known.

The antibiotic or combination of antibiotics given should be bactericidal for the pathogen and, where possible, given in a large dose, preferably intravenously. Although many of the organisms causing IE are very sensitive to antibiotics, access of the antibiotic to the organisms within the vegetations where bacteria are found in large numbers is limited.

Prolonged treatment is necessary to sterilize the vegetations and prevent relapse, yet exactly how long such treatment should be remains ill-defined. The MRC study (Cates and Christie 1951) recommended 'four to six weeks treatment' and since then 6 weeks has been considered the accepted length of antibiotic treatment for any case of endocarditis. Over 20 years ago it was convincingly shown that 2 weeks of intravenous treatment with penicillin plus an aminoglycoside was effective treatment for native valve IE caused by sensitive streptococci (Tan et al. 1971). Old habits die hard, however, and clinicians are not readily persuaded to use such a regimen that is not only very effective but is more acceptable to patients and often enables an earlier discharge from hospital. For most other cases 4 weeks of treatment are usually sufficient. Prolonged courses of antibiotics should be avoided. Detailed guidelines for the treatment of streptococcal, enterococcal and staphylococcal IE are given in the Report from the Working Party in Endocarditis of the British Society for Antimicrobial Chemotherapy

(BSAC) (1985) which has recently been updated (1997).

The choice of antibiotics for the treatment of IE is governed by the susceptibility of the causative organism and it has been conventional practice to rely on the minimum bactericidal concentration (MBC) of the antibiotic rather than disc tests. In practice the MBC is often not easy to interpret and 100% kill may not be achieved in in vitro tests, nor is it known if this is required for successful therapy. In common with the American guidelines, the BSAC Working Party now recommend doing the minimum inhibitory concentration (MIC) and basing therapeutic guidelines on this. Occasionally, tests to find a synergistic combination of antibiotics will be required, especially for enterococcal IE. Although there are recommended regimens for streptococcal, enterococcal and staphylococcal IE (and these organsims account for over 80% of all cases of IE), guidelines for other organisms must inevitably be somewhat anecdotal since far fewer cases are seen.

SERUM BACTERICIDAL TITRES

The serum bactericidal titre was first described 50 years ago by Schlicter and McLean (1947); for many years it has been routine practice in most UK and other laboratories to measure this during the treatment of IE and to alter the antibiotic regimen on the basis of unsatisfactory titres. Remarkably, although these tests have been performed assiduously for many years, until recently there had been few critical evaluations of their efficacy. In their collaborative trial, Weinstein et al. (1985) maintained that the test could accurately predict bacteriological success but not bacteriological failure or clinical outcome; they recommended peak titres of 64 and trough titres of 32 to provide optimal therapy, but this view has been challenged. A UK investigation into laboratory practice (Eykyn 1987) showed that neither the methods used to measure the serum bactericidal titres nor the intrepretation of the results obtained was uniform, yet most microbiologists thought that the tests were helpful, some pointing out that clinicians expected them. This study showed that peak titres of 8 were reasonably predictive of bacteriological cure but not of clinical outcome but that trough titres were of no predictive value at all. It has to be said, however, that bacteriological failure in the treatment of IE is rare. If serum bactericidal titres are estimated, their results should be interpreted in light of the clinical condition of the patient and the antibiotic regimen should never be altered solely on the basis of unsatisfactory titres. The BSAC Working Party has now decided not to recommend them (Report 1997, submitted for publication).

4.8 Prevention of endocarditis in susceptible patients

Since IE is a disease with significant morbidity and mortality, its prevention by prophylactic antibiotics (or other means) is a laudable objective, but how best to achieve this, or indeed whether it can be achieved, is another matter. Although IE results from bacteraemia, many procedures that produce bacteraemia, such as sigmoidoscopy, are rarely, if ever, followed by IE; yet they are very frequently performed, often presumably on patients with undiagnosed susceptible cardiac lesions. There are few reliable data and much anecdote on the subject and we do not even know if antibiotic prophylaxis is effective at all. There have been 2 case-control studies on dental prophylaxis: one found that prophylaxis was effective (Imperiale and Horwitz 1990) and the other (van der Meer et al. 1992b) that it was of marginal value. There are also well documented reports of the apparent failure of appropriate antibiotic prophylaxis to prevent IE after dental procedures (Durack, Kaplan and Bisno 1983). In this study the causative organsims were usually sensitive to the prophylactic antibiotic that had been given. Despite these uncertainties, antibiotic prophylaxis is here to stay, not least alas because of the medicolegal implications of failure to give it. There are numerous national guidelines for prophylaxis and these vary both in their antibiotic regimens and in the range of procedures for which prophylaxis is required. Over the past decade, however, there has been some uniformity of recommendations both within Europe and elsewhere. The diversity of the recommendations serves to emphasize the lack of critical data on which to base them. Compliance with recommended regimens is known to be poor even with the simple single dose general dental recommendation. In addition to failure to give any antibiotics at all, other common errors include starting antibiotics too soon before the procedure, continuing for too long afterwards and using low-dose regimens. In the UK the BSAC Working Party has published its guidelines since 1982 (Report 1982) and these have been regularly updated and are practical; they have been widely adopted throughout the UK.

Prophylaxis is most often given for dental procedures but, as has already been seen, only a minority of patients with IE caused by oral streptococci actually give a history of dental treatment in the preceding weeks. Dental bacteraemia is as likely, or even more likely, to arise from chewing, tooth-brushing or even from the movement of septic or carious teeth. Thus the maintenance of optimum dental health by regular visits to the dentist is probably of more value than antibiotic prophylaxis in the prevention of IE. It is a sobering thought that until about 25 years ago patients who had had an episode of 'viridans' streptococcal IE were advised to have a total dental clearance, irrespective of the condition of their teeth, in the misguided hope that this would prevent further attacks.

If the evidence for efficacy of dental prophylaxis is unconvincing through lack of critical data, that for other procedures for which antibiotic prophylaxis is recommended is even more so. These procedures include various types of instrumentation, particularly of the genitourinary and gastrointestinal tracts. Not only are these procedures performed on very large numbers of susceptible patients, the organisms (enterococci, usually *E. faecalis*) are much more resistant to antibiotics than the 'viridans' streptococci; thus, parenteral regimens are required. A more logical approach would be to restrict such prophylaxis to those with prosthetic valves only but to date no national guidelines have seen fit to do this.

The guidelines for the prevention of late PVE are essentially the same as those outlined for endocarditis on native valves though some differentiate between the regimens for the 2 groups. The prevention of early PVE is a different matter that has already been mentioned briefly and concerns prophylactic antibiotics at the time of valve replacement. This has been a controversial issue for many years and has been plagued by many small poorly conducted trials; the available evidence suggests that antibiotic prophylaxis reduces the postoperative wound infection in cardiothoracic sur-

gery in general (Kreter and Woods 1992) and, by inference, in valve replacement surgery in particular, although prophylactic antibiotics were originally given to reduce PVE before the advent of coronary artery surgery. It is assumed, though never proved, that a reduction in wound infection will equate with a reduction in PVE and this seems a reasonable assumption. Various antibiotics are used and no single regimen has been shown to be superior. The increasing prevalence of methicillin-resistant staphylococci in hospitals, both *S. aureus* (MRSA) and coagulase-negative staphylococci, has led many to use vancomycin rather than, as was usual, a β-lactam such as flucloxacillin or a cephalosporin, and this seems more logical. Whatever antibiotic prophylaxis is used it should not be given for more than 48 h.

REFERENCES

Aronson MD, Bor DH, 1987, Blood cultures, *Ann Intern Med*, **106:** 246–53.

Baskin TW, Rosenthal A, Pruitt BA, 1976, Acute bacterial endocarditis: a silent source of sepsis in the burn patient, *Ann Surg*, **184:** 618–21.

Bayliss R, Clarke C et al., 1983a, The teeth and infective endocarditis, *Br Heart J*, **50:** 506–12.

Bayliss R, Clarke C et al., 1983b, The microbiology and pathogenesis of infective endocarditis, *Br Heart J*, **50:** 513–19.

Belsey MA, 1967, Pneumococcal bacteremia: a report of three cases, *Am J Dis Child*, **113:** 588–9.

Cates JE, Christie RV, 1951, Subacute bacterial endocarditis: a review of 442 patients treated in 14 centres appointed by the Penicillin Trials Committee of the Medical Research Council, *Q J Med (NS)*, **20:** 93–130.

Centers for Disease Control, 1978, Follow-up on mycobacterial contamination of porcine heart valve prostheses, *Morbid Mortal Weekly Rep*, **27:** 92 and 697–8.

Delahaye F, Goulet V et al., 1992, Incidence, caractéristiques démographiques, cliniques, microbiologiques, et évolutives de l'endocardite infectieuse en France en 1990–1991, *Méd Mal Infect*, **22, Spécial:** 975–84.

van Deventer SJH, Büller HR et al., 1988, Endotoxaemia: an early predictor of septicaemia in febrile patients, *Lancet*, **1:** 605–9.

Dismukes WE, Karchmer AW et al., 1973, Prosthetic valve endocarditis: analysis of 38 cases, *Circulation*, **48:** 365–77.

Dorsher CW, Wilson WR, Rosenblatt JE, 1989, Anaerobic bacteremia and cardiovascular infections, *Anaerobic Infections in Humans*, eds Finegold SM, George LW, Academic Press, San Diego, 299–303.

Douglas CWI, Heath J et al., 1993, Identity of viridans streptococci isolated from cases of infective endocarditis, *J Med Microbiol*, **39:** 179–82.

DuPont HL, Spink WW, 1969, Infections due to Gram-negative organisms: an analysis of 860 patients with bacteremia at the University of Minnesota Medical Center, 1958–1966, *Medicine (Baltimore)*, **48:** 307–32.

Durack DT, Kaplan EL, Bisno AL, 1983, Apparent failure of endocarditis prophylaxis: analysis of 52 cases submitted to a national registry, *JAMA*, **250:** 2318–22.

Durack DT, Lukes AS et al., 1994, New criteria for diagnosis of infective endocarditis: utilization of specific echocardiographic findings, *Am J Med*, **96:** 200–8.

Ehrie M, Morgan AP et al., 1978, Endocarditis with the indwelling balloon-tipped pulmonary artery catheter in burn patients, *J Trauma*, **18:** 664–6.

Eskola J, Takala AK et al., 1992, Epidemiology of invasive pneumococcal infections in children in Finland, *JAMA*, **268:** 3323–7.

Espersen F, Frimodt-Møller N et al., 1991, Changing pattern of bone and joint infections due to *Staphylococcus aureus*: study of cases in Denmark, 1959–1988, *Rev Infect Dis*, **13:** 347–60.

Etienne J, Eykyn SJ, 1990, Increase in native valve endocarditis caused by coagulase-negative staphylococci: an Anglo-French clinical and microbiological study, *Br Heart J*, **64:** 381–4.

Eykyn SJ, 1987, The role of the laboratory in assisting treatment – a review of current UK practices, *J Antimicrob Chemother*, **20, Suppl.A:** 51–64.

Eykyn SJ, Gransden WR, Phillips I, 1990, The causative organisms of septicaemia and their epidemiology, *J Antimicrob Chemother*, **25, Suppl.C:** 41–58.

Felner JM, Dowell VR Jr, 1970, Anaerobic bacterial endocarditis, *N Engl J Med*, **283:** 1188–90.

Goodman JS, Crews HD et al., 1969, Bacterial endocarditis as a possible complication of chronic haemodialysis, *N Engl J Med*, **280:** 876–7.

Gransden WR, Eykyn SJ, Phillips I, 1990a, The computerized documentation of septicaemia, *J Antimicrob Chemother*, **25, Suppl. C:** 31–9.

Gransden WR, Eykyn SJ, Phillips I, 1990b, Bacteremia due to *Escherichia coli*: a study of 861 episodes, *Rev Infect Dis*, **12:** 1008–18.

Gruer LD, McKendrick MW, Geddes AM, 1984, Pneumococcal bacteraemia – a continuing challenge, *Q J Med*, **210:** 259–70.

Hardie JM, Whiley RA, 1994, Recent developments in streptococcal taxonomy: their relation to infections, *Rev Med Microbiol*, **5:** 151–62.

Hønberg PZ, Gutschik E, 1987, *Streptococcus bovis* bacteraemia and its association with alimentary-tract neoplasms, *Lancet*, **1:** 163.

Imperiale TF, Horwitz RI, 1990, Does prophylaxis prevent postdental infective endocarditis? A controlled evaluation of protective efficacy, *Am J Med*, **88:** 131–6.

Ispahani P, Pearson NJ, Greenwood D, 1987, Analysis of community and hospital acquired bacteraemia in a large teaching hospital in the United Kingdom, *Q J Med*, **63:** 427–40.

Jumaa PA, Chattopadhyay B, 1994, Pseudobacteraemia, *J Hosp Infect*, **27:** 167–77.

King LH, Bradley KP et al., 1971, Bacterial endocarditis in chronic hemodialysis patients: a complication more common than previously suspected, *Surgery*, **69:** 554–6.

Klein RS, Recco RA et al., 1977, Association of *Streptococcus bovis* with carcinoma of the colon, *N Engl J Med*, **297:** 800–2.

Kreter B, Woods M, 1992, Antibiotic prophylaxis for cardiothoracic operations: metaanalysis of thirty years of clinical trials, *J Thorac Cardiovasc Surg*, **104:** 590–9.

Kuikka A, Syrjänen J et al., 1992, Pneumococcal bacteraemia during a recent decade, *J Infect*, **24:** 157–68.

Leport C, Bure A et al., 1987, Incidence of colonic lesions in

Streptococcus bovis and enterococcal endocarditis, *Lancet*, **1**: 748.

McCabe WR, Jackson GG, 1962, Gram-negative bacteremia I. Etiology and ecology, *Arch Intern Med*, **110**: 847–55.

van der Meer JTM, van Vianen W et al., 1991, Distribution, antibiotic susceptibility and tolerance of bacterial isolates in culture-positive cases of endocarditis in the Netherlands, *Eur J Clin Microbiol Infect Dis*, **10**: 728–34.

van der Meer JTM, Thompson J et al., 1992a, Epidemiology of bacterial endocarditis in the Netherlands 1. Patient characteristics, *Arch Intern Med*, **152**: 1863–8.

van der Meer JTM, van Wijk W et al., 1992b, Efficacy of antibiotic prophylaxis for prevention of native-valve endocarditis, *Lancet*, **339**: 137–9.

Osler W, 1885, The Gulstonian lectures on malignant endocarditis, *Br Med J*, **1**: 467–70, 522–6 and 577–9.

Parker MT, Ball LC, 1976, Streptococci and aerococci associated with systemic infection in man, *J Med Microbiol*, **9**: 275–301.

Phillips I, Eykyn S, Laker M, 1972, Outbreak of hospital infection caused by contaminated autoclaved fluids, *Lancet*, **2**: 1258–60.

Phillips I, Eykyn SJ et al., 1988, Epidemic multiresistant *Escherichia coli* infection in West Lambeth Health District, *Lancet*, **1**: 1038–41.

Phillips I, King A et al., 1990, The antibiotic sensitivity of bacteria isolated from the blood of patients in St Thomas' Hospital, 1969–1988, *J Antimicrob Chemother*, **25, Suppl.C**: 59–80.

Report, 1982, The antibiotic prophylaxis of infective endocarditis. Report of a Working Party of the British Society for Antimicrobial Chemotherapy, *Lancet*, **2**: 1323–6.

Report, 1985, Antibiotic treatment of streptococcal and staphylococcal endocarditis. Report of a Working Party of the British Society for Antimicrobial Chemotherapy, *Lancet*, **2**: 815–17 (1997 version submitted).

von Reyn CF, Levy BS et al., 1981, Infective endocarditis: an analysis based on strict case definitions, *Ann Intern Med*, **94 (part I)**: 505–18.

Roberts FJ, Gaere IW, Coldman A, 1991, Three-year study of positive blood cultures, with emphasis on prognosis, *Rev Infect Dis*, **13**: 34–46.

Rogosa M, Hampp EG et al., 1960, Blood sampling and cultural studies in the detection of post-operative bacteremias , *J Am Dent Assoc*, **60**: 171–80.

Rutledge R, Kim J, Applebaum RE, 1985, Actuarial analysis of the risk of prosthetic valve endocarditis in 1598 patients with mechanical and bioprosthetic valves, *Arch Surg*, **120**: 469–72.

Scheckler WE, 1977, Septicaemia in a community hospital, 1970 through 1973, *JAMA*, **237**: 1938–41.

Scheld WM, Sande MA, 1995, Endocarditis and intravascular infections, *Principles and Practice of Infectious Diseases*, 4th edn, eds Mandell GL, Bennett JE, Dolin R, Churchill Livingstone, New York, 740–83.

Schlicter JG, MacLean H, 1947, A method of determining the effective therapeutic level in the treatment of subacute bacterial endocarditis with penicillin, *Am Heart J*, **34**: 209–11.

Shanson DC, 1989, *Septicaemia and Endocarditis: Clinical and Microbiological Aspects*, Oxford University Press, Oxford, 78.

Skehan JD, Murray M, Mills PG, 1988, Infective endocarditis: incidence and mortality in the North East Thames Region, *Br Heart J*, **59**: 62–8.

Sriskandan S, Cohen J, 1995, The pathogenesis of septic shock, *J Infect*, **30**: 201–6.

Srivastava RK, MacMillan BG, 1979, Cardiac infection in acute burn patients, *Burns*, **6**: 48–54.

Stokes EJ, Ridgway GL, Wren MWD, 1993, *Clinical Microbiology*, 7th edn, Edward Arnold, London, 34–5.

Tan JS, Terhune CA Jr et al., 1971, Successful two-week treatment schedule for penicillin-susceptible *Streptococcus viridans* endocarditis, *Lancet*, **2**: 1340–4.

Tsao MMP, Katz D, 1984, Central venous catheter-induced endocarditis: human correlate of the animal experimental model of endocarditis, *Rev Infect Dis*, **6**: 783–90.

Vandenesch F, Etienne J et al., 1993, Endocarditis due to *Staphylococcus lugdunensis*: report of 11 cases and review, *Clin Infect Dis*, **17**: 871–6.

Washington JA and the International Collaborative Blood Culture Study Group, 1992, An international multicenter study of blood culture practices, *Eur J Clin Microbiol Infect Dis*, **11**: 1115–28.

Weinstein MP, Reller LB et al., 1983, The clinical significance of positive blood cultures: a comprehensive analysis of 500 episodes of bacteremia and fungemia in adults. I. Laboratory and epidemiologic observations and II. Clinical observations, with special reference to factors influencing prognosis, *Rev Infect Dis*, **5**: 35–53 and 54–70.

Weinstein MP, Stratton CW et al., 1985, Multicenter collaborative evaluation of a standardized serum bactericidal test as a prognostic indicator in infective endocarditis, *Am J Med*, **78**: 262–9.

Young SEJ, 1982, Bacteraemia 1975–1980: a survey of cases reported to the PHLS Communicable Surveillance Centre, *J Infect*, **5**: 19–26.

Young SEJ, 1987, Aetiology and epidemiology of infective endocarditis in England and Wales, *J Antimicrob Chemother*, **20, Suppl.C**: 7–14.

Chapter   1 7

BACTERIAL MENINGITIS

K A V Cartwright

1   INTRODUCTION

More than 2000 cases of bacterial meningitis, with at least 150 deaths, are notified each year in the UK and similar data exist for other countries. The emphasis in this chapter will be on the epidemiological, patho-physiological and on diagnostic aspects of the disease. Fuller accounts of the organisms will be found in Volume 2 and the various syndromes are described in Lambert (1991).

In meningitis the membranes that surround the brain and spinal cord become inflamed. Most meningitis is viral, usually with mild illness, but viral and bacterial meningitis may be confused (Maxson and Jacobs 1993).

The commonest cause of bacterial meningitis world wide is *Neisseria meningitidis*, the meningococcus. In unimmunized populations capsulated strains of *Haemophilus influenzae* type b (Hib) may cause as many, or more cases, especially in young children. *Streptococcus pneumoniae* and *Mycobacterium tuberculosis* rank next in order of frequency. Many other microbes, including bacteria, fungi, protozoa and worms, may also cause meningitis or meningeal inflammation.

In neonatal meningitis group B streptococci and *Escherichia coli* predominate, whereas *Listeria monocytogenes* causes meningitis in neonates, during pregnancy and in old age. Fungal meningitis is particularly associated with severe immunosuppression as in the late stages of HIV infection. Many other bacteria including staphylococci (Jensen et al. 1993), coliforms and environmental gram-negative bacilli such as *Pseudomonas aeruginosa* and *Acinetobacter* spp. (Siegman-Ingra et al. 1993) may cause meningitis, often in association with in-patient hospital care, severe immunosuppression, neurosurgery or cranial trauma or infection of cerebrospinal fluid (CSF) reservoirs or shunts.

In economically advanced countries the mortality from bacterial meningitis is less than 10% but it may be 30% or more in developing countries (Greenwood 1987, Bryan et al. 1990, Bijlmer 1991). The epidemiology is changing swiftly with the introduction of effective conjugated polysaccharide vaccines for invasive Hib disease and the imminent availability of similar conjugated vaccines for serogroup A and C meningococcal meningitis and possibly some pneumococcal meningitis (Fig. 17.1). There are good prospects for further reductions in the incidence of bacterial meningitis in the near future.

2   PATHOPHYSIOLOGY

The evolution of bacterial meningitis follows a sequence of exposure to the pathogen, acquisition and then invasion. Invasion can be subdivided into 3 processes: mucosal penetration followed by invasion of the bloodstream, and finally invasion of the meninges (Tunkel and Scheld 1993). The human nasopharynx is the natural habitat of the meningococcus, Hib and the pneumococcus. Exposure is more frequent than acquisition, which is more frequent than bloodstream invasion. Understanding the process of establishment of bacterial meningitis has been assisted greatly by the development of animal models of infection (O'Donoghue et al. 1974, Moxon et al. 1977, Tauber and Zwahlen 1994).

2.1   Exposure

Exposure depends on the frequency and intimacy of interactions between colonized and susceptible individuals and the capacity of colonized individuals to disseminate bacteria from the nasopharynx. Dissemi-

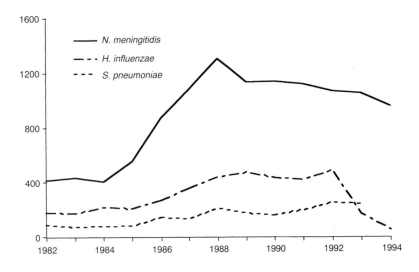

Fig. 17.1 Notifications of selected types of bacterial meningitis, England and Wales, 1982–94. Data for 1994 are provisional; 1994 data for pneumococcal meningitis not available.

nation may be influenced by the intensity of colonization, intercurrent viral infections (Gwaltney et al. 1975) and perhaps by the ambient temperature and humidity.

2.2 Acquisition

Carriage rates reflect acquisitions and the duration of carriage. The duality is important; much evidence suggests that if bacterial invasion is to occur, it follows very shortly after acquisition. Individuals colonized for weeks or months are unlikely to develop invasive disease.

With increasing age, the nasopharynx becomes progressively less susceptible to colonization by meningococci, Hib and pneumococci. This may be due to the development of mucosal immunity.

2.3 Mucosal invasion

Bacterial strains vary in their capacity to invade. Non-capsulate meningococci are essentially avirulent, while strains of serogroups A, B and C are more invasive than strains of serogroups X, Y and W-135 and other groups of meningococci (see Volume 2, Chapter 37). Similarly, non-capsulate strains of *H. influenzae* have little invasive potential, and though there are 6 capsular serotypes of *H. influenzae*, type b strains account for more than 95% of all invasive haemophilus disease in unimmunized populations.

The interaction of bacteria with the nasopharyngeal mucosa has been investigated with tissue explants (Stephens and Farley 1991, Read et al. 1995), cultured epithelial and endothelial cells (Virji et al. 1991) and bacterial transformants. This has allowed comparisons between the behaviour of fully virulent bacteria and strains that differ from them by the deletion of single genes or operons.

Capsulate meningococci bind to epithelial cells by adhesins, including fimbriae and the Opc outer-membrane protein (Virji et al. 1991, 1992). They cross the mucosal barrier by direct invasion of epithelial cells (endocytosis) whereas Hib strains migrate

between epithelial cells by breaking down intercellular tight junctions (Stephens and Farley 1991). Once in the submucosa, the invading bacteria cross the capillary vessel basement membrane and the endothelium to gain access to the bloodstream.

The 3 major bacterial meningitis pathogens produce an IgA1 protease, whereas closely related nasopharyngeal 'commensals', such as *Haemophilus parainfluenzae*, *Neisseria lactamica* and viridans streptococci, do not (Mulks and Plaut 1978, Mulks 1985). Invasion potential and production of IgA1 protease are so closely associated that a causal relationship has long been sought. One hypothesis is that circulating IgA may block binding sites that would otherwise be accessible to lethal, bacteriolytic complement-fixing IgG or IgM antibodies (Griffiss 1982). Bacteria that invade may further be protected by cleavage of the blocking immunoglobulin molecules by IgA protease.

Respiratory viral infections may play a part in precipitating bacterial meningitis (Rolleston 1919, Krasinski et al. 1987, Moore et al. 1990), in particular influenza A, which increases the risk (Cartwright et al. 1991) and the severity (Hubert et al. 1992) of meningococcal disease. The mechanism is probably postviral immune suppression.

2.4 Meningeal invasion

Normal cerebrospinal fluid contains few phagocytic cells and very low levels of complement and antibody; the normal CSF:blood IgG ratio is about 1:800. The integrity of the normal blood–brain barrier, and thus of the subarachnoid space, is maintained by a combination of the tight intercellular junctions between capillary endothelial cells of the cerebral microvasculature, and by the comparative rarity of pinocytosis by these cells.

The cerebral capillary endothelium of the choroid plexus can bind some of the bacteria that cause meningitis. Bound bacteria may then undergo fimbrial phase variation in order to cross the blood–brain barrier (Saukkonen et al. 1988). Bacteria may gain access to the subarachnoid space within host phagocytic cells (Tunkel and Scheldt 1993, McNeil, Virji and Moxon 1994).

Once bacteria are established within the subarachnoid space they are transiently sheltered from the host defences. They can release substances capable of disrupting the blood–brain barrier. In the CSF *H. influenzae* type b lipopolysaccharide (endotoxin) induces the production of inflammatory cytokines including interleukin-1 and tumour necrosis factor. Pneumococcal cell walls, which contain peptidoglycan and teichoic acid, are more potent than capsular polysaccharide in inducing subarachnoid inflammation (Tuomanen et al. 1985). High CSF cytokine concentrations are reached within 1–2 h of the arrival of bacteria in the CSF (Tunkel and Scheldt 1993, Spellerberg and Tuomanen 1994).

Disruption of the blood–brain barrier occurs by a breakdown of the intercellular tight junctions of the cerebral microvascular epithelium, permitting an influx of larger molecules from the bloodstream and migration of phagocytic cells into the CSF.

3 CLINICAL FEATURES

The presenting features of meningitis are determined largely by the age and, to a lesser extent, by the causative organism and the route by which it has reached the meninges. In the great majority of cases, the early signs and symptoms are non-specific. Fever, lassitude, malaise, muscular aches and pains, nausea, vomiting and headache are much more common in viral than in bacterial meningitis. Identification of the symptoms that may give warning of impending serious illness can be very difficult. In Europe and the USA the difficulty is compounded by the fact that influenza, viral respiratory infections and bacterial meningitis all peak in the winter months.

As illness develops, symptoms become more severe; most patients with bacterial meningitis are much more ill than those with viral infections. Most bacterial meningitis occurs in infants and very young children who may not be able to give a verbal account of their symptoms. Familiarity with the symptoms, repeated examinations and a high index of suspicion are the best safeguards for parents and for family doctors. The presence of inconsolable crying, a fit, or any evidence of decreased consciousness in a febrile young child should warrant immediate careful investigation. The combination of fever and a haemorrhagic rash, which may herald meningococcal disease, constitutes a medical emergency.

Tuberculous and fungal meningitis may develop insidiously over days, weeks or even months.

4 DIAGNOSIS OF MENINGITIS

Though bacteria usually gain access to the subarachnoid space via the bloodstream, less frequently they spread directly from adjacent tissues, such as an infected middle ear, or very occasionally from a ruptured cerebral abscess. Bacterial meningitis may follow diagnostic or therapeutic procedures in which the integrity of the subarachnoid space is deliberately breached, as during neurosurgery.

4.1 Cerebrospinal fluid (CSF)

LUMBAR PUNCTURE

Examination of CSF is routine in the investigation of suspected bacterial meningitis (Gray and Fedorko 1992). If intracranial pressure is raised, lumbar puncture may occasionally be followed by herniation of the brain stem through the foramen magnum ('coning'), potentially a fatal event. Papilloedema is an insensitive indicator of raised intracranial pressure and clinicians sometimes avoid lumbar puncture in patients with any evidence of diminished consciousness or fluctuating neurological status. A CT scan is helpful in these circumstances and an increasing proportion of patients with clinical evidence of meningitis are now managed without lumbar puncture.

Despite the hazards, examination of CSF still offers the best chance of observing, isolating and identifying the causative organism in meningitis (Kaplan et al. 1986, British Society for the Study of Infection Research Committee 1995). Lumbar puncture is particularly valuable when an antibiotic has been given before hospital admission. Even when bacteria cannot be recovered on culture, microscopy may confirm the diagnosis and indicate the likely causative organism.

A portion of the CSF sample should be examined promptly to determine the number and type of leucocytes present. Bacterial meningitis is usually accompanied by the presence of neutrophils, but about 5% of CSF samples subsequently found to be culture positive do not contain cells or contain only a few lymphocytes when first examined. The absence of leucocytes should never be used to justify withholding antibiotic treatment if there is reasonable clinical suspicion of bacterial meningitis. The cell population may consist of a mixture of polymorphs and lymphocytes; this is more likely if there has been a long prodrome, or if the patient has been treated with antibiotics. A mixture of cells is sometimes seen in viral meningitis. The CSF leucocyte count may be raised in patients who have had a cerebral haemorrhage a few days earlier and in patients who have had recent fits. In these cases, the cells are predominantly lymphocytes. Other conditions that give rise to a lymphocytic pleocytosis are listed in Table 17.1.

BIOCHEMICAL ANALYSIS

Estimation of CSF glucose and protein can be helpful. The CSF:blood glucose ratio (normally about 70%) is often, though not invariably, reduced in bacterial meningitis, commonly to about 25% (Kaplan et al. 1986) but a normal CSF:blood glucose ratio is common in tuberculous meningitis. The CSF protein is often raised, initially reflecting leakage of blood protein into the CSF; later it may reflect local antibody production. CSF lactate concentration may help to differentiate between bacterial and viral meningitis.

Table 17.1 Conditions causing CSF lymphocytic pleocytosis

Infections
  Viral meningitis
  Partly treated bacterial meningitis
  Syphilis
  Parameningeal infection (e.g. abscess)
  Protozoa (e.g. toxoplasmosis)
  Acute and chronic bacterial meningitis
  Tuberculous meningitis
  Lyme borreliosis
  Fungal meningitis
  Worm infection

Inflammatory processes
  Postictal; post-myelogram
  Post-CNS bleed
  Sarcoidosis; Wegener's granulomatosis
  Malignant hypertension; migraine
  Kawasaki disease
  Post-neurosurgery; intrathecal drugs
  Multiple sclerosis
  SLE; Behçet's syndrome
  Benign intracranial hypertension
  Mollaret's meningitis

Drugs and vaccines
  Trimethoprim; isoniazid
  MMR and polio vaccine
  Ibuprofen; NSAIDs
  Intravenous immunoglobulin

Malignancy
  Meningeal carcinomatosis
  CNS leukaemia and lymphoma

Urine reagent strips have been used for the direct examination of CSF (Moosa, Quortum and Ibrahim 1995) to discriminate accurately between viral and bacterial meningitis. This cheap and simple method may have an important role where laboratory facilities are limited or distant.

MICROSCOPY

Direct microscopy of uncentrifuged or centrifuged CSF may reveal the presence of bacteria or fungi and can provide immediate confirmation of the diagnosis. Staining with acridine orange is more sensitive than the gram stain (Kleinman et al. 1984). The organisms seen on microscopy in antibiotic-treated patients may fail to grow on culture, but the morphology and gram reaction of the organism, the age of the patient and the clinical features often permit an educated guess at the identity of the causative organism.

DETECTION OF BACTERIAL ANTIGEN

Tests for bacterial antigen in CSF can provide a quick diagnosis, but they are less sensitive than the gram stain and do not often alter clinical management (Maxson, Lewno and Schutze 1994). Many tests are based on the agglutination of antibody-coated latex particles and work quite well for pneumococci, meningococci of serogroups A or C, and for group B strepto-

cocci. They are less successful for the detection of serogroup B meningococci. The *Limulus* lysate test is a sensitive test for endotoxin from gram-negative organisms, but has not found wide acceptance.

CULTURE

CSF should be inoculated on to good quality culture media, always including at least Columbia blood agar and a heated blood agar. They should be incubated in 5% CO_2 for a minimum of 48 h. If a ruptured cerebral abscess is suspected, or if meningitis has followed neurosurgery or a history of previous meningeal trauma, a second blood agar plate should be incubated anaerobically for 5–7 days.

POLYMERASE CHAIN REACTION

A polymerase chain reaction (PCR) test for the detection of meningococcal DNA in CSF has been described (Kristiansen et al. 1991) and is specific and sensitive for the diagnosis of meningococcal meningitis (Ni et al. 1992). Amplification of sections of 16S ribosomal RNA, common to most species of pathogenic bacteria, may also prove to be of value (Greisen et al. 1994).

4.2 Peripheral blood

BLOOD CULTURE

Blood cultures are positive in only about half of patients with meningococcal disease who have not previously received parenteral antibiotic therapy and they are almost invariably sterile in those who have. In contrast, in Hib and pneumococcal meningitis the causative organisms are commonly isolated from peripheral blood (British Society for the Study of Infection Research Committee 1995).

MICROSCOPY

When bacteraemia is heavy, meningococci and other bacteria may be detected within polymorphs in Giemsa-stained films of peripheral blood and they can be seen in and grown from tissue fluid obtained from the haemorrhagic skin rash (van Deuren et al. 1993) and from other normally sterile sites such as joints and pericardial fluid.

PCR OF PERIPHERAL BLOOD

A PCR for the detection of meningococcal DNA in blood has recently been developed and validated (Newcombe et al. 1996). The test is of particular value when the patient has received parenteral antibiotic treatment before hospital admission, an increasingly frequent event.

4.3 Serology

Serological tests for meningococcal disease were long hampered by the failure of serogroup B capsular polysaccharide to provoke a good immune response. Second generation serological tests now available in the UK can reliably detect the presence of acute phase

(IgM) meningococcal antibodies in a single serum specimen obtained after the first week of the illness; alternatively, a rising titre of antibody to meningococcal outer-membrane proteins may be sought (Jones and Kaczmarski 1994).

4.4 Nasopharyngeal swabs

Since the main bacterial meningitis pathogens are nasopharyngeal commensals, their isolation from cases of clinical meningitis does not provide evidence of causation. However, when lumbar puncture is not undertaken and blood cultures are negative, a throat swab may give the only chance of an isolate. Meningococci are rarely recovered from healthy infants and the isolation of a well capsulated meningococcus of serogroup B or C from the posterior pharynx of a young child with symptoms of meningitis with or without a haemorrhagic rash is very strong evidence of a meningococcal aetiology. Similarly, the isolation of Hib from a child with meningitis aged 12 months or less is unlikely to be coincidental. However, isolation of a pneumococcus from the nasopharynx does not assist in management.

Swabs of the posterior pharynx are ideally taken through the mouth (Olcén et al. 1979). Patients with clinical meningitis are often too ill to co-operate with peroral swabbing but pernasal swabs are simple to obtain, though an assistant is required to steady the patient's head. A single negative nasopharyngeal swab is an insensitive predictor of freedom from carriage and decisions on the prophylaxis of contacts of meningococcal or Hib disease should never be based on the results of nasopharyngeal swabbing of the contacts.

5 MENINGOCOCCAL DISEASE

5.1 Historical aspects

Vieusseux (1806) described an outbreak of meningococcal disease with 33 deaths in the small community of Eaux Vives, near Lake Geneva in Switzerland in the spring of 1805. Before this, meningococcal disease may have been confused with other spotted fevers, including typhus, which also sometimes occurred in clusters and outbreaks, especially in the military, and was often characterized by a haemorrhagic skin rash. It seems most likely that meningococcal disease has afflicted man for centuries.

August Hirsch (1886) documented many outbreaks of infectious diseases including cerebrospinal fever in Europe and the New World up to 1882. The Italian pathologists Marchiafava and Celli (1884) are credited with the first description of intracellular oval micrococci in a sample of CSF. Three years later Weichselbaum, in Vienna, reported the isolation of an organism he described as *Diplococcus intracellularis meningitidis* from 6 of 8 cases of primary sporadic community-acquired meningitis (Weichselbaum 1887). A period of confusion followed when Jaeger isolated a gram-positive chain-forming coccus from meningitis cases in an outbreak in Stuttgart. Subsequent reports showed that Weichselbaum was correct; Jaeger's gram-positive organism was probably a contaminant.

Eight years later came the first account of lumbar punc-

ture in a living patient (Quincke 1893), and in 1896 meningococci were isolated for the first time from the CSF of patients with meningitis (Heubner 1896). In the same year meningococci were also isolated from human throat cultures (Kiefer 1896), offering an explanation for the spread of the bacteria in human populations.

Before World War I, German and American bacteriologists were developing serum therapy for meningococcal meningitis in an effort to reduce its extremely high mortality (Kolle and Wasserman 1906, Flexner and Jobling 1908). They were able to reduce mortality from about 80% to 25% by repeated intrathecal instillation of immune horse serum (Flexner and Jobling 1908). Not surprisingly, many successfully treated patients developed 'serum disease' (serum sickness) with fever and arthritis.

In Britain, notification of a range of infectious diseases including cerebrospinal fever was introduced in 1912. Two years later, during the first winter of World War I there were several outbreaks of cerebrospinal fever amongst military recruits. Glover (1920) carried out a detailed investigation at the Guards Depot, Caterham, in south London. His report is a masterpiece of early meningococcal epidemiology; he concluded that the disease flared up at times of extreme overcrowding and was preceded by very high nasopharyngeal carriage rates. Effective interventions, including increasing the amount of sleeping accommodation and the space between beds, fixing open windows in huts and shortening of parades, brought the outbreaks to a halt. Later, Dudley and Brennan (1934) and others documented very high nasopharyngeal carriage rates without the occurrence of cases of meningococcal disease.

All the major combatant countries experienced clusters of cases and outbreaks of meningococcal disease in recruit camps but there was little disease in seasoned troops (Rolleston 1919). At the end of the war, French microbiologists published a serogrouping scheme which forms the basis for the current classification system (Nicolle, Debains and Jouan 1918).

In the 1930s Rake and his colleagues showed that freshly isolated meningococci were 'smooth' (capsulate), that they produced a polysaccharide capsule and that such strains produced more potent antisera when used to immunize horses (Rake 1931, Rake and Scherp 1933). Rake also carried out studies on the duration of nasopharyngeal meningococcal carriage and showed that, though very variable, carriage could persist for years.

Rake's work, which was leading towards the development of vaccines, was halted by the discovery of sulphonamides. After their first use in the treatment of human meningococcal infections (Schwentker 1937), sulphonamides were used to treat very large numbers of cases of meningococcal disease at the beginning of World War II. In Britain in 1941 there were 11 000 notified cases and more than 2000 cases in each subsequent year up to 1945 (Fig. 17.2).

Germany, France and the USA also experienced outbreaks of unprecedented size, in each case shortly after becoming a combatant country. These epidemics occurred in association with mobilization (in 1940–41 in the UK, France and Germany, and in 1942–43 in the USA) and usually began among recruits in training, later spilling over into civilian populations. At the same time, most non-combatant countries, such as Sweden, did not experience any great change in the incidence of meningococcal disease.

Sulphonamides transformed the treatment of meningococcal disease – mortality rates fell to about 10–20%. When penicillin became available later in the war it gradually superseded sulphonamides for treatment of invasive disease, but

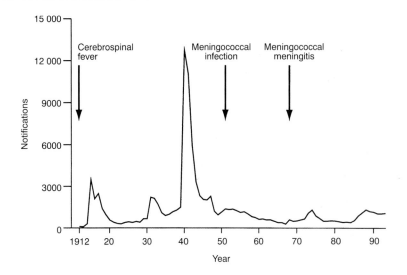

Fig. 17.2 Meningococcal notifications, England and Wales. Data for 1993 are provisional.

sulphonamides continued to be used for the treatment of carriers.

5.2 Epidemiology

Meningococcal disease remains a world-wide problem, occurring sporadically, as clusters of cases and as epidemics. Annual rates of disease in many western countries and in the North American continent are about 1–2 per 100 000 of the total population, though there are wide fluctuations from year to year and from country to country. Even within countries the disease rate can fluctuate remarkably, with clustering of cases in small communities or regions, giving high attack rates (5–25 per 100 000) for months or years. Norway experienced high rates of disease, mainly due to strains of serogroup B (ET-5 clone), for almost 20 years from the 1970s to the 1990s (Lystad and Aasen 1991), whereas the disease incidence in Sweden remained low throughout the same period. At the start of a period of increased disease incidence the average age of cases rises (Peltola, Kataja and Mäkelä 1982) and the severity of disease is greater. These phenomena may reflect the accumulation of susceptible persons in the population.

The 'meningitis belt'

The pattern of disease is quite different in some tropical countries, with large epidemics occurring at irregular intervals, separated by periods of much lower disease activity (Peltola 1983, Moore 1992). Lapeysonnie (1963) drew attention to an area of Africa south of the Sahara and extending almost from coast to coast, where epidemics of meningococcal disease occur every 5–10 years – the 'meningitis belt' (Fig. 17.3). Epidemic waves may last 2 or 3 years.

The boundaries of the meningitis belt are probably defined by climatic factors; continuous high absolute humidity may reduce meningococcal transmission (Cheeseborough et al. 1995). This leads to the situation in sub-Saharan Africa, where countries such as Ghana and Nigeria may experience epidemics of meningococcal disease

in their northern regions, but have low attack rates in their southern coastal areas.

The disease is highly seasonal in the meningitis belt, with an upsurge during the period of dry, dusty winds ('harmattan'), with abrupt cessation of the epidemic with the start of the rainy season. The numbers of cases are staggering by western standards – attack rates of 500 per 100 000 or more have been recorded. The highest attack rate is in the age group 5–15 years; the sexes are equally affected. Multilocus electrophoretic typing (Caugant 1987), which permits identification of meningococcal clones, demonstrates that these epidemics are usually due to the spread of new clones, almost always of serogroup A (Olyhoek, Crowe and Achtman 1987, Achtman 1990, 1995).

Epidemiology in temperate climates

In colder climates the disease is strongly seasonal, with peak rates in the winter months. In Britain, disease rates are highest in December and January, falling to a low point in the autumn months. In western countries the age-specific incidence shows 2 peaks with the first, and larger, in infants and young children. A second smaller, but important peak occurs in late teenage (Fig. 17.4). There is no obvious relationship between the age-specific prevalence of carriage and the incidence of disease. In most western countries affected males outnumber females by up to 1.5:1.

In the UK about 70% of invasive disease is caused by serogroup B meningococci, a further 25% by serogroup C strains and the remainder by a mixture of other serogroups including W-135, Y and X (Jones and Kaczmarski 1994). The large epidemics that occurred during World War I and World War II were caused by strains of serogroup A.

5.3 Carriage

This subject has been dealt with in depth in 2 reviews (Broome 1986, Cartwright 1995). The human nasopharynx is the natural habitat of the meningococcus. Meningococci are not carried by animals, nor are they recovered from the environment. Humans may be selectively colonized because meningococci are only able to acquire iron, an essential nutrient (van Putten

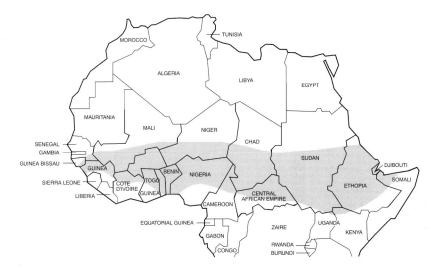

Fig. 17.3 Africa – the meningitis belt.

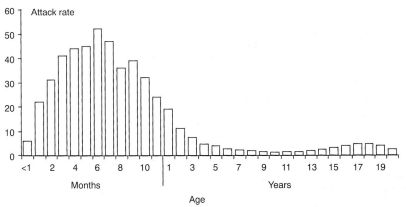

Fig. 17.4 Age-specific incidence of meningococcal disease, England and Wales, 1984–91 (per 10^5 population). (From Jones and Mallard 1993, with permission).

1990), from human transferrin and lactoferrin (Schryvers and Gonzalez 1990). Fimbriae facilitate binding to human epithelial cells, but capsulation reduces adherence. Colonization by a single strain may last for months or even years. Expression of capsule may be downregulated during prolonged carriage.

AGE-SPECIFIC INCIDENCE OF CARRIAGE

Carriage rates are low in infants and young children, but rise with age to peak in late teenage and early adult life (Fig. 17.5). They then decline slowly over the next 20–30 years; carriage is rare after the age of 65 years (Greenfield, Sheehe and Feldman 1971, Cartwright et al. 1987, Caugant et al. 1994).

Most nasopharyngeal meningococci have very low invasive potential. Many express little or no capsular polysaccharide and are non-groupable, or belong to serogroups of low virulence such as X, Y or W-135. Exposure to such strains probably boosts levels of antibody against non-capsular surface antigens.

FACTORS AFFECTING CARRIAGE RATES

Throat swabbing is an insensitive procedure and swabs from individuals and groups underestimate carriage frequency. A single negative throat swab cannot be relied upon as proof of freedom from colonization. Carriage appears to be unaffected by season

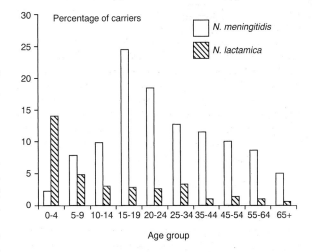

Fig. 17.5 Nasopharyngeal carriage of *N. meningitidis* and *N. lactamica*, Stonehouse, Gloucestershire, November 1986. (From Cartwright et al. 1987, with permission).

(Blakebrough et al. 1982, de Wals et al. 1983), intercurrent viral infection or vaccination with purified capsular polysaccharides.

Smoking has a strong dose-related effect on carriage (Stuart et al. 1989), but contact with a case of meningococcal disease is the most important risk factor for carriage. Rates of carriage are high in family members and close contacts of cases of meningococcal disease (Greenfield and Feldman 1967, Munford et al. 1974). Most such isolates are indistinguishable from the index case strain (Olcén et al. 1981).

5.4   Immunity

The best serological correlate of protection from meningococcal disease is the presence of bactericidal antibodies (Goldschneider, Gotschlich and Artenstein 1969a). For serogroup A and C meningococci, most bactericidal antibody is IgG directed against the capsular polysaccharide and is capable of causing bacterial lysis through the activation of complement (Gotschlich, Goldschneider and Artenstein 1969a). Serogroup B capsular polysaccharide is a very weak antigen for humans, possibly because it shares epitopes with host cell antigens (Finne, Leionen and Mäkelä 1983, Azmi et al. 1995). Antibodies present after serogroup B meningococcal disease are directed against a variety of surface-expressed antigens including outer-membrane proteins and lipopolysaccharide (Kasper et al. 1973, Griffiss et al. 1984).

The role of *Neisseria lactamica*

Bactericidal antibodies are acquired progressively during childhood (Goldschneider, Gotschlich and Artenstein 1969a), beginning at a time when exposure to meningococci is slight. Thus protection is probably first acquired through exposure to other bacteria that express cross-reacting surface antigens (Glode et al. 1977, Guirguis et al. 1985, Devi et al. 1991).

The carriage rate of *Neisseria lactamica* is high when bactericidal meningococcal antibodies are being acquired (see Fig. 17.5). Colonization with *Neisseria lactamica* generates antibody that is bactericidal against a range of serogroups and serotypes of meningococci (Gold et al. 1978). Later in life, exposure to avirulent meningococci induces antibody against a wide range of meningococcal serogroups (Reller, MacGregor and Beaty 1973), indicating that some bactericidal antibody is directed against non-capsular antigens. A number of oral and enteric bacteria also express cross-reactive antigens and probably play a part in generating and maintaining immunity.

Blocking IgA antibodies

Complement-dependent immune lysis is not initiated by IgA. However, secretory or circulating IgA antibodies may block meningococcal surface antigens that would otherwise be accessible to IgG or IgM antibodies that activate complement. Blocking IgA antibodies generated in response to cross-reacting enteric bacteria may be important in some cases of meningococcal disease in older children and adults (Griffiss 1995). The timing of exposure to the meningococcus and the cross-reacting enteric bacterium may be critical (Kilian and Reinholdt 1987, Kilian, Mestecky and Russell 1988).

Complement and properdin deficiencies

Various congenital or acquired immune deficiency syndromes are associated with an increased risk of meningococcal disease (Figueroa and Densen 1991). Deficiency of any of the terminal complement component (C5 to C9) is associated with an increased risk of meningococcal disease, especially of serotypes not normally regarded as invasive, including X, Y and W-135 (Fijen et al. 1989).The risk of second and subsequent attacks is also increased and disease tends to be milder (Ross and Densen 1984). Half the individuals with the very rare deficiency of properdin (factor P) develop meningococcal disease, but this tends to occur in older children or adults and is often overwhelming, with fatality rates greater than 50% (Densen et al. 1987).

Susceptibility at different ages

Meningococcal infection is infrequent in the first 2 months of life, indicating that passively transferred maternal antibodies are important in protection. Subsequently meningococcal disease in infants and young children probably results from exposure of an immunologically virgin child to a virulent meningococcus. This seems less likely in teenagers and young adults in whom there is also a peak of infection (see Fig. 17.4), but at a time when meningococcal carriage is most frequent. Most, if not all, individuals aged 10 years or more will probably on numerous occasions have encountered *Neisseria lactamica*, poorly capsulated meningococci and/or other immunizing bacteria. Therefore meningococcal disease in this age group may result from subversion of pre-existing immunity, inherited increased susceptibility, a high level of exposure to meningococci, or a combination of the 3.

5.5   Meningitis and septicaemia

Meningococcal infection most commonly presents as meningitis (75%) or septicaemia (20%), though the 2 syndromes show considerable overlap; clinical differentiation may be difficult or impossible (Fig. 17.6).

A few patients have other pyogenic infections such as primary septic arthritis, conjunctivitis, pericarditis. The outlook in meningococcal meningitis is very good. Mortality in the UK is less than 5% and the incidence of long-term neurological morbidity, mainly deafness, is low (3–5%). Most meningococcal meningitis occurs in infants and young children in whom the symptoms and signs are similar to those of other types of bacterial meningitis occurring at the same age. A characteristic feature of meningococcal meningitis is the presence of petechiae or purpura in the skin. Though a haemorrhagic skin rash may occur occasionally in Hib or pneumococcal meningitis, it occurs in more than 50% of cases of meningococcal meningitis and in all cases of meningococcal septicaemia. The pathology of the skin lesions resembles a series of localized Shwartzman reactions (DeVoe 1982).

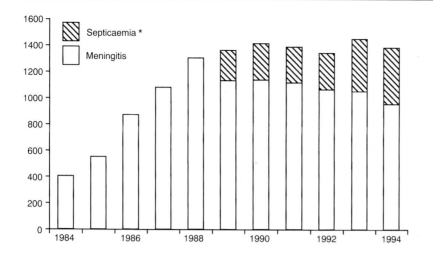

Fig. 17.6 Meningococcal infections in England and Wales: notifications to OPCS, 1984–94. Data for 1994 are provisional. *Meningococcal septicaemia became notifiable in 1989.

Meningococcal meningitis in older patients usually presents with symptoms of malaise, muscular aches and pains, diarrhoea and sometimes vomiting, fever and headache, progressing if unrecognized to confusion, coma, shock and circulatory collapse. In the later stages a haemorrhagic skin rash is almost inevitable. Septicaemia is a far more serious condition with a mortality greater than 20–25%. It can occur with or without evidence of meningitis. Fever, shock and a haemorrhagic skin rash are the hallmarks of this condition. Onset is frequently abrupt, over a few hours. Multisystem failure is common. In addition to antibiotics, inotropes, mechanical ventilation and haemodialysis may be required for considerable periods. Survivors of severe septicaemia may need amputations of necrotic fingers, toes or even limbs.

5.6 Management

ANTIBIOTIC TREATMENT

Benzylpenicillin is the drug of choice in meningococcal disease. The UK Chief Medical Officer recommends that general practitioners and casualty doctors should administer a dose of benzylpenicillin to any patient with suspected meningococcal disease, without awaiting the results of laboratory investigations. This course of action may halve mortality in the more seriously ill, though it makes confirmation of the diagnosis somewhat more difficult (Cartwright et al. 1992). Since the aetiology is not known for certain at the start of in-patient treatment, it is wise to use a broad spectrum antibiotic for the first 24–48 h, especially in young children. Cefotaxime, ceftriaxone or, if cost is a factor, chloramphenicol are suitable alternatives that give high rates of cure; these agents can also be used in patients who are allergic to penicillin. Treatment can be switched to benzylpenicillin when a meningococcal aetiology has been confirmed.

'Penicillin-resistant' meningococci

So-called 'penicillin-resistant' meningococci have been reported in a number of countries and regions including Spain (Saez-Nieto et al. 1992), South Africa, the UK and the North American continent. These strains are better described as showing reduced sensitivity to penicillin and it is likely that it results from acquisition of genetic material from the related *Neisseria flavescens*, an oropharyngeal commensal, leading to production of an altered penicillin-binding protein 2 (Spratt et al. 1989). Illness caused by these strains responds to treatment with adequate doses of benzylpenicillin and there are few reports of treatment failures.

Production of β-lactamase by meningococci isolated from invasive infections has been reported from South Africa and Spain (Botha 1988, Fontanals et al. 1989). Neither strain has survived for detailed investigation.

Duration of treatment

Antibiotic treatment for 7 days may suffice for children with mild illness (McCracken et al. 1987, O'Neill 1993). Longer periods of treatment, of at least 10 days, seem justified in more seriously affected patients, including those with septicaemia.

STEROIDS AND IMMUNOMODULATORS

The role of steroids in meningococcal disease remains controversial. A meta-analysis of recent trials showed a reduction in the incidence of neurological sequelae, mainly deafness, in patients with bacterial meningitis when dexamethasone was given before or with the first dose of antibiotics (Feigin, McCracken and Klein 1992, Schaad et al. 1993, Jafari and McCracken 1994). Most patients had Hib meningitis. Since the pathology of neurological damage is probably similar for the 3 main bacterial pathogens, it seems logical to endorse this addition to treatment in meningococcal and pneumococcal meningitis. Steroids are ineffective in bacterial meningitis if given more than about an hour after the first parenteral dose of antibiotic. A 2 day course is probably as effective as treatment for 4 days (Syrogiannopoulos et al. 1994).

There is no evidence to support the use of dexamethasone in meningococcal septicaemia (Nadel, Levin and Habibi 1995). Various novel therapies for severe meningococcal disease are under consideration including anti-endotoxins, anticytokine response agents, leucocyte activation antagonists, cardiovascular support agents and many others (Nadel, Levin and Habibi 1995).

SECONDARY CASES AND CLUSTERS

Close contacts of cases of meningococcal disease run an increased risk of developing disease in the days and weeks after exposure to an index case, especially a first-degree relative living in the same household. The increased risk may be due to exposure to a known pathogenic strain, an inherited susceptibility to meningococcal infection, transient exposure to a common environmental factor (e.g. influenza virus) (Harrison et al. 1991) or to a combination of these.

The nasopharyngeal carriage rate of meningococci is high in family contacts of cases. Rifampicin, ciprofloxacin and ceftriaxone are all more than 90% successful in eliminating nasopharyngeal colonization in contacts (Cuevas and Hart 1993). They also reduce the incidence of secondary cases of disease in the 30–60 days after the illness of the index case. Though there have been no prospective trials to establish the benefit of chemoprophylaxis, and though there is no evidence to show that the risk of secondary disease is reduced in the longer term, it is accepted policy to offer chemoprophylaxis to defined close contacts (Meningococcal Infections Working Group 1989). If the index case strain was of serogroup A or C, close contacts should be offered A + C vaccine. Regardless of the causative organism, all contacts should be informed about their increased risk of meningococcal disease, which may persist for many months, especially when chemoprophylaxis has been given.

Clusters of cases sometimes occur in playgroups, schools, universities, military establishments and other closed and semi-closed communities. Serogroup C strains are more commonly isolated in such outbreaks. Consideration should be given to the value of chemoprophylaxis with or without vaccination, but each situation must be judged on its merits. The level of public alarm is often at variance with the actual risk.

5.7 Vaccines

The first vaccines for the prevention of meningococcal disease were developed in 1912 (Sophian 1912). Uncontrolled field trials of a whole cell meningococcal vaccine took place in England during World War I (Greenwood 1915). In the 1930s Scherp and Rake (1935) identified capsular material from a meningococcus as a polysaccharide, but work on vaccine development waned when sulphonamides and then penicillin became available. With the emergence of sulphonamide resistance in the 1960s, interest in prevention by vaccination was reawakened. In a series of classical papers Gotschlich, Goldschneider and their colleagues at the Walter Reed Army Institute of Research, Washington, USA, demonstrated the fundamental importance of bactericidal antibodies and went on to develop the first serogroup C polysaccharide vaccine to be properly evaluated in humans (Goldschneider, Gotschlich and Artenstein 1969a, 1969b, Gotschlich, Goldschneider and Artenstein 1969a, Gotschlich, Teh Yung Liu and Artenstein 1969b, Artenstein et al. 1970). Soon after this, a large clinical trial of a serogroup A polysaccharide vaccine was reported from Finland (Peltola et al. 1977) and further serogroup A vaccine studies in Africa followed.

The immunology of meningococcal disease and the major thrust leading to the development of vaccines took place in the USA in the late 1960s. The impetus for this new work was the emergence of sulphonamide resistance, with the resultant inability to reduce the prevalence of carriage in recruit camps.

SEROGROUP A AND C VACCINES

Vaccines containing serogroup A and C polysaccharides are used widely in the UK and quadrivalent A, C, Y and W-135 vaccine is also available. These purified polysaccharide vaccines are not immunogenic in infants, and give only short-term (3–4 years) protection. They are not suitable for universal use and are employed in a more limited set of circumstances (see Table 17.2).

A conjugated serogroup A and C vaccine has undergone preliminary evaluation in the Gambia (Twumasi et al. 1995) and similar conjugate vaccines are currently in clinical trial in infants in the UK (Herbert, Heath and Mayon-White 1995). Such vaccines are expected to be safe and to generate good, long-lasting immunity.

SEROGROUP B VACCINES

Serogroup B polysaccharide is a weak antigen in humans and prospects for effective serogroup B vaccines are more distant (Romero and Outschoorn 1994, Herbert, Heath and Mayon-White 1995). Two serogroup B outer-membrane vesicle vaccines have been developed, in Norway (Bjune et al. 1991) and in Cuba (de Moraes et al. 1992), but neither is effective in infants and there is some evidence that the duration of protection may be limited. Since bactericidal antibody to serogroup B meningococci is directed against surface components other than the capsular polysaccharide, much effort is being invested in the search for stable, surface-expressed serogroup B antigens or epitopes that will provoke the development of human bactericidal antibodies (Poolman, van der Ley and Tommassen 1995). However, meningococci are very well adapted human colonizers and many outer-membrane proteins have hypervariable regions, presumably to evade the host immune response. Among the antigens currently under investigation are the class 1 outer-membrane protein (van der Ley and Poolman 1992, van der Ley et al. 1993) and iron-binding and iron-regulated proteins (Frasch 1995). A further problem with development of serogroup B vaccines is the lack of correlation between the immune responses to candidate antigens in laboratory animals and in man.

Table 17.2 Uses of meningococcal serogroup A + C vaccine

Protection of contacts
Protection of travellers to endemic areas
Control of epidemics
Outbreak control in defined communities
Outbreak control in open communities

6 Pneumococcal meningitis

Unlike Hib meningitis, the incidence of pneumococcal meningitis in the UK has not declined in recent years (Fig. 17.7). In countries that have introduced Hib conjugate vaccines, pneumococci are now the second most common cause of bacterial meningitis. Mortality remains very high at 25% (Sangster, Murdoch and Gray 1982) and is higher still in the elderly. Mortality rates of 40–50% are commonplace in pneumococcal meningitis in tropical Africa (Greenwood 1987). Morbidity is also higher than in meningococcal or Hib meningitis, probably because of the larger numbers of bacteria found in the subarachnoid space in pneumococcal meningitis and their particular capacity to induce a viscid, gelatinous exudate into which antibiotic penetration is poor.

Antibiotic resistance, not only to penicillin but also to chloramphenicol and third generation cephalosporins, is becoming a serious therapeutic problem in many parts of the world (Jacobs and Appelbaum 1995, Tomasz 1995).

Rapid progress in the development of conjugated pneumococcal polysaccharide vaccines offers good prospects for reducing the overall incidence of invasive pneumococcal disease and more modest but still interesting possibilities for reducing the incidence of pneumococcal meningitis. For all these reasons pneumococcal meningitis is an extremely important condition and will remain so for some years.

6.1 Epidemiology

Streptococcus pneumoniae causes bacteraemia and meningitis at all ages, but attack rates are highest in infants, falling to low levels in children and young adults. Bacteraemia rates then rise again to very high levels in the elderly, though rates of meningitis do not.

Meningitis occurs in about one-sixth of all invasive pneumococcal infections. The highest meningitis attack rate occurs in the first week of life, when the invading organisms are probably acquired from the maternal birth canal. Males are affected more often than females and infection is more common in the winter months. In the UK pneumococcal meningitis attack rates have remained fairly constant in recent

years at around 0.5 per 100 000 of the total population per annum (Aszkenasy, George and Begg 1995).

Risk factors

Age is the most important determinant of pneumococcal meningitis, but a number of host conditions predispose to invasive pneumococcal disease. These include splenectomy, thalassaemia, sickle cell disease, alcoholism, myeloma, hypogammaglobulinaemia and complement deficiency. In the USA rates of pneumococcal meningitis are much higher in non-whites. Though pneumococci most frequently gain access to the meninges by blood-borne dissemination, they may also invade directly from an infected middle ear or mastoid cavity, or through a meningeal tear after cranial trauma (Kirkpatrick, Reeves and MacGowan 1994). A distant focus of primary infection, such as pneumonia, otitis media, mastoiditis or sinusitis, is more common in pneumococcal meningitis than in Hib or meningococcal meningitis (Davey et al. 1982). Patients with pneumococcal meningitis often have a pre-existing medical condition (Davey et al. 1982, Kirkpatrick, Reeves and MacGowan 1994).

Only a small number of the 84 pneumococcal serotypes (1–9, 12, 14, 18, 19, 22, 23) are responsible for most invasive pneumococcal disease. Particular serotypes may be associated with central nervous system infection, some with a higher case fatality rate.

6.2 Clinical presentations and outcome

Clinical presentations depend on age, but are similar to other types of acute pyogenic meningitis. Typically the presentation is abrupt but symptoms may develop over several days. At presentation, patients with pneumococcal meningitis tend to be more ill than those with Hib or meningococcal meningitis; fits are commoner (Pederson and Henrichsen 1983) and there may be focal neurological signs, especially cranial nerve palsies. Comatose or semicomatose patients are more likely to have pneumococcal than meningococcal meningitis (Carpenter and Petersdorf 1962). Petechial rashes, though much less frequently encountered than in meningococcal meningitis, may also occur, especially in asplenic patients. In the neonatal

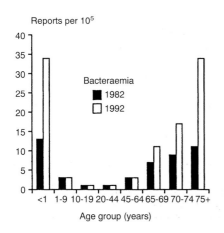

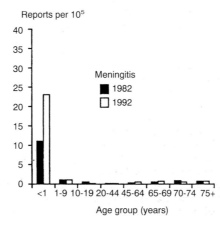

Fig. 17.7 Pneumococcal infections (laboratory reports): bacteraemia and meningitis, England and Wales, 1982 and 1992. (After Aszkenasy, George and Begg 1995).

period clinical presentations are similar to those seen in other types of neonatal bacterial meningitis.

Elderly patients, those with impaired consciousness or with convulsions on admission, or with a distant focus of pneumococcal infection are all more likely to die.

6.3 Treatment

ANTIBIOTICS

Until quite recently, pneumococci were sensitive to penicillin in almost all parts of the world. When the causative strain is fully sensitive (MIC <0.1 μg ml⁻¹), benzylpenicillin in large doses remains the antibiotic treatment of first choice. Schmidt and Sesler (1943) were the first to report penicillin resistance. Multiply antibiotic-resistant strains are now frequently encountered in the USA, Australia, New Guinea and in South Africa (Lister 1995, Schwartz and Tunkel 1995). The prevalence of moderately penicillin-resistant strains (MIC 0.1–1.0 μg ml⁻¹) varies widely from country to country; it is 2% in England and Wales (Aszkenasy, George and Begg 1995), 25% in the USA and 40–45% in Spain and South Africa (Friedland and Klugman 1992a, Tomasz 1995). In most countries the prevalence of moderately resistant and of highly resistant strains (MIC 2.0 μg ml⁻¹ or greater) is increasing (Breiman et al. 1994). Penicillin resistance may have arisen through transfer of genetic material from strains of *Streptococcus mitis* (Coffey et al. 1995).

Pneumococci resistant to third generation cephalosporins have been documented in the USA and in South Africa (Friedland and Klugman 1992a, Tenover, Swenson and McDougal 1992). Detection of resistance to β-lactam antibiotics (Tenover, Swenson and McDougal 1992) is not merely of interest in the laboratory; it is associated with treatment failure (Bradley and Connor 1991, Sloas et al. 1992). In countries with a high prevalence of low-level pneumococcal penicillin resistance, third generation cephalosporins such as cefotaxime and ceftriaxone are widely used as empirical agents of first choice in bacterial meningitis. However, as the level of resistance to penicillin rises, cephalosporins and chloramphenicol lose their efficacy (Friedland and Klugman 1992b, Lister 1995). Antibiotic treatment options for penicillin and cephalosporin-resistant pneumococcal meningitis have recently been reviewed (Jacobs and Appelbaum 1995, Lister 1995, Schwartz and Tunkel 1995). Chloramphenicol should not be used, even though strains may appear sensitive in the laboratory. Vancomycin, with or without the addition of rifampicin, becomes the antibiotic of choice. To cover meningococci, benzylpenicillin should be incorporated into any empirical treatment regimen for bacterial meningitis when the causative organism has not been identified. Though data are scanty, most experts treat pneumococcal meningitis with parenteral antibiotics for at least 10–14 days (McCracken et al. 1987, O'Neill 1993).

STEROIDS

Dexamethasone may reduce mortality and/or morbidity (Girgis et al. 1989, Bhatt et al. 1995), but pneumococcal meningitis is so infrequent that prospective controlled studies of sufficient size have not been carried out. The majority of paediatricians advise its use.

MANAGEMENT OF CONTACTS

Contact with a case of pneumococcal meningitis does not confer an increased risk of disease. Neither antibiotic prophylaxis nor vaccination is necessary to protect intimate contacts of patients with pneumococcal meningitis.

RECURRENT PNEUMOCOCCAL MENINGITIS

The occurrence of a second episode of pneumococcal meningitis in a patient should raise the strong possibility of a dural tear and there is usually, but not always, a history of cranial trauma. Such patients should be referred to a neurosurgeon for evaluation. A few patients with a history of recurrent pneumococcal meningitis but without a dural defect respond poorly to pneumococcal capsular polysaccharides; usually they respond to conjugate pneumococcal vaccines.

6.4 Prevention

PNEUMOCOCCAL VACCINES

Pneumococcal capsular polysaccharides are major virulence determinants and are immunogenic; vaccines based on capsular polysaccharides have been used for more than 20 years. Multivalent vaccines are used because there are more than 80 serotypes and protection is serotype specific. Vaccines containing 6–14 common serotypes were used in the 1970s but were superseded by 23-valent vaccines in the 1980s. Though the frequency with which the different serotypes cause invasive disease varies from country to country, the currently available 23-valent polysaccharide vaccines offer protection in most, if not all countries.

Purified pneumococcal polysaccharides do not make ideal vaccines (Mitchell and Andrew 1995). In common with other bacterial polysaccharides they are high molecular weight compounds with repeating structures that stimulate B lymphocytes directly without stimulating T cells. T cell independent antigens have a number of defects as vaccine candidates (Table 17.3).

Table 17.3 Characteristics of T independent (TI) and T dependent (TD) antibody responses

	TI	TD
T cells required	–	+
Ontogeny of response	Late	Early
Induction of memory	–	+
Isotype restriction	+	–
Affinity maturation	–	+

Purified polysaccharides are converted from TI to TD antigens by conjugation to carrier proteins, e.g. tetanus toxoid.

In older children and adults the antibody induced does not persist, leading to waning of protection over time. The capacity of the 23-valent vaccine to induce good immune responses declines progressively after the age of 60–65 years; immunogenicity is also poor in patient groups at increased risk of invasive disease including those with asplenia, hyposplenism and a variety of immunodeficiency conditions including HIV infection. Patients with AIDS and CD4 counts greater than 500 mm^{-3} respond well; those with lower counts do not respond as well (Rodriguez-Barradas et al. 1992). Thus the groups at highest risk of invasive pneumococcal disease are the same as those in whom purified polysaccharide vaccines are least likely to be effective. Nevertheless, the 23-valent polysaccharide vaccine has been recommended for a wide variety of groups at increased risk of invasive or severe disease. These include patients aged over 2 years with functional or anatomical asplenia or hyposplenism (including sickle cell disease), patients with AIDS (regardless of the stage of illness) and other immunodeficiency states, malignancies, chronic respiratory, renal and liver diseases and some metabolic diseases such as diabetes (Department of Health 1992). It remains unclear whether the 23-valent vaccines protect fit, healthy elderly individuals living in the community. Vaccination does not protect against recurrent pneumococcal meningitis associated with dural tears; repair of the defect is the only effective treatment known. Revaccination with 23-valent pneumococcal polysaccharide vaccine within 18 months of a previous dose is associated with a higher incidence of side effects (Borgono et al. 1978), but there is no evidence that revaccination after 4–6 years causes severe or unacceptable side effects (Kaplan, Sarnaik and Schiffman 1986, Mufson et al. 1991).

Conjugated pneumococcal polysaccharide vaccines are now entering clinical trial. The candidate vaccines so far produced consist of fewer than 10 capsular polysaccharides. These vaccines are expected to be safe and immunogenic in infants; they should give rise to long-lasting, though serotype-specific, protection at almost all ages. They will be expensive and may need to be tailored to the serotypes prevalent in different countries.

Attempts to produce pneumococcal vaccines based on surface-exposed proteins expressed by all pneumococci, regardless of serotype, have so far been unsuccessful. Research is continuing on a number of candidate proteins including pneumolysin, neuraminidase, pneumococcal surface protein A and a 37 kDa outer-membrane protein. Such outer-membrane proteins may become constituents of pneumococcal vaccines in the future, but do not at present look promising candidates on their own (Mitchell and Andrew 1995).

Pneumococcal meningitis in the first month of life is probably not preventable by infant vaccination, even at birth. Alternative strategies, such as maternal immunization during or before pregnancy, or passive protection of newborn infants with immunoglobulin followed by active immunization at a later date, may need to be considered.

ANTIBIOTIC PROPHYLAXIS

Long-term oral penicillin or amoxycillin prophylaxis has been used in an attempt to reduce the risk of invasive pneumococcal disease in patients at increased risk, but there is no evidence that prophylactic antibiotics can reduce the risk of primary or recurrent pneumococcal meningitis.

7 HAEMOPHILUS INFLUENZAE TYPE B (HIB) MENINGITIS

7.1 Epidemiology

Before the widespread introduction of effective vaccines, Hib was the commonest cause of bacterial meningitis in children under the age of 5 in almost all countries; in the USA, Australia, Brazil and Zaire it was the commonest cause of bacterial meningitis in the population as a whole. Within countries, attack rates of invasive Hib disease vary widely. In the UK attack rates of 24–36 per 100 000 children under 5 years were observed in 6 regions in 1990–92 (Anderson et al. 1995), with almost 90% of invasive *H. influenzae* infections occurring in children under 5.

In contrast, attack rates of Hib disease in 'native American' and Australian aboriginal populations of 150–450 per 100 000 children aged under 5 years, i.e. rates 10-fold higher than in Europeans, have been recorded (Bijlmer 1991). In the USA, higher disease rates in blacks than whites may have been due to socioeconomic rather than racial factors (Cochi et al. 1986). Though Hib meningitis has a relatively low case fatality rate in economically advanced countries (3–5%), high fatality rates (20–30%) are common in tropical Africa (Bijlmer 1991).

Before vaccination was introduced, most UK cases of Hib meningitis occurred in infants, with a peak attack rate in the 6–11 month age group (Anderson et al. 1995); in population groups with very high disease attack rates, peak attack rates occurred in children under 6 months old (Bijlmer 1991). A peak of disease at such an early age presented problems in the deployment of vaccines.

The increasing incidence of invasive Hib disease in the USA and the UK in the 1970s and 1980s was probably due to social changes as well as more accurate diagnosis. Attendance at day care centres or preschool nurseries conferred an increased risk of disease; conversely, breast feeding was protective (Redmond and Pichichero 1984, Cochi et al. 1986).

7.2 Bacteriology and immunology

Non-capsulate strains of *H. influenzae* are part of the human nasopharyngeal commensal flora. They are of low pathogenicity and cause mainly localized infections in the respiratory tract in patients with preexisting disease, but they rarely invade.

A small minority of *H. influenzae* strains possess a polysaccharide capsule, which defines 6 serotypes designated a–f. The type b polysaccharide is a polymer of ribose and ribitol phosphate (polyribosephosphate, PRP). Before vaccination was introduced, type b strains (Hib) were responsible for more than 95% of invasive haemophilus disease. Meningitis was the commonest clinical manifestation, followed by epiglottitis, bacteraemia without localizing features, cellulitis, pneumonia and septic arthritis (Anderson et al. 1995). Most, if not all, invasive Hib disease is accompanied by a bacteraemic phase.

Hib is carried mainly by children, but the overall carriage rate in unimmunized populations is only 1% in children under 6 years; the peak of carriage occurs in children aged 24–36 months (Howard, Dunkin and Millar 1988).

The early classical investigations of Fothergill and Wright (1933) showed that blood samples from children aged 3 months to 3 years lacked bactericidal activity against Hib, in contrast to samples from neonates, older children and adults. Subsequently Alexander et al. (1942) showed that administration of Hib antiserum caused a substantial increase in the phagocytosis of Hib bacteria in the subarachnoid space, suggesting the importance of opsonizing type-specific antibodies.

The carriage rate of Hib strains in young children is so low that many who acquire antibodies to PRP must do so without exposure to Hib strains. Their protective antibodies probably result from exposure to heterologous bacteria that produce polysaccharides with antigenic determinants identical to those on PRP. Amongst several other bacterial species, *E. coli* K100 expresses an almost identical polysaccharide and, if fed to adult volunteers or laboratory animals, induces antibodies that show bactericidal and opsonic activity against Hib (Schneerson and Robbins 1975).

Bacteraemia precedes Hib meningitis, epiglottitis and the other invasive Hib syndromes. Why the bacteria localize in the meninges, or other organs, is not well understood (Moxon 1992). Experiments in an infant rat model indicate that the intensity of bacteraemia may be an important factor in the development of meningitis (Moxon and Ostrow 1977).

7.3 Clinical features

The disease may develop insidiously over 24–48 h or it may present more abruptly. Most cases are in infants, who often start by being 'snuffly'. Fever and vomiting are common early but non-specific symptoms (Haggerty and Ziai 1964) that may be accompanied by failure to feed, pallor, irritability and persistent crying. As the infection progresses, shock may supervene, the level of consciousness may become clearly depressed and infants may be extremely ill by the time the diagnosis is made. Seizures occur in a minority of cases (Feigin 1987), more commonly in Hib and pneumococcal meningitis than in meningococcal meningitis.

In older children, the more traditional symptoms of meningitis – headache, neck stiffness and photophobia – may be encountered.

7.4 Treatment

Intravenous chloramphenicol replaced ampicillin when resistance of Hib to the latter due to β-lactamase production began to increase; it is at present 15% in the UK and higher elsewhere. Chloramphenicol fell into disuse partly because of a small but increasing percentage of resistant strains (1–2%), but also because of fears of irreversible bone marrow suppression. It has been replaced by third generation cephalosporins. Cefotaxime and ceftriaxone are superior to cefuroxime; the latter takes longer to sterilize the CSF and is associated with a higher incidence of hearing loss (Schaad et al. 1990). Ceftriaxone may be given as a single daily dose and, in carefully selected patients with milder illness, it is suitable for out-patient completion of a course of parenteral antibiotic treatment for bacterial meningitis. Antimicrobial treatment of Hib meningitis should normally be continued for 7–10 days (McCracken et al. 1987, O'Neill 1993).

Administration of dexamethasone to children with Hib meningitis before, or at the same time as the first dose of antibiotic is given, reduces the incidence of neurological sequelae, principally deafness (Lebel et al. 1988, Feigin, McCracken and Klein 1992, Schaad et al. 1993). Steroids given after the first dose of antibiotic are ineffective. They probably act by blocking the inflammatory cascade induced by the release of endotoxin into the subarachnoid compartment.

Susceptible contacts of cases of invasive Hib disease run a considerably increased risk of developing Hib disease in the weeks after the contact. The degree of increased risk depends on the intimacy of the contact; household contacts are at greater risk than day care centre or preschool playgroup contacts. In the UK, all children up to the age of 4 years should at the time of writing have received Hib vaccine to protect them from infection. Unvaccinated close contacts aged up to 4 years should be offered rifampicin prophylaxis and an immediate course of Hib vaccine: 3 doses if aged under 1 year or one dose if aged 13–48 months. Adult contacts do not need Hib vaccine and require chemoprophylaxis only if an unimmunized contact aged under 4 years is in the household (Cartwright, Begg and Rudd 1994).

7.5 Vaccines

The first Hib vaccines consisted of purified type b capsular polysaccharide (PRP) and suffered from all the defects of T independent antigens (see Table 17.3). In spite of their disadvantages, PRP vaccines were widely used in the USA in the 1980s to immunize children aged over 18 months and they somewhat reduced the incidence of invasive Hib disease.

Conjugated polysaccharides are T dependent antigens and their introduction as vaccines changed the situation dramatically, since such vaccines are immunogenic even in infants under 3 months. They induce high avidity IgG antibodies and long-term immunity that can be boosted with the vaccine.

The impact of Hib vaccination is almost immediate, because almost all invasive Hib disease occurs in infants and very young children. In England and

Wales, Hib vaccines were introduced in October 1992 and by 1994 there was a two-thirds reduction in invasive Hib disease and a continuing falling trend (Fig. 17.8).

Hib vaccine is offered to all UK infants aged 2, 3 and 4 months and to selected at-risk groups such as asplenic adults.

8 NEONATAL MENINGITIS

Neonatal bacterial meningitis is rare but serious, with a mortality up to 30–40% and permanent sequelae in up to 30% of survivors. The causative organisms are different from those of bacterial meningitis at other ages, since most bacterial meningitis in this age group is due to organisms derived from ascending infection in utero or from the birth canal during delivery (de Louvois 1994). Occasionally, outbreaks occur in hospital nurseries. Neonatal bacterial meningitis is almost always preceded by bacteraemia. In the UK the principal causative organisms are gram-negative enteric bacilli and group B streptococci. The latter can cause early onset or late onset disease as long as 3–4 months after birth. Other bacteria, including pneumococci, *L. monocytogenes*, meningococci, other streptococci and *Staphylococcus aureus*, can also cause neonatal meningitis.

The overall rate of infection in the UK is about 0.25 per 1000 live births (de Louvois 1994), whereas in the USA it is probably twice as high (Riley 1972). Twenty years ago gram-negative enteric bacteria were the most frequent cause of neonatal meningitis in the USA, but more recently group B streptococci have predominated. The neonatal sepsis rate with group B streptococci is much higher in the USA than in the UK. In the USA screening late in pregnancy and treatment of carriers has been advocated, but such a policy presents considerable problems (Towers 1995).

Prematurity, low birth weight, prolonged rupture of membranes and prolonged labour all increase the risk of neonatal meningitis. Babies born to mothers who are pyrexial during labour are also at risk and some infections are acquired in utero.

It is unclear why particular babies develop meningitis. Strains of *E. coli* that cause neonatal meningitis almost all express the K1 capsular antigen (Mulder and Zanen 1984). Group B streptococci of type III are more commonly isolated from cases of neonatal meningitis than other group B streptococci and both neonatal and maternal antibody levels to these organisms are lower in affected than in control babies.

Neonates frequently show little specific evidence of meningeal irritation. They may be 'jittery' or may present with listlessness, pallor, crying that may be high-pitched, failure to feed, vomiting and sometimes jaundice; control of respiration, of heart rate and sometimes of temperature becomes unstable. These non-specific symptoms may progress to more obvious depression of consciousness. Raised intracranial pressure, as evidenced by a bulging fontanelle, occurs late, and only in a minority of cases.

Blood cultures are part of the standard investigation of any sick baby. If meningitis is suspected lumbar puncture should be considered at an early stage, though failure to detect an abnormality on initial examination should never lead to the withholding of antibiotic treatment. Infection at another site such as the urinary tract should be excluded.

Once meningitis is confirmed the choice of antibiotics depends on the causative organism. A combination of benzylpenicillin and gentamicin is often used while the results of blood and CSF culture are awaited and can be continued if group B streptococci are isolated. If a gram-negative bacillus is isolated, a combination of a cephalosporin and an aminoglycoside may be appropriate, but treatment should be guided by the antibiotic sensitivity of the particular organism.

9 TUBERCULOUS MENINGITIS

Tuberculous meningitis is rare. In the UK there are fewer than 100 cases each year, the majority in people from the Indian subcontinent. After a steady decline over many years in the incidence of tuberculous disease, there has been a small rise in notifications in the

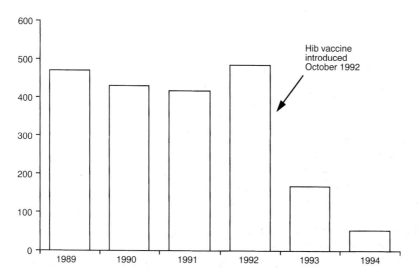

Fig. 17.8 Notifications to OPCS of *H. influenzae* meningitis, England and Wales, 1989–94.

last 3 years. In the USA tuberculous meningitis is a well recognized late complication of AIDS (Bishburg et al. 1986); atypical mycobacteria are sometimes responsible. So far there is little evidence of an overlap between tuberculosis and AIDS in the UK.

Tuberculous meningitis probably always arises as a result of dissemination of tubercle bacilli from a distant focus of infection, often the lung. The disease is caused by liberation of tubercle bacilli from subpial tuberculomata into the subarachnoid space (Rich and McCordock 1933). Postmortem examination confirms the gelatinous nature of the exudate, particularly around the base of the brain, consistent with the high incidence of cranial nerve palsies seen in tuberculous meningitis.

The disease almost always presents insidiously with persistent fever and increasing headache over a period of weeks or months, but, rarely, the presentation may be acute. The cellular exudate in the CSF is most frequently lymphocytic, but may be mixed and the protein concentration is often very high (2–3 g l^{-1}). The CSF:blood glucose ratio is usually, but not always, reduced. In the majority of cases tubercle bacilli are not seen on direct microscopy. The culture of CSF for tubercle bacilli should be extended because about 10% of cultures will become positive only after 6 weeks. There is an obvious place for a CSF mycobacterial PCR test in suspected tuberculous meningitis.

Plain chest and abdominal radiographs may reveal a primary tuberculous focus, so increasing suspicions of tuberculous meningitis. Computed tomography and nuclear magnetic resonance imaging of the cranium are useful investigative techniques (Berger 1994). Since direct microscopy is insensitive, empirical antituberculous treatment may have to be started if the clinical picture is strongly suggestive. Treatment is usually based on a combination of rifampicin, isoniazid and pyrazinamide, but the use of steroids is controversial. In the UK, tuberculous meningitis is usually managed by chest physicians because of their familiarity with antituberculous therapy.

10   OTHER TYPES OF BACTERIAL MENINGITIS

In this brief review it is not possible to list all the more unusual types of bacterial meningitis. Three non-viral causes of aseptic (lymphocytic) meningitis should be briefly mentioned – Lyme borreliosis (Pachner 1995), syphilis (Lukehart et al. 1988) and primary amoebic meningoencephalitis (Carter 1968). These may all present acutely, but all are very rare in the UK. The history, such as that of a tick bite in Lyme meningitis, or of swimming in warm water before amoebic meningoencephalitis, may provide diagnostic clues.

For cryptococcal and fungal meningitis see Volume 4.

REFERENCES

Achtman M, 1990, Molecular epidemiology of epidemic bacterial meningitis, *Rev Med Microbiol*, **1:** 29–38.

Achtman M, 1995, Global epidemiology of meningococcal disease, *Meningococcal Disease*, ed. Cartwright K, John Wiley, Chichester, 159–75.

Alexander HE, Ellis C et al., 1942, Treatment of type-specific *Haemophilus influenzae* infections in infancy and childhood, *J Pediatr*, **20:** 673–98.

Anderson EC, Begg NT et al., 1995, Epidemiology of invasive *Haemophilus influenzae* infections in England and Wales in the pre-vaccination era (1990–2), *Epidemiol Infect*, **115:** 89–100.

Artenstein MS, Gold R et al., 1970, Prevention of meningococcal disease by serogroup C polysaccharide vaccine, *N Engl J Med*, **121:** 372–7.

Aszkenasy OM, George RC, Begg NT, 1995, Pneumococcal bacteraemia and meningitis in England and Wales 1982 to 1992, *Communic Dis Rep Rev*, **5:** R45–50.

Azmi FH, Lucas AH et al., 1995, Human immunoglobulin M paraproteins cross-reactive with *Neisseria meningitidis* group B polysaccharide and fetal brain, *Infect Immun*, **63:** 1906–13.

Berger JRR, 1994, Tuberculous meningitis, *Curr Opin Neurol*, **7:** 191–200.

Bhatt SM, Cabellos C et al., 1995, The impact of dexamethasone on hearing loss in experimental pneumococcal meningitis, *Pediatr Infect Dis J*, **14:** 93–6.

Bijlmer HA, 1991, Worldwide epidemiology of *Haemophilus influenzae* meningitis, *Vaccine*, **9, Suppl.:** S5–9.

Bishburg E, Sunderam G et al., 1986, Central nervous system tuberculosis with the acquired immunodeficiency syndrome and its related complex, *Ann Intern Med*, **105:** 210–13.

Bjune G, Høiby EA et al., 1991, Effect of outer membrane vesicle vaccine against serogroup B meningococcal disease in Norway, *Lancet*, **338:** 1093–6.

Blakebrough IS, Greenwood BM et al., 1982, The epidemiology of infections due to *Neisseria meningitidis* and *Neisseria lactam-ica* in a northern Nigerian community, *J Infect Dis*, **146:** 626–37.

Borgono JM, McLean AA et al., 1978, Vaccination and revaccination with polyvalent pneumococcal polysaccharide vaccines in adults and infants, *Proc Soc Exp Biol Med*, **157:** 148–54.

Botha P, 1988, Penicillin-resistant *Neisseria meningitidis* in southern Africa, *Lancet*, **1:** 54.

Bradley JS, Connor JD, 1991, Ceftriaxone failure in meningitis caused by *Streptococcus pneumoniae* with reduced susceptibility to beta-lactam antibiotics, *Pediatr Infect Dis J*, **10:** 871–3.

Breiman RF, Butler JC et al., 1994, Emergence of drug-resistant pneumococcal infections in the United States, *JAMA*, **271:** 1831–5.

British Society for the Study of Infection Research Committee, 1995, Bacterial meningitis: causes for concern, *J Infect*, **30:** 89–94.

Broome CV, 1986, The carrier state: *Neisseria meningitidis*, *J Antimicrob Chemother*, **18, Suppl. A:** 25–34.

Bryan JP, de Silva HR et al., 1990, Etiology and mortality of bacterial meningitis in northeastern Brazil, *Rev Infect Dis*, **12:** 128–35.

Carpenter RR, Petersdorf RG, 1962, The clinical spectrum of bacterial meningitis, *Am J Med*, **33:** 262–75.

Carter RF, 1968, Primary amoebic meningoencephalitis: clinical, pathological and epidemiological features of six fatal cases, *J Pathol Bacteriol*, **96:** 1–25.

Cartwright K, 1995, Meningococcal carriage and disease, *Meningococcal Disease*, ed. Cartwright K, John Wiley, Chichester, 115–46.

Cartwright KAV, Begg NT, Rudd P, 1994, Use of vaccines and antibiotic prophylaxis in contacts and cases of *Haemophilus influenzae* type b (Hib) disease, *Communic Dis Rep Rev*, **4:** R16–17.

Cartwright KAV, Stuart JM et al., 1987, The Stonehouse survey:

nasopharyngeal carriage of meningococci and *Neisseria lactamica*, *Epidemiol Infect*, **99**: 591–601.

Cartwright KA, Jones DM et al., 1991, Influenza A and meningococcal disease, *Lancet*, **338**: 554–7.

Cartwright K, Reilly S et al., 1992, Early treatment with parenteral penicillin in meningococcal disease, *Br Med J*, **305**: 143–7.

Caugant DA, Mocca LF et al., 1987, Genetic structure of *Neisseria meningitidis* populations in relation to serogroup, serotype, and outer membrane protein pattern, *J Bacteriol*, **169**: 2781–92.

Caugant DA, Høiby EA et al., 1994, Asymptomatic carriage of *Neisseria meningitidis* in a randomly sampled population, *J Clin Microbiol*, **32**: 323–30.

Cheesebrough JS, Morse AP et al., 1995, Meningococcal meningitis and carriage in western Zaire: a hypoendemic zone related to climate?, *Epidemiol Infect*, **114**: 75–92.

Cochi SL, Fleming DW et al., 1986, Primary invasive *Haemophilus influenzae* type b disease: a population-based assessment of risk factors, *J Pediatr*, **108**: 887–96.

Coffey TJ, Dowson CG et al., 1995, Genetics and molecular biology of β-lactam-resistant pneumococci, *Microb Drug Resist*, **1**: 29–34.

Cuevas LE, Hart CA, 1993, Chemoprophylaxis of bacterial meningitis, *J Antimicrob Chemother*, **31 Suppl. B**: 79–91.

Davey PG, Cruikshank JK et al., 1982, Bacterial meningitis – ten years experience, *J Hyg Camb*, **83**: 383–401.

Densen P, Weiler JM et al., 1987, Familial properdin deficiency and fatal meningococcemia. Correction of the bactericidal defect by vaccination, *N Engl J Med*, **316**: 922–6.

Department of Health, 1992, *Immunisation against Infectious Disease*, HMSO, London, 100–3.

van Deuren M, van Dijke BJ et al., 1993, Rapid diagnosis of acute meningococcal infections by needle aspiration of biopsy of skin lesions, *Br Med J*, **306**: 1229–32.

Devi SJN, Schneerson R et al., 1991, Identity between polysaccharide antigens of *Moraxella nonliquefaciens*, group B *Neisseria meningitidis*, and *Escherichia coli* K1 (non-O acetylated), *Infect Immun*, **59**: 732–6.

DeVoe IW, 1982, The meningococcus and mechanisms of pathogenicity, *Microbiol Rev*, **46**: 162–90.

De Wals P, Gilquin C et al., 1983, Longitudinal study of asymptomatic meningococcal carriage in two Belgian populations of schoolchildren, *J Infect*, **6**: 147–56.

Dudley SF, Brennan JR, 1934, High and persistent carrier rates of *Neisseria meningitidis* unaccompanied by cases of meningitis, *J Hyg Camb*, **34**: 525–41.

Feigin RD, 1987, Bacterial meningitis beyond the neonatal period, *Textbook of Pediatric Infections*, 2nd edn, eds Feigin RD, Cherry JD, Saunders, Philadelphia, 439–65.

Feigin RD, McCracken GH, Klein JO, 1992, Diagnosis and management of meningitis, *Pediatr Infect Dis J*, **11**: 785–814.

Figueroa JE, Densen P, 1991, Infectious diseases associated with complement deficiencies, *Clin Microbiol Rev*, **4**: 359–95.

Fijen CAP, Kuijper EJ et al., 1989, Complement deficiencies in patients over ten years old with meningococcal disease due to uncommon serogroups, *Lancet*, **2**: 585–8.

Finne J, Leionen M, Mäkelä H, 1983, Antigenic similarities between brain components and bacteria causing meningitis, *Lancet*, **2**: 355–7.

Flexner S, Jobling JW, 1908, An analysis of four hundred cases of epidemic meningitis treated with the anti-meningitis serum, *J Exp Med*, **10**: 690–733.

Fontanals D, Pineda V et al., 1989, Penicillin resistant beta-lactamase producing *Neisseria meningitidis* in Spain, *Eur J Clin Microbiol Infect Dis*, **8**: 90–1.

Fothergill LD, Wright J, 1933, Influenzal meningitis: the relation of age incidence to the bactericidal power of blood against causal organisms, *J Immunol*, **24**: 273–84.

Frasch CE, 1995, Meningococcal vaccines: past, present and future, *Meningococcal Disease*, ed. Cartwright K, John Wiley, Chichester, 21–34.

Friedland IR, Klugman KP, 1992a, Antibiotic-resistant pneumococcal disease in South African children, *Am J Dis Child*, **146**: 920–3.

Friedland IR, Klugman KP, 1992b, Failure of chloramphenicol therapy in penicillin-resistant pneumococcal meningitis, *Lancet*, **339**: 405–8.

Girgis NI, Farid Z et al., 1989, Dexamethasone treatment for bacterial meningitis in children and adults, *Pediatr Infect Dis J*, **8**: 848–51.

Glode MP, Robbins JB et al., 1977, Cross-antigenicity and immunogenicity between capsular polysaccharides of group C *Neisseria meningitidis* and of *Escherichia coli* K92, *J Infect Dis*, **135**: 94–102.

Glover JA, 1920, Observations of the meningococcus carrier rate and their application to the prevention of cerebro-spinal fever, *Special Report Series of the Medical Research Council (London)*, **50**: 133–65.

Gold R, Goldschneider I et al., 1978, Carriage of *Neisseria meningitidis* and *Neisseria lactamica* in infants and children, *J Infect Dis*, **137**: 112–21.

Goldschneider I, Gotschlich EC, Artenstein MS, 1969a, Human immunity to the meningococcus. I. The role of humoral antibodies, *J Exp Med*, **129**: 1307–26.

Goldschneider I, Gotschlich EC, Artenstein MS, 1969b, Human immunity to the meningococcus. II. Development of natural immunity, *J Exp Med*, **129**: 1327–48.

Gotschlich EC, Goldschneider I, Artenstein MS, 1969a, Human immunity to the meningococcus. IV. Immunogenicity of group A and group C meningococcal polysaccharides in human volunteers, *J Exp Med*, **129**: 1367–84.

Gotschlich EC, Teh Yung Liu, Artenstein MS, 1969b, Human immunity to the meningococcus. III. Preparation and immunochemical properties of the group A, group B and group C meningococcal polysaccharides, *J Exp Med*, **129**: 1349–65.

Gray LD, Fedorko DP, 1992, Laboratory diagnosis of bacterial meningitis, *Clin Microbiol Rev*, **5**: 130–45.

Greenfield S, Feldman HA, 1967, Familial carriers and meningococcal meningitis, *N Engl J Med*, **277**: 498–502.

Greenfield S, Sheehe PR, Feldman HA, 1971, Meningococcal carriage in a population of 'normal' families, *J Infect Dis*, **123**: 67–73.

Greenwood BM, 1987, The epidemiology of acute bacterial meningitis in tropical Africa, *Bacterial Meningitis*, eds Williams JD, Burnie J, Academic Press, London, 61–91.

Greenwood M, 1916, The outbreak of cerebrospinal fever at Salisbury in 1914–15, *Proc R Soc Med*, **10, part 2**: 44–60.

Greisen K, Loeffelholz M et al., 1994, PCR primers and probes for the 16S rRNA gene of most species of pathogenic bacteria, including bacteria found in cerebrospinal fluid, *J Clin Microbiol*, **32**: 335–51.

Griffiss JM, 1982, Epidemic meningococcal disease: synthesis of a hypothetical immunoepidemiologic model, *Rev Infect Dis*, **4**: 159–72.

Griffiss JM, 1995, Mechanisms of host immunity, *Meningococcal Disease*, ed. Cartwright K, John Wiley, Chichester, 35–70.

Griffiss JM, Brandt BL et al., 1984, Immune response of infants and children to disseminated infections with *Neisseria meningitidis*, *J Infect Dis*, **150**: 71–9.

Guirguis N, Schneerson R et al., 1985, *Escherichia coli* K51 and K93 capsular polysaccharides are cross-reactive with the group A capsular polysaccharide of *Neisseria meningitidis*, *J Exp Med*, **162**: 1837–51.

Gwaltney JM, Sande MA et al., 1975, Spread of *Streptococcus pneumoniae* in families. II. Relation of transfer of *S. pneumoniae* to incidence of colds and serum antibody, *J Infect Dis*, **132**: 62–8.

Haggerty RJ, Ziai M, 1964, Acute bacterial meningitis, *Adv Pediatr*, **13**: 129–81.

Harrison LH, Armstrong CW et al., 1991, A cluster of meningococcal disease on a school bus following epidemic influenza, *Arch Intern Med*, **151**: 1005–9.

Herbert MA, Heath PT, Mayon-White RT, 1995, Meningococcal vaccines for the United Kingdom, *Communic Dis Rep Rev*, **5**: R130–5.

Heubner JOL, 1896, Beobachtungen und versuche über den Meningokokkus intracellularis (Weichselbaum-Jaeger), *Jb Kinderheilk*, **43**: 1–22.

Hirsch A, 1886, Epidemic cerebro-spinal meningitis, *Handbook of Geographical and Historical Pathology. Vol. III – Diseases of Organs and Parts*, translated from the German by Creighton C, New Sydenham Society, London, 547–94.

Howard AJ, Dunkin KT, Millar GW, 1988, Nasopharyngeal carriage and antibiotic resistance of *Haemophilus influenzae* in healthy children, *Epidemiol Infect*, **100**: 193–203.

Hubert B, Watier L et al., 1992, Meningococcal disease and influenza-like syndrome: a new approach to an old question, *J Infect Dis*, **166**: 542–5.

Jacobs MR, Appelbaum PC, 1995, Antibiotic-resistant pneumococci, *Rev Med Microbiol*, **6**: 77–93.

Jafari HS, McCracken GH, 1994, Dexamethasone therapy in bacterial meningitis, *Pediatr Ann*, **23**: 83–8.

Jensen AG, Espersen F et al., 1993, *Staphylococcus aureus* meningitis. A review of 104 nationwide, consecutive cases, *Arch Intern Med*, **153**: 1902–8.

Jones DM, Kaczmarski EB, 1994, Meningococcal infections in England and Wales: 1993, *Communic Dis Rep Rev*, **4**: R97–100.

Jones DM, Mallard RH, 1993, Age incidence of meningococcal infection England and Wales, 1984–1991, *J Infect*, **27**: 83–8.

Kaplan J, Sarnaik S, Schiffman G, 1986, Revaccination with polyvalent pneumococcal vaccine in children with sickle cell anaemia, *Am J Pediatr Hematol Oncol*, **8**: 80–2.

Kaplan SL, Smith EO'B et al., 1986, Association between preadmission oral antibiotic therapy and cerebrospinal fluid findings and sequelae caused by *Haemophilus influenzae* type b meningitis, *Pediatr Infect Dis*, **5**: 626–32.

Kasper DL, Winkelhake JL et al., 1973, Antigenic specificity of bactericidal antibodies in antisera to *Neisseria meningitidis*, *J Infect Dis*, **127**: 378–87.

Kiefer F, 1896, Zur Differentialdiagnose des Erregers der epidemischen Cerebrospinal-meningitis und der Gonorrhoe, *Berl Klin Wochenschr*, **33**: 628–30.

Kilian M, Mestecky J, Russell MW, 1988, Defense mechanisms involving Fc-dependent functions of immunoglobulin A and their subversion by bacterial immunoglobulin A proteases, *Microbiol Rev*, **52**: 296–303.

Kilian M, Reinholdt J, 1987, A hypothetical model for the development of invasive infection due to IgA1 protease-producing bacteria, *Adv Exp Med Biol*, **216B**: 1261–9.

Kirkpatrick B, Reeves DS, MacGowan AP, 1994, A review of the clinical presentation, laboratory features, antimicrobial therapy and outcome of 77 episodes of pneumococcal meningitis occurring in children and adults, *J Infect*, **29**: 171–82.

Kleinman MB, Reynolds JK et al., 1984, Superiority of acridine orange versus Gram stain in partially treated bacterial meningitis, *J Pediatr*, **104**: 401–4.

Kolle W, Wasserman A, 1906, Versuche zur Gewinnung und Wertbestimmung eines Meningokokkenserums, *Dtsch Med Wochenschr*, **32**: 609–12.

Krasinski K, Nelson JD et al., 1987, Possible association of mycoplasma and viral respiratory infections with bacterial meningitis, *Am J Epidemiol*, **125**: 499–509.

Kristiansen B-E, Ask E et al., 1991, Rapid diagnosis of meningococcal meningitis by polymerase chain reaction, *Lancet*, **337**: 1568–9.

Lambert HP, 1991, *Infections of the Central Nervous System*, ed. Lambert HP, Arnold, London.

Lapeysonnie L, 1963, La méningite cérébrospinale en Afrique, *Bull W H O*, **28, Suppl.**: 53–114.

Lebel MH, Freij BJ et al., 1988, Dexamethasone therapy for

bacterial meningitis: results of two double-blind, placebo-controlled trials, *N Engl J Med*, **319**: 964–71.

van der Ley P, Poolman JT, 1992, Construction of a multivalent meningococcal vaccine strain based on the class 1 outer membrane protein, *Infect Immun*, **60**: 3156–61.

van der Ley P, van der Biezen J et al., 1993, Use of transformation to construct antigenic hybrids of the class 1 outer membrane protein in *Neisseria meningitidis*, *Infect Immun*, **61**: 4217–24.

Lister PD, 1995, Multiply-resistant pneumococcus: therapeutic problems in the management of serious infections, *Eur J Clin Microbiol Infect Dis*, **14, Suppl. 1**: 18–25.

de Louvois J, 1994, Acute bacterial meningitis in the newborn, *J Antimicrob Chemother*, **34, Suppl. A**: 61–73.

Lukehart S, Hook EW et al., 1988, Invasion of the central nervous system by *Treponema pallidum*. Implications for diagnosis and therapy, *Ann Intern Med*, **109**: 855–62.

Lystad A, Aasen S, 1991, The epidemiology of meningococcal disease in Norway 1975–91, *NIPH Ann*, **14**: 57–65.

McCracken GH, Nelson JD et al., 1987, Consensus report: antimicrobial therapy for bacterial meningitis in infants and children, *Pediatr Infect Dis J*, **6**: 501–5.

McNeil G, Virji M, Moxon ER, 1994, Interactions of *Neisseria meningitidis* with human monocytes, *Microb Pathog*, **16**: 153–63.

Marchiafava E, Celli A, 1884, Spra i micrococchi della meningite cerebrospinale epidemica, *Gazz degli Ospedali*, **5**: 59.

Maxson S, Jacobs RF, 1993, Viral meningitis. Tips to rapidly diagnose treatable causes, *Postgrad Med*, **93**: 153–66.

Maxson S, Lewno MJ, Schutze GE, 1994, Clinical usefulness of cerebrospinal fluid bacterial antigen studies, *J Pediatr*, **125**: 235–8.

Meningococcal Infections Working Group, 1989, The epidemiology and control of meningococcal disease. Internal publication of the Public Health Laboratory Service, London, *Communic Dis Rep*, **8**: 3–6.

Mitchell TJ, Andrew PW, 1995, Vaccines against *Streptococcus pneumoniae*, *Molecular and Clinical Aspects of Bacterial Vaccine Development*, eds Ala'Aldeen DAA, Hormaeche CE, John Wiley, Chichester, 93–117.

Moore PS, 1992, Meningococcal disease in sub-Saharan Africa: a model for the epidemic process, *Clin Infect Dis*, **14**: 515–25.

Moore PS, Hierholzer J et al., 1990, Respiratory viruses and mycoplasma as cofactors for epidemic group A meningococcal meningitis, *JAMA*, **264**: 1271–5.

Moosa AA, Quortum HA, Ibrahim MD, 1995, Rapid diagnosis of bacterial meningitis with reagent strips, *Lancet*, **345**: 1290–1.

de Moraes JC, Perkins BA et al., 1992, Protective efficacy of a serogroup B meningococcal vaccine in São Paolo, Brazil, *Lancet*, **340**: 1074–8.

Moxon ER, 1992, Molecular basis of invasive *Haemophilus influenzae* type b disease, *J Infect Dis*, **165, Suppl. 1**: S77–81.

Moxon ER, Ostrow PT, 1977, *Haemophilus influenzae* meningitis in infant rats: role of bacteremia in pathogenesis of age-dependent inflammatory responses in cerebrospinal fluid, *J Infect Dis*, **135**: 303–7.

Moxon ER, Glode MP et al., 1977, The infant rat as a model of bacterial meningitis, *J Infect Dis*, **136, Suppl.**: S186–92.

Mufson MA, Hughey DF et al., 1991, Revaccination with pneumococcal vaccine of elderly persons 6 years after primary vaccination, *Vaccine*, **9**: 403–7.

Mulder CJJ, Zanen HC, 1984, Neonatal meningitis caused by *Escherichia coli* in the Netherlands, *J Infect Dis*, **150**: 935–9.

Mulks MH, 1985, Microbial IgA proteases, *Bacterial Enzymes and Virulence*, ed. Holder IA, CRC Press, Boca Raton, FL, 81–104.

Mulks MH, Plaut AG, 1978, IgA protease production as a characteristic distinguishing pathogenic from harmless Neisseriaceae, *N Engl J Med*, **299**: 973–6.

Munford RS, Taunay AE et al., 1974, Spread of meningococcal infection within households, *Lancet*, **1**: 1275–8.

Nadel S, Levin M, Habibi P, 1995, Treatment of meningococcal disease in childhood, *Meningococcal Disease*, ed. Cartwright K, John Wiley, Chichester, 207–43.

Newcombe, Cartwright K et al., 1996, PCR of peripheral blood for diagnosis of meningococcal disease, *J Clin Microbiol*, **34:** 1637–40.

Ni H, Knight AI et al., 1992, Polymerase chain reaction for the diagnosis of meningococcal meningitis, *Lancet*, **340:** 1432–4.

Nicolle M, Debains E, Jouan C, 1918, Etudes sur les méningocacciques et les serums anti-méningococciques, *Ann Inst Pasteur*, **32:** 150–69.

O'Donoghue JM, Schweid AI, Beaty HN, 1974, Experimental pneumococcal meningitis. I. A rabbit model, *Proc Soc Exp Biol Med*, **146:** 571–6.

Olcén P, Kjellander J et al., 1979, Culture diagnosis of meningococcal carriers: yield from different sites and influence of storage in transport medium, *J Clin Pathol*, **32:** 1222–5.

Olcén P, Kjellander J et al., 1981, Epidemiology of *Neisseria meningitis*: prevalence and symptoms from the upper respiratory tract in family members to patients with meningococcal disease, *Scand J Infect Dis*, **13:** 105–9.

Olyhoek T, Crowe BA, Achtman M, 1987, Clonal population structure of *Neisseria meningitidis* serogroup A isolated from epidemics and pandemics between 1915 and 1983, *Rev Infect Dis*, **9:** 665–92.

O'Neill P, 1993, How long to treat bacterial meningitis?, *Lancet*, **341:** 530.

Pachner AR, 1995, Early disseminated Lyme disease: Lyme meningitis, *Am J Med*, **98:** 30S–7S.

Parkkinen J, Korhonen TJ et al., 1988, Binding sites in the rat brain for *Escherichia coli* S fimbriae associated with neonatal meningitis, *J Clin Invest*, **81:** 860–5.

Pedersen FK, Henrichsen J, 1983, Pneumococcal meningitis and bacteraemia in Danish children 1969–78, *Acta Pathol Microbiol Immunol Scand*, **91:** 129–34.

Peltola H, 1983, Meningococcal disease: still with us, *Rev Infect Dis*, **5:** 71–91.

Peltola H, Kataja JM, Mäkelä PH, 1982, Shift in the age distribution of meningococcal disease as predictor of an epidemic, *Lancet*, **2:** 595–7.

Peltola H, Mäkelä PH et al., 1977, Clinical efficacy of meningococcus serogroup A capsular polysaccharide vaccine in children three months to five years of age, *N Engl J Med*, **297:** 686–91.

Poolman JT, van der Ley PA, Tommassen J, 1995, Surface structures and secreted products of meningococci, *Meningococcal Disease*, ed. Cartwright K, John Wiley, Chichester, 21–34.

van Putten JPM, 1990, Iron acquisition and the pathogenesis of meningococcal and gonococcal disease, *Med Microbiol Immunol*, **179:** 289–95.

Quincke HI, 1893, Ueber meningitis serosa, *Samml Klin Vort (Leipzig)*, **67:** 655–94.

Rake G, 1931, Biological properties of 'fresh' and 'stock' strains of the meningococcus, *Proc Soc Exp Biol Med*, **29:** 287–9.

Rake G, Scherp HW, 1933, Studies on meningococcus infection. III. The antigenic complex of the meningococcus – a type-specific substance, *J Exp Med*, **58:** 341–60.

Read RC, Fox A et al., 1995, Experimental infection of human nasal mucosal explants with *Neisseria meningitidis*, *J Med Microbiol*, **42:** 353–61.

Redmond SR, Pichichero ME, 1984, *Haemophilus influenzae* type b disease, an epidemiologic study with special reference to day-care centers, *JAMA*, **252:** 2581–4.

Reller LB, MacGregor RR, Beaty HN, 1973, Bactericidal antibody after colonization with *Neisseria meningitidis*, *J Infect Dis*, **127:** 56–62.

Rich AR, McCordock HA, 1933, The pathogenesis of tuberculous meningitis, *Bull Johns Hopkins Hosp*, **52:** 5–37.

Riley HD, 1972, Neonatal meningitis, *J Infect Dis*, **125:** 420–5.

Rodriguez-Barradas MC, Musher DM et al., 1992, Antibody to capsular polysaccharides of *Streptococcus pneumoniae* after vac-

cination of human immunodeficiency virus infected subjects with 23-valent pneumococcal vaccine, *J Infect Dis*, **165:** 553–6.

Rolleston H, 1919, Lumleian lectures on cerebro-spinal fever. Lecture 1, *Lancet*, **1:** 541–9.

Romero JD, Outschoorn IM, 1994, Current status of meningococcal group B vaccine candidates: capsular or non-capsular?, *Clin Microbiol Rev*, **7:** 559–75.

Ross SC, Densen P, 1984, Complement deficiency states and infection: epidemiology, pathogenesis and consequences of neisserial and other infections in an immune deficiency, *Medicine (Baltimore)*, **63:** 243–73.

Sáez-Nieto JA, Lujan R et al., 1992, Epidemiology and molecular basis of penicillin-resistant *Neisseria meningitidis* in Spain: a 5-year history (1985–1989), *Clin Infect Dis*, **14:** 394–402.

Sangster G, Murdoch JMCC, Gray JA, 1982, Bacterial meningitis 1940–79, *J Infect*, **5:** 245–56.

Saukkonnen KM, Nowicki B, Leinonen M, 1988, Role of type 1 and S fimbriae in the pathogenesis of *Escherichia coli* O18:K1 bacteremia and meningitis in the infant rat, *Infect Immun*, **56:** 892–7.

Schaad UB, Suter S et al., 1990, A comparison of ceftriaxone and cefuroxime for the treatment of bacterial meningitis in children, *N Engl J Med*, **322:** 141–7.

Schaad UB, Lips U et al., 1993, Dexamethasone therapy for bacterial meningitis in children, *Lancet*, **342:** 457–61.

Scherp H, Rake G, 1935, Studies on meningococcus infection. VIII. The type I specific substance, *J Exp Med*, **61:** 753–69.

Schmidt LH, Sesler CL, 1943, Development of resistance to penicillin by pneumococci, *Proc Soc Exp Biol Med*, **53:** 353–7.

Schneerson R, Robbins JB, 1975, Induction of serum *Haemophilus influenzae* type b capsular antibodies in adult volunteers fed cross-reacting *Escherichia coli* 075.K100:H5, *N Engl J Med*, **29:** 1093–6.

Schryvers AB, Gonzalez GC, 1990, Receptors for transferrin in pathogenic bacteria are specific for the host's protein, *Can J Microbiol*, **36:** 145–7.

Schwartz MT, Tunkel AR, 1995, Therapy of penicillin-resistant pneumococcal meningitis, *Int J Med Microbiol Virol Parasitol Infect Dis*, **282:** 7–12.

Schwentker FF, 1937, Treatment of meningococci meningitis with sulfanilamide, *J Pediatr*, **11:** 874–80.

Siegman-Ingra Y, Bar-Yosef S et al., 1993, Nosocomial acinetobacter meningitis secondary to invasive procedures: report of 25 cases and review, *Clin Infect Dis*, **17:** 843–9.

Sloas MM, Barrett FF et al., 1992, Cephalosporin treatment failure in penicillin- and cephalosporin-resistant *Streptococcus pneumoniae* meningitis, *Pediatr Infect Dis J*, **11:** 662–6.

Sophian A, Black J, 1912, Prophylactic vaccination against epidemic meningitis, *JAMA*, **59:** 527–32.

Spellerberg B, Tuomanen E, 1994, The pathophysiology of pneumococcal meningitis, *Ann Med*, **26:** 411–18.

Spratt BG, Zhang Q-Y et al., 1989, Recruitment of a penicillin-binding protein gene from *Neisseria flavescens* during the emergence of penicillin resistance in *Neisseria meningitidis*, *Proc Natl Acad Sci USA*, **86:** 8988–92.

Stephens DS, Farley MM, 1991, Pathogenic events during infection of the human nasopharynx with *Neisseria meningitidis* and *Haemophilus influenzae*, *Rev Infect Dis*, **13:** 22–33.

Stuart JM, Cartwright KAV et al., 1989, Effect of smoking on meningococcal carriage, *Lancet*, **2:** 723–5.

Syrogiannopoulos GA, Lourida AN et al., 1994, Dexamethasone therapy for bacterial meningitis in children: 2- versus 4-day regimen, *J Infect Dis*, **169:** 853–8.

Tauber MG, Zwahlen A, 1994, Animal models for meningitis, *Methods Enzymol*, **235:** 93–106.

Tenover FC, Swenson JM, McDougal LK, 1992, Screening for extended spectrum cephalosporin resistance in pneumococci, *Lancet*, **340:** 1420.

Tomasz A, 1995, The pneumococcus at the gates, *N Engl J Med*, **333:** 514–15.

Towers CV, 1995, Group B streptococcus: the US controversy, *Lancet*, **346:** 197–8.

Tunkel AR, Scheld WM, 1993, Pathogenesis and pathophysiology of bacterial meningitis, *Clin Microbiol Rev*, **6:** 118–36.

Tuomanen E, Tomasz A et al., 1985, The relative role of bacterial cell wall and capsule in the induction of inflammation in pneumococcal meningitis, *J Infect Dis*, **151:** 535–40.

Twumasi PA, Kumah S et al., 1995, A trial of a group A plus group C meningococcal polysaccharide-protein conjugate vaccine in African infants, *J Infect Dis*, **171:** 632–8.

Vieusseux G, 1805, Mémoire sur la maladie qui a régné à Genève au printemps de 1805., *J Méd Chir Pharm*, **xi:** 163–82.

Virji M, Kayhty H et al., 1991, The role of pili in the interactions of pathogenic neisseria with cultured human endothelial cells, *Mol Microbiol*, **5:** 1831–41.

Virji M, Makepeace K et al., 1992, Expression of the Opc protein correlates with invasion of epithelial and endothelial cells by *Neisseria meningitidis*, *Mol Microbiol*, **6:** 2785–95.

Weichselbaum A, 1887, Ueber die Aetiologie der akuten Meningitis cerebro-spinalis, *Fortschr Med*, **5:** 573–83, 620–6.

BACTERIAL INFECTIONS OF THE RESPIRATORY TRACT

R C Read and R G Finch

1 INTRODUCTION

Few micro-organisms can colonize the airways and cause disease. This is surprising because of the very large surface area of the respiratory tract and its constant exposure to non-sterile ambient air. It is a tribute to the elaborate host defences of the lung that bacterial infection of the respiratory tract is not much more common. Thousands of micro-organisms are inhaled with the air and aspirated with pharyngeal secretions during sleep (Kikuchi et al. 1994); for each of these there is at least one of 4 possible outcomes. First, the micro-organisms may be rapidly cleared from the lung. Second, they may lodge in the upper respiratory tract and asymptomatically colonize the site. Third, they may persist in regions that are normally sterile, such as below the larynx, as is observed in chronic obstructive pulmonary disease. Finally, they may penetrate epithelium and initiate parenchymal disease, as in pneumonia, or they may invade the bloodstream to cause systemic infection. Microbial load and host defences are the subject of a constant balancing act. Successful microbes have adapted to avoid rapid clearance, gain nutrients, and survive in the respiratory tract sufficiently to grow and disseminate to other hosts. The aim of host defences is to maintain the sterility of the gas exchange areas. Disease results when local defences are overcome and inflammatory cells are recruited to eradicate the infection.

2 PULMONARY DEFENCE MECHANISMS

Pulmonary defence mechanisms are of 2 types (Reynolds 1994), **resident defences**, such as airway architecture and mucociliary clearance, that are constantly operative, and **recruited defences**, that augment the resident defences when the host detects danger, and result in inflammation with resulting disease.

2.1 Resident defences

AIRWAY ARCHITECTURE

Movements of the glottis and epiglottis during swallowing and the cough reflex are important barriers to bacterial invasion of the airway, especially by organisms aspirated from the alimentary tract.

During nose breathing, particles larger than 5 μm are efficiently removed by impaction on the walls of the nose and nasopharynx as a result of airflow rendered turbulent by the nasal turbinates and the configuration of the nasopharynx and oropharynx. Sedimentation is the main mechanism of deposition of particles such as bacteria in the size range 5–0.6 μm and takes place in parts of the lung in which airflow is slow, i.e. between the fifth bronchial division and the terminal lung units. Invasion of the lung by sedimented particles is prevented by the combination of an efficient epithelial barrier, mucociliary clearance, and phagocytic mechanisms.

THE EPITHELIAL BARRIER

The respiratory tract, from the nose to the respiratory bronchiole, is lined by ciliated, pseudostratified, columnar cells interspersed with occasional mucus-secreting cells (see Fig. 18.1). The remainder is lined by non-ciliated epithelium including (1) a small zone of stratified epithelium below the pharyngeal fornix, and (2) non-keratinizing squamous epithelium in the oropharynx, the anterior surface of the epiglottis and the upper half of its posterior surface, the upper half of the aryepiglottic folds and the vocal cords. Tight junctions between epithelial cells provide an efficient barrier to bacterial penetration. This epithelium is continually replenished; if damaged, fully differentiated ciliated cells are replaced within 2–6 weeks, though basal cells continue to protect the basement membrane.

MUCOCILIARY CLEARANCE

Throughout the airway mucus-secreting cells secrete a blanket of mucus that is propelled along by ciliary action towards the larynx where it is coughed up or swallowed. Inhaled bacteria adhere to mucus and are conveyed along this mucociliary escalator (Fig. 18.2). Efficient mucociliary transport of inhaled foreign bodies depends on co-ordinated ciliary beating, the depth and constituents of the periciliary fluid that lies beneath the blanket of mucus, and the rheological qualities of the mucus. Viscid mucus, such as that in cystic fibrosis, is difficult for the cilia to clear. Cilia beat at 12–17 Hz, but the frequency is slightly lower in more peripheral airways. In normal airways, clearance times of inhaled aerosols are 30 min from the lobar bronchi, 4–6 h from 1–5 mm airways, and one day to several months or more, depending on the substance inhaled, from airways distal to the terminal bronchioles. Clearly, disruption of mucociliary clearance leads to stasis of infected mucus and potentially to disease.

SOLUBLE FACTORS IN AIRWAY SECRETIONS

Mucus contains many factors that enhance the clearance of micro-organisms from the airway; most of these are plasma proteins and include α_1-antitrypsin, a low molecular weight chymotrypsin inhibitor. Neutral protease and elastase are secreted by polymorphonuclear leucocytes and alveolar macrophages. α_1-Antitrypsin deficiency is associated with chronic pulmonary disease, probably because of failure to inhibit the neutrophil products during recurrent inflammatory responses to lung infection.

Lysozyme is secreted by neutrophils and found in most mucosal secretions, where it is directly active against some bacteria. Lactoferrin is secreted by mucosal epithelial cells and neutrophils. Like transferrin, it has a high affinity for iron and inhibits bacterial replication within the airway by restricting iron availability.

Surfactant is secreted by pneumocytes within alveoli and has the vital function of reducing surface tension in gas exchange areas and keeping these patent. It also contains non-immune opsonins, notably fibronectin, produced locally by alveolar macrophages. It binds to some bacteria which are then recognized by receptors on the macrophage surface.

Complement

Many of the components of the complement system (see Chapter 4) are present at very low levels in normal bronchial secretions. They are probably derived directly from serum, but alveolar macrophages also secrete a number of the components. In terms of defence against bacteria, complement has 2 broad functions. Deposition of C3b on bacteria ultimately

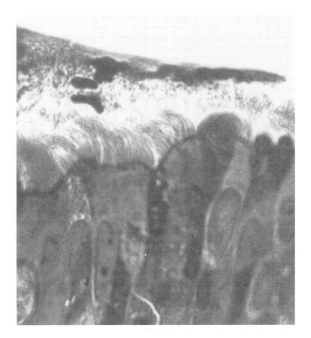

Fig. 18.1 Micrograph of typical human pseudostratified columnar epithelium within the respiratory tract showing ciliated cells interspersed with mucus-secreting (goblet) cells. (Courtesy of A Rutman).

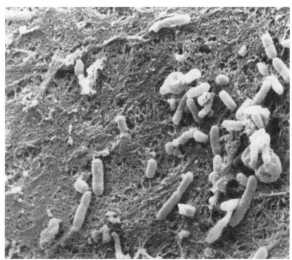

Fig. 18.2 Scanning electron micrograph of airway mucosa showing *H. influenzae* attached to mucus. (A Brain and RC Read).

results in their recognition by macrophage CR1, CR3 and CR4 receptors, and then phagocytosis. Additionally, there is probably sufficient C5 to initiate bacterial lysis by the terminal membrane attack complex. Complement concentrations rise dramatically during periods of lung damage, e.g. during serious infection of the lung, when airways are relatively leaky for serum proteins.

Immunoglobulins

Immunoglobulins IgA, IgG, IgM and IgE, including specific antibody, can be recovered from respiratory tract secretions (Lipscomb et al. 1995). IgM is found in lung washings in only very low concentrations.

Secretory IgA (sIgA) is synthesized by lymphoid cells beneath the basement membrane, predominantly in the upper and middle portions of the respiratory tract. Whereas IgA is the predominant immunoglobulin in the upper airways, lower airway secretions more resemble serum in that the IgG to IgA ratio is much higher. The major function of sIgA is complement-independent neutralization of respiratory viruses. It also opsonizes organisms for phagocytosis by macrophages, but does not contribute to polymorph opsonization; nor does it activate complement. Secretory IgA interacts with lysozyme and complement to augment their bactericidal activity, mediates bacterial adherence to mucus and inhibits bacterial adherence to epithelial surfaces. Once challenged by a given agent, the host produces sIgA in response to homologous challenge. However, the period of immune protection is relatively short in contrast to serum IgG and booster responses are variable after later challenge. Certain bacteria, notably *Streptococcus pneumoniae*, *Haemophilus influenzae* and *Neisseria meningitidis*, secrete IgA proteases capable of inactivating mucosal IgA.

IgG gains access to the airways by transudation from the circulation but it can be produced locally in the lung. It efficiently agglutinates bacteria, mediates bacterial opsonization for macrophages and neutrophils, neutralizes bacterial exotoxins and activates complement. After a primary challenge, specific antibody is released into blood from lung associated lymph nodes and transudes into the airway. Subsequently, memory B cells traffic to the lung and produce specific IgG in response to further specific challenge (Bice, Weissman and Muggenburg 1991).

Alveolar macrophages

Alveolar macrophages are responsible for non-inflammatory clearance of micro-organisms, including those that sediment in the most distal airways beyond mucociliary clearance. They comprise about 80–90% of the cell population of fluid obtained by bronchoalveolar lavage. Four populations of pulmonary macrophages can be distinguished:

1 alveolar macrophages
2 interstitial macrophages
3 dendritic macrophages and
4 intravascular macrophages.

Pulmonary macrophages are derived from peripheral blood monocytes; they differentiate after chemotaxis to pulmonary tissue and can replicate in the lung. Alveolar macrophages reside within the airspace, whereas interstitial macrophages are located in the lung connective tissues. Though alveolar and interstitial macrophages both undertake Fc receptor dependent phagocytosis, they differ in their other functions. Alveolar macrophages are capable of Fc receptor independent phagocytosis and the production of cytokines, such as tumour necrosis factor α (TNF-α) and interferons α and β, that are released in order to recruit an inflammatory response. Production of oxygen radicals is greatest in alveolar macrophages. Interstitial macrophages are adapted for antigen presentation (Lohmann-Matthes et al. 1994), whereas dendritic cells are predominantly non-phagocytic and specialized for antigen presentation. Macrophages in the vascular compartment are located on the capillary endothelium. They are highly phagocytic and probably remove foreign material that enters the lung via the bloodstream.

Alveolar macrophages possess 3 classes of surface receptor that facilitate phagocytosis of bacteria. The Fc receptor, of which there are 4 subclasses with differing affinities, are responsible for the recognition of antibody-coated bacteria. They recognize the Fc region of IgG and IgA on antibody-coated bacteria. The second are complement receptors, CR1, CR3 and CR4, that recognize bacteria coated with C3b. The third are lectin-binding receptors such as the mannose-6-phosphate receptor. After phagocytosis bacteria are enclosed in phagosomes that ultimately acquire the characteristics of lysosomes. Bacteria are killed by a combination of products of the oxidative burst, and bactericidal enzymes and proteins.

The bactericidal activity of alveolar macrophages depends crucially on the inoculum size. Up to about 10^5 bacteria are eliminated by alveolar macrophage phagocytosis alone, whereas the killing of an inoculum of 10^6 requires a modest influx of neutrophils into the alveoli. Inocula greater than 10^8 organisms, however, necessitate activation of local T and B lymphocytes in addition to phagocytosis by macrophages and neutrophils. Apart from the number of micro-organisms, the species of the bacterium can affect the efficiency of killing by macrophages. *Staphylococcus aureus* can be killed adequately by macrophage phagocytosis alone, but *Pseudomonas aeruginosa* and *Klebsiella pneumoniae* additionally require neutrophils to aid intrapulmonary killing. Other bacteria, such as mycobacterial species and *Legionella pneumophila*, are readily phagocytosed by macrophages but cannot be killed. Killing occurs once the macrophage has been activated by T lymphocyte derived macrophage-activating cytokines, e.g. interleukin-1.

2.2 Recruited defences

If the combined effect of mucociliary clearance, complement and macrophage phagocytosis fails to clear an inoculum of bacteria, or if the infecting organism is particularly virulent, for example the type 3 pneumococcus, polymorphonuclear neutrophils and lymphocytes are recruited to augment the host response. Neutrophils migrate from the vascular compartment into the alveolus by chemotaxis. The stimulus for chemotaxis originates within the alveolus and is due to direct generation of chemotactic factors by micro-organisms entering the alveoli, and the release of chemotactic factors from alveolar macrophages after phagocytosis. Leukotriene B4 is an important chemotactic factor that also alters pulmonary capillary permeability. This, together with the secretion of TNF-α by macrophages, promotes the accumulation of neutrophils and fluid and other humoral substances in alveoli. Neutrophils kill ingested bacteria very much faster than macrophages with a combination of oxidative metabolites. This process, together with injury due to proteolytic enzymes, e.g. neutrophil elastase, results in consolidation of the lung.

Bronchoalveolar lavage fluid from the normal resting human lung contains predominantly macrophages but also lymphocytes (20%) including CD4 (helper), CD8 (suppressor) and a few B lymphocytes (Reynolds 1994). There is a complex interplay between lymphocytes, macrophages and neutrophils in the management and termination of inflammation. Lymphocytes can regulate the activation of macrophages and subsequently co-ordinate the inflammatory response in a given infection.

Macrophages infected with organisms capable of intracellular survival, such as *Mycobacterium tuberculosis*, *Pneumocystis carinii*, *Legionella pneumophila*, require cell mediated immunity to eradicate the infection (see Chapter 4).

At the time of primary challenge, antigen is transported to lung-associated lymph nodes either contained within alveolar and dendritic macrophages or recruited neutrophils, or free in the afferent lymphatic fluid (Lipscomb et al. 1995). In the presence of lung inflammation, this process is accelerated. Within lymph nodes, antigen is reprocessed by antigen-presenting cells. Specific T and B cell clones expand and differentiate, and effector T cells and B lymphoblasts migrate out (maximally by 10–14 days), the latter to provide specific antibody locally in lung tissue. Subsequent responses to the same infecting organism are produced by immune memory B cells lodged within the lung parenchyma.

3 PATHOGENESIS OF BACTERIAL RESPIRATORY INFECTIONS

Disease results when the equilibrium between organisms that enter the respiratory tract and resident host defences is disturbed. This may be due to a defect in host defences, an overwhelming microbial challenge, or a combination of the two. A normal host may not be able to deal with the microbial load, due to the large number of organisms or because the organisms possess potent virulence determinants.

3.1 Host defence defects

HOST FACTORS THAT PERMIT INCREASED COLONIZATION OF THE UPPER RESPIRATORY TRACT

Colonization of the upper respiratory tract is probably the first step in the pathogenesis of most bacterial pulmonary infections and adherence of bacteria to epithelial cells is a key event in colonization (Woods 1994). Individuals with poor nutrition, particularly vitamin A deficiency, are more likely to have upper respiratory tract colonization. Epithelial cells from patients with severe or chronic illness appear to be particularly receptive to bacteria, especially gram-negative organisms. This may either be due to a reduction in local IgA, local fibronectin production or to a change in the glycoprotein and glycosphingolipid composition of epithelial cell surfaces.

FAILURE OF EPITHELIAL BARRIERS AND REFLEXES

Bypassing the upper respiratory tract with an endotracheal tube or by tracheostomy vastly increases the host dependence on resident host defences of the lower respiratory tract. The distal airways in intubated patients rapidly become colonized by gram-negative bacteria including *P. aeruginosa* (Johanson et al. 1980). Failure of the swallowing reflex in patients with neurological defects permits aspiration of the commensal oropharyngeal flora and alimentary tract contents.

FAILURE OF MUCOCILIARY CLEARANCE

Ciliary dyskinesia may be due to intrinsic structural abnormalities, including defective dynein arms, defective radial spokes, microtubular transposition and random orientation of the central tubule (Rutland and de Iongh 1990). Such abnormalities can result in complications that range from relatively mild recurrent chest infections and sinusitis to severe clinical problems such as Kartagener's syndrome (sinusitis, bronchiectasis and malrotation of viscera – **situs inversus**). Respiratory viral infection, particularly influenza, can also result in marked depletion of ciliated epithelial cells, reduced mucociliary clearance and secondary bacterial infection, for example with *S. aureus* (Shanley 1995).

Cystic fibrosis is due to abnormalities of chloride ion transport by glandular and ciliated epithelial cells in various tissues, resulting in viscid external secretions. In the airways, this results in inadequate mucociliary clearance, colonization by pathogens with subsequent chronic inflammation and eventual bronchiectasis. These processes lead to virtually continuous inflammation and infection of the respiratory tract of cystic fibrosis patients from infancy onwards.

IMMUNOGLOBULIN DEFICIENCY

Patients with agammaglobulinaemia and dysgammaglobulinaemia produce decreased amounts of some or all of the serum immunoglobulins, notably IgG. They are susceptible to respiratory infections including those due to encapsulated organisms, such as *S. pneumoniae* and *H. influenzae*, and others such as *M. pneumoniae* (Buckley 1992). Chronic respiratory infection due to common variable immunodeficiency can lead to bronchiectasis. Selective IgA deficiency, particularly when associated with deficiency of IgG2, is also associated with recurrent respiratory tract infections. The IgG2 includes antibodies against capsulate organisms such as pneumococcus and *Haemophilus* spp., and also to lipoteichoic acid of *Streptococcus* spp. IgG4 deficiency is also associated with recurrent respiratory tract infection.

REDUCED PHAGOCYTIC ACTIVITY

The commonest cause of failure of the phagocytic response results from iatrogenic immunosuppression. Neutropenia results in a reduced inflammatory response in the lung and an increased incidence of gram-negative bacillary and fungal infection. Macrophages can also be depleted as a result of immunosuppression which results in pneumonia due to intracellular micro-organisms, including *Legionella* spp.

DISTURBED CELLULAR IMMUNITY

Disorders of cell mediated immunity can result from haematological malignancies, e.g. leukaemia, HIV infection, or from drug therapy, e.g. steroids. The consequence for the lung is that an inflammatory response cannot be adequately recruited or controlled, and macrophages cannot be activated to kill intracellular pathogens. The reduction in CD4 (T helper cells) in acquired immune deficiency syndrome (AIDS) is associated with a variety of respiratory infections by intracellular pathogens, notably *P. carinii* and *M. tuberculosis*.

ENVIRONMENTAL INFLUENCES ON THE HOST

Tobacco smoking is the major cause of airway morbidity that leads to recurrent respiratory tract infection. Smoke reduces ciliary clearance by direct toxicity, oxidizes α_1-antitrypsin, increases mucus production, and is a chemoattractant for neutrophils and macrophages in the peripheral airways. These lead to squamous metaplasia of ciliated epithelium, goblet cell hyperplasia and intraepithelial inflammation. The consequences are frequent cough, sputum production and intercurrent infection, particularly with *H. influenzae* and *Moraxella catarrhalis* (Floreani et al. 1994).

The effects of air pollution are far more subtle than those of smoking. Upper respiratory tract infections (coryza and nasal discharge) and lower respiratory infection (pneumonia and purulent sputum production) are more frequently observed in polluted urban areas (Lunn, Knowlden and Handyside 1967). High ambient pollutant levels correlate with upper respiratory infections (Ponka 1990). Pollutants, including sulphur dioxide, nitrogen dioxide, acid aerosols and particulates, reduce mucociliary clearance, damage epithelial cells and impair phagocytosis in vitro (Schlesinger 1990).

3.2 Bacterial virulence mechanisms

Respiratory pathogens produce a variety of virulence factors that promote infection by mechanisms that include:

1 increased adherence to mucosal epithelial cells
2 avoidance of mucociliary clearance
3 increased nutrient acquisition and
4 avoidance of complement deposition and phagocytosis.

Some pathogens produce factors that are directly toxic to the host, such as streptococcal hyaluronidase which allows expansion of the ecological niche and damages host connective tissue.

STREPTOCOCCUS PNEUMONIAE

S. pneumoniae produces a protein adhesin that binds to the *N*-acetylgalactose–galactose component of respiratory tract epithelial cell membrane glycolipids (Krivan, Roberts and Ginsburg 1988). It also produces IgA protease that inactivates respiratory mucosal IgA. Pneumolysin, a 52.8 kDa protein, is a thiol-activated cytotoxin that shares amino acid homology with bacterial thiol-activated toxins and is released on autolysis. In experimental animals it can induce inflammation in the lungs independently of intact pneumococci (Feldman et al. 1991). Virulent pneumococci have an antiphagocytic capsule, which permits evasion of recruited neutrophils, and some capsular serotypes, e.g. serotype 3, are more virulent than others. This may be due to the relative composition of capsules, particularly their choline content (Bruyn et al. 1992). Toxic products of *S. pneumoniae* include hydrogen peroxide (Duane et al. 1993). The cell wall lipoteichoic acid of *S. pneumoniae* is potently pro-inflammatory in the lung by activation of the alternative complement pathway and, like LPS, it elicits production of interleukin-1 (IL-1) and TNF-α (Tuomanen et al. 1995).

HAEMOPHILUS INFLUENZAE

H. influenzae possesses fimbriae that are structurally and serologically related to the P and mannose-sensitive fimbriae of *Escherichia coli* and promote adherence to respiratory epithelium and mucin. *H. influenzae* also appears to bind specifically to GalNAcβ1-4Gal sequences of human lung glycolipids. The organism may also secrete a soluble toxin that reduces ciliary beating and so promotes avoidance of mucociliary clearance (Wilson 1988). Lipo-oligosaccharide of *H. influenzae* is toxic to human respiratory tract epithelium.

BORDETELLA PERTUSSIS

B. pertussis produces several adhesins including a filamentous haemagglutinin (220 kDa), fimbriae and an array of toxins, including pertussis toxin (105 kDa) that binds to respiratory tract ciliated cells and macrophages and is clearly important in airway colonization. Pertussis toxin also causes epithelial cell cytotoxicity by increasing host cell cAMP levels (Masure 1992), an action broadly similar to cholera toxin. Tracheal cytotoxin is a peptidoglycan fragment toxic for ciliated cells that directly induces inflammation in animal models (Wilson et al. 1991). *B. pertussis* can survive in human phagocytes by inhibiting phagosome–lysosome fusion but it does not inhibit the respiratory burst (Steed et al. 1992).

Pseudomonas aeruginosa

P. aeruginosa produces fimbrial and non-fimbrial adhesins that mediate binding to epithelial cell gangliosides after its sialic acid residues have been removed by neuraminidase. It also produces a number of toxins including exotoxin A, which damages respiratory epithelial tissue and inhibits phagocytosis (Coburn 1992), and a number of elastases that act together to damage epithelial cells and blood vessel walls (Galloway 1991). A membrane glycolipid of *P. aeruginosa*, rhamnolipid, can reduce ciliary beating and mucociliary clearance (Read et al. 1992) and secreted pigments including pyocyanin and 1-hydroxyphenazine also reduce ciliary beating (Wilson 1988). Alginate, which forms a viscous gel around bacteria and gives them a mucoid appearance, functions as an adhesin and prevents phagocytosis.

Legionella pneumophila

Little is known of virulence factors of *L. pneumophila* but it appears to survive macrophage phagocytosis. It has a 24 kDa outer-membrane, macrophage invasion protein, that allows invasion of macrophages in the absence of opsonization but this does not appear to improve intracellular survival once the organism is endocytosed. Several bacterial enzymes including acid phosphatase, phospholipase C, protein kinases and superoxide dismutase potentially enhance intracellular survival. *L. pneumophila* proteases cause lung damage and it secretes a metalloproteinase similar to *P. aeruginosa* elastase (Dowling et al. 1992).

4 Respiratory tract commensals

The anterior nares are colonized by staphylococci, micrococci and miscellaneous *Corynebacterium* spp. but the paranasal sinuses are normally sterile.

In the mouth anaerobes colonize periodontal areas and a variety of other organisms including 'viridans' streptococci (e.g. *Streptococcus mitis*, *Streptococcus sanguis*), *Haemophilus* spp., *Neisseria* spp. and diphtheroids are present in saliva. The practical consequence is that sputum can be heavily contaminated and make laboratory interpretation very difficult.

The flora of the oronasopharynx is much more complex; it may be colonized by *Streptococcus* spp., *Neisseria* spp., coliform bacteria, *Bacteroides* spp., fusobacteria, actinomycetes and yeasts. From time to time, however, individuals may be colonized by one or more pathogens, such as β-haemolytic streptococci, *S. pneumoniae*, *H. influenzae*, *N. meningitidis* and *M. catarrhalis*. Periods of asymptomatic colonization may be very short or may last for several months, and although the colonization is asymptomatic it is generally accepted that stable residence at this site is a prerequisite for invasive disease by such organisms as *H. influenzae* and *N. meningitidis*. Point prevalence studies in communities indicate the relative prevalence of these pathogens in the nasopharynx of colonized individuals (Table 18.1).

A number of exogenous factors may disturb the ecology of the mouth and nasopharynx. Antibiotics can suppress oral bacteria and allow yeasts to proliferate and thrush to occur. Smoking and passive smoking increase the prevalence of colonization with pathogens including *N. meningitidis* (Caugant et al. 1994).

The upper respiratory tract is colonized by an abundant resident microbial flora that varies as a result of changing endogenous and exogenous conditions. Below the larynx the lower respiratory tract is sterile in normal individuals because inhaled organisms are rapidly removed by clearance mechanisms.

5 Infections of the upper respiratory tract

5.1 Infections of the oronasopharynx

Sinusitis

The paranasal sinuses are normally sterile. Bacteria recovered by sinus puncture before treatment of acute community-acquired sinusitis include *S. pneumoniae*, *H. influenzae*, anaerobes, *Streptococcus* spp., *M. catarrhalis* and *S. aureus*. In chronic sinusitis, bacteriological cultures are more exotic and polymicrobial than in acute sinusitis and may include anaerobes and *Pseudomonas* spp. (van Cauwenberge, Vander Mijnsbrugge and Ingels 1993). Conservative management of acute sinusitis involves use of appropriate antibiotics such as ampicillin, amoxycillin, trimethoprim–sulphamethoxazole, cefaclor, cefuroxime axetil, amoxycillin–clavulanate and loracarbef (Gwaltney et al. 1992). An alternative strategy is immediate sinus puncture which may permit more rapid resolution and provide material for the determination of antimicrobial sensitivities. Chronic disease should prompt allergic and immunological investigation and prolonged therapy, including antibiotics for anaerobic infection. Ultimately, chronic disease may require surgery to establish free drainage.

Otitis media

Upper respiratory tract infections, often viral, are most commonly responsible for the events that lead to otitis media. Such infections impair the function of the eustachian tube, create a negative pressure and transudation into the middle ear. Bacterial contamination results by reflux from the oropharynx and this leads to further accumulation of fluid and pus.

The 4 stages of otitis media are:

1 **Myringitis** – inflammation of the tympanic membrane
2 **Acute suppurative otitis media** which denotes a

Table 18.1 Point prevalence of nasopharyngeal carriage of pathogens

	Prevalence	
Non-typable *Haemophilus influenzae*	25–48%	(Turk 1984)
Haemophilus influenzae type b	2–4%	(Moxon 1986)
Streptococcus pneumoniae	60–100%	(Austrian 1986)
Neisseria meningitidis	5–10%	(Broome 1986)

middle ear infection behind the reddened tympanic membrane

3 **Secretory (serous) otitis media** which refers to chronic middle ear effusion behind an intact tympanic membrane with acute signs and symptoms and

4 **Chronic suppurative otitis media** – a chronic discharge from the middle ear through a perforation of the tympanic membrane. Chronic disease can lead to loss of aeration of the middle ear cleft and loss of hearing and speech retardation during infancy.

Otitis media primarily affects children but can lead to lifelong sequelae. In acute otitis media the major organisms are *H. influenzae*, *S. pneumoniae* and *M. catarrhalis*. These organisms can also be recovered in chronic otitis media but in addition, *S. aureus*, *E. coli*, *K. pneumoniae*, *P. aeruginosa* and anaerobic bacteria can all be present (Brook and Van der Heyning 1994). Empirical therapy may be given in most cases, including the aminopenicillins and second generation cephalosporins and aminopenicillins in combination with β-lactamase inhibitors where β-lactamase producing organisms are present. About half the patients recover within 10 days with appropriate therapy, whereas most of the remainder have a residual exudate which resolves over 3 months. About 5% develop secretory otitis media.

Chronic otitis media requires surgical correction, drainage and treatment for anaerobic bacteria with agents such as aminopenicillins plus β-lactamase inhibitors. In such cases the microbiological flora should always be determined to rule out the presence of anaerobes or *Pseudomonas* spp.

RHINOSCLEROMA

This is a chronic granulomatous disease of the nose found in eastern Europe and parts of the tropics. It leads to nasal obstruction and marked secretion with postnasal drip. It is due to *Klebsiella pneumoniae* subsp. *rhinoscleromatis* (Volume 2, Chapter 42).

INFECTIONS OF THE PERIORAL AND PERIPHARYNGEAL SPACES

Infections of oral soft tissues are uncommon and caused by endogenous oral bacteria including oral anaerobes. Such infections can lead to pain and swelling of the sublingual and submandibular space (Vincent's angina). An extreme form of this is the rare **Lemierre's syndrome** that consists of oropharyngeal infection and anaerobic bacteraemia, septic thrombophlebitis of the jugular vein with embolization to the lungs and other areas. *Fusobacterium necrophorum* is usually the cause and prolonged treatment with parenteral benzylpenicillin and metronidazole is necessary.

Peritonsillar abscess can occur in patients with recurrent tonsillitis or inadequately treated pharyngotonsillitis. Bacteria that are recovered include *Streptococcus pyogenes*, *Streptococcus milleri*, *H. influenzae* and viridans streptococci. Anaerobes, including *F. necrophorum*, *Prevotella* spp. and *Peptostreptococcus* spp. can also be isolated from peritonsillar abscesses. The clinical features are high fever, intense pain in the throat, voice change and occasionally airway obstruction (Jousimies-Somer et al. 1993). Treatment with needle aspiration and oral penicillin is sufficient for most patients with peritonsillar abscesses (Maharaj, Raja and Hemsley 1991). When incipient airway obstruction is present this is best treated by incision and drainage.

5.2 Laryngotracheal infections

Most laryngitis is due to virus infection but *M. catarrhalis* and *H. influenzae* may be recovered from such patients and some symptoms of laryngitis can be improved with oral erythromycin (Schalen et al. 1992). Tracheitis is usually due to viruses, including respiratory syncytial virus. Bacterial pathogens associated with tracheitis include *H. influenzae*, *S. aureus*, *Streptococcus* spp. including *S. pneumoniae*.

6 PNEUMONIA

This is a general term for disease that includes consolidation of the lung parenchyma. There is acute inflammation in the gas exchange areas of the lung (pneumonitis), with a polymorphonuclear leucocyte exudate in and around alveoli and terminal and respiratory bronchioles. The gross pathology of pneumonia consists of 3 stages. First, there is engorgement in which the lung, when cut, is wet, oedematous and congested. In the second stage (red hepatization), the patient has high fever, cough and a rusty sputum, the lung is dry, red, friable and solid. In the third stage (grey hepatization) there is softening of the cut lung and exudation of yellow purulent fluid.

The most useful clinical classification of pneumonia divides cases into community-acquired or nosocomial. Other considerations include whether the pneumonia results from aspiration or follows from an acute viral infection, is acquired in specific geographical settings, or occurs in the context of immunosuppression, including AIDS.

6.1   Community-acquired pneumonia

The true incidence of community-acquired pneumonia is not easy to determine but approximately one per thousand of the population is admitted to hospital with pneumonia annually in the United Kingdom (Woodhead et al. 1987). In the USA it is estimated that there are approximately 3.3 million episodes of pneumonia per annum (an attack rate of 12 per 1000 persons per year). Each year the bacterial pneumonias account for over 500 000 hospital admissions of patients 15 years or older in the USA (Pennington 1994a). Pneumonia is substantially more common in the winter and affects more males than females (ratio 2–3:1). It is commoner amongst older persons; the annual incidence of pneumonia that requires hospitalization of those older than 75 years is 11.6 cases per 1000, for those aged 35–44 years it is 0.54 cases per 1000 persons (Marrie 1994).

The symptoms include cough, sputum and dyspnoea, and pleuritic pain. Classically the sputum is rusty-coloured in pneumococcal pneumonia but is usually mucoid, scanty or absent, especially at an early stage and in *Mycoplasma* and *Legionella* infections it may be absent. Extrapulmonary symptoms occasionally predominate and patients may present with severe headache, confusion and myalgia. Until recently cases in which these symptoms have predominated have been described as 'atypical pneumonia' and therefore pathognomonic of *Mycoplasma*, *Coxiella* and *Legionella* infection. It is now accepted that atypical presentations may be seen with pneumococcal pneumonia and the distinction is regarded as unhelpful.

Mortality due to community-acquired pneumonia was markedly decreased by the introduction of antibiotics. In the antibiotic era, mortality from ambulatory pneumonia has been of the order of 1% (Woodhead et al. 1987). Mortality in hospitalized patients is about 13–15% (Austrian and Gold 1964, Macfarlane et al. 1982). In patients who need intensive therapy, mortality ranges from 22 to 54% (Woodhead et al. 1985, Torres et al. 1991). The outcome for patients admitted to hospital with pneumonia can be greatly modified by prompt antibiotic therapy. In a large multicentre study none of the patients who died of pneumococcal, staphylococcal, or *M. pneumoniae* pneumonia had received appropriate antibiotics before hospital admission (British Thoracic Society 1987). A number of clinical and laboratory features of community-acquired pneumonia are associated with increased mortality (Table 18.2). Three independent studies have shown a 21-fold increase in the risk of death or the need for intensive therapy when 2 or more of the following factors are present:

1 respiratory rate greater than 30 min^{-1}
2 diastolic blood pressure below 60 mmHg
3 serum urea above 7 mmol l^{-1} (British Thoracic Society 1987, Farr, Sloman and Frisch 1991, Karalus et al. 1991).

Table 18.2   Clinical and laboratory features of community-acquired pneumonia associated with increased risk of death

Clinical features	[a]Respiratory rate >30
	[a]Diastolic BP <60
	Age >60
	Underlying disease
	Confusion
	Atrial fibrillation
	Multilobar involvement
Laboratory features	[a]Urea >7 mmol l^{-1}
	Serum albumin <35 g l^{-1}
	Hypoxaemia Po_2 <8 kPa
	Leucopenia WBC <4000
	Leucocytosis WBC >20 000
	Bacteraemia

[a]21-fold increase in risk of death or requirement of admission to an intensive therapy unit if 2 or 3 of these factors are present.
Data from Farr, Sloman and Frisch (1991), Karulus et al. (1991).

6.2   Community-treated pneumonia

Accurate data for community-treated pneumonia are difficult to obtain. Results of a number of studies in which pathogens were identified in 45–72% of hospitalized patients are summarized in Table 18.3. The predominant organisms are *S. pneumoniae*, which is by far the most common bacterial cause, *M. pneumoniae* and viruses. These series record a preponderance of bacterial causes in hospitalized patients, but it has been estimated that at least half of non-hospitalized cases are due to viruses or mycoplasma (Pennington 1994a).

STREPTOCOCCUS PNEUMONIAE

Epidemiology

S. pneumoniae is frequently isolated from the nasopharynx of asymptomatic individuals (point prevalence – 60–100%). The American serotyping system assigns serotype numbers in sequence from 1 to 83

Table 18.3   Meta-analysis of pathogens causing community-acquired pneumonia

Pathogen	Percentage of cases
Streptococcus pneumoniae	30–54
Haemophilus influenzae	6–15
Influenza A virus	6–9
Mycoplasma pneumoniae	0–18
Legionella pneumophila	2–7
Chlamydia pneumoniae	0–6
Chlamydia psittaci	0–3
Staphylococcus aureus	0–2
Gram-negative bacilli	0–2
Streptococcus spp.	0–1
Coxiella burnetii	0–1
Enterobacteriaceae	0–1
Respiratory syncytial virus	0–1

After Meyer and Finch (1992).

(see Volume 2, Chapter 28). The lower numbered serotypes are most frequently implicated in pneumococcal diseases. In Papua New Guinea, which has a high rate of pneumococcal disease, serotypes 2, 3, 5, 8 and 14 infrequently colonize the nasopharynx but are likely to cause invasive disease. Other serotypes are commonly carried by the population and cause disease in children but not as frequently in adults (serotypes 6, 19F and 23F). The remaining serotypes are relatively rarely carried in the nasopharynx and do not cause disease (Montgomery et al. 1990).

A high incidence of pneumococcal bacteraemia occurs in infants under 2 years of age. The incidence is low in teenage children and young adults, but increases again in men and women in their 70s. The incidence of pneumococcal disease in immunocompetent young adults is 5 per 100 000; the incidence of pneumococcal bacteraemia is 1000 per 100 000 patients with AIDS (Redd et al. 1990). Certain occupational groups, including military recruits, have higher annual rates of infection but the highest recorded incidence is in South African gold miners (Farr and Mandell 1994).

Pathogenesis

The first step in the pathogenesis of pneumococcal disease is believed to be nasopharyngeal colonization. The average duration of carriage is about 6 weeks in adults but some individuals may carry a strain for more than a year. Most infections occur during the first week of carriage, while sensitization and production of IgG proceed (Musher, Watson and Baughn 1990). In normal individuals, with intact mucociliary clearance, there is a much lower risk of pneumococcal disease once colonization is established in comparison with those who have pre-existing pulmonary disease or immunosuppression. However, viral respiratory infections, particularly due to influenza virus, predispose even more individuals to pneumonia. Malnourished individuals, e.g. alcoholics and residents of nursing homes, and those with chronic liver or kidney disease, cancer or diabetes mellitus, are also vulnerable to invasive disease. Splenectomy renders individuals vulnerable to catastrophic pneumococcal bacteraemia.

Highly specific enzyme-linked immunoassay (ELISA) techniques have shown that most healthy young adults lack antibody to the majority of serotype-specific capsular polysaccharides (Musher 1992). Pneumococcal infection probably occurs only in individuals who lack serotype-specific antibody to the capsular polysaccharide of their colonizing serotype.

Clinical features

Pneumococcal pneumonia usually develops over several days with cough and sputum production, dyspnoea, pleuritic chest pain, weakness, malaise and often myalgia. Occasionally a dramatic rigor may be the first symptom; this hyperacute presentation is more common in otherwise healthy young adults. In older patients the presentation is typically more insidious with minimal cough and absence of fever; con-

fusion and hypothermia are often presenting features in this group. Physical examination may reveal evidence of consolidation and chest x-ray commonly reveals an area of infiltration of less than a whole segment (Fig. 18.3), and several areas may be involved (Ort et al. 1983).

Laboratory findings

Most patients have a polymorphonuclear leucocytosis; leucopenia ($<4 \times 10^9 \, 1^{-1}$) is a poor prognostic indicator. There may be hyperbilirubinaemia and elevated liver enzymes.

Examination of sputum requires specimens with at least 15–25 white blood cells and less than 10 epithelial cells in a standard microscopic field. If lancet-shaped gram-positive cocci (i.e. pneumococci) are seen with more than 10 cocci per oil immersion field ($\times 100$), the sensitivity for detection of pneumococci in the sputum is about 60% and the specificity about 85% (Rein et al. 1978). The presence of pneumococci can be confirmed by the capsule swelling (quellung) reaction with polyvalent pneumococcal antiserum but in practice this is rarely used. The success of culture depends on sputum quality – if saliva is present viridans streptococci may outnumber the pneumococci. Transtracheal aspiration and transcutaneous aspiration are more sensitive but are only of value as research tools.

Pneumococcal polysaccharides can be identified rapidly in sputum, blood or urine. Countercurrent immunoelectrophoresis (CIE) is positive in approximately 50% of patients with non-bacteraemic pneumococcal pneumonia when performed on urine and serum, and in 50% of bacteraemic patients when per-

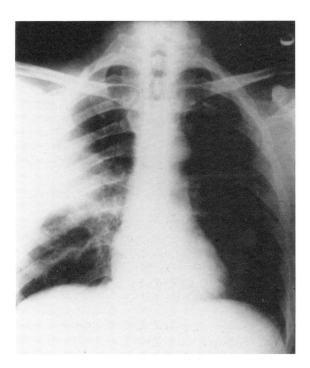

Fig. 18.3 Lobar consolidation in a male, age 25 years, with pneumococcal pneumonia.

formed only on serum. Sputum CIE is positive in approximately 75% of pneumonia patients with positive pneumococcal culture and remains positive after antibiotic therapy. Latex agglutination, coagglutination and ELISA are as reliable as CIE.

Complications

Empyema is the most common complication of pneumococcal pneumonia. A reactive effusion can occur but is trivial; empyema is potentially more serious and is presumably due to bacteria reaching the pleural space via the lymphatics. Clinically, it is signalled by the persistence of fever and leucocytosis after 4–5 days of appropriate antibiotic therapy. Empyema is also suggested by large amounts of pleural fluid seen on the chest x-ray. Empyema should be drained by repeated needle aspiration or a chest tube; thoracotomy is rarely necessary. Complications of pneumococcal bacteraemia such as endocarditis, pericarditis, peritonitis and brain abscess are very uncommon in immunocompetent individuals.

Antimicrobial therapy

Penicillin has long been the mainstay of therapy of pneumococcal disease but *S. pneumoniae* has become more resistant to penicillin over recent years (Markiewicz and Tomasz 1989). Strains with intermediate resistance are now prevalent throughout the world and highly resistant isolates are common in certain geographical areas, e.g. Spain, where more than 40% of isolates are resistant (Garcia-Léon and Cercenada 1992). For this reason an oxacillin disc is used routinely to screen for penicillin-resistant pneumococci. Such strains are often resistant to other antibiotics, such as chloramphenicol, erythromycin and clindamycin, suggesting that the resistance is due to plasmid mediated transfer from other bacterial species. In practice, pneumococcal pneumonia almost always responds to penicillin or cephalosporins in high doses (Friedland and McCracken 1994), in contrast to meningitis. Organisms highly resistant to penicillin are susceptible to vancomycin.

Prevention

The 23-valent pneumococcal vaccine contains antigens from 23 serotypes of pneumococci: 1, 2, 3, 4, 5, 6B, 7F, 8, 9N, 9V, 10A, 11A, 12F, 14, 15B, 17F, 18C, 19A, 19F, 20, 22F, 23F and 33F. These types account for the majority of cases of bacteraemic pneumococcal infection and the vaccine produces antibody responses in approximately 85% of those vaccinated. It is effective in splenectomized individuals though lower antibody levels are achieved (Giebink et al. 1980) but not in children under 2 years of age. Its use is, therefore, recommended in patients with splenic dysfunction or splenectomy and other chronic diseases, including diabetes mellitus, chronic cardiopulmonary disease, renal failure, nephrotic syndrome, liver disease and AIDS, but its use in the immunocompromised is controversial (Hirschmann and Lipsky 1994). A large case-control field study revealed a 56% efficacy in preventing bacteraemic pneumococcal

infection; efficacy in immunocompetent patients (61%) was higher than in immunosuppressed patients (21%) (Shapiro et al. 1991). The vaccines are given by intramuscular or subcutaneous injection. Repeat vaccination is recommended after 3–6 years in certain individuals, e.g. splenectomized adults or children under 10 with nephrotic syndrome or hyposplenism, but local intolerance at the injection site can be a problem.

MYCOPLASMA PNEUMONIAE

M. pneumoniae causes tracheobronchopneumonia with severe constitutional symptoms. The clinical syndrome of primary atypical pneumonia was first described by Reimann (1938). *M. pneumoniae* causes a wide spectrum of clinical disease involving the respiratory tract, skin, central nervous system and blood-forming elements.

Epidemiology

M. pneumoniae spreads with ease in institutions such as schools, universities and military installations. The highest incidence is during the first 2 decades of life. The infection can occur during any season but there is generally a 4 year cycle in which one year of high prevalence is followed by 2 or 3 years of low incidence (Fig. 18.4).

Pathogenesis

The organism is carried in the nasopharynx and infection is transmitted by droplets. *M. pneumoniae* binds to epithelial cells by neuraminic acid receptors and subsequently causes damage to cells locally by hydrogen peroxide production. Once the bronchial mucosa is penetrated a local inflammatory response is initiated. Many of the disease features are a result of a complex immune response to the organism (Tuazon and Murray 1994). Repeated infections result in the generation of sensitized T lymphocytes and autoantibodies, which initiate the pneumonitis. Immune complexes may also contribute to injury of the lung, brain and synovia and elsewhere. The host mediated facets of the disease explain why some patients develop only upper respiratory tract symptoms, whereas others may develop pneumonitis with or without severe extrapulmonary manifestations.

Clinical features

The clinical features are at first similar to influenza except that the onset of *M. pneumoniae* infection tends to be gradual over several days or a week (Clyde 1993). Constitutional symptoms initially include headache, malaise, myalgia and pharyngitis but rigors are uncommon. The cough, which is initially dry and dominates the disease, is the last symptom to clear. Despite antibiotics clinical relapse can occur a week after the initial response. The physical signs are often minimal and include sinus tenderness, pharyngitis without exudate, occasional myringitis. The chest is initially clear but wheezing and rhonchi may develop in the second week. Although the pneumonia is usually self-limited, occasionally adult respiratory distress syndrome asso-

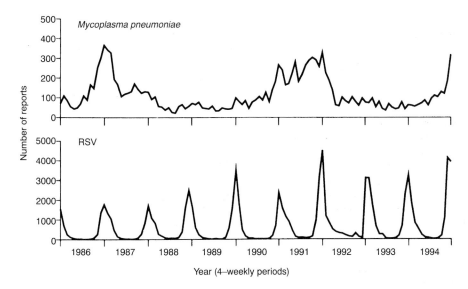

Fig. 18.4 Periodicity of *Mycoplasma pneumoniae* infection, in comparison with respiratory syncytial virus. (Reproduced with permission from CDSC 1995).

ciated with *M. pneumoniae* may develop. Other pulmonary complications are unusual (Tuazon and Murray 1994).

Extrapulmonary manifestations

Pneumonia with rash is most commonly due to *M. pneumoniae*. Stevens–Johnson syndrome in association with *M. pneumoniae* is potentially life-threatening and is probably due to the cell mediated immune response to *M. pneumoniae* but, since the rash often develops after drug therapy, antibiotics, particularly erythromycin, may be responsible (Cherry 1993).

Haemolytic anaemia characteristically occurs 2–3 weeks after the onset of illness, is usually self-limiting and coincides with high cold agglutinin titres. It is complement dependent and involves IgM antibody to the I antigen of red blood cells (Cherry 1993). Although haemolytic anaemia is uncommon, approximately three-quarters of patients with *M. pneumoniae* pneumonia develop high titres of cold agglutinins.

Central nervous system symptoms are present in up to 70% of patients with *M. pneumoniae* infection treated in hospital (Koskiniemi 1993). Encephalitis is the most frequent CNS manifestation, but meningitis, myelitis and polyradiculitis and many other symptoms, including coma, ataxia and stroke due to cerebral infarction, have been reported. *M. pneumoniae* has not been isolated from brain tissue but has been recovered from the cerebrospinal fluid (CSF). In aseptic meningitis the CSF reveals a modest pleocytosis, but occasionally all the white cells are polymorphs.

Laboratory findings

The white blood cell count is usually greater than 10 × 10⁹ per litre and neutrophilia, lymphocytosis and monocytosis can all occur but leucopenia is rare. Routine sputum culture is negative, but *M. pneumoniae* can be grown in broth media in long-term cultures.

A useful bedside test depends on the presence of cold agglutinins. A few drops of blood are placed into a citrate tube and placed in a refrigerator for a few minutes. If cold agglutinins are present agglutination

of red cells will be seen. The IgM cold agglutinins first appear 7–9 days after infection with a peak after 4–6 weeks.

The mainstay of diagnosis is serological. A 4-fold increase in complement fixation titre is diagnostic. Unfortunately serology is frequently negative during the acute phase; even laboratory assay for cold haemagglutinins, the first acute phase marker, is positive in only about 50% of acutely ill patients. ELISA for early IgM does not improve the diagnostic yield (Jacobs 1993). Newer techniques for direct detection of mycoplasma in clinical samples, e.g. sputum and throat, include antigen capture enzyme immunoassay (Ag-EIA), polymerase chain reaction (PCR) and detection of ribosomal RNA genes (Marmion et al. 1993).

Antimicrobial therapy

The mainstays of treatment for *M. pneumoniae* infection are erythromycin and tetracycline. Recovery with erythromycin is quite slow and the antibiotic is often poorly tolerated. Newer macrolides such as azithromycin and clarithromycin are better tolerated and have equivalent activity in vitro. Newer fluoroquinolones, are also active against *M. pneumoniae* (Bébéar et al. 1993).

Prevention

Killed and inactivated vaccines do not evoke effective serum or local respiratory tract immune responses (Tuazon and Murray 1994). Future vaccines may be based on recently discovered peptide adhesins.

LEGIONELLA PNEUMOPHILA

This organism is named after an epidemic of pneumonia in legionnaires who attended the American Legion Convention in Philadelphia in the late summer of 1976 (Fraser et al. 1977). Among the 4500 persons attending, 192 cases were observed and 29 proved fatal. The syndrome was characterized by nonproductive cough, pulse temperature dissociation, abnormalities of liver function, diarrhoea, hyponatraemia, hypophosphataemia, myalgia, confusion and multiple rigors. The condition became known as Legionnaires' disease. A previously unknown pleomorphic gram-negative bacillus was isolated from 4 of the original patients and named *L. pneumophila*. Some 3 years later an acute, short-lived, febrile illness consisting of myalgia but not pneumonia that affected staff and visitors at the County Health Department at Pontiac, Michigan, was shown to be due to *L. pneumophila*. It had a shorter incubation period and there were no deaths (Broome and Fraser 1979). Subsequently devised serological techniques implicated *Legionella* spp. in pneumonia not only in outbreaks associated with the water facilities of large buildings such as hospitals and hotels, but also with sporadic community-acquired infections. *Legionella* are aerobic, fastidious, gram-negative bacilli of which 34 species have been characterized (see Volume 2, Chapter 49). Rarely, infections may be caused by *L. micdadei*, *L. longbeachae*, *L. dumoffii*, *L. bozemanii* and other species (Edelstein and Meyer 1994).

Pathogenesis

Infection results from inhalation of *Legionella*-contaminated aerosols, for example, disseminated by cooling towers, humidifiers, respiratory therapy equipment, showerheads and cooling sprays. *L. pneumophila* is phagocytosed by macrophages but they fail to kill the organism. In macrophages infected in vitro, *Legionella* can multiply between 100 and 1000 times in 48–72 h (Yamamoto et al. 1994). Defence against the infection, therefore, crucially depends on cell mediated immunity, as illustrated by the susceptibility to legionellosis of patients in whom such immunity is deficient; those with neutropenia do not appear to be susceptible.

Epidemiology

Legionella survive in water for prolonged periods. Although infection occurs sporadically in the community (Macfarlane et al. 1982), outbreaks are dramatic and associated with water facilities. Of the 129 cases of Legionnaires' disease reported in England and Wales in 1993, 51% were associated with travel, mainly to Spain, but also to Greece, Turkey, USA and within the UK; 6 were nosocomial and the remainder were sporadic community cases (Joseph et al. 1994a). Outbreaks have occurred in the vicinity of cooling towers (Broome and Fraser 1979), a power station (Morton et al. 1986) and notably, Broadcasting House, London in 1988. The role of air conditioning equipment was demonstrated in Memphis in 1978 (Dondero et al. 1980) and by a large hospital outbreak in Staffordshire, England (Editorial 1986). Showerheads and hot water taps spread aerosols contaminated with *Legionella* (Bolling et al. 1985). This has caused outbreaks in hospitals and is the probable cause of disease in holidaymakers returning from Mediterranean resorts. Contaminated showerheads and tap water led to a prolonged and disastrous outbreak in the VA Wadsworth Medical Center, Los Angeles, with a high rate of nosocomial *Legionella* pneumonia, particularly in immunosuppressed patients. The outbreak was terminated by changing shower-heads and by hyperchlorination of potable water (Shands et al. 1985). Between 1980 and 1992, 218 cases were reported in the UK, of whom 68 patients died. Approximately half were sporadic but 3 hospital outbreaks contributed to the majority of the remaining cases. Hospital domestic water systems were the source of infection in 19 outbreaks. The cooling tower was thought to be the source in one hospital and probably contributed to 2 other outbreaks in which the domestic water system was suspected to be the main source (Joseph et al. 1994b).

Clinical features

The majority of patients with *L. pneumophila* infection have a pneumonia virtually indistinguishable from pneumococcal pneumonia (Edelstein 1993). Clinical features range from asymptomatic infection and non-pneumonic myalgia (Pontiac fever) to Legionnaires' disease with severe pneumonia and extrapulmonary manifestations. After an incubation period of 2–10 days, there is a gradual onset of malaise, lethargy, fever, headache, myalgia, weakness with evolution of a dry non-productive cough after 1–2 days. There may be purulent sputum which can be bloody (Edelstein 1993). In about 25% of patients there may be disorientation, agitation, confusion, hallucinations, ataxia and seizure. The systemic manifestations are probably due to several exotoxins, and possibly endotoxins (Edelstein and Meyer 1994). Extrapulmonary manifestations include pancreatitis, peritonitis, cellulitis, myositis and focal abscesses, and prosthetic valve endocarditis is well recognized. Pneumonia due to species other than *L. pneumophila* is clinically indistinguishable. *Legionella micdadei* infection occurs in immunosuppressed patients and causes nodular pulmonary infiltrates (Pittsburgh pneumonia) (Myerowitz et al. 1979).

Diagnosis

Non-specific laboratory abnormalities include elevated white blood count (usually with neutrophilia), hyponatraemia, elevation of alkaline phosphatase and liver transaminases, and proteinuria. Specific methods of diagnosis include serology, direct fluorescence microscopy, culture, DNA probes and tests for urine antigen (Edelstein and Meyer 1994). Serology is most specific in infections due to *L. pneumophila* of serogroup 1, with seroconversion 6–9 weeks after the acute disease. Antigen can be detected in sputum, bronchoalveolar lavage fluid or lung biopsy material by immunofluorescence with genus-specific monoclonal antibodies, even after several days of chemotherapy. Culture for *L. pneumophila* with supplemented charcoal yeast extract medium (BCYE) succeeds even after the onset of chemotherapy. DNA probes can detect *Legionella* several days after the start of antibiotic therapy. The test for *L. pneumophila* serogroup 1 antigenuria is rapid and highly specific and may be positive for several weeks after recovery from pneumonia.

Antimicrobial chemotherapy

In the Legionnaires' disease outbreak in Philadelphia in 1976, the case fatality rate was highest for patients treated with cephalosporins and lowest with erythromycin. Erythromycin should be given in a dose of 2–4 g per day, initially intravenously in severely ill patients, for at least 3 weeks. Rifampicin should be added for patients who are critically ill. Patients usually respond fairly quickly to erythromycin therapy.

Antimicrobial sensitivity testing is not applicable to *L. pneumophila*. Most of the β-lactam agents are active in vitro against *L. pneumophila*. However, animal models have shown that these agents are ineffective because they do not enter macrophages sufficiently well. Therefore, the potential efficacy of new agents must be based upon their success in intracellular infection and experimental animal models. Azithromycin, clarithromycin, fluoroquinolone antibiotics, trimethoprim–sulphamethoxazole, tetracyclines including doxycycline, and rifampicin are effective in animal models (Edelstein 1993). The latter drugs can be used as second line agents for patients intolerant of erythromycin.

Prevention

Person-to-person transmission of Legionnaires' disease has not been observed. The most important preventive measure is to render water sources safe. Thirty to 80% of hospital cooling towers and water supplies are to some extent contaminated with *Legionella* and in concentrations >10^8 cfu l^{-1} the hazard of infection is increased (Edelstein and Meyer 1994). Chlorination, pasteurization and heating can be used to reduce the *Legionella* burden (Muraca and Stout 1988).

The report of a single case of Legionnaires' disease requires investigation to determine whether it is part of an outbreak, which involves tracing the patient's activities during the incubation period. If hospital-acquired infection is suspected the hospital water maintenance programme must be reviewed and a search made for associated cases, beginning with the immunosuppressed population who are most vulnerable to infection (Saunders, Joseph and Watson 1994).

COXIELLA BURNETII

C. burnetii (see Volume 2, Chapter 36) is the cause of Q fever which was first described in Australia in the 1930s in abattoir workers. The organism spreads between farm animals and man by air-borne transmission, by infected milk, faeces and urine, and is probably also transmitted by tick bite. It is highly resistant to drying and in agricultural facilities contaminates dust, which can cause infection by inhalation. After an incubation period of 2–4 weeks there is abrupt onset of high fever, malaise, headache and neck stiffness. There is dry cough and pleuritic chest pain and on examination there is usually high fever, hepatosplenomegaly but few chest signs. Some patients develop a transient maculopapular rash but the exanthem typical of other rickettsial infections is absent. Most illness resolves within 2 weeks but fever can persist for up to 3 months. Q fever can be complicated by extrapulmonary lesions, including endocarditis. There may be mild hepatitis, occasionally severe and even fulminant. *C. burnetii* may cause blood culture-negative endocarditis many months after the primary infection.

Complement fixation and indirect fluorescent antibody tests reach a peak between 1 and 3 months after original infection. Phase 2 antibodies are raised in acute Q fever; phase 1 antibodies are prominent in patients with chronic Q fever, e.g. endocarditis.

Tetracycline or doxycycline is used to treat acutely ill patients and those with persistent symptoms. Long-term treatment with tetracycline is desirable for patients with Q fever endocarditis, but valve replacement may become necessary.

STAPHYLOCOCCUS AUREUS

Although *S. aureus* pneumonia is usually nosocomial, it accounts for a small proportion of community-acquired pneumonia, particularly during influenza epidemics and in certain patient groups, e.g. diabetics. Though 15–30% of adults are nasal carriers of *S. aureus*, resulting pneumonia is rare and presumably requires an underlying host defect, e.g. diabetes. Staphylococcal pneumonia is also seen in patients with right-sided endocarditis (e.g. in intravenous drug abusers) and in patients with septic thrombophlebitis or an infected vascular prosthesis. Staphylococcal and pneumococcal pneumonia can be differentiated on clinical grounds (Farr et al. 1989). Patients with staphylococcal pneumonia more commonly have pleural effusions and cavitation on chest x-ray and 25% develop abscesses (Waldvogel 1990). Staphylococcal pneumonia secondary to septic embolization from right-sided endocarditis causes multiple small round cavitary lesions.

Clusters of staphylococci seen in the gram stain of sputum is diagnostic. The sputum of patients with suspected *S. aureus* pneumonia should always be examined promptly because a rapid diagnosis may result and a penicillinase-resistant penicillin should be added to the empirical treatment regimen for severe pneumonia. Vancomycin should be used only when pneumonia due to multiple-resistant *S. aureus* is suspected.

HAEMOPHILUS INFLUENZAE

H. influenzae causes community-acquired pneumonia in patients with chronic bronchitis and those with impaired host defences such as smokers or alcoholics. It is also a relatively common cause of pneumonia in children, particularly those aged 4 years and younger. Non-typable *H. influenzae* tends to cause mucosal infections such as those affecting the middle ear and the airway of bronchitics. Capsulate organisms, particularly of type b, cause a significant proportion of invasive parenchymal disease, i.e. pneumonia (Smith 1994). In adults and children the illness tends to be preceded by coryza and sudden onset of pleuritic chest pain is the predominant chest symptom (Crowe and Lavitz 1987). Microbiological diagnosis is notoriously difficult because of sputum contamination by commensal *Haemophilus* spp. and blood culture is usually negative. β-Lactamase production by infecting strains may be very frequent in some areas (Powell et al. 1991). If such strains may be involved, second generation cephalosporins should be used to treat moderately severe pneumonia.

GRAM-NEGATIVE BACILLARY PNEUMONIAS

Although gram-negative bacteria are a prominent cause of nosocomial pneumonia, they may also cause disease in the community, particularly in alcoholics, diabetics, residents of nursing homes and patients with underlying diseases such as malignancy and cardiac or renal failure. The upper respiratory tract becomes colonized followed by aspiration and subsequent pneumonia. The most common gram-negative causes of community pneumonia are *K. pneumoniae*, *E. coli*, *Serratia marcesens*, *Enterobacter* spp. and *Pseudomonas* spp.

K. pneumoniae classically causes pneumonia in debilitated middle-aged males, with sudden fever and rigors, dyspnoea and large volumes of bloody sputum. Often there is a necrotizing process with multiple abscess formation and dramatic lobar consolidation. The sputum contains large numbers of capsulate gram-negative bacilli and blood cultures are often positive. The infection is destructive, often severe and has a high mortality (Feldman et al. 1989).

E. coli is the cause of up to 3% of community pneumonias in American series (Eisenstadt and Crane 1994). It may result by bacteraemic spread from the genitourinary and gastrointestinal tracts and is often bilateral. Other causes of community-acquired gram-negative pneumonia include *Proteus* spp. (*Morganella* and *Providencia* spp.) and *Acinetobacter baumannii*.

Pseudomonas spp. can, rarely, cause dramatic community-acquired pneumonia. *P. aeruginosa* causes pneumonia in patients admitted from nursing homes or individuals with malignancy. The disease is often necrotizing and there is diffuse bilateral consolidation on chest x-ray with occasional multiple abscesses. *Pseudomonas stutzeri* may cause disease in patients with malignancy (Noble and Overman 1994). For a discussion of pneumonia due to *Burkholderia pseudomallei* the reader is referred to Chapter 46.

STREPTOCOCCUS SPP.

Group B streptococcus may cause pneumonia, particularly in elderly, debilitated patients with diabetes mellitus, stroke, dementia and malignancies, and is often associated with other organisms, particularly *S. aureus* and *S. pneumoniae*. Enterococci can cause pneumonia in elderly, debilitated patients with multiple chronic problems, often with nasogastric tubes. Treatment is with high dose penicillin or ampicillin and an aminoglycoside.

RARE CAUSES OF BACTERIAL PNEUMONIA

N. meningitidis can cause a typical pneumonia in the absence of the classic or cutaneous rash and without evidence of meningitis or shock. The disease occurs as outbreaks in military or school dormitories (Koppes et al. 1977). *Bacillus anthracis* may cause pneumonia (wool-sorter's disease) if spores from contaminated animal fur or hair are inhaled (see Chapter 40). The lungs may be involved in up to 20% of cases of brucellosis (Lulu et al. 1988; see Chapter 41). *Pasteurella multocida*, which causes cellulitis after dog bites, can cause a necrotizing pneumonia, usually in patients with pre-existing respiratory disease and with history of exposure to domestic animals. *Yersinia pestis* can cause pneumonia as part of a septicaemic process (see Chapter 44).

THE APPROACH TO PATIENTS WITH COMMUNITY-ACQUIRED PNEUMONIA

In most patients presenting with symptoms and signs of pneumonia the likely cause is *S. pneumoniae*. Routine laboratory investigation should include sputum examination and culture, blood culture, acute and convalescent serology to detect antibodies to viruses, *Mycoplasma*, *Chlamydia*, *Legionella* spp. and *Coxiella burnetii*, antigen detection, and examination of pleural fluid.

ANTIMICROBIAL THERAPY

The British and American thoracic societies have issued guidelines for the management of adult community-acquired pneumonia. The British Thoracic Society (BTS) recommends the use of an aminopenicillin, e.g. oral amoxycillin or intravenous ampicillin or benzylpenicillin, for patients with uncomplicated pneumonia of unknown aetiology without features that indicate severe or non-pneumococcal disease. Suggested alternatives in penicillin-allergic patients include erythromycin or a second or third generation cephalosporin. For severe pneumonia of unknown aetiology the BTS recommends erythromycin plus a second or third generation cephalosporin. Alternatively, the combination of ampicillin, flucloxacillin and erythromycin can be used. If Legionnaires' disease is suspected, treatment with erythromycin is recommended. In severe cases intravenous rifampicin, ciprofloxacin, or both may be added. For suspected staphylococcal pneumonia the recommended treatment is flucloxacillin or nafcillin in combination with fusidic acid or an aminoglycoside. When clinical or epidemiological features suggest mycoplasma pneumonia, erythromycin is added to an aminopenicillin in mild disease (British Thoracic Society 1993).

The American Thoracic Society stratifies therapeutic management according to whether the patient is in hospital or in an out-patient setting, whether there is serious coexisting illness or advanced age, and whether the illness is severe. In out-patient pneumonia without comorbidity in patients 60 years of age or younger empirical treatment with a macrolide or tetracycline is recommended. Treatment recommended for out-patient pneumonia in patients with comorbidity, or in older patients, is with either a second generation cephalosporin, trimethoprim–sulphamethoxazole or a β-lactam with a β-lactamase inhibitor, with a macrolide if legionellosis is suspected.

For hospitalized patients with a community-acquired pneumonia, the recommended treatment is a second or third generation cephalosporin or a β-lactam with a β-lactamase inhibitor with addition of a macrolide if legionellosis is possible. Finally, for hospitalized patients with severe community-acquired pneumonia, the recommended treatment is an intravenous macrolide plus a third generation cephalosporin with anti-*Pseudomonas* activity or other anti-*Pseudomonas* agents such as imipenem or ciprofloxacin (American Thoracic Society 1993).

6.3 Nosocomial pneumonia

Pneumonia is the second most common nosocomial infection after urinary tract infection (Horan et al. 1986), causes considerable mortality and morbidity, and increases hospital stay and its cost. The US Centers for Disease Control have published the following definition of nosocomial pneumonia:

Onset of pneumonia more than 72 h after hospital admission with lung consolidation or an infiltrate on the chest x-ray plus at least one of the following:

(a) infected sputum
(b) solation of a pathogen from the blood, transtracheal aspirate, biopsy or bronchial lavage specimen
(c) isolation of a virus in respiratory secretions
(d) diagnostic antibody titres or
(e) histopathological evidence of pneumonia (CDC 1988).

According to the US National Nosocomial Infection Surveillance (NNIS) system, nosocomial pneumonia occurs at a frequency of 0.6–1.0 episodes per 100 hospitalizations and in 18% of postoperative patients (Horan et al. 1986, Craven, Steager and Barber 1991). Intubated patients may have rates of pneumonia 7–21-fold higher than patients without a respiratory therapy device (Celis et al. 1988). Infection rates are twice as high in large teaching hospitals compared with smaller institutions. Factors that lead to nosocomial pneumonia include older age, chronic lung disease, depressed consciousness, mechanical ventilation, the use of H2 antagonists, frequent changes of ventilator circuits, and the winter season (Celis et al. 1988). Mortality in patients with nosocomial pneumonia is high (20–50%) but only about one-third of fatalities are directly due to pneumonia (Pennington 1994b).

PATHOGENESIS

Most nosocomial pneumonia results from aspiration of pathogens from the upper airways. Patients admitted to intensive care units become colonized with aerobic gram-negative bacilli within 1 week of entering hospital, and of these about 25% develop nosocomial pneumonia; there is a correlation between severity of illness and the likelihood of subsequent colonization with gram-negative organisms (Johanson, Pierce and Sanford 1969). Enterobacteriaceae probably reach the upper respiratory tract by faecal–oral transmission.

However, *P. aeruginosa* and *S. aureus* probably colonize the patient from environmental sources and contamination by attending staff, fomites or supporting equipment (Pennington 1994b).

MICROBIAL AETIOLOGY

The majority of hospital-acquired pneumonias are caused by aerobic gram-negative bacilli; Enterobacteriaceae cause 40% of these pneumonias, *S. aureus* 25% and *P. aeruginosa* 15%; *S. pneumoniae*, *H. influenzae*, fungi, viruses and anaerobic bacteria rarely cause nosocomial pneumonia. The results of 3 large studies of nosocomial pneumonia are shown in Table 18.4. Polymicrobial infections are common. A number of host risk factors can predispose to infection with particular pathogens (reviewed by Niederman 1994). Staphylococcal pneumonia is associated with diabetes, renal failure, a recent history of influenza and recent head injury and trauma, whereas *P. aeruginosa* is seen in malnourished patients, those on steroids or who have chronic structural lung disease or are subject to prolonged mechanical ventilation or tracheostomy. *L. pneumophila* may cause nosocomial pneumonia in hospitals with contaminated water supplies, particularly in patients immunosuppressed by treatment with steroids. Anaerobes are particularly seen in patients with gross aspiration of acid gastric contents and recent thoracoabdominal surgery. Viruses may contribute to nosocomial pneumonia, particularly influenza A, parainfluenza and adenovirus (Dal Nogare 1994). Methods for the diagnosis of nosocomial pneumonia in severely ill patients include transtracheal aspiration, bronchoscopic sampling with or without protective brush and transcutaneous aspiration of lung material, but in many studies these have not proved superior to traditional clinical evaluation (Pennington 1994b). In patients who are conscious, sputum production may yield gram-positive (*S. aureus*) or gram-negative bacteria. In intubated patients, aspirated respiratory secretions and blood cultures may provide a bacteriological diagnosis without the need for bronchoalveolar lavage.

TREATMENT AND PREVENTION

Appropriate therapy should include antibiotics active against *S. aureus* and gram-negative bacteria including *P. aeruginosa*; common regimens include a third generation cephalosporin or fluoroquinolone plus an aminoglycoside.

Prevention of nosocomial pneumonia depends on prevention of colonization and aspiration, and spread of pathogens between patients and staff. Hand washing by staff members should be encouraged. If swallowing is impaired, oral intake should be curtailed and unnecessary nasogastric and endotracheal tubes should be removed. Elevation of the patient's head reduces risk of aspiration (Dal Nogare 1994). Gastric acidity should be maintained by avoidance of H2 antagonists in seriously ill patients and the use of sucralfate to prevent erosive gastritis reduces the incidence of pneumonia (Craven, Steager and Barber 1991).

Table 18.4 Bacteriology from 3 nosocomial pneumonia studies

	Hughes	Bartlett	Bryan
Culture material	Sputum (%)	TTA[a] (%)	Blood (%)
Pseudmonas aeruginosa	17	9	15
Staphylococcus aureus	13	26	27
Enterobacteriaceae[b]	37	48	42
Fungi	6	ND[c]	ND
Anaerobic bacteria	2	35	2
Streptococcus pneumoniae	<3	31	12
Haemophilus influenzae	<3	17	<4
Viruses	<3	ND	ND

[a]TTA, transtracheal aspirate.
[b]Includes *Klebsiella pneumoniae*, *Enterobacter* spp., *Escherichia coli*, *Serratia*, *Proteus*.
[c]ND, not done.
Adapted from Dal Nogare (1994).

6.4 Aspiration pneumonia

Most aspiration pneumonia is polymicrobial and usually includes anaerobes (Finegold 1994). The latter thrive in lungs injured by chemical pneumonitis. Where there is periodontal disease and gingivitis, anaerobic colonization of the mouth is increased. In hospitalized patients and in nursing homes there is increased oropharyngeal colonization with gram-negative bacilli. A full list of potential organisms that may be involved in aspiration pneumonitis is shown in Table 18.5.

Pneumonia in patients with a predisposition to aspiration is insidious and mainly affects dependent zones of the lung. The commonest site is the posterior segment of the right upper lobe, but the apical segments of the lower lobes can be affected. Lung abscess or empyema with high swinging fever may occur, often with foul-smelling sputum and haemoptysis. Microbiological diagnosis is confounded by the normal anaerobic flora of the mouth and the gram stain of the sputum is difficult to interpret. Gram stain of empyema fluid or transtracheal aspirate may reveal the characteristic appearance of *Prevotella* spp., *Porphyromonas* spp. and *Fusobacterium* spp. Bacteraemia is uncommon in aspiration pneumonia.

Treatment of early uncomplicated aspiration or pneumonia in previously normal individuals is relatively straightforward because the majority of oral anaerobes in this situation are sensitive to benzylpenicillin. In patients with underlying disease or who are hospitalized the frequency of infections with non-penicillin-sensitive anaerobes is increased, including the *Bacteroides fragilis* group and gram-negative organisms including *Pseudomonas* spp. The possibility of infection with *S. aureus* should also be covered by administration of clindamycin or an aminoglycoside. Alternatively, combination therapy with a broad spectrum penicillin such as ticarcillin or piperacillin plus an aminoglycoside can be given. Newer antibiotics such as imipenem, or a combination of a broad spectrum antibiotic with a β-lactamase inhibitor are also effective.

6.5 Complications of pneumonia

PLEURAL EFFUSION

Pleural effusions occur very commonly in pneumococcal pneumonia infection. Usually the effusion is sterile and is absorbed spontaneously within a week or 2. Occasionally the effusion is large and requires aspiration. Empyema should be suspected if an effusion persists beyond 2 weeks, especially if there is continuing fever and pain.

EMPYEMA

Pus in the pleural space leads to symptoms of chest pain, fever and general malaise. Most empyemas occur as a complication of pneumonia or lung abscess, but 15–30% occur after thoracic surgery and 10% occur in association with intra-abdominal infection. Empyema following pneumonia is mostly polymicrobial and anaerobes are present in 75% of cases. Empyema after thoracic surgery is more likely to be monomicrobial and due to common nosocomial pathogens such as *S. aureus* and aerobic gram-negative bacilli. Progress of pneumonia to empyema is related to delay in appropriate antimicrobial therapy. Once infection is established the empyema rapidly becomes fibrinopurulent with eventual locule formation in the pleural space and fibrous adhesions between the visceral and parietal pleura. Diagnosis is based on demonstration of purulent pleural fluid. Microbiological diagnosis should include gram and acid-fast stains, wet mount for fungi and culture for aerobic and anaerobic bacteria, *Mycobacterium* spp. and fungi. Once an empyema has developed, the aim should be to sterilize the space with antibiotics and establish early and adequate pleural space drainage. Diffusion of antibiotics into the pleural space is good, but aminoglycosides and some β-lactams may be inactivated in the presence of pus, a low pH, and β-lactamase enzymes (Hughes and van Scoy 1991). Empirical treatment of empyema should include an effective agent against anaerobic bacteria and aerobic gram-negative bacteria. Metronidazole may not be reduced to its active metabolite in a partially oxygenated environment and so clindamycin in

Table 18.5   Potential microbial aetiology of aspiration pneumonitis

Anaerobes
Gram-negative bacilli
  Pigmented *Prevotella* and *Porphyromonas*
  Prevotella aureus, *Prevotella buccae*
  Prevotella oralis group
  Bacteroides ureolyticus group (especially *Bacteroides gracilis*)
  Bacteroides fragilis group
  Fusobacterium nucleatum
  Fusobacterium necrophorum, *Fusobacterium naviforme*, *Fusobacterium gonidiaformans*
Gram-positive cocci
  Peptostreptococcus (especially *Peptostreptococcus magnus*, *Peptostreptococcus asaccharolyticus*, *Peptostreptococcus prevotii*, *Peptostreptococcus anaerobius* and *Peptostreptococcus micros*)
  Micro-aerophilic streptococci (*Streptococcus intermedius*)
Gram-positive non-sporing bacilli
  Actinomyces spp.
  Propionibacterium propionicum
  Bifidobacterium dentium
Gram-positive spore-forming bacilli
  Clostridium (especially *Clostridium perfringens*, *Clostridium ramosum*)
Aerobes
Gram-positive bacilli
  Staphylococcus aureus
  Streptococcus pyogenes
  'viridans' streptococci
Gram-negative bacilli
  Klebsiella pneumoniae
  Enterobacter spp.
  Serratia spp.
  Pseudomonas aeruginosa
  Escherichia coli
  Proteus spp.

Modified after Finegold (1994).

combination with a fluoroquinolone for 4–6 weeks is a suitable combination. Alternatively, imipenem–cilastatin can be used. Drainage of pus is the mainstay of treatment and in the early exudative phase, closed drainage may suffice. If the empyema is loculated, operation can sometimes be avoided by the judicious use of urokinase to break down adhesions (Robinson and Moulton 1994).

Necrotizing pneumonitis and lung abscess

Pus-filled cavities in the lung can evolve when there is suppurative lung infection together with destruction of lung parenchyma. Necrotizing pneumonitis is arbitrarily defined as multiple cavities of less than 2 cm diameter; lung abscesses are larger. Aspiration is the commonest predisposing factor and in such cases the microbial aetiology reflects that seen in aspiration pneumonitis (see Table 18.5). Tooth decay and gingivitis also predispose to necrotizing infections. Abscess may also result in necrotic neoplasms, or in patients with bronchiectasis, during septic embolization from another source (e.g. endocarditis), as a complication of pulmonary embolus and as direct spread from the abdomen (e.g. amoebic abscess).

Pathogenesis

Necrotizing pneumonia after aspiration is common because of the destructive nature of gastric contents and the large microbial load. In the unconscious individual bacteria can replicate in static fluid in dependent lung segments. Some micro-organisms produce necrotizing infections by virtue of their virulence factors, including *F. necrophorum*, *K. pneumoniae* and *S. aureus*. *P. aeruginosa* secretes toxins that create a local vasculitis in addition to pneumonitis. Bronchiectasis can lead to lung abscess by virtue of markedly impaired local airway clearance.

Microbial aetiology

In a study of lung abscess by transtracheal aspiration, the majority of patients had multiple isolates but in every case one or more anaerobes was recovered (Bartlett et al. 1974). The most common were gram-negative bacilli including *Bacteroides* spp. and *Fusobacterium* spp., and also gram-positive cocci including *Peptostreptococcus* spp. and micro-aerophilic streptococci. The aerobic organisms that can cause necrotizing pneumonitis are *S. aureus*, *S. pyogenes*, *K. pneumoniae*, *P. aeruginosa*, *Proteus* spp. and *E. coli*. Occasionally the commoner causes of community-acquired pneumonia such as *S. pneumoniae* and *L. pneumophila* can be involved in a necrotizing process. *Actinomyces* spp., *Arachnia* and *Nocardia* spp. can cause necrotizing pneumonitis as part of a chronic infection. A number of pathogens cause necrotizing pneumonitis in the context of immunosuppression, including *Burkholderia cepacia*, in patients receiving nebulized therapy (Yamagishi et al. 1993). *Legionella* spp. and *Yersinia enterocolitica* can cause necrotizing pneumonias in such patients. Necrotizing pneumonitis is a prominent feature of *Burkholderia pseudomallei* infection (melioidosis) and as part of infection with *B. anthracis* in anthrax and *Y. pestis* in pneumonic plague.

Where multiple abscesses are present in the lung, haematogenous spread from an extrapulmonary focus is the probable cause. *S. aureus* abscesses can complicate right-sided endocarditis particularly in intravenous drug abusers. Enterobacteriaceae can produce multiple abscesses in association with urinary tract or bowel surgery and anaerobes can do so in patients with pelvic infections.

Diagnosis

Microbiological diagnosis can be achieved either by transtracheal aspiration, bronchoscopic alveolar lavage or with a protected brush specimen. Material should be rendered anaerobic as quickly as possible.

Therapy

For patients who are not severely ill, penicillin plus metronidazole or clindamycin is the initial therapy. Treatment must be continued for up to 3 months to achieve cure. In severely ill patients, empirical antibiotic therapy should aim to reduce the burden of β-lactamase producing anaerobes and also *S. aureus* and gram-negative bacilli, including *P. aeruginosa*. Some anaerobic bacteria, including *Actinomyces* spp. and *Propionibacterium* spp., are resistant to metronidazole. Some strains of the *B. fragilis* group are also resistant to the broad spectrum penicillins including piperacillin (Finegold 1994). Severely ill patients with necrotizing pneumonia can be given imipenem or a broad spectrum β-lactam–β-lactamase inhibitor combination.

6.6 Chronic pneumonia

Apart from mycobacteria (see Chapter 21 and Volume 2, Chapter 26), *Actinomyces* spp., notably *Actinomyces israelii* and *Propionibacterium propionicum*, and *Nocardia asteroides* may cause chronic pneumonia (see Chapter 39 and Volume 2, Chapter 20).

6.7 Pneumonia in immunocompromised patients

Most pneumonias in non-HIV immunocompromised patients occur in the context either of neutropenia or T cell defects. These occur in malignancies, particularly haematological malignancies, with and without chemotherapy; they also occur in patients undergoing organ transplantation and attendant immunosuppressive therapy and in other patients receiving steroids. Neutropenic patients are susceptible to pneumonia due to gram-negative organisms, particularly *E. coli*, *Klebsiella* spp., *Enterobacter* spp., *Serratia* spp., *Proteus* spp. and *Pseudomonas*. They are also susceptible to gram-positive infections including *S. aureus* and *Staphylococcus epidermidis* and viridans streptococci (Verhoef 1993). Patients with cellular immune defects such as T cell defects due to cyclosporin, purine antagonists, corticosteroids, or haematological malignancy are vulnerable to pneumonia mainly due to intracellular pathogens such as *Mycobacterium* spp. and *Legionella* spp., but more importantly to viruses, including cytomegalovirus (CMV), commonly derived from the transplanted organ, fungi (*Candida*, *Cryptococcus*) and *P. carinii* (Hughes 1993). It is difficult to distinguish on clinical grounds alone between pneumonia of bacterial or non-bacterial origin, but in general bacterial infections produce a rapidly advancing clinical course with focal infiltrates on chest x-ray (Fanta and Pennington 1994). *P. carinii* pneumonia in the non-HIV setting can also cause a rapidly advancing pneumonia. Bronchoscopy, with bronchoalveolar lavage, is necessary to identify the agents responsible because several may be involved. A number of unusual bacteria cause pneumonia in the immunocompromised host, including *Nocardia* spp., *Bordetella* spp. and *B. cepacia*. Nosocomial outbreaks of pneumonia in immunocompromised patients can be due to *L. pneumophila* (Carratala et al. 1994) and tuberculosis in renal units (Hall et al. 1994). Fanta and Pennington (1994) have proposed a scheme for initiating empirical therapy in immunocompromised patients. Patients with a focal infiltrate should be given antibacterial treatment while results of lung sampling are awaited. A combination of antibiotics to cover staphylococci and resistant gram-negative bacilli, including *Pseudomonas*, should be given, e.g. a third generation cephalosporin and an aminoglycoside, or a combination of broad spectrum penicillin and an aminoglycoside. If *Legionella* is suspected intravenous erythromycin should be added, and if *Aspergillus* is suspected amphotericin B should also be given. The challenging problem of aspergillosis is discussed in Volume 4, Chapter 16.

6.8 Bacterial pneumonia in HIV infection

In late stage HIV infection, particularly in patients with CD4 counts $<0.2 \times 10^9$ per litre, lung disease is dominated by infection with *P. carinii*, *M. tuberculosis*, *Toxoplasma gondii* and *Cryptococcus neoformans*. Patients are also susceptible to conventional bacterial infections. HIV-seropositive individuals have increased susceptibility to bacterial pneumonia, particularly caused by *S. pneumoniae*, *H. influenzae*, *M. catarrhalis*, *K. pneumoniae*, *N. meningitidis*, *Rhodococcus* spp. and *S. aureus* (Mitchell and Miller 1995). This susceptibility is particularly so in patients with a history of intravenous drug abuse (Caiaffa et al. 1994). Smoking of illicit drugs such as marijuana and cocaine are also risk factors. In patients with relatively normal CD4 lymphocyte counts and no other HIV-related symptoms there is an appropriate response to antibiotic therapy. More advanced immunosuppression increases the risk of bacterial pneumonia (Rosen 1994).

Rhodococcus equi has emerged as an important pathogen as a result of the HIV pandemic but is rarely seen in other patients. It is an anaerobic, non-motile, gram-positive organism that causes typical pneumonia which can be necrotizing and associated with pleural effusion. It is sensitive to vancomycin, erythromycin, chloramphenicol and aminoglycosides. Treatment requires prolonged administration of vancomycin and erythromycin (Guerra, Ho and Verghese 1994). Infection with *H. influenzae* in HIV infection is somewhat unusual in that there is a high frequency of capsulate type b organisms in this group (Casadevall et al. 1992).

HIV-positive individuals have an increased incidence of sinusitis. The organisms involved are similar to those in non-HIV infected individuals but *P. aeruginosa* is more frequent in the late stages of HIV disease. Occasionally non-bacterial pathogens such as *Cryptococcus*, *Aspergillus*, *Alternaria* and CMV are responsible. Chronic sinusitis is particularly troublesome in patients with low CD4 counts. Treatment follows general principles.

Patients with HIV infection appear to be more susceptible to chronic bronchitis and bronchiectasis. The most common pathogens responsible for bacterial bronchitis include *H. influenzae* and *S. pneumoniae* though *Pseudomonas* spp. may also be involved (Verghese et al. 1994). Exacerbations respond promptly to appropriate antibiotic therapy but may recur. Bronchiectasis tends to occur as discrete lesions in single lobes.

7 PERTUSSIS

Pertussis (whooping cough) is caused by *Bordetella pertussis*. It causes prolonged paroxysms of cough and in the very young can lead to prolonged apnoea and death; long-term sequelae include bronchiectasis. There is no effective antibiotic treatment for the paroxysmal stage of the disease and prevention is the lynchpin of management.

EPIDEMIOLOGY

B. pertussis is transmitted by droplets and is highly infectious with attack rates in susceptible individuals between 50 and 100%. World wide, there are approximately 50 million cases and 600 000 deaths annually (Henderson 1987). Epidemics occur in cycles of 3–5 years, reflecting the appearance of susceptible individuals in a given population. Since 1950 the incidence of pertussis has been dramatically modified by the introduction of the whole cell vaccine. Vaccination is given to children older than 1 month and provides immunity for approximately 12 years. Before vaccination pertussis was seen mainly in children 1–5 years of age, because of passive protection by maternal antibody in those aged less than 1 year. Adults, including mothers, are generally immune because of natural infection in childhood. In Sweden, where the pertussis programme was terminated in 1979, the incidence of pertussis is 60 cases per 100 000 population, age-specific attack rates per 100 000 have been 630 infants >1 year, 670 in children 1–4 years, and 258 in children 5–9 years (Romanus and Jonsell 1987). In contrast, in Massachusetts, USA, which has an active pertussis programme, the incidence of bacteriologically confirmed pertussis is 0.92 cases per 100 000 population, with a peak incidence in infants aged 1 month (104 per 100 000 population) which then declines to 5 per 100 000 (Marchant et al. 1994). Vaccination limits disease in children but the peak incidence is now in infants aged 1 month probably because of the absence of passive immunity from mothers in whom vaccine-induced immunity has declined. There is evidence of transmission of pertussis from adults to susceptible infants (Mokotoff et al. 1995). During the mid-1970s the general public was alerted by media publicity to the possibility of vaccine-induced brain damage and this led to a decline in vaccine uptake. Subsequently there were 3 large epidemics in the UK at characteristic 4 year intervals in 1977, 1981 and 1985 (Preston 1994). In both Massachusetts (Marchant et al. 1994) and Cincinnati (Christie et al. 1994) there has been a resurgence of pertussis in the last 10 years in the face of vaccination programmes. These are due either to over-reporting or, more worrying, failure of whole cell vaccine efficacy.

PATHOGENESIS

B. pertussis produces a number of virulence factors (see Volume 2, Chapter 38). The first step in *B. pertussis* infection is circumvention of mucociliary clearance by binding to ciliated cells and multiplying on their surfaces. This is achieved by 2 adhesins: filamentous haemagglutinin and pertussis toxin. In addition, *B. pertussis* produces serotype 2 and 3 fimbriae. Colonization of ciliated cells results in their death because of toxin production by the bacterium. This damage to the airway epithelium and direct activity against local neurons by pertussis toxin, is responsible for the paroxysmal cough (Salyers and Whitt 1994). *B. pertussis* survives for long periods in phagocytes. Pertussis toxin inhibits phagocyte killing in vitro and the migration of monocytes. The organism can survive in human polymorphs by inhibiting phagosome–lysosome fusion but it does not inhibit the respiratory burst (Steed et al. 1992). Similarly, *B. pertussis* survives for 3–4 days in human monocyte-derived macrophages (Friedman 1992).

CLINICAL FEATURES

After an incubation period of 1–3 weeks a non-specific catarrhal illness occurs with symptoms of malaise, lethargy, low grade fever, dry cough and poor feeding. A week later paroxysms of coughing occur which increase in pitch before terminating in a deep inspiratory movement accompanied by the typical whoop. Chest examination is usually normal unless pneumonia or lobar collapse have occurred, as it occasionally does in infants. In infants, mortality is due to a combination of apnoea and aspiration of vomitus. In adults, the disease tends to be less severe though typical whooping cough may be seen. Children may be susceptible to bronchial infections for up to a year after pertussis, as the result of reduced host defences of the airway. Bronchiectasis in some adults has been attributed to severe pertussis in childhood.

DIAGNOSIS

In the presence of the typical whoop, diagnosis presents no difficulty but isolation of *B. pertussis* by culture is diagnostic. This is most likely during the late catarrhal and early paroxysmal phases but later becomes progressively less likely. Pernasal pharyngeal swabs should be cultured on Bordet–Gengou agar, supplemented with methicillin or cephalexin to inhibit the normal flora, or patients may be asked to cough directly onto the medium. Cultures must be examined daily for 5–7 days to identify the tiny slow-growing, haemolytic colonies. In nasopharyngeal smears, *B. pertussis* can be detected directly with fluorescent antibody. Serological tests are not used routinely for the diagnosis of pertussis, but agglutinins and complement-fixing antibodies can be detected in serum and anti-pertussis secretory IgA can be detected in nasopharyngeal smears. Laboratory confirmation of pertussis can be difficult, but a cough lasting 2 weeks during community outbreaks is a sensitive and specific marker. Other organisms, including coxsackie viruses, echoviruses, adenoviruses serotypes 1–3, 5 and 7, and *M. pneumoniae*, can cause illness clinically indistinguishable from pertussis.

MANAGEMENT

Treatment during the early stage of the disease can reduce its course and restrict transmission. Erythromycin is recommended for cases and their household contacts, regardless of age or vaccination status. It is important to protect children aged less than 6 months who are too young to vaccinate. Chemoprophylaxis should be given to contacts as early as possible because more than 21 days after first contact it is of limited value (Mokotoff et al. 1995).

PREVENTION

The current vaccine is a killed, whole cell vaccine combined with diphtheria and tetanus toxoids and aluminium-containing adjuvants (DTP vaccine) but an acellular vaccine has been introduced in the USA. The pertussis component contains the 3 major agglutinogens, 1, 2 and 3. It is administered as 3 primary doses at intervals of 2 months beginning at 6–8 weeks of age. Booster doses are given 6–12 months later, and the third dose at 4–6 years of age. The vaccine is believed to have an effectiveness greater than 80% in preventing pertussis but there has been a decline in efficacy in recent years (reviewed by Preston 1994). The duration of protection is limited and wanes by approximately 12 years after immunization. Vaccine failures have been attributed to omission of one of the 3 agglutinogens, or omission of the adjuvant.

A major problem has been public reaction to reports of adverse effects. The most common of these are local reactions at the injection site and high fever; convulsions and brain damage are rare. The risk of permanent neurological damage in normal children given a full course of DTP vaccination is approximately 1 in 100 000, which is less than that of complications from the disease. Vaccination should, however, be avoided in children with a history of convulsions or brain damage in the neonatal period or other neurological disorder and during a febrile illness. A history of idiopathic epilepsy or developmental delay due to neurological disease in first degree relatives is a relative contraindication which should be individually assessed. Those who have had a serious local or systemic reaction to a dose of vaccine should not be given further doses.

These considerations have led to an effort to develop acellular vaccines. Pertussis toxin (PT), filamentous haemagglutinin (FHA), 68 kDa outer-membrane protein (OMP) and fimbrial agglutinogens are the most important antigens that elicit protective immunity against pertussis. FHA and OMP are, together with chemically detoxified PT, the components of some new acellular pertussis vaccines. During a pertussis outbreak in previously immunized children, those with higher serum levels of anti-FHA antibodies remained healthy, whereas those with lower antibody levels developed the disease (He et al. 1994). Formulations of acellular vaccine containing FHA, PT and agglutinogens have been effective since 1981 in Japan in children 24 months of age and older. Pertussis toxoid alone or in combination with FHA has been tested in Swedish children from 6 months of age and gave partial protection against infection and good protection against severe disease (Ad hoc Group for the Study of Vaccines 1988). Acellular vaccines are at present recommended only as boosters. They are expensive and do not give rise to type-specific agglutinins.

INFECTIONS WITH *BORDETELLA* SPP. OTHER THAN *B. PERTUSSIS*

Bordetella parapertussis has been incriminated as a minor cause of whooping cough, particularly a milder form than that caused by *B. pertussis*. Some evidence suggests that *B. parapertussis* may not be a separate species: this includes the isolation of both *B. pertussis* and *B. parapertussis* from whooping cough patients, and the apparent conversion of *B. pertussis* to *B. parapertussis* by loss of a prophage. Doubt has been cast on *Bordetella bronchiseptica* as a possible cause of whooping cough (Woolfrey and Moody 1991).

8 ACUTE BRONCHITIS

Acute bronchitis is manifest as productive cough in a patient without a history of chronic chest disease. The microbial aetiology of acute bronchitis includes viruses, particularly adenovirus, influenza virus, respiratory syncytial virus and parainfluenza virus, the last 2 being particularly common in children. *M. pneumoniae* and the pneumococcus are the prominent bacterial causes of acute bronchitis (Pennington 1994a). On balance, antibiotic therapy is regarded as unnecessary (reviewed by Gonzales and Sande 1995) but the subject is surrounded by controversy. Randomized double blind studies have failed to show a major clinical role for antibiotics in uncomplicated acute bronchitis. Some patients with acute bronchitis experience a prolonged episode of bronchial hyper-reactivity. Antibiotics do not alter this syndrome.

9 CHRONIC BRONCHITIS AND CHRONIC OBSTRUCTIVE PULMONARY DISEASE

Chronic bronchitis is defined as the daily production of sputum for at least 3 consecutive months in 2 consecutive years and its essential feature is chronic bronchial mucin hypersecretion. This may be accompanied by bacterial infection, which causes an increase in the purulence of sputum, and also generalized small airways obstruction. As a result, patients may experience one of 3 entities of increasing severity. These are simple chronic bronchitis with cough productive of non-purulent phlegm, chronic or recurrent mucopurulent bronchitis with cough, and chronic obstructive bronchitis, in which sputum is mostly purulent and there is airways obstruction (Medical Research Council 1965). Each of these is subject to acute exacerbation with a decline in the clinical state of the patient. Although infection is the most common cause of death for people with chronic obstructive pulmonary disease (COPD), it is unclear whether infectious exacerbations are associated with an accelerated loss of lung function during the natural history of chronic bronchitis (Bates 1973).

PATHOGENESIS

Smoking plays a part in the generation of chronic bronchitis (Floreani et al. 1994). Gradually there is increased mucus hypersecretion, depressed ciliary function, and epithelial cell injury. Bacteria that are not normally present in the airway below the larynx are then able to colonize the diseased epithelium (Read et al. 1991) (Fig. 18.5) and this leads to further damage.

BACTERIAL INFECTION AND EXACERBATIONS OF CHRONIC BRONCHITIS

Non-typable *H. influenzae* is most commonly present in acute, purulent exacerbations of chronic bronchitis, but *S. pneumoniae* and *M. catarrhalis* can also be isolated. *H. influenzae* adheres to mucus via fimbriae (Barsum et al. 1995) and galactoside sequences on epithelial cells (Krivan, Roberts and Ginsburg 1988). Soluble products of *H. influenzae* reduce ciliary beat frequency (Wilson et al. 1985) and mucociliary clearance. Non-typable *H. influenzae* are present in the lower respiratory tract of most patients with chronic bronchitis and in all patients at some time, even between exacerbations. Their presence in the sputum

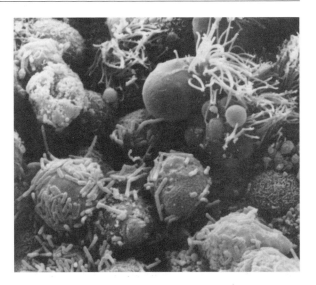

Fig. 18.5 Scanning electron micrograph of non-typable *H. influenzae* adhering to damaged areas of airway mucosa. (A Brain and RC Read).

during periods of increased symptoms does not necessarily imply a pathogenic role, but such a role for *H. influenzae* has been suggested by Musher et al. (1983) who showed that the serum of patients with acute febrile bronchitis contains opsonizing antibody for their own sputum isolates. Virus and mycoplasma infections are responsible for up to a third of the acute exacerbations of chronic obstructive airways disease; the viruses more commonly isolated include influenza A, parainfluenza virus, coronavirus, rhinovirus and herpes simplex virus (reviewed by Floreani et al. 1994). This suggests that bacteria, such as *H. influenzae*, flourish in the airways when viral infection further damages already compromised host defences. The role of *H. influenzae* and *S. pneumoniae* in bacterial infection during chronic obstructive pulmonary disease has been reviewed by Murphy and Sethi (1992).

M. catarrhalis is present in pure culture in some transtracheal aspirates and is a recognized pathogen in chronic bronchitis; improvement is seen with specific treatment for *M. catarrhalis* infection. The organism has also been isolated from the blood and pleural fluid of patients with chronic obstructive airways disease (Murphy and Sethi 1992).

Culture of sputum is of doubtful value because it is likely to be contaminated with the potential pathogens that are also present in oropharyngeal secretions. If such examination is undertaken, care should be taken to ensure that only purulent sputum is examined. This should be homogenized and serial dilutions examined. Examination of mucoid sputum will not yield useful information.

THERAPY OF EXACERBATIONS OF CHRONIC BRONCHITIS

The use of antibiotics in all but the most severely ill patients is controversial. Small studies have either shown a positive effect of antibiotics (Berry et al. 1960, Pines et al. 1968), or no effect (Elmes et al. 1965, Nicotra et al. 1982). In a large placebo-controlled study Anthonisen et al. (1987) found significant benefit from antibiotics in severe but not in mild exacerbations. Airway function also recovered more rapidly with antibiotic treatment.

It is appropriate to treat severe exacerbations of COPD with antibiotics capable of covering *H. influenzae* and *S. pneumoniae*. Rates of resistance to aminopenicillins of sputum isolates of *H. influenzae* are 10–14% in the UK and much higher in tertiary referral centres (Powell et al. 1991). Although antibiotic therapy in patients with mild disease is controversial, appropriate antibiotics include amoxycillin (provided local β-lactamase activity is at low level), co-amoxiclav or the oral cephalosporins and the macrolides, but erythromycin has relatively poor activity against *H. influenzae*. Newer macrolides such as clarithromycin and azithromycin are better orally tolerated and have greater activity against *H. influenzae* in vitro. The fluoroquinolones are highly active against *H. influenzae* and penetrate tissue and sputum well, but pneumococci are only marginally susceptible. New quinolones, with broader activity against gram-positive organisms, and new macrolides and β-lactams that are more active against *H. influenzae* and *S. pneumoniae* are being developed (Wise 1995).

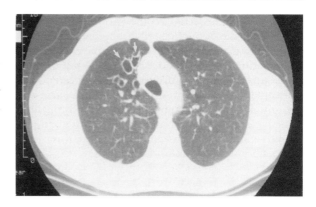

Fig. 18.6   Computed tomography (CT) scan demonstrating dilated airways and bronchial wall thickening in a patient with bronchiectasis. (Courtesy of A Nakielny).

oral cephalosporins or quinolones are effective when β-lactamase-producing strains are isolated. Long-term oral antibiotics are well tolerated and lead to symptomatic improvement but ciprofloxacin-resistant *P. aeruginosa* may be troublesome (Rayner et al. 1995). The use of prophylactic aminoglycosides given by nebulizer is of dubious value. In very severe exacerbations the use of intravenous antibiotics effective against *H. influenzae* and *P. aeruginosa* is indicated.

10   BRONCHIECTASIS

Bronchiectasis is permanent, abnormal dilatation of bronchi accompanied by suppurative inflammation that results in intermittent production of large quantities of purulent sputum. The commonest causes are severe parenchymal infections of the lung including pertussis and measles in childhood and also – most importantly in the developing world – tuberculosis. Foreign bodies, carcinoma, allergic bronchopulmonary aspergillosis and certain congenital abnormalities, including immunoglobulin deficiencies and ciliary abnormalities, can also give rise to bronchiectasis. Cystic fibrosis is associated with bronchiectasis (see section 11). It may also be seen in patients with the α_1-antiprotease deficiencies. Once bronchiectasis is present, repeated infections serve to maintain a vicious circle of inflammation and damage to the already compromised airway, which leads to further infection (Cole and Wilson 1989) (Fig. 18.6).

The sputum flora of such patients often yields a mixed growth but *H. influenzae* is probably the most important in sustaining continued infection and inflammation. *S. aureus* and *S. pneumoniae* are also prominent. In established disease *P. aeruginosa* is associated with a poor prognosis.

MANAGEMENT

The mainstay of treatment of bronchiectasis is drainage, which reduces the frequency of exacerbations, and antibiotic therapy. β-Lactam antibiotics do not penetrate diseased tissue at conventional dosages but high doses of amoxycillin are effective in terminating exacerbations (Cole and Wilson 1989). High doses of

11   CYSTIC FIBROSIS

Cystic fibrosis (CF) is an inherited disease in which there is pancreatic dysfunction and an associated abnormality of airway secretions. The mucins form thick gels which alter their rheological properties. In the airways thick tenacious sputum causes obstruction, leading to recurrent infection. Patients with cystic fibrosis have airway inflammation that commences at birth (Cantin 1995). The carrier rate is about 5% in caucasians; about 6000 people have the disease in the UK.

CLINICAL FEATURES

Infants present with meconium ileus at birth or a little later with diarrhoea or malabsorption, failure to thrive or progressive cough. Patients may also present with recurrent pneumonia. Acute exacerbations occur with increased sputum production, cyanosis, dyspnoea, fever and weight loss. Patients also suffer with nasal polyposis and chronic sinusitis.

ROLE OF MICROBIAL INFECTION

The first pathogen to colonize children with CF is *S. aureus*. This produces α- and δ-toxins that induce bronchial wall injury and abscess formation. The intense inflammatory response to *S. aureus* leads to further tissue destruction.

Staphylococcal airway injury permits colonization by *P. aeruginosa*. Patients are at first colonized with non-mucoid strains but later mucoid variants emerge. The extracellular alginate they produce increases their adherence to ciliated epithelium (Marcus and Baker 1985). Despite the high antibody levels present against such strains and intensive antibiotic therapy, they cannot be completely eradicated. They reappear after treatment but it is not clear whether this is due to recolonization or acquisition of a new strain (Ojeniyi 1994). Alginate also interferes with antibody coating and inhibits phagocytosis of *P. aeruginosa* (Baltimore and Mitchell 1980). Bacterial proteases produced by *P. aeruginosa* cause significant damage to the airways. *Pseudomonas* elastase and alkaline protease are secreted in vivo over prolonged periods in the airways (Suter 1994). *Pseudomonas* elastase increases the permeability of epithelial cells and destroys tight junctions.

The *Pseudomonas* phenazine pigments pyocyanin and 1-hydroxyphenazine interfere with mucociliary function (Wilson et al. 1987); the membrane glycolipid, the haemolysin rhamnolipid, also reduces mucociliary transport in vivo (Read et al. 1992). Exotoxin A produced by most colonizing strains of *P. aeruginosa* causes tissue injury and is highly immunogenic.

Non-capsulate *H. influenzae* is most frequently isolated from infants more than a year old. *B. cepacia* also colonizes CF patients and is transmissible between close contacts. It is occasionally responsible for a fulminating septicaemia. This organism produces a number of virulence factors including adhesins, extracellular polysaccharide, lipopolysaccharide and extracellular enzymes, including proteases and lipases. It is intrinsically highly resistant to antibiotics, including those effective against *P. aeruginosa* (Wilkinson and Pitt 1995), but it is usually sensitive to trimethoprim–sulphamethoxazole and chloramphenicol. Temocillin, a β-lactamase stable antibiotic, may also be useful (Taylor et al. 1992). *Stenotrephomonas* (*Xanthomonas*) *maltophilia* also colonizes patients with CF and can result in disease. A range of other bacteria, including the Enterobacteriaceae, *Candida albicans*, *Aspergillus* spp. and environmental mycobacteria, may also be isolated from these patients but their significance is uncertain.

Although CF patients produced markedly elevated titres of local and systemic antipseudomonal antibodies, the elastase produced by *P. aeruginosa* interferes with their activity by cleaving off the Fab and Fc fragments of immunoglobulins so that they are unable to interact with receptor sites on pulmonary macrophages or neutrophils (Thick et al. 1985).

ANTIMICROBIAL THERAPY

There is continuing controversy over the use of antibiotics in CF. Once disease is established, some physicians attempt to suppress sputum colonization with long-term administration of antibiotics. Such antibiotics include cephalexin, oral chloramphenicol, trimethoprim–sulphamethoxazole, or co-amoxiclav, but

controlled evaluations of this approach are lacking because of obvious methodological problems with such studies (Chartrand and Marks 1994). Most centres treat only acute exacerbations of pulmonary infection, with inclusion of empirical antipseudomonas and *S. aureus* antibiotics. This requires combined antibiotic therapy with a β-lactam plus an aminoglycoside. In principle, antibiotic regimens should be rotated and directed by sputum evaluation and microbial sensitivities. With the genesis of monotherapy capable of activity against both these pathogens, out-patient administration has flourished. Such antibiotics include ceftazidime, the penems, monobactams, and β-lactam–β-lactamase inhibitors. Unfortunately monotherapy can result in the spread of resistant organisms, e.g. *P. aeruginosa*, and this has been demonstrated following the use of ceftazidime (Pedersen et al. 1986). Emergence of *P. aeruginosa* resistance is also seen after monotherapy with imipenem and aztreonam (Chartrand and Marks 1994). The use of oral quinolones has permitted more flexible management of exacerbations. They have been used in children with CF (Schaad et al. 1991) without side effects and their use in moderately severe CF exacerbations can be as effective as traditional intravenous treatment with β-lactams plus aminoglycosides. In vitro susceptibility of isolates returns when the quinolones are withheld for 3 months. The use of aerosolized antibiotics has been advocated but controlled data to support this are limited. Aerosolized tobramycin given by nebulizer has been shown to eradicate *P. aeruginosa* and improve pulmonary function tests (Smith et al. 1989) but emergence of resistance is a problem.

OTHER FORMS OF THERAPY

There is potential to ameliorate the pulmonary disease in cystic fibrosis with somatic gene therapy. The optimal mode of delivery of the normal gene into airway epithelium is under investigation. Adenovirus vectors, DNA–liposome complexes, adeno-associated viral vectors and DNA–ligand complexes have been used effectively in vitro and have been tested in animals. Adenovirus vectors and DNA–liposome complexes are currently in phase 1 clinical trial. There has been transient correction of electrophysiological defects in human CF nasal epithelium (O'Neal and Beaudet 1994). At present, CF patients face the prospect of lung transplantation as their only salvation once extreme disease ensues. Single lung, double lung and heart–lung transplantation have all been used with success in such patients and because the transplanted lung retains the physiological characteristics of the donor, there is no tendency for colonization by *P. aeruginosa* over and above that seen in transplanted lungs in non-CF patients.

REFERENCES

Ad hoc Group for the Study of Pertussis Vaccines, 1988, Placebo-controlled trial of two acellular pertussis vaccines in Sweden – protective efficacy and adverse effects, *Lancet*, **1**: 955–7.

American Thoracic Society, 1993, Guidelines for the initial management of adults with community acquired pneumoniae: diagnosis, assessment of severity, and initial antimicrobial therapy, *Am Rev Respir Dis*, **148**: 1418–26.

Anthonisen NR, Manfreda J et al., 1987, Antibiotic therapy in exacerbations of chronic obstructive pulmonary disease, *Ann Intern Med*, **106**: 196–204.

Austrian R, 1986, Some aspects of the pneumococcal carrier state, *J Antimicrob Chemother*, **18, Suppl. A**: 25–34.

Austrian R, Gold J, 1964, Pneumococcal bacteraemia with special reference to bacteraemic pneumococcal pneumonia, *Ann Intern Med*, **60**: 759–76.

Baltimore RS, Mitchell M, 1980, Immunologic investigations of mucoid strains of *Pseudomonas aeruginosa*: comparison of susceptibility to opsonic antibody in mucoid and non-mucoid strains, *J Infect Dis*, **141**: 238–47.

Barsum W, Wilson R et al., 1995, Interaction of fimbriate and non-fimbriate strains of *H. influenzae* with human airway mucin in vitro, *Eur Respir J*, **8**: 709–14.

Bartlett JG, Gorbach SL et al., 1974, Bacteriology and treatment of primary lung abscess, *Am Rev Respir Dis*, **109**: 510–18.

Bates DV, 1973, The fate of the chronic bronchitic: a report of the 10 year follow-up in the Canadian Department of Veterans' Affairs co-ordinated study of chronic bronchitis, *Am Rev Respir Dis*, **108**: 1043–65.

Bébéar C, Dupon M et al., 1993, Potential improvements in therapeutic options for mycoplasma respiratory infections, *Clin Infect Dis*, **17, Suppl. 1**: S202–7.

Berry DG, Fry J et al., 1960, Exacerbation of chronic bronchitis treatment with oxytetracycline, *Lancet*, **1**: 137–9.

Bice DE, Weissman DN, Muggenburg BA, 1991, Long term maintenance of localised antibody responses in the lung, *Immunology*, **74**: 215–22.

Bolling GE, Plouffe JF et al., 1985, Aerosols containing *Legionella pneumophila* generated by showerheads and hot water fawcetts, *Appl Environ Microbiol*, **50**: 1128–31.

British Thoracic Society, 1987, The hospital management of community acquired pneumonia, *J R Coll Physicians Lond*, **21**: 267–9.

British Thoracic Society, 1993, Guidelines for the management of community-acquired pneumonia in adults admitted to hospital, *Br J Hosp Med*, **49**: 346–50.

Brook I, Van de Heyning PH, 1994, Microbiology and management of otitis media, *Scand J Infect Dis Suppl*, **93**: 20–32.

Broome CV, 1986, The carrier state: *Neisseria meningitidis*, *J Antimicrob Chemother*, **18, Suppl. A**: 25–34.

Broome CV, Fraser DW, 1979, Epidemiologic aspects of legionellosis, *Epidemiol Rev*, **1**: 1–16.

Buckley H, 1992, Immunodeficiency diseases, *JAMA*, **268**: 2797–806.

Bruyn GAW, Zegers BJM et al., 1992, Mechanisms of host defence against infection with *Streptococcus pneumoniae*, *Clin Infect Dis*, **14**: 251–62.

Caiaffa W T, Vlahov D et al., 1994, Bacterial pneumonia among HIV-seropositive injection drug users, *Am J Respir Crit Care Med*, **150**: 1493–8.

Cantin A, 1995, Cystic fibrosis lung inflammation: early, sustained and severe, *Am J Respir Crit Care Med*, **151**: 939–41.

Carratala J, Gudiol F et al., 1994, Risk factors for nosocomial *Legionella pneumophila* pneumonia, *Am J Respir Crit Care Med*, **149**: 625–9.

Casadevall A, Dobroszycki J et al., 1992, *Haemophilus influenzae* type B bacteraemia in adults with AIDS and at risk for AIDS, *Am J Med*, **92**: 587–90.

Caugant DA, Hoiby EA et al., 1994, Asymptomatic carriage of *Neisseria meningitidis* in a randomly sampled population, *J Clin Microbiol*, **32**: 323–50.

van Cauwenberge PB, Vander Mijnsbrugge AM, Ingels KJ, 1993, The microbiology of acute and chronic sinusitis and otitis media: a review, *Eur Arch Otorhinolaryngol*, **250, Suppl. 1**: S3–6.

CDSC, 1995, Current respiratory infections, *Commun Dis Rep*, **5**: 21.

Celis R, Torres A et al., 1988, Nosocomial pneumonia: a multivariate analysis of risk and prognosis, *Chest*, **93**: 318–24.

Centers for Disease Control, 1988, CDC definitions for nosocomial infections 1988, *Am Rev Respir Dis*, **139**: 1058–9.

Chartrand SA, Marks MI, 1994, Pulmonary infections in cystic fibrosis: pathogenesis and therapy, *Respiratory Infections: Diagnosis and Management*, 3rd edn, ed. Pennington JE, Raven Press, New York, 323–48.

Cherry JD, 1993, Anaemia and mucocutaneous lesions due to *Mycoplasma pneumoniae* infections, *Clin Infect Dis*, **17, Suppl. 1**: S47–51.

Christie CDC, Marx ML et al., 1994, The 1993 epidemic of pertussis in Cincinnati: resurgence of disease in a highly immunized population of children, *N Engl J Med*, **331**: 16–21.

Clyde WA, 1993, Clinical overview of typical *Mycoplasma pneumoniae* infections, *Clin Infect Dis*, **17, Suppl. 1**: S32–6.

Coburn J, 1992, *Pseudomonas aeruginosa* exoenzymes, *Curr Top Microbiol Immunol*, **175**: 133–43.

Cole PJ, Wilson R, 1989, Host–microbial interrelationships in respiratory infection, *Chest*, **95**: 2175–83.

Craven DE, Steager KA, Barber TW, 1991, Preventing nosocomial pneumonia: state of the art and perspectives for the 1990s, *Am J Med*, **91, Suppl. 3b**: 44s–53s.

Crowe HL, Lavitz RE, 1987, Invasive *Haemophilus influenzae* disease in adults, *Arch Intern Med*, **147**: 241–4.

Dal Nogare AR, 1994, Nosocomial pneumonia in the medical and surgical patient, *Med Clin North Am*, **78**: 1081–90.

Dondero TJ, Rendtorff RC et al., 1980, An outbreak of legionnaires' disease associated with a contaminated air conditioning cooling tower, *N Engl J Med*, **302**: 365–70.

Dowling JN, Saha AK, Glew RH, 1992, Virulence factors of the family Legionellaceae, *Microbiol Rev*, **56**: 32–60.

Duane PG, Rubins JB et al., 1993, Identification of hydrogen peroxide as a *Streptococcus pneumoniae* toxin for rat alveolar epithelial cells, *Infect Immun*, **61**: 4392–7.

Edelstein PH, 1993, Legionnaires' disease, *Clin Infect Dis*, **16**: 741–9.

Edelstein PH, Meyer RD, 1994, *Legionella* pneumonias, *Respiratory Infections: Diagnosis and Management*, 3rd edn, ed. Pennington JE, Raven Press, New York, 455–84.

Editorial, 1986, Lessons from Stafford, *Lancet*, **327**: 1363–4.

Eisenstadt J, Crane LR, 1994, Gram-negative bacillary pneumonias, *Respiratory Infections: Diagnosis and Management*, 3rd edn, ed. Pennington JE, Raven Press, New York.

Elmes PC, King TKC et al., 1965, Value of ampicillin in the hospital treatment of exacerbations of chronic bronchitis, *Br Med J*, **2**: 904–8.

Fanta CH, Pennington JE, 1994, Pneumonia in the immunocompromised host, *Respiratory Infections: Diagnosis and Management*, 3rd edn, ed. Pennington JE, Raven Press, New York, 275–94.

Farr BM, Mandell GL, 1994, Gram-positive pneumonia, *Respiratory Infections: Diagnosis and Management*, 3rd edn, ed. Pennington JE, Raven Press, New York, 349–67.

Farr BM, Sloman AJ, Frisch MJ, 1991, Predicting death in patients hospitalized for community-acquired pneumonia, *Ann Intern Med*, **115**: 428–36.

Farr BM, Kaiser DL et al., 1989, Prediction of microbial aetiology at admission to hospital for pneumonia from the presenting clinical features, *Thorax*, **44**: 1031–5.

Feldman C, Kallenbach JM et al., 1989, Community-acquired pneumonia of diverse etiology: prognostic features in patients admitted to an intensive care unit and 'severity of illness' score, *Intensive Care Med*, **15**: 302–7.

Feldman C, Munro N et al., 1991, Pneumolysin induces the salient features of pneumococcal infection in the rat lung *in vivo*, *Am J Respir Cell Mol Biol*, **5**: 416–23.

Finegold SM, 1994, Aspiration pneumonia, lung abscess and empyema, *Respiratory Infections: Diagnosis and Management*, 3rd edn, ed. Pennington JE, Raven Press, New York, 311–22.

Floreani AA, Buchalter SE et al., 1994, Chronic bronchitis, *Respiratory Infection: Diagnosis and Management*, 3rd edn, ed. Pennington JE, Raven Press, New York, 149–92.

Fraser DW, Tsai TR et al., 1977, Legionnaires' disease: description of an epidemic of pneumonia, *N Engl J Med*, **297**: 1189–97.

Friedland IR, McCracken GH, 1994, Management of infections caused by antibiotic-resistant *Streptococcus pneumoniae*, *N Engl J Med*, **331**: 377–82.

Friedman RL, Nordensson K et al., 1992, Uptake and intracellular survival of *Bordetella pertussis* in human macrophages, *Infect Immun*, **60**: 4578–85.

Galloway D, 1991, *Pseudomonas aeruginosa* elastase and elastolysis: recent developments, *Mol Microbiol*, **5**: 2315–21.

Garcia-Léon ME, Cercenada E, 1992, Susceptibility of *Streptococcus pneumoniae* to penicillin: a prospective microbiological and clinical study, *Clin Infect Dis*, **14**: 427–35.

Giebink GS, Foker JE et al., 1980, Serum antibody and opsonic responses to vaccination with pneumococcal capsular polysaccharide in normal and splenectomized children, *J Infect Dis*, **141**: 404–12.

Gonzales R, Sande M, 1995, What will it take to stop physicians prescribing antibiotics in acute bronchitis?, *Lancet*, **345**: 665–6.

Guerra LG, Ho H, Verghese A, 1994, New pathogens in pneumonia, *Med Clin North Am*, **78**: 967–85.

Gwaltney JM Jr, Scheld WM et al., 1992, The microbial etiology and antimicrobial therapy of adults with acute community-acquired sinusitis: a fifteen-year experience at the University of Virginia and review of other selected studies, *J Allergy Clin Immunol*, **90**: 457–61.

Hall CM, Willcox PA et al., 1994, Mycobacterial infection in renal transplant recipients, *Chest*, **106**: 435–9.

He Q, Viljanen MK et al., 1994, Antibodies to filamentous haemagglutinin of *Bordetella pertussis* and protection against whooping cough in school children, *J Infect Dis*, **170**: 705–8.

Henderson R, 1987, 'Shots' that save lives, *World Health*, 4–7.

Hirschmann JV, Lipsky BA, 1994, The pneumococcal vaccine after 15 years, *Arch Intern Med*, **154**: 373–7.

Horan TC, White JW et al., 1986, Nosocomial infection surveillance 1984, *MMWR CDS Surveill Summ*, **35**: 17ss–29ss.

Hughes CF, van Scoy RE, 1991, Antibiotic therapy of pleural empyema, *Semin Respir Infect*, **6**: 94–102.

Hughes WT, 1993, Prevention of infection in patients with T cell defects, *Clin Infect Dis*, **17, Suppl. 2**: S367–71.

Jacobs E, 1993, Serological diagnosis of *Mycoplasma pneumoniae* infections: a critical review of current procedures, *Clin Infect Dis*, **17, Suppl. 1**: S79–82.

Johanson WG, Pierce AK, Sanford JP, 1969, Changing pharyngeal bacterial flora of hospitalized patients. Emergence of gram-negative bacilli, *N Engl J Med*, **281**: 1137–40.

Johanson WG, Higuchi JH et al., 1980, Bacterial adherence to epithelial cells in bacillary colonization of the respiratory tract, *Am Rev Respir Dis*, **121**: 55–63.

Joseph CA, Dedman D et al., 1994a, Legionnaires' disease surveillance: England and Wales, 1993, *Commun Dis Rep CDR Rev*, **4 (10)**: R109–11.

Joseph CA, Watson JM et al., 1994b, Nosocomial legionnaires' diseases in England and Wales 1980–1992, *Epidemiol Infect*, **112**: 329–45.

Jousimies-Somer H, Savolainen S et al., 1993, Bacteriologic findings in peritonsillar abscesses in young adults, *Clin Infect Dis*, **6, Suppl. 4**: S292–8.

Karalus NC, Cursons RT et al., 1991, Community-acquired pneumonia: aetiology and prognostic index evaluation, *Thorax*, **46**: 413–18.

Kikuchi R, Watabe N et al., 1994, High incidence of silent aspiration in elderly patients with community acquired pneumonia, *Am J Respir Crit Care Med*, **150**: 251–3.

Koppes GM, Ellenbogen C et al., 1977, Group Y meningococcal disease in United States Airforce recruits, *Am J Med*, **62**: 661–6.

Koskiniemi M, 1993, CNS manifestations associated with *Mycoplasma pneumoniae* infections: summary of cases at the University of Helsinki. A review, *Clin Infect Dis*, **17, Suppl. 1**: S52–7.

Krivan HC, Roberts DD, Ginsburg V, 1988, Many pulmonary pathogenic bacteria bind specifically to the carbohydrate sequence GalNAcβ-1-4 Gal found in some glycolipids, *Proc Natl Acad Sci USA*, **85**: 6157–61.

Lipscomb MF, Bice DE et al., 1995, The regulation of pulmonary immunity, *Adv Immunol*, **59**: 369–455.

Lohmann-Mathes ML, Steinmüller C et al., 1994, Pulmonary macrophages, *Eur Respir J*, **7**: 1678–89.

Lulu AR, Araj GF et al., 1988, Human brucellosis in Kuwait: a prospective study of 400 cases, *Q J Med*, **66**: 39–54.

Lunn JE, Knowlden J, Handyside AJ, 1967, Patterns of respiratory illness in Sheffield infant school children, *Br J Prev Soc Med*, **21**: 7–16.

Macfarlane JT, Finch RG et al., 1982, Study of adult community-acquired pneumonia, *Lancet*, **2**: 255–8.

Maharaj D, Raja V, Hemsley S, 1991, Management of peritonsillar abscess, *J Laryngol Otol*, **105**: 743–5.

Marchant CD, Loghlin AN et al., 1994, Pertussis in Massachusetts 1981–1991: incidence, serologic diagnosis and vaccine effectiveness, *J Infect Dis*, **169**: 1297–305.

Marcus H, Baker NR, 1985, Quantitation of adherence of mucoid and non-mucoid *Pseudomonas aeruginosa* to hamster tracheal epithelium, *Infect Immun*, **47**: 723–9.

Markiewicz AZ, Tomasz A, 1989, Variation in penicillin-binding protein patterns of penicillin-resistant clinical isolates of pneumococci, *J Clin Microbiol*, **27**: 405–10.

Marmion BP, Williamson J et al., 1993, Experience with newer techniques for the laboratory detection of *Mycoplasma pneumoniae* infection: Adelaide 1978–1992, *Clin Infect Dis*, **17, Suppl. 1**: S90–9.

Marrie TJ, 1994, Community acquired pneumonia, *Clin Infect Dis*, **18**: 501–15.

Masure HR, 1992, Modulation of adenylate cyclase toxin production as *Bordetella pertussis* enters human macrophages, *Proc Natl Acad Sci USA*, **89**: 6521–5.

Medical Research Council, 1965, Definition and classification of chronic bronchitis and clinical epidemiological purposes, *Lancet*, **1**: 775–9.

Meyer RD, Finch RG, 1992, Community-acquired pneumonia, *J Hosp Infect*, **22, Suppl. A**: 51–9.

Mitchell DM, Miller RF, 1995, New developments in the pulmonary diseases affecting HIV-infected individuals, *Thorax*, **50**: 294–302.

Mokotoff ED, Dunn RA et al., 1995, Transmission of pertussis from adult to infant – Michigan 1993, *Morbid Mortal Weekly Rep*, **44**: 74–6.

Montgomery JM, Lehmann D et al., 1990, Bacterial colonization of the upper respiratory tract and its association with acute lower respiratory tract infections in highland children of Papua New Guinea, *Rev Infect Dis*, **12, Suppl.**: S1006–16.

Morton S, Bartlett CL et al., 1986, Outbreak of legionnaires' disease from a cooling water system in a power station, *Br J Ind Med*, **43**: 630–5.

Moxon ER, 1986, The carrier state: *Haemophilus influenzae*, *J Antimicrob Chemother*, **18, Suppl. A**: 124.

Muraca PW, Stout JE, 1988, Legionnaires' disease in the working environment. Implications for environmental health, *Am Ind Hyg Assoc J*, **49**: 584–91.

Murphy TF, Sethi S, 1992, Bacterial infection in chronic obstructive pulmonary disease, *Am Rev Respir Dis*, **146**: 1067–83.

Musher DM, 1992, Infections caused by *Streptococcus pneumoniae*: clinical spectrum, pathogenesis, immunity and treatment, *Clin Infect Dis*, **14**: 801–9.

Musher DM, Watson DA, Baughn RE, 1990, Does naturally acquired IgG antibody to cell wall polysaccharide protect human subjects against pneumococcal infection?, *J Infect Dis*, **161** 736–40.

Musher DM, Kubeitschek KR et al., 1983, Pneumonia and acute febrile tracheal bronchitis due to *Haemophilus influenzae*, *Ann Intern Med*, **99**: 444–50.

Myerowitz RL, Pasculle AW et al., 1979, Opportunistic lung infection due to Pittsburgh pneumonia agent, *N Engl J Med*, **301**: 953–8.

Nicotra MB, Rivera M et al., 1982, Antibiotic therapy of acute exacerbations of chronic bronchitis: a controlled study using tetracycline, *Ann Intern Med*, **97**: 18–21.

Niederman MS, 1994, An approach to empiric therapy of nosocomial pneumonia, *Med Clin North Am*, **78**: 1123–41.

Noble RC, Overman SB, 1994, *Pseudomonas stutzeri* infection. A review of hospital isolates and a review of the literature, *Diagn Microbiol Infect Dis*, **19**: 51–64.

Ojeniyi B, 1994, Polyagglutinable *Pseudomonas aeruginosa* from cystic fibrosis patients. A survey, *APMIS Suppl*, **46**: 1–44.

O'Neal WK, Beaudet AL, 1994, Somatogene therapy for cystic fibrosis, *Hum Mol Genet*, **3**: 1497–502.

Ort S, Ryan JL et al., 1983, Pneumococcal pneumonia in hospitalized patients: clinical and radiological presentations, *JAMA*, **249**: 214–18.

Pedersen SS, Koch C et al., 1986, An epidemic spread of multiresistant *Pseudomonas aeruginosa* in a cystic fibrosis centre, *J Antimicrob Chemother*, **17**: 505–16.

Pennington JE (ed.), 1994a, Community-acquired pneumonia, *Respiratory Infections: Diagnosis and Management*, 3rd edn, Raven Press, New York, 193–206.

Pennington JE (ed.), 1994b, Hospital-acquired pneumonia, *Respiratory Infections: Diagnosis and Management*, 3rd edn, Raven Press, New York, 207–27.

Pines A, Raafat H et al., 1968, Antibiotic regimes in severe and acute purulent exacerbations of chronic bronchitis, *Br Med J*, **2**: 735–8.

Ponka A, 1990, Absenteeism and respiratory disease among children and adults in relation to low level air pollution and temperature, *Environ Res*, **52**: 34–46.

Powell M, McVey D et al., 1991, Antimicrobial susceptibility of *Streptococcus pneumoniae*, *Haemophilus influenzae* and *Moraxella catarrhalis* isolated in the UK from sputa, *J Antimicrob Chemother*, **28**: 249–59.

Preston NW, 1994, Pertussis vaccination: neither panic nor complacency, *Lancet*, **344**: 491–2.

Rayner CF, Tillotson G et al., 1995, Efficacy and safety of long-term ciprofloxacin the management of severe bronchiectasis, *J Antimicrob Chemother*, **34**: 149–56.

Read RC, Wilson R et al., 1991, Interaction of non-typable *Haemophilus influenzae* with human respiratory mucosa *in vitro*, *J Infect Dis*, **163**: 549–58.

Read RC, Roberts P et al., 1992, Effect of *Pseudomonas aeruginosa* rhamnolipids on mucociliary transport and ciliary beating, *J Appl Physiol*, **72**: 2271–7.

Redd SC, Rutherford GW III et al., 1990, The role of human immunodeficiency virus infection in pneumococcal bacteremia in San Francisco residents, *J Infect Dis*, **162**: 1012–17.

Reimann HA, 1938, An acute infection of the respiratory tract with atypical pneumonia. A disease entity probably caused by a filterable virus, *JAMA*, **111**: 2377–84.

Rein MF, Gwaltney JM et al., 1978, Accuracy of Gram's stain in identifying pneumococci in sputum, *JAMA*, **239**: 2671–3.

Reynolds HY, 1994, Normal and defective respiratory host defenses, *Respiratory Infections: Diagnosis and Management*, 3rd edn, ed. Pennington JE, Raven Press, New York, 1–34.

Robinson LA, Moulton AL, 1994, Intrapleural fibrinolytic treatment of multi-loculated thoracic empyemas, *Ann Thorac Surg*, **57**: 803–13.

Romanus V, Jonsell R, 1987, Pertussis in Sweden after cessation of general immunization in 1979, *Pediatr Infect Dis J*, **6**: 364–71.

Rosen MJ, 1994, Pneumonia in patients with HIV infection, *Med Clin North Am*, **78**: 1067–79.

Rutland J, de Longh RU, 1990, Random ciliary orientation. A cause of respiratory tract disease, *N Engl J Med*, **323**: 1681–4.

Salyers AA, Whitt DD, 1994, *Bacterial Pathogenesis: a Molecular Approach*, ASM Press, Washington, DC.

Saunders CJP, Joseph CA, Watson JM, 1994, Investigating a single case of legionnaire's disease: guidance for consultants in communicable disease control, *Commun Dis Rep CDR Rev*, **4** (10): R112–14.

Schaad VB, Stoupis C et al., 1991, Clinical, radiological and magnetic resonance monitoring for skeletal toxicity in pediatric patients with cystic fibsosis receiving a three month course of ciprofloxacin, *Pediatr Infect Dis J*, **10**: 723–9.

Schalen L, Eliasson I et al., 1992, Acute laryngitis in adults: results of erythromycin treatment, *Acta Otolaryngol Suppl (Stockh)*, **492**: 55–7.

Schlesinger RB, 1990, The interaction of inhaled toxicants with respiratory tract clearance mechanisms, *Rev Toxicol*, **20**: 257–68.

Shands KN, Ho JL et al., 1985, Potable water as a source of legionnaires' disease, *JAMA*, **253**: 1412–16.

Shanley JD, 1995, Mechanisms of injury by virus infections of the lower respiratory tract, *Rev Med Virol*, **5**: 41–50.

Shapiro ED, Berg AT et al., 1991, The protective efficacy of polyvalent pneumococcal polysaccharide vaccine, *N Engl J Med*, **325**: 1453–60.

Smith AL, 1994, *Haemophilus influenzae*, *Respiratory Infections: Diagnosis and Management*, 3rd edn, ed. Pennington JE, Raven Press, New York, 435–54.

Smith AL, Ramsey BW et al., 1989, Safety of aerosol tobramycin administration for three months to patients with cystic fibrosis, *Pediatr Pulmonol*, **7**: 265–71.

Steed LL, Akporiaye ET et al., 1992, *Bordetella pertussis* induces respiratory burst activity in human polymorphonuclear leucocytes, *Infect Immun*, **60**: 2101–5.

Suter S, 1994, The role of bacterial proteases in the pathogenesis of cystic fibrosis, *Am J Respir Crit Care Med*, **150**: S118–22.

Taylor RFH, Gaya H et al., 1992, Temocillin and cystic fibrosis: outcome of intravenous administration in patients infected with *Pseudomonas cepacia*, *J Antimicrob Chemother*, **29**: 341–3.

Thick RB, Baltimore RS et al., 1985, IgG proteolytic activity of *Pseudomonas aeruginosa* in cystic fibrosis, *J Infect Dis*, **151**: 589–98.

Torres A, Serra-Batilles J et al., 1991, Severe community acquired pneumonia: epidemiology and prognostic factors, *Am Rev Respir Dis*, **144**: 312–18.

Tuazon CU, Murray HW, 1994, Atypical pneumonias, *Respiratory Infections: Diagnosis and Management*, 3rd edn, ed. Pennington JE, Raven Press, New York, 407–34.

Tuomanen EI, Austrian R et al., 1995, Pathogenesis of pneumococcal infection, *N Engl J Med*, **332**: 1280–4.

Turk DC, 1984, The pathogenicity of *Haemophilus influenzae*, *J Med Microbiol*, **18**: 1–16.

Verghese A, Al-Samman M et al., 1994, Chronic bronchitis and bronchiectasis in HIV infection, *Arch Intern Med*, **154**: 2086–91.

Verhoef J, 1993, Prevention of infection in the neutropenic patient, *Clin Infect Dis*, **17, Suppl. 2**: S359–67.

Waldvogel FA, 1990, *Staphylococcal aureus* (including toxic shock syndrome), *Principles and Practice of Infectious Diseases*, 3rd edn, eds Mandell GL, Douglas RG, Bennett J, John Wiley & Sons, New York, 1489–510.

Wilkinson SG, Pitt TL, 1995, *Burkholderia (Pseudomonas) cepacia* pathogenicity and resistance, *Rev Med Microbiol*, **6**: 10–17.

Wilson R, 1988, Secondary ciliary dysfunction, *Clin Sci*, **75:** 113–20.

Wilson R, Roberts DE et al., 1985, The effect of bacterial products on human ciliary function *in vitro*, *Thorax*, **40:** 125–31.

Wilson R, Pitt T et al., 1987, Pyocyanin and 1-hydroxyphenazine produced by *Pseudomonas aeruginosa* inhibit the beating of human respiratory cilia *in vitro*, *J Clin Invest*, **79:** 221–9.

Wilson R, Read RC et al., 1991, Effects of *Bordetella pertussis* infection on human respiratory epithelium *in vivo* and *in vitro*, *Infect Immun*, **59:** 337–45.

Wise R, 1995, New and future antibodies in the treatment of acute respiratory tract infections, *Thorax*, **50:** 223–4.

Woodhead MA, MacFarlane JT et al., 1985, Aetiology and outcome of severe community-acquired pneumonia, *J Infect*, **10:** 204–10.

Woodhead MA, MacFarlane JT et al., 1987, Prospective study of the aetiology and outcome of pneumonia in the community, *Lancet*, **1:** 671–4.

Woods DE, 1994, Bacterial colonization of the respiratory tract: clinical significance, *Respiratory Infections: Diagnosis and Management*, 3rd edn, ed. Pennington JE, Raven Press, New York, 35–41.

Woolfrey BT, Moody JA, 1991, Human infections associated with *Bordetella bronchiseptica*, *Clin Microbiol Rev*, **4:** 243–55.

Yamagishi Y, Fujita J et al., 1993, Epidemic of nosocomial *Pseudomonas cepacia* in immuncompromised patients, *Chest*, **103:** 1706–9.

Yamamoto Y, Cline TW et al., 1994, *Legionella* and macrophages, *Macrophages and Infection*, eds Eisenstein TK and Zwilling B, Marcel Dekker, New York, 329–48.

DIPHTHERIA AND OTHER CORYNEBACTERIAL AND CORYNEFORM INFECTIONS

J E Clarridge, T Popovic and T J Inzana

DIPHTHERIA

1 INTRODUCTION AND HISTORY

The first clear description of diphtheria was that of Aretaeus of Cappadocia in about 100 AD although Hippocrates may have recognized the disease as a clinical entity as early as the fourth century BC. Epidemic diphtheria and the occurrence of palatal paralysis were described by Aetius in the sixth century. In the sixteenth and seventeenth centuries, epidemics swept though the Spanish peninsula, where the disease was termed garrotillo because of the frequency of death from suffocation. A fascinating account of an extensive epidemic of throat distemper in the New England colonies between 1735 and 1740 is given by Caulfield (1939); 5% of the population of New Hampshire died of the disease in 1735. Bretonneau (1826) named the disease diphterite (changing it later to dipht'erie), from the Greek root denoting a prepared skin or hide, because of the leathery appearance of the diphtheritic membrane. Previously, diphtheria had not been clearly distinguished from other ulcerative pharyngeal diseases. The name diphtheria first appeared among the classified causes of death in

England in a report published in 1857, a year that saw the beginning of a noteworthy widespread resurgence of diphtheria in Britain (Creighton 1894, reprinted in 1965). During the 5 decades that followed Bretonneau's publication there was much speculation concerning the aetiology of the disease and Jacobi (1880) presented the various views prevailing immediately before the causative bacterium was described. In 1884, Loeffler's classical paper described the isolation on coagulated serum medium of a bacillus observed microscopically in pseudomembranous material from typical cases of diphtheria. In 1883, Klebs identified the bacillus by microscopic examination of diphtheritic membrane but brought forward no convincing evidence of its aetiological role. *Corynebacterium diphtheriae* was, however, the first bacterium to be established as a specific aetiological agent. Loeffler (1884) not only observed the organism in the throats of 13–22 diphtheria patients and grew it in pure culture from 6 of them, but he also demonstrated its pathogenicity for laboratory animals. Since at necropsy the diphtheria bacilli usually remained localized to the site of inoculation, but organs elsewhere in the body showed major lesions, Loeffler concluded that in the local lesion a potent and probably lethal poison was formed. Since he also isolated it from one healthy child, demonstrating asymptomatic carriage, but failed to isolate it from every clinical case, Loeffler was cautious in claiming that he had determined the aetiology of diphtheria. Further interesting historical details may be found in Dixon, Noble and Smith (1990).

The determination of the role of the exotoxin began in 1888 when Roux and Yersin discovered that sterile filtrates from cultures of the diphtheria bacillus would kill guinea pigs, producing lesions identical with those that resulted from the injection of the living organism. In rabbits inoculated with filtered cultures Roux and Yersin noted the development of paralysis some weeks later.

Also at the end of the nineteenth century, it was discovered that specific immunity could develop in laboratory animals inoculated with small quantities of toxin or diphtheria cultures treated with iodine trichloride and that this immunity could be passively transferred in blood to other animals (von Behring and Kitasato 1890).

Within a few years, antitoxin was being therapeutically, after Behring received assistance from Ehrlich in producing a preparation of suitably high potency (Dolman 1973). Ehrlich subsequently undertook and completed his classical quantitative work which led to internationally accepted methods of standardizing antitoxins and laid the basis for the subsequent development of immunizing agents. An excellent account of these early events is given by Dolman (1973) and Kleinman (1992).

2 DESCRIPTION OF THE DISEASE

2.1 Pathogenesis

The most common disease caused by *C. diphtheriae* is diphtheria, an acute communicable disease manifested by both local infection of the upper respiratory tract and the systemic effects of a toxin, which are most notable in the heart and peripheral nerves. There are 2 phases of diphtheria, the initial local presentation as a severe pharyngitis with tough membranes that can grow over the air passage and cause suffocation and a later systemic phase caused by the effect of circulating exotoxin on tissues of the host.

Diphtheria toxin is the primary virulence factor of *C. diphtheriae*. The structural gene, *tox*, is carried by a family of corynebacteriophages and has been sequenced (Greenfield et al. 1983). It is a 535 residue, 58 kDa exotoxin whose active form consists of 2 polypeptide chains linked by a disulphide bond. Its aminoterminal fragment (A-fragment, 193 residues) contains the catalytic domain with the ADP-ribosyltransferase activity; its carboxyl-terminal fragment (B-fragment, 342 residues) contains the receptor-binding domain including a channel-forming region and the transmembrane domain (Choe et al. 1992, Bennett and Eisenberg 1994, Silverman et al. 1994).

The expression of *tox*, and thus the regulation of exotoxin synthesis, is under the control of a chromosomal iron-dependent repressor, *dtxR*, and a promoter/operator region. The repressor *dtxR* gene encodes a 226-residue protein with slight homology to the *Escherichia coli* Fur protein (25% amino acid homology) (Boyd, Oza and Murphy 1990). This protein consists of at least 3 domains, a transition metal–iron activation domain, a DNA binding domain, and a protein interaction domain (Tao et al. 1994, Qiu et al. 1995). Under high-iron conditions in *C. diphtheriae*, the Fe^{3+}–*dtxR* complex is configured so that it binds to the diphtheria toxin operator and represses toxin biosynthesis. The 3-dimensional structure and sequence of DtxR has been described (Qiu et al. 1995).

The process by which the toxin binds to specific receptors and enters susceptible cells is being defined. Bennett and Eisenberg (1994) describe a 5-step intoxication procedure:

1 the disulphide bridge between the catalytic domain and the transmembrane domain is hydrolysed
2 the receptor domain binds to the diphtheria toxin receptor on the cell
3 the transmembrane domain inserts into the endosomal membrane
4 the catalytic domain is translocated into the cytosol and
5 the catalytic domain stops protein synthesis by inactivating elongation factor 2 via ADP-ribosylation.

All human tissues may be adversely affected by the toxin because all human cells have receptor sites. Accordingly, there is no specific target organ, but clinical consequences generally result from myocardial and neural abnormalities. Death often results from cardiac failure, but necrotic and often haemorrhagic lesions are usually seen in many organs at necropsy. Except for the local site of infection, the lesions are sterile.

Since non-toxigenic strains are also associated with significant invasive disease (Patey et al. 1996) as well as skin lesions, it is probable that *C. diphtheriae* has additional virulence factors causing adherence or invasiveness. The effect of toxigenic and non-toxigenic *C. diphtheriae* on rabbits and guinea pigs was compared by Barksdale, Garmise and Horibata (1960) using 2 strains that differed from each other only by the presence in one of a bacteriophage that determined toxin production. Necrotic local lesions developed in rabbits inoculated intradermally with the toxigenic strain and the animals died from toxaemia, whereas the non-toxigenic strain caused only a local pyogenic lesion which eventually disappeared. In a Swedish study unusually severe disease was associated with strains of one particular DNA homology pattern and it has been suggested that these strains produce secondary factors that account for their high virulence (Karzon and Edwards 1988, Rappuoli, Pergini and Falsen 1988).

The role of β-haemolytic streptococci in potentiating diphtheria infections is not known. However, in both faucial and cutaneous diphtheria, *Streptococcus pyogenes* is often co-isolated from lesions. During an outbreak of respiratory diphtheria in Texas, 32% of patients were simultaneously infected with *C. diphtheriae* and *S. pyogenes*, but the course of the disease and response to treatment were the same as in patients infected only with *C. diphtheriae* (McCloskey et al. 1971). In the Seattle outbreak, 73% of the diphtheritic ulcers harboured *S. pyogenes* (Harnisch et al. 1989), as do ulcers in non-epidemic settings (Hamour et al. 1995). Ramon and Djourichitch (1934) concluded from experimental work in guinea pigs that streptococcal infection lowered the resistance of tissue to invasion by *C. diphtheriae*, but studies in rabbits by Updyke and Frobisher (1947) revealed no such synergic action.

2.2 Modes of transmission

Both asymptomatic carriers and clinical cases are important in the spread of diphtheria. The organism can be carried in the upper respiratory tract of otherwise healthy individuals and appears to have a particular predilection for tonsillar tissue (Wehrle 1982). Transmission occurs in close-contact settings via respiratory droplets or by hand-to-mouth contact with respiratory secretions. Due to the mild clinical presentations and presence of the organisms in the nose as well as in the pharynx, the nasal form of the diseases may favour the spread of the organism. Transmission from cases is believed to be more efficient than from carriers, presumably due to the greater number of organisms present in the upper respiratory tract; in household settings, up to 27% of close contacts may be infected (Farizo et al. 1993). However, in endemic areas, the number of carriers is several-fold higher than the number of cases, emphasizing their role in transmission.

Patients with the cutaneous form of diphtheria have frequently been shown to harbour *C. diphtheriae* in the respiratory tract (Wehrle 1982). The routes of transmission for cutaneous diphtheria are respiratory droplets and direct physical contact (Committee on Infectious Diseases 1994). The organism survives on clothes and dust in the environment of cases; transmission by articles soiled with the discharge from lesions of infected persons may be important, especially when associated with crowding and poor hygiene. Foodborne transmission by infected milk or milk products has occasionally been reported (Goldie and Maddock 1943, Jones et al. 1985, Christenson, Hellstrom and Aust-Kettis 1989).

2.3 Clinical manifestations

C. diphtheriae is only rarely an invasive organism. Clinical manifestations are associated with both the local and systemic effects of the diphtheria toxin that is responsible for local tissue destruction and formation of the membrane (Fischer 1982).

It is convenient to classify diphtheria into several clinical types, depending on the site of the disease (Centers for Disease Control and Prevention 1993b). *C. diphtheriae* infects primarily the upper respiratory tract (respiratory diphtheria), where the organism colonizes the mucosal surface of the nasopharynx and multiplies locally without bloodstream invasion. Following an incubation period of usually 2–5 days, the illness begins gradually with malaise, sore throat, anorexia and fever as a result of substantial systemic absorption of toxin (Committee on Infectious Diseases 1994). Locally, toxin induces tissue necrosis, leucocyte response and formation of a tough, adherent pseudomembrane composed of a mixture of fibrin, dead cells and bacteria (Wehrle 1982). The membrane is tightly adherent and bleedings occur upon attempts to remove it. The membrane usually begins to form on the tonsils or posterior pharynx (pharyngeal diphtheria); in more severe cases it can spread progressively over the pharyngeal wall, fauces and the soft palate all the way to the bronchi. As the membrane spreads the patients may develop significant oedema of the submandibular areas and the anterior neck with the lymphadenopathy, giving them a characteristic 'bullneck appearance'. In severe cases the neck oedema may extend past the clavicles into the chest, accompanied by the erythema. The anterior and lateral neck may be involved. Laryngeal diphtheria can occur as a result of membrane extension, or may be the only site of infection; it presents with hoarseness, stridor and dyspnoea, and rapid diagnosis, intubation or tracheostomy may be required due to the airway obstruction. The disease may progress, if enough toxin enters the bloodstream, causing severe prostration, striking pallor, rapid pulse, stupor and coma. These effects may result in death within a week of onset of symptoms. The absorbed toxin can also cause delayed damage at distant sites; the most frequently affected organs are the heart (myocarditis) and the cranial nerves. These complications may occur from 1 to 12 weeks after disease onset.

Cutaneous diphtheria often appears as a secondary infection of a previous wound. Primary cutaneous diphtheria begins as a tender pustule and enlarges to an oval punched-out ulcer with a membrane and oedematous rolled borders (Lewbow et al. 1946). The infection with *C. diphtheriae* and possibly other organisms can cause a chronic non-healing ulcer. There is often concomitant isolation of *S. pyogenes*. Skin infections may vary in severity, but toxin-induced complications are usually uncommon. Cutaneous diphtheria is reportedly more common in tropical and subtropical areas. *C. diphtheriae* may also cause local infections such as vulvovaginitis, conjunctivitis and primary or secondary otitis media.

Non-toxigenic *C. diphtheriae* has been reported to cause a diphtheria-like membranous tonsillopharyngitis and pharyngitis without a membrane (Edward and Allison 1951, Belsey 1970). Reports have provided support for the association of non-toxigenic *C. diphtheriae* and invasive diseases, including endocarditis and arthritis (Efstratiou, George and Begg 1993, Efstratiou et al. 1993, Gradon, Mayrer and Hayes 1993, Lortholory et al. 1993, Tiley et al. 1993, Patey et al. 1996). Underlying risk factors are commonly observed in these patients (Afgani and Stutman 1993).

Asymptomatic nasopharyngeal infection with *C. diphtheriae* is more frequent than clinical disease. The length of carriage averages 10 days, but chronic carriers may shed the organism for 6 months or more. Antibiotic treatment is effective in terminating shedding (Centers for Disease Control and Prevention 1993b).

2.4 Diagnosis and treatment

The differential diagnosis of respiratory diphtheria includes bacterial (streptococcal, *Arcanobacterium haemolyticum* [Kain et al. 1991]) and viral tonsillopharyngitis, infectious mononucleosis, peritonsillar abscess, Vincent's angina, candidiasis and acute epiglottitis. The imperative in diphtheria treatment is to administer the antitoxin as soon as possible, as it can only neutralize toxin that has not already bound to cells. Therefore, the diagnosis is usually based on clinical presentation (Farizo et al. 1993) before laboratory results are available. Several predisposing factors will make the diagnosis of diphtheria more likely:

1 the patient is unimmunized or has not received the recommended booster immunizations
2 there is a history of contact with a diphtheria case
3 there is a history of recent travel to a region with endemic or epidemic diphtheria
4 the pretreatment antitoxin titre is below 0.01 IU ml^{-1}.

The mainstay of therapy is prompt administration of equine diphtheria antitoxin. Between 20 000 and 100 000 IU, administered intravenously, are recommended depending on the severity and the stage of the disease (Centers for Disease Control and Prevention 1993b).

Although immunization is the most important long-term factor for the prevention of diphtheria, antibiotics play a major role in the treatment and control of diphtheria. They are used to prevent dissemination and toxin production in infected patients, clinical disease in and spread from asymptomatic carriers and colonization of contacts (Maple et al. 1995). Antibiotic therapy (penicillin or erythromycin) will eliminate the organism and consequently prevent further toxin production and its transmission (Krugman et al. 1992, MacGregor 1995). The patient is expected to be non-contagious within 48 h after antibiotics are administered. Recent in vitro susceptibility results on the isolates from the former Soviet Union confirm the older literature: all strains were susceptible to erythromycin, penicillin, ampicillin, cefalothin, chloramphenicol, ciprofloxacin, gentamicin and tetracycline and 97% were susceptible to trimethoprim and rifampicin (Maple et al. 1994).

3 EPIDEMIOLOGY

In the first half of the nineteenth century diphtheria was endemic in Europe and the USA. Between 1850 and 1860 a pandemic with a high mortality rate developed, apparently from a focus in France. After 1885 this began to decline, though the incidence of disease still remained high. In temperate climates the morbidity and mortality rates were highest during the colder months of the year. The age incidence varied but was always highest in the preschool child. The disease was uncommon during the first year of life, but the maximum incidence was reached between the second and fifth years. It gradually declined in the 5–10 year age group, and then fell more rapidly. The probability of disease occurring after the age of 15 years was small (Frost 1928).

At the beginning of this century, diphtheria was one of the major causes of death among children in the USA (Dixon 1984). The case-fatality rate in untreated persons was about 7–10% (highest in infancy and lowest in adolescence) (Munford et al. 1974). However, since the 1920s, when active immunization against diphtheria became available, the number of reported cases in the USA has decreased from about 200 000 in 1921 to only 0–2 cases per year at present (Dixon 1984, Farizo et al. 1993). In Europe, widespread immunization programmes were initiated in the 1940s and the disease was soon eliminated from most countries, eventually reaching an all-time low in 1980 when only 623 cases were reported (Galazka, Robertson and Oblapenko 1995). However, a large-scale and rapidly accelerating diphtheria epidemic that began in Russia in 1990 has made its way to all 15 New Independent States (NIS) of the former Soviet Union (Centers for Disease Control and Prevention 1993a, 1995a). Reported cases in Russia and NIS have increased from 839 in 1989 to 39 703 in 1994 and 35 716 in 1995 (Centers for Disease Control and Prevention 1995a, Hardy, Dittmann and Sutter 1996). In 1994 the case-fatality ratio ranged from 2.8% in the Russian Federation to 23.0% in Lithuania and Turkistan (Centers for Disease Control and Prevention 1995a). The highest age-specific incidence rates were among persons aged 4–10, 15–17 and 40–49 years. The numbers of susceptible people have increased both because fewer people are being vaccinated and because natural immunity decreased as exposure to *C. diphtheriae* declined. Serological studies in the NIS, western Europe and the USA indicate that 20–60% of the adults aged >20 years are susceptible to *C. diphtheriae*. Although the source of the present epidemic in the NIS (Fig. 19.1) is not known, in the southern parts of the NIS, as in many tropical areas throughout the world, there is endemic infection with *C. diphtheriae* associated with cutaneus diphtheria (Hardy, Dittmann and Sutter 1996).

At least 20 imported cases of diphtheria in adults reported in neighbouring European countries, and 2 cases of diphtheria among US citizens, who acquired the disease in the NIS, have occurred since the beginning of the epidemic (Centers for Disease Control and Prevention 1995a). Hence, diphtheria has once again become a cause for global concern (Popovic et al. 1995).

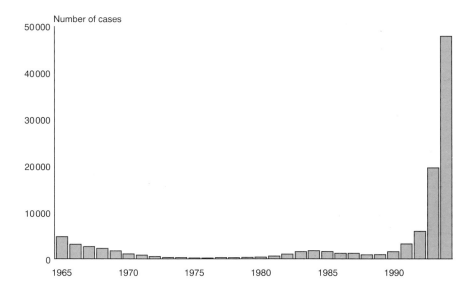

Number of cases

Fig. 19.1 Reported diphtheria cases in the Soviet Union/New Independent States, 1965–94.

3.1 Strain tracking

The isolates of *C. diphtheriae* from different epidemics and geographical regions vary in biotype, proportion that are toxigenic and in clonal origin. For example, during 1959–64, more than 95% of *gravis* strains described in the USA were toxigenic, whereas in the following 3 years the percentage was less than 44 (Brooks, Bennett and Feldman 1974). The variation noted by the same authors in *mitis* strains was even greater; 99% were toxigenic in 1962, 74% in 1969–70 and only 14% in 1971–75. More recently, clinical strains submitted for toxin testing in the UK included 31 non-toxigenic *C. diphtheriae* strains of which there were 19 *C. diphtheriae* var. *gravis*, 9 *C. diphtheriae* var. *belfanti* and 3 *C. diphtheriae* var. *mitis* and 19 toxigenic strains comprising 2 *C. diphtheriae* var. *gravis*, 15 *C. diphtheriae* var. *mitis* and 2 *C. ulcerans* strains (Pallen et al. 1994). However, in Switzerland, all the isolates from drug abusers were non-toxigenic *C. diphtheriae* var. *mitis* (Gruner et al. 1994a), whereas in the former Soviet Union, about 70% of the strains are toxigenic and most are *C. diphtheriae* var. *gravis* (Maple et al. 1994, De Zoysa et al. 1995, Popovic et al. 1995).

There are several useful techniques for strain tracking or the determination of clonal origin that are more discriminatory than colony type or toxin testing. In the past, phage typing and serotyping have been used but were limited as many strains were untypable. They have been superseded by molecular techniques such as whole cell peptide, ribotype and genomic DNA restriction endonuclease fragment polymorphism analysis (Rappuoli, Pergini and Falsen 1988, Coyle et al. 1989, Gruner et al. 1992, 1994a, Krech 1994, De Zoysa et al. 1995). The molecular epidemiology of 106 strains (100 isolated in 1993 from northwestern Russia) of *C. diphtheriae* (81 *C. diphtheriae* var. *gravis* and 25 *C. diphtheriae* var. *mitis*) were examined by ribotyping and genomic DNA restriction endonuclease pattern (De Zoysa et al. 1995) with ribotyping being more discriminatory. They found 7 distinct ribotypes. There was one predominant (64 of 81) *C.*

diphtheriae var. *gravis* ribotype and one predominant (24 of 25) *C. diphtheriae* var. *mitis* ribotype. However, strains with these ribotypes were seen throughout Russia with the same frequency both before the epidemic and during the epidemic (Wachsmuth et al. 1995). In addition, the same study by Wachsmuth et al. showed the emergence of another ribotype, especially in 1993 and 1994. Finally, an excellent correlation exists between ribotyping and multilocus enzyme electrophoresis, which indicated that a distinct clonal group emerged in Russia in 1990 as the epidemic began.

Using pattern analysis of DNA fragments probed with an insertion element, Rappuoli, Pergini and Falsen (1988) showed that the toxigenic *C. diphtheriae* var. *mitis* strains responsible for a Swedish epidemic gave a similar pattern whereas all strains not involved in the epidemic gave unique patterns. Similarly, the strains of non-toxigenic *C. diphtheriae* var. *gravis* associated with sporadic endocarditis occurring in different locations in Australia were not related (Efstratiou et al. 1993, Tiley et al. 1993).

In the Seattle outbreak of predominantly skin infections, toxigenic *C. diphtheriae* var. *intermedius* was the most common isolate although all 3 biotypes were responsible for consecutive, overlapping outbreaks (Coyle et al. 1989). Gruner and colleges found all skin and pharyngeal isolates from a group of intravenous drug abusers were non-toxigenic *C. diphtheriae* var. *mitis*. Each strain was identical by biotyping, resistance patterns and ribotyping, indicating infection by the same clone (Gruner et al. 1992, 1994a, Zuber et al. 1992). Epidemics of cutaneous diphtheria seem to be sporadic; people with poor hygiene and living conditions, such as drug abusers, may be a reservoir for *C. diphtheriae* infection. All biotypes and both the toxigenic (Harmour et al. 1995) and non-toxigenic types of *C. diphtheriae* have been isolated from various sporadic or epidemic cases of cutaneous diphtheria (Coyle et al. 1989, Gruner et al. 1992, Harnisch et al. 1989, De Zoysa et al. 1995).

3.2   Carriage of *C. diphtheriae*

The carriage of *C. diphtheriae* in the absence of symptoms may occur during the incubation period of diphtheria, during convalescence, or in healthy persons. Patients convalescing from diphtheria may harbour *C. diphtheriae* in the throat or nose for many weeks. In a study of 500 patients, one-half of those originally culture-positive became culture-negative during the next 7 days; after 4 weeks over 83% were free of diphtheria bacilli. However, *C. diphtheriae* disappeared more quickly from the throat than from the nose and 90% of those who became carriers were infected in the nose, or nose and throat, whereas the remaining 10% were infected only in the throat. The organisms disappeared more quickly in older than in younger children (Dixon, Noble and Smith 1990).

Before the introduction of universal immunization, diphtheria was typically a disease of households, schools and institutions where children were herded together at susceptible ages. A particular school or institution often became an epidemic centre of the disease for a period of months or years. The closeness and duration of contact seemed to play the major part in determining the spread of the disease. Children sleeping in a single dormitory were much more at risk than those who had casual contact during working hours.

In a prospective study of carriage rates, 117 intravenous drug users were screened for infection with *C. diphtheriae*; non-toxigenic *C. diphtheriae* was found in 5 of 132 throat swab specimens and in 5 of 28 skin ulcer specimens but the disease was not clearly attributable to the isolates. When phenotypic and molecular typing methods were used, these 10 strains were shown to belong to a single clone. In the same study, no *C. diphtheriae* was isolated from 200 controls. In general, carriage rates are low in immunized populations (Mencarelli et al. 1992); these isolations may represent the endemic presence of *C. diphtheriae*.

The epidemiological role of cutaneous infections in the spread of diphtheria in temperate areas was studied by Belsey and colleagues (Belsey et al. 1969, Belsey 1970). They isolated *C. diphtheriae* from clothing, furniture and a variety of environmental sites in households in Louisiana and reported 2 instances of transmission from fomites (Belsey 1970). Persons in contact with diphtheritic skin infections are more likely than contacts of respiratory tract infections to become infected (Belsey and LeBlanc 1975). The great importance of cutaneous spread under certains conditions of poor social hygiene was emphasized by the observations of Jellard (1972). An attempt was made in Seattle by Pedersen et al. (1977) to control a long-standing outbreak of diphtheria, largely cutaneous, by decontaminating the dwellings of infected patients, but the procedures had no apparent beneficial effect. Crosbie and Wright (1941) isolated diphtheria bacilli in large numbers from hospital floor dust near patients with faucial diphtheria and showed that they could remain viable for as long as 5 weeks. It was suspected that dust distributed during floor sweeping and the making of beds played an even more important part in cross-infection in diphtheria wards than direct transmission of droplets from patient to patient. The spread is not zootic as humans are the only host for *C. diphtheriae*.

4   HOST RESPONSE

4.1   Vaccines

Diphtheria antitoxin was discovered in 1890 by von Behring and Kitasato and was first administered to a child in 1891 (Mortimer 1994). Diphtheria was the first bacterial disease for which a toxic cause was identified and the first to be treated successfully with an antitoxin. Initially, balanced mixtures of toxin and antitoxin were successfully used as an immunization agent. In 1913, Ramon introduced a vaccine composed of formalin-treated diphtheria toxin, called anatoxin, which later became known as diphtheria toxoid (Mortimer 1994). Active immunization with diphtheria toxoid became available in the USA in the 1920s and it gradually replaced the toxin–antitoxin combination. In 1926, Glenny and his coworkers found that alum-precipitated toxoid was even more immunogenic, and by the mid 1940s diphtheria toxoid was combined with tetanus toxoid and pertussis vaccine as the now familiar diphtheria–tetanus–pertussis vaccine (DTP) (Mortimer 1994).

Currently, the world-wide production of diphtheria toxoid is fairly standard. It is prepared by treating a sterile toxin filtrate of *C. diphtheriae* with formalin, followed by purification and concentration procedures to achieve the proper dosage (Mortimer 1994). Diphtheria toxoid is unable to fix to mammalian cells and loses its enzymatic activity; thus, it lacks the properties of the toxin but retains the antigenicity and the capacity to react with the antitoxin antibodies. The most commonly used preparation in the USA, DTP, contains between 10 and 20 Lf (limes of flocculation or flocculation units) of diphtheria toxoid per dose. It is recommended for the routine immunization of children under 7 years of age (Centers for Disease Control and Prevention 1995b). A primary series consists of 3 doses, administered at intervals of 4–8 weeks, beginning when the infant is 6–8 weeks old. A fourth dose is given 6–12 months after the third dose and is usually administered at 15–18 months of age. A fifth dose is usually given at 4–6 years of age, before school entry. A preparation with reduced concentration of diphtheria toxoid (adult Td) with a maximum of 2 Lf per dose is used after the seventh birthday because adverse vaccination reactions can increase with age (Mortimer 1994). For previously unimmunized older children and adults, a primary series of 3 doses of Td is given (Centers for Disease Control and Prevention 1995b). The first 2 doses are given at intervals of 4–8 weeks and the third dose is given 6 months to one year after the second. Active adult immunity should be maintained by administering a dose of Td every 10 years and by using Td with tetanus wound prophylaxis.

In the prevaccination era, when diphtheria was

common, natural immunity was commonly acquired by clinical illness or subclinical infection. In addition, carrier rates were high and overcrowded, unhygienic living conditions were common, allowing for almost continuous contact with toxigenic *C. diphtheriae* strains and continuous reinforcement of natural immunity. It is estimated that 80% of all children were immune by the age of 15 (Galazka and Robertson 1995). The group at highest risk was young children over the age of 6 months who recently lost their maternal antibodies. With the introduction of active immunization programmes, however, the number of cases and carriers decreased. Consequently, the opportunities to acquire or to boost natural immunity also decreased. In most developed and developing countries, vaccine coverage of infants and young children continues to rise. Before the widespread use of active immunization, 29% of diphtheria cases were reported in children under the age of 15 years, which was the pattern seen in many developed countries from 1900 to 1940 (Galazka and Robertson 1995). However, with the widespread immunization programme, a shift in the age distribution towards adults has been observed. The proportion of cases among adults rose from 16% in 1958 to 80% in 1977. The current epidemic in Russia and the NIS is characterized by increased incidence in all age groups, with a peak incidence in non-immunized children 5–10 years of age and in adults 30–50 years of age (Centers for Disease Control and Prevention 1995a, Galazka, Robertson and Oblapenko 1995).

The degree to which administration of diphtheria toxoid protects against the disease is defined as the vaccine efficacy. High efficacy signifies that the toxoid potency, vaccine administration and accuracy of a vaccination documentation were mostly adequate. Even if infected, vaccinated persons stand a significantly higher chance of presenting with a mild or inapparent clinical picture; however, no level of antitoxin guarantees complete protection against diphtheria in all persons. Among the diphtheria patients in the USA between 1971 and 1981, only 6.3% of those who were previously fully vaccinated developed a severe form of the disease, compared with 24.7% among non-vaccinated individuals. In addition, none of the fully or partially immunized individuals died (Chen et al. 1985). The clinical efficacy of the vaccine used in Russia and Ukraine has proven to be high (Anonymous 1993). In 1991, the incidence among the unvaccinated children was estimated to be 33 per 100 000 as compared to 5.3 per 100 000 among the vaccinated children. Vaccine efficacy in the Ukrainian children who received 4 or 5 doses of vaccine was 92% and 95%, respectively (Anonymous 1993). Vaccination with diphtheria toxoid protects against the effects of the diphtheria toxin, but it does not prevent infection with *C. diphtheriae*. Therefore, the immunized persons, if infected, can play an important role in transmitting the diseases as carriers. Finally, detectable levels of diphtheria toxin antibodies are not reached in 1–2% of a fully immunized population.

4.2 Measurement of immune response

Given that almost all the damage in patients with diphtheria may be associated with the release of the diphtheria toxin, successful vaccination against diphtheria requires acquisition of diphtheria toxin neutralizing antibodies. A series of antigens present in both A and B subunits of the toxin have been demonstrated. Even though the A subunit is highly immunogenic in humans, antibodies directed at this subunit do not neutralize the toxin's activity (Sesardic and Corbel 1992). On the other hand, antibodies directed at the B subunit act as neutralizing antibodies. Currently, there are several methods available for assessing levels of circulating diphtheria toxin antibodies. Assays based on the ability of the serum to inhibit diphtheria toxin activity in animals or in cell culture will reveal the presence of only those antibodies that are capable of neutralizing the toxin activity and are therefore considered to be protective. In vitro methods will frequently detect non-neutralizing antibodies that arise against toxin regions not essential in the process of receptor binding and neutralization, or against epitopes that become available only following formaldehyde treatment. Methods based on the neutralization of diphtheria toxin are advantageous when the assessment of protective immunity is desired, as the ratio of neutralizing and non-neutralizing antibodies is not constant.

The standard, classic test of immune status against diphtheria has been the Schick test, developed in 1913 (Schick 1913). It served as an acceptable substitute for a more precise measure of immunity for many years (Pappenheimer 1965, Kleinman 1992). Small amounts of diphtheria toxin, injected intracutaneously, will elicit a local inflammatory response in the absence of the antitoxin, peaking at 5 days. Schick positive persons were believed to have a 90% likelihood of protection and, if infected, to manifest a milder disease. In vivo toxin neutralization assays for the determination of serum level of diphtheria toxin antibodies, that uses guinea pigs or rabbits, has been generally recognized as a very sensitive system to detect antibodies capable of neutralizing diphtheria toxin effects (Pappenheimer 1965). A dose of diphtheria toxin antibody necessary to protect the rabbit or a guinea pig against the erythrogenic effect (degree of redness and inflammation at the inoculation site caused by a known dose of diphtheria toxin) is compared to the dose of a standard preparation of diphtheria antitoxin (Efstratiou and Maple 1994). Neutralization of the cytopathic effect of the diphtheria toxin on the tissue culture system, by serum containing diphtheria toxin antibodies, is the basis of the in vitro neutralization assays that use Vero cells (African green monkey kidney cells) (Efstratiou and Maple 1994). Thousands of toxin receptors per cell makes this system an extremely sensitive one (Middlebrook, Dorland and Leppla 1978, Gupta et al. 1994). Currently, other in vitro assays such as ELISA and passive haemagglutination assay are available (Camargo et al. 1984, Melville-Smith and Balfour 1988, Galazka and Kardymowicz

1989, Aggerbeck and Heron 1991); both in vivo and in vitro neutralization assays are used to standardize and verify the sensitivity and specificity of those assays. A significant proportion of IgG antibodies against diphtheria toxin, detected by several ELISA assays, lack the neutralizing capabilities, resulting in poor correlation with the toxin neutralization assays, particularly for sera containing less than 0.1 IU of diphtheria antitoxin per ml.

4.3 Interpretation

The ability of a vaccine to induce a measurable immune response in an individual is defined as the immunogenicity of a vaccine; in the case of diphtheria, it is expressed as the level of diphtheria toxin antibodies. Even though the first methods for assessing the levels of neutralizing antibodies date back to the 1900s, no single replacement for in vivo toxin neutralizing assays has gained general acceptance for all indications for determining levels of diphtheria toxin antibodies. In 1994, at the First International Meeting of the WHO Laboratory Working Group on Diphtheria, it was agreed that in vitro toxin neutralization assay on Vero cells is currently the most appropriate assay for measuring concentrations of diphtheria toxin antibodies in large numbers of human sera (Maple et al. 1995). In vitro assays, such as ELISA and passive haemagglutination assay (PHA), are required to provide direct comparison with the toxin neutralization assay(s), particularly at concentrations below 0.1 IU ml^{-1}. Using these methods, under the agreed upon conditions, several studies have addressed the question of the levels of diphtheria toxin antibodies after administration of varying doses of diphtheria toxoid. It was demonstrated that the same antitoxin level could give different levels of protection in different individuals, and after different degrees of exposure. Levels of diphtheria toxin antibodies >0.01 IU ml^{-1} (basic protection) were detected after the primary vaccination in infancy in over 97% of the recipients (Centers for Disease Control and Prevention 1993a). The immune response to booster vaccination could be demonstrated only 10 days later as a 5–10-fold increase in levels of diphtheria toxin antibodies.

These and other observations and studies, carried out world wide over the past few decades, have resulted in the following internationally accepted interpretations of the measured levels of diphtheria toxin antibodies expressed in IU ml^{-1} (Table 19.1). Depending on the schedule of immunization and incidence of diphtheria, immunity declines in late childhood and adolescence. Even in countries with a long history of high compliance with childhood vaccination, high immunity is not obtained within the adult populations. For example, only 30% of women and 50% of men in Sweden, in the early 1980s, and 27% of all adults in Italy in the late 1990s, had antibody levels higher than 0.01 IU ml^{-1} (Cellesi et al. 1989, Mark et al. 1989). In the USA, between 22 and 62% of adults 18–39 years of age, and 41–84% of those over 60 years of age, lack protective levels of diphtheria toxin antibodies (Sargent et al. 1984, Farizo et al. 1993). Given that it is necessary for at least 70–75% of the total population to have protective antibody levels to confer herd immunity, such a high proportion of susceptible adults world wide represents a significant epidemic potential (Kjeldsen, Simonsen and Heron 1988, Cohen et al. 1991, Miller et al. 1994, Maple et al. 1995). Increased awareness by physicians and other health care workers is necessary to make the diagnosis; continuous epidemiological surveillance of clinical cases and serological surveillance for the identification of high-risk populations are necessary.

5 CONTROL AND PREVENTION

Two recent publications, by the United States Centers for Disease Control and Prevention and by the World Health Organization Regional Office for Europe, provide updated recommendations for the prevention and control of diphtheria (Farizo et al. 1993, Begg 1994). Because most practising clinicians have never seen a case of diphtheria, it is crucial that they remain aware of the possibility of diphtheria, especially in a patient with a nasopharyngeal pseudomembrane. Contact investigations should be initiated immediately upon notification of the health department. The patient must be placed in strict respiratory isolation and the appropriate clinical samples taken for microbiological diagnosis, preferably before antibiotics are commenced. During and after treatment, isolation should be maintained until elimination of the organism is demonstrated by 2 negative cultures obtained at least 24 h apart after completion of antimicrobial therapy. The patient should be immunized with diphtheria toxoid during convalescence, because clinical illness does not necessarily confer natural immunity. Close contacts (which include household members and frequent household visitors, school and work contacts), should, irrespective of vaccination status, be considered at risk. It is now recommended that all close contacts receive antibiotic prophylaxis and be monitored for symptoms and signs of diphtheria for at least 7 days. In cases of assured compliance, a 7–10 day course of erythromycin is recommended; if compliance is doubtful, or there is intolerance to erythromycin, a single intramuscular injection of benzathine penicillin (600 000 units for persons younger than 6 years of age and 1.2 million

Table 19.1 Levels of circulating diphtheria toxin antibodies and their interpretation

Level of diphtheria toxin antibody (IU ml^{-1})	Interpretation
<0.01	Susceptible individual
0.01–0.09	Basic protection
0.1	Full protection
>1.0	Long-term protection

units for persons 6 years of age or older) should be administered. The immunization status of the contacts should be assessed and at least one dose of DTP or Td administered unless they have completed primary immunization and have received a booster within the last 12 months.

It appears that even in highly immunized communities a high level of population immunity, at least 70–75%, is necessary to prevent diphtheria outbreaks. Due to the rarity of natural exposure to toxigenic *C. diphtheriae* nowadays, the necessary levels of immunity can only be obtained by reaching the childhood vaccination coverage of at least 95%, and by achieving high coverage of adults with decennial booster doses of diphtheria toxoid.

6 AETIOLOGY

Diphtheria is caused by *C. diphtheriae* and, rarely, *Corynebacterium ulcerans*. *C. diphtheriae* is a gram-positive, fermentative, somewhat irregular rod which exists as one of 4 biotypes: *gravis*, *mitis*, *intermedius* and *belfanti*. Minimal characteristics for presumptive identification include positive reactions for catalase production, nitrate reduction (except biotype *belfanti*) and glucose and maltose fermentation and negative reactions for urease, sucrose, mannose, xylose and pyrazinamidase. *C. diphtheriae* possesses a large amount (29%) of an unusual cell wall fatty acid: C16:1 w7C. The biotypes of *C. diphtheriae* differ in that *intermedius* is lipophilic (i.e. it needs added lipids for best growth and grows as a small translucent colony on routine media), *gravis* can utilize glycogen and starch and *belfanti* does not reduce nitrate. The association of *C. diphtheriae* subsp. *gravis* with more serious disease than that caused by *C. diphtheriae* subsp. *mitis* has not been confirmed in recent outbreaks. *C. diphtheriae* and, rarely, *C. ulcerans* and *Corynebacterium pseudotuberculosis* can harbour the phage-borne gene for the production of the diphtheria toxin. The isolation of an increasing proportion of non-toxigenic compared to toxigenic *C. diphtheriae* strains is reported. It is not clear whether immunization selectively inhibits growth of the toxigenic strains, or laboratories increasingly identify coryneform organisms involved in diseases other than respiratory diphtheria. It is postulated that the non-toxigenic strains occur more often in people who have been previously immunized.

7 COLLECTION OF SPECIMENS

7.1 Culture and identification

For cases of suspected diphtheria, material for culture is obtained on a swab from the inflamed areas of the membranes that are formed in the throat and nasopharynx. Swabbings of the nasopharynx and throat can also be cultured for the detection of *C. diphtheriae* in suspected carriers. Up to 18% of carriers may be detectable only by nasal culture (Taylor, Tomlinson and Davies 1962, Butterworth et al. 1974). Material

from wounds should be removed by swab or aspiration, taking care to avoid normal skin flora. Smears can be made of the original material for subsequent Neisser or Loeffler's methylene blue stain for observation of metachromatic granules and gram stain for coryneform morphology. This test is, however, unreliable, both in sensitivity and specificity, as *C. diphtheriae* is indistinguishable from many other *Corynebacterium* spp. The specimen should be immediately transported to the laboratory or inoculated onto proper media. If this is not possible, the swab should be sent to a reference laboratory, shipped dry in a sterile tube or in a special packet containing a desiccant such as silica gel. It is reported that *C. diphtheriae* can be isolated from such swabs after delays of up to 9 weeks (Kim-Farley et al. 1987).

Specimens for *C. diphtheriae* should be streaked onto a blood agar plate and onto a tellurite-containing medium (e.g. Hoyle's medium, cystine–tellurite agar or modified Tinsdale medium) (Jellard 1971). The tellurite-containing media have the advantage of being both selective and differential; tellurite inhibits the growth of most nasopharyngeal flora and *C. diphtheriae* has a rare ability (along with a few other corynebacteria, staphylococci and yeasts) to reduce tellurite salt to black-coloured tellurium, rendering the colonies black. The cysteine-containing medium is also differential because only the *C. diphtheriae* group of corynebacteria (*C. diphtheriae*, *C. ulcerans* and *C. pseudotuberculosis*) form a halo surrounding the colony. A Loeffler slant can also be inoculated because *C. diphtheriae* grows most rapidly on this lipid-rich medium and the gram stains from colonies grown on Loeffler medium are best for the demonstration of metachromatic granules. In addition to Tinsdale or tellurite media, inoculation of Loeffler or Pai (1932) slants may increase the sensitivity of culture, and is particularly necessary if no liquid enrichment medium was used for transport. For better recovery, specimens submitted as single swabs should be transferred to a liquid serum or blood-containing medium which can be subcultured after 4 days of incubation onto the media described above. When silica gel is used for transportation, it is essential that desiccated swabs be incubated overnight in a broth supplemented with plasma or blood before they are plated on the routine media recommended. Many clinical laboratories, however, rarely have these special selective media in stock because requests for *C. diphtheriae* culture are rare and media shelf life is short. However, *C. diphtheriae* grow as well on routine blood agar and semiselective media such as CNA (Columbia colistin–naladixic acid) and can be recovered from these plates if there is not overgrowth by contaminating flora (see Volume 2, Chapter 25).

The laboratory diagnosis of unsuspected diphtheria infection is difficult as colonies of *C. diphtheriae* are not distinctive on the agar media usually used for plating throat or wound cultures. Furthermore, the presence of coryneform organisms in mixed culture with other throat or skin flora is usually not reported. Thus the diagnosis of diphtheria in a non-epidemic setting is almost always initially based on clinical observations. Detection of *C. diphtheriae* as an agent of cutaneous diphtheria or endocarditis is related to the completeness of identification of coryneform organisms pursued in the laboratory.

After isolation, identification of *C. diphtheriae* is not difficult. Commercial identification schemes such as Coryne API (bioMérieux, France) allow identification with a high degree of confidence. Tests that are important to distinguish *C. diphtheriae* from other corynebacteria and coryneform organisms are discussed elsewhere (see Volume 2, Chapter 25) and include production of catalase, urease and pyrazinamidase, nitrate reduction, glucose, sucrose, mannose, xylose and maltose fermentation and utilization of starch and glycerol.

7.2 Detection of toxigenicity

A key advance in the diagnosis of diphtheria is the use of polymerase chain reaction (PCR) to detect the toxin gene (Pallen 1991, Hauser et al. 1993, Aravena-Roman et al. 1995). Both Pallen and colleagues and Aravena-Roman and colleagues used the same primer set and found 100% correlation with PCR product detection and guinea pig lethality. Subsequent testing showed it to be useful for rapidly screening clinical *Corynebacterium* spp. isolates with a low (3%) rate of false positives (Pallen et al. 1994). Hauser and colleagues showed excellent correlation between amplification of a 0.9 kb segment of the *tox* gene, ADP-ribosylating activity and guinea pig lethality testing. Mikhailovitch et al. (1995) reported toxin detection by PCR and the standard immunoprecipitation assay (Elek test) (Elek 1949) correlated for all 250 tested isolates from the former Soviet Union. Using another set of primers complementary to sequences within the *tox* gene, Martinetti-Lucchini, Gruner and Altwegg (1992) found the PCR test more accurate than the Elek test when the guinea pig lethality assay was taken as the gold standard. This may be due to false positive precipitate lines in the Elek test. There is also the rare possibility of a false positive PCR assay due to the organism possessing the *tox* gene but without the ability to express it, still being non-toxigenic (Groman et al. 1983, Pallen et al. 1994).

In addition, *C. ulcerans* and *C. pseudotuberculosis* can possess the diphtheria *tox* gene whereas some clinical isolates of *C. diphtheriae* may not (Hauser et al. 1993, Hust et al. 1994, Pallen et al. 1994).

cally important non-diphtheria corynebacteria and other coryneform organisms has greatly increased. The description and relationships of these organisms is given in Volume 2 (see Volume 2, Chapter 25) and in an extensive review (Funke et al. 1997). The coryneform organisms as a group are distinguished from other gram-positive rods in that they have a higher percentage of the guanidine and cytosine bases in their DNA and have a more irregular cell shape, including the ability of some of them to branch. A major taxonomic subdivision within the coryneforms group is based on the organism's type of cell wall and cellular fatty acids (Bernard, Bellefeuille and Ewan (1991). *Corynebacterium*, *Actinomyces* and *Turicella* have primarily straight chained and *Brevibacterium*, *Dermabacter* and *Propionibacterium*, among others, have branched chain cellular fatty acids. Within the genus *Corynebacterium*, distinctions are made on the basis of phenotypic characteristics such as lipophilicity and carbohydrate, urease and nitrate reactions. More recently, 16S RNA sequence comparisons have been used to clarify the confusing situation caused by overlapping, sometimes incorrect and incomplete phenotypic descriptions. For example, Funke et al. (1996) have shown that most clinical isolates that have been called *Corynebacterium xerosis* are in fact *Corynebacterium amycolatum*; this should be kept in mind in the following discussion as the diseases ascribed to *C. xerosis* may actually be caused by *C. amycolatum*. A summary of recent name changes are given in Table 19.2.

The probable clinical significance of the non-diphtheria *Corynebacterium* spp. is dependent on the context in which the organism is isolated. Factors to be assessed include the presence and numbers of the organism in the original gram stain, the pathogenicity and relative numbers of other organisms from the culture, the presence of inflammatory cells and the number of specimens from which the organism is isolated. Even with these observations additional clinical information is often needed to differentiate contamination and colonization from infection.

The important species of non-diphtheritic corynebacteria, the diseases they cause, and their estimated relative importance are shown in Table 19.3. The following text attempts to integrate the newer definitions of species with disease; however, because of the continuing changes in the taxonomy of the organisms and the inadequate description in some literature, the clinical significance of a particular species may have to be revised in the future.

OTHER HUMAN CORYNEBACTERIAL AND CORYNEFORM INFECTIONS

8 INTRODUCTION

In recent years the number of defined groups of medi-

9 DESCRIPTION OF HUMAN DISEASES

9.1 Endocarditis and bacteraemia

Endocarditis, involving both native and prosthetic heart valves, is one of the more commonly reported diseases caused by non-diphtheria corynebacteria. Although all species of *Corynebacterium* may cause endocarditis, the most frequently isolated species are

Table 19.2 Recent taxonomic changes of clinically important coryneforms

Present designation	Former designation
C. afermentans subsp. *afermentans*	Some CDC group ANF-1
C. afermentans subsp. *lipophilum*	
T. otitidis	Some CDC group ANF-1
C. auris	CDC group ANF-1-like
C. propinquum	CDC group ANF-3
C. jeikeium	CDC group JK
C. urealyticum	CDC group D-2
C. glucurolyticum	Previously undescribed
C. accolens	Some CDC group G
C. macginleyi	Some CDC group G
C. amycolatum	Mistakenly most clinical *C. xerosis*, CDC group I2 and F2
C. argentoratense	Previously undescribed
Cellulomonas spp.	Some CDC group A
Microbacterium spp.	Some CDC group A
A. neuii subsp. *neuii*	CDC group 1
A. neuii subsp. *anitratus*	CDC group 1-like
A. bernardiae	CDC group 2
Dermabacter spp.	CDC group 3 and group 5
Brevibacterium casei, Brevibacterium spp.	CDC group B1 and B3

those that are normally found on the skin or in the respiratory tract and include *C. xerosis* (Roder and Frimodt-Moller 1990, Szabo, Lieberman and Lue 1990, Malik and Johar 1995), *Corynebacterium striatum* (Malanoski, Parker and Elipoulos 1992, Rufael and Cohn 1994), *Corynebacterium minutissimum* (Herschorn and Brucker 1985) and *Corynebacterium pseudodiphtheriticum* (Lindner, Hardy and Murphy 1986, Morris et al. 1986, Hatch 1991, Wilson and Shapiro 1992). These organisms are also associated with bacteraemia (Tumbarello et al. 1994). *Corynebacterium jeikeium*, which colonizes skin, particularly in the groin area, may cause endocarditis, often in an immunocompromised patient or those with an indwelling prosthesis (Jackman et al. 1987, Vanbosterhaut et al. 1989, Coyle and Lipsky 1990). *Corynebacterium urealyticum* is infrequently associated with endocarditis (Langs et al. 1988, Ena et al. 1991) and bacteraemia (Soriano et al. 1993). The bacteraemia may be subsequent to a colonized Hickman catheter (Wood and Pepe 1994) or renal transplant (Marshall, Routh and MacGowan 1987). Some genotypes of the lipophilic CDC group G have been associated with endocarditis (Quinn, Comaish and Pedlar 1991), including a fatal case of endocarditis (Austin and Hill 1983). Both *Corynebacterium afermentans* subsp. *lipophilum* and *Corynebacterium propinquum* have been reported to be the causative agent of prosthetic valve endocarditis (Petit et al. 1994, Sewell, Coyle and Funke 1995). As described above, both toxigenic and non-toxigenic *C. diphtheriae* can cause endocarditis.

Other coryneforms reported to cause endocarditis or septicaemia include *Arcanobacterium haemolyticum* (Alos, Barros and Gomez-Garces 1995), *Oerskovia*, '*Corynebacterium aquaticum*' and CDC group 4 (Funke et al. 1997). *Brevibacterium casei*, the most common

clinical isolate among the brevibacteria (Gruner, Pfyffer and von Graevenitz 1993, Gruner et al. 1994b), *Propionibacterium* spp. and *Dermabacter* spp. are common skin bacteria with isolation most often from blood cultures, sometimes associated with sepsis or endocarditis but also as a presumed contaminant (Bernard et al. 1994, Funke et al. 1994b, Gruner et al. 1994c).

Rothia dentocariosa, a member of the normal oral flora, can be a relatively common clinical isolate from oropharyngeal specimens. Although rarely reported as a pathogen, when it is, it is most often associated with endocarditis (Anderson et al. 1993, Weersink et al. 1994).

9.2 Respiratory infections

Some toxigenic strains of *C. ulcerans* can produce disease indistinguishable from diphtheria, as shown by its isolation from the pharyngeal membrane of a patient with laryngeal diphtheria (Hust et al. 1994), as well as less severe nasopharyngeal disease (de Carpentier et al. 1992). The other corynebacteria are only rarely primary pathogens. *C. striatum* (Barr and Murphy 1986, Cowling and Hall 1993, Leonard, Nowowiejski and Warren 1994, Peiris et al. 1994, Martinez-Martinez, Saurez and Ortega 1994), *C. xerosis* (Wallet, Marquette and Courcol 1995) and, rarely, *C. jeikeium* (Waters 1989) have been associated with pneumonia, usually after antibiotic treatment and mechanical ventilation. There can be nosocomial transmission of *C. striatum* with resulting pneumonia (Leonard, Nowowiejski and Warren 1994). Two recent cases of tracheitis and tracheobronchitis caused by *C. pseudodiphtheriticum* in immunocompromised patients have been well documented (Colt et al. 1991, Craig,

Table 19.3   Reported disease association of *Corynebacterium* spp. and other coryneform organisms

Disease and organism	Relative number of reports or strength of association
Endocarditis	
C. diphtheriae toxigenic	+
C. diphtheriae non-toxigenic	+++
C. ulcerans	+
C. xerosis[a]	++
C. striatum	++
C. minutissimum	++
C. macginleyi	+
CDC group G	+
C. afermentans subsp. lipophilum	+
C. jeikeium	++
C. urealyticum	+
C. propinquum	+
C. pseudodiphtheriticum	+++
Brevibacterium	+
Rothia	+++
Oerskovia	+
A. haemolyticum	+
Propionibacterium	+
Bacteraemia	
C. diphtheriae	+
C. xerosis[a]	++
C. striatum	++
C. minutissimum	++
CDC group G	+
C. jeikeium	+++
C. urealyticum	+
C. pseudodiphtheriticum	++
C. afermentans subsp. afermentans	+
'C. aquaticum'	++
Propionibacterium	++
Respiratory	
C. diphtheriae toxigenic	++++
C. diphtheriae non-toxigenic	++
C. ulcerans	+
C. pseudotuberculosis	+
C. xerosis[a]	+
C. striatum	++
C. amycolatum	Probable
C. minutissimum	+
C. argentoratense	+
C. afermentans subsp. lipophilum	+
C. jeikeium	+
C. pseudodiphtheriticum	+++
A. haemolyticum	++++
Urinary tract infection	
C. urealyticum	++++
C. glucuronolyticum	++
CDC group F-1	+
C. jeikeium	+
'C. aquaticum'	+

Macguire and Wallace 1991). Both cases revealed an inflammatory process partially occluding the tracheal lumen and essentially a pure culture of the organism from this material. *C. pseudodiphtheriticum* may also cause pneumonia in an immunointact host (Miller, Rompalo and Coyle 1986).

On rare occasions, *C. pseudotuberculosis* is isolated from humans. It may cause caseous lymphadenitis and

Table 19.3 Continued

Disease and organism	Relative number of reports or strength of association
Skin, ulcer, soft tissue, ostemyelitis	
C. diphtheriae	++++
C. ulcerans	++
C. minutissimum	+
C. jeikeium	++
C. urealyticum	+
A. haemolyticum	++++
Rothia	+
Propionibacterium	++
Infection of prostheses, colonization	
C. xerosis[a]	+++
C. striatum	+++
C. minutissimum	++
C. jeikeium	+++
C. urealyticum	+
C. propinquum	+
C. pseudodiphtheriticum	++
Ear, eye	
C. matruchotii	+
C. macginleyi	++
CDC group F-1	+
CDC group G	++
C. auris	+
Turicella	+

[a]As reported in the literature but may be other species, especially *C. amycolatum*.

pneumonia, particularly in individuals who are immunocompromised or have a close association with infected sheep or goats. Almost all of 12 reports of *C. pseudotuberculosis* infections in humans were cases of caseous lymphadenitis and involved exposure to animals, drinking raw milk, or handling hides (Goldberger, Lipsky and Plorde 1981, Lipsky et al. 1982, Richards and Hurse 1985, House et al. 1986). Recovery from infection required several weeks of antibiotic therapy with erythromycin or tetracycline and surgery. Localized adenopathy and hepatomegaly with fatigue and myalgia have also been reported (Lopez, Wong and Quesada 1966).

A. haemolyticum is associated primarily with pharyngitis, particularly in young adults (Gahrn-Hanson and Frederiksen 1992, Carlson and Kontainen 1994). Clinical significance has been difficult to assess because the organism can be isolated without disease and it is often isolated in association with β-haemolytic streptococci or other pathogens. In a study of 3922 throat cultures, *A. haemolyticum* was recovered from 0.5% of patients over all, but in 2% of those 15–25 years old. It was recovered with β-streptococci in about one-half these patients. Group A β-haemolytic streptococci were recovered as the sole pathogen in 16% of the patients (Carlson and Kontainen 1994). Similarily, MacKenzie et al. (1995), in a study of 11 620 throat cultures, found an incidence of 2.5% in the 15–18 years old group with pharyngitis, whereas there was no isolation of *A. haemolyticum* from healthy controls.

Although a rare cause of infections in healthy humans, *Rhodococcus equi* has become increasingly important as a pathogen of immunosuppressed humans, most commonly AIDS patients, but also those receiving corticosteroids. More than 70 cases of human *R. equi* infections have been reported, most of which involve the lungs and result in pulmonary abscesses (Lipsky et al. 1982, Van Etta et al. 1983, Coyle and Lipsky 1990, Emmons, Reichwein and Winslow 1991, Harvey and Sunstrum 1991, Prescott 1991). Symptoms include fever, fatigue and a chronic, non-productive cough. Cavitary lesions and necrotizing pneumonia due to *R. equi* may resemble infections caused by *Mycobacterium tuberculosis* or *Nocardia* (Brown 1995). Dissemination has also been reported to result in infections of the brain, paraspinal tissues, bone and skin (Prescott 1991) following bacteraemia. Patients usually have a history of contact with animals substantiating this agent as a zoonotic pathogen.

9.3 Urinary tract infection

C. urealyticum is the most important coryneform causing urinary tract infections (UTIs). Rates for significant isolations may vary from essentially zero to 3.5% for UTIs in non-selected populations (France: de Briel et al. 1991; South Africa: Walkden, Klugman and Vally 1993; UK: Marshall and Johnson 1990; USA: Ryan and Murray 1994; Spain: Nebreda-Mayoral et al. 1994).

Alkaline-encrusted cystitis is an ulcerative inflammation of the bladder in which localized ulcers are covered with deposits of struvite ($MgNH_4PO_4.6H_2O$) crystals (Soriano et al. 1985). Starting in 1985, Soriano and colleagues documented the causative role of *C. urealyticum* in alkaline-encrusted cystitis with the phenomenal ability of the organism to split urea, forming ammonia, raise the urine pH and contribute to stone formation as the pathogenic mechanism. The association of *C. urealyticum* with disease characterized by high urine pH, lithiasis and struvite crystals has been confirmed by other workers (de Briel et al. 1991, Nebreda-Mayeral et al. 1994). However, recovery of the organism from urine does not always signify UTI or may indicate less complicated disease (Soriano et al. 1990, de Briel et al. 1991, Nebreda-Mayeral et al. 1994). In a study comparing the recovery from urine of *C. urealyticum* and *C. jeikeium*, both noted for their high antimicrobial resistance, de Briel et al. found *C. urealyticum* was isolated more frequently at 10^5 colony-forming units ml^{-1} with significant disease, whereas *C. jeikeium* was associated with lower densities and less significant disease. They also found that although most patients with either *C. urealyticum* or *C. jeikeium* bacteriuria were positive for the corresponding organism in the inguinal area, none of a sample of healthy people harboured *C. urealyticum* whereas 39% harboured *C. jeikeium*. *C. urealyticum* can spontaneously disappear from urine in the absence of antibiotic therapy and persistent infection is associated with the use of ineffective broad spectrum antibiotics (de Briel et al. 1991). *C. urealyticum* bacteriuria occurs mainly in patients hospitalized for a long period, who are severely immunocompromised, urologically manipulated and elderly, but no deaths have been attributed to *C. urealyticum* (Soriano et al. 1990). *C. urealyticum* has also been associated with pyelonephritis (Aguado, Ponte and Soriano 1987), particularly in immunocompromised, post-renal-transplant patients with surgical complications (Marshall, Routh and MacGowan 1987, Aguado et al. 1993).

Corynebacterium glucuronolyticum (also described as 'Corynebacterium seminale') has been isolated from semen and the male genitourinary tract and may cause prostatitis or urethritis (Funke et al. 1995, Riegel et al. 1995b). It is a strong urease producer. CDC group F1, synonymous with some strains of *Corynebacterium pseudogenitalium* and also a urease producer, has been implicated as a urinary tract pathogen (Soriano and Ponte 1992).

9.4   Infections associated with prostheses, colonization and the compromised host

Corynebacteria are common commensals of human skin and it may be difficult to distinguish whether isolates are primary pathogens, secondary colonizers but pathogens, or merely contaminants. Overgrowth by many corynebacteria, particularly those that are resistant to antimicrobials, may occur after antimicrobial therapy. Infections associated with prostheses are most

frequently caused by organisms colonizing the skin. So-called *C. xerosis* has been associated most often with infections of prostheses such as cerebrospinal fluid (CSF) shunts and post-surgical wounds (Booth, Richards and Chandran 1991, Arisoy, Demmler and Dunne 1993, Lortholary et al. 1993, Wood 1993, Gaskin et al. 1994, King 1994). The rare occasions when *C. xerosis* is a primary pathogen occur in compromised patients (Vettese and Craig 1993). Although *C. striatum* is one of the most commonly isolated corynebacteria (Freney et al. 1991, Gavin et al. 1992), there are few reports unambiguously linking it with infection. In 3 recent reports of *C. striatum* infections (Watkins et al. 1993, Leonard, Nowowiejski and Warren 1994, Peiris et al. 1994), associations involved colonization of indwelling prostheses, feeding tubes or previous chronic wounds (draining elbow sinus, finger granuloma), or eye. *C. pseudodiphtheriticum* has been isolated from draining wounds (LaRocco, Robinson and Robinson 1987), probably as a secondary colonizer. Because of its high level of resistance to antimicrobials and occurrence as skin flora, *C. jeikeium* is one of the more commonly reported corynebacteria involved in infections associated with prostheses, including CSF shunt infections (Coyle and Lipsky 1990, Greene, Clark and Zabramski 1993). Other species found as skin flora and in this setting include *C. amycolatum* (Vanbosterhaut et al. 1989), *C. afermentans* subsp. *lipophilum* (Dealler, Malnick and Cammish 1993) and *C. minutissimum* (Cavendish, Coyle and Ohl 1994).

9.5   Eye and ear infections

C. macginleyi, formerly a portion of CDC group G, is associated with eye infections (Riegel et al. 1995a). *C. (Bacterionema) matruchotii* has also been reported as an isolate from the eye, but the identification schemes employed at that time were not optimum (Wilhelmus, Robinson and Jones 1979). *Turicella otitidis*, *Corynebacterium auris* and lipophilic coryneform bacteria (such as *C. afermentans*) have been isolated from the ear of some patients with otitis media, although a causal relationship is unclear (Funke et al. 1994a, Simonet et al. 1993).

9.6   Skin, soft tissue and other infections

Erythrasma is usually a mild, chronic, localized, superficial infection of the body folds and clefts characterized by well defined areas of dry and scaly or finely wrinkled skin. The scaly erythematous area fluoresces coral pink under long-wave ultraviolet light (Wood's light) due to the production of coproporphyrins. The aetiology and pathogenesis are unknown, but the reduction of bacterial numbers by means of parenteral or topical antibiotic treatment or the use of antibacterial soap results in resolution of the lesions. Although organisms called *C. minutissimum* have been cultured from the disease sites in increased numbers, their identification has not been confirmed by modern methods. In fact the reported fluorescence *of C.*

minutissimum when grown in rich media and viewed under a Wood's light has also not been confirmed (Funke et al. 1997). Erythrasma may be a polymicrobial process (Coyle and Lipsky 1990).

Non-toxigenic *C. ulcerans* has been associated with necrotic granulomas and pulmonary nodules in an immunocompetent host (Dessau et al. 1995). *C. minutissimum* can cause abscess formation. *C. jeikeium* is associated with skin and soft tissue infections and occasionally with meningitis and peritonitis, particularly in the compromised and previously treated host (Johnson, Hulse and Oppenheim 1992). *C. urealyticum* is an infrequent cause of osteomyelitis and wound infections (Soriano and Fernandez-Roblas 1988).

A. haemolyticum is also seen in wound infections. *A. haemolyticum* was isolated with *Fusobacterium* in a fulminant tubo-ovarian soft tissue infection (Batisse-Milton, Gander and Colvin 1995) and with *Staphylococcus* or *Haemophilus influenzae* in 2 cases of surgical wound infection (Esteban, Zapardiel and Soriano 1994). Traumatic wound infections involving *A. haemolyticum* and other organisms continue to be reported (Barker et al. 1992, Ritter et al. 1993).

Actinomyces pyogenes is primarily an animal pathogen, but human isolates associated with wound infections and septicaemia have been reported. However, because of the difficulties stated above, one must be careful in the identification method used before accepting all reports.

There are several organism–disease associations which have been reported but not yet confirmed by modern methods. *Corynebacterium mycetoides* is reported to be associated with tropical ulcers. Although occasionally reported as causing human disease, it is doubtful that the animal pathogens, *Corynebacterium bovis*, *Corynebacterium kutscheri* and *Corynebacterium renale* group were correctly identified (Funke et al. 1997).

10 EPIDEMIOLOGICAL STUDIES

Nosocomial spread of the non-diphtheria corynebacteria mediated through inanimate objects or caretaker hands has been shown, but not person-to-person dissemination of infection. Plasmid analysis, antibiograms and restriction fragment length polymorphism (RFLP) analysis of chromosomal DNA have been used to track strains of *C. jeikeium* (Khabbaz et al. 1986, Pitcher et al. 1990). These studies could not demonstrate that patient-to-patient transmission of *C. jeikeium* occurred. Khabbaz et al. (1986) found ribotyping was not effective as an epidemiological tool to relate urine or skin strain isolates to outbreak clusters.

11 LABORATORY ASPECTS

11.1 Culture and identification

Ambiguities in the taxonomy and definition of many of the *Corynebacterium* spp. and related coryneforms

have hampered appropriate organism identification and thus the disease–organism correlation. Although the use of whole cell fatty acid, the Coryne API strip (bioMérieux Vitek, Hazelwood, MO), cell wall analysis and classical biochemical methods allow microbiologists to correctly identify more fully the coryneform organisms, even with a large number of tests, clinical laboratories may be unable accurately to identify many isolates.

Most *Corynebacterium* spp. grow on blood agar at 35–37°C with or without CO_2 enrichment. Since colonies of some species are small at 24 h (often these are lipophilic or need serum or lipids for best growth), for optimal recovery of coryneform organisms from clinical specimens plates should be incubated for 48 h. Some have suggested that a better rate of isolation of *C. urealyticum* and *C. jeikeium* from potentially contaminated sites can be achieved using selective agar or CNA plates compared to sheep blood agar (SBA) plates (de Briel et al. 1991).

Because *Corynebacterium* organisms and some other coryneform organisms are a significant part of the normal flora of the skin and upper respiratory tract, distinguishing commensal from disease-associated organisms is a major problem. Care must be taken in collecting the specimen.

11.2 Antibiotic susceptibility

Corynebacteria have variable susceptibility patterns. *C. jeikeium* isolates are characteristically multiresistant to antibiotics (Riley, Hollis and Utter 1979, Jackman et al. 1987, Phillipon and Bimet 1990, Pitcher et al. 1990, Williams, Selepak and Gill 1993), but are susceptible to glycopeptide antibiotics and pristinamycin and show variable susceptibility to erythromycin, tetracycline, rifampicin and quinolones (Martinez-Martinez, Ortega and Saurez 1995). *C. urealyticum*, like *C. jeikeium*, is multiresistant to antibiotics, showing resistance to β-lactams and aminoglycosides and variable sensitivity to quinolones norfloxacin, erythromycin, rifampicin and tetracyclines (Aguado, Ponte and Soriano 1987, Vanbosterhaut et al. 1989, Phillipon and Bimet 1990, Soriano et al. 1990, de Briel et al. 1991, Aguado et al. 1993). This intrinsic resistance to antibiotics is thought to be chromosomal rather than plasmid associated (Khabbaz et al. 1986). Some of the newer quinolones were found to be effective in vitro against *C. urealyticum* strains (Martinez-Martinez, Saurez and Ortega 1994). It is less well known that some *C. amycolatum* (but called *C. xerosis*) are multiply resistant, i.e. resistant to β-lactam antibiotics, variably susceptible to aminoglycosides, tetracycline and quinolones, and uniformly susceptible only to vancomycin (Funke, Punter and von Graevenitz 1996). Many *C. striatum* isolates are resistant to the β-lactam antibiotics, but few show high level resistance (sensitive to vancomycin and netilmicin only, Peiris et al. 1994). An increasing number of isolates of CDC group G-1 and G-2, like those of *C. jeikeium* and *C. urealyticum*, are expressing multiresistance to common antibiotics (Williams, Selepak and Gill 1993).

ANIMAL INFECTIONS

12   INTRODUCTION

The *Corynebacterium* spp. of animals are common inhabitants of the skin, mucosal membranes (including conjunctiva), urogenital tract, and gastrointestinal tract. Many species recovered in clinical specimens are commensal isolates and are not well described. Most clinically significant *Corynebacterium* spp. of animals are recovered from livestock. However, occasional infections of companion animals also occur. This section will describe the well established diseases of animals that are caused by corynebacteria and related bacteria, such as *Rhodococcus* and *Eubacterium*. *Actinomyces pyogenes* is probably the most important coryneform isolated in veterinary clinical laboratories. *A. pyogenes* is reviewed elsewhere (see Volume 2, Chapter 20).

There are only a few true *Corynebacterium* spp. that have become established as pathogens of animals and cause specific clinical manifestations. These pathogens and other coryneform or coryneform-like bacteria also cause miscellaneous infections of animals. The coryneform bacteria, diseases with which they have been associated, the clinical presentation of these diseases, and the zoonotic potential of these bacteria for causing human disease are listed in Table 19.4.

13   CLINICAL MANIFESTATIONS

13.1   Caseous lymphadenitis and ulcerative lymphangitis

The aetiological agent of both these diseases, and occasionally other infections, is *C. pseudotuberculosis*, previously known as *Corynebacterium ovis* and Preisz–Nocard bacillus. In the host *C. pseudotuberculosis* is a facultative intracellular pathogen. The pathogenic factors associated with this organism include the exotoxin phospholipase D, which increases vascular permeability, necrosis, pulmonary oedema and shock (Hsu 1984); a heat-stable pyogenic toxin, which attracts leucocytes (Bull and Dickinson 1935); and a large amount of surface lipid ('corynomycolic acid'), which is toxic to phagocytic cells. The lipid is similar to mycolic acid of *Mycobacterium tuberculosis* and probably contributes to survival of the agent in the phagolysosome of phagocytic cells, the chronic nature of the disease, and dissemination to other body sites (Carne, Wickham and Kater 1956).

Caseous lymphadenitis (pseudotuberculosis) is prevalent in sheep and goats in many parts of the world and is characterized by suppuration and necrosis of affected lymph nodes. It is spread from animal to animal, or from a heavily infected environment (such as a resting area) to another animal. *C. pseudotuberculosis* can survive in the environment for extended periods, enhancing transmission. Transmission most commonly occurs when a skin abrasion

on one animal comes in contact with an open abscess on another animal, such as occurs during butting. Female goats and intact males are more commonly afflicted with abscesses than are castrated males and the incidence of abscesses increases with age (Ashfag and Campbell 1979). Pulmonary abscesses can result if *C. pseudotuberculosis* penetrates the buccal mucosa or is inhaled.

The disease begins as a wound infection with inflammation, and is often unnoticed. The agent migrates to the regional lymph node, which enlarges and fills with pus that is initially fluid-like, greenish and odourless, but later becomes thick and caseous, forming concentric, onion-like layers. Infected nodes may enlarge to as much as 10 cm in size.

Ulcerative lymphangitis occurs in horses and mules, usually on the fetlocks, indicating that skin abrasions are important in transmission of the disease. Seasonal incidence of these infections and 'pigeon fever' (see below) suggest that habronemiasis and dermatitis caused by the horn fly may contribute to transmission (Carter, Chengappa and Roberts 1995). Nodules arise and break down to form ulcers, which drain and exude a caseous green pus mixed with blood. The lesions can heal spontaneously, continue to progress for months or years or disseminate to various organs and extremities via the lymphatic system. Haematogenous dissemination may occur, and has been reported to result in abortion (Brumbaugh and Ekman 1981). Rarely, chronic, ulcerative lymphangitis may occur in cattle, buffalo, camels, deer, laboratory mice and other animals in the USA, Europe and Africa (Kariuki and Poulton 1982, Timoney et al. 1988a).

'Pigeon fever' due to *C. pseudotuberculosis* is not uncommon in horses in California. This disease is characterized by large, painful abscesses in the pectoral, lower abdominal and inguinal regions. The lesions typically develop slowly and sometimes recur following surgical drainage. General dissemination may also occur (Timoney et al. 1988a).

Due to the intracellular and chronic nature of *C. pseudotuberculosis* infections, cell mediated immunity is required for clearance of the organism once infection has become established. Killed, whole cell vaccines with various adjuvants are available and reduce the number and size of abscesses, but do not prevent disease (Cameron and Bester 1984, Menzies et al. 1991). Attenuated live vaccines may be required to provide optimum protection against disease (Ayers 1977).

13.2   Urinary tract infections

Infections of the urinary tract, which include cystitis, pyelonephritis and ureteritis that are due to the *C. renale* group of bacteria, occur primarily in cattle and less frequently in sheep and horses. The *C. renale* group includes *C. renale*, *C. pilosum* and *C. cystitidis*, previously known as *C. renale* types I, II and III, respectively. Each species can be distinguished biochemically (Collins and Cummins 1986). Each species is also a distinct antigenic type, which is based on the pilus antigen (Carter, Chengappa and Roberts 1995,

Table 19.4 Coryneforms associated with animals

Organism	Associated with disease	Zoonotic pathogen	Clinical presentation
C. pseudotuberculosis	Sheep, goats, horses; lymph nodes, skin, blood, internal organs	Yes	Abscesses, ulcers, bacteraemia, abortion, pneumonia
C. renale group	Cattle, sheep, horses, swine; urinary tract, kidneys	No	Cystitis, pyelonephritis, ureteritis, abscesses, posthitis
C. kutscheri	Mice, rats, less so guinea pigs; lungs, internal organs	Rare	Respiratory disease, caseous lesions of lungs abscesses of internal organs, septicaemia
C. bovis	Cattle; udder	Rare	Mastitis
C. ulcerans	Cattle; udder	?	Mastitis
R. equi	Horses (esp. foals), swine, sheep, cattle; respiratory tract, lymph nodes, uterus, GI tract, blood	Yes, esp. immunocompromised	Bronchopneumonia, abscesses, lymphangitis, enterocolitis, abortion, lesions of internal organs
C. xerosis[a]	Sheep and goats; urinary tract	?	Ulcerative balanoposthitis, vulvovaginitis, ulcers
C. striatum[a]	Cattle; udder	?	Mastitis
C. minutissimum[a]	Sheep; skin following wounds	?	Skin lesions
E. suis	Female pigs; urinary tract	No	Cystitis, pyelonephritis, haemorrhage
E. tarantellus	Mullets; brain	No	Neurological disease
E. tortuosum	Turkeys; liver, GI tract	No	Granulomas, enteritis

[a]Identification doubtful.
GI, gastrointestinal.

Timoney et al. 1988a). Most infections, particularly pyelonephritis, are caused by *C. renale* and occur in females. Kidney abscesses have also been reported in swine. *C. renale* has also caused osteomyelitis and disseminated infection in a goat without evidence of traumatic wounds, and with caseous lesions similar to those caused by *C. pseudotuberculosis* (Altmaier et al. 1994). Pyelonephritis in the bitch, and enzootic posthitis in castrated male sheep have been caused by *C. renale* and *C. pilosum* (Carter, Chengappa and Roberts 1995). *C. cystitidis* and *C. pilosum* also cause cystitis and pyelonephritis in cows. Although *C. renale* is the most common disease agent of the 3 species, it may also be found in healthy animals in diseased herds. *C. pilosum* occurs in the urine and vagina of up to 4% of healthy cows. By contrast, *C. cystitidis* is widely distributed, causes a more severe, haemorrhagic cystitis than the other species, and is never isolated from healthy cows. It is present on the prepuce of more than 90% of healthy bulls (Hiramune, Murase and Yanagawa 1970) and is transmitted as a venereal disease.

C. renale does not survive long in the environment. The bacteria are shed in the urine and transmission occurs through sexual contact, or when the vulva of a susceptible animal is exposed to infected urine (Timoney et al. 1988a). Bacterial pili, which are antigenically distinct between isolates, are required for adherence to vulvar epithelium (Hayashi, Yanagawa

and Kida 1985). *C. renale* is a strong producer of urease and the ammonia released from urea may be the cause of the inflammation in posthitis and other infections. Infections are ascending and affect the bladder, ureter(s) and one or both kidneys. Infected tissues become thickened and enlarged, with haemorrhage, necrosis and ulceration. Abscesses may be found throughout the kidneys.

Other coryneforms that have been associated with genitourinary tract disease such as ulcerative balanoposthitis and vulvovaginitis include *C. xerosis* (Trichard and Van Tonder 1994) and *Eubacterium suis* but often either the disease association or the identification has been questioned (Jones et al. 1986).

E. suis is a common cause of cystitis and pyelonephritis in breeding sows in Canada, Europe and Australia. Disease isolates in sows have also been reported from Norway, Denmark, Holland, Hong Kong, Switzerland, Malaysia, Germany, Brazil and the USA (Jones et al. 1992). Cystitis is the result of colonization and multiplication of *E. suis* in the bladder. The bacteria are heavily fimbriated, which may enable them to adhere to bladder epithelial cells (Larsen, Hogh and Hovind-Hougen 1986).

Haemorrhage may occur in the bladder mucosa, possibly due to the production of ammonia from urea, resulting in haematuria in acute cases. Non-specific clinical signs may include fever, anorexia, stiffness, arching of back, lameness and weight loss (Blood and Radostits 1989). Ascending infection from the vagina to the bladder occurs initially, and in addition to bacterial adherence, a short and wide urethra may be a factor for those animals that develop infection (Dee 1991). Continued ascending infection to the kidneys results in ureteritis and pyelonephritis. Advanced cases result in weight loss. Sudden death may occur within 12 h due to acute renal failure. In such cases clinical signs may not have been present (Blood and Radostits 1989). The urethra, bladder and ureters may have haemorrhagic or necrotic lesions.

13.3 Respiratory infections

Rhodococcus (*Corynebacterium*) *equi* was first reported as a cause of bronchopneumonia in foals by Magnusson in 1923 in Sweden (Barton and Hughes 1980). It is widely distributed throughout the world in horses and has also caused infections in swine, goats, sheep, cattle and in immunosuppressed humans (Barton and Hughes 1980). *R. equi* is commonly present in the soil, manure and intestines of horses, herbivorous animals and birds. It is very hardy, being relatively resistant to heat and to extremes in pH. Thus, it can survive for long periods in the soil and manure, which are the primary sources of new infections through direct contact, or probably more commonly, inhalation (Carter, Chengappa and Roberts 1995). There is correlation between the incidence of disease and the number of *R. equi* in the stable, but not the pasture (Prescott, Travers and Yager-Johnson 1984).

Normally, *R. equi* is an opportunistic pathogen. During infection, it is a facultative, intracellular parasite of phagocytic cells, particularly alveolar macrophages of horses. Disease primarily occurs in foals as a multifocal, caseonecrotic bronchopneumonia with large abscesses. Greyish-red pus may be present in bronchi and the pulmonary lymph nodes may have a purulent inflammation. Ulcerative enteritis, with focal necrosis and thickening of the intestinal tract, and mesenteric lymphangitis may also occur. Foals 1–5 months of age are usually infected. Disease onset is insidious and mortality may reach 64%. Rarely, ulcerative lymphangitis may occur in young horses, abscesses and arthritis in adult horses, and abortion in pregnant mares (Collett 1994).

The granulomatous nature of the lesions, and the capability of *R. equi* to survive intracellularly suggest that cell mediated immunity is critical for resistance to infection (Prescott, Johnson and Markham 1980). A surface component of *R. equi* has been reported to inhibit the bactericidal activity of polymorphonuclear leucocytes and macrophages (Ellenberger, Kaeberle and Roth 1984), which may account for the capability of the bacteria to survive in granulomatous lesions.

13.4 Pseudotuberculosis of laboratory rodents

C. kutscheri causes a caseous tuberculosis-like disease of the lungs and other organs of mice and rats, and

rarely guinea pigs. Infection has also been reported in voles (Collins and Cummins 1986). Although disease is infrequent, persistent subclinical infections are common in conventionally reared stocks of animals, but rare in barrier-maintained stocks. The bacteria reside in the oropharynx, submaxillary lymph nodes and large intestine. Transmission is by the faecal–oral route (Lindsey et al. 1991).

Disease usually occurs in animals that are immunocompromised due to experimental procedures, dietary deficiency, or concurrent infection with other organisms. Clinical disease in mice is usually characterized by signs of severe septicaemia; animals are often found dead or moribund. Septic emboli are found in many organs. Large emboli lodge in the capillary beds of the kidney and liver. Abscesses occur at the site of infection and other organs. Clinical disease in rats is usually restricted to respiratory infection and includes dyspnoea, râles, weight loss, humped posture and anorexia. Bacterial emboli lodge in the capillaries of the lungs. Large necrotic abscesses occur in the liver, kidneys, subcutis, peritoneal cavity and other sites.

Natural infection often develops after animals are treated with immunosuppressive agents, indicating that latent infections are common and that the cellular immune system probably plays an important role in host resistance.

13.5 Other diseases

C. pseudotuberculosis occasionally causes abortion in ewes and horses, and arthritis and bursitis in lambs. Experimental infection of lambs results in acute fatal infections and chronic infection with development of a carrier state (Girones et al. 1991). Pneumonia, hepatitis, mastitis, orchitis, subcutaneous abscesses, brain abscess and perinatal death have also been reported in sheep and goats (Ameh et al. 1993, Glass, DeLahunta and Jackson 1993, Collett, Bath and Cameron 1994). In Utah and Kenya, bronchopneumonia and skin-lesion tuberculosis due to *C. pseudotuberculosis* have been reported in cattle (Timoney et al. 1988a).

R. equi may cause abscess formation in dogs, cats, cattle and other animals.

C. bovis is considered a commensal of the skin and reproductive tracts of cows and bulls. Rarely, *C. bovis* may be a primary pathogen in mastitis outbreaks (Cobb and Walley 1962, Counter 1981). Overall, however, it is considered a minor mastitis pathogen, causing only minor udder infections. It occurs most commonly in herds where post-milking teat dipping is not practised (du Preez and Giesecke 1994).

Many of the coryneform bacteria that have been isolated from animal specimens are poorly described. They have often been identified based on their microscopic appearance and a few biochemical tests. Therefore the following summary is at best preliminary. *C. minutissimum* has been isolated from wounds of lambs after docking. It has also been isolated from scabs on the brisket and from inflamed interdigital spaces

(Carter, Chengappa and Roberts 1995). As a common commensal of the skin, it is probably present in these lesions as a secondary, opportunistic pathogen. *C. ulcerans* is an uncommon cause of infections in cattle (Ameh, Addo and Hart 1984) and is usually recovered as a pathogen from cases of bovine mastitis. However, it may also be recovered as a commensal in cattle, as well as horses, and therefore its isolation as a pathogen must be proven. *Corynebacterium* spp. have been recovered from 4% of bacteraemic dogs and are not uncommon isolates of dogs with endocarditis of the aortic valve or with pleural infections (Sisson and Thomas 1984). However, the identification of these agents to species level is usually not completed.

Bolo disease is a subacute to chronic, mild dermatitis of wooled sheep caused by an unclassified *Corynebacterium* species (Colly and Lange 1994). The disease is characterized by dark-grey to black discoloration of wool covering affected areas of skin. The species of *Corynebacterium* responsible for Bolo disease has not been identified. Therefore, it has not been confirmed that this disease is caused by a true member of the genus *Corynebacterium*. However, application of the isolated agent to the skin of sheep can reproduce the disease clinically and histopathologically (Colly and Lange 1994).

Eubacterium tarantellus has been isolated from the brains of dead or moribund striped mullet in Biscayne, Florida, that have evidence of neurological disease (Collins and Cummins 1986). *Eubacterium tortuosum* is believed to be the causative agent of turkey liver granulomas and has also been isolated from the faeces of turkeys with enteritis.

14 LABORATORY ASPECTS

14.1 Culture and identification

Isolation of the animal pathogenic coryneforms, *C. pseudotuberculosis*, *C. renale* group, *C. kutscheri* and *R. equi*, is readily accomplished on blood agar under normal atmospheric conditions. *E. suis* grows best under anaerobic conditions.

C. pseudotuberculosis is distinctive as it forms small, translucent colonies that develop a cream to orange colour, and later form dry, scaly, haemolytic colonies on blood agar. The colonies inhibit the activity of the staphylococcal β-toxin (reverse Christie–Atkins–Munch-Petersen [CAMP] test), but cause synergistic haemolysis with *R. equi* (positive CAMP test) (Carter, Chengappa and Roberts 1995). *C. renale* colonies initially are small and dewdrop in shape and later form large moist opaque yellowish colonies. *C. cystitidis* colonies tend to remain small and whitish; growth occurs at 41.5°C. *C. pilosum* colonies are also small, but a pale yellow, and no growth occurs at 41.5°C. Each species can be differentiated by production of acid from xylose and starch: *C. cystitidis* is positive for both reactions, *C. renale* is negative for both reactions, and *C. pilosum* produces acid from starch only (Carter, Chengappa and Roberts 1995).

C. kutscheri colonies are yellow-white and become 1–4 mm in size after 48 h of incubation on blood agar. This species is urease-positive and ferments maltose and sucrose (Carter, Chengappa and Roberts 1995).

Although *C. bovis* has a typical coryneform appearance on gram stain, it is substantially different from other corynebacteria and will probably be transferred to another genus (Carter, Chengappa and Roberts 1995). Colonies are grey, slightly raised and dry. It is lipophilic (containing short-chain mycolic acids and tuberculostearic acid) and grows best on medium enriched with unsaturated, long-chain fatty acids (Collins and Cummins 1986). It grows well on blood agar, particularly the areas containing milk inoculum. *C. bovis* gives variable results for urease, glucose utilization and pyrazinamidase; it is negative in most other biochemical tests.

Key biochemical characteristics for some coryneforms are described here. However, they are not sufficient for confirmed identification and are given in more detail in Volume 2, Chapter 25. For example, the human pathogen *Corynebacterium glucurolyticum* might be confused with *C. renale*. Therefore it is recommended that if the disease–organism link is important (e.g. for publication), a more comprehensive set of tests such as on the Coryne API system be documented. For correct identification, new taxonomic charts must be consulted (Funke et al. 1997).

R. equi grows on blood agar and forms mucoid, spreading colonies, which become pink after 3–4 days of growth. *R. equi* is catalase- and urease-positive and cannot ferment carbohydrates. A selective medium containing nalidixic acid, novobiocin, cycloheximide and potassium tellurite (NANAT) is useful for epidemiology and for isolating the organism from contaminated samples. Colonies of *R. equi* on this medium are black (Woolcock, Multimer and Farmer 1980). A presumptive diagnosis can be made for *R. equi* based on a gram-stained smear of specimens from caseous bronchopneumonia. Large, gram-positive, pleomorphic, coccobacilli, rather than rod shapes, are presumptive evidence of *R. equi* infection. A partially positive acid-fast stain is also a valuable aid to presumptive identification.

E. suis grows best under anaerobic conditions at 37°C, but limited growth occurs in air. Colonies are tiny and shiny after 24 h, enlarge to about 3 mm after 48 h and are flat and grey matte in appearance. Acid is produced from arabinose, xylose and maltose (Timoney et al. 1988a).

14.2 Serology

Serological tests are often highly useful for the diagnosis of diseases caused by *C. pseudotuberculosis*. A large study using a double-antibody ELISA and the exotoxin as antigen has been shown to have a sensitivity and specificity near 100%. In addition, an immunoblot assay using major proteins of *C. pseudotuberculosis* was able to clarify inconclusive test results (ter Laak et al. 1992). Skalka and Literak (1994) reported that the agar gel immunodiffusion test and the toxin neutralization test were useful screening tests for *C. pseudotuberculosis* in herds. In their study, 34.7% of 228 sheep with no clinical evidence of caseous lymphadenitis were serologically positive for antibody to phospholipase D, indicating carriers and chronic infection in sheep are relatively common. Antibodies to *R. equi* can be measured by a variety of assays, including complement fixation, ELISA and agglutination tests. Antibodies are passively transferred from mares to their foals (Timoney et al. 1988b). However, the immune response of foals to *R. equi* may be very poor in both infected animals and those vaccinated with bacterins. It is possible that this poor immune response is due to inhibition by passively acquired antibody, and due to the polysaccharide capsule, which may in itself be poorly immunogenic in young animals. The antibody response to *C. kutscheri* subclinical infections is generally poor, although a serum agglutination test and ELISA test have been used for screening carrier animals (Ackerman, Fox and Murphy 1984, Lindsey et al. 1991, Park et al. 1993). Screening of mice from 3 commercial breeders using the serum agglutination test showed that 5–23% of animals were seropositive (Park et al. 1993).

Immunofluorescent microscopy has been used for rapid confirmatory diagnosis of *E. suis* (Jones et al. 1992).

14.3 Antibiotic susceptibility

C. pseudotuberculosis is sensitive to penicillin, cephalosporins and tetracyclines, but the use of these antibiotics is generally ineffective in established infections because the drugs cannot penetrate abscessed material or enter phagocytic cells.

Synergistic antibiotic therapy for *R. equi* infections can be obtained with a combination of gentamicin and penicillin G, or erythromycin and rifampicin (Prescott and Nicholson 1984). Lincomycin and gentamicin have been reported to be most successful in cats (Elliot, Lawson and Mackenzie 1986). *R. equi* is also susceptible to doxycycline, lincomycin, neomycin and streptomycin (Woolcock and Multimer 1980). Other antibiotics that concentrate intracellularly may also be useful (i.e. clindamycin, clarithromycin, azithromycin, and trimethoprim–sulphamethoxazole) (Brown 1995).

C. bovis isolates are sensitive to erythromycin and rifampicin and of variable sensitivity to penicillins (Brown 1995).

E. suis is sensitive to penicillins, tetracyclines and others. The culling of infected boars is not practical because the colonization rate is so high. During outbreaks control of disease is best accomplished by the prophylactic use of antibiotics and artificial insemination. Antibiotics are effective at eliminating the disease, but recurrence is common.

REFERENCES

Ackerman JI, Fox JG, Murphy JC, 1984, An enzyme linked immunosorbent assay for detection of antibodies to *Corynebacterium kutscheri*, *Lab Anim Sci*, **34**: 38–43.

Afghani B, Stutman HR, 1993, Bacterial arthritis caused by *Corynebacterium diphtheriae*, *Pediatr Infect Dis J*, **12**: 881–2.

Aggerbeck H, Heron I, 1991, Improvement of a Vero cell assay to determine diphtheria antitoxin content in sera, *Biologicals*, **19**: 71–6.

Aguado J, Ponte C, Soriano F, 1987, Bacteriuria with a multiply resistant species of *Corynebacterium* (*Corynebacterium* group D2): an unnoticed cause of urinary tract infection, *J Infect Dis*, **156**: 144–50.

Aguado J, Morales J et al., 1993, Encrusted pyelitis and cystitis by *Corynebacterium urealyticum* (CDC group D2): new and threatening complication following renal transplant, *Transplantation*, **56**: 617–22.

Alos JI, Barros C, Gomez-Garces JL, 1995, Endocarditis caused by *Arcanobacterium haemolyticum*, *Eur J Clin Microbiol Infect Dis*, **14**: 1085–8.

Altmaier KR, Sherman DM et al., 1994, Osteomyelitis and disseminated infection caused by *Corynebacterium renale* in a goat, *J Am Vet Med Assoc*, **204**: 934–7.

Ameh JA, Addo PB, Hart RJC, 1984, *Corynebacterium ulcerans* in humans and cattle in North Devon, *J Hyg*, **92**: 161–4.

Ameh JA, Addo PB et al., 1993, Prevalence of clinical mastitis and of intramammary infections in Nigerian goats, *Prev Vet Med*, **17**: 41–6.

Anderson MD, Kennedy CA et al., 1993, Prosthetic valve endocarditis due to *Rothia dentocariosa*, *Clin Infect Dis*, **17**: 945–6.

Anonymous, 1993, *Proceedings of the Meeting on the Diphtheria Epidemic in Europe*, Foundation Marcel Merieux and the World Health Organization, 1–32.

Aravena-Roman M, Bowman R, O'Neal G, 1995, Polymerase chain reaction for the detection of toxigenic *Corynebacterium diphtheriae*, *Pathology*, **27**: 71–3.

Arisoy ES, Demmler GJ, Dunne WMJ, 1993, *Corynebacterium xerosis* ventriculoperitoneal shunt infection in an infant: a report of a new case and review of the literature, *Pediatr Infect Dis J*, **12**: 536–8.

Ashfag MK, Campbell SG, 1979, A survey of caseous lymphadenitis and its etiology in goats in the United States, *Vet Med/Small Anim Clin*, **74**: 1161–5.

Austin G, Hill E, 1983, Endocarditis due to *Corynebacterium* CDC group G2, *J Infect Dis*, **147**: 1106.

Ayers JL, 1977, Caseous lymphadenitis in goats and sheep: a review of diagnosis, pathogenesis, and immunity, *J Am Vet Med Assoc*, **171**: 1251–4.

Barker KF, Renton NE et al., 1992, *Arcanobacterium haemolyticum* wound infection, *J Infect*, **24**: 214–15.

Barksdale L, Garmise L, Horibata K, 1960, Virulence, toxinogeny and lysogeny in *Corynebacterium diphtheriae*, *Ann N Y Acad Sci*, **88**: 1093.

Barr JG, Murphy PG, 1986, *Corynebacterium striatum*: an unusual organism isolated in pure culture from sputum, *J Infect*, **13**: 297–8 [Letter].

Barton MD, Hughes KL, 1980, *Corynebacterium equi*: a review, *Vet Bull*, **50**: 65–80.

Batisse-Milton SE, Gander RM, Colvin DD, 1995, Tubo-ovarian and peritoneal effusion caused by *Arcanobactericum haemolyticum*, *Clin Microbiol Newslett*, **17**: 118–20.

Begg N, 1994, *Manual for the Management and Control of Diphtheria in the European Region*, Expanded Programme on Immunization WHO European Region, Copenhagen, 1–29.

von Behring E, Kitasato A, 1890, *Dtsch Med Wochenschr*, **16**: 1113, 1145.

Belsey MA, 1970, Isolation of *Corynebacterium diphtheriae* in the environment of skin carriers, *Am J Epidemiol*, **91**: 294–9.

Belsey MA, LeBlanc DR, 1975, Skin infections and the epidemiology of diphtheria: acquisition and persistence of *C. diphtheriae* infections, *Am J Epidemiol*, **102:** 179–84.

Belsey MA, Sinclair M et al., 1969, *Corynebacterium diphtheriae* skin infections in Alabama and Louisiana. A factor in the epidemiology of diphtheria, *N Engl J Med*, **280:** 135–41.

Bennett MJ, Eisenberg D, 1994, Refined structure of monomeric diphtheria toxin at 2.3 A resolution, *Protein Sci*, **3:** 1464–75.

Bernard K, Bellefeuille M, Ewan EP, 1991, Cellular fatty acid composition as an adjunct to the identification of asporogenous, aerobic gram-positive rods, *J Clin Microbiol*, **29:** 83–9.

Bernard K, Bellefeiulle M et al., 1994, Cellular fatty acid composition and phenotypic and cultural characterization of CDC fermentative coryneform groups 3 and 5, *J Clin Microbiol*, **32:** 1217–22.

Blood DC, Radostits OM, 1989, *Veterinary Medicine*, 7th edn, WB Saunders, London, Philadelphia, 573–82.

Booth LV, Richards RH, Chandran DR, 1991, Septic arthritis caused by *Corynebacterium xerosis* following vascular surgery, *Rev Infect Dis*, **13:** 548–9.

Boyd J, Oza MN, Murphy HR, 1990, Molecular cloning and DNA sequence analysis of a diphtheria *tox* iron-dependent regulatory element (dtxR) from *Corynebacterium diphtheriae*, *Proc Natl Acad Sci USA*, **87:** 5968–72.

Bretonneau P, 1826, *Des Inflammations Spéciales du Tissu Muqueux, et en Particulier de la Diphthérite ou Inflammation Pelliculaire, connue sous le Nom de Croup, d'Angine Maligne, d'Angine Gangreneuse, etc.*, Crevot, Paris.

Brooks GF, Bennett JV, Feldman RA, 1974, Diphtheria in the United States, 1959–1970, *J Infect Dis*, **129:** 172–8.

Brown AE, 1995, *Principles and Practice of Infectious Diseases*, 4th edn, Churchill Livingstone, New York, 1872–80.

Brumbaugh GW, Ekman TL, 1981, *Corynebacterium pseudotuberculosis* bacteremia in two horses, *J Am Vet Med Assoc*, **178:** 300–1.

Bull LB, Dickinson CG, 1935, Studies on infection by and resistance to Preisz–Nocard bacillus, *Aust Vet*, **11:** 6–138.

Butterworth A, Abbott JD et al., 1974, Diphtheria in the Manchester area 1967–1971, *Lancet*, **2:** 1558–61.

Camargo ME, Silveira L et al., 1984, Immunoenzymatic assay of anti-diphtheric toxin antibodies in human serum, *Clin Microbiol*, **20:** 772–4.

Cameron CM, Bester FJ, 1984, An improved *Corynebacterium pseudotuberculosis* vaccine for sheep, *Onderstepoort J Vet Res*, **51:** 263–7.

Carlson P, Kontainen S, 1994, Alpha-mannosidase: a rapid test for identification of *Arcanobacterium haemolyticum*, *J Clin Microbiol*, **32:** 854–5.

Carne HR, Wickham N, Kater JC, 1956, A toxic lipid from the surface of *Corynebacterium ovis*, *Nature (London)*, **178:** 701–2.

de Carpentier JP, Flanagan PM et al., 1992, Nasopharyngeal *Corynebacterium ulcerans*: a different diphtheria, *J Laryngol Otol*, **106:** 824–6.

Carter GR, Chengappa MM, Roberts AW, 1995, *Essentials of Veterinary Microbiology*, 5th edn, Williams & Wilkins, Baltimore, 121–6.

Caulfield E, 1939, A true history of the terrible epidemic vulgarly called the throat distemper: which occurred in His Majesty's New England colonies between the years 1735 and 1740, *Yale J Biol Med*, **11:** 219–77.

Cavendish J, Coyle JB, Ohl CA, 1994, Polymicrobial central venous catheter sepsis involving a multiantibiotic-resistant strain of *Corynebacterium minutissimum*, *Clin Infect Dis*, **19:** 204–5.

Cellesi C, Zanchi A et al., 1989, Immunity to diphtheria in a sample adult population from central Italy, *Vaccine*, **7:** 417–20.

Centers for Disease Control and Prevention, 1993a, Diphtheria outbreak – Russian Federation, 1990–1993, *Morbid Mortal Weekly Rep*, **42:** 840–7.

Centers for Disease Control and Prevention, 1993b, Diphtheria, *Epidemiology, Prevention and Control of Vaccine Preventable Diseases*, US Department of Health and Human Services, Atlanta, GA, 3:1–3:10.

Centers for Disease Control and Prevention, 1995a, Diphtheria epidemic – New Independent States of the former Soviet Union, 1990–1994, *Morbid Mortal Weekly Rep*, **44:** 177–81.

Centers for Disease Control and Prevention, 1995b, Recommended childhood immunization schedule, *Morbid Mortal Weekly Rep*, **43:** 51–2.

Chen RT, Broome CV et al., 1985, Diphtheria in the United States, 1971–81, *Am J Public Health*, **75:** 1393–7.

Choe S, Bennett MJ et al., 1992, The crystal structure of diphtheria toxin, *Nature (London)*, **357:** 216–22.

Christenson B, Hellstrom L, Aust-Kettis A, 1989, Diphtheria in Stockholm, with a theory concerning transmission, *J Infect*, **19:** 177–83.

Cobb RW, Walley JK, 1962, *Corynebacterium bovis* as a probable cause of bovine mastitis, *Vet Rec*, **74:** 101–2.

Cohen D, Katzenelson E et al., 1991, Prevalence and correlates of diphtheria toxin antibodies among young adults in Israel, *J Infect*, **23:** 117–21.

Collett MG, 1994, *Eubacterium suis* infections, *Infectious Diseases of Livestock*, eds Coetzer JAW, Thompson GR, Tustin RC, Oxford University Press, Cape Town/Oxford, 1416–18.

Collett MG, Bath GF, Cameron CM, 1994, *Corynebacterium pseudotuberculosis* infections, *Infectious Diseases of Livestock*, eds Coetzer JAW, Thompson GR, Tustin RC, Oxford University Press, Cape Town/Oxford, 1387–95.

Collins MD, Cummins CS, 1986, Genus *Corynebacterium* Lehmann and Newmann 1896, *Bergey's Manual of Systematic Bacteriology*, vol. 2, eds Sneath PHA, Mair NS et al., Williams & Wilkins, Baltimore, 1266–75.

Colly PA, Lange AL, 1994, Bolo disease, *Infectious Diseases of Livestock*, Oxford University Press, Cape Town/Oxford, 1399–401.

Colt HG, Morris JF et al., 1991, Necrotizing tracheitis caused by *Corynebacterium pseudodiphtheriticum*: unique case and review, *J Infect Dis*, **13:** 73–6.

Committee on Infectious Diseases, 1994, Diphtheria, *1994 Red Book: Report of the Committee on Infectious Diseases*, 23rd edn, American Academy of Pediatrics, Elk Grove Village, IL, 177.

Counter DE, 1981, Outbreak of bovine mastitis associated with *Corynebacterium bovis*, *Vet Rec*, **108:** 560–1.

Cowling P, Hall L, 1993, *Corynebacterium striatum*: a clinically significant isolate from sputum in chronic obstructive airways disease, *J Infect*, **26:** 335–6.

Coyle MB, Lipsky BA, 1990, Coryneform bacteria in infectious diseases: clinical and laboratory aspects, *Clin Microbiol Rev*, **3:** 227–46.

Coyle MB, Groman NB et al., 1989, The molecular epidemiology of the three biotypes of *Corynebacterium diphtheriae* in the Seattle outbreak, 1972–1982, *J Infect Dis*, **159:** 670–9.

Craig TJ, Macguire FE, Wallace MR, 1991, Tracheonchitis due to *Corynebacterium pseudodiphtheriticum*, *South Med J*, **84:** 504–6.

Creighton C, 1965, *A History of Epidemics in Britain*, vol. 2, 2nd edn, Frank Cass and Co., London.

Crosbie WE, Wright HD, 1941, Diphtheria bacilli in floor dust, *Lancet*, **1:** 656–9.

De Zoysa A, Efstratiou A et al., 1995, Molecular epidemiology of *Corynebacterium diphtheriae* from northwestern Russia and surrounding countries studied by using ribotyping and pulsed-field gel electrophoresis, *J Clin Microbiol*, **33:** 1080–3.

Dealler S, Malnick H, Cammish D, 1993, Intravenous line infection caused by *Corynebacterium* CDC group ANF-1, *J Hosp Infect*, **23:** 319–20.

Dee SA, 1991, Diagnosing and controlling urinary tract infections caused by *Eubacterium suis* in swine, *Vet Med*, **86:** 231–8.

Dessau RB, Brandt-Christensen M et al., 1995, Pulmonary nodules due to *Corynebacterium ulcerans*, *Eur Respir J*, **8:** 651–3.

Dixon JMS, 1984, Diphtheria in North America, *J Hyg Camb*, **93:** 419–32.

Dixon JMS, Noble WC, Smith GR, 1990, Diphtheria; other corynebacterial and coryneform infections, *Topley and*

Wilson's Principles of Bacteriology, Virology and Immunity, vol. 3, 8th edn, eds Parker MT, Collier LH, Edward Arnold/BC Decker, London/Philadelphia, 56–79.

Dolman CE, 1973, Landmarks and pioneers in the control of diphtheria, *Can J Public Health*, **64**: 317–36.

Edward DG, Allison VD, 1951, Diphtheria in the immunized with observations on diphtheria-like disease associated with nontoxigenic strains of *Corynebacterium diphtheriae*, *J Hyg Camb*, **49**: 205–19.

Efstratiou A, George RC, Begg NT, 1993, Non-toxigenic *Corynebacterium diphtheriae* var. gravis in England, *Lancet*, **341**: 1592–3.

Efstratiou A, Maple PAC, 1994, *Manual for the Laboratory Diagnosis of Diphtheria*, No. ICP-EPI 038(C), World Health Organization, Geneva, 1–82.

Efstratiou A, Tiley SM et al., 1993, Invasive disease caused by multiple clones of *Corynebacterium diphtheriae*, *Clin Infect Dis*, **17**: 136.

Elek SD, 1949, The plate virulence test for diphtheria, *J Clin Pathol*, **2**: 250–8.

Ellenberger MA, Kaeberle ML, Roth JA, 1984, Effect of *Rhodococcus equi* on equine polymorphonuclear leukocyte function, *Vet Immunol Immunopathol*, **7**: 315–24.

Elliot G, Lawson GH, Mackenzie CP, 1986, *Rhodococcus equi* infection of cats, *Vet Rec*, **118**: 693–4.

Emmons W, Reichwein B, Winslow DL, 1991, *Rhodococcus equi* infection in the patient with AIDS: literature review and report of a case, *Rev Infect Dis*, **13**: 91–6.

Ena J, Berenguer J et al., 1991, Endocarditis caused by *Corynebacterium* group D2, *J Infect*, **22**: 95.

Esteban J, Zapardiel J, Soriano F, 1994, Two cases of soft-tissue infection caused by *Arcanobacterium haemolyticum*, *Clin Infect Dis*, **18**: 835–6.

Farizo KM, Strebel PM et al., 1993, Fatal respiratory disease due to *Corynebacterium diphtheriae*: case report and review of guidelines for management, investigation and control, *Clin Infect Dis*, **16**: 59–68A.

Fischer GW, 1982, Diphtheria, *Infections in Children*, Harper & Row, Philadelphia, 652–61.

Freney J, Duperron MT et al., 1991, Evaluation of API Coryne in comparison with conventional methods for identifying coryneform bacteria, *J Clin Microbiol*, **29**: 38–41.

Frost WH, 1928, Infection, immunity and diseases in epidemiology of diphtheria, with special references to some studies in Baltimore, *J Prev Med*, **2**: 325–43.

Funke G, Punter V, von Graevenitz A, 1996, Antimicrobial susceptibility patterns of some recently defined coryneform bacteria, *Antimicrob Agents Chemother*, **40**: 2874–8.

Funke G, Stubbs S et al., 1994a, *Turicella otitidis* gen. nov. sp. nov., a coryneform bacterium isolated from patients with otitis media, *J Syst Bacteriol*, **44**: 270–3.

Funke G, Stubbs S et al., 1994b, Characteristics of CDC group 3 and group 5 coryneform bacteria isolated from clinical specimens and assignment to the genus *Dermabacter*, *J Clin Microbiol*, **32**: 1223–8.

Funke G, Bernard KA et al., 1995, *Corynebacterium glucuronolyticum* sp. nov. isolated from male patients with genitourinary infections, *Med Microbiol Lett*, **4**: 204–15.

Funke G, Lawson PA et al., 1996, Most *Corynebacterium xerosis* strains identified in the routine clinical laboratory correspond to *Corynebacterium amycolatum*, *J Clin Microbiol*, **34**: 1124–8.

Funke G, von Graevenitz A et al., 1997, Clinical microbiology of coryneform bacteria, *Clin Microbiol Rev*, in press.

Gahr-Hansen B, Frederiksen W, 1992, Human infections with *Actinomyces pyogenes* (*Corynebacterium pyogenes*), *Diagn Microbiol Infect Dis*, **15**: 349–54.

Galazka AM, Kardymowicz B, 1989, Immunity against diphtheria among adults in Poland, *Epidemiol Infect*, **103**: 587–93.

Galazka AM, Robertson SE, 1995, Diphtheria: changing patterns in the developing world and the industrialized world, *Eur J Epidemiol*, **11**: 107–17.

Galazka AM, Robertson SE, Oblapenko GP, 1995, Resurgence of diphtheria, *Eur J Epidemiol*, **11**: 95–105.

Gaskin PR, St John MA et al., 1994, Cerebrospinal fluid shunt infection due to *Corynebacterium xerosis*, *J Infect*, **28**: 323–5.

Gavin SE, Leonard RB et al., 1992, Evaluation of the Rapid CORYNE identification system for *Corynebacterium* species and other coryneforms, *J Clin Microbiol*, **30**: 1692–5.

Girones O, Simon MC et al., 1991, Experimental demonstration of the clinical and epidemiological effects of *Corynebacterium pseudotuberculosis ovis* infection in breeding ewes and newborn lambs, *Med Vet*, **8**: 490–503.

Glass EN, DeLahunta A, Jackson C, 1993, Brain abscess in a goat, *Cornell Vet*, **83**: 275–82.

Goldberger AC, Lipsky BA, Plorde JJ, 1981, Suppurative granulomatous lymphadenitis caused by *Corynebacterium ovis* (*pseudotuberculosis*), *Am J Clin Pathol*, **76**: 486–90.

Goldie W, Maddock ECG, 1943, A milk-borne outbreak of diphtheria, *Lancet*, **1**: 285–6.

Gradon JD, Mayrer AR, Hayes J, 1993, *Corynebacterium diphtheriae* endocarditis in France, *Clin Infect Dis*, **17**: 1072.

Greene K, Clark R, Zabramski J, 1993, Ventricular CSF shunt infections associated with *Corynebacterium jeikeium*: report of three cases and review, *Clin Infect Dis*, **16**: 139–41.

Greenfield L, Bjorn MJ et al., 1983, Nucleotide sequence of the structural gene for diphtheria toxin carried by corynebacteriophage beta, *Proc Natl Acad Sci USA*, **80**: 6853–7.

Groman N, Cianciotto N et al., 1983, Detection and expression of DNA homologous to the *tox* gene in nontoxinogenic isolates of *Corynebacterium diphtheriae*, *Infect Immun*, **42**: 48–56.

Gruner E, Pfyffer GE, von Graevenitz A, 1993, Characterization of *Brevibacterium* spp. from clinical specimens, *J Clin Microbiol*, **31**: 1408–12.

Gruner E, Zuber PLF et al., 1992, A cluster of non-toxigenic *Corynebacterium diphtheriae* infections among Swiss intravenous drug abusers, *Med Microbiol Lett*, **1**: 160–7.

Gruner E, Opravil M et al., 1994a, Nontoxigenic *Corynebacterium diphtheriae* isolated from intravenous drug users, *Clin Infect Dis*, **18**: 94–6.

Gruner E, Steigerwalt AG et al., 1994b, Human infections caused by *Brevibacterium casei*, formerly CDC groups B-1 and B-3, *J Clin Microbiol*, **32**: 1511–18.

Gruner E, Steigerwalt A et al., 1994c, Recognition of *Dermabacter hominis*, formerly CDC fermentative coryneform group 3 and group 5 as a potential human pathogen, *J Clin Microbiol*, **32**: 1918–22.

Gupta RK, Higham S et al., 1994, Suitability of the Vero cell method for titration of diphtheria antitoxin in the United States potency test for diphtheria toxoid, *Biologicals*, **22**: 65–72.

Hamour AA, Efstratiou A et al., 1995, Epidemiology and molecular characterisation of toxigenic *Corynebacterium diphtheriae* var. *mitis* from a case of cutaneous diphtheria in Manchester, *J Infect*, **31**: 153–7.

Hardy IR, Dittmann S, Sutter RW, 1996, Current situation and control strategies for resurgence of diphtheria in newly independent states of the former Soviet Union, *Lancet*, **347**: 1739–44.

Harnisch JP, Tronca E et al., 1989, Diphtheria among alcoholic urban adults – a decade of experience in Seattle, *Ann Intern Med*, **111**: 71–82.

Harvey RL, Sunstrum JC, 1991, *Rhodococcus equi* infection in patients with and without human immunodeficiency virus infection, *Rev Infect Dis*, **13**: 139–45.

Hatch SH, 1991, *Corynebacterium pseudodiphtheriticum* endocarditis, *Clin Microbiol Newslett*, **13**: 30–1.

Hauser D, Popoff MR et al., 1993, Polymerase chain assay for diagnosis of potentially toxinogenic *Corynebacterium diphtheriae* strains: correlation with ADP-ribosylation activity assay, *J Clin Microbiol*, **31**: 2720–3.

Hayashi A, Yanagawa R, Kida H, 1985, Adhesion of *Corynebacterium renale* and *Corynebacterium pilosum* to epithelial cells of bovine vulva, *Am J Vet Res*, **46:** 409–11.

Herschorn BJ, Brucker AJ, 1985, Embolic retinopathy due to *Corynebacterium minutissimum* endocarditis, *Br J Ophthalmol*, **69:** 29–31.

Hiramune TM, Murase N, Yanagawa R, 1970, Distribution of the types of *Corynebacterium renale* in cows of Japan, *Jpn J Vet Sci*, **32:** 235–42.

House RW, Schousboe M et al., 1986, *Corynebacterium ovis* (*pseudotuberculosis*) lymphadenitis) in a sheep farmer: a new occupational disease in New Zealand, *N Z Med J*, **99:** 659–62.

Hsu T-Y, 1984, Caseous lymphadenitis in small ruminants: clinical, pathological, and immunological responses to *Corynebacterium pseudotuberculosis* and to fractions and toxins from the micro-organism, *Dissertations Abst Int B*, **45:** 1396.

Hust MH, Metzler B et al., 1994, Toxische Diphtherie durch *Corynebacterium ulcerans*, *Dtsch Med Wochenschr*, **119:** 548–52.

Jackman PJH, Pitcher DG et al., 1987, Classification of corynebacteria associated with endocarditis (group JK) as *Corynebacterium jeikeium* sp. nov., *Syst Appl Microbiol*, **9:** 83–90.

Jacobi A, 1880, *A Treatise on Diphtheria*, William Wood and Co., New York.

Jellard CH, 1971, Comparison of Hoyle's medium and Billings' modification of Tinsdale's medium for the bacteriological diagnosis of diphtheria, *J Med Microbiol*, **4:** 366–9.

Jellard CH, 1972, Diphtheria infection in North West Canada, 1969, 1970, and 1971, *J Hyg*, **70:** 503–10.

Johnson A, Hulse P, Oppenheim B, 1992, *Corynebacterium jeikeium* meningitis and transverse myelitis in a neutropenic patient, *Eur J Clin Microbiol Infect Dis*, **11:** 473–9.

Jones D, Collins MD, 1986, Irregular nonsporeforming gram-positive rods, *Bergey's Manual of Systematic Bacteriology*, vol. 2, eds Sneath PHA, Mair NS et al., Williams & Wilkins, Baltimore, 1261–6.

Jones EE, Kim-Farley RJ et al., 1985, Diphtheria: a possible foodborne outbreak in Hodeida, Yemen Arab Republic, *Bull WHO*, **63:** 287–93.

Jones JET, 1992, *Eubacterium* (*Corynebacterium*) *suis*, *Diseases of Swine*, 7th edn, eds Leman AD, Straw E et al., Iowa State University Press, Ames, Iowa, 643–5.

Kain KC, Noble MA et al., 1991, *Arcanobacterium hemolyticum* infection: confused with scarlet fever and diphtheria, *J Emerg Med*, **9:** 33–5.

Kariuki DP, Poulton J, 1982, Corynebacterial infection of cattle in Kenya, *Trop Anim Health Prod*, **14:** 33–6.

Karzon DT, Edwards KM, 1988, Diphtheria outbreaks in immunized populations, *N Engl J Med*, **318:** 41–3.

Khabbaz RF, Kaper JB et al., 1986, Molecular epidemiology of group JK *Corynebacterium* on a cancer ward: lack of evidence for patient-to-patient transmission, *J Infect Dis*, **154:** 95–9.

Kim-Farley RJ, Soewarso TI et al., 1987, Silica gel as transport medium for *Corynebacterium diphtheriae* under tropical conditions (Indonesia), *J Clin Microbiol*, **25:** 964–5.

King CT, 1994, Sternal wound infection due to *Corynebacterium xerosis*, *Clin Infect Dis*, **19:** 1171–2.

Kjeldsen K, Simonsen O, Heron I, 1988, Immunity against diphtheria and tetanus in the age group 30–70 years, *Scand J Infect Dis*, **20:** 177–85.

Klebs E, 1883, *Verhandlungen des Kongresses fur Innere Medizin*, 36.

Kleinman LC, 1992, Lessons from the history of diphtheria, *N Engl J Med*, **326:** 773–6.

Krech T, 1994, Epidemiological typing of *Corynebacterium diphtheriae*, *Med Micriobiol Lett*, **3:** 1–8.

Krugman S, Katz SL et al., 1992, Diphtheria, *Infectious Diseases of Children*, 9th edn, CV Mosby, St Louis.

ter Laak EA, Bosch J et al., 1992, Double-antibody sandwich enzyme-linked immunosorbent assay and immunoblot analysis used for control of caseous lymphadenitis in goats and sheep, *Am J Vet Res*, **53:** 1125–32.

Langs JC, de Briel D et al., 1988, Endocardite à *Corynebacterium* de groupe D2 à point de départ urinaire, *Med Mal Infect*, **5:** 293–5.

LaRocco M, Robinson C, Robinson A, 1987, *Corynebacterium pseudodiphtheriticum* associated with suppurative lymphadenitis, *Eur J Clin Microbiol*, **6:** 79.

Larsen JL, Hogh P, Hovind-Hougen K, 1986, Hemagglutinating and hydrophobic properties of *Corynebacterium* (*Eubacterium*) *suis*, *Acta Vet Scand*, **27:** 520–30.

Leonard RB, Nowowiejski DJ, Warren JJ, 1994, Molecular evidence of person-to-person transmission of a pigmented strain of *Corynebacterium striatum* in intensive care units, *J Clin Microbiol*, **32:** 164–9.

Lewbow AA, MacLean PD et al., 1946, Tropical ulcers and cutaneous diphtheria, *Arch Intern Med*, **78:** 255–95.

Lindner PS, Hardy DJ, Murphy TF, 1986, Endocarditis due to *Corynebacterium pseudodiphtheriticum*, *N Y State J Med*, **86:** 102–4.

Lindsey JR, Boorman GA et al., 1991, *Companion Guide to Infectious Diseases of Mice and Rats*, National Research Council, Washington, DC, 14–15.

Lipsky BA, Goldberger AC et al., 1982, Infections caused by nondiphtheria corynebacteria, *Rev Infect Dis*, **4:** 1220–35.

Loeffler F, 1884, Medizinal-Statistische Mittheilungen aus dem Kaiserlichen Gesundheitsamte, *The Bacteriology of Diphtheria*, Cambridge University Press, London, 1.

Lopez JF, Wong FM, Quesada J, 1966, *C. pseudotuberculosis*: first case of human infection, *Am J Clin Pathol*, **46:** 562–7.

Lortholary O, Buu-Hoi A et al., 1993, *Corynebacterium diphtheriae* endocarditis in France, *Clin Infect Dis*, **17:** 1072–4.

McCloskey RV, Eller JJ et al., 1971, The 1970 epidemic of diphtheria in San Antonio, *Ann Intern Med*, **75:** 495–503.

MacGregor RR, 1995, *Corynebacterium diphtheriae*, *Principles and Practice of Infectious Diseases*, 4th edn, eds Mandell GL, Bennett JE, Dolin R, Churchill Livingstone, New York, 1865.

Mackenzie A, Fuite LA et al., 1995, Incidence and pathogenicity of *Arcanobacterium haemolyticum* during a 2-year study in Ottawa, *Clin Infect Dis*, **221:** 177–81.

Malanoski GJ, Parker R, Elipoulos GM, 1992, Antimicrobial susceptibilities of a *Corynebacterium* CDC group I1 strain isolated from a patient with endocarditis, *Antimicrob Agents Chemother*, **36:** 1329–31.

Malik AS, Johar MR, 1995, Pneumonia, pericarditis, and endocarditis in a child with *Corynebacterium xerosis* septicemia, *Clin Infect Dis*, **20:** 191–2.

Maple PA, Efstratiou A et al., 1994, The in-vitro susceptibilities of toxigenic strains of *Corynebacterium diphtheriae* isolated in northwestern Russia and surrounding areas to ten antibiotics, *J Antimicrob Chemother*, **34:** 1037–40.

Maple PA, Efstratiou A et al., 1995, Diphtheria immunity in UK blood donors, *Lancet*, **345:** 963–5.

Mark A, Christenson B et al., 1989, Immunity and immunization of children against diphtheria in Sweden, *Eur J Clin Microbiol Infect Dis*, **8:** 214–19.

Marshall FJ, Johnson E, 1990, Corynebacteria: incidence among samples submitted to a clinical laboratory for culture, *Med Lab Sci*, **47:** 36–41.

Marshall RJ, Routh KR, MacGowan AP, 1987, Corynebacterium CDC group D2 bacteremia, *J Clin Pathol*, **40:** 813–15.

Martinetti-Lucchini G, Gruner E, Altwegg M, 1992, Rapid detection of diphtheria toxin by the polymerase chain reaction, *Med Microbiol Lett*, **1:** 276–83.

Martinez-Martinez L, Ortega MC, Suarez AI, 1995, Comparison of E-test with broth microdilution disk diffusion for susceptibility testing of coryneform bacteria, *J Clin Microbiol*, **33:** 1318–21.

Martinez-Martinez L, Suarez AI, Ortega MC, 1994, Fetal pulmonary infection caused by *Corynebacterium striatum*, *Clin Infect Dis*, **19:** 806–7.

Melville-Smith M, Balfour A, 1988, Estimation of *Corynebacterium diphtheriae* antitoxin in human sera: a comparison of an enzyme-linked immunosorbent assay with the toxin neutralization test, *J Med Microbiol*, **25:** 279–83.

Mencarelli M, Zanchi A et al., 1992, Molecular epidemiology of nasopharyngeal corynebacteria in healthy adults from an urban area where diphtheria vaccinations have been extensively practised, *Eur J Epidemiol*, **8**: 560–7.

Menzies PI, Muckle CA et al., 1991, A field trial to evaluate a whole cell vaccine for the prevention of caseous lymphadenitis in sheep and goat flocks, *Can J Vet Res*, **55**: 362–6.

Middlebrook JL, Dorland RB, Leppla SH, 1978, Association of diphtheria toxin with Vero cells: demonstration of a receptor, *J Biol Chem*, **253**: 7325–30.

Mikhailovich VM, Melnikov VG et al., 1995, Application of PCR for detection of toxigenic *Corynebacterium diphtheriae* strains isolated during the Russian diphtheria epidemic, 1990 through 1994, *J Clin Microbiol*, **33**: 3061–3.

Miller E, Rush M et al., 1994, Immunity to diphtheria in adults in England, *Br Med J*, **308**: 598.

Miller RA, Rompalo A, Coyle MB, 1986, *Corynebacterium pseudodiphtheritcum* pneumonia in an immunologically intact host, *Diagn Microbiol Infect Dis*, **4**: 165–71.

Morris AJ, Henderson GK et al., 1986, Relapsing peritonitis in a patient undergoing continuous ambulatory peritoneal dialysis due to *Corynebacterium aquaticum*, *J Infect*, **13**: 151–6.

Mortimer EA Jr, 1994, Diphtheria toxoid, *Vaccines*, 2nd edn, eds Plotkin SA, Mortimer SA, WB Saunders, Philadelphia, 41–56.

Munford RS, Ory HW et al., 1974, Diphtheria deaths in the United States, 1959–1970, *JAMA*, **229**: 1890–3.

Nebreda-Mayoral T, Munoz-Bellido JL, Garcia-Rodriguez JA, 1994, Incidence and characteristics of urinary tract infections caused by *Corynebacterium urealyticum* (*Corynebacterium* group D2), *Eur J Clin Microbiol Infect Dis*, **13**: 600–4.

Pai SE, 1932, A simple egg medium for the cultivation of *Bacillus diphtheriae*, *Chin Med J (Engl Ed)*, **46**: 1203–6.

Pallen MJ, 1991, Rapid screening for toxigenic *Corynebacterium diphtheriae* by polymerase chain reaction, *J Clin Pathol*, **44**: 1025–6.

Pallen MJ, Hay AJ et al., 1994, Polymerase chain reaction for screening clinical isolates of corynebacteria for the production of diphthera toxin, *J Clin Pathol*, **47**: 353–6.

Pappenheimer AM Jr, 1965, The diphtheria bacilli and the diphtheroid, *Bacterial and Mycotic Infections of Man*, 4th edn, eds Dubos RJ, Hirsch JG, JB Lippincott Co, Montreal, 468–89.

Park CK, Yoon YD et al., 1993, Studies on microbiological monitoring of commercial and SPF mice, *J Agric Sci Vet*, **35**: 740–9.

Patey O, Halioua B et al., 1996, *Epidemiological and Molecular Study of Corynebacterium diphtheriae (C.d.) systemic infections in France*, Institut Pasteur, Paris.

Pedersen AH, Spearman J et al., 1977, Diphtheria on skid road, Seattle Wash., *Public Health Rep*, **92**: 336–42.

Peiris V, Fraser S et al., 1994, Isolation of *Corynebacterium striatum* from three hospital patients, *Eur J Clin Infect Dis*, **13**: 36–8.

Petit PLC, Bok JW et al., 1994, Native-valve endocarditis due to CDC coryneform group ANF-3: report of a case and review of corynebacterial endocarditis, *Clin Infect Dis*, **19**: 897–901.

Philippon P, Bimet F, 1990, In vitro susceptibility of *Corynebacterium* group D2 and *Corynebacterium jeikeium* to twelve antibiotics, *Eur J Clin Microbiol Infect Dis*, **9**: 892–5.

Pitcher D, Johnson A et al., 1990, An investigation of nosocomial infection with *Corynebacterium jeikeium* in surgical patients using a ribosomal RNA gene probe, *Eur J Clin Microbiol Infect Dis*, **9**: 643–8.

Popovic T, Wharton M et al., 1995, Are we ready for diphtheria? A report from the diphtheria diagnostic workshop, Atlanta, 11 and 12 July, 1995, *J Infect Dis*, **171**: 765–7.

du Preez JH, Giesecke WH, 1994, Mastitis, *Infectious Diseases of Livestock*, eds Coetzer JAW, Thompson GR, Tustin RC, Oxford University Press, Cape Town/Oxford, 1564–95.

Prescott JF, 1991, *Rhodococcus equi*: an animal and human pathogen, *Clin Microbiol Rev*, **4**: 20–34.

Prescott JF, Johnson JA, Markham RJF, 1980, Experimental stud-

ies on the pathogenesis of *Corynebacterium equi* infection in foals, *Can J Comp Med*, **44**: 280–8.

Prescott JF, Nicholson VM, 1984, The effects of combinations of selected antibiotics on the growth of *Corynebacterium equi*, *J Vet Pharmacol Ther*, **7**: 61–4.

Prescott JF, Travers M, Yager-Johnson JA, 1984, Epidemiological survey of *Corynebacterium equi* infections on five Ontario horse farms, *Can J Comp Med*, **48:** 10–13.

Qiu X, Verlinde CL et al., 1995, Three-dimensional structure of the diphtheria toxin repressor in complex with divalent cation co-repressors, *Structure*, **3**: 87–100.

Quinn A, Comaish J, Pedlar S, 1991, Septic arthritis and endocarditis due to group G-2 coryneform organism, *Lancet*, **338**: 62–3.

Ramon G, Djourichitch M, 1934, L'infection mixte streptodiphtérique: recherches expérimentales, *Ann Inst Pasteur (Paris)*, **53**: 325–40.

Rappuoli R, Pergini M, Falsen E, 1988, Molecular epidemiology of the 1984–1986 outbreak of diphtheria in Sweden, *N Engl J Med*, **318**: 12–14.

Richards M, Hurse A, 1985, *Corynebacterium pseudotuberculosis* abscesses in a young butcher, *Aust N Z J Med*, **15**: 85–6.

Riegel P, Ruimy R et al., 1995a, Genomic diversity and phylogenic relationships among lipid requiring diphtheroids from humans and characterization of *Corynebacterium macginleyi* sp. nov., *Int J Syst Bacteriol*, **45**: 128–33.

Riegel P, Ruimy R et al., 1995b, *Corynebacterium seminale* sp. nov., a new species associated with genital infection in male patients, *J Clin Microbiol*, **33**: 2244–9.

Riley P, Hollis D, Utter G, 1979, Characterization and identification of 95 diphtheroid (group JK) cultures isolated from clinical specimens, *J Clin Microbiol*, **9**: 418–24.

Ritter E, Kaschner A et al., 1993, *Arcanobacterium haemolyticum* from an infected foot wound, *Eur J Clin Microbiol Infect Dis*, **12**: 473–4.

Roder BL, Frimodt-Moller N, 1990, *Corynebacterium xerosis* as a cause of community-acquired endocarditis, *Eur J Clin Microbiol Infect Dis*, **9**: 233–4.

Roux E, Yersin A, 1888, *Ann Inst Pasteur (Paris)*, **2**: 629.

Rufael DW, Cohn SE, 1994, Native valve endocarditis due to *Corynebacterium striatum*: case report and review, *Clin Infect Dis*, **19**: 1054–61.

Ryan M, Murray PR, 1994, Prevalence of *Corynebacterium urealyticum* in urine specimens collected at a university-affiliated medical center, *J Clin Microbiol*, **32**: 1395–6.

Sargent KR, Rossing TH et al., 1984, Diphtheria immunity in Massachusetts – a study of three urban patient populations, *Am J Med Sci*, **287**: 37–9.

Schick B, 1913, Diphtherietoxin-Hautreaktion des Menschen als Vorprobe der prophylaktischen Diphtherieheilseruminjektion, *Munch Med Wochenschr*, **60**: 2608–10.

Sesardic D, Corbel MJ, 1992, Testing for neutralizing potential of serum antibodies to tetanus and diphtheria toxin [letter], *Lancet*, **340**: 737–8.

Sewell DL, Coyle MB, Funke G, 1995, Prosthetic valve endocarditis caused by *Corynebacterium afermentans* subsp. *lipophilum* (CDC coryneform group ANF-1), *J Clin Microbiol*, **33**: 758–64.

Silverman JA, Mindell JA et al., 1994, Structure–function relationships in diphtheria toxin channels: I. Determining a minimal channel-forming domain, *J Membr Biol*, **137**: 17–28.

Simonet M, de Briel D et al., 1993, Coryneform bacteria isolated from middle ear, *J Clin Microbiol*, **31**: 1667–8.

Sisson D, Thomas WP, 1984, Endocarditis of the aortic valve in the dog, *J Am Vet Med Assoc*, **184**: 570–6.

Skalka B, Literak I, 1994, Serodiagnosis of caseous lymphadenitis (pseudotuberculosis) in sheep, *Vet Med Praha*, **39**: 533–9.

Soriano F, Fernadez-Roblas R, 1988, Infections caused by antiobiotic resistant *Corynebacterium* group D2, *Eur J Clin Microbiol Infect Dis*, **7**: 337–41.

Soriano F, Ponte C, 1992, A case of urinary tract infection caused by *Corynebacterium urealyticum* and coryneform group F1, *Eur J Clin Microbiol Infect Dis*, **11:** 62–8.

Soriano F, Ponte C et al., 1985, Corynebacterium group D2 as a cause of alkeline-encrusted cystitis report of four cases and characterization of the organisms, *J Clin Microbiol*, **21:** 788–92.

Soriano F, Aguado J et al., 1990, Urinary tract infection caused by *Corynbacterium* group D2. Report of 82 cases and review, *Rev Infect Dis*, **12:** 1019–34.

Soriano F, Ponte C et al., 1993, Non-urinary tract infections caused by multiply antibiotic-resistant *Corynebacterium urealyticym*, *Clin Infect Dis*, **17:** 890–1.

Szabo S, Lieberman JP, Lue YA, 1990, Unusual pathogens in narcotic associated endocarditis, *Rev Infect Dis*, **12:** 412–15.

Tao X, Schiering N et al., 1994, Iron, DtxR, and the regulation of diphtheria toxin expression, *Mol Microbiol*, **14:** 191–7.

Taylor I, Tomlinson AJH, Davies JR, 1962, Diphtheria control in the 1960's, *R Soc Health J*, **82:** 158–64.

Tiley SM, Kociuba KR et al., 1993, Infective endocarditis due to nontoxigenic *Corynebacterium diphtheriae*: report of seven cases and review, *Clin Infect Dis*, **16:** 271–5.

Timoney JF, Gillespie JH et al., 1988a, The genera *Corynebacterium* and *Eubacterium*, *Hagan and Bruner's Microbiology and Infectious Diseases of Domestic Animals*, 8th edn, Comstock Publishing Associates, Ithaca, 247–54.

Timoney JF, Gillespie JH et al., 1988b, The genus *Rhodococcus*, *Hagan and Bruner's Microbiology and Infectious Diseases of Domestic Animals*, 8th edn, Comstock Publishing Associates, Ithaca.

Trichard CJV, Van Tonder EM, 1994, Ulcerative balanoposthitis and vulvovaginitis of sheep and goats, *Infectious Diseases of Livestock*, eds Coetzer JAW, Thompson GR, Tustin RC, Oxford University Press, Cape Town, 1599–602.

Tumbarello M, Tacconelli E et al., 1994, *Corynebacterium striatum* bacteremia in a patient with AIDS, *Clin Infect Dis*, **18:** 1008–10.

Updyke EL, Frobisher M Jr, 1947, Study of bacterial synergism with reference to etiology of malignant diphtheria, *J Bacteriol*, **54:** 619–32.

Vanbosterhaut B, Surmont I et al., 1989, *Corynebacterium jeikeium* (group JK diphtheroids) endocarditis. A report of five cases, *Diagn Microbiol Infect Dis*, **12:** 265–8.

Van Etta LL, Filice GA et al., 1983, *Corynebacterium equi*: a review of 12 cases of human infection, *Rev Infect Dis*, **5:** 1012–18.

Vettesse TE, Craig CP, 1993, Spontaneous bacterial peritonitis due to *Corynebacterium xerosis*, *Clin Infect Dis*, **17:** 815.

Wachsmuth IK, Mazurova MP et al., 1995, Molecular characterization of *C. diphtheriae* isolates from Russia, *Proceedings of the 95th General Meeting of the American Society for Microbiology*, American Society for Microbiology, Washington, DC, 35.

Walkden D, Klugman K et al., 1993, Urinary tract infection with *Corynebacterium urealyticum* in South Africa, *Eur J Clin Microbiol Infect Dis*, **12:** 18–24.

Wallet F, Marquette CH, Courcol RJ, 1995, Multiresistant *Corynebacterium xerosis* as a cause of pneumonia in a patient with acute leukemia, *Clin Infect Dis*, **18:** 845–6.

Waters BL, 1989, Pathology of culture-proven JK *Corynebacterium* pneumonia. An autopsy case report, *Am J Clin Pathol*, **91:** 616–19.

Watkins DA, Chahine A et al., 1993, *Corynebacterium striatum*: a diphtheroid with pathogenic potential, *Clin Infect Dis*, **17:** 21–5.

Weersink AJ, Rozenbery-Arska M et al., 1994, *Rothia dentocariosa* endocarditis complicated by an abdominal aneurysm, *Clin Infect Dis*, **18:** 489–90.

Wehrle PF, 1982, Diphtheria, *Bacterial Infections of Humans*, Plenum Medical Book Company, New York, 207–18.

Wilhelmus KR, Robinson NM, Jones DB, 1979, *Bacterionema matruchotii* ocular infections, *Am J Ophthalmol*, **87:** 143–7.

Williams DY, Selepak ST, Gill VJ, 1993, Identification of clinical isolates of nondiphtherial *Corynebacterium* species and their antibiotic susceptibility patterns, *Diagn Microbiol Infect Dis*, **17:** 23–8.

Wilson ME, Shapiro DS, 1992, Native valve endocarditis due to *Corynebacterium pseudodiphtheriticum*, *Clin Infect Dis*, **15:** 1059–60.

Wood CA, 1993, Nosocomial infection of a pancreatic pseudocyst due to *Corynebacterium xerosis*, *Clin Infect Dis*, **17:** 934–5.

Wood C, Pepe R, 1994, Bacteremia in a patient with non-urinary tract infection due to *Corynebacterium urealyticum*, *Clin Infect Dis*, **19:** 367–8.

Woolcock JB, Multimer MD, 1980, *Corynebacterium equi*: in vitro susceptibility to twenty-six antimicrobial agents, *Antimicrob Agents Chemother*, **18:** 976–9.

Woolcock JB, Multimer MD, Farmer A-MT, 1980, Epidemiology of *Corynebacterium equi* in horses, *Res Vet Sci*, **28:** 87–90.

Zuber PLF, Gruner E et al., 1992, Invasive infection with nontoxigenic *Corynebacterium diphtheriae* among drug users, *Lancet*, **339:** 1359.

Chapter 20

ORAL INFECTIONS

R P Allaker and J M Hardie

1 INTRODUCTION

The mouth is similar in some respects to other body sites colonized by a characteristic commensal microflora that remains relatively stable as the result of a dynamic balance between interbacterial and host–bacterial interactions (Marsh 1991). More commonly than elsewhere in the body, however, the relationship between the commensal flora and the host can be disrupted in a number of ways that result in the disease of the oral structures.

2 THE NORMAL FLORA OF THE MOUTH

The mouth supports a wide diversity of micro-organisms including bacteria, yeasts, viruses and, on occasions, protozoa. Bacteria are the predominant components of this resident microflora and its high species diversity reflects the wide range of endogenously derived nutrients, the varied types of habitat for colonization and the opportunity to survive on surfaces provided by the plaque biofilm.

Potential habitats in the oral cavity include non-shedding hard tooth surfaces and soft, constantly replaced, epithelial surfaces for attachment. Conditions at these sites vary with respect to oxygen levels and anaerobiosis, availability of nutrients, exposure to salivary secretions or gingival crevicular fluid, masticatory forces and other variables such as oral hygiene. As a result, the composition of the microbial flora of the mouth varies considerably from site to site and at different times (Hardie and Bowden 1974, Marsh and Martin 1992).

The composition of the oral microflora is highly complex and variable. At least 300 different species are known to be associated with the oral cavity but it has been suggested that only half the bacteria found there can be cultured (Duerden et al. 1995).

Three categories of organisms may be unculturable:

1 "Difficult" organisms, i.e. those recovered in some laboratories but not in others, such as the obligate anaerobes *Eubacterium* and *Propionibacterium* spp.
2 Known but uncultivable organisms, e.g. many of the spirochaetes that can be observed microscopically in direct films from oral specimens
3 Unknown and uncultivable organisms.

The use of more stringent tests and modern techniques has allowed many existing oral bacterial species to be reclassified and newly discovered species to be recognized. Such classification procedures have made it possible to discern close associations between individual species and sites in health and disease (Shah and Gharbia 1993).

3 CLASSIFICATION OF ORAL INFECTIONS

Oral infections can be classified in several different ways, as indicated below. Many of the micro-organisms that cause infection in other parts of the body can, on occasions, produce lesions in and around the oral cavity.

3.1   Nature of micro-organisms implicated in the infection

The majority of infections of the oral cavity are bacterial, fungal or viral. Little is known about the role, if any, of mycoplasmas, rickettsiae and protozoa. Most bacterial infections are polymicrobial and it is unusual to find any that are clearly due to a single species. Thus, the relative contribution of different bacterial components in such infections is difficult to determine. This chapter will deal predominantly with bacterial infections of the oral cavity that occur in the developed world. For a more complete picture of oral infections as a whole, reference should be made to other chapters: *Candida* (Volume 4, Chapter 23) and herpesvirus (Volume 1, Chapter 17 and Volume 2, Chapter 11). Fuller accounts of these can also be found in specialized texts on oral conditions (e.g. Sculley and Flint 1989, Samaranayake and McFarlane 1990, Slots and Taubman 1992).

3.2   Origin of infection

Oral infections may arise from an endogenous source, involving micro-organisms normally found in the mouth such as those associated with the plaque-related conditions of caries and periodontal disease. They may also arise from exogenous sources, being caused by micro-organisms not normally found as part of the oral microflora. Exogenous infections, which are less common than endogenous infections, can be further subdivided into primary infections, such as herpes simplex or primary syphilis, and secondary manifestations of systemic infections, such as oral tuberculosis and secondary syphilis.

4   PREDISPOSING FACTORS THAT LEAD TO ORAL INFECTIONS

In health the normal oral microbial ecosystem is remarkably stable in spite of its complexity. Many endogenous and exogenous factors may, however, affect the composition and metabolic activities of the oral microflora (Marsh and Martin 1992). Under normal conditions the equilibrium between the host and the micro-organisms is thought to be mutually beneficial, but disturbances of this steady state can have adverse effects. The oral cavity is a potential portal of entry for organisms into the body, but the commensal oral flora, together with other oral defence mechanisms, plays an important role in protecting the oral cavity from infection by exogenous organisms.

Disturbances to the oral cavity may allow:

1   selective overgrowth of certain endogenous species, such as *Candida albicans*, in patients with HIV infection or AIDS
2   displacement of certain endogenous species, for example *Actinomyces israelii* with resulting actinomycosis after trauma to the mucosa or jaws
3   introduction of exogenous micro-organisms, such

as *Escherichia coli*, that can cause osteomyelitis after radiotherapy.

A large number of local and general predisposing factors can result in oral infections (Table 20.1). Some of these, such as short-term antibiotic therapy, may result in a temporary disturbance, whereas others, such as loss of salivary secretion, may have a permanent effect on susceptibility. Such predisposing factors must be taken into account when treating patients with oral infections.

5   CONDITIONS THAT AFFECT HARD TISSUES

The presence of teeth in the oral cavity is one of the main features that distinguishes the mouth from other body sites. The newborn infant is at first edentulous and the first teeth erupt at about the age of 6 months. The full complement of 20 deciduous teeth is normally in place by 24 months and these start to be replaced by the permanent dentition at around 6 years of age. By the time the child becomes a teenager this process is usually complete, apart from the third molars ('wisdom teeth') that erupt later, unless this is prevented by impaction resulting from insufficient space.

Tooth surfaces are rapidly coated by saliva-derived glycoproteins and then colonized by bacteria to form dental plaque. The metabolic activities of these bacteria are responsible for the 'plaque-related infections', which are the most common conditions that affect the teeth and their supporting structures (MacFarlane 1989).

The crowns of the teeth consist of an outer layer of enamel, an extremely hard and inert material with a high mineral (hydroxyapatite) content that does not contain cells, nerves or blood vessels. Though it is the hardest tissue in the body, dental enamel is susceptible to acid attack, a process that occurs during the initial stages of dental caries. Once the integrity of the tooth has been breached and a carious cavity is formed, the process may progress to involve the underlying dentine and pulp tissue, from which infection may spread by way of the root to involve the periapical area and the surrounding bone.

The bones of the jaw and face may become infected as a result of the progression of dental caries, or by various other routes. Disorders of the supporting structures of the teeth, such as periodontitis, result in resorption of alveolar bone, which ultimately leads to tooth loss. Infection can occur around partially erupted teeth, to cause pericoronitis, and in tooth sockets after extraction. Osteomyelitis of the jaws may follow fractures or develop as a result of other infectious processes in the mouth, and maxillary sinusitis can arise by extension of infection around the upper teeth or after traumatic damage during oral surgery. Some of the conditions that affect the oral hard tissues are considered in greater detail in the following sections.

Table 20.1 Predisposing factors which may result in infections of the oral cavity

Predisposing factors	Possible effect on defence mechanism	Possible resulting oral infection
Physiological		
Elderly	Diminished antibody levels, decrease in salivary flow	Candidosis, root caries
Pregnancy	Unknown	Gingivitis
Trauma		
Local	Tissue integrity loss	Opportunistic infections
General	Debilitation, dehydration	Candidosis
Malnutrition	Deficiencies of iron, vitamin B12	Candidosis
AIDS	Diminished cell mediated immunity	Opportunistic infections, candidosis
Antimicrobial therapy	Loss of colonization resistance, selection of resistant microflora	Opportunistic infections, candidosis
Chemotherapy	Xerostomia	Candidosis, caries
Oral malignancies	Xerostomia, muscular function loss	Candidosis, caries

Modified from Marsh and Martin (1992).

5.1 Dental caries

CLINICAL MANIFESTATIONS

Dental caries (dental decay) is a destructive condition of the dental hard tissues that, if unchecked, can progress to inflammation and death of vital pulp tissue, with eventual spread of infection to the periapical area of the tooth and beyond. In children and young adults, the crown of the tooth is the usual site of attack and lesions most commonly develop in pits and fissures or at approximal sites between the teeth (Kidd and Joyston-Bechal 1987, Thylstrup and Fejerskov 1994). In the more rapid and severe forms of caries (rampant caries), almost any tooth surface may be destroyed, including buccal and lingual smooth surfaces. A particularly rapid and distressing form of caries, sometimes known as 'nursing bottle caries', is associated with the inappropriate use of sweetened comforter bottles or dummies (pacifiers) in infants (Ripa 1978, Brown, Junner and Liew 1985, Milnes and Bowden 1985). This condition may lead to virtually total destruction of the crowns of all erupted deciduous teeth. A similar form of rampant caries has also been reported in small groups of breast-fed children in Tanzania (Matee et al. 1992).

In older individuals, especially those over about 40 years of age, another form of caries is found that leads to the destruction of exposed cementum and dentine around the necks of the teeth. This cemental or root surface caries occurs when there has been loss of attachment of the periodontal tissues, usually due to periodontitis, which results in exposure of the root surface to the oral environment (Vehkalahti and Paunio 1994). This type of caries, which may be difficult to treat, has become an increasing clinical problem in some countries, including the UK, as people tend to live longer and are generally more anxious than in previous generations to keep their natural teeth (McComb 1994, Youngs 1994).

Another form of rampant caries may occur in older individuals after loss of function of the major salivary glands. This sometimes follows radiotherapy of the head and neck for treatment of malignant disease, and is precipitated by the loss of the protective effects of saliva in the mouth (Dreizen et al. 1977). Xerostomia ('dry mouth') due to other causes may also lead to dental caries and other oral problems (Epstein, Stevenson-Moore and Scully 1992).

DIAGNOSIS

Carious lesions in pits, fissures and exposed smooth surfaces (i.e. buccal, labial, lingual and palatal surfaces) can usually be detected visually combined with probing of the suspected lesion. Evidence of early lesions between the teeth, particularly those on mesial and distal surfaces of posterior teeth (premolars and molars) can often only be obtained from radiographs. By the time such lesions are clearly visible they will have extended well into the dentine and may even have reached the pulp of the tooth. The severity of individual carious lesions can be assessed by the amount of hard tissue destruction observed and the depth to which the disease has progressed. Thus, a small initial lesion may involve only a small area of enamel, whereas in more advanced disease there will be destruction of dentine and possible involvement of the pulp. For epidemiological purposes, the amount of caries in an individual is often expressed as a function of the number of teeth or tooth surfaces affected by the disease process. This has given rise to the use of indices such as the DMFT (decayed, missing and filled teeth) and DMFS (decayed, missing and filled surfaces) for scoring permanent teeth; equivalent measures for deciduous teeth being referred to as dmft and dmfs.

EPIDEMIOLOGY

There has been a decrease in the prevalence of coronal caries in many populations in the industrialized world over the last 20–30 years (Bowen and Tabak 1993) but small pockets of 'high risk' groups within such populations may remain. Unfortunately, the reverse trend has been observed in some developing countries, particularly where large numbers of people move from a predominantly rural to an urban environment and, at the same time, radically change their eating and dietary habits (Johnson 1991a). In such situations, where dental manpower may be in short supply or non-existent, dental caries becomes an increasing problem (Bowen and Tabak 1993).

PATHOGENESIS

The initiation of dental caries is by acid demineralization, brought about by the metabolic activities of saccharolytic bacteria on the tooth surface within dental plaque (Van Houte 1994). This process causes loss of mineral from the enamel surface, particularly from the subsurface zone in the early stages, and is to some extent a reversible phenomenon. Thus, it is possible for both demineralization and remineralization to occur sequentially, depending upon local conditions at the enamel–plaque interface (Thylstrup and Fejerskov 1994).

Under conditions that favour continuation of the carious process, which usually prevail when the individual has frequent intakes of fermentable carbohydrate in the diet, the initial enamel lesion develops into a cavity and is no longer reversible by natural processes. At this stage the bacterial flora associated with the lesions may change, becoming more varied and complex, and including a variety of obligate anaerobes (Thylstrup and Fejerskov 1994). Whereas breakdown of enamel seems largely to be by acid demineralization, the destruction of dentine, which has a higher organic matrix content, may be effected by a combination of acid and proteolytic activity.

AETIOLOGY

The bacteria associated with the initiation of dental caries are all acidogenic. In mono-infected gnotobiotic animals, several bacterial genera and species have to varying degrees of severity been shown to have the ability to induce caries (Hardie 1992, Thylstrup and Fejerskov 1994).

Of the various species tested (Table 20.2), strains belonging to the 'Streptococcus mutans group', especially Streptococcus mutans and Streptococcus sobrinus, have most consistently been found to be cariogenic and to cause the most severe destruction of the dentition. The disease does not, however, seem to be caused by one single species, at least in experimental animals.

Studies of the microbial aetiology of dental caries in humans are complicated by the fact that the disease may take months or years to develop in some individuals, and that it is difficult to diagnose clinically in the earliest stages. Thus, by the time lesions are unequivocally recognized the microbial flora responsible for the earliest stages may already have changed as part of the successional changes known to occur during cavitation. Notwithstanding technical difficulties with studies on human caries, however, there is strong evidence for association between the presence of high numbers of mutans streptococci (MS; *S. mutans* and *S. sobrinus*) in the mouth and the development of disease (Loesche 1986, Bowden 1990, Hardie 1992, Thylstrup and Fejerskov 1994). These bacteria can be detected in dental plaque and may also be found in relatively high numbers in the saliva of caries-active individuals.

Another genus frequently implicated in dental caries is *Lactobacillus*. The evidence for the association of lactobacilli with human caries is rather less strong, but these organisms are frequently found in carious lesions and occur in increased numbers in the saliva of caries-active individuals. The possible involvement of other bacteria, including other streptococci and some *Actinomyces* spp., is not at present clear-cut, but it has been suggested that actinomyces may play an important role in root-surface caries (Bowden 1990, Thylstrup and Fejerskov 1994, Schupbach, Osterwalder and Guggenheim 1996).

ASSESSMENT OF CARIES RISK

The observation that high numbers of MS and lactobacilli can be found in saliva of caries-active individuals has led to the use of salivary counts as a means of assessing caries risk. Thus, patients with salivary MS levels of $>2.5 \times 10^5$ per ml may be regarded as 'high risk' and selected for intensive preventive therapy (Krasse 1988, Johnson 1991a, Hardie 1992).

It has been shown that the children of mothers with high salivary MS counts are more likely to acquire these bacteria during the early months of life and are also more likely to develop caries of the deciduous dentition (Köhler, Bratthall and Krasse 1983, Köhler, Andreen and Jonsson 1988). Thus, there is a good case for giving preventive advice and therapy to pregnant and nursing mothers in an attempt to delay or stop colonization of the mouths of their children by potentially cariogenic bacteria.

Studies of the transmission of MS by means of molecular strain-typing methods have shown that children most frequently acquire these bacteria from their mothers (Köhler, Bratthall and Krasse 1983, Caufield, Cutter and Dasanayake 1993). Maternal salivary MS counts can be reduced by a combination of appropriate sugar-controlled diet, good oral hygiene and plaque control, use of topical fluorides, restoration of carious cavities and, if necessary, application of chlorhexidine gluconate as a mouth rinse, toothpaste or topically applied gel (Tenovuo 1991, Tenovuo et al. 1992).

DETERMINANTS OF CARIOGENICITY

The cariogenic activity of MS is thought to be due to a combination of properties. These include ability to produce acid (acidogenicity), ability to survive at low pH (aciduricity), production of extracellular polysaccharides (EPS) from sucrose, production of intracellular polysaccharide (IPS), and ability to survive and grow on the tooth surface (Bowen and Tabak 1993, Thylstrup and Fejerskov 1994). Mutant strains that lack some of these features have been shown to lose cariogenicity in animal model systems. Application of molecular genetic methods to the study of MS has elucidated many of the mechanisms by which these

Table 20.2　Bacteria capable of inducing dental caries in gnotobiotic animals

Genus	Species	Comments
Streptococcus	S. mutans	Associated with human caries
	S. sobrinus	Associated with human caries
	S. rattus	Rarely found in humans
	S. cricetus	Rarely found in humans
	S. ferus	Only isolated from wild rats
	'S. milleri'	One of 'S. milleri group'[a]
	S. oralis	Formerly called 'S. mitior'
	S. salivarius	
	S. sanguis	May include S. gordonii
	'S. faecalis'	
Lactobacillus	L. acidophilus	
	L. casei	
	L. salivarius	
	L. fermentum	
Actinomyces	A. naeslundii	Mainly root surface caries
	A. israelii	Mainly root surface caries
	A. viscosus	Mainly root surface caries

[a] 'S. milleri group' includes S. anginosus, S. constellatus and S. intermedius.

organisms can induce dental caries in susceptible hosts (Bowen and Tabak 1993, Russell 1994).

PREVENTION

Conventional ways of attempting to prevent dental caries include: reduction of dietary sucrose intake, use of systemic and topical fluorides to reduce the acid solubility of the teeth and for their potential antienzymic acid antibacterial effects, regular oral hygiene to reduce levels of dental plaque, and restoration of untreated carious cavities (Kidd and Joyston-Bechal 1987, Bowen and Tabak 1993, Thylstrup and Fejerskov 1994). Chlorhexidine gels and varnishes have also been shown to lower the intraoral levels of mutans streptococci and their application has a place in the management of high risk subjects, although no antimicrobial agent is entirely effective for the prevention of caries (Emilson 1994).

Since the recognition in the early 1960s of the potential role of *S. mutans* and related species in human caries, a number of investigators have explored the possibility of developing an anticaries vaccine based on these streptococci. Various potential antigen preparations have been examined, including whole bacteria, cell walls, glucosyltransferase enzymes, and several purified surface protein antigens, notably antigen I/II or protein B (also known as P1, SpaP and PAc) (Russell 1992). In spite of encouraging results in animal experiments and much useful information about local and systemic responses to these antigens, the vaccines have not so far been tested in human clinical trials. A combination of concerns about potentially damaging side effects and the known efficacy of other, completely safe, caries-preventive measures has inhibited further progress with experiments on active immunization against dental caries (Russell 1992, Bowen and Tabak 1993). The possible use of preformed anti-*S. mutans* antibodies for passive immunization is under investigation and may in future offer an alternative immunological approach to caries prevention (Ma et al. 1990, Ciardi, McGhee and Keith 1992, Russell 1992).

5.2　Dentoalveolar abscesses

Dentoalveolar or periapical abscesses are relatively common manifestations of acute infection in the mouth and may present as dental emergencies. Such abscesses, which usually develop around the apices of teeth with necrotic and infected root canals, result either from the progression and spread of deep carious cavities to involve the pulp chamber or after traumatic pulp exposure. Acute abscesses can also occur in deep periodontal pockets that have become obstructed or traumatized to produce infection alongside the affected tooth.

Dental abscesses may present clinically in different ways, depending on the severity of the infection and the location of the particular tooth involved. In most cases, the presenting features are pain and variable localized swelling that may eventually, if adequate surgical drainage is not achieved, discharge through to the oral mucosa or the skin to produce a fistula. In other situations infection may spread widely along muscle and fascial planes to cause severe soft tissue swelling and cellulitis (Schlossberg 1987). Such spreading odontogenic infections are particularly serious when they involve the orbit (Henry, Hughes and Larned 1992) or the submandibular region, as in Ludwig's angina, in which the airway may be threatened. The degree of fever and other systemic effects that accompany dental abscesses may vary from negligible to severe.

Microbiological studies in recent years have shown that dental abscesses are almost invariably polymicrobial, usually with 3–5 species (range 1–12) present in the pus when good anaerobic culture methods are employed. As with all infections, it is important that appropriate clinical sampling methods are used, and for dental abscesses it is recommended that wherever possible pus is collected by needle and syringe aspiration. Conventional swab samples are more likely to confuse the picture because of contamination with salivary or skin bacteria. Use of appropriate transport media and rapid transfer to the laboratory will also ensure optimum recovery of anaerobes (Dahlen et al. 1993).

It has been well documented since the late 1970s that some 75% of the isolates from periapical abscesses are obligate anaerobes (Hardie 1991, Slots and Taubman 1992). These comprise a variety of genera and species, the majority being either gram-negative rods (particularly *Prevotella*, *Porphyromonas* and *Fusobacterium*) or gram-positive cocci (*Peptostreptococcus*). The remaining 25% include aerobic, facultatively anaerobic, micro-aerophilic and capnophilic species, with α-haemolytic streptococci most frequently found. Unlike abscesses elsewhere, staphylococci are not amongst the most common isolates from odontogenic abscesses. The main groups of bacteria recovered from dental abscesses are summarized in Table 20.3.

Of the streptococci reported from dental abscesses, members of the '*Streptococcus milleri* group' (SMG) are commonly found (Lewis, MacFarlane and McGowan 1990). Few investigators have separated these into *Streptococcus anginosus*, *Streptococcus constellatus* and *Streptococcus intermedius* but it has been suggested that these species may have a predilection for particular body sites (Whiley et al. 1992).

PATHOGENICITY

The bacteria isolated from dental abscesses are usually also part of the normal commensal oral flora, rather than acquired exogenous pathogens. Several of the commonly isolated species have been tested for their ability to produce experimental infections in mice, including SMG streptococci, anaerobic gram-negative rods of various species, and anaerobic gram-positive cocci (Lewis et al. 1988). Although all strains induce some degree of infection in this model, the gram-negative anaerobes produced the most extensive lesions and were recovered in highest numbers from the experimental abscesses. Injection of pairs of bacteria that included either *Prevotella intermedia* or *Fusobacterium nucleatum* and a *Streptococcus* or a *Peptostreptococcus* produced more severe lesions than combinations of the gram-positive cocci. These experiments indicate that the anaerobic gram-negative organisms almost invariably found in dental abscesses may be of major pathogenic significance, but it should not be forgotten that peptostreptococci and the SMG streptococci are also frequently associated with purulent infections in other parts of the body. Capsulate strains of both gram-negative anaerobes and gram-positive cocci are more frequently associated with pus from orofacial abscesses (Brook 1986). However, recent studies of the phagocytosis by human polymorphonuclear leucocytes of dentoalveolar abscess isolates have not revealed any difference between the uptake of capsulate and non-capsulate strains (Lewis et al. 1993). In these experiments, phagocytosis of '*S. milleri*' and anaerobic gram-positive cocci was significantly greater than that observed with *Prevotella intermedia*, *Prevotella oralis* and *Fusobacterium nucleatum*. It remains to be determined why particular combinations of bacteria can resist phagocytosis and other host defence mechanisms during the establishment of dentoalveolar abscesses.

TREATMENT

Well localized dental abscesses with minimal spread of infection and without signs of systemic illness may be treated successfully by surgical drainage alone, without

Table 20.3 Bacteria isolated from dentoalveolar abscesses in studies using modern sampling and anaerobic culture techniques

Aerobic and facultative bacteria	Relative isolation[a] frequency	Obligately anaerobic bacteria	Relative isolation[a] frequency
α-Haemolytic streptococci	+++	*Peptostreptococcus* spp.	+++
β-Haemolytic streptococci	++	*Prevotella* and *Porphyromonas* spp.[b]	+++
Enterococcus spp.	++	*Veillonella* spp.	++
Staphylococcus epidermidis	++	*Propionibacterium* spp.	++
Staphylococcus aureus	++	*Actinomyces* spp.	++
Neisseria spp.	+	*Eubacterium* spp.	++
Corynebacterium spp.	+	*Lactobacillus* spp.	++
Eikenella corrodens	+	*Fusobacterium* spp.	++
Haemophilus spp.	+	*Arachnia propionica*[c]	+
Enterobacteria	+	*Bifidobacterium* spp.	+
Capnocytophaga spp.	+	Spirochaetes	+

[a]+, 0.1–1.0% of reported isolates; ++, 1.1–10% of reported isolates; +++, >10% of reported isolates.
[b]Including black-pigmented anaerobes (formerly classified as *Bacteroides* spp.). Data from Lewis, MacFarlane and McGowan (1990), Hardie (1991), Slots and Taubman (1992), and numerous original publications.
[c]Now classified as *Propionibacterium propionicum*.

the need for antimicrobial chemotherapy. Such drainage may be obtained simply by extracting the offending tooth or by opening the pulp chamber and draining pus through the dental root canal. In many cases, however, symptoms are more severe and adequate drainage may require intraoral mucosal surgical incision or, externally, skin incision. In these situations, systemic antimicrobial treatment is also necessary.

Of the many groups of antimicrobial agents potentially available for treatment of orofacial infections, the penicillins and the nitroimidazoles have been most widely used. Erythromycin has been used as an alternative for penicillin-sensitive patients but resistance to this agent is quite common and clindamycin would appear to be a more effective choice (Heimdahl et al. 1985). It has generally been accepted that, in spite of occasional reports of resistance, the majority of bacteria isolated from dentoalveolar abscesses are sensitive to the commonly used antibiotics, including penicillin, amoxycillin and erythromycin (Lewis, MacFarlane and McGowan 1990). It is, however, apparent that no single antibiotic is likely to be effective against the whole range of bacterial species found in dentoalveolar abscesses. When penicillin is the drug of choice, the conventional approach is to prescribe a 5 day course of phenoxymethylpenicillin for the treatment of acute dentoalveolar abscess. However, a short high dose course of amoxycillin with 2 doses of 3 g, 8 h apart, is equally effective in adults (Lewis, McGowan and MacFarlane 1986) and a similar regimen appears to be preferable for the treatment of acute abscesses associated with primary teeth in children 2–10 years old (Paterson and Curzon 1993). Notwithstanding the widespread recommendation of treatment with penicillin or amoxycillin, it must be borne in mind that 23% of isolates from acute suppurative oral infections are resistant to >1 mg l^{-1} penicillin, 11% are resistant to ampicillin (>2 mg l^{-1}) and 5% to amoxycillin–clavulinic acid (>2 mg l^{-1}) (Lewis et al. 1995). In this study 55% of patients yielded at least one penicillin-resistant isolate and 73% contained a β-lactamase producing strain. Thus, penicillin-resistant bacteria appear to be more commonly present in these infections than was previously thought.

Since antimicrobial therapy for acute dentoalveolar abscesses is usually prescribed empirically before the results of antibiotic susceptibility tests are available, it is common practice to commence treatment with penicillin or amoxycillin, unless there are obvious contraindications. This has the advantage of being effective against most streptococci and many of the anaerobic species likely to be present. Failure to respond within 48 h of commencing penicillin treatment is an indication for adding metronidazole to the regimen (Lewis, MacFarlane and McGowan 1990). In severe cases, a combination of penicillin and metronidazole may be used from the outset. Alternative drugs that may be indicated for penicillin-allergic patients include erythromycin (and other macrolides), clindamycin and tetracycline, other than for children under

13 years of age and pregnant women because of the known effects of tetracycline on developing teeth (Lewis, MacFarlane and McGowan 1990, Karlowsky, Ferguson and Zhanel 1993, Pallasch 1993).

5.3 Sequelae of localized dentoalveolar abscess

As noted above, dentoalveolar abscesses may remain localized around the root of the tooth involved or spread more widely into adjacent tissues. Local spread in mandibular or maxillary bone can produce an acute or chronic osteitis. If a localized periapical abscess is not effectively treated, it may develop into a periapical granuloma and this, in turn, can lead to cyst formation. Acute periapical abscesses may also become chronic with acute exacerbations that lead to sinuses that discharge on mucosal or skin surfaces. Spread along fascial planes may give rise to acute spreading infection, and blood vessel erosion may lead to bacteraemia or septicaemia (Schlossberg 1987, MacFarlane and Samaranayake 1989). Thus, this common form of purulent intraoral infection can range from a relatively innocuous 'gum boil' to a serious life-threatening condition.

5.4 Ludwig's angina

This is an acute, rapid, diffuse, bilateral cellulitis of the floor of the mouth and neck that involves the submental, submandibular and sublingual spaces. It results in severe swelling and induration of the submandibular tissues and elevation of the tongue, often causing obstruction of the airway. In most cases the primary source of infection is of dental origin, such as a dentoalveolar abscess on a lower tooth, but it may also develop from submandibular sialadenitis (salivary gland infection), infected mandibular fractures, oral soft tissue lacerations, and puncture wounds of the floor of the mouth (MacFarlane and Samaranayake, 1989).

Urgent treatment is necessary, with particular attention to maintenance of the airway, surgical drainage and antimicrobial chemotherapy. Only small amounts of pus may be obtained on incision, and these will usually yield a mixture of obligate anaerobes and streptococci (Holbrook 1991). A combination of penicillin and metronidazole is appropriate for initial antimicrobial treatment in most cases, but material obtained at the time of incision and drainage should be cultured to ensure that the causative agents are susceptible.

5.5 Localized alveolar osteitis ('dry socket')

Dry socket is a well recognized painful condition of the jaws that may complicate tooth extraction. Several different terms have been used to describe this condition in the literature, including localized osteitis, alveolar osteitis, alveolitis sicca dolorosa, localized acute alveolar osteomyelitis, postextraction alveolitis, postextraction osteomyelitic syndrome and fibrinolytic alveolitis (Chapnick and Diamond 1992). Dry socket occurs more often after the removal of mandibular (lower) teeth and most frequently with mandibular third molars; the incidence is variously estimated from 0.5% to over 30% of all extractions, with an overall average frequency of around 3%.

The aetiology of dry socket is not fully understood, but is generally considered to be multifactorial. During the process the blood clot, which should normally fill the empty tooth socket and act as the focal point for healing and repair, breaks down and the socket becomes necrotic and infected. In addition to anatomical location, other predisposing factors include the difficulty and amount of trauma sustained during surgery, smoking, age, gender and use of oral contraceptives, local circulation and vasoconstrictors, and fibrinolysis. The repeated observation that dry socket occurs most frequently after removal of mandibular third molars (wisdom teeth), which are often associated with pericoronitis before extraction, suggests that the presence of a locally infected environment is an important contributory factor. Several clinical trials have also shown that prophylactic use of oral antiseptics, such as chlorhexidine or povidone-iodine, and administration of antimicrobial agents locally or systemically, including clindamycin, tetracycline and metronidazole, can reduce the incidence of dry sockets after tooth extraction.

Very little is known about the detailed microbiology of dry socket. It seems probable that the condition represents yet another manifestation of mixed infection in the mouth, involving a variety of obligate and facultative oral anaerobes. It has been suggested that *Treponema denticola* may play a particular role in the aetiology because of its pronounced fibrinolytic activity, but this observation has not been confirmed (Nitzan 1983). Further studies are required to demonstrate whether specific groups of bacteria are involved in the disease process. Patients at particular risk of developing dry socket after third molar surgery include those with a previous history of this complication, those with signs of pericoronitis, smokers, and females taking oral contraceptives. Such patients would benefit from prophylactic use of antimicrobial agents, in addition to meticulous attention to surgical technique to minimize local trauma.

5.6 Osteomyelitis

Acute and chronic forms of osteomyelitis of the jaws can occur, but are relatively uncommon. Osteomyelitis usually develops from a contiguous focus of infection in the oral cavity or after trauma to the jaws, but haematogenous spread is occasionally suspected. Conditions that reduce the bone vascularity, such as radiation therapy, Paget's disease, fibrous dysplasia and bone tumours, may predispose to osteomyelitis. The mandible is affected far more frequently than the maxilla, probably for anatomical reasons.

The onset of acute osteomyelitis of the mandible is characterized by pain, slight fever and paraesthesia or anaesthesia of the lower lip due to increasing pressure on the mental nerve. Later the teeth may become loose and painful to touch and pus may exude from the gingival crevice around affected teeth or discharge through fistulae to the overlying mucosal or skin surfaces. The literature contains some discrepancies with regard to the groups of bacteria found in osteomyelitis of the jaws. Older reports indicate that *Staphylococcus aureus* and *Staphylococcus epidermidis* are the most common causative agents, but more recent studies have revealed the presence of mixtures of anaerobes and other organisms similar to those associated with dentoalveolar abscesses. In addition, there have been reports of osteomyelitis caused by aerobic gram-negative rods, such as *Klebsiella*, *Proteus* and *Pseudomonas aeruginosa*. In view of the wide variety of microorganisms that may be involved, it is important to obtain samples for culture and antibiotic sensitivity to determine the most appropriate therapy.

Treatment of osteomyelitis of the jaws can be complex, particularly if diagnosis is delayed and there is extensive bone destruction. Ideally, appropriate antimicrobial chemotherapy should be started early in the hope of preventing further bone destruction and avoiding the need for surgical intervention. Penicillin G, or clindamycin for penicillin-allergic patients, is usually the drug of choice, but flucloxacillin or other antistaphylococcal drugs may be indicated when β-lactamase producing *S. aureus* is involved (MacFarlane and Samaranayake 1989).

5.7 Maxillary sinusitis

Infection of the maxillary sinus may occur by spread of bacteria from the nose, via the ostium, or from the mouth (see also Chapter 18). Oral bacteria can reach the sinus by direct spread of infection associated with the roots of the upper teeth from the canine to the second molar, which may be in close proximity to the floor of the antrum, as the result of surgical complications after attempts to extract these teeth, or as a result of maxillary fractures (McGowan, Baxter and James 1993). Sinus infections of nasal origin, often following a respiratory virus infection, are commonly caused by *Haemophilus influenzae* or *Streptococcus pneumoniae*, but those originating from the mouth are usually mixed and contain a variety of anaerobes, including anaerobic cocci and *Fusobacterium* spp. (Lundberg et al. 1979, Lundberg 1980).

6 CONDITIONS THAT AFFECT THE SUPPORTING STRUCTURES OF THE TEETH

Periodontal diseases are the most common inflammatory destructive conditions that affect man. They are initiated by components of the dental plaque that develops on the hard tooth surface adjacent to the soft tissues of the supporting periodontium and may be confined to the soft tissues of the gingiva (gingivitis), or extend to the deeper supporting structures with destruction of the periodontal ligament and the alveolar bone that supports the teeth (periodontitis). Such loss of attachment, with associated periodontal pocket formation, may ultimately lead to loosening and loss of the affected teeth.

6.1 Clinical manifestations

The periodontal diseases (Table 20.4) are normally classified according to the age group of the affected person (e.g. prepubertal, juvenile, adult), the rate of progress of the disease (rapid, acute, chronic), the distribution of lesions (localized or generalized), and whether there are any particular predisposing factors (e.g. pregnancy, diabetes, HIV infection) (Slots and Taubman 1992).

6.2 Aetiology

During the past 20 years our understanding of the aetiology and pathogenesis of the periodontal diseases has improved dramatically. Periodontitis is now accepted as following a pattern of discontinuous progression characterized by periods of active disease and remission, rather than a continuous slowly progressive course (Socransky et al. 1984). The biological basis for susceptibility to periodontitis remains unclear; data gathered from young adults suggests that gingivitis is not a risk factor and it has not been proved that obvious gingivitis is a necessary precursor to periodontitis (Prayitno, Addy and Wade 1993). The search for the aetiological agents of destructive periodontal disease has continued for over 100 years (Socransky and Haffajee 1994) but until recently there has been little consensus about the periodontal pathogens. The diversity of bacterial species in the periodontal flora, the variation in composition of the flora from individual to individual and the variation of the host response to different bacterial species are some of the major reasons that a specific microbial aetiology of periodontal disease has not been clearly established. However, *Porphyromonas gingivalis* (formerly *Bacteroides gingivalis*), *Prevotella intermedia* (formerly *Bacteroides intermedius*) and *Actinobacillus actinomycetemcomitans* are at present regarded as major pathogens in advancing periodontitis (Slots et al. 1986). *A. actinomycetemcomitans* is now strongly implicated in juvenile periodontitis

(Slots 1976, Aass, Preus and Gjermo 1992) and *P. gingivalis* has been associated with destructive periodontal lesions in adults (Slots 1977, Tanner et al. 1979). *P. intermedia* has been implicated in the development of chronic gingivitis (Slots 1982), acute necrotizing ulcerative gingivitis (ANUG) (Loesche et al. 1982) and pregnancy gingivitis (Kornman and Loesche 1980). Several other bacteria may also be regarded as possible periodontal pathogens (Table 20.5).

6.3 Epidemiology

Almost all adults in all parts of the world experience gingivitis and some degree of periodontitis. Advanced forms of periodontitis with extensive loss of tooth-supporting connective tissue and alveolar bone occur in approximately 7–15% of the UK adult dentate population (Johnson 1991b).

Evidence for both the vertical and horizontal transmission of periodontal organisms has been provided by means of molecular epidemiology techniques. These have shown that the periodontal pathogens *A. actinomycetemcomitans* and *P. gingivalis* can be transmitted within family groups (Petit et al. 1993, Saarela 1993). Although it is perceived that the oral microflora is relatively stable, it seems probable that new species or different clonal types of the same species can be introduced during the lifetime of an individual. It is also now recognized that not all clonal types of a pathogenic species are equally virulent. Recent studies have demonstrated differences in virulence between isolates of *P. gingivalis*, which suggests that certain isolates found at disease sites may be avirulent (van Steenbergen et al. 1987, Neiders et al. 1989).

6.4 Pathogenesis

The precise mechanisms by which periodontal disease is produced are not fully understood. In order to colonize subgingival sites organisms must be able to attach to one or more surfaces, multiply, compete with other organisms and evade host defence mechanisms. As a consequence a number of potentially toxic products or virulence factors are produced that may cause tissue damage by direct and indirect mechanisms. These include lipopolysaccharide (Daly, Seymour and

Table 20.4 Different types of periodontal diseases

Common	Rare
Chronic marginal gingivitis	HIV-gingivitis and periodontitis
Chronic adult periodontitis	Pregnancy gingivitis
	Acute streptococcal gingivitis
	Acute herpetic gingivitis
	Acute necrotizing ulcerative gingivitis
	Localized juvenile periodontitis
	Prepubertal periodontitis
	Rapidly progressive periodontitis

Table 20.5 Association of suspected bacteria to periodontitis

Very strong	Strong	Moderate	Uncertain
Actinobacillus actinomycetemcomitans *Porphyromonas gingivalis*	*Bacteroides forsythus* *Prevotella intermedia* *Campylobacter rectus* *Eubacterium nodatum* *Treponema* spp.	*Streptococcus intermedius* *Prevotella nigrescens* *Peptostreptococcus micros* *Fusobacterium nucleatum* *Eubacterium* spp. *Eikenella corrodens*	*Selenomonas* spp. *Staphylococcus* spp. *Bacteroides gracilis*

Kieser 1980), cell surface components (Meghji et al. 1994), a range of tissue-damaging enzymes, such as the arginine-specific protease from *P. gingivalis* (Aduse-Opoku et al. 1995) and proline iminopeptidase from *Eikenella corrodens* (Allaker, Young and Hardie 1994a), and metabolic products, such as amines and short-chain carboxylic acids (Greenman, Osborne and Allaker 1988). Indirect toxic effects may be exerted on host cells, for example by neutralizing or modifying host defences through the action of a leucotoxin (Taichman, Dean and Sanderson 1980).

Environmental factors may alter the virulence of periodontal pathogens, as shown by the effect of haemin on the physiology and virulence of *P. gingivalis* (McKee et al. 1986). Physical and chemical interactions between bacteria may also play a role in the nature of the species that colonize a site and ultimately on disease outcome (Socransky and Haffajee 1991).

6.5 Host response

Recent findings emphasize the importance of the interaction between the subgingival plaque flora and various aspects of the host acute inflammatory, humoral and cellular immune responses (Genco 1992, Socransky and Haffajee 1992). Although the inflammatory response to plaque is a basic host defence mechanism against infection, it can also contribute to tissue destruction. A variety of mediators that represent different aspects of the host response to the microbial challenge have been identified in gingival crevicular fluid and serum (Lamster and Novak 1992). Consequently, many of these factors may act as markers of activity and have been examined for their relationship to the clinical course of periodontal disease (Lamster et al. 1994). For example, it has been shown that a number of tissue-derived gingival crevicular fluid protease activities correlate positively with clinical parameters in untreated chronic periodontitis patients (Eley and Cox 1992) and that their levels decrease significantly after treatment (Cox and Eley 1992). Virulence factors may also regulate host cell metabolism and stimulate production of cytokines involved in mediating the inflammatory and immune responses (Takada et al. 1991).

6.6 Diagnosis

Clinical methods for diagnosing periodontal disease include measurement of pocket depth and loss of attachment, estimation of gingival health by observing its colour and swelling, detection of gingival bleeding on probing and visualization of alveolar bone loss in radiographs (Genco, Goldman and Cohen 1990). They are, however, rather crude techniques that are not sufficiently sensitive to allow detection of all stages of disease. Several diagnostic technologies to detect potential periodontal pathogens and their products now exist and these may provide an indicator of future disease activity. These include cultural procedures, microscopy (Loesche 1988), immunological tests (Fine and Mandel 1986), enzyme analysis (Loesche et al. 1990, Allaker, Young and Hardie 1994b) and DNA probes (Loesche 1992). Products of tissue damage have also been examined for their relationship to the clinical course of periodontal disease (see section 6.5).

6.7 Treatment

Plaque control is fundamental to prevent gingivitis, for treatment of established periodontal diseases and to maintain oral health after treatment. Conventional oral hygiene measures, such as tooth brushing and flossing, are normally adequate to control plaque. Various antimicrobial agents that have antiplaque and antigingivitis benefits have also been incorporated into toothpastes and mouthwashes (Marsh and Martin 1992). In more advanced forms of periodontal disease, however, antiplaque agents may not penetrate sufficiently into the pocket to be effective. Professional plaque control, which may require periodontal surgery to gain access to the root surface, is sometimes necessary. After root planing to remove plaque and calculus deposits, topical or systemic antimicrobial agents, such as chlorhexidine, metronidazole or minocycline, may be required to prevent significant recolonization at disease sites (Genco, Goldman and Cohen 1990).

SPECIFIC PERIODONTAL DISEASES

Gingivitis may be localized to one or more specific sites in the mouth, or can occur in a generalized form.

Particular types of gingivitis occur when there is an underlying systemic condition, such as pregnancy, insulin-dependent diabetes or Papillon–Lefèvre syndrome, and in acute necrotizing ulcerative gingivitis. The gingivae may also be susceptible to infections with organisms found only as members of the transient oral flora, including *S. aureus*, *P. aeruginosa* and enteric organisms. Such infections are often related to suppression of the normal subgingival flora by antibiotics, systemic disorders or altered local conditions (Slots and Taubman 1992).

Chronic marginal gingivitis

Chronic marginal gingivitis is a non-specific inflammation in response to dental plaque that involves the dental margins. It is very common in the dentate population and, if proper oral hygiene is restored, the condition is usually eradicated. The microflora associated with gingivitis is more diverse and differs in composition from that found in health (Moore et al. 1987). Apart from an overall increase in plaque mass, there is an initial shift from the plaque dominated by streptococci, that is found in gingival health, to one in which *Actinomyces* spp. predominate. As the condition progresses the plaque microflora becomes more diverse with an increase in the proportions of capnophiles and obligate anaerobes. Although it is difficult to ascertain which organisms are involved directly in the aetiology of gingivitis, certain taxa, including *Actinomyces* spp., spirochaetes, *Prevotella* spp. and *Peptostreptococcus* spp., are known to increase in numbers as the condition progresses.

Acute necrotizing ulcerative gingivitis (ANUG)

Vincent's angina, or acute necrotizing ulcerative gingivitis (ANUG), which mainly occurs in young adults, is a relatively uncommon type of gingivitis in Europe and the USA. It is characterized by a grey gingival pseudomembrane, which is easily removed to reveal a bleeding area, and destruction of the interdental papillae. Patients with ANUG present with marked halitosis, are often debilitated by another illness and suffering from stress. Spirochaetes (*Treponema* spp.), *P. intermedia* and *Fusobacterium* spp. are implicated in the condition (Loesche et al. 1982). Indeed, in smears of affected tissues, organisms are observed to be invasive and resemble spirochaetes and fusiform bacteria. The use of metronidazole is effective in eliminating the causative organisms and is normally accompanied by rapid clinical improvement.

Noma

In underdeveloped countries an extremely severe form of ANUG, noma or cancrum oris, is found in children. Malnutrition, immunodeficiency and concurrent or preceding infection are common underlying features. The initial necrotic lesion spreads from the gingivae into the lips and cheeks, and may extend to the surface of the face to cause extensive tissue loss and severe disfigurement. Antibiotic therapy has dramatically reduced the mortality from noma to 10% but in the related noma neonatorum, the mortality remains high (Holbrook 1991).

Chronic adult periodontitis

Chronic adult periodontitis is the most common form of periodontitis that can affect the general population. Most studies indicate that chronic periodontitis results from the activity of mixtures of interacting bacteria, with very different groups of bacteria able to produce an apparently similar response (Maiden et al. 1990). The majority of these bacteria are obligately anaerobic gram-negative rod and filament-shaped bacteria that are asaccharolytic and proteolytic. In an advanced disease state these mixtures are often dominated by the presence of paticular organisms. *P. gingivalis*, *P. intermedia* and *A. actinomycetemcomitans* are considered to be of special importance, because they are frequently isolated from 'active' periodontitis lesions and are known to possess several potential virulence factors (Haffajee and Socransky 1994).

Localized juvenile periodontitis (LJP)

LJP is a rare condition that usually occurs in adolescents but only 0.1% of the age group are susceptible. The disease is characterized by rapid destruction of the periodontal tissues. The first permanent molars and the incisor teeth are affected with much alveolar bone loss, which may then progress to a more severe and generalized form. In contrast to most other forms of periodontal disease, LJP appears to result from the activity of a relatively specific microflora dominated by *A. actinomycetemcomitans* (Zambon 1985). Some evidence suggests that the disease is familial (Petit et al. 1993) but no convincing defect of host tissues or defence mechanisms has been defined. Rapidly progressive periodontitis (RPP) is a poorly defined clinical condition and may be a late stage of LJP. It is most common in young adults and is characterized by phases of active destruction with marked gingival inflammation and rapid bone loss followed by periods of remission.

RELATED CONDITIONS

Infections around dental implants (peri-implantitis) and infections around partially erupted teeth (pericoronitis) share many clinical characteristics with periodontal pockets (Tanner 1992). The species of bacteria isolated from peri-implantitis and pericoronitis are similar to those isolated from periodontal and gingival infections. It is also recognized that periodontal disease is often associated with oral malodour, which may involve the production of malodorous compounds by the flora associated with periodontal disease (Yaegaki and Sanada 1992).

Pericoronitis

Pericoronitis is an inflammation of the soft tissues that surround the crown of a partially erupted tooth. This may occur in relation to any tooth, at any age, but is most commonly associated with mandibular third molars and usually occurs between the ages of 17 and 25 years. Bacterial infection from the oral cavity is thought to be the initiating factor but local trauma, stress and upper respiratory tract infections may also play a contributory role. Species recognized to be involved in pericoronitis include *P. intermedia, F. nucleatum, Capnocytophaga* spp., *A. actinomycetemcomitans, Peptostreptococcus micros, Veillonella* spp., *S. mitis* and spirochaetes (Mombelli et al. 1990, Wade et al. 1991). There is considerable similarity between the bacteria found in pericoronitis and periodontitis but *P. gingivalis* and *Eubacterium* spp. are often absent from pericoronitis sites. Treatment usually involves appropriate initial antimicrobial chemotherapy, often followed by extraction of the partially erupted tooth. Extraction of the opposing upper third molar is sometimes undertaken to relieve trauma to the infected site during occlusion.

Peri-implantitis

A number of implant systems are now used in humans to replace missing teeth, and most integrate with bone without complications. Small amounts of plaque, comprised mainly of streptococci and *Actinomyces* spp., accumulate on successful implants (Slots and Taubman 1992) but in peri-implantitis anaerobic gram-negative organisms are present. Implants in partially edentulous patients are probably most at risk with infecting organisms that may originate from any remaining natural teeth with periodontal disease. Indeed, implants in partially edentulous patients are more frequently colonized with *P. gingivalis* and *P. intermedia* than those of edentulous patients (George et al. 1994). For the maintenance of dental implants, diagnostic techniques, such as probing pocket depth, radiography and microbial sampling, have been modified from those usually used to measure periodontitis. Bone defects that result from peri-implantitis can be treated by non-surgical and surgical techniques (Jovanovic 1994).

Halitosis (oral malodour)

Periodontal disease is often associated with halitosis. Treatment of periodontal disease with resulting clinical improvement is often accompanied by a reduction in malodorous volatile sulphur compounds (VSC) levels in the breath. VSC may play an important role in the aetiology of periodontal disease and may accelerate the destructive process. Indeed, it has been shown that VSC increase the permeability of the oral mucosa, increase collagen solubility and degradation and reduce protein, collagen and DNA synthesis (Rosenberg 1995).

The main source of oral malodour is now recognized to be as a result of microbial metabolism in the oral cavity. The organisms responsible appear to be proteolytic, anaerobic, gram-negative species that colonize the subgingival plaque associated with periodontal disease (Tonzetich and McBride 1981). Recent studies have shown that the tongue microflora makes a major contribution to oral malodour (Hartley, El-Maaytah and Greenman 1995). The genera *Porphyromonas* and *Prevotella* are prominent among the putative malodorous species, which include spirochaetes, *Fusobacterium* and others. These species produce large amounts of malodorous short-chain fatty acids, such as propionate and butyrate (Greenman,

Osborne and Allaker 1988), and diamines, such as cadaverine and putrescine, and VSC. In vivo, however, oral malodour is due mostly to the micro-organisms that produce VSC, such as hydrogen sulphide (H_2S) and methyl mercaptan (CH_3SH). Other odorous molecules produced by members of the oral flora appear only to modify the quantity and intensity of oral malodour (Tonzeitch 1977). Such odours arise from the microbial degradation of proteins, particularly those that contain cysteine and methionine, peptides and amino acids that are present in saliva, gingival crevicular fluid and in foods that are retained on the teeth.

Various approaches have been made to the control of oral malodour. These include a masking approach, in which a product flavour and corresponding scent masks oral malodour, and an antibacterial approach, to reduce the formation of VSC by controlling the growth or metabolism of gram-negative micro-organisms in the oral cavity (Rosenberg 1995). Treatment and control of periodontal disease, when present, is an essential part of the management of oral malodour; some clinicians also advocate regular tongue cleaning.

7 INFECTIONS OF THE ORAL MUCOSA AND SUBMUCOSA

Mucosal infections in general are caused either by pathogenic micro-organisms of extraoral origin or by members of the normal commensal oral flora. Lesions often develop as opportunistic infections in immunocompromised patients, but also when there is no obvious defect in host defence mechanisms. The presence of an underlying host factor may allow colonization and growth of micro-organisms from the transient flora, such as *S. aureus*. Predisposing factors that lead to oral mucosal infections may be local and include trauma, impaired function of tongue and other oral muscles, inadequate oral hygiene, the presence of dentures and other appliances, and reduced salivary flow. Systemic influences include antibiotic and other drug therapy, impaired immunity, hormonal disturbances and malnutrition.

7.1 Actinomycosis

Actinomycosis is one of the few specific infections that preferentially affects the oral cavity. It can occur at a number of soft tissue body sites, but the cervicofacial region is by far the most common (see also Chapter 39) (Schaal 1981). The formation of a chronic granuloma is characteristic and swelling is also a common feature; in chronic cases multiple discharging sinuses are observed. Actinomyces cells form aggregates that can sometimes be seen by the naked eye as 'sulphur granules'. *A. israelii*, a regular inhabitant of the normal plaque microflora, is most commonly isolated from human actinomycosis, although other species are occasionally reported. Cervicofacial actinomycosis may occur as a consequence of pre-existing periodontal or root canal infection, or surgical trauma (Slots and Taubman 1992). Pus samples almost invariably yield other bacteria in addition to *Actinomyces* spp., including *Propionibacterium propionicus* and on occasions *A. actinomycetemcomitans*, as well as a variety of other facultative and aerobic species. Treatment consists of a combination of surgical drainage and debridement, together with prolonged antimicrobial chemotherapy, usually with penicillin.

7.2 Sialadenitis

Bacterial infections of the salivary glands are most often observed when salivary function is diminished as the result of disease or therapeutic interventions. The parotid is the most common site of acute and chronic bacterial infections of the salivary glands. α-Haemolytic streptococci, *S. aureus* and, increasingly, gram-negative anaerobic organisms, are recognized in the aetiology of sialadenitis (Fox 1991). Infection is particularly likely to occur when a salivary duct is obstructed by a calculus.

7.3 Angular cheilitis

Angular cheilitis can be defined as an erythema with or without a crack or fissures at the angle of the mouth (Ohman 1988). Systemic disorders, including HIV infection, diabetes mellitus and skin diseases, are common among recurrent angular cheilitis patients. Nutritional deficiencies of iron and vitamin B12 are also thought to play a role. Local factors associated with ageing and inadequate dentures also contribute to promote fungal and bacterial growth in skin folds. The microbial flora in angular cheilitis usually involves *Candida* spp., *S. aureus*, or both. Enteric organisms may also play a role in the pathogenesis and maintenance of the condition. In addition to correction of the underlying cause, local antimicrobial treatment with appropriate antifungal or antibacterial agents may be necessary to resolve angular cheilitis.

7.4 Stomatitis

Stomatitis is a rather non-specific term for inflammatory conditions of the oral mucosa. In denture stomatitis, with erythema under a complete or partial denture, *C. albicans* is most often involved. In acute erythematous stomatitis, a rare febrile condition, the causative organism is often *Streptococcus pyogenes*. Bacteria not commonly found as part of the oral flora, including *S. aureus* and *E. coli*, are occasionally associated with inflammatory lesions of the palatal and tongue mucosa. Generally, primary infectious lesions, other than those due to fungi, usually develop only in severely compromised hosts. An example is oral mucositis in elderly, dehydrated patients in which *S. aureus* appears to play a role (Bagg et al. 1995).

8 ORAL MANIFESTATIONS OF SYSTEMIC INFECTIONS

Infections elsewhere in the body may also exhibit lesions in the oral cavity; such infections may lead to additional infections by endogenous oral microorganisms, such as *C. albicans* or exogenous bacteria. Some of these infections are rare and occur only in certain geographical areas.

8.1 Tonsillitis and pharyngitis

The most common cause of infection of the tonsils and pharynx, apart from respiratory viruses, is *Streptococcus pyogenes*, which is not normally found as part of the oral microflora. Acute epiglottitis is sometimes caused by *Haemophilus influenzae*. These infections may occasionally spread into the oral cavity and cause lesions on the oral mucosal surfaces (see also Chapter 18).

8.2 Diphtheria

Diphtheria (see also Chapter 19 and Volume 2, Chapter 25) is a toxin mediated disease due to *Corynebacterium diphtheriae*. The infection is normally limited to the mucosal surfaces of the pharynx, larynx and nasal cavity, and is characterized by formation of pseudomembranes. Occasionally other sites, including the mouth, are involved, with formation of a thick, firmly attached white-yellow membrane on affected mucosal surfaces.

8.3 Gonorrhoea

This is a sexually transmitted infection due to *Neisseria gonorrhoeae* (see also Chapter 33). It occasionally involves the mouth and upper respiratory tract. In oral gonorrhoea painful lesions are found on the soft palate, tongue and gingivae, with white-yellow adherent membranes that on removal leave a bleeding surface.

8.4 Syphilis

Syphilis (see also Chapter 34) is a venereal infection caused by *Treponema pallidum*. The spirochaete is able to penetrate the unbroken oral mucosa and, in primary syphilis, forms an elevated and painless lesion with a marked border (hard chancre), on the lips or tongue. In the secondary stage of the disease small, grey, slightly raised areas, syphilitic patches often referred to as 'snail track ulcers', may be present on the oral mucosal surfaces and the tonsils. In the third syphilitic stage, which is probably related to tissue immune reactions, the characteristic gumma, a granulomatous lesion often surrounded by a fibrous capsule, is often observed. In the mouth, this destructive lesion often affects the hard and soft palates, and the tongue. Since syphilis is one of the less common sexually transmitted diseases, its oral manifestations are rarely seen in the UK.

8.5   Tuberculosis

Tuberculosis (see also Chapter 21) remains a major disease in developing countries and is occurring with increasing frequency in Europe and the USA. It is an important opportunistic infection in the acquired immunodeficiency syndrome (AIDS), as seen particularly in the current epidemic in Africa. Oral tuberculous lesions develop in some patients with pulmonary tuberculosis and may provide the first evidence of a serious underlying condition such as HIV infection. Any oral soft tissue can be infected with *Mycobacterium tuberculosis*, resulting in granulomas or ulcers, often with accompanying lymphadenopathy. Infection of bone also occurs and may progress to tuberculous osteomyelitis. Such infections have been described in tooth sockets after dental extraction and the oral manifestations of tuberculosis are almost invariably secondary to infection elsewhere in the body (Slots and Taubman 1992).

Bacterial infections at oral mucosal sites may also be a consequence of yaws, bejel and pinta (see Chapter 34), leprosy (see Chapter 23), anthrax (see Chapter 40) and tularaemia (see Chapter 49).

9   ORAL INFECTIONS IN THE IMMUNOCOMPROMISED PATIENT

Patients with defective immune function, particularly those infected with human immunodeficiency virus (HIV), often present with oral infections that would be regarded as unusual in healthy subjects (Scully 1992). This reduced ability to combat infection can also be due to inherited defects of the defence mechanisms, or it can result from radiation or cytotoxic drug therapy. Although such patients are particularly susceptible to infection with viruses and yeasts, local and systemic infections with bacteria endogenous to the oral cavity and elsewhere, including Enterobacteriaceae (Schmidt-Westhausen, Fehrenbach and Reichart 1990), are emerging as a serious problem in the management of compromised patients.

The types, presentation, severity and prognosis of oral infections in these groups of patients depend on the interaction of a number of factors. These include the extent of immunosuppression, previous or current antimicrobial treatment, the micro-organisms to which the patient is exposed, and the nature of the immunosuppressive drugs used.

The microbiologically related oral problems in immunocompromised patients include mucositis, ulceration, xerostomia, sialadenitis, osteomyelitis, candidosis, herpes virus infection, periodontal diseases and dental caries (MacFarlane and Samaranayake 1989). Certain clinical conditions and infections are more commonly associated with particular categories of compromised patients than others (MacFarlane and Samaranayake 1989), for example, in acute leukaemia in which the response to dental plaque is exaggerated, with gross inflammatory changes in the adjacent gingival tissues.

9.1   AIDS-related oral infections

Immune deficiency resulting from HIV infection is a predisposing factor to a wide range of oral and non-oral infections (see Volume 1, Chapter 38). HIV-positive patients are particularly susceptible to opportunistic infection with fungi, bacteria and viruses. The resulting oral manifestations include candidosis, herpes, cytomegalovirus (CMV) infection, gingivitis and periodontitis.

Marked gingivitis and rapidly progressive periodontitis are frequently seen in patients with AIDS. Such gingivitis is characterized by a band-like marginal erythema, often accompanied by diffuse redness, which extends into the vestibular mucosa. In contrast to the sites of gingivitis in HIV-negative individuals, affected sites are colonized by *C. albicans* and a range of putative periodontal disease pathogens including *A. actinomycetemcomitans*, *F. nucleatum* and *P. gingivalis* (Zambon, Reynolds and Genco 1990, Rams et al. 1991). An unusually severe and rapidly progressive form of periodontitis is also seen in HIV-positive patients. Deep pocket formation is not necessarily seen at affected sites but severe necrosis of the gingival margin may be observed with interseptal bone sequestration extending to the vestibular area. The microflora at these sites is not markedly different from that at sites of gingivitis but the pathological results are quite distinct. This may be due to differences in the immune status of the 2 groups (Gornitsky et al. 1991).

10   INFECTIONS AT OTHER BODY SITES DUE TO ORAL MICRO-ORGANISMS

As described earlier in this chapter, oral micro-organisms may be present as harmless commensals or become involved as endogenous pathogens in a variety of localized infections. There are also occasions when these bacteria become established at other, more distant, sites in the body and set up serious infections remote from the mouth. An important example of this type of opportunistic infection occurs in infective endocarditis, in which oral bacteria that enter the bloodstream colonize previously damaged heart valves (see Chapter 16). Another potentially life-threatening situation occurs when oral micro-organisms become established as the cause of abscesses at other sites, most significantly in the brain (Chapter 38).

10.1   Infective endocarditis

Many operative procedures in the mouth, particularly tooth extraction, deep subgingival scaling and periodontal surgery, produce an immediate, transient bacteraemia. Almost any oral bacteria may enter the bloodstream in this way, but the bacteria most commonly recovered from such dental bacteraemias are streptococci. In individuals with severe periodontal disease, even more gentle activities such as tooth-brushing and chewing may produce a detectable bacteraemia.

Such short-lived releases of streptococci and other oral bacteria into the circulation are usually of no serious consequence for healthy individuals, but in subjects with pre-existing heart valve lesions there is a considerable risk of infective endocarditis. Predisposing conditions include congenital valve defects, rheumatic fever, prosthetic heart valves and previous episodes of endocarditis.

During the last 30 years changes have been reported in the pattern of endocarditis in the community. Fewer post-rheumatic fever infections have been observed and there has been a shift towards older patients, with a wide variety of identified aetiological agents. Oral or viridans streptococci remain the most common cause and account for more than 60% of isolates (Hardie and Whiley 1992). In a recent study of streptococci isolated from cases of endocarditis 32% were found to be *Streptococcus sanguis*, 30% *Streptococcus oralis* and 13% *Streptococcus gordonii*, with smaller numbers identified as *Streptococcus bovis* (6%), *Streptococcus parasanguis* (4%), *Streptococcus mutans* (4%), *Streptococcus mitis* (4%) and *Streptococcus salivarius* (4%) (Douglas et al. 1993). Earlier studies had shown that the *S. sanguis–S. oralis–S. mitis* group of streptococci were most commonly associated with infective endocarditis, but recent changes in taxonomy and nomenclature of these species renders it difficult to be certain which species were involved (Hardie and Whiley 1994, 1995).

In order to avoid the possibility of precipitating endocarditis as a result of a dental bacteraemia, patients with known cardiac risk factors should be protected by prophylactic administration of antibiotics before oral or dental surgery. Any oral operative procedure during which blood is likely to be drawn should be covered in this way. Specific recommendations, derived from the advice of a Working Party of the British Society for Antimicrobial Chemotherapy (Simmons et al. 1992), are detailed in the *British National Formulary* (British Medical Association 1996) and the *Dental Practitioners' Formulary* (British Medical Association 1994). These are essentially based on the administration of oral amoxycillin 1 h before treatment in patients who are not allergic to penicillin and who are not about to receive a general anaesthetic. Clindamycin is recommended as an alternative agent for patients allergic to penicillin or who have received penicillin more than once in the previous month. Patients at special risk, including those with prosthetic

heart valves or who are allergic to penicillin and require a general anaesthetic, and those who have had a previous attack of endocarditis, should be referred to hospital for dental or oral surgical treatment. In addition to systemically administered antimicrobial agents, local use of antiseptics such as chlorhexidine gel (1%) or chlorhexidine mouthwash (0.2%) help to reduce the severity of any bacteraemia produced during oral surgery.

10.2 Abscesses due to oral bacteria

Bacteria can reach other parts of the body from the mouth by direct spread of infection along tissue planes (Guralnick 1984) or by way of the bloodstream. In the case of the latter, it is not easy with any certainty to establish the source of the organisms, but this may be inferred from their identity if the mouth is known to be their usual habitat.

Streptococci of the SMG, comprising *S. anginosus*, *S. constellatus* and *S. intermedius*, are found in the mouth, gastrointestinal and genitourinary tracts, and have been recognized as significant pathogens in various parts of the body (Gossling 1988, Hardie and Whiley 1992). Recent studies have shown that *S. intermedius*, in particular, is often associated with cerebral abscesses (Whiley et al. 1990, 1992) and the unproven presumption in such cases is that they may have originated from the mouth. Oral anaerobes, such as *Porphyromonas*, *Prevotella* and *Fusobacterium* spp., are also known to spread from infective foci in the mouth to produce abscesses in the brain (Ingham et al. 1978).

As with dentoalveolar abscesses, examination of pus from abscesses in the brain and other organs often reveals a mixed culture of streptococci, obligate anaerobes and other bacteria. The SMG are known to possess tissue-destroying enzymes such as hyaluronidase and chondroitin sulphatase that may contribute to their pathogenic potential (Homer et al. 1993).

In order to establish beyond doubt that any given isolate from an abscess in the brain, or elsewhere in the body, has originated from the mouth, it would be necessary to isolate an identical strain from somewhere in the oral cavity. Appropriate molecular strain-typing techniques are available to compare such isolates, but there are considerable problems in sampling every conceivable ecological niche in the mouth in order to establish the presence of the pathogen. Such detailed studies have not been reported for abscesses but similar techniques have been used to monitor the transmission of various oral species between individuals.

REFERENCES

Aass AM, Preus HR, Gjermo P, 1992, Association between detection of oral *Actinobacillus actinomycetemcomitans* and radiographic bone loss in teenagers. A 4-year longitudinal study, *J Periodontol*, **63**: 682–5.

Aduse-Opoku J, Muir J et al., 1995, Characterisation, genetic analysis, and expression of a protease antigen (PrpRI) of *Porphyromonas gingivalis* W50, *Infect Immun*, **63**: 4744–54.

Allaker RP, Young KA, Hardie JM, 1994a, Production of hydrolytic enzymes by oral isolates of *Eikenella corrodens*, *FEMS Microbiol Lett*, **123**: 69–74.

Allaker RP, Young KA, Hardie JM, 1994b, Rapid detection of proline iminopeptidase as an indicator of *Eikenella corrodens* periodontal infection, *Lett Appl Microbiol*, **19**: 325–7.

Bagg J, Sweeney MP et al., 1995, Possible role of *Staphylococcus aureus* in severe oral mucositis among elderly dehydrated patients, *Microb Ecol Health Dis*, **8**: 51–6.

Bowden GHW, 1990, Microbiology of root surface caries in humans, *J Dent Res*, **69**: 1205–10.

Bowen WH, Tabak LA, 1993, *Cariology for the Nineties*, University of Rochester Press, Rochester, USA.

British Medical Association, 1994, *Dental Practitioners' Formulary*, British Medical Association, London.

British Medical Association, 1996, *British National Formulary*, British Medical Association, London.

Brook I, 1986, Isolation of capsulate anaerobic bacteria from orofacial abscesses, *J Med Microbiol*, **22**: 171–4.

Brown JP, Junner C, Liew V, 1985, A study of *Streptococcus mutans* levels in both infants with bottle caries and their mothers, *Aust Dent J*, **30**: 96–8.

Caufield PW, Cutter GR, Dasanayake AP, 1993, Initial acquisition of mutans streptococci by infants; evidence for a discrete window of infectivity, *J Dent Res*, **72**: 37–45.

Chapnick P, Diamond LH, 1992, A review of dry socket: a double-blind study on the effectiveness of clindamycin in reducing the incidence of dry socket, *J Can Dent Assoc*, **58**: 43–52.

Ciardi JE, McGhee JR, Keith J, 1992, *Genetically Engineered Vaccines: Prospects for Oral Disease Prevention*, Plenum Publishing Corporation, New York.

Cox SW, Eley BM, 1992, Cathepsin B/L-, elastase-, tryptase-, trypsin- and dipeptidyl peptidase IV-like activities in gingival crevicular fluid: a comparison of levels before and after basic periodontal treatment of chronic periodontitis, *J Clin Periodontol*, **19**: 333–9.

Dahlen G, Pipattanagovit P et al., 1993, A comparison of two transport media for saliva and subgingival samples, *Oral Microbiol Immunol*, **8**: 375–82.

Daly CG, Seymour GJ, Kieser JB, 1980, Bacterial endotoxin: a role in chronic inflammatory periodontal disease?, *J Oral Pathol*, **9**: 1–15.

Douglas CWI, Heath J et al., 1993, Identity of viridans streptococci isolated from cases of infective endocarditis, *J Med Microbiol*, **39**: 179–82.

Dreizen S, Daly TE et al., 1977, Oral complications of cancer radiotherapy, *Postgrad Med*, **61**: 85–92.

Duerden BI, Wade WG et al. (eds), 1995, *Medical and Dental Aspects of Anaerobes*, Science Reviews, Northwood, 1–85.

Eley BM, Cox SW, 1992, Correlation of gingival crevicular fluid proteases with clinical and radiological measurements of periodontal attachment loss, *J Dent*, **20**: 90–9.

Emilson CG, 1994, Potential efficacy of chlorhexidine against mutans streptococci and human dental caries, *J Dent Res*, **73**: 682–91.

Epstein JB, Stevenson-Moore P, Scully C, 1992, Management of xerostomia, *J Can Dent Assoc*, **58**: 140–3.

Fine DH, Mandel I, 1986, Indicators of periodontal disease activity, *J Clin Periodontol*, **13**: 533–46.

Fox PC, 1991, Bacterial infections of salivary glands, *Curr Opin Dent*, **1**: 411–14.

Genco RJ, 1992, Host responses in periodontal diseases: current concepts, *J Periodontol*, **63**: 338–55.

Genco RJ, Goldman HM, Cohen DW, 1990, *Contemporary Periodontics*, CV Mosby Company, St Louis.

George K, Zafiropoulos GG et al., 1994, Clinical and microbiological status of osseointegrated implants, *J Periodontol*, **65**: 766–70.

Gornitsky M, Clark DC et al., 1991, Clinical documentation and occurrence of putative periodontopathic bacteria in human immunodeficiency virus-associated periodontal disease, *J Periodontol*, **62**: 576–85.

Gossling J, 1988, Occurrence and pathogenicity of the *Streptococcus milleri* group, *Rev Infect Dis*, **10**: 257–85.

Greenman J, Osborne RH, Allaker RP, 1988, The production of potentially inflammatory compounds by human dental plaque and species of periodontal bacteria, *Microb Ecol Health Dis*, **1**: 245–53.

Guralnick W, 1984, Odontogenic infections, *Br Dent J*, **156**: 440–7.

Haffajee AD, Socransky SS, 1994, Microbial etiological agents of destructive periodontal diseases, *Periodontol 2000*, **5**: 78–111.

Hardie JM, 1991, Dental and oral infection, *Anaerobes in Human Disease*, eds Duerden BI, Drasar BS, Edward Arnold, London, 245–67.

Hardie JM, 1992, Oral microbiology: current concepts in the microbiology of dental caries and periodontal disease, *Br Dent J*, **172**: 271–8.

Hardie JM, Bowden GH, 1974, The normal microbial flora of the mouth, *The Normal Microbial Flora of Man*, eds Skinner FA, Carr JG, Academic Press, London, 47–83.

Hardie JM, Whiley RA, 1992, The genus *Streptococcus* – oral, *The Prokaryotes*, vol. 2, 2nd edn, eds Balows A, Trüper HG et al., Springer-Verlag, New York, 1421–49.

Hardie JM, Whiley RA, 1994, Recent developments in streptococcal taxonomy: their relation to infections, *Rev Med Microbiol*, **5**: 151–62.

Hardie JM, Whiley RA, 1995, The genus *Streptococcus*, *The Genera of Lactic Acid Bacteria*, eds Wood BJB, Holzapfel WH, Chapman & Hall, London, 55–124.

Hartley G, El-Maaytah M, Greenman J, 1995, Tongue microflora of subjects with low and high malodour levels, *J Dent Res*, **74**: 587.

Heimdahl A, von Konow L et al., 1985, Clinical appearance of orofacial infections of odontogenic origin in relation to microbiological findings, *J Clin Microbiol*, **22**: 299–302.

Henry CH, Hughes CV, Larned DC, 1992, Odontogenic infection of the orbit: report of a case, *J Oral Maxillofac Surg*, **50**: 172–8.

Holbrook WP, 1991, Bacterial infections of oral soft-tissues, *Curr Opin Dent*, **1**: 404–10.

Homer KA, Denbow L et al., 1993, Chondroitin sulfate depolymerase and hyaluronidase activities of viridans streptococci determined by a sensitive spectrophotometric assay, *J Clin Microbiol*, **31**: 1648–51.

Ingham HR, High AS et al., 1978, Abscesses of the frontal lobe of the brain secondary to covert dental sepsis, *Lancet*, **2**: 497–9.

Johnson NW, 1991a, *Risk Markers for Oral Diseases. Vol. 1. Dental Caries*, Cambridge University Press, Cambridge.

Johnson NW, 1991b, *Risk Markers for Oral Diseases. Vol. 3. Periodontal Diseases*, Cambridge University Press, Cambridge.

Jovanovic SA, 1994, Diagnosis and treatment of peri-implant disease, *Curr Opin Periodontol*, **1**: 194–202.

Karlowsky J, Ferguson J, Zhanel G, 1993, A review of commonly prescribed oral antibiotics in general dentistry, *J Can Dent Assoc*, **59**: 292–4.

Kidd EAM, Joyston-Bechal S, 1987, *Essentials of Dental Caries*, Wright, Bristol.

Köhler B, Andreen I, Jonsson B, 1988, The earlier the colonisation of mutans streptococci, the higher the caries prevalence at 4 years of age, *Oral Microbiol Immunol*, **3:** 14–17.

Köhler B, Bratthall D, Krasse B, 1983, Preventive measures in mothers influence the establishment of the bacterium *Streptococcus mutans* in their infants, *Arch Oral Biol*, **28:** 225–31.

Kornman KS, Loesche WJ, 1980, The subgingival microbial flora during pregnancy, *J Periodontal Res*, **15:** 111–22.

Krasse B, 1988, Biological factors as indicators of future caries, *Int Dent J*, **38:** 219–25.

Lamster IB, Novak MJ, 1992, Host mediators in gingival crevicular fluid: implications for the pathogenesis of periodontal disease, *Crit Rev Oral Biol Med*, **3:** 31–60.

Lamster IB, Smith QT et al., 1994, Development of a risk profile for periodontal disease: microbial and host response factors, *J Periodontol*, **65:** 511–20.

Lewis MAO, MacFarlane TW, McGowan DA, 1990, A microbiological and clinical review of the acute dentoalveolar abscess, *Br J Oral Maxillofac Surg*, **28:** 359–66.

Lewis MAO, McGowan DA, MacFarlane TW, 1986, Short-course high-dosage amoxycillin in the treatment of acute dento-alveolar abscess, *Br Dent J*, **161:** 299–302.

Lewis MAO, MacFarlane TW et al., 1988, Assessment of the pathogenicity of bacterial species isolated from acute dentoalveolar abscesses, *J Med Microbiol*, **27:** 109–16.

Lewis MAO, Milligan SG et al., 1993, Phagocytosis of bacterial strains isolated from acute dentoalveolar abscess, *J Med Microbiol*, **38:** 151–4.

Lewis MAO, Parkhurst CL et al., 1995, Prevalence of penicillin resistant bacteria in acute suppurative oral infection, *J Antimicrob Chemother*, **35:** 785–91.

Loesche WJ, 1986, Role of *Streptococcus mutans* in human dental decay, *Microbiol Rev*, **50:** 353–80.

Loesche WJ, 1988, The role of spirochetes in periodontal disease, *Adv Dent Res*, **2:** 275–83.

Loesche WJ, 1992, DNA probe and enzyme analysis in periodontal diagnostics, *J Periodontol*, **63:** 1102–9.

Loesche WJ, Syed SA et al., 1982, The bacteriology of acute necrotizing ulcerative gingivitis, *J Periodontol*, **53:** 223–30.

Loesche WJ, Bretz WA et al., 1990, Development of a diagnostic test for anaerobic periodontal infections based on plaque hydrolysis of benzoyl-DL-arginine-naphthylamide, *J Clin Microbiol*, **28:** 1551–9.

Lundberg C, 1980, Dental sinusitis, *Swed Dent J*, **4:** 63–7.

Lundberg C, Carenfelt C et al., 1979, Anaerobic bacteria in maxillary sinusitis, *Scand J Infect Dis*, **19:** 74–6.

McComb D, 1994, Operative dentistry considerations for the elderly, *J Prosthet Dent*, **72:** 517–24.

MacFarlane TW, 1989, Plaque-related infections, *J Med Microbiol*, **29:** 161–70.

MacFarlane TW, Samaranayake LP, 1989, *Clinical Oral Microbiology*, Wright, Bodmin.

McGowan D, Baxter PW, James J, 1993, *The Maxillary Sinus and Its Dental Implications*, Wright, Oxford.

McKee AS, McDermid AS et al., 1986, Effect of hemin on the physiology and virulence of *Bacteroides gingivalis* W50, *Infect Immun*, **52:** 349–55.

Ma JK, Hunjan M et al., 1990, An investigation into the mechanism of protection by local passive immunisation with monoclonal antibodies against *Streptococcus mutans*, *Infect Immun*, **58:** 3407–14.

Maiden MFJ, Carman RJ et al., 1990, Detection of high risk groups and individuals for periodontal diseases: laboratory markers based on the microbiological analysis of subgingival plaque, *J Clin Periodontol*, **17:** 1–13.

Marsh PD, 1991, The significance of maintaining the stability of the natural microflora of the mouth, *Br Dent J*, **171:** 174–7.

Marsh PD, Martin MV, 1992, *Oral Microbiology*, 3rd edn, Chapman and Hall, London.

Matee MN, Mikx FHM et al., 1992, Mutans streptococci and lactobacilli in breast-fed children with rampant caries, *Caries Res*, **26:** 183–7.

Meghji S, Wilson M et al., 1994, Bone resorbing activity of surface-associated material from *Actinobacillus actinomycetemcomitans* and *Eikenella corrodens*, *J Med Microbiol*, **41:** 197–203.

Milnes AR, Bowden GHW, 1985, The microflora associated with development of nursing caries, *Caries Res*, **19:** 289–97.

Mombelli A, Buser D et al., 1990, Suspected periodontopathogens in erupting third molar sites of periodontally healthy individuals, *J Clin Periodontol*, **17:** 48–54.

Moore LVH, Moore WEC et al., 1987, Bacteriology of human gingivitis, *J Dent Res*, **66:** 989–95.

Neiders ME, Chen PB et al., 1989, Heterogeneity of virulence among strains of *Bacteroides gingivalis*, *J Periodont Res*, **24:** 192–8.

Nitzan DW, 1983, On the genesis of 'dry socket', *J Oral Maxillofac Surg*, **41:** 706–10.

Ohman SC, 1988, *Angular Cheilitis: a Clinical, Microbiological and Immuno-histochemical Study*, PhD thesis, University of Gothenburg, Gothenburg.

Pallasch TJ, 1993, Antibiotics for acute orofacial infections, *J Calif Dent Assoc*, **21:** 34–44.

Paterson SA, Curzon MEJ, 1993, The effect of amoxycillin versus penicillin V in the treatment of acutely abscessed primary teeth, *Br Dent J*, **174:** 443–9.

Petit MDA, van Steenbergen TJM et al., 1993, Epidemiology and transmission of *Porphyromonas gingivalis* and *Actinobacillus actinomycetemcomitans* among children and their family members, *J Clin Periodontol*, **20:** 641–50.

Prayitno SW, Addy M, Wade WG, 1993, Does gingivitis lead to periodontitis in young adults?, *Lancet*, **342:** 71–2.

Rams TE, Andriolo M et al., 1991, Microbiological study of HIV-related periodontitis, *J Periodontol*, **62:** 74–81.

Ripa LW, 1978, Nursing habits and dental decay in infants: 'nursing bottle caries', *ASDC J Dent Child*, **45:** 274.

Rosenberg M, 1995, *Bad Breath: Research Perspectives*, Ramot Publishing, Tel Aviv University, Tel Aviv.

Russell MW, 1992, Immunization against dental caries, *Oral Maxillofac Surg Infect*, **2:** 72–80.

Russell RRB, 1994, The application of molecular genetics to the microbiology of dental caries, *Caries Res*, **28:** 69–82.

Saarela M, von Troil-Linden B et al., 1993, Transmission of oral bacterial species between spouses, *Oral Microbiol Immunol*, **8:** 349–54.

Samaranayake LP, MacFarlane TW, 1990, *Oral Candidosis*, Wright, London.

Schaal KP, 1981, Actinomycoses, *Rev Inst Pasteur (Lyon)*, **14:** 279–88.

Schlossberg D, 1987, *Infections of the Head and Neck*, Springer-Verlag, New York.

Schmidt-Westhausen A, Fehrenbach FJ, Reichart PA, 1990, Oral Enterobacteriaceae in patients with HIV infection, *J Oral Pathol Med*, **19:** 229–31.

Schupbach P, Osterwalder V, Guggenheim B, 1996, Human root caries: microbiota of a limited number of root caries lesions, *Caries Res*, **30:** 52–64.

Scully C, 1992, Oral infections in the immunocompromised patient, *Br Dent J*, **172:** 401–7.

Scully C, Flint S, 1989, *An Atlas of Stomatology*, Martin Dunitz, London.

Shah HN, Gharbia SE, 1993, Ecophysiology and taxonomy of *Bacteroides* and related taxa, *Clin Infect Dis*, **16:** 160–7.

Simmons NA, Ball AP et al., 1992, Antibiotic prophylaxis and infective endocarditis, *Lancet*, **339:** 1292–3.

Slots J, 1976, The predominant cultivable organisms in juvenile periodontitis, *Scand J Dent Res*, **84:** 1–10.

Slots J, 1977, The predominant cultivable microflora of advanced periodontitis, *Scand J Dent Res*, **85:** 114–21.

Slots J, 1982, Importance of black-pigmented *Bacteroides* in human periodontal disease, *Host–Parasite Interactions in Periodontal Diseases*, eds Genco RJ, Mergenhagen SE, American Society for Microbiology, Washington, DC, 27–45.

Slots J, Taubman MA, 1992, *Contemporary Oral Microbiology and Immunology*, Mosby Year Book, St Louis.

Slots J, Bragd L et al., 1986, The occurrence of *Actinobacillus actinomycetemcomitans*, *Bacteroides gingivalis* and *Bacteroides intermedius* in destructive periodontal disease in adults, *J Clin Periodontol*, **13:** 570–7.

Socransky SS, Haffajee AD, 1991, Microbial mechanisms in the pathogenesis of destructive periodontal diseases: a critical assessment, *J Periodontal Res*, **26:** 195–212.

Socransky SS, Haffajee AD, 1992, The bacterial etiology of periodontal disease: current concepts, *J Periodontol*, **63:** 322–31.

Socransky SS, Haffajee AD, 1994, Microbiology and immunology of periodontal diseases, *Periodontol 2000*, **5:** 7–25.

Socransky SS, Haffajee AD et al., 1984, New concepts of destructive periodontal disease, *J Clin Periodontol*, **11:** 21–32.

van Steenbergen TJ, Delemarre FG et al., 1987, Differences in virulence within the species *Bacteroides gingivalis*, *Antonie van Leeuwenhoek J Microbiol*, **53:** 233–44.

Taichman NS, Dean RT, Sanderson CJ, 1980, Biochemical and morphological characterisation of the killing of human monocytes by a leucotoxin derived from *Actinobacillus actinomycetemcomitans*, *Infect Immun*, **28:** 258–68.

Takada H, Mihara J et al., 1991, Production of cytokines by human gingival fibroblasts, *Periodontal Disease: Pathogens and Host Immune Responses*, eds Hamada S, Holt SC, McGhee JR, Quintessence, Tokyo, 265–76.

Tanner A, 1992, Microbial etiology in periodontal diseases: Where are we? Where are we going?, *Periodontol Rest Dent*, **1:** 12–24.

Tanner ACR, Haffer C et al., 1979, A study of bacteria associated with advancing periodontal disease in man, *J Clin Periodontol*, **6:** 278–307.

Tenovuo J, 1991, The microbiology and immunology of dental caries in children, *Rev Med Microbiol*, **2:** 76–82.

Tenovuo J, Hakkinen P et al., 1992, Effects of chlorhexidine-fluoride gel treatments in mothers on the establishment of mutans streptococci in primary teeth and the development of dental caries in children, *Caries Res*, **26:** 275–80.

Thylstrup A, Fejerskov O, 1994, *Textbook of Clinical Cariology*, 2nd edn, Munskgaard, Copenhagen.

Tonzetich J, 1977, Production and origin of oral malodour: a review of mechanisms and methods of analysis, *J Periodontol*, **48:** 13–20.

Tonzetich J, McBride BC, 1981, Characterisation of volatile sulphur production by pathogenic and non-pathogenic strains of oral *Bacteroides*, *Arch Oral Biol*, **26:** 963–9.

Van Houte J, 1994, Role of microoorganisms in caries aetiology, *J Dent Res*, **73:** 672–81.

Vehkalahti M, Paunio I, 1994, Association between root caries occurrence and periodontal state, *Caries Res*, **28:** 301–6.

Wade WG, Gray AR et al., 1991, Predominant cultivable flora in pericoronitis, *Oral Microbiol Immunol*, **6:** 310–12.

Whiley RA, Fraser HY et al., 1990, Phenotypic differentiation of *Streptococcus intermedius*, *Streptococcus constellatus*, and *Streptococcus anginosus* strains within the 'Streptococcus milleri group', *J Clin Microbiol*, **28:** 1497–501.

Whiley RA, Beighton D et al., 1992, *Streptococcus intermedius*, *Streptococcus constellatus*, and *Streptococcus anginosus* (the *Streptococcus milleri* group): association with different body sites and clinical infections, *J Clin Microbiol*, **30:** 243–4.

Yaegaki K, Sanada K, 1992, Volatile sulphur compounds in mouth air from clinically healthy subjects and patients with periodontal disease, *J Periodontal Res*, **27:** 233–8.

Youngs G, 1994, Risk factors for and the prevention of root caries in older adults, *Special Care Dent*, **14:** 68–70.

Zambon JJ, 1985, *Actinobacillus actinomycetemcomitans* in human periodontal disease, *J Clin Periodontol*, **12:** 1–20.

Zambon JJ, Reynolds HS, Genco RJ, 1990, Studies of the subgingival microflora in patients with acquired immunodeficiency syndrome, *J Periodontol*, **61:** 699–704.

Chapter 21

TUBERCULOSIS

J M Grange

1 INTRODUCTION

Tuberculosis is a disease of great antiquity and has almost certainly caused more suffering and death than any other infection. Despite the availability of effective chemotherapy, it is still a major health problem in most countries of the world. In the past, tuberculosis was referred to as the 'white plague' and, by John Bunyan, as 'the captain of all of these men of death'. The clinical features of both respiratory and spinal tuberculosis were well described by Hippocrates in about 400 BC (Major 1959); accounts of the disease appeared in the Vedas and other ancient Hindu texts, in which it was termed *rajayakshma* – the king of diseases – and it afflicted neolithic man and pre-Columbian Amerindians (Clark et al. 1987).

The transmissible nature of tuberculosis was established by Villemin (1868) by inoculating rabbits with tuberculous material from humans and cattle. Villemin also established that scrofula (tuberculous lymphadenitis) and pulmonary tuberculosis were manifestations of the same disease process. Villemin's prediction that the causative agent of tuberculosis would be isolated was realized in 1882 when Robert Koch succeeded in cultivating it on inspissated serum. By a large series of inoculations with pure cultures of the bacillus, several generations removed from the primary one, Koch transmitted the disease to many animals of different species. His classical study established without doubt that the bacillus he had isolated was the cause of tuberculosis. The story of Koch's discovery and its sequelae is reviewed by Grange and Bishop (1982).

In addition to cultivating the causative organism, Koch succeeded in staining it by treatment with an alkaline solution of methylene blue for 24 h. Subsequently Ehrlich improved the technique by using a hot solution of carbol fuchsin and it is this technique, slightly modified by Ziehl and Neelsen whose names it bears, that is still widely used today.

Tuberculosis of man and animals is caused by a group of very closely related species forming the *Mycobacterium tuberculosis* complex. These are *M. tuberculosis*, the human tubercle bacillus, *Mycobacterium bovis*, the bovine tubercle bacillus, *Mycobacterium africanum*, a rather heterogeneous group of strains of human origin occurring principally in equatorial Africa, and *Mycobacterium microti*, the vole tubercle bacillus. The complex also contains BCG vaccine, supposedly derived from a strain of *M. bovis*, and occasional isolates, from wild or domesticated animals, which do not fit clearly into the above species. Although divided into these 4 species, on taxonomic grounds they are really variants of a single species.

M. tuberculosis is transmitted almost exclusively in cough spray from patients with open pulmonary tuberculosis and gains access to the body by inhalation of infective droplets usually less than 5 μm across. Consequently, the initial lesion is usually in the lung, from which organisms reach other organs via the lymphatics and the bloodstream. In rural areas where bovine tuberculosis control measures have not been instituted, *M. bovis* is often spread to farm workers by cough spray from diseased cattle whereas town dwellers are infected by the ingestion of infected raw milk or cream. In the latter case the primary lesions are usually in the tonsil or intestinal tract, leading to cervical or mesenteric lymphadenopathy. Human tuberculosis due to *M. bovis* is rare in countries where the disease in cattle is well controlled but occasional cases, principally due to reactivation of old lesions, still occur. Further information can be found in Volume 2 (see Volume 2, Chapter 26).

In the 1970s it was generally expected that tuberculosis would soon be a disease of the past in the developed nations and that, with improvements in living standards, a decline leading to eventual eradication would occur in the developing world. Such expectations have been sadly dashed and, in April 1993, the World Health Organization took the unprecedented step of declaring tuberculosis a 'global emergency' (World Health Organization 1994a).

2   EPIDEMIOLOGY, PREVENTION AND CONTROL

Epidemiological studies on tuberculosis are concerned with the transmission of the disease in the community and the impact of control measures.

2.1   Prevalence in the community

An understanding of the natural history of tuberculosis is essential to determinations of its incidence and prevalence in a community. Not all persons infected by the tubercle bacillus develop overt disease. The proportion of infected persons in whom clinical disease eventually develops is termed the 'disease ratio'. As a general rule, about 10% of non-immunocompromised infected persons eventually develop overt disease. The disease ratio in HIV-positive persons and in those with certain other immunocompromising conditions is much higher (see section 2.5, p. 393).

Tuberculosis is divided into primary and post-primary forms. The immunological basis and clinical features of these 2 types are described elsewhere in this chapter but for practical epidemiological purposes they are defined, respectively, as disease developing within or after 5 years of infection (Styblo 1978). Again, as a general rule, about 5% of infected persons develop primary, and 5% post-primary, disease. The interval between the initial infection and overt disease varies from a few weeks to several decades and post-primary disease may be due to endogenous reactivation of the initial infection or to exogenous reinfection (see section 2.2). Once developed, overt disease may last for over a year unless actively treated. Accordingly the number of cases of active tuberculosis at a given time (the 'point prevalence') is not the same as the number of new cases recorded each year (the 'annual incidence').

Before effective treatment became available the annual death rate from tuberculosis was a useful indicator of the incidence of disease but it is now necessary to rely on active and passive case-finding. Experience has shown that calculations of the incidence of tuberculosis on the basis of case-finding and notification are very unreliable. In Great Britain, where there is a statutory requirement to notify tuberculosis, around 20% of cases are not notified (Sheldon et al. 1992). Accordingly, epidemiological studies are now usually based on determinations of the 'annual infection rate' or 'annual risk of infection'. Infection, for this purpose, is defined as a conversion to tuberculin positivity and the annual risk may be calculated from

the results of tuberculin test surveys of children and young adults (Styblo 1984), provided that they have not had BCG vaccination. Mass miniature radiology (MMR) was a popular case-finding tool but only about 20% of cases of tuberculosis were found in this way and the World Health Organization has recommended that it should no longer be used routinely. It is nevertheless still useful for the screening of certain high risk groups, such as immigrants from high incidence regions and residents in common lodging houses (Capewell et al. 1986).

The annual infection rate gives an indirect indication of the incidence of overt tuberculosis. A 1% annual infection rate indicates that there are about 50 infectious cases for every 100 000 members of the population.

2.2   Endogenous reactivation and exogenous reinfection

For many decades it was dogmatically asserted that primary tuberculosis induced a degree of immunity sufficient to prevent exogenous reinfection. This, in turn, led to the belief that all post-primary tuberculosis is due to endogenous reactivation of a poorly understood 'latent' form of tuberculosis. The fallacy of this dogma became apparent during the conduct of an intensive tuberculosis control campaign in Canadian Eskimo populations (Grzybowski, Styblo and Dorken 1976). This campaign led, as was expected, to a large reduction in the incidence of primary tuberculosis and in the infection rate but also, and unexpectedly, to a reduction of incidence of the disease among older, previously infected persons. This indicated that a significant proportion of cases of post-primary disease was due to exogenous reinfection.

Several studies subsequently confirmed that exogenous reinfection frequently occurs in communities where there are many infectious source cases but that endogenous reactivation is relatively more common in low incidence regions (Styblo 1978, 1984). DNA 'fingerprinting' studies have established that exogenous reinfection occurs more often than previously believed (Stoker 1994).

2.3   Natural trends in the incidence of tuberculosis

In the absence of specific control programmes, the incidence of tuberculosis in the community is affected by many factors, including the density of population, the extent of overcrowding and the general standard of living and health care. The natural trend must be considered when evaluating the impact of BCG vaccination, chemotherapy and other specific antituberculosis control measures, otherwise the impact of these may be overemphasized. In the USA and most European countries there was a decline in the incidence of the disease during the first half of the twentieth century of about 5% annually. In Europe, however, there were temporary increases corresponding with the 2 World Wars. Mass BCG programmes had only a small effect, but the introduction of effective treatment of infectious cases accelerated the decline to 7–8% annually until the mid-1970s. Since that time, the decline rate in many developed countries has slowed and in some there has been an increase (Table 21.1). One of the reasons for the increase is the effect of the HIV pandemic (see section 2.5). Others include immigration from high incidence countries and increasing inner-city deprivation but a key factor is the loss of interest and awareness that resulted from the decline in the incidence of the disease during the previous few decades (Reichmann 1991). In the pre-HIV era, the situation in the developing nations was more variable but in many the annual risk of infection was in slow but steady decline. Owing to the population explosion, however, the absolute number of cases of tuberculosis world wide continually increased.

2.4 The global toll of tuberculosis

According to World Health Organization estimates, one-third of the world's human population (approximately 1700 million persons) has been infected by the tubercle bacillus. This proportion of infected persons is similar in developing and developed countries but in the latter most infected persons are in older age groups. Thus in the USA and UK, for example, only about 12% of persons in the age range principally exposed to HIV, 15–45 years, are infected whereas in sub-Saharan Africa almost 50% of this age group is infected. Each year, 100 million persons enter the infected pool (Kochi 1991).

An estimated 8–10 million people develop overt tuberculosis annually as a result of primary infection, endogenous reactivation or exogenous reinfection (Kochi 1991). The global distribution of these cases is shown in Table 21.2. As the disease is a chronic one which is poorly treated in many parts of the world, there are probably around 20 million patients at any given time. In 1994 about 3 million people (1.1 million children and 1.9 million adults) died of tuberculosis and this mortality rate could rise to 4 million annually by the year 2004 unless there are radical changes in global control initiatives (World Health Organization 1994b). Tuberculosis is the cause of 7% of all deaths and 1 in 4 **preventable** adult deaths, even though it is among the most cost-effective of all adult diseases to treat (Murray, Styblo and Rouillon 1990).

2.5 The impact of the HIV pandemic

The coexistence of HIV infection and tuberculosis has been hailed as one of the most serious threats to human health since the Black Death and has been called 'the Cursed Duet' (Chretien 1990). As explained in section 2.1, persons infected by tubercle bacilli have about a 10% chance of developing tuberculosis during the remainder of their lives; thus they have a less than 0.5% chance of developing overt disease annually. By contrast, an HIV-positive person already infected by the tubercle bacillus has an 8% chance of developing overt disease annually, or up to 50% during the remainder of their relatively short life span (Dolin, Raviglione and Kochi 1994). Thus HIV-positive persons infected by *M. tuberculosis* have a 20-fold higher chance of developing tuberculosis than their HIV-negative counterparts. Put another way, 95% of cases of tuberculosis in the dually infected population are attributable to the effect of the HIV infection whereas the remaining 5% would have occurred if the patients had not been HIV-positive (Dolin, Raviglione and Kochi 1994). In addition, HIV-positive persons are much more likely to develop overt disease after infection or reinfection and the interval between infection and appearance of symptoms is considerably shortened (Edlin et al. 1992, Bouvet et al. 1993).

In mid-1994, there were an estimated 16 million adults (of whom 13–14 million were still alive) and 1 million children infected by HIV world wide (World Health Organization 1994c). From data on the prevalence of both infections at that time it was calculated that about 5.6 million people were dually infected and distributed as shown in Table 21.3. As 8% of dually infected persons develop tuberculosis in one year, HIV was responsible for about 450 000 cases of tuberculosis in 1994, 300 000 of these cases occurring in sub-Saharan Africa. From the global incidence of tuberculosis, it was estimated that about 5% of cases world wide and 20% of cases in Africa were HIV-related.

The impact on medical services of the additional HIV-related cases of tuberculosis has been particularly severely in sub-Saharan Africa. In 4 countries with well organized epidemiological services, Tanzania, Burundi, Malawi and Zambia, increases of 86%, 140%, 180% and 154% respectively were reported between 1984 and 1990 (Narain, Raviglione and Kochi 1992).

The future impact of HIV infection on tuberculosis world wide will depend on changes in the annual tuberculosis infection rate, the prevalence of infection by the tubercle bacillus in the at-risk age group and the prevalence of HIV infection. It has been calculated

Table 21.1 Reported increases in the incidence of tuberculosis in some industrialized countries

Country	Percentage	Time period of increase
Austria	5	1989–1990
Denmark	20	1986–1992
Ireland	9	1988–1991
Italy	27	1988–1992
Netherlands	19	1987–1992
Norway	21	1988–1991
Spain	28	1990–1992
United Kingdom	5	1987–1991
USA	20	1985–1992

Data from World Health Organization (1994a).

Table 21.2   The estimated global toll of tuberculosis in 1991

Region	Persons infected (millions)	New cases	Deaths
Africa	171	1 400 000	660 000
South/Central America	117	560 000	220 000
Eastern Mediterranean	52	594 000	160 000
South East Asia	426	2 480 000	940 000
Western Pacific	574	2 560 000	890 000
Industrialized	382	410 000	40 000
Total	1722	8 004 000	2 910 000

Data from Kochi (1991).

Table 21.3   The estimated numbers and geographical distribution of HIV-infected adults alive in mid-1994 and those dually infected with HIV and *M. tuberculosis*

Geographical region	Total HIV-positive	Dually infected
Sub-Saharan Africa	8 000 000	3 760 000
North Africa/Middle East	100 000	23 000
Western Europe	450 000	49 000
Eastern Europe/Central Asia	50 000	9000
Latin America/Caribbean	1 500 000	450 000
North America	800 000	80 000
East Asia/Pacific	50 000	20 000
South/South East Asia	>2 500 000	>1 150 000
Australia	>20 000	>4000
Total	13 500 000	5 600 000

Data from the World Health Organization (1994b).

that, by the year 2000, the annual incidence of tuberculosis in African cities, given 4 scenarios ranging from optimistic to worst-case, will be between 300 and 4218 per 100 000 (Schulzer et al. 1992). It has also been calculated that by the same year there will be 1 410 000 cases of HIV-related tuberculosis world wide, 604 000 of these in Africa, accounting for about 14% of all cases of tuberculosis (Dolin, Raviglione and Kochi 1994).

Although patients with HIV-related tuberculosis often respond to standard short course chemotherapy, those in Africa are almost 4 times as likely to die of tuberculosis than HIV-negative patients within 13 months of diagnosis, mostly in the first month of therapy (Nunn 1994). Even if therapy induces a bacteriological cure, the patients' subsequent life may be shortened. The reason for this is not fully understood but there is evidence that immune responses in tuberculosis, and in other infections, induce cytokines that enhance the replication of the HIV and thus drive the patient into the full picture of AIDS with considerable shortening of life (reviewed by Festenstein and Grange 1991). Although the details are not clear, there is evidence that TNF-α and other immunological mediators released in tuberculosis lead to transactivation of the HIV provirus and its subsequent replication (Osborn, Kunkel and Nabel 1989). In addition, tuberculosis causes a CD4+ T cell lymphopenia which may synergize with that induced by the HIV (Beck et al. 1985). Whatever the cause, the occurrence of active

tuberculosis in the HIV-positive patient has very serious consequences, demanding strenuous efforts to prevent such disease by programmes of chemoprophylaxis or, preferably, immunoprophylaxis (Stanford et al. 1993a).

2.6   Transmissibility

It is well established that patients with sputum that is positive on direct microscopical examination, and thus contains at least 5000 bacilli in 1 ml, are the principal sources of infection (Rouillon, Perdrizet and Parrot 1976). Smear-negative patients, whether culture-positive or not, are of very low infectivity. There has been considerable debate as to whether this relation between smear positivity and infectivity holds true in the case of HIV-related tuberculosis as such patients are frequently smear-negative. A study in Kenya, however, indicated that pulmonary tuberculosis in HIV-positive persons is, in general, as infectious as in HIV-negative persons (Nunn et al. 1994).

The risk of infection depends greatly on the closeness of contact as well as the infectiousness of the source case. Transmission of tuberculosis occurs principally within households (van Geuns, van Meijer and Styblo 1975) and other groups of people living in close proximity, such as prisoners and residents of common lodging houses. Children under the age of 3 years are particularly susceptible to infection from household source cases, probably owing to closer contact – those exposed to smear-positive and negative source cases have, respectively, a 50% and 6% chance of being infected.

There have been reports of 'explosive' epidemics of tuberculosis in communities after minimal exposure to highly infectious source cases. In one such case 187 of 3764 children aged between 8 and 11 years became infected after use of a swimming pool supervised by an attendant with open tuberculosis (Rao et al. 1980). Explosive epidemics have also occurred in situations, such as hospitals, overcrowded accommodation and prisons, where several HIV-positive persons had been exposed to an infectious source case (Daley et al. 1992, Edlin et al. 1992, Bouvet et al. 1993).

The average number of persons infected by one source case is expressed as the 'transmission or contagious parameter'. The number of persons infected by a source case depends on the length of time that the source patient is infectious. In the absence of therapy, about 65% of patients with open pulmonary tuberculosis die within 4 years of becoming infectious, with an average survival of 14 months (Springett 1971). About a quarter recover spontaneously and a minority become chronic excretors of tubercle bacilli.

In developing countries, where households are often large and health services suboptimal, the contagion parameter is high: each patient with open tuberculosis infects, on average, 20 persons annually. By contrast, patients living under good socioeconomic conditions probably only infect 2 or 3 persons.

2.7 Epidemiological significance of chemotherapy and drug resistance

As tuberculosis is almost always spread from person to person, chemotherapy, by rendering source cases uninfectious, is the main component of control programmes. The impact of chemotherapy on the spread of infection depends on the effectiveness of the therapeutic regimens, the adherence (compliance) of the patients and the percentage of cases that are diagnosed. Patients receiving effective chemotherapy are rapidly rendered non-infectious even though they continue to excrete cultivable tubercle bacilli for several weeks. For practical purposes, patients are usually regarded as being non-infectious from the time that chemotherapy is started (Rouillon, Perdrizet and Parrot 1976) though this is a risky assumption in regions and communities where multidrug resistance is common.

The impact of chemotherapy on disease control also depends on the interval between onset of infectivity and commencement of therapy. The epidemiological impact of chemotherapy is considerably reduced if source cases have infected all their household contacts by the time they commence therapy.

Drug-resistant tuberculosis is on the increase in many parts of the world but the exact extent of the problem and its adverse impact on disease control is poorly documented. Attention was focused on this problem by the occurrence of several outbreaks of HIV-related drug-resistant tuberculosis in the USA

(Dooley and Simone 1994, Morse 1994). In this context, HIV infection is not in itself a cause of drug resistance but it facilitates the rapid dissemination of resistant bacilli in affected populations.

Resistance to one of the drugs that were used in early regimens, streptomycin or isoniazid, is commonly encountered world wide and does not pose a serious threat to tuberculosis control. Resistance to rifampicin is much more serious, especially as most strains resistant to this drug are also resistant to isoniazid. Multidrug resistance (MDR) is usually defined as resistance to isoniazid and rifampicin, with or without additional drug resistance. MDR tuberculosis fails to respond to standard short course chemotherapy and it is necessary to use regimens containing drugs that are considerably less effective, more toxic and more expensive (see section 8.2, p. 409).

It is important to monitor the development and spread of drug resistance but laboratories able to perform drug susceptibility tests of a reliable standard are expensive to establish and maintain and are therefore uncommon in the developing world (World Health Organization 1994d). Thus reports of drug resistance from most developing countries usually give only a crude cross-sectional estimate with little or no information on changing trends (Rieder 1994). The World Health Organization (1994d) has stressed the need for systematic world-wide surveys of drug resistance undertaken by supraregional laboratories.

There are 2 forms of drug resistance. Secondary or acquired resistance is the result of the preferential replication of mutants in patients receiving inadequate therapy. Primary resistant disease occurs when an untreated person is infected by a strain that is already resistant. It is often difficult to be absolutely sure that a person with supposed primary resistant tuberculosis has not previously received antituberculosis therapy. Thus some workers prefer the term initial resistance to primary resistance.

It is important, whenever possible, to distinguish between acquired and initial resistance in the assessment of tuberculosis control services as the continued occurrence of the former indicates that some patients are being inadequately treated.

2.8 Epidemiology of human tuberculosis due to *M. bovis*

Animal reservoirs of *M. bovis* pose a serious threat to human health. Tuberculosis in cattle principally involves the lung and is spread from animal to animal by cough spray. Humans in direct contact with cattle may likewise be infected and develop primary pulmonary lesions. Milk is the principal vector of transmission of *M. bovis* to town dwellers. Such transmission is facilitated by the practice of pooling milk from many cows and herds.

Well executed bovine tuberculosis eradication schemes (see section 9.1, p. 411) result in a rapid decline in the incidence of tuberculosis in cattle followed by a reduction in the incidence of primary manifestations of the disease, such as tuberculous lymphadenitis (scrofula), in the human population.

In countries where tuberculosis has been virtually eradicated in cattle, a few cases continue to occur in the human population. The great majority of such cases occur in persons born before the disease was controlled in cattle and are thus assumed to be due to endogenous reactivation of old lesions. Evidence for human-to-human spread of disease due to *M. bovis* is limited and anecdotal. Whereas primary human tuberculosis of bovine origin is usually non-pulmonary, the lung is involved in about half the cases of post-primary disease (Grange and Yates 1994) and there are reports of cattle being infected by such patients. About a quarter of cases of post-primary human disease involve the genitourinary tract and there have been several reports of farm workers infecting cattle by urinating in cowsheds (see section 9.1, p. 411).

A few cases of HIV-related tuberculosis due to *M. bovis*, and human-to-human spread, have been reported (reviewed by Grange, Daborn and Cosivi 1994). A high incidence of HIV-related tuberculosis due to *M. bovis* in pastoralist communities could lead to increased human-to-animal spread of disease with serious socioeconomic consequences.

For further details of the zoonotic implications of *M. bovis* see Grange and Yates (1994) and Cosivi et al. (1995).

3 PREVENTION AND CONTROL OF HUMAN TUBERCULOSIS

As tuberculosis control programmes are based on the therapy of infectious source cases, their success is dependent on the detection of such cases. Other measures with much less impact include BCG vaccination and prescription of antituberculosis drugs prophylactically to persons exposed to infectious source cases or to healthy but infected persons to prevent reactivation of disease.

The present global emergency of tuberculosis clearly indicates that the available control measures, or our use of such measures, or both, have failed. Control programmes designed by international agencies cannot be effective in the absence of funding and adequate local infrastructures and, as such programmes are inevitably designed by committees, dogma rather than imagination and innovation prevails (Chaulet 1983, Grange and Stanford 1994).

3.1 Case-finding and case-holding

In view of the close relation between sputum smear positivity and infectivity (see section 2.6, p. 394) the provision of reliable microscopy services is of prime importance in control programmes. Infectious persons may be detected passively, i.e. by waiting for those with symptoms to attend the health centres, or actively, by searching for suspects, usually defined as persons with a cough for 1 month or more in duration.

Passive case-finding is very unreliable as, even with good public education, patients often fail to seek medical attention until they are very ill and have probably infected many contacts. One reason for non-presentation is the fear of a long period of hospitalization and loss of earnings. Thus education should stress that, if diagnosed early, therapy of tuberculosis does not interfere with normal employment.

Active case-finding involves a deliberate search for patients and various techniques have been evaluated, notably by Aluoch and his colleagues in Kenya (Aluoch et al. 1985). The most effective was the labour-intensive method of making a direct enquiry to the heads of all households. Enquiries to community leaders and indirect methods, such as enquiries to women attending antenatal or child-care clinics about suspect cases within their families, were less successful. In general, the success of any form of case-finding is inversely proportional to the distance between the suspects' homes and the clinic, stressing the need for the establishment of small clinics in rural areas.

Contact tracing is a key component of tuberculosis control and up to 10% of cases of tuberculosis may be found in this way. Household contacts of patients with smear-positive pulmonary disease should be screened, as should the contacts of patients with non-respiratory smear-negative pulmonary disease as they may prove to be the source cases. DNA 'fingerprinting' of tubercle bacilli is proving to be a useful tool for establishing the way in which tuberculosis is spread in a community and in designing contact tracing procedures (Stoker 1994). For details of contact tracing and the examination of contacts in developed countries see Veen (1992), Etkind (1993) and Report (1994a).

3.2 Problems encountered in chemotherapy

Whereas effective chemotherapy is a key component of tuberculosis control, inadequate regimens or irregularly administered drugs have an adverse effect by prolonging the period of infectivity and generating drug resistance. Inadequate therapy may be the result of poor prescribing practices (Uplekar and Shepard 1991) or the drugs themselves may be at fault. Thus the bioavailability of drugs in combination formulations may be suboptimal (Fox 1990) and drugs may be time-expired before they are used. In some countries it is possible to obtain drugs, including cough mixtures containing isoniazid, without prescription and this may lead to the development of drug resistance.

Even when there is a reliable supply of effective drugs, treatment failure is common and the usual cause is non-adherence. Although the patient is usually blamed for non-adherence, it is much more likely that the medical services are at fault. Strategies for improving adherence include fully supervised or directly observed therapy, combination tablets, blister packs and urine checks but by far the most important strategy is a caring and supportive attitude to the patients and the totality of their problems. Communication and understanding are particularly important in the treatment of patients in ethnic minorities (Grange and Festenstein 1993). Patients usually take their drugs in the initial phase of therapy when they are feeling ill but often fail to do so later on when they are feeling well (Shears 1984). For this reason, the World Health Organization (1995) has stressed the need for directly observed therapy, short course (DOTS; see section 8.1, p. 408). The impact of this strategy is well illustrated by an extensive study by the China Tuberculosis Control Collaboration (1996) in which a cure rate of 50% was increased to almost 90% among new cases and 81% among those previously treated.

3.3 Social factors in disease control

Correct motivation must exist at global, governmental and local levels if tuberculosis is to be controlled effectively. International agencies such as the World Health Organization and the International Union Against Tuberculosis cannot function, except on paper, unless they are adequately funded. It is important not to overemphasize the beneficial effects of 'scientific' medical intervention. The main reason for the decline in the incidence of tuberculosis in the developed nations during the twentieth century was the reduction in overcrowding in the home and in workplaces. Tuberculosis was, and still is, a disease associated with poverty and deprivation. Thus, the last of the '10 commitments' to tuberculosis control proposed by McAdam (1994) demands a reduction of the the social and economic inequalities which allow tuberculosis to flourish. In the same vein, Benatar (1995) has eloquently drawn attention to the need to make progress towards a more just, humane, peaceful and sustainable global community so that tuberculosis and other plagues may be finally eradicated.

It is equally important, however, not to overemphasize 'natural' trends in the behaviour of tuberculosis when considering the final eradication of such disease in low prevalence areas. The belief that the downward trend of tuberculosis observed in the industrially developed nations during most of the twentieth century would continue until the disease was extinct led to a premature loss of interest (Reichman 1991). It is important to remember that tuberculosis is no respector of geographical boundaries and that no person or nation will be safe until the disease is finally conquered.

If the current trends of HIV-related tuberculosis remain unchanged, the situation in the twenty-first century will be exceedingly serious. Prevention of the spread of HIV by education, and control of tuberculosis by use of currently available resources, are having a minimal impact. A ray of hope lies in the development and deployment of therapeutic measures that will correct the immune defect in both tuberculosis and HIV/AIDS (see section 8.7, p. 411). Prophylactic therapy of dually infected persons is fine in principle

but beset with considerable difficulties in practice (see section 8.5, p. 410).

The principles of tuberculosis surveillance and control have been reviewed in detail by Styblo (1986) and a useful practical guide to the organization of control programmes has been prepared by the Oxfam Health Unit (1985).

3.4 Factors affecting the incidence and nature of, and mortality from, tuberculosis

The incidence of tuberculosis within a community varies according to the ethnic origins and socioeconomic status of those affected. In general, the incidence of tuberculosis is higher in men than in women but it is not known whether the latter have a higher innate resistance. There is a particularly high incidence of tuberculosis among the residents of common lodging houses, many of whom are men who smoke and drink excessively (Capewell et al. 1986). A study in China showed that heavy smokers had a high chance of developing tuberculosis and smoking largely accounted for a higher incidence of the disease in males and in the elderly (Yu, Hsieh and Peng 1988).

Certain occupational groups have a higher incidence of tuberculosis than the general population. Workers exposed to metallic or stone dust, including miners, are particularly at risk. Occupational exposure to patients with tuberculosis is a hazard among health care staff. Cases of tuberculosis among clinical laboratory staff have been reported but the risk is minimized by modern safety measures (Collins 1993).

A high incidence of tuberculosis is often found in immigrant communities, particularly among the more recent arrivals from countries where the disease is prevalent. The incidence of non-respiratory forms of tuberculosis, notably cervical lymphadenitis, is relatively more common in immigrant patients although the incidence of genitourinary tuberculosis is similar to that in the indigenous population (Grange, Yates and Ormerod 1995).

Immunosuppressed persons are at risk from tuberculosis. In addition to HIV (see section 2.5, p. 393), predisposing causes include organ transplantation, renal failure and cancer. It is often stated in the literature that steroid therapy predisposes to reactivation tuberculosis but the evidence for this is weak and controversial (Bateman 1993).

4 CLINICAL FEATURES AND NOMENCLATURE OF HUMAN TUBERCULOSIS

4.1 Primary tuberculosis

Human tuberculosis is a disease of numerous different manifestations but there is an underlying pattern which is here briefly depicted. Disease occurring in a person never previously exposed to a tubercle bacillus is termed 'primary tuberculosis'. Infection results in a focus of disease (the Ghon focus) at the site of implantation of the bacillus, usually the lung but occasionally the tonsil, intestine or skin. This focus, together with enlarged, infected regional lymph nodes is termed the 'primary complex'.

In some cases, particularly in tonsillar infections, the primary focus is very small and the enlarged lymph nodes are the only observable manifestations of disease (Fig. 21.1). Lymph node enlargement is often greater in children than in adults.

Haematogenous spread occurs in primary tuberculosis with implantation of bacilli in many organs. In some persons, particularly children under 3 years of age, these foci progress to serious, even fatal, disease principally involving the meninges, kidney, bones and pleurae. Foci developing in the endothelium of major blood vessels may rupture and give rise to widespread small granulomata, a disease termed 'miliary tuberculosis' (Latin: milium, a millet seed).

The primary complex often resolves but it may cause serious local complications. The Ghon focus or a lymph node may erode into a bronchus causing endobronchial lesions or tuberculous pneumonia, or into the pleural or pericardial cavities leading, respectively, to tuberculous pleurisy or empyaema, and pericarditis. A grossly enlarged lymph node may compress a major bronchus, causing a segment or lobe of the lung to collapse (epituberculosis). These complications are reviewed by Miller (1982) and Donald, Fourie and Grange (1996).

Congenital tuberculosis, probably the result of haematogenous infection via the umbilical artery, or of ingestion of infected amniotic fluid, is extremely rare but rapidly fatal if untreated (Snider and Bloch 1984).

Most primary complexes resolve spontaneously but a few tubercle bacilli may enter the poorly understood state of persistence or latency (see section 5.2, p. 400). Such infected but healthy persons are usually, but not invariably, tuberculin-positive.

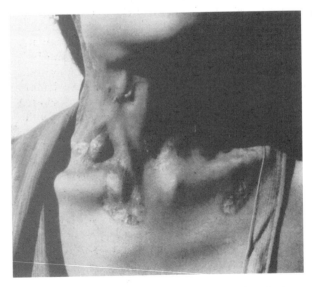

Fig. 21.1 Scrofuloderma: tuberculous cervical lymphadenitis with overlying lupus vulgaris.

Though human tuberculosis is very variable in its manifestations, there is a basic sequence of events referred to by Wallgren (1948) as 'the timetable of tuberculosis'. The original sequence was established by observations on children in the pre-chemotherapeutic era and subsequently modified by Ustvedt (1947). The timetable is shown in Fig. 21.2, but it is of limited usefulness in Europe and the USA where most tuberculosis is post-primary and occurs in adults (Rubilar et al. 1994).

4.2 Post-primary tuberculosis

Post-primary tuberculosis develops in previously infected persons either as a result of endogenous reactivation of latent disease or of exogenous reinfection (see section 2.2, p. 392). It usually occurs 5 years after primary infection although some primary foci, notably in adolescents, progress directly to lesions with the characteristics of post-primary disease: this is termed progressive primary tuberculosis. For poorly understood reasons, the usual site of post-primary disease is the upper part of the lung. The characteristic feature of such disease is extensive tissue necrosis. Very large tumour-like lesions termed tuberculomas may develop and, in common with primary lesions, the conditions within them do not favour mycobacterial growth. The necrotic tissue is softened and eventually liquefied by macrophage-derived proteases and if the lesion erodes into a bronchus, the liquefied contents are discharged and a cavity is formed. In distinct contrast to closed lesions, the well oxygenated cavities are ideal environments for bacillary replication. Thus their walls are lined by numerous bacilli which, in many respects, are behaving more like saprophytes than as primary pathogens. In the absence of treatment, cavities occasionally close spontaneously due to contraction of fibrous scar tissue, with restoration of the previous anoxic conditions and resolution of the disease.

Bacilli escaping from cavities may enter the sputum and be expectorated, thereby infecting other persons. They may also spread through the respiratory tract and cause secondary lesions in the same and contralateral lung and the larynx. Swallowed bacilli may cause tuberculous ulcers to develop in the gastrointestinal tract and the anus. On the other hand, spread of disease to lymph nodes and more distant organs is uncommon in post-primary disease, probably due to the obliteration of draining lymphatics and capillaries by the tissue necrosis and subsequent deposition of scar tissue.

The formation of cavities and localization of the disease process characteristic of post-primary tuberculosis are dependent on immune reactivity. Cavity formation is often limited or absent in immunocompromised persons and dissemination of disease to many organs frequently occurs (Festenstein and Grange 1991).

Various phenomena thought to be immunological in origin occur in tuberculosis. Erythema nodosum and phlyctenular conjunctivitis may be observed at the time of tuberculin conversion 3–8 weeks after primary infection. In a rare

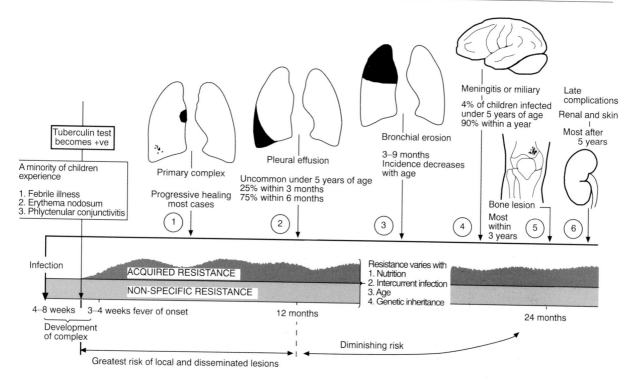

Fig. 21.2 The natural history of untreated primary tuberculosis of childhood. (Based on Wallgren 1948 and reproduced from Miller 1982, with permission).

chronic form of erythema nodosum, termed erythema induratum or Bazin's disease, the lesions may ulcerate. Patients with post-primary tuberculosis occasionally develop crops of skin lesions called tuberculides (reviewed by Grange 1989) or a sterile arthropathy termed Poncet's disease (Wilkinson and Roy 1984). The cause of these uncommon manifestations is unknown.

For general reviews of the clinical features of tuberculosis see Patel and Abrahams (1989), Crofton, Horne and Miller (1992), Davies (1994) and Grange (1996). For descriptions of childhood tuberculosis see Miller (1982) and Donald, Fourie and Grange (1996). The various forms of non-respiratory tuberculosis are reviewed by Kennedy (1989) and Humphries, Lam and Teoh (1994).

5 PATHOGENESIS AND IMMUNOLOGY OF TUBERCULOSIS

The clinical and histological features of tuberculosis are the result of the virulence of the tubercle bacillus and, more critically, the nature and effectiveness of the host's defence mechanisms.

Protective immune reactions in tuberculosis are principally cell mediated. Humoral immune responses are usually, but perhaps rather dogmatically, regarded as having no protective role to play.

Various studies show different pathogen-specific antibody profiles in patients with progressive and resolving tuberculosis (reviewed by Grange 1984) and Bothamley et al. (1989)

described an HLA-linked relation between progressive tuberculosis and antibody to a 38 kDa protein found only in the *M. tuberculosis* complex. It has been postulated that antibody to certain mycobacterial antigens, especially lipoarabinomannan, may limit the dissemination of tuberculosis in childhood (Costello et al. 1992). These reports raise problems of cause and effect; nevertheless, they indicate that a role for antibody in protective immunity to, and pathogenesis of, tuberculosis cannot be dismissed.

There are 2 main types of protective cellular immune responses. Since the first descriptions of the role of the macrophage in cell mediated immunity, it has been widely held that macrophage activation and granuloma formation is the only mechanism by which mycobacterial infections are combated. It is now known that an equally important defence mechanism is the recognition and destruction of exhausted macrophages and other cells in which tubercle bacilli are replicating. Thus, regulated and directed cell destruction is an inevitable and essential part of the protective immune response in tuberculosis (Boom, Wallis and Chervenak 1991, Flynn et al. 1992). By contrast, inappropriate and dysregulated destruction of tissues harbouring disease rather than just infected cells leads to immunopathology and progression of disease. The outcome of infection by the tubercle bacillus depends critically on whether the host responds with a protective or tissue-necrotizing reaction.

5.1 Early immunological events after infection

Tubercle bacilli entering the tissues are taken up by phagocytic cells, such as the alveolar macrophages in the case of pulmonary infection. If the bacilli are not destroyed, they replicate and kill the cell. A local area of inflammation is thus established and more phagocytes are attracted to the site. Some bacilli are transported, probably within phagocytes, to the regional lymph nodes where they are engulfed by antigen-presenting cells (APC). Other bacilli are transported further afield and may cause one of the extrapulmonary forms of primary disease such as tuberculous meningitis (see section 4.1, p. 397).

Epitopes from mycobacteria lying within phagosomes within the APC are presented on the cell surface by the MHC class II (HLA-D) molecules to CD4+ helper T cells which undergo activation and clonal proliferation. These T cells produce a range of cytokines, including interferon-γ (IFN-γ) that activates macrophages. Some T helper cells, however, also produce factors that lead to tissue destroying hypersensitivity, as described below.

If the tubercle bacilli proliferate within the APC and escape from the phagosomes, their epitopes are presented to CD8+ T cells by MHC class I (HLA-A and B) molecules. The CD8+ lymphocyte population contains cytotoxic T cells which are able to lyse any cell presenting antigen in this manner.

5.2 Macrophage activation and granuloma formation

In the early stages of active tuberculosis, most tubercle bacilli are within macrophages that, paradoxically, are the cells best equipped to destroy them by various lysosomal enzymes and reactive oxygen intermediates (ROI). Murine macrophages generate bactericidal reactive nitrogen intermediates (RNI) from L-arginine, but it is doubtful whether human macrophages generate sufficient RNI to kill tubercle bacilli (Rook and Bloom 1994). There are 3 strategies by which mycobacteria survive within macrophages. First, by poorly understood mechanisms, they inhibit fusion of the phagosome to the lysosomes. Second, they neutralize ROI by means of cell wall lipids including peptidoglycolipids (mycosides) and lipoarabinomannan (Chan et al. 1991), and by secreting the enzyme superoxide dismutase. Third, they escape from the phagosome and replicate in the cytoplasm of the cell (McDonough, Kress and Bloom 1993).

Macrophages require activation for their full expression of efficacy against tubercle bacilli. In humans, interferon-γ (IFN-γ) derived from CD4+ helper T cells causes some degree of activation, though not enough to inhibit growth of the tubercle bacillus within the cell, but it also induces a hydroxylase within the macrophage which converts inactive vitamin D into calcitriol. This metabolite further activates the cell (Rook 1988a).

The evidence that a single human macrophage, even when fully activated in this manner, is able to kill tubercle bacilli is elusive. In disease, rather than in experimental in vitro systems, activated macrophages aggregate to form the characteristic lesion of tuberculosis and many other chronic infections, namely, the granuloma. This consists of a compact palisade, many cells thick, of activated macrophages around the area of infection. Microscopically, these activated macrophages resemble epithelial cells and are thus termed epithelioid cells. Some of these fuse together to form multinucleate giant cells which are characteristic of, but not exclusive to, granulomas of tuberculosis. The outer region of the granuloma contains lymphocytes ('round cells') which secrete IFN-γ and other cytokines that activate the macrophages and draw more of these cells to the lesion. Thus, such lesions are termed 'high turnover granulomas of immunogenic origin'.

Activated macrophages produce a cytokine termed tumour necrosis factor (TNF-α; Flesch and Kaufmann 1990). This plays a key role in protective immunity by maintaining the integrity of the granuloma (Rook and Bloom 1994). It is, as described below, also a mediator of tissue-necrotizing immunopathology and it is responsible for the wasting (cachexia, consumption or phthisis) of patients with advanced tuberculosis (Beutler et al. 1985).

Before the induction of high turnover granulomas by the specific immune response, certain mycobacterial components induce low turnover granulomas of the 'foreign body' type which may limit the progression of the disease process. Such granuloma formation may be independent of T cells (Bancroft, Schreiber and Unanue 1991) but there is also evidence that a subpopulation of lymphocytes termed γ/δ T cells may be involved (Kaufmann, Blum and Yamamoto 1993).

It is highly likely that the entire granuloma is much more capable of destroying tubercle bacilli than isolated macrophages (Dannenberg 1993). The palisade of metabolically active macrophages consumes oxygen diffusing into the granuloma so that the centre becomes anoxic and undergoes a type of necrosis which, as it produces material similar in appearance to cottage cheese, is termed caseation. The anoxia and free fatty acids in the caseous centre provide an environment which is highly unfavourable to the tubercle bacilli, many of which die. The granulomas become inactive, fibroblasts surround them with fibrin which then contracts to form scars which may become calcified (Fig. 21.3).

In about 95% of primarily infected persons, these defence mechanisms render the disease quiescent but some bacilli may survive for years or decades in a latent or persister state, the nature of which is not understood (reviewed by Grange 1992). Some workers regard persisting mycobacteria as being in a metabolically dormant state induced by anoxia (Wayne and Lin 1982) whereas others postulate a steady state of replication and killing by immune mechanisms. The latter appears more likely as various forms of immuno-

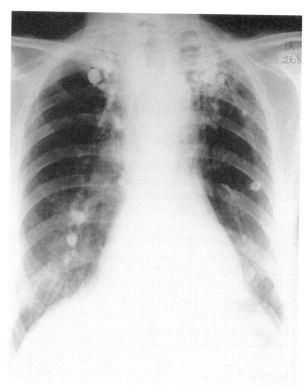

Fig. 21.3 Healed pulmonary tuberculosis with calcification. Anteroposterior chest radiograph showing many radiopaque healed lesions, particularly in the upper zones. (Courtesy of Dr P Ormerod).

suppression predispose to reactivation of latent disease.

5.3 Tuberculin reactivity and delayed hypersensitivity

Tuberculin reactivity was described by Koch (1891) during a search for a remedy for tuberculosis. Koch inoculated tubercle bacilli into the flank of a guinea pig and observed a small nodule at the injection site a week or 2 later. This ulcerated and remained open and contained viable tubercle bacilli, until the animal died. About a month after inoculation local lymph nodes were enlarged and lesions were present in many organs and tissues, leading to death of the animal about 3 months later. When the animal was reinoculated in the opposite flank 1 month after the original challenge, the lesion that developed was quite different. After a day or 2 the skin at the injection site underwent necrosis and then sloughed off, leaving a shallow ulcer. Unlike the primary ulcer, this contained no viable bacilli and it soon healed. A similar reaction, now known as the Koch phenomenon, was induced by injection of either killed tubercle bacilli or a heat concentrated filtrate of the medium in which the bacilli had been grown, a preparation termed Old Tuberculin.

Koch attempted to induce this apparently protective reaction in patients with tuberculosis by systemic injection of Old Tuberculin. Although there were some remarkable cures in patients with disease of the skin or larynx, it appeared to have little or no effect in those with deep lesions. Indeed, there was a worsening of pulmonary disease in some cases and a few fatalities due to allergic reactions ('tuberculin shock'). Thus it appears that if the Koch phenomenon occurs in the skin, larynx or other superficial sites, the bacilli-laden tissue sloughs off but when it occurs in the lung or other internal organ, the bacilli remain in situ and the necrotic process is enhanced.

Old Tuberculin was thus abandoned as a therapeutic agent, but the characteristic dermal reaction induced by it was utilized by von Pirquet (1907) in epidemiological studies as an indicator of past infection by the tubercle bacillus. As Old Tuberculin contained some impurities from the medium, it induced small, non-specific dermal reactions in uninfected persons. This problem was resolved by Seibert (1934) who purified the reagent by precipitating the proteins with acetone and ammonium sulphate. This reagent, Purified Protein Derivative of Tuberculin (PPD), remains the standard skin testing reagent for human and animal use.

Koch also prepared New Tuberculin by grinding whole tubercle bacilli, thereby liberating their cytoplasm. This method of preparing New Tuberculins was later adopted and modified by Stanford and his colleagues who disrupted mycobacteria by ultrasonication (Stanford 1983).

Conversion to a positive response to skin testing with tuberculin occurs between 3 and 8 weeks after primary infection. A reaction is usually evident 24 h after testing and reaches its maximum intensity at 48 or 72 h. Reactions visible 6 h after testing are seen in some patients with active tuberculosis and, more particularly, in healthy hospital workers repeatedly exposed to patients with open tuberculosis (Grange et al. 1986). Biopsies of this reaction show that it is a typical delayed-type hypersensitivity (DTH) reaction of early onset (Gibbs et al. 1991).

The nature of the tuberculin reaction and its relation to protective immunity has been the subject of controversy for several decades. Though often cited as the classical example of a DTH reaction, there are several different DTH reactions, some associated with tissue necrosis and some not. It is now clear that both types, which bear different relations to protective immunity, manifest as positive tuberculin reactions.

Stanford and Lema (1983) observed that some 48 h tuberculin reactions in man are purple coloured, indurated, well demarcated and tender, while others are pink, soft, ill-defined and much less tender. It has been postulated that these reactions correspond to non-necrotizing and necrotizing (Koch-type) reactions described in the mouse (see section 5.5, p. 402). Blood flow studies based on the 2 types of reaction reveal considerable slowing of blood flow in the centre of the more indurated reactions – a phenomenon that could predispose to tissue necrosis (Potts et al. 1992) – and which is possibly due to an action of TNF-α (see section 5.5, p. 402).

The histology of the positive tuberculin test at 48 h has been described by Beck and his colleagues (1986, 1988). There is a dense infiltrate of blood-derived white cells around the capillaries, sweat glands and hair follicles. Macrophages and lymphocytes from the perivascular foci migrate into the interstitial dermis, particularly into the subepidermal region. This migration, particularly that of the monocyte/macrophage cells, is greater in reactions to tuberculin than to leprosin in patients with tuberculosis, and vice versa in leprosy patients, suggesting that this component of the reaction is affected by species-specific antigens.

The diameter of the reaction bears no relation to the density of the cellular infiltrate; indeed, some tuberculin-negative persons have an intense cellular infiltrate. This indicates that the dermal swelling is not caused by the infiltrating cell mass but is a secondary phenomenon, probably due to cytokine release.

5.4 Post-primary tuberculosis and the Koch phenomenon

As outlined in section 4.2 (see section 4.2, p. 398), post-primary tuberculosis, which only develops in a minority of those who successfully overcome the primary lesions, differs in the former in the extensiveness of the necrosis. This is associated with the Koch phenomenon and there is now strong evidence that this reaction is quite distinct in its nature and mechanism to protective immunity. It is therefore necessary to consider the nature of the differences in the immune responses in those who develop post-primary tuberculosis and those who do not and to ask why some people develop an inappropriate reaction that harms their own tissues rather than the invading pathogen.

5.5 Protective immunity and immunopathology in tuberculosis

Though it is now both clear and obvious that tissue-necrotizing hypersensitivity and protective immune reactions in tuberculosis are quite distinct, this has been the subject of much controversy ever since von Pirquet (1907) stated that tuberculin reactivity is a correlate of protective immunity in tuberculosis.

The controversy has been reviewed in detail elsewhere (Bothamley and Grange 1991). The main causes of difficulty were that protective and non-protective responses were both associated with tuberculin positivity, that both were T cell mediated and that there was no place for a distinct tissue-necrotizing hypersensitivity reaction in the classical macrophage-based theory of mycobacterial immunity. Thus there was a strong body of opinion that the various immune reactions were qualitatively identical and that their observed effects reflected the intensity of the reaction.

Resolution of the controversy came with the finding that tuberculin reactions could be divided into non-necrotizing reactions associated with protection and necrotizing reactions associated with immunopathology (Rook and Stanford 1979, Stanford and Lema 1983, Fine 1994).

Tuberculin testing of mice infected with various mycobacteria revealed 2 different reactions (Rook and Stanford 1979). One of these could first be elicited about 10 days after infection and reached maximum intensity about 20 h after testing was non-necrotizing and resembled a skin test reaction demonstrable in mice infected with *Listeria monocytogenes*. The other, peaking at about 40 h and present about 1 month after infection, was thought to be the murine equivalent of the necrotic Koch phenomenon in guinea pigs. Thus the reactions were, respectively, termed 'Listeria-type' and 'Koch-type'. Less virulent strains of BCG and other mycobacteria that do not cause disease in mice elicited the Listeria-type reaction, while more virulent BCG strains and pathogenic mycobacteria elicited the Koch-type reaction. It was also shown that the induction of one type of reaction blocked the subsequent induction of the other.

A great incentive to clarify the relevance of various immune reactions in tuberculosis to protection came from observations that the efficacy of BCG vaccination varies from region to region. A number of studies led to the conclusion that the pattern of immune reactivity to BCG vaccination and infection by a virulent mycobacterium is critically affected by prior exposure of the population to environmental mycobacteria (EM). One explanation, based on experimental studies on guinea pigs (Palmer and Long 1969), was that some communities were highly protected by contact with EM so that BCG vaccination could add little extra protection and thus appeared to be ineffective. The other explanation was that, whereas some species or populations of EM indeed prime for protective responses, others prime for tissue-necrotizing responses (Stanford, Shield and Rook 1981). The effect of BCG is to boost the response that has been primed for. Thus, it would be observed to be effective in regions where it boosted a protective response but not in those where it boosted a tissue-necrotizing response.

Although this appeared a very plausible explanation, it was still difficult to explain how 2 quite different reactions could be mediated by T cells, unless there were functionally very dissimilar populations of these cells.

The dilemma was finally resolved by the demonstration that T helper cells mature into 2 distinct cells, Th1 and Th2, that secrete different, and mutually antagonistic, cytokines (Mosmann and Moore 1991). Building on this key discovery, Bretscher (1992) demonstrated that contact with antigens of a pathogen such as the tubercle bacillus, even if in too small a quantity to induce a detectable immune response, is able to 'imprint' the immune system with information that determines whether subsequent contact with the tubercle bacillus induces a Th1 or Th2 mediated reaction. By this means, the immune system is programmed to respond to a complex antigen such as the tubercle bacillus in a remarkably unified or coherent manner. (The concept of predetermination of immune reactions to mycobacteria was first suggested by Abrahams (1970) in a classic paper entitled 'Original mycobacterial sin'.) Accordingly, the effect of sensitization by environmental mycobacteria on subsequent patterns of immune reactivity in nature and in experimental systems may be seen, and investigated, in terms of the balance between Th1- and Th2-associated cytokine mediated immune responses.

The maturation of T cells to the Th1 and Th2 types is affected by steroid hormones (Daynes, Meikle and Araneo 1991, Rook, Onyebujoh and Stanford 1993). Dehydroepiandrosterone (DHEA) promotes Th1 maturation and glucocorticoids promote Th2 maturation. Thus the hypothalamus–pituitary–adrenal axis, and factors affecting it, may play a crucial role in the outcome of infection by the tubercle bacillus.

The important contribution of tumour necrosis factor (TNF-α) to protective immune responses in tuberculosis has been discussed above. It also, however, plays a key role in the tissue-necrotizing hypersensitivity reaction (the Koch phenomenon) in tuberculosis. The involvement of the same cytokine in the 2 incompatible immune responses is explained by the Th1 and Th2 maturation pathways. It has been shown that, in tuberculosis, tissues containing the tubercle bacillus are rendered extremely sensitive to killing by TNF-α and that the Koch phenomenon is accompanied by a massive systemic release of this cytokine (Al Attiyah, Morino and Rook 1992, Filley et al. 1992). This priming for necrosis only occurs in the presence of cytokines associated with the Th2 T cell maturation pathway (Hernandez-Pando and Rook 1994). Th1-related cytokines, by contrast, do not induce this necrotizing reaction. Thus, the T cell maturation pathway and the factors regulating it are of key importance to the nature of the immune response to infection by the tubercle bacillus.

5.6 Cytotoxic cells and protective immunity

In contrast to the dysregulated tissue destruction in post-primary tuberculosis, targeted destruction of individual cells containing tubercle bacilli is, as described above, of key relevance to protection.

Such lysis may be induced by mycobacterial antigen presented on the cell surface by the class I MHC molecules or by certain 'self' antigens that appear on the surfaces of stressed cells. Some of the latter belong to a class of proteins termed heat shock proteins (HSPs). Most of these are normally present in small quantities within the cell and are involved in the shaping of nascent proteins. Under conditions of stress, such as heat shock, malignant transformation or intracellular parasitism, the amount of these proteins increases and they appear on the cell membrane (Born et al. 1990). The HSPs are found in all nucleate cells and are structurally highly conserved. There is, accordingly, considerable antigenic similarity between HSPs of human beings and mycobacteria. Consequently, HSPs of host or bacterial origin, or both, that are presented on cell surfaces may be targets for cytolytic activity. In this respect, a population of CD4+ cytolytic cells recognizing a predominant mycobacterial HSP has been described (Ottenhoff et al. 1988) and a major

subpopulation of γ/δ cells with cytolytic activity recognize HSPs on the surfaces of infected cells (Orme, Anderson and Boom 1993).

There is also evidence that immune recognition of HSPs and other antigens common to the genus *Mycobacterium* is suppressed in patients with active tuberculosis. Skin testing with a set of new tuberculins prepared from different mycobacterial species reveals 3 categories of reactors (Stanford et al. 1981, Kardjito et al. 1986). Persons in category 1 react to all reagents, even those prepared from mycobacteria that they have never encountered, and are therefore reacting to antigens common to all mycobacteria. Persons in category 2 do not react to any reagents despite previous sensitization by infection or BCG vaccination. Persons in this category, which has a genetic basis (see section 5.8, p. 404), can nevertheless express protective immunity. Persons in category 3 only react to some reagents, indicating that they respond to species-specific but not to common mycobacterial antigens.

Most healthy persons previously infected by the tubercle bacillus are in category 1 but those with active tuberculosis are mostly in category 3, strongly suggesting that their disease process is associated with a reduction in their ability to recognize common mycobacterial antigens. As HSPs are dominant among these common antigens, immune recognition of these is reduced. This phenomenon is not restricted to tuberculosis; it occurs in leprosy, HIV infection and Chagas' disease, all of which are characterized by intracellular parasitism. It has thus been postulated that an immunotherapeutic procedure that could rectify this immune defect could be of value in a range of diseases associated with cell stress (Grange, Stanford and Rook 1995).

In view of the immunodominance of the mycobacterial HSPs and their antigenic similarity to their human counterparts, the possibility that mycobacteria induce autoimmune disease has received much attention (Rook and Stanford 1992). In this context, Freund's complete adjuvant (a suspension of killed mycobacteria in oil) induces an autoimmune arthritis in rats which is adoptively transferable by T cells reacting to the mycobacterial 65 kDa HSP (van Eden et al. 1988). In addition, the HLA-DR4 phenotype is associated with a tendency to develop rheumatoid arthritis and also with strong skin test reactions to tuberculin but not to antigens from other mycobacterial species (Ottenhoff et al. 1986).

In common with tuberculosis, patients with rheumatoid arthritis have elevated levels of an unusual type of immunoglobulin in the IgG class characterized by the absence of a terminal galactose on an oligosaccharide side chain and thus termed agalactosyl IgG or gal(O) (Rook 1988b).

Despite these observations, there is no evidence that autoimmune phenomena contribute to the immunopathology of tuberculosis. Although a sterile arthropathy termed Poncet's disease is associated with tuberculosis, it is uncommon. The usual failure of immunodominant bacterial antigens that cross-react with host antigens, and the latter when expressed in excess, to induce autoimmune phenomena appears to be due to the existence of a powerful regulatory system (Cohen and Young 1991).

5.7 The immune spectrum in tuberculosis

Many attempts have been made to categorize cases of tuberculosis according to an immunological 'spectrum' similar to that clearly evident in leprosy. In general, more differences than similarities have been found between the 2 diseases. In particular, the specific immune defect seen in lepromatous leprosy does not occur in tuberculosis. Anergy in the latter disease is much more generalized and non-specific. In contrast to leprosy, such a categorization in tuberculosis is of little or no clinical value. Ridley and Ridley (1987) divided patients with tuberculosis into 3 histological groups as shown in Table 21.4. Most patients in group 1 had chronic skin tuberculosis, those in group 2 had pulmonary disease whereas those in group 3 had disseminated tuberculosis.

All forms of immunosuppression predispose to tuberculosis due to primary infection, endogenous reactivation or exogenous reinfection and the resulting disease differs from that in the more immunocompetent (Festenstein and Grange 1991). Not only is there a failure to develop the characteristic high turnover granuloma of immunogenic origin in immunosuppressed tuberculosis patients, there is also a suppression of tissue-necrotizing reactions and scar formation that would otherwise limit the spread of infection. Thus, discrete pulmonary lesions and cavity formation are both less common in such patients. Instead, there may be a radiologically rather non-specific spreading pulmonary lesion. Non-pulmonary lesions due to unrestricted bacillary dissemination are frequent in such patients. Dissemination may present as one or more solitary lesions, as widespread lymphadenopathy or as multi-organ involvement. The latter differs from miliary tuberculosis as the discrete granulomas do not develop. Instead, organs contain minute necrotic foci teeming with acid-fast bacilli. These may not be visible radiologically and are only detected by biopsy or at postmortem examination.

Thus, this form of the disease is termed **cryptic disseminated tuberculosis**.

5.8 Genetic factors in mycobacterial immunity

Because not all those exposed to the tubercle bacillus develop overt tuberculosis, some form of genetically determined innate resistance to disease has long been suspected. Early observations on identical and non-identical twins supported this suspicion.

Linkage of susceptibility to tuberculosis and the class I determinants (HLA-A and HLA-B) of the major histocompatibility complex is weak and varies from region to region but significant associations with class II (HLA-D) determinants have been found. Thus the HLA-DR2 gene predisposes to the development of advanced, smear-positive, pulmonary tuberculosis (Khomenko et al. 1990, Brahmajothi et al. 1991). This determinant may affect antigen recognition as it is associated with high levels of antibody to a 38 kDa protein unique to the *M. tuberculosis* complex (Bothamley et al. 1989).

Skin test responses to mycobacterial antigens are affected by the HLA-D phenotype. Thus persons who are unresponsive to all reagents (category 2 nonresponders) lack the HLA-DR3 determinant whereas those with the HLA-DR4 determinant respond strongly to species-specific antigens of *M. tuberculosis* but not to specific antigens of other mycobacterial species (Ottenhoff et al. 1986).

An allele, designated *bcg*, conferring natural macrophage mediated resistance to several intracellular pathogens including BCG, salmonellae and *Leishmania donovani*, has been described in the mouse (Skamene et al. 1982). It codes for a protein termed Nramp (natural-resistance-associated macrophage protein) which is involved in the generation of RNI from L-arginine (Vidal et al. 1993). A closely related protein has been found in humans but, as human macro-

Table 21.4 Grouping of tuberculosis according to histological features

Group	Main cell types	Necrosis	Giant cells	Bacilli
1a	Organized mature epithelioid cells	None	+	None
1b	Unorganized mature and immature epithelioid cells	Patchy fibrinoid	+	Rare
2a	Immature epithelioid cells	Caseation, no nuclear debris	+	Scanty
2b	Immature epithelioid cells and/or undifferentiated histiocytes	Necrosis with nuclear debris and polymorphs	+	+
3a	Scanty macrophages	Extensive, basophilic; coarse nuclear debris	−	++
3b	Very few macrophages	Extensive, eosinophilic; scanty nuclear debris	−	+++

After Ridley and Ridley (1987).

phages appear unable to generate sufficient RNI to kill tubercle bacilli (see section 5.2, p. 400), it may be of less significance to innate immunity in human beings than in mice.

6 VACCINATION STRATEGIES

Koch's isolation of the tubercle bacillus in 1882 was followed by many attempts to prepare a vaccine against tuberculosis, mostly by the various techniques established by Pasteur. During these early studies the concept, held rather dogmatically ever since, arose that an effective vaccine would have to be a living, attenuated one. Such a vaccine was produced by Calmette and Guérin from a tubercle bacillus isolated from a case of bovine mastitis by passaging it 230 times over a period of 11 years, by which time extensive animal studies showed that it had lost its virulence. The vaccine was prepared from a bovine strain rather than a human one on account of a widely held notion that self-limiting tuberculous lesions due to *M. bovis* in childhood provided protection against pulmonary tuberculosis later in life (Marfan's law). This vaccine, bacille Calmette–Guérin (BCG), was given orally to neonates in 1921 but is now given by injection or multipoint inoculation.

The early years of BCG were stormy ones. During the late 1920s and early 1930s there was intense controversy as to whether BCG could revert to virulence. Also, in 1930, the use of the vaccine was dealt a serious blow by a tragic accident in the Hanseatic city of Lubeck where many children were accidentally vaccinated with virulent *M. tuberculosis* and 73 died. This resulted from the practice of growing the vaccine for immediate use in local laboratories and led to the present practice of producing freeze-dried vaccine in well controlled central manufacturing plants. For details of the nature of BCG see Osborn (1983).

The protective efficacy of BCG vaccine has been the subject of considerable controversy as a number of major trials have shown its efficacy to vary from around 80% to none at all (Table 21.5). The various explanations of these discrepancies are outlined elsewhere (see section 5.5, p. 402). A major problem with BCG that greatly limits its use in the control of tuberculosis is that, when given to an uninfected (tuberculin-negative) child, it offers protection against the serious forms of primary infection, especially those due to dissemination of bacilli from the primary complex. It is, however, much less effective in preventing tubercle bacilli from persisting in the tissues and becoming reactivated later in life. For this reason, and because of the risk of severe local reactions, the vaccine should not be given to infected, i.e. tuberculin-positive, persons.

In many infections, the antigens that elicit effective immune responses are species- or strain-specific. There is, however, no theoretical reason, or practical evidence that this is so in the case of intracellular pathogens such as the tubercle bacillus. Indeed, BCG protects equally well against leprosy as against tuberculosis (Brown, Stone and Sutherland 1966) and it protects children against cervical lymphadenitis caused by environmental mycobacteria (Trnka, Dankova and Svandova 1994). Thus there is little doubt that the mycobacterial antigens that induce protective immunity are mostly or entirely among those that are common to all species in the genus.

Many attempts have been, and are being, made to develop a better vaccine and the advent of DNA recombinant technology offers various possibilities such as the identification of the protective antigens of *M. tuberculosis* and inserting multiple copies of these into suitable vectors.

Other workers are investigating the vaccinating potential of environmental mycobacteria that never cause disease and do not elicit severe local reactions if given to tuberculin-positive persons. *Mycobacterium vaccae*, a rapidly growing non-pathogen, can safely be given to such persons and, as there is accumulating evidence that it is an effective immunotherapeutic agent for active tuberculosis (see section 8.7, p. 411), it may well prove equally effective as a vaccine.

7 DIAGNOSIS

7.1 Laboratory methods

Diagnosis of tuberculosis is not easy and the evolution of sensitive, specific and rapid laboratory tests has been a very slow one. World wide, many laboratories only undertake microscopic examinations and those that attempt to isolate the bacillus mostly still employ cultivation techniques that were developed in the early decades of the twentieth century. Rapid radiometric detection of bacterial growth and DNA amplification techniques remain the province of a few privileged centres. Animal inoculation techniques are obsolete.

Specimens for culture must always be collected directly into sterilized containers with care being taken to avoid contamination of the outside of the container. Sputum should ideally be submitted as 3 early-morning specimens but single specimens taken at any time are only slightly less likely to be culture-positive. If sputum is not expectorated, material may be obtained by swabbing the larynx or aspirating the gastric contents after overnight fasting but neither method is as useful as culture of even scanty sputum. Fibreoptic bronchoscopy is increasingly popular, enabling specimens to be obtained from the lung by brushing, biopsy or bronchial washing with relatively little risk to the patient. Care must be taken in cleaning bronchoscopes as 'pseudoepidemics' of mycobacterial disease have resulted from the use of faulty cleaning machines (Gubler, Salfinger and von Graevenitz 1992). There is seldom a need to examine blood, bone marrow and faeces in the routine diagnosis of tuberculosis, although they are examined for other mycobacterial infections in immunocompromised patients.

Excretion of tubercle bacilli in urine is intermittent and collection of early-morning specimens over 3 days is recommended. Pleural, peritoneal and pericardial fluids may be prevented from clotting by the addition of 2 drops of 20% sodium citrate solution to every 10 ml of specimen or, alternatively, the fluids may be directly inoculated at the bedside

Table 21.5 The protective efficacy of BCG vaccine as observed in 9 major studies

Group studied	Year of commencement	Age range	Protection (%)
North American Indian	1935	0–20 years	80
Chicago, USA	1937	3 months	75
Georgia, USA	1947	6–17 years	0
Illinois, USA	1947	Young adults	0
Puerto Rico	1949	1–18 years	31
Georgia, USA	1950	5 years	14
Great Britain	1950	14–15 years	78
South India	1950	All ages	31
South India	1968	All ages	0*

*No protection at 7.5 years but a 15-year follow-up revealed some protection in young persons.

into an equal volume of double strength liquid culture medium.

MICROSCOPIC EXAMINATION

Microscopy provides a simple, sensitive and rapid means of detecting open, infectious cases of pulmonary tuberculosis. To be detected microscopically, there must be between 5000 and 10 000 bacilli in 1 ml of sputum (Rouillon, Perdrizet and Parrot 1976).

Staining techniques are based on the resistance of mycobacteria to decolorization by acid, or a mixture of acid and alcohol after staining by arylmethane dyes, i.e. 'acid fastness'. (It is not possible to distinguish members of the *M. tuberculosis* complex from other mycobacteria by their staining properties. There is no truth in the often-cited statement that the former are acid–alcohol fast while the latter are only acid fast.) The most widely used staining technique is that of Ziehl and Neelsen which employs a hot solution of carbol-fuchsin. Fluorescent methods, employing auramine O, rhodamine B, or both, are based on the same principle. Although requiring more expensive equipment, fluorescence microscopy is more rapid than conventional light microscopy as smears can be screened under low power magnification.

Some workers examine selected purulent or mucopurulent portions of sputum and others concentrate the bacilli by centrifugation of sputum digested by a mucolytic agent (see section on 'Methods for cultivation'). The sensitivity of microscopy is increased by use of the cytocentrifuge to separate and concentrate the bacilli (Saceanu, Pfeiffer and McClean 1993). Care must be taken in microscopy to ensure that specimen containers and staining reagents are not contaminated by saprophytic mycobacteria and other acid-fast material such as bacterial and fungal spores. Tap water is especially likely to contain such mycobacteria (Collins, Grange and Yates 1984). Repeated reports of small numbers acid-fast bacilli in specimens that are culture-negative should raise the suspicion of contamination. Microscopy is also used to detect acid-fast bacilli in urine, cerebrospinal, pleural, peritoneal and pericardial fluids and tissue biopsies. The desirability of examining gastric aspirates microscopically is controversial as saprophytic mycobacteria may be present. For details of microscopical examination see Collins, Grange and Yates (1985).

METHODS FOR CULTIVATION

Cultural techniques are more sensitive than microscopy and may detect as few as 10–100 organisms

per ml of specimen. Löwenstein–Jensen medium, a solid egg-based medium containing glycerol, is widely used for the isolation of *M. tuberculosis* and similar media containing pyruvic acid in place of glycerol are used for the isolation of *M. bovis*. Liquid media are used in the radiometric methods. Biphasic systems containing broth and slides coated with solid agar-based media are commercially available. These permit bacterial growth to be detected more rapidly than by conventional methods but not as rapidly as by radiometric techniques (Salfinger, Demchik and Kafader 1990).

Culture media may be inoculated directly with centrifuge deposits of fluids and homogenized biopsies if it is highly unlikely that they contain non-acid-fast micro-organisms but most other specimens, especially sputum and urine, must first be 'decontaminated'. For this purpose, use is made of the relative resistance of mycobacteria to acids, alkalis and certain disinfectants. Techniques are divisible into 'hard' and 'soft' methods suitable, respectively, for specimens likely to be heavily or lightly contaminated. Differences in resistance between mycobacteria and other organisms is not absolute; hard methods reduce the number of positive isolates. In the UK and USA, the 'hard' 2% NaOH–*N*-acetyl-L-cysteine method is widely used for decontamination of sputum. The *N*-acetyl-L-cysteine is mucolytic and facilitates concentration of bacilli by centrifugation. Other decontaminating agents include sodium dodecyl sulphate (SDS), oxalic acid (for urine and other specimens contaminated by *Pseudomonas* spp.) and trisodium phosphate. For details of methods see Collins, Grange and Yates (1985) and European Society for Mycobacteriology (1991).

An alternative or adjunct to decontamination is the use of media containing 'cocktails' of antimicrobial agents designed to kill virtually all organisms other than mycobacteria (Mitchison, Allen and Manickavasagar 1983). A widely used commercially available cocktail, used particularly in radiometric methods, contains polymyxin, amphotericin, nalidixic acid, trimethoprim and azlocillin (PANTA).

Inoculated culture media are usually incubated for at least 8 weeks and inspected weekly for growth. Most strains of the *M. tuberculosis* complex produce visible colonies within 4 weeks, but growth may be delayed if the patient has received antituberculosis drugs. Cultures should be incubated at 35°C. Colonies appearing on the medium are shown to be mycobacteria by means of Ziehl–Neelsen staining and are usually identified by simple cultural and biochemical tests. Thus, members of the *M. tuberculosis* complex are clearly identifiable by their slow growth rate, lack of pigment, failure to grow at 25°C and sensitivity to *p*-nitrobenzoic acid (Collins, Grange and Yates 1985). Nucleic acid probes for the rapid identification of this complex and, specifically, *M. tuberculosis* are commercially available.

Radiometric techniques

Radiometry enables mycobacterial growth to be detected rapidly, usually within 2–12 days. After appropriate preparation (see above) clinical material is added to bottles containing Middlebrook 12B broth and an antibiotic cocktail (PANTA) and [^{14}C]palmitic acid. If mycobacterial growth occurs, $^{14}CO_2$ is liberated and detected by the appropriate instrumentation. Members of the *M. tuberculosis* complex may be distinguished from other mycobacteria by inoculating 2 bottles, one containing *p*-nitro-α-acetylamino-β-propiophenone (NAP) which inhibits growth of the former. For details of radiometric methods see Heifets (1991).

OTHER TECHNIQUES FOR THE DETECTION OF TUBERCLE BACILLI

Mycobacterial lipids such as tuberculostearic acids are detectable in clinical specimens by the combination of gas chromatography and mass spectroscopy (French et al. 1987). Although very sensitive and specific, the equipment is costly and not widely available.

DNA probes for the direct detection of specific mycobacterial DNA in clinical specimens have been developed but they lack sensitivity. DNA amplification by the polymerase chain reaction (PCR) and related methods are more sensitive and kits for this purpose are commercially available. Amplification techniques for mycobacterial ribosomal RNA, with the advantage that each bacterial cell contains about 2000 copies of the target, are also available (Miller, Hernandez and Cleary 1994). This is a rapidly advancing subject with considerable, and perhaps unnecessary, diversification in techniques driven by patenting legislation. Thus reference to the most recent literature is essential. The state of the art in 1994 was reviewed by Salfinger and Morris (1994) and by Shaw (1994).

Mycobacterial antigen is detectable in clinical specimens by use of specific antibodies in agglutination techniques and ELISA. Development of such tests has been overshadowed by DNA technology but results of the few studies of their use with 'clean' specimens such as cerebrospinal, pleural and peritoneal fluids were encouraging, with high sensitivities and specificities (Wadee, Boting and Reddy 1990). Assays for T cell related enzyme activity, particularly adenosine deaminase (ADA), have been evaluated for the diagnosis of tuberculous meningitis and pleurisy but their use is controversial. In the case of tuberculous meningitis, neither the ELISA nor the ADA assay were as sensitive and specific as the radioactive bromide partition test for meningeal inflammation (Coovadia et al. 1986).

7.2 Tuberculin testing

The tuberculin test is used to determine the annual infection rate of tuberculosis in the community, to assess the effectiveness of control measures, to indicate those requiring BCG vaccination or preventive therapy, and to aid diagnosis.

Weak or negative reactions do not exclude a diagnosis of tuberculosis. Some persons are intrinsically poor reactors (see section 5.8, p. 404) and in others reactivity is depressed due to advanced disease, old age, malnutrition and immunosuppression, including HIV infection. Various skin testing reagents have been developed from Koch's original Old Tuberculin. The most widely used is PPD produced by Seibert and her colleagues (see section 5.3, p. 401).

The dosage of PPD is expressed in International Units (IU) based on a biological standardization against an international standard preparation. Previously, Tuberculin Units, based on weight, were used.

The 3 principal techniques for tuberculin testing are the Mantoux, Heaf and tine tests. In the Mantoux test, an exact amount (usually 0.1 ml) of tuberculin is injected intracutaneously and the diameter of the resulting induration is measured 48–72 h later. This test is the most satisfactory as results can be quantified but it requires some training and skill. It is usually performed with 10 IU of PPD but persons likely to react strongly may first be tested with 1 IU. Opinions differ as to the minimum diameter that should be regarded as 'positive'. In general, reactions of 10 mm or more in diameter may be regarded as positive and those between 5 and 9 mm as doubtful (American Lung Association 1974). These values may require adjustment locally according to the number and extent of small reactions due to sensitization by contact with environmental mycobacteria.

Heaf (1951) introduced a spring-loaded instrument which propels 6 needles into the skin to a depth of 2 mm, the punctures being made through a drop of undiluted PPD (100 000 IU ml^{-1}) placed on the skin. Use of the Heaf test requires very little training but it lacks the precision of the Mantoux test. The test is read after 72 h (although it can be read up to 7 days later) and positive results are recorded as grade 1 (4 or more papules at puncture sites), grade 2 (confluence of the papules into a ring), grade 3 (a single large plaque) and grade 4 (a plaque with vesicle formation or central necrosis).

A major disadvantage of the Heaf test is that the instrument must be properly sterilized between uses: flaming is no longer considered adequate to prevent transmission of viral disease. Instruments with replaceable magnetic heads are available. Alternatively, commercially available tine tests, i.e. disposable multipuncture devices with prongs or tines coated with dried PPD, may be used. Opinions differ as to their reliability. They are suitable for screening purposes but negative reactions should be confirmed by a Mantoux test. It is essential to allow the tines to remain in the skin for several seconds so that the PPD has time to dissolve in the tissue fluids. For a full account of tuberculin testing in clinical practice see Caplin (1980).

7.3 Serodiagnosis

Many attempts have been made to develop serodiagnostic tests for tuberculosis (reviewed by Grange 1984, Wilkins 1994). Despite the huge amount of effort, no serodiagnostic test is widely used clinically. The reason for this is that, although antibodies are undoubtedly produced in mycobacterial disease, the overlap between levels in patients and either healthy persons or those with other diseases is unacceptably large. 'Natural' antibodies are probably due to contact with mycobacteria and related genera in the environment, but the use of purified specific antigens in diagnostic tests has proved disappointing; most of the humoral immune response is directed towards shared antigens. The introduction of monoclonal antibodies made it possible for antibodies to specific epitopes to be detected and assayed. This approach led to high specificity (i.e. very few 'false positives'), but the sensitivity (the ability to diagnose disease when present) was rather low (Wilkins 1994) although the use of several monoclonal antibodies of differing specificities, while making the test rather complex, improved the sensitivity (Hoeppner et al. 1987).

The use of specific antibody to detect mycobacterial antigen in clinical specimens is described in section 7.1 (see section 7.1, p. 405).

7.4 Clinical diagnosis

A high index of clinical suspicion is essential to the early diagnosis of tuberculosis, especially in low incidence regions. A missed or delayed diagnosis of tuberculous meningitis often has very serious consequences. Fibreoptic bronchoscopy, laparoscopy and fine needle aspiration assist in obtaining useful specimens from sites once only accessible by major exploratory surgery. Computerized tomography and magnetic resonance imaging give much clearer images than conventional radiology and often show features that confirm the diagnosis (Figs 21.4 and 21.5; Humphries, Lam and Teoh 1994, Labhard, Nicod and Zellweger 1994).

8 THERAPY

8.1 Standard chemotherapeutic regimens

Effective chemotherapeutic regimens for tuberculosis were developed in the late 1940s and early 1950s. At that time the principal drugs available were streptomycin, isoniazid and *p*-aminosalicylic acid (PAS). Experience with these drugs showed that long periods of therapy (18–24 months) were required to prevent relapse and that, unless multidrug therapy was used, drug-resistant mutants were readily selected.

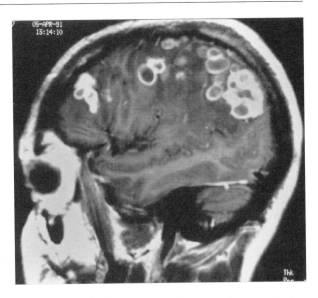

Fig. 21.4 Cerebral computerized tomography scan showing tuberculomas, principally in the left occipital region. (From Labhard, Nicod and Zellweger 1994).

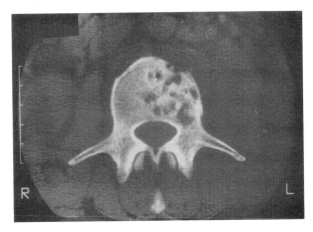

Fig. 21.5 Tuberculosis of the spine. Computerized tomography scan showing erosive lesions in the vertebral body. (Courtesy of Dr M Humphries).

In the early 1970s, the introduction of rifampicin enabled the period of therapy to be reduced from at least 18 months to 6 months. Thus began the era of short course chemotherapy and many studies were undertaken, notably by the British Medical Research Council, to determine the most effective and cost-effective regimens. During these studies, it was shown that, from the point of view of therapy, a tuberculous lesion contains 3 functionally different populations of tubercle bacilli (Mitchison 1985):

A, those freely replicating in the slightly alkaline walls of cavities;

B, those replicating much more slowly in acidic, anoxic closed lesions;

C, near-dormant bacilli which are probably mostly within macrophages.

The efficacy of the antituberculosis drugs varies according to the functional state of the bacilli and this must be taken into account when designing therapeutic regimens.

Most regimens commence with an intensive 2 month phase in which all or most of the bacilli in populations A and B are destroyed and a 4 month continuation phase in which the relatively small number of those in population C are eradicated. Isoniazid is particularly effective at destroying freely replicating bacilli while pyrazinamide sterilizes acidic lesions containing metabolically less active bacilli (pyrazinamide is only active at a low pH). Rifampicin kills bacilli in all 3 populations but its unique action is the eradication of the remaining near-dormant bacilli. For this reason, rifampicin resistance is a very serious and worrying development (see sections 2.7, p. 395 and 8.2).

The standard regimen recommended by the World Health Organization (1994a) for adults is known as directly observed therapy, short course (DOTS) and consists of 2 months of isoniazid, rifampicin, pyrazinamide and ethambutol given daily, followed by 4 months of isoniazid and rifampicin given thrice weekly, all drugs being given under direct supervision. Isoniazid has no effect on near-dormant bacilli but it is included in the continuation phase to prevent the replication of any rifampicin-resistant mutants.

The above, and other regimens advocated by the World Health Organization, are listed in Table 21.6. In the other regimens the drugs are given daily or intermittently throughout. In some countries regimens of longer duration, up to 12 months, and usually based on isoniazid, streptomycin and thiacetazone, are still used on grounds of economy. This, however, is a false economy as the cost for every patient cured is lower if the more expensive, but much more effective, shorter regimens are used.

8.2 Therapy of drug-resistant tuberculosis

The significance of drug resistance, particularly multi-

drug resistance, to tuberculosis control is discussed in section 2.7 (see section 2.7, p. 395).

The US Advisory Council for the Elimination of Tuberculosis recommend that all patients in regions where single- or multidrug resistance is common should receive one of the 4 drug regimens listed in Table 21.6 under direct supervision and that drug susceptibility tests should be performed on all positive cultures, preferably by the rapid radiometric method (Centers for Disease Control 1993). Antituberculosis drugs used to treat multidrug-resistant tuberculosis include ethionamide, rifabutin, amikacin, kanamycin, capreomycin, viomycin, cycloserine and *p*-aminosalicylic acid (PAS). Other agents for which there is anecdotal or in vitro evidence of efficacy include clofazimine (normally used for leprosy), new macrolides (e.g. clarithromycin, azithromycin), fluoroquinolones (e.g. ciprofloxacin, ofloxacin, sparfloxacin) and minocycline. Therapy should continue for 2 years after sputum cultures have become negative.

Regimens for multidrug-resistant tuberculosis are less effective, more toxic and expensive than the standard regimens for drug-susceptible disease. The cure rate in one major survey of directly observed therapy in the USA was 56% among HIV-negative patients but only 20–30% among HIV-positive patients (Goble et al. 1993). For further information on the management of multidrug-resistant tuberculosis see Dooley and Simone (1994) and Morse (1994).

8.3 Therapy of extrapulmonary tuberculosis

The standard short course regimens described above are suitable for all forms of tuberculosis. Physicians tend to treat patients with extrapulmonary tuberculosis, notably tuberculous meningitis, for longer periods although there is no evidence that this is necessary. The drugs used in modern short course therapy cross the blood–brain barrier in sufficient amounts so that intrathecal administration of the drugs is not necessary in cases of tuberculous meningitis.

Surgical intervention may be required for the diagnosis and treatment of extrapulmonary tuberculosis. Examples include excision biopsy of lymph nodes, insertion of shunts for hydrocephalus, relief of obstructions due to scarring in the urinary tract and excision of a scarred, constricted pericardium. Surgery for tuberculosis of the spine is only indicated if there is deformity or evidence of pressure on the spinal cord (Report 1978). If indicated for this condition, surgery may involve simple debridement or more radical excision of the diseased tissues and bone grafting (the Hong Kong operation). Likewise, surgery is only indicated for other forms of skeletal tuberculosis if there is pain, deformity or joint instability.

ADJUNCT STEROID THERAPY

The place for steroids in the therapy of extrapulmonary tuberculosis is controversial. The rationale for their use is that they reduce inflammation and subsequent scarring. They are often given for this reason

Table 21.6 Some drug regimens for tuberculosis recommended by the World Health Organization (1991, 1994a)

Intensive phase: 2 months	Continuation phase: 4 months
Standard regimen: directly observed therapy, short course (DOTS): daily in initial phase and thrice weekly in continuation phase or thrice weekly throughout	
EHRZ	H_3R_3
Daily throughout	
HRZ	HR
SHRZ	HR
EHRZ	HR
Intermittent regimens: thrice weekly throughout	
$S_3H_3R_3Z_3$	$H_3R_3Z_3$
$E_3H_3R_3Z_3$	$H_3R_3Z_3$

H, isoniazid; R, rifampicin; Z, pyrazinamide; S, streptomycin; E, ethambutol. Subscripted 3 indicates thrice weekly administration.

in cases of genitourinary disease and tuberculous pleurisy but there is no clear evidence that the incidence of constrictions and adhesions is reduced. There is, however, evidence that they reduce mortality and subsequent constrictions due to scar formation in tuberculous pericarditis (Strang et al. 1988).

Steroid therapy is essential for relief of cerebral oedema complicating tuberculous meningitis but the evidence for its efficacy when given routinely is conflicting and controversial. Some studies indicate that steroids do not reduce subsequent disability and that they may merely prolong suffering (Escobar et al. 1975) whereas others suggest that residual disabilities are reduced. The evidence either way is weak and further studies are required (Kumarvelu et al. 1994).

Steroids are also used in cases of allergic drug reactions and for the reduction of gross swelling of lymph nodes, due to hypersensitivity reactions, that may occur during chemotherapy of tuberculous lymphadenopathy. For a detailed review of adjunct steroid therapy in tuberculosis see Alzeer and FitzGerald (1993).

8.4 Therapy of tuberculosis in special cases

Patients with renal failure may be treated with rifampicin, isoniazid and pyrazinamide as these are all metabolized or eliminated in the bile. Pyridoxine (vitamin B_6, see section 8.6) reduces the risk of isoniazid-induced encephalopathy which occasionally occurs in such patients.

Patients with reduced liver function may receive isoniazid, ethambutol and streptomycin, although there is no evidence that rifampicin and pyrazinamide are any more hepatotoxic in these patients.

As rifampicin has been shown to be teratogenic in animals it should not be given during the first 3 months of pregnancy. Women on antituberculosis therapy should therefore avoid becoming pregnant and it is important to note that rifampicin reduces the efficacy of oral contraceptives (see section 8.6). Although antituberculosis drugs enter the milk to some extent, mothers on therapy may safely breast-feed their infants.

8.5 Prophylactic and preventive therapy

Originally intended for young children exposed to infectious source cases, preventive therapy has been widely used for adults in countries, especially the USA, where tuberculosis is uncommon and where BCG is not given so that a positive tuberculin test is likely to indicate past infection by *M. tuberculosis*. In general, isoniazid monotherapy is given, on the grounds that there are likely to be very few bacilli and therefore little chance of mutational resistance developing. While of proven efficacy, the justification for giving a potentially hepatotoxic drug to a person with a 1 in 20 chance of developing active disease has been questioned (Israel 1993). In view of the risk of liver damage, which increases with age, such therapy is not

given in the USA to persons aged over 35 years unless there is a particular risk factor, such as transplant surgery. For a review and discussion of isoniazid preventive therapy see O'Brien (1994).

Treatment of HIV-related tuberculosis is often effective but long-term survival is compromised (see section 2.5, p. 393). While preventive therapy is an attractive option in principle, and effective in practice (Pape et al. 1993), its use in countries with high incidences of HIV infection is beset with problems. The World Health Organization and the International Union Against Tuberculosis and Lung Disease (Report 1994b) recommended that persons known to be HIV-positive should be tuberculin tested. Positive reactors with no signs, symptoms and radiological evidence of tuberculosis should be given isoniazid daily, for 6–12 months (those with active tuberculosis should, of course, be fully treated). As facilities for HIV testing in the developing nations are limited, and the establishment of such facilities as a part of tuberculosis control programmes is not recommended by international agencies (Report 1994b), preventive therapy will only be available to a minority of the population and the overall impact is likely to be minimal.

8.6 Drug toxicity and interactions

Drug reactions and toxic effects are uncommon in patients treated with modern short course chemotherapy. Reactions are more frequent among HIV-positive patients. All 3 principal drugs (isoniazid, rifampicin and pyrazinamide) are potentially hepatotoxic. Transient rises in hepatic enzymes often occur during therapy but do not indicate the need to stop treatment. Rifampicin causes a 'flu-like syndrome, particularly if given intermittently rather than daily. Isoniazid may cause peripheral neuropathy and mental disturbance which is preventable by giving pyridoxine (vitamin B_6). This vitamin is particularly indicated for pregnant women, alcoholics and patients with hepatic or renal failure and those who are HIV-positive, malnourished or elderly.

Ethambutol occasionally causes ocular damage. Patients receiving this drug must be informed of this risk and regular checks of visual acuity should be performed during therapy. Streptomycin and other aminoglycosides are nephrotoxic and ototoxic. Thiacetazone is a common cause of skin rashes which, in a minority of cases, proceed to life-threatening exfoliative dermatitis. This is particularly likely to occur in HIV-positive patients who should never knowingly be given this drug. For further details of drug toxicity see Girling (1989).

Clinically significant interactions between the standard antituberculosis drugs are uncommon but interactions with other drugs can have serious consequences. Rifampicin is the usual cause as it is a powerful inducer of cytochrome isoenzymes involved in the metabolism of many drugs, notably steroids, oral contraceptives, antiepileptic drugs and warfarin. Readjustment of drug doses may be required and women taking oral contraceptives should be advised to use other methods of birth control. For a review of clinically significant drug interactions see Grange, Winstanley and Davies (1994).

8.7 Immunotherapy of tuberculosis

As outlined earlier (see sections 5.5 and 5.6, pp. 402 and 403), the human immune response to the tubercle bacillus is usually very effective. In the absence of severe immunosuppression, only 10% of those infected eventually develop clinically evident tuberculosis. In this minority population, the immunological factors responsible for disease are a tissue-necrotizing hypersensitivity reaction associated with type 2 cytokines and, very probably, a suppression of recognition of common mycobacterial antigens that are involved in immune detection and lysis of stressed, bacilli-laden cells. It has been shown in a number of studies (reviewed by Stanford et al. 1994) that an injection of heat-killed *M. vaccae* reverses both these inappropriate immune phenomena.

Clinical trials in several countries have shown that immunotherapy with *M. vaccae* is an effective adjunct to chemotherapy of tuberculosis, especially in cases due to multidrug-resistant bacilli (Etemadi, Farid and Stanford 1992), in HIV-related tuberculosis (Stanford et al. 1993a) and where local factors prevent patients from receiving adequate drug therapy (Onyebujoh et al. 1995). The effect of immunotherapy in the latter situation is shown in Table 21.7. At the time of writing, *M. vaccae* is being subjected to extensive clinical evaluation and should soon be widely available.

9 TUBERCULOSIS IN ANIMALS

Tuberculosis is widespread throughout the animal kingdom and, in mammals, is usually caused by *M. bovis*. The wide range of species in which tuberculosis has been described is shown in Table 21.8. Disease is particularly likely to occur in mammals herded together or kept in captivity.

9.1 Tuberculosis in cattle

This is almost exclusively caused by *M. bovis* and is usually transmitted from animal to animal by the aerogenous route. This results in a pulmonary lesion which, in contrast to human tuberculosis, is usually of the progressive primary type, becoming open and infectious. Disease often spreads to the pleurae and intrathoracic lymph nodes. In some cases, enlarged subpleural lymph nodes resemble clusters of pearls, hence the old German name, *Perlsucht* (pearl disease). Other viscera, including the liver, are sometimes affected. Although milk is an important vector of transmission of the disease to humans, the udder is visibly affected in only 1% of diseased cows although animals may excrete bacilli in their milk in the absence of histologically visible lesions. For details of the pathogenesis of tuberculosis in cattle see Neill et al. (1994).

M. tuberculosis very rarely causes overt disease in cattle, but contact with diseased farm workers may lead to tuberculin conversion. Of greater importance is the ability of farm workers with tuberculosis due to *M. bovis* to infect their herds (Schliesser 1974). This usually occurs by the aerial route, but several cases have resulted from workers with renal tuberculosis urinating in cowsheds (Huitema 1969). The increasing occurrence of HIV-related human tuberculosis due to *M. bovis* may lead to more instances of human-to-cattle transmission of the disease.

DIAGNOSIS OF TUBERCULOSIS IN CATTLE

Tubercle bacilli may be demonstrated in the animals' secretions by microscopy, culture or PCR. Tests based on immune responses, notably release of IFN-γ from peripheral blood lymphocytes in the presence of *M. bovis* antigen, are promising (Wood et al. 1992). In practice, the usual diagnostic tool is tuberculin testing.

The tuberculin test is performed by intradermal injection into the skin of the neck (UK) or the caudal fold (USA) and measurement of the local increase in skin thickness 3–5 days later. As in humans, cross-reactions occur in animals due to contact with environmental mycobacteria, notably *M. avium*.

Table 21.7 Results of a trial of *Mycobacterium vaccae* immunotherapy in Kano, Nigeria, under conditions of very poor antituberculosis drug supply*

	Immunotherapy (n = 34)		Placebo (n = 47)
Mortality	0/34 (0%)	$p < 0.00001$	19/47 (40%)
Mean increase in body weight	7.91 kg	$p < 0.003$	2.04 kg
	(n = 33)		(n = 26)
Mean fall in ESR	42 mm	$p < 0.001$	15 mm
	(n = 33)		(n = 26)
Sputum still positive for AFB	11/33 (33%)	$p < 0.00002$	22/26 (85%)
HIV-seropositive	5/34 (14.7%)		9.47 (19%)
Mortality	0/5 (0%)	$p < 0.03$	6/9 (67%)
Sputum still AFB-positive	0/5 (0%)	$p < 0.018$	3/3 (100%)

*Onyebujoh et al. (1995).

Table 21.8   Some animals (other than cattle) from which *Mycobacterium bovis* has been isolated

African buffalo	*Syncerus caffer*
African elephant	*Loxodonta africana*
Baboon	*Papio cynocephalus anubis*
Bactrian camel	*Camelus bactrianus*
Black rhinoceros	*Diceros bicornis*
Brushtail opossum	*Trichosurus vulpecula*
Cat	*Felis domestica*
Elk	*Cervus elaphus*
Fallow deer	*Dama dama*
Giraffe	*Giraffa camelopardalis*
Goat	*Capra hircus*
Horse	*Equus* spp.
Kudu	*Tragelaphus strepsiceros*
Lechwe	*Kobus lechwe kafuencis*
Lion	*Panthera leo*
Monkey, rhesus	*Macaca mulatta*
Monkey, spider	*Ateles geoffroyi*
Rock hyrax	*Procavia capensis*
Seal	*Neophoca cinerca* and *Arctocephalus fosteri*
Springbok	*Antidorcas marsupialis*
Wart hog	*Phacochoerus aethiopicus*
Wild pig	*Sus scrofa*

Hence, in Great Britain, the single intradermal comparative test, in which 0.1 ml amounts of PPDs prepared from *M. bovis* and *M. avium* are injected into separate sites on the neck, is used. Animals whose reactions are due to sensitization by *M. avium* react more strongly to PPD prepared from this species than that prepared from *M. bovis*. For a comprehensive review of tuberculin testing in cattle see Monaghan et al. (1994).

CONTROL OF TUBERCULOSIS IN CATTLE

Tuberculosis was one of the most serious diseases of cattle in Europe and the USA and it is still a major problem in many parts of the world. In 1945, about 40% of herds in Great Britain contained infected animals (Francis 1947). Early attempts to eradicate bovine tuberculosis based on clinical diagnosis of diseased animals failed because such animals infect many others before they are detected. Effective control requires the use of tuberculin testing to detect infected animals before they become infectious.

The method in general use is to test every animal in a herd and to slaughter all positive reactors. Initially, tuberculin testing must be repeated at intervals of 3 or 6 months to detect any fresh reactors in clean herds. This method, when under statutory control and undertaken by region, and when the co-operation of the farmers is assured by adequate financial compensation, is highly successful. In the USA, the reactor rate was reduced from around 4% in 1971 to 0.06% in 1967 and 0.003% in 1994. This very low incidence may be largely due to the absence of reservoirs of disease in feral and wild mammals in that country (Essey and Koller 1994). In the UK a rate of 18% in 1945, when the eradication programme started, was reduced to 0.16% when the entire country had been covered in 1960, and to 0.038% by 1971. Total eradication of

bovine tuberculosis in the UK and certain other countries has been impeded by the existence of reservoirs in wild animals (see section 9.2) and by human-to-animal transmission. For detailed accounts of bovine tuberculosis control and the problems encountered in many developed countries, see Steele and Thoen (1995).

Control programmes in developing countries are usually minimal and ineffective and data on the extent of the problem in these countries are limited (Cosivi et al. 1995). In Africa, for example, 33 of 41 countries report cases of bovine tuberculosis and only 4 (Kenya, Namibia, Seychelles and Zimbabwe) claim that they are free of the disease. Around 90% of cattle in Africa are in countries where bovine tuberculosis control measures are minimal or non-existent (Report 1993).

9.2   Tuberculosis in other mammals

As shown in Table 21.8, a range of animals other than cattle are susceptible to disease due to *M. bovis*. These pose a risk to humans and domesticated animals. Infection, but not overt tuberculosis, has resulted from exposure of humans to tuberculous elk (Fanning and Edwards 1991) and a rhinoceros (Dalovisio, Stetter and Mikota-Wells 1992).

In some regions of New Zealand, the opossum (*Trichosurus vulpecula*) is a reservoir of tuberculosis due to *M. bovis* and the incidence of reactor cattle is much higher in these regions than in those in which the reservoir has been controlled or is absent (Tweddle and Livingstone 1994). Elimination of opossums in some regions by poisoning led to a reduction of the reactor rate in cattle but total elimination of this reservoir was not considered possible.

In parts of Great Britain, notably the south west, and Ireland, tuberculosis due to *M. bovis* occurs in the badger (*Meles meles*) (Nolan and Wilesmith 1994). Infection occurs by the respiratory route or through bites. The disease develops slowly, with a non-infectious stage lasting several months. Later, disseminated disease develops and numerous bacilli are shed in urine, faeces, respiratory secretions and in pus from infected bite wounds, and readily contaminate pasture land. The first diseased badger in the UK was found in 1971 and a subsequent examination of 6000 carcases showed that 13%, and up to 30% in some areas, had tuberculous lesions (Muirhead, Gallagher and Birn 1974). Despite very strong epidemiological evidence (though no direct proof) of an association between tuberculosis in badgers and cattle, neither public opinion nor practicalities have permitted the eradication of this reservoir which therefore still exists.

Although the rabbit is highly susceptible to experimental *M. bovis* infection, natural disease in regions where cattle and other mammals are affected is rare. The disease is likewise uncommon in other small mammals in such regions. In south west England, where badger tuberculosis is common, the disease was found in 1.3% of moles, 1.2% of rats, 0.9% of foxes and 0.6% of mink (Ministry of Agriculture, Fisheries and Food 1984). Wild and captive deer are susceptible to *M. bovis*, raising problems of diagnosis and control in farmed deer herds (Griffin 1988, Clifton-Hadley and Wilesmith 1991).

The vole bacillus, *M. microti*, is a member of the *M. tuberculosis* complex that has been isolated from voles, shrews and woodmice (Wells 1946) but not in recent years. Bacilli with similar properties have been isolated from the dassie or cape hyrax (*Procavia capensis*; Smith 1960), seals and cats, but their exact taxonomic status and relation to *M. microti* are uncertain.

9.3 Tuberculosis in birds and cold-blooded animals

This disease is almost invariably due to species other than those in the *M. tuberculosis* complex. The relatively high body temperature of birds, 42–43°C, inhibits the growth of tubercle bacilli. Although infection of parrots and, less often, canaries by *M. tuberculosis* has been reported, it only causes superficial lesions.

REFERENCES

Abrahams EW, 1970, Original mycobacterial sin, *Tubercle*, **51**: 316–21 .

Al Attiyah R, Morino C, Rook GAW , 1992, TNF-alpha-mediated tissue damage in mouse footpads primed with mycobacterial preparations, *Res Immunol*, **143**: 601–10.

Aluoch JA, Swai OB et al., 1985, Studies on case-finding for pulmonary tuberculosis in outpatients at 4 district hospitals in Kenya, *Tubercle*, **66**: 237–49.

Alzeer AH, FitzGerald JM, 1993, Corticosteroids and tuberculosis: risks and use as adjunct therapy, *Tuber Lung Dis*, **74**: 6–11.

American Lung Association, 1974, *Diagnostic Standards and Classification of Tuberculosis and Other Mycobacterial Diseases*, American Lung Association, New York, 18.

Bancroft GJ, Schreiber RD, Unanue ER, 1991, Natural immunity: a T-cell-independent pathway of macrophage activation defined in the SCID mouse, *Immunol Rev*, **124**: 5–24.

Bateman ED, 1993, Is tuberculosis prophylaxis necessary for patients receiving corticosteroids for respiratory disease? *Respir Med*, **87**: 485–7.

Beck JS, Potts RC et al., 1985, T4 lymphopenia in patients with active pulmonary tuberculosis, *Clin Exp Immunol*, **60**: 49–54.

Beck JS, Morley SM et al., 1986, The cellular responses of tuberculosis and leprosy patients and of healthy controls in skin tests to new tuberculin and leprosin A, *Clin Exp Immunol*, **64**: 484–9.

Beck JS, Morley SM et al., 1988, Diversity in migration of CD4 and CD8 lymphocytes in different microanatomical compartments of the skin in the tuberculin reaction in man, *Br J Exp Pathol*, **69**: 771–80.

Benatar SR, 1995, Prospects for global health: lessons from tuberculosis, *Thorax*, **50**: 487–9.

Beutler B, Greenwald D et al., 1985, Identity of tumour necrosis factor and the macrophage-secreted factor cachectin, *Nature (London)*, **316**: 552–3.

Boom WH, Wallis RS, Chervenak KA, 1991, Human *Mycobacterium tuberculosis*-reactive CD4+ T-cell clones: heterogeneity in antigen recognition, cytokine production, and cytotoxicity for mononuclear phagocytes, *Infect Immun*, **59**: 2737–43.

Born W, Hall L et al., 1990, Recognition of a peptide antigen by heat shock reactive gd T lymphocytes, *Science*, **249**: 67–9.

Bothamley GH, Grange JM, 1991, The Koch phenomenon and delayed hypersensitivity 1891–1991, *Tubercle*, **72**: 7–12.

Bothamley GH, Beck JS et al., 1989, Association of tuberculosis and *M. tuberculosis*-specific antibody levels with HLA, *J Infect Dis*, **159**: 549–55.

Bouvet E, Casalino E et al., 1993, A nosocomial outbreak of multidrug-resistant *Mycobacterium bovis* among HIV-infected patients. A case-control study, *AIDS*, **7**: 1453–60.

Brahmajothi V, Pitchappan RM et al., 1991, Association of pulmonary tuberculosis and HLA in South India, *Tubercle*, **72**: 123–32.

Bretscher PA, 1992, A strategy to improve the efficacy of vaccination against tuberculosis and leprosy, *Immunol Today*, **13**: 342–5.

Brown JAK, Stone MM, Sutherland I, 1966, BCG vaccination of children against leprosy in Uganda, *Br Med J*, **1**: 7–14.

Capewell S, France AJ et al., 1986, The diagnosis and management of tuberculosis in common hostel dwellers, *Tubercle*, **67**: 125–32.

Caplin M, 1980, *The Tuberculin Test in Clinical Practice: an Illustrated Guide*, Baillière Tindall, London.

Centers for Disease Control, 1993, Initial therapy for tuberculosis in the era of multidrug resistance (Recommendations of the Advisory Council for the Elimination of Tuberculosis), *Morbid Mortal Weekly Rep*, **42 (RR-7)**: 1–8.

Chan J, Fan X et al., 1991, Lipoarabinomannan, a possible virulence factor involved in persistence of *Mycobacterium tuberculosis* within macrophages, *Infect Immun*, **59**: 1755–61.

Chaulet P, 1983, But the emperor has no clothes on! A critique on the report of the joint IUAT/WHO study group, *Bull Int Union Tuberc Lung Dis*, **58**: 153–6.

China Tuberculosis Control Collaboration, 1996, Results of directly observed short-course chemotherapy in 112 842 Chinese patients with smear-positive tuberculosis, *Lancet*, **347**: 358–62.

Chretien J, 1990, Tuberculosis and HIV. The cursed duet, *Bull Int Union Tuberc Lung Dis*, **65 (1)**: 25–8.

Clark G, Kelley M et al., 1987, A re-evaluation of the evolution of mycobacterial disease in human populations, *Curr Anthropol*, **28**: 45–62.

Clifton-Hadley RS, Wilesmith JW, 1991, Tuberculosis in deer: a review, *Vet Rec*, **129**: 5–12.

Cohen IR, Young DB, 1991, Autoimmunity, microbial immunity and the immunological homunculus, *Immunol Today*, **12**: 105–10.

Collins CH, 1993, *Laboratory Acquired Infections*, 3rd edn, Butterworth Heinemann, Oxford.

Collins CH, Grange JM, Yates MD, 1984, Mycobacteria in water, *J Appl Bacteriol*, **57**: 193–211.

Collins CH, Grange JM, Yates MD, 1985, *Organization and Practice in Tuberculosis Bacteriology*, Butterworths, London.

Coovadia YM, Dawood A et al., 1986, Evaluation of adenosine deaminase activity and antibody to *Mycobacterium tuberculosis* antigen 5 in cerebrospinal fluid and the radioactive bromide partition test for the early diagnosis of tuberculous meningitis, *Arch Dis Child*, **61**: 428–35.

Cosivi O, Meslin F-X et al., 1995, The epidemiology of *Mycobacterium bovis* infection in animals and humans, with particular reference to Africa, *Rev Sci Tech*, **14**: 733–46.

Costello AM de L, Kumar A et al., 1992, Does antibody to mycobacterial antigens, including lipoarabinomannan, limit dissemination in childhood tuberculosis?, *Trans R Soc Trop Med Hyg*, **86**: 686–92.

Crofton J, Horne N, Miller F, 1992, *Clinical Tuberculosis*, Macmillan, London.

Daley CL, Small PM et al., 1992, An outbreak of tuberculosis with accelerated progression among persons infected with the human immunodeficiency virus. An analysis using restriction-fragment polymorphisms, *N Engl J Med*, **326**: 231–5.

Dalovisio JR, Stetter M, Mikota-Wells S, 1992, Rhinoceros' rhinorrhea: cause of an outbreak of infection due to airborne *Mycobacterium bovis* in zookeepers, *Clin Infect Dis*, **15**: 598–600.

Dannenberg AM, 1993, Immunopathogenesis of pulmonary tuberculosis, *Hosp Pract*, **28**: 51–8.

Davies PDO, ed., 1994, *Clinical Tuberculosis*, Chapman and Hall, London.

Daynes RA, Meikle AW, Araneo BA, 1991, Locally active steroid hormones may facilitate compartmentalization of immunity by regulating the types of lymphokines produced by helper T cells, *Res Immunol*, **142**: 40–5.

Dolin PJ, Raviglione MC, Kochi A, 1994, Global tuberculosis incidence and mortality during 1990–2000, *Bull W H O*, **72**: 213–20.

Donald PR, Fourie B, Grange JM, eds, 1996, *Tuberculosis in Children*, Van Schaik, Pretoria.

Dooley SW, Simone M, 1994, The extent and management of drug-resistant tuberculosis: the American experience, *Clinical Tuberculosis*, ed. Davies PDO, Chapman and Hall, London, 171–89.

van Eden W, Thole JER et al., 1988, Cloning of the mycobacterial epitope recognised by T lymphocytes in adjuvant arthritis, *Nature (London)*, **331**: 171–3.

Edlin BR, Tokars JL et al., 1992, An outbreak of multidrug resistant tuberculosis in hospitalized patients with the human immunodeficiency virus, *N Engl J Med*, **326**: 1514–21.

Escober JA, Belsey MA et al., 1975, Mortality from tuberculous meningitis reduced by steroid therapy, *Pediatrics*, **56**: 1050–5.

Essey MA, Koller MA, 1994, Status of bovine tuberculosis in North America, *Vet Microbiol*, **40**: 15–22.

Etemadi A, Farid R, Stanford JL, 1992, Immunotherapy for drug-resistant tuberculosis, *Lancet*, **340**: 1360–1.

Etkind S, 1993, Contact tracing in tuberculosis, *Tuberculosis: a Comprehensive International Approach*, eds Reichman LB, Hershfield ES, Marcel Dekker, New York, 275–89.

European Society for Mycobacteriology, 1991, *Manual of Diagnostic and Public Health Mycobacteriology*, 2nd edn, Bureau of Hygiene and Tropical Diseases, London.

Fanning A, Edwards S, 1991, *Mycobacterium bovis* infection in human beings in contact with elk (*Cervus elaphus*) in Alberta, Canada, *Lancet*, **338**: 1253–5.

Festenstein F, Grange JM, 1991, Tuberculosis and the acquired immune deficiency syndrome, *J Appl Bacteriol*, **71**: 19–30.

Filley EA, Bull HA et al., 1992, The effect of *Mycobacterium tuberculosis* on the susceptibility of human cells to the stimulatory and toxic effects of tumour necrosis factor, *Immunology*, **77**: 505–9.

Fine PEM, 1994, Immunities in and to tuberculosis: implications for pathogenesis and vaccination, *Tuberculosis: Back to the Future*, eds Porter JDH, McAdam KPWJ, Wiley, Chichester, 43–78.

Flesch IEA, Kaufmann SHE, 1990, Activation of tuberculostatic macrophage functions by gamma interferon, interleukin-4 and tumour necrosis factor, *Infect Immun*, **58**: 2675–7.

Flynn JL, Goldstein MM et al., 1992, Major histocompatibility complex class I-restricted T cells are required for resistance to *Mycobacterium tuberculosis* infection, *Proc Natl Acad Sci USA*, **89**: 12013–17.

Fox W, 1990, Drug combinations and the bioavailability of rifampicin, *Tubercle*, **71**: 241–5.

Francis J, 1947, *Bovine Tuberculosis*, Staples Press, London.

French GA, Teoh R et al., 1987, Diagnosis of tuberculous meningitis by detection of tuberculostearic acid in cerebrospinal fluid, *Lancet*, **2**: 117–19.

van Geuns HA, Meijer J, Stýblo K, 1975, Results of contact examination in Rotterdam, *Bull Int Union Tuberc Lung Dis*, **50**: 107–21.

Gibbs JH, Grange JM et al., 1991, Early delayed-type hypersensitivity responses in tuberculin skin tests after heavy occupational exposure to tuberculosis, *J Clin Pathol*, **44**: 919–23.

Girling DJ, 1989, The chemotherapy of tuberculosis, *The Biology of the Mycobacteria*, vol. 3, eds Ratledge C, Stanford JL, Grange JM, Academic Press, New York, 285–323.

Goble M, Iseman MD et al., 1993, Treatment of 1712 patients with pulmonary tuberculosis resistant to isoniazid and rifampicin, *N Engl J Med*, **328**: 527–32.

Grange JM, 1984, The humoral immune response in tuberculosis: its nature, biological role and diagnostic usefulness, *Adv Tuberc Res*, **21**: 1–78.

Grange JM, 1989, Tuberculosis and environmental (atypical) mycobacterioses: bacterial, pathological and immunological aspects, *Mycobacterial Skin Diseases*, ed. Harahap M, Kluwer, Dordrecht, 1–32.

Grange JM, 1992, The mystery of the mycobacterial persistor, *Tuber Lung Dis*, **73**: 249–51.

Grange JM, 1996, *Mycobacteria and Human Disease*, 2nd edn, Arnold, London.

Grange JM, Bishop PJ, 1982, 'Über tuberculose'. A tribute to Robert Koch's discovery of the tubercle bacillus, 1882, *Tubercle*, **63**: 3–17.

Grange JM, Daborn C, Cosivi O, 1994, HIV-related tuberculosis due to *Mycobacterium bovis*, *Eur Respir J*, **7**: 1564–6.

Grange JM, Festenstein F, 1993, The human dimension of tuberculosis control, *Tuber Lung Dis*, **74**: 219–22.

Grange JM, Stanford JL, 1994, Dogma and innovation in the global control of tuberculosis, *J R Soc Med*, **87**: 272–5.

Grange JM, Stanford JL, Rook GAW, 1995, Tuberculosis and cancer: parallels in host responses and therapeutic approaches? *Lancet*, **345**: 1350–2.

Grange JM, Winstanley PA, Davies PDO, 1994, Clinically significant drug interactions with antituberculosis agents, *Drug Saf*, **11**: 242–51.

Grange JM, Yates MD, 1994, Zoonotic aspects of *Mycobacterium bovis* infection, *Vet Microbiol*, **40**: 137–51.

Grange JM, Yates MD, Ormerod LP, 1995, Factors determining ethnic differences in the incidence of bacteriologically confirmed genitourinary tuberculosis in south east England, *J Infect*, **30**: 37–40.

Grange JM, Beck JS et al., 1986, The effect of occupational exposure to patients with tuberculosis on dermal reactivity to four new tuberculins among healthy Indonesian adults, *Tubercle*, **67**: 109–18.

Griffin JHT, 1988, The aetiology of tuberculosis and mycobacterial disease in farmed deer, *Irish Vet J*, **42**: 23–6.

Grzybowski S, Styblo K, Dorken E, 1976, Tuberculosis in eskimos, *Tubercle*, **57, Suppl.**: S1–58.

Gubler JGH, Salfinger M, von Graevenitz A, 1992, Pseudoepidemic of non-tuberculous mycobacteria due to a contaminated bronchoscope cleaning machine – report of an outbreak and a review of the literature, *Chest*, **101**: 1245–9.

Heaf F, 1951, Multiple-puncture tuberculin test, *Lancet*, **2**: 151–3.

Heifets L, ed., 1991, *Drug Susceptibility in the Chemotherapy of Mycobacterial Infections*, CRC Press, Boca Raton, 103–9.

Hernandez-Pando R, Rook GAW, 1994, The role of TNF-alpha in T cell-mediated inflammation depends on the Th1/Th2 cytokine balance, *Immunology*, **82**: 591–5.

Hoeppner VH, Jackett P et al., 1987, Appraisal of the monoclonal antibody-based competition test for the serology of tuberculosis in Indonesia, *Serodiag Immunother*, **1**: 69–77.

Huitema H, 1969, The eradication of bovine tuberculosis in cattle and the significance of man as a source of infection in cattle, *Selected Papers, R Netherlands Tuberc Assn*, **12**: 62–7.

Humphries MJ, Lam WK, Teoh R, 1994, Non-respiratory tuberculosis, *Clinical Tuberculosis*, ed. Davies PDO, Chapman and Hall, London, 93–125.

Israel HL, 1993, Chemoprophylaxis for tuberculosis, *Respir Med*, **87**: 81–3.

Kardjito T, Beck JS et al., 1986, A comparison of the responsiveness to four new tuberculins among Indonesian patients with pulmonary tuberculosis and healthy subjects, *Eur J Respir Dis*, **69**: 142–5.

Kaufmann SHE, Blum C, Yamamoto S, 1993, Crosstalk between alpha/beta T cells and gamma/delta T cells in vivo: activation of alpha/beta T cell responses after gamma/delta T cell modulation with the monoclonal antibody GL3, *Proc Natl Acad Sci USA*, **90**: 9620–4.

Kennedy DH, 1989, Extrapulmonary tuberculosis, *The Biology of the Mycobacteria*, vol. 3, eds Ratledge C, Stanford JL, Grange JM, Academic Press, New York, 245–84.

Khomenko AG, Litvinov VI et al., 1990, Tuberculosis in patients with various HLA phenotypes, *Tubercle*, **71**: 187–92.

Koch R, 1891, Weitere Mitteilungen über ein Heilmittel gegen Tuberkulose, *Dtsch Med Wochenschr*, **17**: 101–2.

Kochi A, 1991, The global tuberculosis situation and the new control strategy of the World Health Organization, *Tubercle*, **72**: 1–6.

Kumarvelu S, Prasad K et al., 1994, Randomized controlled trial of dexamethasone in tuberculous meningitis, *Tuber Lung Dis*, **75**: 203–7.

Labhard N, Nicod L, Zellweger JP, 1994, Cerebral tuberculosis in the immunocompetent host: 8 cases observed in Switzerland, *Tuber Lung Dis*, **75**: 454–9.

McAdam KPWJ, 1994, Back to the future: 'the ten commitments', *Tuberculosis: Back to the Future*, eds Porter JDH, McAdam KPWJ, Wiley, Chichester, 267–76.

McDonagh KA, Kress Y, Bloom BR, 1993, Pathogenesis of tuberculosis: interactions of *Mycobacterium tuberculosis* with macrophages, *Infect Immun*, **61**: 2763–73.

Major RH, 1959, *Classic Descriptions of Disease*, 3rd edn, Charles C Thomas, Springfield IL, 52–3.

Miller FJW, 1982, *Tuberculosis in children*, Churchill Livingstone, Edinburgh.

Miller N, Hernandez SG, Cleary TJ, 1994, Evaluation of Gen-Probe Amplified Mycobacterium Tuberculosis Direct Test and PCR for direct detection of *Mycobacterium tuberculosis* in clinical specimens, *J Clin Microbiol*, **32**: 393–7.

Ministry of Agriculture, Fisheries and Food, 1984, *Bovine Tuberculosis in Badgers*, 8th Report, HMSO, London.

Mitchison DA, 1985, Hypothesis: the action of antituberculosis drugs in short course chemotherapy, *Tubercle*, **66**: 219–25.

Mitchison DA, Allen BW, Manickavasagar D, 1983, Selective Kirschner medium in the culture of specimens other than sputum for mycobacteria, *J Clin Pathol*, **36**: 1357–61.

Monaghan ML, Doherty ML et al., 1994, The tuberculin test, *Vet Microbiol*, **40**: 111–24.

Morse DL, 1994, Multidrug resistance. The New York experience, *Tuberculosis: Back to the Future*, eds Porter JDH, McAdam KPWJ, Wiley, Chichester, 225–30.

Mosmann TR, Moore KW, 1991, The role of IL-10 in crossregulation of Th1 and Th2 responses, *Immunol Today*, **12**: A49–53.

Muirhead RH, Gallagher J, Birn KJ, 1974, Tuberculosis in wild badgers in Gloucestershire: epidemiology, *Vet Rec*, **95**: 552–5.

Murray CJ, Styblo K, Rouillon A, 1990, Tuberculosis in developing countries: burden, intervention and cost, *Bull Int Union Tuberc Lung Dis*, **65**: 6–24.

Narain JP, Raviglione MC, Kochi A, 1992, HIV-associated tuberculosis in developing countries: epidemiology and strategies for prevention, *Tuber Lung Dis*, **73**: 311–21.

Neill SD, Pollock JM et al., 1994, Pathogenesis of *Mycobacterium bovis* infection in cattle, *Vet Microbiol*, **40**: 41–52.

Nolan A, Wilesmith JW, 1994, Tuberculosis in badgers (*Meles meles*), *Vet Microbiol*, **40**: 179–91.

Nunn P, 1994, Impact of interaction with HIV, *Tuberculosis: Back to the Future*, eds Porter JDH, McAdam KPWJ, Wiley, Chichester, 49–52.

Nunn P, Mungai M et al., 1994, The effect of human immunodeficiency virus type-1 on the infectiousness of tuberculosis, *Tuber Lung Dis*, **75**: 25–32.

O'Brien RJ, 1994, Preventive therapy for tuberculosis, *Clinical Tuberculosis*, ed. Davies PDO, Chapman and Hall, London, 279–95.

Onyebujoh PC, Abdulmumini T et al., 1995, Immunotherapy with *Mycobacterium vaccae* as an addition to chemotherapy for the treatment of pulmonary tuberculosis under difficult conditions in Africa, *Respir Med*, **89**: 199–207.

Orme IM, Anderson P, Boom WH, 1993, T cell response to *Mycobacterium tuberculosis*, *J Infect Dis*, **167**: 1481–97.

Osborn L, Kunkel S, Nabel GJ, 1989, Tumour necrosis factor and interleukin 1 stimulate the human immunodeficiency virus enhancer by activation of the nuclear factor kappa B, *Proc Natl Acad Sci USA*, **86**: 2236–40.

Osborn TW, 1983, Changes in BCG strains, *Tubercle*, **64**: 1–13.

Ottenhoff THM, Torres P et al., 1986, Evidence for an HLA-DR4 associated immune-response gene for *Mycobacterium tuberculosis*. A clue to the pathogenesis of rheumatoid arthritis, *Lancet*, **2**: 310–12.

Ottenhoff THM, Kale AB et al., 1988, The recombinant 65 KD heat shock protein of *Mycobacterium bovis* BCG/*M. tuberculosis* is a target molecule for CD4+ cytotoxic T lymphocytes that lyse human monocytes, *J Exp Med*, **168**: 1947–52.

Oxfam Health Unit, 1985, *Guidelines for Tuberculosis Control Programmes in Developing Countries*, Oxfam Practical Guide No. 4, Oxfam, Oxford.

Palmer CE, Long MW, 1969, Effects of infection with atypical mycobacteria on BCG vaccination and tuberculosis, *Am Rev Respir Dis*, **94**: 553–68.

Pape JW, Jean SS et al., 1993, Effect of isoniazid prophylaxis on incidence of active tuberculosis and progression of HIV infection, *Lancet*, **342**: 268–72.

Patel AM, Abrahams EW, 1989, Pulmonary tuberculosis, *The Biology of the Mycobacteria*, vol. 3, eds Ratledge C, Stanford JL, Grange JM, Academic Press, New York, 179–244.

von Pirquet C, 1907, Demonstration zur Tuberculindiagnose durch Hautimpfung, *Berl Klin Wochenschr*, **48**: 699.

Potts RC, Beck JS et al., 1992, Measurements of blood flow and histometry of the cellular infiltrate in tuberculin skin test responses of the typical Koch-type and the non-turgid (*Listeria*-type) in pulmonary tuberculosis patients and apparently healthy controls, *Int J Exp Pathol*, **73**: 565–72.

Rao VR, Joanes RF et al., 1980, Outbreak of tuberculosis after minimal exposure to infection, *Br Med J*, **281**: 187–9.

Reichmann LB, 1991, The U-shaped curve of concern, *Am Rev Respir Dis*, **144**: 741–2.

Report, 1978, A controlled trial of anterior spinal fusion and debridement in the surgical management of tuberculosis of the spine in patients on standard chemotherapy: a study in two centres in South Africa (Seventh Report of the Medical Research Council Working Party on Tuberculosis of the Spine), *Tubercle*, **59**: 79–105.

Report, 1993, *Sante Animale Mondiale en 1992*, vols 1 and 2, Office International des Epizooties, Paris.

Report, 1994a, Joint Tuberculosis Committee of the British Thoracic Society. Control and prevention of tuberculosis in the United Kingdom: code of practice, *Thorax*, **49**: 1193–200.

Report, 1994b, International Union against Tuberculosis and Lung Disease/World Health Organization. Tuberculosis preventive therapy in HIV-infected individuals, *Tuber Lung Dis*, **75**: 96–8.

Ridley DS, Ridley MJ, 1987, Rationale for the histological spectrum of tuberculosis. A basis for classification, *Pathology*, **19**: 186–92.

Rieder HL, 1994, Drug-resistant tuberculosis: issues in epidemiology and challenges for public health, *Tuber Lung Dis*, **75**: 321–3.

Rook GAW, 1988a, The role of vitamin D in tuberculosis, *Am Rev Respir Dis*, **138**: 768–70.

Rook GAW, 1988b, Rheumatoid arthritis, mycobacterial antigens and agalactosyl IgG, *Scand J Immunol*, **28**: 487–93.

Rook GAW, Bloom BR, 1994, Mechanisms of pathogenesis in tuberculosis, *Tuberculosis: Pathogensis, Protection, and Control*, ed. Bloom BR, American Society for Microbiology, Washington, DC, 485–501.

Rook GAW, Onyebujoh P, Stanford JL, 1993, TH1/TH2 switching and loss of CD4 cells in chronic infections: an immunoendocrinological hypothesis not exclusive to HIV, *Immunol Today*, **14**: 568–9.

Rook GAW, Stanford JL, 1979, The relevance to protection of three forms of delayed skin test response evoked by *M. leprae* and other mycobacteria in mice: correlation with the classical work in the guinea-pig, *Parasite Immunol*, **1**: 111–23.

Rook GAW, Stanford JL, 1992, Slow bacterial infections or autoimmunity?, *Immunol Today*, **13**: 160–4.

Rouillon A, Perdrizet S, Parrot R, 1976, Transmission of tubercle bacilli: the effects of chemotherapy, *Tubercle*, **57**: 275–99.

Rubilar M, Sime PJ et al., 1994, Time to extend 'the timetable of tuberculosis'?, *Respir Med*, **88**: 481–2.

Saceanu CA, Pfeiffer NC, McLean T, 1993, Evaluation of sputum smears concentrated by cytocentrifugation for detection of acid-fast bacilli, *J Clin Microbiol*, **31**: 2371–4.

Salfinger M, Demchik BS, Kafader FM, 1990, Comparison between the MB Check system, radiometric and conventional methods for recovery of mycobacteria, *J Microbiol Methods*, **12**: 97–100.

Salfinger M, Morris AJ, 1994, The role of the microbiology laboratory in diagnosing mycobacterial disease, *Am J Clin Pathol*, **101, Suppl. 1: Pathology Patterns:** S6–13.

Schliesser T, 1974, Die Bekämpfung der Rindertuberkulose – Tierversuch der Vergangenheit, *Prax Pneumol*, **28, Suppl.:** 870–4.

Schulzer M, Fitzgerald JM et al., 1992, An estimate of the future size of the tuberculosis problem in sub-Saharan Africa resulting from HIV infection, *Tuber Lung Dis*, **73**: 52–8.

Seibert FB, 1934, The isolation and properties of the purified protein derivative of tuberculin, *Am Rev Tuberc*, **30**: 713–20.

Shaw R, 1994, Polymerase chain reaction, *Clinical Tuberculosis*, ed. Davies PDO, Chapman and Hall, London, 381–9.

Shears P, 1984, Tuberculosis control in Somali refugee camps, *Tubercle*, **65**: 111–16.

Sheldon CD, King K et al., 1992, Notification of tuberculosis: how many cases are never reported?, *Thorax*, **47**: 1015–18.

Skamene E, Gros P et al., 1982, Genetic regulation of resistance to intracellular pathogens, *Nature* (London), **297**: 506–9.

Smith N, 1960, The 'dassie' bacillus, *Tubercle*, **41**: 203–12.

Snider DE, Bloch AB, 1984, Congenital tuberculosis, *Tubercle*, **65**: 81–2.

Springett VH, 1971, Ten-year results during the introduction of chemotherapy for tuberculosis, *Tubercle*, **52**: 73–87.

Stanford JL, 1983, Immunologically important constituents of mycobacteria: antigens, *The Biology of the Mycobacteria*, vol. 2, eds Ratledge C, Stanford JL, Academic Press, London, 85–127.

Stanford JL, Lema E, 1983, The use of a sonicate preparation of *Mycobacterium tuberculosis* (new tuberculin) in the assessment of BCG vaccination, *Tubercle*, **64**: 275–82.

Stanford JL, Shield MJ, Rook GAW, 1981, Hypothesis: how environmental mycobacteria may predetermine the protective efficacy of BCG, *Tubercle*, **62**: 55–62.

Stanford JL, Nye PM et al., 1981, A preliminary investigation of the responsiveness or otherwise of patients and staff of a leprosy hospital to groups of shared or species specific antigens of mycobacteria, *Lepr Rev*, **52**: 321–7.

Stanford JL, Onyebujoh PC et al., 1993a, Old plague, new plague and a treatment for both, *AIDS*, **7**: 1275–7.

Stanford JL, Stanford CA et al., 1993b, Chemoprophylaxis for tuberculosis, *Respir Med*, **87**: 398–9.

Stanford JL, Stanford CA et al., 1994, Immunotherapy for tuberculosis. Investigative and practical aspects, *Clin Immunother*, **1**: 430–40.

Steele JH, Thoen C, eds, 1995, Mycobacterium bovis *Infection in Humans and Animals*, Iowa State University Press, Ames, Iowa.

Stoker N, 1994, Tuberculosis in a changing world. Don't stint on surveillance and control, *Br Med J*, **309**: 1178–9.

Strang JG, Kakaza HHS et al., 1988, Controlled clinical trial of complete open surgical drainage and prednisolone in the treatment of tuberculous pericardial effusion in Transkei, *Lancet*, **2**: 1418–22.

Styblo K, 1978, State of the art I: epidemiology of tuberculosis, *Bull Int Union Tuberc Lung Dis*, **53**: 141–52.

Styblo K, 1984, Epidemiology of tuberculosis, *In Infektionskrankheiten und ihre Erreger*, vol. 4/VI, Gustav Fischer, Jena, 77–161.

Styblo K, 1986, Tuberculosis control and surveillance, *Recent Advances in Respiratory Medicine*, No. 4, eds Flenley DC, Petty TL, Churchill Livingstone, Edinburgh, 77–108.

Trnka L, Dankova D, Svandova E, 1994, Six years' experience with the discontinuation of BCG vaccination 4. Protective effect of BCG vaccination against the *Mycobacterium avium–intracellulare* complex, *Tuber Lung Dis*, **75**: 348–52.

Tweddle NE, Livingstone P, 1994, Bovine tuberculosis control and eradication programs in Australia and New Zealand, *Vet Microbiol*, **40**: 23–39.

Uplekar MW, Shepard DS, 1991, Treatment of tuberculosis by private general practitioners in India, *Tubercle*, **72**: 284–90.

Ustvedt HJ, 1947, The relationship between renal tuberculosis and primary infection, *Tubercle*, **28**: 22–5.

Veen J, 1992, Microepidemics of tuberculosis: the stone-in-the-pond principle, *Tuber Lung Dis*, **73**: 73–6.

Vidal SM, Malo D et al., 1993, Natural resistance to infection with intracellular parasites: isolation of a candidate for *Bcg*, *Cell*, **73**: 469–85.

Villemin JA, 1868, *Etudes Experimentales et Cliniqies sur Tuberculose*, Baillière, Paris.

Wadee AA, Boting L, Reddy SG, 1990, Antigen capture assay for detection of a 45-kilodalton *Mycobacterium tuberculosis* antigen, *J Clin Microbiol*, **28**: 2786–91.

Wallgren A, 1948, The time table of tuberculosis, *Tubercle*, **29**: 245–51.

Wayne LG, Lin K-Y, 1982, Glyoxalate metabolism and adaptation of *Mycobacterium tuberculosis* to survival under anaerobic conditions, *Infect Immun*, **37**: 1042–9.

Wells AQ, 1946, *The Murine Type of Tubercle Bacillus*, Medical Research Council Special Report 259, HMSO, London.

Wilkins EGL, 1994, The serodiagnosis of tuberculosis, *Clinical Tuberculosis*, ed. Davies PDO, Chapman and Hall, London, 367–80.

Wilkinson AG, Roy S, 1984, Two cases of Poncet's disease, *Tubercle*, **65**: 301–3.

Wood PR, Corner LA et al., 1992, A field evaluation of serological and cellular diagnostic tests for bovine tuberculosis, *Vet Microbiol*, **31**: 71–9.

World Health Organization, 1991, *WHO Model Prescribing Information. Drugs Used in Mycobacterial Diseases*, World Health Organization, Geneva.

World Health Organization, 1994a, *TB – A Global Emergency*, World Health Organization, Geneva (WHO/TB/94.177).

World Health Organization, 1994b, *The HIV/AIDS and Tuberculosis Epidemics: Implications for TB Control*, World Health Organization, Geneva (WHO/TB/CARG(4)/944).

World Health Organization, 1994c, Acquired immunodeficiency syndrome (AIDS) – data as at 30 June 1994, *Wkly Epidemiol Rec*, **69**: 189–96.

World Health Organization, 1994d, *Guidelines for Surveillance of Drug Resistance in Tuberculosis*, World Health Organization, Geneva (WHO/TB/94.178).

World Health Organization, 1995, *Stop TB at the Source. WHO Report on the Tuberculosis Epidemic, 1995*, World Health Organization, Geneva (WHO/TB/95.183).

Yu G-P, Hsieh C-C, Peng J, 1988, Risk factors associated with the prevalence of pulmonary tuberculosis among sanitary workers in Shanghai, *Tubercle*, **69**: 105–12.

Chapter 22

MYCOBACTERIOSES OTHER THAN TUBERCULOSIS

D B Hornick and L S Schlesinger

1 **General characteristics of non-tuberculous mycobacteria (NTM)**	3 **Extrapulmonary mycobacterioses in the immunocompetent host**
2 **Pulmonary infection in the immunocompetent host**	4 **Mycobacterioses in immunocompromised hosts**

Non-tuberculous mycobacteria (NTM) are the large number of mycobacterial species frequently found in environmental habitats that may colonize and occasionally cause infection in humans and animals. Such infections are termed mycobacterioses (Anon 1989). The terms NTM and mycobacterioses reflect efforts to distinguish these from *Mycobacterium tuberculosis* and tuberculosis. Other terms for NTM are mycobacteria other than tuberculosis (MOTT), potentially pathogenic environmental mycobacteria (PPEM), and the misnomer atypical mycobacteria. NTM are 'typical' mycobacteria but less virulent than *M. tuberculosis* in humans. They may colonize a host without evident tissue invasion and may, at times, be isolated coincidentally as contaminants from the environment. In this case NTM may incorrectly be labelled as colonizers or as the cause of infection. Some NTM are rarely associated with infection (Table 22.1), whereas others can cause significant pulmonary and extra-pulmonary disease in immunocompetent humans, and disseminated infection in immunocompromised hosts. Mycobacterioses are becoming more prevalent with the increasing prevalence of immunocompromised hosts, particularly in relation to the AIDS pandemic. The characteristics of these infections differ from those seen in immunocompetent human hosts as do the organisms involved (Table 22.1). The characteristics of the members of the genus *Mycobacterium* are discussed in Volume 2, Chapter 26.

1 GENERAL CHARACTERISTICS OF NON-TUBERCULOUS MYCOBACTERIA (NTM)

Most NTM are acid-fast bacilli (AFB) and indistinguishable from *M. tuberculosis* except by a negative niacin reaction; other distinguishing characteristics are growth rate and pigmentation. Runyon classified NTM into 4 groups by their growth rate and pigmentation (Runyon 1959). RGM that produce colonies on Lowenstein–Jensen (L–J) slants by 7 days were designated as group IV. Non-pigmented, slow-growing organisms were designated group III, and pigmented species were placed in groups I and II. Some pigmented species that are buff coloured when cultured in the dark, but form a yellow pigment on exposure to light, were called photochromogenic bacteria (group I). Species that form a yellow-orange to orange pigment when grown either in the dark or in light were termed scotochromogenic species (group II). The Runyon classification is now rarely used, because it does not take pathogenicity into account, and modern identification methods rely on a larger array of characteristics. Biochemical methods that yield absolute identifications are complex, time-consuming and best carried out in specialized laboratories (Kent and Kubica 1985). DNA- and RNA-based identification, gas-liquid and thin layer chromatography of cell wall mycolic acids, and other modern tools are more rapid and increasingly used (Kiehn 1993). Molecular biological tools have allowed the identification of previously unrecognized species, such as *Mycobacterium genavense* (Coyle et al. 1992). Modern techniques may eventually reduce the need for extensive biochemical identification schemes.

Table 22.1 NTM with pathogenic potential in immunocompetent versus immunocompromised hosts, and NTM that are most frequently non-pathogenic

NTM that cause infection in immunocompetent hosts	Non-pathogenic NTM in immunocompetent hosts	NTM that cause infection in AIDS patients	NTM that cause infection in immunocompromised hosts (not AIDS)
MAC	*M. gordonae*	MAC	MAC
M. kansasii	*M. terrae*	*M. kansasii*	*M. fortuitum* complex
M. marinum	*M. nonchromogenicum*	*M. genavense*	*M. kansasii*
M. fortuitum complex	*M. triviale*	*M. haemophilum*	*M. xenopi*
M. xenopi	*M. gastri*	*M. malmoense*	*M. haemophilum*
M. simiae	*M. flavescens*	*M. xenopi*	*M. marinum*
M. szulgai	*M. thermoresistibile*	*M. szulgai*	*M. scrofulaceum*
M. malmoense	*N. neoaurum*	*M. simiae*	(*M. neoaurum*)[a]
M. ulcerans		*M. celatum*	(*M. gastri*)[a]
M. smegmatis		*M. marinum*	(*M. thermoresistibile*)[a]
M. haemophilum		(*M. gordonae*)[a]	
M. scrofulaceum			
M. shimoidei			
M. asiaticum			

[a]Generally considered non-pathogens; however, more frequently are implicated as causing disease in immunocompromised hosts.

Since most NTM, and especially the RGM, are killed by sodium hydroxide treatment as used in the preparation of specimens for *M. tuberculosis* (TB) culture, milder methods, such as a modified SDS method, have been described (Salfinger and Kafader 1987). Most NTM grow well on L–J (egg-potato) or Middlebrook 7H10 or 7H11 agar media and Middlebrook 7H9 broth, or its variation 7H12 used in the BACTEC rapid growth system. The radiometric BACTEC-NAP system uses ^{14}C-labelled palmitic acid which, when metabolized by the mycobacteria releases $[^{14}C]O_2$ (Wallace et al. 1990), which can detect growth in as little as 5 days. NAP (*p*-nitro-α-acetylamino-β-propiophenone) selectively inhibits the growth of *M. tuberculosis*, but not of NTM (Laszlo and Siddiqi 1984). Rapid detection can be achieved with DNA probes that hybridize with species-specific ribosomal RNA sequences, and probes to identify *Mycobacterium avium* complex (MAC), *Mycobacterium kansasii*, *Mycobacterium gordonae*, and the *M. tuberculosis* complex, are commercially available.

1.1 NTM that are rarely pathogenic

Some NTM (Table 22.1) are regarded as non-pathogenic because they are not associated with disease in the immunocompetent hosts. Isolation of one of these species from pathological specimens is usually due to contamination. However, the incidence of these bacteria as pathogens in immunocompromised hosts is increasing (see section 4, p. 430) but some regard the evidence of an association as insufficient (Tsukamura 1983, Wayne and Sramek 1992).

M. gordonae, a slow-growing scotochromogen (Runyon group II), is remarkable in that it is commonly isolated from many environments, such as house dust, tap water and hospital water sources. Its pathogenicity is low and less than 40 infections due to it have been reported in the last 30 years, but it is commonly isolated in clinical laboratories (Debrunner

et al. 1992, Wayne and Sramek 1992). A commercially available specific DNA probe allows rapid identification of *M. gordonae* and the disregard of inconsequential isolates.

Less than 20 cases of infection have been attributed to the *M. terrae* complex, but in only 2 cases was the evidence convincing (Wayne and Sramek 1992). Though these organisms are rarely isolated from clinical specimens, they share characteristics with *Mycobacterium malmoense*, which is commonly pathogenic (see section 2.4, p. 425), and it is important to distinguish between these 2 organisms.

1.2 Pseudoinfections

Pseudoinfection is the term used to describe a mistaken diagnosis, because of clinical specimen contamination, that a patient is colonized by NTM or has a mycobacteriosis. Examples of such occurrences include: the contamination of antimicrobial supplements used in the BACTEC culture system (Tokars et al. 1990); the contamination, by *Mycobacterium xenopi*, *Mycobacterium chelonae*, *M. fortuitum* and *M. gordonae*, of hot water used to clean or rinse bronchoscopes after use (Steere, Corrales and von Graevenitz 1979, Nye et al. 1990, Gubler, Salfinger and von Graevenitz 1992, Bennett et al. 1994); and the contamination, by *M. fortuitum*, of ice used to transport bone marrow cultures (Hoy, Rolston and Hopfer 1987). In each case elimination of the contamination resulted in eradication of the pseudoinfections. Clusters of infections by these bacteria without supportive clinical evidence of infection are a clue that the cause may be contamination.

2 PULMONARY INFECTION IN THE IMMUNOCOMPETENT HOST

Surveys of mycobacterioses in the USA, Japan and Switzerland during the 1980s found a similar prevalence of approximately 1.8 per 100 000 (O'Brien, Geiter and Snider 1987, Tsukamura et al. 1988, Debrunner et al. 1992). Pulmonary mycobacterioses caused by MAC predominate and account for 48–70% of infections. In some laboratories NTM are more commonly isolated from respiratory secretions than *M. tuberculosis* and pulmonary mycobacterioses are probably underdiagnosed (Woods and Washington 1987, Cox, Brenner and Bryan 1994, Kennedy and Weber 1994). Human-to-human and animal-to-human transmission has not been documented, and inhalation of contaminated aerosols is the presumed mode of inoculation of the lung. Geographical clustering of infections often matches the environmental distribution of NTM and supports the hypothesis that infections arise from environmental exposure. Host susceptibility is a factor in the development of infections, because in some areas exposure is universal. It is not known whether, as in the case of *M. tuberculosis*, latent infection is part of the pathogenesis. Because of cross-reactivity between shared antigens, species-specific skin tests have not proved reliable to measure immune responses. Active infections in immunocompetent hosts cause granulomatous inflammation of the lung.

Discrimination between colonization and infection by NTM can be difficult. The American Thoracic Society (ATS) criteria for the diagnosis of pulmonary mycobacterioses are as follows:

1 Cavitary or non-cavitary infiltrates (e.g. nodular infiltrates or bronchiectasis) should be present on chest x-ray.
2 Two or more respiratory specimens (sputum or bronchial washings) should demonstrate AFB on smear examination and/or moderate to heavy growth (2+ to 4+) on culture.
3 Other reasonable causes such as fungus (e.g. histoplasmosis, coccidiomycosis) or *M. tuberculosis* must be excluded (Wallace et al. 1990).

The NTM most commonly associated with pulmonary infections are discussed below and their salient features are given in Table 22.2.

2.1 *Mycobacterium avium* complex (MAC) lung infection

The bacteriological and clinical aspects of MAC infections have been reviewed by Inderlied, Kemper and Bermudez (1993) (see also Volume 2, Chapter 26).

EPIDEMIOLOGY OF MAC INFECTIONS

The majority of NTM respiratory isolates are MAC but only about half these are pathogenic, and 90% of the pathogenic strains cause lung disease when immunocompromised hosts are excluded (O'Brien, Geiter and Snider 1987). The ratio of pulmonary to extrapulmonary MAC infections is 2.4, which is similar to that for *M. tuberculosis* (Ellis 1988). In the USA there is a perception that the incidence of pulmonary MAC infections in immunocompetent hosts is rising; but their true prevalence is unknown because mycobacterioses are not reportable (Iseman 1989, Prince et al. 1989). A possible reason for the increase may be that in the past widespread BCG vaccination was cross-protective (Romanus 1983). Animal experiments suggest that BCG vaccination protects against MAC infection (Orme and Collins 1985). Pulmonary MAC infections are endemic in temperate northern regions (e.g. USA, Canada, UK, Europe and Japan), but they also are found in Australia (Dawson 1990) and South Africa (Nel 1981).

MAC have been isolated from bedding material, house dust, soil, plants, swimming pools, hospital water and natural bodies of water (Wolinsky and Rynearson 1968, Reznikov, Leggo and Dawson 1974, Fry, Meissner and Falkinham 1986, Ichiyama, Shimokata and Tsukamura 1988, du Moulin et al. 1988). A water salinity ≤2 g per 100 ml (Gruft, Katz and Blanchard 1975, Falkinham, Parker and Gruft 1980), pH 4.6–6.8 and lower altitudes (Brooks et al. 1984) correlate with the highest recovery of MAC.

The highest reactivity with PPD-B, the specific skin test for MAC, at roughly 70%, is found in the southeast USA, particularly along the gulf coast (Edwards et al. 1969) and the highest rates of active lung infections are in the southeast USA, Atlantic and Pacific coastal regions (O'Brien, Geiter and Snider 1987). Older data suggested that MAC were more often isolated from patients in rural locations (Edwards et al. 1969, Good and Snider 1982).

CHARACTERISTICS OF MAC INFECTION

The first report of MAC as a human pathogen was by Feldman et al. (1943), but how humans become infected remains unknown. Infection is assumed to arise from the environmental reservoir of MAC organisms. MAC is found above contaminated pools of water in small aerosol droplets 0.7–3.3 μm diameter, a size consistent with deposition in human alveoli (Wendt et al. 1980, Parker et al. 1983, Meissner and Falkinham 1986). MAC tend to colonize the respiratory secretions of humans living in close proximity to bodies of water. Poultry, swine and cattle may also be infected by MAC, which gets into the soil by faecal shedding from birds, but not cattle or swine (Inderlied, Kemper and Bermudez 1993). Serovars similar to those from birds have been isolated from humans living in their close proximity, but animal-to-human transmission of infection has not been documented (Meisner and Anz 1977). The predominant serovars in human and animal infections are different (Codias and Reinhardt 1979, Nel 1981). In spite of widespread environmental exposure to MAC in certain geographical regions, the incidence of clinical disease in immunocompetent hosts is extremely low.

The most widely recognized form of lung infection occurs in middle-aged or older white male smokers

Table 22.2 NTM most frequently associated with pulmonary infection, listed in descending order encountered

Aetiological organism	Special characteristics	Most frequent host
M. avium complex	True infection: 47% of isolates;[a] P/E ratio 2.4[b]	Male with COPD; or female, no predisposing lung disease
M. kansasii	Beaded appearance on smear. True infection: 75% of isolates;[a] P/E ratio 18[b]	Elderly male smoker with COPD
M. xenopi	True infection: 25% of isolates;[a] common in UK, Canada, Europe; P/E ratio 25[b]	Elderly male smoker with COPD
M. malmoense	More common in Sweden, UK, Europe; P/E ratio 6.0[b]	Elderly with pre-existing TB, COPD, or lung cancer (M:F, 1.4:1)
M. abscessus	Rapid grower. True infection: 38% of isolates[a]	Elderly non-smoking female; no predisposing lung disease
Less common organisms		
M. fortuitum (rarely *M. peregrinum, M. chelonae*)	Rapid grower. True infection: 18% of isolates[a]	Elderly male smoker with COPD; chronic vomiting
M. bovis[c]	Nearly 100% DNA homology with *M. tuberculosis*	Individuals in areas where infections in beef and dairy cattle not controlled
M. szulgai	True infection: 57% of isolates[a]	Elderly male
M. simiae	True infection: 21% of all isolates[a]	Elderly male. Geographical distribution: Texas, Israel
Others: *M. asiaticum, M. shimoidei*	See text	See text

[a]Data from O'Brien, Geiter and Snider (1987).
[b]P/E ratio, ratio of pulmonary to extrapulmonary infections (Ellis 1988).
[c]Not NTM species, see section 2.6, p. 426.

and lung tissue shows either caseating or non-caseating granulomas. Pre-existing lung disease, including chronic obstructive pulmonary disease (COPD), previous TB, bronchiectasis (including cystic fibrosis), silicosis, chronic aspiration pneumonia and bronchogenic carcinoma, is present in approximately 70% of patients (Bailey et al. 1974, Ahn, Nash and Hurst 1976, Engbaek, Vergmann and Bentzon 1981, Rosenzweig and Schleuter 1981, Hornick et al. 1988, Kilby et al. 1992). These lung diseases have in common substantial impairment of clearance mechanisms, which may allow colonizing bacteria to establish infection. Previous gastrectomy, immunosuppressive therapy, diabetes mellitus and alcoholism are non-pulmonary predisposing factors (Rosenzweig 1979, Wolinsky 1979).

The symptoms of pulmonary MAC infection are generally superimposed on those of the pre-existing chronic lung condition and include chronic productive cough, dyspnoea, malaise, weakness, haemoptysis, weight loss, fever and sweats. Chest x-rays (Fig. 22.1a) shows a cavitary infiltrate in the upper lobe(s) in approximately 50–67% of patients (Tsai, Yue and Duthoy 1968, Christensen et al. 1981). The progression of infection may be indolent or rapid depending on the extent of disease at presentation and the severity of coexisting illness (Ahn, Nash and Hurst 1976, Rosenzweig 1979).

A group of patients with a clinical presentation different from that described above has been described. They were predominantly non-smoking females without identifiable predisposing lung disease (Albelda et al. 1985, Prince et al. 1989). Many were elderly and, less commonly, younger women with pectus excavatum, scoliosis, or mitral valve prolapse (Iseman 1989, Reich and Johnson 1991, Kennedy and Weber 1994). Patients described a chronic productive cough, dyspnoea, malaise and weakness. The disease was referred to as 'Lady Windermere's' syndrome, implying that the pathogenesis was linked to habitual cough suppression (Reich and Johnson 1992), but the true mechanism is unknown. Chest x-ray reveals non-cavitary infiltrates that frequently involves the right middle lobe and lingula (Fig. 22.1b). High resolution computed tomography of the chest reveals characteristic small (<5 mm) nodules with associated bronchiectasis (Swensen, Hartman and Williams 1994). The disease process is indolent and slowly progressive, and patients may have symptoms for up to 10 years. This form of MAC infection may therefore be underdiagnosed. In a substantial proportion of patients the disease is progressive with a mortality as high as 20% (Prince et al. 1989).

A benign form of infection also exists. Of 20 resected benign asymptomatic solitary pulmonary nodules examined by Gribetz et al. (1981), 12 yielded MAC.

(a)

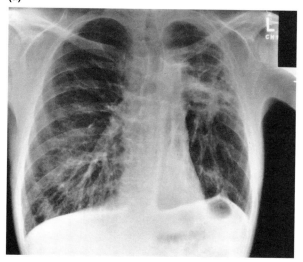

(b)

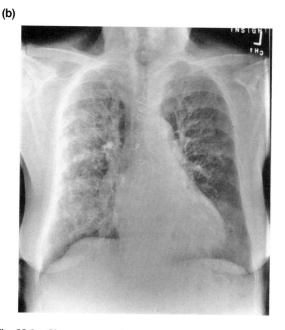

Fig. 22.1 Chest x-rays of patients with MAC pulmonary infection. (a) Male smoker, age 50 years, with COPD. Severe cavitary infiltrate and loss of volume of the left upper lobe are demonstrated. (b) Female non-smoker, age 74 years, without history of lung disease, who has a persistent chronic cough. A reticular nodular infiltrate is seen in both the right middle and upper lobes.

TREATMENT OF MAC PULMONARY INFECTION

Not all persons with sputum cultures positive for MAC require immediate treatment. In patients with severe lung problems or those with a single smear-negative, culture-positive sputum specimen, treatment should be delayed to determine whether the infection is invasive. The guidelines of the ATS (see section 2, p. 421) can be used to determine whether the infection is active (Wallace et al. 1990). The need for treatment should be critically assessed in patients with medication intolerance or allergy, the elderly with indolent

disease, and those in whom previous treatment has failed.

The complex MAC cell wall is a barrier to many antimicrobial agents (Rastogi et al. 1981, Rastogi, Goh and David 1990). MAC isolates are generally resistant in vitro to most antituberculous drugs and in vitro susceptibility correlates poorly with clinical response (Rynearson, Schronts and Wolinsky 1971, Heifets 1988). Long-term treatment failures have been commonplace and only 45–65% of patients responded long term to early multidrug treatment regimens (Dutt and Stead 1979, Davidson et al. 1981, Etzkorn et al. 1986, Hornick et al. 1988), but surgery combined with medical therapy has been effective in highly selected cases (Corpe 1981). This approach has been advocated for patients with adequate cardiopulmonary reserve, in whom the infection is localized to a single lobe (Iseman et al. 1985).

Advances in therapy suggest that better outcomes can be expected with current medical regimens. The extended spectrum macrolide (ESM) drugs (e.g. clarithromycin, azithromycin) are one such promising therapeutic advance (Wallace et al. 1994a, Dautzenberg et al. 1995). These drugs are the first with strong in vitro activity against MAC (Heifets, Lindholm-Levy and Comstock 1992). These macrolides are concentrated in lung tissue and macrophages, have a long half-life, a post-antibiotic effect, and they are well tolerated orally. Availability of ESM antibiotics has led to a re-evaluation of in vitro susceptibility testing to predict the likely clinical response. Resistance to ESM in vitro may develop during monotherapy, and thus predict treatment failure (Albrecht et al. 1994, Heifets, Mor and Vanderkolk 1994, Wallace et al. 1994a).

Another advance is rifabutin, a derivative of rifamycin S, which is more active in vitro against MAC than rifampicin (Saito, Sato and Tomioka 1988). Preliminary data suggest that clinical responses are improved only modestly when rifabutin is used in place of rifampicin (O'Brien, Geiter and Lyle 1990). Side effects unique to rifabutin are also a drawback to its widespread clinical use. Drug combinations, such as ethambutol and rifampicin, are synergistic in vitro and effective in vivo, although MAC are resistant to these agents individually in vitro (Heifets 1982, Zimmer, DeYoung and Roberts 1982).

A regimen of an ESM, ethambutol, rifampicin or rifabutin is recommended in less severe infections. In severe disease the addition of streptomycin for the first 2–4 months of therapy is recommended. Treatment should be continued for 18 months to 2 years or at least 12 months after the last positive sputum culture.

2.2 *Mycobacterium kansasii* lung infection

M. kansasii, first identified as a pulmonary pathogen by Buhler and Pollack (1953), is the second most common cause of pulmonary mycobacteriosis in most parts of the world, including Sweden, Japan, USA, Australia and Switzerland (Sjogren 1981, O'Brien, Geiter and Snider 1987, Tsukamura et al. 1988, Pang

1991, Debrunner et al. 1992). In the USA, Japan and Switzerland, *M. kansasii* accounts for some 25% of pulmonary NTM isolates (O'Brien, Geiter, Snider 1987, Tsukamura et al. 1988, Debrunner et al. 1992).

M. kansasii forms visible niacin-negative, photochromogenic colonies on L–J slants at 2–3 weeks. After 2 weeks in ambient light the colonies turn bright yellow or orange. The 'yellow bacillus', as it was originally called, must be distinguished from other photochromogenic species, such as *Mycobacterium simiae* and *Mycobacterium szulgai*, which also may cause pulmonary mycobacterioses. In sputum smears, *M. kansasii* may appear as distinctive large, cross-barred acid-fast bacilli (Wolinsky 1979). The environmental reservoir of *M. kansasii* is unknown; it has occasionally been isolated from water sources but not from soil (Joynson 1979, Wolinsky 1979).

In contrast to most other pulmonary mycobacterioses, isolation of *M. kansasii* from sputum culture is less likely to represent colonization or contamination (Table 22.2). Colonization is rare, and typically the growth in culture is scanty. Colonization should be suspected in individuals without significant underlying lung disease, or with new or worsening clinical signs (Ahn et al. 1982, Shraufnagel, Leech and Pollak 1986). It is hypothesized that colonization or infection results from inhalation of contaminated aerosols. Patients with active infection are typically male smokers (M:F ratio is 3:1), aged 50 years or older (Ahn et al. 1979, Pang 1991). They usually have coexisting COPD and often live in urban areas (Ahn, Nash and Hurst 1976, O'Brien, Geiter and Snider 1987). *M. kansasii* infections may also coexist with lung cancer, previous TB, or pneumoconiosis (Bailey et al. 1974, O'Brien, Geiter and Snider 1987, Pang 1991). The US geographical distribution of infections forms an inverted 'T' from California to Florida and up from Texas to Illinois (Good and Snider 1982).

The symptoms and clinical characteristics of infection mimic tuberculosis, including cough, fever, night sweats and weight loss. These are superimposed on the persistent symptoms of the coexisting lung disease. In 84–95% of cases the chest x-ray shows apical, cavitary infiltrates (Christensen et al. 1978, O'Brien, Geiter and Snider 1987). *M. kansasii* may also mimic *M. tuberculosis* in that both rarely present as endobronchial lesions identified by bronchoscopy. However, unlike *M. tuberculosis*, the few *M. kansasii* endobronchial lesions that have been reported were in HIV patients and responded well to treatment (Connolly, Baughman and Dohn 1993).

M. kansasii is susceptible to most antituberculous agents except pyrazinamide (PZA) and some strains show intermediate resistance to isoniazid (INH) (Wallace et al. 1990). A recommended regimen is isoniazid, rifampicin and ethambutol daily for 18 months (Wallace et al. 1990). As with most other pulmonary mycobacterioses, large, controlled clinical treatment trials have not been reported. Medication regimens that include rifampicin have relapse rates less than 8% (Ahn et al. 1981) and treatment can be shortened to 12 months if streptomycin is added for the first 3 months (Ahn et al. 1983). Resistance to rifampicin in vitro predicts a poor outcome. Rifampicin resistance has arisen as a result of inadequate initial therapy and has been a greater problem in HIV patients (Wallace et al. 1994b). Newer agents such as the ESMs and fluoroquinolones are active against *M. kansasii* in vitro (Biehle and Cavalieri 1992, Witzig and Franzblau 1993) and may be useful to treat patients infected with rifampicin-resistant bacteria.

2.3   *Mycobacterium xenopi* **lung infection**

The species name derives from the initial isolation from a dermal granuloma of the toad, *Xenopus laevis* (Schwabacher 1959). *M. xenopi* was first identified as a human pulmonary pathogen and a respiratory colonizer by Marks and Schwabacher (1965). Pulmonary *M. xenopi* infections occur more frequently in the UK, Western Europe and Canada (Allen 1982, Smith and Citron 1983, Simor, Salit and Vellend 1984) than in the USA, where *M. xenopi* accounts for less than 0.25% of mycobacteria isolated and reports of pulmonary infections have been more sporadic (Costrini et al. 1981, O'Brien, Geiter and Snider 1987, Hornick et al. 1988). At the Brompton Hospital in London, UK, *M. xenopi* was the most frequent NTM isolate from respiratory secretions (Smith and Citron 1983), and in parts of Canada isolates were second only to MAC (Simor, Salit and Vellend 1984, Thomas, Liu and Weiser 1988). In areas where *M. xenopi* is more endemic, it is most often a colonizer (60–70% of cases), so that the problem of distinguishing pathogens from colonizers of the respiratory tract is similar to that for MAC isolates.

M. xenopi is slow growing, thermophilic and scotochromogenic. It is at least 25 times more frequently isolated from respiratory secretions than from extrapulmonary sites (Ellis 1988). Routine incubation procedures, biochemical and morphological characteristics may result in confusion between *M. xenopi* and MAC. Reliable distinguishing features include formation of spiculated colonies ('X-colonies') early in growth (4–12 days), a positive 3 day arylsulphatase test, and optimal growth at 42–45°C with failure to grow in broth or solid media at 25°C (Marx et al. 1995). Gas and thin layer chromatography analyses of mycolic acids demonstrate 2-docosanol, which is unique to *M. xenopi* (Luquin et al. 1991).

The usual habitat of *M. xenopi* is water. Case clusters have been observed along coastal regions of Europe (e.g. UK, France) and in Ontario, Canada. Nosocomial pseudoinfection (see section 1.2, p. 420) and true infection are associated with contamination of potable water and accumulated organic material at hot water taps in hospitals has also been reported (Costrini et al. 1981, Sniadack et al. 1993).

The ATS guidelines outlined above are useful for identifying patients with invasive infection (Wallace et al. 1990). *M. xenopi* typically causes infection in middle-aged and older males with coexisting pulmonary disease such as COPD or old pulmonary scarring from previous pulmonary TB. The illness is subacute and characterized by cough, sputum production, weight loss and malaise. Chest x-rays show cavitary lesions of the upper lobes in 73–96% of patients and granulomas are seen on lung biopsy (Costrini et al. 1981, Allen 1982, Smith and Citron 1983, Simor, Salit and Vellend 1984). The chest x-ray and histology of pulmonary lesions cannot be distinguished from TB.

Standard antituberculous therapy for treatment of *M. xenopi* infection has been variably successful (Costrini et al. 1981, Allen 1982, Banks et al. 1984). Initial therapy recommended by the ATS is isoniazid, rifampicin, ethambutol and possibly streptomycin (Wallace et al. 1990). In vitro susceptibility suggests that multidrug regimens that include ESM may prove more effective. If initial therapy fails and disease is localized to a single lobe, surgical resection may be considered (Banks et al. 1984, Parrot and Grosset 1988).

2.4 *Mycobacterium malmoense* lung infection

Lung infection due to *M. malmoense* was first described by Schroder and Juhlin (1977) in Malmo, Sweden, where it is the second most common NTM isolate from the respiratory tract, after MAC (Henriques et al. 1994). It is 6 times more likely to cause pulmonary than extrapulmonary infection (Ellis 1988) and is more frequently isolated as a NTM pathogen in Sweden, the UK and northern Europe than the USA (Alberts et al. 1987, Hoffner 1994). For reasons that remain unclear, reports of infection with this bacterium during the last decade have increased substantially in northern Europe and the UK (Henriques et al. 1994, Hoffner 1994).

The clinical features of pulmonary *M. malmoense* and MAC infection are similar. Some 70% of the patients have pre-existing pulmonary disease (e.g. TB, COPD, lung cancer) (Henriques et al. 1994). Radiographic features do not distinguish pulmonary *M. malmoense* infections from those due to other NTM or *M. tuberculosis* (Evans et al. 1993).

The correlation between in vitro susceptibility and clinical response to antituberculous agents is poor (Banks, Jenkins and Smith 1985). Synergy has been demonstrated in vitro for combinations of ethambutol with quinolones, rifampicin and amikacin (Hoffner 1994), but there have been no clinical treatment trials. The outcome of a regimen of isoniazid, rifampicin and ethambutol, continued for 18 months, was good; poor results were attributed to poor patient compliance (Banks, Jenkins and Smith 1985).

2.5 Rapidly growing mycobacteria (RGM) and lung infection

The rare human mycobacterioses due to RGM are almost always caused by members of the *M. fortuitum* complex, which includes subspecies *M. fortuitum*, *M. peregrinum*, *M. chelonae* and *M. abscessus* (Wallace et al. 1991). Specifically, lung infections are most often caused by *Mycobacterium abscessus*. The members of the *M. fortuitum* complex are easily isolated from environmental sites such as water, soil and dust.

An extensive analysis of 154 patients with *M. fortuitum* complex pulmonary infections has been reported (Griffith, Girard and Wallace 1993). *M. abscessus* accounted for approximately 80%, *M. fortuitum* for 12%, and 5% were caused by RGM that defied classification. Most *M. fortuitum* complex lung infections have been reported in the USA clustered along the gulf and southern Atlantic coasts (Wallace et al. 1983). Older studies identified *M. fortuitum* as the predominant species recovered from patients with pulmonary mycobacterioses caused by RGM. These results are, however, questionable because before 1985 it was difficult to distinguish *M. fortuitum* from *M. chelonae* (Griffith, Girard and Wallace 1993). *M. fortuitum* is more frequently isolated from extrapulmonary infections (e.g. skin and soft tissue).

Fewer than half the respiratory isolates of *M. fortuitum* complex represent infection (O'Brien, Geiter and Snider 1987). Typically, patients with invasive infection are elderly, female non-smokers without predisposing lung disease, in contrast to most other causes of pulmonary mycobacterioses. Previous mycobacterial infection (e.g. MAC, *M. tuberculosis*), gastrointestinal disorder associated with recurrent vomiting, cystic fibrosis and other forms of bronchiectasis are encountered. *M. fortuitum* seems to be less pathogenic than *M. abscessus* and is relatively more common in patients with oesophageal disease and other gastrointestinal diseases associated with recurrent vomiting. In this setting, *M. fortuitum* pulmonary infections can be rapidly progressive (Griffith, Girard and Wallace 1993).

The symptoms of pulmonary infection due to *M. fortuitum* complex include chronic productive cough but usually few systemic symptoms. Multilobar infiltrates, localized to the upper lung fields in about 90% of patients, are seen in chest x-rays; cavitation occurs in only 15% of patients. High resolution CT scans show nodular infiltrates associated with bronchiectasis, similar to MAC pulmonary infections in elderly women. Since the clinical setting and x-ray appearances are less typical than those of other pulmonary mycobacterioses, AFB smears and culture are less frequently requested. Furthermore, some isolates may be killed by sodium hydroxide decontamination during sample preparation, and some isolates do not stain well with acid-fast techniques. The disease usually progresses slowly and there is often a long delay between onset of symptoms and diagnosis. More rapid progress may be seen in association with gastrointestinal disease. Mortality from progressive disease approaches 20% (Griffith, Girard and Wallace 1993).

M. fortuitum is susceptible to well tolerated oral agents such as sulphonamides, tetracycline and fluoroquinolones, whereas *M. abscessus* is usually susceptible to agents that must be administered parenterally, such as cefoxitin, amikacin and imipenem (Swenson et al. 1985). Treatment with parenteral agents alone is, however, insufficient in most cases to eliminate disease completely. In combination with antibiotic therapy, surgical resection of the infected area when limited to a single lobe, is usually part of successful treatment (Griffith, Girard and Wallace 1993). ESM drugs may be the first broadly useful oral medications for treating *M. abscessus* (Brown et al. 1992).

2.6   Less common pulmonary mycobacterioses

Though *M. bovis* is more commonly associated with extrapulmonary disease (e.g. genitourinary, bone, joints and CNS), it has recently been cited as an occasional cause of pulmonary infection in Mexican and other Hispanic adult immigrants to the USA. *M. bovis* is discussed throughout this chapter devoted to NTM species in order to be comprehensive. However, *M. bovis* is grouped by convention within the *M. tuberculosis* complex. The microbiology, epidemiology and clinical aspects of infection with this organism have been reviewed by Dankner and colleagues (1993).

Pulmonary infection by *M. bovis* in adults is clinically indistinguishable from that due to *M. tuberculosis*. This makes it important in the laboratory to distinguish between *M. tuberculosis* and *M. bovis*, since the latter is normally resistant to pyrazinamide, which is commonly used for the treatment of tuberculosis. 'Bovine TB' results from cow-to-human and human-to-human aerosol transmission wherever efforts to eliminate infection in domestic beef and dairy cattle have failed. This problem is illustrated by the effect of Hispanic immigration on the spectrum of mycobacterial isolates in the San Diego area of the USA, where up to 3% of these are *M. bovis*.

M. szulgai is uncommonly isolated from pulmonary secretions, but when isolated it is generally pathogenic; one-half to two-thirds of infections are pulmonary (Wolinsky, Gomez and Zimpfer 1972, Maloney et al. 1987). Clinically these resemble those due to *M. tuberculosis* and they generally occur in elderly males. Based on very limited information, *M. szulgai* is usually susceptible to rifampicin, ethambutol, streptomycin and elevated concentrations of isoniazid (Maloney et al. 1987).

An extremely uncommon NTM species is *M. simiae*; it is usually a respiratory colonizer and causes infection in only approximately 20% of cases (Bell et al. 1983, O'Brien, Geiter and Snider 1987). The environmental source of infection and means of transmission have not been clarified. A report from San Antonio, Texas indicates increased isolation from respiratory secretions in that region (Valero et al. 1995). A potential factor is the association of colonization or infection of HIV patients with CD4 counts less than 100. The innate resistance of *M. simiae* to most antituberculous drugs represents a challenge for the treatment of active infection. Limited information suggests that multidrug regimens that include an ESM and a fluoroquinolone may be promising (Valero, Moreno and Graybill 1994).

Fewer than 10 cases of *M. shimoidei* infection have been reported (Tsukamura, Shimoide and Schaefer 1975, Rusch-Gerdes, Wandelt-Freerksen and Schroder 1985). The disease resembles pulmonary tuberculosis and occurs in elderly males, in one case with pre-existing silicosis. Information is insufficient to comment on treatment.

M. asiaticum is also an extremely uncommon respiratory isolate, originally identified as a variant of *M. simiae* (Weiszfeiler, Karasseva and Karczag 1971). Its natural habitat is believed to be the subtropics. The clinical features of active infection and treatment are based on 5 Australian patients (Blacklock et al. 1983). In 2 of these, both elderly male smokers, *M. asiaticum* was definitely only causing progressive pulmonary disease. Though *M. asiaticum* is thought to be only partially susceptible to the conventional drugs, treatment with these led to improvement.

3   EXTRAPULMONARY MYCOBACTERIOSES IN THE IMMUNOCOMPETENT HOST

In the immunocompetent host, NTM can cause infections in cutaneous, deep soft tissues, lymphatics, and other sites (e.g. skeletal, peritoneal catheter-related, ocular). These mycobacterioses are rare, indolent and frequently misidentified. Since an extended period often elapses before a diagnosis is made and more serious and deep infections may result, early diagnosis can prevent significant morbidity.

3.1   Cutaneous and deep soft tissue infections

Mycobacterium ulcerans and *M. marinum* are closely related and the most prevalent NTM that cause cutaneous and deeper tissue infections (Table 22.3). Each is limited to specific types of exposure, geographical location, or both. Other NTM less often cause cutaneous and soft tissue infections and are discussed briefly at the end of this section.

M. marinum is most commonly associated with a superficial cutaneous infection sometimes referred to as 'swimming pool' or 'fish tank' granuloma. In humans it causes deep and superficial infections in the extremities (Fig. 22.2). Almost all infections occur after injuries during activity in contaminated water (e.g. fishing, handling fish, working in an aquarium) (Huminer et al. 1986, Johnston and Izumi 1987), and in many cases the upper extremity is involved. After initial injury the incubation period is generally 2–3 weeks and the earliest lesion is a painless or mildly tender papule that slowly enlarges and eventually begins to drain pus (Collins et al. 1985, Johnston and Izumi 1987, Gluckman 1995). In approximately 20% of cases local or lymphatic spread forms subcutaneous nodules along the regional draining lymphatics in a manner similar to sporotrichosis (Wolinsky, Gomez and Zimpfer 1972, Gluckman 1995). Further extension to regional lymph nodes and systemic infection

Table 22.3 Extrapulmonary infections caused by NTM, listed in descending order encountered

Site of disease	Aetiological organism	Organism characteristics
Cutaneous infection by traumatic inoculation	*M. marinum*	Photochromogen; 28–30°C for optimal growth
	M. ulcerans	Scotochromogen; 28–30°C for optimal growth
	Less common organisms	
	M. fortuitum, M. chelonae, M. abscessus, M. kansasii	See Table 22.2
	M. smegmatis	Rapid grower, 43–45°C for optimal growth
Lymphadenitis (children ages 1–5 years)	*M. avium* complex	See Table 22.2
	M. scrofulaceum	Scotochromogen
	Less common organisms	
	M. malmoense, M. haemophilum, M. bovis,[a] *M. kansasii*	See Tables 22.2 and 22.4
Less common sites		
Musculoskeletal (e.g. tenosynovitis, osteomyelitis)	*M. marinum, M. fortuitum* complex, MAC	See Table 22.2
Catheter-related infection (e.g. peritoneal dialysis)	*M. fortuitum* complex, *M. xenopi, M. kansasii*	See Table 22.2
Other uncommon sites: eye, mastoiditis	See text	See text

[a] Not NTM species, see section 2.6, p. 426.

does not usually occur because of the low temperature required for optimal growth. Progress to deeper involvement is more likely when antigen-specific T cell suppression occurs (Dattwyler, Thomas and Hurst 1987). Reports vary as to whether granulomas are seen in biopsies and mycobacteria are visible by acid-fast stain in only a third of cases. Culture of biopsy specimens at 32°C increases the probability of diagnosis to 70–80% (Collins et al. 1985, Johnston and Izumi 1987, Gluckman 1995).

Most *M. marinum* isolates are susceptible to ethambutol plus rifampicin, and this combination is effective if continued for 6 months or at least 6 weeks after lesions have healed. Sulphamethoxazole–trimethoprim, tetracycline or minocycline can be used for superficial lesions. Surgical debridement is necessary for patients with draining sinus tracts. In contrast to other mycobacterioses, treatment of superficial lesions in AIDS patients is effective and dissemination does not occur, but recurrence after discontinuing treatment is more likely than in the immunocompetent patient (Lambertus and Mathisen 1988). The cure rate for *M. marinum* infections is approximately 80% (Edelstein 1994, Gluckman 1995).

M. ulcerans was first described by MacCallum et al. (1948) in Bairnsdale in Australia and named for the characteristic indolent necrotizing skin ulcer ('Bairnsdale ulcer') it causes. Cutaneous infections also occur in other tropical climates, including Central and South America, South East Asia and West Africa, where the characteristic lesion is called the 'Buruli ulcer', and certain areas have a high prevalence (Muelder and Nourou 1990, Goutzamanis and Gilbert

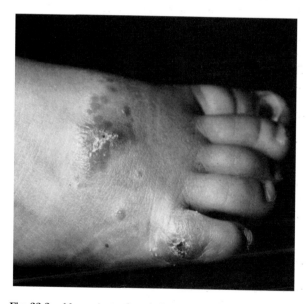

Fig. 22.2 *M. marinum* foot infection in a young boy who injured his fifth toe while swimming and developed a sporotrichoid spread of infection to the top of the foot. (Courtesy of M Stone MD, University of Iowa College of Medicine).

1995). Up to 16.3% of the local population in a rural area of Ivory Coast are infected (Marston et al. 1995).

M. ulcerans is believed to be an environmental saprophyte in tropical regions and has been isolated from swampy water in Uganda, but the natural reservoir has not been clearly identified (Muelder and Nourou 1990, Hayman 1993). The mode of transmission to humans is also uncertain, but traumatic inoculation into the skin is most likely. Most lesions appear on the extremities and the risk of infection can be reduced by wearing protective clothing (Marston et al. 1995). At first a hard, painless, and usually pruritic subcutaneous lump, fixed to the skin, forms. Skin biopsy shows acid-fast bacteria infiltrating the subcutaneous connective tissue (Hayman 1993). The overlying dermal layer becomes necrotic and sloughs to form the characteristic deep ulcer (Fig. 22.3). It has been suggested that an incompletely characterized toxin may explain the necrotizing character of *M. ulcerans* infections. Extracts of culture supernatants are cytotoxic to tissue cultures and cause necrosis when injected subcutaneously into guinea pigs (Hockmeyer et al. 1978).

M. ulcerans infections may remit spontaneously but often leaving significant functional impairment. The response to antituberculous drugs is poor in spite of evidence of susceptibility in vitro (Muelder and Nourou 1990) and treatment of these infections is difficult. Though treatment with sulphamethoxazole–trimethoprim and rifampicin is used, wide surgical excision remains the mainstay of treatment. In some cases raising the temperature of the affected extremity to 40°C is a useful adjunct to therapy (Glynn 1972).

M. fortuitum, M. abscessus and *M. chelonae* of the *M.*

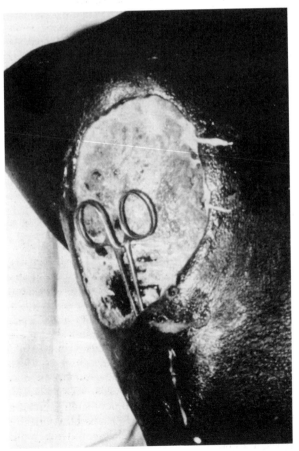

Fig. 22.3   Buruli ulcer on the shoulder caused by *M. ulcerans*. The Spencer Wells forceps are inserted to show the extent of undermining. (Courtesy of the Royal College of General Practitioners).

fortuitum complex most frequently cause skin and soft tissue infections (Wallace et al. 1983). Other species of the *M. fortuitum* complex, such as *M. peregrinum* and 2 biovariants, an unnamed *M. fortuitum* biovar and the *M. chelonae*-like organisms, also very rarely cause skin and soft tissue infections (Wallace et al. 1991, Wallace, Brown and Onyi 1992). Findings include painful, localized cellulitis and abscess formation at a skin site 4–8 weeks after injury, often by a metal object (e.g. nail, blade). Local lymphatic spread in a sporotrichoid fashion has uncommonly been reported (Higgins and Lawrence 1988, Murdoch and Leigh 1989), and systemic symptoms such as fever do not occur. Skin infections associated with a medical procedure or device have also been reported (Wallace et al. 1989).

M. fortuitum is frequently susceptible to tetracyclines, fluoroquinolones, sulphamethoxazole–trimethoprim, amikacin, imipenem and cefoxitin, and susceptibility in vitro correlates well with the results of treatment. Most strains of *M. chelonae* and *M. abscessus*, however, are resistant to doxycycline, fluoroquinolones and sulphamethoxazole–trimethoprim. Limited information shows that cure can be achieved when clarithromycin is used alone for about 6 months (Wallace et al. 1993). In many cases surgical debridement is a necessary adjunct to antibiotic therapy. The proper disinfection of medical devices minimizes the probability of transmitting these mycobacteria in the hospital setting (Brown 1985).

Other RGM not in the *M. fortuitum* complex, such as *Mycobacterium smegmatis, M. flavescens, M. thermoresistibile* and *M. neoaurum*, rarely cause skin and soft tissue infections. Of these, *M. smegmatis*, which is often isolated from the soil (Tsukamura 1976), is the most common. In spite of its name, *M. smegmatis* is not a colonizer or a cause of infection in the lower urinary tract (Wallace et al. 1988). It causes soft tissue infection after skin trauma related to medical procedures in a pattern similar to that seen for organisms of the *M. fortuitum* complex. Human *M. smegmatis* infections are extremely uncommon and treatment experience is limited but in vitro antimicrobial susceptibilities to standard antimicrobial drugs may be a useful guide to therapy (Wallace et al. 1988).

Skin and soft tissue infections due to *M. kansasii* and MAC have rarely been reported in immunocompetent individuals (Love 1987, Breathnach et al. 1995). Such patients have cutaneous abscesses with ulceration and subcutaneous nodules. In most cases skin trauma with exposure to contaminated water was thought to be the mode of inoculation. Subcutaneous nodules and sporotrichoid spread has been described for cutaneous *M. kansasii* infection (Breathnach et al. 1995).

3.2   Lymphadenitis

Painless cervical lymphadenitis of healthy children aged 1–5 years is commonly due to NTM, particularly MAC and *M. scrofulaceum*, whereas in adults it is more commonly due to the *M. tuberculosis* complex (Lai et al. 1984). Mycobacterioses account for some 20% of the infectious causes of cervical lymphadenitis in children (Schaad et al. 1979, Joshi et al. 1989). The other causes include Epstein–Barr virus (EBV), cytomegalovirus (CMV), cat-scratch disease, nocardiosis and tularaemia.

M. tuberculosis complex (e.g. *M. tuberculosis* and *M. bovis*) also causes cervical lymphadenitis in children but the *M. tuberculosis* complex is more frequently responsible where TB is prevalent. Clinical features do not distinguish NTM infections from those due to *M. tuberculosis* complex (Colville 1993). Children become infected with *M. bovis* by ingesting contaminated milk. This problem has been minimized in the USA, Canada and Western Europe by pasteurization of milk and the slaughter of infected cows. In parts of Mexico and Central America, for example, where *M. bovis* remains endemic in beef cattle and dairy herds, transmission to children often occurs (reviewed in Dankner et al. 1993).

Cervical lymphadenitis due to MAC accounts for 63–80% of cases and *M. scrofulaceum* is the next most common (Schaad et al. 1979, Taha, Davidson and Bailey 1985, Joshi et al. 1989). In Swedish children, *M. malmoense* is responsible for a significant proportion of cervical lymphadenitis (Henriques et al. 1994). *M. kansasii* and *M. haemophilum* also cause cervical lymphadenitis, but very infrequently (Wolinsky 1979, Armstrong et al. 1992). *M. genavense*, which is associated with adenopathy in AIDS patients (see section on '*M. genavense* infection', p. 433), has been identified as the cause of abdominal lymphadenopathy and pain in an HIV-negative child (Pechere et al. 1995). An unidentified mycobacterium closely related to *M. genavense* has also been reported to cause cervical lymphadenitis (Bosquee et al. 1995).

Cervical adenitis due to NTM typically causes unilateral painless enlargement of one or more submandibular or preauricular lymph nodes (Fig. 22.4). The overlying skin is usually inflamed and suppurative breakdown occurs in 6% of children (Joshi et al. 1989). Systemic signs of infection or spread of disease to other organs does not occur. Although they are not commonly isolated from the oral flora, it is thought that the NTM organisms enter the lymphatics that drain the oral mucosa as a result of gingival damage when deciduous teeth are lost and permanent teeth erupt, or during episodes of pharyngitis. Granulomatous inflammation is seen on lymph node biopsy; AFB are not always seen but in about 50%, culture of the biopsy specimen or of a needle aspirate yields the NTM species (Alessi and Dudley 1988).

Surgical resection is the most reliable treatment regardless of the NTM isolated (Schaad et al. 1979, Taha, Davidson and Bailey 1985, Joshi et al. 1989). Incision and drainage without resection often results in a persistent sinus tract. The wider resection necessary after spontaneous drainage results in extensive scarring. Although antimicrobial therapy without resection has not been successful in the past, inclusion of an ESM in the medication regimen may be a promising new alternative to surgical resection (Starke and Correa 1995).

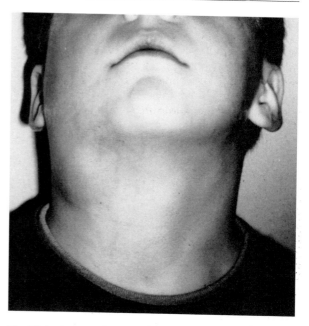

Fig. 22.4 A child, age 5 years, with submandibular cervical lymphadenitis due to MAC. (Courtesy of RJH Smith MD, University of Iowa College of Medicine).

3.3 Other sites of mycobacterioses

Arthritis, tenosynovitis, bursitis, or osteomyelitis may be due to *M. marinum*, MAC, or organisms of the *M. fortuitum* complex, especially *M. abscessus* and *M. fortuitum* (Hoffman et al. 1978, Wallace, Brown and Onyi 1992). In many cases infection is associated with a previous deep puncture wound, joint injection, or other deep trauma in the area of bones or joints. These deep infections may also result from prolonged disease when NTM disease is not suspected until late in the course of infection (Brown and Sanders 1985). When these deep infections are associated with an aquatic-related activity, *M. marinum* is often the cause (Harth, Ralph and Faraawi 1994). Successful treatment consists of drainage with or without surgical resection and specific antimicrobial therapy.

M. fortuitum complex and, less commonly, other NTM (*M. xenopi*, *M. kansasii*) have been implicated in catheter-related infections, particularly the catheter exit site of chronic peritoneal dialysis catheters and peritonitis (Hakim, Hisam and Reuman 1993, White et al. 1993) but they represent less than 3% of such infections. These infections are clinically indistinguishable from other bacterial causes, but should be considered when routine bacterial cultures fail to grow. Effective treatment requires catheter removal (White et al. 1993, Raffalli and Kiehn 1994) and debridement of the exit site. Treatment should include antimicrobial therapy based on the susceptibilities of the mycobacteria isolated (Hakim, Hisam and Reuman 1993).

The *M. fortuitum* complex are rare causes of keratitis associated with contact lens use and other minor ocular trauma (Bullington, Lanier and Font 1992, Broadway et al. 1994, Khooshabeh et al. 1994). Since this infection is rare, misidentification of the causative bacteria is common and appropriate treatment may be delayed. Histological examination, cultures and antibiotic susceptibilities are essential for a diagnosis and selection of appropriate antibiotics (Bullington, Lanier and Font 1992). Even when appropriate antibiotics have been used, surgery may be necessary in some cases to achieve a cure (Broadway et al. 1994, Khooshabeh et al. 1994).

Mastoiditis that fails to respond to standard antibiotics is rarely due to NTM (Moerman et al. 1993). Presence of granulomatous inflammation on biopsy and culture confirm the diagnosis and treatment is with surgery and antibiotic therapy.

4 MYCOBACTERIOSES IN IMMUNOCOMPROMISED HOSTS

Immunocompromised individuals are effective hosts for NTM (Wolinsky 1992, Yates, Pozniak and Grange 1993, Choudhri et al. 1995). Patients with depressed cellular immunity, such as those who have AIDS, lymphoproliferative disorders or transplants, and those on immunosuppressive therapy, are at particular risk. Rarely there may be a genetic basis for disseminated NTM infection (Newport and Levin 1994).

NTM are rarely isolated only from the lungs of immunocompromised patients. AIDS patients differ from other immunocompromised patients in that high numbers of NTM can be recovered from blood. This section deals mainly with the disseminated mycobacterioses associated with AIDS and the mycobacterioses of other immunocompromised hosts. The NTM involved and their salient features are listed in Table 22.4.

4.1 Mycobacteriosis in AIDS patients

Mycobacterioses are increasingly common in AIDS (Wayne and Sramek 1992, Benson and Ellner 1993, Selik, Chu and Ward 1995). In AIDS patients in the USA, mycobacterioses, predominantly due to MAC, are diagnosed in about 25–50% during life and in more than 50% at autopsy (Nightingale et al. 1992, Benson 1994, Henderson and Chapman 1994). This is due mainly to the presence of other superimposed, debilitating or life-threatening illnesses, which obscure mycobacterioses during life. The increased incidence of disseminated MAC infection in AIDS patients is attributable to 2 principal factors: greater surveillance since MAC bacteria were recognized as a potentially treatable cause of morbidity; and the increased survival of patients with AIDS. Besides MAC, *M. kansasii*, *M. xenopi*, *M. gordonae*, *M. malmoense*, *M. haemophilum* and 2 recently identified species, *Mycobacterium genavense* and *Mycobacterium celatum*, cause disseminated infection in HIV patients (see Table 22.1). Rarely, focal extrapulmonary mycobacterioses such as sinusitis (Naguib, Byers and Slater 1994) or spindle cell pseudotumours of the spleen (Suster, Moran and Blanco 1994) are seen in AIDS patients.

MAC and other NTM can cause pulmonary infections in AIDS patients (Rigsby and Curtis 1994). NTM are recoverable from sputum or bronchoalveolar lavage fluid, but true invasion of the lung is difficult to demonstrate and pulmonary symptoms are often minimal. The radiographic appearance of NTM in AIDS differs from that in immunocompetent hosts. The chest x-ray may be normal or show non-specific mediastinal and/or hilar adenopathy or, rarely, patchy alveolar infiltrates. The frequent detection of NTM in blood cultures reflects the disseminated nature of

Table 22.4 NTM associated with disseminated infections in immunosuppressed hosts, listed in descending order encountered

Aetiological organism	Special characteristics	Most frequent host
M. avium complex	*M. avium* serovars predominate	Frequent isolate from AIDS patients; usually extrapulmonary sites
M. kansasii	See Table 22.2	Second most common NTM infection in AIDS patients
Less common organisms		
M. abscessus, M. chelonae, M. fortuitum	See Table 22.2	Risk factor in non-AIDS: long-term steroid Rx; uncommon in AIDS
M. genavense	No growth on solid media; requires liquid media and 6–12 weeks of incubation	AIDS with AFB seen in multiple tissues specimens
M. haemophilum	Non-pigmented, slow grower; growth requires haemin, low temperatures (30–32°C), and CO_2	AIDS

See Table 22.1 for complete list.

infection and the high bacterial burden. The mechanism by which organisms in the blood become recoverable from respiratory secretions is unknown.

MAC INFECTION

M. avium serovars account for more than 90% of typable MAC that cause infection in AIDS, whereas in other patients almost half the isolates are *M. intracellulare* (Guthertz et al. 1989, Raszka et al. 1995). In a study of 216 consecutive cultures of NTM from AIDS patients, *M. avium* was recovered from 77% of positive blood or bone marrow cultures, whereas *M. intracellulare* and other non-*avium* NTM accounted for only 18 and 5% of isolates, respectively. In the USA, for unknown reasons, bacteraemia in AIDS is associated with a limited number of *M. avium* serovars (serovars 1, 4 and 8).

There is no clear association between the environmental prevalence of MAC and disease in the AIDS patients (Von Reyn et al. 1993, Henderson and Chapman 1994). The prevalence of MAC infection in AIDS patients in Africa is very low but this is not due to the absence of MAC in the African environment, although it may be lower than elsewhere (Morrissey et al. 1992, Von Reyn et al. 1993). Indeed, the presence of MAC in the environment may result in a degree of protection against infection (Falkinham 1994).

The smooth transparent (SMT) and smooth domed (SMD) colonial morphologies differ in virulence. SMT are more frequently isolated from blood in AIDS patients (Frothingham and Wilson 1994). Isolates from patients with disseminated MAC often contain mixtures of colony morphologies (Falkinham 1994, Slutsky et al. 1994, Von Reyn et al. 1995). SMT bacteria have greater potential for intracellular multiplication in macrophages, greater virulence in animal models, and are more resistant to antibiotics than SMD bacteria. The morphological difference between SMT and SMD bacteria resides in part in the expression of different glycopeptidolipids.

The most common port of entry and site for dissemination in AIDS patients, in contrast to those who are immunocompetent, is believed to be the gastrointestinal tract. Less often MAC are acquired by inhalation. Infection appears to be primary rather than reactivation of latent disease. The environmental source of MAC in AIDS patients is uncertain but may include potable water (Montecalvo et al. 1994, Von Reyn et al. 1994), hard cheese (Horsburgh et al. 1994a), or soil (Yajko et al. 1995).

AIDS and other immunocompromised patients probably acquire MAC from the environment, followed by bacterial colonization and/or direct tissue invasion and increasing mycobacterial replication and, for a time, intermittent bacteraemia without dissemination. Asymptomatic patients with only intermittent bacteraemia are thought to have a lower burden of tissue infection (Kemper et al. 1994). Continuous bacteraemia with dissemination is usually accompanied by clinical symptoms, and finally death (Torriani et al. 1994, Raszka et al. 1995). The majority

of AIDS patients with symptomatic MAC infection have high grade mycobacteraemia with evidence of disseminated multiple organ, particularly reticuloendothelial organ, disease (Torriani et al. 1994). The organisms are frequently recovered from lymph nodes, liver, spleen, bone marrow and the gastrointestinal tract. MAC infections in the eye, brain, meninges (Dwork, Chin and Boyce 1994, Malessa et al. 1994, Gyure et al. 1995), CSF, skin, tongue, heart, lung, stomach, thyroid, breast, parathyroid, adrenal glands, kidney, pancreas, prostate, testes, skin and soft tissue, abdominal cavity and, more recently, muscle (necrotizing myositis) (Miralles and Bregman 1994) have been documented. At autopsy, MAC is found in virtually every organ system (Torriani et al. 1994). Histopathologically, the infected tissues are filled with large numbers of distended histiocytes packed with acid-fast bacilli, but granulomatous reaction and necrosis may be absent.

The immunological response to MAC is complicated, involving cellular and humoral immune responses (reviewed by Inderlied, Kemper and Bermudez 1993). MAC are facultative intracellular pathogens that enter and multiply primarily in mononuclear phagocytes. Evidence obtained in vitro suggests that *M. avium* replicates more quickly in human macrophages than *M. intracellulare*, but there is no evidence to show that the clinical courses of the 2 infections differ. HIV constituents can directly stimulate the growth of MAC within macrophages. Phagocytes that have ingested MAC produce cytokines, such as tumour necrosis factor (TNF), which activate cellular responses that inhibit the growth of the bacteria. However, MAC of the SMT colony type induce lower levels of TNF production by macrophages, which may explain the greater virulence of these strains. Other strategies for the survival of MAC in macrophages include the ability of bacteria to induce cytokines that deactivate killing by macrophages (Henderson and Chapman 1994) and the inhibition of phagosome–lysosome fusion. In addition to CD4 T lymphocyte-dependent mechanisms for containing MAC infection in immunocompetent individuals, cytotoxic T lymphocytes and natural killer cells also appear to play a role in the cellular immune response.

A potential relationship exists between gastrointestinal or respiratory tract colonization by MAC and bacteraemia with symptomatic disseminated infection, in that positive respiratory tract and stool cultures in asymptomatic patients are reasonably predictive of dissemination; however, cultures are a relatively insensitive screening test (Chin et al. 1994a). Disseminated MAC infection develops in 60–65% of patients with antecedent respiratory colonization, but among all patients who develop disseminated disease, respiratory colonization is detected in only 21–33% before dissemination. Thus, culture is of limited value as a routine screening test.

The strongest single risk factor for disseminated MAC in AIDS is the level of immunosuppression (Horsburgh et al. 1994b) and the risk of MAC infection increases as the CD4 count decreases (Henderson and Chapman 1994). It is most common with a CD4 T lymphocyte count of less than 100 (Benson 1994, Falkinham 1994) and the diagnosis of infection is made a mean of 9 months after the diagnosis of AIDS (Porrman and Katon 1994). Symptomatic HIV-infected patients with CD4 lymphocyte counts of less than 50 are at substantial risk of MAC bacteraemia, which occurs in nearly 45% of patients within one year (Chin et al. 1994a). Differences in infection rate do not correlate with patient age, sex, race or HIV risk factors, nor have significant regional differences in infection rate been noted (Porrman and Katon 1994). Disseminated MAC infection in HIV-negative patients with idiopathic CD4+ T lymphopenia has been described (Thomas et al. 1994).

Disseminated MAC infection in HIV-infected people generally presents as a subacute but progressive syndrome of fever, chills, night sweats, cough, fatigue, diarrhoea and weight loss. Gastrointestinal complaints are particularly common and contribute greatly to morbidity. Diarrhoea is due to small intestinal or colonic involvement and severe abdominal pain is due to enlarged retroperitoneal lymph nodes (Porrman and Katon 1994). Hepatosplenomegaly is detectable on physical examination in 10–50% of patients (Levin 1994). The most common laboratory abnormalities are worsening anaemia and elevated alkaline phosphatase. Pulmonary MAC disease is rare in patients with disseminated MAC infection. Radiographic patterns are non-specific and may include consolidating or nodular infiltrates and cavitation (Kalayjian et al. 1995).

Blood culture by a variety of methods, including lysis centrifugation and BACTEC 12B and 13A broth culture, are highly sensitive (86–98%) in diagnosing disseminated MAC infection (Benson and Ellner 1993, Henderson and Chapman 1994). The level of mycobacteraemia is generally in the range of 10–1000 cfu ml^{-1} of blood. MAC has also frequently been recovered from bone marrow. Recovery of MAC from non-sterile body fluids or tissues, such as the respiratory tract or stool, in the absence of symptoms suggests colonization (see p. 431).

Epidemiological studies indicate that untreated disseminated MAC disease increases morbidity and shortens survival (Chin et al. 1994b, Gleason-Morgan, Church and Ross 1994, Henderson and Chapman 1994, Horsburgh et al. 1994b). Median survival after the diagnosis of MAC is approximately 3–8 months versus approximately 10–16 months in CD4-matched HIV-infected patients without disseminated MAC (Hoover et al. 1995). Based on these data, treatment of MAC infection in AIDS patients, and other severely immunocompromised patients, appears to be justified because it improves symptoms and may increase survival (Horsburgh, Havlik and Ellis 1991, Chin et al. 1994b). Unfortunately, the optimal treatment is not known and long-term therapeutic success is doubtful.

Malabsorption complicates antibiotic regimens in AIDS patients. Placebo-controlled trials show a 50% reduction in MAC bacteraemia in asymptomatic patients with rifabutin prophylaxis, and a US Public Health Service Task Force has recommended rifabutin for all AIDS patients with a CD4 cell count of less than 100 (Masur 1993, Nightingale et al. 1993) but *M. tuberculosis* must first be ruled out. A significant therapeutic advance in the treatment of symptomatic patients are ESM agents with high level activity against MAC. Primary therapy usually includes clarithromycin and ethambutol with or without rifampicin or rifabutin (Havlir 1994, Henderson and Chapman 1994). Though susceptibility tests for MAC have not been standardized, clinical trials in patients with AIDS show a correlation between in vitro susceptibility and clinical response only for clarithromycin (Benson and Ellner 1993, Benson 1994).

A partial response to treatment in terms of diminished symptoms, usually within 2–8 weeks of starting therapy, is seen in 72–95% of patients but blood cultures may remain positive and the required duration of therapy appears to be indefinite (Porrman and Katon 1994, Sullam et al. 1994).

M. KANSASII INFECTION

Pulmonary and disseminated disease due to *M. kansasii* has been reported in patients infected with HIV (Hirasuna 1987, Parenti et al. 1995) and in patients with other immunocompromising conditions (Zvetina et al. 1992). *M. kansasii* is the second most common NTM to affect patients with AIDS in the USA (Bamberger et al. 1994). Data from the CDC indicate that disseminated infection develops in 0.44% of patients in highly endemic areas of the southern and midwestern portions of the USA. Horsburgh and Selik (1989) reported that *M. kansasii* accounts for 2.9% of the NTM that cause disseminated infections in AIDS patients.

The impact of HIV infection on *M. kansasii* infection is shown by 35 patients, all but 2 of whom presented with advanced AIDS and a very low CD4 count (Bamberger et al. 1994). Most of the 22 patients with pulmonary disease presented with fever, cough and dyspnoea, but only 8 of these had radiographic evidence of cavitation or predominantly upper lobe disease. *M. kansasii* was isolated from blood or bone marrow of 10 patients. Most patients with pulmonary or disseminated disease responded to therapy.

The clinical presentation and prognosis of disease due to *M. kansasii* in patients with HIV was examined by Witzig et al. (1995). The patients had CD4 counts of less than 100 and a mean interval of 17 months between the diagnosis of AIDS and isolation of *M. kansasii*; 17 of the 49 patients had disseminated disease. Sputum smears were positive for AFB in 29 patients, and 35 were known cigarette smokers. At the time of initial isolation, 13 patients had other concurrent pulmonary isolates and 15 had other mycobacterial species, mostly MAC, concurrently isolated. It therefore appears that in HIV-infected patients, isolation of *M. kansasii* in sputum is usually associated with disease rather than colonization. Symptoms consisted of fever, weight loss, fatigue, night sweats, chills, cough, sputum production, dyspnoea, chest pain and occasionally haemoptysis. The physical findings were lymphadenopathy and occasionally splenomegaly, hepatomegaly or skin lesions. In contrast to the study of Bamberger et al. (1994), most patients had abnormal chest x-rays, the majority with alveolar infiltrates and a smaller number with cavitation and interstitial infiltrates. Disseminated disease was common and most often diagnosed by blood culture. Patients who received antimycobacterial treatment survived longer than those who did not.

Other types of *M. kansasii* infection in AIDS patients include pericarditis (Moreno et al. 1994), osteomyelitis (Weinroth, Pincetl and Tuazon 1994), tenosynovitis, endobronchial lesions with obstruction (Connolly, Baughman and Dohn 1993) and sinusitis (Li et al. 1994).

Increased resistance of *M. kansasii* to rifampicin, normally a first-line antibiotic against this infection, has been identified in AIDS patients (Wallace et al. 1994b). Of the rifampicin-resistant isolates recovered since 1989, 32% are from HIV-positive patients and treatment failure in AIDS patients, possibly related to the development of rifampicin resistance, has been reported.

M. GENAVENSE INFECTIONS

Hirschel et al. (1990) described an HIV-positive patient who developed a disease clinically resembling that due to MAC. Numerous acid-fast bacilli were found in nearly all tissues examined but cultures were negative. Microscopy and chromatography were consistent with the presence of a mycobacterium and the organism was found to multiply within macrophages. The predominant findings were gastrointestinal symptoms and hepatosplenomegaly. This organism was subsequently identified and named *M. genavense* which is closely related to *M. simiae* (Bottger et al. 1992, Wald et al. 1992).

The organism is probably widespread in the environment (Bessesen et al. 1993, Pechere et al. 1995) and has also been isolated from pet birds with muscle wasting, hepatomegaly and thickening of the small intestine (Hoop et al. 1993). In tissues from humans infected with *M. genavense* pathological changes are seen predominantly in the small intestine, spleen, liver and lymph nodes (Bottger et al. 1992, Maschek et al. 1994). Lungs, myocardium and kidneys are usually not, or only minimally, involved. This led to the view that *M. genavense* is initially harboured in the intestine with rapid dissemination to liver and spleen (Bottger et al. 1992). Histology is similar to that in MAC infection with masses of foamy histiocytes and, depending on the immunological reactivity of the host, poorly formed granulomas, rarely with small areas of necrosis.

M. genavense infection is similar to MAC infection in AIDS and often associated with fever, anorexia, abdominal pain, chronic diarrhoea and massive weight loss; but splenomegaly, hepatomegaly and lymphadenopathy are more prominent (Bessesen et al. 1993, Gaynor et al. 1994, Pechere et al. 1995). A case-control study by Pechere et al. (1995) of 54 patients with disseminated *M. genavense* infection from Europe,

North America and Australia, showed that most were extremely immunocompromised; 87% had fever and weight loss, 72% had anaemia, 44% had diarrhoea, 43% had splenomegaly, and 39% had hepatomegaly.

In 2 series of AIDS patients with disseminated mycobacterial disease, one from an AIDS clinic and one from Europe, North America and Australia, 4% and approximately 10% of cases respectively were due to *M. genavense* (Bessesen et al. 1993, Pechere et al. 1995). In the latter group the median survival was 190 days after *M. genavense* was first isolated. Median survival with treatment was 263 days as compared with 81 days without treatment. In 30% of the patients, *M. genavense* was the first major opportunistic infection and the principal or major contributing cause of death in approximately 56% of the cases that died.

Investigation of patients with suspected *M. genavense* infection should include blood culture, bone marrow biopsy and possibly small bowel biopsy. Nucleic acid-based techniques, such as gene amplification (16S rRNA) by PCR or in situ hybridization with highly specific probes, are advisable for a definitive diagnosis. Treatment has not been standardized (Albrecht et al. 1995a) but a good clinical response has been reported with clarithromycin (Bessesen et al. 1993, Matsiota-Bernard et al. 1995).

4.2 Mycobacteriosis in non-AIDS immunocompromised hosts

Improvements in surgical technique and immunosuppressive drug regimens have contributed to the success of solid organ transplantation, particularly of the kidney and heart, but transplant patients are at risk for a variety of mycobacterioses (Delaney et al. 1993, Patel et al. 1994). NTM infections generally occur late in the post-transplantation period (range 10 days to 269 months; mean 48 months). Most are chronic infections of soft tissues and joints (cutaneous lesions on the extremities, tenosynovitis, arthritis) and osteomyelitis, often with multifocal involvement. Fever, leucocytosis, night sweats, weight loss and lymphadenopathy are usually absent. Skin lesions are often painful erythematous subcutaneous nodules, which can progress to abscess formation. The most commonly involved joints include finger joints, wrists, elbows, ankles and knees, and in these patients diagnosis is often delayed by several months. Pulmonary involvement occurs in approximately a quarter of patients, with radiographic evidence of pulmonary nodules or infiltrates, and over half the patients have concomitant extrapulmonary involvement. Pulmonary involvement is most frequently with *M. kansasii* and skin and joint infections with *M. fortuitum* complex infection. Risk factors for mycobacterioses in solid organ transplant recipients are poorly defined. For heart recipients, they include a history of open heart surgery and immunosuppressive therapy with cyclophosphamide, rather than azathioprine or cyclosporin A (Simpson, Raffin and Remington 1982, Novick, Moreno-Cabral and Stinson 1990). The environment is the likely source in patients with transplant-related immunosuppression and other immunodeficiencies.

Therapy typically includes multidrug antimicrobial therapy, surgical debridement, and/or reduction in doses of immunosuppressive agents, but optimal therapy for mycobacterioses in solid organ transplant recipients has yet to be determined. The outcome is generally favourable, in contrast to such patients with *M. tuberculosis* infection. Important toxic effects related to drug–drug interactions associated with antimycobacterial therapy for solid organ transplant recipients are problematic (Patel et al. 1994). For example, rifampicin increases the catabolism of cyclosporin A.

Patients with the uncommon 'hairy cell' leukaemia appear to have a predilection for mycobacterial infection (approximately 5% of patients), mainly with *M. kansasii* and MAC (Bennett, Vardiman and Golomb 1986, Kramers et al. 1992, Castor, Juhlin and Henriques 1994).

M. AVIUM COMPLEX INFECTION

In the early 1980s before the epidemic of HIV infection and AIDS, disseminated MAC infection was very uncommon; fewer than 40 cases were reported between 1940 and 1984 (Falkinham 1994). More than half the patients were immunocompromised by malignancy or immunodeficient (Horsburgh et al. 1985). These infections remain uncommon other than in HIV-infected patients. Although disseminated disease is more common than focal disease in these patients (Johnson and Kiehn 1994), localized skin infection (Kakinuma and Suzuki 1994), arthritis (Disla et al. 1995) and appendicitis (Livingston et al. 1995) have been described. Disseminated MAC is associated with a high incidence of haematological abnormalities, such as leukaemoid reactions, myelofibrotic changes, the haemophagocytic syndrome, polycythaemia, pancytopenia and myelodysplastic syndrome (Tsukada et al. 1994). In the latter syndrome aggregates of macrophages filled with organisms are seen in the bone marrow without a granulomatous reaction and necrosis, similar to the overwhelming infections seen in late stage AIDS (Tsukada et al. 1994).

M. FORTUITUM COMPLEX INFECTION

Most infections are caused by the 3 species, *M. fortuitum*, *M. chelonae* or *M. abscessus* (Wallace 1994), and predominantly involve skin, soft tissue or bone (Wallace, Brown and Onyi 1992). *M. chelonae* is less widely distributed in the environment than *M. fortuitum*, which may account for the higher incidence of cutaneous disease due to the latter. *M. fortuitum* may, however, be less virulent, since almost all cases of disseminated disease are due to *M. chelonae*. The source of infection can not usually be determined. Swetter, Kindel and Smoller (1993) first reported disseminated *M. chelonae* infection in an immunocompromised host in whom the primary site of infection was the lung.

Disseminated infection, including cutaneous lesions due to *M. chelonae*, have been reviewed by Wallace, Brown and Onyi (1992). Predisposing conditions included organ transplantation, rheumatoid arthritis and autoimmune disorders. Systemic steroid therapy was common to 92% of the patients and appeared to be the most important risk factor for disseminated infection. Disseminated *M. fortuitum* complex infection in AIDS patients appears to be rare (Eichmann, Huszar and Bon 1993). Neutropenia may also be a risk factor for *M. chelonae* infections, which may be underdiagnosed in septic neutropenic patients (McWhinney et al. 1992). Thus, besides cell mediated immunity, other types of host defence may operate to contain *M. fortuitum* complex infections.

The symptoms of infections in immunocompromised patients range from mild to severe. Disseminated infection, with cutaneous manifestations, is usually mild in patients on long-term corticosteroid treatment, and the majority are infected with *M. chelonae* (Wallace, Brown and Onyi 1992). Their systemic symptoms are usually minimal, with negative blood cultures and without serious morbidity and mortality over an extended period.

Patients with leukaemia or lymphoma, on the other hand, can present with a localized catheter-related infection or a more severe disseminated infection with a higher morbidity and mortality. From such patients *M. abscessus* is more often isolated; patients are often also receiving corticosteroids and/or chemotherapy. With disseminated infection, these patients have systemic symptoms, especially fever, and they commonly present with a rash that can range from maculopapular to discrete draining nodules or ulcers. Mycobacteria can often be cultured from skin lesion biopsies and blood cultures. Disseminated infection without skin involvement is rare (Ingram et al. 1993) and antimicrobial agents are generally ineffective in clearing the mycobacterial infection in these patients.

Treatment of *M. fortuitum* complex infection usually involves multiple antibiotics and should be guided by the species isolated. Antimicrobial susceptibility is occasionally a helpful guide when the isolate is not multidrug resistant. Conventional therapy includes amikacin and cefoxitin (Starke and Correa 1995). ESM agents are promising, but resistance develops if they are used alone (Wallace, Brown and Onyi 1992, Wallace et al. 1993, Tebas et al. 1995). Other agents with in vitro activity include fluoroquinolones, sulphonamides, imipenem and tobramycin. *M. chelonae* isolates are often resistant to a broad range of antibiotics (Starke and Correa 1995). Guidelines for the number of antibiotics required or the length of treatment are not available. Less immunocompromised patients may respond to treatment with one or 2 drugs. Prolonged treatment for months to years with 3 or more medications may be appropriate for patients with more severe immune deficiencies. Recovery is enhanced by return of immune function. Ingram et al. (1993) categorized patients to 3 groups according to underlying disease and outcome. Patients with cell mediated immune deficiency, lymphoma or leukaemia presented with widespread multi-organ involvement and severe disease, and survival rate in this group was only 10%. Patients with other underlying diseases had illnesses of intermediate severity and intermediate responses to therapy, whereas the group without a significant immune defect usually presented with more limited skin involvement and responded well to antibiotics, and a survival rate of 90%.

4.3 Less common NTM causing disease in patients with AIDS or other severe immune deficiency states

Infection due to *M. haemophilum* is rare but increasing in prevalence (Dever et al. 1992, Kiehn and White 1994, Straus et al. 1994). The reasons probably include:

1 a greater number of immunocompromised individuals, particularly AIDS patients who are surviving longer with severe CD4 lymphocyte depletion
2 continued prevalence of a behaviour source which increases exposure to *M. haemophilum*
3 increased awareness of infection and
4 implementation of distinct culture methods which enhance isolation.

The organism has never been cultured from the environment, the natural habitat and means of acquisition are unknown, and few data support person-to-person spread. Potential routes of transmission include percutaneous inoculation, inhalation or ingestion. Most patients infected with *M. haemophilum* are immunosuppressed by AIDS, lymphoma, immunosuppressive therapy or organ transplantation (reviewed by Wayne and Sramek 1992, Kiehn et al. 1993). Infection can occur in healthy children and present as cervical and hilar lymphadenitis. In adults, the skin is the most common site of infection with erythematous nodular and ulcerating lesions (Becherer and Hopfer 1992, Darling et al. 1994, Straus et al. 1994). More than 40 cases have been reported since it was first identified by Sompolinsky et al. (1978) as a cause of cutaneous ulcerating lesions in a patient with Hodgkin's disease. The infection should be considered in immunocompromised patients with draining cutaneous ulcers, especially overlying joints in the extremities, which may be related to the lower temperature optimum for growth. Other features may include fever, weight loss, tenosynovitis, septic arthritis, osteomyelitis and respiratory symptoms. *M. haemophilum* has been cultured from skin, bone marrow, blood, lymph nodes, synovial fluid, vitreous fluid, bronchoalveolar lavage fluid, sputum and lung tissue. Histologically, the skin lesions are suppurative granulomas containing acid-fast bacilli. Granuloma formation may not be seen in patients with AIDS.

Treatment of *M. haemophilum* infection includes reduction of the level of immunosuppression, surgical excision of localized disease, and antibiotics. Aminoglycosides, ciprofloxacin, clarithromycin, rifabutin and rifampicin are the most active antimicrobial agents in vitro (Darling et al. 1994, Kiehn and White 1994, Straus et al. 1994). Although infection due to this organism is rarely fatal, it is a cause of significant morbidity. The response to treatment is variable and the progress or recurrence of disease has been documented despite the administration of different regimens (Soubani, Al-Marri and Forlenza 1994).

Disseminated *M. malmoense* infection manifests as fever, night sweats, anorexia, lethargy, weight loss and diarrhoea, in addition to lymphadenitis (Zaugg et al. 1993). Although the infection is similar to MAC, MAC is a very common opportunistic pathogen in late AIDS and *M. malmoense* is only rarely isolated (Chocarro et al. 1994). This discrepancy may be due to differences in the immune response to the 2 mycobacterial species, for example, in their handling by macrophages. The infection of human macrophages with HIV increases the rate of intracellular growth of *M. avium* but not that of *M. malmoense* (Kallenius et al. 1993).

M. celatum, first described in 1993, has been identified as an opportunistic pathogen in AIDS patients (Piersimoni, Tortoli and De Sio 1994, Tortoli et al. 1995). The clinical presentation is similar to infection by MAC and the bacterium appears sensitive to quinolones, clarithromycin and rifabutin (Tortoli et al. 1995).

Pulmonary and extrapulmonary *M. bovis* infection, including lymphadenitis and disseminated infection with meningitis, has been described in patients with AIDS and other immune deficiency states (Dankner et al. 1993, Albrecht et al. 1995b, Stone et al. 1995). Risk factors in a nosocomial outbreak of multidrug-resistant *M. bovis* infection in a group of HIV-infected patients have been described (Bouvet et al. 1993). Rarely, BCG vaccination can lead to disseminated disease in immunocompromised patients (Bohle et al. 1992, Besnard, Sauvion and Offredo 1993, Izes, Bihrle and Thomas 1993, Lallemant-le Coeur et al. 1993, Ryder, Oxtoby and Mvula 1993, Weltman and Rose 1993). Another group at risk are patients treated for bladder cancer who receive bladder instillations of BCG (Lamm et al. 1986, Gupta, Lavengood and Smith 1988, McParland et al. 1992, Hakim et al. 1993, Smith, Alexander and Aranda 1993, LeMense and Strange 1994).

Rare cases of other mycobacteria that can cause localized or disseminated disease in immunocompromised hosts have been described (Wayne and Sramek 1992, Delaporte, Alfandari and Piette 1994, Hoffner 1994). *M. szulgai* is a rare human pathogen (Hoffner 1994, Newshan and Torres 1994) that can cause disseminated disease involving the skin, bones and lungs. *M. neoaurum* is a scotochromogenic RGM that has been identified as a cause of bacteraemia related to central line infections in immunocompromised patients (Holland et al. 1994). It was first isolated from soil, but can be recovered from dust and water.

M. gordonae is generally considered a non-pathogen, but occasional cases of disseminated disease due to it have been reported (Weinberger et al. 1992, Lessnau, Milanese and Talavera 1993). In a study of patients from whom *M. gordonae* was isolated, the 15 HIV-negative patients were only colonized, whereas 12 of 21 HIV-positive patients had probable infection and 2 additional HIV patients had documented disseminated disease. Of the 14 patients with infection, 13 had evidence of cavitary lesions or lymphadenopathy on chest x-ray; the extrapulmonary manifestations were abdominal lymphadenopathy and hepatosplenomegaly (Lessnau, Milanese and Talavera 1993). Antibiotics may improve symptoms and prolong survival.

Disseminated infection with *M. gordonae* may also occur in immunocompetent patients in relation to foreign bodies (Weinberger et al. 1992), but they are not always well documented (Wayne and Sramek 1992).

Pulmonary and disseminated disease due to *M. xenopi* has been reported in patients with AIDS (Eng et al. 1984, Ausina et al. 1988, Jacoby et al. 1995), chronic renal failure, chronic myelogenous leukaemia, diabetes mellitus and transplants and very rarely in immunocompetent patients (Branger et al. 1985, Weber et al. 1989). Extrapulmonary disease alone is rare (Miller et al. 1994, Jones, Schrager and Zabransky 1995). Infection can appear similar to focal pulmonary tuberculosis in patients with early HIV infection and can present as disseminated disease in advanced AIDS.

Rare cases of disseminated *M. scrofulaceum* infection in AIDS patients have been described (Delabie et al. 1991, Wayne and Sramek 1992, Sanders et al. 1995). Typically, primary manifestations are multiple chronic progressive skin lesions, cavitary lung disease and wasting. In a series collected during 28 years, Sanders et al. (1995) found 8 cases of multifocal probable disseminated *M. scrofulaceum* infection; 4 patients had underlying immunodeficiency due to leukaemia, lupus, amyloidosis or immunosuppressive medications, but in 2 cases there was no known immunodeficiency.

For further reports of patients with AIDS or other immunodeficiency states infected with uncommon mycobacterial species, the reader is referred to the following: *M. marinum* (Lambertus and Mathisen 1988, Parent et al. 1995), *M. simiae* (Levy-Frebault et al. 1987), *M. smegmatis* (Young et al. 1986, Peters et al. 1989), *M. thermoresistibile* (Weitzmann et al. 1981, Liu, Andrews and Wright 1984) and *M. conspicuum* (Springer et al. 1995).

REFERENCES

Ahn CH, Nash DR, Hurst GA, 1976, Ventilatory defects in atypical mycobacteriosis: a comparison study with tuberculosis, *Am Rev Respir Dis*, **113:** 273–9.

Ahn CH, Lowell JR et al., 1979, A demographic study of disease due to *Mycobacterium kansasii* or *Mycobacterium intracellulare-avium* in Texas, *Chest*, **75:** 120–5.

Ahn CH, Lowell JR et al., 1981, Chemotherapy for pulmonary disease due to *Mycobacterium kansasii*: efficacies of some individual drugs, *Rev Infect Dis*, **3:** 1028–34.

Ahn CH, McLarty JW et al., 1982, Diagnostic criteria for pulmonary disease caused by *Mycobacterium kansasii* and *Mycobacterium intracellulare*, *Am Rev Respir Dis*, **125:** 388–91.

Ahn CH, Lowell JR et al., 1983, Short-course chemotherapy for pulmonary disease caused by *Mycobacterium kansasii*, *Am Rev Respir Dis*, **128:** 1048–50.

Albelda SM, Kern JA et al., 1985, Expanding the spectrum of pulmonary disease caused by nontuberculous mycobacteria, *Radiology*, **157:** 289–96.

Alberts WM, Chandler KO et al., 1987, Pulmonary disease caused by *Mycobacterium malmoense*, *Am Rev Respir Dis*, **135:** 1375–8.

Albrecht M et al., 1994, Identification of mutations in 23S rRNA gene of clarithromycin-resistant *Mycobacterium intracellulare*, *Antimicrob Agents Chemother*, **38:** 121–2.

Albrecht H, Rusch-Gerdes S et al., 1995a, Treatment of disseminated *Mycobacterium genavense* infection, *AIDS*, **9:** 659–60.

Albrecht H, Stellbrink JJ et al., 1995b, A case of disseminated *Mycobacterium bovis* infection in an AIDS patient, *Eur J Clin Microbiol Infect Dis*, **14:** 226–9.

Alessi DP, Dudley JP, 1988, Atypical mycobacteria-induced cervical adenitis: treatment by needle aspiration, *Arch Otolaryngol Head Neck Surg*, **114:** 664–6.

Allen BW, 1982, *M. xenopi*, *Eur J Respir Dis*, **63:** 291–2.

Anon, 1989, Editor's note, *Am Rev Respir Dis*, **140:** 561.

Armstrong KL, James RW et al., 1992, *Mycobacterium haemophilum* causing perihilar or cervical lymphadenitis in healthy children, *J Pediatr*, **121:** 202–5.

Ausina V, Barrio J et al., 1988, *M. xenopi* infections in the acquired immunodeficiency syndrome, *Ann Intern Med*, **109:** 927–8.

Bailey WC, Brown M et al., 1974, Silico-mycobacterial disease in sandblasters, *Am Rev Respir Dis*, **110:** 115–25.

Bamberger DM, Driks MR et al., 1994, *Mycobacterium kansasii* among patients infected with human immunodeficiency virus in Kansas City, *Clin Infect Dis*, **18:** 395–400.

Banks J, Jenkins PA, Smith AP, 1985, Pulmonary infection with *Mycobacterium malmoense* – a review of treatment and response, *Tubercle*, **66:** 197–203.

Banks J, Hunter AM et al., 1984, Pulmonary infections with *Mycobacterium xenopi*: review of treatment and response, *Thorax*, **39:** 376–82.

Becherer P, Hopfer RL, 1992, Infection with *Mycobacterium haemophilum*, *Clin Infect Dis*, **14:** 793.

Bell RC, Higuchi JH et al., 1983, *Mycobacterium simiae*: clinical features and follow-up of twenty-four patients, *Am Rev Respir Dis*, **127:** 35–8.

Bennett C, Vardiman J, Golomb H, 1986, Disseminated atypical mycobacterial infection in patients with hairy cell leukemia, *Am J Med*, **80:** 891–6.

Bennett SN, Peterson DE et al., 1994, Bronchoscopy-associated *M. xenopi* pseudoinfection, *Am J Respir Crit Care Med*, **150:** 245–50.

Benson C, 1994, Disseminated *Mycobacterium avium* complex disease in patients with AIDS, *AIDS Res Hum Retroviruses*, **10:** 913–16.

Benson CA, Ellner JJ, 1993, *Mycobacterium avium* complex infection and AIDS: advances in theory and practice, *Clin Infect Dis*, **17:** 7–20.

Besnard M, Sauvion S, Offredo C, 1993, Bacillus Calmette–Guérin infection after vaccination of human immunodeficiency virus-infected children, *Infect Dis J*, **12:** 993–7.

Bessesen MT, Shlay M et al., 1993, Disseminated *Mycobacterium genavense* infection: clinical and microbiological features and response to therapy, *AIDS*, **7:** 1357–61.

Biehle J, Cavalieri SJ, 1992, In vitro susceptibility of *Mycobacterium kansasii* to clarithromycin, *Antimicrob Agents Chemother*, **36:** 2039–41.

Blacklock ZM, Dawson DJ et al., 1983, *Mycobacterium asiaticum* as a potential pulmonary pathogen for humans. A clinical and bacteriologic review of five cases, *Am Rev Respir Dis*, **127:** 241–4.

Bohle A, Kirsten D et al., 1992, Clinical evidence of systemic persistence of bacillus Calmette–Guérin: long term pulmonary bacillus Calmette–Guérin infection after intravesical therapy for bladder cancer and subsequent cystectomy, *J Urol*, **148**: 1894–7.

Bosquee L, Bottger EC et al., 1995, Cervical lymphadenitis caused by a fastidious *Mycobacterium* closely related to *Mycobacterium genavense* in an apparently immunocompetent woman: diagnosis by culture-free microbiological methods, *J Clin Microbiol*, **33**: 2670–4.

Bottger EC, Teske A et al., 1992, Disseminated '*Mycobacterium genavense*' infection in patients with AIDS, *Lancet*, **340**: 76–80.

Bouvet E, Casalino E et al., 1993, A nosocomial outbreak of multidrug-resistant *Mycobacterium bovis* among HIV-infected patients. A case control study, *AIDS*, **7**: 1453–60.

Branger B, Gouby A et al., 1985, *Mycobacterium haemophilum* and *Mycobacterium xenopi* associated infection in a renal transplant patient, *Clin Nephrol*, **23**: 46–9.

Breathnach A, Levell M et al., 1995, Cutaneous *Mycobacterium kansasii* infection: case report and review, *Clin Infect Dis*, **20**: 812–17.

Broadway DC, Kerr-Muir MG et al., 1994, *Mycobacterium chelonei* keratitis: a case report and review of previously reported cases, *Eye*, **8, Part1**: 134–42.

Brooks RW, Parker BC et al., 1984, Epidemiology of infection by nontuberculous mycobacteria. V. Numbers of eastern United States soils and correlation with soil characteristics, *Am Rev Respir Dis*, **130**: 630–3.

Brown BA, Wallace RJ Jr et al., 1992, Activities of four macrolides, including clarithromycin, against *Mycobacterium fortuitum*, *Mycobacterium chelonae*, and *Mycobacterium chelonae*-like organisms, *Antimicrob Agents Chemother*, **36**: 180–4.

Brown JW, Sanders CV, 1985, *Mycobacterium marinum* infections: a problem of recognition not therapy, *Arch Intern Med*, **147**: 817–18.

Brown RH, 1985, The rapidly growing mycobacteria – *M. fortuitum* and *M. chelonei*, *Infect Control*, **6**: 283–8.

Buhler VB, Pollack A, 1953, Human infection with atypical acid-fast organisms: report of two cases with pathologic findings, *Am J Clin Pathol*, **23**: 363–74.

Bullington Jr RH, Lanier JD, Font RL, 1992, Nontuberculous mycobacterial keratitis: report of two cases and review of the literature, *Arch Ophthalmol*, **110**: 519–24.

Castor B, Juhlin I, Henriques B, 1994, Septic cutaneous lesions caused by *Mycobacterium malmoense* in a patient with hairy cell leukemia, *Eur J Clin Microbiol Infect Dis*, **13**: 145–8.

Chin DP, Hopewell PC et al., 1994a, *Mycobacterium avium* complex in the respiratory or gastrointestinal tract and the risk of *M. avium* complex bacteremia in patients with human immunodeficiency virus infection, *J Infect Dis*, **169**: 289–95.

Chin DP, Reingold AL et al., 1994b, The impact of *Mycobacterium avium* complex bacteremia and its treatment on survival of AIDS patients – a prospective study, *J Infect Dis*, **170**: 578–84.

Chocarro A, Gonzalez Lopez A et al., 1994, Disseminated infection due to *Mycobacterium malmoense* in a patient infected with human immunodeficiency virus, *Clin Infect Dis*, **19**: 203–4.

Choudhri S, Manfreda J et al., 1995, Clinical significance of nontuberculous mycobacteria isolates in a Canadian tertiary care center, *Clin Infect Dis*, 128–33.

Christensen EE, Dietz GW et al., 1978, Radiographic manifestation of pulmonary *Mycobacterium kansasii*, *Am J Roentgenol*, **131**: 985–93.

Christensen EE, Dietz GW et al., 1981, Initial roentgenographic manifestations of pulmonary *Mycobacterium tuberculosis*, *M. kansasii*, and *Mycobacterium intracellulare* infections, *Chest*, **80**: 132–6.

Codias EK, Reinhardt DJ, 1979, Distribution of serotypes of *Mycobacterium avium-intracellulare-scrofulaceum* complex in Georgia, *Am Rev Respir Dis*, **119**: 965–70.

Collins CH, Grange JM et al., 1985, *M. marinum* infections in man, *J Hyg*, **94**: 135–49.

Colville A, 1993, Retrospective review of culture-positive myco-

bacterial lymphadenitis cases in children in Nottingham 1979–1990, *Eur J Clin Microbiol Infect Dis*, **12**: 192–5.

Connolly MG, Baughman RP, Dohn MN, 1993, *Mycobacterium kansasii* presenting as an endobronchial lesion, *Am Rev Respir Dis*, **148**: 1405–7.

Corpe R, 1981, Surgical management of pulmonary disease due to *Mycobacterium avium-intracellulare*, *Rev Infect Dis*, **3**: 1064–7.

Costrini AM, Mahler DA et al., 1981, Clinical and roentgenographic features of nosocomial pulmonary disease due to *Mycobacterium xenopi*, *Am Rev Respir Dis*, **123**: 104–9.

Cox JN, Brenner ER, Bryan CS, 1994, Changing patterns of mycobacterial disease at a teaching community hospital, *Infect Control Hosp Epidemiol*, **15**: 513–15.

Coyle MB, Carlson LDC et al., 1992, Laboratory aspects of '*Mycobacterium genavense*', a proposed species isolated from AIDS patients, *J Clin Microbiol*, **30**: 3206–12.

Dankner WM, Waecker NJ et al., 1993, *Mycobacterium bovis* infections in San Diego: a clinicoepidemiologic study of 73 patients and a historical review of a forgotten pathogen, *Medicine (Baltimore)*, **72**: 11–37.

Darling TN, Sidhu-Malik N et al., 1994, Treatment of *Mycobacterium haemophilum* infection with an antibiotic regimen including clarithromycin, *Br J Dermatol*, **131**: 376–9.

Dattwyler RJ, Thomas J, Hurst LC, 1987, Antigen-specific T-cell anergy in progressive *M. marinum* infection in humans, *Ann Intern Med*, **107**: 675–7.

Dautzenberg B, Piperno D et al., 1995, Clarithromycin in the treatment of *Mycobacterium avium* lung infections in patients without AIDS, *Chest*, **107**: 1035–40.

Davidson PT, Khanijo V et al., 1981, Treatment of disease due to *Mycobacterium intracellulare*, *Rev Infect Dis*, **3**: 1052–9.

Dawson DJ, 1990, Infection with *Mycobacterium avium* complex in Australian patients with AIDS, *Med J Aust*, **153**: 466–8.

Debrunner M, Salfinger M et al., 1992, Epidemiology and clinical significance of nontuberculous mycobacteria in patients negative for human immunodeficiency virus in Switzerland, *Clin Infect Dis*, **15**: 330–45.

Delabie J, DeWolf-Peeters C et al., 1991, Immunophenotypic analysis of histiocytes involved in AIDS-associated *Mycobacterium scrofulaceum* infection: similarities with lepromatous lepra, *Clin Exp Immunol*, **85**: 214–18.

Delaney V, Sumrani N et al., 1993, Mycobacterial infections in renal allograft recipients, *Transplant Proc*, **25**: 2288–9.

Delaporte E, Alfandari S, Piette F, 1994, *Mycobacterium ulcerans* associated with infection due to the human immunodeficiency virus, *Clin Infect Dis*, **18**: 839.

Dever LL, Martin JW et al., 1992, Varied presentations and responses to treatment of infections caused by *Mycobacterium haemophilum* in patients with AIDS, *Clin Infect Dis*, **14**: 1195–200.

Disla E, Reddy A et al., 1995, Primary *Mycobacterium avium* complex septic arthritis in a patient with AIDS, *Clin Infect Dis*, **20**: 1432–4.

Dutt AK, Stead WW, 1979, Long-term results of medical treatment in *Mycobacterium intracellulare* infection, *Am J Med*, **67**: 449–53.

Dwork AJ, Chin S, Boyce L, 1994, Intracerebral *Mycobacterium avium-intracellulare* in a child with acquired immunodeficiency syndrome, *Pediatr Infect Dis J*, **13**: 1149–51.

Edelstein H, 1994, *Mycobacterium marinum* skin infections. Report of 31 cases and review of the literature, *Arch Intern Med*, **154**: 1359–64.

Edwards LV, Acquaviva FA et al., 1969, An atlas of sensitivity to tuberculin, PPD-B, and histoplasmin in the United States, *Am Rev Respir Dis*, **99**: 1–132.

Eichmann A, Huszar A, Bon A, 1993, *Mycobacterium chelonae* infection of lymph nodes in an HIV-infected patient, *Dermatology*, **187**: 299–300.

Ellis ME, 1988, Mycobacteria other than *M. tuberculosis*, *Curr Opin Infect Dis*, **1**: 252–71.

Eng RHK, Forrester C et al., 1984, *Mycobacterium xenopi* infection in a patient with acquired immunodeficiency syndrome, *Chest*, **86**: 145–7.

Engbaek HC, Vergmann B, Bentzon MW, 1981, Lung disease caused by *Mycobacterium avium/Mycobacterium intracellulare*: an analysis of Danish patients during the period 1962–1976, *Eur J Respir Dis*, **62**: 72–83.

Etzkorn ET, Aldarondo S et al., 1986, Medical therapy of *Mycobacterium avium-intracellulare* pulmonary disease, *Am Rev Respir Dis*, **134**: 442–5.

Evans AJ, Crisp AJ et al., 1993, Pulmonary infections caused by *Mycobacterium malmoense* and *Mycobacterium tuberculosis*: comparison of radiographic features, *Am J Roentgenol*, **161**: 733–7.

Falkinham JO III, 1994, Epidemiology of *Mycobacterium avium* infections in the pre- and post-HIV era, *Res Microbiol*, **145**: 169–72.

Falkinham JO III, Parker BC, Gruft H, 1980, Epidemiology of infection by nontuberculous mycobacteria, *Am Rev Respir Dis*, **121**: 931–7.

Feldman WH, Davis R et al., 1943, An unusual mycobacterium isolate from sputum of a man suffering from pulmonary disease of long duration, *Am Rev Tuberc*, **48**: 82–93.

Frothingham R, Wilson KH, 1994, Molecular phylogeny of the *Mycobacterium avium* complex demonstrates clinically meaningful divisions, *J Infect Dis*, **169**: 305–12.

Fry KL, Meissner PS, Falkinham JO, 1986, Epidemiology of infection by nontuberculous mycobacteria. VI. Identification and use of epidemiologic markers for studies of *Mycobacterium avium*, *M. intracellulare*, and *M. scrofulaceum*, *Am Rev Respir Dis*, **134**: 39–43.

Gaynor CD, Clark RA et al., 1994, Disseminated *Mycobacterium genavense* infection in two patients with AIDS, *Clin Infect Dis*, **18**: 455–7.

Gleason-Morgan D, Church JA, Ross LA, 1994, A comparative study of transfusion-acquired human immunodeficiency virus-infected children with and without disseminate *Mycobacterium avium* complex, *Pediatr Infect Dis J*, **13**: 484–8.

Gluckman SJ, 1995, *Mycobacterium marinum*, *Clin Dermatol*, **13**: 273–6.

Glynn PJ, 1972, The use of surgery and local temperature elevation in *Mycobacterium ulcerans* infection, *Aust N Z J Surg*, **41**: 312–19.

Good RC, Snider DE, 1982, Isolation of non-tuberculosis mycobacterium in the United States, 1980, *J Infect Dis*, **146**: 829–33.

Goutzamanis JJ, Gilbert GL, 1995, *Mycobacterium ulcerans* infection in Australian children: report of eight cases and review, *Clin Infect Dis*, **21**: 1186–92.

Gribetz AR, Damsker B et al., 1981, Solitary pulmonary nodules due to non-tuberculous mycobacteria infection, *Am J Med*, **70**: 39–43.

Griffith DE, Girard WM, Wallace RJ Jr, 1993, Clinical features of pulmonary disease caused by rapidly growing mycobacteria: analysis of 154 patients, *Am Rev Respir Dis*, **147**: 1271–8.

Gruft H, Katz J, Blanchard DC, 1975, Postulated source of *Mycobacterium intracellulare* (Battey) infection, *Am J Epidemiol*, **102**: 311–18.

Gubler JG, Salfinger M, von Graevenitz A, 1992, Pseudoepidemic of nontuberculous mycobacteria due to a contaminated bronchoscope cleaning machine – report of an outbreak and review of the literature, *Chest*, **101**: 1245–9.

Gupta RC, Lavengood Jr R, Smith JP, 1988, Miliary tuberculosis due to intravesical bacillus Calmette–Guérin therapy, *Chest*, **94**: 1296–8.

Guthertz LS, Damsker B et al., 1989, *Mycobacterium avium* and *Mycobacterium intracellulare* infections in patients with and without AIDS, *J Infect Dis*, **160**: 1037–41.

Gyure KA, Prayson RA et al., 1995, Symptomatic *Mycobacterium avium* complex infection of the central nervous system – a case report and review of the literature, *Arch Pathol Lab Med*, **119**: 836–9.

Hakim A, Hisam N, Reuman PD, 1993, Environmental mycobac-

terial peritonitis complicating peritoneal dialysis: three cases and review, *Clin Infect Dis*, **16**: 426–31.

Hakim S, Heaney JA et al., 1993, Psoas abscess following intravesical bacillus Calmette–Guérin for bladder cancer: a case report, *J Urol*, **150**: 188–90.

Harth M, Ralph ED, Faraawi R, 1994, Septic arthritis due to *Mycobacterium marinum*, *J Rheumatol*, **21**: 957–60.

Havlir DV, 1994, *Mycobacterium avium* complex: advances in therapy, *Eur J Clin Microbiol Infect Dis*, **13**: 915–24.

Hayman J, 1993, Out of Africa: observations on the histopathology of *Mycobacterium ulcerans* infection, *J Clin Pathol*, **46**: 5–9.

Heifets L, Lindholm-Levy PJ, Comstock RD, 1992, Clarithromycin minimal inhibitory and bactericidal concentration against *Mycobacterium avium*, *Am Rev Respir Dis*, **145**: 856–8.

Heifets L, Mor N, Vanderkolk J, 1994, *Mycobacterium avium* strains resistant to clarithromycin and azithromycin, *Antimicrob Agents Chemother*, **37**: 2364–70.

Heifets LB, 1982, Synergistic effect of rifampin, streptomycin, ethionamide, and ethambutol on *Mycobacterium intracellulare*, *Am Rev Respir Dis*, **125**: 43–8.

Heifets LB, 1988, Qualitative and quantitative drug susceptibility tests in mycobacteriology, *Am Rev Respir Dis*, **137**: 1217–22.

Henderson HM, Chapman SW, 1994, *Mycobacterium avium-intracellulare*, *Curr Opin Infect Dis*, **7**: 225–30.

Henriques B, Hoffner SE et al., 1994, Infection with *Mycobacterium malmoense* in Sweden: report of 221 cases, *Clin Infect Dis*, **18**: 596–600.

Higgins EM, Lawrence CM, 1988, Sporotrichoid spread of *Mycobacterium chelonei*, *Clin Exp Dermatol*, **13**: 234–6.

Hirasuna JD, 1987, Disseminated *Mycobacterium kansasii* infection in the acquired immunodeficiency syndrome (AIDS), *Ann Intern Med*, **107**: 784.

Hirschel B, Chang HR et al., 1990, Fatal infection with a novel, unidentified mycobacterium in a man with the acquired immunodeficiency syndrome, *N Engl J Med*, **323**: 109–13.

Hockmeyer WT, Krieg RE et al., 1978, Further characterization of *Mycobacterium ulcerans* toxin, *Infect Immun*, **21**: 124–8.

Hoffman GS, Myers RL et al., 1978, Septic arthritis associated with *Mycobacterium-avium*: a case report and literature review, *J Rheumatol*, **5**: 199–209.

Hoffner SE, 1994, Pulmonary infections caused by less frequently encountered slow-growing environmental mycobacteria, *Eur J Clin Microbiol Infect Dis*, **13**: 937–41.

Holland DJ, Chen SCA et al., 1994, *Mycobacterium neoaurum* infection of a Hickman catheter in an immunosuppressed patient, *Clin Infect Dis*, **18**: 1002–3.

Hoop RK, Bottger EC et al., 1993, Mycobacteriosis due to *Mycobacterium genavense* in six pet birds, *J Clin Microbiol*, **31**: 990–3.

Hoover DR, Graham NMH et al., 1995, An epidemiologic analysis of *Mycobacterium avium* complex disease in homosexual men infected with human immunodeficiency virus type 1, *Clin Infect Dis*, **20**: 1250–8.

Hornick DB, Dayton CS et al., 1988, Nontuberculous mycobacterial lung disease: substantiation of a less aggressive approach, *Chest*, **93**: 550–5.

Horsburgh Jr CR, Havlik JA, Ellis DA, 1991, Survival of patients with acquired immune deficiency syndrome and disseminated *Mycobacterium avium* complex infection with and without antimycobacterial chemotherapy, *Am Rev Respir Dis*, **144**: 557–9.

Horsburgh Jr CR, Selik RM, 1989, The epidemiology of disseminated nontuberculous mycobacterial infection in the acquired immunodeficiency syndrome (AIDS), *Am Rev Respir Dis*, **139**: 4–7.

Horsburgh Jr CR, Mason III UG et al., 1985, Disseminated infection with *Mycobacterium avium-intracellulare*: a report of 13 cases and a review of the literature, *Medicine (Baltimore)*, **64**: 36–48.

Horsburgh Jr CR, Chin DP et al., 1994a, Environmental risk factors for acquisition of *Mycobacterium avium* complex in persons with human immunodeficiency virus infection, *J Infect Dis*, **170**: 362–7.

Horsburgh Jr CR, Metchock B et al., 1994b, Predictors of survival in patients with AIDS and disseminated *Mycobacterium avium* complex disease, *J Infect Dis*, **170**: 573–7.

Hoy JK, Rolston L, Hopfer RL, 1987, Pseudoepidemic of *M. fortuitum* in bone marrow cultures, *Am J Infect Control*, **15**: 268–71.

Huminer D, Pitlik SD et al., 1986, Aquarium-borne *Mycobacterium marinum* skin infection: report of a case and review of the literature, *Arch Dermatol*, **122**: 698–703.

Ichiyama S, Shimokata K, Tsukamura M, 1988, The isolation of *Mycobacterium avium* complex from soil, water, and dust, *Microbiol Immunol*, **32**: 733–9.

Inderlied CB, Kemper CA, Bermudez LE, 1993, The *Mycobacterium avium* complex, *Clin Microbiol Rev*, **6**: 266–310.

Ingram CW, Tanner DC et al., 1993, Disseminated infection with rapidly growing mycobacteria, *Clin Infect Dis*, **16**: 463–71.

Iseman MD, 1989, *Mycobacterium avium* complex and the normal host: the other side of the coin, *N Engl J Med*, **321**: 896–8.

Iseman MD, Corpe FR et al., 1985, Disease due to *Mycobacterium avium-intracellulare*, *Chest*, **87, Suppl.**: 139S–49S.

Izes JK, Bihrle III W, Thomas CB, 1993, Corticosteroid-associated fatal mycobacterial sepsis occurring 3 years after instillation of intravesical bacillus Calmette–Guérin, *J Urol*, **150**: 1498–500.

Jacoby HM, Jiva TM et al., 1995, *Mycobacterium xenopi* infection masquerading as pulmonary tuberculosis in two patients infected with human immunodeficiency virus, *Clin Infect Dis*, **20**: 1399–401.

Johnson L, Kiehn TE, 1994, *Mycobacterium avium* complex infections in cancer patients, *Infect Med*, **11**: 184–6.

Johnston JM, Izumi AK, 1987, Cutaneous *Mycobacterum marinum* infection ('swimming pool granuloma'), *Clin Dermatol*, **5**: 68–75.

Jones PG, Schrager MA, Zabransky RJ, 1995, Pott's disease caused by *Mycobacterium xenopi*, *Clin Infect Dis*, **21**: 1352.

Joshi W, Davidson PM et al., 1989, Non-tuberculous mycobacterial lymphadenitis in children, *Eur J Pediatr*, **148**: 751–4.

Joynson DH, 1979, Water: the natural habitat of *Mycobacterium kansasii?*, *Tubercle*, **60**: 77–81.

Kakinuma H, Suzuki H, 1994, *Mycobacterium avium* complex infection limited to the skin in a patient with systemic lupus erythematosus, *Br J Dermatol*, **130**: 785–90.

Kalayjian RC, Toossi Z et al., 1995, Pulmonary disease due to infection by *Mycobacterium avium* complex in patients with AIDS, *Clin Infect Dis*, **20**: 1186–94.

Kallenius G, Melles H et al., 1993, Why *Mycobacterium avium* and not *M. malmoense?*, *Program and Abstracts of the 33rd Interscience Conference on Antimicrobial Agents and Chemotherapy*, Abstract #486: 208.

Kemper CA, Havlir D et al., 1994, Transient bacteremia due to *Mycobacterium avium* complex in patients with AIDS, *J Infect Dis*, **170**: 488–93.

Kennedy TP, Weber DJ, 1994, Nontuberculous mycobacteria, an under-appreciated cause of geriatric lung disease, *Am J Respir Crit Care Med*, **149**: 1654–8.

Kent PT, Kubica GP, 1985, *Public Health Mycobacteriology – A Guide for the Level III Laboratory*, US Department of Health and Human Services, Center for Disease Control, Atlanta, GA.

Khooshabeh R, Grange JM et al., 1994, A case report of *Mycobacterium chelonae* keratitis and a review of mycobacterial infections of the eye and orbit, *Tuber Lung Dis*, **75**: 377–82.

Kiehn TE, 1993, The diagnostic mycobacteriology laboratory of the 1990s, *Clin Infect Dis*, **17**: S447–454.

Kiehn TE, White M, 1994, *Mycobacterium haemophilum*: an emerging pathogen, *Eur J Clin Microbiol Infect Dis*, **13**: 925–31.

Kiehn TE, White M et al., 1993, A cluster of four cases of *Mycobacterium haemophilum* infection, *Eur J Clin Microbiol Infect Dis*, **12**: 114–18.

Kilby JM, Gilligan PH et al., 1992, Non-tuberculous mycobacterial in adult patients with cystic fibrosis, *Chest*, **102**: 70–5.

Kramers C, Raemaekers JMM et al., 1992, Sweet's syndrome as the presenting symptom of hairy cell leukemia with concomitant infection by *Mycobacterium kansasii*, *Ann Hematol*, **65**: 55–8.

Lai KK, Stottmeier KD et al., 1984, Mycobacterial cervical lymphadenopathy: relation of etiologic agents to age, *JAMA*, **251**: 1286–8.

Lallemant-le Coeur S, Lallemant M et al., 1993, Bacillus Calmette–Guérin immunization in infants born to HIV-1-seropositive mothers, *AIDS*, **7**: 149–57.

Lambertus MW, Mathisen GE, 1988, *Mycobacterium marinum* infection in a patient with cryptosporidiosis and the acquired immunodeficiency syndrome, *Cutis*, **42**: 38–40.

Lamm DL, Stogdill VD et al., 1986, Complications of bacillus Calmette–Guérin immunotherapy in 1,278 patients with bladder cancer, *Urology*, **135**: 272–4.

Laszlo A, Siddiqi SH, 1984, Evaluation of a rapid radiometric differentiation test for the *Mycobacterium tuberculosis* complex by selective inhibition with p-nitro-α-acetylamino-β-hydroxy-propiophenone, *J Clin Microbiol*, **19**: 694–8.

LeMense GP, Strange C, 1994, Granulomatous pneumonitis following intravesical BCG: what therapy is needed, *Chest*, **106**: 1624–6.

Lessnau K-D, Milanese S, Talavera W, 1993, *Mycobacterium gordonae*: a treatable disease in HIV-positive patients, *Chest*, **104**: 1779–85.

Levin M, 1994, Acute hypersplenism and thrombocytopenia: a new presentation of disseminated mycobacterial infection in patients with acquired immunodeficiency syndrome, *Acta Haematol*, **91**: 28–31.

Levy-Frebault V, Pangon B et al., 1987, *Mycobacterium simiae* and *Mycobacterium avium-Mycobacterium intracellulare* mixed infection in acquired immune deficiency syndrome, *J Clin Microbiol*, **42**: 154–7.

Li C, Szuba MJ et al., 1994, *Mycobacterium kansasii* sinusitis in a patient with AIDS, *Clin Infect Dis*, **19**: 792–3.

Liu F, Andrews D, Wright DN, 1984, *Mycobacterium thermoresistibile* infection in an immunocompromised host, *J Clin Microbiol*, **19**: 546–7.

Livingston RA, Siberry GK et al., 1995, *Mycobacterium avium* complex in an adolescent infected with the human immunodeficiency virus, *Clin Infect Dis*, **20**: 1579–80.

Love GL, 1987, Nontuberculous mycobacterial skin infection resembling lepromatous leprosy, *South Med J*, **80**: 1060–1.

Luquin M, Ausina V et al., 1991, Evaluation of practical chromatographic procedures for identification of clinical isolates of mycobacteria, *J Clin Microbiol*, **29**: 120–30.

MacCallum P, Tolhurst JC et al., 1948, A new mycobacterial infection in man, *J Pathol Bacteriol*, **60**: 93–122.

McParland C, Cotton DJ et al., 1992, Miliary *Mycobacterium bovis* induced by intravesical bacille Calmette–Guérin immunotherapy, *Am Rev Respir Dis*, **146**: 1330–3.

McWhinney PHM, Yates M et al., 1992, Infection caused by *Mycobacterium chelonae*: a diagnostic and therapeutic problem in the neutropenic patient, *Clin Infect Dis*, **14**: 1208–12.

Malessa R, Diener H-C et al., 1994, Successful treatment of meningoencephalitis caused by *Mycobacterium avium intracellulare* in AIDS, *Clin Investig*, **72**: 850–2.

Maloney JM, Gregg CR et al., 1987, Infections caused by *Mycobacterium szulgai* in humans, *Rev Infect Dis*, **9**: 1120–6.

Marks J, Schwabacher H, 1965, Infection due to *Mycobacterium xenopei*, *Br Med J*, **1**: 32–3.

Marston BJ, Diallo MO et al., 1995, Emergence of Buruli ulcer disease in the Daloa region of Cote d'Ivoire, *Am J Trop Med Hyg*, **52**: 219–24.

Marx CE, Fan K et al., 1995, Laboratory and clinical evaluation of *Mycobacterium xenopi* isolates, *Diagn Microbiol Infect Dis*, **21**: 195–202.

Maschek H, Georgii A et al., 1994, *Mycobacterium genavense*: autopsy findings in three patients, *Am J Clin Pathol*, **101**: 95–9.

Masur H, 1993, Recommendations on prophylaxis and therapy

for disseminated *Mycobacterium avium* complex disease in patients infected with the human immunodeficiency virus, *N Engl J Med*, **329:** 898–903.

Matsiota-Bernard P, Thierry D et al., 1995, *Mycobacterium genavense* infection in a patient with AIDS who was successfully treated with clarithromycin, *Clin Infect Dis*, **20:** 1565–6.

Meisner G, Anz W, 1977, Sources of *Mycobacteriaum avium* complex infection resulting in human disease, *Am Rev Respir Dis*, **116:** 1057–64.

Meissner PS, Falkinham JO, 1986, Plasmid DNA profiles as epidemiologic markers for clinical and environmental isolates of *Mycobacterium avium*, *Mycobacterium intracellulare*, and *Mycobacterium scrofulaceum*, *J Infect Dis*, **153:** 325–31.

Miller WC, Perkins MD et al., 1994, Pott's disease caused by *Mycobacterium xenopi*: case report and review, *Clin Infect Dis*, **19:** 1024–8.

Miralles GD, Bregman Z, 1994, Necrotizing pyomyositis caused by *Mycobacterium avium* complex in a patient with AIDS, *Clin Infect Dis*, **18:** 833–4.

Moerman M, Dierick J et al., 1993, Mastoiditis caused by atypical mycobacteria, *Int J Pediatr Otorhinolaryngol*, **28:** 69–76.

Montecalvo MA, Forester G et al., 1994, Colonisation of potable water with *Mycobacterium avium* complex in homes of HIV-infected patients, *Lancet*, **343:** 1639.

Moreno F, Sharkey-Mathis PK et al., 1994, *Mycobacterium kansasii* pericarditis in patients with AIDS, *Clin Infect Dis*, **19:** 967–9.

Morrissey AB, Aisu TO et al., 1992, Absence of *Mycobacterium avium* complex disease in patients with AIDS in Uganda, *AIDS*, **5:** 477–8.

du Moulin GC, Stottmeier KD et al., 1988, Concentration of *Mycobacterium avium* by hospital hot water systems, *JAMA*, **260:** 1599–601.

Muelder K, Nourou A, 1990, Buruli ulcer in Benin, *Lancet*, **336:** 1109–11.

Murdoch ME, Leigh IM, 1989, Sporotrichoid spread of cutaneous *Mycobacterium chelonei* infection, *Clin Exp Dermatol*, **14:** 309–12.

Naguib MT, Byers JM, Slater LN, 1994, Paranasal sinus infection due to atypical mycobacteria in two patients with AIDS, *Clin Infect Dis*, **19:** 789–91.

Nel EE, 1981, *Mycobacterium-avium-intracellulare* complex serovars isolated in South Africa from humans, swine, and the environment, *Rev Infect Dis*, **3:** 1013–20.

Newport M, Levin M, 1994, Familial disseminated atypical mycobacterial disease, *Immunol Lett*, **43:** 133–8.

Newshan G, Torres RA, 1994, Pulmonary infection due to multi-drug-resistant *Mycobacterium szulgai* in a patient with AIDS, *Clin Infect Dis*, **18:** 1022–3.

Nightingale SD, Byrd LT et al., 1992, Incidence of *Mycobacterium avium-intracellulare* complex bacteremia in human immunodeficiency virus-positive patients, *J Infect Dis*, **165:** 1082–5.

Nightingale SD, Camerson DW et al., 1993, Two controlled trials of rifabutin prophylaxis against *Mycobacterium avium* complex infection in AIDS, *N Engl J Med*, **329:** 828–33.

Novick RJ, Moreno-Cabral CE, Stinson EB, 1990, Nontuberculous mycobacterial infections in heart transplant recipients: a seventeen-year experience, *J Heart Transplant*, **9:** 357–63.

Nye K, Chadha DK et al., 1990, *Mycobacterium chelonei* isolation from bronchoalveolar lavage and its practical implications, *J Hosp Infect*, **16:** 257–61.

O'Brien RJ, Geiter LJ, Lyle MA, 1990, Rifabutin (ansamycin LM427) for the treatment of pulmonary *Mycobacterium avium* complex, *Am Rev Respir Dis*, **141:** 821–6.

O'Brien RJ, Geiter L, Snider DE, 1987, The epidemiology of nontuberculous mycobacterial diseases in the United States, *Am Rev Respir Dis*, **135:** 1007–14.

Orme IM, Collins FM, 1985, Prophylactic effect in mice of BCG vaccination against non-tuberculous mycobacterial infections, *Tubercle*, **66:** 117–20.

Pang SC, 1991, *Mycobacterium kansasii* infections in Western Australia (1967–1987), *Respir Med*, **85:** 213–18.

Parent LJ, Salam MM et al., 1995, Disseminated *Mycobacterium marinum* infection and bacteremia in a child with severe combined immunodeficiency, *Clin Infect Dis*, **21:** 1325–7.

Parenti DM, Symington JS et al., 1995, *Mycobacterium kansasii* bacteremia in patients infected with human immunodeficiency virus, *Clin Infect Dis*, **21:** 1001–3.

Parker BC, Ford MA et al., 1983, Epidemiology of infection by nontuberculous mycobacteria. IV. Preferential aerososlization of *Mycobacterium intracellulare* from natural waters, *Am Rev Respir Dis*, **128:** 652–6.

Parrot RG, Grosset JH, 1988, Post-surgical outcome of 57 patients with *Mycobacterium xenopi* pulmonary infection, *Tubercle*, **69:** 47–55.

Patel R, Roberts GD et al., 1994, Infections due to nontuberculous mycobacteria in kidney, heart, and liver transplant recipients, *Clin Infect Dis*, **19:** 263–73.

Pechere M, Opravil M et al., 1995, Clinical and epidemiologic features of infection with *Mycobacterium genavense*, *Arch Intern Med*, **155:** 400–4.

Peters M, Schurmann D et al., 1989, Immunosuppression and mycobacteria other than *Mycobacterium tuberculosis*: results from patients with and without HIV infection, *Epidemiol Infect*, **103:** 293–300.

Piersimoni C, Tortoli E, De Sio G, 1994, Disseminated infection due to *Mycobacterium celatum* in patient with AIDS, *Lancet*, **344:** 332.

Porrman JC, Katon RM, 1994, Small bowel involvement by *Mycobacterium avium* complex in a patient with AIDS: endoscopic, histologic, and radiographic similarities to Whipple's disease, *Gastrointest Endosc*, **40:** 753–9.

Prince DS, Peterson DD et al., 1989, Infection with *Mycobacterium avium* complex in patients without predisposing conditions, *N Engl J Med*, **321:** 863–8.

Raffalli J, Kiehn TE, 1994, Infections with rapidly growing mycobacteria in patients with cancer, *Infect Med*, **11:** 649–52.

Rastogi N, Goh KS, David HL, 1990, Enhancement of drug susceptibility of *Mycobacterium avium* by inhibitors of cell envelope synthesis, *Antimicrob Agents Chemother*, **34:** 759–64.

Rastogi N, Frehel C et al., 1981, Multiple drug resistance in *Mycobacterium avium*: is the wall architecture responsible for the exclusion of antimicrobial agents?, *Antimicrob Agents Chemother*, **20:** 666–77.

Raszka Jr WV, Skillman LP et al., 1995, Isolation of nontuberculous, non-*avium* mycobacteria from patients infected with human immunodeficiency virus, *Clin Infect Dis*, **20:** 73–6.

Reich JM, Johnson RE, 1991, *Mycobacterium avium* complex pulmonary disease: incidence, presentation, and response to therapy in a community setting, *Am Rev Respir Dis*, **143:** 1381–5.

Reich JM, Johnson RE, 1992, *Mycobacterium avium* complex pulmonary disease presenting as an isolated lingular or middle lobe pattern. The Lady Windermere syndrome, *Chest*, **101:** 1605–9.

Reznikov MJ, Leggo HJ, Dawson DJ, 1974, Investigation by seroagglutination of strains of *Mycobacterium intracellulare-Mycobacterium scrofulaceum* group from house dust and sputum in southeastern Queensland, *Am Rev Respir Dis*, **104:** 951–3.

Rigsby MO, Curtis AM, 1994, Pulmonary disease from nontuberculous mycobacteria in patients with human immunodeficiency virus, *Chest*, **106:** 913–19.

Romanus V, 1983, Childhood tuberculosis in Sweden, *Tubercle*, **64:** 101–10.

Rosenzweig DY, 1979, Pulmonary mycobacterial infections due to *Mycobacterium intracellulare-avium* complex, *Chest*, **75:** 115–19.

Rosenzweig DY, Schleuter DB, 1981, Spectrum of clinical disease in pulmonary infection with *Mycobacterium avium-intracellulare*, *Rev Infect Dis*, **3:** 1046–51.

Runyon EH, 1959, Anonymous mycobacteria in pulmonary disease, *Med Clin North Am*, **43:** 273–90.

Rusch-Gerdes S, Wandelt-Freerksen E, Schroder K-H, 1985,

Occurrence of *Mycobacterium shimoidei* in West Germany, *Zentralbl Bakteriol Mikrobiol Hyg A*, **259**: 146–50.

Ryder RW, Oxtoby MJ, Mvula M, 1993, Safety and immunogenicity of bacille Calmette–Guérin, diphtheria–tetanus–pertussis, and oral polio vaccines in newborn children in Zaire infected with human immunodeficiency virus type 1, *J Pediatr*, **122**: 697–702.

Rynearson TK, Shronts JS, Wolinsky E, 1971, Rifampin: in vitro effect on atypical mycobacteria, *Am Rev Respir Dis*, **104**: 272–4.

Saito H, Sato K, Tomioka H, 1988, Comparative in vitro and in vivo activity of rifabutin and rifampicin against *Mycobacterium avium* complex, *Tubercle*, **69**: 187–92.

Salfinger M, Kafader FM, 1987, Comparison of two pretreatment methods for the detection of mycobacteria from BACTEC and Lowenstein–Jensen slants, *J Microbiol Methods*, **6**: 315–21.

Sanders JW, Walsh AD et al., 1995, Disseminated *Mycobacterium scrofulaceum* infection: a potentially treatable complication of AIDS, *Clin Infect Dis*, **20**: 549–56.

Schaad UB, Votteler TP et al., 1979, Management of atypical mycobacterial lymphadenitis in childhood: a review based on 380 cases, *J Pediatr*, **95**: 356–60.

Schraufnagel DE, Leech JA, Pollak B, 1986, *Mycobacterium kansasii*: colonization and disease, *Br J Dis Chest*, **80**: 131–7.

Schroder KH, Juhlin I, 1977, *Mycobacterium malmoense* sp. nov., *Int J Syst Bacteriol*, **27**: 241–6.

Schwabacher H, 1959, A strain of mycobacterium isolated from skin lesions of a cold-blooded animal, *Xenopus laevis* and its relation to atypical acid-fast bacilli occurring in man, *J Hyg*, **57**: 57–67.

Selik RM, Chu SY, Ward JW, 1995, Trends in infectious diseases and cancers among persons dying of HIV infection in the United States from 1987 to 1992, *Ann Intern Med*, **123**: 933–6.

Simor AE, Salit IE, Vellend H, 1984, The role of *Mycobacterium xenopi* in human disease, *Am Rev Respir Dis*, **129**: 435–8.

Simpson GL, Raffin TA, Remington JS, 1982, Association of prior nocardiosis and subsequent occurrence of nontuberculosis mycobacteriosis in a defined, immunosuppressed population, *J Infect Dis*, **146**: 211–19.

Sjogren I, 1981, Nontuberculous mycobacteria in Sweden: a brief summary, *Rev Infect Dis*, **3**: 1084–6.

Slutsky AM, Arbeit RD et al., 1994, Polyclonal infections due to *Mycobacterium avium* complex in patients with AIDS detected by pulsed-field gel electrophoresis of sequential clinical isolates, *J Clin Microbiol*, **32**: 1773–8.

Smith MJ, Citron KM, 1983, Clinical review of pulmonary disease caused by *Mycobacterium xenopi*, *Thorax*, **38**: 373–7.

Smith RL, Alexander RF, Aranda CP, 1993, Pulmonary granulomata: a complication of intravesical administration of bacillus Calmette–Guérin for superficial bladder carcinoma, *Cancer*, **71**: 1846–7.

Sniadack DH, Ostroff SM et al., 1993, A nosocomial pseudo-outbreak of *Mycobacterium xenopi* due to a contaminated potable water supply: lessons in prevention, *Infect Control Hosp Epidemiol*, **14**: 636–41.

Sompolinsky D, Lagziel D et al., 1978, *Mycobacterium haemophilum* sp. nov., a new pathogen of humans, *Int J Syst Bacteriol*, **28**: 67–75.

Soubani AO, Al-Marri M, Forlenza S, 1994, Successful treatment of disseminated *Mycobacterium haemophilum* infection in a patient with AIDS, *Clin Infect Dis*, **18**: 475–6.

Springer B, Tortoli E et al., 1995, *Mycobacterium conspicuum* sp. nov., a new species isolated from patients with disseminated infections, *J Clin Microbiol*, **33**: 2805–11.

Starke JR, Correa AG, 1995, Management of mycobacterial infection and disease in children, *Pediatr Infect Dis J*, **14**: 455–70.

Steere A, Corrales J, von Graevenitz A, 1979, A cluster of *Mycobacterium gordonae* isolates from bronchoscopy specimens, *Am Rev Respir Dis*, **120**: 214–16.

Stone MM, Vannier AM et al., 1995, Brief report: Meningitis due to Iatrogenic BCG infection in two immunosuppressed children, *N Engl J Med*, **333**: 561–3.

Straus WL, Ostroff SM et al., 1994, Clinical and epidemiologic characteristics of *Mycobacterium haemophilum*, an emerging pathogen in immunocompromised patients, *Ann Intern Med*, **120**: 118–25.

Sullam PM, Gordin FM et al., 1994, Efficacy of rifabutin in the treatment of disseminated infection due to *Mycobacterium avium* complex, *Clin Infect Dis*, **19**: 84–6.

Suster S, Moran CA, Blanco M, 1994, Mycobacterial spindle-cell pseudotumor of the spleen, *Am J Clin Pathol*, **101**: 539–42.

Swensen SJ, Hartman TE, Williams DE, 1994, Computed tomographic diagnosis of *Mycobacterium avium-intracellulare* complex in patients with bronchiectasis, *Chest*, **105**: 49–52.

Swenson JM, Wallace RJ Jr et al., 1985, Antimicrobial susceptibility of five subgroups of *Mycobacterium fortuitum* and *Mycobacterium chelonae*, *Antimicrob Agents Chemother*, **28**: 807–11.

Swetter SM, Kindel SE, Smoller BR, 1993, Cutaneous nodules of *Mycobacterium chelonae* in an immunosuppressed patient with preexisting pulmonary colonization, *J Am Acad Dermatol*, **28**: 352–5.

Taha AM, Davidson PT, Bailey WC, 1985, Surgical treatment of atypical mycobacterial lymphadenitis in children, *Pediatr Infect Dis*, **4**: 664–7.

Tebas P, Sultan F et al., 1995, Rapid development of resistance to clarithromycin following monotherapy for disseminated *Mycobacterium chelonae*, *Clin Infect Dis*, **20**: 443–4.

Thomas D, Leslie D et al., 1994, Disseminated *Mycobacterium avium-intracellulare* infection in an HIV-negative male, *Aust N Z J Med*, **24**: 403.

Thomas P, Liu F, Weiser W, 1988, Characteristics of *Mycobacterium xenopi* disease, *Bull Int Union Tuberc Lung Dis*, **63**: 12–13.

Tokars JI, McNeil MM et al., 1990, *Mycobacterium gordonae* pseudoinfection associated with a contaminated antimicrobial solution, *J Clin Microbiol*, **28**: 2765–9.

Torriani FJ, McCutchan JA et al., 1994, Autopsy findings in AIDS patients with *Mycobacterium avium* complex bacteremia, *J Infect Dis*, **170**: 1601–5.

Tortoli E, Peirsimoni C et al., 1995, Isolation of the newly described species *Mycobacterium celatum* from AIDS patients, *J Clin Microbiol*, **33**: 137–40.

Tsai SH, Yue WY, Duthoy EJ, 1968, Roentgen aspects of chronic pulmonary mycobacteriosis, *Radiology*, **90**: 306–10.

Tsukada H, Chou T et al., 1994, Disseminated *Mycobacterium avium*-intracellulare infection in a patient with myelodysplastic syndrome (refractory anemia), *Am J Hematol*, **45**: 325–9.

Tsukamura M, 1976, Properties of *Mycobacterium smegmatis* freshly isolated from soil, *Jpn J Microbiol*, **20**: 355–6.

Tsukamura M, 1983, Infections due to *Mycobacterium gordonae*, *Iryo*, **37**: 456–62.

Tsukamura M, Shimoide H, Schaefer WB, 1975, A possible new pathogen of group three mycobacteria, *J Gen Microbiol*, **88**: 377–80.

Tsukamura M, Kita N et al., 1988, Studies on the epidemiology of nontuberculous mycobacteriosis in Japan, *Am Rev Respir Dis*, **137**: 1280–4.

Valero G, Moreno F, Graybill JR, 1994, Activities of clarithromycin, ofloxacin, and clarithromycin plus ethambutol against *Mycobacterium simiae* in murine model of disseminated infection, *Antimicrob Agents Chemother*, **38**: 2676–7.

Valero G, Peters J et al., 1995, Clinical isolates of *Mycobacterium simiae* in San Antonio, Texas, *Am J Respir Crit Care Med*, **152**: 1555–7.

Von Reyn CF, Waddell RD et al., 1993, Isolation of *Mycobacterium avium* complex from water in the United States, Finland, Zaire, and Kenya, *J Clin Microbiol*, **31**: 3227–30.

Von Reyn CF, Maslow JN et al., 1994, Persistent colonization of potable water as a source of *Mycobacterium avium* infection in AIDS, *Lancet*, **343**: 1137–41.

Von Reyn CF, Jacobs NJ et al., 1995, Polyclonal *Mycobacterium avium* infections in patients with AIDS: variations in antimicrobial susceptibilities of different strains of *M. avium* isolated from the same patient, *J Clin Microbiol*, **33**: 1008–10.

Wald A, Coyle MB et al., 1992, Infections with a fastidious mycobacterium resembling *Mycobacterium simiae* in seven patients with AIDS, *Ann Intern Med*, **117**: 586–9.

Wallace RJ Jr, 1994, Recent changes in taxonomy and disease manifestations of the rapidly growing mycobacteria, *Eur J Clin Microbiol Infect Dis*, **13**: 953–60.

Wallace RJ Jr, Brown BA, Onyi GO, 1992, Skin, soft tissue, and bone infections due to *Mycobacterium chelonae chelonae*: importance of prior corticosteroid therapy, frequency of disseminated infections, and resistance to oral antimicrobials other than clarithromycin, *J Infect Dis*, **166**: 405–12.

Wallace RJ Jr, Swenson JM et al., 1983, Spectrum of disease due to rapidly growing mycobacteria, *Rev Infect Dis*, **5**: 657–79.

Wallace RJ Jr, Nash DR et al., 1988, Human disease due to *Mycobacterium smegmatis*, *J Infect Dis*, **158**: 52–9.

Wallace RJ Jr, Musser JM et al., 1989, Diversity and sources of rapidly growing mycobacteria associated with infections following cardiac surgery, *J Infect Dis*, **159**: 708–16.

Wallace RJ Jr, O'Brien R et al., 1990, The diagnosis and treatment of disease caused by non-tuberculosis mycobacteria, *Am Rev Respir Dis*, **142**: 940–53.

Wallace RJ Jr, Brown BA et al., 1991, Clinical disease, drug susceptibility, and biochemical patterns of the unnamed third biovariant complex of *M. fortuitum*, *J Infect Dis*, **163**: 598–603.

Wallace RJ Jr, Tanner D et al., 1993, Clinical trial of clarithromycin for cutaneous (disseminated) infection due to *M. chelonae*, *Ann Intern Med*, **119**: 482–6.

Wallace RJ Jr, Brown BA et al., 1994a, Initial clarithromycin monotherapy for *Mycobacterium avium-intracellulare* complex lung disease, *Am J Respir Crit Care Med*, **149**: 1335–41.

Wallace RJ Jr, Dunbar D et al., 1994b, Rifampin-resistant *Mycobacterium kansasii*, *Clin Infect Dis*, **18**: 736–43.

Wasem CF, McCarthy CM, Murray LW, 1991, Multi locus enzyme electrophoresis analysis of *Mycobacterium avium* complex and other mycobacteria, *J Clin Microbiol*, **29**: 264–71.

Wayne LG, Sramek HA, 1992, Agents of newly recognized or infrequently encountered mycobacterial disease, *Clin Microbiol Rev*, **5**: 1–25.

Weber J, Mettang T et al., 1989, Pulmonary disease due to *Mycobacterium xenopi* in a renal allograft recipient: a report of a case and review, *Rev Infect Dis*, **11**: 964–9.

Weinberger M, Berg SL et al., 1992, Disseminated infection with *Mycobacterium gordonae*: report of a case and critical review of the literature, *Clin Infect Dis*, **14**: 1229–39.

Weinroth SE, Pincetl P, Tuazon CU, 1994, Disseminated *Mycobacterium kansasii* infection presenting as pneumonia and osteomyelitis of the skull in a patient with AIDS, *Clin Infect Dis*, **18**: 261–2.

Weiszfeiler JG, Karasseva VT, Karczag E, 1971, A new mycobacterium species: *Mycobacterium asiaticum* n. sp., *Acta Microbiol Acad Sci Hung*, **18**: 247–52.

Weitzmann I, Osadczyi D et al., 1981, *Mycobacterium thermoresistibile*: a new pathogen for humans, *Rev Infect Dis*, **8**: 1024–33.

Weltman AC, Rose DN, 1993, The safety of Bacille Calmette–Guérin vaccination in HIV infection and AIDS, *AIDS*, **7**: 149–57.

Wendt SL, George KL et al., 1980, Epidemiology of infection by nontuberculous mycobacteria. III. Isolation of potentially pathogenic mycobacteria from aerosols, *Am Rev Respir Dis*, **122**: 259–63.

White R, Abreo K et al., 1993, Nontuberculous mycobacterial infections in continuous ambulatory peritoneal dialysis patients, *Am J Kidney Dis*, **22**: 581–7.

Witzig RS, Franzblau SG, 1993, Susceptibility of *Mycobacterium kansasii* to ofloxacin, sparfloxacin, clarithromycin, azithromycin, and fusidic acid, *Antimicrob Agents Chemother*, **37**: 1997–9.

Witzig RS, Fazal BA et al., 1995, Clinical manifestations and implications of co-infection with *Mycobacterium kansasii* and human immunodeficiency virus type 1, *Clin Infect Dis*, **21**: 77–85.

Wolinsky E, 1979, Nontuberculous mycobacteria and associated diseases, *Am Rev Respir Dis*, **119**: 107–59.

Wolinsky E, 1992, Mycobacterial diseases other than tuberculosis, *Clin Infect Dis*, **15**: 1–12.

Wolinsky E, Gomez F, Zimpfer F, 1972, Sporotrichoid *Mycobacterium marinum* infection treated with rifampin–ethambutol, *Am Rev Respir Dis*, **105**: 964–7.

Wolinsky E, Rynearson TK, 1968, Mycobacteria in soil and their relation to disease-associated strains, *Am Rev Respir Dis*, **97**: 1032–7.

Woods GL, Washington JA, 1987, Mycobacteria other than *M. tuberculosis*: review of microbiology and clinical aspects, *Rev Infect Dis*, **9**: 275–94.

Yajko DM, Chin DP et al., 1995, *Mycobacterium avium* complex in water, food, and soil samples collected from the environment of HIV-infected individuals, *J Acquired Immune Defic Syndr*, **9**: 176–82.

Yates MD, Pozniak A, Grange JM, 1993, Isolation of mycobacteria from patients seropositive for the human immunodeficiency virus (HIV) in south east England: 1984–92, *Thorax*, **48**: 990–5.

Young LS, Inderlied CB et al., 1986, Mycobacterial infections in AIDS patients, with an emphasis on the *Mycobacterium avium* complex, *Rev Infect Dis*, **8**: 1024–33.

Zaugg M, Salfinger M et al., 1993, Extrapulmonary and disseminated infections due to *Mycobacterium malmoense*: case report and review, *Clin Infect Dis*, **16**: 540–9.

Zimmer BL, DeYoung DR, Roberts GD, 1982, In vitro synergistic activity or ethambutol, isoniazid, kanamycin, rifampin, and streptomycin against *Mycobacterium avium-M. intracellulare* complex, *Antimicrob Agents Chemother*, **22**: 148–50.

Zvetina JR, Maliwan N et al., 1992, *Mycobacterium kansasii* infection following primary pulmonary malignancy, *Chest*, **102**: 1460–3.

LEPROSY, SARCOIDOSIS AND JOHNE'S DISEASE

M F R Waters

LEPROSY

1 HISTORY AND DISTRIBUTION

Leprosy has been defined as 'a chronic mycobacterial disease, infectious in some cases, primarily affecting the peripheral nervous system and secondarily involving skin and certain other tissues' (Jopling 1978a). The disease is of great antiquity, being well described in written records from India dated 600 BC and from China dated 150 BC. The first objective evidence of leprosy, based on palaeopathology, was obtained from Egyptian mummies of the second century BC, but not earlier (Dzierzykray-Rogalski 1980).

From Egypt, it appears that leprosy spread to Europe; by 150 AD it had reached Greece, and the bones of a skeleton dated fourth century AD, excavated from a Romano-British cemetery in Dorsetshire showed changes diagnostic of leprosy (Reader 1974). By the Middle Ages, it was widespread throughout Europe, and was introduced into the New World, to Central and South America by the Spanish and Portuguese invaders, and subsequently both there and into the southern states of the USA and the Caribbean isles by imported African slaves. It then declined rapidly in Europe, especially in the north, although a mini-epidemic occurred in Norway in the nineteenth century and from around 1850 to 1950 AD it spread widely in Oceania (see Browne 1985 for a detailed history of leprosy). Endemic leprosy died out in the UK by the end of the eighteenth century, although MacLeod (1925) reported 3 isolated indigenous cases, 2 in adolescent boys, who contracted the disease from a parent, elder sibling or spouse suffering from bacilliferous low-resistant 'lepromatous' leprosy infected overseas.

In 1983, the World Health Organization (WHO) estimated that the total number of cases of leprosy in the world was around 10.5 million, with over 5.3 million registered cases (Sansarricq 1983). At that time, treatment with dapsone alone was slow, and had often to be continued for 20 years or for life in 'lepromatous' leprosy and for 5 years in high-resistant 'tuberculoid' leprosy. The relapse rate was significant, especially in lepromatous leprosy. This form of treatment was just beginning to be replaced by multidrug therapy (MDT) (WHO Study Group 1982), analogous to that for the treatment of tuberculosis.

As a result of the introduction of MDT, by early 1996, it was estimated that the total caseload had fallen to 1.3 million, with 926 000 registered cases, 91% of whom were receiving MDT (WHO 1996). Over the previous 14 years, almost 8 million patients had received MDT, with extraordinarily low relapse rates, and the number of endemic countries (defined as having a prevalence of ≥1 : 10 000 population) had fallen to 60 (see Tables 23.1 and 23.2). Nevertheless, the annual case detection rate, which a decade ago was running at around 600 000 per annum was reported

Table 23.1 Estimated number of leprosy cases, by WHO region, 1996

WHO region	Estimated number of cases	Estimated prevalence per 10 000
Africa	170 000	3.2
Americas	170 000	2.2
South East Asia	830 000	6.0
Eastern Mediterranean	40 000	1.0
Western Pacific	50 000	0.3
Total	1 260 000	2.3

as 560 646 in 1994, and 529 376 in 1995. Because of the very long incubation period, it may take 10 years for a new intervention to show its full effect on the leprosy case detection rate (Irgens 1980). And there is some evidence that in many areas cases are being diagnosed on average earlier in the course of their disease. Therefore, it is probable that the true annual incidence is at last falling in areas with well established MDT programmes. But there are also probably between 1.5 and 3 million 'cured' leprosy patients left with significant permanent disability to hands, feet and/or face.

Leprosy is caused by an intracellular acid-fast bacillus, *Mycobacterium leprae*, whose discovery in 1874 by Hansen preceded that of *Mycobacterium tuberculosis* by some 8 years. Although it was the first member of the genus *Mycobacterium* to be described, *M. leprae* is one of the few human bacterial pathogens not yet successfully cultured in vitro. Fortunately, successful transmission of human leprosy to animals was achieved by Shepard in 1960, providing for the first time a means, albeit in vivo, of studying the microbiology of *M. leprae*, and showing that its generation time is 10–11 days. Exploitation and modification of animal infection techniques have done much over the past 4 decades to advance leprosy research. Moreover, to date about two-thirds of the *M. leprae* genome has been mapped, a gene library having been developed by Young et al. in 1985.

2 SPECTRUM OF LEPROSY AND CLINICAL MANIFESTATIONS

Leprosy characteristically displays a great diversity of clinical manifestations, the wide clinical 'spectrum' being related to host ability to develop and to maintain specific cell mediated immunity (CMI). In high resistant **tuberculoid** leprosy, the localized signs are restricted to skin and/or peripheral nerves; it is benign, chronic and often self-healing, and the lepromin reaction (see section 6, p. 449) is strongly positive. Low resistant **lepromatous** leprosy is a severe, generalized, progressive bacteraemic disease, widely and symmetrically involving the skin, peripheral nerves, upper respiratory tract (from the nasal mucosa to the larynx), the reticuloendothelial system, especially the superficial lymph nodes, spleen and Kupffer cells of the liver, the anterior part of the eye, testes and bone marrow; the lepromin reaction is negative.

Early workers emphasized these 2 polar forms, being named respectively 'anaesthetic' and 'nodular' by Danielssen and Boeck (1848) and 'maculoanaesthetic' and 'tuberosa' by Hansen and Looft (1895a). However, the many intermediate or **borderline** forms caused problems in classification, especially as they were often immunologically unstable, tending in the absence of effective treatment to lose CMI and to shift towards lepromatous, or after commencing effective treatment to regain CMI and to shift towards tuberculoid. Therefore many different classifications arose (see Dharmendra 1985), until Ridley and Jopling (1962, 1966) proposed one based on clear clinical, bacteriological (the concentration of bacilli in lesions) and immunohistopathological (the number and nature of lymphocytes in the leprous granuloma and the character of the bacterial host cells of the monocyte-macrophage series) evidence, which is now universally accepted. They divided the spectrum into 5 groups, namely tuberculoid, TT, borderline tuberculoid, BT, mid-borderline, BB, borderline lepromatous, BL, and lepromatous, LL. BT patients have a weak positive lepromin reaction, and BB and BL patients are lepromin-negative. In addition, Ridley and Jopling noted a very early, prespectrum indeterminate (idt) form, usually consisting of a single hypopigmented, hypoaesthetic macule, difficult to diagnose, and self-

Table 23.2 Registered cases of leprosy and coverage with multidrug therapy (MDT), by WHO region, 1996

WHO region	Registered cases	Prevalence per 10 000	Cases on MDT	MDT coverage (%)	Cured with MDT
Africa	95 901	1.77	87 739	91.5	443 610
Americas	123 537	1.64	93 004	75.3	225 450
South East Asia	651 562	4.72	610 669	93.7	7 059 925
Eastern Mediterranean	23 005	0.54	19 083	83.0	52 784
Western Pacific	32 254	0.20	31 943	99.0	206 635
Total	926 259	1.67	842 438	91.0	7 988 404

curing in around 75% of cases, the remainder going on to develop some form of spectrum leprosy.

The names of the 2 polar forms are derived from histopathological features. In the TT form, there are only few acid-fast bacilli (AFB), probably not more than 10^6 in toto, but there is a strong CMI response with numerous epithelioid cells, giant cells and lymphocytes, as in tuberculosis, although caseation only occurs, somewhat infrequently, in nerve trunks. In the LL form there is a striking granulomatous response with many undifferentiated macrophages, often seen as large foamy cells (Virchow cells) packed with AFB. In advanced cases there may be 10^9 *M. leprae* per g of skin, with a patient total bacterial population of up to 10^{12} AFB. In each type of patient the nerves, both sensory, motor and autonomic fibres, are affected, and AFB are present in Schwann and perineurial cells. No other bacterial species has the capacity to invade these nerve cells, even though mild histiocytic infiltrate may occur in nerves around blood vessels in advanced *M. lepraemurium* infection in mice. In tuberculoid infections, the asymmetrically affected nerves are infiltrated by epithelioid cells and lymphocytes, but there is only mild histiocytic infiltration in lepromatous cases. In all forms of leprosy, *M. leprae* organisms invade the nerves and eventually destroy nerve fibres. *M. leprae* invades both dermal nerves in skin lesions and nerve trunks, and occasionally, in TT and BT leprosy, one or more nerve trunks may be involved before the appearance of any skin lesions, so-called polyneuritic or neural leprosy. The most vulnerable sites are, for skin, those parts of the body which tend to remain cool, and for nerve trunks, those subject to trauma close to large joints. The Ridley–Jopling classification, which was originally devised for research purposes, has been used extensively because it contributes to our understanding of the clinical aspects of leprosy, giving guidance especially over prognosis and likely complications. For field use, however, a much simpler classification based on bacterial load has been devised (see p. 448).

Leprosy is an extremely chronic disease, which, if untreated, may be of lifelong duration. In TT and BT leprosy, after a variable length of time it may retrogress as the result of an increase in naturally acquired immunity, sometimes to relapse years later due to a decrease in CMI perhaps associated with intercurrent infection, pregnancy or old age. Even in lepromatous leprosy, disease activity used to vary spontaneously, although most patients died after perhaps 20 years, usually from renal failure due to secondary amyloidosis, intercurrent infection, or secondary pneumonia from laryngeal obstruction. Nowadays the mortality from leprosy itself is negligible, occasional patients dying from secondary amyloidosis or from secondary infection of anaesthetic extremities and neuropathic ulcers.

During the course of the disease, acute immunologically mediated exacerbations, known as 'reactions', commonly occur. There are 2 main varieties. Reversal or type 1 (Jopling 1978b) reaction, which occurs in borderline leprosy and in a minority of the LL patients who have evolved from borderline, is associated with an increase in specific CMI. It is characterized by erythema and swelling of skin lesions, new skin lesions sometimes developing, and by pain and tenderness of swollen nerves. Erythema nodosum leprosum (ENL) or type 2 reaction, which occurs only in LL and a small minority of BL patients, particularly during treatment, is due to an antibody–antigen reaction. Local formation of immune complexes in affected skin results in characteristic crops of small tender erythematous nodules resembling those in erythema nodosum, but more widespread, usually associated with malaise and pyrexia. Other systems may also be involved, leading to neuritis, iridocyclitis, orchitis and immune complex nephritis. Severe chronic ENL may last for years, until the bulk of the dead AFB are removed after 8–10 years in LL leprosy, and if such a reaction is not adequately suppressed, secondary amyloidosis may develop.

3 EPIDEMIOLOGY

In the past, leprosy was subject to few geographical restrictions. At present it occurs mainly in tropical and subtropical areas, between 35° North and 35° South. It has almost died out in Japan and some countries in southern Europe, and the incidence seems to have fallen significantly not only in low endemic areas, such as southern Russia, the Commonwealth of Independent States (CIS), and northern Australia, but also in China, Thailand and Malaysia. The disease is more common among the lower economic classes, associated with overcrowded, dimly lit living conditions (nasally excreted leprosy bacilli can survive for several days in poor light), although malnutrition appears to be much less important than with tuberculosis. After puberty, males are more often affected with 'spectrum' leprosy than females. In high endemic areas, infection seems to occur mainly in children and young adults. In the WHO BCG trial area in central Myanmar, where many children were probably infected by the age of 2 years, the peak incidence of 'tuberculoid' (TT, BT and idt) leprosy was in the age group 5–14 years and that of lepromatous (LL and BL) leprosy was 25–34 years, with a smaller late peak in the over-60 age group (Martinez Dominguez et al. 1980). Leprosy is extremely rare in infants, Brubaker, Meyers and Bourland (1985) being able to identify only 51 undoubted cases reported in children up to 12 months of age. The incubation period is therefore assumed usually to be a matter of years. Studies on patients born and normally resident in non-endemic areas, but who spent relatively brief periods in endemic areas, especially those on American and British servicemen, indicate incubation periods of 2–5 years and 8–12 years for tuberculoid (TT and BT) and lepromatous (BL and LL) leprosy respectively (Feldman and Sturdivant 1976; see Fine 1982). It is usually assumed that adults are far less susceptible than children, a view supported by the infrequency of conjugal leprosy, only around 5% of spouses of lepromatous patients contracting the disease, and by the failure of attempts to infect volunteers experimentally. These data may merely indicate that the majority of adults have already developed significant immunity, either from past exposure to *M. leprae*, or to other mycobacteria with common antigens, whether environmental saprophytes, *M. tuberculosis* or BCG. The infection rate in contacts appears to be high, but the attack rate for clinical disease is low, usually considerably less than the corresponding one for tuberculosis. The absence of a diagnostic skin test of infection, comparable to the Mantoux test, continues to hamper epidemiological studies.

Man is still regarded as the only significant reservoir of *M. leprae*, in spite of recent reports of natural infection with organisms resembling *M. leprae* in armadillos in one part of the USA, and apparently natural infection in a chimpanzee and a sooty mangabey monkey. Lepromatous (LL, BL) patients constitute the main source of infection, most tuberculoid patients being non-infectious. The skin and nasal mucosa are the 2 most heavily infected tissues, but transmission via nasal secretions seems likely in view of the finding that they are responsible in lepromatous patients for a mean daily output of 10^7 viable bacilli (Davey and Rees 1974). Intact skin and the commonly occurring trophic ulcers are meagre sources of bacilli (Weddell, Palmer and Rees 1963, Pedley 1970). Organisms may be shed from ulcerating lepromatous nodules, but these are rare (McDougall and Rees 1973). Infection by inhalation of droplets or droplet nuclei may be more common than infection via the skin. Rees and McDougall (1977) succeeded in transmitting leprosy to immunosuppressed mice by means of aerosols containing *M. leprae*, and Hastings and colleagues were able to infect nude mice through the upper, but not the lower, respiratory tract (Chehl, Job and Hastings 1985). Although *M. leprae* is excreted in the breast milk of an untreated lepromatous mother (Pedley 1967), the numbers of leprosy bacilli inhaled by her baby are likely to exceed greatly the number ingested. Narayanan et al. (1972) showed that mosquitos, which had fed on lepromatous patients, were capable of infecting mice, but the number of bacilli involved was minute, and it is doubtful whether insect transmission is of any importance. Transplacental transmission remains uncertain, although there is evidence that mycobacterial antigen may cross the placenta in untreated lepromatous mothers (Melsom, Harboe and Duncan 1982). Only 29 of the 51 leprous infants reported by Brubaker, Meyers and Bourland (1985) had leprous mothers, of whom only 14 had lepromatous (LL or BL) disease.

There are additional factors, defined or undefined, which are thought to determine the clinical expression of the disease:

3.1 Ethnic factors

It is said that Europeans, Burmese and Chinese are more susceptible than Africans, Indians and Melanesians. In Myanmar, lepromatous leprosy is more common in Burmese than Indians; in Malaysia it was more common in Chinese than in Malays and Indians. How much these different prevalences are due to environmental, cultural or genetic factors is uncertain. In Bangladesh, leprosy remains more common among Hindu tea-estate workers than in the surrounding, ethnically similar Moslem villagers, the former having emigrated several generations ago from a high prevalence area in Bengal.

3.2 Genetic factors

There is no satisfying evidence that genetic factors influence susceptibility to leprosy. But studies from Surinam, India and China have shown that the HLA-DR2 and DR3 alleles are associated with tuberculoid leprosy, whereas the HLA-DQw1 is expressed more frequently in lepromatous patients and in lepromin-negative individuals (Ottenhoff and de Vries 1987), suggesting that genetic influences affect the type of leprosy developed.

3.3 Environmental factors

Of great interest is the low risk of infection in contacts of infected immigrants in northern Europe. Since 1951, around 1300 imported cases of leprosy, including several hundred with untreated or relapsed lepromatous disease, have been notified in the UK, yet no secondary cases have been identified. In the Netherlands, there have been around 2000 imported cases; only a very few children of infected patients have developed clinical disease, and there has been only one case in a Dutchman who had never left the country or had a known contact (Browne 1980, Leiker 1980). The rarity of secondary cases in non-endemic areas suggests that the dose and duration of exposure, likely to be less in countries with good housing conditions and health services, may be important. Dockrell and colleagues (1991) reported evidence for transmission of infection, without development of clinical disease (subclinical infection), in 2 health-care workers tending an undiagnosed case of lepromatous leprosy in an old people's home where they had had close contact with the infectious patient throughout 11 months. Britain, but not the Netherlands, has routinely given BCG as tuberculosis prophylaxis, and also some child household contacts of lepromatous cases were given chemoprophylaxis with dapsone (Jopling, personal communication 1976) and more recently with rifampicin (Waters 1993).

4 DIAGNOSIS

The cardinal signs of leprosy are anaesthesia of the skin lesions, enlargement of nerves and the presence of *M. leprae* in affected skin and nasal mucosa. Leprosy can therefore usually be correctly diagnosed by careful palpation of the peripheral nerves of predilection, with a pen, piece of cotton wool or thermal tester to detect anaesthesia, and a scalpel to remove material for microscopic examination.

The skin provides the most readily available tissue from which to obtain *M. leprae*, by means of the 'slit-skin smear' technique. The chosen site is cleaned with alcohol and allowed to dry. Next a fold is pinched firmly between the thumb and index finger to render it avascular. Using a small sterile scalpel blade, an incision is made about 5 mm long and 3 mm deep, to penetrate well into the infiltrated layer of the dermis. If blood or much tissue juice exudes, it must be wiped off with a dry cotton swab. The scalpel blade is then turned at right angles to the cut and, with its blunt edge, one side of the wound is scraped 2–3 times to obtain tissue pulp from beneath the epidermis. This material is then transferred on the point of the scalpel to a glass microscope slide, where it is spread in a circular motion by the flat side of the blade to produce a uniformly and moderately thick smear over an area 5–7 mm in diameter. Smears are taken from both ear lobes and from the active edge of up to 4 skin lesions, and are positive for acid-fast bacilli in some BT and idt, and all BB, BL and LL untreated patients.

M. leprae is present in the nasal mucosa and nasal secretions of untreated LL and many BL patients. A moistened swab is used for obtaining material from the surface of the inferior turbinate bones. Nasal secretion is collected, preferably early in the morning, by blowing the nose into a polyethylene handkerchief. All samples are examined as smears on glass microscope slides.

All smears are allowed to dry, then are fixed and stained by the Ziehl–Neelsen technique (Fig. 23.1), care being taken not to overheat the carbol-fuchsin, nor, as *M. leprae* is more acid-fast and less alcohol-fast than *M. tuberculosis*, to over-decolorize if acid–alcohol is used. Positive slit-skin smears are scored according to the density of the acid-fast bacilli, the 'bacterial index' (BI; Ridley 1958), which gives an indirect indication of the total bacterial load; serial smears will indicate the response of the patient to chemotherapy. Serial smears can also be used to assess the 'morphological index' (MI; Rees and Waters 1963), which gives a measure of the viability of *M. leprae* on the basis of morphology; uniformly staining bacilli are probably alive, whereas irregularly staining bacilli are dead (Rees 1985).

No completely specific serological or skin test is as yet available despite a number of *M. leprae* antigens having been produced by genetic engineering. Studies of antibody to the species-specific phenolic glycolipid antigen (PGL-I) have proved somewhat disappointing; tuberculoid patients are often PGL-I antibody negative, and although a proportion of contacts and the general population in endemic areas are PGL-I antibody positive, the majority of these remain free of disease, and some negative subjects may later develop leprosy. The lepromin skin test (Mitsuda reaction, see section 6, p. 449) is not a diagnostic test, but is a guide to the resistance of the patient to a leprosy infection.

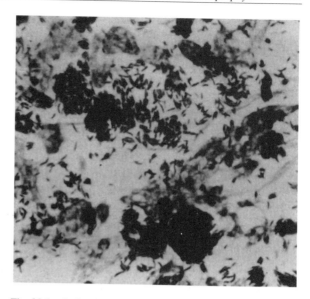

Fig. 23.1 Stained smear of nasal discharge from an untreated lepromatous patient showing *M. leprae* singly and in clumps ('globi') (× 1000).

5 TREATMENT AND PROPHYLAXIS

5.1 Treatment

In view of the antiquity of leprosy, there are surprisingly few historical accounts of treatment. One substance, chaulmoogra oil, had been used to treat leprosy in India for 2000 years and in China from the fifteenth century, and more purified preparations, given by mouth and by injection, were widely used during the period 1850–1900. Hansen and Looft (1895b), in an excellent and nihilistic chapter, described how none of the then recommended remedies, including chaulmoogra oil and Koch's old tuberculin, helped their patients. From about 1900 onwards, derivatives of chaulmoogra oil, especially iodized ethyl esters which could be administered parenterally, were developed, and Lara (1930) claimed that, since 1921 in Culion Leprosarium, 27.1% of 8520 patients became skin-smear negative for acid-fast bacilli following their intradermal use. By and large, it was only the tuberculoid and borderline cases which improved, and relapse rates were high.

In the sulphonamide era, it was found in 1941 that the disubstituted sulphone, sodium glucosulphone (Promin) protected guinea pigs from experimental tuberculosis. It proved inactive in human tuberculosis, but when given intravenously at the US National Leprosarium, Carville, it was shown to be effective against lepromatous leprosy (Faget et al. 1943); laryngitis was controlled, rhinitis improved, incipient blindness was prevented and lepromatous ulcers often healed, even though the dermal infiltrate only slowly resolved, and skin smears remained positive after 2 years. In 1948, the much simpler, cheaper and less toxic sulphone, dapsone (DDS) (Cochrane et al. 1949), which could be given orally as well as parenterally, was introduced, and by the early 1950s was recommended by WHO as the standard drug for the mass treatment of leprosy. The whole prognosis for leprosy was completely changed, although reactions became of greater importance, as they could cause more deformity during successful chemotherapy. However, relapses occurred in lepromatous patients unless treatment was maintained for many years, and from the early 1960s, relapse began to be reported in LL and BL patients who were still receiving treatment. Fortunately, the rapid application of Shepard's (1960) technique of limited bacterial multiplication in mouse foot pads both proved that the latter type of relapse was due to the emergence of drug-resistant strains of *M. leprae* (Pettit and Rees 1964, Pearson, Rees and Waters 1975) and enabled the properties of all available antileprosy drugs to be determined.

The mouse foot pad method provided evidence from more than 25 countries of an ever-increasing prevalence of relapsed lepromatous patients due to 'secondary' DDS resistance; it also demonstrated 'primary' DDS resistance in previously untreated lepromatous patients (Pearson, Haile and Rees 1977). Against this background, WHO convened a Study Group (WHO Study Group 1982) to advise on the catastrophic situation which, if it continued, might destroy the value of dapsone – the least expensive antileprosy drug, with a proved record of efficacy and long-term safety. The Group recommended multidrug therapy (MDT) for all leprosy cases (Table 23.3). The purpose was to ensure that patients with or without DDS resistance would benefit and that no new cases of resistance (to DDS or to the other drugs employed) would arise. It was anticipated that MDT might also shorten the length of treatment, just as the introduction of new and better drug combinations enabled the treatment of tuberculosis to be shortened. Two MDT regimens, designed for field use and based on the patients' bacterial load when untreated, were recommended. Patients were classified as either 'multibacillary', which included all LL, BL and BB patients plus those BT (and rare idt) who had a skin-smear BI reading of 2 or more at any site, or 'paucibacillary', which included all smear-negative BT, TT and idt cases plus those with no smear BI reading greater than 1. Subsequently, for operational reasons (WHO 1988), it was agreed that all smear-positive patients should be classified as 'multibacillary'. A combination of only 2 of 3 drugs (rifampicin, dapsone and clofazimine) was required

for paucibacillary patients, as their bacterial load was too small to contain drug-resistant mutants. The choice of the 3 drugs was made on the basis of their high activity in mice; rifampicin alone was strongly bactericidal (see Rees 1985) and just as effective given monthly as daily (Waters et al. 1978). Monthly visits during the period of MDT ensured supervision for the administration of the most effective and costly drug (rifampicin), and of the 300 mg dose of clofazimine (Table 23.3). The results of MDT therapy have proved outstandingly good. In multibacillary disease, the cumulative risk of relapse on a 9-year follow-up has been 0.77% and in paucibacillary disease 1.07% (WHO 1994), although it is possible that many of the paucibacillary 'relapses' were in fact late type 1 reactions due to recognition of residual antigen rather than multiplication of surviving leprosy bacilli – the differential diagnosis is notoriously difficult. In view of these excellent results, a WHO Study Group (WHO Study Group 1994) recommended that the triple drug multibacillary regimen need only be given for 2 years in all cases; this appears very suitable for mass treatment campaigns, but as subsequently Jamet, Ji and the Marchoux Chemotherapy Study Group (1995) reported a 20% relapse rate among a group of 35 previously untreated LL and BL patients who received this limited duration (2 years) chemotherapy, all the relapses occurring among patients with high bacterial loads, the original advice to continue treatment for 2 years and until skin smears become negative appears wiser for individual patients (see Waters 1995).

Since the introduction of MDT in 1982, 3 new groups of drugs have been found to be bactericidal for *M. leprae*, namely the quinolones pefloxacin and ofloxacin (but not ciprofloxacin), ofloxacin being given in the dosage of 400 mg daily, minocycline 100 mg daily, and clarithromycin 500 mg daily. All are less rapidly bactericidal than rifampicin, but more rapidly so than dapsone and clofazimine. The WHO Study Group (1994) has recommended that ofloxacin or minocycline should be used when patients refuse to accept clofazimine, and has also suggested alternative regimens for those rare patients who suffer from rifampicin resistance or toxicity.

5.2 Prophylaxis

Measures for the control and prevention of leprosy include:

Table 23.3 WHO Study Group's recommended treatments for leprosy

Type of patient[a]	Rifampicin 600 mg once monthly	Dapsone 100 mg daily	Clofazimine 300 mg once monthly + 50 mg daily	Duration (months)
Multibacillary	+[b]	+	+	≥24[c]
Paucibacillary	+	+	−[b]	6

[a]For definitions, see text.
[b]+, Treatment given; −, treatment not given.
[c]Should be continued for at least 2 years and whenever possible until smears become negative.

1 early diagnosis, and treatment with MDT
2 health education to encourage early self-presentation
3 examination of domestic contacts associated with health education, so that any who subsequently develop symptoms of leprosy present rapidly, not waiting for annual surveillance and
4 vaccination of neonates with BCG, the vaccine used for tuberculosis (see Chapter 21).

The advent of successful MDT has increased public awareness and greatly encouraged early self-reporting. WHO is aiming to 'eliminate leprosy as a significant public health problem' (defined as a prevalence of <1:10 000 population) by the year 2000 AD; although some countries will not achieve this objective, the campaign, commenced in 1991, has helped to mobilize the medico-political will, resulting in widespread application of MDT.

There is still need for a fully effective vaccine. Fernandez (1939) observed that over 90% of healthy lepromin-negative children became positive after receiving BCG. There followed a series of field trials of BCG against leprosy in 3 different countries (Myanmar, New Guinea and Uganda) and 2 tuberculosis studies were analysed for their leprosy protection (India and Malawi), all of which showed variable protection from 20 to 80% (see review by Fine 1988). Variable protection is also a feature of the use of BCG vaccine against tuberculosis. A second report from Malawi, based on a randomized controlled trial of single BCG, repeated BCG, or combined BCG and killed *M. leprae* vaccine (Rees 1983) for the prevention of leprosy and tuberculosis (Karonga Prevention Trial Group 1996) showed that, in a population in which a single BCG vaccination affords 50% or more protection against leprosy, but none against tuberculosis, a second vaccination can add appreciably to the protection against leprosy. The addition of *M. leprae* to BCG did not add to the protection provided by BCG alone, although there was some suggestion that it might do so under the age of 15. Further long-term follow-up is required, especially as killed *M. leprae* but not killed BCG will protect mice against experimental foot pad infection (Shepard, Walker and van Landingham 1978). Second-generation vaccines using genetic engineering should quickly become feasible, if and when the protective antigens of *M. leprae* are identified.

Chemoprophylaxis is not currently recommended by WHO in leprosy endemic areas, partly because in the classical dapsone child study in India of Dharmendra and Noordeen (Noordeen 1969) more early cases of leprosy occurred in the dapsone than in the control group during the first year of the study, although thereafter there was highly significant protection. However, in the UK and the USA, chemoprophylaxis is recommended for child household contacts of lepromatous cases, and BCG is also given as immunoprophylaxis in Britain.

6 MITSUDA REACTION

This reaction, also called the 'lepromin reaction', was described by Mitsuda in Japan in 1919. The test is carried out by the intradermal injection of 0.1 ml of an autoclaved extract of *M. leprae* from the skin lesions of lepromatous patients, the extract being referred to as 'integral lepromin'. The crude preparations of Mitsuda's era were standardized on the basis of content of tissue. Modern preparations are standardized according to their *M. leprae* content, and prepared as described in a WHO Memorandum (1979). Standard Mitsuda lepromin contains 4.0×10^7 *M. leprae* per ml and has a shelf-life of 2 years at 4°C. Mitsuda lepromin is increasingly being prepared from armadillo-derived *M. leprae*, such preparations, which are designated '(A)', are likely to replace eventually the lepromin, designated '(H)', derived from human lesions.

A positive reaction takes 2 forms, an early and a late one. The **early reaction** is characterized by an acute localized area of inflammation with congestion and oedema appearing usually in 24–48 h and tending to disappear in 3–4 days. The **late reaction** (Mitsuda reaction) is characterized by local infiltration of the skin starting at about 7 days and proceeding to the formation in 4 weeks of a nodule that may undergo central necrosis and ulceration and take several weeks to heal. The early or 'Fernandez' reaction (Fernandez 1940) is, like the tuberculin reaction, a delayed-type hypersensitivity (DTH). It is, however, usually poorly defined and of little practical use. In contrast, the Mitsuda reaction is not a measure of pre-existing DTH, but is the manifestation of cell mediated immunity, which the Mitsuda lepromin itself can induce. It thus discriminates between persons who are capable of responding to *M. leprae* and those who cannot. It is positive in the majority of healthy adults, even in non-endemic areas, and cannot be used as a diagnostic test. On the other hand, it is of great value in classifying cases of leprosy (see above). Prognostically, the Mitsuda reaction is indicative of resistance to infection. Lepromatous patients are invariably Mitsuda-negative unless or until about 24 or more years have passed since they commenced effective chemotherapy without any relapse. Around this time, when presumably almost all the *M. leprae* antigens have been removed, some develop a weak positive reaction (Waters, Ridley and Lucas 1990). Until then, they are not converted by repeated Mitsuda tests or by BCG, as healthy individuals frequently are. It is a remarkable fact that lepromatous patients, though failing to give a positive skin reaction to the leprosy bacillus, are able to do so in response to antigens of other mycobacteria, indicating that they are anergic both to *M. leprae*-specific antigens and to common mycobacterial antigens, but not to other species-specific antigens.

7 RAT LEPROSY

Rat leprosy is a disease that was first described by Stefansky (1903) in 1901 at Odessa. Rats were being slaughtered in large numbers, consequent on the outbreak of human plague, and rat leprosy was found in 4–5% of them. The incidence reported by other observers varies considerably.

In the USA, McCoy (1913) found rat leprosy in 186 of about 200 000 rats caught in San Francisco, an incidence of 0.093%; Wherry (1908) found it in 20 of 9631 rats caught in Oakland, an incidence of 0.21%. In Japan, Ota and Asami (1932) found the disease in 0.8% of *Rattus norvegicus* and 1.0% of *Rattus rattus;* Yamamoto, Sato and Sato (1936) found it in 1.24% of 2573 rats caught in Tokyo. According to Marchoux (1933), about 5% of the sewer rats in Paris harboured rat leprosy bacilli in the lymph nodes, but in only about 0.6% of the rats were generalized lesions present. In Indonesia 9.3% of about 15 000 rats were said by Lampe and de Moore (1935) to have lesions of the lymph nodes, but not more than 0.23% of the animals had manifest skin leprosy.

The disease in rats exists in 2 forms – the glandular type and the musculocutaneous type – but there appears to be no sharp division between them. In the **glandular type** one or more of the groups of subcutaneous lymph nodes – inguinal, axillary and cervical – is enlarged, hard and whitish. On section the nodes are uniform and hard with no caseation. Microscopically, the capsule and trabeculae are thickened; the sinuses are filled with dense aggregations of irregularly polygonal cells, macrophages, which have a large nucleus and much cytoplasm, the latter packed with acid-fast bacilli, so that the contours of the cell body are often invisible. A few giant cells, with several peripheral nuclei, containing numerous bacilli in their cytoplasm, are also visible. Some organisms may be found free.

In the **musculocutaneous type** the rat is emaciated; the skin presents one or more irregularly round or oval areas of atrophy and alopecia, commonest on the head; occasionally ulcers are seen, about 0.5 cm in diameter, covered with a mealy-looking discharge containing acid-fast bacilli. The subcutaneous tissues are devoid of fat, and show the presence of a greyish-white, granular material, containing numerous acid-fast bacilli. Sometimes nodular masses are found in the muscles covered with patches of stretched atrophic skin. Histologically, numerous acid-fast bacilli are found in the corium and subcutaneous tissue; some are free, but most are situated in the cells of the granulation tissue, and in large cells rich in cytoplasm, which resemble the lepra cells of Virchow, but contain no vacuoles. Acid-fast bacilli invade the muscle fibres, collect around the nuclei, and lead to destruction of the tissue. Lesions of the internal organs are rare, but McCoy (1913) stated that nephritis is very common; the kidneys are enlarged, yellowish-brown, friable and often cystic, but no acid-fast bacilli are found in them. In an examination of 186 leprous rats, McCoy (1913) noted alopecia in 47.5%, cutaneous ulcers in 22%, diffuse subcutaneous infiltration in 97.9%, enlarged lymphatic nodes in 87%, and nephritis in 53.8%.

Inside the cells the bacilli are distributed not in cigar-like bundles as are human leprosy bacilli, but at random like pins in a packet; and instead of displacing the nucleus they arrange themselves around it (Marchoux 1933).

In intravenously infected experimental mice, granulomas appear in the reticuloendothelial system, with gradual enlargement of lymph nodes, liver and spleen; eventually the mouse becomes emaciated and anaemic before dying from the disease.

7.1 As a model of human leprosy

The discovery of a chronic infection due to acid-fast bacilli in a proportion of wild rats throughout the world had no economic or public health importance. Almost immediately, however, infection with the 'Stefansky bacillus' became the focus of intensive study in many countries, especially England, France, Japan and the USA, as an apparent model of human leprosy. The use of the terms rat leprosy for the disease and *M. lepraemurium* for the causative organism unfortunately reinforced the concept of a 'model', even though nerve cells were never infected and infection was not confined to cooler sites. In addition, the causative organism differed in important respects from *M. leprae*.

In vitro culture, including tissue culture, has been used successfully for *M. lepraemurium* but not for *M. leprae*. Thus, *M. lepraemurium* was grown in rat-fibroblast cultures for 500 days at 37°C, with a doubling time of 14–15 days (Rees and Garbutt 1962). It has also been grown on Ogawa's egg-yolk medium, pH 5.8–6.3, at 37°C, though very large inocula were needed (Portaels and Pattyn 1981).

DNA studies (genome size and G + C ratio) showed that of a wide range of mycobacteria, *M. lepraemurium* was the least closely related to *M. leprae*. Close genetic relatedness was shown between *M. lepraemurium* and *M. avium* (Imaeda, Barksdale and Kirchheimer 1982).

8 LEPROSY IN OTHER ANIMALS

8.1 Cat leprosy

Following a brief report from New Zealand (Brown, May and Williams 1962), Lawrence and Wickham (1963) in Australia described a disease in cats characterized by granulomatous lesions of the skin and subcutaneous tissues, often associated with ulceration and enlargement of the lymph nodes. The granulomata contained numerous epithelioid cells packed with acid-fast bacilli and giant cells of the Langhans type. Typical lesions could be reproduced in rats by subcutaneous injection with material from lymph nodes. The cause appears therefore to be the rat leprosy bacillus.

8.2 Lepra bubalorum

Lepra bubalorum is an infectious disease of the buffalo seen in Indonesia. According to Lobel (1934), who studied the disease, it was first noted by Kok and Roesli in 1926. It runs a protracted course and is characterized by multiple cutaneous nodules containing acid-fast bacilli resembling human leprosy bacilli in their appearance and grouping into globular formations. There are no systemic disturbances, and the skin lesions undergo slow resorption. The bacilli have not been cultured, nor has the disease been reproduced experimentally, even in the buffalo itself. Apparently no new cases of the disease have been reported since 1950.

SARCOIDOSIS

Sarcoidosis is a multisystemic disease of man, of uncertain aetiology, characterized by the formation in all of several affected organs or tissues of epithelioid cell tubercles without caseation, though fibrinoid necrosis may be present at the centres of a few, proceeding either to resolution or to conversion into hyaline fibrous tissue (Scadding and Mitchell 1985). Lymphocytes and Langhans giant cells are also present in the follicles. The disease most commonly takes the form of bilateral hilar adenopathy, which usually regresses spontaneously, or there may be associated pulmonary alveolitis or sometimes the lung alone is involved. Other organs most frequently affected are the lymph nodes, skin, eyes, liver, spleen, salivary glands, bones, and occasionally the nervous system.

It is of world-wide distribution, although less commonly diagnosed in the tropics, where skin sarcoid is often mistaken for tuberculoid leprosy despite the differences both in physical signs and histologically, with the former's lack of involvement of dermal nerves. Yet in London sarcoidosis is more common among West Indian and Asian immigrants than among the indigenous white population (Edmondstone and Wilson 1985), a situation similar to that of tuberculosis.

Diagnosis is dependent on positive histological findings from an appropriate tissue biopsy, supported by chest x-ray examination, a negative tuberculin test (two-thirds of patients with sarcoidosis are tuberculin-negative up to a concentration of 1:100), and a positive Kveim–Siltzbach skin test (Kveim 1941, Siltzbach 1966). This last consists of the intradermal injection of a standardized suspension of sarcoid splenic tissue, followed 4–6 weeks later by a biopsy at the site of the reaction to determine if the histological picture is characteristic of the disease. The reaction is positive in about three-quarters of patients with active disease, but in a lower proportion during the stage of late fibrosis (James 1966), although up to 40% of patients with Crohn's disease are also positive (Mitchell et al. 1969); other false positive reactions are few.

The only effective treatment for severe cases is with glucocorticosteroids, which suppress the granuloma formation and, in pulmonary sarcoidosis, the lymphocytic alveolitis, but which may need to be continued perhaps for years as long as disease activity is demonstrable. Indications for commencing steroid therapy are not generally agreed, in pulmonary sarcoidosis Mitchell and Scadding (1974) being influenced by symptoms such as breathlessness whereas de Remee (1977) considered that clinical or biochemical signs of activity were sufficient. Gibson et al. (1996) have shown, in a prospective study, that patients undergoing early spontaneous recoveries have a better prognosis than those requiring immediate steroid therapy, and that regular therapy is better than 'on demand' treatment (see review by Selroos 1996).

Although the cause of sarcoidosis remains unproven, many clinicians, especially Scadding (1971), have provided evidence of an association with mycobacterial infection. This is despite the facts that the prevalence of the disease remains constant in countries in which the tuberculosis death rate is falling; the disease cannot be transmitted to guinea pigs; tubercle bacilli can be demonstrated in only a minority of cases; BCG vaccination affords no protection, and standard anti-tuberculosis chemotherapy has no effect on the course of the disease (see Siltzbach 1969). As early as 1959, Burnet discussed whether sarcoidosis might be caused by a mycobacterial protoplast or L-form, lacking the power to produce the characteristic cell wall, and persisting as an intracellular parasite of mesenchymal cells. Mitchell, Rees and Goswami (1976) and Mitchell and Rees (1983), in a series of experiments lasting a decade, reported the development of disseminated granulomatous lesions in mice inoculated in the footpad with human sarcoid tissue, and the occasional isolation of mycobacteria resembling *M. tuberculosis* from mice passaged with granulomatous material, including filtered supernatant.

Almenoff et al. (1996) have summarized the evidence in favour of sarcoidosis being due to cell wall deficient forms (CWDF) of mycobacteria, including the finding of mycobacterial nucleic acid components using the polymerase chain reaction (PCR) in bronchoalveolar lavage samples, lung tissue, spleen and lymph nodes from patients with sarcoidosis. They also reported the growth of CWDF from the blood of 19 of 20 subjects with sarcoidosis. All isolates stained positively with a monoclonal antibody raised against *M. tuberculosis* (H_{37}RV) whole cell antigen, but no organisms were grown from the blood of 20 controls. They considered that the isolated organisms were mycobacterial in origin, and were similar if not identical to *M. tuberculosis*, but that their role in the pathogenesis of sarcoidosis was as yet unknown (see review by Mitchell 1996).

JOHNE'S DISEASE

Johne's disease (paratuberculosis) is a specific enteritis affecting cattle, sheep, goats and deer, and occasionally other species, both wild and captive, such as yaks, camels and buffaloes (see Chiodini, van Kruiningen and Merkal 1984). Economically, it is one of the most important of the bovine diseases (Benedictus, Dijkhuizen and Stelwagen 1987, Merkal et al. 1987). The causative agent is an acid-fast organism known as Johne's bacillus or *M. paratuberculosis*. The disease was first described by Johne and Frothingham in 1895 at Dresden, who regarded it as a peculiar form of tuberculosis, possibly due to the avian type of bacillus.

Johne's disease occurs in many parts of the world, mainly in the temperate zones but also in the tropics. As the incubation period is lengthy, up to about 18 months, it is uncommon in cows less than 2 years old, the peak incidence being between 3 and 5 years of age. Certain breeds of cattle, such as Jersey, are said to be particularly susceptible. Sheep are less often attacked, though according to McEwen (1939) the disease may exact an annual toll of 5%. Very occasional cases have been reported in horses (see Rankin 1956). In a survey made in the USA by Merkal and his colleagues (1987) *M. paratuberculosis* was isolated from the ileocaecel lymph nodes of 1.6% of 7540 clinically normal cattle at slaughterhouses in 32 states and in Puerto Rico. No recent surveys have been made in the UK, but Taylor (1951a) estimated that 25–30% of cattle were latently infected. The infection may remain latent, but in about 10% of animals it is progressive and proves fatal.

Natural infection usually occurs in calves less than 30 days old, transmission commonly being through the ingestion of fodder or water that has been soiled with faeces of infected animals. It has been shown experimentally that Johne's bacillus may remain alive for several months in infected faeces and ditch water exposed to ordinary atmospheric conditions (Lovell, Levi and Francis 1944). Infection may also occur in fetal life when the placenta of the dam is diseased (Doyle 1958), or in sucklings from the milk of cows with clinical disease.

In cattle, the disease runs a chronic course, subject often to long intermissions, and characterized by failure to thrive, a falling-off in milk yield, excessive thirst, diarrhoea of often varying severity (without blood or mucus) and progressive emaciation despite often normal appetite; there is no fever. Recovery is rare.

9 PATHOLOGY

The main lesions are situated in the last 50 feet of the small intestine, and in the neighbourhood of the ileocaecal junction, but sometimes the whole gut is affected. The intestine is thick and rigid, looking not unlike a hose pipe; the mucosa is greatly thickened and is thrown into regular corrugations, resembling the convolutions of the cerebrum. The mucosa is smooth and pale or pink in colour, and covered with slimy material; on the surface of the corrugations it is dotted with red spots or haemorrhages; between the folds the mucosa often has a warty appearance. Occasionally small nodules are seen, due to enlargement of solitary lymphoid follicles. There is no ulceration of the mucosa, and the peritoneal surface appears normal. The mesenteric lymph nodes are usually enlarged, oedematous and pigmented. Histologically, the mucosa and, to a less extent, the submucosa are infiltrated with lymphoid and epithelioid cells, which are responsible for the thickening. Near the surface of the gut the mucosa is absolutely structureless; all traces of nuclei and cell outlines have disappeared. Giant cells are rare; there is no caseation, ulceration, fibrosis or calcification. Short acid-fast bacilli, often in enormous numbers, are found in the mucosa lying between the glands and in the lymphoid tissue of the solitary follicles; they may invade the submucosa, and very occasionally the underlying muscle layer. The bacilli are arranged in dense clumps, and may be intra- or extracellular. The cellular reaction around the bacilli is diffuse, not localized as in tuberculosis. Bacilli can generally be found microscopically in the mesenteric glands. By cultural methods they can be shown to be widespread throughout the body, being distributed in the liver, spleen, lung and many of the lymph nodes in the cervical and abdominal regions (Taylor 1951a). The reproductive tract may be infected and the organism may be excreted in the semen of bulls (Larsen and Kopecky 1970). In some apparently recovered animals, postmortem examination reveals the presence of intense cellular reactions in the mesenteric glands, which seem to result in the disappearance of the bacilli. Infection in such animals probably remains latent and may never give rise to clinical symptoms. Biochemical aspects of the disease have been reviewed by Patterson and Allen (1972).

In sheep, the clinical and pathological manifestations are more varied than in cattle, corresponding to some extent to the 3 different types of infecting organism (see Taylor 1951b, Stamp and Watt 1954, and Volume 2, Chapter 26). The disease is commonest in animals between 3 and 5 years of age, and is characterized by loss of condition and weight not necessarily accompanied by diarrhoea. Thickening of the intestinal mucous membrane is often only slight in animals infected with the non-pigmented strains; in those infected with pigmented strains the mucosa of the small intestine is bright yellow in colour and the intestinal wall frequently thickened. Calcification of the lesions sometimes occurs in sheep and goats. Infection with pigmented strains has not been reported in goats.

The disease can be reproduced in both cattle and sheep by feeding or by parenteral inoculation with pure cultures of Johne's bacillus (see Volume 2, Chapter 26). After infection some animals clear themselves; some become carriers and excrete the organism; and some carriers eventually become clinical cases. It has recently been claimed that C57BL/6 mice also develop lesions after oral inoculation, and they may prove a useful laboratory model (Veasey et al. 1995).

The bacteriology of the disease is described in Volume 2, Chapter 26.

10 DIAGNOSIS

The antemortem diagnosis of Johne's disease is often difficult. The absence of clinical disease in some infected cattle, and the slow multiplication of the organism (requiring cultivation of 8–16 weeks) contribute to the problem.

None of the available diagnostic tests will detect all

infected animals. Moreover, tests for humoral antibody and cell mediated immunity invariably give some false positive and false negative reactions and are therefore unsuitable as a basis for culling subclinically infected animals.

The definitive diagnosis is based on the finding of *M. paratuberculosis* organisms in the faeces, where they may be demonstrated microscopically in 25–30% of clinical cases, or in the rectal mucosa from a rectal punch biopsy, or occasionally in milk (Smith 1960), and confirmed by culture. Culture may also be positive in cases which are microscopically negative. Faeces are first decontaminated and then inoculated on a medium containing 50% egg yolk, mycobactin and antibiotics (Cameron 1956, Report 1960; see Volume 2, Chapter 26). Decontamination is usually performed with hexadecylpyridinium chloride or benzalkonium chloride, and the mycobactin is preferably prepared from *M. paratuberculosis* rather than *M. phlei* (Riemann and Abbas 1983, Chiodini, van Kruiningen and Merkal 1984, Merkal 1984). With these methods, the period of cultivation is often reduced to 6–8 weeks, and only about 1% of positive specimens require more than 12 weeks. At necropsy the bacilli are best demonstrated in the ileocaecal mucosa and associated lymph nodes, either microscopically or culturally (Taylor 1950).

Immunologically, infected cattle can be divided into 3 main groups, which bear some similarity to the leprosy spectrum. Resistant cases are those which have suppressed the infection, have no clinical signs, and do not shed *M. paratuberculosis* in their faeces, or shed only small numbers intermittently: such cases usually have a positive skin test to **johnin** (see below), their specific lymphocyte transformation test (LTT) (Buergelt et al. 1978) is usually distinctively positive, and their humoral antibody response negative. Advanced clinical cases with multiple clinical signs, and shedding large numbers of bacilli in their faeces, may have weak or negative johnin skin tests and LTT, and a strong positive antibody response. Intermediate cases that are incubating the disease or already have early clinical signs, and are shedding moderate numbers of bacilli, still usually have a positive johnin skin test, and a positive LTT, but have also developed a moderate antibody response.

Johnin is a tuberculin-like substance prepared from glycerine broth cultures of Johne's bacillus (see Twort and Ingram 1912, 1913, Dunkin 1933), usually now used as a purified protein derivative (PPD). In the test, 0.2 ml is injected intradermally in the cervical area and read at 48 h, an avium tuberculin test commonly being performed at the same time; some workers prefer an intravenous johnin test. As already stated, the test may be positive in the absence of lesions demonstrable at necropsy, and often negative due to anergy in the presence of gross lesions (see McEwen 1939, Report 1941, Hole 1958).

The complement-fixation test was the first humoral antibody test to be widely used. It was reported on favourably by Sigurdsson (1945, 1946, 1947) in sheep and by Hole (1958) in cattle. A positive reaction is obtained in a high proportion of clinically affected animals and is therefore useful for confirmatory purposes. Only about 25% of carriers react positively, however, and the test cannot therefore be used for diagnosis of latent infection. Moreover, a positive result is sometimes obtained in apparently healthy animals from non-infected herds (Chandler 1955, Rankin 1961), the false positive reactions being due to cross-reactivity with a number of other infections, including *Corynebacterium renale* (Gilmour and Goudswaard 1972), some other mycobacterial species, with species of *Actinomyces, Dermatophilus, Norcardia* and *Streptomyces*, and with fungi (Chiodini, van Kruiningen and Merkal 1984).

Fluorescent antibody and complement fixation techniques were shown by Goudswaard and his colleagues (1976) to be more sensitive than tests based on haemagglutination, haemagglutination–lysis and immunodiffusion. The numerous serological methods tried, with different degrees of success (Chiodini, van Kruiningen and Merkal 1984), include the enzyme-linked immunosorbent assay (ELISA), the specificity of which is improved by absorption of the serum samples with a suspension of *M. phlei* (Merkal 1984, Yokomizo, Yugi and Merkal 1985, Milner et al. 1987), and an agar gel immunodiffusion test (Sherman, Markham and Bates 1984), which is claimed by some to be the most reliable, at least in clinical cases (see Sockett et al. 1992).

With the development of a gene library of *M. paratuberculosis*, recombinant proteins expressed in *Escherichia coli* are being studied (De Kesel et al. 1993, Elsaatari et al. 1994), PCRs are being developed (Millar et al. 1995), and commercial DNA probes have been compared with faecal culture in the diagnosis of Johne's disease (Sockett, Carr and Collins 1992, Whipple, Kapke and Andersen 1992). Although one such test failed to distinguish between *M. paratuberculosis* and *M. avium* (Thoresen and Saxegaard 1991), the 2 species having close DNA homology, McFadden et al. (1992) claim to have developed probes capable of distinguishing between *M. paratuberculosis* and *M. avium*, both type A and type A/1 (the wood pigeon strain).

11 PROPHYLAXIS

Since the disease appears to be spread mainly by the contamination of water, foodstuffs and pasture land with the faeces of infected animals, preventive measures include the destruction of diseased animals, suitable disposal of their excreta, disinfection of byres, the ploughing-up of infected pasture, a supply of clean piped water, and the segregation of young stock until their first lactation. If this is impracticable, pasture land should be regarded as potentially dangerous for at least a year, and should not be used for the grazing of sheep or cattle. These measures may suffice to eradicate the disease (see Edwards 1947), but cannot be relied on completely. Since in pregnant animals the fetus may become infected, calves from cows suffering from the disease should not be reared. In areas of the world, such as Colorado, where the disease occurs in wild animals – Rocky Mountain big-horn sheep and goats – eradication may prove difficult (Thoen and Muscoplat 1979).

According to Vallee, Rinjard and Vallee (1934), subcutaneous vaccination of non-infected animals with 5–10 mg of a living attenuated culture of Johne's bacillus affords a high degree of protection against the disease. Unfortunately the vaccine sensitizes animals to tuberculin and may interfere with a tuberculosis-eradication scheme. Vaccination also gives rise to positive reactions in serological tests for Johne's disease. Using living non-virulent bacilli suspended in equal parts of olive oil and liquid paraffin to which pumice powder was added as an irritant, Doyle (1964) found during an experience of 20 years that vaccination of calves aged 3–4 weeks, combined with the usual hygienic precautionary measures, afforded a high degree of protection against natural infection. In Norway the same type of vaccine gave comparable results in goats (Saxegaard and Fodstad 1985). Revaccination is probably desirable from time to time, but in sheep, according to Gilmour and Angus (1973), may precipitate a massive cellular response leading to extensive macroscopic lesions. In Iceland a heat-killed phenolized vaccine suspended in mineral oil is said to have reduced the average annual specific mortality in lambs by about 85% (Sigurdsson 1960). The restricted use of a heat-killed vaccine is practised in parts of the USA for controlling the disease in infected herds, but not for prophylaxis in disease-free herds. Vaccination, which does not usually eliminate the disease, reduces the number of deaths, clinical cases and infected animals, and also the faecal shedding of organisms (Chiodini, van Kruiningen and Merkal 1984, Jorgensen 1984, Merkal 1984). Wilesmith (1982) found, however, that in herds in which the calves were vaccinated annually for 4 years paratuberculosis disappeared.

Although no reported treatment of the disease in cattle has so far afforded any promise, administering rifampicin to spontaneously infected macaque monkeys (see below) resulted in the resolution of symptoms and prolongation of life (McClure et al. 1987). In vitro studies suggest that clarithromycin might be a very effective second drug (Rastogi, Goh and Labrousse 1992) in any proposed multidrug regimen.

Reviews of paratuberculosis are given by Doyle (1956), Sigurdsson (1956), Hole (1958), Riemann and Abbas (1983), Chiodini, van Kruiningen and Merkal (1984) and Gilmour (1985).

12 INFECTIONS OF NON-RUMINANT ANIMALS AND HUMANS WITH ORGANISMS RESEMBLING *M. PARATUBERCULOSIS*

Thorel and Desmettre (1982) found that mycobacterial strains from 'tuberculous' infections in wood pigeons (*Columba palumbis*) bore a closer resemblance to *M. paratuberculosis* than to *M. avium*. Wood-pigeon strains produced clinical Johne's disease in experimental calves, and lesions characteristic of *M. avium* infection in chickens (Collins et al. 1985). DNA homology studies at first suggested that both *M. paratuberculosis* and the wood-pigeon strains should be regarded as subspecies of *M. avium*, although McFadden et al. (1987, 1992) have now demonstrated distinctive differences.

Paratuberculosis in 29 of a group of 38 stumptail macaque monkeys (*Macaca arctoides*) was reported by McClure and colleagues (1987). The causative organism, identified as *M. paratuberculosis* by cultural, biochemical and genetic means, was shed by some subclinically infected animals in numbers as high as 2×10^6 cfu g^{-1} of faeces; in animals dying from the disease the numbers sometimes exceeded 10^8 cfu g^{-1} of intestinal tissue.

A slow-growing mycobactin-dependent organism of the genus *Mycobacterium* was isolated by Chiodini et al. (1984) from the intestinal mucosa of human patients with Crohn's disease. This organism resembled *M. paratuberculosis* culturally and biochemically and was considered identical with it as judged by DNA probes (McFadden et al. 1987). In 4 infant goats dosed orally, it produced, after some months, granulomatous lesions of the ileum and more proximal regions of the small intestine, and of the regional lymph nodes (van Kruiningen et al. 1986).

REFERENCES

Almenoff PF, Johnson A et al., 1996, Growth of acid fast L forms from the blood of patients with sarcoidosis, *Thorax*, **51**: 530–3.

Benedictus G, Dijkhuizen AA, Stelwagen, J, 1987, Economic losses due to paratuberculosis in dairy cattle, *Vet Rec*, **121**: 142–6.

Brown LR, May CD, Williams SE, 1962, A non-tuberculoid granuloma in cats, *N Z Vet J*, **10**: 7–9.

Browne SG, 1980, The epidemiological situation of leprosy in Great Britain, *Quad Coop Sanit*, **1**: 34–5.

Browne SG, 1985, The history of leprosy, *Leprosy*, ed. Hastings RC, Churchill Livingstone, Edinburgh, 1–15.

Brubaker ML, Meyers WM, Bourland J, 1985, Leprosy in children one year of age and under, *Int J Lepr*, **53**: 517–23.

Buergelt CD, De Lisle G et al., 1978, In vitro lymphocyte transformation as a herd survey method for bovine paratuberculosis. *Am J Vet Res*, **39**: 591–5.

Burnet FM, 1959, *The Clonal Selection Theory of Acquired Immunity*, Cambridge University Press, Cambridge, 160–3.

Cameron J, 1956, Isolation of *Mycobacterium johnei* from faeces, *J Pathol Bacteriol*, **71**: 223–5.

Chandler RL, 1955, A report on the use in New Zealand of Hole's complement-fixation test for Johne's disease, *N Z Vet J*, **3**: 145–50.

Chehl S, Job CK, Hastings RC, 1985, Transmission of leprosy in nude mice, *Am J Trop Med Hyg*, **34**: 1161–6.

Chiodini RJ, van Kruiningen HJ, Merkal RS, 1984, Ruminant paratuberculosis (Johne's disease): the current status and future prospects, *Cornell Vet*, **74**: 218–62.

Chiodini RJ, van Kruiningen HJ et al., 1984, Characteristics of an unclassified *Mycobacterium* species isolated from patients with Crohn's disease, *J Clin Microbiol*, **20**: 966–71.

Cochrane RG, Ramanujam K et al., 1949, Two and half years'

experimental work on the sulphone group of drugs, *Lepr Rev*, **20**: 4–64.

Collins P, McDiarmid A et al., 1985, Comparison of the pathogenicity of *Mycobacterium paratuberculosis* and *Mycobacterium* spp. isolated from the wood pigeon (*Columba palumbus-L*), *J Comp Pathol*, **95**: 591–7.

Danielssen DC, Boeck CW, 1848, *Traité de la Spedalsked ou Elephantiasis des Grecs*, JB Baillière, Paris.

Davey TF, Rees RJW, 1974, The nasal discharge in leprosy: clinical and bacteriological aspects, *Lepr Rev*, **45**: 121–34.

De Kesel M, Gilot P et al., 1993, Cloning and expression of portions of the 34-kilodalton-protein gene to *Mycobacterium paratuberculosis*: its application to serological analysis of Johne's disease. *J Clin Microbiol*, **31**: 947–54.

Dharmendra, 1985, Classifications of leprosy, *Leprosy*, ed. Hastings RC, Churchill Livingstone, Edinburgh, 88–99.

Dockrell HM, Eascott H et al., 1991, Possible transmission of *Mycobacterium leprae* in a group of UK leprosy contacts. *Lancet*, **338**: 739–43.

Doyle TM, 1956, Johne's disease, *Vet Rec*, **68**: 869–78.

Doyle TM, 1958, Foetal infection in Johne's disease, *Vet Rec*, **70**: 238–41.

Doyle TM, 1964, Vaccination against Johne's disease, *Vet Rec*, **76**: 73–7.

Dunkin GW, 1933, The preparation of Johnin from a synthetic medium without the addition of *B Phlei*. *J Comp Pathol Ther*, **46**: 159–64.

Dzierzykray-Rogalski T, 1980, Palaeopathology of the Ptolemaic inhabitants of the Dakhleh Oasis (Egypt), *J Hum Evol*, **9**: 71–4.

Edmondstone WM, Wilson AG, 1985, Sarcoidosis in Caucasians, Blacks and Asians in London, *Br J Dis Chest*, **79**: 27–36.

Edwards SJ, 1947, Some diseases of dairy cattle, *Vet Rec*, **59**: 211–13.

Elsaatari FAK, Engstrand L et al., 1994, Identification and characterization of *Mycobacterium paratuberculosis* recombinant proteins expressed in *E coli*, *Curr Microbiol*, **29**: 177–84.

Faget GH, Pogge RC et al., 1943, The Promin treatment of leprosy. A progress report, *Public Health Rep*, **58**: 1729–41.

Feldman R, Sturdivant M, 1976, Leprosy in the US, 1950–1969: an epidemiologic review, *South Med J*, **69**: 970–9.

Fernandez JMM, 1939, Estudio comparativo de la reaccion de Mitsuda con las reacciones tuberculericas, *Rev Argent Dermatosifilogia*, **23**: 425–53.

Fernandez JMM, 1940. The early reaction induced by lepromin, *Int J Lepr*, **8**: 1–14.

Fine PEM, 1982, Leprosy: the epidemiology of a slow bacterium, *Epidemiol Rev*, **4**: 161–88.

Fine PEM, 1988, BCG vaccination against tuberculosis and leprosy, *Br Med Bull*, **44**: 691–703.

Gibson GJ, Prescott RJ et al., 1996, British Thoracic Society sarcoidosis study: effects of long term corticosteroid treatment, *Thorax*, **51**: 238–47.

Gilmour NJL, 1985, *Handbuch der bakteriellen Infektionen bei Tieren*, vol. V, eds Blobel H, Schliesser T, VEB Gustav Fischer Verlag, Jena, 281.

Gilmour NJL, Angus KW, 1973, Effect of revaccination on *Mycobacterium johnei* infection in sheep, *J Comp Pathol*, **83**: 437–45.

Gilmour NJL, Goudswaard J, 1972, *Corynebacterium renale* as a cause of reactions to the complement fixation test for Johne's disease, *J Comp Pathol*, **82**: 333–6.

Goudswaard J, Gilmour NJL et al., 1976, Diagnosis of Johne's disease in cattle: a comparison of five serological tests under field conditions, *Vet Rec*, **98**: 461–4.

Hansen GHA, 1874, Undersogelser angraaende spedalskhedens aasager, *Norsk Magazin Laegervidenskaben (Suppl)*, **4**: 76–9.

Hansen GA, Looft C, 1895a, Leprosy: its Clinical and Pathological Aspects, John Wright, Bristol, 2–3.

Hansen GA, Looft C, 1985b, Leprosy: its Clinical and Pathological Aspects, John Wright, Bristol, 105–25.

Hole NH, 1958, Johne's disease, *Adv Vet Sci*, **4**: 341–87.

Imaeda T, Barksdale L, Kirchheimer WF, 1982. Deoxyribo-

nucleic acid of *Mycobacterium lepraemurium*: it genome size, base ratio, and homology with those of other mycobacteria, *Int J Syst Bacteriol*, **32**: 456–8.

Irgens LM, 1980, Leprosy in Norway. An epidemiological study based on a national patient registry, *Lepr Rev*, **51, Suppl. 1**: 1–130.

James DG, 1966, Immunology of sarcoidosis, *Lancet*, **2**: 633–5.

Jamet P, Ji BH, Marchoux Chemotherapy Study Group, 1995, Relapse after long-term follow up of multibacillary patients treated by WHO multidrug regimen, *Int J Lepr*, **63**: 195–201.

Johne HA, Frothingham L, 1895, Ein Eigenthuemlicher Fall von Tuberkulose beim Rind, *Dtsch Z Tiermed Vergleich Pathol*, **21**: 438–54.

Jopling WH, 1978a, *Handbook of Leprosy*, 2nd edn, Heinemann Medical Books Ltd, London, 10.

Jopling WH, 1978b, *Handbook of Leprosy*, 2nd edn. Heinemann Medical Books Ltd, London, 66–71.

Jorgensen JB, 1984, *Paratuberculosis, Diagnostic Methods, their Practical Application, and Experience with Vaccination*, Report EUR 9000EN, eds Jorgensen JB, Aalund O, Commission of the European Community, Luxembourg, 131.

Karonga Prevention Trial Group, 1996, Randomized controlled trial of single BCG, repeated BCG or combined BCG and killed *Mycobacterium leprae* vaccine for prevention of leprosy and tuberculosis in Malawi, *Lancet*, **348**: 17–24.

van Kruiningen HJ, Chiodini RJ et al., 1986, Experimental disease in infant goats induced by a *Mycobacterium* isolated from a patient with Crohn's disease, *Dig Dis Sci*, **31**: 1351–60.

Kveim A, 1941, En ny og specifikk kutans-reaksjon ved Boecks sarcoid, *Nord Med*, **9**: 169–72.

Lampe PHJ, de Moore CE, 1935, Ratten lepra. 1. De diagnostick van de rattenlepra. Het voorkomen van deze rattenziekte te Batavia. De geographsche distributie, *Geneeskd Tijdschr Nederlandsch-Indie Batavia*, **76**: 1618.

Lara CB, 1930, Progress of treatment at Culion, *J Philippine Islands Med Assoc*, **10**: 469–74.

Larsen AB, Kopecky KE, 1970, *Mycobacterium paratuberculosis* in reproductive organs and semen of bulls, *Am J Vet Res*, **31**: 255–7.

Lawrence WE, Wickham N, 1963, Cat leprosy: infection by a bacillus resembling *Mycobacterium lepraemurium*, *Aust Vet J*, **39**: 390–3.

Leiker DL, 1980, Epidemiology of leprosy in the Netherlands, *Quad Coop Sanit*, **1**: 60–4.

Lobel LWM, 1934, Lepra bubalorum, *Nederlandsche Indische Bladen Diergeneeskd*, **46**: no. 5; reprinted in *Int J Lepr*, 1936, **4**: 79–96.

Lovell R, Levi M, Francis J, 1944, Studies on the survival of Johne's bacillus, *J Comp Pathol*, **54**: 120–9.

McClure HM, Chiodini RJ et al., 1987, *Mycobacterium paratuberculosis* infection in a colony of stumptail macaques (*Macaca arctoides*) *J Infect Dis*, **155**: 1011–19.

McCoy GW, 1913, Observations on naturally acquired rat leprosy, *Public Health Bull*, **61**: 27–30.

McDougall AC, Rees RJW, 1973, Ulcerating lepromatous leprosy in a patient with dapsone resistant *Mycobacterium leprae*, *Lepr Rev*, **44**: 59–64.

McEwen AD, 1939, Investigations on Johne's disease of sheep, *J Comp Pathol*, **52**: 69–87.

McFadden JJ, Butcher PD et al., 1987, Crohn's disease-isolated mycobacteria are identical to *Mycobacterium paratuberculosis*, as determined by DNA probes that distinguish between mycobacterial species, *J Clin Microbiol*, **25**: 796–801.

McFadden J, Collins J et al., 1992, Mycobacteria in Crohn's disease – DNA probes identify the wood pigeon strain of *Mycobacterium avium* and *Mycobacterium paratuberculosis* from human tissue, *J Clin Microbiol*, **30**: 3070–3.

MacLeod JMH, 1925, Contact cases of leprosy in the British Isles, *Br Med J*, **1**: 107–8.

Marchoux E, 1933, La lèpre des rats, *Rev Fr Dermatol Vénériol*, **9**: 323–30.

Martinez Dominguez V, Gallego Garbajosa P et al., 1980, Epidemiological information on leprosy in the Singu area of Upper Burma, *Bull WHO,* **58:** 81–9.

Melsom R, Harboe M, Duncan ME, 1982, IgA, IgM and IgG anti-*M leprae* antibodies in babies of leprosy mothers during the first 2 years of life, *Clin Exp Immunol,* **49:** 532–42.

Merkal RS, 1984, Paratuberculosis: advances in cultural, serologic, and vaccination methods, *J Am Vet Med Assoc,* **184:** 939–43.

Merkal RS, Whipple DL et al., 1987, Prevalence of *Mycobacterium paratuberculosis* in ileocecal lymph nodes of cattle culled in the United States, *J Am Vet Med Assoc,* **190:** 676–80.

Millar DS, Withey SJ et al., 1995, Solid-phase hybridization capture of low-abundance target DNA sequences: application to the polymerase chain reaction detection of *Mycobacterium paratuberculosis* and *Mycobacterium avium* subsp *silvaticum, Anal Biochem,* **226:** 325–30.

Milner AR, Lepper AWD et al., 1987, Analysis by ELISA and Western blotting of antibody reactivities in cattle infected with *Mycobacterium paratuberculosis* after absorption of serum with *M. phlei, Res Vet Sci,* **42:** 140–4.

Mitchell DN, 1996, Mycobacteria and sarcoidosis, *Lancet,* **348:** 768–9.

Mitchell DN, Rees RJW, 1983, The nature and physical characteristics of transmissible agents from human sarcoid and Crohn's disease tissues, *Proceedings of the 9th International Conference on Sarcoidosis, Paris, 1981,* eds Chrétien J, Marsac J, Saltier JC, Pergamon Press, Oxford, 132–41.

Mitchell DN, Rees RJW, Goswami KKA, 1976, Transmissible agents from human sarcoid and Crohn's disease tissues, *Lancet,* **2:** 761–5.

Mitchell DN, Scadding JG, 1974, Sarcoidosis: state of the art, *Am Rev Respir Dis,* **110:** 774–802.

Mitchell DN, Cannon P et al., 1969, The Kweim test in Crohn's disease, *Lancet,* **2:** 571–3.

Mitsuda K, 1919, On the value of a skin reaction to a suspension of leprous nodules, *Jpn J Dermatol Urol,* **19:** 697–708. Reprinted in English translation in *Int J Lepr,* 1953, **21:** 347–58.

Narayanan E, Shankara Manja K et al., 1972, Arthropod feeding experiments in lepromatous leprosy, *Lepr Rev,* **43:** 188–93.

Noordeen SK, 1969, Chemoprophylaxis in leprosy, *Lepr India,* **41:** 247–54.

Ota M, Asami S, 1932, Culture du *Mycobacterium leprae muris, C R Soc Biol,* **111:** 287–9.

Ottenhoff THM, de Vries RPP, 1987, HLA class II immune response and suppression genes in leprosy, *Int J Lepr,* **55:** 521–34.

Patterson DSP, Allen WM, 1972, Chronic mycobacterial enteritis in ruminants as a model of Crohn's disease, *Proc R Soc Med,* **65:** 998–1001.

Pearson JMH, Haile GS, Rees RJW, 1977, Primary dapsone resistant leprosy, *Lepr Rev,* **48:** 129–32.

Pearson JMH, Rees RJW, Waters MFR, 1975, Sulphone resistance in leprosy. A review of one hundred proven clinical cases, *Lancet,* **2:** 69–72.

Pedley JC, 1967, The presence of *M. leprae* in human milk, *Lepr Rev,* **38:** 239–42.

Pedley JC, 1970, Composite skin contact smears: a method of demonstrating the non-emergence of *Mycobacterium leprae* from intact lepromatous skin, *Lepr Rev,* **41:** 31–43.

Pettit JHS, Rees RJW, 1964, Sulphone resistance in leprosy. An experimental and clinical study. *Lancet,* **2:** 673–4.

Portaels F, Pattyn SR, 1981, Parameters influencing the in vitro growth of *Mycobacterium lepraemurium, Int J Lepr,* **49:** 194–7.

Rankin JD, 1956, The identification of a strain of *Mycobacterium johnei* recovered from a horse, *J Pathol Bacteriol,* **72:** 689–90.

Rankin JD, 1961, The non-specificity of a complement-fixation test used in the diagnosis of Johne's disease in cattle, *Res Vet Sci,* **2:** 89–95.

Rastogi N, Goh KS, Labrousse V, 1992, Activity of clarithromycin with those of other drugs against *Mycobacterium paratuberculosis* and further enhancement of its extracellular activities by ethambutol, *Antimicrob Agents Chemother,* **36:** 2843–6.

Reader R, 1974, New evidence for the antiquity of leprosy in Early Britain, *J Archaeol Sci,* **1:** 205–7.

Rees RJW, 1983, Progress in the preparation of an antileprosy vaccine from armadillo-derived *Mycobacterium leprae, Int J Lepr,* **51:** 515–18.

Rees RJW, 1985, The microbiology of leprosy, *Leprosy,* ed. Hastings RC, Churchill Livingstone, Edinburgh, 31–52.

Rees RJW, Garbutt EW, 1962, Studies on *Mycobacterium lepraemurium* in tissue culture. I. Multiplication and growth characteristics in cultures of rat fibroblasts, *Br J Exp Pathol,* **43:** 221–35.

Rees RJW, McDougall AC, 1977, Airborne infection with *Mycobacterium leprae* in mice, *J Med Microbiol,* **10:** 63–8.

Rees RJW, Waters MFR, 1963, Applicability of experimental murine leprosy to the study of human leprosy, *Pathogenesis of Leprosy,* Ciba Foundation Study Group, London, Churchill, no. 15, 39–60.

de Remee RA, 1977, The present status of pulmonary sarcoidosis: a house divided, *Chest,* **71:** 388–92.

Report (by the Agricultural Research Council's Committee's on Johne's Disease), 1941, Testing cattle with johnin, *J Hyg,* **41:** 297–319.

Report, 1960, *Animal Health Services in Great Britain,* HMSO, London, p 37.

Ridley DS, 1958, Therapeutic trials in leprosy using serial biopsies, *Lepr Rev,* **29:** 45–52.

Ridley DS, Jopling WH, 1962, A classification of leprosy for research purposes. *Lepr Rev,* **33:** 119–28.

Ridley DS, Jopling WH, 1966, Classification of leprosy according to immunity; a five-group system, *Int J Lepr,* **34:** 255–73.

Riemann HP, Abbas B, 1983, Diagnosis and control of bovine paratuberculosis (Johne's disease), *Adv Vet Sci Comp Med,* **27:** 481–506.

Sansarricq H, 1983, Recent changes in leprosy control, *Lepr Rev,* **54, Suppl.:** 7S–16S.

Saxegaard F, Fodstad FH, 1985, Control of paratuberculosis (Johne's disease) in goats by vaccination, *Vet Rec,* **116:** 439–41.

Scadding JG, 1971, Further observations on sarcoidosis associated with *M. tuberculosis* infection, *Proceedings of the 5th International Conference on Sarcoidosis, Prague, 1969,* eds Levinsky L, Macholda F, University Karlova, Prague, 89–92.

Scadding JG, Mitchell DN, 1985, *Sarcoidosis,* 2nd edn, Chapman and Hall, London, 41.

Selroos O, 1996, Glucocorticosteroids and pulmonary sarcoidosis (editorial), *Thorax,* **51:** 229–30.

Shepard CC, 1960, The experimental disease that follows the injection of human leprosy bacilli into foot pads of mice, *J Exp Med,* **112:** 445–54.

Shepard CC, Walker LL, van Landingham R, 1978, Immunity to *Mycobacterium leprae* infections induced in mice by BCG vaccination at different times before or after challenge, *Infect Immun,* **19:** 391–4.

Sherman DM, Markham RJF, Bates F, 1984, Agar gel immunodiffusion test for diagnosis of clinical paratuberculosis in cattle, *J Am Vet Med Assoc,* **185:** 179–82.

Sigurdsson B, 1945, A specific antigen recovered from tissues infected with *Mycobacterium paratuberculosis* (Johne's disease), *J Immunol,* **51:** 279–90.

Sigurdsson B, 1946, A specific antigen recovered from tissues infected with *Mycobacterium paratuberculosis* (Johne's disease). II. Studies on the nature of the antigen and on methods of demasking it, *J Immunol,* **53:** 127–35.

Sigurdsson B, 1947, A specific antigen recovered from tissues infected with *Mycobacterium paratuberculosis* (Johne's disease). III: Further studies on the nature of the antigen and on methods of demasking it, *J Immunol,* **55:** 131–9.

Sigurdsson B, 1956, Immunological problems in paratuberculosis, *Bacteriol Rev,* **20:** 1–13.

Sigurdsson B, 1960, A killed vaccine against paratuberculosis (Johne's disease) in sheep, *Am J Vet Res,* **21:** 54–67.

Siltzbach LE, 1966, Conferences – Sarcoidosis, *Lancet,* **2:** 695–6.

Siltzbach LE, 1969, Etiology of sarcoidosis, *Practitioner,* **202:** 613–18.

Smith HW, 1960, The examination of milk for the presence of *Mycobacterium johnei, J Pathol Bacteriol,* **80:** 440–2.

Sockett DC, Carr DJ, Collins MT, 1992, Evaluation of conventional and radiometric fecal culture and a commercial DNA probe for diagnosis of *Mycobacterium paratuberculosis* infections in cattle, *Can J Vet Res,* **56:** 148–53.

Sockett DC, Conrad TA et al., 1992, Evaluation of four serological tests for bovine paratuberculosis, *J Clin Microbiol,* **30:** 1134–9.

Stamp JT, Watt JA, 1954, Johne's disease in sheep, *J Comp Pathol,* **64:** 26–40.

Stefansky WK, 1903, *Zentralbl Bakteriol Parasitenkd Infektionskr Hyg,* **33:** 481.

Taylor AW, 1950, Observations on the isolation of *Mycobacterium johnei* in primary culture, *J Pathol Bacteriol,* **62:** 647–50.

Taylor AW, 1951a, Johne's disease – its diagnosis and control, *Vet Rec,* **63:** 776–80.

Taylor AW, 1951b, Varieties of *Mycobacterium johnei* isolated from sheep, *J Pathol Bacteriol,* **63:** 333–6.

Thoen CO, Muscoplat CC, 1979, Recent developments in diagnosis of paratuberculosis (Johne's disease), *J Am Vet Med Assoc,* **174:** 838–40.

Thorel MF, Desmettre P, 1982, Comparative study of mycobacterin-dependent strains of mycobacteria isolated from woodpigeon with *Mycobacterium avium* and *M. paratuberculosis, Ann Microbiol (Paris),* **133B:** 291–302.

Thoresen DF, Saxegaard F, 1991, Gen-probe rapid diagnostic system for the *Mycobacterium avium* complex does not distinguish between *Mycobacterium avium* and *Mycobacterium paratuberculosis, J Clin Microbiol,* **29:** 625–6.

Twort FW, Ingram GLY, 1912, A method for isolating and cultivating the *Mycobacterium enteritidis chronicae pseudotuberculosae bovis Johne,* and some experiments on the preparation of a diagnostic vaccine for pseudo-tuberculous enteritis of bovines, *Proc R Soc Lond [Biol],* **84:** 517–45.

Twort FW, Ingram GLY, 1913, *A Monograph on Johne's Disease,* Baillière, London.

Vallee H, Rinjard P, Vallee M, 1934, Sur la premunisation de l'entérite paratuberculeuse des bovides, *Rev Gen Med Vet,* **43:** 777–9.

Veasey RS, Taylor HW et al., 1995, Histopathology of C57BL/6 mice inoculated with *Mycobacterium paratuberculosis, J Comp Pathol,* **113:** 75–80.

Waters MFR, 1993, Elimination of leprosy, *Lancet,* **341:** 489.

Waters MFR, 1995, Relapse following various types of multidrug therapy in multibacillary leprosy, *Lepr Rev,* **66:** 1–9.

Waters MFR, Ridley DS, Lucas SB, 1990, Positive Mitsuda lepromin reactions in long-term treated lepromatous leprosy, *Lepr Rev,* **61:** 347–52.

Waters MFR, Rees RJW et al., 1978, Rifampicin for lepromatous leprosy: nine years' experience, *Br Med J,* **1:** 133–6.

Weddell G, Palmer E, Rees RJW, 1963, Correspondence – the pathogenesis of leprosy, *Lepr Rev,* **34:** 156–8.

Wherry WB, 1908, Further notes on rat leprosy and on the fate of human and rat leprosy bacilli in flies, *J Infect Dis,* **5:** 507–14.

Whipple DL, Kapke PA, Andersen PR, 1992, Comparison of a commercial DNA probe test and three cultivation procedures for detection of *Mycobacterium paratuberculosis* in bovine feces, *J Vet Diagn Invest,* **4:** 23–7.

WHO, 1988, World Health Organization Expert Committee on Leprosy, Sixth Report, *WHO Tech Rep Ser,* No. 768.

WHO, 1994, WHO Leprosy Unit, Division of Control of Tropical Diseases, Risk of relapse in leprosy, unpublished document number WHO/CTD/LEP/94.1, World Health Organization, Geneva.

WHO, 1996, Progress towards the elimination of leprosy as a public health problem, *Wkly Epidemiol Rec,* **71:** 149–56.

WHO Memorandum, 1979, Recommended safety requirements for the preparation of lepromin: a WHO Memorandum, *Bull W H O,* **57:** 921–3.

WHO Study Group, 1982, Report of the Study Group on chemotherapy of leprosy for control programs *WHO Tech Rep Ser,* No. 675.

WHO Study Group, 1994, Chemotherapy of leprosy, *WHO Tech Rep Ser,* No. 847.

Wilesmith JW, 1982, Johne's disease: a retrospective study of vaccinated herds in Great Britain, *Br Vet J,* **138:** 321–31.

Yamamoto K, Sato M, Sato Y, 1936, Ratten lepra: statistische beobachtungen in Tokyo, *Jpn J Dermatol Urol,* **40:** 28.

Yokomizo Y, Yugi H, Merkal RS, 1985, A method for avoiding false-positive reactions in an enzyme-linked immunosorbent assay (ELISA) for the diagnosis of bovine paratuberculosis, *Jpn J Vet Sci,* **47:** 111–19.

Young RA, Mehra V et al., 1985, Genes for the major protein antigens of the leprosy parasite *Mycobacterium leprae, Nature (London),* **316:** 450–2.

Chapter 24

TYPHOID AND PARATYPHOID

J R L Forsyth

1 INTRODUCTION

Typhoid and paratyphoid represent the classical clinical syndromes associated with those members of the genus *Salmonella* that are most closely and constantly linked to human hosts, and which produce invasive disease. Typhoid, the more important illness, is caused by *Salmonella* Typhi. Paratyphoid is caused by *Salmonella* Paratyphi A, *Salmonella* Paratyphi B and *Salmonella* Paratyphi C (see also Volume 2, Chapter 41). These last 3 tend to have regional distributions. The term 'enteric fever', coined to embrace both typhoid and paratyphoid, has been defined (Levine et al. 1983) as 'a generalized infection of the reticuloendothelial system and intestinal lymphoid tissue accompanied by sustained fever and bacteremia'. The definition encompasses a disease with a range of severity, with typhoid tending to the severe, and paratyphoid to the milder, parts of the spectrum. However, each may range between an asymptomatic infection and a fatal illness. Globally, typhoid is far more common than paratyphoid (Levine et al. 1983) and the picture of enteric fever is only rarely caused by other serovars of *Salmonella enterica* (Rubin and Weinstein 1977).

These conditions, and typhoid in particular, occupy a special place in the list of infective diseases. Affecting both town and country dwellers, enteric fever has been a special obstacle to healthy living in crowded cities. It has also had a major influence in war – often rivalling military malevolence in morbidity and mortality (Leishman 1910). The control of typhoid has represented the paradigm of the sanitary era. Its endemic prevalence represents a divide between the developed and developing worlds. The global burden of typhoid is estimated as some 16 000 000 cases and 600 000 deaths each year (Pang et al. 1995).

Although Thomas Willis in 1643 described a disease strongly suggestive of typhoid and John Hunter's collection included specimens with classical ileal lesions, Gay (1918) believed that the first unambiguous clinical descriptions of enteric fever were by Louis and by Chomel early in the nineteenth century. Diagnostic confusion between typhus and typhoid was only dispelled in the middle of that century by the comparisons by Gerhard, Schoenlein and, finally, Jenner (Parker 1990). At this time, also, William Budd, by his careful observations in Devon and in Bristol, demonstrated convincingly the infectious nature of typhoid; its transmission by contact and by water; and its control by the disinfection and disposal of the faeces of cases (Budd 1873).

In the 1880s, after bacteria became recognized as infectious agents, Eberth detected typhoid bacilli microscopically and Gaffky succeeded in growing them from the spleen in fatal cases. Successful isolation of *S.* Typhi from the faeces, urine and blood followed in 1885 and 1886. Isolation of *S.* Paratyphi A, *S.* Paratyphi B and *S.* Paratyphi C allowed the differentiation of enteric fever into paratyphoid and typhoid (Parker 1990).

2 CLINICAL MANIFESTATIONS

Although the general enteric fever syndrome is well defined, the clinical presentation and course of typhoid and paratyphoid are variable and complicate both diagnosis and management.

2.1 Classical case

In the classical case, the incubation period is about 10–14 days and the onset, with fever, malaise and headache, is slow, insidious and vague. Respiratory symptoms, including bronchitis, are common. During the first week the fever becomes steadily higher on a stepwise pattern, and is about 0.5°C higher in the evening than in the morning. The height of the fever is reached at about 39–39.5°C at the end of the week (Fig. 24.1). The patient is anorexic and becomes progressively more toxic and apathetic. There is abdominal discomfort rather than pain. Constipation, relative bradycardia and mild splenomegaly are common.

During the second week the fever may be steady or may swing. The patient becomes weaker and, mentally, confusion progresses to stupor. In over half the cases, sparse crops of rose spots appear. These occur on the abdomen, lower chest and back and are difficult to see in dark-skinned patients (Huckstep 1962, Wicks, Holmes and Davidson 1971).

Prior to the advent of effective chemotherapy the illness progressed. Stupor worsened and by the third week of the disease the patient became uncomprehending, muttering and disoriented. The tongue became furred and the facies dull. This was the stage for pea-soup diarrhoea and other intestinal complications. Deaths occurred from toxaemia and exhaustion as well as from complications.

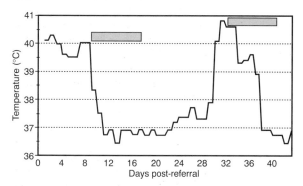

(a) Case with relapse

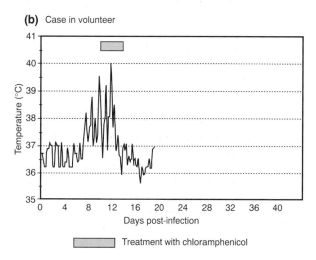

(b) Case in volunteer

Treatment with chloramphenicol

Fig. 24.1 Temperature charts of cases of typhoid illustrating: onset of illness; response to chemotherapy with chloramphenicol; and relapse. The typical delay in the response to chloramphenicol is well shown in the volunteer's chart. (Data by permission from Cook and Marmion 1949 and MM Levine, personal communication 1996).

Recovery usually began by the end of the third week with fever falling steadily, by lysis, but the course could be much prolonged. In any event, patients were profoundly exhausted and a prolonged convalescence could be expected (Hornick 1985). When typhoid occurs in the first trimester of pregnancy, abortion is common (Seoud et al. 1988).

2.2 Mild case

At the other end of the spectrum, active investigation may reveal mild or asymptomatic infections, even with bacteraemia. It has been suggested that only 20% of all those infected with typhoid might have classical disease (Cvjetanovic, Grab and Uemura 1971).

2.3 Typhoid in children

Discrepant views are held on typhoid in children. Some authors stress the mildness of the condition in children, and others the severity. Many point to poor outcomes stemming from delayed diagnosis. In developing countries, views may be coloured by only severely ill children being admitted to hospital. In general, whereas serious and complicated disease occurs, atypical and asymptomatic cases may be disproportionately common among children (Christie 1974, Ferreccio et al. 1984). In the neonate, particularly if infected in utero, typhoid is serious (Reed and Klugman 1994).

2.4 Paratyphoid fever

Typhoid and paratyphoid could only be differentiated when the aetiological agents were isolated (Fig. 24.2, Table 24.1).

Whereas the paratyphoid fevers generally yield milder illness than typhoid (Gadeholt and Madsen 1963), individual cases of enteric fever cannot be diagnosed as typhoid or paratyphoid on clinical grounds alone (Vaughan 1920).

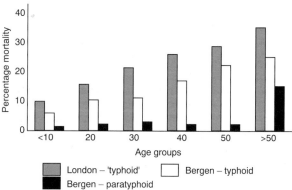

London – 'typhoid'   Bergen – typhoid
Bergen – paratyphoid

Fig. 24.2 Age-specific mortality of typhoid and paratyphoid B before effective chemotherapy: London 1871–94; Bergen 1912–61. Differentiation of these diseases would not have been possible in the earlier series (Goodall and Washbourn 1896, Gadeholt and Madsen 1963).

2.5 Incubation period

The incubation period of typhoid can only be determined when the time of exposure is clearly established, which is often impossible (Stuart and Pullen 1946). It is usually from 8 to 15 days, with wide variations; up to 40 days has been recorded. Long incubation periods tend to follow infection with small doses of organisms (Parker 1990).

2.6 Onset

In about 10% of patients the onset is abrupt, resembling classical septicaemia (Stuart and Pullen 1946). Usually, however, the patient's illness starts with a feeling of vague malaise and restlessness which may go on for days with no clear presenting picture, which explains why the diagnosis may be missed, even by experienced clinicians in endemic areas, especially when other febrile diseases are common (Wicks, Holmes and Davidson 1971, Mishra et al. 1991).

2.7 Complications of enteric fever

RELAPSE

Relapse constitutes the commonest complication of typhoid, occurring in some 10–20% of cases (Table 24.1). In this, the symptoms recur following the end of the initial, classical, attack (Fig. 24.1). After an afebrile interregnum of about 8 or 9 days, but with extremes of 1–70 days, fever and malaise return and rose spots on the trunk of white patients are common. Without treatment, the course of a relapse is normally shorter and milder than the initial attack, but prolonged, severe and even complicated disease may occur.

PERFORATION

Perforation of the bowel occurs in 0.5–5% of cases and continues to be the most dreaded complication of typhoid (van Basten and Stockenbrugger 1994). It may be difficult to recognize clinically and late intervention worsens the prognosis. Perforation is less common in younger children (Butler et al. 1991).

HAEMORRHAGE

Haemorrhage from the bowel ulcerations may occur early in the disease but as the disease progresses larger vessels may be involved and, in pre-antibiotic days, severe haemorrhage occurred in 10–20% of patients. This could be acute and catastrophic (Kearney and Kumar 1993) or more moderate but continued. Intestinal haemorrhage appears to have become substantially less frequent with adequate chemotherapy (Rowland 1961) (Table 24.1).

CARRIER STATE

Continued faecal excretion of *S.* Typhi during convalescence is common, this normally stops within 3 months (Hornick 1985) but may persist for up to a year (Bigelow and Anderson 1933). About 3% of those recovering from typhoid, and somewhat fewer after

paratyphoid B (Vogelsang and Bøe 1948) (Table 24.1), become long-term carriers. Such chronic carriage may even follow asymptomatic infection.

The carrier state occurs disproportionately often following infection in women (Hornick 1985) and in older patients and biliary carriage, with a focus usually in the gall bladder, is far more common than urinary carriage. However, the frequency of urinary carriage in areas in which urinary schistosomiasis is common illustrates the predisposition of damaged organs to harbour persistent infection. Certain other factors, such as failure to produce IgM or other antibodies to *S.* Typhi antigens (Bhaskaram, Sahay and Rao 1990) and non-secretor status (Hofmann et al. 1993), may also predispose. Evidence is accumulating that long-term carriers have an elevated risk of hepatobiliary cancer. Caygill et al. (1995) suggest that this may be mediated by the production of *N*-nitroso compounds by the bacteria.

OTHER SYSTEMS

In typhoid, involvement of the liver is a consistent feature (Morgenstern and Hayes 1991) and, in endemic areas, jaundice with persistent fever may suggest the diagnosis (McKay 1995). Cystitis is rare but *S.* Typhi is often shed in the urine in early stages of the disease and transient renal impairment is common (Khosla and Lochan 1991). A wide range of central nervous system manifestations occur. Typhoid may present as a psychosis (Ali et al. 1992) and cases of ataxia (Trevett et al. 1994) and polyneuritis have been reported. The salmonellas of enteric fever may settle in many sites and may present later as pyogenic lesions with reports of abscesses in cancellous bone, brain and even breast (Stuart and Pullen 1946, Declercq et al. 1994). Occasional asymptomatic individuals have been found to shed typhoid bacilli intravascularly in the absence of excretion in faeces or urine, illustrating the ability of *S.* Typhi to persist in diverse foci (Watson 1967).

2.8 Geographical distribution

Although typhoid is, or has been, world wide, there appear to have been changes in the distribution of the agents of paratyphoid. *S.* Paratyphi C has ceased to be common in Guyana and *S.* Paratyphi A, having disappeared from northern Europe, remains a common cause of disease in South and South East Asia and also in the Middle East and Central and South America. *S.* Paratyphi B has become much less common in Europe and North America and is very rare in the Indian subcontinent. Cases of paratyphoid in travellers reflect these patterns.

3 PATHOGENESIS

Investigation of the pathogenesis of enteric fever has been seriously hampered by the lack of suitable experimental models. Even the chimpanzee exhibits a much modified disease, and only after huge infectious

Table 24.1 Percentage incidence of complications in enteric fever

Author	Goodall[a]	McCrae	Bergen[b]		Rowland	Walker
Year	1896	1913	1948/1963		1961	1965
Disease	Typhoid	Typhoid	Typhoid	Para. B	Typhoid	Typhoid
Cases	506	1500	1119	1528	530	469
					Chemotherapy[c]	
Relapse	13.0	11.4	18.5	3.5	10.8	18.3
Perforation	3.1	2.6	1.7	0.2	0.8	0
Haemorrhage	7.9	7.8	12.4	4.4	1.7	0.2
Chronic carriage	NS[d]	NS	3.3[e]	1.9[e]	NS	1.1
Death	17.4[f]	9.1	12.1	2.3	3.6	0.6

[a]Goodall and Washbourn (1896).
[b]Figures combined from overlapping series published by Vogelsang and Bøe (1948) and Gadeholt and Madsen (1963). These excluded cases which had been treated with specific chemotherapy.
[c]Cases in the series after 1950 were treated with chloramphenicol or ampicillin.
[d]NS, incidence not stated in the series.
[e]Incidence in the subset of the Bergen cases published by Vogelsang and Bøe (1948).
[f]Deaths taken from a large series of 9223 patients admitted between 1871 and 1894.

doses (Warren and Hornick 1979). As a result, direct information has had to come from clinical and pathological observations on patients; from studies on volunteers; and from in vitro studies on cell and tissue cultures.

A systemic disease, analogous to enteric fever in man, is caused in some rodents by *Salmonella* Typhimurium, and to some extent *Salmonella* Enteritidis (Table 24.2), and this model has been used extensively. However, this murine disease is still sufficiently dissimilar to prevent unqualified extrapolation to human enteric fever.

3.1 Site of entry

The evidence that enteric fever is transmitted by food, milk and water and the necropsy findings of ulcerated ileal Peyer's patches suggested an oral route of entry with invasion through the gut. The failure of experimental gargling of virulent *S.* Typhi to cause disease dispelled suspicions that the respiratory tract symptoms, often seen early in enteric fever, related to invasion in the pharynx (Hornick et al. 1970a).

A concept of the general course of invasion came from the distribution of organisms found during natural disease and at necropsy, and from rodent models. The infectious dose is believed to pass through the stomach and pylorus with invasion of epithelium taking place in the small bowel. The bacteria penetrate the cells without causing cellular disruption and pass through to the lamina propria. Here the bacteria are not adequately contained and spread to mesenteric lymph nodes and, by way of the lymphatic system and the thoracic duct, to the bloodstream, giving rise to a transient and usually symptomless primary bacteraemia. The bacteria are arrested and settle largely in spleen, liver and bone marrow and are constrained for the remaining incubation period. At the end of this interval, multiplication of the organisms gives rise to a secondary and persistent bacteraemia along with the signs and symptoms of the disease and bacteria pour into the bowel from the biliary tract. The mesenteric nodes remain infected from the start but the intestinal epithelium may be cleared except at the lymphatic aggregates (Parker 1990).

Table 24.2 Antigenic formulae of *Salmonella* causing enteric fever

	Somatic (O) antigens	Flagellar (H) antigens	
		Phase 1	Phase 2
Enteric fever in man			
Salmonella Typhi	9,12,[Vi][a]	d (j)	−[b](z66)[c]
Salmonella Paratyphi A	1,2,12[d]	a	[1,5]
Salmonella Paratyphi B	1,4,[5],12	b	1,2
Salmonella Paratyphi C	6,7,[Vi]	c	1,5
Enteric fever in mice			
Salmonella Typhimurium	1,4,[5],12	i	1,2
Salmonella Enteritidis	1,9,12	g,m	−

[a][] Antigen variably present.
[b]− Phase 2 antigen normally absent.
[c]() Unusual strains, but common in Indonesia, have these alternative antigens.
[d]Underlining of symbols of somatic antigens indicates these are dependent on lysogenic conversion.
After WHO Collaborating Centre for Reference and Research on *Salmonella*.

3.2 Barriers

The protective role of stomach acid against enteric pathogens is shown by the increased vulnerability of patients who have undergone gastrectomy or who suffer from achlorhydria. A further measure of protection is afforded by the normal flora of the jejunum, as susceptibility is increased by doses of antibiotics before an infective challenge (Hornick et al. 1970a).

3.3 Invasion of the intestinal epithelium

Experimental work has shown how, on the approach of the organisms, the cell surface degenerates and the bacteria enter and traverse the cell, surviving within a membrane-bound vacuole, and emerge in the lamina propria. Despite active reorganization, the cell reconstitutes and can survive the passage of many salmonellas (Francis, Starnbach and Falkow 1992). Direct invasion through M cells is, however, probably more important (Jones, Ghori and Falkow 1994).

The bacteria need intact O antigen to invade and a complex of genes, and their products, governs the ability of the bacteria to adhere to and to internalize within the epithelial cells (Elsinghorst, Baron and Kopecko 1989, Mroczenski-Wildey, DiFabio and Cabello 1989).

3.4 Invasion of macrophages

In the lamina propria, S. Typhi stimulates a predominantly mononuclear response (Mallory 1898) and, when engulfed by the predominant macrophages, many of the bacteria are able to survive and multiply. The process is metabolically complex, with more than 30 salmonella proteins being induced during invasion of the macrophage (Buchmeier and Heffron 1991). The *phoP–phoQ* gene complex in salmonellas appears to determine survival within macrophages (Miller 1991).

It is probable that the enteric bacteria migrate within these macrophages to the regional lymph nodes with continuing proliferation, and thence to the bloodstream and the reticuloendothelial system (Falkow, Isberg and Portnoy 1992). It appears that, within a short time, invasive salmonellas reach safe intracellular havens (Hornick et al. 1970a) which may or may not be macrophages (Dunlap et al. 1992).

3.5 Mediators of clinical manifestations

The results of measurements of the levels of bacteraemia and of circulating endotoxin in patients, as well as experience with typhoid in volunteers previously desensitized to endotoxin, all argue against bacterial endotoxin having an important role in the manifestations of enteric fever (Hornick et al. 1970b, Butler et al. 1978).

On the other hand, there is profound cytokine activity in enteric fever. In the mouse model, it appears that tumour necrosis factor (TNF)-α (Mastroeni et al. 1992), interferon (IFN)-γ and interleukin (IL)-1 (Kita et al. 1992) are involved in terminating the stage of early rapid proliferation. In typhoid, studies in Nepal (Butler et al. 1993) and Indonesia (Keuter et al. 1994) show that increased levels of TNF receptor and lower production of proinflammatory cytokines are markers of severe and complicated cases.

The clinical picture of typhoid is minimally altered either by previous vaccine or by the size of the infecting dose (Glynn et al. 1995) and it is tempting to consider that overt disease follows the accumulation of specific stimuli during incubation to a threshold level; in asymptomatic infection, even with bacteraemia, this threshold is not reached.

3.6 Recovery

Whereas patients receiving successful specific antibacterial treatment show rapid remission of symptoms, in untreated typhoid recovery is generally slow and, in either case, excretion of salmonellas, short of chronic carriage, may be prolonged. These, and the frequency of relapse, indicate the slow and marginal quality of the immunity, probably cell mediated, which reins in the disease.

3.7 Complications

Early after infection the Peyer's patches become hyperplastic and hyperaemic. In some, the overlying tissues become necrotic and ulcerated and create localized areas vulnerable to perforation, whether slow or abrupt. Deep ulceration readily involves large vessels with subsequent major bleeding (Kearney and Kumar 1993).

Chronic biliary carriage is frequently, but not invariably, associated with the presence of gallstones, whether pre-existing or not. S. Typhi can invade stones and thus provide a site capable of constant seeding.

3.8 Host genetics

For 70 years it has been known that, in the mouse model, host susceptibility is under genetic control and the complexity of the determinants has been slowly established (Miller, Hohmann and Pegues 1994). Some observations have also suggested the role of genetic factors in human disease. These include the predisposition of non-secretors of ABH (ABO blood group) substance to become chronic carriers and Naylor's finding of a bi- or trimodal distribution of incubation periods in defined outbreaks of typhoid (Parker 1990).

3.9 Virulence factors

In contrast to the more rapid development of knowledge in mouse typhoid, genetic factors in the enteric fever agents are less well understood. For each of the classical major antigens, flagellar, somatic and capsular (Vi), an association with virulence has been found. Expression of Vi by causative strains has been correlated with virulence in volunteers and with severity of disease in certain outbreaks of typhoid (Hornick 1985). Somatic antigen has been shown to be important in adherence to gut epithelium and in resisting clearance by phagocytes, and flagellar antigen in cell invasion (Finlay and Falkow 1989).

Resistance to the action of polymorphs is mediated, in *S.* Typhi, by failure to trigger the respiratory burst (Hornick 1985). Within macrophages, products of *phoQ* act as detectors (sensor kinases) of environmental status and control the release of *phoP* products, in turn controlling the expression of some 13 different loci, permitting adaptation to a changing intracellular milieu (Belden and Miller 1994). This survival in macrophages represents a marker of virulence and of host specificity.

3.10   Immunity

The nature of immunity to enteric fever is complex. Not even previous systemic disease confers solid immunity. Second attacks of clinical disease, particularly after large infecting doses, have been observed in both natural and experimental disease (Parker 1990). A child has been reported to have caught typhoid twice from the same carrier (Wright et al. 1994). Despite this, carriers appear to show substantial immunity to their own strains. Further systemic disease is exceptional, although the gut of biliary carriers is exposed to high concentrations of demonstrably pathogenic organisms (Thompson 1954).

HUMORAL

Originally, immunity was considered to equate to the development of a specific antibody, as detected by the techniques used. It was shown that mixing virulent bacteria with serum from immunized individuals reduced virulence for experimental animals (Pfeiffer and Kolle 1896a). These findings were extended to relate to particular antigens. In animal models, somatic antigen was a demonstrable virulence factor and flagellar antigen was not. This was taken to mean that antibody to the O antigen was protective but experiments in volunteers revealed little association with antibody levels and vaccine trials indicated an importance of antibody to H and Vi antigens (Cvjetanovic and Uemara 1965, Hornick 1985).

CELLULAR

Against this preoccupation with humoral immunity, it was shown that, irrespective of antibody, infection with a live, avirulent salmonella protected mice against challenge with a virulent strain and that circulating antibody could not stop salmonellas multiplying in liver and spleen. This was felt to indicate that only cell mediated immunity would be relevant in enteric fever (Collins 1974). These experiments, however, in specific, highly susceptible strains of mice ignored the evidence of vaccine trials and were inadequately indicative of enteric fever in humans. Even in the mouse

model, natural killer cells rather than T cells are important in controlling the early stages of infection (Schafer and Eisenstein 1992). Nevertheless, the susceptibility of human patients on steroids or with AIDS to salmonellosis and enteric fever reinforces the importance of the cell mediated arm in these infections (Gotuzzo et al. 1991, Pithie, Malin and Robertson 1993).

The role of different arms of immunity, and aimed against different epitopes, varies with the stage of invasion and infection and the effect is quantitative rather than absolute. It is also clear that the immune response is directed against a much wider range of epitopes than was originally considered but the role of these other entities, which include outer-membrane proteins, in pathogenesis and recovery remains to be elucidated (Blanco et al. 1993).

4   EPIDEMIOLOGY

Historically, typhoid was shown to be a specific infective disease because it only occurred in a particular squalid village when introduced from without, and that its spread was in association with excreta from the site of obvious pathology – the gut (Budd 1873). Hornick's experiments (Parker 1990) suggested that the infectious dose is large, with no volunteer being infected by a dose of 10^3 organisms, but Mossel and Oei (1975) showed how rapid transition through the stomach can explain infection following small doses.

4.1   Sources of infection

Once the causative organism of typhoid was identified, it was possible to discover that infected humans are the only significant ultimate source whereas isolation from other animals is exceptional and from the environment only after human contamination. Budd showed that acute cases of the disease were a potent source of infection to their care givers, but the relevance of convalescent excreters and chronic carriers to the epidemiology of typhoid was not shown until early in the twentieth century (Ledingham and Arkwright 1912).

4.2   Routes of transmission

CONTACT

Transmission from acute cases to care givers is principally by contact. The danger of nursing cases in homes with inferior water supplies and sewage disposal facilities was demonstrated by Ramsey (1934). This factor is likely to be very important in developing countries, with atypical cases and convalescent excreters adding to the hazard (Harvey 1915b).

WATER-BORNE
Drinking water

The efficiency with which typhoid can be spread by the consumption of contaminated water has been demonstrated repeatedly (Holden 1970) and in the late nineteenth century the incidence of typhoid served as an index of the quality of a city's water supply. This led to the adoption of filtration to improve the quality of water, particularly from surface water sources. Delays in implementing this in the USA made the incidence of typhoid in American centres higher than in Europe (Hazen 1903). By 1934, Ramsey could review how reduction in the incidence of typhoid in the USA had followed improvement of water supplies but could also note frequent episodes associated with avoidable failures in treatment and distribution.

Whereas surface waters are readily recognized as dangerously prone to pollution, the need for care in the management of water from apparently pure sources is illustrated by the pollution of bore water either by seepage of sewage through geological imperfections (Murphy, Petrie and Morris 1944) or, as at Croydon, in 1937, by contamination of a well during repairs (Murphy 1938).

Recreation in water

Exposure to contaminated water during recreation carries a much lower risk than drinking it and reports of outbreaks of enteric fever following swimming in water, salt or fresh, have usually involved grossly contaminated environments (Parker 1990). In general, water-associated transmission of paratyphoid seems to be disproportionately rarer than that of typhoid (Savage 1942).

S. Typhi survives poorly in polluted and in warm water, probably due to predation, but survival is extended in sediments (Holden 1970). Whereas these organisms may survive for months in drains and cesspools, storage of water from rivers remains an effective first stage in purification, with a greater than 90% reduction in colony-forming typhoid bacilli in a week.

FOOD-BORNE

Many outbreaks of typhoid and paratyphoid have been food-borne and the contamination of food has occurred under a variety of circumstances. Whereas the population at risk is usually much smaller than in water-borne outbreaks, the organisms may be concentrated in food items or, even more effectively, may multiply in foods under suitable conditions.

Food contaminated by a carrier during preparation

This may result in an extended series of cases with contamination of food giving rise to cases intermittently over weeks or years (Soper 1939). Alternatively, dramatic outbreaks may follow the contamination of a particular dish. In one such, more than 90 people were infected by eating a spaghetti dish and it was shown that the heat of cooking had, in the depth of the dish, favoured multiplication of the pathogens rather than their destruction (Sawyer 1914). In these abrupt outbreaks the problem of locating the source is reduced.

The food vehicle can be unusual. Two major outbreaks in the USA have followed the contamination

of orange juice during preparation (Birkhead et al. 1993).

Food components contaminated at a remote site

Desiccated coconut, prepared under unhygienic conditions in New Guinea, gave rise to cases of typhoid and salmonellosis in Australia when the product was used for decorating confectionery (Wilson and Mackenzie 1955). The salmonellas had survived for months in the dry product.

The consumption of imported canned meats caused a series of epidemics in Britain over some 15 years. This culminated in the large Aberdeen outbreak in 1964. The vehicle was difficult to elucidate because only a few cans were affected and also because an autoclaved can seemed such an improbable source. However, the ability of organisms to penetrate minute flaws in the seams of the retorted cans during cooling in polluted water, and the ability of *S.* Typhi to multiply in the contents without causing spoilage or swelling of cans was finally demonstrated (Anderson and Hobbs 1973). In some episodes, spread was extended by meat from the initial can contaminating a retailer's slicer (Editorial 1973).

Shellfish

Because bivalve shellfish filter particulate matter from the water in which they live, they can concentrate pathogenic micro-organisms and can be a potent source of typhoid, particularly when eaten raw or inadequately cooked. In this way, numerous epidemics, sometimes protracted, have resulted from eating oysters (Mair 1909, Parker 1990).

Milk

Although infection of cattle with *S.* Typhi is exceptional, and with *S.* Paratyphi B most unusual, the circumstances of production, distribution and consumption of milk, as well as its capacity to support the survival and growth of the relevant organisms, have led to many important outbreaks. Cases of typhoid following delivery of milk by a convalescent case were described shortly after Budd's initial publications (Taylor 1858).

The Bournemouth (Shaw 1937) episode is a good example of the complex chain of events that may lead to an outbreak. In this a chronic typhoid carrier contaminated, via a defective cesspool, a stream in which cows waded. From the resulting contamination of the dairy more than 700 cases were infected by consuming raw milk.

Even pasteurization fails to protect when post-processing contamination occurs, as with the notorious Montreal outbreak (Boucher 1927) which led to some 7000 cases.

Dairy products, including cheese, have often been incriminated as vehicles of enteric fever, particularly paratyphoid (Parker 1990).

FLIES AND FOMITES

Firth and Horrocks (1902) found that *S.* Typhi was able to survive when dried on clothing and in soil;

they also showed, in the laboratory, that flies could carry the organism on their feet. Nevertheless, the role of flies in transmission has not been clearly established. Although *S.* Typhi was cultured from 5 of 13 flies captured during a Chicago epidemic, Harvey (1915a) failed to repeat this, despite culturing 500 flies.

4.3 Nosocomial infections

Infections of nursing and medical attendants of cases still occur (Report 1983), but rarely. Similarly, spread in hospitals is unusual although labour wards and neonatal nurseries remain areas of special risk (Ayliffe et al. 1979). Carriers in mental hospitals, however, have long constituted a problem (Grimme 1908) and substantial efforts to detect and treat this group have been made. Frank iatrogenic infection remains a possibility as exemplified by transmission from rectal infusions (Hervey 1929) and by an imperfectly disinfected endoscope (Dean 1977).

4.4 Occupational infection

Occasional infections occur among sewage and sludge workers (Report 1983) but, because of the amplification of bacteria in culture, typhoid is a substantial risk to personnel in diagnostic and research laboratories (Report 1995). Cultures submitted to laboratories for quality assurance have resulted in infection of laboratory workers (Blaser and Lofgren 1981).

4.5 Natural history

Where measured adequately, the distribution and prevalence of typhoid can be shown to have changed dramatically with improving social conditions (see Fig. 24.3).

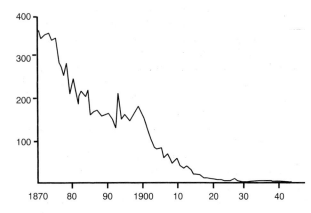

Fig. 24.3 The success of the 'complex web created by modern sanitation'. The fall in standardized death rates from enteric fever, per million, in England and Wales before the advent of effective chemotherapy. (From Bradley 1949, by permission).

IN DEVELOPED COUNTRIES

The building of the 'complex armour created by modern sanitation' in the developed world has been associated with the separation of humans from their sewage, and a steep decline in the incidence of typhoid (Bradley 1949). This impact of modern plumbing was further shown by the massive resurgence of typhoid in parts of Europe following the destruction of facilities and of social organization in the latter phases of the Second World War (Stowman 1948). Since then, the continuing decline in the incidence of enteric fever has resumed, interrupted by sporadic epidemics which have become progressively more rare.

Standards of life-style

The contribution of general standards of living and levels of education to the decline of enteric fevers is shown by the far greater incidence of typhoid in non-volunteers, who were less likely to be health conscious, than in volunteers given only tetanus toxoid, during vaccine trials (Yugoslav Typhoid Commission 1964). Nevertheless, special circumstances may create pockets of high incidence, at variance with general standards of health care and education, as in Santiago, Chile where, for example, inadequately treated sewage was used to irrigate vegetable crops during the dry season (Sears et al. 1984).

Migration and tourism

The extensive immigration to industrialized nations of people from countries in which the enteric fevers are endemic has inevitably introduced chronic carriers as well as some people who must learn and apply the appropriate practices of preventive hygiene (Convery and Frank 1993). Further, travel to and from countries of origin by immigrants and their relatives has contributed extensively to cases of enteric fever in the industrialized countries (Report 1991). To this has been added the enormous growth of tourism, which has included visits to countries with endemic enteric disease. Cases thus acquired abroad now make up a large proportion of all enteric fever notified (Braddick and Sharp 1993, Yew, Goh and Lim 1993).

IN DEVELOPING COUNTRIES

In the developing countries in which the enteric fevers are still endemic, increases in population and urbanization have often been in advance of the ability to create a public health infrastructure, particularly in the face of increasing poverty. Social, economic and military disruptions have also tended to aggravate the incidence of enteric fever (Edelman and Levine 1986). Ashcroft (1964) speculated that, under conditions of intense transmission, subclinical infections occurred very early in life and protected against overt disease later so that modest improvements in hygiene triggered more cases of classical disease. The frequency of severe disease in children in endemic areas, however, indicates that this hypothesis is incomplete.

4.6 Seasonal incidence

Previously, classical typhoid in the USA and in Britain had a peak incidence in summer and autumn (Scott 1941); however, extensive water-borne typhoid created a year-round pattern and seasonal consumption of contaminated shellfish caused a peak in November (Ramsey 1934). Now, sporadic epidemics show no seasonal trend but there is a peak of cases associated with the tourist season in many industrialized countries.

4.7 Age incidence

The series of over 9000 cases reported in London between 1871 and 1894 (Goodall and Washbourn 1896) represented clinical enteric fever in an urban community of all ages (Fig. 24.4) and these data are consistent with the contention that maximum susceptibility lies between the ages of 15 and 25 years. In endemic areas it is probable that many cases occur in children but inadequate diagnostic facilities and surveillance make the proportion uncertain (Hornick 1985).

In epidemics the age incidence is heavily dependent upon the nature of the epidemic and the source of infection (see Fig. 24.5). In Aberdeen, the disproportionate number of cases in women aged between 15 and 29 years was attributed to the popularity of cold meat in dieting schedules (Walker 1965).

5 DIAGNOSIS

5.1 Clinical diagnosis

The clinical diagnosis of enteric fever is difficult and uncertain, particularly in the early stages. Laboratory facilities are essential to ensure optimal diagnosis, appropriate therapy and relevant public health management, but clinical suspicion is necessary before the laboratory assistance can be mobilized.

5.2 Laboratory diagnosis

To determine the aetiology in infective disease, laboratory assistance can take the form of:

1 **cultural isolation** and identification of the organism
2 the recognition of a **specific immunological response** to the agent or
3 the **direct detection** of the aetiological agent, its specific products, antigens or genomic elements – possibly after amplification.

ISOLATION OF THE AETIOLOGICAL AGENT

Over time, improvements in media and laboratory techniques have greatly affected the apparent incidence of the enteric fevers and allowed more thorough epidemiological investigations.

Selective and indicator media

Indicator and selective media are essential to allow the isolation of enteric pathogens from contaminated sites. In most early media, selection was provided by the incorporation of certain dyes and failure to produce acid on the fermentation of lactose was the basis of indication of likely colonies. Variation between the serovars of *S. enterica* requires the use of more than a single medium. Leifson's deoxycholate–citrate agar (DCA), Taylor's xylose–lysine–deoxycholate (XLD) and variants of Wilson and Blair's bismuth sulphite media are all highly effective and remain popular, with the last suffering somewhat from difficulty in preparation and instability in storage (Parker 1990).

Enrichment media

It soon became clear that, for culture from faeces and other contaminated specimens, preliminary specific enrichment of the pathogen in a liquid medium increased the yield after subculture to indicator media. Müller's tetrathionate broth was made more selective by the addition of brilliant green and is still used extensively. However, the selenite broths of Leifson, with variants like strontium selenite (Iveson and Mackay-Scollay 1969), are generally favoured. As with the solid media, however, more than a single broth is essential to recover a full range of serovars of *Salmonella* (Parker 1990).

Standard practice for the isolation of *S.* Typhi from contaminated sites includes the inoculation of one or more enrichment media, with subculture to indicator media the following day, as well as direct inoculation of solid indicator media. Primary pre-enrichment, in a non-selective liquid medium, is important in the resuscitation of damaged organisms, as from dried foods, but needs careful handling to avoid overgrowth of contaminants.

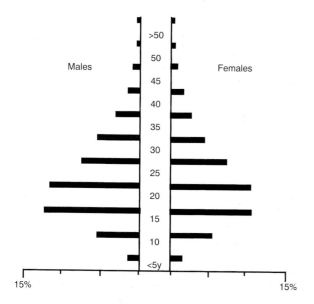

Fig. 24.4 Age- and gender-specific incidence of 'typhoid', London, 1871–94 (Goodall and Washbourn 1896).

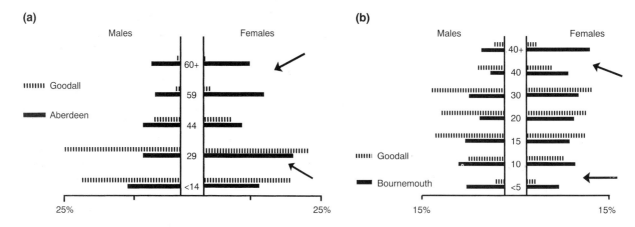

Fig. 24.5 (a) Age- and gender-specific incidence, as percentages of all cases, during the canned-meat associated typhoid outbreak, Aberdeen, 1964, with comparative data from London cases, 1871–94 (data from Goodall and Washbourn 1896, Walker 1965). Arrows point to features of the Aberdeen outbreak. (b) Age- and gender-specific incidence, as percentages of all cases, during the Bournemouth–Poole milk-borne typhoid epidemic, with comparative data from London cases, 1871–94 (data from Goodall and Washbourn 1896, Shaw 1937). Arrows point to special features of the milk-borne outbreak.

SELECTION OF SPECIMENS

The traditional view that *S.* Typhi is maximally isolated from blood in the first week of disease, from faeces in the second and following weeks, and from urine in the third and fourth weeks is generally correct (see Fig. 24.6), but exceptions are frequent. If collected, blood cultures may occasionally be positive in the incubation period and early shedding of the organism in faeces can also occur (Hornick 1985).

Blood

Although the level of bacteraemia is low, blood culture is probably the single most useful diagnostic procedure for the diagnosis of clinical enteric fever. It is often positive during the early ambulant phase of the disease. It continues to be positive until effective treatment is given. It is positive during relapses. With few exceptions, a positive blood culture has a high predictive value for current enteric fever.

The rate of recovery from blood culture, now 70–90%, has improved with advances in technique. For success, taking an adequate volume of blood into a suitable volume of liquid medium (e.g. 10 ml blood to 50 ml liquid medium) and taking cultures on several occasions are more important than the use of additives to combat non-specific inhibitors (Watson 1955).

'Clot culture' in which the serum is removed from a blood specimen and the clot, cut up with sterile scissors or loosened with the use of streptokinase, is incubated with broth for subsequent subculture, has its advocates for the diagnosis of typhoid (Watson 1955). The technique makes use of the residuum of blood submitted for serological or biochemical tests and was of substantial value during the Aberdeen outbreak (Walker 1965).

Faeces

Culture of faeces is a standard diagnostic technique and repeated specimens over 2–3 days should be tested to cope with the variability of timing and profusion of shedding of the organisms. Preliminary dilution of the faeces, even to 1:1000, before inoculation of media has advantages (Parker 1990). Rectal swabs are an inferior option, carrying a lower rate of recovery (Shaughnessy, Friewer and Snyder 1948), but should be used if no other specimen is available.

Urine

During enteric fever, organisms are often shed in the urine, and for diagnosis of cases or carriers 5–20 ml volumes can be mixed with equal volumes of selenite enrichment broth for incubation and subculture.

Bile

Several workers have reported that culture of a duodenal aspirate, rich in bile, has yielded *S.* Typhi when other methods have failed. Both cases and carriers have been diagnosed (Gilman and Hornick 1976,

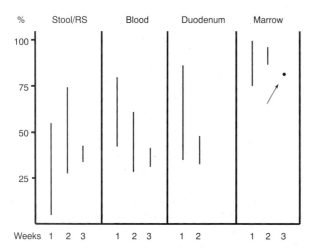

Fig. 24.6 Ranges of rates of isolation of enteric *Salmonella* from different sites during successive weeks of illness (data from Stuart and Pullen 1946, Gilman et al. 1975a, Benavente et al. 1984, Vallenas et al. 1985). Only one author gave data for bone marrow specimens during the third week of illness.

Gilman et al. 1979) using a kit which conveniently samples duodenal mucus with a nylon string, swallowed and later withdrawn.

Bone marrow

For 70 years bone marrow has repeatedly been shown to be the specimen yielding the most positive cultures (Gilman et al. 1975a). Nevertheless, sampling of marrow for culture is not often performed because it requires sterile equipment and skill and is unpleasant for the patients (Vallenas et al. 1985).

IDENTIFICATION OF CULTURES

Presumptive identification is performed by examining the responses of a purified culture to a set of standard biochemical tests. The set chosen usually corresponds with the laboratory's routine and may be from a commercial kit (Vitek, API, etc.) or one or 2 stages of conventional media (Barrow and Feltham 1993, Gray 1995). Standard practice is then to carry out slide agglutination tests for the principal antigens on the presumptively identified culture. Direct agglutination of suspicious colonies off a selective plate is inadvisable as some media reduce the expression of certain surface antigens (Knox, Gell and Pollock 1942) and antigens may be shared between genera. Detailed elucidation of the serovar is usually left to a reference laboratory.

Coagglutination (Mukherjee, Malik and Khan 1993) and enzyme immunoassay (Qadri et al. 1990) tests have been developed to aid preliminary identification of organisms from blood culture broths.

Isolation of a strain allows assessment of antibiotic sensitivity and of strain type, thus aiding patient management, disease surveillance and epidemiological investigation (Salmon and Bartlett 1995).

TYPING

Among the agents of enteric fever, standard schemes for phage typing have been developed for S. Typhi, S. Paratyphi A and S. Paratyphi B. The first of these schemes was developed from the work of Craigie and Yen and the others were developed by Felix and Callow and by Banker, respectively (Anderson and Williams 1956, Parker 1990). All are sourced from the Laboratory of Enteric Pathogens, CPHL, Colindale. These schemes, when carried out by national reference laboratories, have considerable merits in that they are robust; are global in application; have standard interpretation; and a large base of information (IFEPT Report 1982). Molecular methods (Threlfall et al. 1994, Thong et al. 1996), although not yet standard, may fruitfully be used to supplement phage typing.

SEROLOGY

The description by Widal near the end of the nineteenth century (Edelman and Levine 1986), that the sera of typhoid patients developed agglutinating antibodies to S. Typhi, promised an important diagnostic tool but it was half a century before the techniques were standardized (Felix 1950). Agglutinins to the

somatic (TO) antigens (see Table 24.2) develop later in the illness and decline slowly and variably in recovery, but those to flagellar antigens (TH) rise early and persist (Schroeder 1968). The wide distribution of the somatic antigens among related organisms limits the specificity of the relevant reaction. Further, some patients fail to develop demonstrable antibody (Bhaskaram, Sahay and Rao 1990). The Widal test, using those antigen suspensions which are appropriate to the diagnosis of the prevalent enteric fever agents (see Table 24.3), has been used either to compare paired sera to look for specific rises of antibody or to test a single serum taken on admission in the hope that significant antibody levels will already have been reached. The former only provides a late diagnosis and may be modified by treatment. The specificity in both is affected by antibody from previous stimuli, whether from cross-reacting antigens, subclinical disease or vaccine. These deficiencies have led many authors to believe that the test is worthless even in non-endemic areas (Koeleman et al. 1992). Others have felt that the Widal test is useful for cases in children, who have a low prevalence of pre-existing antibody (Choo et al. 1993), or when antibody titres are interpreted in the light of local conditions (Aquino et al. 1991).

Alternative serological techniques

In an attempt to improve specificity and sensitivity, other serological methods have been considered; indirect immunofluorescence, indirect haemagglutination, enzyme immunoassay and counter immunoelectrophoresis have been used (Parker 1990) but have been less promising than tests using outer-membrane proteins as alternative antigens.

A 50–52 kDa protein, felt to be specific to S. Typhi, has been delineated and a dot enzyme immunoassay developed which appears to be as sensitive as the Widal test but with a much better negative predictive value (Ortiz et al. 1989, Ismail, Kader and Kok Hai 1991, Choo et al. 1994).

DIRECT RECOGNITION

Given the frequent need for equipment or reagents too costly or too unstable for those countries of the developing world most affected by typhoid, the value of methods for the direct recognition of specific antigens or nucleic acid is somewhat limited. Slide coagglutination and enzyme immunoassay methods for the detection of antigens of S. Typhi in urine and serum have not been useful (Parker 1990).

For the detection of specific nucleic acid, Rubin et al. (1989) described a probe technique used, with some success, to diagnose typhoid from specimens of blood. Furthermore, several groups have exploited the sensitivity of the polymerase chain reaction (PCR) on clinical specimens (Rahn et al. 1992, Song et al. 1993, Hashimoto et al. 1995).

CARRIER DETECTION

Because the prevalence of carriers in the community is low, their detection, whether to investigate out-

Table 24.3 Antigens used in a representative Widal test

Somatic antigens			
TO		*Salmonella* Typhi	Alcoholized, washed suspensions of fully smooth (S) forms of standard, fully agglutinable strains
AO		*Salmonella* Paratyphi A	
BO		*Salmonella* Paratyphi B	
Flagellar antigens			
TH	d	*Salmonella* Typhi[a]	Formalized suspensions of smooth, motile, forms of standard strains, selected for correct phase[c]
AH	a	*Salmonella* Paratyphi A	
BH	b	*Salmonella* Paratyphi B	
NSH	1,2	*Salmonella* serovar – non-specific phase[b]	

[a]*Salmonella* Virginia may be used as an alternative strain.
[b]*Salmonella* Newport is frequently used.
[c]By passage through Craigie tube or Jameson strip.

breaks or to screen workers in potentially sensitive occupations, demands the use of techniques which are convenient, cheap and have high predictive values. The collection of specimens for culture, although always the definitive step, does not readily meet these criteria, particularly in the routine screening of substantial numbers of workers. The collection of these specimens is inconvenient and prone to substitution; processing is costly and single examinations may miss significant numbers of carriers.

The discovery by Felix that antibody to Vi antigen was closely associated with chronic carriage led to a widely used screening test (Anderson 1961) but one with limited sensitivity and specificity (Bokkenheuser 1964). Attempts to improve the test by coupling extracted Vi antigen to red cells for an indirect haemagglutination test had little success until Wong and colleagues used a gentle extraction procedure to avoid denaturing the antigen (Nolan et al. 1980). This modified test has worked effectively, but not perfectly (Lanata et al. 1983). Screening for antibody to Vi permits cultural tests to be focused upon a smaller proportion of the test population, but isolation is still necessary for confirmation; to determine the route of shedding; and for typing, to determine epidemiological significance.

6 TREATMENT

6.1 Historical

Before the advent of specific antimicrobial chemotherapy, only supportive care was available. Medical debate focused on the importance of nursing care, with a sustaining diet and an adequate fluid intake and on lukewarm baths to reduce fever. The administration of specific antisera, or even inactivated vaccines, proved useless.

6.2 Chemotherapy

EARLY CHEMOTHERAPY

Each group of chemotherapeutic agents discovered has been investigated for its activity in enteric fever and, despite evidence of in vitro sensitivity (Hornick 1985), the aminoglycosides, the tetracyclines, polymyxin and the early cephalosporins were found to be ineffective.

CHLORAMPHENICOL

The efficacy of chloramphenicol was discovered by accident during a therapeutic trial of scrub typhus (Smadel 1950) and was confirmed with a placebo controlled trial (Woodward et al. 1948). Patients showed unprecedented rapid clinical improvement and a dramatic decline in mortality. Nevertheless, it was noted that faecal excretion continued during treatment and that the incidence of relapses was increased (Hornick 1985).

SEMISYNTHETIC PENICILLINS AND CO-TRIMOXAZOLE

Although co-trimoxazole (trimethoprim–sulphamethoxazole) can be a useful second-line drug (Butler, Rumans and Arnold 1982), only the trimethoprim component is effective. Ampicillin proved disappointing in practice (Patel 1964) but amoxycillin is better absorbed when given by mouth and is at least twice as active in vitro (Neu 1974). It was also effective in clinical trials (Gilman et al. 1975b), providing faster defervescence, fewer relapses and fewer residual chronic carriers than in a group treated with chloramphenicol (Scragg and Rubridge 1975).

CEPHALOSPORINS

Cephamandole, cefoperazone and ceftriaxone have been shown to be effective agents. The last has been useful even with 3 day intravenous or intramuscular regimens, but some patients have remained febrile (Acharya et al. 1995).

Fluoroquinolones

The fluoroquinolones are active by mouth, penetrate well in tissues and are concentrated in phagocytes and bile and have been highly effective in treating enteric fever (James 1989). Ciprofloxacin (Gulati et al. 1992) and ofloxacin (Sabbour and Osman 1990) have been most commonly used, and found superior to ceftriaxone (Smith et al. 1994). They represent the drugs of choice in the treatment of enteric fever (DuPont 1993). The fear of serious arthropathy in children has not been upheld in practice (Schaad et al. 1995).

6.3 Drug resistance

Acquired drug resistance came slowly to *S.* Typhi. Initial reports of resistance to chloramphenicol were scattered and isolated. Even the large epidemic in Mexico in 1972, caused by a strain of specific phage type and carrying chloramphenicol resistance on an H_1 plasmid, subsided (Hornick 1985). Continued sensitivity to antibiotics was probably due to the instability of plasmids in this organism (Robins-Browne et al. 1981). However, in the late 1980s the prevalence of chloramphenicol-resistant strains began to rise rapidly in India and Pakistan and, by 1992, 70–80% of strains in many areas were resistant to ampicillin and trimethoprim as well as to chloramphenicol. This stability of resistance-bearing plasmids was new (Pang et al. 1995). Whereas most isolates remain sensitive to the fluoroquinolones, strains with chromosomally mediated resistance are emerging (Rowe, Ward and Threlfall 1995).

6.4 Special treatment regimens

Complicated cases of enteric fever

Hoffman found that augmenting antibiotic treatment of the very toxic cases encountered in Indonesia with high dose dexamethasone reduced mortality from 50% to 10% and, for these severe cases, this has been confirmed elsewhere (Olle Goig and Ruiz 1993). In perforation, prompt surgery, extended antibiotic treatment and vigorous support are needed to cope with the 30% mortality reported in many series (van Basten and Stockenbrugger 1994). For mild cases of intestinal haemorrhage, sedation and transfusion may suffice but, with severe and continuing haemorrhage, modern techniques for angiographic localization and control of bleeding points may need to be supplemented by radical surgery (Kearney and Kumar 1993).

Chronic carrier state

Chronic carriers merit treatment to reduce their chance of malignancy and the constraints upon their life-style as well as to reduce the public health risk. Elective cholecystectomy has been shown to result in lasting cure of the majority of biliary carriers but the procedure bears morbidity and some mortality and a chemotherapeutic option is desirable. Prolonged courses of ampicillin or amoxycillin, with doses at the limit of tolerance, proved successful in curing many carriers who could complete the regimen but the presence of gallstones reduced the chance of success (Parker 1990). The fluoroquinolones have yielded far better results with Gotuzzo et al. (1988) and Ferreccio et al. (1988) achieving apparent cures in more than three-quarters of their subjects. With urinary carriers it is often necessary to treat the underlying lesion first and treatment, where relevant, of underlying schistosomiasis may bring success.

7 Prevention

The enteric fevers are inherently preventable and vulnerable to eradication. Prevention of infective diseases depends on consistently breaking the chain represented by **sources**, **transmission** and **recipients** by appropriate action (Fig. 24.7).

7.1 Limiting the infectivity of sources

The relative importance, as sources, of acute cases, undiagnosed or convalescent excreters, or chronic carriers depends largely on the prevailing state of enteric fever in the community. When enteric fever becomes uncommon, the role of the chronic carrier, often unsuspected and with prolonged infectivity, becomes paramount. However, the importance of identifying all excreters, and of their management with a protocol of suitable enteric precautions, is implicit. This implies the investigation of all individuals who have been exposed to infection.

Tests for the cessation of excretion

All protocols for determining when a case or a carrier can be assumed to have stopped excreting recommend multiple examinations of faeces (and of urine, if relevant) which commence well after the cessation of chemotherapy and with samples taken at such intervals as to improve detection of intermittent excretion (Table 24.4). Braddick, Crump and Yee

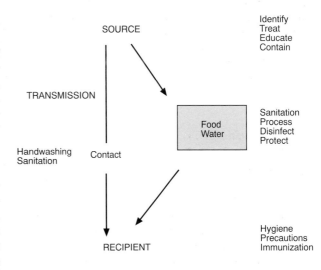

Fig. 24.7 Enteric fever: principles of epidemiology and prevention.

(1991) have reviewed the costs and the efficacy of some standard protocols.

7.2 Preventing transmission

Transmission of the enteric fevers is normally by contact or by oral intake of contaminated food or water. Consistent with a high infectious dose, standard hygienic precautions in hospital or home are very effective if observed. Because some excreters and carriers will inevitably be missed, the importance of everyday hygienic behaviour and of adequate facilities for disposal of excreta and for hand washing is clear.

FOOD-BORNE

The primary prevention of food-borne enteric fever consists in separating excreters from handling food, particularly food which is to be eaten without further cooking. The difficulties of achieving this in countries in which enteric fevers are highly endemic are almost overwhelming. The secondary barrier consists in the management of the production of food components, and of food itself, so as to minimize contamination and the opportunities for the multiplication of food-borne pathogens.

The increasing global trade in salad vegetables (Salmon and Bartlett 1995) and other foods constitutes a heavy responsibility for importers and exporters. In endemic countries, the implementation of suitable techniques for waste water management (Mara and Cairncross 1989) that will allow safe irrigation of crops is a major challenge.

DRINKING WATER

The quality of drinking water can be compromised at any point between the original source and ultimate consumption. Since typhoid represented the paradigm for water-borne disease, the classical methods of selecting the best available source of water, and then providing the barriers of storage, filtration and disinfection, are demonstrably highly effective in prevention, provided the distribution system is also protected and maintained. Nevertheless, in developing countries particularly, the essential infrastructure may be defective in nature or in operational management, and yet remains a priority. For the improvement of small supplies there is an overwhelming need for the implementation of relevant technology (Cairncross and Feachem 1983).

7.3 Recipients

IMMUNIZATION

Inactivated vaccines

The importance of typhoid stimulated both Wright (1896) and Pfeiffer and Kolle (1896b) to develop crude typhoid vaccines from suspensions of inactivated organisms. These vaccines were assessed solely on their ability to elicit antibody. They were initially used extensively, but rarely systematically, in military populations and claims of protection were based on inadequate and unquantifiable assessment (Cockburn 1955). It was clear that protection was imperfect and that, if disease developed, it was not modified by the previous vaccine. Nevertheless, widespread vaccination in the USA army and in the British army in India appeared to result in serovar-specific protection (Harvey 1915b, Batson 1949).

Attempts to improve the vaccine included selection of smooth strains; adding components of *S.* Paratyphi A, *S.* Paratyphi B, or both; producing a freeze-thaw extracted antigen; and attempting to preserve the immunogenicity of the Vi moiety, first in an alcoholized preparation and then by using acetone for killing and drying the component bacteria.

The first well controlled trials were carried out under WHO auspices in the early 1960s and in eastern Europe and Guyana. In these, large numbers of subjects were used, diagnoses were confirmed and randomized controls received unrelated vaccine. The results of these trials eliminated the alcoholized and the freeze-thaw extract vaccines from consideration and showed that whereas the standard heat–phenol vaccine provided significant protection, the acetone-based product was definitely better (see Table 24.5) and that extended protection was possible (Ashcroft et al. 1967). In volunteer experiments, these vaccines gave protection only when the subjects were challenged with a small, ID25 dose of *S.* Typhi. Oral preparations of inactivated vaccines are useless (Parker 1990) and these parenteral whole cell vaccines are associated with high rates of local and even systemic reactions, close to the limits of acceptability. Addition of paratyphoid components was abandoned because of inadequate evidence of extra protection against the increase of reactions (Cvjetanovic and Uemura 1965).

The protective capacity of Vi antigen was greatly enhanced when methods of gentle extraction and purification left immunogenicity intact and reduced reactions. The resulting vaccine, now licensed for use, has shown low rates of reaction and significant protection in trials (Tacket and Levine 1995) (see Table 24.5). As a polysaccharide immunogen, it suffers from being T cell independent. Attempts to prepare protein-conjugated variants are proceeding (Szu et al. 1994).

Oral, live attenuated vaccines

Whereas streptomycin-dependent strains of *S.* Typhi proved impracticable to manage (Levine 1976), the stable *galE* mutant Ty21a strain (Tacket and Levine 1995), isolated after exposing *S.* Typhi Ty2 to *N*-methyl-*N'*-nitrosoguanidine, proved to be highly protective when 3 doses were given in a liquid formulation (Wahdan et al. 1982). This vaccine was licensed and has been used very widely but further trials in Chile and Indonesia have shown disappointing protection, specially when the vaccine was given in enteric coated capsules. Furthermore, the reasons for its attenuation are obscure. Several approaches to attenuation by site-specific genetic deletion have yielded promising candidate strains with well defined genetic lesions. These have included strains with deletions in

Table 24.4 Outlines of 2 sets of guidelines for the management of excreters of enteric *Salmonella* in the community

Guidelines by:	American Public Health Association[a]	Public Health Laboratory Service[b]		
Type of case	Convalescent case Chronic carrier	Convalescent or chronic excreters		
? Differentiate by perceived risk to public	No	Yes		
Grade of risk to public		High: Food handlers[c] Water workers[d]	Medium: Small children Health care workers	Minimal:
?Exclude excreters	Food handlers and patient care HCW[e], from work	From work	From school: from work	Not. Counselling only
Protocols for release after recovery or treatment				
Consecutive negative specimens[f]	3	12	3	
Interval between specimens	1 month	8 × weekly; 4 × monthly	Weekly	
?Post-purgation specimens[g]	No fewer than 1	No fewer than 2		
?Further surveillance	No	6 months		

[a]Benenson (1995).
[b]PHLS Salmonella Sub-Committee (1990). This must be consulted for details.
[c]Handling unwrapped food to be eaten without further cooking.
[d]Workers in direct contact with drinking water.
[e]Health care workers.
[f]Specimens of faeces (urine if indicated).
[g]Specimens of faeces collected following purgation with magnesium sulphate.

Table 24.5   Percentage protection rates from some field trials of typhoid vaccines

	Yugoslav 1[a] 1962	Yugoslav 2[b] 1964	Guyana[c] 1967	S. Africa[d] 1987	Nepal[e] 1987	Egypt[f] 1982	Chile[g] 1989	Indonesia[h] 1991
Heat–phenol	74	54	65					
Alcoholized	50							
Acetone		70	88					
Vi (purified)				64	74			
Ty21a (liquid)[i]						96		53
Ty21a (enteric)[j]							74	42

[a]Yugoslav Typhoid Commission (1962).
[b]Yugoslav Typhoid Commission (1964).
[c]Ashcroft et al. (1967).
[d]Klugman et al. (1987).
[e]Acharya et al. (1987).
[f]Wahdan et al. (1982).
[g]Ferreccio et al. (1989) (3 doses of vaccine, protection at 2 years).
[h]Simanjuntak et al. (1991).
[i]Lyophilized Ty21a, resuspended freshly before ingestion.
[j]Lyophilized Ty21a in enteric coated capsule.

the *phoP* gene, in the *ompR* gene and in *cya* and *crp* but work is most advanced with strains carrying deletions in the *aro* genes (Tacket and Levine 1995). Whereas small-scale trials have shown several candidates to be defective in immunogenicity or in attenuation, CVD 908, a $\Delta aroC \Delta aroD$ strain, is highly promising, far more immunogenic than Ty21a (Pang et al. 1995) and elicits cytotoxic T lymphocytes (Sztein et al. 1995).

TRAVELLERS

For the guidance of travellers to endemic areas, suitable protocols in avoiding infection have been drawn up by WHO and by the health authorities of many industrialized countries. Although questions have been raised about the cost-benefit of immunizing travellers (Behrens and Roberts 1994), the evidence for protective benefit is clear (Schwartz et al. 1990).

7.4   Outbreak investigation in prevention

Even in areas of significant endemicity, recognition and investigation of an outbreak or trend may lead, as with shellfish-associated typhoid in Belfast or the irrigated vegetables in Santiago, to practicable preventive strategies. As the incidence of enteric fever declines, outbreaks are more readily recognized and contribute more to community outrage.

SURVEILLANCE

The recognition of trends requires an appropriate system of surveillance in which both clinical and laboratory data are collected and which functions sufficiently well for timely action. The typing of significant isolates adds value to surveillance by assisting the association of cases, sources and potential vehicles.

Once recognized, a cluster of cases or a trend calls for the definition of the classical factors of *place, time* and *person* in attempting to ascertain potential commonalities of experience and hence exposure.

During investigation, the history of complex pathways of infection and of unlikely vehicles counsel the keeping of an open mind. When numerous individuals have to be screened to find a potential source, it may be found that the ready identification of blood samples and the speed of performing Vi serology may outweigh the known deficiencies of the method (Lanata et al. 1983, Lin et al. 1988). The use of the sewer swab technique has proved invaluable for the location of carriers or the detection of vehicles in many outbreaks (Sears et al. 1984).

Successful investigation of an outbreak may lead to location of the source, the identification of the vehicle and the method of transmission. These then permit rational and targeted public health interventions to eliminate or control the hazard, both in relation to the specific current problem and the potential for future incidents. Reduction of infections leads to fewer sources for the future (Ames and Robins 1943) and this cascade effect has contributed to the rapid reduction in incidence that has occurred in developed countries (see Fig. 24.2).

7.5   Global control

Cvjetanovic's model (Cvjetanovic, Grab and Uemura 1971) favoured improving sanitation over the use of vaccine for the control of typhoid, indicating the added benefits of investment in sanitation. Nevertheless, the preliminary evidence of cost-effectiveness (Shepard et al. 1995) and of herd immunity following widespread use of typhoid vaccine (Bodhidatta et al. 1987, Levine et al. 1989) combine with the economic constraints of developing countries to encourage the adoption of an extensive vaccine strategy, once a suitable agent is available, to bring the problem of endemic typhoid within bounds.

REFERENCES

Acharya IL, Lowe CU et al., 1987, Prevention of typhoid fever in Nepal with the Vi capsular polysaccharide of *Salmonella typhi*. A preliminary report, *N Engl J Med*, **317**: 1101–4.

Acharya G, Butler T et al., 1995, Treatment of typhoid fever: randomized trial of a three-day course of ceftriaxone versus a fourteen-day course of chloramphenicol, *Am J Trop Med Hyg*, **52**: 162–5.

Ali G, Kamili MA et al., 1992, Neuropsychiatric manifestations of typhoid fever, *J Assoc Physicians India*, **40**: 333–5.

Ames WR, Robins M, 1943, Age and sex as factors in the development of the typhoid carrier state, and a method for estimating carrier prevalence, *Am J Public Health*, **33**: 221–30.

Anderson ES, 1961, Report of the P.H.L.S. Working Party on the Bacteriological Examination of Waterworks Employees. The detection of the typhoid carrier state, *J Hyg Camb*, **59**: 231–47.

Anderson ES, Hobbs BC, 1973, Studies of the strain of *Salmonella typhi* responsible for the Aberdeen typhoid outbreak, *Isr J Med Sci*, **9**: 162–74.

Anderson ES, Williams REO, 1956, Bacteriophage typing of enteric pathogens and staphylococci and its use in epidemiology, *J Clin Pathol*, **9**: 94–127.

Aquino RL, Lansang MA et al., 1991, Evaluation of a single Widal test in the diagnosis of enteric fever, *Southeast Asian J Trop Med Public Health*, **22**: 375–9.

Ashcroft MT, 1964, Typhoid and paratyphoid fevers in the tropics, *J Trop Med Hyg*, **67**: 185–9.

Ashcroft MT, Balwant S et al., 1967, A seven-year field trial of two typhoid vaccines in Guyana, *Lancet*, **2**: 1056–9.

Ayliffe GAJ, Geddes AM et al., 1979, Spread of *Salmonella typhi* in a maternity hospital, *J Hyg Camb*, **82**: 353–9.

Barrow GI, Feltham RKA, 1993, *Cowan and Steel's Manual for the Identification of Medical Bacteria*, 3rd edn, Cambridge University Press, London, 128–50.

van Basten JP, Stockenbrugger R, 1994, Typhoid perforation. A review of the literature since 1960, *Trop Geogr Med*, **46**: 336–9.

Batson HC, 1949, Typhoid fever prophylaxis by active immunisation, *Public Health Rep*, **Suppl. 212**: 1–34.

Behrens RH, Roberts JA, 1994, Is travel prophylaxis worth while? Economic appraisal of prophylactic measures against malaria, hepatitis A, and typhoid in travellers, *Br Med J*, **309**: 918–22.

Belden WJ, Miller SI, 1994, Further characterization of the PhoP regulon: identification of new PhoP-activated virulence loci, *Infect Immun*, **62**: 5095–101.

Benavente L, Gotuzzo E et al., 1984, Diagnosis of typhoid fever using a string capsule device, *Trans R Soc Trop Med Hyg*, **78**: 404–6.

Benenson AS (editor in chief), 1995, *Control of Communicable Diseases Manual*, 16th edn, American Public Health Association, Washington, DC, 502–7, 533.

Bhaskaram P, Sahay BK, Rao NS, 1990, Specific immune responses in typhoid fever and after TAB vaccination, *Indian J Med Res*, **91**: 115–19.

Bigelow GH, Anderson GW, 1933, Cure of typhoid carriers, *JAMA*, **101**: 348–52.

Birkhead GS, Morse DL et al., 1993, Typhoid fever at a resort hotel in New York: a large outbreak with an unusual vehicle, *J Infect Dis*, **167**: 1228–32.

Blanco F, Isibasi A et al., 1993, Human cell mediated immunity to porins from *Salmonella typhi*, *Scand J Infect Dis*, **25**: 73–80.

Blaser MJ, Lofgren JP, 1981, Fatal salmonellosis originating in a clinical microbiology laboratory, *J Clin Microbiol*, **13**: 855–8.

Bodhidatta L, Taylor DN et al., 1987, Control of typhoid fever in Bangkok, Thailand, by annual immunization of school-children with parenteral typhoid vaccine, *Rev Infect Dis*, **9**: 841–5.

Bokkenheuser V, 1964, Detection of typhoid carriers, *Am J Public Health*, **54**: 477–86.

Boucher S, 1927, An interim report on the Montreal typhoid fever epidemic, *Med Officer*, **38**: 8.

Braddick MR, Crump BJ, Yee ML, 1991, How long should patients with *Salmonella typhi* or *Salmonella paratyphi* be followed-up? A comparison of published guidelines, *J Public Health Med*, **13**: 101–7.

Braddick MR, Sharp JC, 1993, Enteric fever in Scotland 1975–1990, *Public Health*, **107**: 193–8.

Bradley WH, 1949, The control of typhoid fever, *J Inst Water Engrs*, **3**: 167–78.

Buchmeier NA, Heffron F, 1991, Induction of *Salmonella* stress proteins upon infection of macrophages, *Science*, **248**: 730–2.

Budd W, 1873, *Typhoid Fever: its Nature, Mode of Spreading and Prevention*, Longman Green, London.

Butler T, Rumans L, Arnold K, 1982, Response of typhoid fever caused by chloramphenicol-susceptible and chloramphenicol-resistant strains of *Salmonella typhi* to treatment with trimethoprim-sulfamethoxazole, *Rev Infect Dis*, **4**: 551–61.

Butler T, Bell WR et al., 1978, Typhoid fever: studies of blood coagulation, bacteremia and endotoxemia, *Arch Intern Med*, **138**: 407–503.

Butler T, Islam A et al., 1991, Patterns of morbidity and mortality in typhoid fever dependent on age and gender: review of 552 hospitalized patients with diarrhea, *Rev Infect Dis*, **13**: 85–90.

Butler T, Ho M et al., 1993, Interleukin-6, gamma interferon, and tumor necrosis factor receptors in typhoid fever related to outcome of antimicrobial therapy, *Antimicrob Agents Chemother*, **37**: 2418–21.

Cairncross S, Feachem RG, 1983, *Environmental Health Engineering in the Tropics*, John Wiley, Chichester.

Caygill CP, Braddick M et al., 1995, The association between typhoid carriage, typhoid infection and subsequent cancer at a number of sites, *Eur J Cancer Prev*, **4**: 187–93.

Choo KE, Razif AR et al., 1993, Usefulness of the Widal test in diagnosing childhood typhoid fever in endemic areas, *J Paediatr Child Health*, **29**: 36–9.

Choo KE, Oppenheimer SJ et al., 1994, Rapid serodiagnosis of typhoid fever by dot enzyme immunoassay in an endemic area, *Clin Infect Dis*, **19**: 172–6.

Christie AB, 1974, Typhoid and paratyphoid fevers, *Infectious Diseases: Epidemiology and Clinical Practice*, 2nd edn, Churchill Livingstone, Edinburgh, 55–130.

Cockburn WC, 1955, Large-scale field trials of active immunizing agents with special reference to vaccination against pertussis, *Bull W H O*, **13**: 395–407.

Collins FM, 1974, Vaccines and cell-mediated immunity, *Bacteriol Rev*, **38**: 371–402.

Convery HT, Frank L, 1993, Management issues in a major typhoid fever outbreak, *Am J Public Health*, **83**: 595–6.

Cook AT, Marmion DE, 1949, Chloromycetin in treatment of typhoid fever; 14 cases treated in the Middle East, *Lancet*, **2**: 975–9.

Cvjetanovic B, Grab B, Uemura K, 1971, Epidemiological model of typhoid fever and its use in the planning and evaluation of anti-typhoid immunization and sanitation programmes, *Bull W H O*, **45**: 53–75.

Cvjetanovic B, Uemura K, 1965, The present status of field and laboratory studies of typhoid and paratyphoid vaccines with special reference to studies sponsored by the World Health Organization, *Bull W H O*, **32**: 29–36.

Dean AG, 1977, Transmission of *Salmonella typhi* by fibreoptic endoscopy, *Lancet*, **2**: 134.

Declercq J, Verhaegen J et al., 1994, *Salmonella typhi* osteomyelitis, *Arch Orthop Trauma Surg*, **113**: 232–4.

Dunlap NE, Benjamin WH et al., 1992, A 'safe-site' for *Salmonella typhimurium* is within splenic polymorphonuclear cells, *Microb Pathog*, **13**: 181–90.

DuPont HL, 1993, Quinolones in *Salmonella typhi* infection, *Drugs*, **45, Suppl. 3**: 119–24.

Edelman R, Levine MM, 1986, Summary of an international workshop on typhoid fever, *Rev Infect Dis*, **8**: 329–49.

Editorial, 1973, Aberdeen's typhoid bacillus, *Lancet*, **1**: 645–6.

Elsinghorst EA, Baron LS, Kopecko DJ, 1989, Penetration of human intestinal epithelial cells by *Salmonella*: molecular cloning, expression of *Salmonella typhi* invasion determinants in *Escherichia coli*, *Proc Natl Acad Sci USA*, **86**: 5173–7.

Falkow S, Isberg RR, Portnoy DA, 1992, The interaction of bacteria with mammalian cells, *Annu Rev Cell Biol*, **8**: 333–63.

Felix A, 1950, Standardization of diagnostic agglutination tests: typhoid and paratyphoid A and B fevers, *Bull WHO*, **2**: 643–9.

Ferreccio C, Levine MM et al., 1984, Benign bacteremia caused by *Salmonella typhi* and *paratyphi* in children younger than 2 years, *J Pediatr*, **104**: 899–901.

Ferreccio C, Morris JG Jr et al., 1988, Efficacy of ciprofloxacin in the treatment of chronic typhoid carriers, *J Infect Dis*, **157**: 1235–9.

Ferreccio C, Levine MM et al., 1989, Comparative efficacy of two, three, or four doses of TY21a live oral typhoid vaccine in enteric-coated capsules: a field trial in an endemic area, *J Infect Dis*, **159**: 766–9.

Finlay BB, Falkow S, 1989, Salmonella as an intracellular parasite, *Mol Microbiol*, **3**: 1833–41.

Firth RH, Horrocks-WH, 1902, An inquiry into the influence of soil, fabrics, and flies in the dissemination of enteric infection, *Br Med J*, **2**: 936–43.

Francis CL, Starnbach MN, Falkow S, 1992, Morphological and cytoskeletal changes in epithelial cells occur immediately upon interaction with *Salmonella typhimurium* grown under low-oxygen conditions, *Mol Microbiol*, **6**: 3077–87.

Gadeholt H, Madsen ST, 1963, Clinical course, complications and mortality in typhoid fever as compared with paratyphoid B. A survey of 2647 cases, *Acta Med Scand*, **173**: 753–60.

Gay FP, 1918, *Typhoid Fever: Considered as a Problem of Scientific Medicine*, The Macmillan Company, New York.

Gilman RH, Hornick RB, 1976, Duodenal isolation of *Salmonella typhi* by string capsule in acute typhoid fever, *J Clin Microbiol*, **3**: 456–7.

Gilman RH, Terminel M et al., 1975a, Relative efficacy of blood, urine, rectal swab, bone-marrow and rose-spot cultures for recovery of *Salmonella typhi* in typhoid fever, *Lancet*, **1**: 1211–13.

Gilman R, Terminel M et al., 1975b, Comparison of trimethoprim-sulfamethoxazole and amoxicillin in therapy of chloramphenicol-resistant and chloramphenicol-sensitive typhoid fever, *J Infect Dis*, **132**: 630–6.

Gilman RH, Islam S et al., 1979, Identification of gallbladder typhoid carriers by a string device, *Lancet*, **1**: 795–6.

Glynn JR, Hornick RB et al., 1995, Infecting dose and severity of typhoid: analysis of volunteer data and examination of the influence of the definition of illness used, *Epidemiol Infect*, **115**: 23–30.

Goodall EW, Washbourn JW, 1896, Enteric fever, typhoid fever, *A Manual of Infectious Diseases*, eds Goodall EW, Washbourn JW, HK Lewis, London, 290–329.

Gotuzzo E, Guerra JG et al., 1988, Use of norfloxacin to treat chronic typhoid carriers, *J Infect Dis*, **157**: 1221–5.

Gotuzzo E, Frisancho O et al., 1991, Association between the acquired immunodeficiency syndrome and infection with *Salmonella typhi* or *Salmonella paratyphi* in an endemic typhoid area, *Arch Intern Med*, **151**: 381–2.

Gray LD, 1995, *Escherichia*, *Salmonella*, *Shigella*, and *Yersinia*, *Manual of Clinical Microbiology*, 6th edn, eds Murray PR, Baron EJ et al., ASM Press, Washington, DC, 450–6.

Grimme, 1908, Ueber die Typhusbazillenträger in den Irrenanstalten, *Muench Med Wochenschr*, **55**: 16–19.

Gulati S, Marwaha RK et al., 1992, Multi-drug-resistant *Salmonella typhi* – a need for therapeutic reappraisal, *Ann Trop Paediatr*, **12**: 137–41.

Harvey D, 1915a, The causation and prevention of enteric fever in military service, with special reference to the importance of the carrier: being an account of work done at Naini Tal Enteric Depot, 1908–11. Part 1, *J R Army Med Corps*, **24**: 491–508.

Harvey D, 1915b, The causation and prevention of enteric fever in military service, with special reference to the importance of the carrier: being an account of work done at Naini Tal Enteric Depot, 1908–11. Part 2, *J R Army Med Corps*, **25**: 94–120.

Hashimoto Y, Itho Y et al., 1995, Development of nested PCR based on the ViaB sequence to detect *Salmonella typhi*, *J Clin Microbiol*, **33**: 775–7.

Hazen A, 1903, *The Filtration of Public Water-supplies*, John Wiley, New York.

Hervey CR, 1929, A series of typhoid fever cases infected per rectum, *Am J Public Health*, **19**: 166–71.

Hofmann E, Chianale J et al., 1993, Blood group antigen secretion and gallstone disease in the *Salmonella typhi* chronic carrier state, *J Infect Dis*, **167**: 993–4.

Holden WS, 1970, *Water Treatment and Examination*, J & A Churchill, London, 248–69.

Hornick RB, 1985, Selective primary health care: strategies for control of disease in the developing world. XX. Typhoid fever, *Rev Infect Dis*, **7**: 536–46.

Hornick RB, Greiseman SE et al., 1970a, Typhoid fever: pathogenesis and immunologic control. First of two parts, *N Engl J Med*, **283**: 686–91.

Hornick RB, Greiseman SE et al., 1970b, Typhoid fever: pathogenesis and immunologic control. Second of two parts, *N Engl J Med*, **283**: 739–46.

Huckstep RL, 1962, *Typhoid Fever and Other Salmonella Infections*, Livingstone, Edinburgh.

IFEPT Report, 1982, The geographical distribution of *Salmonella typhi* and *Salmonella paratyphi* A and B phage types during the period 1 January 1970 to 31 December 1973, *J Hyg Camb*, **88**: 231–54.

Ismail A, Kader ZS, Kok Hai O, 1991, Dot enzyme immunosorbent assay for the serodiagnosis of typhoid fever, *Southeast Asian J Trop Med Public Health*, **22**: 563–6.

Iveson JB, Mackay-Scollay EM, 1969, Strontium chloride and strontium selenite enrichment broth media in the isolation of salmonella, *J Hyg Camb*, **67**: 457–64.

James DG, 1989, Therapeutic focus. The fluoroquinolones, *Br J Clin Pract*, **43**: 66–7.

Jones BD, Ghori N, Falkow S, 1994, *Salmonella typhimurium* initiates murine infection by penetrating and destroying the specialized epithelial M cells of the Peyer's patches, *J Exp Med*, **180**: 15–23.

Kearney D, Kumar A, 1993, Massive gastrointestinal haemorrhage in typhoid: successful angiographic localization and embolization, *Australas Radiol*, **37**: 274–6.

Keuter M, Dharmana E et al., 1994, Patterns of proinflammatory cytokines and inhibitors during typhoid fever, *J Infect Dis*, **169**: 1306–11.

Khosla SN, Lochan R, 1991, Renal dysfunction in enteric fever, *J Assoc Physicians India*, **39**: 382–4.

Kita E, Emoto M et al., 1992, Contribution of interferon gamma and membrane-associated interleukin 1 to the resistance to murine typhoid of Ityr mice, *J Leukoc Biol*, **51**: 244–50.

Klugman KP, Gilbertson IT et al., 1987, Protective activity of Vi capsular polysaccharide vaccine against typhoid fever, *Lancet*, **2**: 1165–9.

Knox R, Gell PGH, Pollock MR, 1942, Selective media for organisms of the salmonella group, *J Pathol Bacteriol*, **54**: 469–83.

Koeleman JG, Regensburg DF et al., 1992, Retrospective study to determine the diagnostic value of the Widal test in a non-endemic country, *Eur J Clin Microbiol Infect Dis*, **11**: 167–70.

Lanata CF, Levine MM et al., 1983, Vi serology in detection of chronic *Salmonella typhi* carriers in an endemic area, *Lancet*, **2**: 441–3.

Ledingham JCG, Arkwright JA, 1912, *The Carrier Problem in Infectious Diseases*, Edward Arnold, London.

Leishman WB, 1910, Anti-typhoid inoculation, *J R Inst Public Health*, **18:** 385–401.

Levine MM, Kaper JB et al., 1983, New knowledge on the pathogenesis of bacterial enteric infections as applied to vaccine development, *Microbiol Rev*, **47:** 510–50.

Levine MM, Ferreccio C et al., 1989, Progress in vaccines against typhoid fever, *Rev Infect Dis*, **11, Suppl. 3:** S552–67.

Lin FY, Becke JM et al., 1988, Restaurant-associated outbreak of typhoid fever in Maryland: identification of carrier facilitated by measurement of serum Vi antibodies, *J Clin Microbiol*, **26:** 1194–7.

McCrae T, 1913, Typhoid fever, *Modern Medicine: its Theory and Practice*, vol. 1, 2nd edn, eds Osler W, McCrae T, Lea & Febiger, Philadelphia, 67–199.

McKay S, 1995, Typhoid fever in Cambodia, *Cambodia Dis Bull*, **6:** 52–76.

Mair LWD, 1909, The aetiology of enteric fever in Belfast in relation to water supply, sanitary circumstances, and shellfish, *Proc R Soc Med*, **2:** 187–242.

Mallory FB, 1898, A histological study of typhoid fever, *J Exp Med*, **3:** 611–38.

Mara D, Cairncross S, 1989, *Guidelines for the Safe Use of Wastewater and Excreta in Agriculture and Aquaculture. Measures for Public Health Protection*, World Health Organization/UNEP, Geneva.

Mastroeni P, Villarreal B et al., 1992, Serum TNF alpha inhibitor in mouse typhoid, *Microb Pathog*, **12:** 343–9.

Miller SI, 1991, PhoP/PhoQ: macrophage-specific modulators of *Salmonella* virulence?, *Mol Microbiol*, **5:** 2073–8.

Miller SI, Hohmann EL, Pegues DA, 1994, Salmonella (including *Salmonella typhi*), *Principles and Practice of Infectious Diseases*, eds Mandell GL, Bennett JR, Dolin R, Churchill Livingstone, New York, 2013–33.

Mishra S, Patwari AK et al., 1991, A clinical profile of multidrug resistant typhoid fever, *Indian Pediatr*, **28:** 1171–4.

Morgenstern R, Hayes PC, 1991, The liver in typhoid fever: always affected, not just a complication, *Am J Gastroenterol*, **86:** 1235–9.

Mossel DAA, Oei HY, 1975, Person-to-person transmission of enteric bacterial infection, *Lancet*, **1:** 751.

Mroczenski-Wildey MJ, Di Fabio JL, Cabello FC, 1989, Invasion and lysis of HeLa cell monolayers by *Salmonella typhi*: the role of lipopolysaccharide, *Microb Pathog*, **6:** 143–52.

Mukherjee C, Malik A, Khan HM, 1993, Rapid diagnosis of typhoid fever by co-agglutination in an Indian hospital, *J Med Microbiol*, **39:** 74–7.

Murphy HL, 1938, *Report on a Public Local Enquiry into an Outbreak of Typhoid Fever at Croydon in October and November 1937*, HMSO, London.

Murphy WJ, Petrie LM, Morris JF, 1944, Incidence of typhoid fever – in a population exposed to a contaminated industrial water supply, *Ind Med*, **13:** 995–7.

Neu HC, 1974, Antimicrobial activity and human pharmacology of amoxicillin, *J Infect Dis*, **129, Suppl.:** S123–31.

Nolan CM, Feeley JC et al., 1980, Evaluation of a new assay for Vi antibody in chronic carriers of *Salmonella typhi*, *J Clin Microbiol*, **30:** 1299–306.

Olle Goig JE, Ruiz L, 1993, Typhoid fever in rural Haiti, *Bull Pan Am Health Organ*, **27:** 382–8.

Ortiz V, Isibasi A et al., 1989, Immunoblot detection of class-specific humoral immune response to outer membrane proteins isolated from *Salmonella typhi* in humans with typhoid fever, *J Clin Microbiol*, **27:** 1640–5.

Pang T, Bhutta ZA et al., 1995, Typhoid fever and other salmonellosis: a continuing challenge, *Trends Microbiol*, **3:** 253–5.

Parker MT, 1990, Enteric infections: typhoid and paratyphoid, *Topley & Wilson's Principles of Bacteriology, Virology and Immunity*, vol. 3, 8th edn, eds Parker MT, Collier LH, Edward Arnold, London, 424–46.

Patel KM, 1964, Ampicillin in typhoid fever, *Br Med J*, **1:** 907.

Pfeiffer R, Kolle W, 1896a, Ueber die specifische Immunitäts-reaction der Typhusbacillen, *Z Hyg Infektionskr*, **21:** 203–46.

Pfeiffer R, Kolle W, 1896b, Experimentelle Untersuchungen zur Frage der Schutzimpfung des Menschen gegen Typhus abdominalis, *Dtsch Med Wochenschr*, **22:** 735–7.

PHLS Salmonella Sub-Committee, 1990, *Notes on the Control of Human Sources of Gastrointestinal Infections, Infestations and Bacterial Intoxications in the United Kingdom*, PHLS, London.

Pithie AD, Malin AS, Robertson VJ, 1993, Salmonella and shigella bacteraemia in Zimbabwe, *Cent Afr J Med*, **39:** 110–12.

Qadri A, Ghosh S et al., 1990, Sandwich enzyme immunoassays for detection of *Salmonella typhi*, *J Immunoassay*, **11:** 251–69.

Rahn K, De Grandis SA et al., 1992, Amplification of an *inv*A gene sequence of *Salmonella typhimurium* by polymerase chain reaction as a specific method of detection of *Salmonella*, *Mol Cell Probes*, **6:** 271–9.

Ramsey GH, 1934, What are the essentials of typhoid fever control today?, *Am J Public Health*, **24:** 355–62.

Reed RP, Klugman KP, 1994, Neonatal typhoid fever, *Pediatr Infect Dis J*, **13:** 774–7.

Report, 1983, Typhoid fever, England and Wales, 1978–82; Public Health Laboratory Service, *Br Med J*, **287:** 1205.

Report, 1991, Enteric fever England and Wales 1981–90, *Commun Dis Rep*, **1:** 71.

Report, 1995, *Surveillance of Notifiable Infectious Diseases in Victoria, 1994*, Infectious Disease Unit, Health and Community Services, Melbourne, Australia, 89–90.

Robins-Browne R, Bhamjee A et al., 1981, Acquisition of resistance by *Salmonella typhi* in vivo, *Lancet*, **2:** 148.

Rowe B, Ward LR, Threlfall EJ, 1995, Ciprofloxacin-resistant *Salmonella typhi* in the UK, *Lancet*, **346:** 1302.

Rowland HAK, 1961, The complications of typhoid fever, *J Trop Med Hyg*, **64:** 143–52.

Rubin FA, McWhirter PD et al., 1989, Use of a DNA probe to detect *Salmonella typhi* in the blood of patients with typhoid fever, *J Clin Microbiol*, **27:** 1112–14.

Rubin RH, Weinstein L, 1977, *Salmonellosis: Microbiologic, Pathologic and Clinical Features*, Stratton Intercontinental, New York, 46–58.

Sabbour MS, Osman LM, 1990, Experience with ofloxacin in enteric fever, *J Chemother*, **2:** 113–15.

Salmon RL, Bartlett CLR, 1995, European surveillance systems, *Rev Med Microbiol*, **4:** 267–76.

Savage W, 1942, Paratyphoid fever: an epidemiological study, *J Hyg Camb*, **42:** 393–410.

Sawyer WA, 1914, Ninety-three persons infected by a typhoid carrier at a public dinner, *JAMA*, **63:** 1537–42.

Schaad UB, Salaam MA et al., 1995, Use of fluoroquinolones in pediatrics: consensus report of an International Society of Chemotherapy commission, *Pediatr Infect Dis J*, **14:** 1–9.

Schafer R, Eisenstein TK, 1992, Natural killer cells mediate protection induced by a *Salmonella aro*A mutant, *Infect Immun*, **60:** 791–7.

Schroeder SA, 1968, Interpretation of serologic tests for typhoid, *JAMA*, **206:** 839–40.

Schwartz E, Shlim DR et al., 1990, The effect of oral and parenteral typhoid vaccination on the rate of infection with *Salmonella typhi* and *Salmonella paratyphi* A among foreigners in Nepal, *Arch Intern Med*, **150:** 349–51.

Scott WM, 1941, The enteric fevers, *Lancet*, **1:** 389–93.

Scragg JN, Rubridge CJ, 1975, Amoxycillin in the treatment of typhoid fever, *Am J Trop Med Hyg*, **24:** 860–5.

Sears SD, Ferreccio C et al., 1984, The use of Moore swabs for isolation of *Salmonella typhi* from irrigation water in Santiago, Chile, *J Infect Dis*, **149:** 640–2.

Seoud M, Saade G et al., 1988, Typhoid fever in pregnancy, *Obstet Gynecol*, **71:** 711–14.

Shaughnessy HJ, Friewer F, Snyder A, 1948, Comparative efficiency of rectal swabs and fecal specimens in detecting typhoid and salmonella cases and carriers, *Am J Public Health*, **36:** 670–5.

Shaw WV, 1937, *Report on an Outbreak of Enteric Fever in the County*

Borough of Bournemouth and in the Boroughs of Poole and Christ-church, HMSO, London.

Shepard DS, Walsh JA et al., 1995, Setting priorities for the Children's Vaccine Initiative: a cost-effectiveness approach, *Vaccine*, **13:** 707–14.

Simanjuntak CH, Paleologo FP et al., 1991, Oral immunisation against typhoid fever in Indonesia with Ty21a vaccine, *Lancet*, **338:** 1055–9.

Smadel JE, 1950, Chloramphenicol, Chloromycetin and tropical medicine, *Trans R Soc Trop Med Hyg*, **43:** 555–74.

Smith MD, Duong NM et al., 1994, Comparison of ofloxacin and ceftriaxone for short-course treatment of enteric fever, *Antimicrob Agents Chemother*, **38:** 1716–20.

Song JH, Cho H et al., 1993, Detection of *Salmonella typhi* in the blood of patients with typhoid fever by polymerase chain reaction, *J Clin Microbiol*, **31:** 1439–43.

Soper GA, 1939, The curious career of Typhoid Mary, *Bull N Y Acad Med*, **15:** 698–712.

Stowman K, 1948, Recrudescence of typhoid fever in Europe, *Epidemiol Vital Stat Rep W H O*, **1:** 166–72.

Stuart BM, Pullen RL, 1946, Typhoid fever; clinical analysis of three hundred and sixty cases, *Arch Intern Med*, **78:** 629–61.

Sztein MB, Tanner MK et al., 1995, Cytotoxic T lymphocytes after oral immunization with attenuated vaccine strains of *Salmonella typhi* in humans, *J Immunol*, **155:** 3987–93.

Szu SC, Taylor DN et al., 1994, Laboratory and preliminary clinical characterization of Vi capsular polysaccharide–protein conjugate vaccines, *Infect Immun*, **62:** 4440–4.

Tacket CO, Levine MM, 1995, Human typhoid vaccines – old and new, *Molecular and Clinical Aspects of Bacterial Vaccine Development*, eds Ala'Aldeen DAA, Hormaeche CE, John Wiley, Chichester, 157–78.

Taylor MW, 1858, On the communication of fever by ingesta, *Edinb Med J*, **3:** 993–1004.

Thompson S, 1954, The number of bacilli harboured by enteric carriers, *J Hyg Camb*, **52:** 62–70.

Thong KL, Cordano AM et al., 1996, Molecular analysis of environmental and human isolates of *Salmonella typhi*, *Appl Environ Microbiol*, **62:** 271–4.

Threlfall EJ, Torre E et al., 1994, Insertion sequence IS200 fingerprinting of *Salmonella typhi*: an assessment of epidemiological applicability, *Epidemiol Infect*, **112:** 253–61.

Trevett AJ, Nwokolo N et al., 1994, Ataxia in patients infected with *Salmonella typhi* phage type D2: clinical, biochemical and immunohistochemical studies, *Trans R Soc Trop Med Hyg*, **88:** 565–8.

Vallenas C, Hernandez H et al., 1985, Efficacy of bone marrow, blood, stool and duodenal cultures for bacteriologic confirmation of typhoid fever in children, *Pediatr Infect Dis*, **4:** 496–8.

Vaughan VC, 1920, Typhoid fever in the American expeditionary forces: a clinical study of three hundred and seventy-three cases. The paratyphoids, *JAMA*, **74:** 1145–9.

Vogelsang TM, Bøe J, 1948, Temporary and chronic carriers of *Salmonella typhi* and *Salmonella paratyphi* B, *J Hyg Camb*, **46:** 252–61.

Wahdan MH, Serie C et al., 1982, A controlled field trial of live *Salmonella typhi* strain Ty 21a oral vaccine against typhoid: three-year results, *J Infect Dis*, **145:** 292–8.

Walker W, 1965, The Aberdeen typhoid outbreak of 1964, *Scott Med J*, **10:** 466–79.

Warren JW, Hornick RB, 1979, Immunization against typhoid fever, *Annu Rev Med*, **30:** 457–72.

Watson KC, 1955, Isolation of *Salmonella typhi* from the blood stream, *J Lab Clin Med*, **46:** 128–34.

Watson KC, 1967, Intravascular *Salmonella typhi* as a manifestation of the carrier state, *Lancet*, **2:** 332–4.

Wicks AC, Holmes GS, Davidson L, 1971, Endemic typhoid fever. A diagnostic pitfall, *Q J Med*, **40:** 341–54.

Wilson MM, Mackenzie EF, 1955, Typhoid fever and salmonellosis due to the consumption of infected desiccated coconut, *J Appl Bacteriol*, **18:** 510–21.

Woodward TE, Smadel JE et al., 1948, Preliminary report on the beneficial effect of chloromycetin in the treatment of typhoid fever, *Ann Intern Med*, **29:** 131–4.

Wright AE, 1896, Association of serous haemorrhages with conditions of defective blood coagulability, *Lancet*, **2:** 807–9.

Wright PW, Wallace RJ Jr et al., 1994, A case of recurrent typhoid fever in the United States: importance of the grandmother connection and the use of large restriction fragment pattern analysis of genomic DNA for strain comparison, *Pediatr Infect Dis J*, **13:** 1103–6.

Yew FS, Goh KT, Lim YS, 1993, Epidemiology of typhoid fever in Singapore, *Epidemiol Infect*, **110:** 63–70.

Yugoslav Typhoid Commission, 1962, A controlled field trial of the effectiveness of phenol and alcohol typhoid vaccines: final report, *Bull W H O*, **26:** 357–69.

Yugoslav Typhoid Commission, 1964, A controlled field trial of the effectiveness of acetone-dried and inactivated and heat-phenol-inactivated typhoid vaccines in Yugoslavia, *Bull WHO*, **30:** 623–30.

BACILLARY DYSENTERY

T L Hale

1 INTRODUCTION

Dysentery is an ancient scourge of humans living under conditions allowing faecal–oral transmission. This infectious inflammatory bowel disease is caused by bacteria that invade the mucosa of the large intestine. The defining clinical feature of this infection is passage of bloody, small volume stools with urgency and with rectal tenesmus. In the latter portion of the nineteenth century, *Entamoeba histolytica* (a parasitic amoeba) was identified as an aetiological agent of dysentery. By the turn of the century, however, *Bacillus dysenteriae* was also recognized as a distinct agent of bacterial (bacillary) dysentery. Over the subsequent decades, 3 additional species of dysentery bacilli were identified by systemic epidemiological, physiological and serological investigation of outbreaks. As a result, the 1950 Congress of the International Association of Microbiologists Shigella Commission adopted the generic name of *Shigella*, in honour of Shiga, the Japanese bacteriologist who first described dysentery bacilli in 1898. The Commission also designated species subgroups A (*S. dysenteriae*), B (*S. flexneri*), C (*S. boydii*) and D (*S. sonnei*) (Enterobacteriaceae Sub-committee Reports 1954, Bensted 1956). By the mid-1960s the virulence mechanism of *Shigella* species was characterized as 'enteroinvasive'. This discovery was predicated on bacterial invasion of cultured mammalian cells, invasion of the intestinal epithelium of compromised guinea pigs (LaBrec et al. 1964), invasion of rabbit ileal loops (Voino-Yasenetsky and Khavkin 1964) and invasion of the colonic epithelium of rhesus monkeys (Takeuchi, Formal and Sprinz 1968). In the 1970s it became apparent that some strains which are biochemically and serologically classified as *Escherichia coli* can also express the enteroinvasive phenotype (enteroinvasive *Escherichia coli* or EIEC strains) (DuPont et al. 1971). In the 1980s, *Shigella*–EIEC virulence plasmids were discovered and investigation of the genetic basis of pathogenesis at the molecular level was begun. In the current decade, the interactions between mammalian cells and enteroinvasive pathogens have been explored and the roles of host cell inflammatory elements and cytoskeletal components in the initiation and propagation of *Shigella* infection have been investigated.

2 EPIDEMIOLOGY

2.1 Shigellosis

On the basis of published longitudinal studies performed in developing countries between 1980 and 1986, global diarrhoeal morbidity is estimated at 2.6 episodes per child year (projecting to one billion annual episodes). An estimated average case-fatality ratio of 0.3% supports an extrapolation of 3.3 million deaths each year among individuals under 5 years of age (Bern et al. 1992). Estimates of the prevalence of shigellosis are much less certain since the clinical diagnosis of the infection is ambiguous. For example, gross blood in the stools (the characteristic symptom of dysentery) is often observed inconsistently and mucoid stools, or even watery diarrhoea, can be the sole symptom associated with the laboratory diagnosis of shigellosis (Guerrant et al. 1990, Henry 1991). Since quantification of clinical shigellosis in each study site is imprecise, calculations of global incidence are fraught with uncertainty. By some estimates, however, the annual incidence is 200 million with 650 000 deaths. The public health threat presented by bloody diarrhoea is illustrated by an observed incidence of 0.5 episodes per year in some paediatric populations of Asia and Latin America. Dysentery can account for up to 50% of diarrhoea-associated deaths in these populations, especially during periods of famine when dysentery accounts for almost all increases in diarrhoea-related mortality (Henry 1991).

Shigellae are highly communicable enteric pathogens, as illustrated by the experimentally determined infectious dose of 10–100 organisms for North American adult volunteers (DuPont et al. 1989). In geographical areas that are endemic for shigellosis, the peak incidence of dysentery occurs at 18–24 months of age and the disease persists at relatively high levels until at least 5 years (Stoll et al. 1982, Green et al. 1991, Henry 1991). These age-specific trends suggest that significant risk factors for acquisition of *Shigella* infections include weaning from breast milk and introduction of children into community day-care centres that have an inherent potential for faecal–oral transmission of intestinal bacteria. Secondary transmission of shigellae can also occur at a rate exceeding 50% in households with young children (Wilson et al. 1981). In less developed areas, there is a seasonal trend of increased incidence during the dry season, perhaps reflecting the difficulty of maintaining personal hygiene when water supplies are restricted and also reflecting the peak population of houseflies (*Musca domestica*) that can serve as vectors carrying infectious faecal material on their feet (Levine and Levine 1990).

In the 2 decades after its discovery, *S. dysenteriae* serotype 1 was pandemic in both industrialized and developing countries and the infection was characterized by exceptional severity and considerable mortality. The 'Shiga bacillus' now typically constitutes less than 25% of endemic shigellosis, but epidemic outbreaks of disease by this agent continue to occur in equatorial regions of Africa, Asia and Central America. In Central America, for example, a devastating *S. dysenteriae* serotype 1 epidemic began in 1968. During a 10 month period, 112 000 cases and 8300 deaths were reported in Guatemala (Gangarosa et al. 1970). In total, this 4 year Latin American epidemic resulted in more than 500 000 cases. In the late 1970s, epidemic *S. dysenteriae* serotype 1 disease was detected in eastern Zaire and in 1994 this agent killed up to 15 000 Rwandan refugees in the camps of Goma, Zaire. The underlying reasons for the epidemic spread of *S. dysenteriae* serotype 1 infections are obscure, but it should be noted that, unlike other *Shigella* species, this serotype produces a ricin-like 'Shiga toxin' that is a potent inhibitor of mammalian protein synthesis. Experimental studies in rhesus monkeys, comparing a toxin-negative mutant with a wild-type *S. dysenteriae* serotype 1 strain, suggest that Shiga toxin causes capillary disruption in the colonic mucosa and exacerbates the clinical manifestations of dysentery (Fontaine, Arondel and Sansonetti 1988).

Although the Shiga bacillus continues to be a public health problem of epidemic proportions in some developing countries, the aetiology and clinical prognosis of endemic bacillary dysentery have gradually changed during this century (Green et al. 1991, Finkelman et al. 1994). In the late 1920s, *S. flexneri* became the most frequently isolated *Shigella* species world wide and there was a general shift to milder clinical manifestations and lower case-fatality rates. This species remains the most common *Shigella* isolate in developing countries, while *S. boydii* accounts for less than 10% of isolates in endemic areas (Stoll et al. 1982). *S. sonnei* became the predominant species isolated in western Europe during the war years of 1939–45. A similar shift occurred in North America during hyperendemic periods in the early 1970s and late 1980s (Lee et al. 1991). *S. sonnei* outbreaks are often initiated by contaminated food, especially uncooked vegetables such as iceberg lettuce (Black, Craun and Blake 1978, Frost et al. 1995). Contaminated water can also spread *S. sonnei* during household use (Wharton et al. 1990) or when used to irrigate or wash vegetables (Frost et al. 1995). Subsequent secondary and tertiary person-to-person transmission of *S. sonnei* are also common (Wilson et al. 1981, Wharton et al. 1990).

It has been suggested that the relative proportion of *S. flexneri* and *S. sonnei* in a geographical area is reflective of local hygiene standards (Blaser, Pollard and Feldman 1983, Dan, Michaeli and Treistman 1988). As the general level of personal and environmental hygiene rises, the proportion of *S. flexneri* (group B) isolates falls while the proportion of *S. sonnei* (group D) rises. This 'B:D ratio' also applies to subpopulations within a geographical area. In southern Israel, for example, Jewish and Bedouin populations coexist under different socioeconomic conditions. While the Jewish community enjoys an essentially western standard of living, the Bedouin population is in transition from a nomadic lifestyle to permanent residence. Most Bedouin still live in tents as large family units and the prevalent hygienic conditions are typical of the developing world. During the 1989–92 period of observation, the average B:D ratio for the Jewish population was 0.15 while the ratio for the Bedouin was 3.8 (Finkelman et al. 1994). A similar phenomenon was found in 1974–80 data retrospectively comparing North American Indians (B:D ratio, 2.1–2.9) to the total United States population (B:D ratio, 0.28–0.45) (Blaser, Pollard and Feldman 1983). Indeed, the B:D ratio in some surveys of developing countries is above 10 (Sack et al. 1994). There is no evidence of differential survival of *Shigella* species on environmental surfaces and the infective dose of *S. dysenteriae*, *S. flexneri* and *S. sonnei* is similar in volunteer challenge studies (DuPont et al. 1989). However, transient intestinal colonization of children by *Plesiomonas shigelloides* O17, a common environmental isolate that expresses somatic antigen identical to *S. sonnei* (Rauss et al. 1970, Taylor et al. 1993), may explain the low incidence of *S. sonnei* in developing countries. Colonization with *P. shigelloides* could elicit cross-protection against *S. sonnei* (Sack et al. 1994).

2.2 Enteroinvasive *Escherichia coli*

Since the 1960s, it has been apparent that *E. coli* serotypes O28, O29, O112, O121, O124, O135, O136, O143, O144, O152, O164 and O167 are associated with sporadic outbreaks of infectious colitis. The O antigens of these groups tend to cross-react with those of *S. dysenteriae* or *S. boydii* (Cheasty and Rowe 1983). When experimental challenge studies showed that O143 and O144 isolates from patients with colitis-like symptoms cause bacillary dysentery after ingestion by naive volunteers, it was confirmed that *Shigella*-like virulence phenotypes are expressed by these 'enteroinvasive *E. coli'* (EIEC) (DuPont et al. 1971). Like shigellae, EIEC strains invade mammalian tissue culture cells in vitro (DuPont et al. 1971) and they invade the corneal epithelium of the guinea pig eye, evoking keratoconjunctivitis (Sereny test) (Toledo and Trabulsi 1983). Most EIEC strains are lactose-negative and non-motile, but biochemical or serological criteria are not entirely specific. The largest EIEC outbreak in the United States was caused by an O124 strain contaminating imported cheese (Tulloch et al. 1973) and most other outbreaks are either food- or waterborne (Keyti 1989). The relatively high infectious dose of 1 $\times 10^8$ organisms (DuPont et al. 1971) may explain the rarity of person-to-person EIEC transfer, except in extenuating circumstances such as those pertaining in mental institutions (Harris et al. 1985). This characteristic may also explain the even distribution of these infections among all age groups (Keyti 1989).

3 CLINICAL MANIFESTATIONS

3.1 Symptomatology

Dysentery, the definitive clinical manifestation of shigellosis, is defined as frequent passage of bloody stools with mucus and abdominal pain. Constitutional symptoms such as rectal tenesmus, fever, mild tenderness over the left colon upon palpation and the presence of faecal leucocytes are also suggestive of shigellosis (Mathan and Mathan 1991a). Nevertheless, the specificity of this combination of symptoms is limited. In a survey of hospital admissions at the International Centre for Diarrhoeal Disease Research, Bangladesh (ICDDR,B), for example, only 10% of the *S. sonnei* patients excreted bloody stools whereas 83% and 55% of patients with *S. dysenteriae* 1 and *S. flexneri*, respectively, passed gross faecal blood. In contrast, *S. sonnei* infections were associated with watery diarrhoea in approximately 75% of patients but *S. flexneri* and *S. dysenteriae* type 1 were associated with diarrhoea in only 33% and 22% of patients, respectively (Stoll et al. 1982).

A *S. flexneri* 2a experimental challenge study conducted at the Center of Vaccine Development (CVD) of the University of Maryland (USA) (Kotloff et al. 1995a) gives a detailed profile of clinical shigellosis as experienced by immunologically naive adults. The average time to the first onset of symptoms was 44 h after ingestion of a challenge inoculum of 1000 organisms. Symptoms occurred with the following frequency: 90% diarrhoea (average of 2 litres); 90% dysentery (average of 12 stools); 90% fever (peak of 103°F, 39.4°C); 63% with severe illness. No severe disease was experienced by volunteers ingesting 100 organisms, but 43% had diarrhoea (average of 850 ml) and dysentery (average of 7 stools). Fever (peak of 102.2°F, 39°C) occurred in 28% of the volunteers ingesting the smaller number of shigellae with an average time to onset of any illness of 58 h. Vomiting occurred in about 10% of volunteers regardless of challenge dose.

Shigellosis is usually a self-limiting disease, but retrospective analysis of ICDDR,B hospital admission records revealed fatal infections in 7% of patients (Bennish et al. 1990). Analysis of these data indicated that age (<1 year), altered consciousness (lethargy), abnormally low serum protein level and thrombocytopenia ($<1 \times 10^5$ platelet mm^{-3}) are lethal risk factors. Severe shigellosis (duration of dysentery >10 days) is often associated with stunted growth in children of the developing world (Henry 1991). Haemolytic–uraemic syndrome (HUS) can be a sequela of infection with *S. dysenteriae* serotype 1 that characteristically express the Shiga cytotoxin (Lopez et al. 1989). Reactive arthritis (Reiter syndrome) is a rare sequela of *S. flexneri* infections. The HLA-B27 histocompatibility antigen phenotype is a strong predisposing factor for the latter complication (Bunning, Raybourne and Archer 1988). *Shigella* bacteraemia in HIV-positive patients is an increasingly common complication requiring aggressive antibiotic therapy and prophylaxis (Nelson et al. 1992, Huebner et al. 1993). Shigellaemia may occur in this setting even in the absense of diarrhoea or positive stool culture.

3.2 Histopathology

Colonoscopy of ICDDR,B patients with acute shigellosis, caused by either *S. flexneri* or *S. dysenteriae*, reveals inflammatory changes resembling ulcerative colitis, i.e. diffuse erythema with focal haemorrhages and adherent layers of purulent exudate. Some patients had round aphthoid erosions a few millimetres in diameter, resembling those found in Crohn's disease. In most patients experiencing dysentery for less than 4 days, colitis was confined to the rectosigmoid colon. Proximal involvement of the transverse colon was observed in the majority of patients presenting with dysentery lasting 4 or more days. These findings indicate that the initial lesions occur in the distal colon with retrograde spread of colitis as the infection progresses (Speelman, Kabir and Islam 1984). Rectal biopsy specimens from patients in the Christian Medical College Hospital, Velloer, India illustrate the underlying histopathological changes associated with aphthoid and vascular lesions and with the purulent exudate of shigellosis (Mathan and Mathan 1991b). In patients who had experienced dysenteric symptoms for less than 48 h, aphthoid lesions were found overlying small lymphoid follicles (Fig. 25.1). This clinical finding suggests that *Shigella* infection is initiated in the specialized, follicle-associated, membranous (M) cells. Vascular alterations in the lamina propria appeared to progress from swelling of endothelial cells (with degeneration of mitochondria) to neutrophil margination, intravascular coagulation and vessel dehiscence leading to focal haemorrhages. Focal ulceration of the rectal mucosa was associated with streaming of polymorphonuclear leucocytes (PMNs) into the intestinal lumen (Fig. 25.2) and with extensive epithelial cell detachment. These lesions typically occur in the absence of detectable intracellular bacteria, suggesting that the inflammatory cascade is a primary mediator of the histopathological changes that characterize shigellosis.

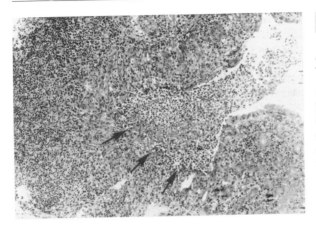

Fig. 25.1 Biopsy specimen of rectal mucosa from a patient experiencing dysentery for <48 h showing an aphthoid ulcer overlying a small lymphoid follicle (arrows) (stain, haematoxylin and eosin; × 71). (Courtesy of MM Mathan).

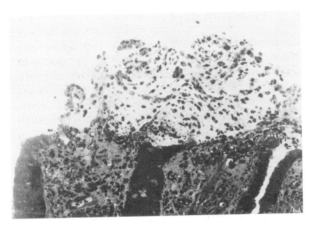

Fig. 25.2 Biopsy specimen of rectal mucosa from a patient with shigellosis that reveals focal ulceration with streaming of polymorphonuclear leucocytes into the lumen (stain, toluidine blue; × 143). (Courtesy of MM Mathan).

Immunohistochemical studies of rectal biopsies obtained from ICDDR,B patients during acute and convalescent stages of infection with *S. flexneri* or *S. dysenteriae* have allowed the characterization of secretion and localization of inflammatory cytokines at the single-cell level (Raqib et al. 1995). This study did not reveal a selective pattern of cytokine production; instead, there was a general upregulation of all cytokines studied including IL-1, IL-4, IL-6, IL-8, TNF and IFN. Severe disease was associated with a relative increase in the number of IL-1β, IL-6, TNF-α, and IFN-γ containing cells. IL-1, IL-4, TNF and IFN activities were localized to mononuclear cells and PMNs, whereas IL-6 and IL-8 were localized in mucosal epithelial cells. Interestingly, cytokine-producing cells were upregulated 30 days after the onset of disease, long after overt symptoms of shigellosis had subsided. These clinical observations suggest that cytokines are acute mediators of tissue damage in this inflammatory bowel disease and that residual cytokine expression may be associated with subclinical manifestations such as growth stunting.

4 PATHOGENIC MECHANISMS

4.1 Diarrhoea

Shigella infections are frequently characterized by a prodrome of watery diarrhoea occurring before the onset of overt dysentery. Indeed, a majority of *S. sonnei* and EIEC infections are manifested solely as watery diarrhoea (Stoll et al. 1982, Taylor et al. 1988). Intestinal perfusion studies have detected active fluid secretion in the small intestine of rhesus monkeys challenged intragastrically with *S. flexneri* (Rout et al. 1975). Since the mucosa of the small intestine is not invaded either in monkeys or in humans ingesting shigellae, this observation suggests that these organisms may elaborate enterotoxin(s) as they transit the small intestine. Recently 2 toxic moieties have been identified by testing the enterotoxic properties of iron-depleted bacterial culture supernatants in Ussing chambers (evaluating ileal tissue electrical response) and in rabbit ileal loops (evaluating fluid accumulation). Both EIEC (Fasano et al. 1990) and *S. flexneri* 2a (Nataro et al. 1993) express an enterotoxin (ShET2) that has been cloned from the respective virulence plasmids. Homologous toxin sequences are found in 75–80% of strains representing all 4 *Shigella* species. Another enterotoxin (ShET1) is apparently unique to the chromosome of *S. flexneri* 2a (Fasano et al. 1995). Both ShET toxins appear to be cytotonic; however, the cytotoxic Shiga toxin of *S. dysenteriae* serotype 1 also has enterotoxic activity in rabbit ileal loops (Eiklid and Olsnes 1983).

The role of enterotoxins in ileal fluid secretion during the early stages of shigellosis remains to be demonstrated using defined toxin-negative mutants. An additional mechanism of fluid secretion is suggested by the clinical observation that patients with acute *Shigella* colitis of the caecum are more likely to experience protracted diarrhoea (Speelman, Kabir and Islam 1984). Perfusion of individuals infected with either *S. flexneri* or *S. dysenteriae* reveals normal ileocaecal flow, net secretion of fluid and electrolyes in the large intestine and impaired colonic fluid absorption (Butler et al. 1986). These studies suggest that the extent of colitis influences clinical manifestations of shigellosis: involvement of the lower colon results in malabsorption and dysentery (scanty, frequent stools reflecting the ileocaecal flow) whereas more extensive inflammation in the upper colon results in diarrhoea (reflecting net colonic secretion in addition to malabsorption). This hypothesis is supported by the observation that indomethacin (an inhibitor of prostaglandin synthesis) decreases fluid secretion in rabbit ileal loops infected with *S. flexneri* (Gots, Formal and Gianella 1974). Fluid accumulation is also inhibited in ileal loops when tissue leucopenia is induced by venous perfusion of rabbits with a monoclonal antibody (anti-CD18) that prevents diapedesis of PMNs (Perdomo et al. 1994). PMNs release hydrogen peroxide and adenosine that can elicit chloride secretion from intestinal crypts and these studies demonstrate that inflammation contributes to intestinal fluid secretion in shigellosis.

4.2 Colitis

The invasive mechanism of *Shigella* pathogenesis has been demonstrated in the guinea pig corneal epithelium (Sereny, 1955), in mammalian tissue cultures (LaBrec et al. 1964), in rabbit ileal loops (Voino-Yasenetsky and Khavkin 1964), in the guinea pig intestinal epithelium (LaBrec et al. 1964) and in the colonic epithelium of the rhesus monkey (Takeuchi, Formal and Sprinz 1968). Recent rabbit ileal loop studies have been especially useful in the experimental analysis of intestinal invasion by shigellae (Wassef, Keren and Mailloux 1989, Perdomo et al. 1994). These studies have demonstrated almost no invasion of the villus epithelium in the static ileal loop during early stages of infection by *S. flexneri* (Fig. 25.3a), but many bacteria are found within follicle-associated M cells (Fig. 25.3b, Fig. 25.4a). The preferential uptake of shigellae by lymphoid tissue was confirmed by quantitative bacterial culture of villous mucosa and Peyer's patches, revealing a 3-fold differential of *Shigella* colony-forming units in the latter tissues 2 hours after challenge (Perdomo et al. 1994). Within a few hours, virulent shigellae transcytose through the follicle-associated epithelium and these organisms are found within the cytoplasm of tissue macrophages, indicating phagocytic uptake (Fig. 25.3c, Fig. 25.4b). Often the bacteria are free in the macrophage cytoplasm, suggesting phagosome lysis, and the cells are heavily vacuolated with perinuclear condensation of chromatin indicative of apoptosis (programmed cell death) (Fig. 25.3d, Fig. 25.4b).

Apoptosis of cultured mouse peritoneal macrophages can be demonstrated after phagocytosis of virulent *S. flexneri*. More central to pathogenesis, however, is the release of the pro-inflammatory cytokine IL-1 before the dissolution of infected macrophages (Zychlinsky et al. 1994a). The pivotal role of this cytokine in shigellosis was demonstrated experimentally by venous perfusion of IL-1ra (receptor antagonist) into rabbits before challenge with *S. flexneri* (Sansonetti et al. 1995). This anti-inflammatory antagonist significantly inhibits ileal loop fluid accumulation and derangement of tissue architecture, reflecting a 40-fold decrease in bacterial invasion of the villous epithelium as documented by quantitative culture of shigellae. A similar amelioration of tissue invasion and symptomatology was associated with tissue leucopenia induced by perfusion anti-CD18 monoclonal antibody that blocks migration of PMNs from blood vessels to foci of infection (Perdomo et al. 1994). These experimental observations indicate that infection of lymphoid follicles with small numbers of shigellae elicits a local leucocytic infiltration that destabilizes intercellular cohesion in adjacent enterocytes and facilitates bacterial invasion of the epithelium beyond the lymphoid structures (Fig. 25.4d). The role of leucocyte transmigration in enterocyte invasion was demonstrated in vitro with polarized T-84 colonic enterocytes grown on permeable filter substrates (Perdomo, Gounon and Sansonetti 1994). Invasion of these T-84 monolayers does not occur when *S. flexneri* is added to apical (brush border) surface. However, transmigration of human PMNs from the basal surface of the monolayer opens paracellular pathways that allow basolateral invasion of the epithelial cells by shigellae. Other experiments show that the IL-8 cytokine is released by cultured T-84 cells after *Shigella* infection (Eckmann, Kagnoff and Fierer 1993). This 'short-range' chemoattractant induces extravasation of PMNs from local villous capillaries (Sansonetti et al. 1995) which may also exacerbate spread of the infection.

Invasion of epithelial cells by shigellae is essentially a process of bacterium-induced phagocytosis involving major cytoskeletal rearrangements (Adam et al. 1995). When cultured HeLa cells are infected with *S. flexneri*, the initial contact of the bacterium with the cell surface induces distinct cytoplasmic actin nucleation zones that radiate tightly bundled filaments organized by the actin-bundling protein T-plastin. These actin/myosin filaments support plasma membrane folds that coalesce to engulf bacteria. The resulting endocytic vacuoles are rapidly lysed by plasmid-encoded proteins (Table 25.1; High et al. 1992) and the shigellae are released into the host cell cytoplasm. In unpolarized HeLa cells, intracellular shigellae associate with actin stress fibres and begin 'organelle-like' movement (Olm) that culminates in perinuclear aggregates of bacteria (Vasselon et al. 1991). In polarized Caco-2 intestinal epithelial cells, Olm causes accumulation of intracellular shigellae at the level of the intermediate junctional actin ring of the zonula adherens (Vasselon et al. 1992) (Fig 25.4d). As shigellae grow in the cytoplasm of cultured mammalian cells, amino acids are scavenged from the host cell pools (Hale and Formal 1981) and host cell energy metabolism is inhibited. In infected cells, there are rapid decreases in lactate and ATP levels, increases in pyruvate and cAMP and morphological alterations of mitochondria (Sansonetti and Mounier 1987). This metabolic derangement may be induced by a plasmid-encoded ATP-hydrolysing apyrase (Bhargava et al. 1995) and it can be postulated that disruption of cellular respiration contributes to necrosis of the colonic epithelium that characterizes bacillary dysentery.

Cell-to-cell spread of intracellular shigellae is initiated by recruitment of host cell actin to form a cytoskeleton-based motor. A plasmid-encoded protein causes the nucleation of filamentous F-actin tails at the distal poles during bacterial cell division (Table 25.1; Vasselon et al. 1992). Constriction of the F-actin tail by the actin-bundling protein plastin pushes the daughter cells toward the host cell plasma membrane (Prevost et al. 1992). The moving organisms impinge on the inner face of the cytoplasmic membrane at the level of the intermediate junction, resulting in rigid protrusions containing one or more shigellae (Fig. 25.4d). Formation of these protrusions requires the participation of cadherins, a family of 'cell adhesion molecules' (CAM) that bundle actin filaments in the intermediate junctions. L-CAM, an intercellular

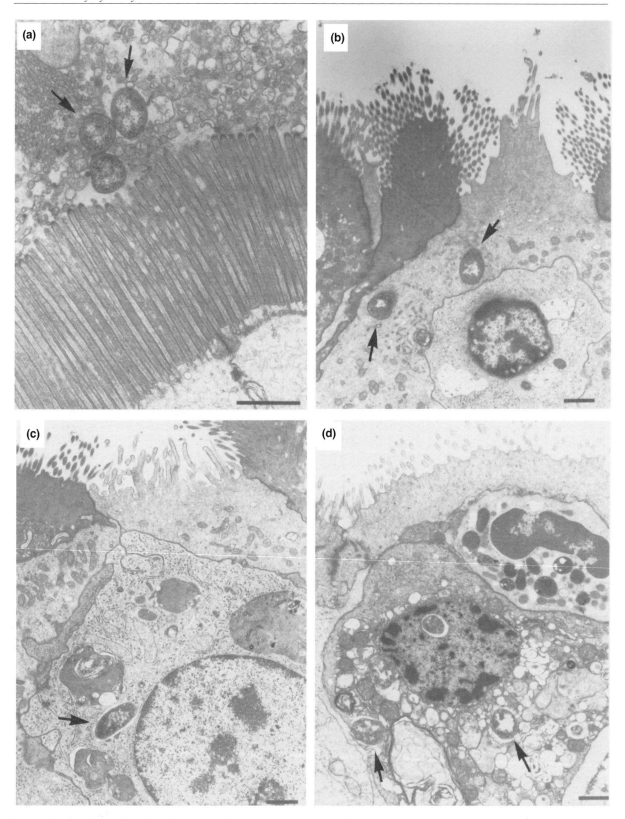

Fig. 25.3 Transmission electron micrographs of rabbit ileal epithelium after injection of *S. flexneri* serotype 5 into ligated intestinal loop. (a) Shigellae (arrows) in the lumen do not infect enterocytes at the apical brush border (8 h). (b) *Shigella* (arrow) ingested by an M cell (4 h). (c) Shigellae (arrows) inside a macrophage underlying an M cell (8 h). (d) Shigellae (arrows) inside a macrophage with perinuclear aggregation of chromatin and vacuolization suggestive of apoptosis (8 h). Note PMN underlying M cell. Bar = 1 μm. (From *J Exp Med* 1994 **180**: 1307).

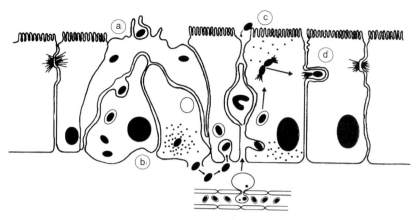

Fig. 25.4 Illustrated stages of colonic epithelium invasion. (a) Ingestion and translocation of shigellae by an M cell. (b) Phagocytosis by macrophage with lysis of phagosomes followed by macrophage apoptosis, release of bacteria and basolateral invasion of adjacent enterocytes. (c) Diapedesis of PMNs from lamina propria capillaries is followed by transmigration of these leucocytes through the epithelium destabilizing intercellular enterocyte cohesion. Retrograde migration of bacteria into the subepithelial space results in basolateral invasion of enterocytes. (d) Intracellular shigellae lyse endocytic vacuoles and use organelle-like movement to migrate to the intermediate junctional ring. Following bacterial septation, polymerized actin tails push the organisms into the cytoplasm of contiguous cells, resulting in intercellular spread.

adhesion molecule that establishes homotypic adhesion with adjacent cells, is also required for internalization of the protrusions by contiguous cells. The requirement for cell-to-cell adhesion suggests active endocytosis of the protrusion (Sansonetti et al. 1994). The double membrane of the internalized protrusion is subsequently lysed by plasmid-encoded proteins (Table 25.1) and the bacteria are released into the cytoplasm of contiguous host cells (Allaoui et al. 1992). Mutant shigellae that cannot recruit and organize an actin motor for intercellular spread are unable to elicit clinical symptoms in rabbit ileal loops or in intragastrically challenged rhesus monkeys (Sansonetti et al. 1991). Thus the active remodelling of the intestinal epithelium for the propagation and spread of shigellae in the intracellular environment is central to the dysenteric manifestations of shigellosis.

5 GENETIC BASIS OF VIRULENCE

5.1 *Shigella* and EIEC virulence plasmids

S. flexneri and *E. coli* are so closely related that the 2 species cannot be distinguished on the basis of polynucleotide hybridization (Brenner et al. 1973). A common system of mating polarities and genetic linkage patterns allows conjugal transfer and incorporation of virtually the entire *Shigella* chromosome into an *E. coli* K-12 recipient, but these matings do not reconstitute the virulence phenotype of the donor. This enigma was resolved by the discovery of a family of large plasmids [(1.2–1.4) $\times$ 10^5 kDa] that carry essentially all the genetic information encoding the virulence attributes of *Shigella* or EIEC (Sansonetti, Kopecko and Formal 1982). The virulence plasmids of *Shigella* species and EIEC are heterogeneous by the criterion of restriction enzyme analysis and incompatibility studies suggest that the plasmids of *S. dysenteriae*, *S. boydii*, *S. flexneri* serotype 6 and EIEC are incompatible with plasmids

of *S. flexneri* serotypes 1–5 and *S. sonnei* (Makino, Sasakawa and Yoshikawa 1988). Nevertheless, these plasmids are interchangeable in their ability to restore virulence to avirulent *Shigella* or *E. coli* recipients. The key role of the virulence plasmid in pathogenesis is illustrated by enhanced Peyer's patch infection in rabbit ileal loops injected with virulent shigellae compared to an avirulent mutant strain that has lost the virulence plasmid (Wassef, Keren and Mailloux 1989, Perdomo et al. 1994). The *S. sonnei* virulence plasmid carries the *rfb* locus encoding the O polysaccharide repeat unit characteristic of species subgroup D. Other *Shigella* species carry this gene on the chromosome.

5.2 Virulence plasmid proteins

The functional similarity of *Shigella* and EIEC virulence plasmids is reflected in a common set of plasmid-encoded proteins, including 4 products that elicit antibody responses as a result of infection (Hale, Oaks and Formal 1985). These Ipa proteins (denoting 'invasion plasmid antigen') include IpaA (70 kDa), IpaB (62 kDa), IpaC (43 kDa) and IpaD (38 kDa) (Buysse et al. 1987). A molecular chaperone, IpgC (denoting 'invasion plasmid gene'), is encoded by the first gene in the *ipa* locus and this 17 kDa protein binds to IpaB and IpaC, preventing the premature association (and degradation) of the 2 chaperoned proteins in the bacterial cytoplasm (Ménard et al. 1994). Neither IpaB nor IpaC has typical signal sequences and translocation of the Ipa proteins to the extracellular milieu is dependent on a complex of plasmid-encoded proteins, 9 of which are transcribed from the *spa* locus (denoting 'surface presentation of antigen') (Venkatesan, Buysse and Oaks 1992) and 6 of which are expressed by the *mxi* locus (denoting 'membrane expression of antigen') (Andrews et al. 1991).

Although a coherent model for formation and transport of the IpaBC complex has yet to be proposed, it is evident that the *mxi-spa* locus encodes components of a highly specialized translocon that has some features found in transport systems of other bacteria. For example, an open reading frame (ORF) of the *spa* operon (Spa47) has significant homology with the ATP binding motif of protein-translocating ATPases found in *Salmonella typhimurium, Bacillus subtilis* and in many eukaryotic cells (Venkatesan, Buysse and Oaks 1992). Four of the *mxi* ORFs have sequence homology with *Yersinia* genes including the *mxiA* ORF, homologous to the LcrD low-calcium response gene (Andrews and Maurelli 1992). *mxiJ* and *mxiH* are homologous to Yop lipoproteins (Allaoui, Sansonetti and Parsot 1992) and *mxiD* is homologous to a putative Yop transport protein (Allaoui, Sansonetti and Parsot 1993). Four of the *mxi* ORFs are periplasmic or outer-membrane proteins and it has been proposed that IpaB and IpaD transiently associate with a *mxi* complex in the bacterial membrane (Ménard, Sansonetti and Parsot 1994). This association of IpaB and IpaD with *mxi-spa* components inhibits the formation and secretion of the IpaBC complex until the bacterium encounters a mammalian host cell, triggering release of the invasin.

Expression of plasmid virulence genes is a metabolic challenge for the bacterium and a regulatory system has evolved to prevent synthesis of these gene products in extraintestinal environments. Co-ordinate induction, or repression, of the *ipa, mxi, spa* regulon is mediated by a 2-component system encoded by *virF* and *virB* plasmid genes (Adler et al. 1989). An obvious environmental cue of the human intestinal tract is elevated temperature, and the virulence regulon is expressed only by bacteria grown at temperatures that exceed 35°C. Low-temperature repression of the virulence regulon is mediated by a chromosomal allele of the *E. coli osmZ* gene, designated *virR* in *Shigella* species. *virR* encodes H-NS, a histone-like protein that represses the synthesis of *virB*, a *trans*-acting inducer of the plasmid virulence regulon (Dagberg and Uhlin 1992). H-NS mediates changes in DNA supercoiling in response to environmental signals (Dorman, Bhriain and Higgins 1990). At human body temperature, the *trans*-acting product of *virF*, a second plasmid regulatory gene, counteracts H-NS repression and allows expression of *virB* (Dagberg and Uhlin 1992). The H-NS histone represses virulence regulon expression at acid pH, precluding invasion of the gastric mucosa. Another environmental cue of the lower intestinal tract is high osmolarity; hypertonic induction of the *Shigella* virulence regulon is mediated by chromosomal *ompR-envZ* alleles expressing a transmembrane osmolarity sensor (Bernardini, Fontaine and Sansonetti 1990).

Mutants of *ipaB* or *ipaC* are non-invasive and the invasive phenotype is restored by clones complementing the genes (Table 25.1, Sasakawa et al. 1989). Additional evidence that IpaBC functions as the *Shigella* invasin can be demonstrated by HeLa cell endocytosis of latex beads coated with the complex, but specific biochemical interactions between IpaBC and mammalian cells remain to be characterized. At the acidic pH characteristic of a phagosome, the IpaBC complex also acts as a membrane-lysing toxin enabling escape of shigellae from endocytic vacuoles in epithelial cells or phagocytic vacuoles in macrophages (Table 25.1, High et al. 1992). Apoptosis of macrophages is apparently induced by IpaB alone (Table 25.1) because an *ipaC ipaD* mutant that expresses IpaB and cloned *E. coli* haemolysin (mediating escape from phagosomes) is able to induce DNA fragmentation characteristic of programmed cell death (Zychlinsky et al. 1994b).

Mutation of a plasmid gene designated *virG* ('G' denoting the seventh *SalI* fragment in a restriction map of the virulence plasmid) (Makino et al. 1986) or, more recently, *icsA* ('ics' denoting **i**ntercellular **s**pread) (Bernardini et al. 1989) negates both intracellular mobility and intercellular spread of shigellae (Table 25.1). Nucleation of F-actin tails to form a cytoskeleton-based motor is dependent upon expression of the 125 kDa *icsA* gene product (Lett et al. 1989, Vasselon et al. 1992). During bacterial cell division, this protein is concentrated at the distal poles, i.e. the protein antigen is excluded from the septal plane of the daughter bacteria (Goldberg et al. 1993). The molecular basis of the unusual unipolar distribution of this outer-membrane protein is unclear, but the LPS matrix may help to orient IcsA since polar localization of this protein occurs only in *S. flexneri* strains that express a smooth O polysaccharide antigen (Rajakumar et al. 1994). F-actin tails form in the immediate vicinity of the unipolar IcsA localization and this antigen is also detected throughout the actin tail. Although a direct effect upon actin has not been demonstrated, this protein does have ATPase activity that may provide energy for cross-linking and stabilization of the actin tail (Goldberg et al. 1993). As the actin tail pushes the shigellae into contiguous cells, lysis of the inner membrane of the double-membrane protrusion is accomplished by the IcsB plasmid-encoded protein (Allaoui et al. 1992). Mutants in the *icsB* gene are avirulent because they do not gain access to the cytoplasm of contiguous cells. It can be speculated that the IpaBC complex may lyse the second membrane (i.e. the plasma membrane of the contiguous cell) (see Fig. 25.1).

6   LABORATORY DIAGNOSIS

6.1   Faecal leucocytes

Patients presenting with diarrhoea and fever, or with dysentery (bloody, mucoid stools), are suspected of having shigellosis. However, the differential diagnosis should include EIEC, *Campylobacter* species, *Salmonella enteritidis, Yersinia enterocolitica* and *Entamoeba histolytica*. Blood in the stools of patients with bacillary dysentery is bright red whereas that of patients infected with *E. histolytica* is usually dark brown. Microscopic examination of stool smears from patients with amoebiasis reveals erythrophagocytic trophozoites with few PMNs. By contrast, shigellosis is characterized by sheets of PMNs with more than 50 faecal leucocytes per high-power microscope field (Speelman et al. 1987). A

Table 25.1　Genetic basis of virulence in *Shigella* species

Tissue	Event	Virulence determinant
Small intestine		
	Diarrhoea	ShET2 (*Shigella* and EIEC plasmid) also ShET1 (*S. flexneri* 2a chromosome) or Shiga toxin (*S. dysenteriae* 1 chromosome)
Large intestine		
M cells	*Shigella* invasion and transcytosis ↓	IpaBC (virulence plasmid)
Macrophage	Phagocytosis of shigellae ↓	IpaBC
	Lysis of phagosome ↓	IpaBC
	Release of IL-1 → (colitis) ↓	
	Apoptosis	IpaB
Enterocyte	*Shigella* invasion (basolateral membrane) ↓	IpaBC
	Lysis of endocytic vacuole ↓	IpaBC
	Intracellular multiplication (organelle-like motility) ↓	?
	Actin nucleation ↓	IcsA
	Intercellular spread ↓ (Colitis)	IcsB (and IpaBC?)

parameter of 10 leucocytes per field can help to differentiate *Shigella* infection from EIEC, *Campylobacter*, *Salmonella*, enterotoxigenic *E. coli* and rotavirus (Echeverria, Sethabutr and Pitarangsi 1991). In the later stages of shigellosis, however, PMNs degenerate, mononuclear cells increase and the exudate loses its diagnostic significance.

6.2　Bacterial culture

A clinical diagnosis of bacillary dysentery should be confirmed by isolation and identification of *Shigella* from the faeces. During the acute phase of the disease, positive cultures are readily obtained from blood-tinged plugs of mucus in freshly passed stool specimens or from rectal swabs. Shigellae can actually be isolated with greater frequency from rectal swabs than from stool specimens (Adkins and Santingo 1987). Stool samples should be processed immediately, but swabs can be held overnight at 4°C if they are suspended in phosphate buffered glycerol saline holding solution (Wells and Morris 1981). Isolation of shigellae in the laboratory is accomplished by streaking of the stool specimen onto a differential and selective medium with subsequent aerobic incubation to inhibit overgrowth of the anaerobic flora. Commonly used primary isolation media include MacConkey agar, Hektoen enteric agar (HEA) and Salmonella–Shigella (SS) agar. These media contain bile salts to inhibit the growth of gram-positive bacteria and pH indicators to differentiate lactose fermenters (coliforms or EIEC) from non-lactose fermenters (shigellae or EIEC). A liquid enrichment medium, such as Hajna gram-negative broth, can also be inoculated with stool and subcultured onto primary isolation media after a short growth period at 37°C. Most laboratories employ both a mildly selective primary medium, such as MacConkey agar, and a highly selective medium, such as HEA or SS. The utility of a mildly selective medium depends on the ability of the microbiologist to isolate small, non-lactose fermenting colonies among the luxuriant coliform colonies. For an experienced technician, MacConkey agar is the most sensitive medium for the isolation of *S. flexneri* whereas HEA is intermediate and SS agar is the least sensitive. However, MacConkey agar and SS agar are more sensitive than HEA for the isolation of *S. sonnei* (Echeverria, Sethabutr and Pitarangsi 1991).

Following overnight incubation of primary isolation media at 37°C, non-lactose fermenting colonies are sampled with an inoculating needle and streaked or stabbed into tubed slants of Kligler's iron agar (KIA) or triple sugar iron (TSI) agar. Isolates producing an alkaline slant and an acid butt are presumptive *Shigella* species. Slide agglutination tests with commercial serogroup and serotype antisera can readily confirm a *Shigella* identification. Phage typing can be useful for epidemiological studies of *Shigella* outbreaks (Frost et al. 1995). A non-agglutinating isolate, with or without gas in the KIA or TSI butt, should be biotyped for possible EIEC identification. Delayed lactose fermenters can be identified as presumptive EIEC on the basis of lysine decarboxylase and acetate fermentation, but even these biochemical reactions are variable in EIEC isolates (Echeverria, Sethabutr and Pitarangsi 1991). Confirmation of an EIEC identification by slide agglutination is impossible for most clinical laboratories since typing sera for EIEC classical serogroups are not commercially available. Unfortunately, many EIEC strains ferment lactose and these colonies are unlikely to be selected for further tests unless they predominate on the primary plate cultures obtained from a severely ill patient.

6.3 DNA–DNA hybridization and polymerase chain reaction (PCR)

Shigella virulence plasmid DNA probes derived from the *mxi-spa* region, or from the multicopy *ipaH* gene, allow the identification of both EIEC and *Shigella* isolates (Sethabutr et al. 1993), but direct probing of stool blots is less sensitive than conventional bacterial culture for the identification of *Shigella* species (Echeverria, Sethabutr and Pitarangsi 1991). In contrast, PCR using *virF* plasmid gene primers is more sensitive than standard culture techniques for the identification of *Shigella* species if the stools are preincubated for 4 h in brain–heart infusion (BHI) broth (Yavzori et al. 1994). These techniques are rapid (less than 8 h) and relatively simple for a well equipped laboratory with experienced technical personnel. PCR is particularly useful for the detection of *Shigella* species in the stools of patients after treatment with bactericidal antibiotics such as ampicillin (Yavzori et al. 1994) or ciprofloxacin (Sethabutr et al. 1993). Since ubiquitous *Shigella* and EIEC virulence plasmid sequences are employed, techniques depending upon these DNA probes or PCR primers lack species specificity.

7 TREATMENT

The first consideration in treating any diarrhoeal disease is correction of isotonic dehydration, potassium loss and metabolic acidosis. Oral rehydration treatment (ORT) is recommended for acute diarrhoea by the World Health Organization, provided that the patient is not vomiting or in shock from severe dehydration. Intravenous fluid replacement is indicated for correction of fluid and electrolyte imbalances in the latter cases. On the other hand, ORT is not likely to have a substantial impact on the clinical prognosis of patients presenting with dysentery, or with persistent diarrhoea incident to malnourishment (Henry 1991). Diphenoxylate–atropine decreases the duration of diarrhoea, but this antagonist of intestinal motility appears to prolong febrile disease and excretion of shigellae (DuPont and Hornick 1973). Loperamide, a synthetic antidiarrhoeal agent, decreases the number of unformed stools in shigellosis by two-thirds provided that an effective antibiotic, such as ciprofloxacin, is included in the regimen (Murphy et al. 1993).

Mild diarrhoea that does not progress to dysentery is not generally recognized as shigellosis and these infections are not treated with antibiotics. However, treatment of persistent *Shigella* diarrhoea is indicated for infants and treatment is also advisable when there is a likelihood of transmission of an infection to contacts. On the other hand, frank dysentery is one of the few enteric infections in which antimicrobial therapy is routinely indicated (Levine 1986). In placebo-controlled experiments, antibiotic treatment decreases the duration of disease from 9 days to 3 days (DuPont and Hornick 1973). Antibiotic resistance in shigellae is now so prevalent that the choice of an effective agent should be based on the sensitivity profile of the patient's isolate. Absorbable drugs such as ampicillin or trimethoprim–sulphamethoxazole quickly eradicate shigellae from the intestine and these agents remain the treatment of choice for sensitive isolates. Nalidixic acid is an effective alternative treatment, but resistance to this antibiotic develops rapidly as a result of extensive usage in the treatment of urinary tract infections, etc. Increasingly, there is multiple resistance to all the commonly recommended drugs, especially in *S. dysenteriae* type 1 isolates. The relatively new absorbable quinolone agents, such as ciprofloxacin, may be superior to ampicillin in eradicating sensitive shigellae from the intestine (Bennish et al. 1990) and ciprofloxacin is one of the few effective treatments for *S. dysenteriae* type 1 infection. A single 1 g dose of ciprofloxacin is an effective therapy for non-Shiga species, but a 5 day regimen of 500 mg every 12 h is recommended for *S. dysenteriae* serotype 1 infections (Bennish et al. 1990). Resistance to quinolones in shigellae occurs at a significantly lower rate than resistance to nalidixic acid, but ciprofloxacin is relatively expensive and difficult to obtain in many endemic areas. In addition, this drug is not approved for use in children by the US Food and Drug Administration because of a theoretical risk of cartilage damage.

8 PREVENTION

8.1 Interrupted transmission of disease

Transmission of shigellosis is readily interrupted by public health measures that preclude contact with contaminated faeces. When clean water and adequate sanitary facilities are available, safe disposal of excreta, protection of food from unwashed hands and extermination of flies are obvious prophylactic measures against single source outbreaks. In endemic areas, however, effective prophylaxis requires a combination of infrastructural and social interventions. In a study of slum areas of Dhaka, Bangladesh, infrastructural improvements (latrines and tube wells) had a significant impact on dysentery in children 5 years of age (Henry 1991). Unfortunately, national strategies for the improvement of environmental services (e.g. safe water and sewage disposal) in developing countries are frequently inadequate or short-lived. On the other hand, educational services encouraging conscious avoidance of faecal contamination, breast feeding and nutritional support for children with dysentery or persistent diarrhoea are proven, cost-effective public health measures reducing the incidence bacillary dysentery (Rohde 1984).

8.2   Vaccination

IMMUNOBIOLOGY OF SHIGELLOSIS

The slow progress of infrastructure improvement and behavioural modification, in addition to the constant challenge of emerging antibiotic resistance in *Shigella* species, has sustained interest in research programmes with the goal of developing safe and effective vaccines. Both epidemiological and experimental observations indicate that clinical shigellosis elicits protective immunity against subsequent infection by the same serotype. In a longitudinal epidemiological study of Chilean children, for example, evidence of prior infection correlates with a 75% reduction in reinfection with the same serotype (Ferreccio et al. 1991). Experimental challenge studies in adult, North American volunteers also indicate that clinical disease elicited by *S. sonnei* or *S. flexneri* serotype 2a gives approximately 75% protection against symptomology after rechallenge with the same strain (Herrington et al. 1990, Kotloff et al. 1995a). In these rechallenge experiments, the volunteers that experienced disease had very mild clinical symptoms compared to the disease experienced by naive controls, i.e. 350 ml diarrhoea versus 2 litres and fever of 100.5°F (38°C) versus 103°F (39.4°C) (see section 3.1, p. 481). All rechallenged volunteers excreted shigellae, but the mean number of organisms isolated from the stools was 10^6, approximately 10-fold less than the average number of colony-forming units isolated from naive controls (Kotloff et al. 1995a). Apparently shigellae are able to colonize the intestine of immune hosts transiently, but colonization (or invasion) is limited to subclinical or mildly infectious levels. These rechallenge studies demonstrate that significant immune protection develops during convalescence from shigellosis, but protection is not uniform and the duration is undetermined.

Human challenge studies have not addressed the specificity of the protective immune response evoked by shigellosis, but experiments with rhesus monkeys show that animals surviving intragastric challenge with *S. flexneri* 2a are not protected against rechallenge with the heterologous *S. sonnei* species (Formal et al. 1991). Epidemiological evidence of serotype specificity is derived from incidence data of Israel Defense Force field camps showing that serum antibody recognizing a specific *Shigella* somatic antigen correlates with diminished risk of subsequent infections involving the homologous serotype (Cohen et al. 1992). The serospecific protection evoked by shigellosis suggests that the immunodominant Ipa proteins (see section 5.2, p. 485) do not evoke antibody neutralizing the IpaBC invasin function.

Passive protection against experimental *Shigella* challenge has been demonstrated in volunteers after ingestion of bovine colostrum containing high titres of immunoglobulin recognizing *S. flexneri* 2a somatic antigen (Tacket et al. 1992). These passive protection studies suggest that antibody against the O-specific polysaccharide somatic antigen protects against shigellosis. Secretory IgA is the predominant antibody present in the stools of convalescent *Shigella* patients (Islam et al. 1995) and secreted monoclonal IgA recognizing *S. flexneri* 2a O polysaccharide gives protection against invasion of the pulmonary epithelium in mice challenged intranasally (Phalipon et al. 1994). The latter studies demonstrate that immune protection of mucosal surfaces is afforded by secretory IgA recognizing the somatic antigen, but the mechanism of protection is unclear. IgG recognizing somatic antigen may also be transudated onto mucosal surfaces and it has been suggested that antibody complement-mediated lysis may eliminate shigellae from the intestine before tissue invasion (Robbins, Chu and Schneerson 1992).

LIVE, ATTENUATED VACCINES

The supposition that avirulent mutant strains can be employed as live, attenuated, oral vaccines has been a guiding principle of *Shigella* vaccine development for 4 decades. In the 1960s, spontaneously arising, avirulent mutants were successfully tested in field trials as oral vaccines (Mel et al. 1971, Meitert et al. 1984). More recent genetic analysis of these mutants indicates that they are non-invasive due to deletions in the virulence plasmid (Venkatesan et al. 1991, Mallett et al. 1993). The major disadvantage of these non-invasive candidates is the impracticality of immunization regimens consisting of 5 oral doses, escalating to 10^{11} cfu. In addition, vomiting or diarrhoea occurs in some vaccinees following ingestion of large numbers of avirulent shigellae (Mel et al. 1971). Partial elucidation of the genetic basis of *Shigella* virulence in the 1980s and 1990s allowed the construction of live, attenuated vaccine candidates that retain the enteroinvasive phenotype. Since these vaccines express the IpaBC invasin, they actively colonize lymphoid follicles in the large intestine of primates, delivering bacteria to the underlying antigen processing cells (Fig. 25.4a,b). Examples of attenuated, enteroinvasive *S. flexneri* vaccine candidates include (1) *icsA* mutants that are unable to spread within the absorptive epithelium (Sansonetti et al. 1991, Noriega et al. 1994), (2) auxotrophic *aro* mutants that are attenuated by a blockage in biosynthesis of aromatic metabolites such as the chorismic acid precursor of *p*-aminobenzoic acid (Karnel et al. 1994) and (3) an *E. coli* K-12 hybrid, *aroD* mutant expressing *S. flexneri* somatic antigen and the plasmid-encoded

Shigella invasive phenotype (Kotloff et al. 1995b). Thus far, clinical trials of these enteroinvasive vaccine candidates have been characterized by a narrow window differentiating immunizing doses from overtly reactogenic intestinal challenge (Hale 1995). The release of inflammatory cytokines during the early stages of *Shigella* infection (see section 3.2, p. 481; Fig. 25.4b; Sansonetti et al. 1995) is probably necessary for an optimal mucosal immune response and these cytokines are also mediators of vaccine reactions such as headache, fever and diarrhoea. Nevertheless, ongoing research with defined enteroinvasive mutants may eventually succeed in establishing the optimal balance between immunogenicity and reactogenicity in live *Shigella* vaccines.

O-SPECIFIC POLYSACCHARIDE VACCINES

Serotype specific immunity suggests that O-specific polysaccharide (O-SP) subunit vaccines could protect against shigellosis (Robbins, Chu and Schneerson 1992). Parenteral injection of subunit vaccines consisting of acid-hydrolysed, detoxified O-SP, covalently conjugated to a protein carrier such as *Pseudomonas aeruginosa* exoprotein A (*r*EPA), evokes only mild local reactions and elicits significant rises in serum antibody (IgG IgM IgA) (Taylor et al. 1993). A *P. shigelloides* O-SP–*r*EPA conjugate was evaluated as a vaccine against *S. sonnei* infection in a recent field trial conducted by the Israel Defence Force Medical Corps and significant protection against diarrhoea was demonstrated (Hale 1995). Alternative subcellular delivery vehicles for O-SP include parenteral ribosomal vaccines (Levenson et al. 1991) and oral or intranasal proteosome-LPS vaccines (Orr et al. 1993, Mallett et al. 1995). Like the chemically haptenated protein–polysaccharide conjugates, these nucleic acid and/or protein carriers elicit T cell dependent immune responses against O-SP. The safety of subunit or subcellular O-SP vaccines facilitates volunteer studies and these products may represent the best hope for the immunoprophylaxis of shigellosis in the near future.

REFERENCES

Adam T, Arpin M et al., 1995, Cytoskeletal rearrangements and the functional role of T-plastin during entry of *Shigella flexneri* into HeLa cells, *J Cell Biol*, **129:** 367–81.

Adkins HJ, Santingo LT, 1987, Increased recovery of enteric pathogens by use of both stool and rectal swab specimens, *J Clin Microbiol*, **25:** 158–9.

Adler B, Sasakawa C et al., 1989, A dual transcriptional activation system for the 230 kb plasmid genes coding for virulence-associated antigens for *Shigella flexneri*, *Mol Microbiol*, **3:** 627–35.

Allaoui A, Sansonetti PJ, Parsot C, 1992, MxiJ, a lipoprotein involved in secretion of *Shigella* Ipa invasions, is homologous to YscJ, a secretion factor of the *Yersinia* Yop proteins, *J Bacteriol*, **174:** 7661–9.

Allaoui A, Sansonetti PJ, Parsot C, 1993, MxiD, an outer membrane protein necessary for the secretion of the *Shigella flexneri* Ipa invasins, *Mol Microbiol*, **7:** 59–68.

Allaoui A, Mounier J et al., 1992, *icsB*: a *Shigella flexneri* virulence gene necessary for the lysis of protrusion during intercellular spread, *Mol Microbiol*, **6:** 1605–16.

Andrews GP, Maurelli AT, 1992, *mxiA* of *Shigella flexneri* 2a, which facilitates export of invasion plasmid antigens, encodes a homolog of the low-calcium response protein, LcrD of *Yersinia pestis*, *Infect Immun*, **60:** 3287–95.

Andrews GP, Hromockyj AE et al., 1991, Two novel virulence loci, *mxiA* and *mxiB*, in *Shigella flexneri* 2a facilitate excretion of invasion plasmid antigens, *Infect Immun*, **59:** 1997–2005.

Bennish ML, Salam MA et al., 1990, Therapy for shigellosis: II. Randomized, double-blind comparison of ciprofloxacin and ampicillin, *J Infect Dis*, **162:** 711–16.

Bensted HJ, 1956, Dysentery bacilli – a brief historical review, *Can J Microbiol*, **2:** 163–74.

Bern C, Martines J et al., 1992, The magnitude of the global problem of diarrhoeal disease: a ten-year update, *Bull W H O*, **70:** 705–14.

Bernardini ML, Fontaine A, Sansonetti PJ, 1990, The two-component regulatory system OmpR-EnvZ controls the virulence of *Shigella flexneri*, *J Bacteriol*, **172:** 6274–81.

Bernardini ML, Mounier J et al., 1989, Identification of *ics*, a plasmid locus of *Shigella flexneri* that governs bacterial intra- and intercellular spread through interaction with F-actin, *Proc Natl Acad Sci USA*, **86:** 3867–71.

Bhargava T, Datta S et al., 1995, Virulent *Shigella* codes for a soluble apyrase: identification, characterization, and cloning of the gene, *Curr Sci*, **68:** 293–300.

Black RE, Craun GF, Blake PA, 1978, Epidemiology of common-source outbreaks of shigellosis in the United States, 1961–1975, *Am J Epidemiol*, **106:** 47–52.

Blaser MJ, Pollard RA, Feldman RA, 1983, *Shigella* infections in the United States, 1974–1980, *J Infect Dis*, **147:** 771–5.

Brenner DJ, Fanning GR et al., 1973, Polynucleotide sequence relatedness among *Shigella* species, *Int J Syst Bacteriol*, **23:** 1–7.

Bunning VK, Raybourne RB, Archer DL, 1988, Foodborne enterobacterial pathogens and rheumatoid disease, *J Appl Bacteriol*, **Symposium Supplement:** 87C–107S.

Butler T, Speelman P et al., 1986, Colonic dysfunction during shigellosis, *J Infect Dis*, **154:** 817–24.

Buysse JM, Stover CK et al., 1987, Molecular cloning of invasion plasmid antigen (*ipa*) genes from *Shigella flexneri*: analysis of *ipa* gene products and genetic mapping, *J Bacteriol*, **169:** 2561–9.

Cheasty T, Rowe B, 1983, Antigenic relationships between the enteroinvasive *Escherichia coli* O antigens O28ac, O112ac, O124, O136, O144, O152, and O164 and *Shigella* O antigens, *J Clin Microbiol*, **17:** 681–4.

Cohen D, Green MS et al., 1992, Natural immunity to shigellosis in two groups with different previous risk of exposure to *Shigella* is only partly expressed by serum antibodies to lipopolysaccharide, *J Infect Dis*, **165:** 785–7.

Dagberg B, Uhlin BE, 1992, Regulation of virulence-associated plasmid genes in enteroinvasive *Escherichia coli*, *J Bacteriol*, **174:** 7606–12.

Dan DM, Michaeli D, Treistman J, 1988, The epidemiology of shigellosis in Israel, *Ann Trop Med Parasitol*, **82:** 159–62.

Dorman C, Bhriain NN, Higgins CF, 1990, DNA supercoiling and environmental regulation of virulence gene expression in *Shigella flexneri*, *Nature (London)*, **344:** 789–92.

DuPont HL, Hornick RB, 1973, Adverse effect of Lomotil therapy in shigellosis, *JAMA*, **13:** 1525–8.

DuPont HL, Formal SB et al., 1971, Pathogenesis of *Escherichia coli* diarrhea, *N Engl J Med*, **285:** 1–9.

DuPont HL, Levine MM et al., 1989, Inoculum size in shigellosis and implications for expected mode of transmission, *J Infect Dis*, **159:** 1126–8.

Echeverria P, Sethabutr O, Pitarangsi C, 1991, Microbiology and diagnosis of infections with *Shigella* and enteroinvasive *Escherichia coli*, *Rev Infect Dis*, **13, Suppl 4:** S220–5.

Eckmann L, Kagnoff MF, Fierer J, 1993, Epithelial cells secrete the chemokine interleukin-8 in response to bacterial entry, *Infect Immun*, **61:** 4569–74.

Eiklid K, Olsnes S, 1983, Animal toxicity for *Shigella dysenteriae* cytotoxin: evidence that the neurotoxic, enterotoxic, and cytotoxic activities are due to one toxin, *J Immunol*, **130:** 380–4.

Enterobacteriaceae Sub-committee Reports, 1954, *Int Bull Bacteriol Nomencl Taxon*, **4:** 1–94.

Fasano A, Kay BA et al., 1990, Enterotoxin and cytotoxin production by enteroinvasive *Escherichia coli, Infect Immun*, **58:** 3717–23.

Fasano A, Noriega FR et al., 1995, Shigella enterotoxin 1: an enterotoxin of *Shigella flexneri* 2a active in rabbit small intestine in vivo and in vitro, *J Clin Invest*, **95:** 2853–61.

Ferreccio C, Prado V et al., 1991, Epidemiologic patterns of acute diarrhea and endemic *Shigella* infections in children in a poor periurban setting in Santiago, Chile, *J Clin Microbiol*, **134:** 614–27.

Finkelman Y, Yagupsky P et al., 1994, Epidemiology of *Shigella* infections in two ethnic groups in a geographic region in southern Israel, *Eur J Clin Microbiol Infect Dis*, **13:** 367–73.

Fontaine A, Arondel J, Sansonetti PJ, 1988, Role of Shiga toxin in the pathogenesis of bacillary dysentery, studied by using a Tox – super mutant of *Shigella dysenteriae* 1, *Infect Immun*, **56:** 3099–109.

Formal SB, Oaks EV et al., 1991, The effect of prior infection with virulent *Shigella flexneri* 2a on the resistance of monkeys to subsequent infection with *Shigella sonnei, J Infect Dis*, **164:** 533–7.

Frost JA, McEvoy MB et al., 1995, An outbreak of *Shigella sonnei* infection associated with consumption of iceberg lettuce, *Emerg Infect Dis*, **1:** 26–9.

Gangarosa EJ, Perera DR et al., 1970, Epidemic Shiga bacillus dysentery in Central America. II. Epidemiologic studies in 1969, *J Infect Dis*, **122:** 181–90.

Goldberg MB, Bârzu O et al., 1993, Unipolar localization and ATPase activity of IcsA, a *Shigella flexneri* protein involved in intracellular movement, *J Bacteriol*, **175:** 2189–96.

Gots R, Formal SB, Gianella RA, 1974, Indomethacin inhibition of *Salmonella typhimurium, Shigella flexneri*, and cholera-mediated rabbit ileal secretion, *J Infect Dis*, **130:** 280–4.

Green MS, Block C et al., 1991, Four decades of shigellosis in Israel: epidemiology of a growing public health problem, *Rev Infect Dis*, **13, Suppl 4:** S248–53.

Guerrant RL, Hughes JM et al., 1990, Diarrhea in developed and developing countries: magnitude, special settings, and etiologies, *Rev Infect Dis*, **12, Suppl 1:** S41–50.

Hale TL, 1995, *Shigella* vaccines, *Molecular and Clinical Aspects of Bacterial Vaccine Development*, eds Ala'Aldeen DAA, Hormaeche CE, John Wiley & Sons Ltd, Chichester, New York, 179–204.

Hale TL, Formal SB, 1981, Protein synthesis in HeLa or Henle 407 cells infected with *Shigella dysenteriae* 1, *Shigella flexneri* 2a, or *Salmonella typhimurium* W118, *Infect Immun*, **32:** 137–44.

Hale TL, Oaks EV, Formal SB, 1985, Identification and antigenic characterization of virulence-associated, plasmid-coded proteins of *Shigella* spp. and enteroinvasive *Escherichia coli, Infect Immun*, **50:** 620–9.

Harris JR, Mariano J et al., 1985, Person to person transmission in an outbreak of enteroinvasive *Escherichia coli, Am J Epidemiol*, **122:** 245–52.

Henry FJ, 1991, The epidemiologic importance of dysentery in communities, *Rev Infect Dis*, **13, Suppl 4:** S238–44.

Herrington DA, VanDeVerg L et al., 1990, Studies in volunteers to evaluate candidate *Shigella* vaccines: further experience with a bivalent *Salmonella typhi–Shigella sonnei* vaccine and protection conferred by previous *Shigella sonnei* disease, *Vaccine*, **8:** 353–7.

High N, Mounier J et al., 1992, IpaB of *Shigella flexneri* causes entry into epithelial cells and escape from the phagocytic vacuole, *EMBO J*, **11:** 1991–9.

Huebner J, Czerwenka W et al., 1993, Shigellemia in AIDS patients: case report and review of the literature, *Infection*, **21:** 122–4.

Islam D, Wretlind B et al., 1995, Immunoglobulin subclass distribution and dynamics of *Shigella*-specific antibody responses in serum and stool samples in shigellosis, *Infect Immun*, **63:** 2054–61.

Karnell A, Li A et al., 1994, Safety and immunogenicity study of the auxotrophic *Shigella flexneri* 2a vaccine SFL 1070 with a deleted *aro*D gene in adult Swedish volunteers, *Vaccine*, **13:** 86–99.

Keyti I, 1989, Epidemiology of the enteroinvasive *Escherichia coli*. Observations in Hungary, *J Hyg Epidemiol Microbiol Immunol*, **33:** 261–7.

Kotloff KL, Losonsky GA et al., 1995a, Evaluation of the safety, immunogenicity, and efficacy in healthy adults of four doses of live oral hybrid *Escherichia coli-Shigella flexneri* 2a vaccine strain EcSf2a-2, *Vaccine*, **13:** 495–502.

Kotloff KL, Nataro JP et al., 1995b, A modified *Shigella* volunteer challenge model in which the inoculum is administered with bicarbonate buffer: clinical experience and implications for *Shigella* infectivity, *Vaccine*, **13:** 1488–94.

LaBrec EH, Schneider H et al., 1964, Epithelial cell penetration as an essential step in the pathogenesis of bacillary dysentery, *J Bacteriol*, **88:** 1503–18.

Lee AL, Shapiro CN et al., 1991, Hyperendemic shigellosis in the United States: a review of surveillance data from 1967–1988, *J Infect Dis*, **164:** 894–900. -

Lett M-C, Sasakawa C et al., 1989, virG, a plasmid-coded virulence gene of *Shigella flexneri*: identification of the virG protein and determination of the complete coding sequence, *J Bacteriol*, **171:** 353–9.

Levenson VI, Egorova TP et al., 1991, Protective ribosomal preparation from *Shigella sonnei* as a parenteral candidate vaccine, *Infect Immun*, **59:** 3610–18.

Levine MM, 1986, Antimicrobial therapy for infectious diarrhea, *Rev Infect Dis*, **8, Suppl 2:** S207–16.

Levine OS, Levine MM, 1990, Houseflies (*Musca domestica*) as mechanical vectors of shigellosis, *Rev Infect Dis*, **13:** 688–96.

Lopez EL, Diaz M et al., 1989, Hemolytic uremic syndrome and diarrhea in Argentine children: the role of Shiga-like toxins, *J Infect Dis*, **160:** 469–75.

Makino S, Sasakawa C, Yoshikawa M, 1988, Genetic relatedness of the basic replicon of the virulence plasmid in shigellae and enteroinvasive *Escherichia coli, Microb Pathog*, **5:** 267–74.

Makino S, Sasakawa C et al., 1986, A genetic determinant required for continuous reinfection of adjacent cells on large plasmid in *Shigella flexneri* 2a, *Cell*, **46:** 267–74.

Mallett CP, VanDeVerg LL et al., 1993, Evaluation of *Shigella* vaccine safety and efficacy in an intranasally challenged mouse model, *Vaccine*, **11:** 190–6.

Mallett CP, Hale TL et al., 1995, Intranasal or intragastric immunization with proteosome – *Shigella* lipopolysaccharide vaccines protects against lethal pneumonia in a murine model of *Shigella* infection, *Infect Immun*, **63:** 2382–6.

Mathan VI, Mathan MM, 1991a, Intestinal manifestations of invasive diarrheas and their diagnosis, *Rev Infect Dis*, **13, Suppl 4:** S311–13.

Mathan MM, Mathan VI, 1991b, Morphology of rectal mucosa of patients with shigellosis, *Rev Infect Dis*, **13, Suppl 4:** S314–18.

Meitert T, Pencu E et al., 1984, Vaccine strain Sh. flexneri T32-ISTRATI. Studies in animals and volunteers. Antidysentery immunoprophylaxis and immunotherapy by live vaccine VADIZEN (Sh. flexneri T32-ISTRATI), *Arch Roum Pathol Exp Microbiol*, **43:** 251–8.

Mel D, Gangarosa EJ et al., 1971, Studies on vaccination against bacillary dysentery. 6. Protection of children by oral immunization with streptomycin-dependent *Shigella* strains, *Bull W H O*, **45:** 457–64.

Ménard R, Sansonetti P, Parsot C, 1994, The secretion of the *Shigella flexneri* Ipa invasions is activated by epithelial cells and controlled by IpaB and IpaD, *EMBO J*, **13**: 5293–302.

Ménard T, Sansonetti P et al., 1994, Extracellular associaton and cytoplasmic partitioning of the IpaB and IpaC invasins of *S. flexneri*, *Cell*, **79**: 515–25.

Murphy GS, Bodhidatta L et al., 1993, Ciprofloxacin and loperamide in the treatment of bacillary dysentery, *Ann Intern Med*, **118**: 582–6.

Nataro JP, Seriwatana J et al., 1993, Cloning and sequencing of a new plasmid-encoded enterotoxin in enteroinvasive *E. coli* and *Shigella*, *29th Joint Conference on Cholera and Related Diseases*, 144–7.

Nelson MR, Shanson DC et al., 1992, *Salmonella, Campylobacter,* and *Shigella* in HIV-seropositive patients, *AIDS*, **6**: 1495–8.

Noriega FR, Wang JY et al., 1994, Construction and characterization of attenuated Δ*aroA* Δ*virG Shigella flexneri* 2a strain CVD 1203, a prototype live oral vaccine, *Infect Immun*, **62**: 5168–72.

Orr N, Robin G et al., 1993, Immunogenicity and efficacy of oral or intranasal *Shigella flexneri* 2a and *Shigella sonnei* proteosome-lipopolysaccharide vaccines in animal models, *Infect Immun*, **61**: 2390–5.

Perdomo JJ, Gounon P, Sansonetti PJ, 1994, Polymorphonuclear leukocyte transmigration promotes invasion of colonic epithelial monolayer by *Shigella flexneri*, *J Clin Invest*, **93**: 633–43.

Perdomo OJJ, Cavaillon JM et al., 1994, Acute inflammation causes epithelial invasion and mucosal destruction in experimental shigellosis, *J Exp Med*, **180**: 1307–19.

Phalipon A, Michetti P et al., 1994, Protection against invasion of the mouse pulmonary epithelium by a monoclonal anitibody directed against *Shigella flexneri* lipopolysaccharide, *Ann N Y Acad Sci*, **730**: 356–8.

Prevost MC, Lesoud M et al., 1992, Unipolar reorganization of F-actin layer at bacterial division and bundling of actin filaments by plastin correlate with movement of *Shigella flexneri* within HeLa cells, *Infect Immun*, **60**: 4088–99.

Rajakumar K, Jost BH et al., 1994, Nucleotide sequence of the rhamnose biosynthetic operon of *Shigella flexneri* 2a and role of lipopolysaccharide in virulence, *J Bacteriol*, **176**: 2362–73.

Rauss K, Kontrohr T et al., 1970, Serological and chemical studies of *Sh. sonnei*, *Plesiomonas shigelloides* and C27 strains, *Acta Microbiol Acad Sci Hung*, **17**: 157–66.

Raqib R, Lindberg AA et al., 1995, Persistence of local cytokine production in shigellosis in acute and convalescent stages, *Infect Immun*, **63**: 289–96.

Robbins JB, Chu C-Y, Schneerson R, 1992, Hypothesis for vaccine development: serum IgG LPS antibodies confer protective immunity to non-typhoidal *Salmonella* and *Shigellae*, *Clin Infect Dis*, **15**: 346–61.

Rohde JE, 1984, Selective primary health care: strategies for control of disease in the developing world. XV. Acute diarrhea, *Rev Infect Dis*, **6**: 840–54.

Rout MR, Formal SB et al., 1975, Pathophysiology of shigella diarrhea in the rhesus monkey: intestinal transport, morphological, and bacteriological studies, *Gastroenterology*, **68**: 270–8.

Sack DA, Hoque ATMS et al., 1994, Is protection against shigellosis induced by natural infection with *Plesiomonas shigelloides*?, *Lancet*, **343**: 1413–15.

Sansonetti PJ, Kopecko DJ, Formal SB, 1982, Involvement of a plasmid in the invasive ability of *Shigella flexneri*, *Infect Immun*, **35**: 852–60.

Sansonetti PJ, Mounier J, 1987, Metabolic events mediating early killing of host cells infected by *Shigella flexneri*, *Microb Pathog*, **3**: 53–61.

Sansonetti PJ, Arondel J et al., 1991, *Omp*B (osmo-regulation) and *ics*A (cell-to-cell spread) mutants of *Shigella flexneri*: vaccine candidates and probes to study the pathogenesis of shigellosis, *Vaccine*, **9**: 416–22.

Sansonetti PJ, Mounier J et al., 1994, Cadherin expression is

required for the spread of *Shigella flexneri* between epithelial cells, *Cell*, **76**: 829–39.

Sansonetti PJ, Arondel J et al., 1995, Role of IL-1 in the pathogenesis of experimental shigellosis, *J Clin Invest*, **96**: 884–92.

Sasakawa C, Adler B et al., 1989, Functional organization and nucleotide sequence of virulence region-2 on the large virulence plasmid of *Shigella flexneri* 2a, *Mol Microbiol*, **3**: 1191–201.

Sereny B, 1955, Experimental *Shigella* keratoconjunctivitis: a preliminary report, *Acta Microbiol Acad Sci Hung*, **2**: 293–6.

Sethabutr O, Venkatesan M et al., 1993, Detection of *Shigella* and enteroinvasive *Escherichia coli* by amplification of the invasion plasmid antigen H DNA sequence in patients with dysentery, *J Infect Dis*, **167**: 458–61.

Speelman P, Kabir I, Islam M, 1984, Distribution and spread of colonic lesions in shigellosis: a colonoscopic study, *J Infect Dis*, **150**: 899–903.

Speelman P, McGlaughlin R et al., 1987, Differences in clinical features and stool finding in shigellosis and amoebic dysentery, *Trans R Soc Trop Med Hyg*, **81**: 549–51.

Stoll BJ, Glass RI et al., 1982, Epidemiologic and clinical features of patients infected with *Shigella* who attended a diarrheal disease hospital in Bangladesh, *J Infect Dis*, **146**: 177–83.

Tacket CO, Binion SB et al., 1992, Efficacy of bovine milk immunoglobulin concentrated in preventing illness after *Shigella flexneri* challenge, *Am J Trop Med Hyg*, **47**: 276–83.

Takeuchi A, Formal SB, Sprinz H, 1968, Experimental acute colitis in the rhesus monkey following peroral infection with *Shigella flexneri*, *Am J Pathol*, **52**: 503–20.

Taylor DN, Echeverria P et al., 1988, Clinical and microbiologic features of *Shigella* and enteroinvasive *Escherichia coli* infections detected by DNA hydridization, *J Clin Microbiol*, **26**: 1362–6.

Taylor DN, Trofa AC et al., 1993, Synthesis, characterization, and clinical evaluation of conjugate vaccines composed of the O-specific polysaccharide of *Shigella flexneri* type 2a and *Shigella sonnei* (*Plesiomonas shigelloides*) bound to bacterial toxoids, *Infect Immun*, **61**: 3678–87.

Toledo MR, Trabulsi LR, 1983, Correlation between biochemical and serological characteristics of *Escherichia coli* and results of the Sereny test, *J Clin Microbiol*, **17**: 419–21.

Tulloch EF, Ryan KJ et al., 1973, Invasive enteropathogenic *Escherichia coli* dysentery; an outbreak in 28 adults, *Ann Intern Med*, **79**: 13–17.

Vasselon T, Mounier J et al., 1991, Stress fiber-based movement of *Shigella flexneri* within cells, *Infect Immun*, **59**: 1723–32.

Vasselon T, Mounier J et al., 1992, Movement along actin filaments of the perijunctional area and de novo polymerization of cellular actin are required for *Shigella flexneri* colonization of epithelial Caco-2 cell monolayers, *Infect Immun*, **60**: 1031–40.

Venkatesan MM, Buysse JM, Oaks EV, 1992, Surface presentation of *Shigella flexneri* invasion plasmid antigens requires the products of the *spa* locus, *J Bacteriol*, **174**: 1990–2001.

Venkatesan MM, Fernandex-Prada C et al., 1991, Virulence phenotype and genetic characteristics of the T32 *Shigella flexneri* 2a vaccine strain, *Vaccine*, **9**: 358–63.

Voino-Yasenetsky MV, Khavkin TN, 1964, A study of intraepithelial localization of dysentery causative agents with the aid of fluorescent antibodies, *J Microbiol*, **12**: 98–100.

Wassef JS, Keren DF, Mailloux JL, 1989, Role of M cells in initial antigen uptake and in ulcer formation in the rabbit intestinal loop model of shigellosis, *Infect Immun*, **57**: 858–63.

Wells JG, Morris GK, 1981, Evaluation of transport methods for isolating *Shigella* spp., *J Clin Microbiol*, **13**: 789–90.

Wharton M, Spiegel RA et al., 1990, A large outbreak of antibiotic-resistant shigellosis at a mass gathering, *J Infect Dis*, **162**: 1324–8.

Wilson R, Feldman RA et al., 1981, Family illness associated with *Shigella* infection: the interrelationship of age of the index patient and the age of household members in the acquisition of illness, *J Infect Dis*, **143**: 130–2.

Yavzori M, Cohen D et al., 1994, Identification of *Shigella* species in stool specimens by DNA amplification of different loci of the *Shigella* virulence plasmid, *Eur J Clin Microbiol Infect Dis*, **13:** 232–7.

Zychlinsky A, Fitting C et al., 1994a, Interleukin 1 is released by murine macrophages during apoptosis induced by *Shigella flexneri*, *J Clin Invest*, **94:** 1328–32.

Zychlinsky A, Kenny B et al., 1994b, IpaB mediates macrophage apoptosis induced by *Shigella flexneri*, *Mol Microbiol*, **11:** 619–27.

Chapter 26

CHOLERA

R V Tauxe

1 INTRODUCTION

Cholera is a severe diarrhoeal illness caused by certain types of *Vibrio cholerae*, which can lead rapidly to dehydration and death. Although other organisms occasionally cause similar illness, the term 'cholera' is reserved for illness caused by infections with toxigenic strains of *V. cholerae* O1 and now O139, whether symptoms are mild or severe. These strains are characterized by their lipopolysaccharide O antigens, of which more than 139 have been described (Shimada et al. 1993). The other O groups do not have the same epidemic potential and are of far less public health significance. Before the advent of serogroup O139, they were referred to collectively as the non-O1 *V. cholerae*. Now 'non-epidemic *V. cholerae*' is a more desirable term than 'non-O1, non-O139 *V. cholerae*'. O1 strains can be further divided into 2 biotypes, El Tor and Classical. Cholera spread throughout the inhabited world in global pandemics until the Sanitary Reform revolution interrupted transmission in many countries by providing safe water and adequate sewage treatment. Mortality associated with typical severe cholera remained high until the more recent widespread use of rehydration therapy reduced the mortality from 25–50% to less than 1%.

The epidemiology of cholera has changed dramatically in the 1990s. The appearance of epidemic cholera in Latin America in 1991 after an absence of over 100 years has stimulated improvements in public health and sanitation throughout the hemisphere but is likely to persist as an important public health threat there for years to come. The deteriorating urban infrastructure in parts of the former Soviet Union has fostered the reappearance of epidemic cholera in Central Asia where it is a marker of the need for basic measures to protect the public health. In 1992 a new strain of *V. cholerae*, called O139 Bengal, appeared in India and caused a major epidemic in a population that was already largely immune to cholera caused by *V. cholerae* O1 strains. While the future of this new epidemic is unknown, it may represent the beginning of a new pandemic. The sudden appearance of this serogroup is a case study in the evolution of bacterial serotypes and in the emergence of new pathogens in general.

2 HISTORY

Epidemic cholera appeared rather recently on the global stage and is linked to the early phases of modern industrialization. Epidemic cholera is not clearly described in early Mediterranean or Middle Eastern medicine though compatible accounts exist in mediaeval India (Pollitzer 1959). The disease has a homeland in the Bengal delta of the Ganges and Brahmaputra Rivers, where the vibrio may have long been established in a natural reservoir, causing infections locally but rarely spreading to other populations, an ecological pattern resembling that of non-epidemic *V. cholerae* now. Beginning in 1817, cholera spread from Bengal to other parts of the world in repeated pandemic waves that affected virtually all of the inhabited world. Precisely when each of these waves began and ended is a matter of historical judgement. The most frequently cited account (Pollitzer 1959) divides them into 6 major pandemics between 1817 and 1923 (Table 26.1). The global spread of cholera was hastened by the establishment of European empires in Asia which led to increased international trade. The Hajj, or annual Muslim pilgrimage to Mecca, helped to disseminate cholera in pandemics 4 through 6. Cholera was likely to have been a regular feature of

Table 26.1 Cholera pandemics since 1817, following Pollitzer (1959)

No.	Years	Origin	Pandemic organism
1	1817–1823	India	?
2	1829–1851	India	?
3	1852–1859	India	?
4	1863–1879	India	?
5	1881–1896	India	*V. cholerae* O1, Classical
6	1899–1923	India	*V. cholerae* O1, Classical
7	1961–Present	Sulawesi, Indonesia	*V. cholerae* O1, El Tor
8?	1992–Present	Madras, India	*V. cholerae* O139

life in Asia in the nineteenth century. However, the impact was particularly severe in the rapidly growing European cities, where huge and highly lethal epidemics were observed. In those cities immigrants from the countryside crowded into new slums seeking employment in the new mills and factories of the industrial revolution. These Dickensian slums bear a striking sociological resemblance to the barrios, favellas and periurban slums that ring cities in the developing world today. In many ways Manila in 1995 may be compared to Manchester, England in 1840 (Sudjik and Redhead 1995). The pandemics had a profound impact on the development of public health itself, leading to the establishment of standing health departments, ongoing infectious disease surveillance, swift and effective public health response to epidemics and modern water and sewage treatment systems.

Investigations of the 1854 epidemic in London by John Snow showed that the cholera death rate in homes served by the Southwark and Vauxhall Water Company was 31 per 1000 houses, 8.5 times higher than the death rate in homes served by the competing company, 3.7 per 1000 houses (Snow 1936). Although neither company provided treated water, the former drew water from the Thames below the city sewage outlet whereas the latter was supplied from the river above the city. An outbreak of cholera was linked to consuming water drawn from one particular and celebrated pump, located in Broad Street. These investigations are classic examples of the application of epidemiological method even in the absence of a defined microbiological cause. In 1890 similar observations were made in Hamburg (Pollitzer 1959). These observations catalysed efforts to provide safe drinking water and adequate sewer systems in Europe and North America.

The aetiology of cholera was described by Robert Koch in 1884, who investigated cholera in Egypt during the fifth pandemic (Koch 1884). The strains he described are what we now refer to as the 'Classical' biotype of *V. cholerae* O1, the cause of pandemics 5 and 6. The cause of pandemics 1 through 4 remains unknown.

In the USA the public health response to cholera became more sophisticated through the nineteenth century (Rosenberg 1987). When the disease first arrived in 1832, the nation responded with prayer and panic and many believed that the disease was a divine

retribution afflicting the wicked. By 1866 a more rational approach prevailed. Temporary boards of health in many cities conducted surveillance, hospitalized cholera cases and took measures to improve the municipal water supply. After 1880, in the fifth and sixth pandemics, resurgent European epidemics again threatened the United States. Laboratory diagnosis was used to identify cases and large municipal aqueducts and protected watersheds were built. Although introductions were documented, sustained epidemic spread did not occur again, suggesting that the public health infrastructure was sufficiently advanced to protect the population.

After the sixth pandemic cholera entered a curious 50 year lull and again was largely restricted to the Bengal homeland. This lull broke in 1961 when epidemic cholera appeared in Sulawezi, Indonesia, with rapid subsequent dissemination (Kamal 1974). This epidemic, caused by the El Tor biotype of *V. cholerae* O1, spread rapidly across Asia and into Africa by 1970 (Fig. 26.1). In 1991 an El Tor strain appeared in Peru in a new epidemic wave that spread swiftly through Latin America (Tauxe and Blake 1992). In the mid-1990s, following the dissolution of the Soviet Union, epidemic cholera again appeared in the decaying cities of central Asia. Thus in 1993 more countries reported cholera than ever before. Epidemic cholera continues to exert a major influence on the global development of society and public health.

3 DESCRIPTION OF THE DISEASE

3.1 Pathogenesis

Cholera follows ingestion of contaminated water or food. The severity of symptoms varies with the dose of bacteria ingested, the effect of gastric acid, and with the patient's blood type (see section 5, p. 504). Following ingestion the vibrios attach to mucosal cells in the small intestine and produce cholera toxin. The organisms do not invade the mucosal cells or damage the integrity of the mucosal surface (Gangarosa et al. 1960). Once toxin is produced the B subunits of the toxin bind to specific ganglioside GM1 receptors on the surface of intestinal mucosal cells (King and van Heyningen 1973). A portion of the A subunit enters the cell and activates adenylate cyclase, producing

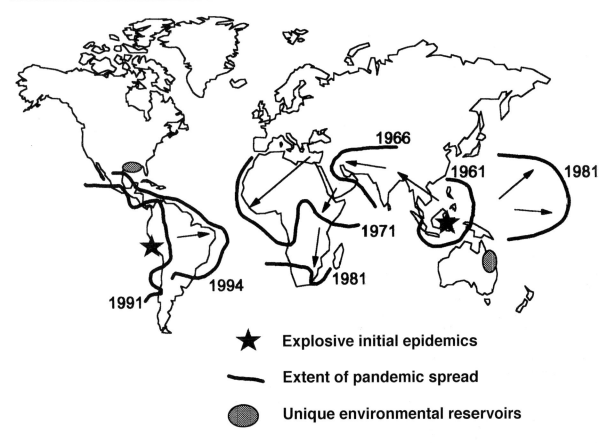

★ **Explosive initial epidemics**

— **Extent of pandemic spread**

⬭ **Unique environmental reservoirs**

Fig. 26.1 Global spread of the seventh cholera pandemic, 1961–94, and recently defined areas with environmental reservoirs of toxigenic El Tor *V. cholerae* O1.

high levels of cyclic AMP in the cells. Cyclic AMP in turn is a secondary messenger that in the crypt cells of the intestine increases the active pumping of chloride ion into the intestinal lumen, while in the villus cells it inhibits the normal absorption of NaCl (Kaper et al. 1994). As electrolytes accumulate in the intestine, potassium, bicarbonate and water follow passively. The intestines fill with alkaline, salty fluid that is isotonic with plasma, an excellent growth medium for *V. cholerae*. Diarrhoea begins when the colon cannot absorb the fluid fast enough, and can exceed 1 litre per hour. For the 70 kg adult this represents a loss of 10% of body weight in 7 h unless fluids and electrolytes are replaced. This loss of fluid and electrolytes produces the characteristic clinical picture as a result of hypovolaemia, hypokalaemia and acidosis.

3.2 Clinical manifestations

The spectrum of symptoms ranges from inapparent infection to life-threatening cholera gravis. In the epidemic setting, 50–75% of infections with El Tor are inapparent, 18–21% produce only a banal diarrhoea, 5–20% are moderate leading to clinical attention and 2–8% are severe (Gangarosa and Mosley 1974, Swerdlow et al. 1994). The clinical features of cholera are the result of a profound loss of intravascular fluids and electrolytes. The illness begins as a watery diarrhoea accompanied by abdominal cramps that typically starts

24–72 h after ingestion of the organisms. The diarrhoea becomes voluminous and in severe cases continuous. The faeces are like clouded water, with flecks of mucus, and are inoffensive smelling. They have been described since Osler's time as 'rice-water' stools but could better be described as thin chicken-rice broth. As electrolyte disturbances become more pronounced, acidosis leads to vomiting and hypokalaemia produces agonizing leg cramps, particularly in older patients. The signs and symptoms of dehydration are apparent once fluid losses exceed 5% of body weight: dry mouth, absence of tears, increasing thirst and loss of skin turgor leading to the so-called 'washerwoman's hands'. As fluid losses reach 10% of body weight the blood pressure drops, the patient becomes obtunded and approaches death from vascular collapse. Fever is rarely pronounced and the patient's sensorium remains clear until the very end. Virtually to the moment of death the disease is reversible if the fluid and electrolyte losses can be vigorously replaced. Transient renal failure may follow rehydration. Cholera can be particularly severe in the pregnant woman and loss of the fetus is likely if infection occurs in the third trimester (Hirschorn, Chowdhury and Lindenbaum 1969). No increase in severity has been described among persons infected with human immunodeficiency virus.

Asymptomatic infections are common in epidemic settings. For example, between 29 and 34% of healthy persons exhibited vibriocidal antibodies early in the course of the Peruvian epidemic, without having experienced diarrhoeal illness and *V. cholerae* O1 was identified in the stool cultures of 2 of 93 healthy persons cultured (Ries et al. 1992, Swerdlow et al. 1992). Patients with symptomatic infections continue to excrete the organisms for several weeks after symptoms resolve in the absence of effective antimicrobial treatment.

Clinical manifestations of infection with *V. cholerae* O139 Bengal are similar to those of *V. cholerae* O1. Several episodes of bacteraemia have been documented with *V. cholerae* O139 as well as a case of subsequent reactive arthropathy (Boyce et al. 1995). It is possible that this organism is more invasive than *V. cholerae* O1, perhaps because of the expression of a capsule in O139 strains.

4 EPIDEMIOLOGY

Modern public health surveillance and reporting was first organized for cholera; thus cholera bears the code 001 in the international classification of diseases and, along with plague and yellow fever, is an internationally notifiable disease. Many countries conduct routine surveillance for cholera and report the results to the World Health Organization. Official global statistics on cholera provide a very incomplete picture. Some countries officially conceal the presence of cholera because of political concerns, fear of inappropriate trade embargoes or loss of tourism and other imagined penalties; they may refer obliquely to 'severe diarrhoeal illness'. In 1993, for example, Bangladesh reported an absurdly low 12 cholera cases and no deaths to the World Health Organization (World Health Organization 1994). In other countries, particularly in Africa, vital statistics are not routinely gathered, disease reporting is limited and many cases and deaths may go unreported.

Where cholera is rare other diarrhoeal illnesses will be more common than cholera. In most industrialized nations the surveillance case definition of cholera depends on laboratory isolation of toxigenic *V. cholerae* O1 or O139 or demonstration of diagnostic antibodies (CDC 1990). In this setting it is important to verify the serogroup as O1 or O139 and the toxigenicity of the organism before calling the illness cholera in the setting of a sporadic case.

Where cholera is common it would be a mistake to restrict case reporting or public health response to laboratory-confirmed cases. The expenditure of scarce laboratory resources confirming many thousands of cases during an epidemic is a gross waste; the most useful roles of the laboratory are to define the beginning of the epidemic, monitor for changes in antimicrobial resistance during the epidemic and establish that an epidemic is over (Bopp, Kay and Wells 1994).

In the developed world when a cholera case is detected it is often important to heighten local surveillance to detect other cases and to establish whether transmission is ongoing. This is done by obtaining cultures from suspected cholera cases coming to medical attention and by testing convalescent sera from severe diarrhoeal cases seen at medical facilities in the preceding weeks (Bopp, Kay and Wells 1994, Mintz et al. 1994). If sewage collection is centralized, placing cotton gauze Moore swabs in the main sewer for 24 h and then culturing them can detect *V. cholerae* in areas drained by the sewer (Barrett et al. 1980). This is an economical way of maintaining surveillance on a population among whom cholera might be introduced (Bopp, Kay and Wells 1994).

4.1 Incidence

In 1993, 78 countries reported cholera to the World Health Organization (World Health Organization 1994). This is the greatest number of countries ever to report cholera, representing the cumulative effects of epidemics in Africa, Latin America and Asia (Fig. 26.2).

The 376 845 cases and 6781 deaths reported in 1993 are only a small fraction of the true total and are largely driven by Latin America where 209 192 cases and 2438 deaths were reported. In the New World, by 15 June 1995, 1 075 372 cases and 10 098 deaths had been reported since the beginning of the Latin American epidemic in 1991 (Pan-American Health Organization 1995). The case-fatality rate varies by continent. In 1993 it was 1.2% in the Americas, 2.0% in Asia and 3.3% in Africa (World Health Organization 1994). These differences reflect differences in reporting and in the delivery of medical care to cholera patients and not an attenuation of the virulence of the organism causing the epidemic in Latin America. In the Amazon where logistics are daunting, cholera case-fatality rates of 13.5% have been reported, nearly as high as observed in some areas of Africa (Quick et al. 1993).

The incidence of cholera depends on the presence of the causative organism, the opportunities available for transmitting it and the immunological experience of the population. Where sanitation is poor and crowded populations are previously uninfected, cholera incidence can be extremely high though even then many infections are asymptomatic. In the first year of the epidemic in Peru, 1.5% of the population was reported with a diagnosis of clinical cholera (Tauxe et al. 1994) and by early 1995 this had risen to 3% (Pan-American Health Organization 1995). It is likely that most Peruvians have been infected. In remote African villages affected by outbreaks, incidence was 1.5 per 100 (Tauxe et al. 1988). In Bangladesh, where cholera has recurred annually for centuries and where infection is likely to be nearly universal and repeated, silent infections may maintain a relatively high level of immunity in the population. Nevertheless the annual incidence of cholera requiring hospitalization ranges from 0.2 to 5 per 1000 (Glass et al. 1982). Along the Gulf Coast of the United States, though the organism is present in the environment, cases are sporadic and rare, ranging from 0 to 20 cases per year without secondary transmission (Blake 1993).

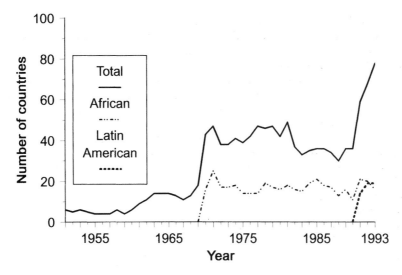

Fig. 26.2 Number of countries reporting cholera to the World Health Organization by year, 1951–93. (Data from World Health Organization).

4.2 Geographical distribution

The seventh cholera pandemic has affected virtually the entire developing world (Fig. 26.1). Developing countries with higher levels of sanitation, such as Chile, Argentina and Thailand, are relatively spared and even in countries affected by epidemics the areas with better sanitation are less likely to be affected. In Mexico the incidence of cholera has a north–south gradient and cases are concentrated in the poorest southern states (Tauxe et al. 1994). Unique strains of *V. cholerae* O1 persist along the US Gulf Coast and in rivers of northeastern Australia. Strains of the Classical biotype of *V. cholerae* O1 which swept the world in earlier pandemics are now limited to coastal Bangladesh while El Tor biotype strains are found further inland in that country, suggesting that the 2 differ in their ecological requirements (Siddique et al. 1991). The relative prevalence of these strains varies unpredictably from year to year, possibly reflecting shifts in their underlying ecology (Glass et al. 1982, Siddique et al. 1991). The impact of *V. cholerae* O139 strains on the balance of types may offer further clues to the ecology of *V. cholerae*.

The new epidemic strain, *V. cholerae* O139 Bengal, which emerged near Madras, remains restricted to Asia (Fig. 26.3) but in the future could be introduced into Africa and other parts of the developing world, truly causing the eighth pandemic.

4.3 Environmental reservoir

Toxigenic *V. cholerae* O1 El Tor strains can persist in rivers and estuaries, indicating they have niches in nature independent of human faecal contamination. This persistence is well demonstrated for the unique strain found along the US Gulf Coast (Blake 1994) where the same unique organisms have been isolated from persons with typical cholera since 1973. These organisms differ from all other strains tested by enzyme

typing (Wachsmuth et al. 1994, Evins et al. 1995), ribotyping (Popovic et al. 1993), pulsed field gel electrophoretic patterns (Cameron et al. 1994) and by the presence of a unique phage marker, VcA-3 (Almeida 1992). These cases have typically consumed undercooked shellfish which presumably acquired the vibrios in their natural habitat (Blake 1993). Other unique strains have been isolated repeatedly from many rivers in northeastern Australia and from persons drinking or swimming in them (Bourke et al. 1986). Other such natural foci are likely to exist but are more difficult to prove where human faecal contamination of the environment is frequent. It is instructive that other vibrios have complex relationships with marine invertebrates. For example, the light-producing *Vibrio fischeri* induces formation of light organs in juveniles of a single species of squid which the bacteria then colonize (McFall-Ngai and Ruby 1991). A specific association between *V. cholerae* and one or more estuarine life forms seems possible and several clues point to an association with plankton. *V. cholerae* O1 produces chitinase, an enzyme that dissolves chitin, the structural protein of invertebrate exoskeletons (Nalin 1976). This suggests they may have a niche in the digestive tracts of marine life that eat crustacea or even a role in the moulting of some crustacea. They attach directly to crustacea, particular to zooplanktonic copepods, apparently without harming them (Huq et al. 1984). They also appear to persist in vitro in association with certain algae (Islam, Drasar and Bradley 1989). Under conditions of extreme starvation they are reported to enter a dormant phase, the so-called 'viable but non-cultivable state' (Colwell and Huq 1994). This state is easy to induce and may be long-lasting but as no reliable means of inducing recovery from this state has been described some would argue it is irreversible and therefore inconsequential.

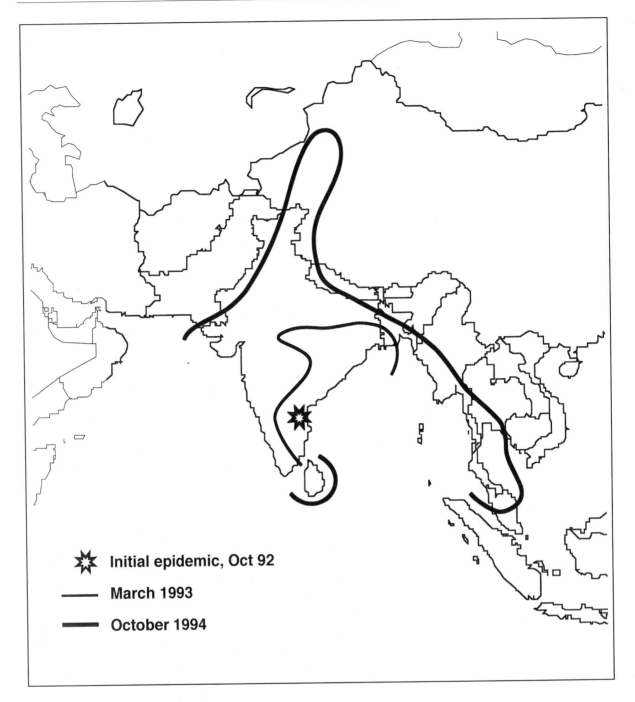

Fig. 26.3 Spread of the epidemic of *V. cholerae* O139 infections in Asia.

4.4 Epidemic behaviour

Cholera can appear as a single isolated case, as focal outbreaks, or in large epidemics. In the developed world the reported occurrence of rare cases is usually the result of travel to the developing world or of consumption of undercooked seafood harvested from a natural reservoir like other vibrio infections. Secondary transmission is unlikely.

In the developing world where sustained transmission is possible, a single case or small outbreak can lead to larger epidemics. In small villages transmission lasts for several weeks. In larger populations an epidemic can persist for many months, slowing in the cooler season and then recurring the following year. Cholera may then disappear or it may recur regularly for many years, perhaps because the organism finds an environmental niche. A long-term carrier state has been described but is extremely rare and plays no defined role in the persistence of the organism (Azurin 1967).

During pandemics 1 through 6 cholera rarely lasted more than a few years in one location. However, in the seventh pandemic cholera has tended to persist or recur once it was introduced. Cholera remains a major threat to health in Africa now 25 years after the seventh pandemic arrived there. This persistence may be related to properties of El Tor strains not shared by the Classical strains that caused pandemics 5 and 6. It may also be a consequence of the far greater density and mobility of human populations now compared to the nineteenth century. It means that cholera will remain an important global public health threat for years to come.

Cholera epidemics occur where breaks in sanitation lead to contaminated water and food consumed by many people. The most characteristic setting is the large periurban slum where people newly arrived from rural areas outstrip the availability of basic urban services. More temporary gatherings also can be affected by cholera outbreaks including religious pilgrimages and refugee encampments. Historically, the Islamic Hajj has played an important role in disseminating pandemics as have the great religious migrations of India (Pollitzer 1959). Cholera has not complicated the Hajj in recent years though pilgrimages in Bangladesh may have accelerated the spread of *V. cholerae* O139.

Refugee camps in Asia and Africa have experienced large epidemics of cholera. These epidemics are most severe when the camps are just being established or are overwhelmed with a new influx of people. The sudden migration of 700 000 Rwandan refugees to fresh lava fields near Goma, Zaire in the summer of 1994, where there were no latrines or wells, led to a catastrophic cholera and dysentery epidemic that killed 5% of the population in the first 3 weeks of the camp (Goma Epidemiology Group 1995). Cholera had recurred in the region for years, suggesting there may be an environmental reservoir in Lake Kivu, the source of water for the camp. In more organized camps of Mozambican refugees in Malawi, epidemic cholera was recurrent though with lower mortality. Cases were most common among the most recent arrivals to the camps who lacked the simplest cooking gear, fuel and water storage pots (Hatch et al. 1994). Cholera is not inevitable among refugees; it was rare among Vietnamese refugees in Thailand and easily controlled once the source was determined (Morris et al. 1982). Epidemic cholera has rarely followed natural disasters except in the Bengal basin. In Bangladesh epidemics of 'severe diarrhoeal disease' occur after typhoons flood coastal regions, though these areas would have had many cholera cases even without unusual flooding.

It is sometimes possible to determine the original source of the infection. This may be a traveller returning from a marketing trip, a visitor who arrives incubating the infection himself, someone bringing contaminated foodstuffs with him, or even the body of a victim being brought back to an ancestral village for burial. It is rare to identify any measure that could have prevented the introduction. *V. cholerae* can also be introduced via ocean freighters that take on ballast water in one harbour and discharge it in the next, which may contaminate shellfish beds near harbours (CDC 1992b). To decrease this risk freighters are now required by the International Maritime Organization to exchange their ballast water while at sea. Throughout the world the tides of humanity that flow from place to place can introduce cholera as long as it persists anywhere.

Cholera is sharply seasonal, becoming rare or undetectable in cooler months. It is not known what determines this seasonality nor how the organism survives from one season to the next. In the Latin American epidemic cholera increases sharply in the early summer and declines slowly in the fall. Attempts to relate seasonality to rain, monsoon or water temperature are inconsistent. In the 1950s, the peak season for cholera in Calcutta was May and June just before the monsoons whereas in Madras, further south on the west coast of India, it was August and September at the end of the monsoons (Pollitzer 1959). In rural Bangladesh the seasonality of El Tor and Classical infections differs: the peak for El Tor is October–November and for Classical biotype it is in December–January (Glass et al. 1982). Seasonal changes in vehicles of transmission or in the biological cycles of an unknown intermediate host could be important but are undocumented.

Year-to-year variation in incidence can be substantial and no general predictive rule is known. In British Colonial India it was noted that the year following a year of drought would tend to have a higher incidence of cholera (Rogers 1957). Along the Gulf Coast the years with highest incidence also happened to be years of drought when salt water incursions moved further inland than usual.

When cholera affects a population that has no pre-existing immunity, the age and sex of cholera patients reflects exposure to infection. In Piura, Peru, where the town water and street-vended beverages made with ice were identified sources, nearly all ages were equally exposed. Incidence in the first 3 weeks of the 1991 epidemic was 1.3% among those aged 5–14 years and 1.8% among those over 15 years of age; males and females were equally affected (Ries et al. 1992). In Italian outbreaks of 1973, transmission occurred through contaminated raw shellfish that were usually eaten by adults, so the median age of cases was 52 years and 60% were male (Baine et al. 1974). Because gastric acidity declines with advancing age, the elderly are often more likely to have severe illness than are younger persons. In Mexico in 1991, the incidence among those over age 65 was 7.1 per 100 000, compared to 2.5 per 100 000 among persons aged 15–24 (Tauxe et al. 1994). Breast-feeding infants are protected, presumably because they do not consume contaminated water or food (Gunn et al. 1979).

In Bangladesh where many adults have natural immunity boosted by re-exposure, cholera caused by *V. cholerae* O1 is more typically an illness of children, though cases in adults are not rare (Glass et al. 1982). Breast-feeding infants are protected because they are not exposed to contaminated water and food and also because of passive protection of antibodies in maternal milk (Glass et al. 1983). When epidemic *V.*

cholerae O139 infections appeared in the Bengal area, pre-existing immunity to O1 strains had little effect and all ages were affected (Cholera Working Group 1993).

Notably absent are cases among health staff caring for cholera cases and among clinical microbiologists. The extreme rarity of such cases underlines the ease with which cholera transmission can be prevented by simple hygienic precautions.

4.5 Modes of transmission

Cholera follows ingestion of food or water contaminated with an infectious dose of the causative organisms. In epidemics the source of contamination is usually the faeces of infected humans. In sporadic cases associated with natural reservoirs the source is independent of faecal contamination.

In the USA, cholera not associated with travel is usually associated with consumption of undercooked crabs, shrimp and oysters harvested on the coast of the Gulf of Mexico (Blake 1993). One outbreak on a Gulf Oil platform followed contamination of rice with seawater which itself was contaminated by the platform's sewage line; in this outbreak it is presumed that faecal contamination played a role (Johnston et al. 1983). Other cases have been related to foods brought from countries where cholera epidemics were occurring, including 2 outbreaks traced to crabs from Ecuador and an outbreak related to fresh frozen coconut milk imported from Thailand (Blake 1993, Taylor et al. 1993).

Cases associated with travel typically occur among 'homeland visitors' who are visiting friends or relatives in their countries of origin in the developing world. They may be exposed to the same risks of cholera as the indigenous population. Cases among more typical tourists or business travellers are extremely rare. The overall infection rate is remarkably low, approximately 1 per million air travellers to affected countries (Weber et al. 1994a).

In the developing world transmission of cholera has been documented through a variety of water- and food-borne mechanisms. During epidemics infections can be spread by more than one mechanism and the dominant source of infection may change. In an epidemic on the Gilbert Islands the initial cases were caused by consumption of partially dried salted fish and a month later illness was associated with eating a variety of raw clams and shrimp as well as salted fish (McIntyre et al. 1979). In 1972 during a cholera epidemic in Portugal an initial wave of cases associated with eating raw shellfish was followed by a sudden surge when a popular brand of bottled water became contaminated, thus infecting those who drank the water precisely to avoid cholera (Blake et al. 1977a, 1977b). In the urban developing world multiple routes may coexist. In Manila cholera was associated with municipal water contaminated at the periphery of the distribution system and with street-vended foods, especially mussel soup (Lim-Quizon et al. 1994). In 8 collaborative investigations into the mechanisms of

transmission of cholera in Latin America, multiple mechanisms of transmission were identified, including different mechanisms in different cities in the same country (Table 26.2).

Water-borne transmission occurs when faeces from an infected person contaminate a stream, lake or shallow well used for drinking water, when municipal water supplies draw from a contaminated source, or when water that was initially clean is contaminated during or after distribution. Water pipes are often laid in the same trench as sewer pipes. If water pressure drops because water supply or pumping power is intermittent, then pressure in the water pipes drops, drawing sewage into the water. Thus, a few cases of cholera that contaminate sewage can multiply rapidly into a city-wide epidemic, while authorities monitoring the initial quality of water going into the piping system at the well head may see no need for chlorination.

Because water is rarely available 24 h a day in the developing world, drinking water is usually stored in the home. If the vessel used to store water has a wide mouth and if water is removed by scooping it out, then the stored water is likely to be further contaminated. Increasing water contamination was measured in Trujillo, Peru, in 1991: faecal coliform counts were 1 per 100 ml in water collected at the well head, 2 per 100 ml at public taps and 20 per 100 ml in water stored in the home (Swerdlow et al. 1992). Protective practices include using a small-mouthed vessel to store water, pouring it out rather than scooping it out, treating water in the home with chlorine or by boiling, or acidifying the water by adding citrus juice (Mujica et al. 1994).

Transmission can also occur through foods contaminated during or after preparation, particularly through moist grains such as rice or millet. When leftover grains are held at ambient temperature a few vibrios can grow to a large dose by the following meal. The risk depends on the sauces that accompany the grain. In Guinea, cholera was associated with the use of a peanut sauce with neutral pH, whereas an acidic tomato sauce was highly protective (St Louis et al. 1990). In Mali, cholera was transmitted by millet, which usually would have been made with acidic fermented goats milk. Because of drought the goats were dry and the millet permitted vibrio survival (Tauxe et al. 1988). Transmission by fruits and vegetables has been documented where they were irrigated with fresh sewage or splashed with sewage on the way to market (Mujica et al. 1994). *V. cholerae* can be transmitted in street-vended foods and beverages which are often prepared in unhygienic ways and then held for many hours at ambient temperatures. In Piura, Peru, street beverages made with contaminated ice were an important source of cholera (Ries et al. 1992). In Guatemala, frozen fruit drinks were the dominant source (Koo et al. 1996).

Seafood can be an important source of cholera in the developing world when shellfish are harvested from contaminated waters and processed with little regard to sanitation. In Guinea-Bissau, cholera was associated with eating small crabs, particularly as left-

Table 26.2 Mechanisms of transmission of epidemic cholera in Latin America, as documented in epidemiological investigations, 1991–1993

	Peru			Ecuador	El Salvador	Bolivia	Brazil	Guatemala
Location	Trujillo	Piura	Iquitos	Guayaquil		Saipina	Fortaleza	Guatemala City
Setting	Urban	Urban	Urban	Urban	Rural	Rural	Rural	Urban
Date	3/91	3/91	7/91	7/91	3/91	2/92	6/93	7/93
Reference	(Swerdlow et al. 1992)	(Ries et al. 1992)	(Mujica et al. 1994)	(Weber et al. 1994b)	(Quick et al. 1995a)	(Gonzales et al. 1992)	*	(Koo 1995)
MECHANISM OF TRANSMISSION								
Water-borne								
Municipal water	+	+						
Surface water			+	+	+	+	+	
Putting hands in water vessel	+	+	+					
Food-borne								
Street-vendors' foods		+						+
Street-vendors' beverages		+						+
Street-vendors' ice/ices		+		+				+
Leftover rice		+	+					+
Fruits/vegetables			+					
Seafood								
Uncooked seafood				+	+			
Cooked seafood				+				

*CDC unpublished data.

overs (Shaffer et al. 1988). In Peru, ice used to ship fish was not made from chlorinated water in 1991 because 'it was not for human consumption' though the fish were typically eaten without cooking (Ries et al. 1992).

Cholera has twice affected air travellers on international flights. One outbreak occurred in 1972 on a flight from Great Britain to Australia and another in 1992 on a flight from Argentina to Los Angeles (Sutton 1974, CDC 1992a). International airlines should stock oral rehydration solutions and avoid serving cold salads or hors d'oeuvres prepared in cities with cholera epidemics.

A high inoculum is required to produce disease so cholera is rarely transmitted directly from one person to another without the intervening contamination of food or water. Health care-givers themselves are very unlikely to become infected. Episodes of nosocomial transmission are likely to be the result of contaminated water or infant formula, not direct person-to-person spread (Blake 1993). Cholera often spreads within households in the developing world. On Truk Island this was particularly likely if the first case in the household was the food-preparer (Holmberg et al. 1984). In Calcutta, secondary cases were more likely if the household stored their drinking water in a large-mouthed container, making it easily contaminated (Deb et al. 1986). Cholera outbreaks have occurred among persons attending the funerals of cholera victims. This is not likely to be due to simple contact with the cadaver, but rather to consuming foods and beverages at a funeral meal that are prepared by bereaved family members after they prepared the corpse for burial (Shaffer et al. 1988).

Transmission of *V. cholerae* O139 has not been well documented but is likely to resemble that of toxigenic *V. cholerae* O1. Repeated isolation from water suggests that water-borne transmission is likely. Food-borne transmission to tourists via rice has been documented (Boyce et al. 1995).

5 VARIATIONS IN HOST RESPONSE

The severity of symptoms varies with the dose of bacteria ingested, the effect of gastric acid and with the patient's blood type. In volunteer feeding trials with *V. cholerae* O1, ingesting 10^6 organisms with bicarbonate buffer or mixed in food regularly results in severe diarrhoeal illness, while doses of 10^9 or more are needed if the vibrios are consumed in water without buffering gastric acidity (Levine et al. 1981). Even lower doses may result in severe illness if the bacteria are protected by the buffering action of food or if little gastric acid is present for other reasons. Of 9 volunteers challenged with 10^6 *V. cholerae* O139 in buffer, 7 developed diarrhoeal illness, suggesting that the infectious dose is similar to that of *V. cholerae* O1 (Morris et al. 1995).

Persons of blood group O are more likely to have severe cholera than are persons of other blood groups. In Bangladesh where blood group O is rela-

tively uncommon, most adults hospitalized with cholera were of blood group O (Glass et al. 1985). This blood group is extremely common throughout Latin America. In Peru, persons with blood group O were no more likely to be infected with *V. cholerae* than others but if infected they were 9-fold more likely to develop life-threatening diarrhoea than were persons with other blood groups (Swerdlow et al. 1994). The reason for the blood group effect is unknown though some have speculated that blood group antigens may inhibit the binding of cholera toxin (Monferran et al. 1990). Curiously, the effect of blood group may be limited to infections with El Tor strains (Clemens et al. 1989).

Because vibrios are sensitive to acid, the state of the patient's gastric acid barrier can determine who gets ill. Gastric acid production is decreased by gastric surgery for ulcer disease, by antacid or anti-ulcer medication and in the youngest infants and people of advanced age. In an Italian outbreak in 1973, 27% of cases had previous gastric surgery (Baine et al. 1974). The possible impact of infection with the gastric bacterium *Helicobacter pylori*, which can induce a state of hypochlorhydria, is less well understood but may be important.

In those patients treated vigorously with fluids, the diarrhoea stops after several days, though toxigenic *V. cholerae* are still present, presumably as a result of secretory immune response. Following infection the patient is typically much more resistant to subsequent challenges with *V. cholerae* O1 but this protection is variable and may not last for more than a few years. Infection with Classical strains provides nearly complete protection against subsequent infection with any *V. cholerae* O1, while infection with El Tor strains provides only 60–70% protection to subsequent infection with either biotype (Clemens et al. 1991). This less solid immunity may help explain why the seventh pandemic has lasted so much longer than pandemics 5 and 6. This is also the reason vaccines are developed from Classical strains even though they are intended to protect against El Tor. Infection with O1 strains appears to provide little subsequent protection from infection with *V. cholerae* O139, although both produce the same toxin. This suggests that antitoxic immunity may play little role in the protective response. Natural infection with *V. cholerae* O139 Bengal also provides less than complete protection; one of 6 volunteers rechallenged after 3 months with the homologous strain developed diarrhoeal illness, compared with 11 of 13 developing diarrhoea after initial challenge; homologous protection was 80% (Morris et al. 1995).

6 AETIOLOGY

V. cholerae is a gram-negative, comma-shaped rod, adapted to life in fresh and brackish water. It has a long terminal flagellum permitting rapid propelling through water and it metabolizes a wide variety of nutrients. *V. cholerae* grows most rapidly at a neutral to somewhat basic pH, in moist environments with traces of salt and organic matter. This includes many foods, such as cooked grains, such as rice or lentils, and cooked shellfish (Kolvin and Roberts 1982). The organism is exquisitely sensitive to drying, sunlight and acid, and dies rapidly at pH of 4.0 or less. *Homo sapiens* is the only vertebrate host.

Like other gram-negative organisms, *V. cholerae* produces lipopolysaccharide O antigen with a variety of terminal sugar groups that can be differentiated serologically; more than 140 serogroups have been defined. The flagellar antigens (H antigens) do not vary within the serogroup and are not used for subtyping (Sakazaki 1992). Until recently only the O1 serogroup had the ability to cause epidemics. *V. cholerae* of non-O1 serogroups can sometimes cause human illness, including diarrhoeal illness and lethal invasive infections, but does not spread in epidemic form. Although often isolated from aquatic environments, most non-O1 *V. cholerae* serogroups are of little importance to public health and care is needed in the interpretation of reports that do not specify the serogroup under discussion. Within the O1 serogroup there are 2 specific antigenic serotypes, Ogawa and Inaba; the serotype Hikojima may represent a mixture of both. Serotype switching has been observed within a given strain, so these are not stable markers (Manning, Stroeher and Morona 1994, Vugia et al. 1994).

A new serogroup, O139, was first detected during epidemics of cholera-like illness in 1992 in India (Ramamurthy et al. 1993). The O139 strains appear to be closely related to O1 strains of biotype El Tor (Berche et al. 1994). Although the nature of the evolutionary event leading to O139 is not known with certainty, a portion of the genome coding for O-antigen synthesis has been deleted from a group of fairly typical El Tor O1 strains and genes have been inserted that code for a different antigen expressed as a polysaccharide capsule, possibly by a phage (Manning, Stroeher and Morona 1994). The epidemic behaviour of these strains shows that the O1 antigen itself is not necessary for the ability to cause epidemics.

6.1 Virulence factors

Cholera toxin is the most critical virulence determinant for *V. cholerae*. Cholera toxin is a protein enterotoxin formed from an active A subunit of 240 amino acids held within a pentamer ring of 5 B subunits, each of which has 103 amino acids (Spangler 1992). Two other enterotoxins produced by *V. cholerae* O1 have been described though the role they play in natural infection is uncertain. These are Zot (zona occludens toxin) (Fasano et al. 1991) and Ace (accessory cholera enterotoxin) (Trucksis et al. 1993). Colonization of the intestinal mucosa is facilitated by pili. The predominant pilus, the toxin co-regulated pilus, is synthesized in conjunction with toxin production and appears to be governed by the same regulatory apparatus (Kaufman and Taylor 1994).

The organism produces varying amounts of toxin depending on the environment in which it finds itself

(Ottemann and Mekalanos 1994). This control occurs through the DNA binding regulatory proteins ToxR and ToxT, the production of which depends on the ToxR regulon. The ToxR regulon and toxin co-regulated pilus has also been identified in *V. cholerae* O139 (Waldor and Mekalanos 1994).

6.2 Strain differentiation

Two biotypes are distinguished among toxigenic O1 strains, El Tor and Classical. Strains of the El Tor biotype agglutinate chicken red cells and lyse sheep red cells while Classical strains do neither; the 2 biotypes can also be separated by phage susceptibility (Kay et al. 1994). Classical strains caused global pandemics in the late nineteenth and early twentieth centuries but since then have disappeared outside of coastal Bangladesh (Siddique et al. 1991). The El Tor strain of *V. cholerae* O1 is named for a Hajj quarantine station in Egypt where it was isolated from an asymptomatic pilgrim early in the twentieth century. Its epidemic potential was debated until the beginning of the seventh pandemic in 1961. There are important epidemiological differences between the 2 strains. Compared to Classical strains, El Tor strains are more likely to produce inapparent infections (Gangarosa and Mosley 1974), persist longer in the environment (Benenson et al. 1965), multiply more rapidly following inoculation into foods (Kolvin and Roberts 1982) and evoke less complete immunity (Clemens et al. 1991).

Molecular methods have revealed a great diversity of subtypes. Multienzyme electrophoresis identified 4 main enzyme types (ET) within El Tor strains, distinguishing the Gulf Coast, Australian, seventh pandemic and Latin American strains; the same method showed that at least 3 subgroups could be distinguished among Classical biotype (Wachsmuth et al. 1994). Ribotyping (RT) identified 9 types among 176 toxigenic El Tor strains tested (Popovic et al. 1993). With pulsed field gel electrophoresis (PFGE), 36 patterns were identified among 142 toxigenic El Tor strains tested, offering a fine grain subtyping that is useful for epidemiological investigations (Cameron et al. 1994). The Latin American epidemic strain that was introduced in Peru in 1991 remains uniform: ET3, RT5 and PFGE pattern 38, a subtype that has yet to be identified elsewhere (Evins et al. 1995). The seventh pandemic in the rest of the world is an overlapping patchwork of strains. Recently, a second strain of *V. cholerae* O1 has spread throughout Central America so that the Latin American epidemic is now polyclonal. This strain resembles strains found elsewhere in Asia and Romania (Evins et al. 1995). Using similar methods, strains of *V. cholerae* O139 isolated early in that epidemic can be divided into at least 2 ribotypes and 4 PFGE types, suggesting that the epidemic of O139 infections is not caused by one uniform 'epidemic strain' (Popovic et al. 1995).

The genes coding for cholera toxin B subunit also show diversity and at least 3 genotypes exist (Olsvik et al. 1993). The significance of this diversity is unclear as all toxin types appear to have the same biological activity. Curiously, the Gulf Coast El Tor strains have the same B subunit type as otherwise unrelated Classical strains, suggesting that toxin genes have been transferred horizontally between unrelated bacterial strains.

7 LABORATORY DIAGNOSIS

Definitive diagnosis is made by isolation and identification of the causative organism or by demonstrating a diagnostic increase or decrease in the antibody response. In the outbreak setting persons with similar illness may be presumed to have cholera once the aetiology of the illness is established for a representative sample. In the industrialized world cholera should be suspected and appropriate stool cultures requested from anyone with severe diarrhoeal illness who recently travelled to the developing world or who has ingested raw shellfish. In the developing world, in the setting of a known or threatened epidemic, presumptive diagnosis is made on clinical grounds. The report of 2 or more adults in the same location with severe watery diarrhoea and vomiting, or the report of an adult dying of watery diarrhoea, may be presumed to be cholera until proved otherwise. Immediate action should be taken to bring adequate supplies for treatment, prevention and diagnosis to that location and to warn surrounding villages of the possibility of cholera. A small number of diagnostic specimens should be collected and transported to a competent laboratory.

7.1 Specimen collection

A sample of fresh faeces is collected by rectal swab or straw directly from the rectum; specimens from bedpan or bucket should be avoided because of the possible presence of residual disinfectant. The specimen should be collected before antimicrobials are administered. The swabs should be immediately placed in a suitable transport medium, such as Cary–Blair, and transported at or below ambient temperature. Freezing is not essential though the specimens should be protected from overheating. In the absence of antimicrobial therapy diagnostic isolation is still possible a week or more after onset.

Environmental samples can be collected by placing a gauze Moore swab in flowing water or sewage for 24 h (Barrett et al. 1980), or by filtering at least 10 litres of standing water through a gauze packed Spira jar (Spira and Ahmed 1981) and then complementing the specimen with alkaline peptone broth for transport and incubation.

7.2 Isolation and identification

V. cholerae is massively excreted in stools of the cholera patient and grows well on several standard bacteriological media. Efficient isolation depends on the use of a selective medium that suppresses other bacterial

species but permits *V. cholerae* to grow. Thiosulphate–citrate–bile salts–sucrose (TCBS) agar is the most widely used medium (Bopp, Kay and Wells 1994). *V. cholerae* produces large translucent yellow colonies on this medium. The organisms ferment sucrose but not lactose. After subculture on media other than TCBS, they can be tested directly with diagnostic antiserum for the presence of O1 antigen. O1 strains will agglutinate in O1 antiserum, producing a coagulated clump on a slide. O139 strains can be identified in the same way with O139 antiserum. Strains that agglutinate in neither O1 nor O139 antiserum may be non-O1, non-O139 strains of *V. cholerae* or other closely related vibrios (such as *Vibrio mimicus*). Definitive identification of such strains may require the services of a reference laboratory and may not be necessary if the only concern is cholera. Strains that agglutinate in O1 antiserum can be further characterized as serotype Inaba or Ogawa using monovalent antisera.

For environmental or food specimens in which the number of *V. cholerae* may be much lower than in stools, an enrichment step is often necessary. Incubating the specimen in alkaline peptone broth for 8 h takes advantage of the affinity *V. cholerae* has for alkaline environments; the broth is subsequently plated on TCBS.

O1 or O139 strains should be further characterized by whether or not they produce cholera toxin. This property was originally defined by the ability of supernatant from a broth culture to induce the outpouring of fluid in the rabbit ileal loop but is more easily detected by tissue culture assay on Chinese hamster ovary cells (Guerrant et al. 1974) or Y1 mouse adrenal cells (Donta et al. 1974), latex bead agglutination (Ito et al. 1983), or by enzyme-linked immunosorbent assay (Almeida et al. 1990). The commercially available latex agglutination assay is the most practical for many laboratories (Almeida et al. 1990). Detection of cholera toxin gene by polymerase chain reaction may permit diagnosis or confirmation of a food vehicle even in the absence of a laboratory isolation (Fields et al. 1992).

Though strains can be further characterized by biotype, the need for biotyping is minimal as only El Tor is found outside of Bangladesh. Within biotype El Tor subtypes can be defined using traditional and molecular techniques (see section 6.2, p. 505). Subtyping is of value in epidemiological investigations to help determine the source of infecting strains.

7.3 Rapid diagnosis

Rapid presumptive diagnostic methods exist. The characteristic darting 'shooting star' motility of the vibrios can be observed by microcopy of a wet mount of fresh faeces and halts immediately if O1 antiserum is added to the slide (Benenson et al. 1964). A rapid diagnostic test based on colorimetric immunoassay detection of the O1 antigen has been marketed; it offers rapid presumptive diagnosis in the field without microscopy (Hasan et al. 1994). The efficiency of this test is approximately the same as that of traditional microbiological methods; using the test provides greater speed of diagnosis at higher cost. A similar assay has been developed for use in detecting O139 strains (Qadri et al. 1994). Rapid methods do not yield a living organism for confirmatory testing or antimicrobial resistance testing. A patient with severe diarrhoea requires rehydration therapy whether or not cholera is confirmed; availability of the rapid test should not affect the management of the individual patient. Rapid diagnosis may prove most useful when it is linked to public health actions that slow spread of an epidemic.

7.4 Serodiagnosis

The human immune response to infection with toxigenic *V. cholerae* O1 infection has been well characterized (Levine et al. 1983). Within 10 days, vibriocidal antibodies appear in serum that rapidly kill target *V. cholerae* O1. This vibriocidal response begins to decline by one month and disappears after a year. There is little difference between antibodies evoked by Ogawa or Inaba strains. In general, Classical strains evoke higher antibody responses than El Tor strains. The somewhat slower antitoxic response peaks by 21–28 days after exposure and remains elevated for several years.

Serodiagnosis of an isolated case depends on demonstration of a 4-fold rise in vibriocidal titres between early and convalescent sera, or a 4-fold fall between convalescent and late convalescent sera (Bopp, Kay and Wells 1994). Detection of antitoxic antibodies is suggestive evidence and is helpful when trying to distinguish between vaccine-induced and natural immunity (if the vaccine does not contain toxin subunits). However, it is difficult to base diagnosis on the presence of antitoxic antibodies alone, as similar antibodies appear after infection with *E. coli* producing heat-labile enterotoxin (ETEC-LT). Methods for distinguishing the 2 responses exist and are applicable in population surveys but may not resolve the isolated case (Svennerholm et al. 1983).

The immune response to infection with toxigenic *V. cholerae* O139 remains incompletely understood (Morris et al. 1995). Neither vibriocidal antibodies nor simple O139 agglutinins are detected though the antitoxic response appears to be similar to that following O1 infection.

8 PRINCIPLES OF TREATMENT

Rapid replacement of lost fluid and electrolytes is the critical life-saving treatment (Swerdlow and Ries 1992). Treatment is the same as for any profoundly dehydrating diarrhoea and should begin as soon as the extent of the dehydration is appreciated, before laboratory diagnosis is confirmed. In severe cases volume replacement requires large volumes of intravenous polyelectrolyte fluids that include adequate sodium, potassium and base, such as Ringer's lactate or Dhaka solution. Use of normal saline will not cor-

rect the potentially lethal acidosis or hypokalaemia and is not by itself adequate treatment. Oral rehydration solution (ORS) using a carefully defined mixture of carbohydrate and electrolytes can be used to replace losses in patients who are able to drink. Rice-based oral rehydration solutions have been developed that may reduce fluid losses further, particularly in children (Molla et al. 1989). Antimicrobial therapy is a useful adjunct that decreases fluid losses and hastens recovery, but it is not sufficient by itself. Effective agents, depending on the antimicrobial resistance of local strains, include tetracycline, doxycycline, trimethoprim–sulphamethoxazole, erythromycin and furazolidone (World Health Organization 1993). Ciprofloxacin given at 250 mg doses once a day for 3 days is as effective as tetracycline (Gotuzzo et al. 1995).

Various adjunctive therapies that have been explored to reduce the volume of diarrhoeal losses without notable success include aspirin, oral antibodies, toxin inhibitors such as free GM1 receptors and cholera phage (Bennish 1994). Opiates and other antiperistaltics are of no benefit and should be avoided. Emesis is best treated by correcting the acidosis; antiemetics are of little use.

9 PREVENTION AND CONTROL

Cholera is not likely to be eradicated. The existence of environmental reservoirs of toxigenic *V. cholerae* O1 means the organism is likely to persist indefinitely. Crowded urban populations in the developing world provide the setting for future epidemics of cholera after the organism is introduced and increasing international mobility makes such introductions likely. As long as the organism persists anywhere, the potential for epidemic cholera exists wherever and whenever conditions are ripe for sustained transmission.

9.1 Chemoprophylaxis

Antimicrobials play a limited role in the control of cholera. Prophylactic treatment of family members of cholera cases in the Philippines was shown to decrease the incidence of infection from 13% in the untreated group to 0% in family members taking 20 doses of tetracycline over 5 days (McCormack et al. 1968). A field trial of ciprofloxacin for chemoprophylaxis among household members of cholera patients in Peru found no significant benefit, though a protective trend was noted (Echevarria et al. 1995). In closed settings such as prisons, ships, or small and isolated villages, the strategy has potential merit. However, chemoprophylaxis on any scale runs the risk of evoking antimicrobial resistance. In Latin America where the practice has been to avoid chemoprophylaxis, the organism remains generally susceptible in 1995 after a million cases have been reported. An instructive exception was in Guayaquil, Ecuador, where a vigorous campaign of family chemoprophylaxis in 1991 was associated with a rapid emergence of multiple resistance which forced the strategy to be abandoned

(Weber et al. 1994b). In addition to the risk of causing the emergence of resistant strains, mass chemoprophylaxis with sulpha or tetracyclines has been associated with severe adverse reactions to the drugs and with the appearance of a folk belief that the antibiotic is a form of vaccine that confers permanent protection.

9.2 Strategies of disinfection and sanitation

In a cholera epidemic, the first priority is to prevent death by assuring adequate treatment and by encouraging the population to seek treatment rapidly once a diarrhoeal episode begins. The success of control efforts depends on knowing the actual mechanisms or vehicles of transmission and having the tools available to block them. Because vehicles may vary, swift epidemiological investigation, including a case-control study, may guide control efforts, especially in the setting of ongoing epidemics refractory to initial control efforts. For example, in 1991 in Santiago, Chile, case investigation suggested that cholera was being transmitted through use of fresh sewage to irrigate cultivated salad vegetables; halting this practice brought an abrupt end to the outbreak and also sharply decreased the incidence of typhoid fever and hepatitis A (Alcayaga et al. 1993). In 1974, in Portugal, successful control followed the identification of 2 sequential vehicles: contaminated raw shellfish and a spring used to make bottled water (Blake et al. 1977a, 1977b). Throughout Latin America, recommendations to boil water, to avoid street-vended foods and to cook seafood followed the identification of these transmission mechanisms early in the epidemic. Such emergency changes are not sustainable and the persisting epidemic demands more fundamental approaches to prevention (Tauxe et al. 1994).

Avenues of sustained transmission have already been closed in many parts of the world. Between 1961 and 1991 there were 56 travel-associated cases in the continental United States, without subsequent spread (Weber et al. 1994a). In the USA and other industrialized nations, when a case of cholera occurs prompt public health action is warranted to determine the source of infection and to ensure the proper disposal of the faeces. Routine sanitation is adequate to prevent further transmission but for some populations, including the homeless, the 'colonias' along the Mexican border and a few Native American reservations, the potential for further transmission still exists. Most populations on the North American and European continents are protected by the large engineering triumphs of the 'sanitary revolution': safe water and sewage treatment systems. Similar efforts now beginning could control cholera by the early twenty-first century in many rapidly developing countries of Asia and Latin America.

Among the least developed countries, large-scale engineering solutions are too costly and there is a critical need for simpler alternatives. Because storage of drinking water in the home is nearly universal in the developing world, modification of the storage vessel

to keep stored water from becoming contaminated is one simple and inexpensive strategy (Mintz et al. 1995). A simple apparatus can produce a chlorine disinfectant solution by the electrolysis of salt water using solar power. With one such machine a village of several thousand people can treat their own drinking water and even make a net profit selling surplus disinfectant to their neighbours (Quick et al. 1995b). Larger ventures to produce a water disinfectant product for routine use in the developing world are of potential commercial interest. Private industry can be a useful partner in the effort to promote domestic water treatment with household bleach (Hospedales et al. 1993). Closer attention to ice production in the developing world can guarantee that treated water is used to make ice, the cheapest of modern luxury goods.

Simple improvements in food preparation may also greatly reduce the risk of cholera. The acidification of sauces should be promoted by public health authorities: tomatoes, tamarind, lemons and yogurt can acidify foods sufficiently to prevent the survival of *V. cholerae* (D'Aquino and Teves 1994). Foods can be made safer by thorough cooking and by heating or at least acidifying leftovers. Street-vendor hygiene can be improved by providing safer carts, promoting the use of clean water, soap and disinfectants, training street vendors in the elements of food safety and by educating consumers to look for vendors who are following simple and visible precautions.

Where raw or undercooked seafood is a dietary staple, precautions that protect harvest waters and that guarantee clean water for processing and clean ice for shipping can help prevent seafood-borne cholera. However, as long as raw shellfish from warm waters are consumed, an irreducible minimum number of cases can still be expected because of the natural estuarine reservoirs of toxigenic *V. cholerae*.

9.3 Immunization

The development of an inexpensive, effective vaccine that provides long-term protection against cholera would be a tremendous public health boon. Efforts to develop such a vaccine have been ongoing for more than a century. Strategies have included vaccines that are based on whole killed bacteria, live attenuated bacteria, toxoids and conjugated lipopolysaccharide O antigen. To date the best vaccines appear to be as good as natural infection with El Tor strains, which itself confers partial and temporary immunity. However, none has shown sufficient long-lasting protection to make it useful as a general tool for public health.

Three vaccines are now commercially available in some countries (Table 26.3). The parenteral killed vaccine tested extensively in the early 1970s is the only vaccine licensed in the USA (CDC 1988). Two oral vaccines are produced and marketed in Europe: a whole cell killed vaccine that includes a B-subunit toxoid, the so-called WC-BS vaccine (Clemens et al. 1988, 1990, Sanchez et al. 1994) and a live attenuated vaccine from the Center for Vaccine Development, CVD

Table 26.3 Characteristics of cholera vaccines now in commercial production

Characteristic	Type	Route	No. of doses	Time to complete primary series	Efficacy	Duration
Cholera vaccine	Extract of killed organisms	Intramuscular injection	2	1 week	50%	3–6 months
Whole cell/B subunit	Killed organisms/B subunit of toxin	Oral	3*	12 weeks	62% at 1 year*†	2 years
CVD 103-HgR	Live attenuated organisms	Oral	1	1 day	59%	At least 6 months

*In Bangladesh field trials. Recent field trial in Peru used 2 doses at 1–2 week intervals, and obtained efficacy at 1–2 months of 86%.
†Against both Classical and El Tor strains. Protection against El Tor alone was reported to be lower.

103-HgR (Levine and Tacket 1994, Lagos et al. 1995). WC-BS was tested extensively in a large Bangladesh field trial with a protective efficacy in the first year of 62% in a location where both El Tor and Classical strains were present (Clemens et al. 1988). Efficacy waned sharply after 2 years and was substantially lower among persons with blood group O (Clemens et al. 1989), among children less than age 5 and against infection with El Tor biotype compared to Classical biotype (Clemens et al. 1990). In a more recent trial in Peruvian military recruits, short-term efficacy in protecting against El Tor cholera in the first 2 months after vaccination was 86% (Sanchez et al. 1994). The efficacy of the CVD 103-HgR vaccine has been measured in volunteer challenge studies conducted in North America. Efficacy is 62–64% against any diarrhoea when challenged with El Tor strains and 100% when challenged with Classical strains (Levine and Tacket 1994). The duration of protection has been documented to 6 months but not tested beyond that. Curiously, the antibody response to CVD 103-HgR is higher in persons with blood group O though it is unclear whether they are better protected (Lagos et al. 1995). Although both vaccines are a substantial improvement over the parenteral vaccine, they are too costly and have too brief an effect for use in protecting the public health in the developing world. These vaccines are primarily marketed to the international traveller, although the risk of cholera is extremely low and no nation currently requires vaccination for entry (CDC 1988). The administration of oral vaccines reconstituted in a cup of water with a buffer could offer particular efficiency in administration and freedom from the hazards of parenteral injection. However, the safety and reliability of this delivery system, which would require large volumes of sterile water for mass immunization, remains to be assessed in the field for any vaccine. Other vaccines are under development including both inactivated and live attenuated vaccines against O1 and O139 Bengal strains (Mekalanos and Sadoff 1994) and lipopolysaccharide-based vaccines (Gupta et al. 1992). A live attenuated *V. cholerae* O139 strain that produces B subunit provided 83% protection against challenge in volunteers one month after immunization similar to that provided by natural infection (Coster et al. 1995).

Cholera vaccine has not been used successfully to control an epidemic. The risk of cholera is immediate whereas the protection afforded by vaccines begins a week or 2 after completion of the primary series. In an extreme example, the cholera epidemic that occurred among refugees at Goma, Zaire, was largely over in 4 weeks, before a 2 dose WC-BS vaccine could have provided protection even had a campaign commenced the day the camp was created (Levine et al. 1995).

Nevertheless, the availability of vaccines leads to pressure to use them. The issue presages what to expect when partially effective vaccines become available for other feared diseases such as AIDS. Humanitarian impulses, coupled with the need for public health departments to 'do something', encourage cholera vaccination campaigns. Long experience has shown that once a campaign is launched, the pressure to vaccinate everyone can be irresistible and scarce public health resources are diverted from other, more important activities. Vaccination is not the only means of preventing cholera, unlike measles or bacterial meningitis. This means that cholera vaccination needs to be shown to be less expensive and more effective than other strategies for preventing the disease before it is adopted as a public health tool (Cvjetanovic 1974).

10 CONCLUSION

Epidemic cholera is an indicator of severe underdevelopment, a sign that the basic sanitary infrastructure of a society fails to guarantee safe water and sewage disposal to its citizens. Communities that make the necessary investments will prevent this and many other diseases that are transmitted through the same routes. Bringing about this sustained world-wide 'sanitary revolution' is a central challenge for global public health in the twenty-first century. The scope of cholera prevention extends beyond public health and clinical medicine to include fisheries, agriculture, shipping and tourism in many nations. Just as cholera spurred the development of sanitary reform and modern public health in Europe and North America so epidemic cholera is likely to be less and less tolerable in the growing democracies of the developing world.

REFERENCES

Alcayaga S, Alcagaya J, Gassibe P, 1993, Changes in the morbidity profile of certain enteric infections after the cholera epidemic, *Rev Chil Infect*, **1**: 5–10.

Almeida RJ, Hickman-Brenner FW et al., 1990, Comparison of a latex agglutination assay and an enzyme-linked immunosorbent assay for detecting cholera toxin, *J Clin Microbiol*, **28**: 128–30.

Almeida RJ, Cameron DN et al., 1992, Vibriophage VcA-3 as an epidemic strain marker for the U.S. Gulf Coast *Vibrio cholerae* O1 clone, *J Clin Microbiol*, **30**: 300–4.

Azurin JC, Kobari K et al., 1967, A long-term carrier of cholera: cholera Dolores, *Bull W H O*, **37**: 745–9.

Baine WB, Zampieri A et al., 1974, Epidemiology of cholera in Italy in 1973, *Lancet*, **2**: 1370–8.

Barrett TJ, Blake PA et al., 1980, Use of Moore swabs for isolating *Vibrio cholerae* from sewage, *J Clin Microbiol*, **11**: 385–8.

Benenson AS, Ahmad SZ, Oseasohn RO, 1965, Person-to-person transmission of cholera, *Proceedings of the Cholera Research Symposium*, US Department of Health, Education and Welfare, Bethesda, MD, 332–6.

Benenson AS, Islam MR, Greenough WB III, 1964, Rapid identification of *Vibrio cholerae* by darkfield microscopy, *Bull W H O*, **30**: 827–31.

Bennish ML, 1994, Cholera: pathophysiology, clinical features, and treatment, *Vibrio cholerae* and Cholera, American Society for Microbiology, Washington DC, 229–55.

Berche P, Poyart C et al., 1994, The novel epidemic strain O139 is closely related to the pandemic strain O1 of *Vibrio cholerae*, *J Infect Dis*, **170**: 701–4.

Blake PA, 1993, Epidemiology of cholera in the Americas, *Gastroenterol Clin North Am*, **22 (3)**: 639–60.

Blake PA, 1994, Endemic cholera in Australia and the United States, *Vibrio cholerae* and Cholera, American Society for Microbiology, Washington DC, 309–19.

Blake PA, Rosenberg ML et al., 1977a, Cholera in Portugal, modes of transmission, *Am J Epidemiol*, **105**: 337–43.

Blake PA, Rosenberg ML et al., 1977b, Cholera in Portugal, transmission by bottled mineral water, *Am J Epidemiol*, **105**: 344–8.

Bopp CA, Kay BA, Wells JG, 1994, *Laboratory Methods for the Diagnosis of Vibrio cholerae*, Centers for Disease Control and Prevention, Atlanta, GA.

Bourke ATC, Cossins YN et al., 1986, Investigation of cholera acquired from the riverine environment in Queensland, *Med J Aust*, **144**: 229–34.

Boyce TG, Mintz ED et al., 1995, *Vibrio cholerae* O139 Bengal infections among tourists to Southeast Asia: an intercontinental foodborne outbreak, *J Infect Dis*, **172**: 1401–4.

Cameron DN, Khambaty FM et al., 1994, Molecular characterization of *Vibrio cholerae* O1 strains by pulsed-field electrophoresis, *J Clin Microbiol*, **32**: 1685–90.

Centers for Disease Control, 1988, Cholera vaccine: recommendations of the Immunization Practices Advisory Committee, *Morbid Mortal Weekly Rep*, **37**: 617–24.

Centers for Disease Control, 1990, Case definitions for public health surveillance, *Morbid Mortal Weekly Rep*, **39**: RR-13.

Centers for Disease Control, 1992a, Cholera associated with an international airline flight, *Morbid Mortal Weekly Rep*, **41**: 134–5.

Centers for Disease Control, 1992b, Isolation of *Vibrio cholerae* O1 from oysters – Mobile Bay, 1991–1992, *Morbid Mortal Weekly Rep*, **42**: 91–3.

Cholera Working Group, 1993, Large epidemic of cholera-like disease in Bangladesh caused by *Vibrio cholerae* O139 synonym Bengal, *Lancet*, **342**: 387–90.

Clemens JD, Harris JR et al., 1988, Field trial of oral cholera vaccines in Bangladesh: results of one year of follow-up, *J Infect Dis*, **158**: 60–9.

Clemens JD, Sack DA et al., 1989, ABO Blood groups and chol-

era: new observations on specificity of risk and modification of vaccine efficacy, *J Infect Dis*, **159**: 770–3.

Clemens JD, Sack DA et al., 1990, Field trial of oral cholera vaccines in Bangladesh: results from three-year follow-up, *Lancet*, **335**: 270–3.

Clemens JD, Van Loon F et al., 1991, Biotype as determinant of natural immunizing effect of cholera, *Lancet*, **337**: 883–4.

Colwell RR, Huq A, 1994, Vibrios in the environment: viable but nonculturable *Vibrio cholerae*, *Vibrio cholerae* and Cholera, American Society for Microbiology, Washington DC, 117–33.

Coster TS, Killeen KP et al., 1995, Safety, immunogenicity, and efficacy of live attenuated *Vibrio cholerae* O139 vaccine prototype, *Lancet*, **345**: 949–52.

Cvjetanovic B, 1974, Economic considerations in cholera control, *Cholera*, WB Saunders, Philadelphia, 435–45.

D'Aquino M, Teves SA, 1994, Lemon juice as a natural biocide for disinfecting drinking water, *Bull Pan Am Health Organ*, **28**: 324–30.

Deb BC, Sircar BK et al., 1986, Studies on interventions to prevent El Tor cholera transmission in urban slums, *Bull W H O*, **64**: 127–31.

Donta ST, Moon HW, Whipp SC, 1974, Detection of heat-labile *Escherichia coli* enterotoxin with the use of adrenal cells in tissue culture, *Science*, **183**: 334–6.

Echevarria J, Seas C et al., 1995, Efficacy and tolerability of ciprofloxacin prophylaxis in adult household contacts of patients with cholera, *Clin Infect Dis*, **20**: 1480–4.

Evins GM, Cameron DN et al., 1995, The emerging diversity of the electrophoretic types of *Vibrio cholerae* in the western hemisphere, *J Infect Dis*, **172**: 173–9.

Fasano A, Baudry B et al., 1991, *Vibrio cholerae* produces a second enterotoxin, which affects intestinal tight junctions, *Proc Natl Acad Sci USA*, **88**: 5242–6.

Fields PI, Popovic T et al., 1992, Use of polymerase chain reaction for detection of toxigenic *Vibrio cholerae* O1 strains from the Latin American cholera epidemic, *J Clin Microbiol*, **30**: 2118–21.

Gangarosa EJ, Mosley WH, 1974, Epidemiology and control of cholera, *Cholera*, WB Saunders, Philadelphia, 381–403.

Gangarosa EJ, Beisel WR et al., 1960, The nature of the gastrointestinal lesion in Asiatic cholera and its relation to pathogenesis. A biopsy study, *Am J Trop Med Hyg*, **9**: 125–35.

Glass RI, Becker S et al., 1982, Endemic cholera in rural Bangladesh, 1966–1980, *Am J Epidemiol*, **116**: 959–70.

Glass RI, Svennerholm A-M et al., 1983, Protection against cholera in breast-fed children by antibodies in breast milk, *N Engl J Med*, **308**: 1389–92.

Glass RI, Holmgren J et al., 1985, Predisposition for cholera of individuals with O blood group; possible evolutionary significance, *Am J Epidemiol*, **121**: 791–6.

Goma Epidemiology Group, 1995, Public health impact of the Rwandan refugee crisis: what happened in Goma, Zaire in July, 1994?, *Lancet*, **345**: 359–61.

Gonzales O, Aguilar A et al., 1992, An outbreak of cholera in rural Bolivia: rapid identification of a major vehicle of transmission, *Program and Abstracts of the 32nd Interscience Conference on Antimicrobial Agents and Chemotherapy, Anaheim, 1992*, American Society for Microbiology, Washington DC, 266.

Gotuzzo E, Seas C et al., 1995, Ciprofloxacin for the treatment of cholera: a randomized double-blind controlled clinical trial of a single daily dose in Peruvian adults, *Clin Infect Dis*, **20**: 1485–90.

Guerrant RL, Brunton LL et al., 1974, Cyclic adenosine monophosphate and alteration of Chinese hamster ovary cell morphology: a rapid, sensitive in vitro assay for the enterotoxins of *Vibrio cholerae* and *Escherichia coli*, *Infect Immun*, **10**: 320–7.

Gunn RA, Kimbal AM et al., 1979, Bottle feeding as a risk factor for cholera in infants, *Lancet*, **2**: 730–2.

Gupta RK, Szu SC et al., 1992, Synthesis, characterization, and some immunologic properties of conjugates composed of detoxified lipopolysaccharide of *Vibrio cholerae* O1 serotype Inaba bound to cholera toxin, *Infect Immun*, **60**: 3201–8.

Hasan JAK, Huq A et al., 1994, A novel kit for rapid detection of *Vibrio cholerae* O1, *J Clin Microbiol*, **32**: 249–52.

Hatch DL, Waldman RJ et al., 1994, Epidemic cholera during refugee resettlement in Malawi, *Int J Epidemiol*, **23**: 1292–9.

Hirschorn N, Chowdhury AKMA, Lindenbaum J, 1969, Cholera in pregnant women, *Lancet*, **1**: 1230–2.

Holmberg SD, Harris JR et al., 1984, Foodborne transmission in Micronesian households, *Lancet*, **1**: 730–2.

Hospedales J, Holder Y et al., 1993, Private sector response against the cholera threat in Trinidad and Tobago, *Bull Pan Am Health Organ*, **27**: 331–6.

Huq A, West PA et al., 1984, Influence of water temperature, salinity, and pH on survival and growth of toxigenic *Vibrio cholerae* serovar O1 associated with live copepods in laboratory microcosms, *Appl Environ Microbiol*, **48**: 420–4.

Islam MS, Drasar BS, Bradley DJ, 1989, Attachment of toxigenic *Vibrio cholerae* O1 to various freshwater plants and survival with a filamentous green algae, *Rhizoclonium fontanum*, *J Trop Med Hyg*, **92**: 396–401.

Ito T, Kuwahara S, Yokota T, 1983, Automatic and manual latex agglutination tests for measurement of cholera toxin and heat-labile enterotoxin of *Escherichia coli*, *J Clin Microbiol*, **17**: 7–12.

Johnston JM, Martin DL et al., 1983, Cholera on a Gulf Coast oil rig, *N Engl J Med*, **309**: 523–6.

Kamal AM, 1974, The seventh pandemic of cholera, *Cholera*, WB Saunders, Philadelphia, 1–14.

Kaper JB, Fasano A, Trucksis M, 1994, Toxins of *Vibrio cholerae*, *Vibrio cholerae* and Cholera, American Society for Microbiology, Washington DC, 145–76.

Kaufman MR, Taylor RK, 1994, The toxin-coregulated pilus: biogenesis and function, *Vibrio cholerae* and Cholera, American Society for Microbiology, Washington DC, 187–202.

Kay BA, Bopp CA, Wells JG, 1994, Isolation and identification of *Vibrio cholerae* O1 from fecal specimens, *Vibrio cholerae* and Cholera, American Society for Microbiology, Washington DC, 1–26.

King CA, van Heyningen WE, 1973, Deactivation of cholera toxin by a sialidase-resistant monosialosylganglioside, *J Infect Dis*, **127**: 639–47.

Koch R, 1884, An address on cholera and its bacillus, *Br Med J*, **2**: 403–7.

Kolvin JL, Roberts D, 1982, Studies on the growth of *Vibrio cholerae* biotype eltor and biotype classical in foods, *J Hyg Camb*, **89**: 243–52.

Koo D, Aragon A et al., 1996, Epidemic cholera in Guatemala, 1993: transmission of a newly introduced epidemic strain by street vendors, *Epidemiol Infect*, **116**: 121–6.

Lagos R, Avendano A et al., 1995, Attenuated live cholera vaccine strain CVD 103-HgR elicits significantly higher serum vibriocidal antibody titers in persons of blood group O, *Infect Immun*, **63**: 707–9.

Levine MM, Tacket CO, 1994, Recombinant live oral vaccines, *Vibrio cholerae* and Cholera, American Society for Microbiology, Washington DC, 395–413.

Levine MM, Black RE et al., 1981, Volunteer studies in development of vaccines against cholera and enterotoxigenic *Escherichia coli*: a review, *Acute Enteric Infections in Children: New Prospects for Treatment and Prevention*, Elsevier, Amsterdam, 443–59.

Levine MM, Kaper JB et al., 1983, New knowledge on pathogenesis of bacterial infections as applied to vaccine development, *Microbiol Rev*, **47**: 510–50.

Levine OS, Swerdlow D et al., 1995, Epidemic cholera and dysentery among Rwandan refugees in Goma, Zaire, 1994. Abstract K72, *Program and Abstracts of the 35th Interscience Conference on Antimicrobial Agents and Chemotherapy, San Francisco, 1995*, American Society for Microbiology, Washington DC, 300.

Lim-Quizon MC, Benabaye RM et al., 1994, Cholera in metropolitan Manila: foodborne transmission via street vendors, *Bull W H O*, **72**: 745–9.

McCormack WM, Chowdhury AM et al., 1968, Tetracycline prophylaxis in families of cholera patients, *Bull W H O*, **38**: 787–92.

McFall-Ngai MJ, Ruby EG, 1991, Symbiont recognition and subsequent morphogenesis as early events in an animal-bacterial mutualism, *Science*, **254**: 1491–4.

McIntyre RC, Tira T et al., 1979, Modes of transmission of cholera in a newly infected population on an atoll: implications for control measures, *Lancet*, **1**: 311–14.

Manning PA, Stroeher UH, Morona R, 1994, Molecular basis for O-antigen biosynthesis in *Vibrio cholerae* O1: Ogawa-Inaba switching, *Vibrio cholerae* and Cholera, American Society for Microbiology, Washington DC, 77–94.

Mekalanos JJ, Sadoff JC, 1994, Cholera vaccines: fighting an ancient scourge, *Science*, **265**: 1387–9.

Mintz ED, Reiff FM, Tauxe RV, 1995, Safe water treatment and storage in the home; a practical new strategy to prevent waterborne disease, *JAMA*, **273**: 948–53.

Mintz ED, Effler P et al., 1994, A rapid public health response to a cryptic outbreak of cholera in Hawaii, *Am J Public Health*, **84**: 1988–91.

Molla AM, Molla A et al., 1989, Food-based oral rehydration salt solution for acute childhood diarrhoea, *Lancet*, **2**: 429–31.

Monferran CG, Roth GA, Cumar FA, 1990, Inhibition of cholera toxin binding to membrane receptors by pig gastric mucin-derived glycopeptides: differential effect depending on the ABO blood group antigenic determinants, *Infect Immun*, **58**: 3966–72.

Morris JG, West GR et al., 1982, Cholera among refugees in Rangsit, Thailand, *J Infect Dis*, **145**: 131–3.

Morris JG, Losonsky GE et al., 1995, Clinical and immunological characteristics of *Vibrio cholerae* O139 Bengal infection in North American volunteers, *J Infect Dis*, **171**: 903–8.

Mujica OJ, Quick RE et al., 1994, Epidemic cholera in the Amazon: the role of produce in disease risk and prevention, *J Infect Dis*, **169**: 1381–4.

Nalin DR, 1976, Cholera, copepods and chitinase, *Lancet*, **2**: 958.

Olsvik O, Wahlberg J et al., 1993, Use of automated sequencing of polymerase chain reaction generated amplicons to identify three types of cholera toxin subunit B in *Vibrio cholerae* O1 strains, *J Clin Microbiol*, **31**: 22–5.

Ottemann KM, Mekalanos JJ, 1994, Regulation of cholera toxin expression in *Vibrio cholerae* and cholera, *Vibrio cholerae* and Cholera, American Society for Microbiology, Washington DC, 177–85.

Pan-American Health Organization, 1995, Cholera in the Americas, *Epidemiol Bull*, **16** (2): 11–13.

Pollitzer R, 1959, History of the disease, *World Health Organization Monograph Series – Cholera*, **43**: 11–50.

Popovic T, Bopp C et al., 1993, Epidemiologic application of a standardized ribotype scheme for *Vibrio cholerae* O1, *J Clin Microbiol*, **31**: 2474–82.

Popovic T, Fields PI et al., 1995, Molecular subtyping of toxigenic *Vibrio cholerae* O139 causing epidemic cholera in India and Bangladesh, 1992–1993, *J Infect Dis*, **171**: 122–7.

Qadri F, Chowdhury A et al., 1994, Development and evaluation of a rapid monoclonal antibody-based coagglutination test for direct detection of *Vibrio cholerae* O139 synonym Bengal in stool samples, *J Clin Microbiol*, **321**: 1589–90.

Quick RE, Vargas R et al., 1993, Epidemic cholera in the Amazon: the challenge of preventing death, *Am J Trop Med Hyg*, **93**: 597–602.

Quick RE, Thompson BL et al., 1995a, Epidemic cholera in rural El Salvador: risk factors in a region covered by a cholera prevention campaign, *Epidemiol Infect*, **114**: 249–55.

Quick R, Venczel L et al., 1995b, Diarrhea prevention in Bolivia through safe water storage vessels and locally produced mixed oxidant disinfectant, *Program and Abstracts of the 35th Interscience Conference on Antimicrobial Agents and Chemotherapy,*

San Francisco, 1995, American Society for Microbiology, Washington DC, 313.

Ramamurthy T, Garg S et al., 1993, Emergence of a novel strain of *Vibrio cholerae* with epidemic potential in southern and eastern India, *Lancet*, **341:** 1347.

Ries AA, Vugia DJ et al., 1992, Cholera in Piura, Peru: a modern urban epidemic, *J Infect Dis*, **166:** 1429–33.

Rogers L, 1957, Thirty years' research on the control of cholera epidemics, *Br Med J* , **2:** 1193–7.

Rosenberg CE, 1987, *The Cholera Years: The United States in 1832, 1849, and 1866*, University of Chicago Press, Chicago IL.

St Louis ME, Porter JD et al., 1990, Epidemic cholera in West Africa: the role of food handling and high-risk foods, *Am J Epidemiol*, **131:** 719–28.

Sakazaki R, 1992, Bacteriology of *Vibrio* and related organisms, *Cholera*, 2nd edn, Plenum, New York, 43.

Sanchez JL, Vasquez B et al., 1994, Protective efficacy of oral whole-cell/recombinant-B-subunit cholera vaccine in Peruvian military recruits, *Lancet*, **344:** 1273–6.

Shaffer N, Mendes P et al., 1988, Epidemic cholera in Guinea-Bissau: importance of foodborne transmission, *Program and Abstracts of the 28th Interscience Conference on Antimicrobial Agents and Chemotherapy, 1988, Los Angeles*, American Society for Microbiology, Washington DC, 370.

Shimada T, Nair GB et al., 1993, Outbreak of *Vibrio cholerae* non-O1 in India and Bangladesh, *Lancet*, **341:** 1346–7.

Siddique AK, Baqui AH et al., 1991, Survival of classic cholera in Bangladesh, *Lancet*, **337:** 1125–7.

Snow J, 1936, Snow on cholera, being a reprint of two papers, *The Commonwealth Fund*, Oxford University Press, London.

Spangler BD, 1992, Structure and function of cholera toxin and the related *Escherichia coli* heat labile enterotoxin, *Microbiol Rev*, **56:** 622–47.

Spira WM, Ahmed QS, 1981, Gauze filtration and enrichment procedures for recovery of *Vibrio cholerae* from contaminated waters, *Appl Environ Microbiol*, **42:** 730–3.

Sudjik D, Redhead D, 1995, The East is big, *Blueprint*, **116:** 27–33.

Sutton RGA, 1974, An outbreak of cholera in Australia due to food served in flight on an international aircraft, *J Hyg Camb*, **72:** 441–51.

Svennerholm A-M, Holmgren J et al., 1983, Serologic differentiation between antitoxin responses to infection with *V. cho-*lerae and enterotoxin-producing *Escherichia coli*, *J Infect Dis*, **147:** 514–21.

Swerdlow DL, Ries AA, 1992, Cholera in the Americas: guidelines for the clinician, *JAMA*, **267:** 1495–9.

Swerdlow DL, Mintz ED et al., 1992, Waterborne transmission of epidemic cholera in Trujillo, Peru: lessons for a continent at risk, *Lancet*, **340:** 28–32.

Swerdlow DL, Mintz ED et al., 1994, Severe life-threatening cholera associated with blood group O in Peru: implications for the Latin American epidemic, *J Infect Dis*, **170:** 468–72.

Tauxe RV, Blake PA, 1992, Epidemic cholera in Latin America, *JAMA*, **267:** 1388–90.

Tauxe RV, Holmberg SD et al., 1988, Epidemic cholera in Mali: high mortality and multiple routes of transmission in a famine area, *Epidemiol Infect*, **100:** 279–89.

Tauxe R, Seminario L et al., 1994, The Latin American epidemic, *Vibrio cholerae* and Cholera, American Society for Microbiology, Washington DC, 321–50.

Taylor JL, Tuttle J et al., 1993, An outbreak of cholera in Maryland associated with imported commercial frozen fresh coconut milk, *J Infect Dis*, **167:** 1330–5.

Trucksis M, Galen JE et al., 1993, Accessory cholera enterotoxin (Ace), the third toxin of a *Vibrio cholerae* virulence cassette, *Proc Natl Acad Sci USA*, **90:** 5267–71.

Vugia DJ, Rodriquez M et al., 1994, Epidemic cholera in Trujillo, Peru 1992: utility of a clinical case definition and shift in *Vibrio cholerae* O1 serotype, *Am J Trop Med Hyg*, **50:** 566–9.

Wachsmuth IK, Olsvik O et al., 1994, The molecular epidemiology of cholera, *Vibrio cholerae* and Cholera, American Society for Microbiology, Washington DC, 357–70.

Waldor MK, Mekalanos JJ, 1994, ToxR regulates virulence gene expression in non-O1 strains of *Vibrio cholerae* that cause epidemic cholera, *Infect Immun*, **62:** 72–8.

Weber JT, Levine WC et al., 1994a, Cholera in the United States, 1965–1991; risks at home and abroad, *Arch Intern Med*, **154:** 551–6.

Weber JT, Mintz ED et al., 1994b, Epidemic cholera in Ecuador: multidrug resistance and transmission by water and seafood, *Epidemiol Infect*, **112:** 1–11.

World Health Organization, 1993, *Guidelines for Cholera Control*, World Health Organization, Geneva.

World Health Organization, 1994, Cholera in 1993, *Wkly Epidemiol Rec*, **69:** 205–11, 213–16.

Diarrhoeal diseases due to *Escherichia coli* and *Aeromonas*

H R Smith and T Cheasty

1 INTRODUCTION

Diarrhoeal disease remains one of the largest health problems in many parts of the world. The disease is often mild and self-limiting but, particularly in the elderly and young children, the symptoms may be very severe. Studies in developing countries have shown that children in the first 2 years of life may have up to 10 separate episodes of diarrhoeal disease, often with significant mortality (Black et al. 1982a). In developed countries diarrhoea remains an important problem in spite of significant advances in water quality, environmental sanitation and agricultural and food hygiene. However, deficiencies in current practices, such as contamination of widely distributed foods, can lead to large outbreaks of disease. The increase in travel between countries has also led to the spread of diarrhoeal disease.

In the last 25 years the importance of *Escherichia coli* as a cause of diarrhoeal disease has increased considerably. This has resulted from advances in knowledge of the mechanisms by which *E. coli* cause diarrhoea; several classes of diarrhoeagenic *E. coli* with distinct virulence factors are now recognized (Table 27.1). The groups described in this chapter are the enteropathogenic (EPEC), enterotoxigenic (ETEC), Vero cytotoxin-producing (VTEC), enteroaggregative (EAggEC) and diffusely adherent *E. coli* (DAEC). The enteroinvasive *E. coli* are very like *Shigella* spp. in their ability to cause a dysentery-like disease and this group

is considered in Chapter 25. Other well studied enteric pathogens that can give rise to diarrhoea are dealt with elsewhere in this volume (*Salmonella*, see Chapters 24 and 28; *Campylobacter*, see Chapter 29; *Staphylococcus aureus*, *Clostridium*, *Bacillus cereus* and *Vibrio*, see Chapter 28; and *Vibrio cholerae*, see Chapter 26).

Over the past 20 years there has been a great deal of interest in the role of members of the genus *Aeromonas* as pathogens in humans and particularly their association with diarrhoeal disease. The role of the motile mesophilic aeromonads as extraintestinal pathogens in man is undisputed. The species most commonly associated with diarrhoeal disease in humans are *Aeromonas hydrophila*, *Aeromonas veronii* biotype sobria (previously reported as *Aeromonas sobria*) and *Aeromonas caviae* (for the current taxonomy and nomenclature see Volume 2, Chapter 45). The role of these 3 species as diarrhoeal pathogens is still highly controversial. However, the volume of published accounts of incidents and outbreaks attributable to these organisms seems to indicate that some strains are involved as causative agents of diarrhoeal disease in man.

Table 27.1 Classes of diarrhoeagenic *E. coli*

Class	Virulence factors	
	Toxins	**Adhesins and other factors**
Enteropathogenic *E. coli* (EPEC)		BFP, AE lesions (intimin)
Enterotoxigenic *E. coli* (ETEC)	ST I, ST IILT I, LT II	CFA/1, CS1, CS2, CS3, CS4, CS5, CS6, CFA/III CS7, CS17, CS18, CS19, PCFO9, PCFO148, PCFO159, PCFO166, 2230, 8786, Longus, K88, K99, 987P, F41, CS31A, CS1541, F17, F42, F141, F165, F107
Vero cytotoxin-producing *E. coli* (VTEC)	VT1, VT2	AE lesions (intimin), E-Hly
Enteroaggregative *E. coli* (EAggEC)	EAST1	AggA (AAF/I, AAF/II)
Diffusely adherent *E. coli* (DAEC)		F1845, AIDA-I

ESCHERICHIA COLI AS A DIARRHOEAL PATHOGEN

E. coli was first described by Escherich (1885) after isolation from the stools of infants with enteritis and it was soon shown that this organism could also be isolated from the stools of healthy infants and adults. This led to the recognition of the importance of distinguishing avirulent strains from those capable of causing diarrhoea. The use of 'serological typing' was used by Goldschmidt (1933) to study the epidemiology of infantile gastroenteritis in institutions. The major advance in this approach was made by Kauffmann (1944, 1947) who developed a comprehensive serotyping scheme for *E. coli*. This allowed the *E. coli* strains associated with outbreaks of infantile enteritis described by Bray (1945) and Giles and Sangster (1948) to be identified serologically. The *E. coli* scheme based on O antigens has been extended and now consists of groups O1 to O173 (Ørskov et al. 1991). Details of the serotyping of *E. coli* are described in Volume 2 (see Volume 2, Chapter 40).

The term enteropathogenic *E. coli* (EPEC), used to describe strains associated epidemiologically with infantile enteritis, was coined by Neter et al. (1955). EPEC strains belonged to particular O:H serotypes but the mechanisms of their pathogenicity were unknown. Some of the factors that contribute to the virulence of EPEC and several distinct groups of diarrhoeagenic *E. coli* are now recognized.

2 CLINICAL MANIFESTATIONS

Strains of *E. coli* that cause diarrhoeal disease are associated with a wide spectrum of symptoms ranging from a mild non-bloody diarrhoea to severe watery or bloody diarrhoea and dysentery. Some patients infected with VTEC may progress to develop haemolytic–uraemic syndrome (HUS). Infections with enteropathogenic *E. coli* usually cause a syndrome of watery diarrhoea; vomiting and fever can occur in infants and children. The clinical illness ranges from self-limiting diarrhoea to a highly protracted syndrome of chronic enteritis accompanied by a failure to thrive and wasting. The clinical severity of EPEC infections has been reported by Clausen and Christie (1982) and Rothbaum et al. (1982). The clinical symptoms caused by enterotoxigenic *E. coli* show considerable variation. In developing countries ETEC causes significant mortality in children under 5 years. The most severe manifestation is a cholera-like disease that is difficult to distinguish clinically from infection with *Vibrio cholerae* O1. This condition can lead to dehydration even in adults. In travellers, diarrhoea caused by ETEC is usually of short duration, often beginning with a rapid onset of loose stools and accompanied by variable symptoms including low grade fever, nausea, vomiting and abdominal cramps.

Infections with VTEC in man cause diarrhoea, haemorrhagic colitis and HUS (Karmali 1989). Haemorrhagic colitis is characterized by grossly bloody diarrhoea, usually with pyrexia. It is frequently preceded by abdominal cramps and watery diarrhoea. HUS is defined by 3 clinical features: acute renal failure, microangiopathic haemolytic anaemia and thrombocytopenia. There are 2 subgroups of HUS. The typical form is associated with a prodromal bloody diarrhoea caused by VTEC infection. The atypical form of HUS does not have a diarrhoeal phase and does not appear to be associated with VTEC infection. Some patients with HUS have features resembling thrombotic thrombocytopenic purpura (TTP) such as neurological disorders and fever.

In developing countries, infection with EAggEC is associated with persistent diarrhoea. The diarrhoea is usually watery and other symptoms include vomiting and dehydration and occasionally abdominal pain. Fever and gross blood in the stools have also been reported in children with diarrhoea associated with EAggEC (Bhan et al. 1989b, Cravioto et al. 1991). Eslava et al. (1993) reported a high mortality in an outbreak due to EAggEC in which the infants had severe diarrhoea; at autopsy destructive lesions of the ileum were seen. An acute watery diarrhoea has been observed in patients infected with DAEC.

3 EPIDEMIOLOGY

Significant differences have been observed in the epidemiology of the groups of diarrhoeagenic *E. coli*. For the recently recognized groups such as EAggEC and DAEC the information from epidemiological studies is very limited. Further well defined prospective studies in different areas of the world are necessary to identify the role of these groups in diarrhoeal disease.

3.1 Enteropathogenic *E. coli*

During the 1940s outbreaks of infantile enteritis occurred with increased frequency in hospitals and nurseries and they were more common in the winter months. These outbreaks were often severe with high attack and fatality rates. Bray (1945) investigated such an outbreak in a London hospital and showed that the epidemic strain of *E. coli* belonged to a serogroup that was subsequently recognized as *E. coli* O111. Similar studies in Aberdeen in 1947 and 1948 implicated 2 serogroups of *E. coli*, O55 and O111, as the causative organisms of epidemics (Giles and Sangster 1948, Smith 1949). In these studies there were 2 peaks in the seasonal incidence; this was highest in March and April, was mainly due to cases in hospital and was accompanied by a high mortality. A smaller peak in July was mainly due to cases in the community. It appeared that an outbreak in the community had occurred before or at the same time as the hospital outbreaks and that cross-infection in the hospital had followed the introduction of the infection by babies admitted while still excreting the causative organism.

During the 1950s many epidemics due to EPEC were reported in Europe and North America. In Britain these outbreaks continued during the 1960s and early 1970s. In late 1967 there was an epidemic in several hospitals in Teeside in which the mortality rate was high (Annotation 1968). Two *E. coli* strains were responsible for these infections, serotypes O119:H6 and O128:H2. A similar outbreak occurred in hospitals in the Manchester area but the causative organism in these cases was O114:H2 (Jacobs et al. 1970). In 1970 and 1971 outbreaks due to O142:H6 occurred in several hospitals in the Glasgow area and also in a Dublin hospital (Love et al. 1972, Hone et al. 1973, Kennedy et al. 1973). In Dublin the infection appeared to be spread by cross-infection after the admission to hospital of infected infants from the community. Retrospective studies of *E. coli* O142 strains isolated from outbreaks in Scotland, England, Northern Ireland, Eire, Indonesia, Canada and the USA suggested that a single enteropathogenic clone may have spread to all those countries (Gross, Rowe and Threlfall 1985). Since the early 1970s few outbreaks of infantile enteritis caused by EPEC have been reported in Britain or the USA. Sporadic cases continue to occur with a peak in the summer months.

In contrast to the situation in Britain and the USA, EPEC strains are among the most frequent causes of diarrhoea in infants in developing countries (Levine and Edelman 1984, Cravioto et al. 1988, Gomes, Blake and Trabulsi 1989, Echeverria et al. 1991, Kain et al. 1991). EPEC infections show a marked seasonality and are associated with warm season peaks. Outbreaks in institutions are often reported but sporadic cases and outbreaks occur very frequently in the general community. Several studies have shown that the peak incidence of enteritis was always in the few months after the beginning of the weaning period (see Gross 1990). Because weaning is often late in developing countries, the age distribution differs from that observed in Europe and North America. Contamination of weaning foods appears to contribute to the transmission of EPEC in developing countries. Most EPEC infections occur in the first 3 years of life but the importance of EPEC as a cause of adult enteritis is difficult to evaluate because few laboratories test for EPEC in patients over 3 years. Outbreaks in the adult population have been reported in the USA and Britain (Schroeder et al. 1968, Vernon 1969).

3.2 Enterotoxigenic *E. coli*

In the developed countries ETEC rarely cause infant or childhood diarrhoea whereas in developing countries these organisms are a major cause of severe disease in young children (Donta, Wallace and Whipp 1977, Black et al. 1981a, Levine 1987).

ETEC INFECTIONS IN DEVELOPED COUNTRIES

Outbreaks of infantile enteritis caused by ETEC in hospitals have been reported. In an outbreak in a hospital nursery in Glasgow 25 babies were affected; the causative organism was *E. coli* O159 that produced heat-stable enterotoxin (ST) (Gross et al. 1976). Fifty-five infants were ill in an outbreak in a special care nursery of a large hospital in the USA; the causative organism was an ST-producing *E. coli* O78 strain (Ryder et al. 1976). The outbreak continued for 9 months and there was heavy contamination with *E. coli* O78 in the patients' environment and the strain was also isolated from milk feeds. Other hospital outbreaks have been reported but the source and routes of transmission of infection were uncertain (Rowe et al. 1978, Moloney et al. 1985). Outbreaks caused by ETEC may also affect adults in developed countries but they are uncommon. More than 2000 staff and visitors at a national park in the USA were affected in an outbreak caused by an *E. coli* O6 strain that produced ST and heat-labile enterotoxin (LT). The source of the outbreak was drinking water contaminated with sewage (Rosenberg et al. 1977). In Japan several outbreaks have been reported, caused mainly by *E. coli* O159 but also, in one case, by *E. coli* O11 (Kudoh et al. 1977). Where the sources were established, outbreaks were caused by contaminated water supplies and some were probably food-borne. A food-borne outbreak occurred in adults in Manchester and the causative organisms were ETEC of serotypes O6:H16 and O27:H20 (Riordan et al. 1985).

ETEC INFECTIONS IN DEVELOPING COUNTRIES

In developing countries the incidence of ETEC infection is highest in the first 2 years of life and diminishes progressively to a low level in older children and adults (Levine et al. 1979, Black et al. 1981b). Prospective village-based studies in Bangladesh showed that in the first 2 years of life each child suffered an average of 6–7 episodes of diarrhoea per year (Black et al. 1982a). About 2 of these attacks of diarrhoea per child per year were thought to be due to ETEC. Another important factor in such studies was that ETEC infections were significantly associated with the development of clinical malnutrition. ETEC infections in endemic areas are most common in warm seasons and contaminated weaning foods and water are important modes of transmission (Black et al. 1981b, 1982b). A study in Thailand suggested that water stored in the home might be a source of ETEC infection but contaminated hands also provided a means of transmission (Echeverria et al. 1987).

TRAVELLERS' DIARRHOEA DUE TO ETEC

Travellers are susceptible to infection by ETEC in countries where ETEC are endemic. Rowe, Taylor and Bettelheim (1970) first demonstrated a relationship between *E. coli* and travellers' diarrhoea in British troops in southern Arabia. About 50% of the diarrhoea cases among new arrivals were due to *E. coli* O148, later shown to produce ST (Rowe, Gross and Scotland 1976). ETEC of serogroup O148 were also found to be a cause of diarrhoea among US soldiers in Vietnam (DuPont et al. 1971). Studies of travellers' diarrhoea in Mexico showed attack rates between 29% and 48% (Gorbach et al. 1975, Merson et al. 1976, DuPont et al. 1983) and ETEC were detected in at least 45% of persons with diarrhoea. Travellers from Europe to tropical countries and also to Mediterranean countries may suffer from diarrhoea caused by ETEC. In Sweden (Bäck, Blomberg and Wadström 1977) and Britain (Gross, Scotland and Rowe 1979) ETEC were found in 11% of people with travellers' diarrhoea. Outbreaks of diarrhoea caused by ETEC have also occurred frequently on cruise ships. Hobbs et al. (1976) isolated a ST-producing *E. coli* O27 strain from 55, 61 and 20% of diarrhoeal cases in 3 successive cruises by the same ship: the evidence suggested that these infections were food-borne. In a later outbreak during a Mediterranean cruise ETEC of several different serotypes were isolated; *E. coli* O27:H7 was the predominant type. It was concluded that the water supply was the source of the infections (O'Mahoney et al. 1986).

3.3 Vero cytotoxin-producing *E. coli*

The role of VTEC as a cause of diarrhoeal disease has been investigated extensively in North America and Europe. However, in developing countries VTEC have not been recognized as a significant cause of diarrhoeal disease. Several surveys in North America and the UK showed VTEC of serogroup O157 in 0.1–2.7%

of non-selected diarrhoeal stools (Griffin and Tauxe 1991). By contrast, few studies have investigated the incidence of VTEC belonging to serogroups other than O157. Pai et al. (1988) in Canada found 0.7% of over 5000 stools contained VTEC other than O157, 2.5% containing O157 VTEC. In a German study, 6.6% of 668 diarrhoeal stools had non-O157 VTEC and 2.7% contained O157 VTEC (Günzer et al. 1992). In cases of haemorrhagic colitis O157 VTEC have been established as major aetiological agents. These organisms have been isolated from 15% to more than 70% of bloody stools in studies in North America and the UK (Griffin and Tauxe 1991). Strains of O157 VTEC were first identified in the UK in the early 1980s (Day et al. 1983). It appears that VTEC belonging to serogroups other than O157 are less frequently associated with bloody stools. A large number of outbreaks of haemorrhagic colitis caused by O157 VTEC have been reported (Table 27.2), sometimes with very significant mortality (Carter et al. 1987). These outbreaks have often been in institutions as well as in the community. The phage typing scheme for O157 VTEC developed by Ahmed et al. (1987) has been very useful in these epidemiological studies (Frost et al. 1993). A small number of outbreaks of diarrhoea or bloody diarrhoea caused by non-O157 VTEC have been documented; the serotypes included O145:H– , O111:H– and O104:H21 (Kudoh et al. 1994). Karmali et al. (1983) first reported the association between VTEC and HUS. Isolation rates of O157 VTEC from cases of HUS range from 19% to over 60% (Griffin and Tauxe 1991). Surveillance of HUS in Britain showed evidence of VTEC infection in 33% of cases; 72% of the VTEC belonged to serogroup O157 (Scotland et al. 1988, Kleanthous et al. 1990). Although O157 VTEC is the major cause of HUS in most studies, community outbreaks of HUS have been associated with VTEC of serogroup O111 (Caprioli et al. 1994, Cameron et al. 1995). HUS is an important paediatric problem in some South American countries such as Chile, Argentina and Uruguay. Evidence of VTEC infection, including O157 VTEC, has been reported (Lopez et al. 1989, Cordovéz et al. 1992). It should also be noted that *Shigella dysenteriae* 1 is an important cause of HUS in countries such as Sri Lanka where the organism is widely distributed.

Diseased and healthy cattle carry VTEC of many different serogroups. Strains of serogroups O5, O26 and O111 can cause severe bloody diarrhoea in calves (Hall et al. 1985, Sherwood, Snodgrass and O'Brien 1985). Although O157 VTEC have been isolated from diarrhoeal calves, their association with disease is not established (Ørskov, Ørskov and Villar 1977, Synge and Hopkins 1992). Tokhi et al. (1993) showed in a longitudinal study in Sri Lanka that VTEC were part of the flora and associated with disease in animals younger than 10 weeks. VTEC of several different serogroups have been isolated from 10–17% of healthy animals, with the higher incidence among younger animals (Montenegro et al. 1990, Willshaw et al. 1993a). In these studies a proportion of the VTEC belonged to O serogroups associated with human dis-

Table 27.2 Examples of outbreaks of haemorrhagic colitis caused by O157 VTEC

Reference	Year	Location	Cases		Fatal	Vehicle
Riley et al. (1983)	1982	Fast food restaurants, Michigan, Oregon, USA	26			Beefburgers
Carter et al. (1987)	1985	Nursing home, Canada	73	(12 HUS)	17	? Sandwiches
Morgan et al. (1988)	1985	Community, East Anglia, UK	49		1	? Vegetables
Salmon et al. (1989)	1987	Christening party, Birmingham, UK	26	(1 HUS)		? Turkey roll
Swerdlow et al. (1992)	1989	Community, Missouri, USA	243	(2 HUS)	4	? Water
Kudoh et al. (1994)	1990	Kindergarten, Japan	319		2	? Well water
Thomas et al. (1993)	1991	Fast food restaurant, Preston, UK	23	(3 HUS)		Beefburgers
Griffin et al. (1994)	1992/3	Fast food restaurants, western USA	732	(55 HUS)	4	Beefburgers
Upton and Coia (1994)	1994	Community, Lothian	100	(9 HUS)	1	Pasteurized milk

ease. O157 VTEC have been isolated from healthy cattle in North America, Britain and Germany. In the USA a study of animals possibly linked to cases of human disease showed that 2.8% of heifers and calves and 0.15% of adult cows had O157 VTEC (Wells et al. 1991). In Britain, up to 3.6% of cattle tested at slaughter carried O157 VTEC (Chapman, Wright and Norman 1989, Chapman et al. 1992, 1993). VTEC have been isolated from 9–25% of samples of meat and meat products (Read et al. 1990, Smith et al. 1991, Willshaw et al. 1993b); in these studies O157 VTEC were not isolated. By contrast, Doyle and Schoeni (1987) reported O157 VTEC in 1.5–3.7% of samples of beef, pork, poultry and lamb. However, in a larger study O157 VTEC were isolated from 0.12% of raw beef samples and 0.06–0.5% of veal kidneys (Griffin and Tauxe 1991). Outbreaks of human infection have been epidemiologically linked to a food product of bovine origin but a causative organism has rarely been isolated. O157 VTEC were isolated from hamburger patties in the first documented outbreak of haemorrhagic colitis (Riley et al. 1983) and from a very large outbreak in the western USA (Bell et al. 1994, Griffin et al. 1994). In Britain, the first isolation of O157 VTEC from a beefburger was associated with a small community outbreak (Willshaw et al. 1994). Unpasteurized milk has also been shown to be a source of VTEC infections. O157 VTEC were isolated from raw milk associated with an outbreak near Sheffield (Chapman, Wright and Higgins 1993). VTEC of serotype O22:H8 were isolated from patients and from milk linked to an outbreak in Germany (Bockemühl et al. 1992). An outbreak of O157 VTEC infection affecting more than 100 people in Scotland was associated with consumption of pasteurized milk. O157 VTEC of the same type were isolated from patients and from the dairy equipment and it was thought that the outbreak resulted from post-pasteurization contamination (Upton and Coia 1994).

Pigs have also been shown to carry VTEC and their presence has been associated with post-weaning diarrhoea and oedema disease in weaned pigs (Marques et al. 1987, Bertschinger and Gyles 1994, Hampson

1994). Some features of oedema disease have been observed in HUS patients with neurological symptoms and peripheral oedema (Karmali et al. 1985a). The main serogroups associated with oedema disease are O138, O139 and O141 (Dobrescu 1983) but they have not been found in cases of human infections. VTEC carriage by other animals has been shown by Beutin et al. (1993) who concluded that healthy domesticated animals were a reservoir of VTEC. Sheep, goats, cats and dogs, as well as cattle and pigs, carried VTEC and some of the serogroups have been found in human infections. By contrast, chickens do not appear to be a source of VTEC.

3.4 Enteroaggregative *E. coli*

The epidemiology of infections caused by EAggEC remains the subject of controversy. In several studies in infants and children in developing countries there was an association with diarrhoea. Studies in India, Mexico and Brazil have reported a strong association with persistent diarrhoea (Bhan et al. 1989a, 1989b, Cravioto et al. 1991, Wanke et al. 1991). In the Mexican study infants in the first 2 years of life were investigated and EAggEC were isolated from 51% of patients with persistent diarrhoea compared with 5% from healthy controls (Cravioto et al. 1991). However, not all studies have found an association of EAggEC with diarrhoea (Gomes, Blake and Trabulsi 1989, Baqui et al. 1992). EAggEC have been isolated in Britain from sporadic cases of diarrhoea (Scotland et al. 1991, 1993). A pilot study of infectious intestinal disease in the community suggested that EAggEC were more common in cases than controls (Roderick et al. 1995). A high proportion of isolates from British children with diarrhoea that belonged to serotypes O44:H18, O111ab:H25 and O126:H27 showed aggregative adherence (Scotland et al. 1991). These serotypes were formerly regarded as 'enteropathogenic' based on epidemiological studies. EAggEC strains of O44:H18 were also isolated from outbreaks affecting young children and elderly patients (Scotland et al. 1991, Smith et al. 1994). The isolation of EAggEC has also been linked with recent foreign travel in studies of diarrhoea in Britain (Brook et al. 1994, Scotland et al. 1994).

3.5 Diffusely adherent *E. coli*

Several epidemiological studies have examined the role of DAEC in developing countries and some have found a significant association between DAEC and diarrhoea (Mathewson et al. 1987, Giron et al. 1991, Baqui et al. 1992). In the majority, however, a significant relationship has not been observed (Levine et al. 1988, Bhan et al. 1989b, Cravioto et al. 1991). Levine et al. (1993) investigated a cohort of Chilean children of ages up to 5 years and found an association of DAEC with diarrhoea that increased with age; children between 4 and 5 years had a relative risk of 2.1 for DAEC diarrhoea. This observation may be relevant to previous studies in which infants were the usual study population.

4 PATHOGENESIS

The distinct classes of pathogenic *E. coli* that cause diarrhoea can be defined on the basis of their virulence properties. The properties of the different classes overlap to a limited extent; this is not surprising because several properties are necessary for the full expression of pathogenesis and there is genetic transfer between strains.

4.1 Enteropathogenic *E. coli*

The ability of EPEC to cause diarrhoea has been confirmed by oral challenge of babies and adults (Ferguson and June 1952, Levine et al. 1978). Early studies demonstrated the adherence of EPEC to intestinal mucosa. Polotsky et al. (1977) examined, by light and electron microscopy, the histopathological lesions in rabbit ligated intestinal loops infected with classical EPEC strains. Lesions were also observed in intestinal biopsies from an infant with diarrhoea caused by *E. coli* O125ac:H21 (Ulshen and Rollo 1980). Rothbaum et al. (1982) observed lesions in infants infected with *E. coli* O119 during a protracted community outbreak; microcolonies of *E. coli* were seen adhering tightly to villus tips. Where there was close attachment of the EPEC to the epithelial cells, 'attaching and effacing' (AE) lesions and destruction of the brush border were observed by electron microscopy (Moon et al. 1983, Knutton, Lloyd and McNeish 1987). Another major advance in the study of EPEC pathogenesis was made when Cravioto et al. (1979) observed that 'classical' EPEC isolated from outbreaks adhered to HEp-2 cells. The bacteria formed clusters and this localized pattern of attachment persisted in the presence of mannose, whereas other types of *E. coli* and those from the normal flora rarely showed mannose-resistant adhesion to HEp-2 cells. Later studies with this model showed that a plasmid, the EPEC adherence factor (EAF) plasmid, was necessary for the full expression of this adhesion

(Baldini et al. 1983). Colostrum-deprived piglets fed wild-type EPEC developed AE lesions whereas piglets fed a plasmid-cured derivative did not. Volunteer studies supported the role of the plasmid in EPEC pathogenesis (Levine et al. 1985). Of 10 individuals fed E2348/69, 9 had clinical diarrhoea compared with only 2 of 9 persons fed the plasmid-cured derivative. The role of chromosomal virulence factors was shown by the observation that 2 volunteers given the plasmid-cured strain had diarrhoea. The factor responsible for HEp-2 adherence was later proposed to be a bundle-forming pilus (Giron, Ho and Schoolnik 1991).

A locus necessary for the production of the attaching and effacing lesion was identified by studies of the chromosomal DNA of EPEC (Jerse et al. 1990). This gene, termed *eaeA*, was shown to encode a 94 kDa outer-membrane protein, termed intimin (Jerse and Kaper 1991). In a volunteer study, all 10 persons fed the wild-type strain developed diarrhoea whereas only 4 of the volunteers given an *eae* mutant strain had diarrhoea (Donnenberg et al. 1992). Recent studies have led to further elucidation of EPEC pathogenesis and it is now proposed as a 3-step process. Adhesion of EPEC to eukaryotic cells is associated with rises in intracellular calcium concentrations and phosphorylation of cytoskeletal proteins (Baldwin et al. 1991, Finlay et al. 1992). Receptor binding of EPEC induces tyrosine protein kinase activity and this leads to release of calcium, which promotes the actin-severing function of villin, the microvillus protein. There is then breakdown of the actin-core microvillus structure and effacement of the microvilli. The overall effect is a dramatic reduction in the absorptive capacity of the brush border and activation of enzymes important in stimulating intestinal secretion (Knutton et al. 1994). Further genetic studies have identified a second locus, *eaeB*, the product of which is necessary for the formation of the attaching and effacing lesion (Donnenberg, Yu and Kaper 1993).

4.2 Enterotoxigenic *E. coli*

The pathogenesis of ETEC involves the ability to colonize the small intestine and produce one or both of the 2 types of enterotoxin, LT and ST.

HEAT-LABILE ENTEROTOXINS

At first only one antigenic type of LT was recognized but in 1983 Green and colleagues reported a second antigenic type of LT, called LT II to distinguish it from the original LT, referred to as LT I. LT I is closely related in its structure, function and antigenicity to cholera toxin (CT) produced by *V. cholerae* (Holmgren 1985, Gyles 1994a). It is a protein complex of one polypeptide A subunit and 5 polypeptide B subunits. The A and B subunits have molecular weights of approximately 30 kDa and 11.5 kDa respectively. X-ray crystallography has shown that the toxin molecule consists of the one A subunit above a central aqueous channel formed by the 5 B subunits, a doughnut-shaped arrangement. The B pentamer constitutes a highly stable arrangement in which the subunits are held together by hydrogen bonds and salt bridges. The A subunit is synthesized as a single polypeptide that consists of a large enzymatically active peptide (A_1) and a small peptide (A_2) which connects the A subunit to the B pentamer. A_1 and A_2 are joined by a single disulphide bond which remains intact until the toxin enters a cell.

The LT IB subunit binds to the lactose-containing oligosaccharide portion of ganglioside GM1, in cell membranes (Griffiths, Finkelstein and Critchley 1986). Unlike CT, LT I also binds a glycoprotein, and can attach weakly to GM2 and asialo-GM1 (Holmgren et al. 1982). Binding is multivalent so that each molecule can bind 5 GM1 molecules. The binding site has been identified by a combination of techniques including x-ray crystallography (Sixma et al. 1993). The toxin is internalized following the binding of all 5 B subunits to the cell membrane but several aspects of the process still require clarification. LT I and CT have the same adenosine diphosphoribosyltransferase activity, transferring adenosine diphosphate (ADP)-ribose from nicotinamide adenine dinucleotide to a major specific target. This enzymatic activity resides in the A_1 fragment of the A subunit. ADP-ribosylation occurs in the brush border membrane of the intestinal epithelial cell and results in activation of adenylate cyclase and a subsequent rise in the level of cyclic adenosine 5'-monophosphate (cAMP). The major clinical effect of LT is diarrhoea and the elevated levels of cAMP are proposed to be the basis for the diarrhoea. Normal intestinal ion-transport mechanisms are maintained by phosphorylation of protein by activation of protein kinases and the excessive stimulation of the protein kinases leads to electrolyte disturbances. The action of LT results in increased secretion of chloride from crypt cells and there is impaired absorption of sodium and chloride by cells at the tips of the villi (Field, Rao and Chang 1989a, 1989b). Water follows the electrolytes because of osmotic effects and a profuse watery diarrhoea results.

The LT I from human ETEC (LT Ih) is closely related to, but distinct from, LT I found in porcine ETEC (LT Ip) (Honda et al. 1981). Both types of LT I are immunologically related to CT. By contrast, LT II differs from LT I in that it is not neutralized by anti-CT or anti-LT I. It has a structure similar to that of LT I (Holmes, Twiddy and Pickett 1986) but LT II binds to a receptor different from GM1; the best binding of LT II is observed with GD1a and GD1b. LT II is similar to LT I in enzymatic activity and mode of activation of adenylate cyclase. However, *E. coli* cells produce LT II at a level about 1% of that of LT I production. Antigenic variation has also been observed with LT II and the LT IIa and LT IIb types have been identified (Gyles 1994a). Although the properties of LT II have to some extent been elucidated, the role of this toxin in disease has not been established.

The structural genes for LT I are on plasmids but chromosomal genes may affect the level of expression by a factor of 100 (Katayama et al. 1990). Sequence analysis has confirmed the relationship between LT Ip and LT Ih (>95% homology) and also between LT I

and CT (Yamamoto and Yokota 1983). In contrast to LT I the structural genes for LT II are chromosomal. The LT IIa and LT I A subunit genes have 57% nucleotide sequence similarity but the B subunit genes lack significant sequence homology (Pickett et al. 1989).

HEAT-STABLE ENTEROTOXINS

Two major types of ST, ST I (or STa) and ST II (or STb), unrelated apart from their heat stability, secretion from the cell and ability to cause diarrhoea, have been reported (Gyles 1994a). ST I has a molecular weight of about 2000 and is resistant to 100°C for 15 min. The molecule is acid-resistant but susceptible to alkaline pH; ST I is completely inactivated by reducing and oxidizing agents that disrupt disulphide bonds (Robertson, Dreyfus and Frantz 1983). Two types of ST I, ST Ia and ST Ib, that share C-terminal antigenic determinants and biologically active sequences have been identified. The central sequence of 11 amino acids is identical with differences at the N-terminal end (Stieglitz et al. 1988). ST I binds to receptors on brush borders of intestinal epithelial cells (De-Sauvage et al. 1992, Hirayama et al. 1992). Although the receptors that bound ST I appeared to be heterogeneous, it has been reported that it is a transmembrane guanylyl cyclase (De-Sauvage, Camerato and Goeddel 1991). Binding of ST I is maximal in villus preparations and decreases from villus to crypt.

ST I activates particulate guanylate cyclase in the brush border of jejunal and ileal epithelial cells leading to elevation of cyclic guanosine 5'-monophosphate (cGMP) levels (Field et al. 1978). ST I does not bind to guanylate cyclase from tissues other than intestinal tissue because these tissues lack the specific receptor. Elevated cGMP causes increased fluid secretion by an unknown mechanism. The end result of ST I action is inhibition of Na^+ coupled chloride absorption in villus tips, plus stimulation of chloride secretion in crypt cells, which lead to excessive fluid in the lumen of the gut (Forte et al. 1992). The concentration of ST I receptors is higher in the colon than in the ileum. Diarrhoea due to ST-producing *E. coli* probably results from the combined effects of fluid secretion in the small intestine and impaired absorption in the colon. ST I acts very rapidly but with a short duration.

ST II is a peptide of 48 amino acids that, unlike LT and ST I, does not alter intracellular levels of cAMP or cGMP; however, the mechanism of action is not known. It has been suggested that ST II acts by opening a receptor-operated calcium channel in the plasma membrane (Dreyfus et al. 1993). ST II is produced by ETEC predominantly of porcine origin but other enterotoxins are often produced by ST II-positive strains (Casey, Herring and Schneider 1993). Casey, Herring and Schneider (1993) concluded that ST II did not contribute significantly to ETEC-induced diarrhoea in neonatal pigs. ST II, like ST I, acts rapidly and for a moderate period with fluid accumulation at a maximal level at about 3 h.

The genes for ST I and ST II are located on plasmids. The ST Ia gene is part of a transposon (So and McCarthy 1980); later studies demonstrated this transposon in ETEC of bovine, porcine and avian origin. DNA sequence analysis showed that the ST Ia gene encoded an 18 amino acid product whereas the gene for ST Ib encoded a product with 19 amino acids. ST Ia is sometimes referred to as STp but is produced by animal and human isolates whereas ST Ib (also termed STh) is produced by human isolates only. Sequence data indicate that ST Ia is synthesized as a 72 amino acid precursor that consists of a 19 amino acid signal peptide, a 35 amino acid pro sequence and the 18 amino acid ST Ia. The function of the pro region is unknown. The DNA sequence for ST II has also been reported (Lee et al. 1983). The structural gene encodes a mature protein of 48 amino acids and a signal peptide of 23 amino acids. Like ST Ia, the ST II gene is part of a transposon.

ADHESIVE FACTORS OF ETEC

Studies of enteritis in pigs first demonstrated that enterotoxin production was not sufficient to enable ETEC to cause diarrhoea (Smith and Linggood 1971). The organism must be able to adhere to the mucosal surface of the intestinal epithelial cells. The majority of ETEC adhesins are non-flagellar, hair-like, rigid filamentous fimbriae that are host-specific and particular fimbriae are found exclusively on either human, bovine or porcine ETEC (de Graaf and Gaastra 1994).

The first colonization factor to be described on human ETEC strains was colonization factor antigen I (CFA/I); its role in disease was demonstrated in volunteer experiments (Evans et al. 1975, 1978). Colonization factor antigen II (CFA/II) was then reported (Evans and Evans 1978) but, unlike CFA/I, was composed of 3 antigenically distinct proteins, coli surface associated antigens CS1, CS2 and CS3 (Cravioto, Scotland and Rowe 1982, Smyth 1982). Strains produced CS1 and CS3, CS2 and CS3 or CS3 alone. Colonization factor antigen IV (CFA/IV) was also shown to comprise 3 antigenic components, CS4, CS5 and CS6. A large number of other colonization factors or putative colonization factors (PCF) have now been documented (Smyth, Marron and Smith 1994). In some cases the serogroup or serotype of the strain has been used to designate ETEC fimbriae; for example, PCFO9, PCFO20, PCFO148, PCFO159:H4 and PCFO166. In other cases the fimbriae have been termed CFA/III, CS7, CS17 and CS19 or they have been named after the strain from which they were characterized, for example, 2230 and 8786. Fimbriae are homopolymers of hundreds of copies of identical protein subunits. CFA/I fimbriae consist of only one type of subunit, of which only that located on the tip is accessible to the receptor (Bühler, Hoschützky and Jann 1991). Not all ETEC adhesins have a fimbrial morphology; some, such as CS3, may be fibrillar structures composed of thin flexible filaments whereas others, such as CS6, are neither fimbrial nor fibrillar. ETEC fimbrial adhesins bind to glycoconjugates, glycoproteins and glycolipids (de Graaf and Gaastra 1994). The adhesin–receptor interaction occurs in a lectin-like fashion with the receptors located in mucus, epithelial membranes and basement membranes. The diversity of these glycoconjugates and their distribution probably explains the host specificity of ETEC. The structural organization of the fimbrial operons of ETEC has been reported. In some cases the location of the structural genes and regulatory genes are non-contiguous. In the case of CFA/I the 2 regions are widely separated on the same plasmid (Smith, Willshaw and Rowe 1982). The CS1 fimbrial operon is also plasmid located whereas that of CS2 is chromosomally determined. The regulatory gene for CS1 and CS2 production is located on a distinct plasmid from that encoding structural genes for CS1 (Smyth, Marron and Smith 1994).

Various colonization factors on ETEC of animal origin have been described. The best studied are K88 and 989P found on porcine, F41 on bovine and K99 on calf, lamb and porcine ETEC. Other adhesins include CS31A, CS1541, F17, F141 and F165 (Smyth, Marron and Smith 1994). The importance of K88 in pathogenesis was demonstrated in feeding experiments in pigs in which it was shown that loss of the plasmid that codes for K88 led to the loss of the ability of the strain to cause diarrhoea. Virulence was restored by reintroduction of the plasmid (Smith and Linggood 1971). These animal ETEC adhesins are either rod-like fimbriae such as 987P, F17, F141 and F165 or fibrillar such as K88, K99, F41, CS31A and CS1541. With the K88 and K99 fibrillar structures adhesive multivalency appears to involve multiple interactions with host receptors. The adhesin of K88 fimbriae is the FaeG protein and regions along the molecules are essential to the receptor binding of the FaeG protein. In the case of K99 FanC is the fimbrial subunit and adhesin of K99 fimbriae. The gene clusters for K88 and K99 fimbriae differ in arrangement compared with those of human ETEC. The structural and regulatory components of K88 and K99 are expressed from one contiguous operon.

4.3 Vero cytotoxin-producing *E. coli*

The pathogenesis of VTEC is not yet clearly understood. The potential virulence factors that have been identified are production of Vero cytotoxins, specific adhesins, formation of attaching and effacing lesions and production of an enterohaemolysin.

VERO CYTOTOXINS

Since Konowalchuk, Speirs and Stavric (1977) described Vero cytotoxin it has been recognized that it is one of a family of related toxins that includes Shiga toxin of *Shigella dysenteriae* 1 (O'Brien et al. 1982, O'Brien and Holmes 1987). O'Brien and LaVeck (1983) purified a toxin from strain H30, serotype O26:H11, and showed that it possessed many of the properties of Shiga toxin; they termed the toxin Shiga-like toxin (SLT). The abbreviations VT and SLT are both in common use and are interchangeable. Two major classes of VT were proposed on the basis of toxin neutralization and DNA hybridization tests (Scotland, Smith and Rowe 1985). VT1 was neutralized by antibodies to Shiga toxin but VT2 was not.

Further studies have demonstrated variants of these 2 types and particularly of VT2. These include VT2c, produced by many O157 VTEC, and VT2e, produced by the majority of VTEC of porcine origin (Smith et al. 1993). All the VT2 variants are neutralized to some extent by polyclonal antiserum against another VT2 but the titres to heterologous toxins may not be as high as to the homologous toxin (Gannon et al. 1990, Hii et al. 1991). VTEC may produce VT1, VT2 or both toxins and strains with genes for more than one form of VT2 have been identified (Schmitt, McKee and O'Brien 1991). It is interesting to note that some VTEC from animal sources also produce heat-labile or heat-stable enterotoxins (Smith et al. 1988). So far this has not been described for VTEC of human origin.

Shiga toxin, VT1 and VT2 are proteins composed of one enzymatically active A subunit and 5 receptor-binding B subunits. X-ray crystallography of the B oligomer revealed a 5-sided assembly of 6-stranded anti-parallel β-sheets similar to the B pentamer of LT (Stein et al. 1992). The biological activities of Shiga toxin and the VTs are the result of the irreversible inhibition of protein synthesis in eukaryotic cells. The toxins cleave a specific N-glycosidic bond at site 4324 in the 28S ribosomal RNA of the 60S ribosomal subunit. This results in the release of a single adenine residue and the failure of elongation factor 1-dependent binding of aminoacyl-tRNA to ribosomes (Igarashi et al. 1987). The A subunit possesses the biological activity. Proteolysis and reduction of a disulphide bond convert the A subunit into a large N-terminal A_1 fragment with enzymatic activity and a small C-terminal A_2 fragment. The B subunit binds the toxin to glycolipids with a common Galα1–4 Gal moiety that is considered to be the functional receptor on cells. The VT2 variants are not identical in binding tests in vitro. VT2, like VT1 and Shiga toxin, binds preferentially to Gb3 (Galα1–4 Galβ1–4 Glc ceramide) in which the galactose is terminal (Lingwood et al. 1987). Although there is some binding of the VT2 variants VT2e and VT2vha to Gb3, binding is preferentially to Gb4 (GalNAcβ1–3 Galα1–4 Galβ1–4 Glc ceramide) in which the disaccharide is internal (Samuel et al. 1990). The susceptibility of a variety of cell lines to VTs is related to presence or absence of the cell surface glycolipid receptor, indicating that these receptors are functionally significant. The distribution and concentration of the specific receptors in various tissues and in different animal species appear to be responsible for differences in target organs (Richardson et al. 1992). Gb3 and related glycolipids are present on erythrocytes and it has been proposed that the binding of VT to erythrocytes may affect the severity of the disease in VTEC infections (Taylor et al. 1990). Newburg et al. (1993) demonstrated that lower erythrocyte Gb3 levels are associated with patients with HUS. However, any role of the binding of VT to erythrocytes in pathogenesis remains to be established (Lingwood 1994). The level of Gb3 expressed by glomerular endothelial cells is increased by the effect of cytokines, tumour necrosis factor-α and interleukin-1 (van de Kar et al. 1992). These cytokines are induced by the action of VT, and also by action of endotoxin, on macrophages and monocytes (Tesh, Ramegowda and Samuel 1994). In vitro activity of VT on primary cell material has been reported. VT was cytotoxic for human umbilical cord cells (Obrig et al. 1987), human vascular endothelial cells (Obrig et al. 1988), human saphenous vein cells (Tesh et al. 1991) and porcine aortic cells (Kavi et al. 1987). Studies on the action of VT at the vascular endothelial cell level have been advanced by the use of human renal (glomerular) microvascular endothelial cells. These are much more sensitive to cytotoxic effects and this results from a 50–150-fold higher level of Gb3 (Obrig et al. 1993).

Several animals have been tested for their susceptibility to VT and experimental infection with VTEC (Gyles 1994b). However, evaluation of the role of VT has been hampered by the lack of an animal model that adequately reproduces the disease seen in man. VT1 and VT2vha caused neurological effects and brain lesions when injected intravenously in pigs. These toxins also caused lesions in the kidney but failed to cause intestinal damage (Gannon, Gyles and Wilcock 1989). In the rabbit ileal loop test VT produced fluid accumulation (O'Brien and LaVeck 1983) and this has also been demonstrated for other VTs. Use of mouse models showed the LD50 of various toxins differed significantly, from 2000 ng for VT1 to 0.9 pg for VT2e. Intravenous injection of VT1 and VT2 into rabbits resulted in anorexia, diarrhoea and neurological symptoms (Richardson et al. 1992). Diarrhoea was accompanied by blood and mucus but in these experiments the kidneys were normal. The binding of toxin to tissues was shown by immunofluorescence and ^{125}I labelling. Binding correlated with the sites of lesions and the location of glycolipid VT receptors.

VT production in several *E. coli* strains is encoded by lysogenic phages (Scotland et al. 1983, Smith, Green and Parsell 1983, O'Brien et al. 1984). VT phages have been isolated from strains of many O serogroups including 26, 29, 111, 119, 128 and particularly 157. By contrast, strains of porcine origin that produce VT2e do not appear to carry VT phages and the VT2e genes are chromosomally located (Smith, Green and Parsell 1983, Rietra et al. 1989). VT1 and VT2 genes were cloned in *E. coli* K12 from phage DNA (Newland et al. 1985, Willshaw et al. 1985) and the VT2e genes were cloned from the genomic DNA of a porcine VTEC strain (Weinstein et al. 1988). Sequence analysis has allowed detailed homology comparisons between different VT genes (Smith et al. 1993). There are only a few nucleotide differences between the genes encoding Shiga toxin and VT1 toxin from several different wild-type strains. The homology between VT1 and VT2 genes is approximately 58% (Jackson et al. 1987). The A and B genes are organized in tandem and both genes appear to be transcribed on a single operon. Translation of the mRNA to yield one A and 5 B subunits is most probably achieved by more efficient initiation of the translation of the B subunit.

ATTACHING AND EFFACING LESIONS

Several observations have indicated that properties other than VT production may be essential for full virulence of VTEC strains. Studies of natural and experimental infection of animals have provided much information. Calves were examined during an outbreak caused by an *E. coli* O5:H−strain that produced VT1; the bacteria were seen closely attached to the surfaces of the colon and the microvilli were effaced and shortened so that bacteria appeared to attach to cups or pedestals (Hall et al. 1985). VTEC of other serogroups isolated from calves with diarrhoea also caused these attaching and effacing (AE) lesions but the disease was often milder than the natural infection (Mainil et al. 1987). The use of gnotobiotic piglets can also demonstrate AE lesions (Francis, Collins and Duimstra 1986, Tzipori et al. 1986,1987). The lesions formed predominantly in the caecum and there was necrosis of up to 80% of the epithelial surface. VTEC of O serogroups 26, 111, 113, 121, 145 and 157 isolated from human infections colonized the caecum, colon and distal ileum of young and weaned rabbits (Pai, Kelly and Meyers 1986). The infections resulted in AE lesions and non-bloody diarrhoea. The histopathological similarity of AE lesions induced by EPEC and VTEC has led to the characterization of the genes necessary for AE lesions in O157 VTEC (Beebakhee et al. 1992, Yu and Kaper 1992). Comparison of the *eaeA* sequences from EPEC and O157 VTEC showed 86% nucleotide homology. However, there was only 59% homology over the 800 base pairs at the C-terminal end of the sequence and it is proposed that this region is associated with binding to receptors on eukaryotic cells and with antigenic variation. The importance of the product of the *eaeA* gene of O157 VTEC, termed intimin O157, was demonstrated in vivo by the failure of an O157 VTEC strain with a mutant *eaeA* locus to attach closely to colonic epithelium of newborn piglets (Donnenberg et al. 1993). The role of chromosomal genes other than *eaeA* was indicated by the isolation of mutant strains that failed to form AE lesions in vitro or in vivo but did not have insertions in *eaeA* (Dytoc et al. 1993). Carriage of the *eae* sequences is serogroup related; VTEC of serogroups O26 and O157 possess *eae* genes (Jerse et al. 1990) but only 18 of 48 VTEC belonging to other serogroups were *eae*-positive (Willshaw et al. 1992).

ADHESION OF VTEC

Many VTEC lack the ability to cause AE lesions but may possess adhesive properties. Studies with a DNA probe for the *eaeA* gene showed that *eae*-negative VTEC were isolated from sporadic cases of haemorrhagic colitis and HUS (Willshaw et al. 1992, de Azavedo et al. 1994). Variable patterns of adhesion to 3 different lines of cultured cells have been observed. VTEC strains that cause oedema disease do not possess *eae* sequences but many produce fimbriae such as F107 that are thought to be important in pathogenesis (Imberechts et al. 1993).

ENTEROHAEMOLYSIN PRODUCTION

An enterohaemolysin (E-Hly) has been described in many VTEC including virtually all O157 strains (Beutin et al. 1988, 1989, Beutin 1991). The production of E-Hly correlated with carriage of a plasmid (Willshaw et al. 1992) and the structural genes encoding production of E-Hly activity were cloned from the pO157 plasmid of strain 933 (Schmidt, Karch and Beutin 1994). Sequence analysis of the cloned fragment showed about 60% homology with the *hlyC* and *hlyA* genes of the α-haemolysin operon (Schmidt, Beutin and Karch 1995). It was also demonstrated that antibodies to E-Hly were present in sera from 19 of 20 patients with O157-associated HUS but only in one control serum. It is interesting to note that α-haemolysin causes release of interleukin-1β from cultured cells. Interleukin-1β increases the cytotoxicity of the VT family of toxins to vascular epithelial cells by stimulating production of Gb3. The role of E-Hly in combination with VT production clearly requires further investigation.

4.4 Enteroaggregative *E. coli*

There have been several investigations of the pathogenic significance of aggregative adhesion including the use of animal models. Studies in rabbit and rat ligated loops and in orally fed gnotobiotic piglets have shown a similar pattern of histopathology in the small bowel. Examination of sections revealed oedematous villi with infiltration of leucocytes and erythrocytes, often with necrosis of the villous tips and haemorrhage (Vial et al. 1988, Tzipori et al. 1992). Autopsy examination of infants following an outbreak in Mexico demonstrated a lesion of the ileum very similar to that observed in animal models. In this outbreak 10 infants died of severe diarrhoea after infection with an enteroaggregative strain (Eslava et al. 1993). Use of cultured human colonic mucosa has demonstrated the aggregative adhesion of a large number of EAggEC strains (Knutton et al. 1992). The strains expressed one or more of 4 morphologically distinct fimbriae and 43 of 44 strains produced fibrillar bundles. Studies of strain 17-2, serotype O3:H2, by Nataro et al. (1992) showed that the aggregative property was located on a 29 kb plasmid fragment; strains carrying this region expressed bundle-forming fimbriae, AAF/I, on the cell surface. The aggregative adhesion phenotype correlated with mannose-resistant haemagglutination as observed in other studies (Scotland et al. 1991, Knutton et al. 1992, Yamamoto et al. 1992). A second fimbrial antigen, AAF/II, has also been reported (Nataro et al. 1995).

Some of the observations on EAggEC infections have suggested that the diarrhoea may, in part, be secretory. An enterotoxic factor produced by some EAggEC has been detected in a rabbit in vitro intestinal model (Savarino et al. 1991). Strain 17-2 produces this low molecular weight heat-stable toxin and the expression is plasmid encoded; it has been termed **enter**oaggregative *E. coli* heat-**s**table enterotoxin (EAST1). The toxin increases enterocyte cGMP levels as observed with STI of enterotoxigenic *E. coli*. The role of EAST1 in EAggEC diarrhoea is not yet elucidated. Baldwin et al. (1992) have reported a 120 kDa protein in supernatants of EAggEC strains with antigenic homology to the *E. coli* haemolysin; the protein caused increases in intracellular calcium in cell cultures. Some *E. coli* strains showing aggregative adhesion have produced diarrhoea in volunteers. When Mathewson et al. (1986) fed strain JM221, serotype O92:H33, to volunteers at a dose of 10^{10} organisms, 5 of 8 subjects became ill. Four different EAggEC strains were fed to volunteers at doses of 10^{10} organisms but only one strain of serotype O44:H18 caused diarrhoea, 4 of 5 subjects suffering diarrhoea (Nataro et al. 1995). These experiments suggest there are differences in the virulence of EAggEC strains.

4.5 Diffusely adherent *E. coli*

The pathogenesis of DAEC is poorly understood. Bilge et al. (1989) described a fimbrial structure (F1845) present in approximately 75% of DAEC strains but the role of these fimbriae has not been demonstrated. Another adhesin associated with diffuse adherence has been reported (Benz and Schmidt 1993). In this case a plasmid gene encoded the adhesin which appeared to be afimbrial and was genetically distinct from the gene determining F1845. Adult volunteers have been challenged with DAEC of serogroups O15 and O75 (Tacket et al. 1990) but none of the 43 volunteers developed diarrhoea and the role of DAEC in disease remains in doubt.

5 HOST RESPONSE

The host response to infection with *E. coli* was demonstrated in early studies when Lesage (1897) observed that serum from patients with infantile enteritis agglutinated *E. coli* isolated from other sufferers in the same outbreak but not those from healthy subjects. Studies of EPEC infection showed that about 50% of children had acquired haemagglutinating antibody to EPEC by the age of 1 year (Neter et al. 1955). Serum and milk antibody to EPEC O antigens is common in nursing mothers and may provide immunity (Cravioto et al. 1988). The host response to EPEC infection was also examined in volunteers (Levine et al. 1985). Of 10 volunteers who developed diarrhoea, 9 produced antibody to a 94 kDa protein detected by SDS-PAGE in outer-membrane preparations of EPEC with the EAF plasmid. The only volunteer who failed to develop diarrhoea had antibody against this 94 kDa protein before challenge, which suggested that it may be an important protective antigen. The development of immunity to infection with ETEC has also been proposed (Black et al. 1981a). In a study in Bangladesh high titres of serum antibody to LT were found, especially in young children (Black et al. 1981b). Persons with ETEC diarrhoea had a significant rise in LT antitoxin but pre-existing high levels of antitoxin did not predict protection from ETEC diarrhoea. Similar

age-specific patterns with peak LT antitoxin titres in children younger than 5 years have been found in Thailand, Panama and other developing countries (Ryder et al. 1982, Echeverria et al. 1983). Serum and intestinal secretory IgA antibody responses to the homologous O antigen occur in approximately 90% of persons with clinical ETEC infections (Levine et al. 1979). The serum O antibody is predominantly IgM and peaks about 8–10 days after onset of infection. Rises in serum IgG and intestinal secretory IgA antibody to CFA/I have been detected following infection with CFA/I-positive ETEC strains (Evans et al. 1978, Levine et al. 1982). In contrast to these significant antibody responses to CFAs and LT, the appearance of neutralizing or binding antitoxin to ST after ETEC infection has not been reported.

Host responses have been examined following VTEC infection and particularly in cases of HUS. Rising antibody titres to VT have been shown in man and animals and were shown to protect against systemic effects during VTEC infection in animal trials but diarrhoea was not prevented. Only about 10% of healthy humans have VT1-IgG and during HUS less than a third of patients develop neutralizing antibodies to VT1 (Karmali et al. 1994). Specific antibodies to VT2 and the VT2 variant, VT2c, were very infrequently seen in cases and controls. VT interacts with human B cells, leading to partial B cell depletion, especially in the B cell germinal centres (Lingwood 1994). This may explain why most HUS patients fail to develop antibodies to VT. During infection with VTEC humans develop specific antibodies against the lipopolysaccharide (LPS) of O157 and other O groups (Chart, Scotland and Rowe 1989, Chart and Rowe 1990). Little work has been done on the host response to infection with EAggEC and DAEC.

6 LABORATORY DIAGNOSIS

Many of the tests for the different groups of diarrhoeagenic *E. coli* are performed only in research and reference laboratories. Several assays are being developed commercially and this should lead to a much wider laboratory investigation of diarrhoeal disease caused by *E. coli*.

6.1 Enteropathogenic *E. coli*

Laboratory tests for EPEC serogroups are carried out with commercially available antisera and O:H typing is performed in certain national reference laboratories. Strains are tested for the localized pattern of adhesion typical of 'classical' EPEC (Cravioto et al. 1979), in the presence of D-mannose with HEp-2 cells in a 6 h test (Scotland et al. 1989a). Cells are washed after incubation for 3 h at 37°C followed by a further incubation for 3 h before washing, fixing and staining. The pattern of adhesion is then recorded (Fig. 27.1). Some laboratories have reported difficulties in distinguishing between localized, diffuse and aggregative patterns of attachment. In part this seems to be due to the use of a shorter primary incubation period (Scaletsky et al. 1984) and it is recommended that the 6 h assay should be employed. EPEC cause an accumulation of actin in HEp-2 cells beneath the attaching bacteria. This is the basis of the in vitro fluorescence actin-staining (FAS) assay (Knutton et al. 1989). The cell monolayer is fixed, made permeable and at the end of the adhesion assay it is treated with phalloidin labelled with fluorescein isothiocyanate. Using phase contrast microscopy, areas of fluorescence and their position are compared with the site of attached bacteria.

An ELISA for the detection of EPEC that show localized adherence has been described (Albert et al. 1991). The classical EPEC strain, E2348/69 serotype O127:H6, was used to prepare an antiserum absorbed with a plasmid-negative derivative (see section 4.1, p. 518). The ELISA detected all strains that showed good localized adherence whereas EPEC strains that did not show adhesion were negative. A DNA probe (EAF) has been prepared from the plasmid pMAR2 present in strain E2348/69 (Baldini, Nataro and Kaper 1986). The EAF plasmid encodes a bundle-forming pilus and a DNA probe has been developed from the DNA sequence (Giron et al. 1993). A probe has also been prepared from a chromosomal gene necessary for the attaching and effacing ability of EPEC (Jerse et al. 1990). This is the *eaeA* probe for *E. coli* **a**ttaching and **e**ffacing. The *eaeA*, EAF and *bfp* probes can be used to test strains belonging to EPEC serogroups as well as other *E. coli*. Classical EPEC outbreak strains are positive with all 3 probes whereas most EPEC serogroup strains isolated in recent years in the UK are *eae*-positive but negative with the EAF probe (Smith et al. 1990, Scotland et al. 1991, 1993). The importance of the *eae*+ EAF− strains in human disease has yet to be established.

6.2 Enterotoxigenic *E. coli*

Toxin production by ETEC was originally demonstrated in animal models. In the standard test for ST I, sterile culture filtrates are tested for their ability to cause fluid accumulation in the intestines of infant mice (Dean et al. 1972). Alternative methods have been developed and shown to be satisfactory after comparison with the infant mouse test. An enzyme immunoassay with synthetic toxin detects both ST Ia and ST Ib in culture filtrates (Scotland et al. 1989b); this test is commercially available. Various DNA probes and PCRs have been developed for the detection of ST I genes (Scotland et al. 1989b, Sommerfelt 1991, Wray and Woodward 1994). The probes are labelled radioactively or preferably with non-radioactive reporter molecules such as biotin, digoxigenin or fluorescein.

The standard assay for the LTI is to test culture filtrates on Chinese hamster ovary (CHO), Yl mouse adrenal or Vero cells grown in tissue culture (Donta, Moon and Whipp 1974, Scotland, Gross and Rowe 1985). LTI causes elongation of CHO cells and rounding of Yl and Vero cells. Many immunological tests have been described for the detection of LTI including some available as kits such as a reversed passive latex agglutination (Scotland, Flomen and Rowe 1989) and a coagglutination test (Chapman and Daly 1989). Polynucleotide and oligonucleotide probes and PCRs for LTI genes have been reported (Sommerfelt 1991, Wray and Woodward 1994). The LTII toxin can be detected by neutralization and immunological methods with an antiserum specific for LTII; a DNA probe has been developed for LTII genes (Pickett et al. 1986).

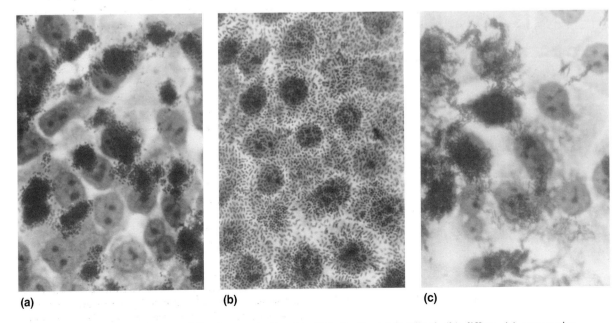

(a)   **(b)**   **(c)**

Fig. 27.1 Patterns of attachment of diarrhoeagenic *E. coli* to HEp-2 cells: (a) localized, (b) diffuse, (c) aggregative.

6.3   Vero cytotoxin-producing *E. coli*

Evidence of VTEC infection can be provided by the isolation of VTEC including O157 VTEC, demonstration of specific VT in faecal specimens or by the presence of antibodies to VTEC LPS. Most clinical laboratories test for O157 VTEC by plating faecal specimens directly on MacConkey agar plates with 1% D-sorbitol instead of lactose since, unlike most *E. coli*, O157 VTEC do not ferment sorbitol within 24 h (Farmer and Davis 1985, March and Ratnam 1986). Non-sorbitol fermenting colonies are tested for agglutination with an O157 antiserum or with an O157 latex agglutination kit. Modifications of sorbitol MacConkey (SMAC) agar have been described to improve selectivity for O157 VTEC. These include incorporation of cefixime and rhamnose into SMAC agar (Chapman et al. 1991) and SMAC agar containing derivatives of glucuronide to detect production of β-glucuronidase. Unlike most *E. coli*, O157 VTEC do not produce β-glucuronidase. The use of SMAC agar with cefixime and tellurite or SMAC agar with cefixime, rhamnose and tellurite has also been described (Zadik, Chapman and Siddons 1993, Hindle et al. 1995). Atypical O157 VTEC strains that ferment sorbitol in 24 h and produce β-glucuronidase have been reported in Germany (Günzer et al. 1992). They have not been detected in the UK but would not have been identified using the above methods. Faecal specimens are examined for the presence of VTEC by testing colonies for VT production or the presence of VT genes. Presumptive O157 VTEC should also be confirmed in these tests as there have been a few isolations of *E. coli* O157 with all the characteristics of O157 VTEC except for the presence of VT genes. VT production is usually detected by the cytotoxic effect of culture supernatants on Vero cell monolayers in tissue culture (Scotland, Day and Rowe 1980). Cytotoxic effects on Vero cells should be confirmed by neutralization with antisera against VT1 or VT2. An alternative to testing individual colonies is to examine sweeps from growth and the sensitivity of this test can be increased by use of polymyxin B to release VT (Karmali et al. 1985b). Several ELISAs have been described for the detection of VT (Basta, Karmali and Lingwood 1989, Downes et al. 1989). In these tests glycolipid Gb3 or monoclonal antibodies are used to bind the VT and the bound toxin is detected with monoclonal or polyclonal antisera against VT. These tests are not as sensitive as Vero cell tests but they are rapid and convenient and are available commercially. The presence of VT genes can be detected by DNA probes in hybridization experiments or by amplification using PCR (Willshaw et al. 1987, Karch and Meyer 1989a, 1989b, Pollard et al. 1990). Non-radioactive probes for VT genes make this approach available to a wider range of laboratories. Purified *E. coli* isolates or a large number of colonies from a faecal specimen can be tested by DNA hybridization.

6.4   Enteroaggregative *E. coli*

Serogrouping is of little value for the identification of EAggEC since these strains belong to a large number of different serogroups including some EPEC O groups such as 44, 55, 111 and 126 (Scotland et al. 1991). EAggEC are identified by testing for attachment to HEp-2 cells (Nataro et al. 1987, Scotland et al. 1989a) and a 6 h test is recommended. Aggregative adhesion is plasmid mediated in most strains and a DNA probe has been developed from a plasmid in *E. coli* strain 17-2 (Baudry et al. 1990). The enterotoxin EAST1 can be demonstrated in a rabbit intestinal model in vitro (Savarino et al. 1991). The gene encoding this toxin has been sequenced and a DNA probe has been developed (Savarino et al. 1993).

6.5   Diffusely adherent *E. coli*

DAEC are identified by testing for attachment to HEp-2 cells in a 6 h assay (Scotland et al. 1989a). Two DNA probes for diffuse adhesion that do not cross-hybridize have been developed from 2 different *E. coli* strains (Bilge et al. 1989, Benz and Schmidt 1993). This suggests that different gene sequences may determine the same phenotype of diffuse adhesion.

7   CONTROL AND PREVENTION

Some of the factors affecting the control of infections caused by diarrhoeagenic *E. coli* have been described in section 3 (see section 3, p. 515). In this section general preventive measures and studies on vaccine development are considered.

7.1   Preventive measures

Spread of *E. coli* infections in hospitals and nurseries is mainly from patient to patient and by contaminated infant feeds. Very strict hygiene procedures are required to prevent this spread and barrier nursing with isolation of infected patients is required. Control of outbreaks may require ward closure with thorough cleaning and disinfection of the ward or nursery and screening of personnel before they are reopened. Contaminated foods and water are probably the main vehicles by which ETEC are transmitted in developing countries. Thus, the provision of safe water supplies and hygienic practice in the handling and preparation of foods are of great importance. These factors are particularly important for recently weaned children. Travellers to countries where ETEC infections are common should eat hot foods and bottled drinks or water. Salads, unwashed fruit and unheated milk should be avoided. Two major modes of infection with VTEC in man have been identified. The first is consumption of contaminated foods of animal origin, cross-contaminated foods or contaminated water; the second is contact with infected persons and asymptomatic carriers who may play a role. As with other enteric pathogens measures that reduce faecal cross-contamination are beneficial for the reduction of VTEC infection. The use of Hazard Analysis Critical Control Point (HACCP) techniques, animal identification and good management practices may be essential to reduce the spread of these organisms. Little information about specific risk factors for VTEC carriage and spread in cattle is available. Some evidence suggests that farm management practices affect the prevalence of VTEC in herds. Future prevention programmes will require further study of these risk factors.

7.2 Vaccines

A vaccine for diarrhoea caused by EPEC is not available but work in this area has continued since the 1960s. Several oral vaccines were tested in infants for safety and immunogenicity and 2 similar vaccines were evaluated in field trials. A sodium deoxycholate Boivin extract vaccine was produced from O111, O55 and O86 by Rauss et al. (1972). Infants up to 1 year old were randomized to receive 3 doses of vaccine or placebo orally over 6 days followed by boosters. The vaccine had an efficacy of 41% in a trial with 1687 subjects but the least protection was seen in the neonate age group that suffered most severely from EPEC enteritis. A second vaccine prepared by Mochmann et al. (1974) from O111 and O55 strains was given a field trial in East Germany in 1970–72. There were 3 cases of O111 or O55 related disease in 3 of 6255 vaccinated children compared with 15 of 12870 unimmunized infants. These vaccines are not in routine use and future approaches to EPEC vaccines are likely to be based on knowledge of the adhesive mechanisms such as the bundle-forming pili and intimin.

Vaccine candidates for control of infection with ETEC include non-living antigen vaccines and several live vaccines. Toxoids and mixtures of inactivated whole cells and purified surface antigens have been included in the non-living vaccines. The killed whole cell *V. cholerae* plus CTB subunit oral vaccine tested in Bangladesh confirmed about 65% cross-protection against diarrhoea due to LT-positive *E. coli* in the 3 months following vaccination (Clements et al. 1988). Purified colonization factor fimbriae have been encapsulated into polyactide–polyglycolide microspheres (Reid et al. 1993). In volunteer studies 3 doses of this preparation confirmed 30% protection against challenge with a homologous strain (Tacket et al. 1993). Inactivated ETEC cells given alone or with toxoids have also been investigated in oral vaccines. Volunteers were protected with a colicin-inactivated whole cell oral vaccine (Evans et al. 1988). An alternative oral vaccine consists of formalin-inactivated ETEC with different CFAs in combination with the B subunit of CT (Svennerholm, Holmgren and Sack 1989). Adult volunteers have been protected against ETEC infection with an orally administered preparation of milk immunoglobulin enriched for antibodies against ETEC (Tacket et al. 1988). The preparation contained 45% immunoglobulin and none of the immunized volunteers developed diarrhoea whereas 9 of 10 controls had diarrhoea. Effective vaccines against VTEC, EAggEC and DAEC infection in man have not been developed.

8 TREATMENT

Early correction of fluid and electrolyte imbalance is the most important factor in preventing fatal cases of *E. coli* related diarrhoea.

A range of antimicrobial agents has been used for the treatment of diarrhoea caused by *E. coli*. However, the widespread use of this approach has been criticized on the grounds of drug toxicity and the risk of an increase and spread of antimicrobial resistance. Specific antimicrobial therapy against EPEC may be indicated in certain clinical situations and orally administered non-absorbable antibiotics such as neomycin have been used (Gomez and Cleary 1994). Other antimicrobial regimens have been used, for example, mecillinam or trimethoprim–sulphamethoxazole. High levels of antimicrobial resistance have been reported among EPEC strains. The role of antibiotics for the treatment of ETEC infections is also debatable. There is evidence that the diarrhoea is reduced in duration following treatment with co-trimoxazole or trimethoprim (Black et al. 1982c, DuPont et al. 1982). Ciprofloxacin was as effective as co-trimoxazole in a study in Mexico (Ericsson et al. 1987). The fluoroquinolones have good in vitro activity against *E. coli* but are not recommended for children and growing adolescents because of their toxic effects on cartilage in young animals (see Wood 1990). There has been much debate on the use of antimicrobial therapy for illness caused by VTEC of serogroup O157 but the information is limited. Recommendations on the avoidance of antimicrobial therapy for O157 VTEC infection are based on studies that suggested first, that the duration of symptoms was not reduced and, secondly, that there may be an increased risk of development of HUS. The latter suggestion was based on possible eradication of other bowel flora and an increase in release of Vero cytotoxin in the presence of antibiotics (Wood 1990). Experiments in vitro have shown increased cytotoxic activity in the presence of co-trimoxazole or trimethoprim but there was a reduction with ciprofloxacin. The conclusion based on the available evidence was that the data fail to support the use of antimicrobial therapy to reduce the duration of acute O157 VTEC diarrhoea but it is not known if this applies to all antibiotics.

The use of antimotility agents for O157 VTEC infections has also been investigated. There was a significant association with progression to HUS and therefore these agents should not be used for bloody diarrhoea (Cimolai et al. 1990). Evidence suggests that resistance to antimicrobial agents is becoming more prevalent in O157 VTEC strains. Between 1984 and 1987, all 56 isolates examined in Washington State were sensitive to antibiotics whereas between 1989 and 1991, 13 of 176 strains were resistant (Kim et al. 1994).

A similar situation prevails in England and Wales where the proportion of O157 VTEC resistant to at least one antimicrobial agent has increased from 10% in 1992 to 20% in 1994. The increasing resistance of O157 VTEC could complicate future treatment trials.

Colonization with EAggEC was prevented in volunteers who took prophylatic ciprofloxacin but this was not observed with those who received placebo or trimethoprim–sulphamethoxazole (Cohen et al. 1993). Multiple drug resistance has been reported in EAggEC and quinolone treatment has been recommended for treatment of EAggEC-associated diarrhoea (Yamamoto et al. 1992). These findings support the need for diagnosis of diarrhoea caused by different groups of *E. coli* and sensitivity testing when appropriate.

MESOPHILIC *AEROMONAS* SPP. AS DIARRHOEAL PATHOGENS

The first report of *Aeromonas* spp. associated with diarrhoeal disease is believed to be by Caselitz (1958) in Jamaica. He repeatedly isolated a strain of *Aeromonas* from a child with diarrhoea and demonstrated the agglutinins to the strain in the child's serum. Further reports from around the world of *Aeromonas* spp. associated with diarrhoeal disease and implicated as intestinal pathogens followed. As the interest in this group of organisms increased, serious problems arose. The first area of concern was with the taxonomy of this group of organisms which has changed frequently over the years and appears to be quite complex. The early reports on the motile mesophilic aeromonads frequently referred to this group as the '*Aeromonas hydrophila* group' but the isolates were never accurately speciated. Popoff (1984), using a phenotypic classification based on biochemical tests, identified the motile mesophilic *Aeromonas* species as *A. hydrophila*, *A. sobria* and *A. caviae*. Since then 14 DNA hybridization groups (HG) have now been identified and names have been given to most of these groups (Carnahan, Behram and Joseph 1991, Zywno et al. 1992). Most laboratories, using phenotypic methods, now identify the mesophilic *Aeromonas* species as *A. caviae*, *A. hydrophila* and *A. veronii* biotype sobria.

The second problem area concerned the identification of the virulence mechanisms associated with the 3 species isolated from cases of diarrhoeal disease. There have been reports linking virulence factors produced by these *Aeromonas* species to pathogenicity in humans. Many of these virulence factors appear to be similar to those previously described above for *E. coli*, such as production of adhesins, cytotoxins, enterotoxins and haemolysins. However, there has been no animal model in which *Aeromonas*-associated diarrhoea has been successfully demonstrated.

The third area of concern has been the lack of an internationally accepted standardized and comprehensive serotyping scheme and this has hindered the study of the epidemiology of *Aeromonas*-associated diarrhoea. There are, however, schemes for the typing of the somatic antigens of the mesophilic *Aeromonas* species (Sakazaki and Shimada 1984, Guinee and Jansen 1987).

Nevertheless, over the past decade increasing clinical and epidemiological evidence has indicated that mesophilic aeromonads should be regarded as enteric pathogens despite the non-fulfilment of Koch's postulates, that is, no animal model and no well documented outbreaks of *Aeromonas*-associated diarrhoea.

9 CLINICAL MANIFESTATIONS

Aeromonas spp. associated with diarrhoeal disease produce symptoms similar to those identified with *E. coli*, which range from a mild diarrhoea to a febrile dysentery-like illness. The most common is a mild, self-limiting, watery diarrhoea of short duration. The frequency of other clinical features, including bloody or mucoid stools, abdominal cramps, fever and vomiting, varies considerably. A chronic persistent diarrhoea, lasting for several months, has also been attributed to *Aeromonas* spp.

Clinical evidence indicates that *Aeromonas*-associated diarrhoea, although affecting all age groups, is more common in children under 5 years and in the elderly (Gracey, Burke and Robinson 1982, Millership, Curnow and Chattopadhyay 1983, Agger, McCormick and Gurwith 1985, San Joaquin and Pickett 1988). In a study of 1156 children with *Aeromonas*-associated diarrhoea 3 patterns of illness were reported; watery diarrhoea of up to 1 week in duration, chronic watery diarrhoea lasting 2–3 months and diarrhoea with blood and mucus, both acute and chronic (Gracey, Burke and Robinson 1982). Campsauer and Andremont (1982) reported the isolation of *A. sobria* from patients with cholera-like illness, with one patient requiring 21 litres of intravenous fluids. Both Pitarangsi et al. (1982) and Deodhar, Saraswathi and Varudkar (1991) reported on the severity of the illness with 10–12 stools being passed in some cases of diarrhoea during a period of 24 h.

The acute diarrhoeal illness associated with *Aeromonas* species has been observed more frequently in children, particularly those from developing countries, whereas the chronic form is seen mainly in adults from developed countries (Altwegg and Geiss 1989). *Aeromonas* spp. have also been implicated in travellers' diarrhoea (Echeverria et al. 1981, Gracey et al. 1984).

The 3 species *A. hydrophila*, *A. veronii* biotype sobria and *A. caviae* have all been isolated from faeces. Goodwin et al. (1983), Agger, McCormick and Gurwith (1985) and Gracey and Burke (1986) failed to correlate *A. caviae* with diarrhoeal disease. However, Altwegg (1985) and Megraud (1986) showed *A. caviae* to be the most common species isolated from cases of diarrhoea. One report of haemolytic–uraemic syndrome associated with a case of *A. hydrophila*-associated diarrhoea has been published (Bogdanovic et al. 1991).

10 EPIDEMIOLOGY

Numerous reports and surveys have appeared from all 5 continents regarding the isolation of the mesophilic *Aeromonas* species from the faeces of patients with diarrhoea (Sanyal, Singh and Sen 1975, Wadström et al. 1976, Echeverria et al. 1981, Gracey, Burke and Robinson 1982, Millership, Curnow and Chattopadhyay 1983, Agger, McCormick and Gurwith 1985, Figura et al. 1986, Megraud 1986, Old, Gordon and Hill 1986, Figueroa et al. 1988, Kuijper et al. 1989, Deodhar, Saraswathi and Varudkar 1991). They vary considerably in the reported frequency of isolation of these species from cases of diarrhoea as compared with the frequency of isolation from asymptomatic individuals. In Thailand Echeverria et al. (1981) showed, in a study of Peace Corps volunteers, a significant difference in isolation rates, 31% from cases of diarrhoea and 9% from healthy controls. Another study in Thailand by Pitarangsi et al. (1982) recorded no difference in the isolation rates of *Aeromonas* species among the general population, 27% in cases with diarrhoea and 24% from those with no diarrhoea. Gracey, Burke and Robinson (1982) in a 1 year study in Australia reported an isolation rate of 10% from children with diarrhoea and <1% in children without diarrhoea. In the USA Challapalli et al. (1988) in a 2 year study isolated *Aeromonas* from 7% of children with diarrhoea and from 2% of controls. In Italy Figura et al. (1986) and in England Millership, Stephenson and Tabaqchali (1987) both showed a higher isolation rate from cases than from controls but the differences in isolation rates were not statistically significant. Generally, the association between *Aeromonas* spp. and diarrhoea is found to be most prevalent in children younger than 2 years, adults over 50 years of age and amongst the immunocompromised (Gracey, Burke and Robinson 1982, Burke et al. 1983, San Joaquin and Pickett 1988, Kuijper et al. 1989). Studies that have indicated a seasonal peak in the isolation rates of *Aeromonas* spp. associated with diarrhoea have all shown the peak to be in the late summer months (Gracey, Burke and Robinson 1982, Agger, McCormick and Gurwith 1985, Old, Gordon and Hill 1986, Megraud 1986, Wilcox et al. 1992).

Water is believed to be the main source of infection and the mesophilic *Aeromonas* species have readily been found in all forms of water including chlorinated supplies. In water as in humans the isolation rates of these organisms exhibit a seasonality, their numbers rising during the summer months with the increase in temperature (Hazen et al. 1978, Burke et al. 1984a, 1984b, Williams and LaRock 1985, Picard and Goullet 1987, Kooij 1988, Havelaar et al. 1992). Gray (1984) isolated *Aeromonas* spp. not only from drinking water but also from 12% of the livestock, cows, horses, pigs and sheep, that drank from the supply. Foods are also a source of potential infection for man; the mesophilic aeromonads have been found in a wide variety of foods including fish, seafood, poultry, red meat and raw milk (Callister and Agger 1987, Palumbo et al. 1989).

11 PATHOGENESIS

The mesophilic aeromonads produce a variety of virulence factors including adhesins, enterotoxins, haemolysins and proteases that are potential virulence factors. Some strains may also possess an enteroinvasive factor detectable in tissue culture using HEp-2 cells (Watson et al. 1985).

Pitarangsi et al. (1982) fed a cytotoxic *Aeromonas* strain from a patient with acute diarrhoea to 5 rhesus monkeys and failed to produce diarrhoea at a challenge dose of 10^9 organisms per ml. In a human challenge experiment, Morgan et al. (1985), using a panel of 5 *Aeromonas* strains possessing the putative virulence properties of production of cytotoxin, enterotoxin and haemolysin, observed diarrhoea in only 2 of 57 volunteers fed with doses ranging between 10^4 and 10^{10} organisms per ml.

11.1 Haemolysins

Two types of haemolysin have been described, α- and β-haemolysins (Ljung, Eneroth and Wadström 1981). The weak α-haemolysin produces partial haemolysis of erythrocytes and a reversible cytotoxic effect in tissue culture and is not considered to be significant. The β-haemolysin, aerolysin, is irreversibly cytotoxic in tissue culture, is not immunologically cross-reactive with cholera toxin, and causes fluid accumulation in suckling mice (Asao et al. 1984).

11.2 Enterotoxins

Two non-haemolytic enterotoxins have been described. Ljung, Eneroth and Wadström (1981) reported a heat-labile, cytotonic enterotoxin that produced fluid accumulation in rabbits and rats but not suckling mice and was immunologically unrelated to cholera toxin. Chakraborty et al. (1984) cloned the gene for the production of this toxin into *E. coli*. The second non-haemolytic, cytotonic enterotoxin was first described by Campbell and Houston (1985). This enterotoxin caused fluid accumulation in infant mice and was also cross-reactive with cholera toxin.

Until recently it was believed that toxins were produced only by isolates of *A. hydrophila* and *A. veronii* biotype sobria and not by isolates of *A. caviae*. Namdari and Bottone (1990) reported on strains of *A. caviae*, isolated from cases of diarrhoea in children, that adhered to HEp-2 cells and produced a cytotoxin that caused fluid accumulation in suckling mice. Singh and Sanyal (1992) demonstrated similar properties in both human and environmental isolates of *A. caviae* after consecutive passages through the rabbit intestinal loop.

11.3 Adherence

Aeromonas strains adhere to erythrocytes, rabbit brush border and human buccal cells (Atkinson and Trust 1980, Levett and Daniel 1981, Burke, Cooper and Robinson 1986). Clark et al. (1989), using cultured mouse adrenal cells, observed that *A. sobria* and *A. hydrophila* isolates showed a greater ability to bind to the adrenal cells than isolates of *A. caviae* and that optimal attachment occurred after 30 min of incubation at 37°C. In a study of 273 *Aeromonas* isolates from faeces, food and the environment, Nishikawa, Kimura and Kishi (1991) reported mannose-resistant adhesion of 8 faecal isolates, 6 *A. sobria* and 2 *A. hydrophila* to INT407 cells.

11.4 Invasive ability

There have been very few studies on the invasive ability of the motile *Aeromonas* spp. and its pathogenic potential. Using HEp-2 cells Lawson, Burke and Chang (1985) reported human faecal isolates of *A. hydrophila* to be invasive and Figura et al. (1988) showed invasion by isolates of *A. sobria*; however, Watson et al. (1985) failed to find invasive *A. caviae* in their study. Gray, Stickler and Bryant (1990), in a study of *Aeromonas* spp. isolated from livestock, reported isolates of *A. sobria* that were capable of HEp-2 cell invasion.

12 HOST RESPONSE

Little is known about the host response to intestinal infection with *Aeromonas* strains. Caselitz (1958) observed that serum from a patient with diarrhoea agglutinated the *Aeromonas* strain isolated from the patient's faeces. Jiang et al. (1991) demonstrated a 4-fold increase in secretory IgA among travellers with diarrhoea shedding *A. hydrophila* and *A. sobria* and no IgA response from those with diarrhoea shedding *A. caviae*. Further work is necessary on the immune response to intestinal infection to provide additional evidence of the enteropathogenicity of the mesophilic *Aeromonas* species in man.

13 LABORATORY DIAGNOSIS

No single medium is accepted world wide for the isolation of *Aeromonas* from faeces. The organisms grow on most enteric media including MacConkey agar, xylose–sodium deoxycholate–citrate agar and cefsulodin–Irgasan–novobiocin agar. Blood agar containing ampicillin is also widely used but ampicillin-sensitive strains have been reported. On most enteric media *Aeromonas* spp. appear to be morphologically very similar to members of the Enterobacteriaceae and therefore the oxidase test is of great importance and should be used routinely on all suspect colonies.

14 TREATMENT

Most incidents of *Aeromonas*-associated diarrhoea are believed to be self-limiting and rehydration therapy rather than specific antimicrobial treatment may be all that is required. However, antimicrobial therapy may be indicated in cases of severe, bloody or chronic diarrhoea or in immunocompromised patients. Most *Aeromonas* isolates are resistant to ampicillin and the drugs of choice are chloramphenicol, co-trimoxazole and tetracycline (Janda and Duffey 1988). Treatment with ciprofloxacin was successful in 3 patients who were hospitalized with severe or persistent diarrhoea (Nathwani et al. 1991). Although there have been no controlled clinical trials on patients with *Aeromonas*-associated diarrhoea, observational studies and in vitro susceptibility studies have led Mathewson and DuPont (1991) to postulate that the use of antibacterial drugs shortens the duration of clinical disease.

REFERENCES

Agger WA, McCormick JD, Gurwith MJ, 1985, Clinical and microbiological features of *Aeromonas* associated diarrhea, *J Clin Microbiol*, **21:** 909–13.

Ahmed R, Bopp C et al., 1987, Phage-typing scheme for *Escherichia coli* O157:H7, *J Infect Dis*, **155:** 806–9.

Albert MJ, Ansaruzzaman M et al., 1991, An ELISA for the detection of localized adherent classic enteropathogenic *Escherichia coli* serogroups, *J Infect Dis*, **164:** 986–9.

Altwegg M, 1985, *Aeromonas caviae*: an enteric pathogen, *Infection*, **13:** 228–31.

Altwegg M, Geiss HK, 1989, *Aeromonas* as a human pathogen, *Crit Rev Microbiol*, **16:** 253–86.

Annotation, 1968, Gastroenteritis due to *Escherichia coli*, *Lancet*, **1:** 32.

Asao T, Kinoshita Y et al., 1984, Purification and some properties of *Aeromonas hydrophila* hemolysin, *Infect Immun*, **46:** 122–7.

Atkinson HM, Trust TJ, 1980, Hemagglutination properties and adherence ability of *Aeromonas hydrophila*, *Infect Immun*, **27:** 938–46.

de Azavedo J, McWhirter E et al., 1994, *EAE*-negative verotoxin-producing *Escherichia coli* associated with hemolytic uremic syndrome and hemorrhagic colitis, *Recent Advances in Verocytotoxin-producing Escherichia coli* Infections, eds Karmali MA, Goglio AG, Elsevier Science, Amsterdam, 265–8.

Bäck E, Blomberg S, Wadström T, 1977, Enterotoxigenic *Escherichia coli* in Sweden, *Infection*, **5:** 2–5.

Baldini MM, Kaper JB et al., 1983, Plasmid-mediated adhesion in enteropathogenic *Escherichia coli*, *J Pediatr Gastroenterol Nutr*, **2:** 534–8.

Baldini MM, Nataro JP, Kaper JB, 1986, Localization of a determinant for HEp-2 adherence by enteropathogenic *Escherichia coli*, *Infect Immun*, **52:** 334–6.

Baldwin TJ, Ward W et al., 1991, Elevation of intracellular free calcium levels in HEp-2 cells infected with enteropathogenic *Escherichia coli*, *Infect Immun*, **59:** 1599–604.

Baldwin TJ, Knutton S et al., 1992, Enteroaggregative *Escherichia coli* strains secrete a heat-labile toxin antigenically related to *E. coli* hemolysin, *Infect Immun*, **60:** 2092–5.

Baqui AH, Sack RB et al., 1992, Enteropathogens associated with acute and persistent diarrhea in Bangladeshi children <5 years of age, *J Infect Dis*, **166:** 792–6.

Basta M, Karmali M, Lingwood C, 1989, Sensitive receptor-specified enzyme-linked immunosorbent assay for *Escherichia coli* verocytotoxin, *J Clin Microbiol*, **27:** 1617–22.

Baudry B, Savarino SJ et al., 1990, A sensitive and specific DNA probe to identify enteroaggregative *E. coli*, a recently discovered diarrheal pathogen, *J Infect Dis*, **161:** 1249–51.

Beebakhee G, Louie M et al., 1992, Cloning and nucleotide sequence of the *eae* gene homologue from enterohemorrhagic *Escherichia coli* serotype O157:H7, *FEMS Microbiol Lett*, **91:** 63–8.

Bell BP, Goldoft M et al., 1994, A multi state outbreak of *Escherichia coli* O157:H7-associated bloody diarrhea and hemolytic uremic syndrome from hamburgers: the Washington experience, *JAMA*, **272:** 1349–53.

Benz I, Schmidt MA, 1993, Diffuse adherence of enteropathogenic *Escherichia coli* strains – processing of AIDA-I, *Zentrabl Bakteriol*, **278:** 197–208.

Bertschinger HU, Gyles CL, 1994, Oedema disease of pigs, *Escherichia coli* in Domestic Animals and Humans, ed. Gyles CL, CAB International, Wallingford, UK, 193–219.

Beutin L, 1991, The different haemolysins of *Escherichia coli*, *Med Microbiol*, **180:** 167–82.

Beutin L, Prada J et al., 1988, Enterohaemolysin, a new type of haemolysin produced by some strains of enteropathogenic *E. coli* (EPEC), *Zentralbl Bakteriol Mikrobiol Hyg*, **267:** 576–88.

Beutin L, Montenegro MA et al., 1989, Close association of verotoxin (Shiga-like toxin) production with enterohemolysin production in strains of *Escherichia coli*, *J Clin Microbiol*, **27:** 2559–64.

Beutin L, Geier D et al., 1993, Prevalence and some properties of verotoxin (Shiga-like toxin) producing *Escherichia coli* in seven different species of healthy domestic animals, *J Clin Microbiol*, **31:** 2483–8.

Bhan MK, Khoshoo V et al., 1989a, Enteroaggregative *Escherichia coli* and *Salmonella* associated with nondysenteric persistent diarrhea, *Pediatr Infect Dis J*, **8:** 499–502.

Bhan MK, Raj P et al., 1989b, Enteroaggregative *Escherichia coli* associated with persistent diarrhea in a cohort of rural children in India, *J Infect Dis*, **159:** 1061–4.

Bilge SS, Clausen S et al., 1989, Molecular characterisation of a fimbrial adhesin, F1845, mediating diffuse adherence of diarrhea-associated *Escherichia coli* to HEp-2 cells, *J Bacteriol*, **171:** 4281–9.

Black RE, Merson MH et al., 1981a, Incidence and severity of rotovirus and *E. coli* diarrhoea in rural Bangladesh. Implications for vaccine development, *Lancet*, **1:** 141–3.

Black RE, Merson MH et al., 1981b, Enterotoxigenic *E. coli* diarrhea: acquired immunity and transmission in an endemic area, *Bull W H O*, **59:** 253–8.

Black RE, Brown KH et al., 1982a, Longitudinal studies of infectious diseases and physical growth of children in rural Bangladesh. II Incidence of diarrhea and association with known pathogens, *Am J Epidemiol*, **115:** 315–24.

Black RE, Brown KH et al., 1982b, Contamination of weaning foods and transmission of enterotoxigenic *Escherichia coli* diarrhoea in children in rural Bangladesh, *Trans R Soc Trop Med Hyg*, **76:** 259–64.

Black RE, Levine MM et al., 1982c, Treatment of experimentally induced enterotoxigenic *Escherichia coli* diarrhea with trimethoprim, trimethoprim–sulfamethoxazole or placebo, *Rev Infect Dis*, **4:** 540–5.

Bockemühl J, Aleksic S et al., 1992, Serological and biochemical properties of Shiga-like toxin (verocytotoxin)-producing strains of *Escherichia coli*, other than O-group O157, from patients in Germany, *Zentralbl Bakteriol*, **276:** 189–95.

Bogdanovic R, Cobeljic M et al., 1991, Haemolytic–uraemic syndrome associated with *Aeromonas hydrophila* enterocolitis, *Pediatr Nephrol*, **5:** 293–5.

Bray J, 1945, Isolation of antigenically homogeneous strains of *Bact coli neapolitanum* from summer diarrhoea in infants, *J Pathol Bacteriol*, **57:** 239–47.

Brook MG, Smith HR et al., 1994, Prospective study of verocytotoxin-producing, enteroaggregative and diffusely adherent

Escherichia coli in different diarrhoeal states, *Epidemiol Infect*, **112:** 63–7.

Bühler T, Hoschützky H, Jann K, 1991, Analysis of colonization factor antigen I, an adhesin of enterotoxigenic *Escherichia coli* O78:H11: fimbrial morphology and location of the receptor-binding site, *Infect Immun*, **59:** 3876–82.

Burke V, Cooper M, Robinson J, 1986, Haemagglutination patterns of *Aeromonas* spp. related to species and source of strains, *Aust J Exp Biol Med Sci*, **64:** 563–70.

Burke V, Gracey M et al., 1983, The microbiology of childhood gastroenteritis: *Aeromonas* species and other infective agents, *J Infect Dis*, **148:** 68–74.

Burke V, Robinson J et al., 1984a, Isolation of *Aeromonas hydrophila* from a metropolitan water supply: seasonal correlation with clinical isolates, *Appl Environ Microbiol*, **48:** 361–6.

Burke V, Robinson J et al., 1984b, Isolation of *Aeromonas* spp. from an unchlorinated domestic water supply, *Appl Environ Microbiol*, **48:** 367–70.

Callister SM, Agger WA, 1987, Enumeration and characterization of *Aeromonas hydrophila* and *Aeromonas caviae* isolated from grocery store produce, *Appl Environ Microbiol*, **53:** 249–53.

Cameron S, Walker C et al., 1995, Enterohaemorrhagic *Escherichia coli* outbreak in South Australia associated with the consumption of mettwurst, *Commun Dis Intell*, **19:** 70–1.

Campbell JD, Houston CW, 1985, Effect of cultural conditions on the presence of a cholera toxin cross-reactive factor in culture filtrates of *Aeromonas hydrophila*, *Curr Microbiol*, **12:** 101–6.

Campsauer H, Andremont A, 1982, Cholera-like illness due to *Aeromonas sobria*, *J Infect Dis*, **145:** 248–54.

Caprioli A, Luzzi I et al., 1994, Community outbreak of hemolytic uremic syndrome associated with non-O157 Vero cytotoxin-producing *Escherichia coli*, *J Infect Dis*, **169:** 208–11.

Carnahan AM, Behram S, Joseph SW, 1991, Aerokey II: a flexible key for identifying clinical *Aeromonas* species, *J Clin Microbiol*, **29:** 2843–9.

Carter AO, Borczyk AA et al., 1987, A severe outbreak of *Escherichia coli* O157:H7 associated hemorrhagic colitis in a nursing home, *N Engl J Med*, **317:** 1496–500.

Caselitz FH, 1958, Zur Frage von *Pseudomonas aeruginosa* und verwandten Mikroorganismen als Enteritiserreger, *Z Tropenmed Parasitol*, **9:** 269–75.

Casey TA, Herring CJ, Schneider RA, 1993, Expression of STb enterotoxin by adherent *E. coli* is not sufficient to cause severe diarrhea in neonatal pigs, *Abstracts 93rd Mtg ASM Washington DC*, 44.

Chakraborty T, Montenegro MA et al., 1984, Cloning of enterotoxin gene from *Aeromonas hydrophila* provides conclusive evidence of the production of a cytotonic enterotoxin, *Infect Immun*, **46:** 435–41.

Challapalli M, Tess BR et al., 1988, *Aeromonas*-associated diarrhea in children, *Pediatr Infect Dis J*, **7:** 693–8.

Chapman PA, Daly CM, 1989, Comparison of Y1 mouse adrenal cell and coagglutination assays for detection of *Escherichia coli* heat-labile enterotoxin, *J Clin Pathol*, **42:** 755–8.

Chapman PA, Wright DJ, Higgins R, 1993, Untreated milk as a source of verotoxigenic *E. coli* O157, *Vet Rec*, **133:** 171–2.

Chapman PA, Wright DJ, Norman P, 1989, Verotoxin-producing *Escherichia coli* infections in Sheffield: cattle as a possible source, *Epidemiol Infect*, **102:** 439–45.

Chapman PA, Siddons CA et al., 1991, An improved selective medium for the isolation of *Escherichia coli* O157, *J Med Microbiol*, **35:** 107–10.

Chapman PA, Siddons CA et al., 1992, Cattle as a source of verotoxigenic *Escherichia coli* O157, *Vet Rec*, **131:** 323–4.

Chapman PA, Siddons CA et al., 1993, Cattle as a possible source of verocytotoxin-producing *Escherichia coli* O157 infections in man, *Epidemiol Infect*, **111:** 439–47.

Chart H, Rowe B, 1990, Serological identification of infection by Vero cytotoxin-producing *Escherichia coli* in patients with haemolytic uraemic syndrome, *Serodiag Immunother Infect Dis*, **4**: 413–18.

Chart H, Scotland SM, Rowe B, 1989, Serum antibodies to *Escherichia coli* serotype O157:H7 in patients with hemolytic uremic syndrome, *J Clin Microbiol*, **27**: 285–90.

Cimolai N, Carter JE et al., 1990, Risk factors for the progression of *Escherichia coli* O157:H7 enteritis to hemolytic–uremic syndrome, *J Pediatr*, **116**: 589–92.

Clark RB, Knoop FC et al., 1989, Attachment of mesophilic aeromonads to cultured mammalian cells, *Curr Microbiol*, **19**: 97–102.

Clausen CR, Christie DL, 1982, Chronic diarrhea in infants caused by adherent enteropathogenic *Escherichia coli*, *J Pediatr*, **100**: 358–61.

Clements JD, Harris J et al., 1988, Field trial of oral cholera vaccines in Bangladesh: results of one year of follow-up, *J Infect Dis*, **158**: 60–9.

Cohen MB, Hawkins JA et al., 1993, Colonization by enteroaggregative *Escherichia coli* in travelers with and without diarrhea, *J Clin Microbiol*, **31**: 351–3.

Cordovéz A, Prado V et al., 1992, Enterohemorrhagic *Escherichia coli* associated with hemolytic–uremic syndrome in Chilean children, *J Clin Microbiol*, **30**: 2153–7.

Cravioto A, Scotland SM, Rowe B, 1982, Hemagglutination activity and colonization factor antigens I and II in enterotoxigenic and non-enterotoxigenic strains of *Escherichia coli* isolated from humans, *Infect Immun*, **36**: 189–97.

Cravioto A, Gross RJ et al., 1979, An adhesive factor found in strains of *Escherichia coli* belonging to the traditional infantile enteropathogenic serotypes, *Curr Microbiol*, **3**: 95–9.

Cravioto A, Reyes RE et al., 1988, Prospective study of diarrhoeal disease in a cohort of rural Mexican children: incidence and isolated pathogens during the first two years of life, *Epidemiol Infect*, **101**: 123–34.

Cravioto A, Tello A et al., 1991, Association of *Escherichia coli* HEp-2 adherence patterns with type and duration of diarrhoea, *Lancet*, **337**: 262–4.

Day NP, Scotland SM et al., 1983, *Escherichia coli* O157:H7 associated with human infections in the United Kingdom, *Lancet*, **1**: 825.

Dean AG, Ching Y-C et al., 1972, Test for *Escherichia coli* enterotoxin using infant mice. Application in a study of diarrhea in children in Honolulu, *J Infect Dis*, **15**: 407–11.

Deodhar LP, Saraswathi K, Varudkar A, 1991, *Aeromonas* spp. and their association with human diarrheal disease, *J Clin Microbiol*, **29**: 853–6.

De-Sauvage FJ, Camerato TR, Goeddel DV, 1991, Primary structure and functional expression of receptor for *Escherichia coli* heat-stable enterotoxin, *J Biol Chem*, **266**: 17912–18.

De-Sauvage FJ, Horuk R et al., 1992, Characterization of the recombinant human receptor for *Escherichia coli* heat-stable enterotoxin, *J Biol Chem*, **267**: 6479–82.

Dobrescu L, 1983, New biological effect of edema disease principle (*Escherichia coli*-neurotoxin) and its use as an *in vitro* assay for this toxin, *Am J Vet Res*, **44**: 31–4.

Donnenberg MS, Yu J, Kaper JB, 1993, A second chromosomal gene necessary for intimate attachment of enteropathogenic *Escherichia coli* to epithelial cells, *J Bacteriol*, **175**: 4670–80.

Donnenberg MS, Tacket CO et al., 1992, The role of the *eae* gene in experimental human enteropathogenic *Escherichia coli* (EPEC) infection, *Clin Res*, **40**: 214A.

Donnenberg MS, Tzipori S et al., 1993, The role of the *eae* gene of enterohemorrhagic *Escherichia coli* in intimate attachment *in vitro* and in a porcine model, *J Clin Invest*, **92**: 1418–24.

Donta ST, Moon HW, Whipp SC, 1974, Detection of heat-labile *Escherichia coli* enterotoxin with the use of adrenal cells in tissue culture, *Science*, **183**: 334–6.

Donta ST, Wallace RB, Whipp SC, 1977, Enterotoxigenic *Escherichia coli* and diarrheal disease in Mexican children, *J Infect Dis*, **155**: 482–5.

Downes FP, Green JH et al., 1989, Development and evaluation

of enzyme-linked immunosorbent assays for detection of Shiga-like toxin I and Shiga-like toxin II, *J Clin Microbiol*, **27**: 1292–7.

Doyle MP, Schoeni JL, 1987, Isolation of *Escherichia coli* O157:H7 from retail fresh meats and poultry, *Appl Environ Microbiol*, **53**: 2394–6.

Dreyfus LA, Harville B et al., 1993, Calcium influx mediated by the *Escherichia coli* heat-stable enterotoxin b (STb), *Proc Natl Acad Sci USA*, **90**: 3202–6.

DuPont HL, Formal SB et al., 1971, Pathogenesis of *Escherichia coli* diarrhea, *N Engl J Med*, **285**: 1–9.

DuPont HL, Reves RR et al., 1982, Treatment of travelers' diarrhea with trimethoprim/sulfamethoxazole and with trimethoprim alone, *N Engl J Med*, **307**: 841–4.

DuPont HL, Galindo E et al., 1983, Prevention of travelers' diarrhea with trimethoprim/sulfamethoxazole and trimethoprim alone, *Gastroenterology*, **84**: 75–80.

Dytoc M, Soni R et al., 1993, Multiple determinants of verotoxin-producing *Escherichia coli* O157:H7 attachment-effacement, *Infect Immun*, **61**: 3382–91.

Echeverria P, Blacklow NR et al., 1981, Travelers diarrhea among American Peace Corps volunteers in rural Thailand, *J Infect Dis*, **145**: 767–71.

Echeverria P, Burke DS et al., 1983, Age-specific prevalence of antibody to rotavirus, *Escherichia coli* heat-labile enterotoxin, Norwalk virus, and hepatitis A virus in a rural community in Thailand, *J Clin Microbiol*, **17**: 923–5.

Echeverria P, Taylor DN et al., 1987, Potential sources of enterotoxigenic *Escherichia coli* in homes of children with diarrhoea in Thailand, *Bull W H O*, **65**: 207–15.

Echeverria P, Orskov F et al., 1991, Attaching and effacing enteropathogenic *Escherichia coli* as a cause of infantile diarrhea in Bangkok, *J Infect Dis*, **164**: 550–4.

Ericsson CD, Johnson PC et al., 1987, Ciprofloxacin or trimethoprim–sulfamethoxazole as initial therapy for traveler's diarrhea. A placebo-controlled, randomized trial, *Ann Intern Med*, **106**: 216–20.

Escherich T, 1885, Die Darmbacterien des Neugeborenen und säuglings, *Fortschr Med*, **3**: 515–22.

Eslava C, Villaseca J et al., 1993, Identification of a protein with toxigenic activity produced by enteroaggregative *Escherichia coli*, *Abstracts 93rd Mtg ASM, Washington DC*, 44.

Evans DG, Evans DJ, 1978, New surface-associated heat-labile colonization factor antigen (CFA/II) produced by enterotoxigenic *Escherichia coli* of serogroups O6 and O8, *Infect Immun*, **21**: 638–47.

Evans DG, Silver RP et al., 1975, Plasmid controlled colonization factor associated with virulence in *Escherichia coli* enterotoxigenic for humans, *Infect Immun*, **12**: 656–67.

Evans DG, Satterwhite TK et al., 1978, Differences in serological responses and excretion patterns of volunteers challenged with enterotoxigenic *E. coli* with and without the colonization factor antigen, *Infect Immun*, **19**: 883–8.

Evans DJ, Evans DG et al., 1988, Immunoprotective oral whole cell vaccine for enterotoxigenic *Escherichia coli* diarrhoea prepared by *in situ* destruction of chromosomal and plasmid DNA with colicin E2, *FEMS Microbiol Immunol*, **47**: 9–18.

Farmer JJ, Davis BR, 1985, H7 antiserum-sorbitol fermentation medium: a single tube screening medium for detecting *Escherichia coli* O157:H7 associated with hemorrhagic colitis, *J Clin Microbiol*, **22**: 620–5.

Ferguson WW, June RC, 1952, Experiments on feeding adult volunteers with *Escherichia coli* 111, B4, a coliform organism associated with infant diarrhea, *Am J Hyg*, **55**: 155–69.

Field M, Rao MC, Chang EB, 1989a, Intestinal electrolyte transport and diarrheal disease I, *N Engl J Med*, **321**: 800–6.

Field M. Rao MC, Chang EB, 1989b, Intestinal electrolyte transport and diarrheal disease II, *N Engl J Med*, **321**: 879–83.

Field M, Graf LH et al., 1978, Heat-stable enterotoxin of *Escherichia coli*, *in vitro* effects on guanylate cyclase activity, cyclic

GMP concentration, and with transport in small intestine, *Proc Natl Acad Sci USA*, **75**: 2800–4.

Figueroa G, Galeno H et al., 1988, Enteropathogenicity of *Aeromonas* species isolated from infants: a cohort study, *J Infect*, **17**: 205–13.

Figura N, Marri L et al., 1986, Prevalence, species differentiation and toxigenicity of *Aeromonas* strains in cases of childhood gastroenteritis and in controls, *J Clin Microbiol*, **23**: 595–9.

Finlay BB, Rosenshine I et al., 1992, Cytoskeletal composition of attaching and effacing lesions associated with enteropathogenic *Escherichia coli* adherence to HeLa cells, *Infect Immun*, **60**: 2541–3.

Forte LR, Thorne PK et al., 1992, Stimulation of intestinal Cl-transport by heat-stable enterotoxin: activation of cAMP-dependent protein kinase by cGMP, *Am J Physiol*, **263**: C607–15.

Francis DH, Collins JE, Duimstra JR, 1986, Infection of gnotobiotic pigs with an *Escherichia coli* O157:H7 strain associated with an outbreak of hemorrhagic colitis, *Infect Immun*, **51**: 953–6.

Frost JA, Cheasty T et al., 1993, Phage typing of Vero cytotoxin-producing *Escherichia coli* O157 isolated in the United Kingdom: 1989–1991, *Epidemiol Infect*, **110**: 469–76.

Gannon VPJ, Gyles CL, Wilcock BP, 1989, Effects of *Escherichia coli* Shiga-like toxins (verotoxins) in pigs, *Can J Vet Res*, **53**: 306–12.

Gannon VPJ, Teerling C et al., 1990, Molecular cloning and nucleotide sequence of another variant of the *Escherichia coli* Shiga-like toxin II family, *J Gen Microbiol*, **136**: 1125–35.

Giles C, Sangster G, 1948, An outbreak of infantile gastro-enteritis in Aberdeen. The association of a special type of *Bact. coli* with the infection, *J Hyg*, **46**: 1–9.

Giron JA, Ho ASY, Schoolnik GK, 1991, An inducible bundle forming pilus of enteropathogenic *Escherichia coli*, *Science*, **254**: 710–13.

Giron JA, Jones T et al., 1991, Diffuse-adhering *Escherichia coli* (DAEC) as a putative cause of diarrhea in Mayan children in Mexico, *J Infect Dis*, **163**: 507–13.

Giron JA, Donnenberg MS et al., 1993, Distribution of the bundle-forming pilus structural gene (*bfpA*) among enteropathogenic *Escherichia coli*, *J Infect Dis*, **168**: 1037–41.

Goldschmidt R, 1933, Untersuchungen zur ätiologie der durchfallserkrankungen des säuglings, *Jahrb Kinderheilkd Phys Erz*, **139**: 318–58.

Gomes TAT, Blake PA, Trabulsi LR, 1989, Prevalence of *Escherichia coli* strains with localized, diffuse, and aggregative adherence to HeLa cells in infants with diarrhea and matched controls, *J Clin Microbiol*, **27**: 266–9.

Gomez HF, Cleary TG, 1994, *Escherichia coli* as a cause of diarrhea in children, *Semin Pediatr Infect Dis*, **5**: 175–82.

Goodwin CS, Harper WES et al., 1983, Enterotoxigenic *Aeromonas hydrophila* and diarrhoea in adults, *Med J Aust*, **1**: 25–6.

Gorbach SL, Kean BH et al., 1975, Travelers' diarrhea and toxigenic *Escherichia coli*, *N Engl J Med*, **292**: 933–5.

de Graaf FK, Gaastra W, 1994, Fimbriae of enterotoxigenic *Escherichia coli*, *Fimbriae: Adhesion, Genetics, Biogenesis and Vaccines*, ed. Klemm P, CRC Press, Boca Raton, FL, 57–88.

Gracey M, Burke V, 1986, Characteristics of *Aeromonas* species and their association with human diarrhoeal disease, *J Diarrhoeal Dis Res*, **4**: 70–3.

Gracey M, Burke V, Robinson J, 1982, *Aeromonas*-associated gastroenteritis, *Lancet*, **2**: 1304–6.

Gracey M, Burke V et al., 1984, *Aeromonas* spp. in travellers' diarrhoea, *Br Med J*, **289**: 658.

Gray SJ, 1984, *Aeromonas hydrophila* in livestock: incidence, biochemical characteristics and antibiotic susceptibility, *J Hyg*, **92**: 365–75.

Gray SJ, Stickler DJ, Bryant TN, 1990, The incidence of virulence factors in mesophilic *Aeromonas* species isolated from farm animals and their environment, *Epidemiol Infect*, **105**: 277–94.

Green BA, Neill RJ et al., 1983, Evidence that a new enterotoxin of *Escherichia coli* which activates adenylate cyclase in eucaryotic target cells is not plasmid mediated, *Infect Immun*, **41**: 383–90.

Griffin PM, Tauxe RV, 1991, The epidemiology of infections caused by *Escherichia coli* O157:H7, enterohemorrhagic *E. coli*, and the associated hemolytic uremic syndrome, *Epidemiol Rev*, **13**: 60–98.

Griffin PM, Bell BP et al., 1994, Large outbreak of *Escherichia coli* O157:H7 infections in the Western United States: the big picture, *Recent Advances in Verocytotoxin-producing Escherichia coli Infections*, eds Karmali MA, Goglio AG, Elsevier Science, Amsterdam, 233–40.

Griffiths SL, Finkelstein RA, Critchley DR, 1986, Characterization of the receptor for cholera toxin and *Escherichia coli* heat-labile toxin in rabbit intestinal brush borders, *Biochem J*, **238**: 313–22.

Gross RJ, 1990, *Escherichia coli* diarrhoea, *Topley and Wilson's Principles of Bacteriology, Virology and Immunity*, 8th edn, vol. 3, eds Parker MT, Collier LH, Edward Arnold, London, 470–87.

Gross RJ, Rowe B, Threlfall EJ, 1985, *Escherichia coli* O142.H6: a drug resistant enteropathogenic clone?, *J Hyg*, **94**: 181–91.

Gross RJ, Scotland SM, Rowe B, 1979, Enterotoxigenic *Escherichia coli* causing diarrhoea in travellers returning to the United Kingdom, *Br Med J*, **1**: 1463.

Gross RJ, Rowe B et al., 1976, A new *Escherichia coli* O group O159, associated with outbreaks of enteritis in infants, *Scand J Infect Dis*, **8**: 195–8.

Guinee PAM, Jansen WH, 1987, Serotyping of *Aeromonas* species using passive haemagglutination, *Zentralbl Bakteriol Hyg*, **265**: 305–13.

Günzer F, Böhm H et al., 1992, Molecular detection of sorbitol-fermenting *Escherichia coli* O157 in patients with hemolytic–uremic syndrome, *J Clin Microbiol*, **30**: 1807–10.

Gyles CL, 1994a, *Escherichia coli* enterotoxins, *Escherichia coli in Domestic Animals and Humans*, ed. Gyles CL, CAB International, Wallingford, UK, 337–64.

Gyles CL, 1994b, VT toxaemia in animal models, *Recent Advances in Verocytotoxin-producing Escherichia coli Infections*, eds Karmali MA, Goglio AG, Elsevier Science, Amsterdam, 233–40.

Hall GA, Reynolds DJ et al., 1985, Dysentery caused by *Escherichia coli* (S102-9) in calves: natural and experimental disease, *Vet Pathol*, **22**: 156–63.

Hampson DJ, 1994, Postweaning *Escherichia coli* diarrhoea in pigs, *Escherichia coli in Domestic Animals and Humans*, ed. Gyles CL, CAB International, Wallingford, UK, 171–91.

Havelaar AH, Schets FM et al., 1992, Typing of *Aeromonas* strains from patients with diarrhoea and from drinking water, *J Appl Bacteriol*, **72**: 435–44.

Hazen TC, Fliermans CB et al., 1978, Prevalence and distribution of *Aeromonas hydrophila* in the United States, *Appl Environ Microbiol*, **36**: 731–8.

Hii JH, Gyles C et al., 1991, Development of verotoxin 2- and verotoxin 2 variant (VT2v)-specific oligonucleotide probes on the basis of the nucleotide sequence of the B cistron of VT2v from *Escherichia coli* E32511 and B2F1, *J Clin Microbiol*, **29**: 2704–9.

Hindle MA, Bolton EJ et al., 1995, Improved detection of Vero cytotoxin-producing *Escherichia coli* O157 in faecal samples by enrichment culture, *PHLS Microbiol Dig*, **12**: 71–3.

Hirayama T, Wada A et al., 1992, Glycoprotein receptors for a heat-stable enterotoxin (STh) produced by enterotoxigenic *Escherichia coli*, *Infect Immun*, **60**: 4213–20.

Hobbs BC, Rowe B et al., 1976, *Escherichia coli* O27 in adult diarrhoea, *J Hyg*, **77**: 393–400.

Holmes RK, Twiddy EM, Pickett CL, 1986, Purification and characterization of type II heat-labile enterotoxin of *Escherichia coli*, *Infect Immun*, **53**: 464–73.

Holmgren J, 1985, Toxins affecting intestinal transport processes, *The Virulence of Escherichia coli: Reviews and Methods*, ed. Sussman M, Academic Press, London, 177–91.

Holmgren J, Fredman P et al., 1982, Rabbit intestinal glycoprotein receptors for *Escherichia coli* heat-labile enterotoxin lacking affinity for cholera toxin, *Infect Immun*, **38**: 424–33.

Honda T, Tsuji T et al., 1981, Immunological nonidentity of heat-labile enterotoxins from human and porcine enterotoxigenic *Escherichia coli*, *Infect Immun*, **34**: 337–40.

Hone R, Fitzpatrick S et al., 1973, Infantile enteritis in Dublin caused by *Escherichia coli* O142, *J Med Microbiol*, **6**: 505–10.

Igarashi K, Ogasawara T et al., 1987, Inhibition of elongation factor 1-dependent aminoacyl-tRNA binding to ribosomes by Shiga-like toxin 1 (VT1) from *Escherichia coli* O157:H7 and by Shiga-toxin, *FEMS Microbiol Lett*, **44**: 91–4.

Imberechts H, de Greve H et al., 1993, The role of adhesive F107 fimbriae and of SLT-IIv toxin in the pathogenesis of edema disease in pigs, *Zentralbl Bakteriol*, **278**: 445–50.

Jackson MP, Neill RJ et al., 1987, Nucleotide sequence analysis and comparison of the structural genes for Shiga-like toxin I and Shiga-like toxin II encoded by bacteriophages from *Escherichia coli* 933, *FEMS Microbiol Lett*, **44**: 109–14.

Jacobs I, Holzel A et al., 1970, Outbreak of infantile gastro-enteritis due to *Escherichia coli* O114, *Arch Dis Child*, **45**: 656–63.

Janda JM, Duffey PS, 1988, Mesophilic aeromonads in human disease: current taxonomy, laboratory identification and infectious disease spectrum, *Rev Infect Dis*, **10**: 980–7.

Jerse AE, Kaper JB, 1991, The *eae* gene of enteropathogenic *Escherichia coli* encodes a 94-kilodalton membrane protein, the expression of which is influenced by the EAF plasmid, *Infect Immun*, **59**: 4302–9.

Jerse AE, Yu J et al., 1990, A genetic locus of enteropathogenic *Escherichia coli* necessary for production of attaching and effacing lesions on tissue culture cells, *Proc Natl Acad Sci USA*, **87**: 7839–43.

Jiang ZD, Nelson AC et al., 1991, Intestinal secretory response to infection with *Aeromonas* species and *Plesiomonas shigelloides* among students from the United States in Mexico, *J Infect Dis*, **164**: 979–82.

Kain KC, Barteluk RL et al., 1991, Etiology of childhood diarrhea in Beijing, China, *J Clin Microbiol*, **29**: 90–5.

van de Kar NCAJ, Monnens LAH et al., 1992, Tumor necrosis factor and interleukin-1 induce expression of the Vero cytotoxin receptor globotriaosylceramide on human endothelial cells: implications for the pathogenesis of the hemolytic uremic syndrome, *Blood*, **80**: 2755–64.

Karch H, Meyer T, 1989a, Evaluation of oligonucleotide probes for identification of Shiga-like-toxin-producing *Escherichia coli*, *J Clin Microbiol*, **27**: 1180–6.

Karch H, Meyer T, 1989b, Single primer pair for amplifying segments of distinct Shiga-like-toxin genes by polymerase chain reaction, *J Clin Microbiol*, **27**: 2751–7.

Karmali MA, 1989, Infection by verocytotoxin-producing *Escherichia coli*, *Clin Microbiol Rev*, **2**: 15–38.

Karmali MA, Steele BT et al., 1983, Sporadic cases of haemolytic–uraemic syndrome associated with faecal cytotoxin and cytotoxin-producing *Escherichia coli* in stools, *Lancet*, **1**: 619–20.

Karmali MA, Petric M et al., 1985a, The association between idiopathic hemolytic uremic syndrome and infection by verotoxin-producing *Escherichia coli*, *J Infect Dis*, **151**: 775–82.

Karmali MA, Petric M et al., 1985b, Sensitive method for detecting low numbers of verotoxin-producing *Escherichia coli* in mixed cultures by use of colony sweeps and polymyxin extraction of verotoxin, *J Clin Microbiol*, **22**: 614–19.

Karmali MA, Petric M et al., 1994, Enzyme-linked immunosorbent assay for detection of immunoglobulin G antibodies to *Escherichia coli* Vero cytotoxin 1, *J Clin Microbiol*, **32**: 1457–63.

Katayama S, Ninomiya M et al., 1990, Transcriptional control plays an important role for the production of heat-labile enterotoxin in enterotoxigenic *Escherichia coli* of human origin, *Microbiol Immunol*, **34**: 11–24.

Kauffmann F, 1944, Zur serologie der coli-gruppe, *Acta Pathol Microbiol Scand*, **21**: 20–45.

Kauffmann F, 1947, The serology of the coli group, *J Immunol*, **57**: 71–100.

Kavi J, Chant I et al., 1987, Cytopathic effect of verotoxin on endothelial cells, *Lancet*, **2**: 1035.

Kennedy DH, Walter GH et al., 1973, An outbreak of infantile gastro-enteritis due to *E. coli* O142, *J Clin Pathol*, **26**: 731–7.

Kim HH, Samadpour M et al., 1994, Characteristics of antibiotic resistant *Escherichia coli* O157:H7 in Washington State, 1984–1991, *J Infect Dis*, **170**: 1606–9.

Kleanthous H, Smith HR et al., 1990, Haemolytic uraemic syndromes in the British Isles, 1985–8: association with Vero cytotoxin producing *Escherichia coli*. Part 2: microbiological aspects, *Arch Dis Child*, **65**: 722–7.

Knutton S, Lloyd DR, McNeish AS, 1987, Adhesion of enteropathogenic *Escherichia coli* to human intestinal enterocytes and cultured human intestinal mucosa, *Infect Immun*, **55**: 69–77.

Knutton S, Baldwin T et al., 1989, Actin accumulation at sites of bacterial adhesion to tissue culture cells: basis of a new diagnostic test for enteropathogenic and enterohemorrhagic *Escherichia coli*, *Infect Immun*, **57**: 1290–8.

Knutton S, Shaw RK et al., 1992, Ability of enteroaggregative *Escherichia coli* strains to adhere in vitro to human intestinal mucosa, *Infect Immun*, **60**: 2083–91.

Knutton S, Baldwin TJ et al., 1994, Intracellular changes in 'attaching and effacing' adhesion, *Recent Advances in Verocytotoxin-producing Escherichia coli* Infections, eds Karmali MA, Goglio AG, Elsevier Science, Amsterdam, 215–22.

Konowalchuk J, Speirs JI, Stavric S, 1977, Vero response to a cytotoxin of *Escherichia coli*, *Infect Immun*, **18**: 775–9.

Kooij N, Fainstein V, 1988, Properties of aeromonads and their occurrence and hygienic significance in drinking waters, *Zentralbl Bakteriol Hyg B*, **187**: 1–17.

Kudoh Y, Zen-Yogi H et al., 1977, Outbreaks of acute enteritis due to heat-stable enterotoxin-producing strains of *Escherichia coli*, *Microbiol Immunol*, **21**: 175–8.

Kudoh Y, Kai A et al., 1994, Epidemiological surveys on verocytotoxin-producing *Escherichia coli* infections in Japan, *Recent Advances in Verocytotoxin-producing Escherichia coli* Infections, eds Karmali MA, Goglio AG, Elsevier Science, Amsterdam, 53–6.

Kuijper EJ, Bol P et al., 1989, Clinical and epidemiologic aspects of members of *Aeromonas* DNA hybridization groups isolated from human feces, *J Clin Microbiol*, **27**: 1531–7.

Lawson MA, Burke V, Chang BJ, 1985, Invasion of HEp-2 cells by fecal isolates of *Aeromonas hydrophila*, *Infect Immun*, **47**: 680–3.

Lee CH, Moseley SL et al., 1983, Characterization of the gene encoding heat-stable toxin II and preliminary molecular epidemiological studies of enterotoxigenic *Escherichia coli* heat-stable toxin II, *Infect Immun*, **42**: 264–8.

Lesage AA, 1897, Contribution á l'étude des entérites infantiles; séro-diagnostic; des races de *Bactérium coli*, *C R Soc Biol (Paris)*, **49**: 900–1.

Levett PN, Daniel RR, 1981, Adhesion of vibrios and aeromonads to isolated rabbit brush borders, *J Gen Microbiol*, **125**: 167–72.

Levine MM, 1987, *Escherichia coli* that cause diarrhea: enterotoxigenic, enteropathogenic enteroinvasive, enterohemorrhagic and enteroadherent, *J Infect Dis*, **155**: 377–89.

Levine MM, Edelman R, 1984, Enteropathogenic *Escherichia coli* of classic serotypes associated with infant diarrhea: epidemiology and pathogenesis, *Epidemiol Rev*, **6**: 31–51.

Levine MM, Bergquist EJ et al., 1978, *Escherichia coli* strains that cause diarrhoea but do not produce heat-labile or heat-stable enterotoxins and are non-invasive, *Lancet*, **1**: 1119–22.

Levine MM, Nalin D et al., 1979, Immunity to enterotoxigenic *Escherichia coli*, *Infect Immun*, **23**: 729–36.

Levine MM, Black RE et al., 1982, Reactogenicity, immunogenicity and efficacy studies of *Escherichia coli* type 1 somatic pili parenteral vaccine in man, *Scand J Infect Dis Suppl*, **33**: 83–95.

Levine MM, Nataro JP et al., 1985, The diarrheal response of humans to some classic serotypes of enteropathogenic *Escherichia coli* is dependent on a plasmid encoding enteroadhesiveness factor, *J Infect Dis*, **152:** 550–9.

Levine MM, Prado V et al., 1988, Use of DNA probes and HEp-2 cell adherence assay to detect diarrheagenic *Escherichia coli*, *J Infect Dis*, **158:** 224–8.

Levine MM, Ferreccio C et al., 1993, Epidemiologic studies of *Escherichia coli* diarrheal infections in a low socioeconomic level periurbal community in Santiago, Chile, *Am J Epidemiol*, **138:** 849–68.

Lingwood CA, 1994, Verotoxin recognition of its glycolipid receptor, globotriaosylceramide: role in pathogenesis, *Recent Advances in Verocytotoxin-producing Escherichia coli* Infections, eds Karmali MA, Goglio AG, Elsevier Science, Amsterdam, 131–7.

Lingwood CA, Law H et al., 1987, Glycolipid binding of natural and recombinant *Escherichia coli* produced verotoxin *in-vitro*, *J Biol Chem*, **262:** 8834–9.

Ljungh A, Eneroth P, Wadström T, 1981, Separation and characterization of enterotoxin and two hemoysins from *Aeromonas hydrophila*, *Acta Pathol Microbiol Scand Sect B*, **89:** 787–94.

Lopez EL, Diaz M et al., 1989, Hemolytic uremic syndrome and diarrhea in Argentine children: the role of Shiga-like toxin, *J Infect Dis*, **160:** 469–75.

Love WC, Gordon AM et al., 1972, Infantile gastroenteritis due to *Escherichia coli* O142, *Lancet*, **2:** 355–7.

Mainil JF, Duchesnes CJ et al., 1987, Shiga-like toxin production and attaching effacing activity of *Escherichia coli* associated with calf diarrhea, *Am J Vet Res*, 743–8.

March SB, Ratnam S, 1986, Sorbitol–MacConkey medium for detection of *Escherichia coli* O157:H7 associated with hemorrhagic colitis, *J Clin Microbiol*, **23:** 869–72.

Marques LRM, Peiris JSM et al., 1987, *Escherichia coli* strains isolated from pigs with edema disease produce a variant of Shiga-like toxin II, *FEMS Microbiol Lett*, **44:** 33–8.

Mathewson JJ, DuPont HL, 1991, *Aeromonas* species: role as human pathogens, *Curr Clin Top Infect Dis*, **12:** 26–36.

Mathewson JJ, Johnson PC et al., 1986, Pathogenicity of enteroadherent *Escherichia coli* in adult volunteers, *J Infect Dis*, **154:** 524–7.

Mathewson JJ, Oberhelman RA et al., 1987, Enteroadherent *Escherichia coli* as a cause of diarrhea among children in Mexico, *J Clin Microbiol*, **25:** 1917–19.

Megraud F, 1986, Incidence and virulence of *Aeromonas* species in faeces of children with diarrhoea, *Eur J Clin Microbiol*, **5:** 787–94.

Merson MH, Morris GK et al., 1976, Travelers' diarrhea in Mexico, *N Engl J Med*, **294:** 1299–305.

Millership SE, Curnow SR, Chattopadhyay B, 1983, Faecal carriage rate of *Aeromonas hydrophila*, *J Clin Pathol*, **380:** 920–3.

Millership SE, Stephenson JR, Tabaqchali S, 1987, Epidemiology of *Aeromonas* species in a hospital, *J Hosp Infect*, **11:** 169–75.

Mochmann H, Ocklitz HW et al., 1974, Oral immunization with an extract of *E. coli* enteritidis, *Acta Microbiol Acad Scient Hung*, **21:** 193–6.

Moloney AC, Corbett-Feeney G et al., 1985, Gastroenteritis associated with enterotoxigenic *Escherichia coli* O78:H12, *Irish J Med Sci*, **154:** 23–6.

Montenegro MA, Bülte M et al., 1990, Detection and characterization of fecal verotoxin-producing *Escherichia coli* from healthy cattle, *J Clin Microbiol*, **28:** 1417–21.

Moon HW, Whipp SC et al., 1983, Attaching and effacing activities of rabbit and human enteropathogenic *Escherichia coli* in pig and rabbit intestines, *Infect Immun*, **41:** 1340–51.

Morgan DR, Johnson PC et al., 1985, Lack of correlation between known virulence properties of *Aeromonas hydrophila* and enteropathogenicity for humans, *Infect Immun*, **50:** 62–5.

Morgan GM, Newman C et al., 1988, First recognised community outbreak of haemorrhagic colitis due to verotoxin-producing *Escherichia coli* O157:H7 in the UK, *Epidemiol Infect*, **101:** 83–91.

Namdari H, Bottone EJ, 1990, Cytotoxin and enterotoxin production as factors delineating enteropathogenicity of *Aeromonas caviae*, *J Clin Microbiol*, **28:** 1796–8.

Nataro JP, Kaper JB et al., 1987, Patterns of adherence of diarrheagenic *Escherichia coli* to HEp-2 cells, *J Pediatr Infect Dis*, **16:** 829–31.

Nataro JP, Deng Y et al., 1992, Aggregative adherence fimbriae I of enteroaggregative *Escherichia coli* mediate adherence to HEp-2 cells and hemagglutination of human erythrocytes, *Infect Immun*, **60:** 2297–304.

Nataro JP, Yikang D et al., 1995, Heterogeneity of enteroaggregative *Escherichia coli* virulence demonstrated in volunteers, *J Infect Dis*, **171:** 465–8.

Nathwani D, Robert BS et al., 1991, Treatment of symptomatic enteric *Aeromonas hydrophila* infection with ciprofloxacin, *Scand J Infect Dis*, **23:** 653–4.

Neter E, Westphal O et al., 1955, Demonstration of antibodies against enteropathogenic *Escherichia coli* in sera of children of various ages, *Pediatrics*, **16:** 801–7.

Newburg DS, Chaturvedi P et al., 1993, Susceptibility to hemolytic–uremic syndrome relates to erythrocyte glycosphingolipid patterns, *J Infect Dis*, **168:** 476–9.

Newland JW, Strockbine NA et al., 1985, Cloning of Shiga-like toxin structural genes from a toxin converting phage of *Escherichia coli*, *Science*, **230:** 179–81.

Nishikawa Y, Kimura T, Kishi T, 1991, Mannose-resistant adhesion of motile *Aeromonas* to INT407 cells and the differences among isolates from humans, food and water, *Epidemiol Infect*, **107:** 171–9.

O'Brien AD, Holmes RK, 1987, Shiga and Shiga-like toxins, *Microbiol Rev*, **51:** 206–20.

O'Brien AD, LaVeck GD, 1983, Purification and characterization of a *Shigella dysenteriae* 1-like toxin produced by *Escherichia coli*, *Infect Immun*, **40:** 675–83.

O'Brien AD, LaVeck GD et al., 1982, Production of *Shigella dysenteriae* type 1-like cytotoxin by *Escherichia coli*, *J Infect Dis*, **146:** 763–9.

O'Brien AD, Newland JW et al., 1984, Shiga-like toxin-converting phages from *Escherichia coli* strains that cause hemorrhagic colitis or infantile diarrhea, *Science*, **226:** 694–6.

Obrig TG, Del Vecchio PJ et al., 1987, Pathogenesis of haemolytic uraemic syndrome, *Lancet*, **2:** 687.

Obrig TG, Del Vecchio PJ et al., 1988, Direct cytotoxic action of Shiga toxin on human vascular endothelial cells, *Infect Immun*, **56:** 2373–8.

Obrig TG, Louise CB et al., 1993, Endothelial heterogeneity in Shiga toxin receptors and responses, *J Biol Chem*, **268:** 15484–8.

Old DC, Gordon DP, Hill A, 1986, A one-year study of the incidence of motile *Aeromonas* among Dundee patients with gastroenteritis, *Comm Dis Scot*, **51:** 7–10.

O'Mahoney MC, Noah ND et al., 1986, An outbreak of gastroenteritis on a passenger cruise ship, *J Hyg*, **97:** 229–36.

Ørskov F, Ørskov I, Villar JA, 1977, Cattle as reservoir of verotoxin-producing *Escherichia coli* O157:H7, *Lancet*, **2:** 276.

Ørskov I, Wachsmuth IK et al., 1991, Two new *Escherichia coli* O groups: O172 from Shiga-like toxin II-producing strains (EHEC) and O173 from enteroinvasive *E. coli* (EIEC), *Acta Pathol Microbiol*, **99:** 30–2.

Pai CH, Kelly JK, Meyers GL, 1986, Experimental infection of infant rabbits with verotoxin-producing *Escherichia coli*, *Infect Immun*, **51:** 16–23.

Pai CH, Ahmed N et al., 1988, Epidemiology of sporadic diarrhea due to Vero cytotoxin-producing *Escherichia coli*: a two year prospective study, *J Infect Dis*, **157:** 1054–7.

Palumbo SA, Bencivengo MM et al., 1989, Characterization of the *Aeromonas hydrophila* group isolated from retail foods of animal origin, *J Clin Microbiol*, **27:** 854–9.

Picard B, Goullet P, 1987, Seasonal prevalence of nosocomial *Aeromonas hydrophila* infection related to *Aeromonas* in hospital water, *J Hosp Infect*, **10:** 152–5.

Pickett CL, Twiddy EM et al., 1986, Cloning of genes that encode a new heat-labile enterotoxin of *Escherichia coli*, *J Bacteriol*, **165**: 348–52.

Pickett CL, Twiddy EM et al., 1989, Cloning, nucleotide sequence, and hybridization studies of the type IIb heat-labile enterotoxin gene of *Escherichia coli*, *J Bacteriol*, **171**: 4945–52.

Pitarangsi C, Echeverria P et al., 1982, Enteropathogenicity of *Aeromonas hydrophila* and *Plesiomonas shigelloides*: prevalence among individuals with and without diarrhea in Thailand, *Infect Immun*, **35**: 666–73.

Pollard DR, Johnson WM et al., 1990, Rapid and specific detection of verotoxin genes in *Escherichia coli* by the polymerase chain reaction, *J Clin Microbiol*, **28**: 540–5.

Polotsky YE, Dragunskaya EM et al., 1977, Pathogenic effect of enterotoxigenic *Escherichia coli* and *Escherichia coli* causing infantile diarrhoea, *Acta Microbiol Acad Scient Hung*, **24**: 221–36.

Popoff MY, 1984, *Bergey's Manual of Systematic Bacteriology*, 9th edn, Williams and Wilkins, Baltimore, 545–8.

Rauss K, Ketyi I et al., 1972, Specific oral prevention of infantile enteritis. 3. Experiments with corpuscular vaccine, *Acta Microbiol Acad Scient Hung*, **19**: 19–28.

Read SC, Gyles CL et al., 1990, Prevalence of Vero cytotoxigenic *Escherichia coli* in ground beef, pork and chicken in South Western Ontario, *Epidemiol Infect*, **105**: 11–20.

Reid RH, Boedeker EC et al., 1993, Preclinical evaluation of microencapsulated CFA/II oral vaccine against enterotoxigenic *E. coli*, *Vaccine*, **11**: 159–67.

Richardson SE, Rotman TA et al., 1992, Experimental verocytotoxemia in rabbits, *Infect Immun*, **60**: 4154–67.

Rietra PJGM, Willshaw GA et al., 1989, Comparison of Vero-cytotoxin-encoding phages from *Escherichia coli* of human and bovine origin, *J Gen Microbiol*, **135**: 2307–18.

Riley LW, Remis RS et al., 1983, Hemorrhagic colitis associated with a rare *Escherichia coli* serotype, *N Engl J Med*, **308**: 681–5.

Riordan T, Gross RJ et al., 1985, An outbreak of food-borne enterotoxigenic *Escherichia coli* diarrhoea in England, *J Infect*, **11**: 167–71.

Robertson DC, Dreyfus LA, Frantz JC, 1983, Chemical and immunological properties of *Escherichia coli* heat-stable enterotoxins, *Prog Food Nutr Sci*, **7**: 147–56.

Roderick P, Wheeler J et al., 1995, A pilot study of infectious intestinal disease in England, *Epidemiol Infect*, **114**: 277–88.

Rosenberg ML, Koplan JP et al., 1977, Epidemic diarrhea at Crater Lake from enterotoxigenic *Escherichia coli*, *Ann Intern Med*, **86**: 714–18.

Rothbaum R, McAdams AJ et al., 1982, A clinico pathologic study of enterocyte-adherent *Escherichia coli*: a cause of protracted diarrhea in infants, *Gastroenterology*, **83**: 441–54.

Rowe B, Gross RJ, Scotland SM, 1976, Serotyping of *E. coli*, *Lancet*, **2**: 37–8.

Rowe B, Taylor J, Bettelheim KA, 1970, An investigation of travellers' diarrhoea, *Lancet*, **1**: 1–5.

Rowe B, Gross RJ et al., 1978, Outbreak of infantile enteritis caused by enterotoxigenic *Escherichia coli* O6H16, *J Clin Pathol*, **31**: 217–19.

Ryder RW, Wachsmuth IK et al., 1976, Infantile diarrhea produced by heat-stable enterotoxigenic *Escherichia coli*, *N Engl J Med*, **295**: 849–53.

Ryder RW, Greenberg H et al., 1982, Seroepidemiology of heat-labile enterotoxigenic *Escherichia coli* and Norwalk virus infections in Panamanians, Canal Zone residents, Apachi Indians and United States Peace Corps volunteers, *Infect Immun*, **37**: 903–6.

Sakazaki R, Shimada T, 1984, O-serogrouping scheme for mesophilic *Aeromonas* strains, *Jpn J Med Sci Biol*, **37**: 247–55.

Salmon RL, Farrell ID et al., 1989, A christening party outbreak of haemorrhagic colitis and haemolytic uraemic syndrome associated with *Escherichia coli* O157:H7, *Epidemiol Infect*, **103**: 249–54.

Samuel JE, Perera LP et al., 1990, Comparison of the glycolipid receptor specificities of Shiga-like toxin type II and Shiga-like toxin type II variants, *Infect Immun*, **58**: 611–18.

San Joaquin VH, Pickett DA, 1988, *Aeromonas*-associated gastroenteritis in children, *Pediatr Infect Dis J*, **7**: 53–7.

Sanyal SC, Singh JC, Sen PC, 1975, Enteropathogenicity of *Aeromonas hydrophila* and *Plesiomonas shigelloides*, *J Med Microbiol*, **8**: 195–8.

Savarino SJ, Fasano A et al., 1991, Enteroaggregative *Escherichia coli* elaborate a heat-stable enterotoxin demonstrable in an in vitro rabbit intestinal model, *J Clin Invest*, **87**: 1450–5.

Savarino SJ, Fasano A et al., 1993, Enteroaggregative *Escherichia coli* heat-stable enterotoxin 1 represents another subfamily of *E. coli* heat-stable toxin, *Proc Natl Acad Sci USA*, **90**: 3093–7.

Scaletsky ICA, Silva MLM et al., 1984, Distinctive patterns of adherence of enteropathogenic *Escherichia coli* to HeLa cells, *Infect Immun*, **45**: 534–6.

Schmidt H, Beutin L, Karch H, 1995, Molecular analysis of the plasmid-encoded hemolysin of *Escherichia coli* O157:H7 strain EDL 933, *Infect Immun*, **63**: 1055–61.

Schmidt H, Karch H, Beutin L, 1994, The large-sized plasmids of enterohaemorrhagic *Escherichia coli* O157 strains encode hemolysins, which are presumably members of the *E. coli*-α hemolysin family, *FEMS Microbiol Lett*, **117**: 189–96.

Schmitt CK, McKee ML, O'Brien AD, 1991, Two copies of Shiga-like toxin II-related genes common in enterohemorrhagic *Escherichia coli* strains are responsible for the antigenic heterogeneity of the O157:H- strain E32511, *Infect Immun*, **59**: 1065–73.

Schroeder S, Caldwell JR et al., 1968, A water-borne outbreak of gastro-enteritis in adults associated with *Escherichia coli*, *Lancet*, **2**: 737–40.

Scotland SM, Day NP, Rowe B, 1980, Production of a cytotoxin affecting Vero cells by strains of *Escherichia coli* belonging to traditional enteropathogenic serogroups, *FEMS Microbiol Lett*, 15–17.

Scotland SM, Flomen RH, Rowe B, 1989, Evaluation of a reversed passive latex agglutination test for the detection of *Escherichia coli* heat-labile toxin in culture supernatants, *J Clin Microbiol*, **27**: 339–40.

Scotland SM, Gross RJ, Rowe B, 1985, Laboratory tests for enterotoxin production, enteroinvasion and adhesion in diarrhoeagenic *Escherichia coli*, *The Virulence of Escherichia coli. Reviews and Methods*, ed. Sussman M, Academic Press, London, 395–405.

Scotland SM, Smith HR, Rowe B, 1985, Two distinct toxins active on Vero cells from *Escherichia coli* O157, *Lancet*, **2**: 885–6.

Scotland SM, Smith HR et al., 1983, Vero cytotoxin production in strain of *Escherichia coli* is determined by genes carried on bacteriophage, *Lancet*, **2**: 216.

Scotland SM, Rowe B et al., 1988, Vero cytotoxin-producing strains of *Escherichia coli* from children with haemolytic uraemic syndrome and their detection by specific DNA probes, *J Med Microbiol*, **25**: 237–43.

Scotland SM, Willshaw GA et al., 1989a, Adhesion to cells in culture and plasmid profiles of enteropathogenic *Escherichia coli* isolated from outbreaks and sporadic cases of infant diarrhoea, *J Infect*, **19**: 237–49.

Scotland SM, Willshaw GA et al., 1989b, Identification of *Escherichia coli* that produces heat-stable enterotoxin ST$_A$ by a commercially available enzyme-linked immunoassay and comparison of the assay with infant mouse and DNA probe tests, *J Clin Microbiol*, **27**: 1697–9.

Scotland SM, Smith HR et al., 1991, Identification of enteropathogenic *Escherichia coli* isolated in Britain as enteroaggregative or as members of a subclass of attaching-and-effacing *E. coli* not hybridizing with the EPEC adherence-factor probe, *J Med Microbiol*, **35**: 278–83.

Scotland SM, Willshaw GA et al., 1993, Virulence properties of *Escherichia coli* strains belonging to serogroups O26, O55, O111 and O128 isolated in the United Kingdom in 1991 from patients with diarrhoea, *Epidemiol Infect*, **111**: 429–38.

Scotland SM, Willshaw GA et al., 1994, Association of enteroaggregative *Escherichia coli* with travellers' diarrhoea, *J Infect*, **29:** 115–16.

Sherwood D, Snodgrass DR, O'Brien AD, 1985, Shiga-like toxin production from *Escherichia coli* associated with calf diarrhoea, *Vet Rec*, **116:** 217–18.

Singh DV, Sanyal SC, 1992, Haemolysin and enterotoxin production by *Aeromonas caviae* isolated from diarrhoeal patients, fish and environment, *J Diarrhoeal Dis Res*, **1:** 16–20.

Sixma TK, Kalk KH et al., 1993, Refined structure of *Escherichia coli* heat-labile enterotoxin, a close relative of cholera toxin, *J Mol Biol*, **230:** 890–910.

Smith HR, Willshaw GA, Rowe B, 1982, Mapping of a plasmid, coding for colonization factor antigen I and heat-stable enterotoxin production, isolated from an enterotoxigenic strain of *Escherichia coli*, *J Bacteriol*, **149:** 264–75.

Smith HR, Scotland SM et al., 1988, Vero cytotoxin production and presence of VT genes in *Escherichia coli* strains of animal origin, *J Gen Microbiol*, **134:** 829–34.

Smith HR, Scotland SM et al., 1990, Examination of strains belonging to enteropathogenic *Escherichia coli* serogroups for genes encoding EPEC adherence factor and Vero cytotoxins, *J Med Microbiol*, **31:** 234–40.

Smith HR, Cheasty T et al., 1991, Examination of retail chickens and sausages in Britain for Vero cytotoxin-producing *Escherichia coli*, *Appl Environ Microbiol*, **57:** 2091–3.

Smith HR, Willshaw GA et al., 1993, Properties of Vero cytotoxin-producing *Escherichia coli* isolated from human sources, *Zentralbl Bakteriol*, **278:** 436–44.

Smith HR, Scotland SM et al., 1994, Isolates of *Escherichia coli* O44:H18 of diverse origin are enteroaggregative, *J Infect Dis*, **170:** 1610–13.

Smith HW, Green P, Parsell Z, 1983, Vero cell toxins in *Escherichia coli* and related bacteria: transfer by phage and conjugation and toxic action in laboratory animals, chickens and pigs, *J Gen Microbiol*, **129:** 3121–37.

Smith HW, Linggood MA, 1971, Observations on the pathogenic properties of the K88, Hly and Ent plasmids of *Escherichia coli* with particular reference to porcine diarrhoea, *J Med Microbiol*, **4:** 467–85.

Smith J, 1949, The association of certain types (α and β) of *Bact. coli* with infantile gastroenteritis, *J Hyg*, **47:** 221–6.

Smyth CJ, 1982, Two mannose-resistant haemagglutinins of enterotoxigenic *Escherichia coli* of serotype O6:K15:H16 or H- isolated from travellers and infantile diarrhoea, *J Gen Microbiol*, **128:** 2081–96.

Smyth CJ, Marron M, Smith SGJ, 1994, Fimbriae of *Escherichia coli*, *Escherichia coli* in Domestic Animals and Humans, ed. Gyles CL, CAB International, Wallingford, UK, 399–435.

So M, McCarthy BJ, 1980, Nucleotide sequence of the bacterial transposon Tn1681 encoding a heat-stable (ST) toxin and its identification in enterotoxigenic *Escherichia coli* strains, *Proc Natl Acad Sci USA*, **77:** 4011–15.

Sommerfelt H, 1991, Nucleic acid hybridization for the identification of enterotoxigenic *Escherichia coli*, *Rev Med Microbiol*, **2:** 138–46.

Stein PE, Boodhoo A et al., 1992, Crystal structure of the cell-binding B oligomer of verotoxin-1 from *E. coli*, *Nature (London)*, **355:** 748–50.

Stieglitz H, Cervantes L et al., 1988, Cloning sequencing and expression in Ficoll generated minicells of an *Escherichia coli* heat stable enterotoxin gene, *Plasmid*, **20:** 42–53.

Svennerholm A-M, Holmgren J, Sack DA, 1989, Development of oral vaccines against enterotoxigenic *Escherichia coli* diarrhoea, *Vaccine*, **7:** 196–8.

Swerdlow DL, Woodruff A et al., 1992, A waterborne outbreak in Missouri of *Escherichia coli* O157:H7 associated with bloody diarrhea and death, *Ann Intern Med*, **117:** 812–19.

Synge BA, Hopkins GF, 1992, Verotoxigenic *Escherichia coli* O157 in Scottish calves, *Vet Rec*, **130:** 583.

Tacket CO, Losonsky G et al., 1988, Protection by milk immunoglobulin concentrate against oral challenge with enterotoxigenic *Escherichia coli* diarrhea, *N Engl J Med*, **318:** 1240–3.

Tacket CO, Moseley SL et al., 1990, Challenge studies in volunteers using *Escherichia coli* strains with diffuse adherence to HEp-2 cells, *J Infect Dis*, **162:** 550–2.

Tacket CO, Losonsky GA et al., 1993, Phase 1 study of an ETEC vaccine consisting of CFA/II in biodegradable polymer microspheres, *Abstracts 93rd Mtg ASM, Washington DC*, 153.

Taylor CM, Milford DV et al., 1990, The expression of blood group P1 in post-enteropathic haemolytic uraemic syndrome, *Pediatr Nephrol*, **4:** 59–61.

Tesh VL, Ramegowda B, Samuel JE, 1994, Purified Shiga-like toxins induce expression of proinflammatory cytokines from murine peritoneal macrophages, *Infect Immun*, **62:** 5085–94.

Tesh VL, Samuel JE et al., 1991, Evaluation of the role of Shiga and Shiga-like toxins in mediating direct damage to human vascular endothelial cells, *J Infect Dis*, **164:** 344–52.

Thomas A, Chart H et al., 1993, Vero cytotoxin-producing *Escherichia coli*, particularly serogroup O157, associated with human infections in the United Kingdom: 1989–91, *Epidemiol Infect*, **110:** 591–600.

Tokhi AM, Peiris JSM et al., 1993, A longitudinal study of Vero cytotoxin producing *Escherichia coli* in cattle calves in Sri Lanka, *Epidemiol Infect*, **110:** 197–208.

Tzipori S, Wachsmuth IK et al., 1986, The pathogenesis of hemorrhagic colitis caused by *Escherichia coli* O157:H7 in gnotobiotic piglets, *J Infect Dis*, **154:** 712–16.

Tzipori S, Karch H et al., 1987, Role of a 60 megadalton plasmid and Shiga-like toxins in the pathogenesis of infection caused by enterohemorrhagic *Escherichia coli* O157:H7 in gnotobiotic piglets, *Infect Immun*, **55:** 3117–25.

Tzipori S, Montanaro J et al., 1992, Studies with enteroaggregative *Escherichia coli* in the gnotobiotic piglet gastroenteritis model, *Infect Immun*, **60:** 5302–6.

Ulshen MH, Rollo JL, 1980, Pathogenesis of *Escherichia coli* gastroenteritis in man – another mechanism, *N Engl J Med*, **302:** 99–101.

Upton P, Coia JE, 1994, Outbreak of *Escherichia coli* O157 infection associated with pasteurised milk supply, *Lancet*, **344:** 1015.

Vernon E, 1969, Food poisoning and Salmonella infections in England and Wales 1967, *Public Health (London)*, **83:** 205–23.

Vial PA, Robins-Browne R et al., 1988, Characterization of enteroadherent–aggregative *Escherichia coli*, a putative agent of diarrheal disease, *J Infect Dis*, **158:** 70–9.

Wadström T, Aust-Kettis A et al., 1976, Enterotoxin-producing bacteria and parasites in stools of Ethiopian children with diarrhoeal disease, *Arch Dis Child*, **51:** 865–70.

Wanke CA, Schorling JB et al., 1991, Potential role of adherence traits of *Escherichia coli* in persistent diarrhea in an urban Brazilian slum, *Pediatr Infect Dis J*, **10:** 746–51.

Watson IM, Robinson JO et al., 1985, Invasiveness of *Aeromonas* spp. in relation to biotype, virulence factors and clinical features, *J Clin Microbiol*, **22:** 48–51.

Weinstein DL, Jackson MP et al., 1988, Cloning and sequencing of a Shiga-like toxin type II variant from an *Escherichia coli* strain responsible for edema disease of swine, *J Bacteriol*, **170:** 4223–30.

Wells JG, Shipman LD et al., 1991, Isolation of *Escherichia coli* serotype O157:H7 and other Shiga-like toxin-producing *E. coli* from dairy cattle, *J Clin Microbiol*, **29:** 985–9.

Wilcox MH, Cook AM et al., 1992, *Aeromonas* spp. as a potential cause of diarrhoea in children, *J Clin Pathol*, **45:** 959–63.

Williams LA, LaRock PA, 1985, Temporal occurrence of *Vibrio* species and *Aeromonas hydrophila* in estuarine sediments, *Appl Environ Microbiol*, **50:** 1490–5.

Willshaw GA, Smith HR et al., 1985, Cloning of genes determining the production of Vero cytotoxin by *Escherichia coli*, *J Gen Microbiol*, **131:** 3047–53.

Willshaw GA, Smith HR et al., 1987, Heterogeneity of *Escherichia coli* phages encoding Vero cytotoxins: comparison of cloned sequences determining VT1 and VT2 and development of specific gene probes, *J Gen Microbiol*, **133:** 1309–17.

Willshaw GA, Scotland SM et al., 1992, Properties of Vero cytotoxin-producing *Escherichia coli* of human origin of O serogroups other than O157, *J Infect Dis*, **166:** 797–802.

Willshaw GA, Cheasty T et al., 1993a, Vero cytotoxin-producing *Escherichia coli* in a herd of dairy cattle, *Vet Rec*, **132:** 96.

Willshaw GA, Smith HR et al., 1993b, Examination of raw beef products for the presence of Vero cytotoxin producing *Escherichia coli*, particularly those of serogroup O157, *J Appl Bacteriol*, **75:** 420–6.

Willshaw GA, Thirlwell J et al., 1994, Vero cytotoxin-producing *Escherichia coli* O157 in beefburgers linked to an outbreak of diarrhoea, haemorrhagic colitis and haemolytic uraemic syndrome, *Lett Appl Microbiol*, **18:** 304–7.

Wood MJ, 1990, The use of antibiotics in infections due to *Escherichia coli* O157:H7, *PHLS Microbiol Dig*, **8:** 18–22.

Wray C, Woodward MJ, 1994, Laboratory diagnosis of *Escherichia coli* infections, *Escherichia coli* in Domestic Animals and Humans, ed. Gyles CL, CAB International, Wallingford, UK, 595–628.

Yamamoto T, Yokota T, 1983, Sequence of heat-labile enterotoxin of *Escherichia coli* pathogenic for humans, *J Bacteriol*, **155:** 728–33.

Yamamoto T, Koyama Y et al., 1992, Localized, aggregative and diffuse adherence to HeLa cells, plastic, and human small intestines by *Escherichia coli* isolated from patients with diarrhea, *J Infect Dis*, **166:** 1295–310.

Yu J, Kaper JB, 1992, Cloning and characterization of the *eae* gene of enterohaemorrhagic *Escherichia coli* O157:H7, *Mol Microbiol*, **6:** 411–17.

Zadik PM, Chapman PA, Siddons CA, 1993, Use of tellurite for the selection of Vero cytotoxigenic *Escherichia coli* O157, *J Med Microbiol*, **39:** 155–8.

Zywno SR, Arceneaux El et al., 1992, Siderophore production and DNA hybridization groups of *Aeromonas* species, *J Clin Microbiol*, **30:** 619–20.

Food-borne Bacterial Gastroenteritis

R J Gilbert and T J Humphrey

Consumption of unwholesome food may give rise to bacterial, mycotic, viral or helminthic infections, or to poisoning caused by toxins present in the food before ingestion. In the latter type of disease a distinction must be made between toxins of bacterial or chemical origin. Though this chapter deals with bacterial gastroenteritis, chemical poisoning will be considered briefly for purposes of differential diagnosis.

1 Chemical food poisoning

Certain foods may inherently be poisonous, such as toadstools, cereals infected with the fungus *Claviceps purpurea* that forms the poison responsible for ergotism, and incorrectly stored scombroid fish. Heavy metals, particularly lead, arsenic, zinc, cadmium and mercury and their compounds, may contaminate foods and powders such as nicotinic acid and sodium fluoride may be mistaken for flour. Mussels and some fish, mainly in warm latitudes, that have fed on marine dinoflagellates may be capable of causing paralytic shellfish and ciguatera poisoning. Foods may also contain aflatoxin.

In the UK, chemical food poisoning is probably responsible for less than 1% of all food-poisoning episodes, but in eastern countries it is said to be more common. In Spain a very large outbreak of chemical food poisoning was attributed to the consumption of olive oil adulterated with chemically contaminated rape-seed oil (Anon 1983). There were c. 20 000 cases of poisoning and more than 350 deaths. Apart from one or 2 neurotoxins, such as *ortho*-tricresyl phosphate, the main characteristic of chemical food poisoning is vomiting within a few minutes to half an hour of ingestion. In this respect it differs strikingly from poisoning of bacterial origin, which rarely manifests itself in under 2 h and usually not until much later. Recovery

is usually more rapid, but with certain poisons the case-fatality rate may be quite high.

2 Bacterial gastroenteritis

Food-borne disease has been defined by the World Health Organization (WHO) as disease of an infectious or toxigenic nature caused by or thought to be caused by the consumption of food or water. For the purposes of this chapter the term 'bacterial gastroenteritis' is restricted to acute gastroenteritis due to the presence in food of bacteria, usually in large numbers, or their products. Gastroenteritis may be of the following types:

1 **infection type** due to the multiplication of bacteria in vivo of bacteria ingested with the food, e.g. salmonellae or *Vibrio parahaemolyticus*
2 **toxin type** due to ingestion of food in which a toxin, e.g. staphylococcal enterotoxin or *Bacillus cereus* emetic toxin, has already been formed and
3 **intermediate type** due to the release of enterotoxin by bacteria in the bowel, e.g. by *Clostridium perfringens*, that does not readily produce the toxin in food.

It is customary, in the UK, to exclude from food-poisoning statistics incidents of the infection type caused by *Shigella* spp. (see Chapter 25) or by *Salmonella* Typhi and Paratyphi B (see Chapter 24), though these may be clinically indistinguishable from those due to 'food-poisoning' salmonellae. Several other organisms that give rise to diarrhoea in humans may from time to time cause outbreaks clearly associated with the consumption of a particular item of food and these are considered elsewhere in this volume: *Campylobacter* spp. in Chapter 29, *Yersinia enterocolitica* and *Escherichia coli* in Chapter 27 and *Vibrio cholerae* in

Chapter 26. Botulism, in which bacteria multiply in food and form a toxin which, when ingested, acts on the central nervous system, is described in Chapter 37. For food-borne listeriosis see Chapter 31.

For general accounts of food poisoning and other food-borne infections and intoxications see Cliver (1990), Hui et al. (1994) or Mossel et al. (1995).

2.1 Symptomatology

Some types of gastroenteritis can be recognized clinically by their typical symptoms. The clinical and epidemiological features of the more common forms of bacterial gastroenteritis are summarized in Table 28.1. Those caused by organisms that multiply in the body, such as salmonella infection, do not give rise to symptoms for several hours or even days. They are characterized by fever, abdominal pain, diarrhoea and to a lesser extent by nausea and vomiting, and their duration is usually 2–5 days. Forms in which toxin is preformed in the food or is produced soon after ingestion have a shorter incubation period of 2–6 h and are non-febrile. These are characterized by nausea and vomiting and to a lesser extent by diarrhoea. Recovery is usually complete within 24 h. However, serious illness and death may occur from several types of bacterial gastroenteritis, e.g. salmonellae, shigellae and *E. coli*.

2.2 Epidemiology

INCIDENCE

It is difficult to assess the true incidence of gastroenteritis. Data for England and Wales for the years 1981–1994 are given in Table 28.2. Before 1939, only the larger outbreaks reached the notice of the authorities, and much of the apparent increase observed between 1941 and 1955 may be attributed to more frequent reporting of outbreaks and sporadic infections by medical practitioners and to the growth of a comprehensive bacteriological service during these years. It is believed, however, that some increase did occur associated with the growth of communal feeding, the use of precooked foods and made-up dishes, and the bulk handling of foodstuffs. The upward trend of notifications reached a peak in 1955 followed by a modest improvement with the total number of reported incidents falling from 8961 in 1955 to 3744 in 1966. From then until the late 1970s and early 1980s there was a gradual increase in the number of reported incidents, particularly those caused by salmonellae. Thereafter, there was a marked rise in the incidence of human salmonellosis in many countries. This was largely associated with *Salmonella* Enteritidis as a consequence of the infection of poultry flocks both nationally and internationally. This will be discussed below (see section on 'Chickens', p. 542).

Information is becoming increasingly available about gastroenteritis in countries other than the UK. For example, Todd (1994) has provided details about food-borne disease in a number of countries. He showed that whereas in England and Wales between 1985 and 1989 the mean rate was 65.4 per 100 000 population, it was 105.8 in Germany and 458.6 in Turkey. Analysis of data from different countries also highlights differences in the importance of certain pathogens between countries. Thus, whereas salmonellae and campylobacter are most frequently isolated from cases of food-borne disease in the majority of developed countries, *V. parahaemolyticus* is more important in Japan (Todd 1994). This undoubtedly reflects high rates of consumption of fish and fish products. WHO data are also available (Schmidt 1995) and these will be noted below in relation to salmonellae (see section 3, p. 541). Food-borne illness of all types is under extensive surveillance in the USA and is an important public health activity of the Centers for Disease Control and Prevention (CDC), as well as the State health departments.

The incidence of gastroenteritis in the UK parallels the atmospheric temperature. Much food becomes contaminated with potentially pathogenic organisms but if these are not permitted to grow the risk of gastroenteritis is small. The 3 main classes of gastroenteritis due to specific organisms vary in their seasonal incidence, but staphylococcal gastroenteritis is more strictly confined to the warmer months of the year.

The real distribution of bacterial gastroenteritis cannot be determined with certainty. The methods of recording tend to exaggerate the frequency of salmonella gastroenteritis relative to that due to other agents because it is easily recognized by bacteriological methods and is frequently classified as gastroenteritis even when it cannot be attributed to the consumption of a particular food. A single outbreak is therefore often recorded as a large number of separate sporadic 'incidents'. Other forms of bacterial gastroenteritis, such as those caused by *Staphylococcus aureus*, *C. perfringens* and *B. cereus*, are more difficult to recognize in the absence of an obvious outbreak, and sporadic attacks are seldom recorded. In 1987, for example, salmonella infection accounted for 99% of all incidents but for only 89% of cases. Staphylococcal and clostridial poisoning, which each caused less than 1% of incidents, resulted in 1 and 7% of cases respectively. Of 169 outbreaks that affected members of more than one family, 57% were due to salmonellae, 28% to clostridia, 9% to *B. cereus* and other *Bacillus* spp., and 6% to staphylococci. A number of incidents occur in which none of the recognized bacterial agents can be found. Some of these, particularly those with a longer incubation period of up to 48 h, are undoubtedly of viral origin (Appleton, Palmer and Gilbert 1981).

2.3 Morbidity and mortality

The attack rate varies greatly in different outbreaks, owing partly to the uneven distribution of the infecting organism or toxin in the food and partly to variation in the individual susceptibility of those exposed to risk, but on the whole it tends to be high. Hobbs (1971) listed a number of outbreaks associated with the consumption of poultry, with attack rates of

Table 28.1 Some clinical and epidemiological features of bacterial food poisoning

Organism	Incubation period (h)	Duration and symptoms	Sources of organisms
Salmonella	6–48 (usually 12–36)	1–7 days Diarrhoea, abdominal pain, vomiting, fever nearly always present	Human and animal excreta Raw meat and poultry, feeding meals, etc. Unpasteurized milk, eggs
Clostridium perfringens	8–20	12–24 h Diarrhoea, abdominal pain, nausea but vomiting uncommon, no fever	Dust, soil, human and animal excreta Raw meat and poultry, dried foods, herbs and spices
Staphylococcus aureus	2–6	6–24 h Nausea, vomiting, diarrhoea and abdominal pain, but no fever. Collapse and dehydration in severe cases	Anterior nares and skin of man and animals; septic lesions, e.g. boils, carbuncles, whitlows; raw milk of cows, sheep and goats; cream and cheese made from raw milk
Vibrio parahaemolyticus	2–48 (usually 12–18)	2–5 days Profuse diarrhoea often leading to dehydration, abdominal pain, vomiting and fever	Raw and cooked seafoods, e.g. fish, prawns, crabs and other shellfish
Bacillus cereus	(a) 8–16, diarrhoeal syndrome	(a) 12–24 h Abdominal pain, diarrhoea and sometimes nausea	Common in soil and vegetation (a) Meat products, soups, vegetables, puddings and sauces
	(b) 1–5, vomiting syndrome	(b) 6–24 h Nausea and vomiting, and sometimes diarrhoea	(b) Rice

8–86% (mean 20%) for salmonella, 17–100% (mean 25%) for *C. perfringens*, and 6–92% (mean 23%) for *S. aureus*. In a recent investigation of 47 salmonella outbreaks that involved a number of vehicles and 5 different serotypes, the mean attack rate was 56% (Glynn and Bradley 1992). In outbreaks of unknown aetiology in which the agent is possibly a virus, the attack rates can be higher, with a range of 20–86%. In 10 outbreaks cited by Appleton, Palmer and Gilbert (1981) the mean attack rate was 47%. The case-fatality rate is generally low. In the mid-1980s *S*. Enteritidis epidemic in the USA, less than 0.5% of those infected died (Miller, Hohmann and Pegues 1995) and between 1989 and 1991 there were 191 registered deaths due to salmonellosis in England and Wales (Sockett et al. 1993). This is equivalent to a rate of 0.12–0.13 per 100 000 population, which is 27% higher than for the period 1986–88.

Sex apparently has little effect on case-fatality rates, but age is of importance; most deaths occur in the very young and the old.

3 BACTERIOLOGY AND EPIDEMIOLOGY OF SALMONELLA GASTROENTERITIS

The salmonellae are now regarded as serotypes of a single genospecies *Salmonella enterica* (syn. *choleraesuis*) (see Volume 2, Chapter 41). Almost all of the serotypes with which we are concerned in this chapter belong to subspecies 1 and these are designated by names that are printed in Roman type. We shall omit the specific and subspecific designations and use only the serotype names preceded by the word 'serotype' or *Salmonella*. Many different serotypes are involved in gastroenteritis. Table 28.3 lists those most commonly

Table 28.2 Bacterial food poisoning in England and Wales[a]

| Year | Number of reported cases caused by | | |
	Salmonella	*Staphylococcus aureus*	*Clostridium perfringens*
1981	10 251	143	918
1982	12 322	89	1455
1983	15 155	160	1624
1984	14 727	181	1716
1985	13 330	118	1466
1986	16 976	76	896
1987	20 532	178	1266
1988	27 478	111	1312
1989	29 998	104	901
1990	30 112	55	1442
1991	27 693	61	733
1992	31 355	112	805
1993	30 650	28	562
1994	30 559	74	446

[a]Based on reports to the Public Health Laboratory Service Communicable Disease Surveillance Centre.

encountered in England and Wales and the USA from 1987 to 1995.

When surveillance systems were first established, relatively few salmonellae were identified as being associated with human infection. The situation has become more complex. In principle, a large number of salmonella serotypes have the capacity to cause human illness. In practice, however, the epidemiological pattern is dominated by relatively few serotypes. Discussion will be largely confined to England and Wales and the USA as trends of infection in these countries are indicative of those found in many, although not all, other parts of the world. Table 28.3 shows data for 1987–95. There are clear similarities between the 2 countries in that Enteritidis and Typhimurium dominate the epidemiological pattern although in England and Wales a far greater proportion of cases are caused by Enteritidis. This may be associated with differences in phage types (PTs) prevalent in the 2 countries and is discussed below. Serotype Typhimurium was predominant until the middle to late 1980s when the pandemic of infections caused by serotype Enteritidis (Rodrigue, Tauxe and Rowe 1990) began. The upward trend in Enteritidis infections started earlier in the USA and peaked in the mid-1980s but has never reached the high incidence seen in many western European countries, including England and Wales (Fig. 28.1). Until recently, there were also differences in the distribution of Enteritidis PTs between different geographical regions. PT4 predominated in western Europe, PT1 in eastern Europe and PTs 8 and 13a in North America. Although this pattern is still generally observed, there have been some changes, particularly with regard to PT4. This phage type is becoming increasingly important in human infections in some parts of the USA (Boyce et al. 1996) and would appear to be spreading (Gomez, personal communication 1996).

Infections with Enteritidis are associated with the contamination of eggs and poultry meat and this is discussed in detail below (see section on 'Chickens'). Other serotypes can become temporarily important. For example, in England and Wales between 1977 and 1980 S. Hadar, a serotype seldom identified before 1971, became the second most commonly isolated serotype. The main reservoir of the organism was turkeys. In 1981 the number of isolations of S. Hadar fell dramatically and this is thought to be associated with the removal of infected flocks.

3.1 Animal reservoirs of salmonellae

Though human infection with *Salmonella* is widespread and frequent, the majority of food-poisoning outbreaks due to this group of organisms follow the consumption of food directly or indirectly associated with infection in some animal. Except for the host-specific serotypes, Dublin in cattle, Choleraesuis in pigs, Abortusovis in sheep, Gallinarum-Pullorum in chickens, and Typhi and Paratyphi B in man, and some phage types of Enteritidis and Typhimurium, the sequence of events for salmonella gastroenteritis is: contaminated animal feed→animal→food→man.

The role of animals, particularly food animals, in the salmonella cycle (animals → food → environment → man) has long been recognized (Palmer and Rowe 1986). It is well established that pigs and poultry are major reservoirs for salmonellae and that cattle are the main source of S. Typhimurium. Most salmonella infections in animals are symptomless. This prevalence in animals is reflected by the frequency with which the organism can be detected in products of animal origin. However, food animals are not the only source; salmonella infection occurs quite frequently in wildlife and in a variety of pet animals including terrapins, frogs and fish, and can be transmitted either directly or by means of contaminated food. Such sources are probably of less importance than food animals, and the risk they present is more easily controlled. The incidence of salmonella infection in food and other animals has been reviewed by Gilbert and Roberts (1986) and Ziprin (1994).

Chickens

Chickens and other poultry, like wild birds, are often infected with salmonellae. Apart from serotype Gallinarum-Pullorum, which has a fairly high degree of specificity for chickens (see Volume 2, Chapter 41), numerous other serotypes can give rise to acute fatal infections in chicks; adult birds are seldom ill but may suffer from chronic or latent infection (Smith and Buxton 1951). Various serotypes are associated with commercially reared chickens. In the UK in 1994, for example, 32 serotypes were identified in 982 salmonellae isolated from chickens (Anon 1995a). The most common was serotype Enteritidis, which accounted for 339 (35%). The next most common were S. mbandaka and S. senftenberg with 8% and 14% respectively. Salmonellae may become endemic in poultry units and come to attention only when an outbreak of human

Table 28.3 The 5 most common salmonella serotypes isolated from human sources 1987–95

Year	England and Wales[a]			USA[b]		
	Total	Order of frequency	Serotype (%)	Total	Order of frequency	Serotype (%)
1987	20 532	1	Typhimurium (37)	46 359	1	Typhimurium (23)
		2	Enteritidis (33)		2	Enteritidis (15)
		3	Virchow		3	Heidelberg
		4	Thompson		4	Hadar
		5	Heidelberg		5	Newport
1988	27 478	1	Enteritidis (56)	45 410	1	Typhimurium (21)
		2	Typhimurium (23)		2	Enteritidis (16)
		3	Virchow		3	Heidelberg
		4	Infantis		4	Newport
		5	Heidelberg		5	Hadar
1989	29 998	1	Enteritidis (53)	43 321	1	Typhimurium (20)
		2	Typhimurium (24)		2	Enteritidis (20)
		3	Virchow		3	Heidelberg
		4	Hadar		4	Newport
		5	Infantis		5	Hadar
1990	30 112	1	Enteritidis (63)	42 338	1	Enteritidis (21)
		2	Typhimurium (18)		2	Typhimurium (20)
		3	Virchow		3	Heidelberg
		4	Infantis		4	Hadar
		5	Heidelberg		5	Newport
1991	27 693	1	Enteritidis (63)	40 443	1	Enteritidis (22)
		2	Typhimurium (19)		2	Typhimurium (21)
		3	Virchow		3	Heidelberg
		4	Newport		4	Hadar
		5	Agona		5	Newport
1992	31 355	1	Enteritidis (64)	34 688	1	Typhimurium (22)
		2	Typhimurium (17)		2	Enteritidis (19)
		3	Virchow		3	Heidelberg
		4	Newport		4	Hadar
		5	Hadar		5	Newport
1993	30 650	1	Enteritidis (66)	36 917	1	Typhimurium (23)
		2	Typhimurium (16)		2	Enteritidis (22)
		3	Virchow		3	Heidelberg
		4	Newport		4	Newport
		5	Hadar		5	Hadar
1994	30 559	1	Enteritidis (57)	37 522	1	Enteritidis (26)
		2	Typhimurium (18)		2	Typhimurium (21)
		3	Virchow		3	Heidelberg
		4	Hadar		4	Newport
		5	Newport		5	Hadar
1995	28 791	1	Enteritidis (52)	41 222	1	Enteritidis (25)
		2	Typhimurium (21)		2	Typhimurium (22)
		3	Virchow		3	Newport
		4	Hadar		4	Heidelberg
		5	Newport		5	Hadar

[a]Data supplied by the Public Health Laboratory Service Communicable Disease Surveillance Centre.
[b]Salmonella Surveillance Document, annual tabulation summary, 1993–95, US Department of Health and Human Services.

infection is associated with consumption of contaminated chicken meat.

The above data are evidence of the importance of serotype Enteritidis in commercial poultry. Incidents of infection with serotype Enteritidis in fowls increased in frequency in the UK and elsewhere during the 1980s. There were 8 reports under the Zoonoses Order (1975) in 1981 and 111 in 1987. By 1991 this had increased to 1340 reports (PHLS/SVS 1992) partly as a result of flock monitoring. Infection with Enteritidis PT4 can cause clinical disease, including yolk-sac infections and pericarditis in young chicks, occasionally accompanied by septicaemic lesions in the liver.

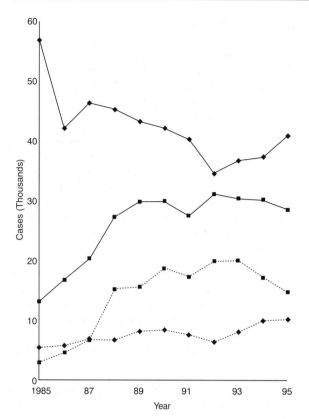

Fig. 28.1   Recent trends in human salmonellosis in England and Wales and the USA: –◆–, total confirmed cases in the USA; –■–, total confirmed cases in England and Wales; ···◆···, Enteritidis cases in the USA; ···■···, Enteritidis cases in England and Wales.

A mortality of 20% has been reported at 3–5 weeks of age (Lister 1988). In mature broilers a mucopurulent pericarditis may be seen (Lister 1988, Rampling et al. 1989).

Other commercial poultry

All poultry has the potential to be infected with salmonellae. In the UK in the 1950s duck eggs were an important vehicle for human infection with serotype Typhimurium (Hobbs and Gilbert 1978). Contamination was the result of systemic infection (Marthedal 1977). This serotype is still found in commercial ducks and geese in the UK and accounted for 50 (32%) of the isolations in 1994. In all, 20 different serotypes were isolated and the most common after *S.* Typhimurium was serotype Enteritidis, which was isolated on 37 (23%) occasions (Anon 1995a). Nevertheless, duck eggs and meat are now only very rarely implicated in cases of human salmonellosis in the UK. An identical situation exists in the great majority of countries in Eastern and Western Europe (Schmidt 1995).

Turkey poults can be seriously affected by salmonella infection. A variety of serotypes can be involved but serotypes Enteritidis and Typhimurium are probably the most important. These 2 salmonellae are, however, currently of little importance in UK turkeys. In 1994 there were 552 isolations from commercial turkeys comprising 30 serotypes, of which *S.* Newport

represented 34%. There were very few isolations of *S.* Typhimurium, but 15% were serotype Enteritidis, a marked increase on 1993 (Anon 1995a).

Other birds

Other birds may also be infected with salmonellae and pigeons, gulls and sparrows have been shown to excrete the organisms. Gulls that feed in polluted estuaries may excrete typhoid, paratyphoid and other salmonellae (Johnston, Maclachlan and Hopkins 1979). Fenlon (1981) reported that 12.9% of 1242 samples of seagull faeces contained salmonellae, the number of positive samples being significantly higher than that from the faeces of other small birds near sewage outfalls. Gulls that feed around refuse tips or slaughterhouses may also show a raised incidence of salmonella carriage (Fenlon 1983). Infection of cattle after pasture contamination with gull faeces has been described (Coulson, Butterfield and Thomas 1983) but the significance of gulls as vectors of salmonellae has been questioned (Girdwood et al. 1985). Sparrows that gained access to a hospital kitchen were the source of salmonellae that caused outbreaks of gastroenteritis in a large mental hospital (Penfold, Amery and Morley Peet 1979).

Eggs

The infection of laying hens with serotype Enteritidis is currently of great importance in the international pandemic of human infections (Rodrigue, Tauxe and Rowe 1990, Schmidt 1995). Salmonellae can be isolated from egg shells and contents. Various different serotypes have been recovered from shells and are probably present as a consequence of intestinal carriage in the bird but infection of the lower oviduct with serotype Enteritidis may also be important (Humphrey et al. 1991a). Salmonellae on egg shells can contaminate egg contents by migration through the shell and associated membranes. This is more likely when egg shells are damaged (Vadehra, Baker and Naylor 1969), when a warm, newly laid egg comes into contact with faecal material (Sparks and Board 1985, Padron 1990), or a combination of these events. Salmonellae present on egg shells may also contaminate the contents when eggs are broken and may grow in broken out egg if stored at ambient temperature. This route of contamination was believed to have contributed to 2 large outbreaks of human salmonellosis in North America in 1962 and 1963 (Thatcher and Montford 1962, Ager et al. 1967). The recent and continuing pandemic of *S.* Enteritidis infection (Rodrigue, Tauxe and Rowe 1990) appears to be associated with the contamination of egg contents before the egg is laid (see section 3.3, p. 547).

Pigs

The prevalence of salmonella infection in pigs varies from country to country. In England and Wales, for example, there were 423 isolations of salmonella from commercial pigs in 1994 (Anon 1995a). *S.* Typhimurium accounted for 64% of these and phage types DT104, 193 and 208 predominated; there was only one isolate of *S.* Choleraesuis. In contrast, *S.* Choleraesuis infection in pigs remains an important problem in the USA (Ziprin 1994). It is a known porcine pathogen that is invasive in pigs and can establish a carrier state. Other serotypes such as Heidelberg, Newport and Typhimurium are also invasive in pigs (Wood 1989, Pospischil, Wood and Anderson 1990, Wood et al. 1991). Carrier animals are a potential public health threat and contaminated pork products such as sausages are frequently salmonella-positive (Roberts et al. 1975, Nichols and de Louvois 1995). Sausages and processed meats often contain mechanically recovered meat. This is derived from bone by crushing and extraction after the main meat component has been removed from the bone; it frequently contains chicken and may be contaminated with salmonella.

Cattle

Bovine salmonellosis is dominated by serotypes Dublin and Typhimurium (Ferris and Miller 1990). For example, in the UK in 1994, Dublin accounted for 40% of salmonella isolates from adult cattle and 27% of those from calves. The corresponding figures for Typhimurium were 42 and 59%, respectively. Of particular concern is the rapid rise in bovine infection caused by serotype Typhimurium DT104, because this organism is resistant to a wide range of antibiotics (Threlfall et al. 1994a). This bacterium is being isolated from an increasing number of other animals, including sheep, pigs and chickens. The increased incidence of DT104 in food animals is matched by a marked increase in the number of reported human cases in England and Wales (Wall et al. 1994). There have also been large outbreaks in Washington State, USA (T Gomez, personal communication 1996), Germany and Austria (P G Wall, personal communication 1996).

Previously important multi-resistant phage types of Typhimurium such as DT193 and 204C have shown a marked decline in recent years (Anon 1995a). In serotype Typhimurium, resistance is usually plasmid mediated (Threlfall, Rowe and Ward 1993, Threlfall et al. 1994b) and such strains may be selected by antimicrobial drugs extensively used to combat salmonella infections in cattle. In Typhimurium DT104, however, the resistance genes are chromosomal. This is of particular concern because it may permit the maintenance of antimicrobial resistance in the absence of selection pressures (Brown 1991).

Other animals

All animals can be colonized or infected with salmonellae. Serotype Abortusovis used to be a problem in sheep where it caused abortion in ewes. This serotype was not isolated in the UK in 1993 or 1994 (Anon 1995a). Some other serotypes such as Dublin and Typhimurium can cause severe infection in lambs (Prost and Riemann 1967, Gitter and Sojka 1970) but these are not common.

Dogs and other pets

Cats and dogs can be asymptomatic carriers of a wide range of salmonella serotypes. Carriage rates in cats varies between 1 and 18% and in dogs between 0.6 and 28% (Ziprin 1994). In 1976 in the USA 53 salmonella serotypes were isolated from 8000 dogs (Shimi, Keyhani and Bolurchi 1976) and serotype Typhimurium was recovered from 40% of these. In early surveillance studies many of the serotypes in dog faeces could also be recovered from dehydrated dogmeal (Galton, Harless and Hardy 1955). In the USA, various dehydrated dogfoods were found to be salmonella-negative (Ziprin 1994), which suggested that cats and dogs probably acquire salmonellae from meat or their environment. Survival of salmonellae in dog faeces can be prolonged and serotype Ohio persists for over 3 months (Choudhary et al. 1985).

In a few companion animals, salmonella infection can become manifest as clinical illness. In cats, salmonellosis may present as a chronic febrile illness or occasionally as conjunctivitis or bacteraemia. Infected dogs can have diarrhoea with or without fever but more severe cases may involve haemorrhagic colitis.

Rats and mice

Rats and mice may have natural infections with Typhimurium, Enteritidis and other salmonella serotypes. Surveys of carrier rates in rat populations have given results varying from 4 to 7%, with serotype Enteritidis, usually of the Danysz biotype, as the commonest organism (Brown and Parker 1957). Rodents that gain access to farms may spread salmonellae to and from animal feeds via their droppings (Edel et al. 1973). Ludlam (1954) observed that the proportion of infected rats caught in and around a meat factory at one time rose to 40% and that many different serotypes were present. House mice were thought to be to blame for sporadic cases of salmonellosis in an old people's home in the Netherlands, and after eradication of the mice no further cases arose (Beckers et al. 1982). Mice are important in the dissemination of serotype Enteritidis to laying hens (Eckroade, Davison and Benson 1991) and the artificial infection of wild mice with a strain of Enteritidis resulted in the excretion of the bacterium for over 6 months (Davies and Wray 1994).

Salmonellae have been isolated from water courses and farm-associated wild animals (Davies and Wray 1994). Various biting and non-biting arthropods, including fleas (Jadin 1951), ticks (Floyd and Hoogstraal 1956), human lice (Liu, Zia and Chung 1937), animal lice (Milner, Jellison and Smith 1957) and cockroaches (Mackerras and Pope 1948), have been shown to be salmonella-positive. Flies and other insects can introduce salmonellae into the farm environment and play a part in their dissemination (Edel et al. 1978). Hobbs and Roberts (1987) cited an outbreak of salmonellosis among children in a hospital in Australia, in which flies, cockroaches and mice were all found to be carriers of the organism responsible for the infection. It was not suggested that they were the original source but that they had picked up the bacteria from the contaminated environment and conveyed them on their feet and bodies.

3.2 Epidemiology of salmonella infections among domestic animals

Many domestic animals suffer from salmonella infection, but the number of serotypes causing illness in a particular species at any time and in any country is usually small. These indigenous salmonella infections, for example *S.* Dublin in cattle and *S.* Typhimurium in calves, appear to behave like human enteric infection. They are probably acquired from a rather small dose and many animals become severely ill, whereas others become permanent carriers. Good animal husbandry is necessary to minimize the spread of infection, particularly on farms practising intensive rearing. Once infection has been introduced into a herd or flock, rapid spread can occur by faecal–oral and other routes. Transmission may also occur when susceptible and infected animals are brought into contact with each other: for example, when they are mixed in pens; at service; by contact with the faeces of infected animals; when stock is placed in inadequately disinfected pens; by the transfer of contamination from pen to pen by the movement of animals or other means (Linton 1979); or by cross-infection between animals during transport to market or in lairages awaiting slaughter. The cleaning of contaminated market and farm buildings can be difficult; salmonellae were isolated from 8% of floor-swab samples taken from a calf-rearing unit after cleaning and disinfection (Wray et al. 1990). These authors also showed that salmonellae could be isolated from 50% of samples taken from calf markets and 21 and 7% of samples taken from transport vehicles before and after cleaning, respectively (Wray et al. 1991).

Animals that graze on pasture recently sprayed with slurries of animal wastes can become infected from this source (Jack and Hepper 1969). The degree of infectivity of such pasture will depend on the persistence and concentration of the organisms and the interval between spraying and grazing (Taylor and Burrows 1971, Taylor 1973) but salmonellae are capable of prolonged survival in faecal material, slurry and on pasture (Wray 1975).

The routes of salmonella infection of commercial poultry varies with the serotype. The principal route with serotype Enteritidis is from infected breeding stock and the organism can be transmitted vertically as a consequence of infection of reproductive organs in a manner similar to serotypes Pullorum and Gallinarum. Various other serotypes may also be invasive in poultry and can be transmitted vertically, but this does not occur at the same frequency as with Enteritidis – a fact recognized by the European Union Zoonoses Directive (Anon 1992). The farm environment may also be important and it has been demonstrated that infection can be perpetuated by polluted drinking water and inadequate cleaning of poultry houses and associated equipment. The re-use of litter

can also lead to the infection of replacement flocks (Fanelli, Sadler and Brownell 1970).

With the exception of vertical transmission, the above routes of infection are less important than contaminated feedstuffs as a source of salmonellae in farm livestock. This is particularly true with poultry (Williams 1981). Various exotic salmonellae have been demonstrated in animal feed and many appear in the animal and human population. In a number of well documented instances a particular serotype responsible for infection in humans has been traced back to feed given to food animals: Typhimurium in pork (Miller et al. 1969), Virchow in spit-roasted poultry (Pennington et al. 1968), and Agona in chickens and pigs originating from contaminated fish meal (Clark et al. 1973). The events that lead from the use of contaminated animal feed to human infection have been described for many serotypes (Lee 1973).

In the UK legislation has been introduced to control the contamination of home-produced and imported animal feedstuffs with salmonellae, and animal feeds may only be tested in authorized laboratories. These measures have been remarkably successful and the contamination rates in UK-produced processed animal protein and fishmeal has declined from 10% in 1986 to 3% in 1994 (Anon 1995a).

The use of feeding meals that contain low concentrations of antibiotic and chemotherapeutic agents allows pigs, poultry and calves to be fattened more quickly and economically. However, past indiscriminate use of such agents, including penicillins, tetracyclines and sulphonamides, for growth promotion or prophylactic purposes has resulted in the appearance of strains resistant to these agents. The emergence of multi-resistant strains of serotype Typhimurium over this period was reviewed by Anderson (1968). The resistance spectrum and the proportion of drug-resistant strains increased dramatically in the early 1960s. The Swann Committee (Report 1969) examined the use of antibiotics in veterinary medicine and animal husbandry. It and a WHO working party (World Health Organization 1974) recommended that only antimicrobial agents that do not have a therapeutic value, e.g. bacitracin, bambermycin (Flavomycin) and virginiamycin, should be used as growth-promoting agents in animal feeds. Despite these recommendations multi-resistant strains, notably of serotype Typhimurium, continue to appear and to infect animals and man (Threlfall, Rowe and Ward 1993, Threlfall et al. 1994a, 1994b, Frost, Threlfall and Rowe 1995).

There can be wide variations in the carriage rate of salmonellae in food animals especially by red meat animals. For example, salmonellas are rarely isolated from well adult sheep and cattle in the UK (Mackey 1989). In parts of Australia and the USA, however, high levels of intestinal carriage have been demonstrated (Samual et al. 1980). The prevalence of salmonella-positive red meat animals will increase as a result of mixing at markets (Wray et al. 1991) and the stress of transportation can also lead to the recrudescence of latent infections (Williams and Spencer

1973). Salmonellae also spread rapidly during transportation or in the lairage prior to slaughter. Grau and Smith (1974) demonstrated that the prevalence of salmonella-positive lamb carcasses is related to holding time before animals are slaughtered.

3.3 Source of infection in man

TYPE OF FOOD

It can be difficult to identify vehicles of infection in salmonella outbreaks by microbiological examination of food remnants because these are usually discarded before the onset of symptoms, 12–36 h after the meal. For this reason vehicle identification has often depended on epidemiological methods. Usually case-control studies have been used to identify vehicles in individual outbreaks or clusters of sporadic cases over a wider area in which a particular salmonella is involved. In such investigations infected persons and matched controls are interrogated about recent food consumption patterns. This has made it possible in the USA (St Louis et al. 1988) and the UK (Cowden et al. 1989a) to identify contaminated poultry meat and eggs as important, national vehicles for *S.* Enteritidis infection. Similar investigations in the UK also identified *S.* Typhimurium DT124 in salami sticks (Cowden et al. 1989b) and *S.* Saintpaul in mung bean sprouts (O'Mahony et al. 1990) as vehicles for widespread sporadic infection. Improvements in epidemiological surveillance in the UK made it possible in 1989–91 to identify vehicles in 56% of general salmonella outbreaks compared with 44% between 1986 and 1988 (Sockett et al. 1993).

Any foodstuff may be a vehicle for salmonella infection. In practice, however, the epidemiological pattern of human infection is dominated by relatively few foods. In many countries contaminated poultry meat and eggs are most important, particularly where *S.* Enteritidis is the dominant serotype (Rodrigue, Tauxe and Rowe 1990). For example, in the late 1980s early 1990s data from 22 European countries (Schmidt 1995) showed that foods containing eggs or egg products were the vehicles in 25.4% of gastroenteritis outbreaks and meat and meat products, principally poultry, in 23.4%. In most of these outbreaks salmonellae were the causative agent. Data from England and Wales are typical of the pattern; in 1988–91, food vehicles were identified in 430 general salmonella outbreaks (Humphrey, Threlfall and Cruickshank 1997). Eggs and poultry meat were implicated in 41% and 26% respectively of these incidents and the majority of outbreaks were due to *S.* Enteritidis PT4. The importance of this organism in contaminated poultry products was even more clear cut and of 233 outbreaks in which a vehicle was identified, 78% involved either eggs or poultry meat. Though these figures are striking, they may underestimate the importance of poultry products because many of other foods implicated in some outbreaks contained poultry meat, eggs or both.

The multinational importance of *S.* Enteritidis is, in part, a consequence of the increased centralization of the poultry industry (Hunter 1994), since world wide only a few specialist firms supply breeding stock. However, many countries have yet to experience an upsurge in infections with *S.* Enteritidis and, as the result of control measures by the poultry industry, they may not occur. In such countries poultry meat is still of importance and a range of serotypes and foods, such as red meat or milk, may be involved.

In the developed world most milk is pasteurized before consumption and this has led to a marked reduction in milk-associated salmonellosis. Where outbreaks occur, raw or improperly pasteurized milk or milk products are usually implicated. For example, a very large multi-state outbreak in the USA was caused by consumption of pasteurized milk contaminated during the bottling process with raw milk containing *S.* Typhimurium (Ryan et al. 1987). Salmonellae can survive in some cheeses and these have been implicated in some large outbreaks, such as in Canada, where 1500 people were infected with *S.* Typhimurium after consuming contaminated cheddar-type cheese (D'Aoust 1985). More recently, in the UK, an outbreak of infection with *S.* Dublin was associated with soft unpasteurized cows' milk cheese (Maguire et al. 1992) and in France an outbreak of serotype Paratyphi B that involved 273 people was caused by contaminated cheese made from unpasteurized goats' milk (Desenclos et al. 1996).

The risks associated with other foods have been reviewed by Gilbert and Roberts (1979). Canned foods are now only occasionally associated with gastroenteritis and very rarely with salmonella gastroenteritis. Gilbert, Kolvin and Roberts (1982) cited 169 outbreaks of gastroenteritis and food-borne infections associated with freshly opened canned food between 1929 and 1980. Of these only 16 were caused by salmonellae, 8 were outbreaks of typhoid fever and 8 were salmonella food poisoning. All occurred before 1970 and all but one were associated with meat products.

MODES OF FOOD CONTAMINATION

Food of animal origin may contain salmonellae because:

1. it was derived from an infected animal
2. an animal was slaughtered in close proximity to infected animals
3. it was contaminated with salmonellae from a source such as raw meat on the same work surface
4. it was contaminated with salmonellae from meat processors with salmonellosis.

It is often difficult to distinguish between intrinsically and extrinsically contaminated animal products.

Meat

The frequency with which salmonellae are found in meat varies widely from place to place, between different species of animals, and at different times. Many surveys, in various countries, have been carried out on the occurrence of salmonellae in meat animals on the farm and at the slaughterhouse, and in meat at the abattoir, processing plant and retail shop. The wide variation in the prevalence of salmonella-positive samples between and in different surveys makes the direct comparison of data difficult. There is no doubt, however, that comminuted meat and offal can be heavily contaminated. A PHLS survey in England and Wales revealed that 17% of sausage samples were salmonella-positive and contaminated sausage meat was implicated in 12 outbreaks of salmonellosis in England and Wales in 1988–94 (Nichols and de Louvois 1995). Sausages from restaurants and take-aways have also been linked to sporadic cases of *S.* Typhimurium DT104 infection (Wall et al. 1994).

The international importance of poultry meat as a vector of human salmonellosis is reflected in the generally high prevalence of contaminated carcasses; typical data are the results of a PHLS survey in England and Wales in 1987. In this study 64% of frozen chicken and 54% of chilled chicken carcasses, respectively, were salmonella-positive (Roberts 1991). The study was repeated in 1994 and contamination rates had fallen to 41% for frozen chickens and 33% for fresh chicken (Anon 1996). This improvement reflects the impact of improved control by the UK poultry industry and the effect of the European Union Zoonoses directive. The general lack of authoritative data from other countries makes comparison difficult, but in a study in Scotland conducted at about the time of the above study a contamination rate of 20% of carcasses was found with little difference between frozen and chilled birds (Anon 1996). Quite different results were obtained in a survey in the Czech Republic in 1990, where 3.2% of 1510 samples of raw poultry were found positive for salmonella, but this had declined to 1.7% in 1991 (Schmidt 1995).

Poultry carcass contamination rates frequently exceed carriage rates in the live animal as the result of cross-contamination during processing. Evisceration, when gut contents spill onto carcasses, and immersion scalding, to loosen feathers before automatic plucking, are of particular importance. Salmonellae can build up in scald-tank water, especially during soft scalding for fresh chickens, where the water is at 50–52°C and scalding can result in contamination of carcass surfaces and deep tissues (Lillard 1973, Mulder, Dorresteijn and van der Broek 1978). Scalding is inefficient at killing or removing salmonellae attached to chicken skin (Notermans and Kampelmacher 1975), and those that survive are more difficult to remove during the later stages of processing.

Cross-contamination also occurs during red meat slaughter but it is less intensive and provides more opportunities for control. Carcass contamination of food animals is usually confined to surfaces and, for example, examination of deep muscle tissues from beef carcasses does not yield potential human pathogens (Gill 1979). This is not the case with chicken and, in 2 independent investigations in the UK (Humphrey 1991, Rampling, personal communication 1993) *S.* Enteritidis PT4 was isolated from aseptically collected muscle samples from chickens purchased at retail outlets. The public health implications of such isolations have yet to be fully assessed but a case-control study in the UK found that PT4 infection was associated with the consumption of hot, cooked take-away chicken (Cowden et al. 1989a). The organism was probably present in tissues either as a result of invasive disease (Lister 1988) or the ingress of contaminated scald-tank water (Lillard 1973).

Milk and milk products

Salmonellae may be excreted in the milk by cows with septicaemic infection or udder lesions, or they may enter the milk by contamination from faeces or from a human case or carrier. Of 132 outbreaks of milk-borne salmonella gastroenteritis between 1951 and 1980, 22 were attributed to excretion of the organisms in the milk, 49 to faecal contamination and 16 to infection in calves. In 7 outbreaks in previously symptomless herds the source of infection was suggested as contaminated animal feed (4), water (1), and pasture flooded with effluent (1) and 7 outbreaks were thought to be due to human infection (Galbraith, Forbes and Clifford 1982). In one outbreak in Scotland in which *S.* Dublin was isolated from the milk, at least 700 persons were affected (Small and Sharp 1979). In the USA in 1985 an outbreak of over 16 000 culture-confirmed cases of infection with an antibiotic-resistant strain of Typhimurium was observed and traced to a pasteurized low-fat milk produced by a single dairy plant (Ryan et al. 1987). Salmonella carriage by dairy cows can be prolonged and Giles, Hopper and Wray (1989) noted that Typhimurium DT49a persisted in a dairy herd for over 3 years. Proper pasteurization is the only effective control measure and prohibition of the sale of unpasteurized milk in Scotland in 1983 has almost eliminated milk-borne salmonella outbreaks in that country.

Eggs

At times in the past, duck, hen and pigeon eggs have been responsible for gastroenteritis (PHLS 1989). Past problems with hens' eggs particularly involved products such as bulk liquid raw egg and spray-dried egg powder which were responsible for the introduction of a range of different salmonellae into the UK during and immediately after World War II. The widespread rise in human salmonellosis due to *S.* Enteritidis in the 1980s was associated with contamination of egg contents. Strong evidence suggests that this is the result of infection of the reproductive tissue (Hoop and Pospischil 1993). Examination of naturally contaminated eggs revealed that there was no association between shell and contents contamination (Humphrey, Cruickshank and Rowe 1989, Mawer, Spain and Rowe 1989, Humphrey et al. 1991b), and *S.* Enteritidis was almost always present in pure culture (Humphrey 1994). This may be further evidence for the involvement of reproductive tissue in the transmission of salmonellas. There is, as yet, no indication that *S.* Enteritidis can pass more effectively than other competing faecal organisms through egg shells and the underlying membranes. Indeed, recent work by

Dolman and Board (1992) has shown that the bacterium does not compete effectively with other potential contaminants in the shell membranes or in the albumen in eggs stored at room temperature. The apparent predilection of *S.* Enteritidis for reproductive tissue means that it can be isolated from such tissue even in the absence of faecal carriage (Lister 1988, Bygrave and Gallagher 1989) and this can create problems in flock surveillance.

Before the recent problems with *S.* Enteritidis and eggs, there had been few surveys of the prevalence of hens' eggs with salmonella-positive contents. Philbrook, MacCready and van Roekel (1960) isolated *S.* Typhimurium from the contents of 0.3% of a sample of 1137 eggs but Chapman, Rhodes and Rylands (1988) were unable to detect *S.* Typhimurium in the contents of 1000 eggs taken from infected flocks. Recent work in the USA suggested that *S.* Enteritidis survives better than *S.* Typhimurium in the contents of eggs during formation (Keller, personal communication 1996). Much work has been done on eggs from flocks known or thought to be infected with *S.* Enteritidis. The observed prevalence of eggs with salmonella-positive contents has been very variable. A survey of 8700 eggs from 22 naturally infected flocks, by the Exeter Public Health Laboratory between 1988 and 1991, revealed an overall prevalence of 0.6% and results from individual flocks were in the range 0.1–10%. Perales and Audicana (1989) examined eggs from Spanish flocks implicated in *S.* Enteritidis PT4 outbreaks and 0.1% were contents-positive. In the UK, Paul and Batchelor (1988) isolated *S.* Enteritidis PT4 from the contents of 5 of 10 eggs from a small free-range flock.

Almost all currently available evidence about the numbers of *S.* Enteritidis in the contents of clean, intact eggs from naturally (Humphrey, Cruickshank and Rowe 1989, Humphrey et al. 1989a, 1991b, Mawer, Spain and Rowe 1989) or artificially infected hens (Timoney et al. 1989, Gast and Beard 1990) indicates that fresh eggs contain few salmonellae, but the organism can grow in eggs that have been stored. There is a close relationship between egg age and the numbers of *S.* Enteritidis present in naturally contaminated eggs, and eggs held at 20°C for longer than 3 weeks are significantly more heavily contaminated than those examined earlier (Humphrey et al. 1991b). Eggs purchased from retail outlets and stored at 20–21°C for 5 weeks before examination showed essentially the same pattern with approximately 50% of the eggs heavily contaminated (de Louvois 1994). The principal site of contamination of eggs is the outside of the vitelline (yolk) membrane (Humphrey 1994). The few cells of Enteritidis present in this environment are unable to overcome the strong iron-binding systems of egg albumen and thus are unable to grow until they gain access to the iron-rich yolk contents. The vitelline membrane of the fresh egg does not permit yolk invasion, which only occurs when storage-related changes to membrane permeability has taken place. The rate of vitelline membrane breakdown can be accelerated by exposure to high temperatures, high humidity and fluctuating temperatures. Once inside the yolk, growth of *S.* Enteritidis is rapid and an inoculum of only 5 cells can reach 10^{11} cells per egg within 24 h at 20°C (Humphrey et al. 1989b). After purchase eggs should be refrigerated (Anon 1988). The microbiology of eggs and egg products has been reviewed by Humphrey (1994).

Contamination of egg contents is a manifestation of the vertical transmission of *S.* Enteritidis; this will also occur with fertile eggs produced by poultry breeding flocks. The recognition of this feature of the bacterium led to the European Union Zoonosis Directive (Anon 1992) which requires the regular monitoring of breeding flocks and the slaughter of those found to be infected with serotypes Enteritidis or Typhimurium. The Directive and concerted action by the UK poultry industry are probably responsible for the improvement in poultry carcass contamination rates seen in the UK between 1990 and 1994 (Anon 1996).

Other products

Certain animal products administered orally as medicaments may contain salmonellae and may result in outbreaks of infection; these include dried thyroid powder (Kallings et al. 1966), pancreatin (Glencross 1972) and carmine dye (Lang et al. 1967, Rowe et al. 1971).

Chocolate products, which normally give little cause for concern because of their low water activity (a_w), have caused a few outbreaks of salmonellosis. More than 170 cases of infection with serotype Eastbourne were reported in Canada and the USA in 1973–74 after the consumption of chocolate products (Craven et al. 1975), and in 1982 imported Italian chocolate that contained serotype Napoli gave rise to many cases of disease in England and Wales (Gill et al. 1983). The interesting feature in both outbreaks was that the dose sufficient to cause illness was low, probably not more than 1000 organisms in the Eastbourne outbreak. Numbers of *S.* Napoli found in the Italian chocolate ranged from 2 to 23 or more per g (Greenwood and Hooper 1983).

CONTAMINATION OF FOOD FROM EXTRANEOUS SOURCES

A food may be derived from a source free from salmonellae but become contaminated in the course of manufacture, transport or sale. Sometimes the source of bacteria is another foodstuff; cooked meats may be contaminated from raw meat, or even from egg products (Graham, Payne and Taylor 1958, Humphrey, Martin and Whitehead 1994), either by direct contact or via utensils, work surfaces, or hands. Fish and shellfish from polluted rivers and estuaries may also contain salmonellae (Floyd and Jones 1954, Gulasekharam, Velaudapillai and Niles 1956) and several dried vegetable products, including herbs and spices, have been shown to contain salmonellae in small numbers (Roberts, Watson and Gilbert 1982).

Outbreaks of typhoid and paratyphoid fevers and of other salmonellosis have been attributed to the consumption of a number of products of plant origin, including salad vegetables (celery, watercress, lettuce, endive, bean sprouts), rhubarb, water melon, desiccated coconut and pepper. The organisms that contaminate these foods may come from sources such as soil, water and fertilizers and from faeces, particularly when poor hygiene is practised (Roberts, Watson and Gilbert 1982). These products do not, however, lead to many outbreaks of gastroenteritis. Before 1961, desiccated coconut was responsible for a number of outbreaks (Galbraith et al. 1960). In 1959–60 a survey of this product imported into Britain from Sri Lanka showed that 9% of samples were contaminated with salmonellae. Hygiene regulations were then introduced in Sri Lanka (Anon 1961) to improve the production methods. The contamination rates of this product are now low (0.9%; Gilbert and Roberts 1979).

Salmonellae may be introduced into food by infected animals. Rats and mice have always been considered as vectors (see p. 545), not because they are more susceptible to salmonella infection than other animals but because of their habits in feeding and defaecation. In an outbreak of salmonellosis in which pasteurized milk was the vehicle, the bottle tops were found to be contaminated with mouse faeces (Galbraith and Pusey 1984).

Infection from human sources

The part played by the human excreter is difficult to evaluate. Savage (1932) investigated 121 outbreaks of food-borne salmonella infection and concluded that there were only 5 in which a human carrier seemed to have been responsible. Similarly, a study by Roberts (1982) showed that, although infected food handlers were discovered in 126 of 396 salmonella outbreaks in England and Wales between 1970 and 1979, in only 9 was there evidence to suggest that they were the original source of the contaminating organisms. These food handlers had either recently returned from holidays abroad or had continued to prepare food while suffering symptoms of gastroenteritis.

It is now widely held that food is less often contaminated from human than from animal sources. In most incidents of salmonella gastroenteritis the food handlers are victims, not sources, and they become infected through their frequent contact with contaminated raw food, from tasting during preparation, or from eating left-over contaminated food. Patients who have suffered from salmonella infection usually excrete the causative organism for several weeks. Half have ceased to do so by the end of the fourth week, and about 90% by the eighth week (Kwantes 1952). According to Lennox, Harvey and Thomson (1954) the proportion of patients who excrete the organism shows little change for the first 3 weeks, and then falls steeply until the middle of the seventh week. After this, the rate of fall again becomes slow. The disappearance of salmonellae from the faeces during convalescence is thus described by a sigmoid curve. Excretion tends to last longer in infants than in older persons (Szanton 1957). Many excreters of salmonellae give no history of recent gastrointestinal illness: such symptomless

excretion is of similar duration to convalescent excretion. True chronic carriage (see Chapter 24) is very rare. In England and Wales the Public Health [Infectious Diseases] Regulations 1968 laid down that workers whose jobs include the handling of food and who are shown to be carriers of infection may be excluded from work until 3 negative stool samples have been obtained. However, Pether and Scott (1982) suggested that clinically recovered food handlers with formed stools should be allowed to return to work, because they do not present a hazard, provided that normal hygienic practices are observed. In this respect it has been demonstrated that salmonellae are readily removed by hand washing (Pether and Gilbert 1971). Cruickshank and Humphrey (1987) concurred with this view and suggest that priority should be accorded to improving hygienic practice rather than the search for symptomless excreters; food handlers should be excluded from work only for the duration of their illness. Those with diarrhoea do, however, constitute a significant risk and should be excluded from work for 48 h after recovery (Anon 1995b).

Although the direct involvement of carrier food handlers as disseminators of salmonellae is doubtful, their potential role in food cross-contamination is beyond dispute. Salmonella-contaminated raw products, principally meat and poultry, bring about extensive contamination of the kitchen environment (de Wit, Broekhuizen and Kampelmacher 1979, de Boer and Hahne 1990). The homogenization of contaminated egg contents also resulted in the production of contaminated droplets which distributed *S. Enteritidis* widely in the environment around the mixing bowl (Humphrey, Martin and Whitehead 1994). Survival at 20°C was prolonged (>24 h) in small egg droplets and smears.

Many salmonella outbreaks have resulted from poor kitchen practice and Roberts (1986) estimated that in approximately 14% cross-contamination was an important contributory factor. Salmonellae also grow well on a variety of cooked or raw foods (Ingham, Alford and McCown 1990, Golden, Rhodehamel and Kutter 1993) and storage at non-refrigeration temperatures is important in many outbreaks (Roberts 1986). For example, Luby, Jones and Horan (1993) reported a large outbreak in which customers became infected with *S. Agona* or *S. Hadar* because cooked turkey was held unrefrigerated in a small restaurant kitchen for several hours, rinsed with water to remove offensive odour and was incompletely reheated before serving.

Many workers who deal with contaminated raw food ingredients become symptomless excreters of salmonellae. Carriage of salmonellae may be intermittent and the serotype may change with different batches of raw food. Contamination of workers' hands by raw materials, especially of animal origin, is of much greater importance than human faecal contamination. De Wit and Kampelmacher (1981) isolated salmonellae from the hands of 5–36% of workers in factories in which raw materials of animal origin were processed. In factories that deal with 'clean' food ingredients the same authors found low rates of contamination with *E. coli* only; in those not dealing with food *E. coli* was absent.

The infecting dose

In spite of the widespread occurrence of infection in domestic animals and in animal products used for food, salmonella gastroenteritis is still relatively infrequent in man although the incidence of infection is increasing in many countries. The relatively low levels of human illness may be associated with the fact that with many serotypes large doses of salmonellae are usually required for human infection. The dose necessary and the types of illness vary, however, with the invading species and serotype. This statement is supported by human volunteer experiments (McCullough and Eisele 1951a, 1951b, 1951c). Some volunteers became ill after ingesting 125 000 *S.* Bareilly or 152 000 *S.* Newport organisms; others resisted doses of 1 700 000 and 1 350 000 organisms, respectively. Infection with *S.* Derby required an infecting dose of 15 000 000 organisms. One strain of *S.* Anatum had an infecting dose of less than a million, whereas for another strain the dose required was about 50 000 000 organisms. There is increasing evidence from the analysis of outbreaks and the implicated foods that in foodstuffs in which the bacteria are protected from gastric acidity, lower numbers can initiate infection. Investigations by Blaser and Newman (1982) suggested that in 6 of 11 outbreaks of human salmonellosis the ingested doses were small – less than 1000 organisms; outbreaks in which the doses were larger showed high attack rates and short periods of incubation (Stevens et al. 1989). Roberts (1988) cited a number of outbreaks in which the infectious dose was low. Foods with a high fat content or good buffering capacity may protect small numbers of salmonellae during their passage through the acid regions of the stomach, thus permitting a lower dose of organisms to initiate infection. Examples of such foods associated with salmonella outbreaks are chocolate (Gill et al. 1983), cheddar cheese (D'Aoust 1985) and salami sticks (Cowden et al. 1989b). Minimal infective doses vary with age and state of health; in the young they are very low. Analysis of a large number of outbreaks demonstrated that, for non-typhoid salmonellosis, there was a relationship between infecting dose and the severity of illness (Glynn and Bradley 1992, Mintz et al. 1994).

Antibiotic treatment

The treatment of non-typhoidal salmonellosis is usually confined to fluid and electrolyte replacement, because the infection is usually self-limiting. Treatment with antibiotics in uncomplicated cases is not usual and has been shown to have little effect on symptoms or duration in children (Nelson et al. 1980) or adults (Carlstedt et al. 1990). Relapse is more common in health care workers treated with a fluoroquinolone (Neill et al. 1991). Treatment may also prolong the period of faecal excretion of the organism (Dixon 1965, Aserkoff and Bennett 1969).

4 OTHER FORMS OF GASTROENTERITIS

4.1 *Clostridium perfringens* type A gastroenteritis

Clostridium perfringens type A is widely distributed in soil. It is commonly found in the faeces of man and animals and in a variety of foods, particularly meat, poultry and their products. Spores of *C. perfringens* survive cooking; and during slow cooling and unrefrigerated storage they germinate to form vegetative cells that multiply rapidly. Under optimal growth conditions at temperatures between 43 and 47°C the organism has a generation time of only 10–12 min.

Although the first account of a suspected outbreak of *C. perfringens* gastroenteritis was reported by Klein (1895), it was not until Knox and Macdonald (1943) described outbreaks that affected children after the consumption of school meals that serious consideration was given to the organism as a cause of foodborne disease. McClung (1945) described 3 outbreaks in the USA associated with chicken dishes cooked the day before consumption and Osterling (1952) reported 15 outbreaks in Sweden. Conclusive proof that *C. perfringens* caused gastroenteritis came from Hobbs and her colleagues (1953) who investigated 18 outbreaks in great detail. Volunteer feeding studies and serological typing of isolates by means of 8 antisera prepared against some of the outbreak strains provided the proof.

C. perfringens gastroenteritis is characterized by the onset of diarrhoea and abdominal pain usually 8–20 h after the ingestion of food containing large numbers of vegetative cells. Vomiting is uncommon and pyrexia, shivering and headache are rare. The duration of the illness is short and symptoms usually disappear within 10–24 h. Fatalities are rare but have occurred among debilitated persons, particularly the elderly.

Outbreaks are almost invariably caused by meat and poultry dishes that have been cooked hours in advance and then cooled slowly, or even allowed to stand at room temperature for several hours before serving. Large masses of cooked meat provide a favourable anaerobic medium for the proliferation of the organism from any spores that survive cooking. High viable counts ($\geq 10^6$ g^{-1}) are reached in a few hours. After the ingestion of large numbers of vegetative cells of *C. perfringens* in a food, multiplication occurs in the intestine for a brief period followed by sporulation and the production of an enterotoxin.

It was at first assumed that only the 'heat-resistant' strains, i.e. those whose spores survived heating at 100°C for 60 min, were capable of causing gastroenteritis. Later it became apparent that 'heat-sensitive' isolates were equally capable of causing outbreaks (Sutton and Hobbs 1965, Taylor and Coetzee 1966). The presence of large numbers ($> 10^5$ g^{-1}) of *C. perfringens* in the majority of faeces of those suffering from diarrhoea and suspected of being affected in an outbreak is an important diagnostic feature. In the faeces of normal healthy persons counts are usually of the order of 10^3–10^4 g^{-1}, but numbers increase with age and can be 10^8–10^9 g^{-1} in elderly institutionalized patients (Yamagishi et al. 1976, Stringer, Watson and Gilbert 1985).

Viable counts of *C. perfringens* (spores and vegetative cells) should be carried out on samples of suspected foods associated with outbreaks. Similar counts should also be made on faecal specimens collected from ill persons. In addition, counts of *C. perfringens* spores alone should be determined on faecal suspensions diluted 1 in 10 and heated at 80°C for 10 min. Methods for the isolation and enumeration of *C. perfringens* in food and faeces have been the subject of 2 comprehensive studies by the International Commission on Microbiological Specifications for Foods (Hauschild et al. 1977, 1979).

Isolates of *C. perfringens* from suspected foods and the faeces of patients can be typed serologically; the type-specific antigens reside in the capsular polysaccharide. The original scheme of antisera in the UK against 75 strains was expanded to include 36 Japanese strains and 33 strains from the USA (Stringer, Turnbull and Gilbert 1980). One or more specific serotypes were shown to be responsible in 75% of 1451 outbreaks in the UK (Brett, personal communication 1996). Other typing methods that have been described include bacteriocin typing (Mahony 1974, Watson 1985), enzyme typing (Pons, Combe and Leluan 1994) and plasmid profiling (Mahony et al. 1987, Eisgruber, Wiedmann and Stolle 1995).

The enterotoxin produced by *C. perfringens* is thought to be a spore-related toxin that is formed in the intestine at the time of sporulation. In some strains, however, enterotoxin production has been detected in the apparent absence of sporulation (Goldner et al. 1986). In the laboratory, enterotoxin is produced in sporulation media but not in ordinary growth media. The toxin produces fluid accumulation in the ligated rabbit-ileal loop (Duncan, Sugiyama and Strong 1968), erythema in the skin of guinea pigs when injected intradermally (Stark and Duncan 1971), increased capillary permeability in guinea pig skin (Stark and Duncan 1972), and diarrhoea when fed orally to monkeys, rabbits and human volunteers (Duncan and Strong 1969, 1971, Skjelkålé and Uemura 1977b). The biological responses in animals have been used to measure the concentrations of enterotoxin in culture filtrates or fractions.

The enterotoxin has been purified by a variety of methods (see Labbé 1989), including a large-scale technique (Reynolds, Tranter and Hambleton 1986). This has led to the determination of its molecular weight (34–35 kDa) and amino acid sequence (Richardson and Granum 1985) and to the development of numerous methods for its detection (Bartholomew et al. 1985, Harmon and Kautter 1986, Berry, Stringer and Uemura 1986). Berry et al. (1988) compared an ELISA, a Vero-cell assay and a method in which reversed passive latex agglutination was measured by a commercially available kit. Identification of

strains which produce enterotoxin is difficult because *C. perfringens* sporulates poorly in ordinary culture media. van Damme-Jongsten et al. (1990) have shown that DNA hybridization is a suitable method for the identification of strains of *C. perfringens* that have the potential to produce enterotoxin.

Skjelkålé and Uemura (1977a) investigated 2 episodes of gastroenteritis and were unable to detect *C. perfringens* enterotoxin in the sera of acutely ill patients, but a rising antitoxin titre was detected during the following 2 months. In a later study these workers (Skjelkålé and Uemura 1977b) showed that a dose of 8 mg of purified enterotoxin administered orally was necessary to cause diarrhoea in volunteers. A dose of more than 10 mg resulted in a measurable concentration of enterotoxin (2 µg g^{-1}) in faeces. Studies on serum before and after dosing indicated that the measurement of anti-enterotoxin titres was of little diagnostic value.

The administration of cell extracts of an enterotoxigenic strain of *C. perfringens* to various animals led Niilo (1971) to conclude that enterotoxin caused increases in capillary permeability, vasodilation and intestinal mobility. McDonel and Duncan (1975) showed that, in the presence of enterotoxin at concentrations capable of causing fluid accumulation in the ligated rabbit-ileal loop, epithelium was denuded from the tips of the intestinal villi. The mode of action of *C. perfringens* enterotoxin has been reviewed by McDonel (1980) and McClane (1992).

In addition to *C. perfringens* type A strains, enterotoxin production has been reported for type C (Skjelkålé and Duncan 1975) and type D strains (Uemura and Skjelkålé 1976). The chemical, physical and immunological properties of the enterotoxins produced by the type A, C and D organisms are identical. For a description of enteritis necroticans or **pigbel**, caused by *C. perfringens* type C in New Guinea, see Chapter 35.

C. perfringens and its enterotoxin have also been implicated as a cause of non-food-related diarrhoea associated with antibiotic treatment (Borriello et al. 1984), person-to-person transmission in hospital patients (Borriello et al. 1985, Jackson et al. 1986) and occurring as sporadic cases (Brett et al. 1992, Mpamugo, Donovan and Brett 1995).

4.2 *Staphylococcus aureus* gastroenteritis

The ability of some staphylococcal strains to produce a toxic substance capable of causing vomiting and diarrhoea was reported in Belgium (1894), the USA (1907) and the Philippines (1914) but attracted little attention until Dack and coworkers (1930) in Chicago described it for a fourth time after their studies on volunteers. During the next 30 years little was added to this basic information mainly because a reliable and widely applicable assay method was not available. Nevertheless, the study of epidemics of staphylococcal gastroenteritis by orthodox epidemiological and bacteriological methods, supplemented by a limited number of experiments – none of them strictly quantitative – on volunteers and monkeys, had provided a general picture of the conditions under which staphylococci multiply and form enterotoxin in food. After 1960, several immunological methods of detecting and measuring enterotoxin were devised and their use confirmed and extended the conclusions reached earlier.

Seven serologically distinct enterotoxins A, B, C, D, E, G and, most recently, H (Su and Wong 1995) have so far been recognized; of these, enterotoxin A is by far the most often incriminated in outbreaks of gastroenteritis. The enterotoxins are simple proteins with a disulphide bridge, are resistant to most proteolytic enzymes and, to some extent, to heat (see below). Bergdoll et al. (1981) described a toxin produced by staphylococci isolated from cases of toxic shock syndrome (see Chapter 14). The toxin was named enterotoxin F because of its apparent emetic activity in monkeys. The emetic action could not be confirmed, however, and the toxin was renamed toxic shock syndrome toxin-1 (TSST-1) (Bergdoll and Schlievert 1984).

Although heating at 100°C lessens the toxicity of the enterotoxins, normal boiling of foods is insufficient to inactivate them completely. A high pH protects enterotoxin activity and reactivation can occur (Schwabe et al. 1990). The temperature and times used for processing canned foods will, however, usually destroy any enterotoxin present. Despite the relative stability of the enterotoxins, heated foods are seldom implicated in outbreaks unless recontamination and multiplication of the organism occur. The enterotoxins may also be resistant to irradiation (Modi, Rose and Tranter 1990).

The presence of other organisms in the food affects the production of enterotoxin, apparently by limiting the multiplication of the staphylococcus. In addition to being affected by temperature and time, enterotoxin production is affected by food composition, pH, moisture content and atmospheric conditions (Smith, Buchanan and Palumbo 1983). The degree of initial contamination and the type of enterotoxin produced are additional factors. Although enterotoxin is believed to be produced only by coagulase-positive staphylococci (*S. aureus*), there are a few reports of coagulase-negative enterotoxin-positive variants of the organism (Lotter and Genigeorgis 1975, 1977, Evans et al. 1983, Crass and Bergdoll 1986). A large outbreak of gastroenteritis has also been associated with a coagulase-positive strain of *Staphylococcus intermedius* which produced enterotoxin A (Khambaty, Bennett and Shah 1994).

Staphylococcal gastroenteritis occurs in many countries and is associated with a wide range of foods whose only common property appears to be the ability to support vigorous bacterial growth. The optimum temperature for the production of enterotoxin is 35–40°C and the lower the temperature the smaller the amount of enterotoxin produced.

The main clinical signs are nausea, vomiting, abdominal pain and diarrhoea, developing 2–6 h after the ingestion of contaminated food. Clinically, the illness closely resembles severe sea sickness. The incubation time and the severity of symptoms depend on the amount of enterotoxin consumed and the sensitivity of the person; in severe cases, dehydration and collapse can occur and intravenous therapy may be necessary. Recovery is rapid, usually within 24 h.

The foods most often implicated in outbreaks depend on the food habits of the country. About 70% of the outbreaks in England and Wales are associated with meat and poultry. The products, which are usually eaten cold, include ham, meat pies and chicken. Cold sweets, such as trifle and cream cakes, have also been incriminated on many occasions. In the USA baked ham is often implicated and in Japan hand-prepared rice balls have caused many outbreaks.

Outbreaks associated with canned foods and meat pastes in jars also occur. Most of these are due to contamination of the contents after the can or jar has been opened, but staphylococcal gastroenteritis sometimes follows the consumption of food from freshly opened cans. The evidence suggests that the staphylococci enter the can during the cooling process through minute defects in the seam. Large numbers of *S. aureus* can usually be isolated from the remainder of the contents of the can, but sometimes the organism is present in only small numbers, or may have disappeared entirely.

In some countries, especially those with a warm climate, raw milk and raw milk products such as cheese continue to be responsible for many outbreaks. These outbreaks are the only ones in which the staphylococcus may come directly from a source other than the human carrier. It is usual to find that at least one cow in a dairy herd is excreting *S. aureus* from the udder, often without clinical evidence of mastitis (Steede and Smith 1954). In a few outbreaks the organism may have reached the milk from a human source.

Humans are the most important source of *S. aureus* implicated in gastroenteritis. It is usually the food handler who contaminates the food, and under favourable conditions the staphylococcus will multiply and produce enterotoxin in the product. Food handlers may be nasal carriers or carry the organism on their hands. Between 20 and 50% of the population are carriers of *S. aureus* (Williams 1963) and about 15% carry enterotoxigenic strains. Lesions such as boils, carbuncles and whitlows are also foci of staphylococcal infection. In only a small proportion of hand-carriers are septic lesions present on the hands. Many, however, have apparently non-septic cuts and abrasions from which the organism can be isolated in much greater numbers than from the rest of the hand (Hobbs and Thomas 1948).

In a typical outbreak of staphylococcal gastroenteritis the strains of *S. aureus* isolated from specimens of vomitus and faeces are identical with those from the implicated food, and from the hands and often the nose of a food handler. The incriminated food often contains more than 10^6 organisms per g and the strains are identified by phage typing and by testing for enterotoxin production. Strains implicated in gastroenteritis are usually lysed by phages of group III or groups I and III. Because many strains of *S. aureus* are enterotoxigenic, tests for the production of enterotoxin will not alone be sufficient to identify the strain responsible for an outbreak. When sufficient food is available, a sample of 20–100 g can be tested for the presence of enterotoxin. As little as 0.1–1.0 µg of enterotoxin can be sufficient to produce illness in humans. ELISA and reversed passive latex agglutination (RPLA) kits for the detection of staphylococcal enterotoxins in foods are commercially available. ELISA is more sensitive than RPLA; enterotoxin was detected by ELISA in 15 foods from separate outbreaks in the UK but by RPLA in only 12 of these (Wieneke and Gilbert 1987).

Information from various countries indicates that strains of *S. aureus* that produce enterotoxin A, or both enterotoxins A and D, are responsible for about 70% of outbreaks of staphylococcal gastroenteritis (Bergdoll 1979). Investigations by Wieneke, Roberts and Gilbert (1993) on strains from 387 separate outbreaks in the UK between 1969 and 1994 showed enterotoxin production as follows: type A, 223 (58%); type B, 8; type C, 5; type D, 17; type E, 3; types A and D, 56 (14%), types C and D, 28; other combinations, 31. The remaining 16 strains did not produce enterotoxins A to E. In addition there were 2 outbreaks in which enterotoxin A was detected in the implicated food, cheese in both cases, in the absence of viable *S. aureus*.

Reports from many countries indicate that between 15 and 70% of strains of *S. aureus* isolated from various sources, including a wide variety of foods, produce one or more enterotoxins (Wieneke 1974). All studies agree, however, that production of enterotoxin A predominates only among strains from gastroenteritis.

For reviews of staphylococcal gastroenteritis, staphylococcal enterotoxins and detailed information on the characters of *S. aureus* and its behaviour in food, see Genigeorgis (1989), Halpin-Dohnalek and Marth (1989), Bergdoll (1992) and Tranter and Brehm (1994).

4.3   *Bacillus cereus* gastroenteritis

Reports of food-borne disease attributed to anthracoid *Bacillus* spp. resembling *B. cereus* have appeared in the European literature since 1906 (Goepfert, Spira and Kim 1972). However, *B. cereus* was first conclusively implicated as an aetiological agent by Hauge (1950).

B. cereus is now well established as a cause of food-borne illness, accounting for 1–23% of the total number of outbreaks of known bacterial origin reported by countries throughout the world (Kramer and Gilbert 1989). Two distinct clinical forms of gastroenteritis result from the consumption of foods heavily contaminated with this organism. The **diarrhoeal syndrome** is characterized by an incubation period ranging from 8 to 16 h, abdominal pain, profuse watery diarrhoea and rectal tenesmus, occasionally accompanied by nausea and vomiting; the symptoms persist for between 12 and 24 h. By contrast, the **emetic syndrome** is

characterized by a short incubation period (1–5 h), nausea, vomiting and stomach cramps; diarrhoea, occurring later, may also occur. The symptoms of the diarrhoeal syndrome are similar to those of *C. perfringens* gastroenteritis and those of the emetic syndrome to *S. aureus* gastroenteritis.

The classical description of the diarrhoeal syndrome was based on 4 outbreaks in Norway that affected some 600 persons and were attributed to a vanilla sauce prepared and stored for 24 h at room temperature before being served (Hauge 1955). Samples of sauce taken after one episode contained $(25–110) \times 10^6$ *B. cereus* organisms per g. The heating used during preparation had been insufficient to destroy all the spores in one of the ingredients, corn starch, leaving those surviving to germinate and multiply when conditions became favourable. Similar outbreaks were subsequently reported throughout Europe, USA, Canada, Asia and Australia (Goepfert, Spira and Kim 1972, Gilbert 1979, Kramer and Gilbert 1992), with a notably higher incidence of disease in northern and eastern European countries, attributed in part to the widespread culinary use of spices, which are often heavily contaminated with *B. cereus*, and, in part, to unsatisfactory hygiene (Ormay and Novotny 1969). An additional feature of the diarrhoeal syndrome is the great diversity of foods implicated, which include casseroles, sausages, other cooked meat and poultry dishes, cooked vegetables, fish, soups, sauces, various dessert dishes, pasta and milk and dairy products. *B. cereus* has been demonstrated in such foods in numbers ranging from 500 000 to 10^9 g^{-1} (Kramer and Gilbert 1989).

The emetic syndrome was first described in detail by Mortimer and McCann (1974), who investigated 6 incidents associated with cooked rice. Between 1971 and 1987, 234 outbreaks affecting more than 1200 persons were reported in Britain, mainly during the warmer months (Kramer and Gilbert 1989). This illness is usually quite mild and transient but some patients have been admitted to hospital because of excessive vomiting. Gutkin (1975) described a case with periorbital oedema. Some 85% of outbreaks of the emetic syndrome have been associated with boiled or fried rice, served in oriental restaurants and 'takeaways', and can be attributed to the practice of preparing rice in bulk too far in advance of requirement. These are then held for long periods at room temperature before being reheated. The endospores of certain strains found on raw rice survive boiling and stir-frying procedures (Gilbert, Stringer and Peace 1974); they then germinate under favourable conditions. Vegetative cell growth is rapid in cooked rice stored at room temperature and may be enhanced by the addition of beef, chicken or egg (Morita and Woodburn 1977). In most outbreaks *B. cereus* can be isolated in large numbers $(10^5–10^9)$ from the implicated food and from the faeces of sufferers within 72 h of the onset of illness. Similar outbreaks in many parts of the world are increasingly being recognized. A small proportion of these has been caused by foods other than cooked rice, including cooked noodles and spaghetti, filled sweet pastries, dairy products and infant feeds (Gilbert 1979, Kramer and Gilbert 1989).

The rapid onset of symptoms, the afebrile nature of the illness, and its short duration indicate that *B. cereus* gastroenteritis is an intoxication rather than an infection. Several studies, reviewed by Turnbull (1986) and Drobiniewski (1993) have been made on the nature and properties of the toxic factors concerned. The toxin responsible for diarrhoeal symptoms is a true enterotoxin capable of causing fluid accumulation in rabbit ileal loops, altering vascular permeability in rabbit skin, and killing mice when injected intravenously. It is synthesized and released during the exponential growth phase of the organism (Spira and Goepfert 1975). Oral administration of crude preparations to rhesus monkeys caused diarrhoea (Goepfert 1978). The enterotoxin is a thermolabile antigenic protein with a multicomponent structure of MWs 38–45 kDa (Turnbull et al. 1979b, Thompson et al. 1984, Shinagawa et al. 1991). Its dermonecrotic property and necrotizing effect on the intestinal epithelium are believed to be of relevance also to the pathogenesis of non-gastrointestinal *B. cereus* infections (Turnbull et al. 1979a).

Melling and colleagues (1976) carried out feeding trials with rhesus monkeys to determine whether a separate enterotoxigenic factor was responsible for the emetic syndrome. Only strains isolated from vomiting outbreaks were capable of causing vomiting; furthermore, this response could be elicited only if the test strains were grown in rice culture. The toxin has been characterized as a highly stable molecule of low molecular weight (Melling and Capel 1978). Culture filtrates of *B. cereus* strains and extracts of food that have given rise to the emetic syndrome have been shown to elicit a specific vacuolation response from HEp-2 cells (Hughes et al. 1988, Szabo, Speirs and Akhtar 1991). The toxin appears to be a novel dodecadepsipeptide (Agata et al. 1994, 1995).

B. cereus belongs to the morphological group 1 of Smith, Gordon and Clark (1952) and grows within the temperature range of 10–48°C, with an optimum between 28 and 35°C. The spores and vegetative cells are ubiquitous and may be readily isolated from the air, soil, natural waters, vegetation and many kinds of food, including milk, cereals, spices, meat and poultry (Goepfert, Spira and Kim 1972, Norris et al. 1981). Ghosh (1978) isolated *B. cereus* in low numbers from 14% of single faecal specimens obtained from 711 adults in the general population. Turnbull and Kramer (1985) compared the faecal carriage rates of *B. cereus* in different population groups. The isolation rates reported (0–43%) were thought to depend mainly on diet and season. Association of a particular food-borne illness with *B. cereus* requires the isolation of large numbers ($>10^5$ g^{-1}) of this organism from the implicated food together with its detection in acute-phase specimens of faeces or vomitus from affected persons. Enrichment procedures are generally of little value in the laboratory diagnosis of *B. cereus* gastroenteritis.

Methods for the detection and identification of *B.* *cereus* in foods and clinical specimens have been reviewed by Kramer et al. (1982) and van Netten and Kramer (1992). Most of the selective media advocated (Mossel, Koopman and Jongerius 1967, Kim and Goepfert 1971, Holbrook and Anderson 1980, Szabo, Todd and Rayman 1984) contain polymyxin B for the suppression of gram-negative organisms, and also egg yolk, mannitol and a pH indicator. *B. cereus* colonies are lecithinase-positive and mannitol-negative.

A serological typing scheme has been devised to facilitate the epidemiological investigation of *B. cereus* gastroenteritis (Taylor and Gilbert 1975, Gilbert and Parry 1977). Based on the type specificity of the flagellar (H) antigens the scheme comprises 40 agglutinating antisera prepared against prototype strains from selected foods and clinical specimens. In 90% of outbreaks the causative serotype can be established. Of 200 episodes of the emetic syndrome in various parts of the world, 63.5% were caused by *B. cereus* type H.1 (Kramer and Gilbert 1992). Endospores of type H.1 strains differ from those of other serotypes in possessing a strikingly greater resistance to heat (Parry and Gilbert 1980). Plasmid analysis (de Buono et al. 1988, Nishikawa et al. 1996) and phage typing (Ahmed et al. 1995) have also been described.

4.4 Gastroenteritis associated with the *Bacillus subtilis* group

The '*Bacillus subtilis* group' embraces 4 closely related species: *B. subtilis*, *B. licheniformis*, *B. pumilus* and *B. amyloliquefaciens*. These sporogenic organisms commonly occur in soil and plant material and occupy most environmental habitats. Because of their ubiquitous nature, isolates from food or clinical specimens are usually considered of little or no clinical significance. Since 1974, however, more than 160 incidents of *B. subtilis* group gastroenteritis involving some 900 cases have been reported in the UK (Kramer and Gilbert 1989, Gilbert unpublished). In most incidents, high levels of the organism were isolated from the implicated food [range (8×10^4)–(8×10^9) g^{-1}], often in almost pure culture, and from acute-phase faecal specimens. The principal food vehicles were meat and/or vegetable products such as sausage rolls, pies, curries and various ethnic rice dishes, and occasionally bread, crumpets and pizzas. Illness associated with *B. subtilis* is characterized by acute-onset vomiting (median 2.5 h, <1 h in a third of cases) often accompanied by diarrhoea; with *B. licheniformis*, diarrhoea is more common than vomiting and the median incubation period is 8 h. Similar outbreaks have been described by Tong et al. (1962), Nielsen and Pedersen (1974), Turnbull (1979) and Todd (1982).

4.5 *Vibrio parahaemolyticus* gastroenteritis

The halophilic vibrio *V. parahaemolyticus* (see Volume 2, Chapter 45) was first recognized as a cause of gastroenteritis in Japan in 1950 and was responsible for c. 70% of the cases of bacterial gastroenteritis in that country in the 1960s (Sakazaki 1979). Outbreaks have subsequently been reported from many countries throughout the world. The illness is characterized by acute diarrhoea, abdominal pain and nausea; headache, vomiting and fever are less common symptoms. Illness usually begins about 12–24 h after the ingestion of contaminated food although the interval may be as short as 4 h or as long as 96 h. A more severe dysentery-like form of illness with mucoid or sanguineous faeces has been described in several countries. Hospitalization is rare, unless severe fluid loss has occurred, and the illness is usually self-limiting after a few days.

Unique among the pathogenic vibrios is the correlation between pathogenicity of *V. parahaemolyticus* and β-haemolysis of human erythrocytes in an agar medium – the Kanagawa phenomenon. The association between the ability of an isolate to produce the thermostable haemolysin responsible for the Kanagawa phenomenon and its ability to cause gastroenteritis is well established. Marine strains of *V. parahaemolyticus* are predominantly Kanagawa-negative whereas isolates from patients with diarrhoea are almost exclusively Kanagawa-positive. Selective multiplication of the few strains of Kanagawa-positive *V. parahaemolyticus* in the aquatic environment probably occurs in the human intestine during infection and these predominate in faecal specimens once diarrhoeal symptoms develop (Joseph, Colwell and Kaper 1982).

V. parahaemolyticus has been isolated from estuarine and inshore coastal waters throughout the world. Outbreaks of gastroenteritis are almost exclusively associated with consumption of contaminated fish and shellfish. There is a pronounced seasonal incidence with outbreaks occurring mostly during warmer months when *V. parahaemolyticus* is most prevalent in the aquatic environment. In volunteer feeding tests levels of 10^{10} cells of Kanagawa-negative strains failed to elicit symptoms, whereas the minimum infective dose for Kanagawa-positive strains ranged from 2×10^5 to 3×10^7 cells (Sanyal and Sen 1974).

A serological typing scheme based on 11 thermostable somatic O antigens and 65 thermolabile capsular K antigens can be used in the investigation of outbreaks. Culture media for the isolation and enumeration of pathogenic *Vibrio* spp. including *V. parahaemolyticus* have been reviewed by Donovan and van Netten (1995).

For reviews on *Vibrio cholerae* see Chapter 26 and Kaysner (1992); for *V. parahaemolyticus* see Twedt (1989) and Chai and Pace (1994); for *Vibrio vulnificus* see Oliver (1989) and Levine and Griffin (1993) and for *Vibrio* spp. see Volume 2, Chapter 45, Janda et al. (1988) and West (1989).

4.6 Other forms of bacterial gastroenteritis

Outbreaks have been described in which known food poisoning bacteria were not isolated, but a food eaten by the sufferers contained large numbers of another organism. Taken alone, evidence of this sort should not be accorded undue significance. Samples are often collected many hours after the suspected meal was eaten and the food may have been left at room temperature in the meantime. The claims of each organism must be considered separately. The repeated isolation of a particular bacterium from foods thought to have caused illness, especially when the cultures are almost pure, coupled with the isolation of the same agent from the faeces or vomitus of the patients, strengthens the suspicion that it is a pathogen. The final proof, however, must depend upon the production of the disease in volunteers. Bryan (1979) and Stiles (1989) have reviewed extensively the evidence incriminating a wide range of these other bacteria in episodes of gastroenteritis.

Non-bacterial agents clearly play a part in some types of gastroenteritis, such as viral gastroenteritis, scombrotoxic fish poisoning, ciguatera poisoning, paralytic and diarrhoeic shellfish poisoning and poisoning by red kidney beans.

5 INVESTIGATION OF OUTBREAKS OF GASTROENTERITIS

The immediate objectives of the investigation of an outbreak of gastroenteritis are as follows:

1 to verify that there is an outbreak of illness and that the causative agent was food-borne
2 to determine the nature of the agent and the foodstuff or foodstuffs by which it was transmitted
3 to determine the way in which the food was contaminated
4 to ensure that all cases or carriers of the agent are identified
5 to stop the outbreak if it is continuing.

The procedures to be followed are:

1 to secure a complete list of sufferers, with clinical histories and a full list of the foods consumed in the previous 2–3 days
2 to record details of the origin, and the mode of preparation and storage, of the suspected foods
3 to collect specimens for laboratory examination (below) and subsequently
4 to endeavour to find out how the food or foods thought to have been responsible were contaminated and to find the reservoir of the causative organism.

To identify the vehicle of infection it may be necessary to supplement the examination and questioning of sufferers by parallel studies of control groups either of non-sufferers or of randomly selected members of the same population. Suitable epidemiological techniques for this are discussed in Chapter 9. Materials collected for examination should include:

1 the actual food consumed
2 the faeces and vomitus of patients and
3 the blood, spleen, liver and intestine of fatal cases.

As soon as sufficient evidence has been obtained, either from the clinical investigation or from the preliminary bacteriological examination, to indicate the probable vehicle and the causal agent, it will be possible to decide what further specimens are required. These may include, according to circumstances, specimens from contacts or food handlers, samples of food ingredients, and swabs and washings from the premises in which the food was prepared.

5.1 Salmonella outbreaks

In salmonella outbreaks the organisms can frequently be demonstrated in the faeces of patients; vomited matter is much less satisfactory. If the incriminated food is available it may be possible to demonstrate the presence of the organisms here also, but in a large proportion of outbreaks the food vehicle is not determined, often because symptoms did not appear before the food remnants were discarded. The occurrence of uncommon serotypes of salmonella often affords a strong indication of the probable vehicle or reservoir of infection; with more common serotypes, such as Typhimurium and Enteritidis, even phage typing may not be sufficient to discriminate between strains. In these cases isolates will be subjected to additional tests which include the determination of drug resistance patterns and the ability to transfer resistance and genotypic methods such as ribotyping, insertion sequence (IS) 200 typing and pulse field gel electrophoresis (PFGE) of the DNA partially digested with different restriction enzymes (see Volume 2, Chapter 41).

After an attack of salmonella gastroenteritis about 50% of patients excrete the causative organism in the faeces for 4–5 weeks or longer. It is, therefore, always worthwhile attempting to make a retrospective diagnosis by examining the faeces of convalescents.

It is possible to isolate salmonellae from foods, particularly those that have caused illness, using the same techniques as those for faecal samples. This is not the usual procedure, however, and food and environmental samples are almost always examined using techniques capable of detecting low levels of contamination. There is a wealth of published information on salmonella isolation techniques and these have been summarized by Mossel et al. (1995). A disadvantage with salmonella isolation methodologies for foods is the time taken to complete the procedure which can often exceed 4 days. A range of 'rapid' methods has been explored and continues to be developed. Current knowledge has been summarized by Patel (1994).

5.2 *Clostridium perfringens* outbreaks

When investigating these outbreaks it should be remembered that, after multiplying in food, *C. perfringens* is mainly in the vegetative state. Unheated material should therefore be cultured on blood agar or neomycin blood agar. Qualitative tests for *C. perfringens* in faeces are of limited diagnostic significance

and counts of viable organisms should therefore be performed.

At least one of the following criteria should be satisfied for the laboratory confirmation of an outbreak:

1 the incriminated food, correctly stored after the incident, contains $>10^5$ *C. perfringens* per g
2 the median faecal spore count of *C. perfringens* is $>10^5 \ g^{-1}$
3 strains isolated from the incriminated food and faecal specimens belong to the same serotype
4 isolates from the faeces of most of the patients belong to the same serotype
5 enterotoxin is detected in faecal specimens.

Although still valuable, criteria 1–4 may sometimes not be helpful when:

1 the incriminated food has been stored frozen or for more than 48 h resulting in a decrease in viable vegetative cells
2 faecal specimens have been collected several days after onset of symptoms resulting in a decrease in the faecal spore count, and re-establishment of the patients' own serotypes
3 the isolated strains are non-typable and
4 dealing with geriatric long-stay hospital or institution patients, who may carry large numbers of the same serotype in the absence of diarrhoea (Berry et al. 1987).

It is because of these problems, together with the time required for isolation, purification and serotyping, and the availability of a commercial RPLA kit, that demonstration of the enterotoxin in faeces has become the most common procedure in the confirmation of outbreaks of *C. perfringens* gastroenteritis.

5.3 *Staphylococcus aureus* outbreaks

Vomitus and faecal specimens from the patients should be examined for the presence of *S. aureus* within 24 h of the onset of illness. Suspected foods and hand and nose swabs from food handlers should also be tested for *S. aureus*. All strains should be phage typed and when possible examined for the ability to produce enterotoxin. The mere presence of *S. aureus* in the faeces of sufferers or in the nose or on the hands of a food handler is of no significance. A particular food handler cannot be incriminated with any certainty unless a staphylococcal strain from his hands or nose is identical with one present in the suspect food. Detection of enterotoxin in an incriminated food is convincing evidence of staphylococcal gastroenteritis. If the food is not available for examination, however, the finding of the same enterotoxigenic strain in the faeces or vomitus of several patients with typical symptoms may also be sufficient evidence.

In most staphylococcal outbreaks the organism is present in large numbers (10^6–$10^9 \ g^{-1}$) in the food. The presence of less than $10^4 \ g^{-1}$ is of little significance unless a food, such as pasteurized or spray-dried milk, was heated before it was consumed or a matured cheese was kept for a long period after manufacture.

5.4 *Bacillus cereus* outbreaks

Since the spores of *B. cereus* are so widely distributed in the environment, the presence of the organism in small numbers in many types of food and in some faecal specimens is to be expected. It follows, therefore, that the mere detection of *B. cereus* in a food sample is insufficient to implicate either the food or the organism as the cause of an outbreak.

At least one of the following criteria should be satisfied for the laboratory confirmation of an outbreak:

1 *B. cereus* strains of the same serotype are present in the epidemiologically incriminated food and in the faeces or vomitus of the affected persons
2 large numbers ($>10^5$ g^{-1}) of *B. cereus* of an established food poisoning serotype are isolated from the incriminated food, or faeces or vomitus of the affected persons
3 large numbers ($>10^5$ g^{-1}) of *B. cereus* are isolated from the incriminated food, and organisms are detected in the faeces, vomitus, or both, of the affected persons
4 detection of the emetic toxin or the diarrhoeal enterotoxin in the incriminated food.

5.5 *Vibrio parahaemolyticus* outbreaks

In outbreaks of gastroenteritis associated with fish or shellfish, halophilic vibrios should be borne in mind. These organisms can easily be recognized on various selective media (Donovan and van Netten 1995) or media used for the detection of *V. cholerae*, and one of these should be included as a routine when faecal specimens from outbreaks or sporadic cases of diarrhoea of uncertain cause are examined. On thiosulphate citrate bile-salt sucrose agar *V. parahaemolyticus* appears as colonies 2–3 mm in diameter with a green or blue centre. Isolates from faeces and the incriminated food, invariably fish or shellfish, should be sent to a Reference Laboratory for confirmation, serotyping and Kanagawa tests.

6 PREVENTION

The risk of food poisoning, especially with the types where the multiplication of micro-organisms is an essential prerequisite for illness to occur, would be substantially reduced if all foods were cooked while fresh and eaten immediately. This is not always possible in practice, particularly when large numbers of people are being catered for at the same time. Analysis of factors that contributed to the occurrence of 1918 outbreaks of gastroenteritis in the USA, 1961–82 (Bryan 1988) and 1479 outbreaks in England and Wales, 1970–82 (Roberts 1986) showed that the most common problems were storage of food at ambient temperature, inadequate cooling or reheating, warm holding and undercooking. The analysis demonstrated that foods were often held for considerable periods at temperatures that permitted rapid bacterial multiplication. Much can be done by an intelligent combination of refrigeration, cooking and hot storage, but the complete safety of all potentially dangerous foods is difficult to ensure by these means alone. For this reason, attempts should also be made to reduce the frequency with which pathogens gain access to food, particularly to food in bulk, and to find a means of freeing contaminated foods of bacteria without impairing their quality. Green foods that are to be eaten raw should be thoroughly washed; molluscan shellfish such as oysters and mussels should be cultivated in biologically clean water and, where appropriate, subject to cleansing (depuration) in UV light- or chlorine-disinfected water. Zoonotic infections caused by salmonellae may be most effectively controlled by on-farm intervention measures as has been discussed earlier. Despite the routine inspection of meat – which cannot, of course, detect carrier animals – and an understanding of the relevant cycles of infection, too much material contaminated with salmonella and other pathogens still enters the kitchen in the form of raw ingredients.

All non-spore-forming food poisoning organisms are killed by thorough cooking, although this can be difficult to define; there is a possibility that other foods, which are to be eaten without further heating, may become cross-contaminated by hands, surfaces and utensils used for preparing both raw and cooked foods. All meat should be regarded as potentially dangerous and should not be eaten raw. To protect the vulnerable, hen eggs should be boiled for 7 min; frying that does not ensure coagulation of the yolk is insufficient to destroy all salmonellae. All cooking utensils should be thoroughly dried after cleaning before they are put away.

It can be difficult to make foods safe by heating without impairing their palatability. The penetration of heat into a large joint of meat or a large turkey is slow, and the interior may not reach or be kept long enough at a temperature sufficient to kill all pathogens. Though most food poisoning organisms are not specially heat-resistant, apart from sporing forms such as *C. perfringens* and *B. cereus*, there is variation in this respect between strains. The degree of heat necessary to destroy them is also affected by the nature of the medium in which they are contained. The safety of a food to the consumer will depend not only on the effectiveness of the cooking procedure but also on the handling and storage of food after cooking. Heat-resistant spores of *C. perfringens* may be activated by the cooking process and begin to germinate rapidly during long, slow cooling or warm holding periods.

Canning of food needs careful supervision. Not only must the heat treatment be sufficient to destroy all pathogenic organisms, but the water in which the cans are cooled should be of drinking standard. Otherwise pathogenic organisms may enter the can through the seams, which tend to gape during autoclaving and to allow organisms to be sucked in as cooling proceeds.

The regular bacteriological examination of food handlers contributes little to the control of salmonella gastroenteritis. A strict code of personal hygiene should be enforced in all catering establishments and

Table 28.4 Numbers of food poisoning organisms in foods incriminated in outbreaks in the UK

Number of viable organisms per g of food	Number (%) of outbreaks caused by		
	Bacillus cereus[a]	*Clostridium perfringens*[b]	*Staphylococcus aureus*[c]
$<10^4$	5 (1.8)	58 (19.9)	14 (5.2)
$10^4–<10^5$	11 (4.1)	47 (16.0)	11 (4.1)
$10^5–<10^6$	60 (22.0)	65 (22.3)	28 (10.3)
$10^6–<10^7$	76 (28.0)	58 (19.9)	48 (17.7)
$10^7–<10^8$	59 (21.7)	35 (12.0)	64 (23.6)
$10^8–<10^9$	43 (15.8)	26 (8.9)	62 (22.9)
$10^9–<10^{10}$	13 (4.8)	2 (0.7)	42 (15.4)
$>10^{10}$	5 (1.8)	1 (0.3)	2 (0.8)
TOTAL	272	292	271

The median counts per g in all outbreaks were: *B. cereus* 5×10^6; *C. perfringens* 4×10^5; *S. aureus* 4×10^7.
[a]In years 1971–94.
[b]In years 1967–94.
[c]In years 1962–94.

particular attention paid to the washing of hands after each visit to the lavatory and after handling raw foods such as meat and poultry. Thorough cleaning and disinfection of food utensils and surfaces after use will reduce the risk of cross-contamination between foods. In a large catering establishment separate areas and staff should be allocated for the preparation of raw and cooked foods.

Strains of *S. aureus* implicated in staphylococcal gastroenteritis are usually of human origin. Control of this type of gastroenteritis, therefore, depends on 'no-handling' techniques for the preparation or processing of the foods usually associated with the disease, together with adequate refrigeration.

Current methods of processing make it inevitable that spores of *C. perfringens* will often be present in meat and poultry; they will also be found on a wide range of other ingredients, such as herbs, spices, vegetables and soup mixes. However, this organism is dangerous only when ingested in large numbers; thus, prevention is concerned not only with its destruction, but also with the control of spore germination and of the subsequent multiplication of vegetative cells in cooked foods. Such control can be achieved either by serving food hot immediately after cooking, or by cooling rapidly and storing in a refrigerator until required, when it should be served cold. If required hot it should be thoroughly reheated to boiling point.

Rapid cooling of large bulks of food is often difficult, and special plant employing forced draughts of cold air, or cold rooms with extraction fans, may be necessary. Large quantities of food will cool more rapidly if broken down into smaller portions or, if liquid, into shallow layers. The same precautions are required with foods associated with outbreaks of *B. cereus* gastroenteritis, for example large quantities of cooked rice.

In summary, Table 28.4 shows that foods incriminated in outbreaks due to *B. cereus*, *C. perfringens* and *S. aureus* are usually found to be contaminated with large numbers of these organisms. This emphasizes the need for the widespread adoption of practices aimed at preventing the introduction and multiplication of pathogens in food.

Application of a hazard analysis critical control points (HACCP) programme is now widely recommended in many countries for all food production processes, irrespective of scale. Once the sources of contamination (the hazards) and the important points at which, and by how, they can be controlled (critical control points) are identified, and controls introduced, then the greater assurance of a safe product. The final line of defence in the prevention of most types of bacterial gastroenteritis is good kitchen hygiene and this requires education of all those in the preparation, processing and service of food both on the commercial and the domestic scale.

REFERENCES

Agata N, Mori M et al., 1994, A novel dodecadepsipeptide, cerulide, isolated from *Bacillus cereus* causes vacuole formation in Hep-2 cells, *FEMS Microbiol Lett*, **121**: 31–4.

Agata N, Ohta M et al., 1995, A novel, dodecadepsipeptide, cerulide, is an emetic toxin of *Bacillus cereus*, *FEMS Microbiol Lett*, **129**: 17–20.

Ager EA, Kenrad E et al., 1967, Two outbreaks of eggborne salmonellosis and implications for their prevention, *J Am Med Assoc*, **199**: 372–8.

Ahmed R, Sankar-Mistry P et al., 1995, *Bacillus cereus* phage typing as an epidemiological tool in outbreaks of food poisoning investigations, *J Clin Microbiol*, **33**: 636–40.

Anderson ES, 1968, Drug resistance in *Salmonella typhimurium* and its implications, *Br Med J*, **3**: 333.

Anon, 1947, *Special Report Series*, No. 360, Medical Research Council, London.

Anon, 1961, *Desiccated Coconut (Manufacture and Export) Regulations 1961*, Coconut Products Ordinance.

Anon, 1983, Toxic oil syndrome, *Lancet*, **1**: 1257–8.

Anon, 1988, *Raw Shell Eggs*, EL/88/P136, Department of Health, London.

Anon, 1992, *Report Council of the European Communities Directive*, 92/117/EEC. 17 December 1992.

Anon, 1995a, *Salmonella in Animal and Poultry Production 1994*, Ministry of Agriculture, Fisheries and Foods, London.

Anon, 1995b, The prevention of human transmission of gastrointestinal infection and bacterial intoxication. Report of a Working Party of the PHLS Salmonella Committee, *CDR Rev*, **5**: 157–72.

Anon, 1996, *Report on Poultry Meat. Advisory Committee on the Microbiological Safety of Food*, HMSO, London, 110.

Appleton H, Palmer SR, Gilbert RJ, 1981, Foodborne gastroenteritis of unknown aetiology: a virus infection?, *Br Med J*, **282:** 1801–2.

Aserkoff B, Bennet JV, 1969, Effect of antibiotic therapy in acute salmonellosis on the faecal excretion of salmonellae, *N Engl J Med*, **281:** 636–40.

Bartholomew BA, Stringer MF et al., 1985, Development and application of an enzyme-linked immunosorbent assay for *Clostridium perfringens* type A enterotoxin, *J Clin Pathol*, **38:** 222–8.

Beckers HJ, van Leusden FM et al., 1982, Sporadic cases of salmonellosis associated with mice in a home for aged persons, *J Appl Bacteriol*, **53:** xiv.

Bergdoll MS, 1979, *Foodborne Infections and Intoxications*, 2nd edn, eds Riemann H, Bryan FL, Academic Press, New York and London, 443–94.

Bergdoll MS, Schlievert PM, 1984, Toxic shock syndrome toxin, *Lancet*, **2:** 691.

Bergdoll MS, Crass BA et al., 1981, A new staphylococcal enterotoxin, enterotoxin F, associated with toxic-shock-syndrome, *Lancet*, **1:** 1017–21.

Bergdoll MS, 1992, Staphylococcal intoxication in mass feeding, *Food Poisoning Handbook of Natural Toxins*, vol. 7, ed. Tu AT, Marcel Dekker, New York, 25–47.

Berry PR, Stringer MF, Uemura T, 1986, Comparison of latex agglutination and ELISA for the detection of *Clostridium perfringens* type A enterotoxin in faeces, *Lett Appl Microbiol*, **2:** 101–2.

Berry PR, Wieneke AA et al., 1987, Use of commercial kits for the detection of *Clostridium perfringens* and *Staphylococcus aureus* enterotoxins, *Immunological Techniques in Microbiology*, Society for Applied Bacteriology Technical Series No. 24, eds Grange JM, Fox A, Morgan NL, Blackwell Scientific Publications, Oxford, 245–54.

Berry PR, Rodhouse JC et al., 1988, An evaluation of ELISA, RPLA and Vero cell assay for the detection of *Clostridium perfringens* enterotoxin in faecal specimens, *J Clin Pathol*, **41:** 458–61.

Blaser MJ, Newman LDS, 1982, A review of human salmonellosis. I. Infective dose, *Rev Infect Dis*, **4:** 1096–106.

de Boer E, Hahne M, 1990, Cross-contamination with *Campylobacter jejuni* and *Salmonella* spp., *J Food Prot*, **53:** 1067–8.

Borriello SP, Larson HE et al., 1984, Enterotoxigenic *Clostridium perfringens*: a possible cause of antibiotic-associated diarrhoea, *Lancet*, **1:** 305–7.

Borriello SP, Barclay FE et al., 1985, Epidemiology of diarrhoea caused by enterotoxigenic *Clostridium perfringens*, *J Med Microbiol*, **20:** 363–72.

Boyce TG, Koo D et al., 1996, Recurrent outbreaks of *Salmonella* Enteritidis infections in a Texas restaurant: phage type 4 arrives in the United States, *Epidemiol Infect*, **117:** 29–34.

Brett MM, Rodhouse JC et al., 1992, Detection of *Clostridium perfringens* and its enterotoxin in cases of sporadic diarrhoea, *J Clin Pathol*, **45:** 609–11.

Brown CM, 1991, Instability of multiple resistance plasmids in *Salmonella typhimurium* isolated from poultry, *Epidemiol Infect*, **106:** 247–57.

Brown CM, Parker MT, 1957, Salmonella infections in rodents in Manchester with special reference to *Salmonella enteritidis* var. Danysz, *Lancet*, **2:** 1277–9.

Bryan FL, 1979, Infections and intoxications caused by other bacteria, *Foodborne Infections and Intoxications*, 2nd edn, eds Riemann H, Bryan FL, Academic Press, New York, 211–97.

Bryan FL, 1988, Risks associated with practices, procedures and processes that lead to outbreaks of foodborne diseases, *J Food Prot*, **51:** 663–73.

de Buono BA, Brondrum J et al., 1988, Plasmid, serotypic, and enterotoxin analysis of *Bacillus cereus* in an outbreak setting, *J Clin Microbiol*, **26:** 1571–4.

Bygrave AC, Gallagher J, 1989, Transmission of *Salmonella enteritidis* in poultry, *Vet Rec*, **124:** 333.

Carlstedt G, Dahl P et al., 1990, Norfloxacin treatment of salmonellosis does not shorten carrier state, *Scand J Infect Dis*, **22:** 553.

Chai T, Pace J, 1994, *Vibrio parahaemolyticus*, *Foodborne Disease Handbook*, vol.1, eds Hui YH, Gorham JR et al., Marcel Dekker, New York, 395–425.

Chapman PA, Rhodes P, Rylands W, 1988, *Salmonella typhimurium* phage type 141 infections in Sheffield during 1984 and 1985: association with hens' eggs, *Epidemiol Infect*, **101:** 75–82.

Choudhary SP, Kalimuddin M et al., 1985, Observations on natural and experimental salmonellosis in dogs, *J Diarrhoeal Res*, **3:** 149–53.

Clark GMcC, Kaufmann AF et al., 1973, Epidemiology of an international outbreak of *Salmonella agona*, *Lancet*, **2:** 490–3.

Cliver DO (ed.), 1990, *Foodborne Diseases*, Academic Press, New York.

Coulson JC, Butterfield J, Thomas C, 1983, The herring gull, *Larus argentatus*, as a likely transmitting agent of *Salmonella montevideo* to sheep and cattle, *J Hyg*, **91:** 437–43.

Cowden JM, Lynch D et al., 1989a, Report of a national case control study of *Salmonella enteritidis* phage type 4 infection, *Br Med J*, **299:** 771–3.

Cowden JM, O'Mahony M et al., 1989b, A national outbreak of *Salmonella typhimurium* DT124 caused by contaminated salami sticks, *Epidemiol Infect*, **103:** 219–25.

Crass BA, Bergdoll MS, 1986, Involvement of coagulase-negative staphylococci in toxic shock syndrome, *J Clin Microbiol*, **23:** 43–5.

Craven PC, Mackel DC et al., 1975, International outbreak of *Salmonella eastbourne* infection traced to contaminated chocolate, *Lancet*, **2:** 788–92.

Cruickshank JG, Humphrey TJ, 1987, The carrier food-handler and non-typhoid salmonellosis, *Epidemiol Infect*, **98:** 223–30.

Dack GM, Cary WE et al., 1930, An outbreak of food poisoning proved to be due to a yellow haemolytic staphylococcus, *J Prev Med*, **4:** 167–75.

van Damme-Jongsten M, Rodhouse J et al., 1990, Synthetic DNA probes for detection of enterotoxigenic *Clostridium perfringens* strains isolated from outbreaks of food poisoning, *J Clin Microbiol*, **28:** 131–3.

D'Aoust JY, 1985, Infective dose of *Salmonella typhimurium* in cheese, *Am J Epidemiol*, **122:** 717–20.

Davies RH, Wray C, 1994, Salmonella pollution in poultry units and associated enterprises, *Pollution in Livestock Production Systems*, CAB International, 137–65.

Desenclos J-C, Bouvet P et al., 1996, Large outbreak of *Salmonella enterica* serotype *paratyphi* B infection caused by a goats milk cheese, France, 1993: a case finding and epidemiological study, *Br Med J*, **312:** 91–4.

Dixon JMS, 1965, Effect of antibiotic treatment on duration of excretion of *Salmonella typhimurium* by children, *Br Med J*, **2:** 1343–5.

Dolman J, Board RG, 1992, The influence of temperature on the behaviour of mixed bacterial contamination of the shell membrane of hens' eggs, *Epidemiol Infect*, **108:** 115–21.

Donovan TJ, van Netten P, 1995, Culture media for the isolation and enumeration of pathogenic *Vibrio* species in foods and environmental samples, *Int J Food Microbiol*, **26:** 77–91.

Drobiniewski FA, 1993, *Bacillus cereus* and related species, *Clin Microbiol Rev*, **6:** 324–38.

Duncan CL, Strong DH, 1969, Ileal loop fluid accumulation and production of diarrhoea in rabbits by cell-free products of *Clostridium perfringens*, *J Bacteriol*, **100:** 86–94.

Duncan CL, Strong DH, 1971, *Clostridium perfringens* type A food poisoning. I. Response of the rabbit ileum as an indication of enteropathogenicity of strains of *Clostridium perfringens* in monkeys, *Infect Immun*, **3:** 167–70.

Duncan CL, Sugiyama H, Strong DH, 1968, Rabbit ileal loop

response to strains of *Clostridium perfringens*, *J Bacteriol*, **95:** 1560–6.

Eckroade RJ, Davison S, Benson CE, 1991, Enviromental contamination of pullet and layer houses with *Salmonella enteritidis*, *Proceedings of the Symposium on Diagnosis and Control of Salmonella, San Diego, California, USA*, 14–17.

Edel W, van Schothorst M et al., 1973, Mechanism and prevention of salmonella infection in animals, *Microbiological Safety of Food*, eds Hobbs BC, Christian JHB, Academic Press, London, 247.

Edel W, van Schothorst M et al., 1978, Epidemiological studies on salmonella in a certain area ('Walcheren project'). III. The presence of salmonella in man, insects, seagulls and in foods, chopping-block scrapings from butchers' shops, effluent of sewage treatment plants and drains of butchers' shops, *Zentralbl Bakteriol Parasitenkd Infektionskr Hyg Abt Orig A*, **242, part 4:** 468–80.

Eisgruber H, Wiedmann M, Stolle A, 1995, Use of plasmid profiling as a typing method for epidemiologically related *Clostridium perfringens* isolates from food poisoning cases and outbreaks, *Lett Appl Microbiol*, **20:** 290–4.

Evans JB, Ananaba GA et al., 1983, Enterotoxin production by atypical *Staphylococcus aureus* from poultry, *J Appl Bacteriol*, **54:** 257–61.

Fanelli MJ, Sadler WW, Brownell JR, 1970, Preliminary studies of persistence of salmonella in poultry litter, *Avian Dis*, **14:** 131–41.

Fenlon DR, 1981, Seagulls (*Larus* spp.) as vectors of salmonellae: an investigation into the range of serotypes and numbers of salmonellae in gull faeces, *J Hyg*, **86:** 195–202.

Fenlon DR, 1983, A comparison of salmonella serotypes found in the faeces of gulls feeding at sewage works with serotypes present in the sewage, *J Hyg*, **91:** 47–52.

Ferris KE, Miller DA, 1990, *Salmonella* serotypes from animal and related sources reported during July 1989–June 1990, *Proceedings of the 94th Annual Meeting of the United States Animal Health Association*, 463–88.

Floyd TM, Hoogstraal H, 1956, Isolation of salmonella from ticks in Egypt, *J Egypt Public Health Assoc*, **31:** 119–28.

Floyd TM, Jones GB, 1954, Isolation of *Shigella* and *Salmonella* organisms from Nile fish, *Am J Trop Med Hyg*, **3:** 475–80.

Frost JA, Threlfall EJ, Rowe B, 1995, Antibiotic resistance in salmonellas from humans in England and Wales: the situation in 1994, *PHLS Microbiol Dig*, **12:** 131–3.

Galbraith NS, Pusey JJ, 1984, Milkborne infectious disease in England and Wales 1939–1982, *Health Hazards of Milk*, ed. Freed DLJ, Baillière and Tindall, London, 27–59.

Galbraith NS, Forbes P, Clifford C, 1982, Communicable disease associated with milk and dairy products in England and Wales 1951–1980, *Br Med J*, **1:** 1761–5.

Galbraith NS, Hobbs BC et al., 1960, Salmonellae in desiccated coconut. An interim report, *Monthly Bull Min Health Public Health Lab Serv*, **19:** 99–106.

Galton MM, Harless M, Hardy AV, 1955, Salmonella isolations from dehydrated dog meals, *J Am Vet Med Assoc*, **126:** 57–8.

Gast RK, Beard CW, 1990, Production of *Salmonella enteritidis*-contaminated eggs by experimentally infected hens, *Avian Dis*, **34:** 438–46.

Genigeorgis CA, 1989, Present state of knowledge on staphylococcal intoxication, *Int J Food Microbiol*, **9:** 327–60.

Ghosh AC, 1978, Prevalence of *Bacillus cereus* in the faeces of healthy adults, *J Hyg Camb*, **80:** 233–6.

Gilbert RJ, 1979, *Bacillus cereus* gastroenteritis, *Foodborne Infections and Intoxications*, 2nd edn, eds Riemann H, Bryan FL, Academic Press, New York, 495–518.

Gilbert RJ, Kolvin JL, Roberts D, 1982, Canned foods – the problems of food poisoning and spoilage, *Health Hyg*, **4:** 41–7.

Gilbert RJ, Parry JM, 1977, Serotypes of *Bacillus cereus* from outbreaks of food poisoning and from routine foods, *J Hyg Camb*, **78:** 69–74.

Gilbert RJ, Roberts D, 1979, Food poisoning associated with foods other than meat and poultry – outbreaks and surveillance studies, *Health Hyg*, **3:** 33–40.

Gilbert RJ, Roberts D, 1986, Salmonella special – food hygiene aspects and laboratory methods, *PHLS Microbiol Dig*, **3:** 32–4.

Gilbert RJ, Stringer MF, Peace TC, 1974, The survival and growth of *Bacillus cereus* in boiled and fried rice in relation to outbreaks of food poisoning, *J Hyg Camb*, **73:** 433–44.

Giles N, Hopper SA, Wray C, 1989, Persistence of *Salmonella typhimurium* in a large dairy herd, *Epidemiol Infect*, **103:** 235–41.

Gill CO, 1979, A review: intrinsic bacteria in meat, *J Appl Bacteriol*, **47:** 367–78.

Gill ON, Sockett PN et al., 1983, Outbreak of *Salmonella napoli* infection caused by contaminated chocolate bars, *Lancet*, **1:** 574–7.

Girdwood RWA, Fricker CR et al., 1985, Incidence and significance of salmonella carriage by gulls (*Larus* spp.) in Scotland, *J Hyg*, **95:** 229–41.

Gitter M, Sojka WJ, 1970, *S. dublin* abortion in sheep, *Vet Rec*, **87:** 775–8.

Glencross EJG, 1972, Pancreatin as a source of hospital-acquired salmonellosis, *Br Med J*, **2:** 376–8.

Glynn JR, Bradley DJ, 1992, The relationship between dose and severity of disease in reported outbreaks of salmonella infection, *Epidemiol Infect*, **109:** 371–88.

Goepfert JM, 1978, Monkey feeding trials in the investigation of the nature of *Bacillus cereus* food poisoning, *Proceedings of the 4th International Congress of Food Science and Technology*, **3:** 178–81.

Goepfert JM, Spira WM, Kim HU, 1972, *Bacillus cereus*: a food poisoning organism. A review, *J Milk Food Technol*, **35:** 213–27.

Golden DA, Rhodehamel EJ, Kutter DA, 1993, Growth of *Salmonella* spp. in cantaloupe, watermelon and honeydew melons, *J Food Prot*, **56:** 194–6.

Goldner SB, Solberg M et al., 1986, Enterotoxin synthesis by nonsporulating cultures of *Clostridium perfringens*, *Appl Environ Microbiol*, **52:** 407–12.

Graham JM, Payne DJH, Taylor CED, 1958, *Salmonella irumu* infection indirectly associated with South African frozen egg, *Monthly Bull Min Health Public Health Lab Serv*, **17:** 176–9.

Grau FH, Smith MG, 1974, Salmonella contamination of sheep and mutton carcases related to pre-slaughter holding conditions, *J Appl Bacteriol*, **37:** 111–16.

Greenwood MH, Hooper WL, 1983, Chocolate bars contaminated with *Salmonella napoli*: an infectivity study, *Br Med J*, **286:** 1394.

Gulasekharam J, Veludapillai T, Niles GR, 1956, The isolation of salmonella organisms from fresh fish sold in a Colombo fish market, *J Hyg Camb*, **54:** 581–4.

Gutkin BJ, 1975, *Bacillus cereus* intoxication followed by periorbital oedema, *Br Med J*, **4:** 24.

Halpin-Dohnalek MI, Marth EH, 1989, *Staphylococcus aureus*: production of extracellular compounds and behaviour in foods – a review, *J Food Prot*, **52:** 267–82.

Harmon SM, Kautter DA, 1986, Evaluation of a reversed passive latex agglutination test kit for *Clostridium perfringens* enterotoxin, *J Food Prot*, **49:** 523–5.

Hauge S, 1950, *Bacillus cereus* as a cause of food poisoning, *Nord Hyg Tidskrift*, **31:** 189–206.

Hauge S, 1955, Food poisoning caused by aerobic spore-forming bacilli, *J Appl Bacteriol*, **18:** 591–5.

Hauschild AHW, Gilbert RJ et al., 1977, ICMSF methods studies. VIII. Comparative study for the enumeration of *Clostridium perfringens* in foods, *Can J Microbiol*, **23:** 884–92.

Hauschild AHW, Desmarchelier P et al., 1979, ICMSF methods studies. XII. Comparative study for the enumeration of *Clostridium perfringens* in faeces, *Can J Microbiol*, **25:** 953–63.

Hobbs BC, 1971, Food poisoning from poultry, *Poultry Disease and World Economy*, eds Gordon RF, Freeman BM, Longman, Edinburgh, 65–80.

Hobbs BC, Gilbert RJ, 1978, *Food Poisoning and Food Hygiene*, 4th edn, Edward Arnold, London, 54–7.

Hobbs BC, Roberts D, 1987, *Food Poisoning and Food Hygiene*, 5th edn, Edward Arnold, London.

Hobbs BC, Thomas MEM, 1948, Staphylococcal food poisoning from infected lambs' tongues, *Monthly Bull Min Health Public Health Lab Serv*, **7:** 261–6.

Hobbs BC, Smith ME et al., 1953, *Clostridium welchii* food poisoning, *J Hyg Camb*, **51:** 75–101.

Holbrook R, Anderson JM, 1980, An improved selective and diagnostic medium for the isolation and enumeration of *Bacillus cereus* in foods, *Can J Microbiol*, **26:** 753–9.

Hoop RK, Pospischil A, 1993, Bacteriological, serological, histological and immuno-histochemical findings in laying hens with naturally acquired *Salmonella enteritidis* phage type 4 infection, *Vet Rec*, **133:** 391–3.

Hughes S, Bartholomew B et al., 1988, Potential application of a HEp-2 assay in the investigation of *Bacillus cereus* emetic syndrome food poisoning, *FEMS Microbiol Lett*, **52:** 7–12.

Hui YH, Gorham JR et al. (eds), 1994, Diseases caused by bacteria, *Foodborne Disease Handbook*, vol. 1, Marcel Dekker, New York.

Humphrey TJ, 1991, Food poisoning – a change in patterns?, *Vet Annu*, **31:** 32–7.

Humphrey TJ, 1994, Contamination of egg shell and contents with *Salmonella enteritidis*: a review, *Int J Food Microbiol*, **21:** 31–40.

Humphrey TJ, Cruickshank JG, Rowe B, 1989, *Salmonella enteritidis* phage type 4 and hens' eggs, *Lancet*, **1:** 281.

Humphrey TJ, Martin K, Whitehead A, 1994, Contamination of hands and work surfaces with *Salmonella enteritidis* PT4 during the preparation of egg dishes, *Epidemiol Infect*, **113:** 403–9.

Humphrey TJ, Threlfall EJ, Cruickshank JG, 1997, Salmonellosis, *Textbook on Zoonoses Control*, eds Palmer SR, Soulsby L, Simpson D, Oxford University Press, Oxford, in press.

Humphrey TJ, Baskerville A et al., 1989a, *Salmonella enteritidis* PT4 from the contents of intact eggs: a study involving naturally infected hens, *Epidemiol Infect*, **103:** 415–23.

Humphrey TJ, Greenwood M et al., 1989b, The survival of salmonella in shell eggs under simulated domestic conditions, *Epidemiol Infect*, **103:** 35–45.

Humphrey TJ, Chart H et al., 1991a, The influence of age on the response of SPF hens to infection with *Salmonella enteritidis* PT4, *Epidemiol Infect*, **106:** 33–45.

Humphrey TJ, Whitehead A et al., 1991b, Numbers of *Salmonella enteritidis* in the contents of naturally contaminated hen's eggs, *Epidemiol Infect*, **106:** 32–7.

Hunter PR, 1994, Epizootics of salmonella infection in poultry may be the result of modern selective breeding practices, *Eur J Epidemiol*, **8:** 851–5.

Ingham SC, Alford RA, McCown AP, 1990, Comparative growth rates of *Salmonella typhimurium* and *Pseudomonas fragii* on cooked crab meat stored under air and modified atmosphere, *J Food Prot*, **53:** 566–7.

Jack EJ, Hepper PJ, 1969, An outbreak of *Salmonella typhimurium* infection in cattle associated with the spreading of slurry, *Vet Rec*, **84:** 196–9.

Jackson SG, Ypi-Chuck DA et al., 1986, Diagnostic importance of *Clostridium perfringens* enterotoxin analysis in recurring enteritis among elderly, chronic care psychiatric patients, *J Clin Microbiol*, **23:** 748–51.

Jadin J, 1951, Contribution à l'étude des intoxications alimentaires au Ruanda-Urundi, *Rev Belge Pathol Med Exp*, **21:** 8–10.

Janda JM, Powers C et al., 1988, Current perspectives on the epidemiology and pathogenesis of clinically significant *Vibrio* spp., *Clin Microbiol Rev*, **1:** 245–67.

Johnston WS, Maclachlan GK, Hopkins GF, 1979, Possible involvement of seagulls (*Larus* spp.) and transmission of salmonella in dairy cattle, *Vet Rec*, **105:** 526–7.

Joseph SW, Colwell RR, Kaper JB, 1982, *Vibrio parahaemolyticus* and related halophilic vibrios, *Crit Rev Microbiol*, **10:** 77–124.

Kallings LO, Ringertz O et al., 1966, Microbiological contamination of medical preparations, *Acta Pharm Suecica*, **3:** 219–28.

Kaysner CA, 1992, Cholera infection and poisoning, *Food Poisoning Handbook of Natural Toxins*, vol. 7, ed. Tu AT, Marcel Dekker, New York, 155–70.

Khambaty FM, Bennett RW, Shah DB, 1994, Application of pulsed-field gel electrophoresis to the epidemiological characterisation of *Staphylococcus intermedius* implicated in a food-related outbreak, *Epidemiol Infect*, **113:** 75–81.

Kim HV, Goepfert JM, 1971, Enumeration and identification of *Bacillus cereus* in foods, *Appl Microbiol*, **22:** 581–7.

Klein E, 1895, Ueber einen pathogenen anaeroben Darmbacillus, *Bacillus enteritidis sporogenes*, *Zentralbl Bakteriol Parasitenkd Infektionskr Hyg I Abt Orig*, **18:** 737–43.

Knox R, Macdonald EK, 1943, Outbreaks of food poisoning in certain Leicester institutions, *Med Officer*, **69:** 21–2.

Kramer JM, Gilbert RJ, 1989, *Bacillus cereus* and other *Bacillus* species, *Foodborne Bacterial Pathogens*, ed. Doyle MP, Marcel Dekker, New York, 21–70.

Kramer JM, Gilbert RJ, 1992, *Bacillus cereus* gastroenteritis, *Food Poisoning Handbook of Natural Toxins*, vol. 7, ed. Tu AT, Marcel Dekker, New York, 119–53.

Kramer JM, Turnbull PCB et al., 1982, Identification and characterisation of *Bacillus cereus* and other *Bacillus* species associated with foods and food poisoning, *Isolation and Identification Methods for Food Poisoning Organisms*, eds Corry JEL, Roberts D, Skinner FA, Academic Press, London, 261–86.

Kwantes W, 1952, An explosive outbreak of *Salmonella typhimurium* food poisoning in Llanelly, *Monthly Bull Min Health Public Health Lab Serv*, **11:** 239–48.

Labbé RG, 1989, *Clostridium perfringens*, *Foodborne Bacterial Pathogens*, ed. Doyle MP, Marcel Dekker, New York, 191–234.

Lang DJ, Kunz LS et al., 1967, Carmine as a source of nosocomial salmonellosis, *N Engl J Med*, **276:** 829–32.

Lee JA, 1973, Salmonellae in poultry in Great Britain, *The Microbiological Safety of Food*, eds Hobbs BC, Christian JHN, Academic Press, London, 197–207.

Lennox M, Harvey RWS, Thomson S, 1954, Outbreak of food poisoning due to *Salmonella typhimurium* with observations on duration of infection, *J Hyg*, **42:** 311–14.

Levine WC, Griffin PM, 1993, The Gulf Coast *Vibrio* Working Group 1993. *Vibrio* infections on the Gulf Coast: the results of a first year of regional surveillance, *J Infect Dis*, **167:** 479–83.

Lillard HS, 1973, Contamination of blood system and edible parts of poultry with *Clostridium perfringens* during water scalding, *J Food Sci*, **38:** 151–4.

Linton AH, 1979, Salmonellosis in pigs, *Br Vet J*, **135:** 109–12.

Lister SA, 1988, *Salmonella enteritidis* infection in broiler and broiler-breeders, *Vet Rec*, **123:** 350.

Liu PY, Zia SH, Chung HL, 1937, Report, *Proc Soc Exp Biol Med*, **37:** 17.

Lotter LP, Genigeorgis CA, 1975, Deoxyribonucleic acid base components and biochemical properties of certain coagulase-negative enterotoxigenic cocci, *Appl Microbiol*, **29:** 152–8.

Lotter LP, Genigeorgis CA, 1977, Isolation of coagulase-positive variants from coagulase-negative enterotoxigenic staphylococci, *Zentralbl Bakteriol Parasitenkd Infektionskr Hyg Abt I Orig*, **A239:** 18–30.

de Louvois J, 1994, Salmonella contamination of stored hens' eggs, *PHLS Microbiol Dig*, **11:** 203–5.

Luby SP, Jones JL, Horan JM, 1993, A large salmonellosis outbreak associated with a frequently penalised restaurant, *Epidemiol Infect*, **110:** 31–9.

Ludlam GB, 1954, Salmonella in rats, with special reference to findings in a butcher's by-products factory, *Monthly Bull Min Health Public Health Lab Serv*, **13:** 196.

McClane B, 1992, *Clostridium perfringens* enterotoxin: structure, action and detection, *J Food Safety*, **12:** 237–52.

McClung LS, 1945, Human food poisoning due to growth of *Cl. perfringens* (*Cl. welchii*) in freshly cooked chicken: preliminary note, *J Bacteriol*, **50:** 229–31.

McCullough NB, Eisele CW, 1951a, Experimental human salmonellosis; pathogenicity of strains of *Salmonella meleagridis* and *Salmonella anatum* obtained from spray-dried whole egg, *J Infect Dis*, **88:** 278–89.

McCullough NB, Eisele CW, 1951b, Experimental human salmonellosis; pathogenicity of strains of *Salmonella newport, Salmonella derby* and *Salmonella bareilly* obtained from spray-dried whole egg, *J Infect Dis*, **89:** 209–13.

McCullough NB, Eisele CW, 1951c, Experimental human salmonellosis; pathogenicity of strains of *Salmonella pullorum* obtained from spray-dried whole egg, *J Infect Dis*, **89:** 259–65.

McDonel JL, 1980, *Clostridium perfringens* toxins (type A, B, C, D, E), *Pharmacol Ther*, **10:** 617–55.

McDonel JL, Duncan CL, 1975, Histopathological effect of *Clostridium perfringens* enterotoxin in the rabbit ileum, *Infect Immun*, **12:** 1214–18.

Mackerras IM, Pope P, 1948, Experimental salmonella infections in Australian cockroaches, *Aust J Exp Biol Med Sci*, **26:** 465–70.

Mackey BM, 1989, The incidence of food poisoning bacteria on red meat and poultry in the United Kingdom, *Food Sci Technol Today*, **3:** 246–9.

Maguire H, Cowden JM et al., 1992, An outbreak of *Salmonella dublin* infection in England and Wales associated with a soft unpasteurised cows' milk cheese, *Epidemiol Infect*, **109:** 380–96.

Mahony DE, 1974, Bacteriocin susceptibility of *Clostridium perfringens*: a provisional typing schema, *Appl Microbiol*, **28:** 172–6.

Mahony DE, Stringer MF et al., 1987, Plasmid analysis as a means of strain differentiation in *Clostridium perfringens*, *J Clin Microbiol*, **25:** 1333–5.

Marthedal HE, 1977, Report, *Proceedings of the International Symposium on Salmonella and Prospects for Control* University of Guelph, Guelph, Ontario, 78.

Mawer SL, Spain GE, Rowe B, 1989, *Salmonella enteritidis* phage type 4 and hens' eggs, *Lancet*, **1:** 280–1.

Melling J, Capel BJ, 1978, Characteristics of *Bacillus cereus* emetic toxin, *FEMS Microbiol Lett*, **4:** 133–5.

Melling J, Capel BJ et al., 1976, Identification of a novel enterotoxigenic activity associated with *Bacillus cereus*, *J Clin Pathol*, **29:** 938–40.

Miller AR, Elias-Jones TF et al., 1969, *Salmonella typhimurium* phage type 32 infection in Glasgow and the west central area of Scotland, *Med Officer*, **121:** 223–7.

Miller SI, Hohmann EL, Pegues DA, 1995, Salmonella (including *Salmonella typhi*), *Principles and Practice of Infectious Diseases*, eds Mandell GL, Bennett JE, Dolin R, Churchill Livingstone, New York, 2013.

Milner KC, Jellison WL, Smith B, 1957, The role of lice in transmission of *Salmonella*, *J Infect Dis*, **101:** 181–92.

Mintz ED, Carter ML et al., 1994, Dose-response effects in an outbreak of *Salmonella enteritidis*, *Epidemiol Infect*, **112:** 13–23.

Modi NK, Rose SA, Tranter HS, 1990, The effects of irradiation and temperature on the immunological activity of staphylococcal enterotoxin A, *Int J Food Microbiol*, **11:** 85–92.

Morita TN, Woodburn MJ, 1977, Simulation of *Bacillus cereus* growth by protein in cooked rice combinations, *J Food Sci*, **42:** 1232–5.

Mortimer PR, McCann G, 1974, Food poisoning episodes associated with *Bacillus cereus* in fried rice, *Lancet*, **1:** 1043–5.

Mossel DAA, Koopman MJ, Jongerius E, 1967, Enumeration of *Bacillus cereus* in foods, *Appl Microbiol*, **15:** 650–3.

Mossel DAA, Corry JEL et al., 1995, *Essentials of the Microbiology of Foods: a Textbook for Advanced Studies*, John Wiley & Sons, Chichester.

Mpamugo O, Donovan T, Brett MM, 1995, Enterotoxigenic *Clostridium perfringens* as a cause of sporadic cases of diarrhoea, *J Med Microbiol*, **43:** 442–5.

Mulder RWAW, Dorresteijn LWJ, van der Broek J, 1978, Cross-contamination during the scalding and plucking of broilers, *Br Poult Sci*, **19:** 61–70.

Neill MA, Opal SM et al., 1991, Failure of ciprofloxacin to eradicate convalescent faecal excretion after acute salmonellosis: experience during an outbreak in health care workers, *Ann Intern Med*, **114:** 195.

Nelson JD, Kusmiesz H et al., 1980, Treatment of salmonella gastroenteritis with ampicillin, amoxacillin or placebo, *Pediatrics*, **65:** 1125.

van Netten P, Kramer JM, 1992, Media for the detection and enumeration of *Bacillus cereus* in foods: a review, *Int J Food Microbiol*, **17:** 85–99.

Nichols GL, de Louvois J, 1995, The microbiological quality of raw sausages sold in the UK, *PHLS Microbiol Dig*, **12:** 236.

Nielsen SF, Pedersen HO, 1974, Studier over bakterieforekomsten i roraeg, *Dansk Veterinartidsskrift*, **57:** 756–9.

Niilo L, 1971, Mechanism of action of the enteropathogenic factor of *Clostridium perfringens* type A, *Infect Immun*, **3:** 100–6.

Nishikawa Y, Kramer JM et al., 1996, Evaluation of serotyping, biotyping, plasmid analysis and HEp-2 vacuolation factor assay in the epidemiological investigation of *Bacillus cereus* emetic syndrome food poisoning, *Int J Food Microbiol*, **31:** 149–59.

Norris JR, Berkeley RCW et al., 1981, The genera *Bacillus* and *Sporolactobacillus, The Prokaryotes – A Handbook on Habitats, Isolation and Identification of Bacteria*, vol. 2, eds Starr MP, Stolp H et al., Springer-Verlag, Berlin, 1711–42.

Notermans S, Kampelmacher EH, 1975, Heat destruction of some bacterial strains attached to broiler skin, *Br Poult Sci*, **16:** 351–61.

Oliver JD, 1989, *Vibrio vulnificus, Foodborne Bacterial Pathogens*, ed. Doyle MP, Marcel Dekker, New York, 569–600.

O'Mahony M, Cowden JM et al., 1990, An outbreak of *Salmonella saint paul* infection associated with bean sprouts, *Epidemiol Infect*, **104:** 229–35.

Ormay L, Novotny T, 1969, The significance of *B. cereus* food poisoning in Hungary, *Microbiology of Dried Foods. Proceedings of the 6th International Symposium on Food Microbiology, Bilthoven*, eds Kampelmacher EH, Ingram M, Mossel DAA, Haarlem, Grafische Industrie, 279–85.

Osterling S, 1952, Food poisoning caused by *Clostridium perfringens (welchii)*: preliminary note, *Nord Hyg Tidskrift*, **33:** 173.

Padron M, 1990, *Salmonella typhimurium* penetration through the eggshell of hatching eggs, *Avian Dis*, **34:** 463–5.

Palmer SJ, Rowe B, 1986, Trends in salmonella infections, *PHLS Microbiol Dig No. 2*, **3:** 18.

Parry JM, Gilbert RJ, 1980, Studies on the heat resistance of *Bacillus cereus* spores and growth of the organisms in boiled rice, *J Hyg Camb*, **84:** 77–82.

Patel P (ed.), 1994, *Rapid Analysis Techniques in Food Microbiology*, Blackie Academic and Professional, London.

Paul J, Batchelor B, 1988, *Salmonella enteritidis* phage type 4 and hens' eggs, *Lancet*, **2:** 1421.

Penfold JB, Amery HCC, Morley Peet PJ, 1979, Gastroenteritis associated with wild birds in a hospital kitchen, *Br Med J*, **2:** 802.

Pennington JH, Brooksbank NH et al., 1968, *Salmonella virchow* in a chicken-packing station and associated rearing units, *Br Med J*, **4:** 804–6.

Perales I, Audicana A, 1989, The role of hens' eggs in outbreak of salmonellosis in North Spain, *Int J Food Microbiol*, **8:** 175–80.

Pether JVS, Gilbert RJ, 1971, The survival of salmonellas on finger-tips and transfer of the organisms to food, *J Hyg Camb*, **69:** 673–81.

Pether JVS, Scott RJD, 1982, Salmonella carriers; are they dangerous? A study to identify finger contamination with salmonellas by convalescent carriers, *J Infect*, **5:** 81–8.

Philbrook FR, MacCready RA, van Roekel H, 1960, Salmonellosis spread by a dietary supplement of avian source, *N Engl J Med*, **263:** 713–18.

Pons JL, Combe ML, Leluan G, 1994, Multilocus enzyme typing of human and animal strains of *Clostridium perfringens*, *FEMS Microbiol Lett*, **121:** 25–30.

Pospischil A, Wood RL, Anderson TD, 1990, Peroxidase-antiperoxidase and immunogold labelling of *Salmonella typhi-*

murium and *Salmonella choleraesuis* var *kunzendorf* in tissues of experimentally infected swine, *Am J Vet Res*, **51:** 619–24.

Prost E, Riemann H, 1967, Food-borne salmonellosis, *Annu Rev Microbiol*, **21:** 495–528.

Public Health Laboratory Service, 1989, Salmonella in eggs. PHLS evidence to Agriculture Committee, *PHLS Microbiol Dig*, **6, No. 1:** 1.

Rampling A, Anderson JR et al., 1989, *Salmonella enteritidis* phage type 4 infection of broiler chicken: a hazard to public health, *Lancet*, **2:** 436–8.

Report, 1969, *Joint Committee on the Use of antibiotics in Animal Husbandry and Veterinary Medicine*, Cmnd 4190, HMSO, London.

Reynolds D, Tranter HS, Hambleton P, 1986, Scaled-up production and purification of *Clostridium perfringens* type A enterotoxin, *J Appl Bacteriol*, **60:** 517–25.

Richardson M, Granum PE, 1985, The amino acid sequence of the enterotoxin from *Clostridium perfringens* type A, *FEBS Lett*, **182:** 479–84.

Roberts D, 1982, Factors contributing to outbreaks of food poisoning in England and Wales, 1970–1979, *J Hyg Camb*, **89:** 491–8.

Roberts D, 1986, Factors contributing to outbreaks of foodborne infection and intoxication in England and Wales 1970–1982, *Safe Food for All. Proceedings of the 2nd World Congress on Foodborne Infections and Intoxications, Berlin*, vol. 1, Institute of Veterinary Medicine, Berlin, 157–9.

Roberts D, 1988, Trends in food poisoning, *Food Sci Technol Today*, **2:** 28–34.

Roberts D, 1991, Salmonella in chilled and frozen chicken, *Lancet*, **337:** 984–5.

Roberts D, Watson GN, Gilbert RJ, 1982, Contamination of food plants and plant products with bacteria of public health significance, *Bacteria and Plants*, eds Rhodes-Roberts M, Skinner FA, Academic Press, London, 169–95.

Roberts D, Boag K et al., 1975, The isolation of salmonellas from British pork sausages and sausage meat, *J Hyg Camb*, **75:** 173–84.

Rodrigue DC, Tauxe RV, Rowe B, 1990, International increase in *Salmonella enteritidis*: a new pandemic, *Epidemiol Infect*, **105:** 21–7.

Rowe B, Hall MLM et al., 1971, *S. cubana* and carmine dye, *Br Med J*, **2:** 401.

Ryan CA, Nickels MK et al., 1987, Massive outbreak of antimicrobial-resistant salmonellosis traced to pasteurized milk, *JAMA*, **258:** 3269–774.

Sakazaki R, 1979, Vibrio infections, *Foodborne Infections and Intoxications*, 2nd edn, eds Riemann H, Bryan FL, Academic Press, New York, 173–209.

Samual JL, O'Boyle PA et al., 1980, Distribution of salmonella in the carcases of normal cattle at slaughter, *Res Vet Sci*, **28:** 368–72.

Sanyal SC, Sen PC, 1974, Human volunteer study on the pathogenicity of *Vibrio parahaemolyticus*, *Proceedings of 2nd US-Japan Conference on Toxic Micro-organisms, Tokyo*, Saikon Publishing Co., Tokyo, 227–30.

Savage WG, 1932, Some problems of salmonella food poisoning; tenth William Thompson Sedgwick memorial lecture, *J Prev Med*, **6:** 425–51.

Schmidt K (ed.), 1995, *WHO Surveillance Programme for Control of Foodborne Infections and Intoxications in Europe*, Federal Institute for Health Protection, Berlin.

Schwabe M, Notermans S et al., 1990, Inactivation of staphylococcal enterotoxins by heat and reactivation by high pH treatment, *Int J Food Microbiol*, **10:** 33–42.

Shimi A, Keyhani M, Bolurchi M, 1976, Salmonellosis in apparently healthy dogs, *Vet Rec*, **98:** 110–11.

Shinagawa K, Sugiyama J et al., 1991, Improved methods for purification of an enterotoxin produced by *Bacillus cereus*, *FEMS Microbiol Lett*, **80:** 1–6.

Skjelkåle R, Duncan CL, 1975, Enterotoxin formation by different toxigenic types of *Clostridium perfringens*, *Infect Immun*, **11:** 563–75.

Skjelkåle R, Uemura T, 1977a, Detection of enterotoxin in faeces and anti-enterotoxin in serum after *Clostridium perfringens* food poisoning, *J Appl Bacteriol*, **42:** 355–63.

Skjelkåle R, Uemura T, 1977b, Experimental diarrhoea in human volunteers following oral administration of *Clostridium perfringens* enterotoxin, *J Appl Bacteriol*, **43:** 281–6.

Small RG, Sharp JCM, 1979, A milk-borne outbreak due to *Salmonella dublin*, *J Hyg*, **82:** 95–100.

Smith HW, Buxton A, 1951, Isolation of salmonellae from faeces of domestic animals, *Br Med J*, **1:** 1478–83.

Smith JL, Buchanan RL, Palumbo SA, 1983, Effect of food environment on staphylococcal enterotoxin synthesis: a review, *J Food Prot*, **46:** 545–55.

Smith NR, Gordon RE, Clark FE, 1952, *Aerobic Sporeforming Bacteria*, Report Agriculture Monograph no.16, United States Department of Agriculture, Washington, DC.

Sockett PN, Cowden JM et al., 1993, Foodborne disease surveillance in England and Wales: 1989–1991, *CDR Rev*, **3:** R159–73.

Sparks NHC, Board RG, 1985, Bacterial penetration of the recently oviposited shell of hens' eggs, *Aust Vet J*, **62:** 169–70.

Spira WM, Goepfert JM, 1975, Biological characteristics of an enterotoxin produced by *Bacillus cereus*, *Can J Microbiol*, **21:** 1236–46.

St Louis ME, Morse DL et al., 1988, The emergence of grade A eggs as a major source of *Salmonella enteritidis* infections: new implications for the control of salmonellosis, *JAMA*, **259:** 2103–7.

Stark RL, Duncan CL, 1971, Biological characteristics of *Clostridium perfringens* type A enterotoxin, *Infect Immun*, **4:** 89–96.

Stark RL, Duncan CL, 1972, Transient increase in capillary permeability induced by *Clostridium perfringens* type A enterotoxin, *Infect Immun*, **5:** 147–50.

Steede FDF, Smith HW, 1954, Staphylococcal food poisoning due to infected cows' milk, *Br Med J*, **2:** 576–8.

Stevens A, Joseph C et al., 1989, A large outbreak of *Salmonella enteritidis* phage type 4 associated with eggs from overseas, *Epidemiol Infect*, **103:** 425–33.

Stiles ME, 1989, Less recognised or presumptive foodborne pathogenic bacteria, *Foodborne Bacterial Pathogens*, ed. Doyle MP, Marcel Dekker, New York, 673–733.

Stringer MF, Turnbull PCB, Gilbert RJ, 1980, Application of serological typing to the investigation of outbreaks of *Clostridium perfringens* food poisoning, 1970–1978, *J Hyg*, **84:** 443–56.

Stringer MF, Watson GN, Gilbert RJ, 1985, Faecal carriage of *Clostridium perfringens*, *J Hyg Camb*, **95:** 277–88.

Su YC, Wong ACL, 1995, Identification and purification of a new staphylococcal enterotoxin, H, *Appl Environ Microbiol*, **61:** 1438–43.

Sutton RGA, Hobbs BC, 1965, Food poisoning caused by heat-sensitive *Clostridium welchii*. A report of five recent outbreaks, *J Hyg Camb*, **66:** 135–46.

Szabo RA, Speirs JI, Akhtar M, 1991, Cell culture detection and conditions for production of a *Bacillus cereus* heat-stable toxin, *J Food Prot*, **54:** 272–6.

Szabo RA, Todd ECD, Rayman MK, 1984, Twenty-four hour isolation and confirmation of *Bacillus cereus* in foods, *J Food Prot*, **47:** 856.

Szanton VL, 1957, A 30-month study of 80 cases of *Salmonella oranienburg* infection, *Pediatrics*, **20 (5):** 794–808.

Taylor AJ, Gilbert RJ, 1975, *Bacillus cereus* food poisoning: a provisional serotyping scheme, *J Med Microbiol*, **8:** 543–50.

Taylor CED, Coetzee EFC, 1966, Range of heat resistance of *Clostridium welchii* associated with suspected food poisoning, *Monthly Bull Min Health Public Health Lab Serv*, **25:** 142–4.

Taylor RJ, 1973, A further assessment of the potential hazard for calves allowed to graze pasture contaminated with *Salmonella dublin* in slurry, *Br Vet J*, **129:** 354–8.

Taylor RJ, Burrows MR, 1971, The survival of *Escherichia coli* and

Salmonella dublin in slurry on pasture and the infectivity of *S. dublin* for grazing calves, *Br Vet J*, **127**: 536–43.

Thatcher FS, Montford J, 1962, Egg products as a source of salmonellae in processed foods, *Can J Public Health*, **53**: 61–9.

Thompson NE, Ketterhagen MJU et al., 1984, Isolation and some properties of an enterotoxin produced by *Bacillus cereus*, *Infect Immun*, **43**: 887–94.

Threlfall EJ, Rowe B, Ward LR, 1993, A comparison of multiple antibiotic resistance from humans and food animals in England and Wales 1981–1990, *Epidemiol Infect*, **111**: 189–97.

Threlfall EJ, Frost JA et al., 1994a, Epidemic in cattle and humans of *Salmonella typhimurium* DT104 with chromosomally integrated multiple drug resistance, *Vet Rec*, **134**: 577.

Threlfall EJ, Hampton MD et al., 1994b, Identification of a conjugative plasmid carrying antibiotic resistance and salmonella plasmid virulance (*spv*) genes in epidemic strains of *Salmonella typhimurium*, *Lett Appl Microbiol*, **18**: 82–5.

Timoney JF, Shivaprasad HL et al., 1989, Egg transmission after infection of hens with *Salmonella typhimurium* phage type 4, *Vet Rec*, **125**: 600–1.

Todd ECD, 1982, Food and waterborne disease in Canada – 1977 Annual Summary, *J Food Prot*, **45**: 865–73.

Todd ECD, 1994, Surveillance of foodborne disease, *Foodborne Disease Handbook*, vol. 1, eds Hui YH, Gorham JR et al., Marcel Dekker, New York, 461–536.

Tong JL, Engle HM et al., 1962, Investigation of an outbreak of food poisoning traced to turkey meat, *Am J Public Health*, **52**: 976–90.

Tranter HS, Brehm RD, 1994, The detection and aetiological significance of staphylococcal enterotoxins, *Rev Med Microbiol*, **5**: 56–64.

Turnbull PCB, 1979, *Bacillus subtilis, Communicable Disease Report No.31.*

Turnbull PCB, 1986, *Bacillus cereus* toxins, *J Pharmacol Ther*, **13**: 453–505.

Turnbull PCB, Kramer JM, 1985, Intestinal carriage of *Bacillus cereus*: faecal isolation studies in three population groups, *J Hyg Camb*, **95**: 629–38.

Turnbull PCB, Jørgensen K et al., 1979a, Severe clinical conditions associated with *Bacillus cereus* and the apparent involvement of exotoxins, *J Clin Pathol*, **32**: 289–93.

Turnbull PCB, Kramer JM et al., 1979b, Properties and production characteristics of vomiting, diarrhoeal and necrotizing toxins of *Bacillus cereus*, *Am J Clin Nutr*, **32**: 219–28.

Twedt RM, 1989, *Vibrio parahaemolyticus, Foodborne Bacterial Pathogens*, ed. Doyle MP, Marcel Dekker, New York, 543–68.

Uemura T, Skjelkålé R, 1976, An enterotoxin produced by *Clostridium perfringens* type D. Purification by affinity chromatography, *Acta Pathol Microbiol Scand Sect B*, **84**: 414–20.

Vadehra DV, Baker RC, Naylor HB, 1969, Salmonella infection of cracked eggs, *Poult Sci*, **48**: 954–7.

Wall PG, Morgan D et al., 1994, A case control study of infection with an epidemic strain of multiresistant *Salmonella typhimurium* DT104 in England and Wales, *CDR Rev*, **4**: R130.

Watson GN, 1985, The assessment and application of a bacteriocin typing scheme for *Clostridium perfringens*, *J Hyg Camb*, **94**: 69–79.

West PA, 1989, The human pathogenic vibrios – a public health update with environmental perspectives, *Epidemiol Infect*, **103**: 1–34.

Wieneke AA, 1974, Enterotoxin production by strains of *Staphylococcus aureus* isolated from foods and human beings, *J Hyg Camb*, **73**: 255–62.

Wieneke AA, Gilbert RJ, 1987, Comparison of four methods for the detection of staphylococcal enterotoxin in foods from outbreaks of food poisoning, *Int J Food Microbiol*, **4**: 135–43.

Wieneke AA, Roberts D, Gilbert RJ, 1993, Staphylococcal food poisoning in the United Kingdom, 1969–1990, *Epidemiol Infect*, **110**: 519–31.

Williams EF, Spencer R, 1973, Abattoir practices and their effect on the incidence of salmonella in meat, *The Microbiological Safety of Food*, eds Hobbs BC, Christian JHB, Academic Press, London, 41–6.

Williams JE, 1981, Salmonellas in poultry feeds – a worldwide review. Part 1, *World Poult Sci J*, **37**: 16–19.

Williams REO, 1963, Healthy carriage of *Staphylococcus aureus*: its prevalence and importance, *Bacteriol Rev*, **27**: 56–71.

de Wit JC, Broekhuizen G, Kampelmacher EH, 1979, Cross-contamination during the preparation of frozen chickens in the kitchen, *J Hyg Camb*, **83**: 27–32.

de Wit JC, Kampelmacher EH, 1981, Some aspects of microbial contamination of hands of workers in food industries, *Zentralbl Bakteriol Mikrobiol Hyg I Abt Orig B*, **172**: 390–400.

Wood RL, 1989, Swine as a reservoir of salmonella. Persistent infection with *Salmonella typhimurium* and *Salmonella newport* to market age, *Proceedings of 93rd Annual Meeting of the United States Animal Health Association*, United States Animal Health Association, 513–16.

Wood RL, Rose R et al., 1991, Experimental establishment of persistent infection in swine with a zoonotic strain of *Salmonella newport*, *Am J Vet Res*, **52**: 813–19.

World Health Organization, 1974, *The Public Health Aspects of Antibiotics in Feedstuffs*, WHO, Copenhagen.

Wray C, 1975, Survival and spread of pathogenic bacteria of veterinary importance within the environment, *Vet Bull*, **45**: 543–50.

Wray C, Todd N et al., 1990, The epidemiology of salmonella infection of calves: the role of dealers, *Epidemiol Infect*, **105**: 295–305.

Wray C, Todd N et al., 1991, The epidemiology of salmonella in calves: the role of markets and vehicles, *Epidemiol Infect*, **107**: 521–5.

Yamagishi T, Serikawa T et al., 1976, Persistent high numbers of *Clostridium perfringens* in the intestines of Japanese aged adults, *Jpn J Microbiol*, **20**: 397–403.

Ziprin RL, 1994, Salmonella, *Foodborne Disease Handbook*, vol. 1, eds Hui YH, Gorham JR et al., Marcel Dekker, New York, 253–318.

Chapter 29

INFECTION WITH *CAMPYLOBACTER* AND *ARCOBACTER*

M B Skirrow

The main importance of campylobacters lies in their role as enteropathogens of man. In most industrialized countries *Campylobacter jejuni* and *Campylobacter coli* are together the most frequently identified cause of acute infective diarrhoea and in developing countries they contribute significantly to the burden of diarrhoeal disease in young children. Thus, the emphasis in this chapter is on campylobacter enteritis. The type species of the genus, *Campylobacter fetus*, is a common cause of abortion and infectious infertility in sheep and cattle, but it only occasionally causes disease in man. Other campylobacter species are associated with human periodontal disease, avian hepatitis and porcine proliferative enteropathy (PPE), but their precise role in these diseases is uncertain.

The pathogenicity of arcobacters is less well defined, but they have been isolated from aborted cattle, pig and sheep fetuses, animals with diarrhoea, and children with diarrhoea, mainly in developing countries.

1 CAMPYLOBACTER ENTERITIS

1.1 Historical background

The earliest record of what was presumptively campylobacter enteritis was made over 100 years ago by Theodor Escherich (Escherich 1886). He described organisms resembling *C. jejuni* in smears made from the colonic contents of babies who had died of 'cholera infantum', but he was unable to culture them and considered they had a prognostic rather than causative role in the disease. There followed numerous articles, mainly in German, on 'non-culturable' spiral bacteria in dysenteric disease (reviewed by Kist 1985), but interest in them waned. Some 30 years later, Jones

and Little (1931a, 1931b) isolated 'vibrios', now regarded as *C. jejuni*, from calves with enteritis and cattle with epidemic 'winter scours'.

The first isolation of campylobacters from man came in 1938, when an organism, presumptively *C. jejuni*, was isolated from the blood of 13 victims of a milk-borne outbreak of acute diarrhoea affecting 357 inmates of 2 state institutions in the USA (Levy 1946). Elizabeth King (1957, 1962) was the first to give a proper description of these enteric campylobacters, or 'related vibrios' as she called them, and point out that they were associated with bloody diarrhoea. Further progress depended on devising a method for isolating these fastidious bacteria from faeces. This vital breakthrough was made in Belgium by Butzler and Dekeyser, who applied a differential filtration method used in veterinary microbiology for the isolation of *C. fetus* from abortion material (Dekeyser et al. 1972). Yet Butzler's startling report of the isolation of campylobacters from 5% of children with diarrhoea in Brussels (Butzler et al. 1973) received no recognition until Skirrow (1977) confirmed and extended these findings in the UK.

1.2 Bacteriology

C. jejuni (*C. jejuni* subsp. *jejuni*) and *C. coli* are the species most frequently isolated from patients with campylobacter enteritis. In general, *C. coli* accounts for only 5–10% of infections, but higher proportions have been reported from some parts of the world, notably 55% in the Central African Republic (Georges-Courbot et al. 1990) and 35% in former Yugoslavia (Popović-Uroić 1989). In the latter region (now Croatia), the proportion of *C. coli* infections rose to 75% during the autumn when home slaughtered and processed pigs are traditionally eaten. *Campylobacter lari* makes up less than 0.1% of campylobacter infections. It has occasionally been found causing invasive infection in patients with immune deficiency and it has been indirectly incriminated as a cause of a waterborne outbreak of enteritis in Canada (Borczyk et al. 1987).

At least 8 other *Campylobacter*, or former *Campylobacter*, species are associated with diarrhoeal disease, but they are much less common than *C. jejuni* or *C. coli* and their roles are less well defined, mainly because their detection requires special isolation methods that are not in general use (Bolton, Hutchinson and Parker 1988, Albert et al. 1992). In general, they are more prevalent in developing than industrialized countries. In the latter, they are usually isolated from patients who have recently returned from abroad, or from the blood of patients with immune deficiency.

Campylobacter upsaliensis is the most important of these 'lesser' campylobacters. In a South African study, it accounted for 22% of all campylobacter infections detected in children admitted to hospital with chronic diarrhoea, many with anaemia, kwashiorkor, or pneumonia (Lastovica and Le Roux 1993). A similar figure was found in a study of mainly aboriginal children in central Australia (Albert et al. 1992). In a large study in Belgium, *C. upsaliensis* comprised 13% of campylobacters isolated over 3 years (Goossens et al. 1990), but many of the patients were immigrants from Morocco and Turkey. A survey in the UK gave an equivalent figure of 3.4% (Bolton, Hutchinson and Parker 1988).

C. jejuni subsp. *doylei*, which is slow growing and fastidious compared with subspecies *jejuni*, has been found in 32% of campylobacter infections in aboriginal children in central Australia (Albert et al. 1992) and in 10.5% of children in South Africa (Lastovica and Le Roux 1993), but in less than 1% of patients in Europe (Goossens et al. 1990, Bolton, Hutchinson and Parker 1988). *Campylobacter concisus* has been isolated from patients with diarrhoea, but its significance is not clear. There have been occasions when *C. concisus* has been misidentified as *Campylobacter mucosalis*, as these species are almost indistinguishable by phenotypic methods; at the time of writing there are no substantiated reports of human infection with *C. mucosalis* (On 1994). *Campylobacter hyointestinalis* has been found occasionally in patients with diarrhoea (Albert et al 1992, Salama et al. 1992).

Arcobacter butzleri (formerly *Campylobacter butzleri*) was found by Taylor et al. (1991) in 2.4% of Thai children with diarrhoea (16% of campylobacters isolated). It has been found in a few patients in the USA (Kiehlbauch et al. 1991) and it has been linked with an outbreak of recurrent abdominal cramps, without diarrhoea, in 10 schoolchildren in Italy (Vandamme et al. 1992a). *Arcobacter cryaerophilus* (formerly *Campylobacter cryaerophila*) subgroup 2 has also been found in patients with diarrhoea, though less frequently than *A. butzleri*. *Helicobacter cinaedi* and *Helicobacter fennelliae* (formerly *Campylobacter cinaedi* and *Campylobacter fennelliae*) are associated with proctocolitis and diarrhoea, particularly in practising male homosexuals (see Chapter 30).

An account of human infections caused by campylobacters other than *C. jejuni* and *C. coli* is given by Mishu Allos, Blaser and Lastovica (1995). The following text describes campylobacter enteritis as caused by *C. jejuni* subsp. *jejuni* and *C. coli*.

1.3 Clinical manifestations

The average incubation period of campylobacter enteritis is 3 days. Mean incubation periods in point-source outbreaks and volunteer experiments range from 1.5 to 5.0 days, but in individual patients apparent incubation periods ranging from 18 h to 8 days have been recorded. Not all infections are accompanied by clinical illness. A prospective study of children attending day nurseries in the UK showed that half the infections were symptomless (Riordan 1988) and symptomless excreters are commonly found among family contacts of cases.

Abdominal pain and diarrhoea are the presenting symptoms in most cases, but about one-third of patients ill enough to seek medical advice suffer prodromal influenza-like symptoms (fever, myalgia, malaise) lasting from a few hours to one or more days. More severely affected patients may have rigors, high fever and delirium; children may suffer febrile seizures. In general, the disease is clinically indistinguishable from enteritis due to salmonella, shigella, or other bacterial enteropathogen, but abdominal pain tends to be more severe in campylobacter enteritis (Jewkes et al. 1981, Mattila 1994). Indeed, it can be severe enough to mimic acute appendicitis, often before diarrhoea has become apparent. Liquid stools may become profuse, watery and later contain blood. The colon may be particularly affected and colitic symptoms may predominate from the outset, thereby mimicking acute ulcerative colitis. Whatever the pattern of infection, spontaneous resolution within a few days is the rule. Campylobacters may be passed in the faeces for several more weeks. In a study using sensitive culture methods, they could be detected for a mean period of 37 days, with a maximum of 69 days (Kapperud et al. 1992a).

COMPLICATIONS

Acute complications are generally rare and are the result of a local extension of infection, such as cholecystitis and genuine acute appendicitis, but there are 3 notable late complications. The most frequent is reactive arthritis, which is indistinguishable from the reactive (aseptic) arthritis seen after salmonella, yersinia and other gut infections. It has been estimated to occur in about 1% of cases. It is troublesome but ultimately benign. Less benign is the haemolytic–uraemic syndrome (HUS), which has been reported as arising 3–10 days after the onset of symptoms in at least 9 patients, 5 of them children under the age of 5 years.

The most serious complication is Guillain–Barré syndrome (GBS) or postinfective polyneuropathy, which is particularly associated with strains possessing the O19 (Penner) antigen. It has been estimated that 14–44% of GBS episodes are attributable to campylobacter infection, which makes it the most frequently identified antecedent event in GBS. The pathogenesis of the condition is unknown, but there is evidence of immunological cross-reactivity between certain campylobacter antigens and peripheral nerve myelin proteins, which could result in an autoimmune reaction. The subject is reviewed by Rees et al. (1993).

A full account of the clinical aspects of campylobacter enteritis is given by Skirrow and Blaser (1995).

1.4 Epidemiology

INCIDENCE AND DEMOGRAPHY

In most industrialized countries campylobacter enteritis is the most frequent form of acute infective diarrhoea. Laboratory reports give incidences in the order of 50–100 cases per 100 000 population per year. In the UK almost 50 000 infections were reported by laboratories in 1994, representing an annual incidence of about 90 per 100 000. This figure has increased 4-fold in the last 15 years, but much of this rise is due to increased sampling. No such increase has been reported in the USA. As laboratory diagnosed cases represent only a fraction of all infections, the true incidence is much higher and certainly more difficult to measure. A survey of patients attending a single practice in England gave an incidence of 1.1% per year (Kendall and Tanner 1982). This figure is close to the estimate of 1% per year in the USA calculated from isolation and consultation rates in a waterborne outbreak of campylobacter enteritis (Sacks et al. 1986, Tauxe 1992). According to these figures, some 500 000 infections in the UK and 2.3 million infections in the USA occur annually. Death is rare and often due to underlying disease, but in the USA estimates have ranged from 200 to 700 deaths per year (Tauxe 1992). In general, incidences are higher in rural than urban areas (Sibbald and Sharp 1985, Popović-Uroić 1989).

Although the incidence of around 1% per year is high, it is below the level necessary for the development of population immunity. Thus, in industrialized countries the disease affects adults as well as children. It has an unusual bimodal age distribution with a peak incidence in children aged 0–4 years and a secondary peak in young adults aged 20–24 years (Fig. 29.1).

A study in the UK showed that this pattern is partly distorted by inflated sampling rates in young children (Skirrow 1987). By taking the number of faecal samples tested in each age group as the denominator, instead of the population sampled, the highest rates were shown to be in young adults. The same study also showed an increased male to female ratio in young adults (1.7:1) compared with the average for all ages (1.3:1). Moreover, this ratio was exaggerated during peak incidence in the summer (2.1:1); indeed, the isolation rate in young men with diarrhoea at this time reached 32%. The reasons for these patterns of age- and sex-specific incidence are unknown.

Seasonal trends

In temperate regions incidence changes in a remarkably constant manner in relation to season. There is a sharp rise in early summer followed by a gradual decline to winter base levels. In the UK this pattern has remained constant over a decade (Fig. 29.2). A smaller rise is sometimes seen in autumn and in the USA this rise is caused by isolations associated with outbreaks (Tauxe 1992).

Travellers' diarrhoea

Owing to the high prevalence of campylobacter infection in developing countries (see p. 570), it is not surprising that campylobacters are a leading cause of travellers' diarrhoea (Taylor 1992). Its incidence may vary with the season. In a study of Finnish tourists (Mattila et al. 1992), campylobacter enteritis was found to be the leading cause of travellers' diarrhoea in winter (28% of cases) but not in autumn (7%). Imported infections account for at least 50% of campylobacter infections in Scandinavia, but only 10–25% in the UK.

Costs

The economic costs of campylobacter enteritis are high. A detailed survey in the UK in 1986 showed that the hard costs of health care and lost productive output averaged £265 (about $400) per patient; the intangible costs of 'pain and suffering' were placed at £310 per patient (Sockett and Pearson 1988). The average cost of a patient admitted to hospital is at least £750

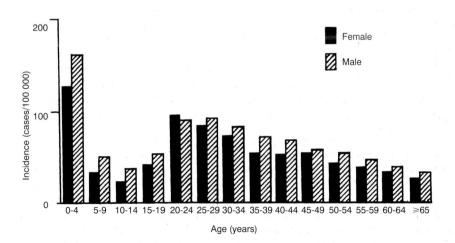

Fig. 29.1 Incidence of campylobacter enteritis by age and sex showing bimodal pattern. (Laboratory isolations England and Wales 1989 and 1990 reported to the Public Health Laboratory Service Communicable Disease Surveillance Centre, London).

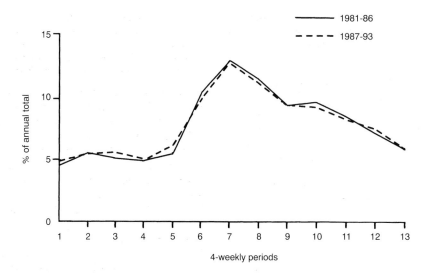

Fig. 29.2 Seasonal pattern of campylobacter infection (England and Wales) showing stability over several years. Mean values 1981–86 and 1987–93. (Data from the Public Health Laboratory Service Communicable Disease Surveillance Centre, London).

(Sockett and Pearson 1988, Rao and Fuller 1992). Thus, in the UK, the hard costs of laboratory diagnosed cases alone amounts to some 13 million per year and the true cost of all cases is many times higher.

Developing countries

Poor quality drinking water, poor sanitation and close contact with animals in the home combine to make campylobacter infection hyperendemic in developing countries. This gives rise to a pattern of disease very different from that in industrialized countries. Several episodes of infection are likely to be experienced by children during the first 2 years of life. Infants derive some protection from maternal antibody, including specific IgA in breast milk (Ruiz-Palacios et al. 1990). Diarrhoea is a feature of about half of all initial infections, but an increasing proportion of subsequent infections are asymptomatic (Calva et al. 1988, Georges-Courbot et al. 1990). Older children and adults are largely unaffected. Infection with more than one strain or species of campylobacter is a frequent finding. There are no clear seasonal trends in tropical countries. Morbidity is difficult to assess, but despite the high frequency of subclinical infection, there is little doubt that campylobacters make a substantial contribution to childhood diarrhoea in developing countries. The subject is explored in more detail by Taylor (1992).

SOURCES AND TRANSMISSION OF INFECTION

Campylobacter enteritis is a zoonosis. *C. jejuni* and *C. coli* are widely distributed in nature as inhabitants of the intestinal tract of a wide variety of birds and to a lesser extent mammals. Their high optimum growth temperature reflects their adaptation to the avian gut. Gulls (*Larus* spp.) are a particularly rich source of campylobacters and they are the main hosts of *C. lari.* Shedding of campylobacters by wild birds causes contamination of open waters and pastures, even in

remote places, and these act as sources of infection for domestic animals.

Campylobacters can survive in water for many weeks, even months, at temperatures below 15°C; the lower the temperature, the longer the survival. Many of the strains isolated from wild sources are of serotypes not encountered in man. The strains causing human disease, and there are many, probably represent a selected population that have become adapted to living in domestic animals. There is some correlation between campylobacter serotypes and host species, but there is a considerable mix. It is possible that more discriminatory typing techniques will show more specific associations. *C. coli* is particularly associated with pigs.

Indirect transmission via food, milk and water

Less than 1% of reported infections in the UK are part of known outbreaks; most infections are apparently single sporadic cases. The sources of most of these infections are undetermined, but they are probably food-borne. Apart from raw milk, raw meats, especially poultry, are the main source of campylobacters entering the food chain. The occurrence of campylobacters in food-producing animals and their products is shown in Table 29.1. It will be seen that broiler chickens stand out as by far the largest potential source of the bacteria. Campylobacter counts of up to 10^6 per carcase are commonplace in broilers, whereas counts are much lower in red meats, a difference that is accentuated after freezing.

Unlike salmonellas, campylobacters do not multiply in food so they seldom cause explosive outbreaks of food poisoning. Some 48 food-borne outbreaks have been reported world wide, almost half of them in Japan. The incriminated or suspect food item was identified in 21 cases (Table 29.2). In the remainder, only the meal could be identified as the common factor.

Table 29.1 The prevalence of campylobacters in food-producing animals and their products. Mean percentage positive (number of surveys from which data taken shown in parentheses)

	Live animal	Retailed product	
		Fresh	Frozen
Broiler chickens	60 (20)	59 (25)	43 (6)
Cattle/beef	21 (12)	3.1 (10)	0 (1)
Sheep/lamb	22 (8)	5.8 (5)	2.0 (1)
Pigs/pork	82 (14)	3.0 (10)	0 (1)
Offal[a]	NA	22 (8)	1.8 (3)

[a]Mostly liver, kidney, heart from cattle, sheep and pigs.
NA, not applicable.

Table 29.2 Foods (excluding milk) incriminated or suspected as vehicle of infection in food-borne outbreaks of campylobacter enteritis

Food	Number of recorded outbreaks
Chicken	9
Turkey	3
Red meat	4
Raw shellfish	2
Egg	2[a]
Cake icing	1
Specific meal (item of food undetermined)	27

[a]Frozen, 1; undercooked, 1.

Similar foods have been identified as carrying an increased risk of infection in case-control studies: raw milk, chickens, raw fish, raw shellfish, mushrooms. In a major case-control study in the Seattle area in the USA, it was calculated that 48% of infections were due to the home consumption (and by inference handling) of chickens (Harris, Weiss and Nolan 1986). A similar figure has been reported in the UK (Neal and Slack 1995), although in another case-control study handling chicken in domestic kitchens was found to carry less risk of infection than in controls (Adak et al. 1995). One explanation for this surprising result is that the controls included people who were symptom free because their frequent handling of chickens made them immune.

There are 3 ways in which infection can be acquired from raw meats.

1 Bacteria may be transferred unwittingly from fingers to mouth when handling the raw product in the kitchen. This is especially likely with inexperienced food handlers.
2 The product may be consumed raw or undercooked, either by choice or accident. Conventional cooking readily kills campylobacters, but fondue and barbecue cooking may not (Mouton et al. 1982, Kapperud et al. 1992b).
3 Bacteria may be transferred from raw meats to 'innocent' ready-to-eat foods on fingers or utensils. This is almost certainly a frequent mode of transmission, but it is diffi-

cult to demonstrate (de Boer and Hahne 1990). Campylobacters have been isolated from flies (Rosef and Kapperud 1983, Khalil et al. 1994) and cockroaches (Umunnabuike and Irokanulo 1986), but the extent to which these insects contaminate food is unknown.

Raw milk is an important source of campylobacter infection. Campylobacters have been isolated from 2.5–12.3% of bulked raw milk samples in the UK, The Netherlands and the USA (Humphrey and Hart 1988, Rohrbach et al. 1992). Numerous outbreaks of campylobacter enteritis have arisen from the consumption of raw or inadequately treated milk, some of them on a grand scale, notably one in England affecting about 2500 schoolchildren (Table 29.3). Campylobacters get into the milk either through faecal contamination at the time of milking, or through excretion in the milk of a cow with campylobacter mastitis (Orr et al. 1995). Goats' milk has also been implicated in outbreaks of infection (Harris et al. 1987). An unusual cause of sporadic milk-borne infection in the UK is the contamination of doorstep delivered milk by magpies (*Pica pica*), jackdaws (*Corvus monedula*) and crows (*Corvus corone*), that in some areas have developed the habit of pecking through the foil tops of bottles (Southern, Smith and Palmer 1990, Phillips 1995).

Untreated water is another important source of campylobacter infection. Sporadic infection is common in persons who drink water from streams or pools while trekking or camping (Taylor et al. 1983). The accidental ingestion of seawater may also cause infection. More important are major community outbreaks from contaminated public water supplies. There have been at least 10 such outbreaks, the largest affecting about one-fifth of a town's population of 16 000 in the USA (Table 29.3). In all such cases the water was from a source considered clean enough not to need chlorination, or else there had been a defect in the chlorination or distribution system.

Direct transmission from animals and man

Direct transmission accounts for a minority of infections and is mainly occupational in people who work in close contact with animals or their products, such as farmers, veterinarians, slaughterhouse workers and butchers. Jones and Robinson (1981) showed that 18% of veterinary assistants, 36% of cattle abattoir workers and 27–68% of poultry processors had serological evidence of past infection, compared with only 2% of urban antenatal patients.

Direct transmission may also occur in the home through contact with infected pets. The most frequent circumstance is the arrival into a household of a new puppy or kitten that becomes ill with campylobacter enteritis. The victim is often a young child or the person caring for the sick animal. From a case-control study in the USA it was estimated that about 6% of infections could be attributed to exposure to domestic animals with diarrhoea (Saeed, Harris and DiGiacomo 1993). In a UK study, this exposure was found to carry a relative risk of infection of 2.39 compared with controls (Adak et al. 1995).

In general, the risk of direct person-to-person

Table 29.3 Some notable water-borne and milk-borne outbreaks of campylobacter enteritis

Place	Number of cases	Attack rate (%)	Suspected cause	Reference
Water-borne				
Sweden	2000	17	Backflow from river into distribution system	Mentzing (1981)
USA	3000	19	Fault in distribution system	Vogt et al. (1982)
England (boarding school)	257	54	Open-topped cold-water storage tank	Palmer et al. (1983)
USA	865	56	Chlorination failure	Sacks et al. (1986)
Norway	680	68	Unchlorinated supply contaminated by flooding	Melby et al. (1991)
Milk-borne				
Scotland	616	50	Pasteurization failure (failed power supply)	Wallace (1980)
England	2500 (school children)	Not known	Incorrect use of bypass valve in pasteurizer	Jones et al. (1981)

spread of campylobacter infection is low. Point-source outbreaks are usually notable for the scarcity of secondary cases. The main exception is when the primary case is a young child. Patients with campylobacter diarrhoea in hospital can be safely nursed under simple 'excretion precautions' without strict isolation. Infants born to mothers who are excreting campylobacters are at risk of infection at the time of birth and 5 outbreaks of infection in neonatal units have been recorded, one with cases of meningitis (Butzler and Goossens 1988). Indirect vehicles of infection, such as communally used rectal thermometers, were likely causes. Practising homosexual men are at increased risk of infection.

1.5 Pathology and pathogenesis

The jejunum, small intestine, colon and rectum may all be affected to some degree; thus the disease might be more accurately termed campylobacter enterocolitis. The terminal ileum is probably the most frequently affected site. Mesenteric adenitis is a regular feature. Histological examination shows acute inflammation of the mucosa, with oedema and infiltration of the lamina propria with neutrophil leucocytes and mononuclear cells. Crypt abscesses may be present. The appearances are indistinguishable from those seen in salmonella, shigella, or yersinia infection, but they are distinct from those of inflammatory bowel disease, unless the campylobacter infection has become prolonged (Skirrow 1990). In keeping with the acute inflammation of the mucosa, leucocytes and erythrocytes are present in the faeces.

INFECTIVE DOSE

Infection has been established with a dose of 500 organisms taken in a glass of milk (Robinson 1981). Other volunteer experiments showed increasing rates of infection as doses were raised from 800 (in effect 400, as half of the bacteria were aflagellate) to 2×10^9 bacteria (Black et al. 1988). However, there was no

clear relation between dose and illness or incubation period. The establishment of infection with low doses is consistent with the high attack rates observed in milk- and water-borne outbreaks of campylobacter enteritis (Table 29.3). Campylobacters are susceptible to acid conditions, so factors governing gastric acidity and transit time strongly influence infectivity. For example, organisms ingested in milk or water are more likely to reach the duodenum intact because of the buffering action of milk or the washing through of stomach contents by water.

INITIAL COLONIZATION

Once campylobacters reach the bile-rich environment of the duodenum and upper ileum they are able to multiply. Active motility is an essential factor for colonization of the mucosa. Powered by long polar flagella, their spiral shape enables them to corkscrew their way through the mucus gel covering the mucosa. The role of adherence to epithelial cells is less well defined. A pattern of diffuse adherence and internalization has been observed in tissue culture systems (e.g. HeLa and Caco-2 cell monolayers) with many strains, but there is only a partial relation between this feature and the type and severity of clinical illness (Everest et al. 1992). Intact flagella appear to be necessary for internalization but not for adherence (Grant and Konkel 1993), although they play an essential role in bringing the bacteria into contact with the mucosa.

PATHOGENIC MECHANISMS

Tissue invasion

Many campylobacter strains are able to invade tissue culture cell lines and there are indications that tissue invasion forms part of the pathogenesis of campylobacter enteritis. However, their invasive ability is less than that of shigellae and other classically invasive bacteria. Campylobacters are invariably negative in the Sereny test. Bacteraemia has been recorded in 0.15% of cases (0.6% in patients aged over 65 years), but transient bacteraemia early in the infection is probably much more frequent (Skirrow et al. 1993). Unlike *C. fetus*, most strains of *C. jejuni* and *C. coli* are susceptible to the non-specific complement-mediated bactericidal activity of normal human serum (Blaser, Smith and Kohler 1985).

Toxins

A cholera-like enterotoxin and several types of cytotoxic activity in cell monolayer cultures have been described in cultures of some campylobacter strains (see Volume 2, Chapter 54), but their significance in relation to pathogenesis is far from clear. The amount of enterotoxin produced is generally much less than that produced by enterotoxigenic *Escherichia coli*. Antibodies to the various toxins have not been found in patients infected with 'toxigenic' strains and apparently non-toxigenic strains are capable of causing disease. Kita and colleagues (1990) describe a hepatotoxic factor (or factors) in whole-cell lysates of some *C. jejuni* strains and clinical hepatitis has occasionally been reported in patients (Skirrow and Blaser 1995).

1.6 Host response

HUMORAL RESPONSE

Specific antibodies to campylobacter antigens appear in the serum from about the fifth day of illness, peak within 2–4 weeks and then decline over several months (Blaser and Duncan 1984). All 3 classes of immunoglobulin (IgA, IgG, IgM) are produced. IgA antibody is also secreted in the gut (Nachamkin and Yang 1992) and in the breast milk of immune mothers (Ruiz-Palacios et al. 1990, Nachamkin et al. 1994). The most important campylobacter immunogens are flagellar and major outer-membrane proteins, and a group of 28–32 kDa proteins designated PEB. These PEB proteins are conserved and not serotypically variable among *C. jejuni* and *C. coli* strains, so they are potential vaccine candidates. Antibodies to campylobacter lipopolysaccharide (LPS) are also produced and they are both strain and species specific. Strain-specific antibodies are important because at least one LPS type (O19) shows cross-reactivity with host glycolipid, which is probably the mechanism whereby some patients infected with O19 strains develop Guillain–Barré syndrome (see p. 568). The humoral response is an essential element of immunity, as patients with hypogammaglobulinaemia are prone to develop persistent and sometimes severe campylobacter infection.

CELLULAR RESPONSE

Little is known about the cellular response to infection. Campylobacters are phagocytosed by mononuclear cells, macrophages and polymorphonuclear granulocytes. Phagocytosis is much enhanced by opsonization, but properties of the infecting strain also influence the reaction (Bär, Glenn-Calvo and Krausse 1991). The fact that patients with AIDS are more prone to campylobacter enteritis than usual indicates that cell mediated immunity plays some part

in defence against infection (Sorvillo, Lieb and Waterman 1991), although in advanced cases secondary hypogammaglobulinaemia may add to this effect.

CLINICAL EXPRESSION OF IMMUNITY

Experiments in volunteers and in non-human primates clearly show that campylobacter infection confers immunity to early rechallenge with a homologous strain (Black et al. 1988), but we do not know how long immunity lasts, nor how much protection is afforded against heterologous strains. Immunity from a single episode of infection is certainly not complete, as natural infections arising 6–18 months apart in otherwise healthy subjects are not unusual; the strains in such cases are invariably of different serotypes. On the other hand, people regularly exposed to infection acquire general immunity to the many hundreds of existing strains without suffering more than a few clinical attacks of enteritis. This has been reported in newcomers to commercial poultry handling (Christenson et al. 1983) and in habitual drinkers of raw milk. For example, in a milk-borne outbreak of campylobacter enteritis in Oregon, USA, there was a 76% attack rate among those exposed to infection for the first time, but no-one was ill among those who habitually drank raw milk (Blaser, Sazie and Williams 1987). Similar findings were reported by Jones, Robinson and Eldridge (1981).

Children in developing countries, where infection is hyperendemic, acquire general immunity to campylobacter enteritis after only a few episodes of infection. Symptomatic infections give way to asymptomatic infections as children enter their second and third years of life (Calva et al. 1988) and this correlates with the appearance of specific antibody (Martin et al. 1989). IgG antibodies in such children rise to a maximum at 2–4 years of age and then decline, whereas IgA antibody rises steadily and is maintained into adult life (Blaser, Taylor and Echeverria 1986). The explanation put forward for the transient IgG response is that as IgA rises it prevents invasive infection, thus removing the stimulus for further IgG production. Breast feeding helps to protect against campylobacter enteritis, mainly through the action of specific secretory IgA, which is particularly plentiful in colostrum (Ruiz-Palacios et al. 1990). It is not known whether cessation of exposure to infection results in a gradual loss of immunity.

1.7 Diagnosis

As campylobacter enteritis cannot be distinguished clinically from other forms of infectious diarrhoea, diagnosis depends on identifying the bacteria in a laboratory. Faecal specimens should be delivered to the laboratory within 24 h of collection and if possible stored in a refrigerator. If longer delays are likely, faeces should be placed in a transport medium recommended by the testing laboratory.

It is often possible to make a rapid presumptive diagnosis by direct microscopy, as campylobacters can be recognized by their characteristic rapid jerking motility in wet preparations, or spiral morphology in stained smears. This can provide a quick provisional result where urgent action, such as surgery for suspected appendicitis, is contemplated. Other direct methods, such as latex agglutination or DNA probing, are not sufficiently developed to detect campylobacters in faeces, although they can detect them in young cultures, or identify the species of bacterial colonies.

CULTURE

The culture and isolation of campylobacters from faeces is the conventional method of diagnosing infection. Originally this was achieved by selective filtration, which took advantage of the small size of campylobacters to separate them from other faecal flora, but it was not long before selective media were developed which allowed specimens to be plated directly without the need for filtration. Although the early blood-containing selective media, such as Skirrow's and Butzler's media, are still used, there is an increasing trend to use charcoal-based blood-free media with cefoperazone as a sole selective agent (Endtz et al. 1991). Plates are incubated micro-aerobically in closed jars, usually at 42–43°C, which gives a selective advantage to *C. jejuni* and *C. coli*. Results are available within 2 days.

Membrane filtration

Several species of campylobacter and arcobacter associated with enteritis are sensitive to some of the antimicrobial agents contained in campylobacter selective media. Such species are usually slower growing and more fastidious than *C. jejuni* or *C. coli* and some are unable to grow at 42°C. Where such strains are prevalent, which is mainly in developing countries, membrane filtration methods have come back into use. All species of campylobacter can be isolated by this method, but most workers find that it is less sensitive than selective agars for *C. jejuni* and *C. coli* (Bolton, Hutchinson and Parker 1988, Albert et al. 1992).

Enrichment and pre-enrichment culture

Preliminary enrichment culture in a selective broth, such as that of Bolton and Robertson (1982), increases sensitivity, but it has only marginal advantage for the culture of stools from patients with diarrhoea. Its chief use is for detecting small numbers of campylobacters in formed stools, or in specimens that have been excessively delayed in transit, but it prolongs the time of final reporting to 3 or 4 days. However, enrichment culture is essential for the isolation of campylobacters from food and environmental samples. Pre-enrichment for a few hours in plain broth at 37°C is necessary for bacteria that have been sublethally injured by freezing, or heating (Humphrey 1986).

Full accounts of the isolation of campylobacters from clinical material and foods are given by Goossens and Butzler (1992) and Corry et al. (1995), respectively.

SERODIAGNOSIS

A retrospective serological diagnosis is sometimes required for patients thought to have a late compli-

cation of campylobacter infection, but in whom a bacteriological diagnosis was not made at the time of the original illness. Tests are designed to detect group antigens common to all strains of *C. jejuni* and *C. coli*. The first such test was a complement-fixation test (Jones, Eldridge and Dale 1980), but it is not very sensitive. An enzyme-linked immunosorbent assay (ELISA) using an acid–glycine extract of the bacteria as antigen is a more sensitive method and it can detect specific classes of antibody (IgA, IgM, IgG) (Rautelin and Kosunen 1987). Sera from patients with campylobacter infection may give false positive reactions in serological tests for legionella infection (Marshall, Boswell and Kudesia 1994).

Tests that detect strain-specific antigens can be invaluable for the retrospective detection of cases in outbreaks (Jones, Robinson and Eldridge 1981). They are also useful for the detection of specific antigens, for example the presence of O19 antigen in patients with GBS. Agglutination, bactericidal, ELISA and immunoblotting tests have been used for this purpose.

1.8 Control

GENERAL MEASURES

The provision of safe water supplies and safe disposal of sewage are basic to the control of any infection spread by the faecal–oral route and campylobacter enteritis is no exception. The public need to be educated on the importance of good hygiene, in particular the need to wash the hands after handling sick animals and before handling food. Both domestic and professional food handlers should be instructed on good hygienic practice in food preparation, especially the importance of handling and storing raw meats separately from other foods. All milk sold to the public should be pasteurized or otherwise heat treated.

CONTROL OF INFECTION IN FOOD-PRODUCING ANIMALS

Because there is a large natural reservoir of campylobacters in wild animals and natural water, complete control of infection in domestic animals is unattainable. In the case of larger animals, steps can be taken to minimize the contamination of carcases with gut contents at slaughter, but there is a limit to what is practicable. Fortunately, blast chilling greatly reduces the numbers of campylobacters through surface drying.

Broiler chickens and other poultry are more of a problem. Most broiler flocks are heavily colonized with campylobacters and mass mechanized processing ensures that many birds from uncolonized flocks end up contaminated. There seems to be no practicable way of reducing cross-contamination during mass processing, so the remedy must be to prevent, or at least reduce, the initial colonization of flocks (Humphrey 1989). This should be possible, as almost all birds are raised in closed buildings and infection is not transmitted vertically via eggs (Jacobs-Reitsma et al. 1995). Several experimental interventions have been successful. They include the application of strict hygienic measures and the exclusion of birds and rodents from chicken houses, but the most promising seems to be the installation of water supply systems that ensure the exclusion of campylobacters (Pearson et al. 1993, Kapperud et al. 1993). The principle of competitive exclusion by feeding normal gut flora or a specific mix of organisms to chicks is another promising approach (Humphrey, Lanning and Mead 1989, Schoeni and Wong 1994). Terminal irradiation is a certain way to make poultry safe from all pathogens, but there is public disquiet over such a policy. The control of campylobacter infection in poultry is likely to have a greater impact on the incidence of campylobacter enteritis in industrialized countries than any other measure.

VACCINATION

No vaccine against campylobacter enteritis is currently available, but vaccination would be an appropriate approach for the control of the disease in children in developing countries and for others at increased risk of infection. Several antigens are vaccine candidates, notably the 28–32 kDa PEB proteins referred to previously (p. 573). A vaccine consisting of inactivated campylobacter whole cells given with *Escherichia coli* LT enterotoxin as adjuvant has shown promise in animal models and is being developed for human trials in the USA (Harberberger and Walker 1994).

1.9 Treatment

Most patients with campylobacter enteritis require no more than simple supportive treatment in the form of fluid and electrolyte replacement. Antimicrobial therapy is effective if given early in the disease, but as most victims are recovering by the time a bacteriological diagnosis is made, it is seldom appropriate. However, if at that time a patient is still acutely ill, it is reasonable to give a short course of an appropriate antimicrobial agent. Erythromycin remains the best choice as resistance rates remain generally low, although there are areas, for example Thailand, where rates are high. In general, erythromycin resistance is much more frequent in *C. coli* than *C. jejuni*. Fluoroquinolones are highly effective against sensitive strains of both species, but resistance has increased alarmingly since the late 1980s. Ciprofloxacin resistance rates as high as 50% have been reported in Spain and The Netherlands. The widespread use of enrofloxacin in poultry has been blamed for this trend (Jacobs-Reitsma, Kan and Bolder 1994). Gentamicin is effective in rare invasive life-threatening infections.

2 OTHER CAMPYLOBACTER INFECTIONS OF MAN

2.1 Systemic campylobacteriosis

Systemic campylobacteriosis is the term used for a variety of primary bacteraemic or septicaemic infections, usually caused by *C. fetus*, in immunodeficient patients. This is distinct from the transient bacteraemia sometimes seen in campylobacter enteritis due to *C. jejuni* or *C. coli*. The condition is uncommon. Only 22 cases of *C. fetus* bacteraemia were reported over an 11 year period in England and Wales (Skirrow et al. 1993). Typical predisposing conditions are malignant disease (e.g. leukaemia, lymphoma, Hodgkin's disease), alcoholic cirrhosis, chronic renal failure, hypogammaglobulinaemia and AIDS. Infection probably arises from intestinal colonization, but intestinal symptoms occur in only about one in 4 infections. Some patients have focal infection elsewhere in the body and the high incidence of thrombophlebitis and endocarditis suggests that *C. fetus* has an affinity for endovascular surfaces. Other forms of focal infection are pericarditis, septic arthritis, spontaneous peritonitis, meningitis and septic abortion (Schmidt et al. 1980, Mishu Allos, Blaser and Lastovica 1995). Septic abortion merits special consideration as it affects apparently healthy women.

2.2 Campylobacter abortion

The first bacteriologically proven case of human campylobacter infection was that of a French woman aged 39 years who aborted a 6-month-old fetus 5 weeks after an influenza-like bacteraemic illness with what was then called '*Vibrio fetus*' (Vinzent, Dumas and Picard 1947). Some 29 cases of campylobacter abortion, or premature labour with early infant death, have been described, 12 due to *C. fetus*, 16 to *C. jejuni* and one to *C. coli*. Gestation at the time of infection ranged from 13 to 32 weeks (Simor et al. 1986). The essential pathology appears to be a placentitis that causes fetal death through placental insufficiency, a picture similar to that seen in campylobacter abortion in sheep (see section 3.1, p. 576). As in sheep, placental infection probably arises by haematogenous spread from the gut, but the affinity of campylobacters for the human placenta is clearly far less than it is for the sheep placenta. The pathology is described more fully by Skirrow (1994).

2.3 Periodontal disease

Campylobacters of several species are found in human gingival flora: *Campylobacter sputorum, Campylobacter concisus, Campylobacter rectus, Campylobacter curvus, Campylobacter showae, Campylobacter gracilis*, [*Bacteroides*] *ureolyticus* (which is probably a campylobacter). Some are found in large numbers in the periodontal pockets of diseased gums, usually in association with anaerobic bacteria, but their role in pathogenesis or maintenance of the disease state is not clear. Attention has been focused mainly on *C. rectus* (Rams, Feik and Slots 1993).

3 CAMPYLOBACTER AND ARCOBACTER INFECTIONS OF ANIMALS

3.1 Campylobacter abortion and infertility

OVINE ABORTION

On 6 February 1906, McFadyean and Stockman (1913) obtained pure cultures of 'a vibrio' (*C. fetus*) from a ewe and the stomach contents of her dead fetus. This was the first recorded isolation of a campylobacter of any species. The organism was named '*Vibrio fetus*' by Smith and Taylor (1919) and for many years the disease became known as 'vibrionic abortion'. It is found in most sheep farming areas of the world. In the UK campylobacters rank third as a cause of outbreaks of ovine abortion (4–13%), exceeded only by *Chlamydia psittaci* (15–24%) and *Toxoplasma gondii* (12–22%) (Allsup 1985). *C. fetus* is the species classically associated with ovine abortion, but in Allsup's study 43% of outbreaks were caused by *C. jejuni* and 21% by *C. coli*. Arcobacter species, notably *A. cryaerophilus*, have occasionally been isolated from sporadic cases of ovine abortion.

Abortion usually occurs in the late stages of pregnancy and, exceptionally, abortion rates may exceed 60%. Campylobacters are commonly carried in the intestines and gall bladders of healthy sheep and it is thought that placental infection is initiated through bacteraemia arising from these sites. Bacteraemia has been observed following oral inoculation of pregnant ewes and Lowrie and Pearce (1970) showed that a strain of '*V. fetus*' from an outbreak had a strong predilection for ovine placental and chorionic tissue. Increased faecal carriage rates have been observed, often with concomitant mild diarrhoea, in flocks suffering high abortion rates. The interval between infection and abortion ranges from 13 to 113 days.

It is unusual for a flock to suffer campylobacter abortion in successive years, which indicates that at least medium-term immunity is acquired. Vaccines can be effective (Hansen et al. 1990) and losses can be reduced if vaccination is applied immediately after the detection of excess abortions in a flock.

BOVINE ABORTION AND INFECTIOUS INFERTILITY

Although McFadyean and Stockman (1913) had observed 'vibrionic abortion' in cows, it was Theobald Smith (1918) who established that '*Vibrio fetus*' was a cause of sporadic abortion in cattle. As in epizootic abortion of sheep, the infection is transmitted intestinally. *C. fetus* is the species typically associated with the disease, but *C. jejuni* has also been implicated (Van Donkersgoed et al. 1990). In addition, *A. cryaerophilus* and *Arcobacter skirrowii* have been isolated from aborted bovine fetuses (Vandamme et al. 1992b).

Nearly 30 years after Smith's work, it was observed that '*V. fetus*' infection was associated with lowered conception rates in cows and that bulls had serological evidence of infection (Plastridge, Williams and Petrie

1947). This was the first stage in the discovery of the more serious form of campylobacter infection of cattle, namely infectious infertility, in which infection is transmitted venereally by carrier bulls. The bacteriology was clarified by Florent (1959) who showed that sporadic abortion and infectious infertility were caused by distinct organisms ('*V. foetus* var. *intestinalis*' and '*V. foetus* var. *venerealis*') now known as *C. fetus* subsp. *fetus* and *C. fetus* subsp. *venerealis*, respectively. Infected bulls carry *C. fetus* subsp. *venerealis* on the mucous membranes of the prepuce and sometimes urethra without visible signs. The bacteria are transmitted to the cow during coitus, causing mild vaginitis, cervicitis, endometritis and salpingitis. As a result, embryos die within 15–21 days of conception, oestrus becomes irregular and the number of matings required to produce a viable conception is greatly increased. The pathogenesis of embryo death is unknown, but it has been suggested that endometritis prevents implantation, or that the growth of *C. fetus* restricts the supply of oxygen to the embryo at a time when it is most vulnerable (Ware 1980). Infertility lasts for up to 10 months. Bulls can be infected from contaminated bedding and equipment as well as through coitus with infected cows.

Infection is diagnosed by detecting *C. fetus* in the vaginal mucus of cows or fresh preputial washings of bulls. Care must be taken not to confuse *C. fetus* with *C. sputorum* biotype *bubulus*, a harmless commensal of the bovine preputial sac. Screening large herds for infection can be more conveniently done by the demonstration of specific antibody in vaginal mucus (Hewson, Lander and Gill 1985).

The disease is of world-wide distribution and major economic importance. Substantial control can be achieved by artificial insemination (AI) programmes in which semen from bulls is tested and certified to be free from campylobacters. In industrialized countries these programmes are usually protected by legislation. However, pockets of infection can still arise through the persistence of traditional practices, as happened in Scotland in the mid-1970s (MacLaren and Wright 1977). In developing countries without controlled AI programmes widespread infection persists. Vaccines prepared against high molecular weight surface (S-layer) proteins of *C. fetus* are effective both for prevention and the treatment of infected cows and carrier bulls. Campylobacter infertility in cattle is described more fully elsewhere (Lawson 1959, Dekeyser 1984).

CAMPYLOBACTER AND ARCOBACTER ABORTION IN OTHER ANIMALS

There are isolated reports of *C. jejuni* abortion in goats, mink, dogs and cynomolgus monkeys. Abortion has been produced experimentally in ferrets with *C. jejuni* and in rodents with *C. jejuni* or *C. fetus*. *C. fetus* has been isolated from an aborted foal from a thoroughbred horse. Arcobacters have been isolated from up to 43% of aborted piglets, but their significance is in doubt as they can also be isolated from the internal organs of healthy piglets. *A. cryaerophilus* is the species most frequently recorded, but *A. butzleri* and

A. skirrowii are also represented (Vandamme et al. 1992b). The subject is reviewed by Skirrow (1994).

3.2 Miscellaneous campylobacter and arcobacter infections of animals

CAMPYLOBACTER ENTERITIS IN ANIMALS

It is difficult to assess the enteropathogenicity of campylobacters in animals, because they are often found equally in both sick and well animals. Most animals are exposed to infection from birth and develop immunity early. Moreover, the timing of first infections may be such that their effects are mitigated by passively acquired maternal antibody. The situation is analogous to that of children in developing countries.

Monkeys are susceptible to campylobacter enteritis in much the same way as man. Recently imported monkeys are especially vulnerable (Tribe and Fleming 1983). Dogs are also susceptible, but immunity has been shown to develop at an early age (Newton et al. 1988). Occasional severe infections have been reported (Slee 1979). Experimental infection of pups produces only mild disease (Macartney et al. 1988).

Experimental infection of calves and lambs suggests they are not particularly susceptible to campylobacter enteritis, but Stansfield, Hunt and Kemble (1986) described a severe outbreak of scouring, with a 12% mortality, apparently due to *C. jejuni*, in fattening lambs. A severe disease known as weaner colitis in lambs has been associated with an unidentified catalase-negative campylobacter in Australia (Stephens et al. 1984).

Whether *C. coli* alone or with other agents causes diarrhoea in pigs has long been a subject of debate. Experimental infection of colostrum-deprived piglets with a porcine strain of *C. coli* was found to produce mild ileitis and diarrhoea (Olubunmi and Taylor 1982).

Poultry appear to be little affected by campylobacter infection. Neill, Campbell and Greene (1984) observed that wet litter, indicative of diarrhoea, coincided with the appearance of *C. jejuni* in broiler flocks and that deaths occurred when infection was introduced before the birds were 2 weeks old. Experimental infection of newly hatched chicks has given conflicting results. 'Vibrios' resembling *C. jejuni* were described by Truscott and Morin (1964) as an apparent cause of transmissible enteritis (bluecomb disease) in turkeys.

The subject of campylobacter enteritis in animals is reviewed by Skirrow (1994).

CAMPYLOBACTER MASTITIS IN COWS

This infection, which has obvious public health implications, was induced experimentally with *C. jejuni* by Lander and Gill (1980) before natural infection had been detected (Morgan et al. 1985, Orr et al. 1995). Clinical signs of mastitis may be minimal yet infection can persist for at least 12 weeks. Moreover, in experimental infection the highest bacterial counts were observed early in the infection before the milk had become obviously abnormal. Bovine mastitis due to *A. cryaerophilus* has also been observed and reproduced experimentally (Logan, Neill and Mackie 1982).

AVIAN HEPATITIS

In the late 1950s a form of avian hepatitis was described, attributed to 'vibrios' conforming to the description of *C. jejuni*. The disease was widespread in continental Europe and North America and diarrhoea was a frequent clinical feature (Peckham 1972). The disease remains something of a mystery, as it has disappeared spontaneously and attempts to reproduce it by the inoculation of pure cultures of current strains of *C. jejuni* have failed.

PORCINE PROLIFERATIVE ENTEROPATHY (PPE)

The proliferative enteropathies are a group of puzzling diseases characterized by enterocyte proliferation affecting pigs, hamsters and, to a lesser extent, ferrets and rabbits. *C. mucosalis* and *C. hyointestinalis* can be found in large numbers in the lesions, but not commonly in the intestines of normal pigs. Yet inoculation of healthy pigs with pure cultures of either organism fails to reproduce the disease. New light was shed on the problem when a curved obligate intracellular bacterium was identified in the proliferating epithelial cells characteristic of the lesions (reviewed by Lawson and McOrist 1993). Gebhart and colleagues (1993) claim that it is closely related to *Desulfovibrio desulfuricans*, a sulphate-reducing proteobacterium, to which they gave the provisional name 'ileal symbiont intracellularis'. It is capable of reproducing the disease in conventional but not germ-free pigs. On the other hand, Alderton and colleagues (1995) claim that the organism is a new campylobacter species, *Campylobacter hyoilei*.

REFERENCES

Adak GK, Cowden JM et al., 1995, The Public Health Laboratory Service national case-control study of primary indigenous sporadic cases of campylobacter infection, *Epidemiol Infect*, **115:** 15–22.

Albert MJ, Tee W et al., 1992, Comparison of a blood-free medium and a filtration technique for the isolation of *Campylobacter* spp. from diarrhoeal stools of hospitalized patients in central Australia, *J Med Microbiol*, **37:** 176–9.

Alderton MR, Korolik V et al., 1995, *Campylobacter hyoilei* sp. nov., associated with porcine proliferative enteritis, *Int J Syst Bacteriol*, **45:** 61–6.

Allsup TN, 1985, Ovine campylobacter abortion, *Agriculture. Campylobacter*, ed Lander KP, Commission of the European Communities, Luxembourg, 93–107.

Bär W, Glenn-Calvo E, Krausse R, 1991, Phagocytosis of enteric *Campylobacter* by human and murine granulocytes, *FEMS Microbiol Lett*, **76:** 143–9.

Black RE, Levine MM et al., 1988, Experimental *Campylobacter jejuni* infection in humans, *J Infect Dis*, **157:** 472–9.

Blaser MJ, Duncan DJ, 1984, Human serum antibody response to *Campylobacter jejuni* infection as measured in an enzyme-linked immunosorbent assay, *Infect Immun*, **44:** 292–8.

Blaser MJ, Sazie E, Williams P, 1987, The influence of immunity on raw milk-associated *Campylobacter* infection, *JAMA*, **257:** 43–6.

Blaser MJ, Smith PF, Kohler PA, 1985, Susceptibility of *Campylobacter* isolates to the bactericidal activity in human serum, *J Infect Dis*, **151:** 227–35.

Blaser MJ, Taylor DN, Echeverria P, 1986, Immune response to *Campylobacter jejuni* in a rural community in Thailand, *J Infect Dis*, **153:** 249–54.

de Boer E, Hahne M, 1990, Cross-contamination with *Campylobacter jejuni* and *Salmonella* spp. from raw chicken products during food preparation, *J Food Prot*, **53:** 1067–8.

Bolton FJ, Hutchinson DN, Parker G, 1988, Reassessment of selective agars and filtration techniques for isolation of *Campylobacter* species from faeces, *Eur J Clin Microbiol Infect Dis*, **7:** 155–60.

Bolton FJ, Robertson L, 1982, A selective medium for isolating *Campylobacter jejuni/coli*, *J Clin Pathol*, **35:** 462–7.

Borczyk A (here spelled 'Broczyk'), Thompson S et al., 1987, Water-borne outbreak of *Campylobacter laridis*-associated gastroenteritis, *Lancet*, **1:** 164–5.

Butzler J-P, Goossens H, 1988, *Campylobacter jejuni* infection as a hospital problem: an overview, *J Hosp Infect*, **11, Suppl. A:** 374–7.

Butzler J-P, Dekeyser P et al., 1973, Related vibrio in stools, *J Pediatr*, **82:** 493–5.

Calva JJ, Ruiz-Palacios GM et al., 1988, Cohort study of intestinal infection with campylobacter in Mexican children, *Lancet*, **1:** 503–6.

Christenson B, Ringner Å et al., 1983, An outbreak of campylobacter enteritis among the staff of a poultry abattoir in Sweden, *Scand J Infect Dis*, **15:** 167–72.

Corry JEL, Post DE et al., 1995, Culture media for the isolation of campylobacters, *Int J Food Microbiol*, **26:** 43–76.

Dekeyser J, 1984, Bovine genital campylobacteriosis, *Campylobacter Infections in Man and Animals*, ed. Butzler J-P, CRC Press, Boca Raton, FL, 181–91.

Dekeyser P, Gossuin-Detrain M et al., 1972, Acute enteritis due to related vibrio: first positive stool cultures, *J Infect Dis*, **125:** 390–2.

Endtz HP, Ruijs GJHM et al., 1991, Comparison of six media, including a semisolid agar, for the isolation of various *Campylobacter* species from stool specimens, *J Clin Microbiol*, **29:** 1007–10.

Escherich T, 1886, Beiträge zur Kenntniss der Darmbacterien. III. Ueber das Vorkommen von Vibrionen im Darmcanal und den Stuhlgängen der säuglinge. [Articles adding to the knowledge of intestinal bacteria. III. On the existence of vibrios in the intestines and faeces of babies], *Münch Med Wochenschr*, **33:** 815–17, 833–5.

Everest PH, Goossens H et al., 1992, Differentiated Caco-2 cells as a model for enteric invasion by *Campylobacter jejuni* and *C. coli*, *J Med Microbiol*, **37:** 319–25.

Florent A, 1959, Les deux vibrioses génitales de la bête bovine: la vibriose vénérienne, due à *V. foetus venerialis*, et la vibriose d'origine intestinale due à *V. foetus intestinalis*, *Proceedings of the 16th International Veterinary Congress, Madrid*, **2:** 953–7.

Gebhart CJ, Barns SM et al., 1993, Ileal symbiont intracellularis, an obligate intracellular bacterium of porcine intestines showing a relationship to *Desulfovibrio* species, *Int J Syst Bacteriol*, **43:** 533–8.

Georges-Courbot MC, Cassel-Beraud AM et al., 1990, A cohort study of enteric campylobacter infection in children from birth to two years in Bangui (Central African Republic), *Trans R Soc Trop Med Hyg*, **84:** 122–5.

Goossens H, Butzler J-P, 1992, Isolation and identification of *Campylobacter* spp., *Campylobacter jejuni*: Current Status and Future Trends, eds Nachamkin I, Blaser MJ, Tompkins LS, American Society for Microbiology, New York, 93–109.

Goossens H, Vlaes L et al., 1990, Is '*Campylobacter upsaliensis*' an unrecognised cause of human diarrhoea?, *Lancet*, **335:** 584–6.

Grant CCR, Konkel ME, 1993, Role of flagella in adherence, internalization, and translocation of *Campylobacter jejuni* in nonpolarized and polarized epithelial cell cultures, *Infect Immun*, **61:** 1764–71.

Hansen DE, Hedstrom OR et al., 1990, Efficacy of a vaccine to prevent *Chlamydia*- or *Campylobacter*-induced abortion in ewes, *J Am Vet Med Assoc*, **196:** 731–4.

Harberberger RL, Walker RI, 1994, Prospects and problems for development of a vaccine against diarrhea caused by *Campylobacter*, *Vaccine Res*, **3:** 15–22.

Harris NV, Weiss NS, Nolan CM, 1986, The role of poultry and meats in the etiology of *Campylobacter jejuni/coli* enteritis, *Am J Public Health*, **76:** 407–11.

Harris NV, Kimball TJ et al., 1987, *Campylobacter jejuni* enteritis associated with raw goat's milk, *Am J Epidemiol*, **126:** 179–86.

Hewson PI, Lander KP, Gill KPW, 1985, Enzyme-linked immunosorbent assay for antibodies to *Campylobacter fetus* in bovine vaginal mucus, *Res Vet Sci*, **38:** 41–5.

Humphrey TJ, 1986, Injury and recovery in freeze- or heat-damaged *Campylobacter jejuni*, *Lett Appl Microbiol*, **3:** 81–4.

Humphrey TJ, 1989, Salmonella, campylobacter and poultry: possible control measures, *Abstr Hyg Commun Dis*, **64:** R1–8.

Humphrey TJ, Hart RJC, 1988, Campylobacter and salmonella contamination of unpasteurized cows' milk on sale to the public, *J Appl Bacteriol*, **65:** 463–7.

Humphrey TJ, Lanning DG, Mead GC, 1989, Inhibition of *Campylobacter jejuni* in vitro by broiler chicken caecal contents, *Vet Rec*, **125:** 272–3.

Jacobs-Reitsma WF, Kan CA, Bolder NM, 1994, The induction of quinolone resistance in *Campylobacter* bacteria in broilers by quinolone treatment, *Lett Appl Microbiol*, **19:** 228–31.

Jacobs-Reitsma WF, van de Giessen AW et al., 1995, Epidemiology of *Campylobacter* spp. at two Dutch broiler farms, *Epidemiol Infect*, **114:** 413–21.

Jewkes J, Larson HE et al., 1981, Aetiology of acute diarrhoea in adults, *Gut*, **22:** 388–92.

Jones DM, Eldridge J, Dale BAS, 1980, Serological response to *Campylobacter jejuni/coli* infection, *J Clin Pathol*, **33:** 767–9.

Jones DM, Robinson DA, 1981, Occupational exposure to *Campylobacter jejuni/coli* infection, *Lancet*, **1:** 440–1.

Jones DM, Robinson DA, Eldridge J, 1981, Serological studies in two outbreaks of *Campylobacter jejuni* infection, *J Hyg*, **87:** 163–70.

Jones FS, Little RB, 1931a, The etiology of infectious diarrhea (winter scours) in cattle, *J Exp Med*, **53:** 835–43.

Jones FS, Little RB, 1931b, Vibrionic enteritis of calves, *J Exp Med*, **53:** 845–51.

Jones PH, Willis AT et al., 1981, Campylobacter enteritis associated with the consumption of free school milk, *J Hyg*, **87:** 155–62.

Kapperud G, Lassen J et al., 1992a, Clinical features of sporadic campylobacter infections in Norway, *Scand J Infect Dis*, **24:** 741–9.

Kapperud G, Skjerve E et al., 1992b, Risk factors for *Campylobacter* infections: results of a case-control study in southeastern Norway, *J Clin Microbiol*, **30:** 3117–21.

Kapperud G, Skjerve E et al., 1993, Epidemiological investigation of risk factors for campylobacter colonization in Norwegian broiler flocks, *Epidemiol Infect*, **111:** 245–55.

Kendall EJC, Tanner EI, 1982, Campylobacter enteritis in general practice, *J Hyg*, **88:** 155–63.

Khalil K, Lindblom G-B et al., 1994, Flies and water as reservoirs for bacterial enteropathogens in urban and rural areas in and around Lahore, Pakistan, *Epidemiol Infect*, **113:** 435–44.

Kiehlbauch JA, Brenner DJ et al., 1991, *Campylobacter butzleri* sp. nov. isolated from humans and animals with diarrheal illness, *J Clin Microbiol*, **29:** 376–85.

King EO, 1957, Human infections with *Vibrio fetus* and a closely related vibrio, *J Infect Dis*, **101:** 119–28.

King EO, 1962, The laboratory recognition of *Vibrio fetus* and a closely related *vibrio* isolated from cases of human vibriosis, *Ann N Y Acad Sci*, **98:** 700–11.

Kist M, 1985, The historical background to campylobacter infection: new aspects, *Campylobacter III*, eds Pearson AD, Skirrow MB et al., Public Health Laboratory Service, London, 23–7.

Kita E, Oku D et al., 1990, Hepatotoxic activity of *Campylobacter jejuni*, *J Med Microbiol*, **33:** 171–82.

Lander KP, Gill KPW, 1980, Experimental infection of the bovine udder with *Campylobacter coli/jejuni*, *J Hyg*, **84:** 421–8.

Lastovica AJ, Le Roux E, 1993, Prevalence and distribution of *Campylobacter* spp. in the diarrhoeic stools and blood cultures of paediatric patients, *Acta Gastroenterol Belg*, **56, Suppl.:** 34.

Lawson GHK, McOrist S, 1993, The enigma of the proliferative enteropathies: a review, *J Comp Pathol*, **84:** 41–6.

Lawson JR, 1959, Vibriosis, *Infectious Diseases of Animals. Diseases due to Bacteria*, eds Stableforth AW, Galloway IA, Butterworths, London, 745–84.

Levy AJ, 1946, A gastro-enteritis outbreak probably due to a bovine strain of vibrio, *Yale J Biol Med*, **18:** 243–58.

Logan EF, Neill SD, Mackie DP, 1982, Mastitis in dairy cows associated with an aerotolerant campylobacter, *Vet Rec*, **110:** 229–30.

Lowrie DB, Pearce JH, 1970, The placental localisation of *Vibrio fetus*, *J Med Microbiol*, **3:** 607–14.

Macartney L, Al-Mashat RR et al., 1988, Experimental infection of dogs with *Campylobacter jejuni*, *Vet Rec*, **122:** 245–9.

McFadyean J, Stockman S, 1913, *Report of the Departmental Committee appointed by the Board of Agriculture and Fisheries to inquire into Epizootic Abortion. Part III. Abortion in Sheep*, HMSO, London.

MacLaren APC, Wright CL, 1977, *Campylobacter fetus* (*Vibrio fetus*) infection in dairy herds in South-West Scotland, *Vet Rec*, **101:** 463–4.

Marshall LE, Boswell TCJ, Kudesia G, 1994, False positive legionella serology in campylobacter infection: campylobacter serotypes, duration of antibody response and elimination of cross-reactions in the indirect fluorescent antibody test, *Epidemiol Infect*, **112:** 347–57.

Martin PMV, Mathiot J et al., 1989, Immune response to *Campylobacter jejuni* and *Campylobacter coli* in a cohort of children from birth to 2 years of age, *Infect Immun*, **57:** 2542–6.

Mattila L, 1994, Clinical features and duration of traveler's diarrhea in relation to its etiology, *Clin Infect Dis*, **19:** 728–34.

Mattila L, Siitonen A et al., 1992, Seasonal variation in etiology of traveler's diarrhea, *J Infect Dis*, **165:** 385–8.

Melby K, Gondrosen B et al., 1991, Waterborne campylobacteriosis in northern Norway, *Int J Food Microbiol*, **12:** 151–6.

Mentzing L-O, 1981, Waterborne outbreaks of campylobacter enteritis in central Sweden, *Lancet*, **2:** 352–4.

Mishu Allos B, Blaser MJ, Lastovica AJ, 1995, Atypical campylobacters and related microorganisms, *Infections of the Gastrointestinal Tract*, eds Blaser MJ, Smith PD et al., Raven Press, New York, 849–65.

Morgan G, Chadwick P et al., 1985, *Campylobacter jejuni* mastitis in a cow: a zoonosis-related incident, *Vet Rec*, **116:** 111.

Mouton RP, Veltkamp JJ et al., 1982, Analysis of a small outbreak of campylobacter infections with high morbidity, *Campylobacter: Epidemiology, Pathogenesis and Biochemistry*, ed. Newell DG, MTP Press, Lancaster, 129–34.

Nachamkin I, Yang X-H, 1992, Local immune responses to the *Campylobacter* flagellin in acute *Campylobacter* gastrointestinal infection, *J Clin Microbiol*, **30:** 509–11.

Nachamkin I, Fischer SH et al., 1994, Immunoglobulin A antibodies directed against *Campylobacter jejuni* flagellin present in breast milk, *Epidemiol Infect*, **112:** 359–65.

Neal KR, Slack RCB, 1995, The autumn peak in campylobacter gastro-enteritis. Are the risk factors the same for travel- and UK-acquired campylobacter infections, *J Public Health Med*, **17:** 98–102.

Neill SD, Campbell JN, Greene JA, 1984, *Campylobacter* species in broiler chickens, *Avian Pathol*, **13:** 777–85.

Newton CM, Newell DG et al., 1988, Campylobacter infection in a closed dog breeding colony, *Vet Rec*, **123:** 152–4.

Olubunmi PA, Taylor DJ, 1982, Production of enteritis in pigs by the oral inoculation of pure cultures of *Campylobacter coli*, *Vet Rec*, **111:** 197–202.

On SLW, 1994, Confirmation of human *Campylobacter concisus* isolates misidentified as *Campylobacter mucosalis* and suggestions for improved differentiation between the two species, *J Clin Microbiol*, **32:** 2305–6.

Orr KE, Lightfoot NF et al., 1995, Direct milk excretion of *Campylobacter jejuni* in a dairy cow causing cases of human enteritis, *Epidemiol Infect*, **114:** 15–24.

Palmer SR, Gully PR et al., 1983, Water-borne outbreak of campylobacter gastroenteritis, *Lancet*, **1:** 287–90.

Pearson AD, Greenwood M et al., 1993, Colonization of broiler chickens by waterborne *Campylobacter jejuni*, *Appl Environ Microbiol*, **59:** 987–96.

Peckham MC, 1972, Vibrionic hepatitis, *Diseases of Poultry*, 6th edn, eds Hofstad MS, Calnek BW et al., Iowa State University Press, Ames IA, 322–44.

Phillips CA, 1995, Bird attacks on milk bottles and campylobacter infection, *Lancet*, **346:** 386.

Plastridge WN, Williams LF, Petrie D, 1947, Vibrionic abortion in cattle, *Am J Vet Res*, **8:** 178–83.

Popović-Uroić T, 1989, *Campylobacter jejuni* and *Campylobacter coli* diarrhoea in rural and urban populations in Yugoslavia, *Epidemiol Infect*, **102:** 59–67.

Rams TE, Feik D, Slots J, 1993, *Campylobacter rectus* in human periodontitis, *Oral Microbiol Immunol*, **8:** 230–5.

Rao GG, Fuller M, 1992, A review of hospitalized patients with bacterial gastroenteritis, *J Hosp Infect*, **20:** 105–11.

Rautelin HI, Kosunen TU, 1987, *Campylobacter* etiology in human gastroenteritis demonstrated by antibodies to acid extract antigen, *J Clin Microbiol*, **25:** 1944–51.

Rees JH, Gregson NA et al., 1993, *Campylobacter jejuni* and Guillain–Barré syndrome, *Q J Med*, **86:** 623–34.

Riordan T, 1988, Intestinal infection with campylobacter in children, *Lancet*, **1:** 992.

Robinson DA, 1981, Infective dose of *Campylobacter jejuni* in milk, *Br Med J*, **282:** 1584.

Robinson DA, Jones DM, 1981, Milk-borne campylobacter infection, *Br Med J*, **282:** 1374–6.

Rohrbach BW, Draughon FA et al., 1992, Prevalence of *Listeria monocytogenes*, *Campylobacter jejuni*, *Yersinia enterocolitica*, and *Salmonella* in bulk tank milk: risk factors and risk of human exposure, *J Food Prot*, **55:** 93–7.

Rosef O, Kapperud G, 1983, House flies (*Musca domestica*) as possible vectors of *Campylobacter fetus* subsp. *jejuni*, *Appl Environ Microbiol*, **45:** 381–3.

Ruiz-Palacios GM, Calva JJ et al., 1990, Protection of breast-fed infants against *Campylobacter* diarrhea by antibodies in human milk, *J Pediatr*, **116:** 707–13.

Sacks JJ, Lieb S et al., 1986, Epidemic campylobacteriosis associated with a community water supply, *Am J Public Health*, **76:** 424–8.

Saeed AM, Harris NV, DiGiacomo RF, 1993, The role of exposure to animals in the etiology of *Campylobacter jejuni/coli* enteritis, *Am J Epidemiol*, **137:** 108–14.

Salama SM, Tabor H et al., 1992, Pulsed-field gel electrophoresis for epidemiologic studies of *Campylobacter hyointestinalis* isolates, *J Clin Microbiol*, **30:** 1982–4.

Schmidt U, Chmel H et al., 1980, The clinical spectrum of *Campylobacter fetus* infections: report of five cases and review of the literature, *Q J Med*, **49:** 431–42.

Schoeni JL, Wong ACL, 1994, Inhibition of *Campylobacter jejuni* colonization in chicks by defined competitive exclusion bacteria, *Appl Environ Microbiol*, **60:** 1191–7.

Sibbald CJ, Sharp JCM, 1985, Campylobacter infections in urban and rural populations in Scotland, *J Hyg*, **95:** 87–93.

Simor AE, Karmali MA et al., 1986, Abortion and perinatal sepsis associated with campylobacter infection, *Rev Infect Dis*, **8:** 397–402.

Skirrow MB, 1977, Campylobacter enteritis: a 'new' disease, *Br Med J*, **2:** 9–11.

Skirrow MB, 1987, A demographic survey of campylobacter, salmonella and shigella infections in England, *Epidemiol Infect*, **99:** 647–57.

Skirrow MB, 1990, Campylobacter, salmonella, shigella and other acute bacterial disorders, *Inflammatory Bowel Diseases*, 2nd edn, eds Allan RN, Keighley MRB et al., Churchill Livingstone, Edinburgh, 595–607.

Skirrow MB, 1994, Diseases due to *Campylobacter, Helicobacter* and related bacteria, *J Comp Pathol*, **111:** 113–49.

Skirrow MB, Blaser MJ, 1995, *Campylobacter jejuni, Infections of the Gastrointestinal Tract*, eds Blaser MJ, Smith PD et al., Raven Press, New York, 825–48.

Skirrow MB, Jones DM et al., 1993, Campylobacter bacteraemia in England and Wales, 1981–91, *Epidemiol Infect*, **110:** 567–73.

Slee A, 1979, Haemorrhagic gastroenteritis in a dog, *Vet Rec*, **104:** 14–15.

Smith T, 1918, Spirilla associated with disease of the fetal membranes in cattle (infectious abortion), *J Exp Med*, **28:** 701–19.

Smith T, Taylor M, 1919, Some morphological and biological characters of the spirilla (*Vibrio fetus*, n. sp.) associated with disease of the fetal membranes in cattle, *J Exp Med*, **30:** 299–311.

Sockett PN, Pearson AD, 1988, Cost implications of human campylobacter infections, *Campylobacter IV*, eds Kaijser B, Falsen E, University of Göteborg, Göteborg, 261–4.

Sorvillo FJ, Lieb LE, Waterman SH, 1991, Incidence of campylobacteriosis among patients with AIDS in Los Angeles County, *J Acquired Immune Defic Syndr*, **4:** 598–602.

Southern JP, Smith RMM, Palmer SR, 1990, Bird attack on milk bottles: possible mode of transmission of *Campylobacter jejuni* to man, *Lancet*, **336:** 1425–7.

Stansfield DG, Hunt B, Kemble PR, 1986, Campylobacter gastroenteritis in fattening lambs, *Vet Rec*, **118:** 210–11.

Stephens LR, Browning JW et al., 1984, Colitis in sheep due to a *Campylobacter*-like bacterium, *Aust Vet J*, **61:** 183–7.

Tauxe RV, 1992, Epidemiology of *Campylobacter jejuni* infections in the United States and other industrialized nations, *Campylobacter jejuni*: Current Status and Future Trends, eds Nachamkin I, Blaser MJ, Tompkins LS, American Society for Microbiology, Washington, 9–19.

Taylor DN, 1992, *Campylobacter* infections in developing countries, *Campylobacter jejuni*: Current Status and Future Trends, eds Nachamkin I, Blaser MJ, Tompkins LS, American Society for Microbiology, New York, 20–30.

Taylor DN, McDermott KT et al., 1983, Campylobacter enteritis from untreated water in the Rocky Mountains, *Ann Intern Med*, **99:** 38–40.

Taylor DN, Kiehlbauch JA et al., 1991, Isolation of group 2 aerotolerant *Campylobacter* species from Thai children with diarrhea, *J Infect Dis*, **163:** 1062–7.

Tribe GW, Fleming MP, 1983, Biphasic enteritis in imported cynomolgus (*Macaca fascicularis*) monkeys infected with *Shigella, Salmonella* and *Campylobacter* species, *Lab Anim*, **17:** 65–9.

Truscott RB, Morin EW, 1964, A bacterial agent causing bluecomb disease in turkeys II. Transmission and studies of the etiological agent, *Avian Dis*, **8:** 27–35.

Umunnabuike AC, Irokanulo EA, 1986, Isolation of *Campylobacter* subsp. *jejuni* from oriental and American cockroaches caught in kitchens and poultry houses in Vom, Nigeria, *Int J Zoon*, **13:** 180–6.

Vandamme P, Pugina P et al., 1992a, Outbreak of recurrent abdominal cramps associated with *Arcobacter butzleri* in an Italian school, *J Clin Microbiol*, **30:** 2335–7.

Vandamme P, Vancanneyt M et al., 1992b, Polyphasic taxonomic study of the emended genus *Arcobacter* with *Arcobacter butzleri* comb. nov. and *Arcobacter skirrowii* sp. nov., an aerotolerant bacterium isolated from veterinary specimens, *Int J Syst Bacteriol*, **42:** 344–56.

Van Donkersgoed J, Janzen ED et al., 1990, *Campylobacter jejuni* abortions in two beef cattle herds in Saskatchewan, *Can Vet J*, **31:** 373–7.

Vinzent R, Dumas J, Picard N, 1947, Septicémie grave au cours de la grossesse, due à un vibrion. Avortement consécutif, *Bull Acad Nat Med*, **131:** 90–2.

Vogt RL, Sours HE et al., 1982, Campylobacter enteritis associated with contaminated water, *Ann Intern Med*, **96:** 292–6.

Wallace JM, 1980, Milk-associated campylobacter infection, *Health Bull*, **38:** 57–61.

Ware DA, 1980, Pathogenicity of *Campylobacter fetus* subsp. *venerealis* in causing infertility in cattle, *Br Vet J*, **136:** 301–3.

Wood RC, MacDonald KL, Osterholm MT, 1992, *Campylobacter* enteritis outbreaks associated with drinking raw milk during youth activities, *JAMA*, **268:** 3228–30.

Chapter 30

INFECTION WITH *HELICOBACTER*

Y Glupczynski

1 HISTORICAL BACKGROUND

Spiral gastric bacteria are not new. The existence of gastric spiral organisms colonizing the mucus and glands of the stomach of healthy dogs was first reported by Bizzozero in 1893. Salomon (1896) confirmed their presence in dogs and also found them in cats and rats, but not in man. It is unlikely that these organisms were *Helicobacter pylori*, particularly as they were associated with parietal rather than mucus-secreting cells. The first observation of spiral-shaped organisms in the human stomach may have been by Krienitz (1906) who described 3 different types of 'spirochaetes' in the stomach of a patient with carcinoma of the lesser curve, one of which may have been *H. pylori*. In 1938, Doenges observed spiral bacteria that he also reported as 'spirochetes' in the gastric mucosa of about 50% of human stomachs examined at routine necropsies from accident victims, but he was unable to correlate their presence with gastric diseases. Freedberg and Baron (1940) reported similar organisms in 37% of gastrectomy specimens from patients with peptic ulcer or carcinoma. Following the introduction of flexible fibreoptic gastroscopy during the 1970s, Steer and Colin-Jones (1975) came near to identifying *H. pylori* and its association with gastritis in a large study of biopsy specimens, but misinterpretation of culture results led to the wrong conclusion that the organisms seen were *Pseudomonas aeruginosa*.

In 1982, Warren and Marshall were the first to culture and identify *H. pylori* (initially called *Campylobacter pyloridis* and then *Campylobacter pylori*) and to establish the association between the presence of this organism in the human gastric mucosa and the occurrence of histological gastritis (Warren and Marshall 1983, 1984). Within a few years of the publication of Warren and Marshall's work many reports appeared world wide, confirming the close association between *H. pylori* and chronic active gastritis as well as with gastric

and duodenal ulcers. The development of sensitive and specific diagnostic methods, and the application of therapies that can eliminate the infection have resulted in more precise appreciation of the clinical relevance of *H. pylori* in various gastroduodenal diseases.

2 EPIDEMIOLOGICAL ASPECTS

H. pylori is responsible for one of the world's most common bacterial infections. It is usually acquired without knowledge of the time of exposure, the source or the magnitude of the infecting dose. *H. pylori* infection persists silently in most infected individuals and causes superficial gastritis that persists for years, leading to chronic inflammation. In developing countries the organism is acquired early in childhood, with infection rates of 50–60% by the age of 10 and up to 90% in adults (Megraud et al. 1989). By contrast, in developed countries few infections occur during childhood and a gradual increase in prevalence is observed with age (at a rate of about 0.5–1% per year), leading to infection rates of 20–30% by the age of 20 and of about 50% at 50–60 years. Prevalence also varies between populations of different ethnic origin. In the USA, healthy adult Hispanic and black populations have seropositivity rates several-fold higher than non-Hispanic white populations, independently of age, gender, geographical location (urban versus rural), educational level and current income (Graham et al. 1991b). The reasons for these highly significant differences in seroprevalence rates among ethnic groups are not well understood, but socioeconomic conditions during childhood, such as crowding, poor sanitation and close contact with infected persons, appear to be important risk factors. A twin study from Scandinavia comparing the rates of infection in monozygotic and dizygotic twin pairs reared apart or together has suggested a large inherited susceptibility to infection in addition to environment-related factors (Malaty et al. 1994).

2.1 Sources and transmission of infection

The natural hosts for *H. pylori* are humans. Closely similar but distinguishable organisms have been isolated in primates (Goodwin et al. 1989b). *H. pylori* has been isolated from the stomachs of domestic cats, raising the possibility that the organism may be a zoonotic pathogen with transmission occurring from cats to humans (Handt et al. 1994). There is no primary environmental reservoir and person-to-person transmission is probably the dominant mode of transmission, although controversy exists over whether faecal–oral or oral–oral spread predominates. From its protected niche in the gastric mucosa *H. pylori* could either be transmitted by the oral–oral route with episodes of gastro-oesophageal reflux permitting access to the mouth, or be excreted in the faeces. *H. pylori* has now been isolated from the faeces (Thomas et al. 1992, Kelly et al. 1994), from dental plaque (Shames et al. 1989) and from saliva (Ferguson et al. 1993), albeit on few occasions, but it has been detected by polymerase chain reaction (PCR) at both sites in a greater proportion of infected subjects by Mapstone et al. (1993), suggesting that transmission by both routes can indeed occur. The increased rates of infection among children of West African mothers who premasticate their infants' food (Albenque et al. 1990) and among Chinese who share eating utensils favours oral–oral transmission. An increased rate of infection has also been reported among endoscopists not wearing gloves (Mitchell, Lee and Carrick 1989).

However, rates of infection among dental workers were not elevated compared to age-matched control groups (Malaty et al. 1992). The main epidemiological evidence supporting faecal–oral transmission is the similarity of the seroepidemiology with that of hepatitis A (Graham et al. 1991a). Whether by oral–oral route or by faecal–oral transmission, intrafamilial spread appears to occur in western populations (Drumm et al. 1990). When a parent or a child is infected, the other family members are usually more likely to be infected than family members from uninfected index cases (parent or children). Cross-sectional studies have shown that both a high density of living and limited access to sanitary facilities are significantly associated with higher infection rates, especially when promiscuous living conditions prevailed during childhood (Mendall et al. 1992). Likewise, *H. pylori* seropositivity rates are also notoriously higher in persons living in institutions. For example, at a Bangkok orphanage *H. pylori* seropositivity was 74% in children 2–4 years old, well above the rates in children living in rural Thailand (Perez-Perez et al. 1990). In another study from Australia, Berkowicz and Lee (1987) found 3 times the expected prevalence of antibody among inmates of an institution for the mentally retarded. Transmission of *H. pylori* in the endoscopy suite can occasionally occur. Patient-to-patient

transmission by an endoscope is a potential threat which has been reported at a frequency of 3 infections for every 1000 gastroduodenoscopies in one study from The Netherlands (Langenberg et al. 1990). Contact with secretions from infected patients may also subject endoscopists to risk of infection and accidental infections as well as epidemics of gastritis transmitted by infected gastric secretions have been reported in detail (Gledhill et al. 1985, Sobala et al. 1991a). The prevalence of *H. pylori* infection was significantly higher in a group of Australian gastroenterologists than in an age-matched group of control subjects (Lin et al. 1994).

There is little evidence for transmission between couples (Perez-Perez et al. 1991). Nor is there any correlation with sexual preference, number of sexual partners, history of sexually transmitted diseases, or infection with human immunodeficiency virus among those infected with *H. pylori* compared with those who were not infected (Polish et al. 1991).

3 BACTERIOLOGY AND PATHOGENESIS

Helicobacter pylori is the type species of the genus *Helicobacter* that was proposed by Goodwin et al. (1989a). This genus originally contained 2 species: *H. pylori*, the human gastric pathogen, and *H. mustelae*, a similar bacterium found in the stomach of ferrets. Helicobacter organisms are curved or spiral-shaped, gram-negative, strictly microaerophilic and motile by means of sheathed flagella, the general characteristics of most mucus-associated intestinal bacteria. Although these 2 species had several campylobacter-like characters, they were separated from the genus *Campylobacter* on the basis of their unique specific fatty acid profile, specific ultrastructure, respiratory quinones, growth requirements, enzyme characteristics and a very different RNA sequence (see Volume 2, Chapter 54). As of 1995, there are at least 14 species within the genus *Helicobacter*. These species, their hosts and habitat are detailed in Table 30.1. *H. pylori* and '*H. heilmanii*' are the only 2 species which have been associated with human gastric disease. *H. cinaedi* and *H. fennelliae* are causes of enteritis and proctocolitis, especially in homosexual men, and they may sometimes also cause bacteraemia. Distinguishing features of 4 important members of the *Helicobacter* genus are compared in Table 30.2.

H. pylori has the peculiarity of being a remarkably homogeneous species phenotypically while showing considerable genomic diversity. Characterization of the protein profiles, lipopolysaccharides or surface antigens have been proposed as typing criteria in order to differentiate *H. pylori* strains isolated in different parts of the world. Unfortunately, most of the strains display little heterogeneity and fall into few different groups so that these techniques are not useful for strain differentiation. In contrast, analysis of the *H. pylori* genome by newer methods of molecular fingerprinting (e.g. restriction fragment length poly-

Table 30.1 *Helicobacter* species and their hosts (as of 1995)

Species	Hosts	Primary site
H. pylori	Humans (? monkey, ? pig, cat)	Gastric mucosa
H. mustelae	Ferrets	Gastric mucosa
H. felis	Cats, dogs	Gastric mucosa
H. nemestrinae	Macaque monkeys	Gastric mucosa
H. acinonyx	Cheetah	Gastric mucosa
H. muridarum	Mice, rats	Intestinal mucosa
H. cinaedi	Humans, rodents	Intestinal mucosa
H. fennelliae	Humans	Intestinal mucosa
'H. rappini'[a]	Sheep, dogs, humans	Liver, stomach, faeces
H. canis	Dogs	Faeces
'H. heilmanii'[b]	Cats, dogs, humans	Gastric mucosa
H. hepaticus	Mice	Liver, intestinal mucosa
H. bilis	Mice	Liver, bile, intestine
H. pullorum	Poultry, humans	Duodenum, intestine (poultry), faeces (humans)

[a]Previously known as *Flexispira rappini*. A proposal has been made to place the organism within the genus *Helicobacter*.
[b]Unculturable helix-shaped organism previously known as *Gastrospirillum hominis*. RNA sequencing analysis has placed the organism in the genus *Helicobacter*, and the name 'H. heilmanii' has been proposed (Solnick et al. 1993).

Table 30.2 Important members of the genus *Helicobacter*

Name	Host	Features	Disease associations and comments
H. pylori	Human	Multiple (4–6) sheathed flagella at one end	Causes gastritis in humans. Also found sometimes in domesticated or caged animals, e.g. monkeys, pigs, cats
H. heilmanii[a]	Cats, dogs, humans (rarely)	Corkscrew appearance with between 4 and 20 turns, at least 12 sheathed flagella at one end, no axial periplasmic fibres noted by electron microscopy	About 1% of human gastritis cases are caused by this bacterium, presumably acquired from cats and dogs
H. mustelae	Ferret	Several randomly placed flagella	Gastritis and ulcerations commonly develop in ferrets, useful model for studying pathogenic mechanisms
H. felis	Cats and dogs	Differs only from *H. heilmanii* by the presence of axial periplasmic fibres noted by electron microscopy	Isolated from cats, can be propagated in mice, useful in screening trials for anti-*H. pylori* chemotherapeutic agents, studies of pathogenic mechanisms and for development of a vaccine model

[a]Previously known as *Gastrospirillum hominis*.

morphism (RFLP), pulse field gel electrophoresis (PFGE), randomly amplified polymorphic DNA (RAPD), PCR) has brought to light the extreme heterogeneity of *H. pylori*, each infecting strain displaying an almost unique fingerprint (Megraud 1994). It has not yet been possible to assign a particular genovar to specific gastric diseases (e.g. chronic gastritis versus peptic ulcer or gastric cancer) nor to a phenotypic characteristic; the molecular fingerprint methods have proved useful mainly for tracing the intrafamilial spread of *H. pylori* (Bamford et al. 1993) or for differentiating between recrudescence and reinfection after attempts to eradicate *H. pylori* (Rautelin et al. 1994).

3.1 Location of the organism and nature of the infection

The bacteria live in and beneath the layer of mucus that covers the gastric mucosa; in this situation the pH is near neutrality. The vast majority of *H. pylori* are located adjacent to surface and pit gastric epithelial cells (Fig. 30.1).

Any part of the stomach may become colonized, but the mucus-secreting epithelium of the antrum is the favoured site. Areas of gastric metaplasia in the duodenum or elsewhere in the digestive tract may also become colonized, but *H. pylori* does not colonize areas of intestinal metaplasia in the stomach. The electron microscope shows adherence of *H. pylori* to human gastric mucus cells and in some cases involves the formation of pedestal attachments. At such sites there is effacement of microvilli, flattening of cells, with loss of mucin granules, disruption of cytoskeletal elements and alteration of intercellular complexes (Goodwin, Armstrong and Marshall 1986). Colonization of the mucosa by *H. pylori* is almost invariably associated with the histological pattern of chronic active gastritis or antral type-B gastritis (Price 1991), which is clearly distinct from type-A autoimmune inflammation of the acid-secreting mucosa of the body of the stomach, found in pernicious anaemia. This pattern is usually characterized by mononuclear cell infiltration associated with superficial infiltration of polymorphonuclear leucocytes of the epithelium (Robert and Weinstein 1993). The amount of inflammation may be highly variable, ranging from minimal inflammatory infiltration of the lamina propria with intact glandular architecture, to severe dense

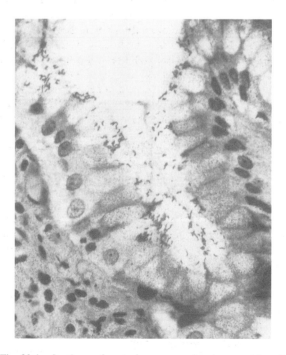

Fig. 30.1 Section of antral mucosa showing gastric pit colonized with *Helicobacter pylori*. Warthin–Starry silver stain (× 560).

inflammation with microabscess formation, reactive epithelial atypia and the presence of intraepithelial neutrophils. In general, there is a correlation between the number of *H. pylori* organisms present and the degree of polymorph infiltration. On average, bacteria are present in less than 5% of biopsy specimens that are histologically normal and, when present, are located most commonly in the gastric body. Since the distribution of bacteria may be patchy, occasional cases of chronic superficial gastritis with neutrophil activity may fail to show *H. pylori* organisms due to sampling errors (Bayerdörffer et al. 1989). If left untreated the infection does not usually resolve spontaneously but persists for life. Over the course of years or decades, there is extension of the inflammatory process into the deeper portions of the mucosa, partial loss of the pyloric glands and endocrine cells (i.e. atrophy) of the antrum, and a progressive replacement of the mucosa by intestinal metaplasia (Sipponen, Kekki and Siurala 1991).

3.2 Pathogenesis of *H. pylori* infection

The success of *H. pylori* as a gastric pathogen appears to be dependent on both colonization and maintenance factors as well as pathogenic mechanisms. Several putative virulence factors have now been identified. The spiral shape and polar flagella of *H. pylori* provide its motility in gastric juice and gastric mucus (Hazell et al. 1986). Urease enzyme, by breaking down the urea in gastric juice, appears to generate enough bicarbonate and ammonia around *H. pylori* to allow its safe migration through the gastric acid barrier and its arrival at the protective mucus layer. Motility and urease have been shown to be essential factors for colonization in an animal model using gnotobiotic piglets (Eaton, Morgan and Krakowka 1989). Other adaptative enzymes that may facilitate the survival of *H. pylori* in the gastric mucosa include catalase and superoxide dismutase (both of which protect bacteria against the toxic effects of reactive oxygen metabolites released by gastric neutrophils) and the presence of various specific bacterial adhesins and mucosal cell receptors (Lee, Fox and Hazell 1993). In addition to these colonization- and maintenance-promoting factors, *H. pylori* produces a variety of toxic substances such as ammonia, urease, mucinase, phospholipase A, haemolysin and cytotoxins, all of which may cause direct injury to the gastric mucosa barrier. Urease, LPS and a platelet-activating factor (paf-acether) are potent inflammatory mediators capable of stimulating neutrophils, monocytes and macrophages in vitro (Mai et al. 1991); such factors may thus indirectly contribute to the decreased mucosal integrity by inducing chronic inflammation. Moreover, the expression by *H. pylori* of a conserved heat shock protein (Hsp60) sharing extensive homology with gastric epithelial antigens has been suggested to play a role in *H. pylori* pathogenesis by inducing an autoimmune response (Macchia et al. 1993). One of the most interesting aspects of *H. pylori* pathogenicity is the so-called 'vacuolating cytotoxin'. This toxin is expressed in about 50% of *H.*

pylori strains and is responsible for inducing vacuoles in a variety of eukaryotic cell lines (Leunk et al. 1988). It has been characterized and purified as an 87 kDa protein which shows limited homology with other known bacterial toxins (Cover and Blaser 1992). The gene encoding this cytotoxin is called *vacA* and has been cloned by Cover et al. (1994). The *vacA* gene is present in all *H. pylori* strains, regardless of whether they express toxin activity in vitro. However, the *vacA* sequences of tox + and tox - strains present large dissimilarities (Cover et al. 1994). Oral administration of purified cytotoxin to mice causes ulceration and gastric lesions bearing some similarities with the pathology observed in humans (Telford et al. 1994). In naturally infected humans, this vacuolating cytotoxin may be an important virulence factor. Cytotoxic activity is significantly more prevalent in isolates of *H. pylori* from individuals with peptic ulcer than from those with gastritis only (Figura et al. 1989) and a more intense mucosal polymorphonuclear leucocyte infiltration is present in gastric biopsy specimens from patients infected with tox + strains (Cover et al. 1993). A second gene (*cagA*), encoding a 120–130 kDa protein associated with the expression of cytotoxin activity, has been identified (Covacci et al. 1993). Contrary to the toxin gene, this gene is only present when the cagA protein is present. The cagA protein appears as a marker for vacuolating toxin effect but mutation of the *cagA* gene indicates that it is not necessary for cytotoxin activity (Tummuru, Cover and Blaser 1994). Serum and gastric mucosal anti-cagA antibodies are present in nearly all duodenal ulcer disease and are found significantly more frequently in patients with peptic ulcer or with gastric cancer than in individuals with *H. pylori* gastritis alone (Crabtree et al. 1991, 1993). The presence of *cagA* or *vacA* has no clinical usefulness at this time and the exact function of *cagA* is still unknown.

4 CLINICAL CONSEQUENCES OF H. PYLORI INFECTION

4.1 Epidemic hypochlorhydria and acute gastritis

Two outbreaks of mild gastrointestinal illness with abdominal pain, nausea and vomiting were reported in previously healthy people who, in a study on stomach secretions underwent gastric instrumentation (Ramsey et al. 1979, Gledhill et al. 1985). All suffered profound hypochlorhydria which lasted for several months. Retrospective histological examination of material from these outbreaks showed *H. pylori*-like bacteria and active gastritis; moreover, analysis of stored sera from one study demonstrated rising titres of *H. pylori* antibodies. It was presumed that the 2 outbreaks resulted from cross-infection by instruments passed into the stomach. In 2 volunteer experiments similar acute manifestations occurred after the ingestion of pure cultures of *H. pylori* (Marshall et al. 1985, Morris et al. 1987).

4.2 Chronic gastritis

Most frequently *H. pylori* infection presents as a chronic infection and results in an asymptomatic superficial gastritis. There is now much evidence for a causal relationship between *H. pylori* and chronic superficial gastritis:

1 accidental and voluntary ingestion of *H. pylori* has resulted in sporadic cases or in epidemics of gastritis
2 natural infection and experimental challenges in various animals simulate human infection with resulting chronic gastritis (Fox and Lee 1993)
3 antimicrobial therapy to eradicate infection results in resolution of gastritis (Glupczynski et al. 1988)
4 *H. pylori* only overlies the gastric epithelium and its infection is associated with only certain types of gastroduodenal inflammation (Ormand et al. 1991)
5 there is a universal local and systemic immune response to *H. pylori* that can be detected serologically (mainly IgG and IgA antibodies) and
6 the levels of *H. pylori* specific antibodies decrease with therapy, concomitant with diminution in inflammation (Rauws et al. 1988).

4.3 Peptic ulceration

A causal relationship between *H. pylori* and peptic ulceration is more difficult to establish as there are no satisfactory animal models and because only a small proportion of infected individuals develops peptic ulcer. However, there is a close association between *H. pylori* and peptic ulceration. Over 95% of patients with duodenal ulcer have *H. pylori* gastritis. Thus infection with *H. pylori* may be a prerequisite for the occurrence of almost all duodenal ulcers in the absence of other precipitating factors such as non-steroidal anti-inflammatory drug (NSAID) use or Zollinger–Ellison syndrome (Nensey et al. 1991). The association between *H. pylori* and gastric ulcer is slightly less strong, about 80% of patients with non-NSAID-induced gastric ulcers being infected. Longitudinal case-control studies over a 3–10 year period have shown that patients with *H. pylori* infection have a 4–13-fold increase in the risk of developing duodenal or gastric ulcers (Sipponen et al. 1990, Nomura et al. 1994). The strongest evidence for the pathogenic role of *H. pylori* in peptic ulcer is the marked decrease in recurrence rates of ulcers following *H. pylori* eradication (Hentschel et al. 1993). Our knowledge of the exact role of *H. pylori* in the pathogenesis of this disease is still incomplete and it is probable that certain host or organism characteristics, not yet characterized, as well as environmental factors, play a role in the development of peptic ulcer.

4.4 Gastric malignancy

Descriptive epidemiological studies have shown a higher frequency of gastric cancer in populations with higher prevalences of *H. pylori* infection and a geographical correlation has been found between *H. pylori* infection and gastric cancer death rate (Eurogast Study Group 1993). More importantly, several prospective case-control serological studies have detected a 3–6-fold increased gastric cancer risk in individuals infected with *H. pylori* and an attributable risk of at least 50% of all gastric cancers (Forman et al. 1991, Nomura et al. 1991, Parsonnet et al. 1991). One recent prospective study has shown that *H. pylori* chronic diffuse gastritis did significantly increase the risk of developing intestinal metaplasia and atrophic gastritis over a mean follow-up of 10 years (Kuipers et al. 1995); these pathological lesions are widely accepted as precursors of gastric carcinoma. Since gastric cancer develops only in a small proportion of infected subjects and because it may also occur without evidence of past *H. pylori* infection, other environmental cofactors may be important in determining the gastric cancer risk.

Epidemiological data suggest that *H. pylori* may be associated with non-Hodgkin's lymphoma and with mucosa-associated lymphoid tissue (MALT) lymphoma (Wotherspoon et al. 1991, Parsonnet et al. 1994). Successful eradication of *H. pylori* by specific antimicrobial treatment has resulted in the complete or partial tumour regression in 27 out of 33 (82%) patients with low-grade MALT gastric lymphoma (Bayerdörffer et al. 1995). However, long-term follow-up will be needed to clarify whether the remission is lasting.

5 Diagnosis

Various tests are available to diagnose *H. pylori* infection. These tests can be categorized into those that are based on direct assessment of gastric biopsies and indirect tests that detect an immunological response (i.e. antibodies against *H. pylori*) or metabolic products (i.e. urease activity) of *H. pylori*.

The gold standard for the detection of *H. pylori* has been defined as culture, histopathological examination of gastric biopsies, or serology, depending on the experience of the investigator. In order to optimize the diagnosis of *H. pylori*, it is usually recommended that several tests be used together. The choice of particular tests will depend on locally available facilities, cost considerations and clinical circumstances in which the diagnosis of *H. pylori* is to be made. The different tests for the detection of *H. pylori* are briefly described in the following section and are summarized in Table 30.3.

5.1 Microscopy

The morphology of *H. pylori* is sufficiently distinctive for diagnosis to be made by light microscopy. The conventional histological haematoxylin–eosin (HE) stain at high magnification is able to detect most cases of *H. pylori* infection unless the number of organisms is very low. The organisms are best seen in or near

adherent mucus on the luminal side of the gastric surface and pit epithelial cells. There are more sensitive staining methods for the diagnosis of *H. pylori*, including the modified Giemsa or Warthin–Starry silver stain (Madan et al. 1988). The Warthin–Starry stain as originally used by Warren (Warren and Marshall 1983) gives excellent results but it is quite labour-intensive, costly and requires experienced technicians for reliable performance. The modified Giemsa stain is simpler and less labour-intensive. Other stains that have been recommended for the diagnosis of *H. pylori* include acridine orange (fluorescence), cresyl-fast violet, Gimenez, or Brown–Hopps. Phase-contrast microscopy of a wet preparation of crushed tissue is convenient and quick. Gram staining of mucus smears or of biopsy imprints can also be used but is generally considered to be less sensitive than the other stains. The sensitivity and specificity of histology for the diagnosis of *H. pylori* are over 95% in experienced hands and when multiple gastric biopsies are obtained.

5.2 Culture

The most specific method to diagnose infection is culture of *H. pylori* from tissue biopsies. However, relying on culture alone can mean missing a substantial proportion of infected cases for technical reasons, including overgrowth of other bacteria and low bacterial load. Attention to transport conditions of the biopsies is particularly crucial for an adequate diagnostic yield. When suspended in saline solution or distilled water, biopsy specimens must be cultured within 4 and 6 h of being taken. Specimens can be kept in Stuart semi-solid transport medium for 24 h if stored at 4°C (Soltesz, Zeeberg and Wadstrom 1992). Selective media that suppress nasopharyngeal flora and other potential contaminants are available commercially (Dent and McNulty 1988) and should be used together with a non-selective fresh blood-based agar in order to ensure optimal recovery of *H. pylori*. Plates are incubated at 37°C under humid microaerophilic conditions with an optimal O_2 concentration of 5–10% for at least 5–7 days before being discarded. The sensitivity of culture ranges from 75 to 90%, even in expert hands. Currently the main value of culture is for epidemiological typing as well as for determination of antibiotic resistance, which is becoming an increasing problem (Glupczynski 1992).

5.3 Biopsy urease test

H. pylori produces such abundant urease that the enzyme can be detected in specimens of infected gastric mucosa placed directly in a solution of urea with phenol red as an indicator. In the original test, Christensen's urea broth was used (McNulty and Wise 1985, 1986), but unbuffered urea solutions, if freshly prepared, and the use of gels instead of broth give quicker results (Marshall et al. 1987, Arvind et al. 1988). A number of modifications have been described and kits are now available from several commercial sources (e.g. Campylobacter-like organism

Table 30.3 Summary of tests for detection of *H. pylori*

Test	Sensitivity[a] (%)	Specificity[a] (%)	Cost[b]	Endoscopy required	Comments
Histology	90->95	95-99	++	Yes	Multiple antral biopsies recommended because of the irregular distribution of the organisms, allows evaluation of the degree of inflammation
Culture	75-90	100	+++	Yes	Variable results depending on the expertise of the laboratory; required for susceptibility testing and epidemiological studies
Rapid urease test (e.g. CLO test)	85-95	90->95	+	Yes	Can be performed rapidly; decreased sensitivity immediately after antimicrobial treatment
Gastric biopsy PCR	≥95	100	+++	Yes	Technically very demanding; not yet available in clinical practice
^{13}C breath test (non-radioactive)	≥95	98-100	+++	No	Preferred in pregnant women, childen; not widely available; well suited to early follow-up of antimicrobial treatment
^{14}C breath test (radioactive)	≥95	90-100	++	No	Small radiation exposure; well suited to follow-up of antimicrobial therapy
Serology	80-95	85->95	+	No	Widely available; useful tool for screening patients before endoscopy and also for seroepidemiological studies; not appropriate for short-term treatment monitoring

[a]Average estimates from data reported in the literature.
[b]+, least expensive; ++, moderately expensive; +++, most expensive.

(CLO) test). The test can have a sensitivity of at least 80% and a specificity approaching 100% when the reaction is positive within 1 h. In clinical practice, biopsy urease testing has the advantage of diagnosing *H. pylori* status in most cases soon after endoscopy, which is helpful for the clinician planning therapeutic interventions. This test is widely available and it is also much less expensive than histology or culture of gastric biopsies.

5.4 Molecular tests

Molecular techniques may become more relevant in the future for the diagnosis of *H. pylori* infection. The method with the potential for greatest sensitivity is detection of *H. pylori*-specific DNA using PCR. Using gastric biopsy material and gastric juice aspirates, various target DNA sequences have been used for PCR diagnosis, including a portion of the 16S rRNA gene (Hoshina et al. 1990), a gene encoding for a urease subunit (Westblom et al. 1993) and a portion of a gene encoding a species-specific 26 kDa protein (Hammar et al. 1992). Initial results with all these PCR tests have yielded high sensitivities and specificities.

5.5 Urea breath tests

Urea breath tests are based on the principle that urea that has been labelled with a carbon isotope is administered orally and is hydrolysed by urease produced by viable *H. pylori* in the stomach, if present. As a result, ammonia is produced and bicarbonate is excreted in the breath as CO_2. The amount of labelled CO_2 in breath is indicative of the amount of urease activity and can be used as a marker of *H. pylori* infection. Two types of isotopically labelled urea are utilized: [^{13}C]urea (Graham et al. 1987) and [^{14}C]urea (Marshall and Surveyor 1988). Both tests measure active infection, have the great advantage of being non-invasive and are useful in making a primary diagnosis as well as monitoring response to therapy. The [^{13}C]urea breath test is more costly and is not yet widely available in clinical practice because it requires mass spectrometry equipment for measuring the excretion of the ^{13}C non-radioactive isotope. On the other hand, the [^{14}C]urea breath test, which is simpler to perform than the ^{13}C test, only requires a scintillation counter (available at many hospitals) for measuring the excreted labelled CO_2. The ^{14}C test is thus less expensive, but it involves exposure to a long-lived radioactive isotope, albeit at a very low dose; therefore, testing with ^{13}C is preferred for use in children and in pregnant women. The sensitivity and specificity of breath testing to detect *H. pylori* infection is generally over 95%. Breath tests have also proved very reliable in indicating cure or therapeutic failure one month after antibiotic therapy (Logan et al. 1994).

5.6 Serology

H. pylori infection results in a systemic as well as local immune response characterized by an elevation of specific IgG and IgA in serum, elevated secretory IgA and low-level gastric IgM (Rathbone et al. 1986), phenomena that have permitted development of a variety of serological tests for the detection of *H. pylori*. Several serological techniques have been used for the study of *H. pylori* infection (e.g. complement fixation, haemagglutination, immunoblot, fluoroimmunoassay) but enzyme-linked immunosorbent assay (ELISA) is currently considered the optimal serological method. Various antigens have been employed for detection of *H. pylori*-specific antibodies, including whole cells and whole-cell sonicates, acid-glycine extracts and heat-stable antigens, or more purified enriched antigen fractions such as urease and a 120 kDa protein. Tests using a mixture of the more purified antigen preparations have generally been more sensitive and specific than tests using whole-cell or sonicated extracts (Hirschl et al. 1990). Many kits using the enriched antigens for detecting specific *H. pylori* IgG are available commercially. The best of these serum ELISA tests generally yield sensitivities and specificities around 90% and 95%, respectively, compared to histology or urease testing (Goossens et al. 1992). Rapid office-based tests using whole blood or salivary secretions have been developed but methodological problems currently preclude their use as diagnostic tests. Since elevated IgG antibody levels may persist for years in untreated individuals, serology has been very useful for epidemiological studies and also for screening individual dyspeptic patients before endoscopy (Megraud et al. 1989, Sobala et al. 1991b). After successful bacterial eradication, antibody titres tend to decrease to approximately 50% of pretreatment levels at about 6 months (Kosunen et al. 1992). There are, however, large person-to-person variations in changes in antibody titres after successful therapy and in some individuals low levels of IgG may persist for years after *H. pylori* eradication (Glupczynski et al. 1992). Serological assays may be of limited value for short-term monitoring of antimicrobial therapy and use of the urea breath tests (^{13}C or ^{14}C tests) may be more appropriate in this setting.

6 GENERAL TREATMENT APPROACHES

Several studies have shown the favourable impact of *H. pylori* eradication on the long-term clinical course of peptic ulcer disease. Cure of the infection heals duodenal and gastric ulcers refractory to antisecretory drugs, speeds up ulcer healing, heals ulcers without concomitant gastric acid suppression and, most importantly, virtually prevents recurrences and ulcer complications (Hosking et al. 1994, Sung et al. 1995). Available studies have all demonstrated a substantial reduction in the risk of gastric and duodenal ulcer recurrence to <10% within a year when *H. pylori* has been successfully eradicated (Tytgat 1994). Consequently, the US National Institutes of Health Consensus Conference (NIH Consensus Conference 1994) has recently recommended that all ulcer patients infected with *H. pylori* should be treated with antimicrobial agents.

6.1 Treatment regimens

Because of its unique location in the gastric mucosa and mucus, the treatment of *H. pylori* infection has proved to be difficult. Many antimicrobial agents are poorly secreted in the gastric mucosa or are inactivated in the acid environment of the stomach. This means that in vitro activity of various agents usually does not translate into success in vivo. Routine testing of *H. pylori* susceptibility to metronidazole has been recommended, since in vitro resistance is often predictive of eradication failure (Glupczynski 1992). Initial monotherapy with bismuth or with a single antibiotic has resulted in low success rates and in most cases recrudescence of infection was observed within one month of stopping treatment. Therefore, eradication of *H. pylori* is currently defined as the absence of infection at least 4 weeks after stopping treatment. A 14 day triple therapy including a bismuth preparation, metronidazole and either amoxicillin or tetracycline has been very effective with eradication rates of around 90% (Tytgat 1994). A substantial decrease in efficacy has been noted, however, with triple therapy regimens when primary metronidazole-resistant strains are detected; success rates dropped from 95 to 60% (Burette et al. 1992). A 2 week dual therapy containing omeprazole – a potent pump inhibitor of gastric epithelial cells – and amoxycillin or clarithromycin has also been effective with eradication rates ranging between 60 and 80%. The latter regimens have the great advantage of being simpler and much better tolerated than the conventional triple therapy and they are currently frequently used as the first-line treatment option. One week triple therapies combining omeprazole and a low dose of 2 antibiotics (metronidazole or amoxycillin plus clarithromycin) have yielded very promising results with eradication rates constantly above 90% (Goddard and Logan 1995). Such treatment regimens may become the method of choice in the near future.

6.2 Prevention

With our lack of knowledge concerning the exact sources, reservoirs and modes of transmission of *H. pylori*, there is currently no possibility of preventing this infection. Primary prevention of infection in childhood may be in the future the most effective way to eliminate gastric cancer in high-risk populations, but this must await the development of an effective vaccine. The potential for *H. pylori* antigens such as urease and vacA as candidate vaccine components is being assessed in various animal models (Michetti et al. 1994, Marchetti et al. 1995).

REFERENCES

Albenque M, Tall F et al., 1990, Epidemiological study of *Helicobacter pylori* transmission from mother to child in Africa, *Rev Esp Enferm Dig*, **78 (Suppl.1):** 48–9.

Arvind AS, Cook RS et al., 1988, One-minute endoscopy room test for *Campylobacter pylori*, *Lancet*, **1:** 704.

Bamford KB, Bickley J et al., 1993, *Helicobacter pylori*: comparison of DNA fingerprints provides evidence for intrafamilial infection, *Gut*, **34:** 1348–50.

Bayerdörffer E, Oertel H et al., 1989, Topographic association between active gastritis and *Campylobacter pylori* colonisation, *J Clin Pathol*, **42:** 834–9.

Bayerdörffer E, Neubauer A et al., 1995, Regression of primary gastric lymphoma of mucus-associated lymphoid-tissue type after cure of *Helicobacter pylori* infection, *Lancet*, **345:** 1591–4.

Berkowicz J, Lee A, 1987, Person-to-person transmission of *Campylobacter pylori*, *Lancet*, **2:** 680–1.

Bizzozero G, 1893, Ueber die Schlauchfoermingen drusen des Magendarmkanals und die Beziehungen ihres Epithels zu dem oberfachen Epithel der Schleimhaut, *Arch Mikr Anat*, **42:** 82.

Burette A, Glupczynski Y, De Prez C, 1992, Evaluation of various multi-drug eradication regimens for *Helicobacter pylori*, *Eur J Gastroenterol Hepatol*, **4:** 817–23.

Covacci A, Censini S et al., 1993, Molecular characterization of the 128-kDa immunodominant antigen of *Helicobacter pylori* associated with cytotoxicity and duodenal ulcer, *Proc Natl Acad Sci USA*, **90:** 5791–5.

Cover TL, Blaser MJ, 1992, Purification and characterization of the vacuolating toxin from *Helicobacter pylori*, *J Biol Chem*, **267:** 10570–5.

Cover TL, Cao P et al., 1993, Correlation between vacuolating cytotoxin production by *Helicobacter pylori* isolates in vitro and in vivo, *Infect Immun*, **61:** 5008–12.

Cover TL, Tummuru MK et al., 1994, Divergence of genetic sequences for the vacuolating cytotoxin among *Helicobacter pylori* strains, *J Biol Chem*, **269:** 10566–73.

Crabtree JE, Taylor JD et al., 1991, Mucosal IgA recognition of *Helicobacter pylori* 120 kDa protein, peptic ulceration, and gastric pathology, *Lancet*, **338:** 332–5.

Crabtree JE, Wyatt JI et al., 1993, Systemic and mucosal humoral responses to *Helicobacter pylori* in gastric cancer, *Gut*, **34:** 1339–43.

Dent JC McNulty CA, 1988, Evaluation of a new selective medium for *Campylobacter pylori*, *Eur J Clin Microbiol Infect Dis*, **7:** 555–8.

Drumm B, Perez Perez GI et al., 1990, Intrafamilial clustering of *Helicobacter pylori* infection, *N Engl J Med*, **322:** 359–63.

Eaton KA, Morgan DR, Krakowka S, 1989, *Campylobacter pylori* virulence factors in gnotobiotic piglets, *Infect Immun*, **57:** 1119–25.

Eurogast Study Group, 1993, An international association between *Helicobacter pylori* infection and gastric cancer, *Lancet*, **341:** 1359–62.

Ferguson DA Jr, Li C et al., 1993, Isolation of *Helicobacter pylori* from saliva, *J Clin Microbiol*, **31:** 2802–4.

Figura N, Guglielmetti P et al., 1989, Cytotoxin production by *Campylobacter pylori* strains isolated from patients with peptic ulcers and from patients with chronic gastritis only, *J Clin Microbiol*, **27:** 225–6.

Forman D, Newell DG et al., 1991, Association between infection with *Helicobacter pylori* and risk of gastric cancer: evidence from a prospective investigation, *Br Med J*, **302:** 1302–5.

Fox JG, Lee A, 1993, Gastric *Helicobacter* infection in animals: natural and experimental infections, *Helicobacter pylori* – Biology and Clinical Practice, eds Goodwin CS, Worsley BW, CRC Press, Boca Raton, 407–30.

Freedberg AS, Barron LE, 1940, The presence of spirochaetes in human gastric mucosa, *Am J Dig Dis*, **7:** 443–5.

Gledhill T, Leicester RJ et al., 1985, Epidemic hypochlorhydria, *Br Med J*, **290:** 1383–6.

Glupczynski Y, 1992, Results of a multicentre European survey in 1991 of metronidazole resistance in *Helicobacter pylori*, *Eur J Clin Microbiol Infect Dis*, **11:** 777–81.

Glupczynski Y, Burette A et al., 1988, *Campylobacter pylori* associated gastritis: a double-blind placebo-controlled trial with amoxycillin, *Am J Gastroenterol*, **83:** 365–72.

Glupczynski Y, Burette A et al., 1992, Effect of antimicrobial therapy on specific serologic response to *Helicobacter pylori* infection, *Eur J Clin Microbiol Infect Dis*, **11:** 583–8.

Goddard A, Logan R, 1995, One-week low-dose triple therapy: new standards for *Helicobacter pylori* treatment, *Eur J Gastroenterol Hepatol*, **7:** 1–3.

Goodwin CS, Armstrong JA, Marshall BJ, 1986, *Campylobacter pyloridis*, gastritis, and peptic ulceration, *J Clin Pathol*, **39:** 353–65.

Goodwin CS, Armstrong JA et al., 1989a, Transfer of *Campylobacter pylori* and *Campylobacter mustelae* to *Helicobacter* gen. nov. as *Helicobacter pylori* comb. nov. and *Helicobacter mustelae* comb. nov., respectively, *Int J Syst Bacteriol*, **39:** 397–405.

Goodwin CS, McConnell W et al., 1989b, Cellular fatty acid composition of *Campylobacter pylori* from primates and ferrets compared with those of other campylobacters, *J Clin Microbiol*, **27:** 938–43.

Goossens H, Glupczynski Y et al., 1992, Evaluation of a commercially available second-generation immunoglobulin G enzyme immunoassay for detection of *Helicobacter pylori* infection, *J Clin Microbiol*, **30:** 176–80.

Graham DY, Klein PD et al., 1987, *Campylobacter pylori* detected noninvasively by the ^{13}C-urea breath test, *Lancet*, **1:** 1174–7.

Graham DY, Adam E et al., 1991a, Seroepidemiology of *Helicobacter pylori* infection in India. Comparison of developing and developed countries, *Dig Dis Sci*, **36:** 1084–8.

Graham DY, Malaty HM et al., 1991b, Epidemiology of *Helicobacter pylori* in an asymptomatic population in the United States. Effect of age, race, and socioeconomic status, *Gastroenterology*, **100:** 1495–501.

Hammar M, Tyszkiewicz T et al., 1992, Rapid detection of *Helicobacter pylori* in gastric biopsy material by polymerase chain reaction, *J Clin Microbiol*, **30:** 54–8.

Handt LK, Fox JG et al., 1994, *Helicobacter pylori* isolated from the domestic cat: public health implications, *Infect Immun*, **62:** 2367–74.

Hazell SL, Lee A et al., 1986, *Campylobacter pyloridis* and gastritis; association with intercellular spaces and adaptation to an environment of mucus as important factors in colonization of the gastric epithelium, *J Infect Dis*, **153:** 658–63.

Hentschel E, Brandstatter G et al., 1993, Effect of ranitidine and amoxycillin plus metronidazole on the eradication of *Helicobacter pylori* and the recurrence of duodenal ulcer, *N Engl J Med*, **328:** 308–12.

Hirschl AM, Rathbone BJ et al., 1990, Comparison of ELISA antigen preparations alone or in combination for serodiagnosing *Helicobacter pylori* infections, *J Clin Pathol*, **43:** 511–13.

Hoshina S, Kahn SM et al., 1990, Direct detection and amplification of *Helicobacter pylori* ribosomal 16S gene segments from gastric endoscopic biopsies, *Diagn Microbiol Infect Dis*, **13:** 473–9.

Hosking SW, Ling TK et al., 1994, Duodenal ulcer healing by eradication of *Helicobacter pylori* without anti-acid treatment: randomised controlled trial, *Lancet*, **343:** 508–10.

Kelly SM, Pitcher MC et al., 1994, Isolation of *Helicobacter pylori* from feces of patients with dyspepsia in the United Kingdom, *Gastroenterology*, **107:** 1671–4.

Kosunen TU, Seppala K et al., 1992, Diagnostic value of decreasing IgG, IgA, and IgM antibody titres after eradication of *Helicobacter pylori*, *Lancet*, **339:** 893–5.

Krienitz W, 1906, Ueber das Auftreten von Spirochaeten verschiedener form im mageninhalt bei Carcinoma ventriculi, *Dtsch Med Wochenschr*, **28:** 872.

Kuipers EJ, Uyterlinde AM et al., 1995, Long-term sequelae of *Helicobacter* pylori gastritis, *Lancet*, **345:** 1525–8.

Langenberg W, Rauws EA et al., 1990, Patient-to-patient transmission of *Campylobacter pylori* infection by fiberoptic gastroduodenoscopy and biopsy, *J Infect Dis*, **161:** 507–11.

Lee A, Fox JG, Hazell SL, 1993, Pathogenicity of *H.pylori* – a perspective, *Infect Immun*, **61:** 1601–10.

Leunk RD, Johnson PT et al., 1988, Cytotoxic activity in broth-culture filtrates of *Campylobacter pylori*, *J Med Microbiol*, **26:** 93–9.

Lin SK, Lambert JR et al., 1994, *Helicobacter pylori* prevalence in endoscopy and medical staff, *J Gastroenterol Hepatol*, **9:** 319–24.

Logan RP, Gummett PA et al., 1994, Eradication of *Helicobacter pylori* with clarithromycin and omeprazole, *Gut*, **35:** 323–6.

McNulty CA, Wise R, 1985, Rapid diagnosis of *Campylobacter*-associated gastritis, *Lancet*, **1:** 1443–4.

McNulty CA, Wise R, 1986, Rapid diagnosis of *Campylobacter pyloridis* gastritis, *Lancet*, **1:** 387.

Macchia G, Massone A et al., 1993, The Hsp60 protein of *Helicobacter pylori*: structure and immune response in patients with gastroduodenal diseases, *Mol Microbiol*, **9:** 645–52.

Madan E, Kemp J et al., 1988, Evaluation of staining methods for identifying *Campylobacter pylori*, *Am J Clin Pathol*, **90:** 450–3.

Mai UE, Perez Perez GI et al., 1991, Soluble surface proteins from *Helicobacter pylori* activate monocytes/macrophages by lipopolysaccharide-independent mechanism, *J Clin Invest*, **87:** 894–900.

Malaty HM, Evans DJ Jr et al., 1992, *Helicobacter pylori* infection in dental workers: a seroepidemiology study, *Am J Gastroenterol*, **87:** 1728–31.

Malaty HM, Engstrand L et al., 1994, *Helicobacter pylori* infection: genetic and environmental influences. A study of twins, *Ann Intern Med*, **120:** 982–6.

Mapstone NP, Lynch DA et al., 1993, Identification of *Helicobacter pylori* DNA in the mouths and stomachs of patients with gastritis using PCR, *J Clin Pathol*, **46:** 540–3.

Marchetti M, Arico B et al., 1995, Development of a mouse model of *Helicobacter pylori* infection that mimics human disease, *Science*, **267:** 1655–8.

Marshall BJ, Surveyor I, 1988, Carbon-14 urea breath test for the diagnosis of *Campylobacter pylori* associated gastritis, *J Nucl Med*, **29:** 11–16.

Marshall BJ, Armstrong JA et al., 1985, Attempt to fulfil Koch's postulates for pyloric *Campylobacter*, *Med J Aust*, **142:** 436–9.

Marshall BJ, Warren JR et al., 1987, Rapid urease test in the management of *Campylobacter pyloridis*-associated gastritis, *Am J Gastroenterol*, **82:** 200–10.

Megraud F, 1994, *H. pylori* species heterogeneity, *Helicobacter pylori*: Basic Mechanisms to Clinical Cure, eds Hunt RH, Tytgat GNJ, Kluwer Academic, Dordrecht, 28–40.

Megraud F, Brassens Rabbe MP et al., 1989, Seroepidemiology of *Campylobacter pylori* infection in various populations, *J Clin Microbiol*, **27:** 1870–3.

Mendall MA, Goggin PM et al., 1992, Childhood living conditions and *Helicobacter pylori* seropositivity in adult life, *Lancet*, **339:** 896–7.

Michetti P, Corthesy-Theulaz I et al., 1994, Immunization of BALB/c mice against *Helicobacter felis* infection with *Helicobacter pylori* urease, *Gastroenterology*, **107:** 1002–11.

Mitchell HM, Lee A, Carrick J, 1989, Increased incidence of *Campylobacter pylori* infection in gastroenterologists: further evidence to support person-to-person transmission of *C. pylori*, *Scand J Gastroenterol*, **24:** 396–400.

Morris A, Nicholson G, 1987, Ingestion of *Campylobacter pyloridis* causes gastritis and raised fasting gastric pH, *Am J Gastroenterol*, **82:** 192–9.

Nensey YM, Schubert TT et al., 1991, *Helicobacter pylori*-negative duodenal ulcer, *Am J Med*, **91:** 15–18.

NIH Consensus Conference, 1994, *Helicobacter pylori* in peptic ulcer disease, *JAMA*, **272:** 65–9.

Nomura A, Stemmermann GN et al., 1991, *Helicobacter pylori* infection and gastric carcinoma among Japanese Americans in Hawaii, *N Engl J Med*, **325:** 1132–6.

Nomura A, Stemmermann GN et al., 1994, *Helicobacter pylori* infection and the risk for duodenal and gastric ulceration, *Ann Intern Med*, **120:** 977–81.

Ormand JE, Talley NJ et al., 1991, Prevalence of *Helicobacter pylori* in specific forms of gastritis. Further evidence supporting a pathogenic role for *H. pylori* in chronic nonspecific gastritis, *Dig Dis Sci*, **36:** 142–5.

Parsonnet J, Friedman GD et al., 1991, *Helicobacter pylori* infection and the risk of gastric carcinoma, *N Engl J Med*, **325:** 1127–31.

Parsonnet J, Hansen S et al., 1994, *Helicobacter pylori* infection and gastric lymphoma, *N Engl J Med*, **330:** 1267–71.

Perez Perez GI, Taylor DN et al., 1990, Seroprevalence of *Helicobacter pylori* infections in Thailand, *J Infect Dis*, **161:** 1237–41.

Perez Perez GI, Witkin SS et al., 1991, Seroprevalence of *Helicobacter pylori* infection in couples, *J Clin Microbiol*, **29:** 642–4.

Polish LB, Douglas JM Jr et al., 1991, Characterization of risk factors for *Helicobacter pylori* infection among men attending a sexually transmitted disease clinic: lack of evidence for sexual transmission, *J Clin Microbiol*, **29:** 2139–43.

Price AB, 1991, The Sydney system: histological division, *J Gastroenterol Hepatol*, **6:** 209–22.

Ramsey EJ, Carey KV et al., 1979, Epidemic gastritis with hypochlorhydria, *Gastroenterology*, **76:** 1449–57.

Rathbone BJ, Wyatt JI et al., 1986, Systemic and local antibody responses to gastric *Campylobacter pyloridis* in nonulcer dyspepsia, *Gut*, **27:** 642–7.

Rautelin H, Tee W et al., 1994, Ribotyping patterns and emergence of metronidazole resistance in paired clinical samples of *Helicobacter pylori*, **32:** 1079–82.

Rauws EA, Langenberg W et al., 1988, *Campylobacter pyloridis*-associated chronic active antral gastritis. A prospective study of its prevalence and the effects of antibacterial and antiulcer treatment, *Gastroenterology*, **94:** 33–40.

Robert ME, Weinstein WM, 1993, *Helicobacter pylori*-associated gastric pathology, *Gastroenterol Clin North Am*, **22:** 59–72.

Salomon H, 1896, Über das Spirillum des saugetiermagens und sein verhalten zu den belegzellen, *Zentralbl Bakteriol Parasitenkd Infektionskr*, **19**.

Shames B, Krajden S et al., 1989, Evidence for the occurrence of the same strain of *Campylobacter pylori* in the stomach and dental plaque, *J Clin Microbiol*, **27:** 2849–50.

Sipponen P, Kekki M, Siurala M, 1991, The Sydney System: epidemiology and natural history of chronic gastritis, *J Gastroenterol Hepatol*, **6:** 244–51.

Sipponen P, Varis K et al., 1990, Cumulative 10-year risk of symptomatic duodenal and gastric ulcer in patients with or without chronic gastritis – a clinical follow-up study of 454 outpatients, *Scand J Gastroenterol*, **25:** 966–73.

Sobala GM, Crabtree JE et al., 1991a, Acute *Helicobacter pylori* infection: clinical features, local and systemic immune response, gastric mucosal histology, and gastric juice ascorbic acid concentrations, *Gut*, **32:** 1415–18.

Sobala GM, Crabtree JE et al., 1991b, Screening dyspepsia by serology to *Helicobacter pylori*, *Lancet*, **338:** 94–6.

Solnick JV, O'Rourke J et al., 1993, An uncultured gastric spiral organism is a newly identified *Helicobacter* in humans, *J Infect Dis*, **168:** 379–85.

Soltesz V, Zeeberg B, Wadstrom T, 1992, Optimal survival of *Helicobacter pylori* under various transport conditions, *J Clin Microbiol*, **30:** 1453–6.

Steer HW, Colin-Jones DG, 1975, Mucosal changes in gastric ulceration and their response to carbenoxolone sodium, *Gut*, **16:** 590–7.

Sung JJ, Chung SC et al., 1995, Antibacterial treatment of gastric ulcers associated with *Helicobacter pylori*, *N Engl J Med*, **332:** 139–42.

Telford JL, Ghiara P et al., 1994, Gene structure of the *Helicobacter pylori* cytotoxin and evidence of its key role in gastric disease, *J Exp Med*, **179:** 1653–8.

Thomas JE, Gibson GR et al., 1992, Isolation of *Helicobacter pylori* from human faeces, *Lancet*, **340:** 1194–5.

Tummuru MK, Cover TL, Blaser MJ, 1994, Mutation of the cytotoxin-associated *cagA* gene does not affect the vacuolating cytotoxin activity of *Helicobacter pylori*, *Infect Immun*, **62:** 2609–13.

Tytgat GN, 1994, Review article: treatments that impact favourably upon the eradication of *Helicobacter pylori* and ulcer recurrence, *Aliment Pharmacol Ther*, **8:** 359–68.

Warren JR, Marshall BJ, 1983, Unidentified curved bacilli on gastric epithelium in chronic active gastritis, *Lancet*, **1:** 1273–5.

Warren JR, Marshall BJ, 1984, Unidentified curved bacilli in the stomach of patients with gastritis and peptic ulceration, *Lancet*, **1:** 1311–15.

Westblom TU, Phadnis S et al., 1993, Diagnosis of *Helicobacter pylori* infection by means of a polymerase chain reaction assay for gastric juice aspirates, *Clin Infect Dis*, **16:** 367–71.

Wotherspoon AC, Ortiz Hidalgo C et al., 1991, *Helicobacter pylori*-associated gastritis and primary B-cell gastric lymphoma, *Lancet*, **338:** 1175–6.

INFECTIONS CAUSED BY *LISTERIA MONOCYTOGENES* AND *ERYSIPELOTHRIX RHUSIOPATHIAE*

W F Schlech III

LISTERIA MONOCYTOGENES

Listeriosis is a generic term for a variety of syndromes caused by *Listeria monocytogenes*, a gram-positive motile bacterium first isolated in 1926 by EGD Murray (Murray et al. 1926). The bacterium, initially called *Bacterium monocytogenes*, has had other names including *Listerella hepatolytica* (Pirie 1927) and *Listerella hominis*. The bacterium was renamed *Listeria monocytogenes* in 1940. Other *Listeria* species including *Listeria ivanovii* (Cummins et al. 1994) and *Listeria seeligeri* (Rocourt et al. 1986) have caused isolated cases of human disease but are more generally considered to be veterinary pathogens.

Although the first description of the organism occurred during an epizootic in laboratory rabbits that developed a characteristic monocytosis, naturally acquired infection in wild and domestic animals is relatively frequent. Pirie described a plague-like disease of gerbils in South Africa as early as 1927 (Pirie 1927) and the organism has been isolated in a wide variety of wild and domestic animals since that time (Gray and Killinger 1966).

1 EPIDEMIOLOGY

Listeriosis is primarily a zoonotic disease with humans as an accidental but important host. Direct transmission can occur to veterinarians and others working with infected animals (Cain and McCann 1986). Most transmission, however, is indirect and the most important mode of transmission is food-borne infection for both animals and humans (Schlech 1992). The organism is commonly found in soil, standing water and other vegetation and can be identified in the faeces of humans and animals. Gut colonization leads to shedding of the organism in the environment with contamination of crops designated for animal and human consumption. The association of silage feeding with listeriosis in animals is well established (Low and Renton 1985). Anecdotal transmission to people by milk from cows with *Listeria* mastitis has been noted (Potel 1953–54) but it was not until 1981 that a large outbreak of neonatal and adult listeriosis in Nova Scotia was attributed to contaminated cole slaw (Schlech et al. 1983). Subsequent outbreaks have been caused by a wide variety of foodstuffs including dairy products (Fleming et al. 1985, Linnan et al. 1988) and processed meats (McLauchlin et al. 1991, Goulet et al. 1993). Soft cheeses and pâtés appear to be particularly good vehicles for infection. The ability of the organism to proliferate at refrigerator temperatures probably contributes to high levels of contamination in implicated food products. Secondary contamination of other foods may occur where a contaminated item is introduced to a 'delicatessen' environment where the organism proliferates in biofilms and contaminates other foods in close proximity.

Cross-contamination in the hospital environment appears to be rare. In the few cases described, an 'early-onset' neonatal infection has caused 'late-onset' infection in an infant who had indirect contact in the delivery suite (Karchel and Leonard 1981). However, some instances of cross-infection may be attributable to small clusters of food-borne infection in the community affecting pregnant women from the same geographical area. Recently a dramatic example of cross-infection occurred in Costa Rican babies who were bathed in contaminated mineral oil with subsequent development of 'late-onset' neonatal meningitis (Schuchat et al. 1991a). The source was an early-onset case of neonatal sepsis who was bathed in the oil that was subsequently used to bathe other infants.

Identification of cross-infection and food-borne outbreaks has been enhanced by the development of new methods of identifying strains of *L. monocytogenes* from clinical and environmental specimens. Early typing systems identified serovars 1/2a, 4a and 4b as the most common isolates from animal and human sources (Seeliger and Hohne, 1979). Serotyping alone may not separate epidemic from endemic cases of listeriosis and more discrete methods of typing have therefore been developed for use in outbreak investigation. Phage typing has been helpful (McLauchlin et al. 1986) but may be supplanted in the future by multilocus enzyme electrophoresis (Bibb et al. 1989), ribosomal RNA fingerprinting (Graves et al. 1994), restriction fragment length polymorphism (RFLP) analysis (Carriere et al. 1991) and randomly amplified polymorphic DNA analysis (RAPD) (Czajka and Batt 1994). These techniques can be highly discriminating and have helped separate background cases from epidemic cases in more recent outbreaks.

1.1 Listeriosis in animals: domestic ruminants

Listeriosis is an uncommon but troublesome infection in the agricultural industry. Several syndromes in ruminants have been described including encephalitis, abortion and stillbirth, septicaemia, mastitis, diarrhoea and keratoconjunctivitis. The most common are encephalitis and abortion and stillbirth. Gill described 'circling disease' in a flock of sheep in New Zealand (Gill 1937) and identified the most characteristic features of *Listeria* encephalitis. *L. monocytogenes* has a particular predilection for infecting the hindbrain with production of facial paralysis, blindness, ataxia, dullness and 'circling'. The disease is invariably fatal, but has a varying course of between 2 and 14 days, depending on the species.

The mode of transmission of the organism from the environment is debated. Some investigators feel that the organism travels from the oral mucosal membrane via the trigeminal nerve to the hindbrain with production of typical encephalitic features (Charlton and Garcia 1977). A more common view is that most infections are caused by ingestion of spoiled silage whose high pH promotes the growth of *L. monocytogenes*. The organism translocates from the gastrointestinal tract, causing sepsis and secondary encephalitis; encephalitis is the common presenting feature.

Abortion in cattle and sheep is the second most common clinical presentation in animals. Cattle in western North America have acquired the infection through ingestion of *L. monocytogenes* on pine needles, a syndrome described as 'pine needle abortion' (Adams, Neff and Jackson 1979). Ingestion of the organism leads to sepsis and secondary placental infection with death and expulsion of a macerated fetus or premature birth and death with typical granulomatous lesions found in the viscera. The adult animals rarely show symptoms but *L. monocytogenes* may be isolated in milk with or without signs of mastitis in these animals.

This occult mastitis may be responsible for a syndrome of septicaemia in unweaned lambs although this may be due to initial intrauterine infection. Calves do not seem to develop a sepsis syndrome as frequently as lambs. The organism may be carried in the uterus of infected cattle for up to 3 years.

The gastrointestinal mode of transmission has also resulted in diarrhoea and septicaemia in sheep with fatal outcome. This has been attributed to ingestion of poor quality silage with very high levels of *L. monocytogenes* (Low and Renton 1985).

OTHER DOMESTIC ANIMALS

Listeriosis in other domestic species is much less common than in sheep and cattle. Isolated case reports and small epizootics have been described in swine, rabbits, horses and poultry. Both encephalitis and generalized infection with septicaemia have been described pathologically in these animals. Laboratory animals such as guinea pigs, mice and rats can be infected experimentally and are occasionally the victims of small epizootics. Experimental infections of these animals have been instrumental in defining the immune response to this archetypal intracellular pathogen. Another important observation from experimental infection is the presence of 'natural' resistance to *Listeria* infection. 'Natural' resistance, which may be genetically defined, may help predict susceptibility or resistance in otherwise immunologically competent hosts.

NON-DOMESTICATED ANIMALS

Case reports of infection in other animals have been frequently described, the organism being isolated from brain, blood, or viscera after death in the wild from unknown causes. The organism has been isolated from birds, fish, crustaceans, ticks and mammals. It appears to be an uncommon cause of natural death in the wild although epizootics have been described in lemmings and gerbils.

1.2 Listeriosis in man

The spectrum of human infections due to *L. monocytogenes* is remarkably similar to that in animal species. Perinatal infection is the most common clinical syndrome and includes abortion, stillbirth and neonatal sepsis and meningitis. In adults, meningitis and encephalitis are most common but a wide variety of other clinical syndromes have been reported

(Schuchat et al. 1991b) including cutaneous infection, endocarditis, osteomyelitis, septic arthritis, peritonitis and a self-limited food-borne diarrhoeal illness occasionally complicated by sepsis (Riedo et al. 1994).

NEONATAL OR PERINATAL LISTERIOSIS

Perinatal listeriosis is best understood in the context of the mother–infant pair. Infection or colonization of the gastrointestinal tract of the mother may result in an acute febrile illness mimicking pyelonephritis or influenza. In early pregnancy premature labour and abortion results with delivery of a macerated infant with pathological evidence of widespread miliary granulomatous infection. The maternal infection is self-limited, although the organism can be cultured from the blood. If the maternal infection occurs late in pregnancy the infant may be stillborn or septic at birth with significant subsequent mortality and morbidity. Collectively these syndromes are termed 'early-onset' perinatal listeriosis (Albritton, Wiggens and Feely 1976).

Colonization of the maternal gastrointestinal tract may also result in contamination of a healthy infant delivered at birth with subsequent development of neonatal meningitis 7–14 days later. A recent review of perinatal listeriosis has been published by McLauchlin (1990).

LISTERIOSIS IN ADULTS

Two-thirds of adult cases of listeriosis present as meningitis or meningoencephalitis. The course tends to be subacute and symptoms include headache, fever, nausea and vomiting. An encephalitic picture with cranial nerve palsies and seizures is more common than is seen in other forms of bacterial meningitis. The presence of ataxia and tremors reflects the peculiar predilection of the organism for the brain stem and cerebellum, remarkably similar to the 'circling disease' seen in animals (Dee and Lorber 1986, Bach and Davis 1987).

Central nervous system infection can develop in immunocompetent adults but most cases occur in patients with underlying disorders of cell mediated immune function. These include haematological and non-haematological malignancies treated with chemotherapy and patients undergoing solid organ and bone marrow transplantation. Cirrhosis secondary to haemochromatosis or alcoholic liver disease are also predisposing factors, as is HIV infection (Berenguer, Soleva and Diaz 1991).

One-third of adult cases present as a bacteraemic syndrome. *Listeria* sepsis in adults is almost always found in immunocompromised hosts. Whereas brain stem or cerebellar symptoms may suggest the diagnosis of listeriosis in the central nervous system, *Listeria* sepsis is a non-specific syndrome and is indistinguishable from other forms of sepsis in this host population. Metastatic infection after sepsis can occur and case reports of endocarditis, hepatic and splenic abscess, ophthalmitis and osteomyelitis have been described. Cases of endocarditis usually occur in

patients with a prosthetic valve and carries a high mortality rate (50%) (Lifshitz et al. 1993).

Cutaneous listeriosis is an occupational hazard for veterinarians who handle infected animals, particularly during parturition (Owen et al. 1960). A pustular rash with or without fever has been described. *Listeria* pneumonitis from aspiration of contaminated food is uncommon and is usually found in patients with a predisposition for aspiration and a positive blood culture for *L. monocytogenes*.

Recurrence of a *Listeria* infection is very rare and in a large series reported in Britain only 2 adults and a child had recurrent disease (McLauchlin et al. 1986). These appeared to be relapsed infection rather than reacquisition from the environment. *L. monocytogenes* is not a cause of chronic abortion or failure to conceive despite early reports to the contrary.

Most recently, *L. monocytogenes* has been implicated in cases of severe food poisoning. Several outbreaks of mild to severe gastroenteritis have been attributed to contaminated food (Reido et al. 1994) with *Listeria* sepsis as a consequence in a few patients. In the food-borne outbreaks so far described, chocolate milk, soft cheese, shrimp salad and rice salad have been implicated as vehicles.

2 DIAGNOSIS

The diagnosis of listeriosis depends on isolation of the organism from a normally sterile site, usually blood or cerebrospinal fluid. There are no characteristic clinical features to confirm the diagnosis without culture. The CT scan may be helpful if multiple small abscesses are found in the central nervous system, particularly the hindbrain, but these are not pathognomonic. Further information can be found in Volume 2 (see Volume 2, Chapter 30).

3 CULTURAL METHODS

L. monocytogenes grows well in broth culture including brain–heart infusion, trypticase soy and thioglycollate broths. Primary isolation from normally sterile sites can be made on blood agar. The 'cold enrichment' technique described by Gray and Killinger (1966) is not necessary for clinical specimens although it may be helpful in isolating the organism from the environment.

Selective media are necessary for isolation of the organism from food and environmental samples as well as from stool and vaginal secretions. Several selective media such as Oxford agar, modified Oxford agar and PALCAM (polymyxin–acroflavin–lithium chloride–ceftazidime–aesculin–mannitol) agar are useful (van Netten et al. 1989).

Identification of the organism after primary culture is straightforward. All strains of *L. monocytogenes* are motile, distinguishing the organism from *Erysipelothrix* and most *Corynebacterium* spp. 'Tumbling motility' is seen in hanging drop preparations of primary cultures. Organisms are more motile at room temperature than at 37°C as the organism does not express flagellar protein at the higher temperature.

On sheep blood agar narrow zones of β-haemolysis can be found but the colony may have to be moved to confirm the presence of haemolysis. *L. seeligeri* and *L. ivanovii* are also β-haemolytic but are not human pathogens. The CAMP (Christie–Atkins–Munch-Petersen) test with *Staphylococcus aureus* for *L. monocytogenes* and *L. seeligeri* and *Rhodococcus equi* for *L. ivanovii* help distinguish the 3 species.

Diagnosis of infection without culture is difficult. Serological studies have been unhelpful because of cross-reactions with other *Listeria* species, staphylococci, enterococci and corynebacteria. Seroreactivity may be common in the population because of frequent gastrointestinal exposure and even specific antibody responses may not define an acute infection. New techniques to detect antibody to the haemolysin of *L. monocytogenes* have been developed and were helpful in defining exposure to chocolate milk in one outbreak.

Blood cultures may be positive in a third of patients with central nervous system infection. Examination of the CSF in patients with meningitis usually reveals a profile similar to that seen with tuberculous or cryptococcal meningitis. Cell counts are usually less than 500 with a prominent lymphocytosis. The protein is elevated and the glucose is variably low. The organism can be seen on gram stain, often in pairs with a 'hinged' morphology. A positive gram stain is infrequent in comparison to more common causes of bacterial meningitis. The peripheral blood usually demonstrates a granulocytosis; the monocytosis originally found in rabbit models of infection is not characteristic of human infection.

Faecal carriage rates vary between 1 and 5% of the general population and isolation of *L. monocytogenes* in stool is possible (Bojsen-Moller 1972). Isolation of the organism from stool has also helped to identify outbreaks of *Listeria* gastroenteritis when other pathogens have not been found.

In invasive listeriosis biopsy specimens often show a mixed histological pattern. The placenta of infected infants with 'early-onset' disease have a typical granulomatous pattern and micro-organisms can be seen by gram stain. Hepatic granulomatosis may also be seen in infants with early-onset listeriosis (granulomatosis infantiseptica) but suppurative changes are more common in meningitic infections and reflect the acute onset of this illness.

4 TREATMENT

Because listeriosis is such an uncommon disease, no controlled clinical trials of appropriate antibiotic therapy have been carried out. The organism, however, is sensitive to a variety of antibiotics and resistance patterns have not substantially changed over time. Ampicillin and penicillin are the drugs of choice; ampicillin is preferred because of its bactericidal activity and penetration into the central nervous system (Schlech

1990). In vitro and in vivo data from animal models suggest that aminoglycosides may be synergistic with ampicillin and aminoglycosides are usually included in therapy. The duration of treatment is uncertain but should be for at least 14 days. Patients who are severely immunocompromised (such as those with AIDS) probably should have much longer courses of 3–4 weeks and lifelong suppressive therapy in AIDS patients should be considered.

For patients who are allergic to penicillin, the combination of trimethoprim and sulphamethoxazole is a good alternative. The organism is, however, susceptible to erythromycin, tetracycline and chloramphenicol. The newer macrolides and quinolones appear to be active in vitro but have not been extensively studied in patients.

It is important to remember that cephalosporins are uniformly inactive against *L. monocytogenes*. This makes them unsuitable as single agents for the empirical treatment of neonatal meningitis, as listeriosis is a relatively common cause of this disorder. Ampicillin should always be included in the empirical therapy of neonatal meningitis if cephalosporins are included for activity against other species.

If *Listeria* sepsis can be identified early in pregnancy therapy can prevent infection in the infant and a subsequent normal delivery of a healthy infant may result. However, because the symptoms of *Listeria* sepsis in the mother are non-specific, it may not be possible to diagnose the condition empirically in the absence of a community-wide outbreak of listeriosis. Blood cultures should be seriously considered in all pregnant women who show obscure or ill-defined symptoms of an illness.

Because *Listeria* are present in many 'ready-to-eat' foods the prevention of the illness from food-borne sources is difficult. The introduction of HACCP (hazard analysis of critical control points) programmes in the food industry has been identified as an important factor in diminishing the environmental contamination by *L. monocytogenes* in 'ready-to-eat' foods not subject to further processing. Vaccines for veterinary listeriosis have been developed but their efficacy even in sheep and cattle is uncertain and no vaccine is available for human populations. For immunocompromised patients a number of recommendations have been made to decrease the risk of food-borne listeriosis (Table 31.1). The use of trimethoprim sulphamethoxazole for the prophylaxis of *Pneumocystis carinii* infection in AIDS patients may also help to prevent *Listeria* infection in this well defined population.

ERYSIPELOTHRIX RHUSIOPATHIAE

Erysipelothrix rhusiopathiae is a gram-positive bacillus which causes both veterinary disease (swine erysipelas) and human infection (erysipeloid). The organism was

Table 31.1 Dietary recommendations for preventing food-borne listeriosis[a]

For all persons
Thoroughly cook raw food from animal sources (e.g. beef, pork and poultry)
Thoroughly wash raw vegetables before eating
Keep uncooked meats separate from vegetables, cooked foods and ready-to-eat foods
Avoid consumption of raw (unpasteurized) milk or foods made from raw milk
Wash hands, knives and cutting boards after handling uncooked foods
Additional recommendations for persons at high risk[b]
Avoid soft cheeses (e.g. Mexican-style, feta, brie, camembert, and blue-veined cheeses). (There is no need to avoid hard cheeses, cream cheese, cottage cheese or yogurt).
Leftover foods or ready-to-eat foods (e.g. hot dogs) should be reheated until steaming hot before eating.
Although the risk for listeriosis associated with foods from delicatessen counters is relatively low, pregnant women and immunosuppressed persons may choose to avoid these foods or to thoroughly reheat cold cuts before eating.

[a]From Centers for Disease Control Update: foodborne listeriosis–United States, 1988–1990, *Morbid Mortal Weekly Rep* **41**: 251, 1992.
[b]Persons immunocompromised by illness or medications, pregnant women and the elderly.

first isolated by Koch (1880) and then described as a cause of human disease by Rosenbach (1909). The related species *Erysipelothrix tonsillarum* does not appear to be a human pathogen but has been isolated from cases of endocarditis in dogs (Takahashi 1993).

5 EPIDEMIOLOGY

Erysipeloid, like listeriosis, is an incidental zoonotic infection of humans. Swine erysipelas, on the other hand, is a common disease in animals and *Erysipelothrix* has been isolated from a wide variety of animal species (Reboli and Farrar 1989). Unlike *L. monocytogenes*, *Erysipelothrix* does not persist in soil or vegetation and carriage by swine in the upper respiratory tract and faeces appears to cause subsequent spread of sporadic and epidemic disease in swine (Wood and Shuman 1974). The infection is more common in the summer and autumn and may have a periodic cycle of 4–5 years, possibly related to waxing and waning immunity in animal populations. Although the economic impact of the disease is primarily in swine, sheep and poultry may also be affected.

Human infection is almost always acquired by direct handling of infected animal tissues and fomites. The disease is an occupational hazard for individuals handling meat, fish and crustaceans and for those in any occupation involved with handling the byproducts of animal husbandry. Sporadic cases are more commonly seen, although outbreaks of the infection among fish handlers or abattoir workers have been described. Classical reported outbreaks include those reported by Stefansky and Grunfeld (1930) in fish workers in Odessa and in workers manufacturing bone buttons (Lawson and Stinett 1933). The incidence in the general population is unknown although one serological study (Molin et al. 1989) found antibodies to the organism in 16% of a group of 138 abattoir workers. The incidence of serious *Erysipelothrix* infection does not seem to be increased among immunocompromised patients although alcoholism may be a risk factor in some cases of *Erysipelothrix* bacteraemia.

5.1 *Erysipelothrix* in animals

Four clinical types of erysipelas have been described in swine: acute septicaemia, urticaria, endocarditis and chronic arthritis. Cutaneous involvement may be seen in all forms of the disease with the most characteristic being the quadrangular or rhombic patches in the mild urticarial form ('the diamonds'). Acute septicaemic erysipelas has a case fatality rate of 80% within 3 or 4 days. Endocarditis also ends fatally but with a more delayed course of weeks. The urticarial form of the disease usually resolves spontaneously whereas the chronic arthritic form is characterized by crippling and growth retardation. In wild animals, autopsy evidence usually suggests the acute septicaemic form of disease with widespread organ involvement (Campbell et al. 1994). Septicaemic infections are also characteristic of outbreaks or sporadic cases in poultry (Mutalib et al. 1993).

5.2 Human infection with *Erysipelothrix rhusiopathiae*

Rosenbach (1909) described the most typical form of the disease in humans. The erysipeloid of Rosenbach is a localized cellulitis caused by direct inoculation of the organism into the skin. From the time of exposure the incubation period is 1–2 weeks with development of a typical painful papule followed by peripheral spread with occasional central clearing. Development of localized abscess is uncommon. The lesion is very painful but can resolve spontaneously. Systemic symptoms are infrequent but lymphangitis and lymphadenopathy occur in a third of patients. In some patients a systemic illness does develop with fever and formation of bullae at the site of infection.

In its most severe form, *Erysipelothrix* sepsis and endocarditis may develop. About a third of the patients will have cutaneous lesions in addition to the systemic infection. Cutaneous disease does not appear to predispose to sepsis but when bacteraemia is found it is usually in association with endocarditis, similar to the disease seen in swine. Some history of occupational exposure can usually be determined in reported cases of endocarditis. Localized abscess, glomerulonephritis, meningitis and brain abscess have been described as complications of the bacteraemia. The chronic arthritis seen in swine is not found in human infection, although localized osteomyelitis may occur at the time of the acute infection.

6 DIAGNOSIS

E. rhusiopathiae grows well in blood and chocolate agar in 5–10% CO_2. For patients with bacteraemia, isolation using automated blood culture systems works well. The best specimen for culture in cutaneous disease is usually a biopsy from the leading edge of the area of cellulitis. The biopsy should be held in 1% glucose prior to primary culture. Serotyping systems have been described for *Erysipelothrix* but are not helpful clinically or epidemiologically (Jones 1986). Multilocus enzyme electrophoresis is also being developed as a typing system for *Erysipelothrix* (Chooromoney and Hampson 1994). Non-cultural methods of identification including polymerase chain reaction (PCR) have been developed and may be useful for screening of environmental specimens (Makino et al. 1994). An antibody response to *Erysipelothrix* does occur but is

not useful for clinical diagnosis. Further information can be found in Volume 2 (see Volume 2, Chapter 30).

7 TREATMENT

In the pre-antibiotic era most cases of erysipeloid resolved spontaneously. However, an early report on the usefulness of penicillin G in therapy suggested that treatment with penicillin G will hasten recovery and is mandatory for the more severe forms of disease (Stiles 1947). The organism is broadly sensitive to a wide range of β-lactams, including the penicillins and cephalosporins, and newer agents, including quinolones and macrolides. Unlike most other aerobic gram-positive bacteria, the organism is not susceptible to vancomycin; clindamycin or erythromycin may be used in patients with severe penicillin allergy or where a β-lactam is otherwise contraindicated. For patients with prosthetic valve endocarditis, valve replacement should be carried out at some point during antibiotic therapy. Despite these interventions the mortality rate of *Erysipelothrix* endocarditis approaches 50% (Gorby and Peacock 1988).

REFERENCES

Adams CJ, Neff TE, Jackson LL, 1979, Induction of *Listeria monocytogenes* infection by the consumption of Ponderosa pine needles, *Infect Immun*, **24**: 117–20.

Albritton WL, Wiggens GL, Feely JC, 1976, Neonatal listeriosis: distribution of serotypes in relation to age at onset of disease, *J Pediatr*, **88**: 41.

Bach MC, Davis KM, 1987, *Listeria* rhombencephalitis mimicking tuberculosis meningitis, *Rev Infect Dis*, **9**: 130.

Berenguer J, Soleva J, Diaz MD, 1991, Listeriosis in patients infected with human immunodeficiency virus, *Rev Infect Dis*, **13**: 115–19.

Bibb WF, Schwartz B et al., 1989, Analysis of *L. monocytogenes* by multilocus enzyme electrophoresis and application of the method to epidemiologic investigations, *J Food Microbiol*, **8**: 233–9.

Bojsen-Moller J, 1972, Human listeriosis: diagnostic, epidemiologic and clinical studies, *Acta Pathol Microbiol Scand*, **229**: 72–92.

Cain DB, McCannVL, 1986, An unusual case of cutaneous listeriosis, *J Clin Microbiol*, **23**: 976–7.

Campbell GD, Addison EM et al., 1994, *Erysipelothrix rhusiopathiae* serotype 17, septicemia in moose (*Alces alces*) from Algonquin Park, Ontario, *Wildl Dis*, **30**: 436–8.

Carriere C, Allardet-Servent A et al., 1991, DNA polymorphism in strains of *Listeria monocytogenes*, *J Clin Microbiol*, **29**: 1351–5.

Charlton AM, Garcia MM, 1977, Spontaneous listeria encephalitis and neuritis in sheep. Light microscopic studies, *Vet Pathol*, **24**: 297A.

Chooromoney KN, Hampson DJ, 1994, Analysis of *Erysipelothrix rhusiopathiae* and *Erysipelothrix tonsillarum* by multilocus enzyme electrophoresis, *J Clin Microbiol*, **134**: 371–6.

Cummins AJ, Fielding AK et al., 1994, *Listeria ivanovii* infection in a patient with AIDS, *J Infect*, **28**: 89–91.

Czajka J, Batt CA, 1994, Verification of causal relationships between *Listeria monocytogenes* isolates implicated in foodborne outbreaks of listeriosis by randomly amplified polymorphic DNA patterns, *J Clin Microbiol*, **32**: 1280–7.

Dee RR, Lorber B, 1986, Brain abscess due to *Listeria monocytogenes*: case report and literature review, *Rev Infect Dis*, **8**: 1968.

Fleming DW, Cochi SL et al., 1985, Pasteurized milk as a vehicle

of infection in an outbreak of listeriosis, *N Engl J Med*, **312**: 404–7.

Gill DA, 1937, Ovine bacterial encephalitis (circling disease) and the bacterial genus *Listerella*, *Aust Vet J*, **13**: 46–56.

Gorby GL, Peacock JE, 1988, *Erysipelothrix rhusiopathiae* endocarditis: microbiologic, epidemiologic and clinical features of an occupational disease, *Rev Infect Dis*, **10**: 317–25.

Goulet V, Lepoutre A et al., 1993, Epidémie de listériose en France. Bilan final et résultats de l' enquête épidémiologique, *Bull Epidemiol Heb*, **4**: 13–14.

Graves LM, Swaminathan B et al., 1994, Comparison of ribotyping and multilocus ezyme electrophoresis for subtyping of *L. monocytogenes* isolates, *J Clin Microbiol*, **32**: 2936–43.

Gray ML, Killinger AH, 1966, *Listeria monocytogenes* and listeric infections, *Bacteriol Rev*, **30**: 309–82A.

Jones D, 1986, Genus *Erysipelothrix*, *Bergey's Manual of Systematic Bacteriology*, vol. 2, eds Sneath PHA, Mair MS et al., Williams and Williams, Baltimore, 1245–9.

Kachel W, Leonard HG, 1981, Babies cross-infected with *L. monocytogenes*, *Lancet*, **2**: 939–40.

Koch R, 1880, *Investigations into the Aetiology of Traumatic Infectious Diseases*, New Sydenham Society, London.

Lawson GB, Stinett MS, 1933, Erysipeloid occurring among workers in a button factory, *South Med J*, **26**: 1068–70.

Lifschitz A, Fadilah R et al., 1993, *Listeria monocytogenes* endocarditis in a patient with a prosthetic aortic valve, *Israel J Med Sci*, **29**: 49–50.

Linnan MJ, Mascola L et al., 1988, Epidemic listeriosis associated with Mexican-style cheese, *N Engl J Med*, **319**: 823–8.

Low JC, Renton CP, 1985, Septicemia, encephalitis and abortions in a housed flock of sheep caused by *Listeria monocytogenes* type 1/2, *Vet Rec*, **116**: 147–50.

McLauchlin J, 1990, A summary of 722 cases 1. Listeriosis during pregnancy and in the newborn, *Epidemiol Infect*, **104**: 181–9.

McLauchlin J, Audurier A et al., 1986, The evaluation of a phage-typing system for *L. monocytogenes* for use in epidemiological studies, *J Med Microbiol*, **22**: 357–65.

McLauchlin J, Hall SM et al., 1991, Human listeriosis and paté: a possible association, *Br Med J*, **303**: 773–5.

Makino S, Okada Y et al., 1994, Direct and rapid detection of

Erysipelothrix rhusiopathiae DNA in animals by PCR, *J Clin Microbiol*, **32:** 1526–31.

Molin G, Soderlind O et al., 1989, Occurence of *Erysipelothrix rhusiopathiae* on pork and pig slurry, and the distribution of specific antibodies in abattoir workers, *J Appl Bacteriol*, **67:** 347–P.

Murray EGD, Webb RA et al., 1926, A disease of rabbits characterized by a large mononuclear leucocytosis, caused by a hitherto undescribed bacillus, *Bacterium monocytogenes, J Pathol Biol,* **29:** 407–39.

Mutalib AA, King JM et al., 1993, Erysipelas in caged laying chickens in suspected erysipeloid in animal caretakers, *J Vet Diagn Invest,* **5:** 198–201.

van Netten P, Perales I et al., 1989, Liquid and solid selective differential media for the detection and enumeration of *Listeria monocytogenes* and other *Listeria* spp., *Int J Food Microbiol,* **8:** 299–316.

Owen CR, Meis A et al., 1960, A case of primary cutaneous listeriosis, *N Engl J Med,* **262:** 1026–8.

Pirie JHH, 1927, A new disease of veld rodents 'Tiger river disease', *Pub S Afr Inst Med Res,* **3:** 163–86.

Potel J, 1953–54, *Wiss Z Martin Luther Univ,* **3:** 341–64.

Reboli AC, Farrar WE, 1989, *Erysipelothrix rhusiopathiae*: an occupational pathogen, *Clin Microbiol Rev,* **2:** 354–9.

Riedo FX, Pinner RW et al., 1994, A point-source foodborne listeriosis outbreak: documented incubation period and possible mild illness, *J Infect Dis,* **170:** 693–6.

Rocourt J, Hof H et al., 1986, Méningite purulente aiguë à *Listeria seeligerii* chez un adulte immunocompétent, *Schweiz Med Wochenschr,* **116:** 248–51.

Rosenbach FJ, 1909, Experimentalle morphologische and klinische Studie uber die krankheitserregenden Mikroorganismen des Schweinerotlaufs, des Erysipeloids und der Mausesepsis, *Zentralbl Hyg Infektionskr,* **63:** 343–69.

Schlech WF, 1990, Listeriosis, *Current Therapy in Infectious Diseases,* 3rd edn, eds Kass EH, Platt R, B C Decker, Toronto, 297–304.

Schlech WF, 1992, Expanding the horizons of foodborne listeriosis, *JAMA,* **267:** 2081–2.

Schlech WF, Lavigne PM et al., 1983, Epidemic listeriosis: evidence for transmission by food, *N Engl J Med,* **308:** 203–6.

Schuchat A, Lizano C et al., 1991a, Outbreak of neonatal listeriosis associated with mineral oil, *Pediatr Infect Dis J,* **10:** 183–9.

Schuchat A, Swaminathan B et al., 1991b, Epidemiology of human listeriosis, *Clin Microbiol Rev,* **4:** 169–83.

Seeliger HPR, Hohne K, 1979, Serotyping of *L. monocytogenes* and related species, *Methods in Microbiology,* vol. 13, eds Bergand T, Norris JR, Academic Press, New York, 31–49.

Stefansky WK, Grunfeld AA, 1930, Eine epidemine des erysipeloids in Odessa, *Zentralbl Bakteriol Parasitenkd,* **117:** 376–8.

Stiles GW, 1947, Chronic erysipeloid (swine *Erysipelothrix*) in a man: the effect of treatment with penicillin, *JAMA,* **134:** 953–5.

Takahashi T, Tamura Y et al., 1993, *Erysipelothrix tonsillarum* isolated from dogs with endocarditis in Belgium, *Res Vet Sci,* **54:** 264–5.

Wood RL, Shuman RD, 1974, Swine erysipelas, *Diseases of Swine,* 4th edn, eds Dunne HW, Leaman AD, Iowa State University Press, Ames, Iowa, 565–620.

Chapter 32

URINARY TRACT INFECTIONS

M Sussman

1 INTRODUCTION

The urinary tract is the second most common site of bacterial infection in humans. It has been estimated that in their lifetime 10–20% of women in the USA may be expected suffer a urinary tract infection and that each year up to 3% of women will have more than one episode of such infection (Patton, Nash and Abrutyn 1991, Ronald and Pattulo 1991). Stamey (1980a) has estimated that once a woman has had a urinary tract infection she has a 25% chance of a recurrence. Though urinary tract infections are responsible for much illness and great misery, only a small proportion lead to chronic renal failure or death. The infected urinary tract is, however, the commonest source of the organisms responsible for septicaemia.

The urinary tract is in communication with the outside world only by way of the urethra and this renders the common occurrence of urinary tract infection a matter for some surprise. Under normal conditions, the constant flow of urine through the upper part of the tract and the intermittent emptying of the bladder is an efficient washout mechanism that should remove micro-organisms that gain entry. It has become evident that uropathogenic organisms possess specific means for the colonization of the uroepithelium but the means by which subsequent damage is brought about remain for the greater part little understood. When the smooth flow of urine is disturbed by anatomical or functional abnormalities, particularly if some urine remains in the bladder at the end of micturition, colonization of the urinary tract is to be

expected and bacterial virulence factors play a subsidiary part in the genesis of disease.

It is accepted that most uropathogens originate from the host microbial flora and most commonly from the faecal flora, but they may be 'exogenous', as when introduced during diagnostic or therapeutic instrumentation of the urinary tract. The ascending route by way of the urethra is the most usual by which micro-organisms enter the urinary tract. Such infections always begin as a colonization of the uroepithelium. Less commonly, blood-borne infection may lead to metastatic tissue infection of the kidney, such as staphylococcal renal abscess or renal tuberculosis (see Chapter 21). There is no persuasive evidence that urinary tract infection ever arises by the lymphatic route.

2 HISTORICAL BACKGROUND

A reference in the Hearst papyrus (1550 BC) to 'sending forth heat from the bladder' may be a reference to urinary tract infection (Asscher 1980). In the tradition of Galen (131–201 AD) visual observation of the urine (uroscopy) was part of routine medical practice and it would be surprising if the early uroscopists did not correlate dysuria and turbid urine. The Persian physician Rhazes (860–932) in his great encyclopaedia of medicine, the *El hawi*, gives a clear description of pyelitis (Browne 1962). The early history of urinary tract infection is reviewed by Asscher (1980) and Haber (1988).

The properties of urine as a bacterial growth medium were recognized by Pasteur (1863) and somewhat later the relationship between bacteriuria and symptoms was recognized (Roberts 1881). The observations that turned out to be of major significance for an understanding of urinary tract infections was the development of quantitative urine bacteriology. By comparing the viable bacterial counts of catheter and voided urine it became possible to make a clear distinction between contamination and infection. This for the first time made it possible to study the epidemiology of urinary tract infections.

3 THE URINARY ECOSYSTEM

The urinary tract may be regarded as a specialized ecosystem akin to a chemostat in which urine continuously produced by the kidney is intermittently voided through the urethra. Its behaviour in health and during infective processes is determined by anatomical and functional factors. The bacterial flora of the urethra and periurethral area may also play a part in resistance and susceptibility to infection. Finally, the composition of the urine in part determines the rate of bacterial growth in the urinary tract.

3.1 Anatomical and functional factors

The urinary tract consists of the kidneys from which urine drains through the ureters to the bladder. The vesicoureteric junction is controlled by functional valves that allow urine into the bladder but normally prevent reflux from the bladder into ureters. The urine is retained in the bladder until it is voided through the urethra.

The smooth mucosal surface of the urinary tract and its anatomy allow the unimpeded flow of urine so that at the end of micturition only a fine film of urine is retained on the surface of the empty bladder. The normally continuous flow of urine exercises a powerful effect that tends to prevent infection and organisms that gain entrance are rapidly washed out of the bladder from which they cannot reach the ureters and kidneys. Congenital abnormalities, such as urethral valves, and acquired abnormalities, such as outflow obstruction, may interfere with the 'smooth' flow and drainage of urine and may lead to the retention within the system of variable volumes of urine (residual urine) that may become infected and then represent a permanently retained bacterial inoculum that tends to perpetuate the infection. An important example is infection of the residual urine retained in the bladder when micturition is impeded, as by prostatic hypertrophy. When the vesicoureteric valves are incompetent, reflux occurs and may lead to residual urine with the maintenance of infection. Infection is more probable in women because of their rather short urethra in which backflow may occur (Hinman 1966).

3.2 Bacterial flora

The normal urinary tract is sterile. Since most urinary tract infections are ascending in nature, the urethral, periurethral, introital, vaginal and faecal flora may be of significance in pathogenesis and resistance. In males, the preputial flora may be important. This bacterial flora may also play a part in either preventing or permitting uropathogens to colonize before ascent into the urinary tract.

The distal urethra has a sparse but complex and variable flora that is mainly of significance for the contamination it may introduce into urine collected for examination. The population consists of aerobic and anaerobic bacteria, including coagulase-negative staphylococci, streptococci, enterococci, diphtheroids, non-pathogenic *Neisseria* spp., *Bacteroides, Fusobacterium, Peptostreptococcus, Eubacterium* and *Clostridium* spp. (Bowie et al. 1977, Summanen et al. 1993). Commensal mycobacteria and mycoplasmas may also be present.

The mature vagina, under oestrogenic influence, is an acidic environment (c. pH 5) in which *Lactobacillus* spp. predominate but aerobic cocci, non-sporing anaerobic bacilli and clostridia may also be present. The pH of prepubertal and postmenopausal vagina is close to neutrality and has a bacterial flora that may include enterobacteria (Hooton and Stamm 1996). Lactobacilli may prevent vaginal colonization by uropathogens (see section 12.2, p. 615).

3.3 Multiplication of bacteria in urine

The infected urinary tract is a dynamic culture system in which bacteria multiply, urine is continuously added by the kidneys and from which urine is drained by micturition. The bacterial population in the system is determined by its growth rate and the balance between urine production and the volume of the system (O'Grady and Cattell 1966). The bacterial growth rate varies within wide limits according to bacterial species and urine composition (Roberts and Beard 1965, Asscher et al. 1966). Urine flow may be affected by diuresis or dehydration, and the volume of the urinary drainage system may be markedly increased by the anatomical changes that accompany pregnancy.

The capacity of urine to support bacterial growth depends on its chemical composition, pH and osmolality. Whereas some chemical constituents, such as glucose and amino acids, serve as bacterial nutrients, others, such as urea and organic acids, act as growth inhibitors. The growth rate is optimal in a pH range of 6.0–7.0 and an osmolality below 200–1100 mosm kg^{-1} (Asscher et al. 1966). Urine osmolality is an index of renal concentrating power; intrarenal infection is associated with reduced osmolality, which encourages bacteriuria (Winberg 1959, Kaitz 1961), and its eradication corrects the impairment of urinary concentrating ability (Norden and Tuttle 1965).

Glucose present in normal urine is the main energy source for the growth of urinary pathogens and its concentration is normally sufficient to support maximal growth rates. The number of bacteria in the urine of diabetic patients is significantly higher than in that of non-diabetic controls (O'Sullivan et al. 1961). This is consistent with experimental observations that increased urine glucose concentrations prolong exponential growth and give rise to higher final bacterial populations; competitors of glucose utilization, such as 2-deoxy-D-glucose and 6-deoxy-D-glucose, reduce bacterial counts in urine (Weiser, Asscher and Sussman 1969).

Though the amino acid composition of urine may vary considerably and affect bacterial growth (Roberts, Clayton and Bean 1968), it is unlikely that they are important in urinary tract infection. The organic acids normally present in urine may be bacteriostatic according to the degree of their dissociation, which is pH-dependent. Urea in high concentration is bactericidal for uropathogens (Schlegel, Cuellar and O'Dell 1961, Kaye 1968), but its effect is mainly due to an increase in osmolality; the addition of salts to a high osmolality also results in growth inhibition (Asscher, Sussman and Weiser 1968).

4 SIGNIFICANT BACTERIURIA

Bacteriuria is defined as the presence of multiplying bacteria within the urinary drainage system. A central problem in the diagnosis of bacteriuria by the examination of voided urine is to distinguish between contamination and bacteriuria. Kass (1956) observed that some healthy women have bacteriuria; on the basis of a large number of observations he was able to define 'significant' bacteriuria as the presence of more than 100 000 organisms per ml in a carefully collected sample of clean-voided or midstream urine. If this number of organisms is found in a single urine sample from a given individual, the probability of true bacteriuria is about 80%, and if the observation is repeated the probability rises to about 96%. The definition made it possible to distinguish true bacteriuria from urine contamination.

Significant bacteriuria in a given sample correlates 95% with results obtained by examining catheter specimens of urine. This relationship is not, however, valid in all circumstances. It is less valid under conditions of water loading, low urinary pH, high urea concentration or hyperosmolarity. High fluid intake increases the rate of bladder emptying and lowers the bacterial count; inadequate chemotherapy may do the same. Similarly, alkalinizing or acidifying agents may reduce the bacterial growth rate and give rise to a low bacterial count.

The observations that formed the basis for the definition of significant bacteriuria were made in asymptomatic women (Kass 1956, see also section 7.1, p. 608). It is recognized, however, that, of women with symptoms of acute lower urinary tract infection characterized by frequency and dysuria, 30–50% have counts of less than 100 000 organisms per ml (Gallagher, Montgomerie and North 1965, O'Grady et al. 1970, Tapsall et al. 1975). This is also true of specimens obtained by suprapubic bladder aspiration (Mabeck 1969, Kraft and Stamey 1977).

Significant bacteriuria is usually due to a single bacterial strain; the presence of more than one species usually, but not always, indicates contamination. Freeman, Sisson and Burdess (1996) have shown, however, that what appear to be pure bacterial growths on routine culture may in fact be heterogeneous.

5 URINARY PATHOGENS

Only a few species can initiate infection in the normal urinary tract but a wide range of organisms may cause infection in patients with structural or functional abnormalities of the urinary tract. The same is true of patients with urinary catheters. The source of the infecting organisms is usually the faecal flora of the patient (Vosti, Goldberg and Rantz 1965, Grüneberg, Leigh and Brumfitt 1968) but when infection occurs in patients with catheters or after instrumentation of the urinary tract the source of infecting organisms is commonly exogenous.

Much evidence suggests that the perineum is the source of organisms that cause urinary tract infection and that they can be found there before infection occurs (Stamey et al. 1971, Bollgren and Winberg 1976, Pfau and Sacks 1981) but in recurrent infection this is probably not an important predisposing factor (Cattell et al. 1974, Kunin, Polyak and Postel 1980, Brumfitt, Gargan and Hamilton-Miller 1987).

Escherichia coli is the commonest cause of all urinary tract infections. It accounts for about 90% of community-acquired infections and a smaller proportion of infections in other situations. It is a general rule that the more complicated the background in which a urinary tract infection occurs the lower the probability that it is due to *E. coli* but even then it is the predominant uropathogen (Table 32.1). The majority of urinary *E. coli* isolates belong to a small number of O serogroups, particularly O1, O2, O4, O6, O7 and O75. This led to the suggestion that these serogroups have special uropathogenic potential (Rantz 1962), but these are also the predominant serogroups in the faeces of both infected and non-infected patients (Turck and Petersdorf 1962, Anderson et al. 1965, Grüneberg, Leigh and Brumfitt 1968). It is clear, therefore, that serotype alone cannot explain the uropathogenicity of *E. coli*. Various other factors are necessary for the virulence of *E. coli* in the urinary tract but the limited number of serotypes is related to the clonal origin of pathogenic strains (see section 8.1, p. 610).

Proteus spp. are important primary uropathogens; about 80% of *Proteus* infections are due to *Proteus mirabilis* and the rest to *Proteus vulgaris*. These infections are particularly common in uncircumcised boys (Naylor 1984) and it has been suggested that this is due to colonization of the preputial sac (Hallett, Pead and Maskell 1976). The powerful urease of *Proteus* spp. (see Volume 2, Chapter 43) leads to a marked rise in urine pH, the precipitation of phosphates and stone formation. In patients with catheters or urinary obstruction, *Proteus* spp. may cause chronic infection.

Streptococci seldom cause primary infections of the urinary tract. Enterococci are common contaminants in urine because they are present in normal faeces, are commonly found on the perineum and grow at low temperatures. *Enterococcus faecalis* occasionally causes infection after invasive procedures on the urinary tract. *Streptococcus agalactiae* (group B) is part of the normal vaginal and perineal flora and is an

Table 32.1 Prevalence of microbial causes of urinary tract infection[a]

Site of infection	Organism	Community-acquired (%)	Nosocomial infections (%)
Bladder	*Escherichia coli*	90	50
	Proteus mirabilis	5–8	
	Indole +ve *Proteus* spp.		} 10–12
	Klebsiella spp.	1–2	15–20
	Coagulase-negative staphylococci[b]	1–2	1–2
	Enterococcus faecalis	<1	10–12
	Streptococcus spp.	<1	
	Staphylococcus aureus		<1
	Enterobacter spp.		2–5
	Pseudomonas aeruginosa		10–15
	Citrobacter spp.		<1
	Acinetobacter spp.		<1
Prostate	*Escherichia coli*		
	Corynebacterium spp.		
	Anaerobes		
Urethra	*Escherichia coli*		
	Coagulase-negative staphylococci		
	Streptococcus spp.		
	Neisseria gonorrhoeae		
	Chlamydia trachomatis		
	Ureaplasma urealyticum		

[a]The percentages in the above table are based on c. 2000 samples of infected urine examined in 1987 and 1988 in the microbiology laboratory of a District General Hospital in the United Kingdom.
[b]The prevalence of *Staphylococcus saprophyticus* in young women is higher.

occasional primary uropathogen in women but it may not grow on some media used for routine urine examination.

Staphylococcus saprophyticus, which is novobiocin-resistant (see Chapter 14 and Volume 2, Chapter 27) is a primary uropathogen and is responsible for about 20% of urethritis and cystitis in sexually active but otherwise healthy women aged 16–25 (Hovelius, Colleen and Mardh 1984, Pead, Maskell and Morris 1985). *S. saprophyticus* may also be responsible for infections in sexually abused children (Goldenring, Fried and Tames 1988). Various other staphylococci, including *Staphylococcus epidermidis*, may cause mild urinary tract infections after instrumentation or urological operations (see Chapter 14). *S. epidermidis* and micrococci are members of the normal skin flora and are often present as contaminants in urine. Ascending urinary tract infections due to *Staphylococcus aureus* are rare but the organisms may be found in the urine of patients with staphylococcal septicaemia (see Chapter 14); usually they are contaminants derived from the perineum.

Though *E. coli* is also the commonest uropathogen in hospitalized patients, many other gram-negative bacilli are also frequent causative organisms. These include *Klebsiella*, *Enterobacter*, indole-positive *Proteus* and *Citrobacter*. Such organisms may be selected in the hospital setting by antimicrobial use, cross-infection or colonization of patients.

Infections due to *Pseudomonas aeruginosa* are particularly associated with major urological abnormalities, open urinary drainage systems and long-term indwelling catheters. The strains responsible almost always show multiple resistance to antimicrobial agents; profuse slime production may lead to catheter blockage. Infection with *P. aeruginosa* may be asymptomatic but instrumentation or even catheterization of such patients can lead to bacteraemia with potentially disastrous consequences.

The significance of anaerobes and other fastidious bacteria such as *Gardnerella vaginalis*, *Haemophilus* spp., *Corynebacterium* spp., *Streptococcus milleri*, lactobacilli, micro-aerophilic streptococci and *Ureaplasma urealyticum* in urinary tract infection is the subject of controversy (Finegold et al. 1965, Maskell 1986). Such organisms are unlikely to be isolated by routine urine culture but they may be found after prolonged culture of urine specimens under micro-aerophilic or anaerobic conditions, particularly in specimens that give low or negative counts by routine methods. These organisms may cause infection of the urethra, prostate and paraurethral glands but there is little evidence that they cause cystitis.

6 DIAGNOSIS

6.1 Urine collection

The accurate diagnosis of urinary tract infection requires urine specimens free from contamination and they must be examined in the laboratory before bacterial multiplication has taken place. Since the urine stream flushes out the potentially contaminating urethral flora, midstream urine is satisfactory for most diagnostic purposes. Nevertheless, special co-operation is necessary to collect satisfactory specimens of urine from women and young children. If urine is difficult to obtain, suprapubic aspiration may be necessary; there is no case for the use of catheters.

Women must be carefully instructed to swab the vulva thoroughly with water or a solution of a bland soap free from antiseptics. Though it has been conventional to instruct men to retract the foreskin and cleanse the glans penis, this is probably unnecessary (Lipsky 1989).

For the diagnosis of urethritis or infection in the para-urethral glands, midstream urine is unhelpful and the first 5–10 ml of voided urine should be collected. If there is a discharge, a smear and swab may prove adequate. The comparison of a urethral specimen with a midstream specimen is useful to identify the site of infection. Methods for the diagnosis of bacterial prostatitis are described below (see section 16, p. 616).

In the case of catheterized patients, urine should be collected through the drainage tubing and never from the collection bag.

In infants and children it is difficult to collect uncontaminated urine via the urethra but it may be possible to obtain 'clean-catch' specimens after careful cleansing of the genitalia. The use of collection bags may be an alternative but special care is necessary when interpreting the results obtained with such specimens. Suprapubic aspiration of urine is safe and easy to perform in the newborn, infants and young children (Abbott 1978), and accurate laboratory results are obtained. This technique can also be used in adult women when uncontaminated specimens cannot be obtained by other methods (Bailey and Little 1969). The differential diagnosis of upper urinary tract infection by urine culture is considered below (see section 6.3, p. 607).

Bacteria grow rapidly in urine at room temperature and above. If specimens cannot be examined within 2 h they must be stored at 4°C. Examination should not be unduly delayed because, even with refrigeration, some species may grow, and leucocytes, erythrocytes and casts may become degraded. If refrigeration cannot be provided, the use of boric acid as a preservative can be helpful but leucocytes are rapidly degraded in such specimens.

Delays before reception in the laboratory are inevitable with urine collected in the community. In this case careful collection techniques and efficient transport systems serve to reduce the number of unsatisfactory specimens. Methods suitable for use in the physician's surgery include the dip-slide and reagent strips for the detection of nitrite (Kunin 1987; see also p. 606).

6.2 Laboratory methods

The laboratory examination of urine for the diagnosis of infection seen superficially appears initially to be simple and straightforward. This is a misconception because a number of confounding factors interfere first in the collection of specimens, then in their testing, and finally in the interpretation of results. The main available test procedures are listed in Table 32.2.

MICROSCOPY

Microscopy is an important part of the laboratory examination of urine and can be carried out on uncentrifuged urine or the deposit obtained by centrifugation. Centrifuge deposits are useful for the identification of cells, casts and other solid elements such as crystals. The examination of a fresh specimen of uncentrifuged urine can be helpful for the rapid presumptive diagnosis of urinary tract infections provided that more than c. 30 000 bacteria per ml are present (Kunin 1961).

Table 32.2 Methods for the examination of urine

Culture
Quantitative
Pour-plate
Surface viable count
Semiquantitative
Dip-spoon
Standard loop
Filter paper strip
Swab inoculation
Chemical
Nitrite detection
Tetrazolium reduction
Glucose assay
Catalase detection
Leucocyte
Count
Leucocyte esterase
Staining
Gram's method
Filtration and staining
Automated
Photometry (turbidity)
Bioluminescence (ATP assay)
Electrical impedance
Limulus amoebocyte assay
(lipopolysaccharide)
Microcalorimetry
Particle counting and sizing
Radiometry (^{14}C release)

Leucocytes

An increase in the number of leucocytes (pyuria) does not necessarily indicate the presence of inflammation. Though pyuria is present in most clinical infections, it may be absent in covert bacteriuria. Gross contamination of the urine with leucocytes may occur where there is a genital tract infection or urethritis. Inflammation of the bladder, such as trigonitis, or trauma, surgery or urethral catheterization, may increase the number of leucocytes in the urine; in tuberculosis there may be pyuria without bacteriuria.

Since the urine leucocyte count is highly variable and can be misleading, the leucocyte excretion rate is the most precise method of measuring pyuria. Urine is collected over a defined period and the number of leucocytes is counted. An excretion rate of more than 4×10^5 leucocytes per hour correlates with symptomatic urinary tract infection (Little 1964, Brumfitt 1965). Alternatively, the leucocyte count in centrifuged urine can be determined with a haemocytometer and the result calculated; the same can be done with a known volume of uncentrifuged urine. A leucocyte count of more than 10 mm^{-3} represents an excretion rate of more than 4×10^5 leucocytes per hour (Brumfitt 1965). Less than 10% of patients with covert bacteriuria have pyuria, whereas this is present in 96% of patients with bacteriuria and symptoms. Urine flow and the physicochemical composition of the urine may affect the white cell excretion rate and it may continue to be raised for a time after a urinary tract infection has cleared.

Pyuria can also be determined with reagent strips (see p. 607).

CULTURE

The count of viable bacteria in a correctly collected sample of urine is the 'gold standard' for the diagnosis of bacteriuria. The most accurate methods of counting bacteria are the pour-plate and the surface viable count but they are time-consuming and for routine purposes semiquantitative techniques are used. These are useful for examining large numbers of urine specimens; the most commonly used techniques are the standard loop (Hoeprich 1960), filter-paper strip (Leigh and Williams 1964), dip-spoon (Mackey and Sandys 1965) and dip-slide (Guttmann and Naylor 1967). Semiquantitative methods for the examination of urine have been reviewed by Sussman and Asscher (1979).

Coliform counts of less than 100 organisms per ml should be considered significant in women with symptoms, particularly in the presence of pyuria (Stamm et al. 1980, 1982), though the validation of such low counts is difficult in routine practice. In men with urinary symptoms, counts of less than 100 000 organisms per ml can occasionally be significant and counts as low as 150 organisms per ml may constitute evidence of infection (Stamey, Govan and Palmer 1965). Colony counts for the diagnosis of various types of urinary tract infection are shown in Table 32.3.

Any bacterial colony count obtained from specimens collected by catheterization, renal biopsy, suprapubic aspiration (Monzon et al. 1958) and post-prostatic massage (Meares and Stamey 1968) is significant because of the low probability of contamination. 'First-catch' (urethral) urine or the first voided 5 ml may provide useful information for the diagnosis of urethritis or urethral syndrome, but the assessment of such samples is complicated (Stamey 1980b).

Multiple strains more frequently become established in patients with indwelling urethral catheters. Infections associated with the urethra, para-urethral glands and kidney may also be polymicrobial and include anaerobic or fastidious organisms.

For routine urine culture 2 media are conventionally used. One of these is a non-selective medium, which serves partly to identify the degree of contamination, whereas the other, e.g. cystine lactose electrolyte-deficient (CLED) medium (Mackey and Sandys 1966), is selective for the most common urinary pathogens. Other media are used for special purposes.

CHEMICAL AND ENZYMATIC METHODS

A number of chemical and enzyme-based tests have been described for the examination of urine. These include the triphenyltetrazolium chloride reduction test (Simmons and Williams 1962), detection of low urine glucose concentration (Schersten and Fritz 1967), detection of nitrite (Males, Bartholomew and Amsterdam 1983), bacterial ATP (Thore et al. 1975) and of endotoxin (Nachum and Shanbrom 1981). Pyuria may be detected by leucocyte esterase activity (Perry, Matthews and Weesner 1982). The detection of nitrite and leucocyte esterase has been incorporated in reagent strip screening tests (see p. 607).

The examination of urine for protein and glucose plays little part in the diagnosis of bacterial infection. Though proteinuria is an indicator of renal disease, it may be due to inflammatory exudates or vaginal secretions. Quantitative estimation in a timed urine specimen is necessary for accurate evaluation.

AUTOMATED METHODS

The heavy load in clinical microbiology laboratories represented by urine examination has prompted the design of a number of automated methods. **Photometric methods** measure light scattered by bacteria but, because they depend on growth rate and incubation time, they are unreliable for slow-growing organisms (Pezzlo et al. 1982). **Bioluminescence methods** measure bacterial ATP by a method that depends on the firefly luciferin–luciferase system. These methods are rapid but because more than 15% of specimens give false positive results, their specificity is poor (Thore et al. 1975). Other automated methods depend on calorimetry, electrical impedance, filtration, flow cytometry, fluorescence and radiometry of $^{14}CO_2$ released by bacterial metabolism from isotope-labelled substrates. Most of these methods are more widely used in the USA than in the UK. These methods have been reviewed by Eisenstadt and Washington (1996).

Table 32.3 Diagnostic colony counts for the diagnosis of bacteriuria

	Colony count per ml	
	Enterobacteria	Other organisms
Asymptomatic infections[a]		
Men	$\geq 10^5$	$\geq 10^5$
Women	$\geq 10^5$	$\geq 10^5$
Symptomatic infections		
Men	$\geq 10^3$	$\geq 10^3$
Women	$\geq 10^2$	$\geq 10^5$

[a]Counts in 2 consecutive urine specimens.
After Johnson (1991).

SCREENING

Great efforts have been made to devise screening tests for the diagnosis of urinary tract infection. The ideal of a screening test with a specificity and sensitivity of 100% has not been achieved. The many putative screening procedures include microscopy for bacteria and leucocytes. Tests for bacterial catalase have been proposed but streptococci and enterococci do not produce catalase, whereas host cells in the urine do. Screening methods based on filtration and bioluminescence have unsatisfactory positive predictive values, but their negative predictive values are high.

Commercially available reagent strips ('dipsticks') allow rapid colorimetric assays for a number of urine constituents and pH. For the diagnosis of urinary tract infection the tests for nitrite and leucocyte esterase are the most important. Most, but not all, uropathogens reduce the nitrate in urine to nitrite, which is not normally present. Provided the infected urine has had a sufficient residence time in the bladder, the presence of nitrite is evidence of infection. Similarly, a positive test for leucocyte esterase is indicative of infection. Individually the tests for nitrite and leucocyte esterase have too low a positive predictive value for them to be useful for diagnosis. When used in combination, the 2 tests have a high sensitivity and specificity, but their positive predictive value is too low to be reliable for diagnosis. Under carefully controlled conditions they can, however, be used to screen for urine specimens that do not require further examination (see Table 32.4).

6.3 Localization of infection

Clinical signs and symptoms are often a poor guide to distinguish between upper and lower urinary tract infections. The means of localization of urinary tract infections can be divided into:

1 non-invasive methods, in which only blood and urine are examined and
2 invasive methods, in which investigative procedures are performed on the patient (Table 32.5).

The value of invasive procedures is limited to a selected group of patients, such as women with recurrent infection or symptoms that may represent upper tract infection. In men, in whom the prevalence of urinary infection is low, persistent or recurrent symptoms referable to the urinary tract or prostate may require investigation to find the site of infection.

NON-INVASIVE METHODS

The use of differential urine culture to detect infections of the urethra and its associated glands is discussed on p. 616.

Infections of the upper urinary tract may be made by the detection of antibody-coated bacteria in the urine (Thomas, Shelokov and Forland 1974). In renal bacteriuria the organisms are coated with antibody, which is detected with fluorescein-labelled anti-IgG, whereas in infections localized to the bladder this coating is not observed. Though this method is of

Table 32.4 Typical results of screening tests for nitrite and leucocyte esterase[a]

	Sensitivity (%)	Specificity (%)	Predictive value Positive (%)	Negative (%)
Leucocyte esterase	83	81	55	91
Nitrite	57	91	59	91
Leucocyte esterase + nitrite	51	85	66	91
Leucocyte esterase or nitrite	93	75	38	98

[a]Means of the results reported by Audurier et al. (1988), Goldstein et al. (1991), Yeni (1991).

Table 32.5 Methods for the localization of urinary tract infection

Non-invasive methods	Invasive methods
Differential culture of urethral and midstream urine	Bladder washout
Antibody-coated bacteria	Pyelography
Serum antibody titration	Micturating cystography
Urinary enzyme assay	Urethrocystography
Renal biopsy	Ureteric catheterization
β_2-Microglobulin assay	Stamey test[a]
Renal concentrating ability	
Circulating Tamm–Horsfall antibody	

[a]See Stamey and Pfau (1963).

theoretical value for distinguishing between renal and bladder bacteriuria (Harding et al. 1978, Stamey 1980b), it is difficult to interpret and it is less accurate in children than in adults. Confusion may also arise from bacteria of vaginal and prostatic origin which may also be coated with antibody.

The production of serum antibodies against the O antigens of gram-negative bacteria, particularly *E. coli*, has been used in the diagnosis of upper urinary tract infection. Patients with acute pyelonephritis or symptomless renal parenchymal infection tend to have raised titres, whereas absent or lower titres are associated with bladder infections. Two techniques have been described for the detection of antibody: indirect haemagglutination detects IgM antibodies (Needell et al. 1955) and direct bacterial agglutination detects mainly IgG antibodies (Percival, Brumfitt and de Louvois 1964). IgG is particularly associated with recurrent and chronic infections. The results may, however, be difficult to read, antigen production is variable, and the antibody is strain-specific. Detection of antibody is limited to the strain isolated from the current infection, but this may not be the actual cause of the renal infection. Preparations of group antigens do not give satisfactory results. In addition, antibody production is poor in children, in the elderly and in symptomless infections. Titres of IgM depend on the phase of the infection and the correlation with the test for antibody-coated bacteria is poor (Hanson et al. 1978).

Urinary β_2-microglobulin and urinary enzymes of renal origin have been used to detect renal damage, but they are of little value (Sandberg et al. 1986). The measurement of serum C-reactive protein is a simple and efficient test to distinguish between upper and lower tract infection. Since concentrations rapidly fall to normal after cure, it can be used as an indicator of successful treatment (Jodal and Hanson 1975). IgG antibodies to Tamm–Horsfall protein may also be useful to discriminate between pyelonephritis and cystitis (Hanson et al. 1978). Renal concentrating ability and osmolality are impaired during renal infection (Ronald, Cutler and Turck 1969), but the causal relationship has not been established and renal function may be normal (Turck 1978). Impairment may also be present without upper tract infection or even bacteriuria.

INVASIVE METHODS

Excretion urography shows anatomical and some physiological abnormalities but does not establish the site of infection. Cystoscopy may be necessary to exclude bladder and urethral abnormalities and micturating cystography may show bladder dysfunction and vesicoureteric reflux. An abnormal excretion urogram with bacteriuria that persists in spite of appropriate antimicrobial chemotherapy requires further investigation. Upper tract infection can be distinguished from lower tract infection by methods in which urine is cultured before and after prolonged bladder washout (Fairley et al. 1971). This will show whether bacteria are present only in the bladder or are in the ureteric urine and derived from the kidney. This method does not allow localization of the infection to an individual kidney, and in the presence of reflux renal bacteriuria is not detectable. Catheterization of individual ureters can be difficult but has the advantage of identifying the infected kidney (Stamey and Pfau 1963). When renal biopsy is performed the tissue removed should be cultured, though the results may be unreliable because of the patchy nature of the infected areas and small size of the sample (Reeves and Brumfitt 1968). A positive culture provides a definitive bacteriological diagnosis.

7 CLINICAL URINARY TRACT INFECTION

7.1 Asymptomatic, covert or symptomless bacteriuria

The observation by Kass (1956), now regarded as classical, showed that some women have significant bacteriuria without symptoms, a state described as 'asymptomatic significant bacteriuria'. The condition has variously been termed symptomless or covert bacteriuria. Since in most women asymptomatic bacteriuria is in reality part of a continuum punctuated by symptomatic episodes (Sussman et al. 1969), **covert bacteriuria** is a better term than asymptomatic bacteriuria. Covert bacteriuria is, however, not limited to women but occurs in males other than healthy adult men. The prevalence of covert bacteriuria at various ages is shown in Table 32.6. In the otherwise healthy normal adult, covert bacteriuria is benign and there is no indication for its treatment (Asscher et al 1969). The suggestion that covert bacteriuria in the elderly is associated with excess mortality (Dontas et al. 1981) has not been confirmed (Nordenstam et al. 1986).

Covert bacteriuria in pregnancy is associated with high incidence of acute urinary tract infection (see section 7.5).

7.2 Acute cystitis

Cystitis is the commonest presentation of urinary tract infection. It is characterized by dysuria, frequency of micturition, suprapubic discomfort and a cloudy urine. In women the incidence of cystitis increases at puberty and continues throughout adult life, whereas in men the condition is uncommon until later life, unless there are underlying conditions. Particularly in younger women, cystitis is associated with sexual activity (Remis and Gurwith 1987) and the use of contraceptive diaphragms (Fihn and Latham 1985). About one-third of women with cystitis experience a recurrence of the infection. Symptoms similar to those of cystitis may be observed in a number of sexually transmitted diseases.

7.3 Urethral syndrome

A striking proportion of women (30–50%) who present with symptoms suggestive of a urinary tract infection do not have significant bacteriuria (Gallagher, Montgomerie and North 1965, O'Grady et al. 1970). Culture of urine obtained by suprapubic aspiration shows that some of these women have cystitis with a low bacterial count, but in the remainder the urine is sterile or contains small numbers of contaminants (Stamm et al. 1981). Such patients are described as having the **urethral syndrome** (abacterial cystitis). The aetiology of the condition continues to be debated, but a single cause for it is unlikely (Tait et al. 1985). In some cases the cause is *Chlamydia trachomatis* (Stamm et al. 1980, 1981) but Gillespie and his colleagues (1989) found no evidence of bacterial or chlamydial infection in urethral syndrome. It has been suggested that fastidious bacteria are responsible (Maskell 1986) and other microbial and non-microbial aetiologies have also been suggested.

Table 32.6 The prevalence of covert bacteriuria[a]

	Age (years)	Prevalence (mean %)
Neonates		
male		2.7
female		<0.4
Schoolboys	5–12	0.03
Schoolgirls	5–12	2
Adult men	16–65	0.5
Adult women	16–65	4

[a]Figures assembled from Lincoln and Winberg (1964), Kass, Savage and Santamarina (1965), Kunin and Paquin (1965).

Despite the controversy about the aetiology and pathogenesis of the urethral syndrome, it appears that most patients benefit from antimicrobial therapy.

A urethral syndrome may also be observed in young men and usually this is due to non-specific urethritis.

7.4 Acute pyelonephritis

The main clinical features of acute pyelonephritis include loin pain, fever and a positive urine culture, but many renal infections are symptomless. The commonest infecting organism is *E. coli* but in the presence of abnormalities of the urinary tract, such as congenital deformities, stone or hydronephrosis, other bacteria, such as *P. mirabilis, Klebsiella* spp. and enterococci may be responsible. *P. aeruginosa* is particularly associated with gross abnormality and obstructive uropathy. Acute pyelonephritis is common in pregnant women with previously untreated covert bacteriuria, most frequently in the second trimester, at delivery or in the postpartum period (Whalley 1967). In patients with diabetes, upper urinary tract infection is common (Forland, Thomas and Shelokov 1977) and severe complications such as necrotizing papillitis may occur.

7.5 Bacteriuria of pregnancy

In the first trimester of pregnancy the prevalence of covert bacteriuria is about 5% (Savage, Hajj and Kass 1967) but by term it may reach about 10%, and up to about one-third of these women develop acute pyelonephritis. The incidence is related particularly to increasing parity and a past history of urinary tract infection (Whalley 1967). Acute pyelonephritis in pregnant women can to a great extent be prevented by the treatment of symptomless bacteriuria with antimicrobial agents (Condie et al. 1968). The effect of bacteriuria on fetal health is the subject of much controversy; prematurity, low birth weight and fetal mortality appear to be increased, but the effect of bacteriuria is probably small. Long-term follow-up of women with pregnancy bacteriuria shows a high incidence of radiological abnormalities and these may affect the response to treatment (Leigh, Grüneberg and Brumfitt 1968). The association between bacteriuria and acute pyelonephritis and other risk factors justifies urinary screening programmes for antenatal bacteriuria. However, since symptomatic infection tends to occur later in pregnancy, such women would not be identified by early screening. The subject has been reviewed by MacLean (1996).

7.6 Infection in diabetes mellitus

Urinary tract infection is up to 3 times more common in diabetic than in non-diabetic women and increases with age; this is not the case in men or school-age diabetics (Vejlsgaard 1966, Mackie and Drury 1996). In adults, levels of glycosuria are not significant but failure to control the blood sugar may be a contributory factor for the development of infection (Rayfield et al. 1982). Diabetics are particularly predisposed to develop acute pyelonephritis and renal papillary necrosis (Eknoyan et al. 1982). Bacterial counts tend to be high in diabetic urine because of increased glucose content (O'Sullivan et al. 1961, Weiser, Asscher and Sussman 1969) and may favour the development of severe urinary complications. Progressive renal damage is more related to the metabolic effects of the diabetes than to superimposed infection (Forland and Thomas 1985). The subject has been reviewed by Mackie and Drury (1996).

7.7   Chronic pyelonephritis

Chronic pyelonephritis is the second most common cause of end-stage renal failure after chronic glomerulonephritis. There is no evidence that urinary tract infection in adults causes progressive renal damage except occasionally in adults with obstructive uropathy. The origin of chronic pyelonephritis is to be found in urinary infections of infancy and early childhood, particularly those associated with vesicoureteric reflux. When adult patients with clinical and subclinical urinary tract infection are followed, progressive kidney damage is not observed. Progressive kidney damage was not observed in a 24 year follow-up of pregnant women with urinary tract abnormalities, including chronic pyelonephritis, in whom bacteriuria could not be eradicated (Leigh, Grüneberg and Brumfitt 1968). Hypertension is often the earliest indication of kidney damage, but the evidence is not persuasive that symptomless bacteriuria or acute lower urinary tract infection are associated with hypertension (Nicolle 1996). Antimicrobial therapy and blood pressure control may prevent progress of the renal damage in chronic pyelonephritis but most patients with chronic pyelonephritis do not have bacteriuria.

7.8   Other upper urinary tract infections

Renal carbuncle due to *S. aureus* is a haematogenous infection that may follow a skin infection, staphylococcal septicaemia or colonization of an intravenous line. The lesion is localized in the renal cortex and urine culture can be negative even in the presence of pyuria. In that case the diagnosis may be made radiologically or by ultrasound, and blood cultures may be positive.

Perinephric abscess does not involve the renal parenchyma, but it may complicate acute pyelonephritis, in which case the causative pathogen derives from the urinary tract.

Pyonephrosis is usually unilateral and results from a bacterial infection that arises in an obstructed ureter. It may follow investigative procedures and be due to secondary infection, often by less common urinary pathogens. The patient may become seriously ill from gram-negative bacteraemia and shock; the diagnosis may be made by culture of blood culture or pus obtained from the affected kidney. Urine culture is positive only if there is drainage into the bladder.

The management of all these conditions is predominantly surgical, with appropriate antimicrobial chemotherapy for which bacteriological data are essential.

7.9   Infections associated with bladder dysfunction

Severe bladder dysfunction often leads to chronic and recurrent urinary tract infection. The mechanisms have been noted above (see section 3.1, p. 602). Neurological disorders, including spinal cord injury, multiple sclerosis or cerebrovascular accidents, and malignant disease of the bladder and prostate, as well as bladder disturbances after prostatectomy and other surgical procedures, may be responsible. They often necessitate intermittent or permanent urethral catheterization. Acute pyelonephritis that results from ascending infection is rare, but many patients have symptomless infection which probably indicates bladder colonization. The organisms responsible are often hospital-associated and may show multiple antimicrobial resistance. It may be difficult to obtain uncontaminated urine specimens for examination and mixed cultures are common. *P. aeruginosa* is a frequent pathogen in catheterized patients (see p. 604). Bacteriuria should always be confirmed in such patients but treatment should be given only if there are constitutional symptoms or difficulties in maintaining free drainage. Systemic antimicrobial therapy is ineffective in the presence of a catheter, and bladder washouts with antiseptic or antimicrobial agents may be the best method of treatment.

8   PATHOGENESIS

Uropathogens may enter the urinary tract spontaneously by the ascending route and such organisms are derived from the host faecal flora. In women the periurethral area is colonized first, followed by the urethra and finally the bladder. Alternatively, exogenous bacteria may be introduced during catheterization or surgical instrumentation and in this case infection may be due to a wider range of organisms. Once within the urinary tract the organisms may ascend from the bladder to infect the kidney.

In view of the concordance between the serotypes of *E. coli* present in the faeces and those that cause urinary tract infection (Grüneberg 1969) it was at one time believed that their pathogenicity is incidental ('**prevalence theory**'). It has become clear, however, that to overcome the natural defence mechanisms of the urinary tract, uropathogenic strains of *E. coli* possess a number potent specific virulence factors that are responsible in the first place for colonization and subsequently for tissue damage ('**special pathogenicity theory**').

8.1   Colonization

In healthy adult women the introitus and the periurethral area are colonized by *S. epidermidis*, lactobacilli, corynebacteria and streptococci. Before puberty and after the menopause *Bacteroides* spp. predominate (Bollgren et al. 1979, Marrie, Swantee and Hartlen 1980), particularly in young girls susceptible to urinary tract infection (Bollgren et al. 1981). Periurethral colonization by enterobacteria is unusual except in the presence of urinary tract infection, except in women susceptible to recurrent urinary tract infection (Cox et al. 1968, Bailey et al. 1973). In males the preputial mucosa tend to become colonized with bacteria (Fussell et al. 1988), and there is evidence that in the first year of life infection is related to the prepuce and that circumcision reduces susceptibility (Herzog 1989, Winberg et al. 1989).

Much evidence has accumulated to show that the adherence of *E. coli* to uroepithelium is crucial to counteract the natural clearance of the urinary tract and to allow its colonization (Reid and Sobel 1987). These adherence properties were originally recognized in terms of the haemagglutination of the erythrocytes of various animal species and they correlate with the presence of fimbriae on the bacterial surface (Duguid et al. 1955). Apart from erythrocytes, fimbriae adhere to many other cell types, which suggests that they play an important role in the colonization of epithelia (Ofek and Doyle 1994).

Two classes of fimbriae can be recognized on the surface of *E. coli* and these carry ligands (**adhesins**) that bind to receptors present on cells. Haemagglutination by common or type 1 fimbriae, termed mannose-sensitive (MS), is inhibited by D-mannose and various mannosides. Such fimbriae are also widely distributed amongst gram-negative bacilli and they bind to mannose-containing receptors (Sharon and Ofek 1986). Haemagglutination by the second, heterogeneous, class of fimbriae, which are termed mannose-resistant (MR), is not inhibited by D-mannose or mannosides, and these bind to a variety of receptors.

MANNOSE-RESISTANT FIMBRIAE

In clinical urinary tract infection (Ofek, Mosek and Sharon 1981, Pere et al. 1987) and in experimental animal models (van den Bosch et al. 1980) the presence of MR fimbriae on *E. coli* correlates with virulence. A number of different MR fimbriae can be distinguished on the basis of the specific receptors to which they bind. The best studied of these are P fimbriae that bind to neutral globoseries glycolipids, including globotetraosylceramide and trihexosylceramide, which are antigens of the P blood group system (Leffler and Svanborg-Edén 1980). The minimal receptor to which these fimbriae bind is α-D-Gal-(1→4)-β-D-Gal (Gal-Gal) (Källenius et al. 1981a).

P fimbriae are expressed in vivo by *E. coli* in urinary tract infections (Kiselius et al. 1989) but strains that can express P fimbriae are uncommon in normal faeces. Occasionally, however, the P-fimbriated strain responsible for a urinary infection can be detected in the patient's faeces (Källenius et al. 1981b). P receptors are widely distributed in the kidney and bladder (Johnson 1997). Most strains of *E. coli* isolated from children with acute pyelonephritis are P-fimbriate (Väisänen et al. 1981) and the same is true for adults.

There is, however, a lower prevalence of P-fimbriate *E. coli* in lower urinary tract infections.

A number of MR fimbriae that do not recognize the Gal-Gal receptor are known as X adhesins or non-P MR adhesins (Johnson 1997). Thus, S fimbriae bind to sialyl glycosides (Hanisch, Hacker and Schroten 1993) and G fimbriae bind to *N*-acetylglucosamine (Väisänen-Rhen, Korhonen and Finne 1983). Binding sites for S fimbriae are widely distributed in the urinary tract but S-fimbriate *E. coli* are probably more important in neonatal meningitis than in urinary tract infection.

A number of MR adhesins are not associated with fimbriae and are termed non-fimbrial adhesins (NFA). Of these NFA-3 binds to the N blood group antigen (glycophorin A^{NN}) and NFA-4 binds to the M blood group antigen (glycophorin A^{MM}). These adhesins are uncommon and their significance in the pathogenesis of urinary infections is unknown.

TYPE 1 FIMBRIAE

The majority of strains of *E. coli* and most other Enterobactriaceae possess type 1 fimbriae (Duguid and Old 1980). Since adhesion by these fimbriae is inhibited by D-mannose and mannosides, it is thought that mannose forms part of the receptors to which they attach. Such receptors are present on most epithelia and may play a part in their colonization. Type 1 fimbriae also attach to uromucoid (Tamm–Horsfall glycoprotein), which is produced by the renal tubules and is excreted in the urine. Receptors for type 1 fimbriae are less widely distributed in the urinary tract than are P receptors. Type 1 fimbriae attach to unidentified receptors on polymorphonuclear leucocytes. This may lead to non-opsonic phagocytosis, depending on the hydrophobicity of the organism, and cell activation with the release granule contents, generation of a respiratory burst and the release of cytokines (Steadman and Topley 1997).

ADHERENCE AND THE GENESIS OF URINARY TRACT INFECTION

Strains of *E. coli* isolated from patients with urinary infections produce type 1 fimbriae in vivo (Kiselius et al. 1989). Their importance in the pathogenesis of the infection is, however, difficult to determine because of their wide distribution including on non-pathogenic strains. They attach poorly to renal tissue (Hagberg et al. 1986) and in a mouse experimental model infected with a mixture of type 1 fimbriate and their homologous non-fimbriate variants, the former are present mainly in the bladder (Hagberg et al. 1983a, 1983b). It may be, therefore, that these fimbriae are significant in periurethral, urethral and possibly bladder colonization. The presence of Tamm–Horsfall glycoprotein in the human bladder makes it difficult to be certain whether attachment of type 1 fimbriae is truely to the epithelium or merely to the glycoprotein attached to it. Evidence against the significance of these fimbriae in the pathogenesis of urinary tract infection comes from the ineffectiveness of type 1 fimbrial vaccines (O'Hanley 1990).

Overwhelming evidence confirms the importance of MR fimbriae, particularly P fimbriae, in urinary tract infection. They are produced in vivo during infections (Kiselius et al. 1989) and they are present on more than 80% of *E. coli* isolated from children with acute pyelonephritis but only on about 10% of faecal strains (Väisänen et al. 1981); in adults with pyelonephritis the prevalence of P fimbriae is lower (O'Hanley et al. 1985b). In pregnancy, infection with MR-fimbriate *E. coli* is significantly correlated with a history of urinary tract infection and those with such a history have a 7-fold greater chance that their current infection is due to an MR-fimbriate strain (Parry et al. 1983).

In the lower urinary tract infections of adults and children the significance of P fimbriae is uncertain. Similarly, the significance of X adhesins in all urinary tact infection has yet to be determined but they are more common in adult lower urinary tract infection.

Ørskov, Ferencz and Ørskov (1980) have suggested that in the colon, where mucus is plentiful, type 1 fimbriae actively maintain colonization of *E. coli* including potentially uropathogenic strains, whereas in the urinary tract mucus plays a dual role. Organisms that produce only type 1 fimbriae are flushed out with the mucus, whereas those that produce P and other MR adhesins will colonize the epithelium. The on–off switches ('**phase variation**') that control fimbrial expression may be part of this process and it is conceivable that *E. coli* express fimbriae and other virulence factors in response to the environments they encounter.

As in the case of other pathogenic types of *E. coli*, uropathogenic strains of *E. coli* may be derived from clones (Achtman and Pluschke 1986). It is known that in uropathogenic *E. coli* groups of virulence factors are located close together in so-called 'pathogenicity-associated islands' in which the genes are coordinately controlled.

8.2   Survival and invasion

Once colonization has been established, a separate range of virulence factors determine whether the organisms can invade the host and survive. Most of the evidence for the function of these factors is circumstantial but it is persuasive, particularly because it appears that they act additively (Johnson 1997).

Somatic antigens and serum sensitivity

Uropathogenic strains of *E. coli* express group II K antigens rather than the group I antigens of nonpathogenic strains (Jann and Jann 1983) and a high proportion of urinary strains express K antigens. These antigens are antiphagocytic and are in part responsible for serum resistance because of their anticomplementary activity (Ørskov and Ørskov 1985).

A restricted range of O serogroups of *E. coli*, usually concordant with those in the faeces of patients, is responsible for urinary tract infections. The concordance is less in individuals with covert bacteriuria (Roberts et al. 1975), which provides indirect evidence that O antigens are virulence factors. In part this may

be due to changes in the faecal serogroup, but rough strains with shorter polysaccharide side chains are more common in covert bacteriuria than in symptomatic infection (Hanson et al. 1975). It may be that during prolonged colonization *E. coli* strains with reduced virulence are selected, possibly as the result of selective pressures due to urinary antibodies. Such serological changes may also occur in the course of chronic infections (Bettelheim and Taylor 1969). Conversely, when patients become infected with a new serotype of *E. coli*, after antimicrobial therapy, symptomatic infection often follows (Asscher et al. 1969). O antigenic lipopolysaccharides are powerful virulence factors (Hull 1997) directly involved in the pathogenesis of urinary tract infection. They induce the shedding of uroepithelial cells (Aronson et al. 1988) and are probably responsible for interference with ureteral motility (Teague and Boyarsky 1968, Thuselius and Araj 1987). Lipopolysaccharides also cause renal damage by the activation of granulocytes (Steadman and Topley 1997).

Classical and alternative pathway complement-dependent bacteriolysis are important antibacterial defence mechanisms (Taylor 1985; see also Chapter 4). The susceptibility of organisms depends on their surface characteristics and particularly their O antigens. Strains of *E. coli* from cases of covert bacteriuria are more serum-sensitive than those from acute urinary tract infections and, similarly, serum resistance appears to be an important factor in invasive infections such as pyelopnephritis (Lomberg et al. 1984) and in urinary tract-derived septicaemia (McCabe et al. 1978).

Haemolysin production

Iron is an essential bacterial nutrient that in the human host is tightly bound to protein carriers, such as transferrin. Normal urine contains sufficient iron, probably derived from the breakdown of various cells, to allow bacterial growth but during tissue-invasive processes iron availability becomes limiting and under these conditions 2 mechanisms for iron scavenging are available. Haemolysin releases haemoglobin from erythrocytes and bacterial siderophores compete for iron with host iron-binding proteins. When bound by siderophore, the iron is taken up by special bacterial surface receptors and can be utilized by the pathogen.

The association between haemolysin production and uropathogenicity has long been recognized. A high proportion of *E. coli* strains isolated from urinary tract infections produce haemolysin (Minshew et al. 1978) and such strains are more virulent in animals than non-haemolytic strains (van den Bosch, Emödy and Kétyi 1982). Haemolysin production is also related to virulence in experimental haematogenous pyelonephritis (van den Bosch, de Graaff and MacLaren 1979). For a review of *E. coli* haemolysins see Ludwig and Goebel (1997).

Enterobacteria secrete enterochelin (enterobactin) during growth under conditions of iron limitation; iron enterochelin has a formation constant (10^{52}) sufficiently high to abstract iron in vivo and it is known to be produced during *E. coli* infections (Griffiths and Humphreys 1980). Under the control of the chromosome or the plasmid pCoIV, many strains of *E. coli* associated with urinary tract infections produce aerobactin, another siderophore. Some 75% of uropathogens associated with septicaemia produce aerobactin (Montgomerie et al. 1984). For details of the part iron scavenging plays in infections see Griffiths (1985, 1997).

UREASE

A number of uropathogens, particularly *P. mirabilis* and *P. vulgaris*, produce a urease that is active within the urinary tract. By raising the urine pH it leads to the precipitation of phosphates, particularly magnesium ammonium phosphate ($MgNH_4PO_4.6H_2O$, struvite) which tends to aggregate and form 'staghorn' calculi within the renal pelvis. The urease inhibitor acetohydroxamic acid prevents invasion of the kidney by *Proteus* and confirms the function of urease as a virulence factor (Musher et al. 1975). Acetohydroxamic acid is too toxic for clinical use but the urease inhibitor hydroxyurea has been shown clinically to reduce stone growth (Smith 1984) and may have a role to play in conjunction with lithotripsy in the management of some renal calculi. Some strains of *Klebsiella* also produce a urease.

Urease is also a significant virulence factor in bladder invasion by *S. saprophyticus* (Gatermann, John and Marre 1989).

9 SUSCEPTIBILITY FACTORS

A number of factors render individuals susceptible to urinary tract infection (Table 32.7) but frequently in individual patients none can be identified. Often, for unknown reasons, when such factors are present, infection does not occur. The explanations probably lie in the balance between host resistance and bacterial virulence.

Table 32.7 Susceptibility factors for urinary tract infection

Innate
Secretor status
Anatomical
Congenital abnormalities
Acquired structural defects
Functional
Outflow obstruction
Residual urine
Vesicoureteric reflux
Pregnancy
Pathological
Diabetes mellitus
Calculi
Surgery
Instrumentation

9.1 Urinary catheterization

The risks of catheterization have long been recognized (Beeson 1958) and render it unjustifiable to collect urine for examination in this way. The incidence of infection associated with a single urethral catheterization is 1–5% (Turck, Goffe and Petersdorf 1962, Walter and Vejlsgaard 1978). As the duration of catheterization increases so does the risk of infection; over 90% of closed drainage systems (Kass 1956) and some 50% of closed systems in place for 4–7 days become infected (Kunin and McCormack 1966). Bacteria that cause catheter-associated infection adhere to catheter materials and produce a biofilm that consists of bacteria embedded in an extracellular matrix (Roberts, Kaack and Fussell 1993). These biofilm-embedded bacteria are resistant to phagocytosis and to antibiotics that may appear to be effective by laboratory testing (Zimmerli, Lew and Waldvogel 1984).

When a catheter is removed after a short period of catheterization, bacteriuria can be expected to resolve very quickly but this becomes less likely the longer the catheter has been in place. Attempts to treat catheter-associated bacteriuria with antimicrobial agents is unlikely to succeed and bears the risk of selection of resistant organisms.

Special risk groups, such as pregnant women (Brumfitt, Davies and Rosser 1961), elderly or debilitated patients and diabetics, have a risk of infection of about 20% for each catheterization. For each day that the catheter is retained the risk of developing bacteriuria is 3–10%. More than 20% of nosocomial infections are those of the urinary tract and about 75% of these follow the use of instruments in the urinary tract (Turck and Stamm 1981).

Most infections that follow catheterization are not associated with complications but a small proportion of patients (1–2%) develop bacteraemia (McGowan, Barnes and Finland 1975) and the frequency of hospital-acquired bacteraemia in catheterized patients is said to be 3 times greater than in non-catheterized patients (Jepsen et al. 1982). Bacteraemia occurs most frequently when a catheter is changed or removed and may be followed by serious metastatic infection such as osteomyelitis. Catheterized patients should be regularly monitored for bacteriuria with careful specimen collection to avoid contamination. Catheter-induced urinary tract infections may be due to unusual pathogens and mixed cultures are not uncommon. Catheter insertion and removal must be carried out with full aseptic technique.

Advances in the technique of catheterization have not significantly reduced the incidence of catheter-induced bacteriuria. Catheterization should be carried out only when it is absolutely necessary and catheters should be removed at the earliest opportunity.

For a fuller account of the prevention of infection in catheterized patients, see Chapter 13.

10 DEFENCE AND IMMUNITY

Little is known about the non-specific and specific mechanisms that protect the urinary tract. Although the system is open to the environment and the urine creates a 'fluid bridge', uropathogens appear, nevertheless, to have highly effective virulence factors, which suggests that there is a correspondingly effective system of defences.

The mucosal defence mechanisms consist of secreted substances that inhibit the adhesion of bacteria or kill them (Vivaldi et al. 1965). The bladder epithelium is covered by a hydrophilic layer of sulphated polysaccharides (glycosaminoglycan) that may act as a barrier to adhesion. The role of mucosal defence mechanisms is, however, unclear; they may be significant in eliminating small numbers of bacteria, even though phagocytosis is impaired in urine (Chernew and Braude 1962), but their effect on established infection is probably small. Since neither phagocytosis nor antibody can account for the antibacterial action of the bladder, it has been suggested that mucosal defence is due to locally produced bactericidal organics (Norden, Green and Kass 1968).

Urine contains IgG and secretory IgA (sIgA) (Hanson et al. 1970) and their concentration may be increased in urinary tract infection (Jodal et al. 1970). The information about IgM is conflicting (Kaufman, Katz and McIntosh 1970, Uehling and Stiehm 1971) but it probably arises from proteinuria and leakage of inflammatory exudate. The sIgA present in normal urine is derived mainly from the urethra (Burdon 1971) and may be a barrier to the ascent of bacteria into the bladder. The concentration of sIgA but not that of IgG increases with age and during infection (Kaufman, Katz and McIntosh 1970). The maturation of IgA production which occurs in later childhood may in part account for spontaneous recovery from recurrent urinary tract infections (Uehling and Stiehm 1971, Burdon 1975).

In animal experimental models of infection antibodies are produced locally in renal tissue and may have a protective role. In ascending infections infiltration with T cells takes place in the kidney (Hjelm 1984) and at a later stage suppressor T cells appear and may play a part in the persistence of bacteria in the kidney (Miller, Marshall and Nelson 1983).

An immune response occurs in adults and children with renal infection (Needell et al. 1955, Winberg et al. 1963, Percival, Brumfitt and de Louvois 1964), and strain-specific antibodies directed against *E. coli* O, K and fimbrial antigens can be demonstrated in the circulation. At first these are IgM but in long-standing or recurrent infections IgG antibodies appear. The part these antibodies play in resistance and recovery is not clear.

11 EPIDEMIOLOGY OF URINARY INFECTIONS

The prevalence of covert bacteriuria varies between the sexes and with age (see Table 32.6). It increases with age and parity (Kass, Savage and Santamarina 1965), and spontaneous remissions and new acquisitions of infection are common (Asscher et al. 1973a). The development of certain pathological conditions also favours urinary tract infection (Kunin 1987).

In the first months of life bacteriuria affects between 1% and 2% of babies (Lincoln and Winberg 1964, Wettergren, Jodal and Jonasson 1985) and is significantly more common in boys than girls (Stansfeld 1966, Abbott 1972). This may be related to congenital or functional abnormalities of the urinary tract. Later in infancy and in preschool children the prevalence of bacteriuria is higher in girls than boys. In the school years it occurs in 1–3% of girls but in less than 0.1% of boys (Kunin, Deutscher and Paquin 1964, Savage et al. 1969, Asscher et al. 1973b). Most of the affected children have symptomless bacteriuria that can be detected only by screening. Further rises in the prevalence in schoolgirls and adult women to about 5% are associated with sexual activity and pregnancy. The prevalence in nuns and unmarried women is lower than in married women (Kunin and McCormack 1968).

In schoolboys the prevalence of bacteriuria is very low (0.03%, Kunin, Zacha and Paquin 1962), and symptomatic episodes are rare. The prevalence in young adult males is less than 1% but in middle-aged and elderly men it rises to about 15% as prostatic hypertrophy becomes common. At all ages the prevalence of symptomless bacteriuria considerably exceeds that of symptomatic infection, but the difference is less apparent in elderly patients and those infected in hospital than in young adults in the general population.

The frequency of significant bacteriuria is increased in various disease states. In adult diabetics the frequency is about 20% but there is no difference between that in diabetic and non-diabetic schoolchildren. Hypertension, congenital renal disease, renal calculi, hydronephrosis and urethral catheterization are all associated with increased rates of bacteriuria (Jackson et al. 1962). Hospital-acquired urinary tract infections account for a significant proportion (20–40%) of all infections acquired in hospital (Jepsen 1987); most follow some form of instrumentation to the urinary tract (Garibaldi et al. 1974).

12 PREVENTION

12.1 Prophylaxis

Some women tend to suffer recurrences of urinary tract infection, particularly after sexual intercourse, and these can often be prevented by the non-specific measures of encouraging an ample intake of fluids and personal hygiene. The use of contraceptive diaphragms, but not other devices, is also associated with an increased risk of infection. When non-specific measures fail, low dose antimicrobial prophylaxis may be effective. This consists of nitofurantoin (50 mg), trimethoprim (100 mg), co-trimoxazole (240 mg) or norfloxacin (200 mg) last thing at night after the bladder has been emptied (Ohkoshi and Naber 1992, Bailey 1994). Prophylaxis can be limited to alternate nights or only after intercourse.

Pregnant women with covert bacteriuria are at substantial risk of developing acute pyelonephritis (Little 1965) and this can be prevented in the majority with suitable antimicrobial chemotherapy (see section 7.5, p. 609).

12.2 Competitive exclusion

Lactobacilli and their cell wall fragments inhibit the adherence of uropathogens to uroepithelial cells in vitro, possibly by their own ability to adhere (Chan et al. 1985). Some strains produce hydrogen peroxide that may be inhibitory. The introduction of *Lactobacillus casei* into the bladder of rats and swabbing of the introitus with the organism prevents urinary tract infection (Reid et al. 1985). It has been suggested that introduction of lactobacilli into the vagina may prevent urinary tract infection in women but adequate trials have yet to be carried out.

12.3 Vaccines

The high incidence of urinary tract infections and the expense they incur on health services have led to the search for effective vaccines but early attempts to develop these were confounded by the unnatural animal models used for vaccine evaluation. Advancing knowledge of the virulence characteristics of uropathogenic *E. coli* and the receptors present on human and animal uroepithelia have made it possible to define the necessary characteristics of experimental animal models suitable for vaccine evaluation. BALB/c mice appear to be similar to humans in the kinds and distribution of receptors on their uroepithelium and, when immunized with a vaccine of purified P fimbriae, they are protected against renal infection with uropathogenic *E. coli* (O'Hanley et al. 1985a). Though P fimbriae are heterogeneous, they possess common antigens that may turn out to be the basis for useful vaccines (O'Hanley 1990). Serious attempts to design vaccines against urinary tract infections appear to have been made only with *E. coli*.

13 TREATMENT

Incidentally discovered covert bacteriuria in adults should not be treated except in pregnancy. Diabetics and those about to have surgery or other instrumentation of the urinary tract should be treated because bacteriuria is a major risk factor for serious complications. Since in young children the symptoms of urinary tract infection tend to be non-specific, bacteriuria may be significant and its cause should be investigated.

Antimicrobial therapy plays a key role in the treatment of symptomatic urinary tract infection. In choosing an antimicrobial agent, its pharmacokinetic properties must be considered as well as the susceptibility of the causative organism. Most compounds active against urinary pathogens are excreted in the urine at high concentrations, but their concentration in the substance of the kidney is related to that in the blood rather than that in the urine. Treatment should be adjusted to the needs of the individual patient, but 2 major principles should be followed:

1 the dose of an antimicrobial agent should produce therapeutic concentrations at the site of infection and

2 the course of treatment should not be significantly longer than is necessary to sterilize the urine.

This aproach limits the possible unwanted effects of treatment and reduces the risk of bacterial resistance, superinfection and drug toxicity.

For simple acute community-acquired infections, a short treatment course of not more than 3 days is usually sufficient to effect a cure. Symptoms usually resolve after the first few doses and longer courses of treatment offer no advantages. Single dose therapy is often effective in uncomplicated urinary tract infection but even with a high dose the cure rates are less than with conventional treatment regimens. If single dose treatment is chosen it should be taken last thing at night to maintain a high overnight concentration of antimicrobial agent in the bladder.

Recurrent infection in the absence of an underlying abnormality should be treated according to the probable precipitating cause. In women, recurrence may be associated with sexual intercourse and prophylaxis may be appropriate (see section 12.1, p. 614). In men with recurrent infection due to prostatic dysfunction in whom surgical operation is undesirable or not possible, a single daily dose may prevent recurrence. A similar regimen may be used in women with stress incontinence, pelvic-floor weakness and disturbance of bladder emptying, or when persistence of the infection may lead to progressive renal damage. In long-term therapy, the dose should be the minimum to maintain sterility of the urine and prevent side effects; regular monitoring of the urine is necessary.

Complicated urinary tract infections are often difficult to treat and the pathogens may show a wide spectrum of antimicrobial resistance. A prolonged course of therapy is often necessary and high doses should be given when there is renal involvement.

Many different antimicrobial agents are available for the treatment of urinary tract infection. Their usefulness is limited only by resistance in the urinary pathogens and unwanted effects in the patient. Oral agents such as trimethoprim, co-trimoxazole, sulphonamides, ampicillin and amoxycillin are widely used and resistance to them remains uncommon in the community. Nitrofurantoin, nalidixic acid and mandelamine are also valuable for long-term suppressive therapy, but their concentration in renal tissue is low. In hospitals, an increasing percentage of urinary pathogens are resistant to β-lactam drugs. The organisms responsible for hospital-acquired urinary tract infection are often resistant to a variety of antimicrobial agents, and systemic treatment with an aminoglycoside or one of the newer penicillins or cephalosporins may be necessary. The quinolones provide an effective means of oral therapy for infections caused by multi-resistant bacteria.

Excellent accounts of the management of urinary tract infection are given by Bailey (1996) for women and by Riden and Schaeffer (1996) for men.

14 OTHER URINARY TRACT INFECTIONS

The prevalence of tuberculosis of the urinary tract and kidney has in recent years declined in Britain but it may represent about one-third of non-pulmonary tuberculosis (Kennedy 1989). The availability of effective treatment justifies efforts to establish an early diagnosis. This is based on the presence of persistent sterile pyuria and culture of tubercle bacilli often in small numbers. Detection of acid-fast bacilli by microscopy may be misleading because saprophytic mycobacteria such as *Mycobacterium smegmatis* may be present in normal urine.

Many viruses, including human immunodeficiency virus (HIV) (Volume 1, Chapter 38), Hantaan virus (Volume 1, Chapter 30), hepatitis B virus (Volume 1, Chapter 36) and cytomegalovirus (Volume 1, Chapter 19), may play a role in renal disease. Virus lesions in the genital tract, such as those of herpes, may give rise to urinary tract symptoms but there is no evidence that viruses are significant causes of ordinary urinary tract infection.

Fungal infections of the kidney may mimic renal tuberculosis and may be important in immunosuppressed patients. Bladder colonization with *Candida albicans* may be associated with urinary catheters (see also Volume 4, Chapter 23). Candidiasis of the genital tract is a common cause of the contamination of poorly collected specimens of urine.

Parasitic infections of the urinary tract, such as schistosomiasis (Volume 5, Chapter 25), trypanosomiasis (see Volume 5, Chapters 14 and 15), filariasis (Volume 5, Chapter 32) and hydatid disease (Volume 5, Chapter 28) and may cause various types of pathological lesion in the urinary tract.

15 URETHRITIS

The commonest types of urethritis in men are sexually transmitted diseases, gonococcal and non-gonococcal (NGU), associated with inflammation and urethral discharge (see Chapters 33 and 54). Urethritis may rarely also be associated with bacterial prostatitis (see section 16). In such cases urinary pathogens will be present in urethral urine and the same organism will be present in the urine obtained after prostatic massage. In women, comparison of urethral and midstream specimens of urine occasionally reveals urinary pathogens or fastidious organisms in low counts and confined to the urethra. The exact site of infection in such patients is not clear but it may be in the paraurethral glands. Commonly the urethra in cath-

eterized patients becomes colonized with gram-negative bacilli; men may also acquire these organisms through sexual intercourse (Stamey 1980a).

16 BACTERIAL PROSTATITIS

The prostatic secretions of humans and dogs have antibacterial activity (Stamey et al. 1968). The antibacterial factor is associated with the presence of zinc (Fair, Couch and Wehner 1976) and prostatic fluid zinc levels are reduced in men with chronic bacterial prostatitis. However, little is known of the pathogenesis of prostatic infections.

Bacterial prostatitis may be acute or chronic and is the most common urinary tract infection of men. It may be complicated by abscess formation. In acute prostatitis the distribution of causative organisms is broadly similar to that of other urinary tract infections, with *E. coli* and other Enterobacteriaceae the most common pathogens. Mixed infections may occur but the significance of gram-positive organisms is doubtful.

In older men prostatitis is commonly related to outflow obstruction due to prostatic hypertrophy or urinary instrumentation but in younger men there may be no such predisposing cause. The bacteria responsible for prostatitis originate from the urethra or the urinary tract and there is evidence that intraprostatic reflux of urine can occur (Kirby et al. 1982).

In young men, prostatic infection causes frequency, dysuria and perineal or testicular pain; in acute cases there may be more general symptoms, including high fever. A urethral discharge is not usually present and on examination the prostate may be enlarged, boggy and painful. Massage of the enlarged prostate usually yields copious volumes of fluid.

The differential diagnosis of bacterial from nonbacterial prostatitis may be made by the quantitative bacteriological study of separate urine and prostatic secretions (Meares and Stamey 1968) in the following sequence. The first 10 ml of voided bladder urine (VB1) are collected followed, after about 200 ml, by a midstream specimen (VB2). Then prostatic massage is carried out to collect the expressed prostatic secretions (EPS) and immediately a further 10 ml of urine (VB3) are collected. Bacterial growth limited to EPS and VB3 is diagnostic of bacterial prostatitis, whereas a 10-fold higher count in EPS and VB3 as compared with VB1 is suggestive of such infection. The method has a diagnostic yield of up to 70% but it may be confounded by previous antimicrobial therapy. In addition to the common urinary pathogens, anaerobes, fastidious bacteria, *Chlamydia* and *Ureaplasma* should be sought.

Chronic prostatitis is uncommon and runs a course characterized by intermittent bacteriuria. The diagnosis can reliably be made only by the quantitative bacteriological method described above. In addition to the usual pathogens, *E. faecalis* and *Pseudomonas* spp. may be found, often in relatively small numbers. Gram-positive organisms are less often found and only rarely cause the characteristic intermittent bacteriuria. The possible part in chronic prostatitis played by *Chlamydia* and *Ureaplasma* remains uncertain.

Non-bacterial (abacterial) prostatitis is a more common syndrome than bacterial prostatitis. A history of urinary tract infection is uncommon and its aetiology remains the subject of controversy but it has been suggested that some cases may be due to *Chlamydia* or *Ureaplasma*. *U. urealyticum* has been isolated from the prostatic secretions of these patients and they responded to treatment with tetracycline (Brunner, Weidner and Schiefer 1983). Other observations cast doubt on the possible role of *Chlamydia* and *Ureaplasma* (Mardh and Collen 1975, Mardh et al. 1978, Berger et al. 1989).

The treatment of prostatitis is difficult because many antimicrobial agents poorly penetrate the gland and persistence of bacteria in the prostate may be a cause of recurrent infection. The most important factors that determine penetration are ionization in the plasma and lipid solubility (Winningham et al. 1968, Meares 1982). To pass into the prostate, agents must be non-ionized and lipid-soluble but not protein-bound; fluoroquinolones have these characteristics. Thus, ciprofloxacin reaches concentrations in the prostate higher than those in the plasma (Hoogkamp-Korstanje, van Oort and Schipper 1984) and high cure rates of chronic bacterial prostatitis have been achieved with this drug (Childs 1990).

REFERENCES

Abbott GD, 1972, Neonatal bacteriuria: a prospective study in 1,460 infants, *Br Med J*, **1**: 267–9.

Abbott GD, 1978, Neonatal bacteriuria – the value of bladder puncture in resolving problems of interpretation arising from voided urine specimens, *Aust Paediatr J*, **14**: 83–6.

Achtman M, Pluschke G, 1986, Clonal analysis of descent and virulence among selected *Escherichia coli*, *Annu Rev Microbiol*, **40**: 185–210.

Anderson HJ, Lincoln K et al., 1965, Studies of urinary tract infections in infancy and childhood. V. A comparison of the coli antibody titer in pyelonephritis measured by means of homologous urinary and fecal *E. coli* antigens, *J Pediatr*, **67**: 1073–9.

Aronson M, Medalia O et al., 1988, Endotoxin-induced shedding of viable uroepithelial cells is an antimicrobial defense system, *Infect Immun*, **56**: 1615–17.

Asscher AW, 1980, *The Challenge of Urinary Tract Infections*, Academic Press, London.

Asscher AW, Sussman M, Weiser R, 1968, Bacterial growth in human urine, *Urinary Tract Infections*, eds O'Grady F, Brumfitt W, Oxford University Press, London, 3–13.

Asscher AW, Sussman M et al., 1966, Urine as a medium for bacterial growth, *Lancet*, **2**: 1037–41.

Asscher AW, Sussman M et al., 1969, Asymptomatic significant bacteriuria in the non-pregnant woman. II. Response to treatment and follow-up, *Br Med J*, **1**: 804–6.

Asscher AW, Chick S et al., 1973a, Natural history of asymptomatic bacteriuria (ASB) in non-pregnant women, *Urinary Tract Infections*, eds Brumfitt W, Asscher AW, Oxford University Press, London, 51–60.

Asscher AW, McLachlan MSF et al., 1973b, Screening for asymptomatic urinary tract infection in schoolgirls, *Lancet*, **2**: 13–14.

Audurier A, Burdin JC et al., 1988, Evaluation d'un test de dépistage de l'infection urinaire, *Pathol Biol*, **36**: 921–4.

Bailey RR, 1994, Management of uncomplicated urinary tract infections, *Int J Antimicrob Agents*, **4**: 95–100.

Bailey RR, 1996, Management of uncomplicated urinary tract infection in women, *Infections of the Kidney and Urinary Tract*, ed. Cattell WR, Oxford University Press, Oxford, 129–57.

Bailey RR, Little PJ, 1969, Suprapubic bladder aspiration in diagnosis of urinary tract infection, *Br Med J*, **1**: 293–4.

Bailey RR, Gower PE et al., 1973, Urinary tract infection in non-pregnant women, *Lancet*, **2**: 275–7.

Beeson PB, 1958, The case against the catheter, *Am J Med*, **24**: 1–36.

Berger RE, Krieger JN et al., 1989, Case-control study of men with suspected chronic idiopathic prostatitis, *J Urol*, **141**: 328–31.

Bettelheim K, Taylor J, 1969, A study of *Escherichia coli* isolated from chronic urinary tract infections, *J Med Microbiol*, **2**: 225–36.

Bollgren I, Winberg J, 1976, The periurethral aerobic flora in girls highly susceptible to urinary infections, *Acta Paediatr Scand*, **65**: 81–7.

Bollgren I, Källenius G et al., 1979, Periurethral anaerobic flora of healthy young girls, *J Clin Microbiol*, **10**: 419–23.

Bollgren I, Nord CE et al., 1981, Periurethral flora of girls highly susceptible to urinary tract infections, *J Urol*, **125**: 715–20.

van den Bosch JF, Emödy L, Kétyi I, 1982, Virulence of haemolytic strains of *Escherichia coli* in various models, *FEMS Microbiol Lett*, **13**: 427–30.

van den Bosch JF, de Graaff J, MacLaren DM, 1979, Virulence of *Escherichia coli* in experimental haematogenous pyelonephritis in mice, *Infect Immun*, **25**: 68–74.

van den Bosch JF, Verboom-Sohmer U et al., 1980, Mannose-sensitive and mannose-resistant adherence to human uroepithelial cells and urinary virulence of *Escherichia coli*, *Infect Immun*, **29**: 226–33.

Bowie WR, Pollock HM et al., 1977, Bacteriology of the urethra in normal men and men with nongonococcal urethritis, *J Clin Microbiol*, **6**: 482–8.

Browne EG, 1962, *Arabian Medicine*, Cambridge University Press, Cambridge.

Brumfitt W, 1965, Urinary white cells and their value, *J Clin Pathol*, **18**: 550–5.

Brumfitt W, Davies BI, Rosser E ap I, 1961, Urethral catheter as a cause of urinary infection in pregnancy and puerperium, *Lancet*, **2**: 1059–62.

Brumfitt W, Gargan RA, Hamilton-Miller JMT, 1987, Periurethral enterobacterial carriage preceding urinary infection, *Lancet*, **1**: 824–7.

Brunner H, Weidner W, Schiefer HG, 1983, Studies of the role of *Ureaplasma urealyticum* and *Mycoplasma hominis* in prostatitis *J Infect Dis*, **147**: 807–13.

Burdon DW, 1971, Immunoglobulins of normal human urine and urethral secretions, *Immunology*, **21**: 363–8.

Burdon DW, 1975, Immunological reactions to urinary infection: the nature and function of secretory immunoglobulins, *Scientific Foundation in Urology*, vol. 1, eds Innes-Williams D, Chisholm GD, Heineman, London, 192–6.

Cattell WR, McSherry MA et al., 1974, Periurethral enterobacterial carriage in pathogenesis of recurrent urinary infection, *Br Med J*, **4**: 136–9.

Chan RCY, Reid G et al., 1985, Competitive exclusion of uropathogens from human uroepithelial cells by *Lactobacillus* whole cells and cell wall fragments, *Infect Immun*, **47**: 84–9.

Chernew I, Braude AI, 1962, Depression of phagocytosis by solutes in concentrations found in kidney and urine, *J Clin Invest*, **41**: 1945–53.

Childs SJ, 1990, Ciprofloxacin in the treatment of chronic bacterial prostatitis, *Urology*, **35, Suppl.**: 15–18.

Condie AP, Williams JD et al., 1968, Complications of bacteriuria in pregnancy, *Urinary Tract Infections*, eds O'Grady F, Brumfitt W, Oxford University Press, London, 148–59.

Cox CE, Lucy SS et al., 1968, The urethra and its relationship to urinary tract infection, *J Urol*, **99**: 632–8.

Dontas AS, Kasviki-Charvati P et al., 1981, Bacteriuria and survival in old age, *N Engl J Med*, **304**: 939–43.

Duguid JP, Old DC, 1980, Adhesive properties of Enterobacteriaceae, *Bacterial Adherence*, ed. Beechey EH, Chapman and Hall, London, 187–217.

Duguid JP, Smith IW et al., 1955, Non-flagellar filamentous appendages ('fimbriae') and haemagglutinating activity in *Bacterium coli*, *J Pathol Bacteriol*, **70**: 335–48.

Eisenstadt J, Washington JA, 1996, Diagnostic microbiology for bacteria and yeasts causing urinary tract infections, *Urinary Tract Infections: Molecular Pathogenesis and Clinical Management*, eds Mobley HLT, Warren JW, ASM Press, Washington, DC, 27–66.

Eknoyan G, Qunibi WY et al., 1982, Renal papillary necrosis: an update, *Medicine (Baltimore)*, **61**: 55–73.

Fair WR, Couch J, Wehner N, 1976, Prostatic antibacterial factor. Identity and significance, *Urology*, **7**: 169–77.

Fairley KF, Carson NE et al., 1971, Site of infection in acute urinary tract infection in general practice, *Lancet*, **2**: 615–18.

Fihn SD, Latham RH, 1985, Association between diaphragm use and urinary tract infection, *JAMA*, **254**: 240–5.

Finegold SM, Miller LG et al., 1965, Significance of anaerobic and capnophilic bacteria isolated from the urinary tract, *Progress in Pyelonephritis*, ed. Kass EH, FA Davis, Philadelphia, 159–78.

Forland M, Thomas V, 1985, The treatment of urinary tract infections in women with diabetes mellitus, *Diabetes Care*, **8**: 499–506.

Forland M, Thomas V, Shelokov A, 1977, Urinary tract infections in patients with diabetes mellitus, *JAMA*, **238**: 1924–6.

Freeman R, Sisson PR, Burdess B, 1996, Heterogeneity within apparently pure cultures of *Escherichia coli* freshly isolated from significant bacteriuria, *J Med Microbiol*, **45**: 349–52.

Fussell EN, Kaack MB et al., 1988, Adherence of bacteria to human foreskins, *J Urol*, **140**: 997–1001.

Gallagher DJA, Montgomerie JL, North JDK, 1965, Acute infections of the urinary tract and the urethral syndrome in general practice, *Br Med J*, **1**: 622–6.

Garibaldi RM, Burke JP et al., 1974, Meatal colonisation and catheter-associated bacteriuria, *N Engl J Med*, **303**: 316–18.

Gatermann S, John J, Marre R, 1989, *Staphylococcus saprophyticus* urease: characterization and contribution to uropathogenicity in unobstructed urinary tract infection in rats, *Infect Immun*, **57**: 110–16.

Gillespie WA, Henderson EP et al., 1989, Microbiology of the urethral (frequency and dysuria) syndrome. A controlled study with 5-year review, *Br J Urol*, **64**: 270–4.

Goldenring JM, Fried DC, Tames SM, 1988, *Staphylococcus saprophyticus* urinary tract infection in a sexually abused child, *Pediatr Infect Dis J*, **7**: 73–4.

Goldstein F, Georges E et al., 1991, Rapid detection of urinary tract infection, *Clinical Advances in Urinalysis*, ed. Sussman M, Bayer Diagnostics, Paris, 33–7.

Griffiths E, 1985, Candidate virulence markers, *The Virulence of Escherichia coli: Reviews and Methods*, ed. Sussman M, Academic Press, London, 193–226.

Griffiths E, 1997, Iron and the virulence of *Escherichia coli*, *Escherichia coli: Mechanisms of Virulence*, ed. Sussman M, Cambridge University Press, Cambridge, 331–72.

Griffiths E, Humphreys J, 1980, Isolation of enterochelin from the peritoneal washings of guinea-pigs lethally infected with *Escherichia coli*, *Infect Immun*, **28**: 286–9.

Grüneberg RN, 1969, Relationship of infecting urinary organisms to the faecal flora in patients with symptomatic urinary infection, *Lancet*, **2**: 766–8.

Grüneberg RN, Leigh DA, Brumfitt W, 1968, *Escherichia coli* serotypes in urinary tract infection: studies in domiciliary, ante-natal and hospital practice, *Urinary Tract Infections*, eds O'Grady F, Brumfitt W, Oxford University Press, London, 68–79.

Guttman DE, Naylor GRE, 1967, Dip-slide: an aid to quantitative urine culture in general practice, *Br Med J*, **3**: 343–5.

Haber MH, 1988, Pisse prophecy: a brief history of urinalysis, *Clin Lab Med*, **8**: 415–30.

Hagberg L, Lam J et al., 1986, Interaction of a pyelonephritogenic *Escherichia coli* strain with tissue components of the mouse urinary tract, *J Urol*, **136**: 165–72.

Hagberg L, Engberg I et al., 1983a, Acending unobstructed urinary tract infection in mice caused by pyelonephritogenic *Escherichia coli* of human origin, *Infect Immun*, **40**: 273–83.

Hagberg L, Hull R et al., 1983b, Contribution of adhesion to bacterial persistence in the mouse urinary tract, *Infect Immun*, **40**: 265–72.

Hallett RJ, Pead L, Maskell R, 1976, Urinary infection in boys, *Lancet*, **2**: 1107–10.

Hanisch F-G, Hacker J, Schroten H, 1993, Specificity of S fimbriae on recombinant *Escherichia coli*: preferential binding to gangliosides expressing NeuGca(2-3)Gal and NeuAca(2-8)NeuAc, *Infect Immun*, **61**: 2108–15.

Hanson LA, Holmgren J et al., 1970, Immunoglobulins in urines of children with urinary tract infection, *The Secretory Immunologic System*, eds Dayton DH, Small PA et al., US Department of Health, Education and Welfare, Bethesda MD, 367–83.

Hanson LA, Ahlstedt S et al., 1975, The host parasite relationship in urinary tract infection, *Kidney Int*, **8**: S28–34.

Hanson LA, Ahlsedt S et al., 1978, Immunology of urinary tract infection, *Infections of the Urinary Tract*, eds Kass EH, Brumfitt W, University of Chicago Press, Chicago, 105–12.

Harding GKM, Marrie TJ et al., 1978, Urinary tract infection localization in women, *JAMA*, **240**: 1147–50.

Herzog LW, 1989, Urinary tract infection and circumcision. A case control study, *Am J Dis Child*, **143**: 348–50.

Hinman F, 1966, Mechanism for the entry of bacteria and the establishment of urinary infection in female children, *J Urol*, **96**: 546–50.

Hjelm EM, 1984, Local cellular immune response in ascending urinary tract infection: occurrence of T-cells, immunoglobulin-producing cells and Ia-expressing cells in rat urinary tract infection, *Infect Immun*, **44**: 627–32.

Hoeprich PD, 1960, Culture of the urine, *J Lab Clin Med*, **56**: 899–907.

Hoogkamp-Korstanje JAA, van Oort HJ, Schipper JJ, 1984, Intraprostatic concentration of ciprofloxacin and its activity against urinary pathogens, *J Antimicrob Chemother*, **14**: 641–5.

Hooton TM, Stamm WE, 1996, The vaginal flora and urinary tract infections, *Urinary Tract Infections: Molecular Pathogenesis and Clinical Management*, eds Mobley HLT, Warren JW, American Society for Microbiology, Washington, DC, 67–94.

Hovelius B, Colleen S, Mardh PA, 1984, Urinary tract infections in men caused by *Staphylococcus saprophyticus*, *Scand J Infect Dis*, **16**: 37–41.

Hull S, 1997, *Escherichia coli* lipopolysaccharide in pathogenesis and virulence, *Escherichia coli: Mechanisms of Virulence*, ed. Sussman M, Cambridge University Press, Cambridge, 145–68.

Jackson GG, Arana-Sialer JA et al., 1962, Profiles of pyelonephritis, *Arch Intern Med*, **110**: 663–75.

Jann K, Jann B, 1983, The K antigens of *Escherichia coli*, *Prog Allergy*, **33**: 53–79.

Jepsen OB, 1987, Urinary tract infections: an overview, *Chemioterapia*, **6**: 179–83.

Jepsen OB, Larsen SO et al., 1982, Urinary tract infection and bacteraemia in hospitalized medical patients – a European multicentre prevalence survey on nosocomial infection, *J Hosp Med*, **3**: 241–52.

Jodal U, Hanson LA, 1975, Sequential determination of C-reactive protein in acute childhood pyelonephritis, *Acta Paediatr Scand*, **65**: 319–22.

Jodal U, Hanson LA et al., 1970, Studies of antibodies and immunoglobulin levels in urine from children with urinary tract infections caused by *E. coli*, *Acta Paediatr Scand Suppl*, **206**: 78–9.

Johnson CC, 1991, Definitions, classification, and clinical presentation of urinary tract infection, *Med Clin North Am*, **75**: 241–52.

Johnson JR, 1997, Urinary tract infection, Escherichia coli: *Mechanisms of Virulence*, ed. Sussman M, Cambridge University Press, Cambridge, 495–549.

Kaitz A, 1961, Urinary concentrating ability in pregnant women with asymptomatic bacteriuria, *J Clin Invest*, **40**: 1331–8.

Källenius G, Mollby R et al., 1981a, Occurrence of P fimbriated *Escherichia coli* in urinary tract infection, *Lancet*, **2**: 1369–72.

Källenius G, Svenson SB et al., 1981b, Structure of carbohydrate part of receptor on human uroepithelial cells for pyelonephritogenic *Escherichia coli*, *Lancet*, **2**: 604–6.

Kass EH, 1956, Asymptomatic infections of the urinary tract, *Trans Assoc Am Physicians*, **69**: 56–64.

Kass EH, Savage W, Santamarina BAG, 1965, The significance of bacteriuria in preventive medicine, *Progress in Pyelonephritis*, ed. Kass EH, FA Davis, Philadelphia, 3–10.

Kaufman DB, Katz R, McIntosh RWW, 1970, Secretory IgA in urinary tract infections, *Br Med J*, **4**: 463–5.

Kaye D, 1968, Antibacterial activity of human urine, *J Clin Invest*, **47**: 2374–90.

Kennedy DH, 1989, Extrapulmonary tuberculosis, *The Biology of the Mycobacteria*, vol. 3, eds Ratledge C, Stanford J, Grange JM, Academic Press, New York, 245–84.

Kirby, RS Low D et al., 1982, Intraprostatic urinary reflux: an aetiological factor in abacterial prostatitis, *Br J Urol*, **54**: 729–31.

Kiselius PV, Schwan WR et al., 1989, In vivo expression and variation of *Escherichia coli* type 1 and P pili in the urine of adults with acute urinary tract infections, *Infect Immun*, **57**: 1656–62.

Kraft JK, Stamey TA, 1977, The natural history of symptomatic recurrent bacteriuria in women, *Medicine (Baltimore)*, **56**: 55–60.

Kunin CM, 1961, The quantitative significance of bacteria visualized in the unstained urinary sediment, *N Engl J Med*, **265**: 589–90.

Kunin CM, 1987, *Detection, Prevention and Management of Urinary Tract Infections*, 4th edn, Lea and Febiger, Philadelphia.

Kunin CM, Deutscher R, Paquin AJ, 1964, Urinary tract infection in schoolchildren: an epidemiological, clinical and laboratory study, *Medicine (Baltimore)*, **43**: 91–130.

Kunin CM, McCormack RG, 1966, Prevention of catheter-induced urinary tract infections by sterile closed drainage, *N Engl J Med*, **274**: 1115–61.

Kunin CM, McCormack RG, 1968, An epidemiologic study of bacteriuria and blood pressure among nuns and working women, *N Engl J Med*, **278**: 635–42.

Kunin CM, Paquin AJ, 1965, Frequency and natural history of urinary tract infection in schoolchildren, *Progress in Pyelonephritis*, ed. Kass EH, FA Davis, Philadelphia, 33–44.

Kunin CM, Polyak F, Postel E, 1980, Periurethral bacterial flora in women. Prolonged intermittent colonization with *Escherichia coli*, *JAMA*, **243**: 134–9.

Kunin CM, Zacha E, Paquin AJ, 1962, Urinary tract infections in schoolchildren. I. Prevalence of bacteriuria and associated urologic findings, *N Engl J Med*, **266**: 1287–96.

Leffler H, Svanborg-Edén C, 1980, Chemical identification of a glycosphingolipid receptor for *Escherichia coli* attaching to human urinary tract epithelial cells agglutinating human erythrocytes, *FEMS Microbiol Lett*, **8**: 127–34.

Leigh DA, Grüneberg RN, Brumfitt W, 1968, Long-term follow-up of bacteriuria in pregnancy, *Lancet*, **1**: 603–5.

Leigh DA, Williams JD, 1964, Method for the detection of significant bacteriuria in large groups of patients, *J Clin Pathol*, **17**: 498–503.

Lincoln K, Winberg J, 1964, Studies of urinary infections in infancy and childhood. II. Quantitative estimation of bacteriuria in undetected neonates with special reference to the occurrence of asymptomatic infections, *Acta Paediatr Scand*, **53**: 307–16.

Lipsky BA, 1989, Urinary tract infection in men: epidemiology, pathophysiology, diagnosis and treatment, *Ann Intern Med*, **110**: 138–50.

Little PJ, 1964, A comparison of the urinary white cell concentration with white cell excretion rate, *Br J Urol*, **36**: 360–3.

Little PJ, 1965, Prevention of pyelonephritis of pregnancy, *Lancet*, **1**: 567–9.

Lomberg H, Hellström M et al., 1984, Virulence-associated traits in *Escherichia coli* causing first and recurrent episodes of urinary tract infection in children with and without vesico-ureteric reflux, *J Infect Dis*, **150**: 561–9.

Ludwig A, Goebel W, 1997, Haemolysins of *Escherichia coli*, Escherichia coli: *Mechanisms of Virulence*, ed. Sussman M, Cambridge University Press, 281–330.

Mabeck CE, 1969, Studies in urinary tract infections. I. The diagnosis of bacteriuria in women, *Acta Med Scand*, **186**: 35–8.

McCabe WR, Kaijser B et al., 1978, *Escherichia coli* in bacteremia: K and O antigens and serum sensitivity of strains from adults and neonates, *J Infect Dis*, **138**: 33–41.

McGowan JE, Barnes MW, Finland M, 1975, Bacteremia at Boston City Hospital: occurrence and mortality during 12 selected years (1935–1972) with special reference to hospital-acquired cases, *J Infect Dis*, **132**: 316–35.

Mackey JP, Sandys GH, 1965, Laboratory diagnosis of infections of the urinary tract in general practice by means of a dip-inoculum transport medium, *Br Med J*, **2**: 1286–8.

Mackey JP, Sandys GH, 1966, Diagnosis of urinary infections, *Br Med J*, **1**: 1173.

Mackie ADR, Drury PL, 1996, Urinary tract infection in diabetes mellitus, *Infections of the Kidney and Urinary Tract*, ed. Cattell WR, Oxford University Press, Oxford, 218–33.

MacLean AB, 1996, Urinary tract infection and pregnancy, *Infections of the Kidney and Urinary Tract*, ed. Cattell WR, Oxford University Press, Oxford, 205–17.

Males BM, Bartholomew WR, Amsterdam D, 1983, Leukocyte esterase-nitrite and bioluminescence assays as urine screens, *J Clin Microbiol*, **22**: 531–4.

Mardh PA, Collen S, 1975, Search for uro-genital tract infections in patients with symptoms of prostatitis. Studies on aerobic and strictly anaerobic bacteria, mycoplasma, fungi, trichomonads and viruses, *Scand J Urol Nephrol*, **9**: 8–16.

Mardh PA, Ripa KT et al., 1978, Role of *Chlamydia trachomatis* in non-acute prostatitis, *Br J Vener Dis*, **54**: 330–4.

Marrie TJ, Swantee CA, Hartlen M, 1980, Aerobic and anaerobic urethral flora in healthy females in various physiological age groups and of females with urinary tract infection, *J Clin Microbiol*, **11**: 654–9.

Maskell R, 1986, Are fastidious organisms an important cause of dysuria and frequency? – the case for, *Microbial Diseases in Nephrology*, eds Asscher AW, Brumfitt W, Wiley, Chichester, 1–18.

Meares EM, 1982, Prostatitis: review of parmacokinetics and therapy, *Rev Infect Dis*, **4**: 475–83.

Meares EM, Stamey TA, 1968, Bacteriologic localization patterns in bacterial prostatitis and urethritis, *Invest Urol*, **5**: 492–518.

Miller TE, Marshall E, Nelson J, 1983, Infection-induced immunosuppression in pyelonephritis: characteristics of suppressor cells, *Kidney Int*, **24**: 313–22.

Minshew BH, Jorgensen J et al., 1978, Some characteristics of *Escherichia coli* strains isolated from extra-intestinal infections in humans, *J Infect Dis*, **137**: 648–54.

Montgomerie JL, Bindereif A et al., 1984, Association of hydroxamate siderophore (aerobactin) with *Escherichia coli* isolated from patients with bacteremia, *Infect Immun*, **46**: 835–8.

Monzon OT, Ory EM et al., 1958, A comparison of bacterial counts of the urine obtained by needle aspiration of the bladder, catheterization and mid-stream voided methods, *N Engl J Med*, **259:** 764–7.

Musher DM, Griffith DP et al., 1975, Role of urease in pyelonephritis resulting from urinary tract infection with *Proteus*, *J Infect Dis*, **131:** 177–81.

Nachum R, Shanbrom E, 1981, Rapid detection of Gram-negative bacteriuria by *Limulus* amoebocyte lysate assay, *J Clin Microbiol*, **13:** 158–62.

Naylor GRE, 1984, A 16-month analysis of urinary tract infection in children, *J Med Microbiol*, **17:** 31–6.

Needell MH, Neter E et al., 1955, Antibody (haemagglutinin) in response of patients with infections of the urinary tract, *J Urol*, **74:** 674–82.

Nicolle LE, 1996, Uncomplicated urinary tract infection in women, *Infections of the Kidney and Urinary Tract*, ed. Cattell WR, Oxford University Press, Oxford, 115–28.

Norden CW, Gree GM, Kass EH, 1968, Antibacterial mechanisms of the urinary bladder, *J Clin Invest*, **47:** 2689–700.

Norden CW, Tuttle EP, 1965, Impairment of urinary concentrating ability in pregnant women with asymptomatic bacteriuria, *Progress in Pyelonephritis*, ed. Kass EH, FA Davis, Philadelphia, 73–80.

Nordenstam GR, Brandberg CA et al., 1986, Bacteriuria and mortality in an elderly population, *N Engl J Med*, **314:** 1152–6.

Ofek I, Doyle RJ, 1994, *Bacterial Adhesion to Cells and Tissues*, Chapman and Hall, New York.

Ofek I, Mosek A, Sharon N, 1981, Mannose-specific adherence of *Escherichia coli* freshly excreted in the urine of patients with urinary tract infections and of isolates subcultured from infected urine, *Infect Immun*, **34:** 708–11.

O'Grady F, Cattell WR, 1966, Kinetics of urinary tract infection. II. The bladder, *Br J Urol*, **38:** 156–62.

O'Grady FW, Richards B et al., 1970, Introital enterobacteria, urinary infection and the urethral syndrome, *Lancet*, **2:** 1208–10.

O'Hanley P, 1990, Vaccines against *Escherichia coli* urinary tract infections, *New Generations of Vaccines*, eds Woodrow GC, Levine MM, Marcel Dekker, New York, 631–48.

O'Hanley P, Lark D et al., 1985a, Molecular basis of *Escherichia coli* colonization of the upper urinary tract in BALB/c mice, *J Clin Invest*, **75:** 347–60.

O'Hanley P, Low D et al., 1985b, Gal-Gal binding and haemolysin phenotypes and genotypes associated with uropathogenic *Escherichia coli*, *N Engl J Med*, **313:** 414–20.

Ohkoshi M, Naber KG, 1992, International consensus discussion on clinical evaluation of drug efficacy in urinary tract infection, *Infection*, **20, Suppl. 3:** S135–42.

Ørskov I, Ferencz A, Ørskov F, 1980, Tamm–Horsfall protein or uromucoid is the normal urinary slime that traps Type 1 fimbriated *Escherichia coli*, *Lancet*, **1:** 887.

Ørskov I, Ørskov F, 1985, *Escherichia coli* in extraintestinal infections, *J Hyg Camb*, **95:** 551–75.

O'Sullivan DJ, Fitzgerald MG et al., 1961, Urinary tract infection: a comparative study in the diabetic and general populations, *Br Med J*, **1:** 786–8.

Parry SH, Boonchai S et al., 1983, A comparative study of the mannose-resistant and mannose-sensitive haemagglutinins of *Escherichia coli* isolated from urinary tract infection, *Infection*, **11:** 123–8.

Pasteur L, 1863, Examen de role attribué au gaz oxygène atmosphérique dans la destruction de matières animales et végétales après la mort, *C R Acad Sci*, **56:** 734.

Patton JP, Nash DB, Abrutyn E, 1991, Urinary tract infection: economic considerations, *Med Clin North Am*, **75:** 495–513.

Pead L, Maskell R, Morris J, 1985, *Staphylococcus saprophyticus* as a urinary pathogen: a six-year prospective survey, *Br Med J*, **291:** 1157–9.

Percival A, Brumfitt W, de Louvois J, 1964, Serum antibody levels as an indication of clinically inapparent pyelonephritis, *Lancet*, **2:** 1027–33.

Pere A, Nowicki B et al., 1987, Expression of P, type-1 and type 1C fimbriae on *Escherichia coli* in the urine of patients with acute urinary tract infection, *J Infect Dis*, **156:** 567–74.

Perry JL, Matthews JS, Weesner DE, 1982, Evaluation of leukocyte esterase activity as a rapid screening technique for bacteriuria, *J Clin Microbiol*, **15:** 852–4.

Pezzlo MT, Tan GL et al., 1982, Screening of urine by three automated methods, *J Clin Microbiol*, **15:** 468–74.

Pfau A, Sacks TG, 1981, The bacterial flora of the vaginal vestibule, urethra and vagina in premenopausal women with recurrent urinary tract infection, *J Urol*, **126:** 630–4.

Rantz LA, 1962, Serological grouping of *Escherichia coli*. Study in urinary tract infection, *Arch Intern Med*, **109:** 37–42.

Rayfield EJ, Ault MJ et al., 1982, Infection and diabetes: the case for glucose control, *Am J Med*, **72:** 439–50.

Reeves DS, Brumfitt W, 1968, Localization of urinary tract infection, *Urinary Tract Infection*, eds O'Grady F, Brumfitt W, Oxford University Press, London, 53–67.

Reid G, Sobel JD, 1987, Bacterial adherence in the pathogenesis of urinary tract infection, *Rev Infect Dis*, **9:** 470–87.

Reid G, Chan RCY et al., 1985, Prevention of urinary tract infection in rats with an indigenous *Lactobacillus casei* strain, *Infect Immun*, **49:** 320–4.

Remis RS, Gurwith MJ, 1987, Risk factors for urinary tract infection, *Am J Epidemiol*, **126:** 685–94.

Riden DJ, Schaeffer AJ, 1996, Urinary tract infection in men, *Infections of the Kidney and Urinary Tract*, ed. Cattell WR, Oxford University Press, Oxford, 265–90.

Roberts AP, Beard RW, 1965, Some factors affecting bacterial invasion of bladder during pregnancy, *Lancet*, **1:** 1133–6.

Roberts AP, Clayton SG, Bean HS, 1968, Urine factors affecting bacterial growth, *Urinary Tract Infection*, eds O'Grady F, Brumfitt W, Oxford University Press, London, 14–23.

Roberts AP, Linton JD et al., 1975, Urinary and faecal *Escherichia coli* O-serotypes in symptomatic urinary tract infection and asymptomatic bacteriuria, *J Med Microbial*, **8:** 311–18.

Roberts JA, Kaack MB, Fussell EN, 1993, Adherence to urethral catheters by bacteria causing nosocomial infections, *Urology*, **41:** 338–42.

Roberts W, 1881, On the occurrence of micro-organisms in fresh urine, *Br Med J*, **2:** 623–5.

Ronald AR, Cutler RE, Turck M, 1969, Effect of bacteriuria on renal concentrating mechanisms, *Ann Intern Med*, **70:** 723–33.

Ronald AR, Pattullo AL, 1991, The natural history of urinary infection in adults, *Med Clin North Am*, **75:** 299–312.

Sandberg T, Bergmark J et al., 1986, Diagnostic potential of urinary enzymes and β_2-microglobulin in acute urinary tract infection, *Acta Med Scand*, **219:** 489–95.

Savage DCL, Wilson MI et al., 1969, Asymptomatic bacteriuria in girl entrants to Dundee primary schools, *Br Med J*, **3:** 75–80.

Savage WE, Hajj SN, Kass EH, 1967, Demographic and prognostic characteristics of bacteriuria in pregnancy, *Medicine (Baltimore)*, **46:** 385–407.

Schersten B, Fritz H, 1967, Subnormal levels of glucose in urine: a sign of urinary tract infection, *JAMA*, **201:** 949–52.

Schlegel JU, Cuellar J, O'Dell RM, 1961, Bactericidal effect of urea, *J Urol*, **86:** 819–22.

Sharon N, Ofek I, 1986, Mannose specific surface lectins, *Microbial Lectins and Agglutinins: Properties and Biological Activities*, ed. Mirelman D, Wiley, New York, 55–81.

Simmons NA, Williams JD, 1962, A simple test for significant bacteriuria, *Lancet*, **1:** 1377–8.

Smith A, 1984, New treatment for struvite urinary stones, *N Engl J Med*, **311:** 792–4.

Stamey TA, 1980a, Some observations on the pathogenesis of recurrent bacteriuria in women and children, *Pathogenesis and Treatment of Urinary Tract Infections*, Williams & Wilkins, Baltimore, MD, 210–89.

Stamey TA, 1980b, The diagnosis, localization and classification of urinary infections, *Pathogenesis and Treatment of Urinary Tract Infections*, Williams & Wilkins, Baltimore, MD, 1–51.

Stamey TA, Govan DE, Palmer JM, 1965, The localization and treatment of urinary tract infections: the role of bactericidal urine levels as opposed to serum levels, *Medicine (Baltimore)*, **44**: 1–36.

Stamey TA, Pfau A, 1963, Some functional, pathologic and chemotherapeutic characteristics of unilateral pyelonephritis in man. II. Bacteriologic and chemotherapeutic characteristics, *Invest Urol*, **1**: 162–72.

Stamey TA, Fair R et al., 1968, Antibacterial nature of prostatic fluid, *Nature* (London), **218**: 444–7.

Stamey TA, Timothy M et al., 1971, Recurrent urinary infections in adult women. The role of introital enterobacteria, *California Med*, **115**: 1–19.

Stamm WE, Wagner KF et al., 1980, Causes of the acute urethral syndrome in women, *N Engl J Med*, **303**: 409–15.

Stamm WE, Running K et al., 1981, Treatment of urethral syndrome, *N Engl J Med*, **304**: 956–8.

Stamm WE, Counts GW et al., 1982, Diagnosis of coliform infection in acutely dysuric women, *N Engl J Med*, **307**: 463–8.

Stansfeld JM, 1966, Clinical observations relating to incidence and aetiology of urinary tract infections in children, *Br Med J*, **1**: 631–5.

Steadman R, Topley N, 1997, Cellular activation by uropathogenic *Escherichia coli*, Escherichia coli: *Mechanisms of Virulence*, ed. Sussman M, Cambridge University Press, Cambridge, 553–78.

Summanen P, Baron EJ et al., 1993, *Wadsworth Anaerobic Bacteriology Manual*, Star Publishing Co., Belmont, CA.

Sussman M, Asscher AW, 1979, Urinary tract infection, *Renal Disease*, eds Black D, Jones NF, Blackwell Scientific Publications, Oxford, 400–36.

Sussman M, Asscher AW et al., 1969, Asymptomatic significant bacteriuria in the non-pregnant woman. I. Description of a population, *Br Med J*, **1**: 799–803.

Tait J, Peddie BA et al., 1985, Urethral syndrome (abacterial cystitis) – search for a pathogen, *Br J Urol*, **57**: 552–6.

Tapsall TW, Taylor TC et al., 1975, Relevance of 'significant bacteriuria' to aetiology and diagnosis of urinary tract infection, *Lancet*, **1**: 637–9.

Taylor PW, 1985, Measurement of the bactericidal activity of serum, *The Virulence of* Escherichia coli: *Reviews and Methods*, ed. Sussman M, Academic Press, London, 445–56.

Teague N, Boyarsky S, 1968, Further effects of coliform bacteria on ureteral peristalsis, *J Urol*, **99**: 720–4.

Thomas V, Shelokov A, Forland M, 1974, Antibody-coated bacteria in urine and the site of urinary tract infection, *N Engl J Med*, **290**: 588–90.

Thore A, Ansehn S et al., 1975, Detection of bacteriuria by luciferase assay of adenosine triphosphate, *J Clin Microbiol*, **1**: 1–8.

Thuselius O, Araj G, 1987, The effect of uropathogenic bacteria on ureteral motility, *Urol Res*, **15**: 273–6.

Turck M, 1978, Importance of localization of urinary tract infections in women, *Infections of the Urinary Tract*, eds Kass EH, Brumfitt W, University of Chicago Press, Chicago, 114–21.

Turck M, Goffe B, Petersdorf RG, 1962, The urethral catheter and urinary tract infection, *J Urol*, **88**: 834–7.

Turck M, Petersdorf RG, 1962, The epidemiology of non-enteric *Escherichia coli* infections: prevalence of serological groups, *J Clin Invest*, **41**: 1760–5.

Turck M, Stamm WE, 1981, Nosocomial infection of the urinary tract, *Am J Med*, **70**: 651–4.

Uehling DT, Stiehm ER, 1971, Elevated urinary secretory IgA in children with urinary tract infection, *Pediatrics*, **47**: 40–6.

Väisänen V, Elo J et al., 1981, Mannose-resistant haemagglutination and P antigen recognition are characteristic of *Escherichia coli* causing primary pyelonephritis, *Lancet*, **2**: 1366–9.

Väisänen-Rhen V, Korhonen TK, Finne J, 1983, Novel cell-binding activity for *N*-acetyl-D-glucosamine in an *Escherichia coli* strain, *Science*, **159**: 233–6.

Vejlsgaard R, 1966, Studies on urinary infection in diabetics. I. Bacteriuria in patients with diabetes mellitus and in control patients, *Acta Med Scand*, **179**: 173–82.

Vivaldi E, Munoz J et al., 1965, Factors affecting the clearance of bacteria within the urinary tract, *Progress in Pyelonephritis*, ed. Kass EH, FA Davis, Philadelphia, 531–5.

Vosti KL, Goldberg LM, Rantz LA, 1965, Host–parasite interactions amongst infections caused by *Escherichia coli*, *Progress in Pyelonephritis*, ed. Kass EH, FA Davis, Philadelphia, 103–10.

Walter S, Vejlsgaard R, 1978, Diagnostic catheterisation and bacteriuria in women with urinary incontinence, *Br J Urol*, **50**: 106–8.

Weiser R, Asscher AW, Sussman M, 1969, Glycosuria and the growth of urinary pathogens, *Invest Urol*, **6**: 650–6.

Wettergen B, Jodal U, Jonasson G, 1985, Epidemiology of bacteriuria during the first year of life, *Acta Paediatr Scand*, **74**: 925–33.

Whalley P, 1967, Bacteriuria of pregnancy, *Am J Obstet Gynecol*, **97**: 723–38.

Winberg J, 1959, Renal function studies in infants and children with acute non-obstructive urinary tract infections, *Acta Paediatr Scand*, **48**: 577–89.

Winberg J, Andersen HJ et al., 1963, Studies on urinary infections in infants and children. I. Antibody response in different types of urinary tract infections caused by coliform bacteria, *Br Med J*, **2**: 524–7.

Winberg J, Bollgren I et al., 1989, The prepuce: a mistake of nature, *Lancet*, **1**: 598–9.

Winningham DG, Nemoy NJ et al., 1968, Diffusion of antibiotics from plasma into prostatic fluid, *Nature* (London), **219**: 139–43.

Yeni P, Tournot F et al., 1991, An evaluation of screening for urinary infection in hospital patients, *Clinical Advances in Urinalysis*, ed. Sussman M, Bayer Diagnostics, Paris, 38–41.

Zimmerli W, Lew PD, Waldvogel FA, 1984, Pathogenesis of foreign body infection. Evidence for a local granulocyte defect, *J Clin Invest*, **73**: 1191–200.

Chapter 33

Gonorrhoea, chancroid and granuloma venereum

A E Jephcott

1 Gonorrhoea	3 Granuloma venereum
2 Chancroid	

1 Gonorrhoea

1.1 History

Gonorrhoea has a history stretching back into antiquity and is mentioned in biblical writings. In Leviticus there is reference to the 'running issue' and in Numbers of Moses's orders for quarantine, personal hygiene and even slaughter of all Midianite women 'that have known man by lying with him'. The first scientific observations on the disease are attributed to Hippocrates (460–355 BC), who dissected inflamed urethrae; the name 'gonorrhoea' is attributed to Galen (120–200 AD).

The causal agent, the gonococcus (*Neisseria gonorrhoeae*), was discovered by Neisser in 1879 who saw it in 35 cases of gonorrhoea, but not in nongonorrhoeal pus, such as that accompanying chancres and buboes, or in simple vaginal discharges; he demonstrated its presence in 7 cases of ophthalmia neonatorum and in 2 cases of adult ophthalmia. Though unable through illness to complete his investigation, he placed the aetiological role of the gonococcus on a footing that has never since been seriously challenged. It was left to Bumm (1885) to cultivate the organism and, by inoculation experiments on human subjects, to demonstrate its pathogenicity in pure culture. The history of gonorrhoea has been reviewed by Morton (1977) (see also Volume 2, Chapter 37).

1.2 Clinical aspects

Gonorrhoea in adults

Gonorrhoea is an acute infectious disease generally characterized by primary invasion of the genitourinary tract and sometimes complicated by secondary disturbances of greater or lesser severity.

In men the anterior urethra is first attacked. Classical descriptions report that after an incubation period of 2–7 days a mucoid discharge appears that often becomes purulent. This is accompanied by dysuria and frequency of micturition. The gonococci seen in the discharge lie predominantly within the pus cells. Infections in men may be symptomless, as were up to 60% of infections in US servicemen (Handsfield et al. 1974), but rates of symptomless infection vary with populations studied and are usually much lower than this (McMillan and Pattman 1979). However, Sherrard and Barlow (1993) observed that only 51% of their patients experienced discharge and dysuria and noted an increasing incubation period with a median of 7.9 days. Symptomless men represent a particularly dangerous source of infection as they can remain undetected for long periods and, moreover, they are responsible for an excess of complicated infections in females (Handsfield et al. 1974).

In women the endocervix is the primary site of infection. The urethra may also become infected, but in premenopausal women positive vaginal cultures result from contamination from an infected cervix, because the glycogen-rich mucosa of the vagina is inimical to the growth of gonococci. There may be increased vaginal discharge, dysuria and frequency of micturition, as well as lower abdominal and pelvic pain. Up to 50% of patients may be symptom-free (Barlow and Phillips 1978), but in one study 80% of infected women reported symptoms on direct questioning (Donegan 1985).

Anorectal infection may occur in either sex. In men this follows rectal intercourse but is otherwise rare; it is far more common in women. Thin and Shaw (1979) found that over 50% of infected women had positive rectal cultures. This can follow rectal intercourse but may also arise as a result of auto-inoculation of the rectal mucosa with infected vaginal discharge (Kilpatrick 1972). The cells affected are those of the transitional zone between the anus and the rectum and the columnar cells of the rectal crypts. The clinical picture in both sexes varies from the symptomless to the severe with profuse discharge of mucus or pus, pain and tenesmus.

Pharyngeal infection may follow orogenital contact in either sex, and occasionally follows auto-inoculation with infected genital secretions; it is usually symptomless and only rarely associated with exudative pharyngitis (Sherrard and Barlow 1993). It has followed the eating of a diagnostic culture plate (Lipsitt and Parmett 1984).

Complications of gonorrhoea in adults

The infection may remain localized or may affect the glands that drain into the genitourinary tract and reach the more distant parts of the genital tract by retrograde spread. In women, Bartholin's and Skene's glands may become inflamed. In men, infection of Littré's glands and the subepithelial tissues of the urethra may lead to periurethal abscess and stricture. Infection may also spread to the prostate, the seminal vesicles and Cowper's glands, and this was largely responsible for the chronicity of the disease before the advent of antibiotic therapy. The epididymes may become affected and inflammation of these may result in sterility. In the female, gonococci may spread to the fallopian tubes or further to cause salpingitis or even perihepatitis (the Fitz-Hugh–Curtis syndrome). The latter is now known also to be caused by *Chlamydia trachomatis*. Salpingitis, too, may be caused by *C. trachomatis*, but a significant proportion of it, probably higher in North America than in Europe, is caused by the gonococcus (Mårdh 1980). One legacy of an attack of salpingitis is a 7–10-fold increase in the risk of ectopic pregnancy. Infertility after one episode of salpingitis occurs in 10–20% of women, rising to 60% after more than 3 episodes (Weström 1980). The economic costs of these complications in developed countries are very great (Curran 1980); in parts of Africa they are a major cause of ill health and have produced subfertile populations (World Health Organization 1978a, Arya, Taber and Nsanze 1980).

Disseminated gonococcal infection (DGI) occurs in 1–3% of patients with gonorrhoea by spread through the bloodstream (Knapp and Holmes 1975), but its frequency varies with locality. It is more common in women than men, occurring most frequently at the onset of menstruation or during pregnancy. In men it usually follows a symptomless infection. The common form of this condition is known as the 'arthritis dermatitis syndrome', in which there is fever with flitting arthritis or tenosynovitis and frequently a characteristic sparse rash. Myopericarditis commonly accompanies DGI, but acute endocarditis is now a rare complication. However, before the use of antimicrobial therapy it was a major cause of acute endocarditis (Thayer 1922) and meningitis, too, is still occasionally caused by *N. gonorrhoeae*. Recovery from DGI is usually rapid and complete after antimicrobial therapy (for review see Holmes, Counts and Beatty 1971).

Neonatal gonorrhoea

Ophthalmia neonatorum results from contamination of the eyes during birth. Gonococci are responsible for less than 30% of cases and these tend to occur during the first 12 days of life. Gonococcal ophthalmia responds rapidly to antibiotics, but if untreated will lead to permanent damage to the eye and blindness. During the first decade of this century gonococcal ophthalmia was responsible for one-quarter of admissions to schools for the blind in the USA (Bassam 1966) and for a similar proportion in Europe. It can readily be prevented by the instillation of antibacterial drops or ointment into the eyes at birth. Originally 1% silver nitrate was used but this has been superseded by antibiotics. Whilst this practice continues in the USA it is now considered necessary in the UK only in deliveries known to involve an infected mother. Babies born to infected mothers are frequently premature. They may develop gonococcal bacteraemia, arthritis and infections of the umbilicus, anogenital area and the nasopharynx as well as of the eye (Israel, Rissing and Brooks 1975). Skin infections do not occur but gonococcal abscesses at the sites of scalp monitoring electrodes have been reported (Plavidal and Werch 1976).

In the UK 11 cases of gonococcal ophthalmia were reported in 1991 whereas in parts of sub-Saharan Africa best estimates place rates between 0.9% and 5% of all births (Schultz, Cates and O'Mara 1987).

Gonorrhoea in children

Infection rates in prepubertal children increase with age (Branch and Paxton 1965). Transmission to younger children may be by fomites such as infected linen and in older children by voluntary sexual activity (Branch and Paxton 1965), but in all age groups sexual abuse almost certainly plays the major role.

In little girls the disease often takes the form of gonococcal vulvovaginitis. The gonococcus attacks columnar rather than squamous epithelium. Lactic acid produced by lactobacilli from glycogen in the stratified squamous epithelium protects the adult vagina against gonococci. Before puberty the vagina and vulva are lined by an immature squamous epithelium which lacks glycogen and so is not protected. Thus vulvovaginitis occurs much more commonly in children than in adults, whereas complications that affect the internal genital organs are seen more often in adults. Acute gonococcal pelvic peritonitis may, however, occur in children. The urethral and rectal mucosae are susceptible throughout life. Hence, both in adult gonorrhoea in the female and in vulvovaginitis in children, the rectum is frequently affected.

1.3 Epidemiology and sociology

The incidence of gonorrhoea reflects the adaptation of the organism to the human host and the life-style of the human community. Gonorrhoea is a social as well as a microbial disease. The organism has no animal reservoir and relies entirely on human behaviour for its successful transmission. The dynamics of the transmission of gonorrhoea in their simplest form can be modelled by the equation $R_0 = \beta CD$ (Brunham and Plummer 1990) where R_0 is reproductive rate (i.e. the number of new infections engendered by a prior infection); β is the probability of transmission per partnership; C is the rate of partner change; and D is the duration the patient remains infective.

When R_0 is less than one the infection will die out in a community; the amount greater than one R_0 is, the larger the number of cases that will occur. Clearly, an increasing number of partners increases R_0, but it can be reduced by diminishing the probability of transmission (β), for example by the use of barrier contraceptives, and by active case finding and treatment which will reduce D. Calculations reveal that endemicity in the developed world is maintained by the heightened transmission within small groups rather than by diffuse infection of the whole community (Potterat, Dukes and Rothenberg 1987).

In England and Wales the end of both World Wars was accompanied by dramatic surges in gonorrhoeal infection rates. These rapidly fell back to pre-existing levels but were followed by steady sustained rises that after World War II eventually greatly exceeded the immediately post-war peak (see Fig. 33.1).

This resulted from the major social changes that took place at that time. It was a period of greater emancipation and education, with consequent questioning and frequent rejection of traditional values and a climate of changing attitudes to homosexual and extramarital sexual relationships prevailed. There was greater population mobility and affluence and the constraints of fear of infection or of pregnancy (Guthe 1961) receded with the advent of effective antimicrobials and oral contraceptives. All these tended to increase the number and frequency of change of sexual partners to the level necessary to produce an explosion of gonorrhoea.

Similar rises were recorded in most western countries and caused international alarm. Countermeas-

ures aimed mainly at D were generally ineffective until recognition of the emerging AIDS epidemic forced widespread changes in sexual practice with greater awareness of β and C. This has been dramatically effective in western countries. Thus, from a peak of almost 59 000 cases reported in 1977 only 11 803 cases were recorded in England during 1993; in Sweden rates fell from 487 per 100 000 in 1970 to 14 per 100 000 in 1990. In the USA efforts have been less successful – rates have fallen from 456 per 100 000 in 1976 but remained at 201 per 100 000 in 1992, as a result of the persistence of high rates in disadvantaged black populations.

Data on infection rates in the developing world are far less complete, but in many areas infection rates are very high and have been so for a long time. Figures in sub-Saharan Africa have revealed between 7 and 20% of pregnant women to be infected, with known complications of gonorrhoea accounting for 50% of all cases of infertility (Bergström 1990). Rates for ophthalmia neonatorum have already been mentioned (see section on 'Neonatal gonorrhoea, p. 624).

Gonorrhoea is predominantly a disease of the young and sexually active; those prone to infection tend to have certain other characteristics in common. Ekstrøm (1966, 1970) noted that infected Danish youths tended to have had poor home backgrounds, left school early and had poor job records. They were usually unskilled, showed evidence of emotional disturbance, made frequent changes of sex partner and had high rates of pregnancy, abortion, alcohol abuse and criminal offences. Other workers have found similar patterns.

Prostitutes not unexpectedly show high infection rates (Meheus, De Clercq and Prat 1974). Thus 40% of 44 female and 6 male prostitutes in Toronto in 1987 had gonorrhoea (Read, Cave and Goldberg 1988). Their relative importance in the spread of gonorrhoea varies with geographical locality (World Health Organization 1978b). In the western Pacific, prostitutes account for 80–90% of male gonococcal infections, whereas in post-war USA and Europe 'good time girls' replaced them (Guthe 1961, Pemberton et al.

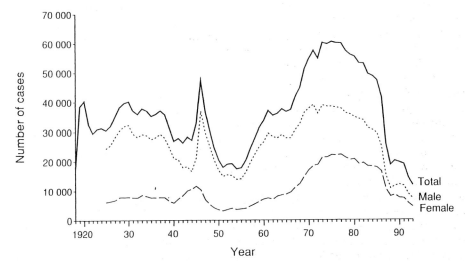

Fig. 33.1 Gonorrhoea – cases seen in Sexually Transmitted Disease Clinics, England and Wales 1918–1993 (figures obtained from CDSC London).

1972), but this trend has now reversed and a prostitution 'drugs for sex' culture is currently responsible for pockets of high gonorrhoea rates in North America and to a lesser extent in the UK.

Homosexual activities are often associated with high sexually transmitted disease (STD) infection rates (Sandholzer 1983). The vulnerability of male homosexuals to infection with human immunodeficiency virus is now generally recognized and the resulting drastic changes in practice have been mirrored in significant decreases in gonorrhoea rates in many groups of these persons (Carne et al. 1987); alarmingly, a return towards earlier rates has been detected in some more recent surveys (Riley 1991).

The effect of more modern contraceptive practice on the incidence of gonorrhoea is complex and controversial. The frequency of intercourse and the number of partners have been seen to be high amongst women who use oral contraception (Juhlin and Lidén 1969). Moreover, the steep rise in gonorrhoea rates in Norway occurred 5 years after that in Sweden. In both countries it was temporally related to the licensing of oral contraception (Danielsson 1990). Intrauterine devices offer the same convenience and will probably have the same effect; moreover, these devices are associated with increased risk of salpingitis. By contrast, oral contraception appears to protect against this complication, possibly by plugging the cervical os with mucus. Barrier methods are less convenient, but are known to protect against gonorrhoea (Barlow 1977, Weller 1993). A massive fall in gonorrhoea rates in Sweden followed an active publicity campaign aimed at encouraging the use of condoms. This predated AIDS-related campaigns as the graphs published by Danielsson (1990) confirm.

1.4 Pathogenesis

By far the commonest method of infection is by sexual intercourse. The risk of men contracting infection varies with the number of exposures to infectious females. Hooper and coworkers (1978) estimated a rate of 10% for one exposure, rising to 57% for 4 exposures or more. This study was not fully controlled, but it appeared that black American males were at greater risk (53% for one exposure) than their white compatriots. Holmes, Johnson and Trostle (1970) estimated the risk at 22% and considered that males were probably at greatest risk from menstruating females. Challenge experiments suggest that over 10^3 colony-forming units (cfu) are required reliably to infect the male urethra (Brinton et al. 1978). The number of gonococci present in the vagina seems to be highly variable. Lowe and Kraus (1976) isolated numbers ranging from 4.0×10^2 to 1.8×10^7 cfu. The risk of infection for women exposed to infected men has not been as thoroughly investigated, but those who may have been exposed on more than one occasion have infection rates of between 92% and 59% (Thin, Williams and Nicol 1970, Wright and Daunt 1973).

Once transferred, the gonococci rapidly attach to mucosal cells; micturition after intercourse will not remove them. Clearly the organisms show a marked ability to adhere to human cells, especially the squamocolumnar cells of the uterine cervix. Considerable evidence has accumulated that pili facilitate the adhesion of gonococci to a range of human cells in vitro (Punsalang and Sawyer 1973, Ward, Watt and Roberston 1974, Mårdh and Weström 1976). It seems that pili on infectious gonococci can overcome the electrostatic forces of repulsion between the negatively charged bacterial surface and the sialic acid on the surface of the host cell, and can bind the organism loosely to the cell surface (Heckels et al. 1976). Each pilus consists of up to 10 000 identical, predominantly hydrophobic protein subunits of c. 20.3 kDa, which contain many conserved areas and a small number of highly variable sites (Robertson, Vincent and Ward 1977, Brinton et al. 1978). Shifts in expressed pilus antigens occur during the course of infection (Seifert et al. 1994), allowing the organisms to move from one tissue location to another by altering their tropisms (Jonsson et al. 1994). These result from shuffling and recombination of multiple silent incomplete copies of *pilS* genes with a single intact pilin gene complete with promoter sequence (Bergström et al. 1986). In laboratory culture pilated gonococci produce small domed colonies classified as type 1 and type 2 by Kellogg et al. (1963) or P^+ and P^{++} colonies by Swanson (1978), who refined Kellogg's classification. On laboratory subculture pilated gonococci give rise to non-pilated variants. These produce flatter colonies which were classified as type 3 and type 4 by Kellogg and as P^- by Swanson. Non-pilated strains of gonococci are more susceptible to phagocytosis and are unable to infect human volunteers (Kellogg et al. 1968), but loss of pili may be of advantage to gonococci once within their host. This variation is known as phase change. It occurs in vitro at a frequency of 1×10^{-3}. Two recently recognized associated high molecular weight (c. 110 kDa) proteins, $PilC_1$ and $PilC_2$, are coded by 2 closely related genes. These may take part in pilus adhesion or may be involved in phase variation (Jonsson, Nyberg and Normark 1991).

When the organisms are loosely attached to host cells other factors come into play. These include non-specific mechanisms such as the mutual attraction of hydrophobic moieties on cell and bacterial surfaces and also more specific mechanisms. Gonococcal outer-membrane protein II (opacity protein or Opa) occurs on the cell wall and appears to be concerned in this process (Bessen and Gotschlich 1986). Its presence is associated with opaque colonial (Opa$^+$) forms. A single strain of gonococcus may produce many different variants of the protein during the course of an infection but at times may form none at all (Swanson 1982) and then gives rise to transparent (Opa$^-$) colonies. Kellogg's type 2 and 3 colonial forms are opaque. These correspond to O^+ and O^{++} colonies of Swanson, whereas types 1 and 4 correspond to Swanson's O^- (transparent) classification. There are 11 complete copies of the *opa* genes in each gonococcal cell, each with unique sequences and its own intact promoter sequence. Expression of a particular Opa protein results from slipped-strand mispairing during DNA replication of pentameric repeat (CTCTT) codons that result in a translational frame shift (Murphy et al. 1989). Any number of genes may be expressed at a given moment, depending of whether they have shifted into or out of frame, so that a cell may produce several different Opa proteins at the same time or none at all. Presence of the protein correlates with ability to adhere to host cells, the ligands involved being asiolectins, and different antigenic variants of the protein appear to impart abilities to adhere to different cell types (Lambden et al. 1979). Gonococci isolated during different phases of the menstrual cycle and from different anatomical sites in the same patient may show differences in protein II content and composition (Swanson 1983) and during the course of an infection different proteins II will be expressed sequentially. These findings suggest that variations that occur within an infecting strain help it to spread to different tissues as it colonizes its host. Antibodies to this protein correlate with a reduced risk of salpingitis (Plummer et al. 1994). For a review see Nassif and Magdalene (1995).

The outer layers of gonococci include much endotoxin. This incorporates a lipo-oligosaccharide that is clearly toxic to host cells. This also undergoes antigenic variation during the course of an infection, varying in molecular weight from 3.6 to 4.8 kDa with corresponding changes in antigenicity (Yamasaki et al. 1994). Different molecular weights of this substance also alter the spatial arrangements of other structures on the gonococcal surface, so altering exposed molecules and susceptibilities. The 4.8 kDa form can be chemically modified (sialylated) by bacterial 2,3-sialyltransferase acting on CMP′N′-acetylneuraminic acid present in host tissues. This protects it from the killing action of normal human serum (Smith, Cole and Parsons 1992) and generates an epitope that mimics one present on host cells, so aiding virulence (Mandrell et al. 1990, Schneider et al. 1991) and offering a possible explanation of the differing susceptibilities to gonorrhoea of persons of different blood groups (Kinane et al. 1983).

Some host cells are probably damaged by gonococcal endotoxin in their local environment (Gregg, Melly and McGee 1980), but others are invaded by the organism. The organisms become attached to the microvilli of the cell membrane (Ward, Watt and Robertson 1974, McGee, Johnson and Taylor-Robinson 1981) and it is possible that the major outer-membrane protein (protein I) may insert into the host cell membrane (Blake 1985). The organisms then enter the cells as a result of a phagocytic process (endocytosis) and multiply. This causes cell death and the organisms are released into the subepithelial tissue. Shifts in the antigenic structure of the outer layer of the organism during this process assist in the tissue tropism requirements and in evading immune and phagocytic defences.

It is clear that gonococci can survive and multiply within epithelial cells but their fate in polymorphs is less certain. Phagocytosed gonococci abound in urethral and cervical pus. They are present within phagosomes in these cells and degranulation into these phagosomes has been demonstrated, with dead organisms present in the vacuoles. However, some polymorphs can be found that contain large numbers of organisms, apparently damaged and releasing viable gonococci. Experiments in vitro reveal that the vast majority of phagocytosed organisms are killed (Drutz 1978) and it is to be expected that most die in vivo. However, it has been shown that some will survive phagocytosis (Casey, Shafer and Spitzangel 1986) and Novotny and colleagues (1977) demonstrated so-called 'infectious units' that may represent surviving gonococci in the remains of dead polymorphonuclear cells; these are protected from host attack and can invade epithelial cells.

Spread to the fallopian tube seems to occur mainly at the time of menstruation. Whether this is due to hormonal or epithelial changes is unknown. However, strains isolated from the salpinges tend to be of phenotypes that lack protein II, but also genetically similar, being of relatively non-fastidious auxotypes, and that carry protein I of subgroup WI (Buchanan et al. 1980). In these respects they differ from strains that tend to produce overt lower genital tract inflammation with discharge; they are usually of subgroup WII/III and are very sensitive to the killing action of human serum.

Normal human serum contains antibodies produced as a result of exposure to commensal Enterobacteriaceae. These bind to gonococcal lipo-oligosaccharide and, by fixing complement, lyse the cells. Certain strains of gonococci have particular abilities to resist this action and to spread to distant sites, so producing the DGI syndromes. Organisms isolated from such sites are of the transparent-colony phenotype and usually form a particular protein I of subgroup WI (Hildebrandt et al. 1978). They are highly susceptible to penicillin (Wiesner et al. 1973) and require arginine, hypoxanthine and uracil for growth (Knapp and Holmes 1975). They are resistant to the killing action of normal serum (Schoolnik, Buchanan and Holmes 1976) in the presence of a 'blocking antibody' in serum which acts by preventing the complement fixing bactericidal antibodies from gaining access to gonococcal oligosaccharides by binding with an antigenically constant porin protein (protein III) present on the cell surface.

Host factors also play a part in dissemination of the gonococcus. Acquired specific antibody to protein I prevents repeated attacks of salpingitis due to the same type of protein I-containing gonococci and also protects against DGI by these strains (Buchanan et al. 1980). Complement and natural non-specific antibodies also have a significant role in preventing dissemination. Thus, families with deficiencies of the terminal components of the complement pathway show a significant liability to develop bacteraemia caused by gonococci or meningococci (Petersen et al. 1979, Forster et al. 1987). Hormonal influences must play a part in spread within the body, but these are probably indirect. Direct effects on the organisms have been demonstrated, with oestrogens enhancing growth and testosterone and progesterone inhibiting it. Because the inhibiting agents have more effect on Opa⁺ than on Opa⁻ colonies, the latter should predominate in the second half of the menstrual cycle. The quantities of hormone used in making these observations were higher than physiological levels and their relevance to human infection is not clear (Salit 1982). Similarly the effects of race are apparent but are difficult to interpret. Afro-Caribbean races seem more prone to infection than caucasians, but this may be due solely to increased frequency of blood group B amongst blacks, which seems to confer vulnerability to infection (Kinane et al. 1983). In addition, however, the auxotypes of gonococci that circulate in the respective communities seem to be different. Whilst temporal variations occur, auxotypes associated with symptomless and disseminated infection are common in white populations and those associated with overt genital infections are more common in black populations (Noble and Parekh 1983).

REPRODUCTION OF THE DISEASE IN MAN AND ANIMALS

Bumm (1885) produced infection in man by instilling a pure culture of gonococci into the urethra but others have not always been successful. Mahoney and colleagues (1946) obtained unpredictable results and they were more successful in reproducing the disease in male volunteers with gonococcal pus than with cultures. Gonococci change on subculture. In 1904 Lipschütz reported changes in the colonial morphology on subculture and these were investigated in great detail by Raven in 1934. The changes were known as 'dissociation' of the gonococci and Hill (1948) associated them with loss of virulence. It was, however, left to Kellogg and his coworkers (1963, 1968) to demonstrate that gonococci from clinical cases produced small colonies and were able to give rise to infection in volunteers. These were later shown to be pilated by Jephcott, Reyn and Birch-Andersen (1971).

The male chimpanzee can be infected intraurethrally with gonococci of the small colony type and can then transmit gonorrhoea sexually to a female cage mate (Brown, Lucas and Kuhn 1972), but convenient and inexpensive means of reproducing gonococcal infection of the mucosae are not available. Much use has therefore been made of animal models with a less close resemblance to the natural disease. The successful use of subcutaneous chambers in guinea pigs and mice was described by Arko (1973). Fertile hens' eggs inoculated intravenously or into the allantoic space and intracerebral inoculation of mice have been employed but difficulties in distinguishing toxic effects from true infection limit their usefulness.

1.5   Bacteriological diagnosis

The diagnosis of gonorrhoea rests on demonstrating the presence of the causative organisms. In acute infections, typical clusters of gram-negative intracellular diplococci in smears taken from genital exudate afford a good presumptive diagnosis. By this means it is possible to detect about 95% of infections in males but only 50–60% of those in females (Barlow and Phillips 1978). Cultural methods are therefore usually employed in addition; these are slower but have the advantage of making it possible to test strains for their antibiotic susceptibility. Other methods of direct detection of gonococci are increasingly becoming available. These do not require viable gonococci and are particularly appropriate where speed of diagnosis is required or prolonged transit of specimens is necessary.

Sites to be examined should include the urethra and cervix in the female and the urethra in the male. Repeated culture tests may be required, but Jephcott and Raschid (1978) found that 99% of cases could be diagnosed by means of 2 culture tests. Inclusion of a rectal swab increases isolation rates in women (Thin and Shaw 1979) and is necessary in the male homosexual; the pharynx should be examined in either sex if this is thought appropriate. Koch (1948) reported that cervical cultures were most likely to be positive during the oestrogenic phase of the menstrual cycle when the cervical mucus is almost neutral in reaction, but Falk and Krook (1967) found no such relationship. In men, first-voided urine is more easily obtained, gives excellent results and is a socially acceptable substitute for the urethral swab (Feng, Medeiros and Murray 1977).

Gonococci are particularly sensitive to desiccation and oxidation in air. Hence swabs should either be plated out immediately, or they should be placed in Stuart's or Amies's transport medium in which they will remain viable for 12 h and frequently for much longer. Reyn, Korner and Bentzon (1960) recovered gonococci from artificially infected swabs in Stuart's medium after storage for 72 h at 23–25°C. Wooden swab sticks should be boiled in Sørensen's buffer (pH 7.4) and the swabs should be coated with charcoal to absorb toxic substances (probably fatty acids) present in the transport medium (Moffett, Young and Stuart 1948). Inoculated plates may be incubated immediately or transported before incubation.

METHODS OF CULTURE

Gonococci require humid conditions, an atmosphere containing between 3 and 10% carbon dioxide and a temperature of incubation of 35–36°C (Reyn 1965). Media should be nutritious. The choice of basal medium is not critical but it should be enriched with 5–10% heated or freeze-thaw lysed blood. Serum, yeast extract or IsoVitaleX (Difco) alone or in combination may be added.

Antibiotics may be incorporated to render the medium selective for gonococci. Their usefulness depends on the degree of contamination likely to be encountered. This in turn reflects the site of sampling. Thus rectal and pharyngeal swabs must be plated on to selective media. The degree of contamination also reflects the skill with which swabs are taken and the degree of colony separation obtained during the plating-out process. The usual antibiotics added are vancomycin 3 μg ml^{-1}, colistin 7.5 μg ml^{-1}, trimethoprim 3–8 μg ml^{-1} and nystatin 12.5 μg ml^{-1}. Addition of these antibiotics is the basis of the traditional Thayer–Martin medium for the isolation of gonococci (Thayer and Martin 1966).

The *env* mutant gonococci will not grow on selective media. Reyn and Bentzon (1972) reported that some 5% of strains were susceptible to the concentration of vancomycin used and recommended the use of a non-selective plate in parallel. Jephcott (1977) showed that if a single medium is employed it should be only moderately selective. Lincomycin 1 μg ml^{-1} in place of vancomycin is used in modified New York Medium (Young 1978) and similar media are gaining popularity because this antibiotic appears to be less toxic to gonococci. For comparative studies of the efficacies of isolation and of transport media see Taylor and Phillips (1980).

Direct inoculation of culture plates in the clinic is advocated as the method of choice to avoid premature death of gonococci on swabs. This can present logistical problems and transport-cum-culture systems have been designed to overcome the disadvantages of conventional direct plating systems while retaining their advantages. The original system, which employed a pregassed bottle (Transgrow) was described by Martin and Lester (1971). Developments that use small plates (Martin and Jackson 1975) or slides (Till-u-Test) (Donald 1980), with a citric acid–sodium bicarbonate tablet to produce carbon dioxide and which retain this in a gas-impermeable plastic envelope, are more popular. They are expensive and at present find little use in clinic practice in the United Kingdom but they are widely used in the USA.

IDENTIFICATION OF CULTURED GONOCOCCI

Plates should be examined after 24–48 h of incubation. Gonococci appear as small greyish-white oxidase-positive colonies. The bacteria show their diplococcal appearance to a far lesser extent than in vivo. Organisms with these characteristics grown from genital sites on selective culture media have been designated 'presumptive gonococci' by Schroeter and Pazin (1970). They have a very high probability of being gonococci. For a review of cultural diagnosis see Young (1981) and Knapp and Rice (1995).

Carbohydrate degradation tests

The tests used may depend on changes in the substrate during growth of the organism or they may be rapid methods in which a very heavy inoculum of bacteria containing preformed enzymes is added to lightly buffered solutions of sugars with an indicator of pH change. In the latter, acid production can usually be detected after incubation for 2–3 h. Comparative studies of various methods have been reported by Shtibel and Toma (1978). Dillon, Carballo and Pauze (1988) evaluated many commercially available test kits based on these principles.

Immunofluorescence staining

This method was described by Deacon and colleagues (1960). Young cultures should be examined and brilliant fluorescence of the periphery of individual gonococci can be seen. Results are rapid and compare favourably with slower sugar degradation tests (Lind 1969); pure cultures are not essential. Tests by blind sampling of 18 h cultures give satisfactory results (Danielsson 1963). The use of monoclonal antibodies (Welch and Cartwright 1988) originally improved sensitivity and specificity but with time it has become apparent that certain strains currently circulating are not detected by these antibodies. Thus Beebe and colleagues (1993) observed that 4.6% of strains of *N. gonorrhoeae* that reacted with a polyclonal reagent failed to react with the monoclonal antibodies; Turner, Gough and Jephcott (1995) found up to 20% of isolates to be unreactive. Both groups of authors concluded that this test was unsuitable as the sole means of identifying cultured gonococci in their localities.

Coagglutination

Identification of cultured gonococci by coagglutination of antibody-coated staphylococci on a slide, originally described by Danielsson and Kronvall in 1974, is simple and quick. Young and Reid (1984) and Anand, Gubash and Shaw (1988) compared polyclonal and monoclonal variants of the test and found the original monoclonal and the polyclonal systems both gave over 97.5% agreement; however, they noted that one pool of monoclonal antibodies no longer detected all circulating strains, whereas another retained its high sensitivity. The problem of varying responses to serological reagents was addressed by Evins et al. (1988).

Chromogenic enzyme substrates

D'Amato and colleagues (1978) developed a system of chromogenic substrates that identified cultured gonococci within a few hours. This has now been refined as the basis of the Gonochek II (E Y Laboratories Inc, San Mateo CA. USA) and was found to give 100% agreement with 80 neisserial isolates tested by Brown and Thomas (1985). This method is in widespread use in diagnostic laboratories but reactions obtained are not unique to gonococci. For this reason the system must be used only for specimens isolated on selective media (*Neisseria sicca* and *Neisseria mucosa* give misleading results). The enzymes detected are γ-glutamyl aminopeptidase, prolyl aminopeptidase and β-galactosidase.

Nucleic acid hybridization

A synthetic oligonucleotide probe specific for gonococcal rRNA has been developed by Rossau and colleagues (1990) and a biotinylated DNA probe (Ortho Diagnostic Systems, Neckargemund FRG) evaluated by Näher, Kohl and Petzoldt (1989) was found to identify 100% of test strains of gonococci but to be insufficiently specific for routine use.

Direct detection of gonococci in women

Cultural methods are reliable and sensitive but require several days to yield an answer. In men almost all cases can be diagnosed rapidly by a gram-stained film and other rapid techniques are therefore hard to justify. However, large numbers of infections in women remain undiagnosed by this method (Thin and Shaw 1979) and accordingly other techniques have been investigated. Antigen has been sought directly by fluorescent antibody techniques, but even the most effective monoclonal antibody system detected only 65–72% of infected sites in women (Ison et al. 1985). Antigen has also been sought directly by the enzyme-linked immunosorbent assay (ELISA) method (Gonozyme, Abbott Laboratories, Chicago, IL, USA). In men, results are no better than with a gram film, but in women, Danielsson, Moi and Forslin (1983) found results almost as good as those obtainable by culture. They suggested that the test might have a place as a rapid alternative to culture in women, especially where transport delays are a problem. Possible cross-reactions limit its usefulness for examining material from rectal and pharyngeal sites and the proportion of false-positive results produced by this test in low prevalence populations limits its usefulness in such groups (Nachamkin et al. 1984).

Nucleic acid hybridization by ribosomal RNA probing is now available commercially as the Gen-Probe PACE 2 system (Gen Probe Inc, San Diego, CA, USA). Vlaspolder and colleagues (1993) found it very quick and more sensitive and reliable than culture. The system uses chemiluminescence rather than radioactivity and will undoubtedly find a place where cost is not the limiting factor. A radioactive system for DNA plasmid probing was described by Perine and coworkers (1985). This worked admirably as a reference laboratory system for screening populations on a different continent, but is not a practicable proposition for a diagnostic laboratory.

Serological diagnosis of gonorrhoea

In the pre-antibiotic era, chronic or complicated gonorrhoea was common and serological tests were widely used as aids to diagnosis. With the introduction of effective therapy infections are cut short before much antibody is formed. As a result of this and of improved selective media for the isolation of the gonococci, serological tests have been relegated to a minor place or abandoned completely in many laboratories.

After the original observations of Müller and Oppenheim (1906), complement-fixation tests with suspensions or crude extracts of gonococci were used for many years. These presented a wide array of antigens but were not very sensitive in uncomplicated infections (ranging from 10 to 50%) and also gave non-specific results; in complicated infections sensitivity rose to approximately 60%. More recent experience with the test is reviewed by Young, Henrichsen and McMillan (1980). Much work has since been directed to the use of defined gonococcal antigens, including pilus (Buchanan et al. 1973, Reimann and Lind 1977) and outer-membrane protein antigens in radioimmunoassay, ELISA and haemagglutination tests (Glynn and Ison 1978). Serum IgG, IgM and IgA antibodies are produced during gonococcal infection; their detection as an aid to diagnosis has been studied by immunofluorescence (Welch and O'Reilly 1973, McMillan et al. 1979a) and by ELISA tests (Ison and Glynn 1979). Other approaches have been directed to the detection of IgA antibody in secretions (McMillan et al. 1979b, 1980) which occur together with local IgG. IgM antibodies are found less often and then only in very recent infections (McMillan et al. 1979a).

Many of these new methods are much more sensitive than the original complement-fixation test and may give useful results in high-risk groups, but they are not entirely satisfactory. They do not distinguish present from past infections and may cross-react with antibodies to meningococci. Toshach (1978), for example, obtained positive serological results in flocculation and immunofluorescence tests for gonorrhoea in 35% of meningococcal carriers who gave no clinical or bacteriological evidence of gonorrhoea. This limits the value of these tests as screening methods for detecting unsuspected latent infections. They may be of use in the investigation of patients with suspected complications of gonorrhoea, such as salpingitis or disseminated infection, if a rise in titre can be demonstrated. However, their role is subordinate to the isolation of gonococci in culture and, despite the advantage they offer of diagnosing gonorrhoea without the need for a genital examination, the only current need for a serological test is to monitor antibody production by potential vaccines. For a review of serological tests see Ison (1987).

1.6   Chemotherapy and resistance

Treatment of gonorrhoea was revolutionized by the introduction of the sulphonamides (Dees and Colston 1937) but resistant strains emerged rapidly and within less than a decade these agents were almost invariably ineffective (Campbell 1944). They were replaced by penicillin which had then just become available. At first all strains were susceptible to small doses of penicillin but in 1959 Reyn, Korner and Bentzon (1958) found strains 20 times less sensitive than the most resistant encountered in 1944, with a 200-fold variation between the most sensitive and most resistant strains. In parts of the world where antibiotic therapy was not closely regulated, notably the Far East and Africa, this increase in resistance continued, so that by 1969 decreased sensitivity (minimum inhibitory concentration (MIC) >0.1 mg 1^{-1}) was detected in 77% of isolates in the Philippines by Keys, Halverson and Clarke (1969) and 18% showed an MIC >0.5 mg 1^{-1}. At about the same time, only c. 35% of strains from England and Norway had a MIC >0.1 mg 1^{-1} and MICs exceeding 1 mg 1^{-1} were very rare (Gundersen, Ødegaard and Gjessing 1969, Seth, Kolator and Wilkinson 1979). This insensitivity to penicillin was often associated with increased resistance to streptomycin, tetracycline, erythromycin, rifampicin and chloramphenicol. It was the result of additive effects of a number of chromosomal mutations, including those at the *penA*, *penB* and *mtr* loci (Sparling, Sarubbi and Blackman 1975). Mutations at the *env* locus have the reverse effect, increasing sensitivity and cell wall permeability and are unlinked, but resistance mutations to other drugs occur at loci close together on the chromosome. For a review of this subject see Johnson and Morse (1988). Gonococci that show this form of resistance have been designated 'chromosomally resistant *Neisseria gonorrhoeae*' (CMRNG); the MIC of penicillin for these strains rarely exceeds 1 mg l^{-1}, but Shtibel (1980) reported the isolation of strains in Canada with an MIC of 30 mg l^{-1}. In the USA CMRNG strains represented 6.4% of all gonococci in a 1991 survey (Gorwitz et al. 1993). In non-metropolitan United Kingdom they are responsible for approximately 1% of infections, but are more frequent in the capital where imported strains are more common (Ison et al. 1994).

Strains of gonococci totally resistant to penicillin through the production of a β-lactamase (PPNG) were first reported in American servicemen returning from the Far East (Ashford, Golash and Hemming 1976) and in a patient from West Africa (Phillips 1976). The origin of PPNG is obscure but evidence suggests that they arose in the Philippines in early 1976. Such strains have since been found to be very prevalent in the Philippines, Singapore, Thailand and West Africa; they have been carried to the rest of the world but have not become universally established. Lower levels of infection with PPNG have been experienced in western countries where effective alternative therapies are available. Numbers of PPNG detected in the UK reached a peak at 1223 in 1983 and have fallen steadily since; fewer than 200 strains were detected in 1993 (Communicable Diseases Surveillance Centre, London, unpublished data). Imported cases represent less than half the infections currently seen in the United Kingdom. In the USA rates appear to be higher: 13.1% of strains produced penicillinase in a 1991 survey (Gorwitz et al. 1993).

Penicillinase production is plasmid-mediated. Originally strains from the Far East carried a 4400 kDa plasmid and were of prototrophic or proline-requiring auxotypes, whereas those from Africa carried a 3200 kDa plasmid and were of arginine-requiring auxotypes (Siegel et al. 1978). Both plasmids have a non-transposable region homologous to part of the TnA transposon, including that coding for the TEM1 β-lactamase. The 3200 kDa plasmid represents a deletion of non-TnA elements of the larger plasmid (Dickgeisser, Bennett and Richmond 1982) which probably originates from a TnA transposon insertion into a cryptic plasmid from *Haemophilus parainfluenzae* (Brunton, Clare and Meir 1986). In addition, one-half of the Far Eastern strains carried a 24 500 kDa transfer plasmid. As time has passed these distinct patterns have become blurred. Strains that carry plasmids of 3200 and 24500 kDa have been recognized (Dillon and Pauze 1981, van Embden et al. 1981) and the strict

relationships of auxotype and plasmid pattern have been lost, which suggests considerable evolution among strains. Subsequently plasmids of 2900 and 3050 kDa, the so-called Rio and Toronto plasmids, were reported, respectively from Holland and Canada (van Embden, Dessens-Kroon and van Klingeren 1985, Yeung et al. 1986). These appear to be deletion mutants of the 4400 kDa plasmid. Similarly, an insertion mutant of the 3200 kDa plasmid, the Nimes plasmid, was identified by Gouby, Bourg and Ramuz (1986). These remain uncommon but other variants may well be detected (for review see Dillon and Yeung 1989).

Treatment is usually given before sensitivity test results are known, if indeed they are carried out. It is recommended that agents are used that will be successful in over 95% of cases (Handsfield et al. 1992). In non-metropolitan Britain resistant strains are relatively uncommon and oral amoxycillin 3.5 g remains effective. In the capital, where resistance rates are higher, oral ciprofloxacin 0.5 g is often used. The regimens recommended by the USA Department of Health and Human Services are ceftriaxone 125 mg, or cefixime 400 mg, ciprofloxacin 500 mg or ofloxacin 400 mg orally (Centers for Disease Control 1993).

Infections with known or suspected penicillinase-producing or penicillin-resistant strains can be treated with the β-lactamase-stable cephalosporins (cefuroxime, cefotaxime, or ceftriaxone) or with ciprofloxacin or spectinomycin. Resistance to spectinomycin occurs as a result of a single major mutation; pencillinase-producing strains that are resistant to spectinomycin have been detected (Ashford et al. 1981) but no recent isolates resistant to spectinomycin have been reported. Some CMRNG show a reduced sensitivity to some second generation cephalosporins; this may in the future become clinically significant.

Chromosomally mediated resistance to tetracycline may be of the order of 2–4 mg l^{-1} and occasionally higher. Strains with a MIC >16 mg l^{-1} were reported by Knapp et al. (1987). Such strains carry plasmids of 25 200 kDa that appeared to be recombinants of the 24 500 kDa plasmid with the *tetM* determinant from streptococci (Morse et al. 1986), but this has been disputed by Gascoyne, Heritage and Hawkey (1990) who demonstrated major differences between these plasmids. Detection of these strains emphasizes the need for frequent monitoring of antibiotic sensitivities and of treatment failure rates. Two types of this plasmid now are recognized, so-called American and Dutch, representing 2 different mosaics of the pre-existing *tetM* plasmid. Whereas these strains are relatively uncommon in the UK, they accounted for 7.8% of strains examined in the USA in 1991; of these, approximately one-third also carried a penicillinase plasmid (Gorwitz et al. 1993).

Ciprofloxacin has become the preferred drug in many areas of the world where penicillin and tetracycline resistance are common. Unfortunately this has created a selection pressure for resistance to this drug and increasing levels of chromosomally mediated resistance are seen. As a result strains resistant to the current dose of ciprofloxacin are being encountered in the UK (Birley, McDonald and Fletcher 1994).

1.7 Prevention

The current world-wide epidemic of gonorrhoea is showing signs of successful control, at least in the developed world. Active measures are aimed at rapid detection and treatment of cases and the prompt and energetic tracing of their contacts, both the primary (source) contact and secondary contacts who have subsequently been exposed to infection. Contact tracing must be put in place in conjunction with campaigns to reduce the frequency of indiscriminate unprotected sexual intercourse between casual or multiple sex partners. Active case finding and treatment of these and their contacts have been practised for many years, but it was not until the more recent campaigns to alter behaviour, promoted in response to the emerging AIDS pandemic, that it was possible to achieve significant reductions in gonorrhoea figures. These measures when combined have proved dramatically successful in western Europe and in the bulk of the population in the USA. In these groups gonorrhoea is now a very uncommon infection.

Vaccination

To be of value a vaccine would have to confer some immunity against a wide range of strains of gonococci and prevent the establishment of symptomless infections. It need not necessarily, however, entirely prevent infection; prevention of transmissibility or complications such as salpingitis might be more easily accomplished and could justify vaccination of certain risk groups. No current vaccine fulfils even these desiderata. Moreover, even if an effective vaccine could be developed, it is debatable whether its benefits would be outweighed by the increased levels of other sexually transmitted diseases that might follow vaccine protection against one specific venereal infection.

Strain-specific immunity to challenge after the use of a whole-cell vaccine in 4 chimpanzees was demonstrated by Arko et al. (1976). An autolysed whole-cell vaccine was tried in man by Greenberg and coworkers (1974); though it produced a good antibody response it gave no protection in a field trial. Since this survey, major ethical difficulties have prevented adequate clinical trials in man and, at best, laboratory-based trials have shown an increase in dose needed to infect (Brinton et al. 1982).

The outer layers of the gonococcus have now been intensively studied; because they are exposed to the host defences they seem likely vaccine candidates. Pilus vaccines have been investigated but their likelihood of success is not high because Tramont et al. (1979) showed that pilus antigens alter considerably as the organism passes from person to person and also within the same host. Pilus vaccine has been shown to induce measurable strain-specific immunity to challenge in human volunteers (Brinton et al. 1980, 1982) and a promise of success was obtained by Rothbard et al. (1985) who showed that synthetic peptides can produce a polyclonal antibody that inhibits homologous and heterologous gonococcal attachment to epithelial cells in vitro. However, a clinical trial with purified pili from a single strain that produced significant levels of cross-reactive antibody failed to show protection in men (Tramont et al. 1985). Protein I (PI) is the predominant outer-membrane constituent, comprising about 60% of the weight of the membrane fraction. There are limited numbers of serotypes of this protein. It is known that natural infection protects against repeated attacks of salpingitis due to gonococci with the same PI type (Buchanan et al. 1980). For these reasons it remains a preferred candidate for vaccine production. Purified PI is only weakly immunogenic (Buchanan et al. 1980) but monoclonal antibodies directed against conserved epitopes have proved protective in bactericidal and opsonic assays in vitro (Virji et al. 1987). Studies reported to the World Health Organization (1983) demonstrated production of specific antibody in volunteers.

Three other proteins that appear to be antigenically constant and occur only in pathogenic neisseriae offer themselves as protective antigens. These are: IgA protease (Mulks and Plaut 1978); H.8, a heat-modifiable protein of 30–31 kDa (Cannon et al. 1984); and an iron-binding protein of 37 kDa (Meitzner et al. 1987). Protein III, a porin component that forms a complex with protein I (Blake 1985), has also been considered as it is immunogenic and does not show antigenic heterogeneity. There is major doubt as to the wisdom of including this agent as it would induce 'blocking antibody' that would protect gonococci against the killing action of normal serum, such that a vaccine containing protein III might render the vaccinee more vulnerable to systemic spread of the gonococcus.

Gonococcal lipo-oligosaccharide antibody is bactericidal and could play an important role in vaccine protection (Rice and Kasper 1977). Seid and colleagues (1985) have shown that detoxified gonococcal lipo-oligosaccharide is not only immunogenic but will act as an adjuvant if coupled to pilus proteins in experimental vaccines. However, as with the other surface components, considerable antigenic shifts take place during the course of an infection, once again casting doubt on its suitability in practice.

The current status of gonorrhoeal vaccines was reviewed by Tramont (1989).

For general reviews of gonorrhoea, its incidence, epidemiology, pathogenesis, diagnosis and treatment, the reader is referred to Brooks and Donegan (1985), Sparling, Tsai and Cornelissen (1990) and Easmon and Ison (1991).

2 Chancroid

Chancroid is characterized by painful, soft, non-indurated ulcers that become covered with purulent exudate. They occur singly or in groups on the external genitalia and neighbouring regions. In about 30% of sufferers, inguinal buboes develop; these are very painful and can break down to produce deep, ragged-edged craters. Secondary lesions are frequent but further systemic spread does not occur. Occasionally superinfection with *Fusobacterium* spp. or *Bacteroides* spp. can lead to gangrenous phagedenic ulceration and extensive destruction of the external genitalia. Synonyms for the disease are chancre mou, soft sore, soft chancre and ulcus molle.

This disease is caused by *Haemophilus ducreyi*, a small gram-negative bacillus first described in smears by Ducrey (1890) at the University of Naples. He transferred infections in 3 patients from genital ulcer to forearm. It was cultured by Petersen in 1895 (see Himmel 1901). Istmanov and Akopiantz in 1897 (quoted in Himmel 1901) successfully reproduced the disease in human subjects with cultured organisms, and ulcerative lesions followed inoculation into monkeys and rabbits of cultures several generations removed from the primary isolation (Reenstierna 1921, Nicolle 1923). Recent observations suggest that lesions were the result of microbial toxicity rather than growth and that the body temperature of animals is too high to support growth in the tissues. Totten and colleagues (1994) reported successful infection of the foreskins of adult pigtailed macaques.

Infection is transmitted by sexual intercourse, probably through damaged areas of the skin, and ulcers are usually located at sites of genital trauma. In the United Kingdom approximately 60 cases are reported annually. The disease in the western hemisphere is primarily associated with travellers returning from Asia and Africa (Nayyar, Stolz and Michel 1979) where chancroid is considered to be endemic (Kibukamusoke 1965, Nsanze et al. 1981). Nevertheless, outbreaks are recognized from time to time in temperate climates (Lykke-Olesen et al. 1979, Hammond et al. 1980). It is clear that a changing pattern of infection is being experienced in the southern states of North America where an increasing incidence, from approximately 800 cases in 1967, to a peak of almost 5000 cases per annum in 1988, has been recognized. It is nevertheless still regarded as under-reported in the USA (Schulte, Martich and Schmid 1992) where it is associated with underprivileged populations, prostitution and drug abuse. Studies in the UK by McEntegart, Hafiz and Kinghorn (1982) suggested that the organism may be present in a wide variety of ulcerative genital conditions in temperate climates and may not necessarily be the primary pathogen but this has not been confirmed. American studies have, however, shown that over 10% of genital ulcers in which *H. ducreyi* was demonstrated also yielded evidence of *Treponema pallidum* or herpes simplex virus infection (Webb et al. 1995). There is also controversy about the symptomless carriage of the organism. Older studies suggested that *H. ducreyi* might be carried in the absence of lesions (Brams 1924, Saelhof 1925). More recent work failed to confirm this (Plummer et al. 1983, Messing et al. 1983), but suggested that symptomless females may form a significant source of infection (Taylor et al. 1984). The wheel has turned full circle and the organisms have now been detected in genital secretions of symptomless African prostitutes by polymerase chain reaction (PCR) technology (Hawkes et al. 1995). Chancroid is the commonest cause of genital ulceration in sub-Saharan Africa and plays a significant role in the epidemiology of human immunodeficiency virus infection in this part of the world (Piot and Laga 1989), being an important risk factor in its heterosexual transmission (Wasserheit 1992).

2.1 Bacteriological diagnosis

Part of the uncertainty about the epidemiology of chancroid results from difficulties in culturing the organism. Traditionally media heavily enriched with blood or serum, or consisting entirely of these, were used. Borchardt and Hoke (1970) even recommended the use of the patient's own serum as a culture medium and Deacon and colleagues (1956) recommended fresh clots of human or rabbit blood. These media were very vulnerable to contaminants; indeed, production of a secondary lesion on the patient's arm or thigh by auto-inoculation of genital secretions was commonly practised in order to obtain a pure culture. Matters were placed on a more certain footing by Hammond and colleagues (1978a) who developed a medium that was selective and did not rely solely on blood products. This consisted of gonococcal agar base with haemoglobin, IsoVitaleX 1% and vancomycin 3 mg l^{-1}. Nsanze et al. (1981) reported the isolation of *H. ducreyi* from 70% of patients with clinical chancroid in Kenya on this medium modified by the addition of 5% fetal calf serum. Sottnek et al. (1980) compared the efficacies of 5 isolation media and found vancomycin (3 mg l^{-1}) and fetal calf serum to be important, but Taylor and colleagues (1984) found horse blood with IsoVitaleX 1% most helpful. Serum may act by absorbing inhibiting substances and can be replaced with activated charcoal; haem may be replaced by catalase (Lockett et al. 1991, Totten and Stamm 1994). Moreover, it seems that differences in the peptone nitrogen source are of considerable importance (Ajello et al. 1956). It is clear that different formulations should be assessed for efficacy by any prospective user. Plates should be incubated at 35°C in moist conditions and with added CO_2.

The organisms can sometimes be identified by a characteristic 'school of fish' arrangement in smears from lesions and also from culture plates, but reliance on this as the sole means of diagnosis is responsible for much of our ignorance of the prevalence of the disease in the developing world. Colonies on solid culture medium are highly characteristic; up to 2 mm in size, domed and firmly cohesive, so that they may be pushed intact over the surface of the medium. This is a result of close intercellular adhesion (Morse 1989). Starch granules aggregate in the immediate vicinity of colonies; this can be helpful in recognizing the organisms on clear media (Sturm and Zanen 1984). Minimal criteria for identification include a requirement for haemin (X factor) which should be confirmed by the porphyrin test of Hammond et al. (1978b). Colonies are oxidase-positive when tested with *NNNN*-tetramethyl-*p*-phenylenediamine dihydrochloride, but are not so with the *NN* compound, and they are nitrate-positive. A positive test for alkaline phosphatase and negative tests for catalase, indole, urease and carbohydrate utilization will also be obtained. DNA probing has now been used to identify cultures.

A direct immunofluorescence test based on monoclonal antibodies directed against outer-membrane polypeptides of *H. ducreyi* was reported as an alternative to cultural diagnosis by Karim and colleagues (1989); Finn, Karim and Easmon (1990) described characterization of polyclonal and monoclonal antibodies that could be used as the basis for diagnostic reagents. Many polyclonal antisera cross-react with other bacterial species but the apparent poor specificity of antibody-based tests probably resulted from insensitive culture methods. Molecular techniques have also been applied experimentally to the direct detection of the organisms. DNA probes have been investigated by Parsons et al. (1989, 1990) but these do not seem to be sufficiently sensitive to detect the organism reliably in clinical materials. PCR techniques appear more specific (Chui et al. 1993) and a commercial kit is likely to become available in the near future (Orle et al. 1994).

The host immune response has been used in diagnosis. Thus, a delayed hypersensitivity skin test (the Ito–Reenstierna test) was used to aid diagnosis (Ito 1913, Reenstierna 1924, Cole and Levin 1935). A 0.2 ml injection of a killed bacterial suspension gave rise to a positive reaction in two-thirds of cases. Its usefulness was limited because the test tended to become positive late in primary infections and once positive remained so for life. Improved culture techniques have rendered it obsolete and the reagent is no longer commercially available. Numerous serological test have been devised, including several effective ELISA systems (see, for example, Desjardins et al. 1992). Persisting IgG antibodies make the tests unhelpful in the diagnosis of current infections (Alfa et al. 1992), but IgM antibodies appear more relevant.

2.2 Antibiotic treatment

Many isolates of *H. ducreyi* possess β-lactamase, which MacLean, Bowden and Albritton (1980) reported to be a TEM1 β-lactamase derived from a Tn*2* transposon. Brunton et al. (1979) described a 6000 kDa plasmid that codes for this. Handsfield et al. (1981) reported plasmids of 7300, 5700 and 3200 kDa, originating from different parts of the world. Brunton et al. (1982) showed that the larger plasmids are identical to the 2 types of *N. gonorrhoeae* plasmid except in that they carry the complete Tn*A* sequence. In certain areas of Africa all strains tested have been reported to produce penicillinase (Fast et al. 1982) and resistance to other antibiotics appears to be common. The *tet*M resistance factor has been detected in *H. ducreyi* (Roberts 1989), as in other genitourinary pathogens. It is located on a conjugative plasmid of 34 000 kDa similar to that of *N. gonorrhoeae* but this last lacks cer-

tain sequences and so is unlikely to be its source (Roberts 1990).

Sulphonamides and tetracyclines are most widely used for treatment but with variable results. Failures have been most common in infections originating in Asia. For these, Hart (1975) recommended streptomycin, kanamycin and cephalothin. Nayyar, Stolz and Michel (1979) obtained good results with trimethoprim and considered this the drug of choice; their findings were confirmed by Fast et al. (1982). The guidelines issued by the US Department of Health and Human Services (Centers for Disease Control 1993) advocate azithromycin, erythromycin or ceftriaxone, with ciprofloxacin or amoxycillin plus clavulanic acid as less well evaluated alternatives. Current World Health Organization recommendations include ceftriaxone, erythromycin and co-trimoxazole.

For extensive reviews of chancroid and *H. ducreyi* the reader is referred to Albritton (1989), Morse (1989) and Trees and Morse (1995).

3 GRANULOMA VENEREUM

This is a chronic, destructive, granulomatous condition of the superficial tissue of the genital region. It should not be confused with lymphogranuloma venereum but has many synonyms: the most widely used are granuloma inguinale and granuloma venereum; others include donovanosis, granuloma donovani, granuloma contagiosa, granuloma tropicum, granuloma pudendi tropicum and sclerosing granuloma.

The disease was probably first described in 1882 by McLeod (see Hart 1983) and the causative organism was first recognized by Donovan (1905) who described the characteristic intracellular bodies in smears from the ulcerated lesions, which he regarded as parasites. They have now been recognized as capsulated gram-negative bacilli. The organism defied attempts at culture until Anderson (1943) succeeded in growing it in the chick-embryo yolk sac. Subsequently, Dulaney, Guo and Packer (1948) grew the organism on slopes of heated Locke's solution and egg yolk, and Rake and Oskay (1948) succeeded with modified Levinthal agar. It was last successfully cultured in 1962 by Goldberg.

The cultured organism is a sometimes capsulated, moderately pleomorphic, large gram-negative rod with unipolar or bipolar staining. The electron microscopic appearance is that of a gram-negative rod (Davis 1970). Antigens are shared with *Escherichia* (Packer and Goldberg 1950). In tissue smears the organism occurs in multiple vacuoles inside large histiocytes and occasionally in polymorphonuclear or plasma cells (Dodson et al. 1974). These are known as Donovan bodies; they consist of bipolar staining rods measuring 1–2 μm × (0.5–0.7) μm surrounded by a capsule of variable size. Vacuoles may contain up to 30 bacteria before these are liberated by cell rupture. The correct name of the organism is *Calymmatobacterium granulomatis* (Aragao and Vianna 1913).

The incubation period is ill-defined and probably

varies between a few days and 2–3 years, but most infections manifest themselves within 3–40 days of exposure (Clarke 1947). The initial subcutaneous nodules break down to give ulcers that, unlike those of chancroid, are painless; they exhibit beefy red granulations. The ulcers slowly enlarge and may produce daughter lesions and result in much local tissue loss and scarring. Spread to the inguinal region can mimic lymphadenitis by producing a periadenitis (pseudobubo), but true bubo formation does not occur. Extensive scarring and pelvic fibrosis can result. Primary oral infection can occur (Garg et al. 1975) and distant spread to the face and involvement of the liver, thorax and bones (Kirkpatrick 1970) have been reported.

The venereal nature of transmission of this infection has been disputed; auto-infection from faecally carried organisms may play a part (Goldberg 1964). The disease appears to be only mildly contagious and repeated exposures are necessary for infection. Anal lesions occur after rectal intercourse (Marmell 1958). It may be difficult to distinguish the lesions clinically from carcinoma, amoebiasis and secondary syphilis, and a clinical form of chancroid closely resembles this condition (Verdich 1984).

Granuloma venereum is associated with a warm climate and poor personal hygiene. It is rarely reported in the UK and is uncommon in other developed countries but is frequently encountered in New Guinea, India, Africa and in the Caribbean islands (Kiraly 1973). It is reported to be increasing in South Africa (Freinkel 1990) but has all but disappeared from the southern states of the USA where it once was commonplace. A skin test with a reagent made from yolk sac cultures was described by Anderson, Goodpasture and de Monbreun (1945); a complement-fixation test was described by Rake (1948), who obtained positive results in 87% of clinical cases of granuloma inguinale, but also from 14% of patients with varicose or decubitus ulcers. These tests have little place today. Diagnosis is made by microscopic demonstration of Donovan bodies in biopsy specimens; these are best stained by the Leishman or Giemsa stains and can be seen in 60–80% of cases (von Haam 1938). Recently, immunofluorescent and immunoperoxidase reactions with patients' serum have been described (Afrika 1990). It is important to establish a firm diagnosis in cases of granuloma venereum, not only for its own sake, but to avoid misdiagnosing one of the conditions, mentioned above, that it may resemble clinically.

Spontaneous resolution has been reported (Pradinaud et al. 1981) but active treatment should be undertaken. The use of antimony has given way to antibiotics but sensitivity tests for these are not available and assessments have been empirical. Penicillin, ampicillin and cephalosporins are ineffective against the causal organism but can eliminate significant secondary infection. Tetracyclines are probably the most widely favoured drugs (World Health Organization 1981), with their more recent derivatives minocycline and doxycycline (Velasco, Miller and Zaias 1972), but chloramphenicol and thiamphenicol are also very effective. Erythromycin (Robinson and Cohen 1953), gentamicin and streptomycin (Greenblatt 1953) have been used successfully. Most recently, co-trimoxazole (Latif, Mason and Paraiwa 1988) and norfloxacin (Ramanan et al. 1990) have been found very effective.

The importance of this disease, in addition to the chronic ill health and disfigurement it can cause, has been redoubled by its role, along with other ulcerative venereal disease (Wasserheit 1992), as a major co-factor in the transmission of HIV infection. For a recent review see Richens (1991).

REFERENCES

Afrika DJ, 1990, Demonstration of Donovan bodies in lesions of granuloma inguinale using an immunoperoxidase method, *Med Technol S Afr*, **4:** 294–6.

Ajello GW, Deacon WE et al., 1956, Nutritional studies of a virulent strain of *Haemophilus ducreyi*, *J Bacteriol*, **72:** 802–8.

Albritton WL, 1989, Biology of *Haemophilus ducreyi*, *Microbiol Rev*, **53:** 377–89.

Alfa MJ, Olsen N et al., 1992, Use of an absorption enzyme immunoassay to evaluate the *Haemophilus ducreyi* specific and cross-reactive humoral immune response of humans, *Sex Transm Dis*, **19:** 309–14.

Anand CM, Gubash SM, Shaw H, 1988, Serologic confirmation of *Neisseria gonorrhoeae* by monoclonal antibody-based co-agglutination procedures, *J Clin Microbiol*, **26:** 2283–6.

Anderson K, 1943, The cultivation from granuloma inguinale of a microorganism having the characteristics of Donovan bodies in the yolk sac of chick embryos, *Science*, **97:** 560–1.

Anderson K, Goodpasture EW, de Monbreun WA, 1945, Immunologic relationship of *Donovania granulomatis* to granuloma inguinale, *J Exp Med*, **81:** 41–50.

Aragao H de B, Vianna G, 1913, Pesquizas sobre o granuloma venereo, *Mem Inst Oswaldo Cruz*, **5:** 211–38.

Arko RJ, 1973, Implantation and use of a subcutaneous culture chamber in laboratory animals, *Lab Anim Sci*, **23:** 105–6.

Arko RJ, Duncan WP et al., 1976, Immunity in infection with *Neisseria gonorrhoeae*, duration and serological response in the chimpanzee, *J Infect Dis*, **133:** 441–7.

Arya OP, Taber SR, Nsanze H, 1980, Gonorrhoea and female infertility in rural Uganda, *Am J Obstet Gynecol*, **138:** 929–32.

Ashford WA, Golash RG, Hemming VG, 1976, Penicillinase-producing *Neisseria gonorrhoeae*, *Lancet*, **2:** 657–8.

Ashford WA, Potts DW et al., 1981, Spectinomycin-resistant penicillinase producing *Neisseria gonorrhoeae*, *Lancet*, **2:** 1035–7.

Barlow D, 1977, The condom and gonorrhoea, *Lancet*, **2:** 811–12.

Barlow D, Phillips I, 1978, Gonorrhoea in women. Diagnostic clinical and laboratory aspects, *Lancet*, **1:** 761–4.

Bassam PC, 1966, Specific prophylaxis for gonorrhoeal ophthalmia neonatorum. A review, *N Engl J Med*, **274:** 731–4.

Beebe JL, Rau MP et al., 1993, Incidence of *Neisseria gonorrhoeae* isolates negative by Syva direct fluorescent antibody test but positive by Gen-Probe Accuprobe test in sexually transmitted disease clinic population, *J Clin Microbiol*, **31:** 2535–7.

Bergström S, 1990, Genital infections and reproductive health: infertility and morbidity of mother and child in developing countries, *Scand J Infect Dis*, **69, Suppl.:** 99–105.

Bergström S, Robbins K et al., 1986, Pilation control mechanisms in *Neisseria gonorrhoeae*, *Proc Natl Acad Sci USA*, **83:** 3890–4.

Bessen D, Gotschlich EC, 1986, Interactions of gonococci with HeLa cells: attachment, detachment, replication, penetration, and role of protein II, *Infect Immun*, **54:** 154–60.

Birley H, McDonald P, Fletcher J, 1994, High level ciprofloxacin resistance in *Neisseria gonorrhoeae*, *Genitourin Med*, **70**: 292–3.

Blake MS, 1985, Implications of the active role of gonococcal porins in disease, *The Pathogenic Neisseriae*, ed. Schoolnik GK, American Society for Microbiology, Washington, DC, 251–8.

Borchardt KA, Hoke AW, 1970, Simplified laboratory technique for the diagnosis of chancroid, *Arch Dermatol*, **102**: 188–92.

Brams J, 1924, Isolation of the Ducrey bacillus from the smegma of thirty men, *Trans Chicago Pathol Soc 1923–4*, **xii**: 84.

Branch G, Paxton R, 1965, A study of gonococcal infection among infants and children, *Public Health Rep*, **80**: 347–52.

Brinton CC, Bryan J et al., 1978, Uses of pili in gonorrhoea control, *Immunobiology of* Neisseria gonorrhoeae, eds Brooks CF, Gotschlich EC et al., American Society for Microbiology, Washington, DC, 155–78.

Brinton CC, Brown A et al., 1980, Preparation, testing, safety, antigenicity, immunogenicity and serological specificity of a purified gonococcal pilus vaccine for gonorrhea, *Current Chemotherapy and Infectious Diseases*, eds Nelson JD, Grassi C, American Society for Microbiology, Washington, DC, 1242.

Brinton CC, Wood SW et al., 1982, The development of a neisserial pilus vaccine for gonorrhea and meningococcal meningitis, *Semin Infect Dis*, **4**: 140.

Brooks GF, Donegan EA, eds, 1985, *Gonococcal Infection*, Edward Arnold, London.

Brown JD, Thomas KR, 1985, Rapid enzyme system for the identification of pathogenic *Neisseria* spp., *J Clin Microbiol*, **21**: 857–8.

Brown WJ, Lucas CT, Kuhn USG, 1972, Gonorrhoea in the chimpanzee. Infection with laboratory-passed gonococci and by natural transmission, *Br J Vener Dis*, **48**: 177–8.

Brunham RC, Plummer FA, 1990, A general model of sexually transmitted disease epidemiology and its implications for control, *Med Clin North Am*, **74**: 1339–52.

Brunton J, Clare D, Meier MA, 1986, Molecular epidemiology of antibiotic resistance plasmids of *Haemophilus* species and *Neisseria gonorrhoeae*, *Rev Infect Dis*, **8**: 713–24.

Brunton JL, MacLean I et al., 1979, Plasmid mediated ampicillin resitance in *Haemophilus ducreyi*, *Antimicrob Agents Chemother*, **15**: 294–9.

Brunton J, Meier M et al., 1982, Molecular epidemiology of beta-lactamase-specifying plasmids of *Haemophilus ducreyi*, *Antimicrob Agents Chemother*, **21**: 857–63.

Buchanan TM, Eschenbach DA et al., 1980, Gonococcal salpingitis is less likely to recur with *Neisseria gonorrhoeae* of the same outer membrane protein antigenic type, *Am J Obstet Gynecol*, **138**: 978–80.

Buchanan TM, Swanson J et al., 1973, Quantitative determination of antibody to gonococcal pili. Changes in antibody levels with gonococcal infection, *J Clin Invest*, **52**: 2896–909.

Bumm E, 1885, Menschliches Blutserum als Nahrboden für pathogene Microorganismen, *Dtsch Med Wochenschr*, **2**: 910–11.

Campbell DJ, 1944, Gonorrhoea in North Africa and Central Mediterranean, *Br Med J*, **2**: 44.

Cannon JG, Black WJ et al., 1984, Monoclonal antibody which recognizes an outer membrane antigen common to pathogenic *Neisseria* species but not most non-pathogenic *Neisseria* species, *Infect Immun*, **43**: 994–9.

Carne CA, Weller IVD et al., 1987, Prevalence of antibodies to human immunodeficiency virus, gonorrhoea rates and changed sexual behaviour in homosexual men in London, *Lancet*, **1**: 656–8.

Casey SG, Shafer WM, Spitzangel JK, 1986, *Neisseria gonorrhoeae* survives intraleukocytic oxygen independent antimicrobial capacities of anaeroic and aerobic granulocytes in the presence of pyocin lethal to extracellular gonococci, *Infect Immunol*, **52**: 384–9.

Centers for Disease Control, 1993, 1993 Sexually transmitted diseases treatment guidelines, *Morbid Mortal Weekly Rep*, **42 RR14**: 20–2 and 57–60.

Chui L, Albritton W et al., 1993, Development of the polymerase chain reaction for diagnosis of chancroid, *J Clin Microbiol*, **31**: 659–64.

Clarke CW, 1947, Notes on the epidemiology of granuloma inguinale, *J Vener Dis Inf*, **28**: 189–94.

Cole HN, Levin EA, 1935, Intradermal reaction for chancroids with chancroidal bubo pus, *JAMA*, **105**: 2040–4.

Curran JW, 1980, Economic consequences of pelvic inflammatory disease in the United States, *Am J Obstet Gynecol*, **138**: 848–51.

D'Amato RF, Eriquez LA et al., 1978, Rapid identification of *Neisseria gonorrhoeae* and *Neisseria meningitidis* by using enzymatic profiles, *J Clin Microbiol*, **7**: 77–81.

Danielsson D, 1963, The demonstration of *N. gonorrhoeae* with the aid of fluorescent antibodies, *Acta Derm Venerol (Stockh)*, **43**: 511–21.

Danielsson D, 1990, Gonorrhoea and syphilis in Sweden – past and present, *Scand J Infect Dis*, **69**: 69–76.

Danielsson D, Kronvall G, 1974, Slide agglutination method for the serological identification of *Neisseria gonorrhoeae* with anti-gonococcal antibodies absorbed to protein A-containing staphylococci, *Appl Microbiol*, **27**: 368–74.

Danielsson D, Moi H, Forslin L, 1983, Diagnosis of urogenital gonorrhoea by detecting gonococcal antigen with solid phase enzyme immunoassay (Gonozyme), *J Clin Pathol*, **36**: 674–7.

Davis CM, 1970, Granuloma inguinale. A clinical, histological and ultrastructural study, *JAMA*, **211**: 632–6.

Deacon WE, Albritton DC et al., 1956, V.D.R.L. Chancroid studies. 1. A simple procedure for the isolation and identification of *Haemophilus ducreyi*, *J Invest Dermatol*, **26**: 399–406.

Deacon WE, Peacock WL et al., 1960, Fluorescent antibody tests for the detection of the gonococcus in women, *Public Health Rep Washington*, **75**: 125–9.

Dees JE, Colston JAC, 1937, Use of sulfanilimide in gonococcic infections: preliminary report, *JAMA*, **108**: 1855–8.

Desjardins M, Thompson CE et al., 1992, Standardisation of enzyme immunoassay for human antibody to *Haemophilus ducreyi*, *J Clin Microbiol*, **30**: 2019–24.

Dickgeisser N, Bennett PM, Richmond MH, 1982, Penicillinase-producing *Neisseria gonorrhoeae*: a molecular comparison of 5.3 kb and 7.4 kb beta-lactamase plasmids, *J Bacteriol*, **151**: 1171–5.

Dillon J-A, Yeung K-H, 1989, β-Lactamase plasmids and chromosomally mediated antibiotic resistance in pathogenic *Neisseria* species, *Clin Microbiol Rev*, **2**: S125–33.

Dillon JR, Carballo M, Pauze M, 1988, Evaluation of eight methods for identification of pathogenic *Neisseria* species, *J Clin Microbiol*, **26**: 493–7.

Dillon JR, Pauze M, 1981, Appearance in Canada of *Neisseria gonorrhoeae* strains with a 3.2 megadalton pencillinase plasmid and a 24.5 megadalton transfer plasmid, *Lancet*, **2**: 700.

Dodson RF, Fritz GS et al., 1974, Donovanosis: a morphologic study, *J Invest Dermatol*, **62**: 611–14.

Donald WH, 1980, Assessment of the Till-u-Test GC slide, *Br J Vener Dis*, **56**: 81–2.

Donegan EA, 1985, Epidemiology of gonococcal infection, *Gonococcal Infection*, eds Brooks GF, Donegan EA, Edward Arnold, London, 186.

Donovan C, 1905, Ulcerating granuloma of the pudenda, *Indian Med Gaz*, **40**: 411–14.

Drutz DJ, 1978, Intracellular fate of *Neisseria gonorrhoeae*, *Immunobiology of* Neisseria gonorrhoeae, eds Brooks GF, Gotschlich EC et al., American Society for Microbiology, Washington, DC, 232–5.

Ducrey A, 1890, Recherches expérimentales sur la nature intime du principe contagieux du chancre mou, *Ann Dermatol Syphil (sér. 3)*, **1**: 56.

Dulaney AD, Guo K, Packer H, 1948, *Donovania granulomatis*: cultivation, antigen preparation and immunological tests, *J Immunol*, **59**: 335–40.

Easmon CSF, Ison CA, 1991, Current trends in the diagnosis and treatment of gonorrhoea, *Recent Advances in STD and AIDS*, 4th edn, eds Harris JWR, Forster SM, Churchill Livingstone, Edinburgh, 159–82.

Ekstrøm K, 1966, One hundred teenagers in Copenhagen infected with gonorrhoea, *Br J Vener Dis*, **42**: 162–6.

Ekstrøm K, 1970, Patterns of sexual behaviour in relation to venereal disease, *Br J Vener Dis*, **46**: 93–5.

van Embden JD, Dessens-Kroon M, van Klingeren B, 1985, A new beta-lactamase plasmid in *Neisseria gonorrhoeae*, *J Antimicrob Chemother*, **15**: 247–50.

van Embden JDA, van Klingeren B et al., 1981, Emergence in the Netherlands of penicillinase-producing gonococci carrying 'Africa' plasma in combination with transfer plasmid, *Lancet*, **1**: 938.

Evins GM, Pigott NE et al., 1988, Panel of reference strains for evaluation of reagents used to identify gonococci, *J Clin Microbiol*, **26**: 354–7.

Falk V, Krook G, 1967, Do results of culture for gonococci vary with sampling phase of menstrual cycle?, *Acta Derm Venereol (Stockh)*, **47**: 190–3.

Fast MV, Nsanze H et al., 1982, Treatment of chancroid by clavulanic acid with amoxycillin in patients with β-lactamase positive *Haemophilus ducreyi* infection, *Lancet*, **2**: 509–11.

Feng WC, Medeiros AA, Murray ES, 1977, Diagnosis of gonorrhoea in male patients by culture of uncentrifuged first-voided urine, *JAMA*, **237**: 896–7.

Finn GY, Karim QN, Easmon CSF, 1990, The production and characterisation of rabbit antiserum and murine monoclonal antibodies to *Haemophilus ducreyi*, *J Med Microbiol*, **31**: 219–24.

Forster GE, Pinching AJ et al., 1987, New microbial and host factors in disseminated gonococcal infection: case report, *Genitourin Med*, **63**: 169–71.

Freinkel AL, 1990, The enigma of granuloma inguinale in South Africa, *S Afr Med J*, **77**: 301–3.

Garg BR, Lal S et al., 1975, Donovanosis (granuloma inguinale) of the oral cavity, *Br J Vener Dis*, **51**: 136–7.

Gascoyne DM, Heritage J, Hawkey PM, 1990, The 25.2 MDa tetracycline-resistance plasmid is not derived from the 24.5 MDa conjugative plasmid of *Neisseria gonorrhoeae*, *J Anitmicrob Chemother*, **25**: 39–47.

Glynn AA, Ison C, 1978, Serological diagnosis of gonorrhoea by an enzyme-linked immunosorbent assay, *Br J Vener Dis*, **54**: 97–102.

Goldberg J, 1962, Studies on granuloma inguinale V. Isolation of a bacterium resembling *Donovania granulomatis* from the faeces of a patient with granuloma inguinale, *Br J Vener Dis*, **38**: 99–102.

Goldberg J, 1964, Studies on granuloma inguinale VII. Some epidemiological consideratons, *Br J Vener Dis*, **40**: 140–5.

Gorwitz R, Nakashima AK et al., 1993, Sentinel surveillance for antimicrobial resistance in *Neisseria gonorrhoeae* – United States 1988–91, *Morbid Mortal Weekly Rep*, **42 (3)**: 29–39.

Gouby A, Bourg G, Ramuz M, 1986, Previously undescribed 6.6 kilobase R plasmid in penicillinase producing *Neisseria gonorrhoeae*, *Antimicrob Agents Chemother*, **29**: 1095–7.

Greenberg L, Diena BB et al., 1974, Gonococcal vaccine studies in Inuvik, *Can J Public Health*, **65**: 29–33.

Greenblatt RD, 1953, *Management of Chancroid, Granuloma Inguinale and Lymphogranuloma Venereum*, Publication No. 225, US Public Health Service, Washington, DC.

Gregg CR, Melly MA, McGee ZA, 1980, Gonococcal lipopolysaccharide: a toxin for human fallopian tube mucosa, *Am J Obstet Gynecol*, **138**: 981–4.

Gundersen T, Ødegaard K, Gjessing HC, 1969, Treatment of gonorrhoea by one oral dose of ampicillin and probenecid combined, *Br J Vener Dis*, **45**: 235–7.

Guthe T, 1961, Failure to control gonorrhoea, *Bull W H O*, **24**: 297–306.

von Haam E, 1938, The laboratory diagnosis of venereal lesions, *Urolog Cutan Rev*, **42**: 412–22.

Hammond GW, Lian CJ et al., 1978a, Comparison of specimen collection and laboratory techniques for isolation of *Haemophilus ducreyi*, *J Clin Microbiol*, **7**: 39–43.

Hammond GW, Lian CJ et al., 1978b, Determination and haemin requirement of *Haemophilus ducreyi*. Evaluation of the Porphyrin Test Media used in the satellite growth test, *J Clin Microbiol*, **7**: 243–6.

Hammond GW, Slutchuk M et al., 1980, Epidemiology, clinical, laboratory and therapeutic features of an urban outbreak of chancroid in North America, *Rev Infect Dis*, **2**: 867–79.

Handsfield HH, Lipman TO et al., 1974, Asymptomatic gonorrhoea in men. Diagnosis, natural course prevalence and significance, *N Engl J Med*, **290**: 123–30.

Handsfield HH, Totten PA et al., 1981, Molecular epidemiology of *Haemophilus ducreyi* infections, *Ann Intern Med*, **95**: 315–18.

Handsfield HH, Ronald AR et al., 1992, Evaluation of new anti-infective drugs for the treatment of sexually transmitted chlamydial infections and related clinical syndromes, *Clin Infect Dis*, **15, Suppl. 1**: S131–9.

Hart G, 1975, Venereal disease in a war environment: incidence and management, *Med J Aust*, **1**: 808–10.

Hart G, 1983, Chancroid, donovanosis and lymphogranuloma venereum, *Dermatologic Clinics*, ed. Felman YM, WB Saunders, Philadelphia, 75–84.

Hawkes S, West B et al., 1995, Asymptomatic carriage of *Haemophilus ducreyi* confirmed by the polymerase chain reaction, *Genitourin Med*, **71**: 224–7.

Heckels JE, Blackett B et al., 1976, The influence of surface charge on the attachment of *Neisseria gonorrhoeae* to human cells, *J Gen Microbiol*, **96**: 359–64.

Hildebrandt JF, Mayer LW et al., 1978, *Neisseria gonorrhoeae* acquire a new principal outer membrane protein when transformed to resistance to serum bactericidal activity, *Infect Immun*, **20**: 267–73.

Hill JH, 1948, Fundamental problems for laboratory research on *Neisseria gonorrhoeae* and gonococcal infection, *Am J Syph Gon Vener Dis*, **32**: 165–89.

Himmel J, 1901, Contribution à l' étude de l'immunité des animaux vis à vis du bacille du chancre mou, *Ann Inst Pasteur*, **15**: 928–40.

Holmes KK, Counts GW, Beatty HN, 1971, Disseminated gonococcal infection, *Ann Intern Med*, **74**: 979–93.

Holmes KK, Johnson DW, Trostle HJ, 1970, An estimate of the risk of men acquiring gonorrhoea by sexual contact with infected females, *Am J Epidemiol*, **91**: 170–4.

Hooper RR, Reynolds GH et al., 1978, Cohort study of venereal disease I: the risk of gonorrhoea transmission from infected women and men, *Am J Epidemiol*, **108**: 136–44.

Ison CA, 1987, Immunology of gonorrhoea, *Immunology of Sexually Transmitted Diseases*, ed. Wright DJM, Kluwer Academic Publishers, Dordrecht, Boston and London, 95–116.

Ison CA, Glynn AA, 1979, Classes of antibodies in acute gonorrhoea, *Lancet*, **1**: 1165–8.

Ison CA, McClean K et al., 1985, Evaluation of a direct immunofluorescence test for diagnosing gonorrhoea, *J Clin Pathol*, **38**: 1142–5.

Ison CA, Woodford N et al., 1994, Surveillance of antibiotic resistance in *Neisseria gonorrhoeae*, *Pathology and Immunobiology of Neisseriaceae*, eds Conde-Glez CJ, Morse S et al., Instituto Nacional De Salud Publica, Cuernavaca, Mexico, 71–6.

Israel KS, Rissing KB, Brooks GF, 1975, Neonatal and childhood gonococcal infections, *Clin Obstet Gynecol*, **18**: 143–51.

Ito T, 1913, Klinische und bakteriologisch-serologische Studien über Ulcus molle Ducreysche Streptobazillen, *Archiv Dermatol Syphilis Wien Leipzig*, **116**: 341–74.

Jephcott AE, 1977, Laboratory diagnosis of gonorrhoea, MD Thesis, University of Sheffield, 49–56.

Jephcott AE, Raschid S, 1978, Improved management in the diagnosis of gonorrhoea in women, *Br J Vener Dis*, **54**: 155–9.

Jephcott AE, Reyn A, Birch-Andersen A, 1971, *Neisseria gonorrhoeae*. III. Demonstration of presumed appendages to cells from different colony types, *Acta Pathol Microbiol Scand*, **B79:** 437–9.

Johnson SR, Morse SA, 1988, Antibiotic resistance in *Neisseria gonorrhoeae*: genetics and mechanisms of resistance, *Sex Transm Dis*, **15:** 217–24.

Jonsson A-B, Nyberg G, Normark S, 1991, Phase variation of gonococcal pili by frameshift mutation in *pilC* a novel gene for pilus assembly, *EMBO J*, **10:** 477–88.

Jonsson A-B, Liver D et al., 1994, Sequence changes in the pilus subunit lead to tropism variation of *Neisseria gonorrhoeae* to human tissue, *Mol Microbiol*, **13:** 407–16.

Juhlin L, Lidén S, 1969, Influence of contraceptive gestagen pills on sexual behaviour and the spread of gonorrhoea, *Br J Vener Dis*, **45:** 321–4.

Karim QN, Finn GY et al., 1989, Rapid detection of *Haemophilus ducreyi* in clinical and experimental infections using monoclonal antibody: a preliminary evaluation, *Genitourin Med*, **65:** 361–5.

Kellogg DS, Peacock WL et al., 1963, *Neisseria gonorrhoeae*. I. Virulence genetically linked to clonal variation, *J Bacteriol*, **85:** 1274–9.

Kellogg DS, Cohen IR et al., 1968, *Neisseria gonorrhoeae*. II. Colonial variation and pathogenicity during 35 months in vitro, *J Bacteriol*, **96:** 596–605.

Keys TF, Halverson CW, Clarke EJ, 1969, Single-dose treatment of gonorrhea with selected antibiotic agents, *JAMA*, **210:** 857–61.

Kibukamusoke JW, 1965, Venereal disease in East Africa, *Trans R Soc Trop Med Hyg*, **59:** 642–8.

Kilpatrick ZM, 1972, Current concepts, *N Engl J Med*, **287:** 967–9.

Kinane DF, Blackwell CC et al., 1983, Blood group, secretor status and susceptibility to *Neisseria gonorrhoeae*, *Br J Vener Dis*, **59:** 44–6.

Kiraly K, 1973, The venereal disease problem around the world, *J Reprod Med*, **11:** 119–22.

Kirkpatrick DJ, 1970, Donovanosis (granuloma inguinale) a rare cause of osteolytic bone lesions, *Clin Radiol*, **21:** 101–5.

Knapp JS, Holmes KK, 1975, Disseminated gonococcal infections caused by *Neisseria gonorrhoeae* with unique nutritional requirements, *J Infect Dis*, **132:** 204–8.

Knapp JS, Rice RJ, 1995, *Neisseria* and *Branhamella, Manual of Clinical Microbiology*, eds Murray PR, Baron EJ et al., ASM Press, Washington, DC, 324–40.

Knapp JS, Zenilman JM et al., 1987, Frequency and distribution in the United States of strains of *Neisseria gonorrhoeae* with plasmid-mediated high-level resistance to tetracycline, *J Infect Dis*, **155:** 819–22.

Koch ML, 1948, Pancreatic digest chocolate blood agar for the isolation of the gonococcus, *J Bacteriol*, **56:** 83–7.

Lambden PR, Heckels JE et al., 1979, Variations in surface protein composition associated with virulence properties in opacity types of *Neisseria gonorrhoeae*, *J Gen Microbiol*, **114:** 305–12.

Latif A, Mason PR, Paraiwa E, 1988, The treatment of donovanosis (granuloma inguinale), *Sex Transm Dis*, **15:** 27–9.

Lind I, 1969, Combined use of fluorescent antibody technique and culture on selective medium for the identification of *Neisseria gonorrhoeae*, *Acta Pathol Microbiol Scand*, **76:** 279–87.

Lipschütz B, 1904, Ueber einen einfachen Gonokokken-nährboden, *Zentralbl Bakteriol Parasitenkd Infektionskr Hyg Jena*, **36:** 743–7.

Lipsitt HJ, Parmett AJ, 1984, Non-sexual transmission of gonorrhoea to a child, *N Engl J Med*, **311:** 470.

Lockett AE, Dance DAB et al., 1991, Serum-free media for the isolation of *Haemophilus ducreyi*, *Lancet*, **338:** 326.

Lowe TL, Kraus SJ, 1976, Quantitation of *Neisseria gonorrhoeae* from women with gonorrhoea, *J Infect Dis*, **133:** 621–6.

Lykke-Olesen L, Larsen L et al., 1979, Epidemic chancroid in Greenland 1977–78, *Lancet*, **1:** 654–6.

McEntegart MG, Hafiz S, Kinghorn GR, 1982, *Haemophilus ducreyi* infections – time for reappraisal, *J Hyg*, **89:** 467–78.

McGee AZ, Johnson AP, Taylor-Robinson D, 1981, Pathogenic mechanisms of *Neisseria gonorrhoeae*: observations on damage to human fallopian tubes in organ culture by gonococci of colony type 1 or type 4, *J Infect Dis*, **143:** 413–22.

MacLean IW, Bowden GHW, Albritton WL, 1980, TEM-type β-lactamase production of *Haemophilus ducreyi*, *Antimicrob Agents Chemother*, **17:** 897–900.

McMillan A, Pattman RS, 1979, Evaluation of urethral culture for *Neisseria gonorrhoeae* in the routine investigation of men attending a STD clinic, *Br J Vener Dis*, **55:** 271–3.

McMillan A, McNeillage G et al., 1979a, Serum immunoglobulin response in uncomplicated gonorrhoea, *Br J Vener Dis*, **55:** 5–9.

McMillan A, McNeillage G et al., 1979b, Secretory antibody response of the cervix to infection with *Neisseria gonorrhoeae*, *Br J Vener Dis*, **55:** 265–70.

McMillan A, McNeillage G et al., 1980, Detection of gonococcal IgA in cervical secretions by indirect immunofluorescence, *Br J Vener Dis*, **56:** 223–6.

Mahoney JF, van Slyke CJ et al., 1946, Experimental gonococcic urethritis in human volunteers, *Am J Syph Gon Vener Dis*, **30:** 1–39.

Mandrell RG, Lesse AJ et al., 1990, In vitro and in vivo modification of *Neisseria gonorrhoeae* lipooligosaccharide epitope structure by sialylation, *J Exp Med*, **171:** 1649–64.

Mårdh P-A, 1980, An overview of infectious agents of salpingitis, their biology, and recent advances in methods of detection, *Am J Obstet Gynecol*, **138:** 933–51.

Mårdh P-A, Weström L, 1976, Adherence of bacterial to vaginal epithelial cells, *Infect Immun*, **13:** 661–6.

Marmell M, 1958, Donovanosis of the anus in the male: an epidemiological consideration, *Br J Vener Dis*, **34:** 213–18.

Martin JE, Jackson RL, 1975, A biological environmental chamber for the culture of *Neisseria gonorrhoeae*, *J Am Vener Dis Assoc*, **2:** 28–30.

Martin JE, Lester A, 1971, Transgrow: a medium for transport and growth of *Neisseria gonorrhoeae* and *Neisseria meningitidis*, *Health Serv Ment Health Admin Health Rep*, **86:** 30–3.

Meheus A, De Clercq A, Prat R, 1974, Prevalence of gonorrhoea in prostitutes in a central African town, *Br J Vener Dis*, **50:** 50–2.

Meitzner TA, Bolan G et al., 1987, Purification and characterization of the major iron-regulated protein expressed by pathogenic Neisseriae, *J Exp Med*, **165:** 1041–57.

Messing M, Sottnek FO et al., 1983, Isolation of haemophilus species from the genital tract, *Sex Transm Dis*, **10:** 56–61.

Moffet M, Young JL, Stuart RD, 1948, Centralised gonococcus culture for dispersed clinics, *Br Med J*, **2:** 421–4.

Morse SA, 1989, Chancroid and *Haemophilus ducreyi*, *Clin Microbiol Rev*, **2:** 137–57.

Morse SA, Johnson SR et al., 1986, High level tetracycline resistance in *Neisseria gonorrhoeae* is result of acquisition of streptococcal tet M determinant, *Antimicrob Agents Chemother*, **30:** 664–70.

Morton RS, 1977, *Gonorrhoea*, WB Saunders, London.

Mulks MH, Plaut AG, 1978, IgA protease production as a characteristic distinguishing pathogenic from harmless Neisseriaceae, *N Engl J Med*, **299:** 973–6.

Müller R, Oppenheim M, 1906, Ueber den Nachweis von Antikorpern im Serum eines an Arthritis gonorrhoica Erkrankten mittels Komplementablenkung, *Wien Klin Wochenschr*, **19:** 894.

Murphy G, Connel T et al., 1989, Phase variation of gonococcal protein II: regulation of gene expression by lipped-strand misparing of a repetitive DNA sequence, *Cell*, **56:** 539–47.

Nachamkin I, Sondheimer SJ et al., 1984, Detection of *Neisseria gonorrhoeae* in cervical swabs using Gonozyme enzyme immunoassay. Clinical evaluation in a university family planning clinic, *Am J Clin Pathol*, **82:** 461–5.

Näher H, Kohl PK, Petzoldt D, 1989, Evaluation of a non-radioactive DNA probe for confirmatory identification of *Neisseria gonorrhoeae*, *Zentralbl Bakteriol*, **272:** 181–5.

Nassif X, Magdalene S, 1995, Interaction of pathogenic neisseriae with nonphagocytic cells, *Clin Microbiol Rev*, **8**: 376–88.

Nayyar KC, Stolz E, Michel MF, 1979, Rising incidence of chancroid in Rotterdam, *Br J Vener Dis*, **55**: 439.

Nicolle C, 1923, Isolement culture et conservation dans les laboratoires du streptobacille du chancre mou, *C R Soc Biol*, **88**: 871–3.

Noble RC, Parekh MC, 1983, Bactericidal properties of urine for *Neisseria gonorrhoeae*, *Sex Transm Dis*, **14**: 221–6.

Novotny P, Short JA et al., 1977, Studies on the mechanism of pathogenicity of *Neisseria gonorrhoeae*, *J Med Microbiol*, **10**: 347–65.

Nsanze H, Fast MV et al., 1981, Genital ulcers in Kenya: clinical and laboratory study, *Br J Vener Dis*, **57**: 378–81.

Orle KA, Martin DH et al., 1994, Multiplex PCR detection of *Haemophilus ducreyi*, *Treponema pallidum* and herpes simplex viruses types 1 and 2 from genital ulcers, *Abstr 94th Annu Meet Am Soc Microbiol*, **Abstr C437**: 568.

Packer H, Goldberg J, 1950, Studies of antigenic relationship of *D. granulomatis* to members of the tribe Eschericheae, *Am J Syph Gon Vener Dis*, **34**: 342–50.

Parsons LM, Shayegani M et al., 1989, DNA probes for the identification of *Haemophilus ducreyi*, *J Clin Microbiol*, **27**: 1441–5.

Parsons LM, Shayegani M et al., 1990, Construction of DNA probes for the identification of *Haemophilus ducreyi*, *Gene Probes of Bacteria*, eds Macario AJ, Conway de Macario E, Academic Press, New York, 69–94.

Pemberton J, McCann JS et al., 1972, Socio-medical characteristics of patients attending a VD clinic and the circumstances of infection, *Br J Vener Dis*, **48**: 391–6.

Perine PL, Totten PA et al., 1985, Evaluation of a DNA-hybridization method for detection of African and Asian strains of *Neissseria gonorrhoeae* in men with urethritis, *J Infect Dis*, **152**: 59–63.

Petersen BH, Lee TJ et al., 1979, *Neisseria meningitidis* and *Neisseria gonorrhoeae* bacteremia associated with C6, C7, or C8 deficiencies, *Ann Intern Med*, **90**: 917–20.

Phillips I, 1976, β-Lactamase-producing penicillin-resistant gonococcus, *Lancet*, **2**: 656–7.

Piot P, Laga M, 1989, Genital ulcers, other sexually transmitted diseases and the sexual transmission of HIV, *Br Med J*, **298**: 623–4.

Plavidal FJ, Werch A, 1976, Fetal scalp abscess secondary to intrauterine monitoring. A case report, *Am J Obstet Gynecol*, **125**: 65–70.

Plummer FA, D'Costa LJ et al., 1983, Epidemiology of chancroid and *Haemophilus ducreyi* in Nairobi, Kenya, *Lancet*, **2**: 1293–5.

Plummer FA, Chubb H et al., 1994, Antibodies to opacity proteins (Opa) correlate with a reduced risk of gonococcal salpingitis, *J Clin Invest*, **93**: 1748–55.

Potterat JL, Dukes RL, Rothenberg RB, 1987, Disease transmission by heterosexual men with gonorrhoea: an empiric estimate, *Sex Transm Dis*, **14**: 107–10.

Pradinaud R, Grosshans E et al., 1981, Etude de 24 cas de donovanose en Guyane Francaise, *Bull Soc Pathol Exot Filiales*, **74**: 30–6.

Punsalang AP, Sawyer WD, 1973, Role of pili in the virulence of *Neisseria gonorrhoeae*, *Infect Immun*, **8**: 255–63.

Rake G, 1948, The antigenic relationships of *Donovania granulomatis* (Anderson) and the significance of this organism in granuloma inguinale, *Am J Syph Gon Vener Dis*, **32**: 150–8.

Rake G, Oskay JJ, 1948, Cultural characteristics of *Donovania granulomatis*, *J Bacteriol*, **55**: 667–75.

Ramanan C, Sarma PSA et al., 1990, Treatment of donavanosis with norfloxacin, *Int J Dermatol*, **29**: 298–9.

Raven C, 1934, Dissociation of gonococcus, *J Infect Dis*, **55**: 328–39.

Read SE, Cave C, Goldberg E, 1988, STD's including HIV in teenage prostitutes, *IV International Conference on AIDS Stockholm*, **Abstr 4554**.

Reenstierna J, 1921, Chancre mou expérimental chez le singe et le lapin, *Acta Derm Venereol*, **2**: 1–7.

Reenstierna J, 1924, Untersuchungen über den Bacillus Ducrey. I. Heterstellung und Eigenshaften eines Antistreptobacillenserums. II Cutireaction beim ulcus molle, *Arch Inst Pasteur Tunis*, **55**: 273.

Reimann K, Lind I, 1977, An indirect haemagglutination test for demonstrating gonococcal antibodies using gonococcal pili as antigen, *Acta Pathol Microbiol Scand*, **C85**: 155–62.

Reyn A, 1965, Laboratory diagnosis of gonocccal infections, *Bull W H O*, **32**: 449–69.

Reyn A, Bentzon MW, 1972, Comparison of a selective and a non-selective medium for the diagnosis of gonorrhoea to ascertain the sensitivity of *Neisseria gonorrheae* to vancomycin, *Br J Vener Dis*, **48**: 363–8.

Reyn A, Korner B, Bentzon MW, 1958, Effects of penicillin, streptomycin and tetracycline on *N. gonorrhoeae* isolated in 1944 and 1957, *Br J Vener Dis*, **34**: 227–39.

Reyn A, Korner B, Bentzon MW, 1960, Transportation of material for the cultivation of the gonococcus, *Br J Vener Dis*, **36**: 243–56.

Rice PA, Kasper DI, 1977, Characterization of gonococcal antigen responsible for induction of bactericidal antibodies in disseminated infection, *J Clin Invest*, **60**: 1149–58.

Richens J, 1991, The diagnosis and treatment of donovanosis (granuloma inguinale), *Genitourin Med*, **67**: 441–52.

Riley VC, 1991, Resurgent gonorrhoea in homosexual men, *Lancet*, **337**: 183.

Roberts MC, 1989, Plasmid mediated Tet M in *Haemophilus ducreyi*, *Antimicrob Agents Chemother*, **33**: 1611–13.

Roberts MC, 1990, Characterisation of the Tet M determinants in urogential and respiratory bacteria, *Antimicrob Agents Chemother*, **34**: 476–8.

Robertson JN, Vincent P, Ward ME, 1977, The preparation and properties of gonococcal pili, *J Gen Microbiol*, **102**: 169–77.

Robinson HM, Cohen MM, 1953, Treatment of granuloma inguinale with erythromycin, *J Invest Dermatol*, **20**: 407–9.

Rossau R, Duhamel M et al., 1990, Evaluation of an rRNA-derived oligonucleotide probe for culture confirmation of *Neisseria gonorrhoeae*, *J Clin Microbiol*, **28**: 944–8.

Rothbard JB, Fernandez R et al., 1985, Antibodies to peptides corresponding to a conserved sequence of gonococcal pilins block bacterial adhesion, *Proc Natl Acad Sci USA*, **82**: 915–19.

Saelhof CC, 1925, Can normal persons be carriers of the Ducrey bacillus?, *J Urol*, **13**: 485–7.

Salit IE, 1982, The differential susceptibility of gonococcal opacity variants to sex hormones, *Can J Microbiol*, **28**: 301–6.

Sandholzer TA, 1983, Factors affecting the incidence and management of sexually transmitted diseases in homosexual men, *Sexually Transmitted Diseases in Homosexual Men*, eds Ostrow DG, Sandholzer TA, Felman YM, Plenum Medical Book Co., New York, 3–12.

Schoolnik GK, Buchanan TM, Holmes KK, 1976, Gonococci causing disseminated infection are resistant to the bactericidal action of normal serum, *J Clin Invest*, **58**: 1163–73.

Schneider H, Griffis MJ et al., 1991, Expression of paragloboside-like lipopolisaccharides may be a necessary component of gonococcal pathogenesis in man, *J Exp Med*, **174**: 1601–5.

Schroeter AL, Pazin GJ, 1970, Gonorrhoea, *Ann Intern Med*, **72**: 553–7.

Schulte JM, Martich FA, Schmid GP, 1992, Chancroid in the United States 1981–1990: evidence for under-reporting of cases, *Morbid Mortal Weekly Rep*, **41, No. SS-3**: 57–61.

Schultz KF, Cates W, O'Mara PR, 1987, Pregnancy loss, infant death and suffering: legacy of syphilis and gonorrhoea in Africa, *Genitourin Med*, **63**: 320–5.

Seid RC, Schneider H et al., 1985, Enhanced antigenicity and immunogenicity of gonococcal pilus–lipopolysaccharide conjugates, *The Pathogenic Neisseriae*, ed. Schoolnik GK, American Society for Microbiology, Washington, DC, 309–15.

Seifert HS, Wright CJ et al., 1994, Multiple gonococcal pili variants are produced during experimental human infections, *J Clin Invest*, **93**: 2744–9.

Seth AD, Kolator B, Wilkinson AE, 1979, Sensitivity of *Neisseria gonorrhoeae* to antibiotics in London 1976–78, *Br J Vener Dis*, **55**: 325–8.

Sherrard J, Barlow D, 1993, Gonorrhoea in men, *Lancet*, **341**: 245.

Shtibel R, 1980, Non-beta-lactamase producing *Neisseria gonorrhoeae* highly resistant to pencillin, *Lancet*, **2**: 39.

Shtibel R, Toma S, 1978, *Neisseria gonorrhoeae*: evaluation of some methods used for carbohydrate utilisation, *Can J Microbiol*, **24**: 177–81.

Siegel MS, Perine PL et al., 1978, Epidemiology of pencillinase-producing *Neisseria gonorrhoeae*, *Immunobiology of* Neisseria gonorrhoeae, eds Brooks GF, Gotschlich EC et al., American Society for Microbiology, Washington, DC, 75–9.

Smith H, Cole JA, Parsons NJ, 1992, The sialylation of gonococcal lipopolysaccharide by host factors: a major impact on pathogenesis, *FEMS Microbiol Lett*, **79**: 287–92.

Sottnek FO, Biddle JW et al., 1980, Isolation and identification of *Haemophilus ducreyi* in a clinical study, *J Clin Microbiol*, **12**: 170–4.

Sparling PF, Sarubbi FA, Blackman E, 1975, Inheritance of low-level resistance to pencillin, tetracycline and chloramphenicol in *Neisseria gonorrhoeae*, *J Bacteriol*, **124**: 740–9.

Sparling PF, Tsai J, Cornelissen CN, 1990, Gonococci are survivors, *Scand J Infect Dis Suppl*, **69**: 125–36.

Sturm AH, Zanen HC, 1984, Characteristics of *Haemophilus ducreyi* in culture, *J Clin Microbiol*, **19**: 672–4.

Swanson J, 1978, Outer membrane variants of *Neisseria gonorrhoeae*, *Immunobiology of* Neisseria gonorrhoeae, eds Brooks GF, Gotschlich EC et al., American Society for Microbiology, Washington, DC, 130–7.

Swanson J, 1982, Colony opacity and protein II compositions, *Infect Immun*, **37**: 359–68.

Swanson J, 1983, Gonococcal adherence: selected topics, *Rev Infect Dis*, **5**: S678–84.

Taylor DN, Duangmani C et al., 1984, The role of *Haemophilus ducreyi* in penile ulcers, *Sex Transm Dis*, **11**: 148–51.

Taylor E, Phillips I, 1980, Assessment of transport and isolation methods for gonococci, *Br J Vener Dis*, **56**: 390–3.

Thayer JD, Martin JE, 1966, Improved medium selective for cultivation of *N. gonorrhoeae* and *N. meningitidis*, *Public Health Rep*, **81**: 559–62.

Thayer WS, 1922, On the cardiac complications of gonorrhoea, *Johns Hopkins Hosp Bull*, **33**: 361–72.

Thin RN, Shaw EJ, 1979, Diagnosis of gonorrhoea in women, *Br J Vener Dis*, **55**: 10–13.

Thin RNT, Williams IA, Nicol CS, 1970, Direct and delayed methods of immunofluorescent diagnosis of gonorrhoea in women, *Br J Vener Dis*, **47**: 27–30.

Toshach S, 1978, Effects of meningococcal carriage on serological tests for gonorrhoea, *Can J Public Health*, **69**: 127–9.

Totten PA, Stamm WE, 1994, Clear broth and plate media for culture of *Haemophilus ducreyi*, *J Clin Microbiol*, **32**, 2019–23.

Totten PA, Morton WR et al., 1994, A primate model for chancroid, *J Infect Dis*, **169**: 1284–90.

Tramont EC, 1989, Gonococcal vaccines, *Clin Microbiol Rev*, **2**: S74–7.

Tramont EC, Hodge WC et al., 1979, Differences in attachment antigens of gonococci in reinfection, *J Lab Clin Med*, **93**: 730–5.

Tramont EC, Boslego JW et al., 1985, Parenteral gonococcal pilus vaccine, *The Pathogenic Neisseriae*, ed. Schoolnik GK, American Society for Microbiology, Washington, DC, 316–22.

Trees DL, Morse SA, 1995, Chancorid and *Haemophilus ducreyi*: an update, *Clin Microbiol Rev*, **8**: 357–75.

Turner A, Gough KR, Jephcott AE, 1995, A comparison of three methods for the culture confirmation of *Neisseria gonorrhoeae* currently circulating in the UK. Internal PHLS document.

Velasco JE, Miller E, Zaias N, 1972, Minocycline in the treatment of venereal disease, *JAMA*, **22**: 1323–5.

Verdich J, 1984, *Haemophilus ducreyi* infection resembling granuloma inguinale, *Acta Derm Venereol*, **64**: 452–5.

Virji M, Fletcher JN et al., 1987, The potential protective effect of monoclonal antibodies gonococcal outer membrane protein IA, *J Gen Microbiol*, **133**: 2639–46.

Vlaspolder F, Mutsaers JAEM et al., 1993, Value of DNA probe assay (Gen-Probe) compared with that of culture for the diagnosis of gonococcal infection, *J Clin Microbiol*, **31**: 107–10.

Ward ME, Watt PJ, Robertson JN, 1974, The human fallopian tube: a laboratory model for gonococcal infection, *J Infect Dis*, **129**: 650–9.

Wasserheit JN, 1992, Epidemiological synergy: interrelationships between human immunodeficiency virus infection and other sexually transmitted diseases, *Sex Transm Dis*, **19**: 61–77.

Webb EM, Hotchkiss R et al., 1995, Chancroid detected by polymerase chain reaction – Jackson Mississippi 1994/5, *Morbid Mortal Weekly Rep*, **44**: 567–74.

Welch BG, O'Reilly RJ, 1973, An indirect fluorescent-antibody technique for the study of uncomplicated gonorrhoea, *J Infect Dis*, **127**: 69–76.

Welch WD, Cartwright G, 1988, Fluorescent monoclonal antibody compared with carbohydrate utilization for the rapid identification of *Neisseria gonorrhoeae*, *J Clin Microbiol*, **26**: 293–6.

Weller SC, 1993, A meta-analysis of condom effectiveness in reducing sexually transmitted HIV, *Soc Sci Med*, **36**: 1635–44.

Weström L, 1980, Incidence, prevalence and trends of acute pelvic inflammatory disease and its consequences in industrialized countries, *Am J Obstet Gynecol*, **138**: 880–92.

Wiesner PJ, Tronca E et al., 1973, Clinical spectrum of pharyngeal gonococcal infection, *N Engl J Med*, **288**: 181–5.

World Health Organization, 1978a, *Neisseria gonorrhoeae* and gonococcal infection, *W H O Tech Rep Ser*, **616**: 43 and 56.

World Health Organization, 1978b, *Neisseria gonorrhoea* and gonococcal infection, *W H O Tech Rep Ser*, **616**: 39–40.

World Health Organization, 1981, Non-gonococcal urethritis and other sexually transmitted diseases of public health importance, *W H O Tech Rep Ser*, **660**: 55.

World Health Organization, 1983, Unpublished document WHO/VDT83/434, 15.

Wright DJM, Daunt O, 1973, How infectious is gonorrhoea?, *Lancet*, **1**: 208.

Yamasaki R, Kerwood D et al., 1994, The structure of lipooligosaccharide produced by *Neisseria gonorrhoeae* strain 15253 isolated from a patient with disseminated infection, *Neisseria 94: Proceedings of Ninth International Pathogenic Neisseria Conference*, eds Evans JS, Yost SE et al., Winchester, Hampshire, UK, 13–14.

Yeung K-H, Dillon JR et al., 1986, A novel 4.9 kilobase plasmid associated with an outbreak of penicillinase-producing *Neisseria gonorrhoeae*, *J Infect Dis*, **153**: 1162–5.

Young H, 1978, Cultural diagnosis of gonorrhoea with modified New York City (MNYC) medium, *Br J Vener Dis*, **54**: 36–40.

Young H, 1981, Advances in routine laboratory procedures for the diagnosis of gonorrhoea, *Recent Advances in Sexually Transmitted Diseases – 2*, 2nd edn, ed. Harris JRW, Churchill Livingstone, Edinburgh, 59–71.

Young H, Henrichsen C, McMillan A, 1980, The diagnostic value of a gonococcal complement fixation test, *Med Lab Sci*, **37**: 165–70.

Young H, Reid K, 1984, Immunological identification of *Neisseria gonorrhoeae* with monoclonal and polycolonal antibody coagglutination reagents, *J Clin Pathol*, **37**: 1276–81.

Chapter 34

Syphilis and related treponematoses

S A Larsen, S J Norris, B M Steiner and A H Rudolph

1 INTRODUCTION

Sexually acquired syphilis is the best known of the diseases caused by the members of the genus *Treponema*. The origin of syphilis is unclear because syphilis is a disease of many manifestations and definitive paleopathological findings are absent. Three theories related to the origin of syphilis exist: pre-Columbian, Columbian and evolutionary. Each school has certain elements that support its conclusions, but none can be totally proved or totally refuted.

1.1 Pre-Columbian school

In support of the pre-Columbian theory that syphilis existed in the Old World before Columbus's discovery of America is the discussion in medical literature of leprosy (1200s–1300s) that was believed to be sexually transmitted (Hirsch 1883). This form of leprosy was also thought to be inheritable and some believe that syphilis may be one of the skin diseases described as leprosy in the Bible. Today, leprosy is not known to be inherited or transmitted from casual sexual contact, but takes prolonged exposure for infection to occur (Nakamura 1988). Further supporting the theory that syphilis was misidentified as leprosy are the reports of 'temporary leprosy' cured by the use of mercurial ointments and, more effectively, by the oral administration of mercury. Mercury was later used to treat syphilis and had been used by the ancient Chinese to treat 'yinshih', a sore due to 'unclean sexual intercourse'.

1.2 Columbian school

Documentation for the Columbian school for the origin of syphilis is better than for the pre-Columbian school. The finding of crania and other bone relics with indications of treponemal damage throughout the Americas and the lack of paleopathological documentation that syphilis was present in the Old World both support the Columbian school. Egyptian mummies examined in the 1900s showed no evidence of syphilitic injuries to bones or teeth, whereas cranial periostitis in skulls dated by carbon methods back to AD 834 has been described in relics from the western Pacific (Goff 1967).

1.3 Evolutionary school

The more contemporary approach is the evolutionary school postulated by Hudson in 1946, based on a single organism responding to changes in the environmental temperature, and by Hackett in 1963, based on a single organism developing in the Euro–Afro–Asian land mass sometime before 20 000 BC and evolving to the distinct species and subspecies located in various geographical areas (Table 34.1). Today, yaws caused by *Treponema pallidum* subspecies *pertenue* is found in equatorial regions. Endemic syphilis, caused by *T. pallidum* subspecies *endemicum*, is found in hot, dry climates, whereas venereal syphilis, caused by *T. pallidum* subspecies *pallidum*, although now found world wide, in the sixteenth century was limited to temperate zones. Another treponemal disease, pinta, caused by *Treponema carateum*, is limited to northern South America and Central America and, according to Hackett, was relegated to the Americas when the Behring Strait flooded in or about 10 000 BC as a result of global warming.

Support for the evolutionary school

Researchers over the years have been able to modify experimental syphilis in rabbits by adjusting the temperature of the environment, thus supporting the hypothesis of one species and the belief that the differ-

Table 34.1 Characteristics of the human treponematoses[a]

	T. pallidum subsp. *pallidum*	*T. pallidum* subsp. *pertenue*	*T. pallidum* subsp. *endemicum*	*T. carateum*
Disease	Syphilis	Yaws (frambesia, pian)	Endemic syphilis (bejel, dichuchwa)	Pinta (carate, cute)
Distribution	World wide	Tropical areas, of both hemispheres	Arid areas, Africa, Middle East, Former Yugoslavia	Semiarid, Central and South America
Age of onset	Adolescents, adults	Children	Children to adults	Children, adolescents
Transmission	Sexual contact	Skin contact	Mucous membrane	Skin contact
Congenital infection	Yes	No	Rarely	No

[a]See references: US Public Health Service 1968, Perine et al. 1984, 1985, Engelkens et al. 1991a, 1991b.

entiation of the treponemal diseases depends on environmental factors rather than on differences among treponemal species (Turner and Hollander 1957, Hollander 1981). Adding further support to this hypothesis is the fact that none of the current scientific techniques distinguishes the other pathogenic treponemes from each other or from subspecies *pallidum*. The standard serological tests for syphilis are uniformly reactive in yaws, pinta and non-venereal endemic syphilis. Western blotting assays do not differentiate the antibodies formed in response to syphilis from those formed in response to yaws or pinta (Fohn et al. 1988, Noordhoek et al. 1991a). Most molecular approaches, such as DNA sequencing, DNA probes and polymerase chain reaction (PCR) techniques also have failed to distinguish the pathogenic treponemes (Noordhoek et al. 1991a, 1991b). Even though none of the current tests distinguishes between the organisms, animal studies indicate differences in susceptibility of the hamster and the rabbit to infection with *T. pallidum* subspecies *pallidum*, *pertenue*, or *endemicum* (Schell et al. 1979, 1981).

1.4 Challenges to the diagnosis of the treponemal diseases

Not only is the origin of syphilis unclear, the diagnosis of sexually acquired syphilis and of the related treponematoses offers the clinical laboratory challenges not associated with most other bacterial infections. The lack of a culture system (Fieldsteel, Cox and Moeckli 1981, Norris 1982) that allows for the growth of the organism from clinical specimens has necessitated the use of alternative methods for detection of the treponemes or antibody against *T. pallidum* subspecies. Many of these techniques were developed 20 or more years ago and have been refined over the years. There are now available various new tests that offer either greater ease of performance or the ability to diagnose difficult cases such as congenital syphilis. With the development of PCR and other molecular techniques, new and potentially more sensitive techniques may soon be available, at least to the reference laboratory.

2 EPIDEMIOLOGY

By 1958, with the general use of penicillin, syphilis in the USA had been almost eliminated. However, periodically after this time the levels of syphilis increased, then decreased (Fig. 34.1). Frequently the increases correlated with behavioural changes, such as the use of birth control pills in the 1960s, gay bath houses in the 1970s and 1980s and crack cocaine in the 1990s (Brandt 1988, Finelli, Budd and Spitalny 1993). In 1990 in the USA, the rate of primary and secondary cases was 20.3 per 100 000, the highest rate since 1952. Since 1991, the male-to-female ratio has approached 1, suggesting that much of the transmission of syphilis is heterosexual (Fig. 34.1). With acquired syphilis in the heterosexual population there was an increase in the number of infants born with congenital syphilis to a rate of 107.2 per 100 000 live births in 1991. The rates of sexually acquired syphilis for 1994 and 1995 declined to approximately 8 cases per 100 000 population (Centers for Disease Control and Prevention 1995). Likewise, the rate of congenital syphilis began to decline in 1992 and has continued to decline to a rate of approximately 55 per 100 000 live births in 1994. Another report indicates that syphilis dramatically increased in Estonia, Latvia, Lithuania and Russia between 1992 and 1993 to rates of greater than 18 cases per 100 000 population (Linglof 1995). In comparison to the USA and the Baltic States, rates of syphilis have progressively declined since the advent of penicillin therapy in other industrialized countries. In 1993, only 312 cases of syphilis were reported for England and Wales (Nakashima et al. 1996). In the non-industrialized nations, syphilis remains a significant health problem.

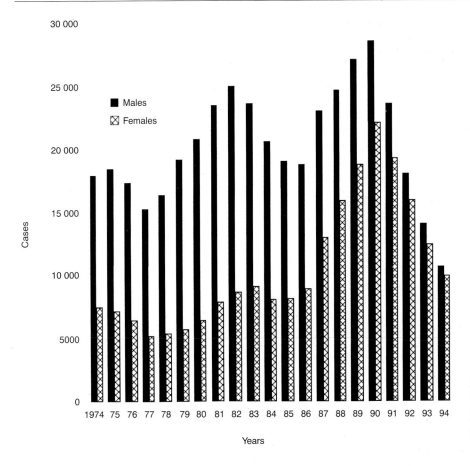

Fig. 34.1 Number of cases of syphilis 1974–94 in the USA by gender.

3 PATHOLOGY AND MANIFESTATIONS OF SYPHILIS

Untreated syphilis is a chronic disease that progresses through a variety of stages, each with distinct manifestations and pathology, as shown in Table 34.2.

3.1 Early syphilis

Sexual transmission of syphilis requires direct contact with infectious lesions. Approximately 30% of persons who have sex with an infected partner will develop syphilis (Sparling 1990). Within hours after initial con-

Table 34.2 Stages of infection for sexually acquired syphilis

Stage	Time post-infection	Symptom	Site
Primary	10–90 days (avg 21 days)	Chancre, single or multiple, regional lymphadenopathy	Skin or mucous membranes
Secondary	6 weeks–6 months	Multiple lesions, lymphadenopathy, fever, malaise, condylomata lata	Skin or mucous membranes
		Alopecia	Hair, eyebrows
		Asymptomatic or symptomatic CNS involvement	Meninges
Latent	Early, ≤1 year; late, >1year	Asymptomatic	
Late	Months to years		
Benign		Gummatous lesion	Tissue, any organ
Cardiovascular		Aortic aneurysm, tree barking	Aorta
Neurosyphilis		Paresis, tabes dorsalis, dementia,	Meningovascular
		Optical atrophy	Eye

tact with the organism, treponemes disseminate throughout the body; however, preferential multiplication occurs at the site of entry (Table 34.2). The skin surrounding the primary lesion or chancre is oedematous and infiltrated with inflammatory cells. The chancre centre is mucoid, containing hyaluronic acid and chondroitin sulphate surrounded by a cellular infiltrate of primarily mononuclear cells; the base of the chancre is fibrotic with neovascularization. The lesions, once present, may spontaneously resolve in 1–5 weeks. During the primary stage, the inguinal lymph nodes may be slightly enlarged, but are rarely tender. Serous fluids from the lesion contain numerous treponemes. Humoral antibodies, as detected by the standard non-treponemal and treponemal serological tests for syphilis, usually do not appear until 1–4 weeks after the chancre has formed.

By the secondary stage of syphilis, the organism has invaded every organ of the body and virtually all body fluids. Non-specific symptoms develop 1–5 weeks after the primary lesion has healed and may include fever, headache, sore throat, arthralgias and anorexia (Table 34.2). However, a generalized rash, mucous patches and condylomata lata are the most characteristic symptoms of secondary syphilis. Epithelial changes for these lesions include infiltration of leucocytes, necrosis of keratinocytes, some thickening of the epithelial cells and various degrees of hyperkeratosis (Chiu and Radolf 1994). These manifestations spontaneously resolve, usually within 2–6 weeks, but may recur during the first year of infection if the patient is not treated. Circulating immune complexes composed of IgG and C3 (Chiu and Radolf 1994), detected in approximately 80% of the secondary cases, may lead to immune complex deposition in the kidneys and subsequent renal damage.

In the early latent stage, the disease progresses from an acute to a chronic infection. During the latent period, following the secondary stage, a relapse to the secondary stage may occur. Duration of infection of <1 year, which is asymptomatic, is arbitrarily defined for epidemiological purposes as 'early latent stage'. Because lesions are not usually present after the first year, the disease is not considered infectious and the term late latent is assigned to this stage. However, in pregancy, *T. pallidum* can still be transmitted to the fetus up to 4 years after the initial infection, if the initial infection is not treated.

3.2 Late syphilis

The pathogenesis of the various forms that the late or tertiary stage of syphilis may take is not completely understood. Often, symptoms of late stage syphilis occur 10–20 years after the initial infection (Table 34.2).

An unusual form of late syphilis is benign late. The gumma (lesions) of this stage were previously reported to occur in 16% of the cases of untreated syphilis from 2 to more than 40 years after the initial infection (United States Public Health Service 1968). The gummas resemble the granuloma of tuberculosis

and may occur in the skin, bones, mucosae, viscera, muscles and ocular structure. With osseous gummas, reactive new bone formation and osteolysis are characteristic (Chiu and Radolf 1994). Because organisms are rare and the lesions are characteristic of an inflammatory response, some have suggested that the gummas are a result of hypersensitivity to the few treponemes or *T. pallidum* antigens remaining in foci of long-standing infections.

Older literature states that cardiovascular syphilis occurred in 10% of the patients with untreated syphilis (United States Public Health Service 1968). The lesions in the aorta in cardiovascular syphilis are related to the multiplication of treponemes (Fitzgerald 1981). Apparently treponemes spread via the lymphatics and lodge preferentially in the proximal aorta, producing endarteritis, which may also involve the coronary arteries near the ostia. This inflammatory process may last for years and eventually affect all 3 layers of the aortic wall. Degeneration of the intima with atherosclerotic plaque formation results in 'tree barking' (Bulkley 1984).

In the pre-antibiotic era, neurosyphilis was reported to occur in 6.5% of the cases. The lesions in the central nervous system in neurosyphilis are also related to the multiplication of treponemes (Fitzgerald 1981). Although neurological forms of syphilis (e.g. syphilitic meningitis) may develop during the secondary stage, neurosyphilis is usually a complication of late syphilis but may occur as early as 2 years after initial infection. Neurosyphilis may take many forms. All forms have in common chronic meningitis, producing vascular or parenchymatous sequelae in the cerebrum and spinal cord (Swartz 1984). In acute syphilitic meningitis, granular ependymitis and endarteritis may develop, which may lead to thrombosis, vascular occlusion and cerebral infarction. As a result of obstruction of the cerebrospinal fluid (CSF) flow, several forms of hydrocephalus result. In generalized paresis, gross findings include cerebral atrophy, demyelinization of the cortical white matter and varying degrees of thickening of the meninges consistent with chronic meningitis. Cerebral atrophy, particularly of the frontal poles and tips of the temporal lobes, is prominent. Whorls of subependymal astrocytes forming granular ependymitis are a characteristic finding on microscopic examination. Treponemes can be demonstrated in brain tissue or CSF by direct immunofluorescence, PCR (Gordon et al. 1994) or Dieterle silver stain. Nevertheless, symptoms consistent with neurosyphilis may not always be present (Hook and Marra 1992, Rudolph and Larsen 1993), i.e. asymptomatic neurosyphilis. Asymptomatic neurosyphilis usually is recognized as a disease entity when a lumbar puncture is performed on a person with a reactive serological test for syphilis and no history of treatment (Centers for Disease Control and Prevention 1993).

3.3 Congenital syphilis

In congenital syphilis, a primary stage does not occur because the organisms directly infect the fetal circulation. Necrotizing funisitis may or may not be present (Schwartz et al. 1995). Treponemes, or the effects thereof, are detectable in almost every tissue of the infant. The standard serological tests for syphilis, based on the measurement of IgG, reflect passively transferred antibodies from the mother to the infant, rather than IgM antibodies produced during gestation. Currently, the diagnosis of neonatal congenital syphilis depends on a combination of results from physical, radiographic, serological and direct microscopic examinations (Zenker and Berman 1990). Clinical signs of congenital syphilis include hepatosplenomegaly, cutaneous lesions, osteochondritis and snuffles (Kaufman et al. 1977). Although some clinical manifestations may be present at birth, they are more often seen at 3 weeks to 6 months. At birth, up to 50% of the infants with congenital syphilis are asymptomatic (Kaufman et al. 1977); other stigmata that may develop later include teeth and bone malformation, deafness, blindness and learning disabilities.

4 LABORATORY DIAGNOSIS

Various test methods for the diagnosis of syphilis have been developed. These tests for syphilis fall into 4 categories:

1 direct microscopic examination, used when lesions are present
2 non-treponemal tests, used for screening
3 treponemal tests that are confirmatory and
4 direct antigen detection tests currently used in research settings and as gold standards for test evaluation.

4.1 Direct microscopic methods

The first association of *Spirochaeta pallida*, as *T. pallidum* was then known, with the disease syphilis was made in 1904–5 by Schaudinn and Hoffmann using a modified Giemsa stain to examine lesion material from individuals with chancres. Coles in 1909 described the use of darkfield illumination for the examination of *S. pallida*, noting especially the motility of the organism (Table 34.3). Today, darkfield examination is still a viable method for the diagnosis of syphilis. In the mid-1960s, the direct fluorescent antibody test for *T. pallidum* (DFA-TP) was developed (Yobs, Brown and Hunter 1964) and later modified for use with monoclonal antibodies (Hook et al. 1985, Ito et al. 1992) and tissue sections in the direct fluorescent antibody tissue test for *T. pallidum* (DFAT-TP) (Hunter et al. 1984, Ito et al. 1992) (Table 34.3).

When lesions are present, direct detection of the organism is the most specific and easiest means of diagnosing syphilis. A positive result on microscopic examination is definitive evidence of syphilis, if infection with other pathogenic treponemes can be excluded. Also, primary syphilis can be diagnosed by darkfield several days to several weeks before the appearance of reactive serological tests. However, a negative direct microscopic finding does not exclude

the diagnosis of syphilis. Too few organisms may be present to be observed because the lesion may be in the healing stage, or the spirochaete may have been altered by systemic or topical treatment. In addition, the sample may be reported as unsatisfactory because an accurate reading may be prevented by the presence of too many blood cells, air bubbles, or tissue fragments. The reported sensitivities of the direct microscopic methods range from 73% to 100% (Daniels and Ferneyhough 1977, Romanowski et al. 1987, Ito et al. 1992).

Direct microscopic methods are suitable for rapid screening if the tests are performed by experienced laboratory personnel. When direct microscopic results are negative, other diseases, such as herpes and chancroid, should be considered because other sexually transmitted diseases are also characterized by lesions.

DARKFIELD

Because of their narrow width, treponemes cannot be observed with the ordinary light microscope. Microscopes equipped with a double-reflecting or single-reflecting darkfield condenser are needed to perform the darkfield examination. Illumination for darkfield microscopy is obtained when light rays strike the object in the field at an oblique angle so that no direct light rays, but only the rays that are reflected from the object, enter the microscope. Therefore, the object itself appears to be illuminated against a dark background. For details of the test see Creighton 1990.

T. pallidum is distinguished from other spiral organisms by the tightness of the spirals and characteristic corkscrew movement. However, *T. pallidum* subspecies *pallidum* cannot be distinguished from the other pathogenic treponemes. *T. pallidum* is a delicate, corkscrew-shaped organism with rigid, uniform, tightly wound, deep spirals. The characteristic motion of *T. pallidum* is a deliberate forward and backward movement with rotation about the longitudinal axis. Organisms easily confused with *T. pallidum* are *Treponema refringens* and *Treponema denticola*. Adequate training and experience are necessary to make an accurate diagnosis by darkfield microscopy. The untrained observer may be deceived by artefacts such as cotton fibres and Brownian motion.

Darkfield examination is most productive during primary, secondary, infectious relapsing and early congenital syphilis when moist lesions containing large numbers of treponemes (e.g. chancres, condylomata lata, or mucous patches) are present. Enlarged regional lymph nodes can also serve as a specimen source if the involved node is aspirated and the material obtained is examined. Darkfield examination of lesions of the cervix and vagina are possible if special techniques are used for collection of the specimen.

Because viability of the treponeme is necessary to distinguish *T. pallidum* from morphologically similar saprophytic spirochaetes within and near the genitalia, darkfield examination must be accomplished immediately after the specimen is obtained. Equipment and personnel for darkfield examination must be readily available, or the patient must be sent to a facility where the procedure can be performed.

The proper specimen for darkfield microscopy consists of serous fluid that contains *T. pallidum*, but is free of erythrocytes, other organisms and tissue debris. The lesion should be cleansed only if encrusted or obviously contaminated and only a minimal amount of tap water or physiological saline (without antibacterial additives) should be used. Even the experienced observer may find it difficult or impossible to differentiate *T. pallidum* from saprophytic spirochaetes in the mouth; thus, darkfield microscopy should not be used for the examination of samples from oral lesions.

DIRECT FLUORESCENT ANTIBODY TECHNIQUES

The DFA-TP detects and differentiates pathogenic treponemes from non-pathogenic treponemes by an antigen–antibody reaction; thus, the organism is not required to be motile. In addition, because the conjugates used are specific for pathogenic strains of *Treponema*, the DFA-TP is applicable to samples collected from oral, rectal, or intestinal lesions. Because the organism need not be motile, an additional advantage of the DFA-TP over the darkfield is that specimens collected from patients in clinic settings can be submitted to a reference laboratory for examination. Smears may be stained with fluorescein–isothiocyanate (FITC)-labelled anti-*T. pallidum* globulin prepared from the serum of humans or rabbits with syphilis absorbed with Reiter treponemes, or with FITC-conjugated or with a mouse monoclonal antibody to *T. pallidum* (Romanowski et al. 1987, Hunter 1990, Ito et al. 1991, 1992). However, even though monoclonal antibodies are used, the test cannot distinguish between the pathogenic strains of *Treponema*. The DFA-TP method has been used to detect the presence of *T. pallidum* subspecies in tissues (Wilkinson and Cowell 1971, Hunter et al. 1984, Ito et al. 1991, 1992), body fluids (Smith and Israel 1967, Wilkinson 1973), secretions and lesion exudates (Kellogg and Mothershed 1969, Ito et al. 1991, 1992).

A combination of the direct fluorescent antibody tissue test for *T. pallidum* (DFAT-TP) and histological stains may be used to examine biopsy and autopsy material for the presence of pathogenic *Treponema*. Any tissue can be used, but most frequently tissues for paraffin-embedded sections are collected from the brain, gastrointestinal tract, placenta, umbilical cord,

or skin. Often DFAT-TP is used to diagnose late stage or congenital syphilis or to distinguish skin lesions of secondary or late syphilis from those of Lyme disease (Ito et al. 1992). Slides prepared from sections are stained with a FITC-labelled monoclonal conjugate as for the DFA-TP, or by an indirect method by using first either an antibody to *T. pallidum* prepared from human serum or from an immunized rabbit or a mouse monoclonal antibody, followed by an FITC-labelled antihuman, antirabbit, or antimouse globulin. A testicular tissue section from a rabbit infected with *T. pallidum* is used as the control. The condition of the initial biopsy specimen or autopsy sample and the thickness of the tissue sections affect the outcome of the test. When the DFAT-TP test and the Steiner stain (Swisher 1987), a silver stain, were used to examine umbilical cords, agreement between the 2 tests was found to be 100% (Schwartz et al. 1995).

4.2   Serological tests

The most common methods for the diagnosis of syphilis are serological tests. These tests detect either antibodies to lipoidal antigens indicative of an infection (non-treponemal methods) or antibodies against specific treponemal antigens (treponemal methods). Those tests that are considered as standard tests for syphilis in the USA are shown in Table 34.4. Details of test performance for each of the standard tests and the methods for specimen collection are found in *A Manual of Tests for Syphilis* (Larsen, Hunter and Kraus 1990). Serum is the specimen of choice for all serological tests. However, plasma samples also may be used in the macroscopic non-treponemal card tests. The technician must check the product insert that accompanies the commercial test reagents to be sure that the plasma sample has not exceeded the recommended storage time and that the blood was collected in the specified anticoagulant.

NON-TREPONEMAL TESTS

The non-treponemal tests are fast, easy to perform and excellent for screening purposes. The non-treponemal (reagin) tests measure IgM and IgG antibodies to lipoidal material released from damaged host cells; to lipoprotein-like material; and possibly to cardiolipin released from the treponemes (Matthews, Yang and Jenkin 1979, Belisle et al. 1994). The antilipoidal antibodies are not only produced as a consequence of syphilis and other treponemal diseases, but also may

Table 34.3   History of tests for syphilis: direct antigen detection tests

Date	Author	Accomplishment
1905	Schaudinn and Hoffmann	Linked *Spirochaeta pallida* (*Treponema pallidum*) with syphilis
1909	Coles	Described use of darkfield illumination
1964	Yobs, Brown and Hunter	Developed the direct fluorescent antibody (DFA-TP) test
1991	Grimprel et al.	Described polymerase chain reaction (PCR) for the diagnosis of congenital syphilis
1991b	Noordhoek et al.	Applied PCR to the diagnosis of neurosyphilis

Table 34.4 The standard serological tests for syphilis in the USA

Non-treponemal	Treponemal

Microscopic tests
   Venereal Disease Research Laboratory (VDRL) slide
   Unheated serum reagin (USR)
	Microscopic tests
	   Fluorescent treponemal antibody absorption (FTA-ABS)
	   FTA-ABS double staining (DS)

Macroscopic tests
   Rapid plasma reagin (RPR) 18 mm circle card
 	
   Toluidine red unheated serum test (TRUST)
	Macroscopic test
	   Microhaemagglutination assay for antibodies to *T. pallidum* (MHA-TP)

be produced in response to non-treponemal diseases of an acute and chronic nature in which tissue damage occurs (Catterall 1972). Without some other evidence for the diagnosis of syphilis, a reactive non-treponemal test does not confirm *T. pallidum* infection.

Around the same time that the aetiological agent of syphilis was being observed, the first non-treponemal test for syphilis was also being developed (Table 34.5). In 1906, Wassermann, Neisser, and Brück adapted the complement fixation test, previously introduced by Bordet and Gengou in 1901, to serological testing for syphilis. Although the complement fixation tests contributed immensely to the diagnosis of syphilis, they were complicated. Subsequent work by Michaelis in 1907 and Meinicke in 1917, using distilled water or sodium chloride extracts of liver, resulted in the first precipitation tests that did not require complement (Eagle 1937). In 1922, Kahn introduced a flocculation test without complement that could be read macroscopically in a few hours. Many modifications of the Kahn test appeared (Kampmeier 1983). However, because of the crudely derived extracts of tissue serving as antigens, the tests varied in quality, sensitivity and specificity. A major breakthrough in antigen standardization occurred in 1941 when Pangborn successfully isolated from beef heart the active antigenic component, cardiolipin. Cardiolipin, when combined with lecithin and cholesterol, forms a serologically active antigen for the detection of syphilitic antibodies. In contrast to the crude tissue extract antigens, the pure cardiolipin–cholesterol–lecithin antigens could be standardized chemically as well as serologically, thus ensuring greater reproducibility of test results both within and between laboratories. With the advent of these new purified antigens, microflocculation tests, such as the Venereal Disease Research Laboratory (VDRL) test (Harris, Rosenberg and Riedel 1946), were developed. These flocculation tests, in which commercially available standardized reagents were used, yielded reproducible results, could be rapidly performed, gave acceptable levels of sensitivity and specificity and were soon converted to methods for mass screening. The addition of choline chloride and EDTA to the VDRL antigen enhanced the reactivity of the test and stabilized the antigen suspension (Portnoy et al. 1961). In the resulting unheated serum reagin (USR) test, as the name implies, the need for heating serum was eliminated and plasma was also

found to be an acceptable test sample source. The next modification in the late 1950s was the incorporation of charcoal particles into the USR antigen to aid in reading the reaction (Portnoy, Carson and Smith 1957). The resulting test was the rapid plasma reagin (RPR) test performed on a plastic coated card. Additional modifications of the RPR card test resulted in the reagin screen test (RST) (March and Stiles 1980) and the toluidine red unheated serum test (TRUST) (Pettit et al. 1983) and numerous other variations on the RPR test.

Flocculation tests

The 4 non-treponemal flocculation tests currently considered as standard tests in the USA and elsewhere (see Table 34.4) are based on an antigen composed of an alcoholic solution containing measured amounts of cardiolipin, cholesterol and sufficient purified lecithin to produce standard reactivity. In these non-treponemal tests, the liposomes formed in the cardiolipin–cholesterol–lecithin emulsion are barely visible. In agglutination, precipitin and flocculation reactions, antigen–antibody recognition occurs first, followed by the aggregation and antigen–antibody lattice formation. Because the reaction in the non-treponemal tests stays suspended and the 2 reactants themselves are not readily visible, the term flocculation, rather than agglutination, is used to describe this type of reaction. Based on the 1995 College of American Pathologists Syphilis Serology Survey, the RPR card test is the most widely used non-treponemal test in the USA.

The 4 standard non-treponemal tests can be used as qualitative tests for initial screening or as the quantitative tests to follow treatment (Fiumara 1978, 1979, 1980a, 1980b, Pettit et al. 1981, Brown et al. 1985, Romanowski et al. 1991). In the qualitative non-treponemal tests, undiluted serum from a patient is used to measure the presence or absence of antibodies. In the quantitative non-treponemal tests, serial 2-fold dilutions are made and the serum is diluted until an end point is reached. Quantitative reactions are reported in terms of the highest (last) dilution in which the specimen is fully reactive. Quantitative tests are more informative than qualitative tests alone. Quantitative tests establish a baseline of reactivity from which change can be measured; recent infection can be demonstrated by a 4-fold rise in titre and reinfection or relapse can be detected among persons with a

Table 34.5 History of tests for syphilis: non-treponemal tests

Date	Author	Accomplishment
1906	Wassermann, Neisser and Brück	Developed complement-fixation test
1907	Michaelis	Developed first precipitation test without need for complement
1922	Kahn	Introduced a flocculation test that required no complement
1941	Pangborn	Isolated and purified cardiolipin
1946	Harris, Rosenberg and Riedel	Developed Venereal Disease Research Laboratory (VDRL) test
1957	Portnoy, Carson and Smith	Modified the VDRL to create the unheated serum reagin (USR)
1961	Portnoy et al.	Modified the USR to create the rapid plasma reagin (RPR)
1980	March and Stiles	Developed reagin screen test (RST)
1983	Pettit et al.	Modified USR to create toluidine red unheated serum test (TRUST)
1987	Pedersen, Orum and Mouritsen	Developed non-treponemal enzyme-linked immunosorbent (ELISA)

persistently reactive (serofast) test for syphilis. All serum samples exhibiting any degree of reactivity or roughness should be diluted. Although all 4 tests have the same level of sensitivity and specificity (Table 34.6), the levels of reactivity vary. These different levels of reactivity are reflected in the different end point titres obtained when the same serum specimen is tested in the 4 tests (Pettit et al. 1981, 1983). Because success or failure of treatment is based on just a 2-dilution decrease in titre, the serum sample used as the baseline should be drawn the day treatment is begun (Mahoney, Arnold and Harris 1949). Because reactivity levels vary among the tests, the test used in the initial testing should also be used to monitor treatment.

ELISA non-treponemal antibody tests

In 1987, Pedersen, Orum and Mouritsen developed a VDRL–enzyme-linked immunosorbent assay (ELISA) to detect IgG antibodies. The newest of the non-treponemal tests, VISUWELL Reagin, is based on the Pedersen method (White and Fuller 1989). In the indirect ELISA procedure, VDRL antigen coats the wells of a microtitre plate. The patient's serum is added and non-treponemal antibodies attach to the VDRL antigen. These antibodies are then detected with an antihuman immunoglobulin conjugate lab-

elled with an enzyme. Finally, at a specified time a stop solution is added and results are read spectrophoto-metrically. Studies (Pedersen, Orum and Mouritsen 1987, White and Fuller 1989) have shown the test to have a sensitivity of 97% in untreated syphilis and a specificity of 97% (Table 34.6). Like the other non-treponemal tests, the reactivity of the VISUWELL Reagin test usually disappears with treatment of the patient. The major disadvantage of VISUWELL Reagin test is the inability to quantitate the reactivity of a patient's serum to an end point titre in order to assess the efficacy of treatment. Using the VISUWELL Reagin test, several hundred tests can be performed in a day.

PROBLEMS ENCOUNTERED WITH THE NON-TREPONEMAL TESTS

Three major problems are encountered with the non-treponemal tests: the prozone phenomenon, false positive reactions and test interpretation. Serum samples containing large amounts of non-treponemal antibody occasionally demonstrate a prozone reaction in the non-treponemal serological tests. Prozone reactions occur in 1–2% of patients with secondary syphilis (Spangler et al. 1964, Jurado, Campbell and Martin 1993). A prozone occurs when an antibody is in excess, incomplete, or blocks the normal antigen–anti-

Table 34.6 The sensitivities and specificities of the non-treponemal tests

Test	% Sensitivity Stage of infection				% Specificity
	Primary	Secondary	Latent	Late	Non-syphilis
VDRL	78 (74–87)[a]	100	95 (88–100)	71 (37–94)	98 (96–99)
RPR	86 (77–100)	100	98 (95–100)	73	98 (93–99)
USR	80 (72–88)	100	95 (88–100)		99
TRUST	85 (77–86)	100	98 (95–100)		99 (98–99)
VDRL/ELISA	90	100	100		98

[a]Range of sensitivity in CDC studies.

body reaction. Initially, these strongly reactive serum samples may show a weakly reactive, atypical, or on rare occasions, a negative rough reaction or grainy appearance in undiluted serum. Upon dilution of a serum exhibiting the prozone reaction, the reactivity will increase and then decrease as the end point titre is approached. Dilution of the antibody to 1:16 is usually adequate to obtain the proper optimal concentration and a readily detectable reaction. All tests with a 'rough' appearance should be quantitated. A serologist may not detect a prozone reaction because of a lack of reading experience. When fresh serum samples are tested, some exhibit innate roughness. Many serologists compensate for this roughness in their reading and fail to quantitate all serum samples exhibiting a grainy appearance (negative roughs). A second reason that the prozone reaction may not be detected is that the antigen is added to the serum before the sample is spread to fill the circle. The physical spreading of the serum first, before adding the antigen, dilutes the antibodies slightly and frequently prevents the prozone reaction.

The incidence of false positive reactions depends on the test used and the population studied. False positive reactions occurring with the non-treponemal tests can be divided into 2 groups: those that are acute false positive reactions of <6 months' duration and those that are chronic false positive reactions that persist for >6 months (Jaffe and Musher 1990). Acute false positive non-treponemal reactions have been associated with hepatitis, infectious mononucleosis, viral pneumonia, chickenpox, measles, other viral infections, malaria, immunizations, pregnancy and laboratory or technical error (Table 34.7). Chronic false positive reactions have been associated with connective tissue diseases such as systemic lupus erythematosus or diseases associated with immunoglobulin abnormalities which are more common in women; thus, chronic false positive reactions are more common in women than in men. Other conditions associated with chronic false positive reactions are narcotic addiction, ageing (Tuffanelli 1966), leprosy and malignancy (Jaffe and Musher 1990) (Table 34.7). HIV infection has not been associated with an increase in false positive non-treponemal test results in individuals with a low risk of drug addiction (Rusnak et al. 1994). At one time, titre was used to distinguish between false and true positive results, titres of >8 considered as true positives and those <8 as possible false positives. The titre of false positive reactions is usually low, but on rare occasions can be extremely high; therefore, the quantitative titre cannot be used to differentiate between a false positive reaction and syphilis. This is especially true for persons who inject illegal drugs. More than 10% of intravenous drug users have false positive test results with titres >8 (Larsen 1983).

The interpretation of non-treponemal test results depends on the population being tested. The predictive value of the non-treponemal tests is increased when combined with a reactive treponemal test. Therefore, when the non-treponemal tests are used as screening tests in a low risk population, all reactive results should be confirmed with a treponemal test. In some low risk populations, every reactive result may be a false positive result. Non-treponemal test results also must be interpreted according to the stage of syphilis suspected. A reactive or weakly reactive result can be seen in all stages of syphilis. These results can also indicate a person who is serofast or could represent a false positive reaction. A non-reactive result generally excludes active infection. However, serological tests may be non-reactive during incubating disease.

A major source of error in the non-treponemal tests is improper temperature of the laboratory, specimens, or reagents. If the temperature of any one of these is <23°C, test reactivity is decreased; if the temperature is >29°C, test reactivity is increased. Other sources of errors include the testing of haemolysed specimens (especially in the VDRL-CSF) or contaminated or lipoidal specimens, improper rotation time or speed and incorrect antigen delivery (Larsen, Hunter and Kraus 1990).

TREPONEMAL TESTS

All treponemal tests use *T. pallidum* or the components thereof as the antigen and are based on the detection of antibodies directed against treponemal components. Treponemal tests are used primarily to verify reactivity in the non-treponemal tests. The treponemal tests may also be used to confirm a clinical impression of syphilis in which the non-treponemal test is non-reactive, but there is evidence of syphilis, such as might occur in late syphilis. Treponemal tests are technically more difficult and costly to perform than non-treponemal tests and preferably should not be used to screen for syphilis. When treponemal tests are used for screening purposes, about 1% (Goldman and Lantz 1971) of the general population will have false positive results. However, a reactive treponemal test result on a sample that is also reactive in a non-treponemal test is highly specific. Since treponemal tests remain reactive despite therapy, they cannot be used to monitor response to treatment. Only 3 tests are considered standard treponemal test techniques in the USA (see Table 34.4).

Initial attempts to develop a test using an antigen derived from the treponeme were unsuccessful until 1949 when Nelson and Mayer developed the first treponemal antibody test, the *Treponema pallidum* immobilization (TPI) test (Table 34.8). The TPI test used *T. pallidum* (Nichols strain) grown in rabbit testes as the antigen and was based on the ability of patients' antibody and complement to immobilize living treponemes, as observed by darkfield microscopy. The TPI test was rapidly accepted as a specific test for syphilis. However, because the TPI test was complicated, technically difficult, time-consuming and expensive to perform, a simpler procedure was sought. In addition, studies (Hedersted 1976, Rein et al. 1980) in the 1970s found that the TPI test was less sensitive and specific than the treponemal tests developed in the 1960s. As with the non-treponemal tests, an array of treponemal tests was later developed, some of which enjoyed short

Table 34.7 Causes of acute and chronic false positive reactions in the non-treponemal tests

Acute	Chronic
Hepatitis	Connective tissue diseases
Viral pneumonia	Immunoglobulin abnormalities
Measles	Narcotic addiction
Malaria	Ageing
Pregnancy	Leprosy
Infectious mononucleosis	Malignancy
Chickenpox	
Other viral infections	
Immunizations	
Laboratory or technical error	

periods of popularity (Table 34.8). However, a significant proportion of false positive reactions occurred with these tests and subsequent evaluation proved them to be less specific and sensitive than the TPI test (Sparling 1971).

Fluorescent treponemal antibody tests

In 1957, a major advance in treponemal antigen tests occurred with the development of the fluorescent treponemal antibody (FTA) test (Deacon, Falcone and Harris 1957). The original FTA procedure used a 1:5 dilution of the patient's serum in saline solution, reacted with a suspension of killed treponemes. Non-specific reactions were encountered in approximately 25% of normal serum specimens (Wallace and Norins 1969). To eliminate these false positive reactions, the test was modified by diluting the patient's serum to 1:200 (called the FTA-200) (Deacon, Freeman and Harris 1960). However, the FTA-200 test, although highly specific, was not very sensitive. The non-specific reactions of the original FTA test were found to arise because of shared antigens common to *T. pallidum* and the non-pathogenic treponemes that occur as part of the normal bacterial flora of humans. Deacon and Hunter (1962), by preparing a sonicate from cultures of the Reiter spirochaete, removed by absorption the common antigens. Their work led to the development of the more specific and sensitive fluorescent trepone-

mal antibody absorption (FTA-ABS) test (Hunter, Deacon and Meyer 1964). The FTA-ABS and its counterpart, the FTA-ABS double-staining (DS) test, used with incident light microscopes (Hunter et al. 1979), remain the standard treponemal tests for syphilis today.

The FTA-ABS test is an indirect fluorescent antibody technique. In this procedure, the antigen used is subspecies *pallidum* (Nichols strain). Plasma cannot be used in the FTA-ABS tests. The patient's serum is first diluted to 1:5 in sorbent (an extract from cultures of the non-pathogenic Reiter treponeme) to remove group treponemal antibodies that are produced in some persons in response to non-pathogenic treponemes. Next, the serum is layered on a microscope slide to which *T. pallidum* has been fixed. If the patient's serum contains antibody, it coats the treponeme. FITC-labelled antihuman immunoglobulin is added and combines with the patient's antibodies adhering to *T. pallidum*, resulting in FITC-stained spirochaetes that are visible when examined by a fluorescence microscope. A modification of the standard FTA-ABS test is the FTA-ABS DS test (Hunter 1990). The FTA-ABS DS technique employs a tetramethylrhodamine isothiocyanate-labelled, antihuman IgG globulin and a counterstain with FITC-labelled anti-*T. pallidum* conjugate. The counterstain was developed for use with microscopes with incident

Table 34.8 History of tests for syphilis: treponemal tests

Date	Author	Accomplishment
1949	Nelson and Mayer	Developed the first treponemal antibody test, the *Treponema pallidum* immobilization (TPI) test
1953	D'Allesandro and Dardanoni	Developed the Reiter complement fixation test
1957	Deacon, Falcone and Harris	Developed the fluorescent treponemal antibody (FTA) test
1964	Hunter, Deacon and Meyer	Modified the FTA by the addition of sorbent, FTA-ABS test
1965	Rathlev	Developed the haemagglutination test for syphilis (TPHA)
1969	Cox, Logan and Norins	Modified TPHA to a micromethod (MHA-TP)
1975	Veldekamp and Visser	Developed treponemal enzyme-linked immunosorbent test (ELISA)
1982	Hanff et al.	Applied the Western blot technique to the diagnosis of syphilis
1989	Schouls et al.	First to use a cloned antigen in a serological test for syphilis

illumination to eliminate the need to locate the treponemes by darkfield when the patient's serum did not contain antibodies to *T. pallidum*. Therefore, counterstaining the organism ensures that the non-reactive result is due to the absence of antibodies and not to the absence of treponemes on the slide when it is read with incident illumination. Reactive results of both FTA-ABS tests cover a range of staining intensities from 1+ (reactive minimal) to 4+. Because beaded fluorescence (atypical staining) has been observed in serum from patients with active systemic lupus erythematosus and from patients with other autoimmune diseases, this observation should also be reported.

IgM variations on the FTA test

Several variations on the FTA-ABS test have been used for the diagnosis of congenital syphilis by replacing the IgG conjugate with an IgM conjugate. The FTA IgM and the FTA-ABS IgM were reported to be both non-specific and lacking in sensitivity (Alford et al. 1969, Mamunes et al. 1970, Johnston 1972a, Kaufman et al. 1977, Muller 1986, Larsen and Zenker 1990). The specificity of the FTA-ABS IgM test for neonatal congenital syphilis, as well as other indirect immunofluorescent IgM tests for prenatal infections, has been questioned by the observation that newborns may produce IgM antibodies in response to passively transferred maternal IgG antibody rather than in response to the infectious agent itself (Reimer et al. 1975). The fractionation of the infant's serum in the FTA-ABS 19S IgM test appears to eliminate the majority of the problems with the specificity of the test. The FTA-ABS 19S IgM test is not available in kit form and matching the reagents to be used in the test is extremely difficult. False positive reactions in the current version of the FTA-ABS IgM test with the 19S fraction of IgM have been reported in normal infants, but they are infrequent and the test may be a useful confirmatory procedure to differentiate passive transfer of maternal antibody from active infection (Muller 1986, Stoll et al. 1993). Still the major drawback of the FTA-ABS IgM 19S test for neonatal congenital syphilis lies in its insensitivity (Reimer et al. 1975, Stoll et al. 1993). Therefore, while the FTA-ABS 19S IgM test for congenital syphilis may be useful as a confirmatory test, it should not be used as a screening procedure and, at this time, cannot replace careful repeated clinical assessment combined with serial quantitative non-treponemal tests in the evaluation of the newborn with possible congenital syphilis.

CSF variations on the FTA test

Another variation on the FTA-ABS procedure is the FTA-ABS CSF test for the diagnosis of neurosyphilis. FTA tests used for CSF examination have included techniques that used undiluted CSF (the CSF-FTA) (Harris et al. 1960, Escobar, Dalton and Allison 1970, Garner and Backhouse 1971, Duncan, Jenkins and Parham 1972, Wilkinson 1973, Jaffe et al. 1978b, Larsen et al.1985) and tests that used CSF diluted to 1:5 with sorbent (the CSF-FTA-ABS test). FTA tests on

CSF are more sensitive than the CSF-VDRL slide test. However, the clinical significance of this greater sensitivity remains to be established, because the test may be reactive as a result of antibodies remaining in the CSF of patients who had been adequately treated for early or latent syphilis rather than as a result of neurosyphilis (Jaffe et al. 1978b). False positive results have been reported with the CSF-FTA tests (Escobar Dalton and Allison 1970, Larsen et al. 1985) that appear to be eliminated by diluting the CSF in sorbent. The results of 3 studies appear to support the use of a non-reactive result with the FTA-ABS CSF test to rule out neurosyphilis (Jaffe et al 1978b, Luger, Marhold and Schmidt 1988, Marra et al. 1995).

The sources for errors are numerous with the FTA-ABS tests and its variations because they are multi-component tests and each component must be matched with another. Conjugates must be properly titrated and controls for reactive, reactive minimal, non-reactive and non-specific staining, and sorbent must be included. Slides must be evaluated to ensure that the antigen is adhering. In addition, the microscope must be in proper operating condition with the appropriate filters in place.

Haemagglutination methods

In 1965, Rathlev reported the first reliable application of haemagglutination techniques to the serological diagnosis of syphilis. The antigen used in her procedure was formalinized, tanned sheep erythrocytes sensitized with ultrasonicated material from *T. pallidum* (Nichols strain). The presence of treponemal antibodies in the patient's serum was detected by the indirect agglutination of the sensitized erythrocytes and the subsequent formation of a mat of erythrocytes upon their settling. In 1967 Rathlev published the results of her experience with this method on 300 serum samples. Modifications of Rathlev's procedure followed, including the use of an improved reaction medium (Tomizawa and Kasamatsu 1966) and a sorbent much like the one used in the FTA-ABS test for removal of group treponemal antibodies (Tomizawa, Kasamatsu and Yamaya 1969). The haemagglutination procedure was first a tube test known as the *T. pallidum* haemagglutination (TPHA) test. Subsequently, reagents for a microvolume haemagglutination test (Cox, Logan and Norins 1969), the microhaemagglutination assay for antibodies to *T. pallidum* (MHA-TP), became commercially available. Other haemagglutination tests for syphilis, based on the use of sensitized turkey, sheep or chicken cells and performed in microtitre plates, are currently available world wide. The haemagglutination tests are simpler to perform than the fluorescent antibody tests; one haemagglutination method, the PK-*T. pallidum* (PK-TP), has recently been automated.

The microhaemagglutination reagents, manufactured by Fujirebio in Japan and sold as the MHA-TP or TPHA, are the most widely used reagents. The antigen used in the procedure is formalinized, tanned sheep erythrocytes sensitized with ultrasonicated material from *T. pallidum* (Nichols strain). The patient's serum is first mixed with absorbing diluent made from non-pathogenic Reiter treponemes and other absorbents and stabilizers. The serum is then placed in a microtitre plate and sensitized sheep red cells are added. Unsensitized cells are used as a control for non-specific reactivity. Reactive results are reported over a range of agglutination patterns, from a smooth mat of agglutinated cells surrounded by a smaller red circle of unagglutinated cells with haemagglutination outside the circle (1+), to a smooth mat of agglutinated cells covering the entire bottom of the well (4+). Inconclusive results are reported when a heterophile reaction that cannot be diluted out is observed.

Because the test is based on agglutination, quantitation of treponemal antibodies is possible, but has not proved to be useful. Most studies demonstrate no practical relationship between the titre and either the progression of the disease or the clinical stage of syphilis diagnosed; unlike the quantitative non-treponemal tests, the quantitative haemagglutination test does not seem to be useful in post-treatment evaluation (Cox, Logan and Stout 1971, Buist, Pertile and Morris 1973, Johnston 1972b). The sources for error with the haemagglutination tests are usually associated with the use of dusty or improper plates, pipetting errors and vibrations in the laboratory.

An automated haemagglutination test is the Olympus PK-TP. This test was developed mainly for use in blood banking. The instrument used is a PK7100 or 7200, an automated pretransfusion blood testing system, which is the basic equipment for blood grouping and typing used by the American Red Cross. The instrument is capable of running 240 samples per hour. The PK-TP reagent is composed of chicken erythrocytes that have been fixed, then sensitized with components of sonicated *T. pallidum*. In the USA, the use of the test as a screening test is restricted at this time to blood banking organizations. Early experience with the PK-TP in blood banks (Forbes, Rutter and Abraham 1991) indicates that the PK-TP is at least twice as specific as the RPR card test.

ELISA treponemal antibody tests

The ELISA was first applied to the area of syphilis serology in 1975 (Veldekamp and Visser 1975) (Table 34.8). Since that time many other tests using the ELISA format have been developed and evaluated as treponemal tests (Pedersen et al. 1982, Pope, Hunter and Feeley 1982, Farshy et al. 1985, Burdash et al. 1987, Moyer, Hudson and Hausler 1987, Young et al. 1992, Nayar and Campos 1993). Of the commercial ELISA tests designed to replace the FTA-ABS and haemagglutination tests as confirmatory tests for syphilis, initial evaluations have found all to have sensitivities and specificities similar to those of the other treponemal tests (Nayar and Campos 1993), but more extensive evaluation is necessary (Norgard 1993). Many of the ELISA tests are based on the use of cloned antigens. The first cloned antigen to be used in the development of a serological test for the diagnosis of syphilis was the TmpA protein (Schouls et al.

1989). This protein has since been shown to be a membrane-localized lipoprotein. It is found closely associated with another membrane protein (TmpB), and the 2 genes may be transcriptionally coupled since the start ATG of one overlaps with the termination codon of the other. The gene yields a mature protein of approximately 42 kDa. When used for an ELISA, this protein proved to be both sensitive and specific; results were almost exactly the same as those seen with the MHA-TP and FTA-ABS tests. The authors (Schouls et al. 1989) found a significant correlation between the antibody titre against this antigen and efficacy of treatment of patients. Therefore, they suggested that the test could be of significance in monitoring treatment for syphilis with antibiotics. The test is not yet available on the US market.

Several other recombinant proteins have been used to develop ELISAs since, the most prominent being the TmpB and TmpC proteins. The protein on which the greatest amount of work has been done is the 47 kDa protein (Jones et al. 1984), which is now thought to be a penicillin-binding protein. This protein has been shown to be immunodominant, produced in large quantities by the treponemes and does not cross-react to any extent with similar proteins from the commensal treponemes. The ELISA system that uses this protein is the VISUWELL syphilis test and is available in Canada and the USA.

Limitations of the ELISA tests are time and costs when small numbers of samples are to be processed. The main advantages are the capacity to process large numbers of samples and the automated readout. No longer is the reading of the test subjective, as for the FTA-ABS and haemagglutination tests, but a spectrophotometric determination is made and an objective reading provided as a printout.

IgM variation on the ELISA test

A variation on the ELISA test is the Captia syphilis M test (Ijsselmuiden et al. 1989, Lefèvre Bertrand and Bauriaud 1990, Stoll et al. 1993) for the detection of congenital syphilis in the newborn. Because infected infants can produce IgM in utero after 3 months of gestation and the fetus can be infected with *T. pallidum* at any time during gestation, an IgM ELISA test has been developed. The test is based on using anti-human IgM antibody to capture IgM in the patient's serum, followed by the addition of a purified *T. pallidum* antigen to detect those IgM antibodies in the patient's serum directed toward *T. pallidum* (Ijsselmuiden et al. 1989). One study (Stoll et al. 1993) found that the IgM capture ELISA was more sensitive than the FTA-ABS 19S IgM test in detecting probable cases of congenital syphilis; however, another study (Bromberg, Rawstron and Tannis 1993) found the test to be equal in sensitivity to the IgM Western immunoblot in neonatal congenital syphilis, but less sensitive than the Western blot in detecting delayed onset congenital syphilis. Current interpretations of the IgM capture test results are given in Table 34.9. The interpretation of the test result is linked to the treatment status of the mother and her stage of syphilis.

Immunoblotting

The Western blot technique developed by Hanff et al. (1982) for *T. pallidum* can be used to detect either IgG (Byrne et al. 1992, Norgard 1993) or IgM (Sanchez et al. 1989, Meyer, Eddy and Baughn 1994) antibodies. Performance of the Western blot techniques for syphilis is similar to the techniques used for confirmation of antibodies to the human immunodeficiency virus (HIV). To prepare the strips for *T. pallidum* immunoblotting, initially a boiled sodium dodecyl sulphate (SDS) extract of the organism is electrophoresed through a gradient gel. After electrophoresis, a sheet of nitrocellulose is placed on top of the gel and the protein immunodeterminants are electrophoretically transferred to the blot. The blot is cut into strips and incubated with the patient's serum sample. If a commercial test kit is used, the starting point is the nitrocellulose strip. After incubation of the strips with the patient's serum, antibodies are detected using a second antibody as in an indirect test, labelled with either an enzyme and substrate or a radioactive material. To date, many investigators (Norris and the *Treponema pallidum* Polypeptide Research Group 1993) and the manufacturer of at least one commercial product agree that detected antibodies to the immunodeterminants with molecular masses of 15.5 kDa, 17 kDa, 44.5 kDa and 47 kDa appear to be diagnostic for acquired syphilis. The test using IgG conjugate appears to be at least as sensitive and specific as the FTA-ABS tests (Byrne et al. 1992) and efforts have been made to standardize the procedure (George, Pope and Larsen 1991). In addition, various groups have reported the use of cloned proteins that are secreted from the cytoplasm for Western blotting (Strugnell, Cockayne and Penn 1990, Norris and the *Treponema pallidum* Polypeptide Research Group 1993).

PROBLEMS ENCOUNTERED WITH THE TREPONEMAL TESTS

Although false positive results in the treponemal tests are often transient and their cause is unknown, a definite association has been made between false positive FTA-ABS test results and the diagnosis of systemic discoid (Shore and Faricelli 1977, Anderson and Stillman 1978) and drug-induced varieties of lupus erythematosus (Kraus, Haserick and Lantz 1970, Kraus et al. 1971, McKenna, Schroeter and Kierland 1973, Monson 1973) (Table 34.10). Patients with systemic lupus erythematosus can have false positive FTA-ABS tests that exhibit an 'atypical beading' fluorescence pattern. To resolve these types of false positive reactions, absorption with calf thymus DNA can be used to remove the anti-DNA antibodies in the serum (Kraus et al. 1971). Unexplained reactive serological results may also occur, in elderly patients. Further, some false positive reactions may be due to the failure of the sorbent used in the tests to remove all cross-reacting group, genus, or family antibodies (e.g. Lyme disease) (Hunter et al. 1986, Magnarelli et al. 1990). In these instances, absorption with *Treponema phagedenis* or the use of the haemagglutination test or immunoblotting may be the only means of differentiating between syphilis and a false positive reaction.

Of the 2 standard treponemal test systems (fluorescent antibody and haemagglutination) currently in use, the haemagglutination methods give fewer false positive test results (Jaffe et al. 1978a, Wentworth et al. 1978, Larsen et al. 1981). In general, the occurrence of false positive haemagglutination tests is rare in 'healthy' persons (<1%). Inconclusive haemagglutination tests have been reported for patients with infectious mononucleosis, especially in the presence of a high heterophile antibody level (Johnston 1972b). Presumably, false positive haemagglutination tests also occur in samples from drug addicts, patients with collagen disease, patients with leprosy and in patients with other miscellaneous con-

Table 34.10 Causes of chronic false positive reactions in the treponemal tests

Systemic lupus erythematosus
Drug-induced lupus erythematosus
Narcotic addiction
Ageing

Table 34.9 Interpretation of Captia Syphilis M results for the diagnosis of congenital syphilis

Infant's result	Clinical signs/ symptoms in infant	Mother's treatment history	Serodiagnosis
Non-reactive	Present	Untreated or inadequately treated	Congenital syphilis
Non-reactive	Absent	Untreated or inadequately treated early syphilis	Possible incubating congenital syphilis
Non-reactive	Absent	Untreated or inadequately treated latent syphilis	Unknown risk of congenital syphilis
Reactive	Present	Untreated or inadequately treated	Congenital syphilis
Reactive	Absent	Untreated or inadequately treated	Suggestive of congenital syphilis

ditions (Wentworth et al. 1978, Rein et al. 1980, Larsen et al. 1981). In some cases, the results are difficult to assess because syphilis may coexist with these other conditions. If both the FTA-ABS and haemagglutination tests are reactive, the sample is most likely (95%) from a person who has or has had syphilis (Rein et al. 1980). However, the diagnosis rests with clinical judgement.

Treponemal tests vary in their reactivity in early primary syphilis (Table 34.11); the varied sensitivities of the treponemal tests in primary syphilis are related to the time of serum collection after lesion development. For 85% of persons successfully treated, test results can remain reactive for years, for some people a lifetime (Schroeter et al. 1972). In addition, for the diagnosis of late untreated syphilis, reactivity in the treponemal test may be the only indication of a previous treponemal infection.

4.3 Direct antigen detection methods

The shortcomings of the standard tests for syphilis for the diagnosis of early primary, congenital and neurosyphilis make techniques based on the detection of treponemal DNA or antigens very appealing (see Table 34.3, p. 646). In order to determine the sensitivity and specificity of these newer techniques, rabbit infectivity testing (RIT) is used as the gold standard (Grimprel et al. 1991, Sanchez et al. 1993).

ANIMAL INOCULATION

The oldest method for detecting infection with *T. pallidum* is animal infectivity testing. This technique probably offers the most sensitive method for detecting infectious treponemes. Numerous animal species, from hamsters to chimpanzees, have been used either to maintain treponemes or to determine infectivity (Wilcox and Guthe 1966). However, not all animals develop visible signs of infection or reactive serological tests. The rabbit is the most practical animal because a local lesion can be produced at the site of inoculation, the tissues remain infective for the life of the animal, infection can be transferred from one animal to another using minced lymph nodes or testes, and serological tests for syphilis become reactive. Any specimen can be used for RIT as long as the material was collected less than 1 h before inoculation or is flash-frozen immediately after collection

and maintained in liquid nitrogen or at temperatures of $-78°C$ or below (Turner and Fleming 1939). Rabbits are usually inoculated intratesticularly or intradermally with the samples suspected of being infective; ocular, intravenous, or scrotal inoculation may also be used. Detailed methods for the maintenance and passage of *T. pallidum* in rabbits are available from CDC (Centers for Disease Control and Prevention 1994). The incubation period in rabbits from inoculation to the formation of lesions is inversely proportional to the size of the inoculum (Magnuson, Eagle and Fleishman 1948). The sensitivity of RIT approaches 100% if the number of organisms in the inoculum exceeds 23 (Magnuson et al. 1956) and the patient has not received antibiotic treatment.

DNA PROBES

The greatest difficulty with the DNA approach to syphilis diagnosis is the lack of understanding of the biology of the organism, which complicates the selection of target antigens or DNA sequences. Despite these difficulties some progress has been made in treponemal diagnosis using techniques based on molecular biology. All these techniques are presently experimental but they offer the possibility of great sensitivity and, in some cases, increased potential for automation of syphilis testing.

DNA probes have already found clinical application for the identification of a number of clinically important pathogens (Wilkinson, Sampson and Plikaytis 1986, Viscidi and Yolken 1987). Experience with other spirochaetes indicates the possible applicability of this methodology in the identification of *T. pallidum* (Terpstra, Schoone and Ter Schegget 1986). Dot blot assays based on DNA probes appear to lack sufficient sensitivity to serve as clinical tests, but no attempt has been made to optimize the assay by determining what sequences would be most suitable; thus, the potential of this method is still undetermined. In many of the problem areas in syphilis diagnosis (neurosyphilis, congenital syphilis), only rarely are large numbers of treponemes seen in clinical samples (Schwartz et al. 1995) and, thus, the sensitivity of the dot blot would have to be considerably enhanced to make this a viable method of diagnosis for syphilis.

Table 34.11 The sensitivities and specificities of treponemal tests

Test	% Sensitivity Stage of infection				% Specificity
	Primary	**Secondary**	**Latent**	**Late**	**Non-syphilis**
FTA-ABS	84 (70–100)[a]	100	100	96	97 (94–100)
MHA-TP	79 (69–90)	100	99 (97–100)	94	99 (98–100)
FTA-ABS DS	86 (69–93)	100	100		98 (97–100)
EIA-47kDa	90	100	100		94
Western blot	90	100	100		98

[a]Range in CDC studies.

PCR

Because of the low sensitivity of DNA probes as cited above, PCR-based methods might offer better possibilities for clinical applications. PCR-based tests have been developed by several laboratories either as potential diagnostic tests or to identify *T. pallidum*-infected animals in experimental systems (Burstain et al. 1991, Grimprel et al. 1991, Noordhoek et al. 1991b, Wicher et al. 1992, Sanchez et al. 1993). Most of the tests have been based on the genes encoding membrane lipoproteins of which a large number have been cloned and sequenced. This work has been significantly aided by the fact that *T. pallidum* is extremely genetically conserved. Whereas variation in membrane and surface-associated proteins is common among many species of bacteria, this variation has never been shown with *T. pallidum*; even the different subspecies show essentially identical patterns by one-dimensional SDS-PAGE (Strugnell, Cockayne and Penn 1990). This extreme genetic stability is probably related to the apparent lack of significant DNA repair capacity in *T. pallidum* (Steiner et al. 1984) and the possible absence of the recA gene product (Stamm, Parrish and Gherardine 1991), which would indicate little or no recombinational capacity in this spirochaete.

Two PCR-based techniques were described almost simultaneously (Grimprel et al. 1991, Noordhoek et al. 1991b). Since sensitive and inexpensive serological tests are available for most stages of syphilis in adults, the investigators in these 2 papers concentrated on problem areas in which definitive diagnosis is beyond the abilities of most clinical laboratories. The first of these techniques was based on the amplification of a 658 base pair segment of the gene for the 47 kDa surface antigen; this is a lipoprotein that is antigenically dominant in the human immune response to *T. pallidum* (Jones et al. 1984). The test was performed on clinical specimens (amniotic fluid, neonatal sera and neonatal CSF) for use in the diagnosis of congenital syphilis in neonates (Grimprel et al. 1991, Norgard 1993, Sanchez et al. 1993). The test results were verified with the RIT. In the various tissue fluids examined (Grimprel et al. 1991, Sanchez et al. 1993), the overall sensitivity was 78% when compared with results obtained in the RIT. The major difficulty with the test was one that has hindered the application of PCR in other clinical settings: lack of sensitivity in detecting positive specimens. False positive results, caused by the improper handling of the specimens and resulting in contamination with extraneous treponemal DNA, did not seem to be a problem (Kwok and Higuchi 1989). Of the samples that were negative by RIT, none was positive by PCR.

Only in the amniotic fluid samples was the PCR sufficiently sensitive to be considered as a diagnostic test; CSF and serum results correlated approximately 60–67% with positive results by the RIT. The lack of sensitivity has generally been found to be related to non-specific inhibitors of the PCR reaction. To eliminate inhibition, Grimprel et al. (1991) used 4 different methods to isolate DNA from the samples: a boiling method, a low-spin separation, an alkaline lysis and a spin separation method. The low-spin and alkaline lysis methods seemed to give the best correlations with rabbit infectivity. The alkaline lysis methods showed better results with small volumes of sample usually obtained from the clinical specimens than did the other methods.

Several studies have indicated that *T. pallidum* can persist for long periods in the central nervous system, even in patients who have received adequate antibiotic treatment (Berry et al. 1987, Hay et al. 1990). Serological tests have proved inadequate in the diagnosis of patients with CNS syphilis; their results commonly remain positive in the treponemal tests whether they are still infected or not (Jaffe et al. 1978b, Larsen et al. 1985, Marra et al. 1995). Thus, a method that could detect the presence of *T. pallidum* in small volumes of CSF could prove extremely valuable, especially in determining whether treatment was sufficient in cases where neurosyphilis is suspected or known to have occurred. Noordhoek et al. (1991b) used as their target the gene coding for a 39 kDa basic membrane protein. Primers derived from this gene showed a lack of specificity but the authors were able largely to overcome this problem by using a second pair of nested primers within the sequence used in the first round of amplification. A very serious difficulty developed in this series of tests, which is analogous to problems found in the serological diagnosis of neurosyphilis, namely, the inability to differentiate between patients with active infections and patients who no longer appeared to harbour living treponemes. All patients who had been previously infected with *T. pallidum* were positive by PCR regardless of previous treatment status. Because there is considerable controversy over whether the present treatment regimens successfully eliminate *T. pallidum* from the central nervous system (Berry et al. 1987, Johns, Tierney and Felsenstein 1987, Lukehart et al. 1988, Musher 1991), it was not possible to evaluate these results with certainty. Positive PCR results could indicate either the persistence of small numbers of viable treponemes or of dead organisms containing DNA which could be amplified.

At least 2 other groups have used PCR to detect *T. pallidum* either in clinical samples or in experimental animals (Hay et al. 1990, Wicher et al. 1992). The first group (Hay et al. 1990) used primers derived from the gene sequence of *tmpA* (codes for a 45 kDa membrane protein) and the 4D antigen (an oligomeric protein with multiple forms) as primers. They found a sensitivity of detection equivalent to 65 organisms in non-clinical specimens but did not determine the sensitivity in CSF. They indicated that PCR could be used for determination of treatment success, but this was before the report by Noordhoek et al. (1991b); they also did not evaluate the PCR against known serological tests so the reported sensitivity could not be compared with that of standard clinical methods. The second group (Wicher et al. 1992) used a primer sequence derived from basic membrane protein, a cloned membrane protein with a basic pH. The specimens tested were from a rabbit model of congenital syphilis. An interesting result of these experiments was that only whole blood proved to be positive by PCR; serum samples were uniformly negative with the exception of a single sample that was partially haemolysed. No inhibitory effect was seen with heparin, although this polysaccharide is known to cause inhibition of PCR in other systems (Holodniy et al. 1991). The system as described would seem to have fewer difficulties, in most cases; for example, specimens can be frozen and there are fewer problems with inhibitory materials in the sample. The reason for the inconsistencies with results of other systems is difficult to identify because the animals and samples involved, as well as the PCR target sequence, were different. Because of the controversy over sample source (i.e. whole blood, lesion material, CSF, serum, or amniotic fluid), the appropriate sample source is still under consideration.

PCR could be extremely valuable in diagnosing infection in congenital syphilis (passively transferred antibodies now confuse the diagnosis), in diagnosing neurosyphilis (the only serological test is only 50% sensitive), in diagnosing early primary syphilis (the only tests available are microscopic) and, finally, in distinguishing new infections from old infections (now only a rise in titre can be used). Few clinical studies that compare PCR results with direct microscopic examination have been reported. Results from one study (Jethwa et al. 1995) comparing DFA-TP with PCR using a primer encoding for the 47 kDa protein found a concordance of 95.5% when touch preparations of genital lesions were examined.

5 USE AND INTERPRETATION OF SEROLOGICAL TESTS

5.1 Sexually acquired syphilis

For the laboratory diagnosis of sexually acquired syphilis, each stage has a particular testing requirement. In the USA, the routine testing scheme is direct microscopic examination of lesion exudates, followed by a non-treponemal test that, if reactive, is confirmed with a treponemal test (Table 34.12).

EARLY SYPHILIS

Criteria for the diagnosis of syphilis are divided into 3 categories: definitive, presumptive and suggestive (Centers for Disease Control 1991). These criteria are given in Table 34.12 for the diagnosis of early syphilis. In primary syphilis, the MHA-TP is less sensitive than the FTA-ABS test and probably is less sensitive than the non-treponemal tests, when used to confirm reactivity in the non-treponemal test (Jaffe et al. 1978a, Larsen et al. 1981). As the disease reaches the secondary stage, with few if any exceptions, all serological tests for syphilis are reactive and treponemes may be found in lesions by direct microscopic examination. Serological tests are reactive in the early latent stage, but the reactivity in the non-treponemal tests decreases with increasing latency.

Patients with late latent syphilis, i.e. with reactive non-treponemal and treponemal tests, no clinical and historical findings and an unknown history of treatment or non-reactive serological results, should be evaluated for potential asymptomatic neurosyphilis.

LATE SYPHILIS

Even when the patient has not received treatment, the non-treponemal tests may be only weakly reactive or even non-reactive in the late stages of syphilis. Because results for approximately 30% of patients with late syphilis will be non-reactive in the non-treponemal tests, treponemal test results should be obtained if syphilis in these stages is suspected and the non-treponemal tests are non-reactive. However, the sensitivity of the treponemal tests also declines somewhat in the late stages of syphilis (see Table 34.11, p. 654).

In the lesions (gummas) of benign late syphilis, few treponemes are found by direct microscopic examination. However, if gummas are present, then a definitive diagnosis is based on the observation of *T. pallidum* in biopsy samples by DFAT-TP or by a reactive PCR result (Horowitz et al. 1994) (Table 34.13). Presumptive diagnosis is based on a reactive treponemal test and no known history of treatment for syphilis. Diagnosis of cardiovascular syphilis is made on the bases of symptoms indicative of aortic insufficiency or aneurysm, reactive treponemal test results and no known history of treatment for syphilis.

5.2 Neurosyphilis

CSF examinations, such as the VDRL-CSF slide test, total protein and white cell counts, should be performed on the spinal fluid of patients with late latent syphilis and those with clinical symptoms and signs consistent with neurosyphilis (Table 34.13). Diagnosis of neurosyphilis requires a reactive treponemal test result with a serum sample and a CSF cell count of >5 mononuclear cells per cubic centimetre and CSF total protein in excess of 40 mg dl^{-1}.

The VDRL-CSF test should be performed only if the patient's serum treponemal test is reactive. The VDRL is the only test that should be used for testing CSF (Larsen et al. 1985). The results of the VDRL-CSF test are reported as either reactive or as non-reactive. A quantitative test is performed to determine the titre of the antibodies in the CSF by preparing 2-fold serial dilutions in saline. False positive VDRL-CSF test results have been reported infrequently (Cutler et al. 1954). Because of a lack of sensitivity and specificity the RPR and TRUST card tests cannot be used to test CSF (Larsen et al. 1985). A non-reactive result in the FTA-ABS CSF test (Jaffe et al. 1978b, Marra et al. 1995) may be used to rule out neurosyphilis.

5.3 Congenital syphilis

The control of congenital syphilis can be accomplished by treating pregnant women who are infected. Since false positive non-treponemal test results have been reported in samples from pregnant

Table 34.12 Criteria for diagnosis of early syphilis

Primary
Definitive
  Direct microscopic identification of *T. pallidum* in lesion material, lymph node aspirate, or biopsy
  section
Presumptive (requires 1 **and** either 2 or 3)
  1 Typical lesion
  2 Reactive non-treponemal or treponemal test and no history of syphilis
  3 For persons with a history of syphilis a 4-fold increase in titre on a quantitative non-treponemal test
    when results of past tests are compared with the most recent test results
Suggestive (requires 1 and 2)
  1 Lesion resembling a chancre
  2 Sexual contact within the preceding 90 days with a person who has primary, secondary, or early
    latent syphilis

Secondary
Definitive
  Direct microscopic identification of *T. pallidum* in lesion material, lymph node aspirate or biopsy
  section
Presumptive (requires 1 **and** either 2 or 3)
  1 Skin or mucous membrane lesions typical of secondary syphilis
    (a) Macular, papular, follicular, papulosquamous, or pustular
    (b) Condylomata lata (anogenital region or mouth)
    (c) Mucous patches (oropharynx or cervix)
  2 Reactive non-treponemal test titre ≥ 8, a reactive treponemal test and no previous history of syphilis
  3 For persons with a history of syphilis, a 4-fold increase in the most recent titre when compared with
    previous test results
Suggestive (requires 1 and 2, and is made only when serological tests are not available)
  1 Presence of clinical manifestations as described above
  2 Sexual exposure within the past 6 months to a person with early syphilis

Early latent
Definitive
  A definitive diagnosis does not exist because lesions are not present in the latent stage
Presumptive (requires 1, 2 **and** 3 or 4)
  1 Absence of signs and symptoms
  2 Reactive non-treponemal and treponemal test results
  3 A history of a non-reactive non-treponemal test the prior year
  4 A 4-fold increase in titre compared with the previous test results for persons with a history of
    syphilis or a history of symptoms compatible with early syphilis
Suggestive (requires 1 **and** 2)
  1 A reactive non-treponemal test result
  2 A history of sexual exposure within the preceding year

women (Buchanan and Haserick 1970), it is especially important to confirm reactive results and, if reactive, the patient should be treated. Also in pregnancy, non-treponemal titres remaining from previous treatment of syphilis tend to increase non-specifically. This increase in titre may be confused with the diagnosis of reinfection or relapse. An increase in titre may be considered non-specific if previous treatment can be documented and if positive lesions, a 4-fold increase in titre and a history of recent sexual exposure to a person with infectious syphilis are absent.

When screening for congenital syphilis at delivery, CDC recommends the testing of the mother's serum rather than cord blood (United States Public Health Service 1968). Recent studies (Chhabra et al. 1993, Stoll et al. 1993) compared the reactivity of the mother's serum, cord blood and infant's serum and found that the maternal sample is the best indicator of infection, followed by neonatal serum; cord blood is the least reactive. Infant's serum is the specimen of choice for the IgM specific tests. The standard serological tests for syphilis, based on the measurement of IgG, reflect passively transferred antibodies from the mother to the infant, rather than IgM antibodies produced during gestation. Previously, the difference in the mother's non-treponemal test titre and the infant's titre at delivery was thought to be a means of distinguishing infected from uninfected infants. If the infant's titre was higher than that of the mother's, then the infant had congenital syphilis (Stokes, Beerman and Ingraham 1944). However, the converse has not been found to be true. A lower titre in the infant's serum than in that of the mother does not rule out congenital syphilis (Stoll et al. 1993). Examination of

Table 34.13 Criteria for the diagnosis of late syphilis and neonatal congenital syphilis

Benign and cardiovascular
Definitive
   Observation by direct microscopic examination of treponemes in tissue sections by direct fluorescent antibody tissue test for *T. pallidum* (DFAT-TP)
Presumptive
   1 A reactive treponemal test
   2 No known history of treatment for syphilis
   3 Characteristic symptoms of benign or cardiovascular syphilis

Neurosyphilis
Definitive (requires 1 **and** either 2 or 3)
   1 A reactive serum treponemal test
   2 A reactive VDRL-CSF on a spinal fluid sample
   3 Identification of *T. palladum* in CSF or tissue by microscopic examination or animal inoculation
Presumptive (requires 1 **and** either 2 or 3)
   1 A reactive serum treponemal test
   2 Clinical signs of neurosyphilis
   3 Elevated CSF protein or leucocyte count in the absence of other known causes

Neonatal congenital syphilis
Definitive
   Demonstration of *T. pallidum* by direct microscopic examination of umbilical cord, placenta, nasal discharge or skin lesion material
Presumptive (requires 1, 2 **and** 3)
   1 Determination that the infant was born to a mother who had untreated or inadequately treated syphilis at delivery regardless of findings in the infant
   2 An infant who has a reactive treponemal test result
   3 One of the following additional criteria
      (a) Clinical sign or symptoms of congenital syphilis on physical examination
      (b) An abnormal CSF finding without other cause
      (c) Reactive VDRL-CSF test result
      (d) A reactive IgM antibody test specific for syphilis

serum sample pairs from mothers and infants in cases of congenital syphilis indicated that only in 22% of the cases did the infant have a titre higher than that of the mother. The passively transferred antibodies should be catabolized and undetectable among non-infected infants between the ages of 12 and 18 months (Ingraham 1951, Chang et al. 1995). Criteria for the diagnosis of neonatal congenital syphilis are given in Table 34.13.

5.4 HIV-infected persons with syphilis

In the 1980s, studies showed that 70% of serum specimens from homosexual men with acquired immuno-deficiency syndrome (AIDS) reacted in the treponemal test for syphilis (Rogers et al. 1983). More recent studies in the heterosexual population indicate that approximately 60% of HIV-infected females have reactive syphilis serological test results (Castro et al. 1988); 15% of adolescents with reactive serological tests for syphilis are also positive for HIV antibodies (McCabe, Jaffe and Diaz 1993). Although most HIV-infected persons who are also infected with *T. pallidum* appear to respond normally in the serological tests for syphilis and have typical clinical signs (Gourevitch et al. 1993, Rolfs et al. 1993), several exceptions have been published (Dawson, Evans and Lawrence 1988,

Lanska, Lanska and Schmidley 1988, Radolf and Kaplan 1988) or reported to CDC. The problems in the diagnosis of syphilis are:

1 confusing clinical signs and symptoms
2 lack of serological response in a patient with a clinically confirmed case of active syphilis (Hicks et al. 1987, Gregory, Sanchez and Buckness 1990)
3 failure of non-treponemal test titres to decline after treatment with standard regimens
4 unusually high titres in non-treponemal tests (Musher 1991), perhaps as the result of B cell activation (Lane et al. 1983)
5 rapid progression to late stages of syphilis and neurological involvement even after treatment of primary or secondary syphilis (Berry et al. 1987, Johns, Tierney and Felsenstein 1987, Fernandez-Guerrero et al. 1988, Kase et al. 1988, Musher 1991, Gordon et al. 1994) and
6 the disappearance of treponemal test reactivity over time (Haas et al. 1990).

Whether these problems in the diagnosis of syphilis occur more frequently in HIV-seropositive persons than in HIV-seronegative persons with syphilis is unclear. Aberrant results in the serological tests for syphilis appear to be related to abnormally low absolute CD4 cell counts and are relatively rare (Hicks et al. 1987, Gregory, Sanchez and Buchness 1990). The diagnosis of syphilis in these cases was supported either by an observation of *T. pallidum* in material from typical lesions or by the appearance of serological reactivity after treatment. The delay in development of a response to syphilis, theoretically, should be expected in persons with abnormal lymphocyte counts; however, the frequency of this occurrence appears to be low (Rolfs et al. 1993). In addition, recent studies (Gourevitch et al. 1993, Jurado, Campbell and Martin 1993, Rolfs et al. 1993) found that end point titres in the non-treponemal tests are higher among HIV-infected persons than among individuals not infected with the HIV.

The failure of non-treponemal test titres to decline after treatment with standard therapy has been documented for HIV-seronegative persons treated during latent stage or late stage syphilis and in persons treated for reinfection (Fiumara 1979, 1980a, Romanowski et al. 1991). Therefore, the failure of titres to decline with treatment for syphilis in HIV-infected persons is probably related to the stage of syphilis rather than to HIV status.

Previously, infection with *T. pallidum* has been reported to be immunosuppressive (Jensen and From 1982, Pavia, Folds and Baseman 1976). Recently, Pope and colleagues (1994) reported that although the percentages of CD4 and CD8 lymphocyte subsets for persons with syphilis were within the range of those percentages found in uninfected persons, the percentage of CD4 cells were significantly lower ($p < 0.001$) and CD8 cells higher ($p = 0.03$) among patients with syphilis than in the uninfected population. Early findings in the study by Rolfs et al. (1993) indicated that infection with *T. pallidum* in the HIV-positive person exacerbates the depletion of CD4 receptor cells.

The disappearance of reactivity in the treponemal tests after treatment and over time has been reported in the past, before the identification of HIV-1. Schroeter et al. (1972) reported that 14% of the patients with early syphilis lost their reactivity in the FTA-ABS test within 2 years after treatment. Further studies (Haas et al. 1990) found that specimens from 40% of men with AIDS and 7% of asymptomatic HIV-seropositive men with histories of treatment for syphilis became non-reactive in the treponemal tests, whereas the treponemal test results of the HIV-seronegative men remained reactive. Loss of reactivity in the treponemal tests was related to decreased total CD4 lymphocytes and CD4:CD8 ratios, and a non-treponemal test titre of less than 1:32 at the time of treatment. In the study of Haas et al. (1990), none of the persons had active syphilis. On the other hand, when persons being treated for active syphilis (with and without HIV infection) were followed up over time (Gourevitch et al. 1993), 16% of the patients lost treponemal test reactivity after treatment. The loss of reactivity could not be related to HIV, CD4 count, or stage of syphilis. However, initial low non-treponemal test titre was weakly associated with the loss of treponemal test reactivity.

The literature abounds with descriptions of syphilis in so-called late stage forms in relatively young persons who are HIV-seropositive (Johns, Tierney and Felsenstein 1987, Dawson, Evans and Lawrence 1988, Fernandez-Guerrero et al. 1988, Kase et al. 1988, Lanska, Lanska and Schmidley 1988, Radolf and Kaplan 1988), but neurological symptoms may be present among patients with secondary syphilis who are also HIV-seronegative (Merritt, Adams and Solomon 1946). One study (Lukehart et al. 1988) found indications of *T. pallidum* in the central nervous system of 40% of patients with early syphilis. However, no correlation was found between HIV infection and the invasion of the central nervous system by *T. pallidum*. *T. pallidum* was isolated from 27% of HIV-infected persons and 32% of those in the study who were not infected with HIV.

6 TREATMENT AND ANTIMICROBIAL SUSCEPTIBILITIES

The syphilis treatment guidelines recommended by CDC in 1993 are provided in Table 34.14 (Centers for Disease Control and Prevention 1993). Penicillin and its derivatives are the preferred antimicrobial agents for the treatment of syphilis and the other treponematoses. Early syphilis in immunologically normal patients can be treated effectively with a single dose of benzathine penicillin G. Neurosyphilis should be treated with either aqueous crystalline penicillin G or procaine penicillin, because benzathine penicillin does not achieve treponemicidal concentrations in the central nervous system. In immunologically normal patients, the remaining organisms following treatment are apparently cleared by the host, because the incidence of a relapse is low in these patients. Even though most HIV-seropositive persons treated with standard regimens for syphilis appear to respond to treatment (Gourevitch et al. 1993, Rolfs et al. 1993), one cannot totally disregard the role of cell mediated immunity in protecting the person against the progression of syphilis (Metzger 1976) or the interaction of an intact immune system with therapeutic agents (Fernandez-Guerrero et al. 1988). HIV-infected individuals may be susceptible to neurological or ocular complications of syphilis following benzathine penicillin treatment (Berry et al. 1987). Therefore, some authors have recommended that therapy appropriate for neurosyphilis (aqueous penicillin G or procaine penicillin with probenecid) be used for all patients coinfected with *T. pallidum* and HIV, and that HIV-positive patients be examined carefully for clinical signs of neurological involvement (e.g. CSF examination) before and after therapy (Berry et al. 1987, Hook 1989). Late stage syphilis patients with evidence of neurosyphilis or other forms of active syphilis should have a CSF examination; if neurological involvement is not indicated, prolonged treatment with benzathine penicillin is recommended.

Effective therapy of early syphilis may result in a Jarisch–Herxheimer reaction consisting of fever and

Table 34.14 Recommended treatment regimen for acquired adult syphilis

---

Primary or secondary syphilis
  Benzathine penicillin G, 2.4 million units i.m., in a single dose

Early latent syphilis (normal CSF examination, if performed)
  Benzathine penicillin G, 2.4 million units i.m. in a single dose

Late latent syphilis or latent syphilis of unknown duration
  Benzathine penicillin G, 7.2 million units total, administered at 3 doses of 2.4 million units i.m.
    each, administered at intervals of 1 week

Late syphilis
  (Late [tertiary] syphilis refers to patients with gumma and patients with cardiovascular syphilis, but
    not to neurosyphilis. Non-allergic patients without evidence of neurosyphilis should be treated with
    the following regimen.)
  Benzathine penicillin G, 7.2 million units total, given as 3 doses of 2.4 million units i.m.,
    administered at intervals of 1 week

Neurosyphilis[a]
Recommended regimen
  12–24 million units aqueous crystalline penicillin G daily, administered as 2–4 million units i.v. every
    4 h, for 1–14 days
Alternative regimen (if compliance can be assured)
  2.4 million units procaine penicillin i.m. daily, plus probenecid 500 mg orally 4 times a day, both for
    10–14 days

---

[a]The duration of these regimes is shorter than that of the regimen used for late syphilis in the absence of neurosyphilis. Therefore, some experts administer benzathine penicillin, 2.4 million units i.m., after completion of these neurosyphilis treatment regimens, to provide a comparable total duration of therapy.

local intensification of lesions. This reaction, thought to result from the rapid release of treponemal antigens, occurs within the first 12 h of the initiation of therapy and usually resolves within 24 h.

Doxycycline and tetracycline can be used as alternative therapies for the treatment of penicillin-allergic individuals. Erythromycin is no longer recommended because of the occurrence of treatment failures and the possible existence of erythromycin-resistant strains (Stapleton, Stamm and Bassford 1985); the macrolides are contraindicated in pregnant women. In these cases, it is suggested that a penicillin allergy be documented by thorough questioning regarding the patient's history and by skin testing. If necessary, the patient may be desensitized to permit use of penicillin therapy (Centers for Disease Control and Prevention 1993). A Jarisch–Herxheimer reaction occurring in pregnant women may cause premature labour, fetal distress, or (rarely) stillbirth. However, the high probability of fetal damage resulting from syphilitic infection in the absence of adequate therapy outweighs this risk.

Antimicrobial susceptibility testing is not straightforward because there is no method for the continuous culture of *T. pallidum*. Various approaches have been used to determine the susceptibilities of representative strains (e.g. the Nichols strain) to antimicrobial agents, including in vitro loss of motility or infectivity, treatment of experimental animal infections, human trials and examination of the susceptibility of non-pathogenic, cultivable treponemes (Rein 1976). Inhibition of protein synthesis and of in vitro multiplication in a tissue culture system has been shown to be an effective means of determining susceptibility

(Stapleton, Stamm and Bassford 1985, Norris and Edmondson 1988). In common with other spirochaetes, *T. pallidum* was relatively insensitive to 7 quinolones tested and to rifampicin. *T. pallidum* strains appear to be uniformly susceptible for penicillin and other β-lactams. There is no evidence for the development of resistance to penicillin, as has occurred with *Neisseria gonorrhoeae* and other pathogens. Penicillin G provides greater inhibitory activity than do cephalosporins and other β-lactams tested. Ceftriaxone, amoxycillin and ampicillin are active against *T. pallidum* in vitro and also appear to be effective in the treatment of early syphilis. Amoxycillin and ampicillin offer no theoretical advantage over benzathine penicillin G. Ceftriaxone has a long serum half-life and reaches high levels in the central nervous system. However, the cost is high, multiple doses are required and there is a 3–7% risk of adverse reactions in penicillin-allergic individuals; in addition, the data on efficacy in patients are limited. Therefore, ceftriaxone is not currently recommended as an alternative therapy for early syphilis.

6.1 Evaluation after treatment

To follow the efficacy of therapy, patients should be monitored to ensure that signs and symptoms have resolved and that titre has declined. To monitor the efficacy of treatment, quantitative non-treponemal tests should be performed on the patient's serum samples, which are drawn at intervals of 3 months for at least 1 year. Following adequate therapy for initial episodes of primary and secondary syphilis, there should be at least a 4-fold decline in the VDRL titre by the third or fourth month and an 8-fold decline in titre by the sixth to eight month (Brown et al. 1985). When the RPR card test is used to monitor treatment, the initial 4-fold decline in titre may not be observed until the sixth or eighth month after treatment (Romanowski et al. 1991). For most patients treated in early syphilis, the titres decline until little or no reaction is detected after the first 3 years (Fiumara 1978, 1980b, Romanowski et al. 1991). Patients treated in the latent or late stages, or who have had multiple episodes of syphilis, may show a more gradual decline in titre (Fiumara 1979, 1980a). Low titre will persist in approximately 50% of these patients after 2 years. As far as can be determined, this persistent seropositivity does not signify treatment failure or reinfection and these patients are likely to remain serofast even if they are retreated.

7 RELATED TREPONEMES

Yaws, endemic syphilis (bejel) and pinta were common infections before the World Health Organization eradication programme that began in 1948. In the early 1950s, it was estimated that more than 200 million people had been exposed to yaws. Areas where the non-venereal treponematoses are endemic are now more restricted, but decreased surveillance has led to a return of disease in many areas. Therefore, the clinical appearance of the lesions formed by *T. pallidum* subspecies *pertenue*, *pallidum*, *endemicum* and *Treponema carateum*, the anatomical location of the lesion, the mode of transmission, the age of the individual and the geographical location of the infected individual are the only criteria that can be used to diagnose these infections as separate entities (Perine et al. 1984, Benenson 1990).

7.1 Bejel

The lesions of bejel (endemic syphilis) develop after an incubation period of 2 weeks to 3 months. Mucous patches of the mouth usually occur first, followed by moist papules in folds of the skin and drier lesions of the trunk and extremities. A primary sore is rarely evident. Both depigmentation and hyperpigmentation are common. The late manifestations include destructive lesions of skin, long bones and nasopharynx similar to the gummas of late syphilis (Perine et al. 1984, Benenson 1990). However, neurological, cardiovascular and congenital forms are rarely reported. The disease was once common among children living in poor socioeconomic conditions in the arid regions of the eastern Mediterranean, Asia and Africa. Bejel still persists in Chad, Sudan and Ethiopia but the occurrence of the disease is not well established in southern Africa (Meheus and Antal 1992).

7.2 Yaws

The primary lesion of yaws, commonly referred to as the mother yaw, occurs after an incubation period of 2 weeks to 3 months. This initial lesion is a papilloma located on the face or extremities. The lesion may slowly proliferate to form a frambesial or raspberry-like lesion or the initial lesion may ulcerate. Secondary lesions of disseminated or satellite papillomata (daughter yaws) form in successive eruptions (crops) with the first crop appearing either before or shortly after the mother yaw has resolved. Other symptoms accompanying the secondary lesions include aching of long bones and inflammation of the fingers and toes. Papillomata and hyperkeratoses that form on the soles and palms are usually very painful and disabling. These lesions heal spontaneously but relapses may occur during the secondary or late phases. The late stage develops in approximately 10% of untreated patients. The stage is characterized by destructive lesions of the skin and bones (Perine et al. 1984, Benenson 1990). Congenital yaws has not been documented; controversy exists over the occurrence of neurological and cardiovascular forms (Engelkens et al. 1991a). Today, yaws is primarily a disease of children living in the tropical areas of Central and West Africa (Meheus and Antal 1992). Some small foci of disease remain in the Americas and on the islands of the Caribbean (Meheus and Antal 1992).

7.3 Pinta

Perhaps the most distinctive lesions of the pathogenic treponematoses are observed in pinta. First, a primary scaling papule forms 1–8 weeks after infection on the hands, legs, or the back of the foot. Within 3 months to 1 year, a maculopapular, erythematous secondary rash appears that may evolve into tertiary splotches of altered skin pigmentation. Initially the macules are blue, progressing to violet, then brown and finally becoming depigmented after months to years. Treponemes are found in the pigmented lesions; the achromic scars are usually free of treponemes. The lesions of the secondary rash most commonly progressing to the late form are frequently found on the face and extremities; lesions in different stages of pigmentation can be observed simultaneously (Perine et al. 1984, Benenson 1990). Systemic infection with organ or bone involvement apparently does not occur. Pinta is predominantly a disease found among older children and adults living in the Indian tribes of Mexico and the Amazon basin (Meheus and Antal 1992). Because of the location of the primary lesion, trauma is suspected of providing the portal of entry for the treponemes. Direct and prolonged contact with initial, secondary and early tertiary lesions appears to be necessary for transmission to take place; however, the mode of transmission is not entirely clear (Engelkens et al. 1991b).

Because yaws, pinta and non-venereal syphilis are often childhood diseases, the non-treponemal test titres of adults are expected to be ≤8 for those from a geographical region where endemic treponematoses were virtually eliminated by mass campaigns in the 1950s and 1960s (Antal and Causse 1985, Meheus and Antal 1992). Therefore, any titre >8 is suggestive of venereal syphilis for adults from these regions (Gershman et al. 1992, McDermott et al. 1993). Likewise, a titre of ≥8 in a child suggests a resurgence of yaws in these particular areas (Perine et al. 1985).

7.4 Other human host associated spirochaetes

In addition to *T. pallidum* and related pathogens, various anaerobic treponemes and other spirochaetes are parasites of humans (see also Volume 2, Chapter 55). These include separate groups of spirochaetes found in the oral cavity (particularly the gingival crevices), in sebaceous secretions in the genital region and in the colon and rectum. In general these spirochaetes are considered commensal organisms. However, there is evidence that spirochaetes are involved in gingivitis and periodontal disease and that overgrowth of intestinal spirochaetes may correlate with the occurrence of diarrhoea or other bowel disorders.

ORAL SPIROCHAETES

Various spirochaetes inhabit supragingival and subgingival plaque in humans; only a small proportion of these have been cultured in vitro and characterized (Choi et al. 1994). Those that have been cultivated and identified to species level are within the genus *Treponema*. Although the species differ from one another slightly in terms of cell diameter and helical configuration, it is generally not possible to identify them on morphological grounds; biochemical parameters such as growth requirements, carbohydrate fermentation and enzymatic activities are used for identifying species (Smibert, Johnson and Ranney 1984).

The oral spirochaetes are difficult to isolate from healthy gingiva, but they increase both in prevalence and in numbers of organisms present in patients with gingivitis or periodontal disease. Treponemes are detected in subgingival plaque of 88–97% of patients with periodontal disease (Moore et al. 1987). *Treponema socranskii* is the most common isolate, followed by *T. denticola* and *Treponema pectinovorum*. The procedures for isolation and characterization of oral spirochaetes have been described previously (Smibert and Burmeister 1983, Smibert 1984, Smibert, Johnson and Ranney 1984, Moore et al. 1987, Miller, Smibert and Norris 1992). Pathogen-related oral spirochaetes (PROS) were found in plaque samples from 11 of 17 patients with necrotizing ulcerative gingivitis and from 10 of 19 patients with periodontitis, but were absent from 24 healthy subjects (Riviere et al. 1991a, 1991b, 1991c, Simonson et al. 1993). PROS have not been cultured in vitro and are identified by their reactivity with monoclonal antibodies specific for *T. pallidum* antigens, including the 35 kDa flagellar sheath protein and a major 47 kDa lipoprotein. Gingivitis and periodontitis patients also expressed IgG antibodies reactive with 47, 27, 14 and 12 kDa *T. pallidum* subspecies *pallidum* antigens, whereas a smaller proportion of healthy subjects had detectable antibodies against only the 47 and 37 kDa antigens (Riviere et al. 1991a). PROS were found in periodontal tissues of

ulcerative patients (Riviere et al. 1991a, 1991c) and were capable of migrating through a mouse abdomen wall barrier, an invasive property shared with *T. pallidum* but not with the cultivable oral treponemes (Riviere et al. 1991b). Oral spirochaetes reactive with anti-*T. pallidum* monoclonal antibodies were also detected in gorillas and dogs (Simonson et al. 1993). Further studies to establish the taxonomic relationship between PROS and other spirochaetes and to determine whether PROS represent frank pathogens are in progress.

NON-PATHOGENIC SPIROCHAETES OF THE GENITAL REGION

T. phagedenis, T. refringens and *Treponema minutum* are treponemal species that inhabit smegma (sebaceous secretions and desquamated epithelial cells), which is found beneath the prepuce and in other epithelial folds of the genital region. Although *T. phagedenis* and *T. refringens* have been shown by DNA–DNA hybridization to have ≤5% homology with *T. pallidum* (Fieldsteel 1983), comparison of 16S rRNA sequences indicates that they are related to the pathogenic treponemes. These harmless flora could potentially be misidentified as *T. pallidum* in darkfield preparations from skin sites. Unlike the pathogenic treponemes, these non-pathogenic treponemes are readily cultured (Miller, Smibert and Norris 1992).

INTESTINAL SPIROCHAETES

The presence of spirochaetes in the colon, rectum and faeces of humans has been recognized for over a 100 years (Ruane et al. 1989). Since the description of 'human intestinal spirochaetosis' in 1967 (Harland and Lee 1967), there has been a resurgence of interest in the possible involvement of intestinal spirochaetes in diarrhoea and other gastrointestinal diseases, as well as in the apparently high prevalence of these organisms in homosexual males and HIV-infected individuals (Ruane et al. 1989). Despite this history, the taxonomy, prevalence, distribution and possible disease associations of these organisms are still unclear.

The human intestinal spirochaetes have not yet been classified and appear to be a heterogeneous group rather than a single species. Although it has been suggested (Coene et al. 1989) that the human spirochaetes are related to *Serpulina hyodysenteriae* (the causative agent of swine dysentery) and *Serpulina innocens* (an apathogenic swine organism), recent multilocus enzyme electrophoresis, DNA–DNA hybridization and morphological analyses (Lee et al. 1993) have indicated that human isolates are more closely related to a different group of pig intestinal isolates. Similar organisms are also present in mice, rats and dogs (Koopman et al. 1993). The human intestinal spirochaete *Brachyspira aalborgi* (Hovind-Hougen et al. 1982) appears to be distinct from the majority of human and animal strains (Koopman et al. 1993). Restriction fragment length polymorphism indicates sequence heterogeneity both among the human isolates and in comparison with isolates from other animals. Further analysis of the taxonomy and pathobiology of these organisms will be necessary to clarify their phylogenetic relationships and possible role in human disease.

When observed in association with rectal or colonic tissue, these organisms are typically attached by the tip to the apical surface of the columnar epithelial cells. Although the spirochaetes can form a dense layer visible by light microscopy (using silver staining or other staining techniques), signs of tissue damage or inflammation are usually absent.

A clear association between intestinal spirochaetes and disease has not been established (Ruane et al. 1989). Spirochaetes can be present in healthy individuals as well as in those with diarrhoea or other gastro-intestinal symptoms. In the early 1900s, several studies examined spirochaetes in human stool specimens by light microscopy. In those studies with over 100 patients, the percentage of subjects with spirochaetes ranged from 3.3% to 61%. Recent light and electron microscopic examinations and culture of rectal biopsy samples from heterosexual patients have indicated the presence of spirochaetes in 1.9–6.9% of subjects and helical organisms were found to be associated with healthy and inflamed appendixes. Higher proportions of homosexual males have been reported to have intestinal spirochaetes. At present, there is no clear evidence for an association between intestinal spirochaetosis and HIV infection.

REFERENCES

Alford CA Jr, Polt SS et al., 1969, Gamma-M-fluorescent treponemal antibody in the diagnosis of congenital syphilis, *N Engl J Med*, **280:** 1086–91.

Anderson B, Stillman MT, 1978, False-positive FTA-ABS in hydralazine-induced lupus, *JAMA*, **239:** 1392–3.

Antal GM, Causse G, 1985, The control of endemic treponematoses, *Rev Infect Dis*, **7 (S2):** S220–6.

Belisle JT, Brandt ME et al., 1994, Fatty acids of *Treponema pallidum* and *Borrelia burgdorferi* lipoproteins, *J Bacteriol*, **176:** 2151–7.

Benenson AS, ed., 1990, *Control of Communicable Diseases in Man*, 15th edn, American Public Health Association, Washington, DC, 323–4, 425–4, 483–6.

Berry CD, Hooten TM et al., 1987, Neurologic relapse after benzathine penicillin therapy for secondary syphilis in a patient with HIV infection, *N Engl J Med*, **316:** 1587–9.

Bordet J, Gengou O, 1901, Sur l'existence de substances sensigilisatrice dans la plupart des serums antimicrobiens, *Ann Inst Pasteur*, **15:** 289.

Brandt AM, 1988, The syphilis epidemic and its relation to AIDS, *Science*, **239:** 375–80.

Bromberg K, Rawstron S, Tannis G, 1993, Diagnosis of congenital syphilis by combining *Treponema pallidum*-specific IgM detection with immunofluorescent antigen detection for *T. pallidum*, *J Infect Dis*, **168:** 238–42.

Brown ST, Zaidi A et al., 1985, Serological response to syphilis treatment: a new analysis of old data, *JAMA*, **253:** 1296–9.

Buchanan CS, Haserick JR, 1970, FTA-ABS test in pregnancy. A probably false-positive reaction, *Arch Dermatol*, **102:** 322–5.

Buist DGP, Pertile R, Morris GJ, 1973, Evaluation of the *T. pallidum* haemagglutination test, *Pathology*, **5:** 249–52.

Bulkley BH, 1984, Cardiovascular syphilis, *Sexually Transmitted Diseases*, eds Holmes K, Mardh P-A et al., McGraw-Hill, New York, 334–8.

Burdash NM, Hinds KK et al., 1987, Evaluation of the syphilis Bio-EnzaBead assay for the detection of treponemal antibody, *J Clin Microbiol*, **25:** 808–11.

Burstain JM, Grimprel E et al., 1991, Sensitive detection of *Treponema pallidum* by using the polymerase chain reaction, *J Clin Microbiol*, **29:** 62–9.

Byrne RE, Laske S et al., 1992, Evaluation of a *Treponema pallidum* Western immunoblot assay as a confirmatory test for syphilis, *J Clin Microbiol*, **30:** 115–22.

Castro KG, Lieb S et al., 1988, Transmission of HIV in Belle Glade, Florida: lessons for other communities in the United States, *Science*, **239:** 193–7.

Catterall RD, 1972, Presidential address to the M.S.S.V.D.: systemic disease and the biological false-positive reaction, *Br J Vener Dis*, **48:** 1–12.

Centers for Disease Control, 1991, *Sexually Transmitted Diseases Clinical Practices Guidelines*, US Department of Health and Human Services, Public Health Services, Atlanta, GA, III-36–41.

Centers for Disease Control and Prevention, 1993, Sexually transmitted diseases treatment guidelines, *Morbid Mortal Weekly Rep*, **42 (RR-14):** 27–46.

Centers for Disease Control and Prevention, 1994, *Passage and maintenance of* Treponema pallidum *by intratesticular infection of rabbits*, US Department of Health and Human Services, Public Health Services, Atlanta, GA, 1–12.

Centers for Disease Control and Prevention, Division of STD Prevention, 1995, *Sexually Transmitted Disease Surveillance, 1994*, US Department of Health and Human Services, Public Health Services, Atlanta, GA, 17–23, 76–94.

Chang SN, Chung K et al., 1995, Seroconversion of the serologic tests for syphilis in the newborns born to treated syphilitic mothers, *Genitourin Med*, **71:** 68–70.

Chhabra RS, Brion LP et al., 1993, Comparison of maternal sera, cord blood and neonatal sera for detection of presumptive congenital syphilis: relationship with maternal treatment, *Pediatrics*, **91:** 88–91.

Chiu MJ, Radolf JD, 1994, Syphilis, *Infectious Diseases: a Treatise of Infectious Processes*, 5th edn, eds Hoeprich PD, Jordan MC, Ronald AR, JB Lippincott, Philadelphia, 694–714.

Choi BK, Paster BJ et al., 1994, Diversity of cultivable and uncultivable oral spirochetes from a patient with severe destructive periodontitis, *Infect Immun*, **62:** 1889–95.

Coene M, Agliano AM et al., 1989, Comparative analysis of the genomes of intestinal spirochetes of human and animal origin, *Infect Immun*, **57:** 138–45.

Coles AC, 1909, *Spirochaeta pallida*: methods of examination and detection, especially by means of the dark-ground illumination, *Br Med J*, **1:** 1117–20.

Cox PM, Logan LC, Norins LC, 1969, Automated, quantitative microhemagglutination assay for *Treponema pallidum* antibodies, *Appl Microbiol*, **18:** 485–9.

Cox PM, Logan LC, Stout GW, 1971, Further studies of a quantitative automated microhemagglutination assay for antibodies to *Treponema pallidum*, *Public Health Lab*, **29:** 43–50.

Creighton ET, 1990, Darkfield microscopy for the detection and identification of *Treponema pallidum*, A Manual of Tests for Syphilis, 8th edn, eds Larsen SA, Hunter EF, Kraus SJ, American Public Health Association, Washington, DC, 49–62.

Cutler JC, Bauer TJ et al., 1954, Comparison of spinal fluid findings among syphilitic and nonsyphilitic individuals, *Am J Syph Gonorrhea Vener Dis*, **38:** 447–58.

D'Alessandro G, Dardanoni L, 1953, Isolation and purification of the protein antigen of the Reiter treponeme. A study of its serologic reactions, *Am J Syph*, **37:** 137–50.

Daniels KC, Ferneyhough HS, 1977, Specific direct fluorescent antibody detection of *Treponema pallidum, Health Lab Sci,* **14:** 164–71.

Dawson S, Evans BA, Lawrence AG, 1988, Benign tertiary syphilis and HIV infection, *AIDS,* **2:** 315–16.

Deacon WE, Falcone VH, Harris A, 1957, A fluorescent test for treponemal antibodies, *Proc Soc Exp Biol Med,* **96:** 477–80.

Deacon WE, Freeman EM, Harris A, 1960, Fluorescent treponemal antibody test. Modification based on quantitation (FTA-200), *Proc Soc Exp Biol Med,* **103:** 827–9.

Deacon WE, Hunter EF, 1962, Treponemal antigens as related to identification and syphilis serology, *Proc Soc Exp Biol Med,* **110:** 352–6.

Duncan WP, Jenkins TW, Parham CE, 1972, Fluorescent treponemal antibody-cerebrospinal fluid (FTA-CSF) test, *Br J Vener Dis,* **48:** 97–101.

Eagle H, 1937, Introduction, *The Laboratory Diagnosis of Syphilis,* CV Mosby, St Louis, 21–8.

Engelkens HJH, Judanarso J et al., 1991a, Endemic treponematoses. I. Yaws, *Int J Dermatol,* **30:** 77–83.

Engelkens HJH, Niemel PLA et al., 1991b, Endemic treponematoses. II. Pinta and endemic syphilis, *Int J Dermatol,* **30:** 231–8.

Escobar MR, Dalton HP, Allison MJ, 1970, Fluorescent antibody tests for syphilis using cerebrospinal fluid: clinical correlation in 150 cases, *Am J Clin Pathol,* **53:** 886–90.

Farshy CE, Hunter EF et al., 1985, Four-step enzyme-linked immunosorbent assay for detection of *Treponema pallidum* antibody, *J Clin Microbiol,* **21:** 387–9.

Fernandez-Guerrero ML, Miranda C et al., 1988, The treatment of neurosyphilis in patients with HIV infection, *JAMA,* **259:** 1495–6.

Fieldsteel AH, 1983, Genetics, *Pathogenesis and Immunology of Treponemal Infection,* eds Schell RF, Musher DM, Marcel Dekker, New York, 39–54.

Fieldsteel AH, Cox DL, Moeckli RA, 1981, Cultivation of virulent *Treponema pallidum* in tissue culture, *Infect Immun,* **32:** 908–15.

Finelli L, Budd J, Spitalny KC, 1993, Early syphilis relationship to sex, drugs, and changes in high-risk behavior from 1987–1990, *Sex Transm Dis,* **20:** 89–95.

Fitzgerald TJ, 1981, Pathogenesis and immunology of *Treponema pallidum, Annu Rev Microbiol,* **35:** 29–54.

Fiumara NJ, 1978, Treatment of early latent syphilis of less than one year's duration, *Sex Transm Dis,* **5:** 85–8.

Fiumara NJ, 1979, Serologic responses to treatment of 128 patients with late latent syphilis, *Sex Transm Dis,* **6:** 243–6.

Fiumara NJ, 1980a, Reinfection primary, secondary and latent syphilis. The serologic response after treatment, *Sex Transm Dis,* **7:** 111–15.

Fiumara NJ, 1980b, Treatment of primary and secondary syphilis; serological response, *JAMA,* **243:** 2500–2.

Fohn MJ, Wignall FS et al., 1988, Specificity of antibodies from patients with pinta for antigens of *Treponema pallidum* subspecies *pallidum, J Infect Dis,* **157:** 32–7.

Forbes G, Rutter P, Abraham C, 1991, Significant cost savings with an automated syphilis screening test, *Transfusion,* **31, Suppl.:** 75S.

Garner MF, Backhouse JL, 1971, Fluorescent treponemal antibody tests on cerebrospinal fluid, *Br J Vener Dis,* **47:** 356–8.

George RW, Pope V, Larsen SA, 1991, Use of the Western blot for the diagnosis of syphilis, *Clin Immunol Newslett,* **8:** 124–8.

Gershman KA, Rolfs RT et al., 1992, Seroepidemiological characterization of a syphilis epidemic in the Republic of the Marshall Islands, formerly a yaws endemic area, *Int J Epidemiol,* **21:** 599–606.

Goff CW, 1967, Syphilis, *Diseases of Antiquity,* eds Brothwell D, Sandison AT, Charles C Thomas, Springfield IL, 279–94.

Goldman JN, Lantz MA, 1971, FTA-ABS and VDRL slide test reactivity in a population of nuns, *JAMA,* **217:** 53–5.

Gordon SM, Eaton ME et al., 1994, Response of symptomatic neurosyphilis to high-dose intrvenous penicillin G in persons infected with the human immunodeficiency virus, *N Engl J Med,* **331:** 1469–73.

Gourevitch MN, Selwyn PA et al., 1993, Effects of HIV infection on the serologic manifestation and response to treatment of syphilis in intravenous drug users, *Ann Intern Med,* **118:** 350–5.

Gregory N, Sanchez M, Buchness MR, 1990, The spectrum of syphilis in patients with human immunodeficiency virus infection, *J Am Acad Dermatol,* **22:** 1061–7.

Grimprel E, Sanchez PJ et al., 1991, Use of polymerase chain reaction and rabbit infectivity testing to detect *Treponema pallidum* in amniotic fluid, *J Clin Microbiol,* **29:** 1711–18.

Haas J, Bolan G et al., 1990, Sensitivity of treponemal tests for detecting prior treated syphilis during human immunodeficiency virus infection, *J Infect Dis,* **162:** 862–6.

Hackett CJ, 1963, On the origin of the human treponematoses (pinta, yaws, endemic syphilis and venereal syphilis), *Bull W H O,* **29:** 7–41.

Hanff PA, Fehniger TE et al., 1982, Humoral immune response in human syphilis to polypeptides of *Treponema pallidum, J Immunol,* **129:** 1287–91.

Harland WA, Lee FD, 1967, Intestinal spirochaetosis, *Br Med J,* **3:** 718–19.

Harris A, Rosenberg AA, Riedel LM, 1946, A microflocculation test for syphilis using cardiolipin antigen: preliminary report, *J Vener Dis Inform,* **27:** 159–72.

Harris AD, Bossak HM et al., 1960, Comparison of the fluorescent treponemal antibody test with other tests for syphilis on cerebrospinal fluids, *Br J Vener Dis,* **36:** 178–80.

Hay PE, Clarke JR et al., 1990, Use of the polymerase chain reaction to detect DNA sequences specific to pathogenic treponemes in cerebrospinal fluid, *FEMS Microbiol Lett,* **68:** 233–8.

Hedersted B, 1976, Studies on the *Treponema pallidum* immobilizing activity in normal human serum. 2. Serum factors participating in the normal serum immobilization reaction, *Acta Pathol Microbiol Scand Sect C,* **84:** 135–41.

Hicks CD, Benson PM et al., 1987, Seronegative secondary syphilis in a patient infected with the human immunodeficiency virus (HIV) with Kaposi sarcoma, *Ann Intern Med,* **107:** 492–5.

Hirsch A, 1883, *Handbook of Geographical and Historical Pathology, Vol. 2 Chronic Infective, Toxic, Parasitic, Septic and Constitutional Diseases,* Charles Creighton, trans., The New Sydenham Society, London.

Hollander DH, 1981, Treponematosis from pinta to venereal syphilis revisited: hypothesis for temperature determination of disease patterns, *Sex Transm Dis,* **8:** 34–7.

Holodniy M, Kim S et al., 1991, Inhibition of human immunodeficiency virus gene amplification by heparin, *J Clin Microbiol,* **29:** 676–9.

Hook EW III, 1989, Treatment of syphilis: current recommendations, alternatives, and continuing problems, *Rev Infect Dis,* **11, Suppl. 6:** S1511–17.

Hook EW III, Marra CM, 1992, Acquired syphilis in adults, *N Engl J Med,* **326:** 1060–9.

Hook EW III, Roddy RE et al., 1985, Detection of *Treponema pallidum* in lesion exudate with a pathogen-specific monoclonal antibody, *J Clin Microbiol,* **22:** 241–4.

Horowitz H, Wicher K et al., 1994, Cerebral syphilitic gumma confirmed by PCR in an HIV infected patient, *N Engl J Med,* **331:** 1488–91.

Hovind-Hougen K, Birch-Andersen A et al., 1982, Intestinal spirochetosis: morphological characterization and cultivation of the spirochete *Brachyspira aalborgi* gen. nov., sp. nov., *J Clin Microbiol,* **16:** 1127–36.

Hudson EH, 1946, A unitarian view of treponematosis, *Am J Trop Med,* **26:** 135–9.

Hunter EF, 1990, Fluorescent treponemal antibody-absorption (FTA-ABS) test, *A Manual of Tests for Syphilis,* 8th edition, eds Larsen SA, Hunter EF, Kraus SJ, American Public Health Association, Washington, DC, 129–40.

Hunter EF, Deacon WE, Meyer PE, 1964, An improved FTA test for syphilis: the absorption procedure (FTA-ABS), *Public Health Rep,* **79:** 410–12.

Hunter EF, McKenney RM et al., 1979, Double-staining procedure for the fluorescent treponemal antibody-absorption (FTA-ABS) test, *Br J Vener Dis*, **55**: 105–8.

Hunter EF, Greer PW et al., 1984, Immuno-fluorescent staining of *Treponema* in tissues fixed with formalin, *Arch Pathol Lab Med*, **108**: 878–80.

Hunter EF, Russell H et al., 1986, Evaluation of sera from patients with Lyme disease in the fluorescent treponemal antibody-absorption tests for syphilis, *Sex Transm Dis*, **13**: 232–6.

Ijsselmuiden OE, van der Sluis JJ et al., 1989, An IgM capture enzyme-linked immunosorbent assay to detect IgM antibodies to treponemes in patients with syphilis, *Genitourin Med*, **65**: 79–83.

Ingraham NR Jr, 1951, Section II: Syphilis in pregnancy and congenital syphilis, *J Acta Dermatovenereol*, **31 (S24)**: 60–88.

Ito F, Hunter EF et al., 1991, Specific immunofluorescence staining of *T. pallidum* in smears and tissues, *J Clin Microbiol*, **29**: 444–8.

Ito F, George RW et al., 1992, Specific immunofluorescent staining of pathogenic treponemes with a monoclonal antibody, *J Clin Microbiol*, **30**: 831–8.

Jaffe HW, Larsen SA et al., 1978a, Hemagglutination tests for syphilis antibody, *Am J Clin Pathol*, **70**: 230–3.

Jaffe HW, Larsen SA et al., 1978b, Tests for treponemal antibody in CSF, *Arch Intern Med*, **138**: 252–5.

Jaffe HW, Musher DM, 1990, Management of the reactive syphilis serology, *Sexually Transmitted Diseases*, 2nd edn, eds Holmes KK, Mårdh P-A et al., McGraw-Hill Information Services Company, New York, 935–9.

Jensen JR, From E, 1982, Alterations in T-lymphocytes and T-lymphocyte subpopulations in patients with syphilis, *Br J Vener Dis*, **58**: 18–22.

Jethwa HS, Schmitz JL et al., 1995, Comparison of molecular and microscopic techniques for detection of *Treponema pallidum* in genital ulcers, *J Clin Microbiol*, **33**: 180–3.

Johns DR, Tierney M, Felsenstein D, 1987, Alteration in the natural history of neurosyphilis by concurrent infection with the human immunodeficiency virus, *N Engl J Med*, **316**: 1569–72.

Johnston NA, 1972a, Neonatal congenital syphilis: diagnosis by the absorbed fluorescent treponemal antibody (IgM) test, *Br J Vener Dis*, **48**: 464–9.

Johnston NA, 1972b, *Treponema pallidum* haemagglutination test for syphilis: evaluation of a modified micro-method, *Br J Vener Dis*, **48**: 474–8.

Jones SA, Marchitto KS et al., 1984, Monoclonal antibody with haemagglutination, immobilization, and neutralization activities defines an immunodominant, 47,000 mol. wt., surface-exposed immunogen of *Treponema pallidum* (Nichols), *J Exp Med*, **160**: 1404–20.

Jurado RL, Campbell J, Martin PD, 1993, Prozone phenomenon in secondary syphilis: has its time arrived? *Arch Intern Med*, **153**: 2496–8.

Kahn RL, 1922, A simple quantitative precipitation reaction for syphilis, *Arch Dermatol Syphilol*, **5; 6**: 570–8, 734–43; 332–41.

Kampmeier RH, 1983, The evolution of the flocculation screening test for syphilis, *Sex Transm Dis*, **10**: 156–9.

Kase CS, Levitz SM et al., 1988, Pontine pure motor hemiparesis due to meningovascular syphilis in human immunodeficiency virus-positive patients, *Arch Neurol*, **45**: 832.

Kaufman RE, Jones OG et al., 1977, Questionnaire survey of reported early congenital syphilis, problems in diagnosis prevention and treatment, *Sex Transm Dis*, **4**: 135–9.

Kellogg DS Jr, Mothershed SM, 1969, Immunofluorescent detection of *Treponema pallidum*: a review, *JAMA*, **107**: 938–41.

Koopman MBH, Kasbohrer A et al., 1993, Genetic similarity of intestinal spirochetes from humans and various animal species, *J Clin Microbiol*, **31**: 711–16.

Kraus SJ, Haserick JR, Lantz MA, 1970, Fluorescent treponemal antibody-absorption test reactions in lupus erythematosus. Atypical beading pattern and probably false-positive reactions, *N Engl J Med*, **282**: 1287–90.

Kraus SJ, Haserick JR et al., 1971, Atypical fluorescence in the fluorescent treponemal antibody-absorption (FTA-ABS) test related to deoxyribonucleic acid (DNA) antibodies, *J Immunol*, **106**: 1665–9.

Kwok S, Higuchi R, 1989, Avoiding false positives with PCR, *Nature (London)*, **339**: 237–8.

Lane HC, Masur H et al., 1983, Abnormalities of B-cell activation and immunoregulation in patients with the acquired immunodeficiency syndrome, *N Engl J Med*, **309**: 453–8.

Lanska MJ, Lanska DJ, Schmidley FW, 1988, Syphilitic polyradiculopathy in an HIV-positive man, *Neurology*, **38**: 1297–301.

Larsen SA, 1983, Current status of laboratory tests for syphilis, *Diagnostic Immunology: Technology Assessment*, eds Rippey J, Nakamura R, American College of Pathologists, Skokie, Illinois, 162–70.

Larsen SA, Hunter EF, Kraus SJ, eds, 1990, *A Manual of Tests for Syphilis*, 8th edn, American Public Health Association, Washington, DC, 2–191.

Larsen SA, Zenker PN, 1990, Congenital syphilis: past, present, and future, *Clin Microbiol Newslett*, **12**: 181–2.

Larsen SA, Hambie EA et al., 1981, Specificity, sensitivity, and reproducibility among the fluorescent treponemal antibody absorption test, the microhemagglutination assay for *Treponema pallidum* antibodies, and the hemagglutination treponemal test for syphilis, *J Clin Microbiol*, **14**: 441–5.

Larsen SA, Hambie EA et al., 1985, Cerebrospinal fluid serologic test for syphilis: treponemal and nontreponemal tests, *Advances in Sexually Transmitted Diseases*, eds Morisset R, Kurstak E, VNU Science Press, Utrecht, The Netherlands, 157–62.

Lee JI, McLaren AJ et al., 1993, Human intestinal spirochetes are distinct from *Serpulina hyodysenteriae*, *J Clin Microbiol*, **31**: 16–21.

Lefèvre JC, Bertrand MA, Bauriaud R, 1990, Evaluation of the Captia enzyme immunoassays for detection of immunoglobulins G and M to *Treponema pallidum* in syphilis, *J Clin Microbiol*, **28**: 1704–7.

Linglof T, 1995, Rapid increase of syphilis and gonorrhea in parts of the former USSR, *Sex Transm Dis*, **22**: 160–1.

Luger A, Marhold I, Schmidt BL, 1988, Laboratory support in the diagnosis of neurosyphilis, *WHO/VDT/RES*, **379**: 1–25.

Lukehart SA, Hook EW III et al., 1988, Invasion of the central nervous system by *Treponema pallidum*: implications for diagnosis and treatment, *Ann Intern Med*, **109**: 855–62.

McCabe E, Jaffe LR, Diaz A, 1993, Human Immunodeficiency virus seropositivity in adolescents with syphilis, *Pediatrics*, **92**: 695–8.

McDermott J, Steketee R et al., 1993, Syphilis-associated perinatal and infant mortality in rural Malawi, *Bull W H O*, **71**: 773–80.

McKenna CH, Schroeter AL, Kierland RR, 1973, The fluorescent treponemal antibody absorbed (FTA-ABS) test beading phenomenon in connective tissue diseases, *Mayo Clin Proc*, **48**: 545–8.

Magnarelli LA, Miller JN et al., 1990, Cross-reactivity of nonspecific treponemal antibody in serologic tests for Lyme disease, *J Clin Microbiol*, **28**: 1276–9.

Magnuson HJ, Eagle H, Fleischman R, 1948, The minimal infectious inoculum of *Spirochaeta pallida* (Nichols strain) and a consideration of its rate of multiplication in vivo, *Am J Syph*, **32**: 1–18.

Magnuson HJ, Thomas EW et al., 1956, Inoculation syphilis in human volunteers, *Medicine (Baltimore)*, **35**: 33–82.

Mahoney JF, Arnold RC, Harris A, 1949, Penicillin treatment of early syphilis – first four patients after six years, *J Vener Dis Inform*, **30**: 350–5.

Mamunes P, Cave VG et al., 1970, Early diagnosis of neonatal syphilis: evaluation of a gamma-M-fluorescent treponemal antibody test, *Am J Dis Child*, **120**: 17–21.

March RW, Stiles GE, 1980, The reagin screen test: a new reagin card test for syphilis, *Sex Transm Dis*, **7**: 66–70.

Marra CM, Critchlow CW et al., 1995, Cerebrospinal fluid treponemal antibodies in untreated early syphilis, *Arch Neurol*, **52**: 68–72.

Matthews HM, Yang TK, Jenkin HM, 1979, Unique lipid composition of *Treponema pallidum* (Nichols virulent strain), *Infect Immun*, **24**: 713–19.

Meheus A, Antal GM, 1992, The endemic treponematoses: not yet eradicated, *World Health Stat Q*, **45**: 228–37.

Meinicke E, 1917, Ueber eine neue methode der seologischen lues diagnose, *Berl Klin Wochenschr*, **54**: 613–14.

Merritt HH, Adams RD, Solomon HC, 1946, Asymptomatic neurosyphilis, *Neurosyphilis*, Oxford University Press, New York, 68–82.

Metzger M, 1976, The role of immunologic responses in protection against syphilis, *The Biology of Parasitic Spirochetes*, ed. Johnson RC, Academic Press, New York, 327–37.

Meyer MP, Eddy T, Baughn RE, 1994, Analysis of Western blotting (immunoblotting) technique in diagnosis of congenital syphilis, *J Clin Microbiol*, **32**: 629–33.

Michaelis L, 1907, Präcipitinreaktion bei syphilis, *Berl Klin Wochenschr*, **44**: 1477–8.

Miller JN, Smibert RM, Norris SJ, 1992, The genus *Treponema*, *The Prokaryotes. A Handbook on the Biology of Bacteria, Ecophysiology, Isolation, Identification, and Applications*, 2nd edn, eds Balows A, Truper HG et al., Springer-Verlag, New York, 3537–59.

Monson RA, 1973, Biologic false-positive FTA-ABS test in drug-induced lupus erythematosus, *JAMA*, **24**: 1028–30.

Moore LVH, Moore WEC et al., 1987, Bacteriology of human gingivitis, *J Dent Res*, **66**: 989–95.

Moyer NP, Hudson JD, Hausler WJ Jr, 1987, Evaluation of the Bio-EnzaBead Test for syphilis, *J Clin Microbiol*, **25**: 619–23.

Muller F, 1986, Review: specific immunoglobulin M and G antibodies in the rapid diagnosis of human treponemal infections, *Diagn Immunol*, **4**: 1–9.

Musher DM, 1991, Syphilis, neurosyphilis, penicillin and AIDS, *J Infect Dis*, **163**: 1201–6.

Nakamura K, 1988, Leprosy, *Laboratory Diagnosis of Infectious Diseases, Principles and Practices. Vol. 1 Bacterial, Mycotic and Parasitic Diseases*, eds Balows A, Hausler WJ Jr et al., Springer-Verlag, New York, 333–43.

Nakashima AK, Rolfs RT et al., 1996, Epidemiology of syphilis in the United States, 1941–1993, *Sex Transm Dis*, **23**: 16–23.

Nayar R, Campos JM, 1993, Evaluation of the DCL Syphilis-G enzyme immunoassay test kit for the serologic diagnosis of syphilis, *Am J Clin Pathol*, **99**: 282–5.

Nelson RA Jr, Mayer MM, 1949, Immobilization of *Treponema pallidum in vitro* by antibody produced in syphilitic infection, *J Exp Med*, **89**: 369–93.

Noordhoek GT, Engelkens HJH et al., 1991a, Yaws in West Sumatra, Indonesia: clinical manifestations, serological findings, and characterisation of new treponema isolates by DNA probes, *Eur J Clin Microbiol Infect Dis*, **10**: 12–19.

Noordhoek GT, Wolters EC et al., 1991b, Detection by polymerase chain reaction of *Treponema pallidum* DNA in cerebrospinal fluid from neurosyphilis patients before and after antibiotic treatment, *J Clin Microbiol*, **29**: 1976–84.

Norgard MV, 1993, Clinical and diagnostic issues of acquired and congenital syphilis encompassed in the current syphilis epidemic, *Curr Opin Infect Dis*, **6**: 9–16.

Norris SJ, 1982, In vitro cultivation of *Treponema pallidum*: independent confirmation, *Infect Immun*, **36**: 437–9.

Norris SJ, Edmondson DG, 1988, In vitro culture system to determine the MICs and MBCs of antimicrobial agents against *Treponema pallidum* subsp. *pallidum* (Nichols strain), *Antimicrob Agents Chemother*, **32**: 68–74.

Norris SJ and the *Treponema pallidum* Polypeptide Research Group, 1993, Polypeptides of *Treponema pallidum*: progress toward understanding their structural, functional and immunologic roles, *Microbiol Rev*, **57**: 750–79.

Pangborn MC, 1941, A new serologically active phospholipid from beef heart, *Proc Soc Exp Biol Med*, **48**: 484–6.

Pavia CS, Folds JD, Baseman JB, 1976, Depression of lymphocyte response to concanavalin A in rabbits infected with *Treponema pallidum* (Nichols strain), *Infect Immun*, **14**: 320–2.

Pedersen NS, Orum O, Mouritsen S, 1987, Enzyme-linked immunosorbent assay for detection of antibodies to venereal disease research laboratory (VDRL) antigen in syphilis, *J Clin Microbiol*, **25**: 1711–16.

Pedersen NS, Petersen CS et al., 1982, Serodiagnosis of syphilis by an enzyme-linked immunosorbent assay for IgG antibodies against the Reiter treponema flagellum, *Scand J Immunol*, **15**: 341–8.

Perine PL, Hopkins DR et al., 1984, *Handbook of Endemic Treponematoses: Yaws, Endemic Syphilis and Pinta*, World Health Organization, Geneva, 1–26.

Perine PL, Nelson JW et al., 1985, New technologies for use in the surveillance and control of yaws, *Rev Infect Dis*, **767 (S2)**: S295–9.

Pettit DE, Larsen SA et al., 1981, Unheated serum reagin test as a quantitative test for syphilis, *J Clin Microbiol*, **15**: 238–42.

Pettit DE, Larsen SA et al., 1983, Toluidine red unheated serum test, a nontreponemal test for syphilis, *J Clin Microbiol*, **18**: 1141–5.

Pope V, Hunter EF, Feeley JC, 1982, Evaluation of the microenzyme-linked immunosorbent assay with *Treponema pallidum* antigen, *J Clin Microbiol*, **15**: 630–4.

Pope V, Larsen SA et al., 1994, Flow cytometric analysis of peripheral blood lymphocyte immunophenotypes in persons infected with *Treponema pallidum*, *Clin Diagn Lab Immunol*, **1**: 121–4.

Portnoy J, Carson W, Smith CA, 1957, Rapid plasma reagin test for syphilis, *Public Health Rep*, **72**: 761–6.

Portnoy J, Bossak HW et al., 1961, A rapid reagin test with unheated serum and new improved antigen suspension, *Public Health Rep*, **76**: 933–5.

Radolf JD, Kaplan RP, 1988, Unusual manifestations of secondary syphilis and abnormal humoral immune response to *Treponema pallidum* antigens in a homosexual man with asymptomatic human immunodeficiency virus infection, *J Am Acad Dermatol*, **18**: 423–8.

Rathlev T, 1965, Haemagglutination tests utilizing antigens from pathogenic and apathogenic *Treponema pallidum*, *WHO/VDT/RES*, **77**: 65.

Rathlev T, 1967, Haemagglutination test utilizing pathogenic *Treponema pallidum* for the serodiagnosis of syphilis, *Br J Vener Dis*, **43**: 181–5.

Reimer CB, Black CM et al., 1975, The specificity of fetal IgM: antibody or anti-antibody?, *Ann NY Acad Sci*, **254**: 77–93.

Rein MF, 1976, Biopharmacology of syphilotherapy, *J Am Vener Dis Assoc*, **3**: 109–27.

Rein MF, Banks GW et al., 1980, Failure of the *Treponema pallidum* immobilization test to provide additional diagnostic information about contemporary problem sera, *Sex Transm Dis*, **7**: 101–5.

Riviere GR, Wagoner MA et al., 1991a, Identification of spirochetes related to *Treponema pallidum* in necrotizing ulcerative gingivitis and chronic periodontitis, *N Engl J Med*, **325**: 539–43.

Riviere GR, Weisz KS et al., 1991b, Pathogen-related oral spirochetes from dental plaque are invasive, *Infect Immun*, **59**: 3377–80.

Riviere GR, Weisz KS et al., 1991c, Pathogen-related spirochetes identified within gingival tissue from patients with acute necrotizing ulcerative gingivitis, *Infect Immun*, **59**: 2653–7.

Rogers MF, Morens DM et al., 1983, National case control study of Kaposi's sarcoma and *Pneumocystis carinii* pneumonia in homosexual men. Part 2, laboratory results, *Ann Intern Med*, **99**: 151–8.

Rolfs RT, Hindershot E et al., 1993, Treatment of early syphilis in HIV-infected and HIV-uninfected patients – preliminary results of the syphilis and HIV study, Abstracts of the ISSTDR Meeting, Helsinki, Finland.

Romanowski B, Forsey E et al., 1987, Detection of *Treponema pallidum* by a fluorescent monoclonal antibody test, *Sex Transm Dis*, **22:** 156–9.

Romanowski B, Sutherland R et al., 1991, Serologic response to treatment of infectious syphilis, *Ann Intern Med*, **114:** 1005–9.

Ruane PJ, Nakata MM et al., 1989, Spirochete-like organisms in the human gastrointestinal tract, *Rev Infect Dis*, **11:** 184–96.

Rudolph AH, Larsen SA, 1993, Laboratory diagnosis of syphilis, *Clinical Dermatology*, Unit 16–22A, JB Lippincott, Philadelphia, 1–16.

Rusnak JM, Butzin C et al., 1994, Incidence and cause of false-positive rapid plasma reagin test in patients with HIV infection, *J Infect Dis*, **169:** 1356–9.

Sanchez PJ, McCracken GH et al., 1989, Molecular analysis of the fetal IgM response to *Treponema pallidum* antigen: implications for improved serodiagnosis of congenital syphilis, *J Infect Dis*, **159:** 508–17.

Sanchez PJ, Wendel GD et al., 1993, Evaluation of molecular methodologies and rabbit infectivity testing for the diagnosis of congenital syphilis and neonatal central nervous system invasion by *Treponema pallidum*, *J Infect Dis*, **167:** 148–57.

Schaudinn F, Hoffmann P, 1904–5, Vorläufiger bericht über das vorkommen von Spirochäten in syphilitischen krandkheitprodukten und bei papillomen, *Arb Gesundhtsamte (Berl)*, **22:** 527–34.

Schell RF, LeFrock JF et al., 1979, Use of CB hamsters in the study of *Treponema pertenue*, *Br J Vener Dis*, **55:** 316–19.

Schell RF, LeFrock JF et al., 1981, LSH hamster model of syphilitic infection and transfer of resistance with immune T cells, *Hamster Immune Responses in Infectious and Oncologic Diseases*, eds Streilein J, Hart DA et al., Plenum Publishing, New York, 291–300.

Schouls LM, Ijsselmuiden OE et al., 1989, Overproduction and purification of *Treponema pallidum* recombinant DNA-derived proteins TmpA and TmpB and their potential use in serodiagnosis of syphilis, *Infect Immun*, **57:** 2612–23.

Schroeter AL, Lucas JB et al., 1972, Treatment of early syphilis and reactivity of serologic tests, *JAMA*, **221:** 471–6.

Schwartz DA, Larsen SA et al., 1995, Pathology of the umbilical cord in congenital syphilis, *Hum Pathol*, **26:** 784–91.

Shore RN, Faricelli JA, 1977, Borderline and reactive FTA-ABS results in lupus erythematosus, *Arch Dermatol*, **113:** 37–41.

Simonson L, Braswell L et al., 1993, Human oral spirochete antigen in certain animal populations, 93rd General Meeting American Society for Microbiology, Abstr D-133, 118.

Smibert RM, 1984, Genus III. *Treponema* Schaudinn 1905, *Bergey's Manual of Systematic Bacteriology*, vol. 1, eds Krieg NR, Holt JG, Williams & Wilkins, Baltimore, 49–57.

Smibert RM, Burmeister JA, 1983, *Treponema pectinovorum* sp. nov. isolated from humans with periodontitis, *Int J Syst Bacteriol*, **33:** 852–6.

Smibert RM, Johnson JL, Ranney RR, 1984, *Treponema socranskii* sp. nov., *Treponema socranskii* subsp. *socranskii* subsp. nov., *Treponema socranskii* subsp. *paredis* subsp. nov. isolated from the human periodontia, *Int J Syst Bacteriol*, **34:** 457–62.

Smith JL, Israel CR, 1967, Spirochetes in the aqueous humor in seronegative ocular syphilis: persistence after penicillin therapy, *Ophthalmology*, **77:** 474–7.

Spangler AS, Jackson JH et al., 1964, Syphilis with a negative blood test reaction, *JAMA*, **189:** 87–90.

Sparling PF, 1971, Diagnosis and treatment of syphilis, *N Engl J Med*, **284:** 642–53.

Sparling PF, 1990, Natural history of syphilis, *Sexually Transmitted Diseases*, 2nd edn, eds Holmes KK, Mardh P-A et al., McGraw-Hill Information Services Co., New York, 213–19.

Stapleton JT, Stamm LV, Bassford PJ Jr, 1985, Potential for development of antibiotic resistance in pathogenic treponemes, *Rev Infect Dis*, **7:** S314–17.

Stamm LV, Parrish EA, Gherardini FC, 1991, Cloning of the *recA* from a free-living leptospire and distribution of RecA-like protein among spirochetes, *Appl Environ Microbiol*, **57:** 183–9.

Steiner BM, Wong GHW et al., 1984, Oxygen toxicity in *Treponema pallidum*: deoxyribonucleic acid single-stranded breakage induced by low doses of hydrogen peroxide, *Can J Microbiol*, **30:** 1467–76.

Stokes JH, Beerman H, Ingraham NR Jr, 1944, Familial and prenatal syphilis (congenital or heredosyphilis), *Modern Clinical Syphilology*, 3rd edn, ed. Stokes JH, WB Saunders, Philadelphia, 1068–112.

Stoll BJ, Lee FK et al., 1993, Improved serodiagnosis of congenital syphilis with combined assay approach, *J Infect Dis*, **167:** 1093–9.

Strugnell R, Cockayne A, Penn CW, 1990, Molecular and antigenic analysis of treponemes, *Crit Rev Microbiol*, **17:** 231–50.

Swartz MN, 1984, Neurosyphilis, *Sexually Transmitted Diseases*, eds Holmes K, Mardh P-A et al., McGraw-Hill, New York, 318–34.

Swisher BL, 1987, Modified Steiner procedure for microwave staining of spirochetes and nonfilamentous bacteria, *J Histotechnol*, **10:** 241–3.

Terpstra WJ, Schoone GJ, Ter Schegget J, 1986, Detection of leptospiral DNA by nucleic acid hybridisation with ^{32}P and biotin-labelled probes, *J Med Microbiol*, **22:** 23–8.

Tomizawa T, Kasamatsu S, 1966, Hemagglutination tests for diagnosis of syphilis. A preliminary report, *Jpn J Med Sci Biol*, **19:** 305–8.

Tomizawa T, Kasamatsu S, Yamaya S, 1969, Usefulness of the hemagglutination test using *Treponema pallidum* antigen (TPHA) for the serodiagnosis of syphilis, *Jpn J Med Sci Biol*, **22:** 341–50.

Tuffanelli DL, 1966, Aging and false-positive reactions for syphilis, *Br J Vener Dis*, **42:** 40–1.

Turner TB, Fleming WJ, 1939, Prolonged maintenance of spirochetes and filtrable viruses in the frozen state, *J Exp Med*, **67:** 620–37.

Turner TB, Hollander DH, 1957, *Biology of the Treponematoses*, Monograph Series No. 35, World Health Organization, Geneva.

United States Public Health Service, 1968, *Syphilis a Synopsis*, Publication No. 1660, US Government Printing Office, Washington, DC.

Veldekamp J, Visser AM, 1975, Application of the enzyme-linked immunosorbent assay (ELISA) in the serodiagnosis of syphilis, *Br J Vener Dis*, **51:** 227–31.

Viscidi RP, Yolken RG, 1987, Molecular diagnosis of infectious diseases by nucleic acid hybridization, *Mol Cell Probes*, **1:** 3–14.

Wallace AL, Norins LC, 1969, Syphilis serology today, *Progress in Clinical Pathology*, vol. 2, ed. Stefanini M, Grune & Stratton, New York, 198–215.

Wassermann A, Neisser A, Brück C, 1906, Eine serodianostische reaktion bei syphilis, *Dtsch Med Wochenschr*, **32:** 745–6.

Wentworth BB, Thompson MA et al., 1978, Comparison of a hemagglutination treponemal test for syphilis (HATTS) with other serologic methods for the diagnosis of syphilis, *Sex Transm Dis*, **5:** 103–11.

White TJ, Fuller SA, 1989, Visuwell Reagin, a nontreponemal enzyme-linked immunosorbent assay for the serodiagnosis of syphilis, *J Clin Microbiol*, **27:** 2300–4.

Wicher K, Noordhoek GT et al., 1992, Detection of *Treponema pallidum* in early syphilis by DNA amplification, *J Clin Microbiol*, **30:** 497–500.

Wilcox RR, Guthe T, 1966, *Treponema pallidum*, a bibliographical review of the culture and survival of *T. pallidum* and associated organisms, *Bull W H O*, **35 (S):** 91–3.

Wilkinson AE, 1973, Fluorescent treponemal antibody tests on cerebrospinal fluid, *Br J Vener Dis*, **49:** 346–9.

Wilkinson AE, Cowell LP, 1971, Immunofluorescent staining for the detection of *T. pallidum* in early syphilitic lesions, *Br J Vener Dis*, **47:** 252–4.

Wilkinson HW, Sampson JS, Plikaytis BB, 1986, Evaluation of a commercial gene probe for identification of *Legionella* cultures, *J Clin Microbiol*, **23:** 217–20.

Yobs AR, Brown L, Hunter EF, 1964, Fluorescent antibody technique in early syphilis, *Arch Pathol*, **77:** 220–5.

Young H, Moyes A et al., 1992, Enzyme immunoassay for antitreponemal IgG: screening or confirmatory test?, *J Clin Pathol*, **45:** 37–41.

Zenker PN, Berman SM, 1990, Congenital syphilis: reporting and reality, *Am J Public Health*, **80:** 271–2.

Chapter 35

GAS GANGRENE AND OTHER CLOSTRIDIAL INFECTIONS

M Sussman, S P Borriello and D J Taylor

1   INTRODUCTION

Members of the genus *Clostridium* (see Volume 2, Chapter 32) including its pathogenic species are found principally in the soil and some species are present as a very small component of the bowel flora of humans and animals. From the soil and from faeces clostridia may reach other sites, and they are present in dust. The clostridia are not normally invasive but they produce a number of toxins and enzymes that are responsible for their pathogenic effects. Pathogenic clostridia may cause 2 general types of infection: histotoxic infections, such as gas gangrene, after traumatic implantation into ischaemic tissues; and toxin-induced disease in various target tissues, including the bowel and the nervous system. This chapter deals with the histotoxic and related infections, clostridial bacteraemia, necrotizing jejunitis and *Clostridium difficile* infections. Food poisoning due to *Clostridium perfringens* is dealt with in Chapter 28. Tetanus, which is due to *Clostridium tetani*, is considered in Chapter 36 and botulism, which is due to *Clostridium botulinum*, is considered in Chapter 37.

Infections of animals due to clostridia are considered below because of some striking parallels with certain infection of humans (see section 5, p. 679).

2   GAS GANGRENE

2.1   History

Gas gangrene (clostridial myonecrosis) became prominent during World War I. Its incidence was extremely high in battle wounds sustained during the campaigns in France and Belgium and the results were devastating. Since gas gangrene had been uncommon in earlier wars (Keen 1915, Bowlby 1919) and was uncommon in civilian injuries, it came to be regarded as a disease of modern war associated with extensive and heavily contaminated wounds.

The 'hospital gangrene' recorded before the introduction of antiseptic surgical techniques by Lister was anaerobic necrotizing fasciitis rather than clostridial myonecrosis (Bowlby 1919). Conditions recognizable as gas gangrene were rarely recorded in antiquity (Millar 1932, Sussman 1958).

2.2   Incidence

INCIDENCE IN MILITARY PRACTICE

The incidence of gangrene in World War I wounds seems to have depended on the distribution of clostridia in the soil of the battlefield. It was common in the agricultural fertile battlefields of northern Europe but uncommon in Iraq, Egypt and the Gallipoli peninsula. This is consistent with the observation that the clostridia responsible for gas gangrene reflect their presence in the soil (MacLennan 1943b, 1962).

In the first year of World War I the incidence of gas gangrene among casualties in the British expeditionary force was about 12% and the mortality rate some 25%. The incidence fell to 1% later in the war when the importance of early wound excision and other prophylactic measures were recognized (Report 1919) and by 1918 the incidence in base hospitals had fallen to 0.3% (Bowlby 1919). During World War II the incidence of gas gangrene in British troops was 0.3–0.8% depending on the theatre of operations (MacLennan 1962). The incidence in US forces was from 0 to 4.5% and a higher incidence was associated with land battles (Smith 1949, Smith and Gardner 1949). In aerial combat the incidence of clostridial wound infection was 1.8% (Cutler and

Sandusky 1944), probably related to contaminated clothing. During the Korean War, when early evacuation and treatment of casualties was practised, the incidence of gas gangrene was 0.08% without mortality (Howard and Inui 1954). By the time of the Vietnam War gas gangrene was rare and it was suggested that as a disease of war it was almost extinct (Unsworth 1973). Confirmation of this conclusion comes from the Falklands campaign and Operation Desert Storm during which gas gangrene was not observed in British troops or those under western command. The availability of appropriate medical services appears to be crucial, because in these wars it was observed in other troops.

Incidence in civilian practice

In the 1970s in the developed world a civilian incidence of gas gangrene of 0.1–1.0 per 10^6 population per year was calculated (Roding, Groeneveld and Boerema 1972, Hart et al. 1975). Wounds of the magnitude seen in war are uncommon in civilian practice and early appropriate surgical treatment and prophylaxis are usually readily available. This may not be the case in developing areas, where gas gangrene after accidental trauma is said to be common.

Though gas gangrene is characteristically associated with serious accidental trauma, it may follow clean elective surgery (Morton 1967, Parker 1967, Braithwaite et al. 1982, Gledhill 1982, Wells et al. 1985). It is a rare but serious complication that may follow the injection of adrenaline (Anon 1968, Teo and Balasubramanian 1983, Hallagan et al. 1992) or insulin (Chin, Martinez and Garmel 1993), usually into the lower parts of the body. The causative organism is *C. perfringens*, which contaminates the skin of the perineum, buttocks and thighs, and originates from the bowel. Clostridial infection of the myometrium, usually due to *C. perfringens*, is particularly related to criminal instrument-induced abortion but it is rare after normal childbirth (Butler 1945, Hill 1964). *C. perfringens* is not often present in the vagina, and then only in small numbers (Lindner et al. 1978, Thadepalli et al. 1978) and is derived from the bowel via perineum. Spontaneous or metastatic gas gangrene is rare in humans (Willis 1969, Engeset et al. 1973, Gatt 1985, Narula and Khatib 1985, Mulier, Morgan and Fabry 1993, Norgaard et al. 1993); it may be associated with diabetes mellitus (Gliemroth, Heise and Missler 1996, Hengster and Pernthaler 1996).

Histotoxic clostridia may also be involved in many other types of infection. Some of these are considered later in the present chapter. Useful discussions of clostridial soft tissue infections have been provided by Gorbach (1992) and Lorber (1995). Detailed reviews of gas gangrene and related infections have been published by MacLennan (1962), Willis (1991) and Finegold and George (1989).

2.3 Bacteriology

Clostridial wound infections may be of 3 types (MacLennan 1943b, 1962) with increasing severity. The first is **simple contamination**, when clostridia are present in injured tissues but without evidence of infection. Such contamination is common and the

wounds heal by first intention without sequelae. The second is **clostridial cellulitis**, in which the infection is limited to local fascia, muscle is not involved and toxaemia is minimal. Finally, in **clostridial myonecrosis** healthy muscle is affected and toxaemia is severe. In the presence of tissue anoxia simple contamination may rapidly progress to cellulitis and myonecrosis.

Anaerobic cellulitis is characterized by a foul, seropurulent infection of the depths of the wound without muscle involvement and toxaemia is insignificant. The organisms responsible are proteolytic and non-toxigenic clostridia, and strains of *C. perfringens* of low toxigenicity. In gas gangrene, on the other hand, the important pathogens are *C. perfringens*, *Clostridium novyi*, *Clostridium septicum* and *Clostridium histolyticum*; *Clostridium sordellii*, *Clostridium fallax* and *Clostridium carnis* are less important. The most frequently encountered non-pathogens include *Clostridium sporogenes*, *Clostridium bifermentans* and *Clostridium tertium*. Since anaerobic infections are due to wound contamination, they are almost always polymicrobial; it is rare for gas gangrene to be monomicrobial. Surveys of the clostridial flora of gas gangrene in battle casualties have shown that *C. perfringens* and *C. novyi* are of major importance (MacLennan 1943b, Hamilton 1944–45, Cooke et al. 1945, Smith and George 1946, Stock 1947).

The prevalence of individual clostridial species in gas gangrene and the incidence of infection largely depend on the number and distribution of the organisms in the environment of the patient. Missiles may cause contamination at the time of injury by implanting soil and clothing, and from their own flora (Thoresby 1966, Thoresby and Darlow 1967, Thoresby and Watts 1967); bullets are not sterilized by firing. The dense and diverse distribution of clostridia in the soil of the Somme and Ypres battlefields was responsible for the high incidence of infection in these battlefields (Keen 1915), whereas the rarity of gas gangrene in the Western Desert campaigns of World War II was probably due to the negligible anaerobic flora of desert sands (MacLennan 1943b). The clostridial flora of clothing consists mainly of *C. perfringens* and *C. sporogenes*, derived from contamination by bowel flora.

The bacterial flora present in gas gangrene commonly includes non-clostridial anaerobes and various facultative aerobes (Weinberg and Séguin 1918, MacLennan 1943a, 1943b, Strawitz et al. 1955). Though this 'associated flora' plays no direct part in myonecrosis, it may facilitate tissue invasion by synergy with histotoxic clostridia.

C. botulinum may be present in wounds (Hall 1945) but rarely gives rise to clinical botulism (wound botulism). When wound botulism occurs it is usually due to *C. botulinum* type A or B, and most cases have been reported from the USA (Davis, Mattman and Wiley 1951, Thomas, Keleher and McKee 1951, Merson and Dowell 1973). The incubation period from wounding to the onset of neurological symptoms is 4–14 days (see Chapter 37).

2.4 Pathogenesis

Clostridia cannot multiply and produce disease in normal tissues because the high oxidation–reduction potential (*E*h) of the circulating blood (+126–+246 mV) and of the tissues is above that necessary for the initiation of anaerobic bacterial growth (+74 mV for *C. perfringens*) (Oakley 1954, Futter and Richardson 1971).

Broth cultures of *C. perfringens*, *C. septicum* or *C. novyi* injected into guinea pigs produce a disease similar to gas gangrene; washed bacilli free of toxins are pathogenic only in large doses. However, mixtures of small doses of toxin-free bacilli and sublethal doses of culture filtrate are highly virulent (de Kruif and Bollman 1917). The filtrate acts by allowing the bacilli to proliferate in the tissues, produce fresh toxin, and finally kill the animal. It may be concluded that in gas gangrene clostridial toxins and other substances break down tissue defences and allow otherwise harmless, potentially toxigenic bacilli to multiply.

Anaerobic bacterial infections of humans are typically associated with locally damaged tissues and commonly also with a 'compromised' host. Once an anaerobic infection is established, toxinogenesis by the infecting organisms leads to a progressive weakening of host defences. There is a spectrum of interaction between bacterial pathogenicity and host resistance. At one end of this spectrum the ubiquity of clostridia ensures that most accidental wounds are exposed to the risk of contamination at the time of injury, but contamination of the wound does not make gas gangrene inevitable; anaerobic conditions must exist in the lesion if the organisms are to multiply. In the absence of an anaerobic environment toxigenic clostridia remain dormant and are eliminated by the local defence mechanisms. Post-cholecystectomy bacteraemia due to *C. perfringens* is an example of the other extreme of the spectrum. Before host defence mechanisms can react to the challenge, toxaemia rapidly causes gross intravascular haemolysis and death. The predisposing factors have been discussed by Willis (1977, 1985, 1991) and Finegold and George (1989).

The central factor that allows anaerobes to grow in wounds is tissue anoxia. Trauma frequently reduces tissue perfusion and initiates the sequence of events that lead to tissue colonization by contaminating anaerobes. High-velocity missiles destroy soft tissues by 'cavitation' (Thoresby 1966) and reduce local tissue perfusion; the shock wave damages more distant blood vessels. Vascular damage is the most important event that predisposes to anaerobic infections (Lowry and Curtis 1947, North 1947).

Foreign material implanted into a wound at the time of injury usually carries potential pathogens that contaminate the damaged tissues. The cavitational effect of high-velocity missiles, by sucking in soil, clothing and skin, brings about deep-seated contamination to which the missile also contributes. The resulting haemorrhage into the tissues potentiates the increasing tissue hypoxia, which may be aggravated by blood loss and shock. It is for these reasons that the use of

tourniquets and tight plasters is contraindicated in the early treatment of such wounds, and delayed primary suture is the correct course of action. The local build-up of pressure in the tissues due to extravasation of blood and tissue fluids is prevented by wide wound incision. Foreign bodies and soil present in the wound favours the establishment of anaerobiosis. Facultative anaerobes, such as *Escherichia coli* and *Proteus* spp., that may also be present in the wound, contribute to the reduction of the local *E*h by utilizing any remaining oxygen. An account of infection in missile wounds has been published by Matheson (1968).

The course of events in *C. perfringens* infections that complicate clean elective surgery is similar to that associated with accidental trauma, but there are differences in the nature and degree of the initiating determinants. The infecting organisms are endogenous on the skin of the patient and are implanted by the surgical procedures. Mid-thigh amputation for obliterative arterial disease is associated with particular risk as is lower-limb surgery in which foreign materials are implanted, such as pinning and plating of femoral fractures (Knutsdon 1983, Laszlow and Elo 1983). The application of tourniquets or use of bloodless field techniques during limb surgery, poor haemostasis, excessive use of diathermy or prolonged use of retractors may favour colonization by anaerobes. Even though surgical trauma is localized, the wound may be heavily contaminated with skin commensals. Particularly in elderly patients, tissue perfusion may be greatly reduced by arterial disease or poor circulation. Foreign bodies, the effects of anaesthesia and surgical trauma are major contributory factors that add to postsurgical anaerobic sepsis.

Gas gangrene after injections into the buttock or thigh is due to the implantation of endogenous anaerobes into the muscle and the irritant or vasoconstrictor action of drugs, which reduce or abolish the local circulation in tissues that may already be subject to poor perfusion, with resulting profound reduction of tissue *E*h. Adrenaline with its vasoconstrictive effect is particularly notorious in this connection (Evans, Miles and Niven 1948, Bishop and Marshall 1960).

A series of changes occurs in the damaged and anoxic tissues that lead to a rapidly falling *E*h and establish an ideal environment for the growth of clostridia (see Oakley 1954, Willis 1969). The production of bacterial toxins and products of bacterial metabolism promotes the growth of the organisms so that gas gangrene becomes established. Defences are further compromised, since neither phagocytes nor antibodies can enter the necrotic zone, and absence of perfusion prevents antimicrobial agents from reaching the affected tissues.

Culture filtrates of broth cultures of clostridia contain toxins, enzymes and other substances that 'activate' the infection. Thus, young cultures of *C. perfringens* contain a non-toxic antigen that activates washed bacilli, and whose aggressive effect is neutralized by the corresponding antibody (Fredette and Frappier 1946). Older culture filtrates of *C. perfringens* type A contain several substances including α and θ toxins, collagenase (κ), hyaluronidase (μ), deoxyribonuclease (ν), and a fibrinolysin. Two other antigenic substances whose action is neutralized by antitoxic sera are recognized. The first sensitizes blood vessels to the action of adrenaline, and the other inhibits phagocytosis (Ganley, Merchant and Bohr 1955). Injection of toxic filtrates into animals simulates the lesions in naturally infected human muscle (Kettle 1919, Govan 1946), which are characterized by oedema, necrosis, and capillary and venous thrombosis. These are accompanied by proteolysis, lipolysis, release of lipid-derived phosphorus, and the tissues disintegrate as the result of the actions of bacterial collagenase, lecithinase and hyaluronidase (Frazer et al. 1945, Robb-Smith 1945).

2.5 The role of clostridial toxins in gas gangrene

The onset of clinical gas gangrene coincides with toxin production, which initiates the extension of the syndrome, in which histotoxic necrosis is followed by bacterial invasion of necrosing tissue. Toxin also enters the circulation and contributes to the increasing toxaemia and shock.

Three kinds of evidence indicate that biologically active clostridial products participate in gas gangrene:

1 the association of pathogenicity with ability to produce these substances
2 mimicry of the disease by injection of these substances into susceptible tissue and
3 the protective or curative effect of antibodies to the substances.

The pathogenicity of strains of *C. perfringens* type A is associated with production of α toxin, and hyaluronidase is produced by about half the toxigenic strains (Robertson and Keppie 1941, McClean, Rogers and Williams 1943, Keppie and Robertson 1944, Evans 1945, Kass, Lichstein and Waisbren 1945). Production of collagenase (Evans 1947a) and θ toxin (Stevens et al. 1993a) are also associated with the virulence of *C. perfringens*. However, this simple association does not constitute proof of a causal link. Better proof is provided by the fact that the natural lesion can be reproduced by toxic filtrates that contain a number of active components. The more stringent immunological evidence is meagre, that antibodies are protective. Thus, of the antibodies against α and θ toxin, hyaluronidase and collagenase, only α antitoxin protects guinea pigs (Evans 1943a, 1943b, 1947b). The importance of α toxin is supported by the efficacy of active immunization with a toxoid, whereas the part played by hyaluronidase and collagenase in the genesis of gas gangrene appears to be less important.

The role of collagenase in causing proteolytic damage to uninfected muscle and in this way supplying amino acids and peptides for bacterial growth was postulated by Smith (1949). The spread of the infection may be facilitated by the hyaluronidase of *C. perfringens* or by hyaluronidase produced by other organisms present in the wound (McClean and Rogers 1944). Hyaluronidase itself cannot to any significant extent penetrate intercellularly (Hechter 1946), but with its assistance infected fluid under the pressure of oedema may move more readily. One of the reasons for the success of early surgical treatment in gas gangrene may be the relief of such pressure. This is illustrated by the observation that simple incision of 4 h old *C. perfringens* lesions of the thigh muscles of guinea pigs allows their survival as compared with control animals not so treated (Hartley and Evans 1946).

The part the lecithinase (α toxin) plays in the myonecrosis is more readily understood than its role in the toxaemia of gas gangrene. Filtrates of *C. perfringens* type A have an acute action on heart muscle and the isolated heart perfused with α toxin is killed and phosphoryl choline is released (Kellaway, Trethewie and Turner 1940a, 1940b, Wright 1950). The toxic action of lecithinase can be neutralized by mixing it with lecithin before it is injected (Wright and Hopkins 1946). Similarly, dogs and mice can be protected against toxaemia by the intravenous injection of lecithin isolated from human and animal tissue (Zamecnik, Folch and Brewster 1945, Gordon, Turner and Dmochowski 1954). However, toxin is rapidly fixed to muscle (Wright and Hopkins 1946) and little or no free toxin is detectable in the blood or tissues of humans or animals with toxaemia (Balch and Ganley 1957, Linsey 1959). High concentrations of antitoxin in the blood do not protect against toxaemia even if given early in the infection, and intravascular α toxin does not necessarily produce toxaemia, though it induces haemolysis. This led MacLennan and Macfarlane (1945) and Macfarlane and MacLennan (1945) to question whether toxaemia is due directly to α toxin. They suggested that, as in traumatic shock, the toxaemia is due to the release of products of tissue injury secondary to the local effects of toxin (Zamecnik, Nathanson and Aub 1947, Berg and Levinson 1955, 1957, 1959). Nevertheless, the absence of detectable α toxin in lesions and in the circulation in natural and experimental gas gangrene does not exclude its participation in local or general disease. In myonecrosis, disruption of sarcolemma and fragmentation of muscle fibres (Robb-Smith 1945) and oedema are compatible with intoxication, and toxin may have a profound effect on the membranes of cells or cell particles (Macfarlane and Datta 1954). Hyaluronidase, deoxyribonuclease, collagenase and fibrinolysin may play a role but this has been difficult to prove. Thus, Aikat and Dible (1956) found no evidence that *C. perfringens* collagenase causes damage to connective tissue, which they suggested was due mainly to α toxin and hyaluronidase. They also concluded that in infections due to *C. novyi* the α toxin produces disruptive oedema and muscle changes, and that ε toxin causes lipolysis. There is no evidence for an effect of the hyaluronidase of *C. novyi* or *C. septicum* in myositis (Aikat and Dible 1960).

The disease in rabbits infected experimentally with *C. perfringens* alone or together with *C. sporogenes* proceeds in 2 stages. First, capillaries are destroyed by α toxin and then the organisms give rise to a general bacteraemia. The local lesion is the source of toxin and bacteria (Katitch et al. 1964).

The toxins of *C. novyi* and *C. septicum* have not been separated to allow study of their effects in vivo. Immunological evidence for the part that the toxins of *C. perfringens*, *C. novyi* and *C. septicum* plays in the genesis of gas gangrene comes from the protection afforded by toxoids prepared from the α toxins of these organisms, whereas passively administered antitoxin is ineffective in the presence of infected muscle, but this is true only for local myonecrosis. The toxaemia associated with the natural disease remains unexplained. The systemic effects of *C. perfringens* α toxin are discussed by MacLennan (1962).

C. perfringens type A antitoxins are bactericidal for the bacteria in tissue fluids. Though the bactericidin does not agglutinate the organisms and is not a recognized antitoxin, it can be absorbed by *C. perfringens* suspensions. It appears to be responsible for the protective effect of antitoxin in experimental infection in the chick embryo, guinea pig and mouse. It is notable that the bactericidal effect of this factor is most evident at relatively high *E*h, but it is known that antitoxin is generally ineffective in established experimental myonecrosis (Bullen and Cushnie 1962).

The pathology of gas gangrene has been described by Favata et al. (1944), Frazer et al. (1945), Govan (1946) and Aikat and Dible (1956, 1960).

2.6 Clinical presentation

The incubation period of gas gangrene after injury varies from 7 h to 7 days. Pain develops early in the region of the wound and increases in intensity with progressive swelling and oedema. The pulse rate increases markedly, is feeble and often impalpable and there is a mild to moderate pyrexia.

The wound is oedematous, tender and exudes a profuse serous or serosanguinous discharge. As the disease progresses, bubbles of gas appear in the discharge, crepitus may become evident in the tissues and the skin becomes white and marbled. The patient is collapsed, profoundly toxaemic and shocked, but remains mentally alert and anxious. The blood pressure falls and peripheral venous collapse often makes venepuncture impossible. The syndrome usually terminates with sudden death due to circulatory failure. The presence of gas may not be obvious and is often a late development. Moreover, infections due to other organisms such as *Prevotella melaninogenica*, *E. coli* or even *Bacillus cereus* sometimes show copious gas formation (Bessman and Wagner 1975, Lewis et al. 1978, Fitzpatrick et al. 1979). Interstitial gas sometimes represents pockets of air that have been forced into the tissues during wounding. Radiological examination may identify gas in the muscle planes and helps to determine the extent of the infection (Kemp 1945).

Bacteraemia is a rare, late and usually agonal complication of clostridial myonecrosis. *C. perfringens* bacteraemia is commonly associated with intravascular haemolysis and is more likely to be found in uterine gas gangrene that may follow abortion or childbirth, and as a rare complication of biliary tract surgery (Brown et al. 1948, Pyrtek and Bartus 1962, Hill 1964, Plimpton 1964, Turner 1964, Yudis and Zucker 1967).

It is essential to distinguish clinically between gas gangrene, clostridial cellulitis and anaerobic streptococcal myositis, because of the important differences in their prognosis, and surgical and therapeutic management (Lowry and Curtis 1947, Anderson, Marr and Jaffe 1972). Apart from pseudomembranous colitis (PMC) due to *C. difficile*, clostridial infections are not transmissible from person to person and do not pose problems of hospital cross-infection.

Accounts of gas gangrene have been published by MacLennan (1943b, 1962), Macfarlane and MacLennan (1945) and Weinstein and Barza (1973).

2.7 Diagnosis

Gas gangrene is essentially a clinical diagnosis. The presence of pathogenic clostridia in a wound, and particularly of *C. perfringens*, is of little pathognomonic significance. Anaerobic bacteriology cannot provide timely confirmatory evidence in a disease with an incubation period that may be as short as 4 h, and is on the average 1–2 days. However, direct examination of the wound material must not be omitted, because it may yield valuable information, especially for the diagnosis of anaerobic streptococcal myositis (see MacLennan 1943a, Memorandum 1943, Hayward 1945). In obstetric infection the presence of capsulated *C. perfringens*-like bacilli in gram-stained smears is almost diagnostic of pathogenic *C. perfringens* (Butler 1945).

Rapid enzymological tests have been proposed for the identification of clostridial products in wound exudates. A species-specific sialidase-inhibition test gives results in 2–6 h and agrees well with the results of bacteriological examination for *C. perfringens* infection but not for *C. septicum* or *C. sordellii* (Roggentin et al. 1991). In an alternative approach, sialidases in exudates are bound in microtitre plates to immobilized polyclonal antibodies and the sialidase activity assayed against a fluorogenic substrate (Roggentin et al. 1993).

Apart from examination of smears, full bacteriological examination must include direct culture to assess the relative numbers of the various bacilli present and the inoculation of cooked meat broth for enrichment purposes and subsequent plating. The media used should include those that contain substrates such as egg yolk and blood agar to allow identification of various toxins. If suitable antitoxic sera are available they may for convenience be prepared as half-antitoxin plates. Selective agar media facilitate early recognition and isolation of relevant organisms. Schemes for the bacteriological study of clostridial sepsis have been described by Hayward (1945) and Willis and Phillips (1988).

2.8 Prophylaxis and treatment

PREVENTION AND TREATMENT

The most important prophylactic measure is early and adequate surgery (Latta 1951, Howard and Inui 1954, Lindberg et al. 1955, Strawitz et al. 1955, Wheatley 1967, Altemeier 1979, Anon 1984). Damaged muscle must be excised to leave only healthy, well vascularized tissue and the area irrigated to reduce numbers of contaminating micro-organisms. Management is by delayed primary closure; the importance of this technique has repeatedly been emphasized by military experience (Ogilvie 1944, Shouler 1983, Anon 1984).

Incision of the gangrenous muscle along its length improves the survival rate of guinea pigs experimentally infected with *C. perfringens* (Hartley and Evans 1946), probably by reducing tension in the oedematous muscle and improving the blood supply. In experimental *C. novyi* gas gangrene in sheep, wound incision alone fails to delay the onset of gas gangrene and has no effect on survival, but adequate excision greatly improves survival (Thoresby and Matheson 1967a, 1967b). In humans, when formal wound excision for prophylactic purposes is not possible, the skin wound can be enlarged and the deep fascia incised to relieve tension and allow free drainage. Further excision can then be carried out at a later stage (Memorandum 1943).

Parenteral antimicrobial therapy must be started as soon as possible after wounding to ensure that therapeutic drug concentrations are present in the tissues at the time of surgery. Benzylpenicillin was recommended by Garrod et al. (1973) but metronidazole is now regarded as the prophylactic antimicrobial compound of choice (Bartlett 1982, Brazier et al. 1985, Eggleston 1986, Stevens, Maier and Mitten 1987a, 1987b). Metronidazole is given intravenously before surgery and then every 8 h for 24 h, followed by a 12-hourly schedule. In sheep with experimental high-velocity missile wounds contaminated with clostridia, penicillin alone given within 9 h of wounding and challenge is effective prophylaxis (Owen-Smith and Matheson 1968). In humans, antimicrobial prophylaxis alone is of no value, but its use together with surgery, particularly if this is carried out soon after wounding, reduces the risk of anaerobic infection (Altemeier, McMurrin and Alt 1951, Garrod 1958, MacLennan 1962, Barber and Garrod 1963). Antitoxin is prophylactically and therapeutically ineffective and is no longer available.

Elective surgery in the hip and thigh region in elderly patients carries a significant risk of postoperative gas gangrene due to endogenous *C. perfringens* (Taylor 1960, Parker 1967). Prophylaxis in such patients consists of meticulous preoperative skin preparation (Ayliffe and Lowbury 1969) and peroperative prophylaxis with metronidazole or benzylpenicillin, continued for 48 h after surgery.

HYPERBARIC OXYGEN

Hyperbaric oxygen therapy has revolutionized the treatment of gas gangrene (Brummelkamp, Hogendijk and Boerema 1961, Brummelkamp, Boerema and Hoogendyk 1963, Roding, Groeneveld and Boerema 1972, Hirn 1993, Thom 1993). Before its introduction, successful management of gas gangrene required radical excision of the affected muscle. Muscles were excised from origin to insertion, or the limb amputated. Though controlled trials of hyperbaric oxygen have not been carried out, its effectiveness is supported by experimental (Boerema and Brummelkamp 1960) and clinical evidence (Brown et al. 1994). Over a period of 12 years in the Netherlands, Roding, Groeneveld and Boerema (1972) treated 130 patients, of whom 29 died (22.3%), only 14 from gas gangrene. The death rate in cases due to civilian trauma was only 12.2%, compared with 45.2% in postoperation cases. Often the use of hyperbaric oxygen led to the saving of limbs that would otherwise have been amputated. The disease was most effectively controlled in patients who survived for 48 h after the start of hyperbaric oxy-

gen treatment. Hyperbaric oxygen treatment consists in exposure to oxygen at 2.5–3 atm pressure for 1.5–2 h as soon as possible after admission and is accompanied by resuscitation and intravenous metronidazole or penicillin. A single-patient chamber may be used, or a larger chamber that also accommodates medical staff. The larger chambers are pressurized with air and the patient is given oxygen by means of a face mask. Since hyperbaric oxygen does not revive necrotic tissue, surgical toilet, rather than radical excision, is carried out as soon as the patient's general condition has improved. Subsequent treatments in the chamber are given at intervals of about 8 h for the first 24 h and then at intervals of 12 h. Since many infections are mixed a broad spectrum antibiotic may be given in addition to metronidazole (Hart et al. 1975, Darke, King and Slack 1977, Skiles, Covert and Fletcher 1978). An appropriate combination is metronidazole, gentamicin and amoxycillin. Patients must be transferred early and speedily to a hyperbaric oxygen unit, because untreated gas gangrene runs a fulminating course and leads rapidly to fatal intoxication. Hyperbaric oxygen therapy has been reviewed by Rudge (1993).

Hyperbaric oxygen directly impairs the growth of clostridia (Hopkinson and Towers 1963, Bullen, Cushnie and Stoner 1966) and also prevents production of *C. perfringens* α toxin (van Unnik 1965, Kaye 1966) and vegetative bacilli are killed. Thus, *C. perfringens* implanted into untreated mice in agar discs inoculated with c. 10^3 viable organisms, multiplies about 10^4-fold in 48 h without causing illness. However, only few viable organisms can be recovered from such discs in mice exposed 4 times to 3 atm of oxygen for 90 min (Hill and Osterhout 1972). The part that hyperbaric oxygen, antimicrobial agents and surgery play in the treatment of clostridial myositis has been examined in experimental animal models (Hirn, Niinikoski and Lehtonen 1992, Stevens et al. 1993b). The effects of hyperbaric oxygen on micro-organisms, and the factors that affect the response of clostridial infection to hyperbaric oxygen therapy have been reviewed by Gottlieb (1971). Hyperbaric oxygen may also promote the viability of tissues to which the blood supply is impaired.

ANTIMICROBIAL AGENTS

Histotoxic clostridia associated with wound infections are susceptible to several antimicrobial agents (Martin, Gardner and Washington 1972, Savage 1974, Dornbusch, Nord and Dahlback 1975). *C. septicum* and *C. perfringens* are highly susceptible to benzylpenicillin (Brazier et al. 1985), but some clostridia are resistant to benzylpenicillin (Rosenblatt 1984, Brazier et al. 1985).

The activity of other penicillins against clostridia in decreasing order is amoxycillin, carbenicillin, flucloxacillin and mecillinam. The combination of amoxycillin plus clavulanic acid (Augmentin) is active in vitro. The cephalosporins, cephamycins and monobactams are poorly active against clostridia (Selwyn 1980, Brogden and Heel 1986), but imipenem (a carbapenem of the thienamycin class) has good activity in vitro (Wexler and Finegold 1985). The 4-quinolones are only moderately to poorly active against clostridia (Goldstein and Citron 1985, Delmee and Avesani 1986, King and Phillips 1986, Watt and Brown 1986). With some exceptions, metronidazole, chloramphenicol, benzylpenicillin and erythromycin are the most effective anticlostridial drugs. Tetracyclines and clindamycin are less effective and the aminoglycosides much less so (Staneck and Washington 1974, Sutter and Finegold 1976, Brazier et al. 1985, Robbins et al. 1987, Stevens, Laine and Mitten 1987, Stevens, Maier and Mitten 1987a, 1987b). The drugs of choice for the prevention and treatment of clostridial wound infections are metronidazole and benzylpenicillin.

3 OTHER CLOSTRIDIAL INFECTIONS OF HUMANS

The histotoxic clostridia may participate in infective conditions other than myonecrosis. Penetrating wounds may rarely result in brain abscess, acute purulent meningitis, panophthalmitis, endocarditis, septic arthritis and intrapleural infections. *C. perfringens* is the organism most commonly responsible. These infections have been reviewed by Willis (1969, 1977, 1991) and Finegold and George (1989).

3.1 Bacteraemia

C. perfringens is present on the skin over the antecubital fossa in 20% of subjects (Ahmad and Darrell 1976) and its presence in routine blood cultures is due to contamination from the skin; contaminated skin may rarely be responsible for clinically significant bacteraemia due to *C. perfringens* (Rose 1979).

Clostridia may invade the bloodstream late in gas gangrene. This is most commonly due to *C. perfringens* and *C. septicum* (Weinberg and Séguin 1918, Report 1919). *C. septicum* bacteraemia may spontaneously complicate malignant disease of the colon and 'neutropenic enterocolitis' (see section 3.2). *C. perfringens* bacteraemia is rare after surgery on the gastrointestinal tract, or after the perforation of peptic ulcers. It is an uncommon complication of acute emphysematous cholecystitis (Willis 1969, Gorbach and Thadepalli 1975). Most idiopathic bacteraemias are probably secondary to covert, often intra-abdominal, pathological abnormalities.

Clinically significant bacteraemia is dramatic in its onset and follows an overwhelmingly rapid course with intravascular haemolysis, shock, haemoglobinuria, renal failure, and rapidly deepening jaundice and cyanosis. The clostridium can be isolated by blood culture and is sometimes visible in gram-stained blood films. Endocarditis due to clostridia is rare (Case, Goforth and Silva 1972, Alvarez-Elcoro and Sifuentes-Osorio 1984). Clostridial bacteraemia in patients with gas gangrene has a grave prognosis, but early or transient bacteraemia, probably due to mechanical causes rather than invasion, is of little significance (Butler 1937, Gorbach and Thadepalli 1975).

3.2 *Clostridium septicum* bacteraemia

This has long been recognized, sometimes associated with spontaneous gas gangrene in which *C. perfringens* or *C. septicum* entered the circulation through a malignant lesion of the colon (Valentine 1957, Cabrera, Tsukada and Pickren 1965, Francois et al. 1994). Boggs, Frei and Thomas (1958) observed clostridial bacteraemia in patients with leukaemia and thought that it was due to invasion of infected leukaemic infiltrates of the caecum and colon. The association of *C. septicum* bacteraemia with ileocaecal neoplasia is now well recognized.

The primary ileocaecal syndrome has had a variety of names (typhlitis, ileocaecal syndrome, necrotizing enteropathy) and is now usually known as neutropenic enterocolitis because of its association with severe neutropenia. The disease is frequently complicated by a severe and progressive sepsis due to invasion by *C. septicum* (Bignold and Harvey 1979, Rifkin 1980, King et al. 1984, Hiew, Silberstein and Hennessy 1993). *C. septicum* probably plays the leading primary role in most cases of neutropenic colitis (Rifkin 1980, King et al. 1984). Most patients with *C. septicum* bacteraemia have malignant disease including haematological malignancies (Koransky, Stargel and Dowell Jr 1979, Lorimer and Eidus 1994). Neutropenic patients who present with pyrexia, abdominal symptoms and hypotension should raise the suspicion of endogenous clostridial infection (Warren and Mason 1970, Gorse et al. 1984, Pelfrey et al. 1984). The portal of entry for the organism is probably ulceration of the bowel. The organism proliferates locally to produce an enterocolitic lesion with submucosal oedema, haemorrhage and necrosis, which allows invasion of the bloodstream. *C. septicum* is relatively sparse in the human intestine and it is not known why it, rather than *C. perfringens*, behaves in this way.

Clostridial bacteraemia has been reviewed by Spencer (1991) and Stevens et al. (1990).

3.3 Enteric infections

A mild diarrhoea associated with the consumption of communal meals was for some time attributed to *C. perfringens* present in the food. In 1953 Hobbs and her colleagues established that certain strains of *C. perfringens* type A were responsible for this disease, which is described in Chapter 28.

Severe bowel disease due to *C. perfringens* type C was first described in 1946 in Germany as enteritis necroticans ('Darmbrand'). It was characterized by a diffuse sloughing enteritis of the jejunum, ileum and colon. In 1963 a similar disease was identified in the native population of Papua New Guinea (Murrell and Roth 1963). The aetiological association between *C. difficile* and PMC was established by Bartlett et al. (1977) (see section 4, p. 676).

3.4 Necrotizing jejunitis (enteritis necroticans; pigbel)

This is a severe and often fatal disease due to *C. perfringens* type C. It was first recorded by Zeissler and Rassfeld-Sternberg (1949) in northwest Germany (Fick and Wolken 1949). Severe lower abdominal pain and diarrhoea developed some hours after individuals had eaten rabbit, tinned meat or fish paste. Blood and mucosal sloughs were present in the stools in some cases and there were deaths due to peripheral circulatory collapse or intestinal obstruction due to massive mucosal oedema of the intestinal mucosa. The jejunum was principally affected.

Sporadic cases of necrotizing jejunitis have been recorded (Calnan 1950, Govan and MacIntosh 1951, Patterson and Rosenbaum 1952, Wright and Stanfield 1967, Severin, de la Fuente and Stringer 1984). A second major outbreak was reported from New Guinea (Murrell and Roth 1963, Murrell et al. 1966a, 1966b, Murrell 1967), in which *C. perfringens* type C was again identified as the probable pathogen (Egerton and Walker 1964). Subsequently, the syndrome was seen in other parts of the world (Foster 1966, Sekabunga 1966, Wright and Stanfield 1967, Gurovsky and Samuel 1972 from East Africa; Headington et al. 1967, Welch and Sumitswan 1975, Johnson et al. 1987 from Thailand; Narayan and Rao 1970, Pujari and Deodhare 1980 from India). It has been suggested that *C. perfringens* type A may occasionally also cause the disease (van Kessel et al. 1985).

In New Guinea, necrotizing jejunitis was referred to as the 'pigbel' syndrome (New Guinea pidgin English, *pig-bel* = abdominal discomfort after a large pork meal), because of its relationship to the widespread practice of pork feasting in the locality. Murrell et al. (1966b) defined pigbel as an acute, patchy, necrotizing and inflammatory disease of the small bowel in Highland Melanesians in New Guinea. The disease is predominantly one of children, males more commonly affected than females. It is characterized by anorexia, severe upper abdominal pain, bloody diarrhoea and vomiting and has been classified into 4 clinical types:

1 an acute form with fulminating toxaemia and shock, with a mortality rate of around 85%
2 an acute surgical form in which there may be mechanical and paralytic ileus, acute strangulation, and perforation and peritonitis, with a mortality rate of about 40%
3 a subacute surgical form in which there may be acute and chronic small bowel obstruction, intestinal fistulae, ulcerative jejunitis and peritoneal adhesions, with a mortality rate of about 40% and
4 a mild form without complications and progressing to complete recovery.

The pathology of pigbel has been described by Cooke (1979). Treatment includes resuscitation with blood transfusion, bowel decompression and resection, and antimicrobial therapy (Smith 1969, Pujari and Deodhare 1980, Millar 1981).

PATHOGENESIS

Pigbel in New Guinea is due to *C. perfringens* and its β toxin. The organism is widely distributed in the village environment and is present in the faeces of more than 70% of normal persons (Lawrence et al. 1979b). After ingestion, *C. perfringens* type C proliferates in the intestine and releases its β toxin, which under normal circumstances is destroyed by intestinal proteinases to which it is highly sensitive. A number of factors may operate in Papua New Guinea to preserve the intra-luminal activity of the β toxin, with resulting severe toxic intestinal damage (Lawrence and Walker 1976, Lawrence 1979, Walker 1985).

Though frank malnutrition is uncommon among native New Guineans, the diet is very low in protein, which markedly reduces production of intestinal proteinase enzymes. The staple diet is sweet potato, which provides up to 90% of dietary calories and contains heat-stable trypsin inhibitors. In addition, infestation with the roundworm *Ascaris lumbricoides*, which secretes a trypsin inhibitor, may contribute to reduction of proteinase activity. The occurrence of pigbel, particularly in children, is due to their poor immunity to β toxin. When a high protein diet is eaten together with sweet potato, the conditions are ideal for the growth of *C. perfringens* type C and the production of β toxin, which is then less likely to be degraded by proteolytic enzymes.

Damage by the toxin occurs some time before symptoms are evident, by which time administration of antitoxin is ineffective (Rooney, Shepherd and Suebu 1979), but active immunization with *C. perfringens* type C β toxoid confers a high degree of lasting protection (Lawrence et al. 1979a, Walker et al. 1979, Davis et al. 1982). The pathogenesis of the disease and the effectiveness of immunization have been demonstrated by Lawrence and Cooke (1980).

An account of pigbel is given by Davis (1984).

4 CLOSTRIDIUM DIFFICILE INFECTION

Clostridium difficile is most commonly associated with infections of the large bowel. It is the cause of many cases of antibiotic-associated diarrhoea and nearly all cases of pseudomembranous colitis (PMC). As such, it is the most common identifiable bacterial cause of nosocomial diarrhoea, and one of the most common anaerobic infections. However, infection is not restricted to the gut, and rare cases of extra-intestinal infection have been reported (Feldman, Kallich and Weinstein 1995).

The importance of *C. difficile* as a pathogen is put in perspective by Willis (1988) who wrote: 'Among all of the many advances that have been made in our understanding of anaerobic bacteria and anaerobic bacterial disease during the last 40 years, elucidation of the syndrome of antibiotic-associated pseudomembranous colitis ranks as a major triumph.'

4.1 History

PMC was first described by Finney (1893) as a postoperative complication of gastroenterostomy. Over the years its aetiology was variously ascribed to such causes as gastrointestinal surgery ('postoperative enterocolitis'), antibiotic therapy ('antibiotic-associated enterocolitis'), clindamycin therapy ('clindamycin-associated colitis') and staphylococcal sepsis ('staphylococcal enterocolitis') (Gorbach and Bartlett 1977).

This, and other cases, preceded the use of antibiotics but interest in the disease was stimulated in the 1950s and 1960s because cases were associated with the administration of tetracycline and chloramphenicol (Reiner, Schlesinger and Miller 1952, Hummel, Altmeier and Hill 1964) and again in the 1970s because of an association with the administration of clindamycin (Tedesco, Barton and Alpers 1974). These observations encouraged the development of an extremely active, though relatively short, period of research, which, together with a number of earlier, sometimes unrelated observations, culminated in the discovery of *C. difficile* as an aetiological agent of antibiotic-associated PMC. In the course of a search for a possible viral cause of PMC, Larson et al. (1977), at the Clinical Research Centre, Harrow in England, reported the detection of a cytopathic agent in filtrates of faeces from 5 patients with histologically proven disease. They concluded that the agent was probably a bacterial protein toxin. Animal model studies, largely in the USA, established that the toxin was clostridial in origin (Bartlett et al. 1977, Rifkin et al. 1977). These studies showed that disease in antibiotic pretreated hamsters could be transferred serially by intracaecal injection of caecal contents from diseased animals, and that filtrates of these caecal contents were cytopathic for cells in tissue culture. More importantly, the cytopathic activity could be neutralized by *C. sordellii* antitoxin, though *C. sordellii* was not present in diseased animals. This dilemma was quickly resolved by the identification of *C. difficile* as the dominant *Clostridium* species in this material, that it produced disease in antibiotic pretreated hamsters, and further that it produced a cytopathic toxin that could be neutralized by *C. sordellii* antitoxin (Bartlett et al. 1977, 1978a, 1978b, Rifkin et al. 1977). The final cornerstone of proof was put in place by the isolation of *C. difficile* from the faeces of patients with PMC (Bartlett et al. 1978c, George RH et al. 1978, George WL et al. 1978, Larson et al. 1978).

4.2 Pathology

The disease is well defined histopathologically (Goulston and McGovern 1965, Price and Davies 1977, Price 1984) and almost invariably restricted to the colon. The mucosa becomes necrotic and, in fulminating cases, an exudative membrane forms, which resembles that seen in diphtheria. The pseudomembrane forms in multiple, friable yellow-white plaques that vary in size from a few centimetres to about 2 mm in diameter and are attached to the mucosal surface; they may become confluent. Between the mucosal plaques only congestion may be apparent. Microscopically, the membrane appears as a fibrinous exudate that contains leucocytes, epithelial cells and mucin; the underlying intestinal submucosa shows a varying degree of necrosis and inflammation.

In the earliest stages of the disease 'summit-lesions', tiny superficial intercryptal erosions, may be found (Price and Davies 1977). However, for accurate diagnosis the adjacent mucosa must show no more than oedema and focal clusters of polymorphs. Where there is full thickness mucosal necrosis the features are no longer diagnostic and may resemble other conditions that have a stage of complete mucosal necrosis, e.g. ischaemia or radiation damage.

The association of infection with antibiotic use is due to the requirement for disruption of the normal stable gut microbiota (microflora) before *C. difficile* can establish and produce toxins. The barrier effect afforded by the normal microbiota is frequently referred to as colonization resistance. This barrier effect to infection with *C. difficile* and its disruption with antibiotics has been demonstrated in animals (Larson, Price and Borriello 1980, Larson and Borriello 1990) and in vitro with human and animal faecal or caecal material (Borriello and Barclay 1986, Borriello Barclay and Welch 1988). A variety of antibiotics can predispose to *C. difficile* infection (Borriello and Larson 1981, Tedesco 1984, George 1988), the frequency of association being related to the route of administration, frequency of use and the impact on the bacterial components of the gut microbiota. For example, McFarland, Surawicz and Stamm (1990) found that the short-term use of high dose cephalosporins (<1 week; >10 g cumulative), or the use of broad spectrum penicillin for longer than 7 days, was associated with *C. difficile* infection. Although it is difficult to extrapolate the relative risk of infection associated with a given antibiotic from frequency of association of particular antibiotics, there is evidence from the hamster model of the disease that the major difference between oral antibiotics is the duration, rather than the degree, of susceptibility induced (Larson and Borriello 1990). It is possible that the higher incidence of infection in the elderly is due in part to their poorer colonization resistance (Borriello and Barclay 1986), so that a smaller effect by antibiotics is required to induce susceptibility to colonization with *C. difficile*. Neonates, who are in the process of developing a complex gut microbiota, are the other age group with a poor barrier effect. Indeed, *C. difficile* was first isolated from the faeces of neonates (Hall and O'Toole 1935), in whom it is commonly present (Larson et al. 1982). *C. difficile* toxins are also commonly present in such faeces (Libby, Donta and Wilkins 1983, Borriello 1990). Why infants usually appear to be unaffected by the toxins remains unknown. Rarely, antibiotic-associated PMC occurs in older children (Viscidi and Bartlett 1981), and even more rarely in infancy (Scopes, Smith and Beach 1980, Donta, Stuppy and Myers 1981, Richardson et al. 1981, Price et al. 1990).

4.3 Pathogenesis

Once *C. difficile* is established in the bowel, disease is a consequence of the production of 2 large protein toxins, toxins A and B, both of which have been cloned and sequenced (Barroso et al. 1990, Dove et al. 1990). Non-toxigenic strains of *C. difficile* are known and may be present with toxigenic strains in patients with antibiotic-associated diarrhoea (Borriello and Honour 1983). Earlier studies with toxigenic isolates indicated that toxins A and B are always present together (Lyerly, Sullivan and Wilkins 1983). However, a rare cytotoxic isolate of *C. difficile* that lacks most of the gene for toxin A, but which is lethal in the hamster model of disease, has been described (Borriello et al. 1992b, Lyerly et al. 1992). The possibility that toxin A may be responsible for the enterocolitis is supported by the observations of Lyerly et al. (1985). In a series of animal feeding experiments they showed that the culture filtrates from a strain of *C. difficile* caused intestinal lesions and diarrhoea, but filtrate from which toxin A had been removed was inactive. Moreover, although toxin B was inactive, the 2 toxins appeared to act synergistically. Various studies (Mitchell et al. 1986, 1987, Ketley et al. 1987, Triadafilopoulos et al. 1987) have shown that toxin A has both histotoxic and 'enterotoxic' activity and that the toxin is of major importance in the causation of tissue damage and luminal fluid accumulation in experimental animals. In rabbits with ileal and colonic loops, they showed that fluid secretion occurred when the toxin had penetrated to the deeper tissues of the bowel wall, and that this was probably the outcome of repeated cycles of toxin uptake and tissue damage. Gross haemorrhage occurred in the ileal tissues and villus architecture was severely damaged, giving rise to a bloody protein-rich luminal fluid. There was damage to the surface epithelium in the colon, with interstitial haemorrhages and a watery luminal fluid containing little protein. Interestingly, there is evidence that the tissue damage is a consequence of toxin A-induced recruitment of neutrophils (Triadafilopoulos et al. 1987). Toxin A does not appear to stimulate active secretion; rather, the diarrhoea may be due to increased permeability and reduced absorption. The increased permeability is probably due to loss of cell tight junction integrity, as a consequence of the cytopathic activity of toxin A. Until recently the mechanism of the potent cytopathic effect of both toxins, which results from disruption of the cell cytoskeleton, was unknown. It is now known, however, that for toxin B this is due to glucosylation of Rho proteins (Just et al. 1995). Since both toxins are cytotoxic, it is difficult to explain the lack of 'enterotoxic'-like activity of purified toxin B in animals. This may be due to a lack of specific surface-exposed receptors. These are still unknown for toxin B, though for toxin A there is evidence that Lewis X, Y and I antigens can serve as receptors (Tucker and Wilkins 1991). Whether these are functional receptors in the gut is difficult to determine, particularly because they are not universally expressed by colonic epithelial cells. There is recent evidence that in humans, toxin B may independently cause tissue damage (Reigler et al. 1995).

In addition to the toxins, other factors produced by *C. difficile* may contribute to colonization of the gut and pathology. These have been reviewed (Borriello 1990, Borriello et al. 1990) and include secretion of proteases, adhesion to mucus and production of fimbriae.

4.4 Clinical manifestations

C. difficile infection is almost always associated with recent or current administration of antibiotics and most commonly occurs in hospitalized elderly patients (Borriello and Larson 1981, McFarland, Surawicz and Stamm 1990). Disease is mainly restricted to the colon and may be associated with a spectrum of disease severity, ranging from trivial diarrhoea, through moderately severe disease with watery diarrhoea, abdominal pain and systemic upset, to life-threatening PMC. The latter may be accompanied by toxic megacolon (rare), electrolyte imbalance and occasional bowel perforation. Frank blood in the stool is not common. The onset of symptoms is frequently abrupt with explosive watery foul-smelling diarrhoea (Bennett, Allen and Millard 1984, Bartlett 1992) accompanied by abdominal pain, fever in some patients, and a raised blood leucocyte count.

Very rarely, reactive arthritis may occur as a consequence of gut infection (Cope, Anderson and Wilkins 1992). In total 14 such cases have been reported, and 6 of 10 cases tested were HLA-B27 positive.

4.5 Diagnosis

Diagnosis of *C. difficile* infection is based on detection of toxin in the faeces (Report 1994a). This can be achieved by application of faecal filtrates to cells such as African green monkey kidney (Vero) cells in tissue culture and observation of cytopathic effects that can be neutralized with specific antiserum (Chang, Lauermann and Bartlett 1979, Borriello and Welch 1984), or by use of commercial enzyme immunoassays, the majority of which detect toxin A (Borriello et al. 1992a, Doern, Coughlin and Wu 1992, Mattia et al. 1993). Such kits make it possible for laboratories without tissue culture facilities to offer a same-day diagnosis. Stool samples that cannot be processed for toxin assay on the day of receipt should be refrigerated. An advantage of tissue culture for toxin detection is that other toxins can be detected, for example the enterotoxin of *C. perfringens*, another cause of nosocomial diarrhoea (Borriello et al. 1984, Jackson et al. 1986, Larson and Borriello 1988).

Isolation of toxigenic *C. difficile* from samples of faeces is not in itself diagnostic, but is essential for typing as part of the epidemiological investigations of outbreaks. The organism can usually be cultured by exploiting the selective action of cycloserine and cefoxitin (George et al. 1979, Willey and Bartlett 1979), by selection of its spores by alcohol treatment (Borriello and Honour 1981, Levett 1985), or by a combination of both (Borriello and Honour 1984). Recognition of *C. difficile* colonies on primary isolation is facilitated by their characteristic yellow-green fluorescence under long-wave ultraviolet light (George et al. 1979). Various methods have been used for typing or fingerprinting. Though no single standard method is at present accepted for this organism, many have been reviewed by Tabaqchali and Wilks (1992).

The presence of *C. difficile* toxin in faeces is diagnostic of *C. difficile* infection, but this is not necessarily diagnostic of PMC, which can only be confirmed by detection of typical lesions on sigmoidoscopy and histological examination of tissue. Unfortunately, negative findings at sigmoidoscopy do not exclude the diagnosis, because the rectosigmoid may be spared (Seppälä, Hjelt and Sipponen 1981).

4.6 Epidemiology and control

The incidence of the disease is uncertain. Published reports show a wide variation between studies and suggest that episodes of locally increased prevalence occur. These may be attributable to predisposing causes that affect particular groups, such as general surgical patients (Testore et al. 1988), oncology patients (Gerard et al. 1988), those with chronic renal disease (Bruce et al. 1982), or to hospital-acquired infection. Undoubtedly the latter is often a factor together with other predisposing causes. The recognition that case clustering occurs, that the hospital environment may become contaminated with *C. difficile*, and that the organism can be detected in the faeces of some in contact with infected patients, supports the view that *C. difficile* infection results from cross-infection in hospitals (Greenfield et al. 1981, Burdon 1982, Larson et al. 1982, Walters et al. 1982, Cumming et al. 1986, Heard et al. 1986, McFarland et al. 1989). It is recommended that infected patients should be isolated (Mulligan et al. 1980, Kim et al. 1981, Report 1994b) but efforts to limit dissemination of the organism in chronic-care and other long-stay wards may meet with little success (Bender et al. 1986). The 'carrier state' and its epidemiological associations have been reviewed by George (1986) and Mulligan (1988). Attempts to clear the organism from asymptomatic excreters are of no value, though various workers have attempted to achieve this (Johnson et al. 1992).

The spores of *C. difficile* are highly resistant and can survive on inanimate surfaces for many months (Fekety et al. 1981). Attempts to eradicate *C. difficile* from the hospital environment have not been very successful (Katz et al. 1988, Struelens et al. 1991). Most of the reduction achieved is more consistent with the physical removal of bacterial spores than with chemical disinfection. Where an acceptable level of reduction was achieved (Katz et al. 1988) the concentration and pH of the hypochlorite solution used would be unsuitable for long-term use. Fortunately, an exposure for 10 min to 2% alkaline buffered glutaraldehyde is suitable for the decontamination of medical equipment that cannot be steam sterilized (Rutala, Gergen and Weber 1993).

Community cases of *C. difficile* gastrointestinal infection are rare, even though the organism can be recovered from a wide variety of environmental sites, including soil (Hafiz and Oakley 1976), domestic animals (Princewell and Agba 1982) and household pets (Borriello et al. 1983, Riley et al. 1991).

There is little doubt that the most important factor in preventing infection with *C. difficile* is strict control

of antibiotic use. This should be coupled with good enteric infection control practices, such as handwashing, equipment sterilization, environmental cleaning and isolation of patients with diarrhoea (Report 1994b). The same approach is important for the control of outbreaks.

4.7 Treatment and management

When diarrhoea develops during a course of antimicrobial therapy, withdrawal of the offending agent often leads to early resolution of symptoms, even in some cases of established PMC. Since fluid loss may be considerable, attention to fluid replacement and electrolyte balance is necessary. Antimicrobial therapy in the management of *C. difficile*-associated diarrhoea and PMC should be reserved for patients with severe infections or for those in whom diarrhoea fails to improve spontaneously within 48 h. A number of antibiotics, in particular vancomycin (Keighley et al. 1978, Tedesco et al. 1978) and metronidazole (Pashby, Bolton and Sherriff 1979, Teasley et al. 1983), have been used successfully and are reviewed by Wilcox and Spencer (1992). Vancomycin is poorly absorbed from the gastrointestinal tract and high concentrations are readily attained in the bowel after oral administration; this agent may thereby be looked upon as providing essentially topical therapy within the gut. Metronidazole, on the other hand, is rapidly absorbed from the upper gastrointestinal tract, but also produces therapeutic concentrations in diarrhoeal stools. These 2 agents appear to have similar efficacy and relapse rates and are both well tolerated.

The use of ion-exchange resins as binding agents for *C. difficile* toxin has not been attended with much benefit and anti-diarrhoeal agents such as loperamide and codeine may prolong or exacerbate symptoms by delaying toxin elimination.

The optimum treatment for relapse or reinfection is less certain. In general, repeat courses of vancomycin or metronidazole are successful (Fekety et al. 1984, Bartlett 1985). A regimen of tapering doses, followed by pulsed treatment with vancomycin, has also proved effective (Tedesco, Gordon and Fortson 1985). For very resistant cases, various bacteriotherapeutic approaches have been tried (Schwan et al. 1984, Gorbach, Chang and Goldin 1987, Seal et al. 1987, Surawicz et al. 1989, Schellenberg et al. 1994), ranging from rectal infusion of normal faeces to use of a nontoxigenic avirulent strain of *C. difficile*.

5 CLOSTRIDIAL INFECTIONS OF ANIMALS

Clostridia have been identified in the gut contents of most mammals and birds in which they have been sought and they cause infections in other tissues under conditions of reduced oxygen tension. These include wounds and trauma that arise from the behaviour or management of the species concerned and to a lesser extent from procedures such as castration, injection and surgical operations. The behaviour of clostridia in many animals and bird species and the development of clostridial disease is critically affected by specific immunity and its transfer. Maternal antibody does not cross the placenta of the major farm animal species but is transferred in the colostrum soon after birth. It is absorbed by the neonate during a short period that in most species lasts only a few hours, after which the neonatal intestine loses the ability to absorb colostral antibody. Levels of systemic antibody absorbed in this way decline with age and it has generally disappeared 12 weeks after birth. Most farm animals are suckled for a variable period and additional local protection is provided by antibody in the milk. This protection is withdrawn at weaning when there may also be a dramatic change in the nature of the food, which provides an important substrate for the development of enteric clostridial disease. Passive immunity in birds is transmitted from mother to offspring in the egg yolk and systemic immunity declines gradually from hatching onwards.

Populations of most farm animals kept for meat consist of young animals under the age of sexual maturity with a sexually mature breeding population. Birth often occurs at a specific time (sheep) or in specialized accommodation (pigs and some cattle) and large numbers of neonates may be present, presenting opportunities for clostridial disease. Young animals may be moved to new environments (chicks and calves) where they will encounter contamination with clostridial species or strains to which they do not have immunity, and they will be mixed with other animals of the same species that may be carriers. Companion animals, such as dogs, cats and horses, have a population structure more closely resembling that of humans and are usually kept in smaller numbers. Where they are kept in larger numbers, similar problems may arise (Struble et al. 1994).

Vaccination against clostridial disease is almost universal in sheep populations as, in most developed countries, is vaccination against tetanus in horses. Vaccination is less commonly carried out in other species, but it means that many of the classical diseases of sheep and other farm livestock are now rare and seen only in populations that have not been vaccinated or where, for some reason, antibody has not been transferred from mother to offspring. The widespread use of vaccination against animal clostridial diseases and its success in preventing these suggests that such protection may be valuable in the management of these infections in all species, including humans.

Another significant way in which clostridial disease in animals differs from that in humans is that enteric clostridia are profoundly affected by the use of growth-permitting antimicrobial agents in the rations of some farm livestock (De Vries et al. 1993, Kyriakis et al. 1995). They may be included in the rations of chickens and pigs and, to a lesser extent, lambs and calves not maintained at pasture. In Europe, but not in other parts of the world such as the USA, these substances are licensed for use only if unrelated to the major therapeutic antimicrobial agents. They may prevent enteric clostridial colonization or disease while in use. Therapeutic antimicrobial agents have exactly the same value. Their limitations and side effects in animals are the same as in humans, and post-antimicrobial colitis associated with *C. difficile* occurs, particularly in dogs, cats and small rodents such as hamsters and rabbits, but this is not always the case (Struble et al. 1994, Perkins et al. 1995). Similar conditions also occur in horses with *Clostridium cadaveris* (Staempfli, Prescott and Brash 1992).

The discovery of the major clostridial diseases of animals and early work on these has been reviewed in detail in previous editions of this book. The earlier work will be referred to here only where it illustrates matters of importance in the biology of the organisms or the features of the diseases.

C. tetani and *C. botulinum* relatively frequently cause clinical disease in animals and birds. The pathogenesis of infection is similar to that in humans (see Chapters 36 and 37).

5.1   **Infections due to *Clostridium perfringens***

C. perfringens causes a number of well defined conditions of animals in which the organism multiplies in the gut and produces toxins that give rise to disease. Some of these diseases are sufficiently well known to merit common names and they have been studied for many years. Others have been identified more recently after the introduction of such techniques as the polymerase chain reaction (PCR) to detect the presence of the toxin genes (Havard, Hunter and Titball 1992) and ELISA and latex agglutination tests (Martin and Naylor 1994) for the toxins in pathological material. These tests and cell culture methods (Borrmann and Schulze 1995) have largely replaced mouse protection tests, which are now only a requirement for vaccine safety evaluation.

CLOSTRIDIUM PERFRINGENS TYPE A

C. perfringens type A is increasingly recognized as a cause of enteric disease in animals and the syndromes it causes are in the course of being defined. The organism colonizes neonates soon after birth and may cause disease if specific colostral antibody has not been ingested. Soon after weaning, the change in diet from milk to carbohydrate coincides with the decline of passive immunity and infection may take place when animals are mixed. Finally, the development of inflammation of the gastrointestinal tract for any reason results in colonization of the lesion by *C. perfringens* type A. Both vegetative cells, which produce large amounts of α toxin, and sporulating strains that produce enterotoxin may be isolated from enteritis in piglets, chickens, calves and foals. They have been used to reproduce the syndromes from which they were isolated. The colonization of enteric lesions caused by other agents and syndromes in adult animals, such as post-calving *C. perfringens* type A enteritis in cows, have been documented on the basis of diagnostic findings but have not been reproduced experimentally. Acute diarrhoea can be reproduced in horses by feeding *C. perfringens* type A (Wierup 1977).

Enteritis in piglets is well documented and can be reproduced experimentally with strains that produce a toxin or enterotoxin (Estrada Correa 1986). In piglets aged 36–48 h the former causes a creamy, rarely-fatal diarrhoea tinted with blood that resolves in 5–7 days (Olubunmi and Taylor 1985). Affected piglets become dehydrated and there is perineal faecal staining. Animals about to die develop reduced rectal temperatures and abdominal discoloration before they become unconscious. The abdominal skin is discoloured and decay is rapid. The intestines, particularly in chronic cases, are mildly inflamed with thickened walls and distended with creamy contents and their mucosa is necrotic with pronounced villous atrophy in the small intestine. It is difficult to reproduce the condition with pure α toxin, but the mucosa in gut loops becomes inflamed. Piglets may be protected by antiserum to α toxin and the disease may be prevented in the field by vaccinating sows with formalin-killed *C. perfringens* type A that contains inactivated α toxin; commercial vaccines have been produced. Enterotoxigenic strains produce a more watery diarrhoea of shorter duration in piglets (Estrada Correa and Taylor 1986). They can cause a non-fatal diarrhoea lasting 3–5 days in weaned non-immune piglets accompanied by loss of condition and a depressed growth rate. Enterotoxin and sporulated organisms can be detected in the faeces of pigs with diarrhoea and antibody to enterotoxin develops in the serum (Jestin, Popoff and Mahe 1985, Estrada Correa and Taylor 1988). This syndrome is prevented in pigs that receive the growth-permitting antimicrobial agents avoparcin (Taylor and Estrada Correa 1988), salinomycin and virginiamycin.

Enteritis in chickens (necrotic enteritis), which is due to vegetative strains of *C. perfringens* type A, can be reproduced experimentally (Prescott, Sivendra and Barnum 1978). Affected birds may die and there is inflammation and necrosis of the small intestine.

Similar infections have been reproduced in calves, which confirms the pathogenicity of α toxin-producing strains isolated from clinical cases of creamy diarrhoea in calves.

Vegetative and sporulating strains of *C. perfringens* type A have been isolated from dogs and cats and enterotoxin has been demonstrated in their faeces.

Gangrene

The principal organism found in gangrenous wounds of animals is *C. perfringens* type A, but it is accompanied by a wide range of other organisms such as *C. septicum*, *C. novyi* type A, *C. sordellii* and a variety of other clostridia. Other genera of aerobic bacteria and anaerobes may also be present.

Lamb dysentery

Lamb dysentery is a severe and often fatal haemorrhagic enteritis of lambs that occurs within the first few days of life. It is caused by *C. perfringens* type B which infects lambs soon after birth and multiplies in the intestine. Disease does not result in animals exposed to a light challenge and that have ingested adequate colostrum which contains specific antibody to the organism and its toxins. The organism multiplies and causes disease in animals born into heavily infected environments such as unhygienic lambing pens towards the end of the season, or those with less than adequate levels of colostrum. This is particularly likely in the first few days of life because adult levels of trypsin are not produced until 4 days of age and the β toxin is not inactivated. Disease may continue if trypsin levels are reduced; the organism may invade and persist where there are lesions from some other cause. This may rise to disease in slightly older animals.

Affected lambs may be found dead or appear dull with a hunched back and perineal staining with reddish faeces that contain altered blood and necrotic material; they usually collapse and die within 24 h. In affected lambs in moderate condition with perineal staining, the changes are confined largely to the small intestine. A variable length of the small intestine is dark in colour, ulcerated and intensely inflamed with blood in the lumen. In chronically affected or older animals there is necrosis of the mucosal lesions. Large numbers of large gram-positive bacilli can be seen in smears of the ulcerated areas and in the contents; *C. perfringens* type B can be recovered in profuse culture from the lesions. Preformed toxin may be demonstrated in the bowel contents by ELISA with monoclonal antibody to the β toxin. The gene for the toxin may be detected by PCR. Histology shows an ulcerated and inflamed mucosa with the presence of large numbers of gram-positive bacilli adherent to the eroded lamina propria. Such observations are only of marginal diagnostic value in animals that have been found dead.

In some countries, *C. perfringens* type B may not be present, but where it is common, as in the UK, the clinical signs of the disease in young lambs are suggestive and the ulcerative intestinal lesions confirm the disease as being a clostridial enteritis. The demonstration of preformed β toxin by ELISA or cell culture methods (Borrmann and Schulze 1995), or by mouse protection tests where ELISA is not available, and identification of isolated organisms as *C. perfringens* type B confirms the diagnosis. The use of ELISA and PCR have shown that *C. perfringens* types C and D may also be present in this syndrome.

Treatment is rarely successful. The severe damage to the lamina propria before clinical signs develop means that affected animals rarely respond to treatment with oral ampicillin. Prevention in groups at risk depends on improving hygiene at lambing, administration of oral ampicillin soon after birth to prevent intestinal infection, and protecting the lamb with parenteral horse antiserum to β and ε toxins. It is important that lambs receive colostrum. Where ewes are vaccinated at mating with the aluminium hydroxide formalized toxoid vaccine before lambing, the colostral antibody alone should be protective.

Enterotoxaemia due to *C. perfringens* type C (synonym: struck of sheep)

C. perfringens type C is the cause of 2 potentially recognizable clinicopathological syndromes: an enterotoxaemia of sheep known as 'struck', which occurs locally in sheep on rich feed, and a haemorrhagic enteritis of neonatal piglets.

The disease in sheep is associated with adults and was first described on the Romney Marsh in England, but it occurs world wide. The disease has a short course and animals are often found dead. The major feature that differentiates this condition from pulpy kidney in sheep is haemorrhagic enteritis with ulceration of the intestinal mucosa and abundant blood-stained peritoneal fluid. The carcass decays rapidly and the muscles become oedematous. The organism also affects lambs 0–4 days of age in areas of the world where *C. perfringens* type B does not occur and it may occur in some areas with classic lamb dysentery. The major toxin in this disease is the β toxin, which can be demonstrated in the peritoneal fluid and in the gut contents.

The disease in piglets is more common and occurs in piglets 2–4 days old; it causes sudden death or haemorrhagic diarrhoea. Affected piglets are in good condition, pass blood-stained faeces, rapidly develop dark discoloration of the abdominal skin, a subnormal temperature, pass into a coma and die. In large herds outbreaks may last for months; affected piglets and all members of an affected litter usually die. Animals 7–10 days of age may have chronic diarrhoea that contains necrotic material but little blood, and these animals may recover completely or remain stunted. The carcasses of affected piglets are in good condition but may have abdominal discoloration. The striking feature of the pathology is a heavily inflamed red small intestine that contains fluid blood and the mucosa is red or blackened. Large gram-positive rods are present in large numbers in smears and in stained or frozen sections viewed by immunofluorescence or immunoperoxidase; they may be shown to adhere to the denuded villi. Profuse cultures of *C. perfringens* type C can be isolated, β toxin can be demonstrated in the gut contents by ELISA and the gene can be demonstrated by PCR.

Treatment of affected piglets is not practical because the clinical signs do not develop until fatal intestinal damage has occurred, but treatment of at-risk piglets with oral ampicillin within 12 h of birth stops the development of the disease at the stage of colonization and prevents mortality. Hyperimmune serum may be given parenterally, but long-term protection against struck and piglet enterotoxaemia is by vaccination. In the case of struck, the ewe must be protected, whereas in the case of piglets, the sow must be immunized and then again within 2–4 weeks of parturition, to ensure that sufficient antibody is present in the colostrum. Piglets must ingest adequate colostrum to be protected.

Other species such as calves, goats and foals may develop similar syndromes from which *C. perfringens* types C and B may be isolated. Affected animals may be found dead but in the case of calves it is more common for animals aged 7–10 days to become depressed, develop diarrhoea, dysentery and abdominal pain, and they often die in convulsions. A similar disease occurs in foals, and chickens may also be affected. It is necessary to identify the type of *C. perfringens* involved.

PULPY KIDNEY DISEASE OF SHEEP

Pulpy kidney disease of sheep is a fatal enterotoxaemia of non-immune lambs due to the growth of *C. perfringens* type D in the intestine and the systemic effects of its ∈ toxin, which is absorbed. In sucking lambs it is associated with high milk intake and in weaned animals with excess food or a change of diet. The macerated kidney from which the common name of the disease derives is relatively frequently found in animals that have died from the disease. *C. perfringens* type D enters the body from the udder, through the investigative behaviour of young lambs, in contaminated feed after weaning, or from soil in grazing animals. The organism may be destroyed in the rumen (forestomach) but spores and vegetative cells pass through the immature rumen of young sucking lambs and when rumen function is disturbed as in ruminal acidosis. Organisms may also be protected by milk casein. Once in the intestine, the organisms multiply to reach high numbers with undigested carbohydrate as substrate, and enterotoxaemia may occur in lambs as early as 4–5 days of age. Systemic immunity to the ∈ toxin determines whether disease develops. Lambs are susceptible when antibody is absent because of lack of colostrum, if the ewe is non-immune, and again when passive antibody has declined towards weaning. The ∈ prototoxin is produced in the intestine and is split to the active toxin by proteolytic gut enzymes such as trypsin. The disease is therefore uncommon in animals aged less than 4 days when trypsin secretion begins. The active toxin increases intestinal permeability and is absorbed to cause a profuse mucoid diarrhoea and central nervous system depression. Vascular permeability is increased by an effect on endothelium, and fluid extravasation occurs throughout the body. The toxin increases the permeability of the renal tubules in life and causes a characteristic autolysis after death. Marked hyperglycaemia occurs as a result of the mobilization of hepatic glycogen stores.

The disease runs its course in less than 12 h and animals are usually found dead. Affected animals move away from the flock, are depressed, stagger, become recumbent, develop clonic convulsions and die, but those that survive longest may have a greenish diarrhoea. Hyperglycaemia and glycosuria are major features. Animals that have died from the disease are generally in good condition but there may be perineal faecal staining. Gross lesions may not be evident, particularly in recently dead animals, but clear fluid is often present in the pericardial, peritoneal and pleural cavities. Petechial haemorrhages may be seen on the epicardium, endocardium, lungs, pleura and mesentery and often there is pulmonary oedema. Other abdominal organs may appear normal but the small intestine is often flaccid with pasty contents; patchy inflammation may be seen on the abomasal and small intestinal mucosae. The kidneys appear normal in very fresh carcasses, but within a few hours of death they appear soft and, when rinsed, disintegrate to leave strands of fibrous material; the bladder urine contains glucose. Focal symmetrical haemorrhage is seen in the cerebral basal ganglia in animals that have died after lengthy clinical signs; microscopic evidence of symmetrical encephalomalacia may be seen in the base of the brain. The carcass decays rapidly and lesions

become less distinct. Large gram-positive rods are common in smears of the small intestinal contents and ∈ toxin may be demonstrated by ELISA in the intestinal contents and fluid transudates from body cavities. *C. perfringens* type D may be isolated in profuse culture from the small intestine.

Diagnosis depends on the age of the animal, the history, brief clinical signs and the presence of hyperglycaemia. The presence of the characteristic renal lesions at necropsy and clear fluid in the body cavities are also suggestive. Further presumptive evidence comes from the identification of *C. perfringens* type D in the intestinal contents, but confirmation depends upon the demonstration of ∈ toxin in the intestines or extravasated fluids. Effective treatment is not available but for prevention it is necessary to ensure that lambs ingest colostrum, that dietary changes are gradual and that hygiene is practised in lambing pens. Animals at risk may be given hyperimmune horse serum against β and ∈ toxins. Protection is afforded by active vaccination with formolized whole cultures or toxoid in aluminium hydroxide adjuvants, if given prior to the period of risk. Lambs must be protected by vaccination of the ewe, which is given vaccine at intervals of 2 weeks and a booster dose 2–6 weeks before lambing. Ingestion of colostrum is essential.

5.2 Blackleg (synonym: blackquarter)

Blackleg is an acute, frequently fatal disease of cattle that occurs to a lesser extent in sheep and rarely in pigs. It is caused primarily by *Clostridium chauvoei* acquired from spores in the soil that enter the body by a route that is not clear. Clinical disease arises when the spores germinate in tissues such as the larger muscle masses. Germination takes place when oxygen levels fall in the tissues after trauma, such as at sites of injection of antimicrobial agents or vaccines, or after exertion. Spores can be isolated from spleen, liver and alimentary tract but most lesions originate in muscle. Vegetative organisms grow at anoxic sites and in the first instance lesions are frequently limited to the affected muscles; the lesion is a clostridial myonecrosis. Fresh lesions are blackened and have a rancid odour. There is cavitation of muscle fibres and small bubbles of gas produced by the organism are present. The odour is due to butyric acid produced by the organism. The lesions are surrounded by varying degrees of oedema. Enzymes and toxins produced by the organism later diffuse throughout the body to cause effects in other areas. After death organisms may be found in lesions and many parts of the body.

Blackleg affects cattle in good condition between 6 months and 2 years of age and is most common in animals at grass in the summer. The disease presents as lameness associated with large, hot, painful, crackling swellings over the large muscle masses, especially the gluteals. Affected animals may be febrile and usually die within 12–36 h of the onset of clinical signs and most animals are found dead. If the disease is treated successfully, or in the rare cases of natural recovery, lesions rapidly become cold and the overlying skin becomes necrotic. After recovery, there are sunken, cold, frequently hairless areas on the surface of the affected muscle mass. Function is not regained in the affected muscle mass and animals may remain lame. In sheep the disease may also affect the skin of the head and the vulva.

Pathological findings are complicated by the rapid decay of the carcass. The characteristic dark muscle masses surrounded by oedema may be disguised by the processes of decay associated with the spread of the organism from the original lesion and colonization of the body by clostridia from the gut. Histological findings in recently dead animals include a bacterial myositis with eosinophilic muscle fibres, neutrophils and large gram-positive bacilli limited to individual affected muscles; similar lesions may be found in the heart. Lesions in recovered animals consist of liquefaction of the originally affected muscle mass and its eventual replacement by a cavity or fibrous tissue, whereas adjacent muscles appear normal.

The disease should be suspected when young cattle in previously good condition are seen to be stiff and lame after introduction to 'blackleg fields' contaminated with spores from past cases, river flooding or after ditching operations during which spores in the soil may be disturbed. Examination of the animal may confirm the presence of lesions and postmortem examination reveals the characteristic lesions in freshly dead animals. Decay may make lesions more difficult to identify in animals that have been dead for some time. The organism can be demonstrated in the lesions as a large gram-positive rod with a central or subterminal spore and with specific fluorescent antibody. Antibody labelled with other dyes or immunoperoxidase methods (Giraudo Cornesa, Vannelli and Uzal 1995) may be used to identify *C. septicum* that is frequently present in the lesions and *C. novyi*, which occurs more rarely. *C. chauvoei* can be isolated from affected tissues, but it is very oxygen-sensitive and is rapidly overgrown by the *C. septicum* that is frequently also present. Treatment with penicillin and other antimicrobial agents may compromise recovery of the organism.

In its earliest stages the disease can be treated with penicillin and other antimicrobial agents active against clostridia, but the affected muscle group is rarely saved and the animal usually remains lame. On affected farms prevention is essential and consists of prophylactic antimicrobial injection to prevent disease during procedures such as vaccination against the disease with inactivated adjuvanted vaccines. Most commercial vaccines contain killed whole culture and adjuvant or alum precipitated toxoid and they protect for up to a year. Dead animals should be buried or burned to prevent pasture contamination with spores; animals at risk but not yet fully vaccine protected may be moved to clean pasture.

5.3 Braxy

Braxy is a disease of sheep that occurs mainly in northwest Europe. It is generally fatal and runs a short course, characterized by inflammation of the wall of the abomasum (fourth stomach) due to infection with *C. septicum*. The disease occurs mainly in young, unvaccinated and hence non-immune sheep in their first winter and is associated with the ingestion of frozen forage during severe frost. It is assumed that such feed results in damage to the abomasal wall with colonization by *C. septicum*, but direct experimental evidence for this mechanism of pathogenesis is lacking. The organism is commonly found in the sheep gastrointestinal tract and in the soil. The disease is rarely diagnosed because vaccination is widespread and the historical levels of mortality (35% of the age group at risk) are no longer seen.

The clinical signs of braxy are not pathognomonic. In the acute disease death is sudden whereas in the subacute form there is a sudden onset of illness with weakness, anorexia and inability to keep up with the group. Affected animals may have a high fever (42°C), abdominal pain and distension, rapidly become comatose, dyspnoeic and die within a few hours of the onset of clinical signs. Postmortem examination of freshly dead animals shows excess turbid peritoneal fluid and a few petechiae on the epicardium, but the most prominent changes are present in the abomasum and less frequently in the duodenum and proximal small intestine. The walls of these organs are thickened and oedematous; the abomasal mucosa is intensely reddened and inflamed

and sometimes appears black. *C. septicum* may be seen as chains of large gram-positive bacilli in smears made directly from the affected mucosa and can be isolated from the lesions and from the heart blood. It may be identifiable by culture, immunofluorescence in smears, and by immunoperoxidase in tissue sections. The *C. septicum* α toxin may be demonstrated in body cavity exudates.

Diagnosis is based on the appearance of the lesions, demonstration of *C. septicum* in the lesion and identification of the toxin in transudates. The pathological findings are best observed in recently dead animals because decay is rapid and the appearances rapidly becomes less specific. Decay also makes the bacteriological diagnosis more difficult because the organism may be recovered from animals that have died from other causes and its tendency to swarming on blood agar means that even a few colonies may lead to its identification as the cause of lesions that have another origin. The clinical signs are rarely seen and they are insufficiently distinctive for a diagnosis.

The short course of the disease makes treatment impracticable and control depends primarily on vaccination with formalin-killed alum adjuvanted whole cultures or toxoid before exposure is likely. The vaccine is usually available only as part of a multicomponent clostridial vaccine. Restriction of access to frosty vegetation by housing reduces the likelihood of disease.

5.4 Black disease of sheep (synonym: infectious necrotic hepatitis)

Black disease is an acute toxaemia of non-immune sheep caused by the toxins of *C. novyi* produced in infected foci of liver tissue damaged by fascioliasis. Similar conditions occur in cattle, pigs and horses (infectious necrotic hepatitis) but in these species, and especially in pigs, the disease is not always associated with fascioliasis. The spores of *C. novyi* type B are present in the tissues, and particularly the liver, of sheep in infected areas; invasion of the liver by migrating immature liver fluke (*Fasciola hepatica*) damages the tissues and results in reduction of the oxygen tension that allows the germination and growth of the organism. The clostridium remains restricted to the damaged areas, which become necrotic, but its α toxin diffuses from the lesion to cause systemic effects and death. Spores of *C. novyi* type B survive on infected pasture and are ingested to reach the liver by way of the lymphatics (Bagadi and Sewell 1973, 1974). Liver fluke infection causes lesions of sufficient severity to induce black disease only when heavy infections occur at one time, such as during drought or on irrigated pastures and after the introduction of susceptible sheep to heavily contaminated pasture. Disease occurs up to 6 weeks after exposure because the flukes must reach the stage of development necessary to cause the liver damage and initiate the disease. As a consequence of this delay, disease may occur when sheep have been moved from affected to clean pasture. Such carrier sheep may introduce the organism to previously uninfected areas and spores may be exposed after flooding or soil disturbance such as ditching. Disease ceases soon after frost kills metacercariae on the pasture. The pathogenesis of *C. novyi* type B infection in cattle generally resembles that in sheep, but in horses and pigs the factors that result in lowered levels of oxygen in the liver are not clear.

Few clinical signs are observed in sheep and pigs, because the animals are generally found dead, but during life there may be fever up to 42°C in sheep and this falls rapidly as the animal dies in sternal recumbency. In cattle, there may be sudden depression, coldness of the skin, abdominal pain and suppressed rumen (forestomach) sounds and semifluid faeces with death after 24 h. In horses, the disease presents as a peritonitis leading to depression, straining and recumbency, resulting in death after 2–3 days. Dead animals decay rapidly and are often found with blood-stained froth on the nostrils. In sheep, surface blood vessels are congested to such an extent that the skin appears dark or black, giving rise to the name 'black disease'. There is gelatinous oedema of the subcutaneous tissues and fascial planes and clear amber fluid is present in the body cavities. In all species there is congestion and darkening of the liver; in cattle and sheep areas of necrosis may be identified as pale, bile-stained patches 1–2 cm in diameter, sometimes with a reddish halo of venous congestion. There may be blood-filled areas with immature flukes and the lesions continue into the substance of the liver. In pigs, small bubbles of gas are found in the liver but foci of necrosis are uncommon. The lesions contain large numbers of very large gram-positive bacilli that may be isolated and identified as *C. novyi* under strictly anaerobic conditions. Preformed β toxin is present in body cavity fluid and the liver lesion. Diagnosis is based on the postmortem findings of a congested carcass and the presence of the liver lesions and must be confirmed by the identification of *C. novyi* in the lesions by immunofluorescence and by demonstration of preformed toxin in the lesions or peritoneal fluid by ELISA. Demonstration of the organism in the liver or tissues of animals that have been dead for more than a few hours is not significant because the organism may be present in animals that have not died from the disease, but demonstration of preformed toxin is confirmatory. Without experience culture is extremely difficult and isolation by culture is usually impossible in animals that have been treated.

Since disease is rarely seen in its clinical stages, treatment is usually ineffective; parenteral penicillin may be of value in cattle, whereas in pigs, success has been reported with parenteral penicillin and trimethoprim plus sulphonamide.

Control in sheep is largely by the use of vaccination. Vaccines usually contain formolized whole cultures of *C. novyi* type B or toxoid with an aluminium hydroxide adjuvant; they are given as part of a multicomponent clostridial vaccine before possible exposure. Restricting access to fluke-infested pasture and care in the disposal of carcasses to avoid pasture contamination may reduce the incidence of the disease.

5.5 Bacilliary haemoglobinuria in cattle (synonym: redwater)

This disease is due to *Clostridium haemolyticum* (formerly *C. novyi* type D). It is a fatal infectious toxaemia of cattle and sometimes sheep, principally in the western USA, but occasionally in other parts of the world including the UK and Ireland. The pathogenesis resembles that of black disease, but liver fluke is only one cause of the necrosis that allows germination of spores in the liver. *Fusobacterium necrophorum* abscesses, *Cysticercus tenuicollis* cysts and telangiectasis may each initiate the anaerobic conditions that commonly result from portal vein thrombosis. The haemolysin is elaborated in the infarct and leads to intravascular haemolysis. Abdominal pain, dullness and low fever may be present, but animals may be found dead. The faeces are brownish and the urine is dark red. At postmortem examination there may be blood-stained faeces on the perineum, subcutaneous oedema, some jaundice, fluid in the body cavities and haemorrhagic lesions in the abomasum (fourth stomach). The condition is suggested by the characteristic infarcts in the liver and haemoglobinuria. *C. haemolyticum* can be demonstrated in the lesions by immunofluorescence or immunoperoxidase (Uzal et al. 1992). Control is similar to that for black disease, by reducing exposure to infected pastures and parasites that can initiate the lesion and protection by vaccination with formolized whole cultures or toxoids.

REFERENCES

Ahmad FJ, Darrell JH, 1976, Significance of the isolation of *Clostridium welchii* from routine blood cultures, *J Clin Pathol*, **29:** 185–6.

Aikat BK, Dible JH, 1956, Pathology of *Clostridium welchii* infection, *J Pathol Bacteriol*, **71:** 461–76.

Aikat BK, Dible JH, 1960, Local and general effects of cultures and culture-filtrates of *Clostridium oedematiens*, *Cl. septicum*, *Cl. sporogenes* and *Cl. histolyticum*, *J Pathol Bacteriol*, **79:** 227–41.

Altemeier WA, 1979, Principles in the management of traumatic wounds and in infection control, *Bull NY Acad Sci*, **55:** 123–38.

Altemeier WA, McMurrin JA, Alt MP, 1951, Chloramphenicol and aureomycin in experimental gas gangrene, *JAMA*, **145:** 440.

Alvarez-Elcoro S, Sifuentes-Osorio J, 1984, *Clostridium perfringens* bacteraemia in prosthetic valve endocarditis, *Arch Intern Med*, **144:** 849–50.

Anderson CB, Marr JJ, Jaffe BM, 1972, Anaerobic streptococcal infections simulating gas gangrene, *Arch Surg*, **104:** 186–9.

Anon, 1968, Gas gangrene from adrenaline, *Br Med J*, **1:** 721.

Anon, 1984, Remembering gas gangrene, *Lancet*, **2:** 851–2.

Ayliffe GAJ, Lowbury EJL, 1969, Sources of gas gangrene in hospital, *Br Med J*, **2:** 333–7.

Bagadi HO, Sewell MHH, 1973, Experimental studies on infectious necrotic hepatitis (Black Disease) of sheep, *Res Vet Sci*, **15:** 53–61.

Bagadi HO, Sewell MHH, 1974, A study of the route of dissemination of orally administered spores of *Clostridium novyi* type B in guinea pigs and sheep, *Res Vet Sci*, **17:** 179–81.

Balch HH, Ganley OH, 1957, Observations on the pathogenesis of *Clostridium welchii* myonecrosis, *Ann Surg*, **146:** 86–97.

Barber M, Garrod LP, 1963, *Antibiotic and Chemotherapy*, Livingstone, Edinburgh.

Barroso LA, Wang SZ et al., 1990, Nucleotide sequence of *Clostridium difficile* toxin B gene, *Nucleic Acids Res*, **18:** 4004.

Bartlett JG, 1982, Anti-anaerobic antibacterial agents, *Lancet*, **2:** 478–81.

Bartlett JG, 1985, Treatment of *Clostridium difficile* colitis, *Gastroenterology*, **89:** 1192–5.

Bartlett JG, 1992, Antibiotic-associated diarrhea, *Clin Infect Dis*, **15:** 573–81.

Bartlett JG, Onderdonk AB et al., 1977, Clindamycin-associated colitis due to a toxin producing species of *Clostridium* in hamsters, *J Infect Dis*, **135:** 701–5.

Bartlett JG, Chang T-W et al., 1978a, Antibiotic-induced entercolitis in hamsters: studies with eleven agents and evidence to support the pathogenic role of toxin producing clostridia, *Am J Vet Res*, **39:** 1525–30.

Bartlett JG, Chang T-W et al., 1978b, Antibiotic-associated pseudomembranous colitis due to toxin-producing clostridia, *N Engl J Med*, **298:** 531–4.

Bartlett JG, Moon N et al., 1978c, Role of *Clostridium difficile* in antibiotic-associated pseudomembranous colitis, *Gastroenterology*, **75:** 778–82.

Bender BS, Laughon BE et al., 1986, Is *Clostridium difficile* endemic in chronic care facilities?, *Lancet*, **2:** 11–13.

Bennett GCT, Allen E, Millard PH, 1984, *Clostridium difficile* diarrhoea: a highly infectious organism, *Age Ageing*, **13:** 363–6.

Berg M, Levinson SA, 1955, Nephrotic damage by *Clostridium perfringens* toxin: protective effect of amino acids against hyperglycemia and renal damage by *C. perfringens* toxin, *Arch Pathol*, **59:** 656–68.

Berg M, Levinson SA, 1957, Hyperglycemia induced in dogs by *Clostridium perfringens* toxin, *Arch Pathol*, **64:** 633–42.

Berg M, Levinson SA, 1959, Hyperglycemia and histochemical changes induced in frogs by *Clostridium perfringens* toxin, *Arch Pathol*, **68:** 83–93.

Bessman AN, Wagner W, 1975, Nonclostridial gas gangrene: report of 48 cases and review of the literature, *JAMA*, **233:** 958–63.

Bignold LP, Harvey HPB, 1979, Necrotising enterocolitis associated with invasion by *Clostridium septicum* complicating cyclic neutropenia, *Aust NZ J Med*, **9:** 426–9.

Bishop RF, Marshall V, 1960, The enhancement of *Clostridium welchii* infection by adrenaline-in-oil, *Med J Aust*, **2:** 656–7.

Boerema I, Brummelkamp WH, 1960, Treatment of anaerobic infections by inhalation of oxygen under a pressure of three atmospheres, *Ned Tijdschr Geneeskd*, **104:** 2548–50.

Boggs DR, Frei E, Thomas LB, 1958, Clostridial gas gangrene and septicemia in four patients with leukemia, *N Engl J Med*, **259:** 1255–8.

Borriello SP, 1990, Pathogenesis of *Clostridium difficile* infection of the gut, *J Med Microbiol*, **33:** 207–15.

Borriello SP, Barclay FE, 1986, An in-vitro model of colonisation resistance to *Clostridium difficile* infection, *J Med Microbiol*, **21:** 299–309.

Borriello SP, Barclay FE, Welch AR, 1988, Evaluation of the predictive capability of an in vitro model of colonisation resistance to *Clostridium difficile* infection, *Microb Ecol Health Dis*, **1:** 61–4.

Borriello SP, Honour P, 1981, Simplified procedure for the routine isolation of *Clostridium difficile* from faeces, *J Clin Pathol*, **34:** 1124–7.

Borriello SP, Honour P, 1983, Concomitance of cytotoxigenic and non-cytotoxigenic *Clostridium difficile* in stool specimens, *J Clin Microbiol*, **18:** 1006–7.

Borriello SP, Honour P, 1984, Detection, isolation and identification of *Clostridium difficile*, *Antibiotic associated Diarrhoea and Colitis*, ed. Borriello SP, Martinus Nijhoff, Boston, 38–47.

Borriello SP, Larson HE, 1981, Antibiotic and pseudomembranous colitis, *J Antimicrob Chemother*, **7, Suppl. A:** 53–62.

Borriello SP, Welch AR, 1984, Detection of *Clostridium difficile* toxins, *Antibiotic associated Diarrhoea and Colitis*, ed. Borriello SP, Martinus Nijhoff, Boston, 49–56.

Borriello SP, Honour P et al., 1983, Household pets as a potential reservoir for *Clostridium difficile* infection, *J Clin Pathol*, **36:** 84–7.

Borriello SP, Larson HE et al., 1984, Enterotoxigenic *Clostridium perfringens*: a possible cause of antibiotic-associated diarrhoea, *Lancet*, **1:** 305–7.

Borriello SP, Davies HA et al., 1990, Virulence factors of *Clostridium difficile*, *Rev Infect Dis*, **12, Suppl. 2:** S185–91.

Borriello SP, Vale T et al., 1992a, Evaluation of a commerical enzyme immunoassay kit for the detection of *Clostridium difficile* toxin A, *Eur J Clin Microbiol Infect Dis*, **11:** 360–3.

Borriello SP, Wren BW et al., 1992b, Molecular immunological and biological characterization of a toxin A-negative, toxin B-positive strain of *Clostridium difficile*, *Infect Immun*, **60:** 419–29.

Borrmann E, Schulze F, 1995, Nachweis von *Clostridium perfringens* toxinen und zellkulturen, *Munch Tierarzt Wochenschr*, **108:** 466–70.

Bowlby A, 1919, British military surgery in the time of Hunter and in the Great War, *Br Med J*, **1:** 285–93.

Braithwaite PA, Challis DC et al., 1982, Clostridial myonecrosis after resection of skin tumours in an immunosuppressed patient, *Med J Aust*, **1:** 515–19.

Brazier JS, Levett PN et al., 1985, Antibiotic susceptibility of clinical isolates of clostridia, *J Antimicrob Chemother*, **15:** 181–5.

Brogden RN, Heel RC, 1986, Aztreonam. A review of its antibacterial activity, pharmacokinetic properties and therapeutic use, *Drugs*, **31:** 96–130.

Brown DR, Davis NL et al., 1994, A multicenter review of the treatment of major truncal necrotizing infections with and without hyperbaric oxygen, *Am J Surg*, **167:** 485–9.

Brown RK, Milch E et al., 1948, Gallbladder gas gangrene, *Gastroenterology*, **10:** 626–33.

Bruce D, Ritchie C et al., 1982, *Clostridium difficile*-associated colitis: cross-infection in predisposed patients with renal failure, *NZ Med J*, **95:** 265–7.

Brummelkamp WH, Boerema I, Hoogendyk L, 1963, Treatment of clostridial infections with hyperbaric oxygen drenching. A report of 26 cases, *Lancet*, **1:** 235–8.

Brummelkamp WH, Hogendijk J, Boerema I, 1961, Treatment of anaerobic infections (clostridial myositis) by drenching the tissues with oxygen under high atmospheric pressure, *Surgery*, **49:** 299–302.

Bullen JJ, Cushnie GH, 1962, Experimental gas gangrene: the effect of antiserum on the growth of *Clostridium welchii* type A, *J Pathol Bacteriol*, **84:** 177–92.

Bullen JJ, Cushnie GH, Stoner HB, 1966, Oxygen uptake by *Clostridium welchii* type A: its possible role in experimental infections in passively immunised animals, *Br J Exp Pathol*, **47:** 488–506.

Burdon DW, 1982, *Clostridium difficile*: the epidemiology and prevention of hospital-acquired infection, *Infection*, **10:** 203–4.

Butler HM, 1937, *Blood Cultures and their Significance*, Churchill, London.

Butler HM, 1945, Bacteriological studies of *Clostridium welchii* infections in man, *Surg Gynecol Obstet*, **81:** 475–86.

Cabrera A, Tsukada Y, Pickren JW, 1965, Clostridial gas gangrene and septicemia in malignant disease, *Cancer*, **18:** 800–6.

Calnan CD, 1950, Enteritis necroticans, *Br Med J*, **1:** 228.

Case DB, Goforth JM, Silva J, 1972, A case of *Clostridium perfringens* endocarditis, *Johns Hopkins Med J*, **130:** 54–6.

Chang T-W, Lauermann M, Bartlett JG, 1979, Cytotoxicity assay in antibiotic-associated colitis, *J Infect Dis*, **140:** 765–70.

Chin RL, Martinez R, Garmel G, 1993, Gas gangrene from subcutaneous insulin administration, *Am J Emerg Med*, **11:** 622–5.

Cooke R, 1979, The pathology of pig-bel, *P N G Med J*, **22:** 35–8.

Cooke WT, Frazer AC et al., 1945, Clostridial infections in war wounds, *Lancet*, **1:** 487–93.

Cope A, Anderson J, Wilkins E, 1992, *Clostridium difficile* toxin-induced reactive arthritis in a patient with chronic Reiter's syndrome, *Eur J Clin Microbiol Infect Dis*, **11:** 40–3.

Cumming AD, Thomson BJ et al., 1986, Diarrhoea due to *Clostridium difficile* associated with antibiotic treatment in patients receiving dialysis: the role of cross-infection, *Br Med J*, **292:** 238–9.

Cutler EC, Sandusky WR, 1944, Treatment of clostridial infections with penicillin, *Br J Surg*, **32:** 168–76.

Darke SG, King AM, Slack WK, 1977, Gas gangrene and related infection: classification, clinical features and aetiology, management and mortality. A report of 88 cases, *Br J Surg*, **64:** 104–12.

Davis JB, Mattman LH, Wiley M, 1951, *Clostridium botulinum* in fatal wound infection, *JAMA*, **146:** 646–8.

Davis M, Lawrence G et al., 1982, Longevity of protection by active immunisation against necrotising enteritis in Papua New Guinea, *Lancet*, **2:** 389–90.

Davis MW (ed.), 1984, *Pigbel – Necrotizing Enteritis in Papua New Guinea*, Monograph Series No. 6, Papua New Guinea Institute of Medical Research, New Guinea, Goroka.

Delmee M, Avesani V, 1986, Comparative in vitro activity of seven quinolones against 100 clinical isolates of *Clostridium difficile*, *Antimicrob Agents Chemother*, **29:** 374–5.

De Vries LA, Daube G et al., 1993, In vitro susceptibility of *Clostridium perfringens* isolated from farm animals to growth enhancing antibiotics, *J Appl Bacteriol*, **75:** 55–7.

Doern GV, Coughlin RT, Wu L, 1992, Laboratory diagnosis of *Clostridium difficile*-associated gastrointestinal disease: comparison of monoclonal antibody enzyme immunoassay for toxins A and B with a monoclonal antibody enzyme immunoassay for toxin A only and two cytotoxicity assays, *J Clin Microbiol*, **30:** 2042–6.

Donta ST, Stuppy MS, Myers MG, 1981, Neonatal antibiotic-associated colitis, *Am J Dis Child*, **135:** 181–2.

Dornbusch K, Nord CE, Dahlback A, 1975, Antibiotic suscepti-bility of *Clostridium* species isolated from human infections, *Scand J Infect Dis*, **7:** 127–34.

Dove CH, Wang S-Z et al., 1990, Molecular characterisation of the *Clostridium difficile* toxin A gene, *Infect Immun*, **58:** 480–8.

Egerton JR, Walker PD, 1964, The isolation of *Clostridium perfringens* type C from necrotic enteritis of man in Papua New Guinea, *J Pathol Bacteriol*, **88:** 275–8.

Eggleston M, 1986, Metronidazole, *Infect Control*, **7:** 514–18.

Engeset J, MacIntyre J et al., 1973, *Clostridium welchii* infection: an unusual case, *Br Med J*, **2:** 91–2.

Estrada Correa A, 1986, *Studies of* Clostridium perfringens *Type A Enteritis in the Pig*, PhD thesis, University of Glasgow.

Estrada Correa A, Taylor DJ, 1986, Enterotoxigenic *Clostridium perfringens* type A as a cause of diarrhoea in pigs, *Proc Int Pig Vet Soc*, **9:** 171.

Estrada Correa A, Taylor DJ, 1988, Enterotoxigenic *Clostridium perfringens* type A as a cause of diarrhoea in weaned pigs, *Proc Int Pig Vet Soc*, **10:** 138.

Evans DG, 1943a, The protective properties of the alpha anti-toxin and theta-anti haemolysin occurring in *Cl. welchii* type A antiserum, *Br J Exp Pathol*, **24:** 81–8.

Evans DG, 1943b, Protective properties of alpha antitoxin and anti hyaluronidasae occurring in *Cl. welchii* type A antiserum, *J Pathol Bacteriol*, **55:** 427–34.

Evans DG, 1945, The in vitro production of alpha-toxin, theta-toxin and hyaluronidase by strains of *Cl. welchii* type A and the relationship of in-vitro properties to virulence for guinea-pigs, *J Pathol Bacteriol*, **57:** 75–85.

Evans DG, 1947a, Anticollagenase in immunity to *Cl. welchii* type A infection, *Br J Exp Pathol*, **28:** 24–30.

Evans DG, 1947b, The production by certain species of *Clostridium* of enzymes disintegrating hide powder, *J Gen Microbiol*, **1:** 378–84.

Evans DG, Miles AA, Niven JF, 1948, The enhancement of bac-terial infections by adrenaline, *Br J Exp Pathol*, **29:** 20–39.

Favata BV, Dowdy AH et al., 1944, The pathology of experi-mental clostridial infections in dogs, *Surg Gynecol Obstet*, **79:** 660–8.

Fekety R, Kim K-H et al., 1981, Epidemiology of antibiotic-associated colitis: isolation of *Clostridium difficile* from the hos-pital environment, *Am J Med*, **70:** 906–8.

Fekety R, Silva J et al., 1984, Treatment of antibiotic-associated colitis with vancomycin, *J Antimicrob Chemother*, **14, Suppl. D:** 97–102.

Feldman RJ, Kallich M, Weinstein MP, 1995, Bacteremia due to *Clostridium difficile*: case report and review of extraintestinal *C. difficile* infections, *Clin Infect Dis*, **20:** 1560–2.

Fick KA, Wolken AP, 1949, Necrotic jejunitis, *Lancet*, **1:** 519–21.

Finegold SM, George WL, 1989, *Anaerobic Bacteria in Humans*, Academic Press, New York.

Finney JMT, 1893, Gastroenterostomy for cicatrizing ulcer of the pylorus, *Bull John Hopkins Hosp*, **4:** 53–5.

Fitzpatrick DJ, Turnbull PCB et al., 1979, Two gas-gangrene-like infections due to *Bacillus cereus*, *Br J Surg*, **66:** 577–9.

Foster WD, 1966, The pathology of necrotising jejunitis in Uganda, *East Afr Med J*, **43:** 550–3.

Francois B, Delaire L et al., 1994, Gas gangrene and purulent pericarditis during *Clostridium* septicemia revealing a cecal carcinoma, *Intensive Care Med*, **20:** 309.

Frazer AC, Elkes JJ et al., 1945, Effects of *Cl. welchii* type A toxin on body tissues and fluids, *Lancet*, **1:** 457–60.

Fredette V, Frappier A, 1946, Recherches sur l'immunité dans la gangrène gazeuse: action déchaînante de filtrats non-toxiques de cultures de *Cl. perfringens* dans la gangrène gazeuse expérimentale, *Rev Can Biol*, **5:** 436–41.

Futter BV, Richardson G, 1971, Anaerobic jars in the quantitative recovery of clostridia, *Isolation of Anaerobes*, eds Shapton DA, Board RG, Academic Press, London, 81–91.

Ganley OH, Merchant DJ, Bohr DF, 1955, The relationship of toxic fractions of a filtrate of *Clostridium perfringens* type A to the pathogenesis of clostridial myonecrosis, *J Exp Med*, **101:** 605–15.

Garrod LP, 1958, The chemoprophylaxis of gas gangrene, *J R Army Med Corps*, **104:** 209–15.

Garrod LP, Lambert HP et al., 1973, *Antibiotic and Chemotherapy*, 4th edn, Churchill Livingstone, Edinburgh.

Gatt D, 1985, Non-traumatic metastatic clostridial myonecrosis in a seventeen-year-old, *Br J Surg*, **72:** 240–1.

George RH, 1986, The carrier state: *Clostridium difficile*, *J Anti-microb Chemother*, **18, Suppl. A:** 47–58.

George RH, Symonds JM et al., 1978, Identification of *Clostridium difficile* as a cause of pseudomembranous colitis, *Br Med J*, **1:** 695.

George WL, 1988, Antimicrobial agent-associated diarrhea in adult humans, Clostridium difficile*: its Role in Intestinal Disease*, eds Rolfe RD, Finegold SM, Academic Press, San Diego, 31– 44.

George WL, Sutter VL et al., 1978, Aetiology of antimicrobial-agent-associated colitis, *Lancet*, **1:** 802–3.

George WL, Sutter VL et al., 1979, Selective and differential medium for isolation of *Clostridium difficile*, *J Clin Microbiol*, **9:** 214–19.

Gerard M, Defresne N et al., 1988, Incidence and significance of *Clostridium difficile* in hospitalized cancer patients, *Eur J Clin Microbiol Infect Dis*, **7:** 274–8.

Giraudo Cornesa LC, Vannelli SA, Uzal FA, 1995, Detection of *Clostridium chauvoei* in formalin fixed paraffin embedded tissues of sheep by the peroxidase-antiperoxidase (PAP) tech-nique, *Vet Res Commun*, **19:** 451–6.

Gledhill T, 1982, Gas gangrene following cholecystectomy, *Br J Clin Pract*, **36:** 23–5.

Gliemroth J, Heise S, Missler U, 1996, A 64-year-old man with diabetes and ascending paraplegia, *Lancet*, **347:** 516.

Goldstein EJC, Citron DM, 1985, Comparative activity of the qui-nolones against anaerobic bacteria isolated in community hospitals, *Antimicrob Agents Chemother*, **27:** 657–9.

Gorbach SL, 1992, Gas gangrene and other clostridial skin and soft tissue infections, *Infectious Diseases*, eds Gorbach SL, Bart-lett JG, Blacklow NR, Saunders, Philadelphia, 764–70.

Gorbach SL, Bartlett JG, 1977, Pseudomembranous entero-colitis: a review of its diverse forms, *J Infect Dis*, **135:** 589–94.

Gorbach SL, Chang TW, Goldin B, 1987, Successful treatment of relapsing *Clostridium difficile* colitis with lactobacillus GG, *Lancet*, **2:** 1519.

Gorbach SL, Thadepalli H, 1975, Isolation of *Clostridium* in human infections: evaluation of 114 cases, *J Infect Dis*, **131, Suppl.:** S81–5.

Gordon J, Turner GC, Dmochowski L, 1954, Inhibition of alpha and theta toxins of *Clostridium welchii* by lecithin, *J Pathol Bac-teriol*, **67:** 605–9.

Gorse GJ, Slater LM et al., 1984, CNS infection and bacteremia due to *Clostridium septicum*, *Arch Neurol*, **41:** 882–4.

Gottlieb SF, 1971, Effect of hyperbaric oxygen on micro-organisms, *Annu Rev Microbiol*, **25:** 111–52.

Goulston SJM, McGovern VJ, 1965, Pseudomembranous colitis, *Gut*, **6:** 207–12.

Govan ADT, 1946, Account of pathology of some cases of *Cl. welchii* infection, *J Pathol Bacteriol*, **58:** 423–30.

Govan ADT, MacIntosh AD, 1951, Enteritis necroticans com-plicating pregnancy, *J Obstet Gynaecol Br Empire*, **58:** 1935–8.

Greenfield C, Burroughs A et al., 1981, Is pseudomembranous colitis infectious?, *Lancet*, **1:** 371–2.

Gurovsky A, Samuel I, 1972, Case report: acute necrotising enter-itis, *Ethiop Med J*, **10:** 23–8.

Hafiz S, Oakley CL, 1976, *Clostridium difficile*: isolation and characteristics, *J Med Microbiol*, **9:** 129–36.

Hall IC, 1945, Occurrence of *Bacillus botulinus* types A and B, in accidental wounds, *J Bacteriol*, **50:** 213–17.

Hall IC, O'Toole E, 1935, Intestinal flora in new-born infants with a description of a new pathogenic anaerobe *Bacillus difficilis*, *Am J Dis Child*, **49:** 390–402.

Hallagan LF, Scott JL et al., 1992, Clostridial myonecrosis resulting from subcutaneous epinephrine suspension injection, *Ann Emerg Med*, **21:** 434–6.

Hamilton J, 1944–45, Anaerobic infection in war wounds, *Can Med Serv J*, **2:** 387–407.

Hart GB, Cave RH et al., 1975, Clostridial myonecrosis: the constant menace, *Milit Med*, **140:** 461–3.

Hartley P, Evans DG, 1946, Discussion on the toxaemia of gas gangrene, *Proc R Soc Med*, **39:** 295–6.

Havard HL, Hunter SEC, Titball RW, 1992, Comparison of the nucleotide sequence and development of a PCR test for the epsilon toxin gene of *Clostridium perfringens* type B and type D, *FEMS Microbiol Lett*, **97:** 77–81.

Hayward NJ, 1945, The examination of wounds for clostridia, *Proc Assoc Clin Pathol (London)*, **1:** 5–17.

Headington JT, Sathornsumathi S et al., 1967, Segmental infarcts of the small intestine and mesenteric adenitis in Thai children, *Lancet*, **1:** 802–6.

Heard SR, O'Farrell S et al., 1986, The epidemiology of *Clostridium difficile* with use of a typing scheme: nosocomial acquisition and cross-infection among immunocompromised patients, *J Infect Dis*, **153:** 159–62.

Hechter O, 1946, Mechanism of hyaluronidase action in skin, *Science*, **104:** 409–10.

Hengster P, Pernthaler H, 1996, Gas gangrene: necropsy is imperative, *Lancet*, **347:** 553.

Hiew CY, Silberstein M, Hennessy OF, 1993, Fatal *Clostridium septicum* myonecrosis, *Australas Radiol*, **37:** 399–400.

Hill AM, 1964, Why morbid? Paths of progress in the control of obstetric infection, 1931 to 1960, *Med J Aust*, **1:** 101–11.

Hill GB, Osterhout S, 1972, Experimental effects of hyperbaric oxygen on selected clostridial species. II. In-vitro studies in mice, *J Infect Dis*, **125:** 26–35.

Hirn M, 1993, Hyperbaric oxygen in the treatment of gas gangrene and perineal necrotizing fasciitis. A clinical and experimental study, *Eur J Surg Suppl*, **570:** 1–36.

Hirn M, Niinikoski J, Lehtonen OP, 1992, Effect of hyperbaric oxygen and surgery on experimental gas gangrene, *Eur Surg Res*, **24:** 356–62.

Hobbs BC, Smith ME et al., 1953, *Clostridium welchii* food poisoning, *J Hyg*, **51:** 75–101.

Hopkinson WI, Towers AG, 1963, Effects of hyperbaric oxygen on some common pathogenic bacteria, *Lancet*, **2:** 1361–3.

Howard JM, Inui KK, 1954, Clostridial myositis-gas gangrene. Observations of battle casualties in Korea, *Surgery*, **36:** 1115–18.

Hummel RP, Altmeier WA, Hill EO, 1964, Iatrogenic staphylococcal enterocolitis, *Ann Surg*, **160:** 551–60.

Jackson SG, Deborah A et al., 1986, Diagnostic importance of *Clostridium perfringens* enterotoxin analysis in recurring enteritis among elderly, chronic care psychiatric patients, *J Clin Microbiol*, **23:** 748–51.

Jestin A, Popoff MR, Mahe S, 1985, Epizootiological investigations of a diarrhoeic syndrome in weaned pigs, *Am J Vet Res*, **46:** 2149–51.

Johnson S, Echeverria P et al., 1987, Enteritis necroticans among Khemer children at an evacuation site in Thailand, *Lancet*, **2:** 496–500.

Johnson S, Homan SR et al., 1992, Treatment of asymptomatic *Clostridium difficile* carriers (faecal excretors) with vancomycin or metronidazole. A randomised, placebo-controlled trial, *Ann Intern Med*, **117:** 297–302.

Just I, Selzer J et al., 1995, Glucosylation of Rho proteins by *Clostridium difficile* toxin B, *Nature (London)*, **375:** 500–3.

Kass EH, Lichstein HC, Waisbren BA, 1945, Occurrence of hyaluronidase and lecithinase in relation to virulence of *Clostridium welchii*, *Proc Soc Exp Biol Med*, **58:** 172–5.

Katich R, Voukitchevitch Z et al., 1964, Recherches sur la pathogénie de la gangrène gazeuse lors d'infection provoquée par *W. perfringens* A, seul ou en association avec *Cl. sporogenes* et avec *Cl. sporogenes* et *Staphylococcus aureus*, *Rev Immunol*, **28:** 63–74.

Katz GW, Gitlin SD et al., 1988, Acquisition of *Clostridium difficile* from the hospital environment, *Am J Epidemiol*, **127:** 1289–94.

Kaye D, 1966, Effect of hyperbaric oxygen on clostridia in vitro and in vivo, *Proc Soc Exp Biol Med*, **124:** 360–6.

Keen WW, 1915, The contrast between the surgery of the Civil War and that of the present war, *NY Med J*, **150:** 817–24.

Keighley MRB, Burdon DW et al., 1978, Randomised controlled trial of vancomycin for pseudomembranous colitis and post-operative diarrhoea, *Br Med J*, **2:** 1667–9.

Kellaway CH, Trethewie ER, Turner AW, 1940a, Neurotoxic and circulatory effects of the toxin of *Cl. welchii* type D, *Aust J Exp Biol Med Sci*, **18:** 225–52.

Kellaway CH, Trethewie ER, Turner AW, 1940b, The liberation of histamine and of adenyl compounds by the toxin of *Cl. welchii* type D, *Aust J Exp Biol Med Sci*, **18:** 253–64.

Kemp FH, 1945, X-rays in diagnosis and location of gas gangrene, *Lancet*, **1:** 332–6.

Keppie J, Robertson M, 1944, In vitro toxigenicity and other characters of strains of *Cl. welchii* type A from various sources, *J Pathol Bacteriol*, **56:** 123–32.

van Kessel LJP, Verbrugh HA et al., 1985, Necrotising enteritis associated with toxigenic type A *Clostridium perfringens*, *J Infect Dis*, **151:** 974–5.

Ketley JM, Mitchell TJ et al., 1987, The effects of *Clostridium difficile* crude toxins and toxin A on ileal and colonic loops in immune and non-immune rabbits, *J Med Microbiol*, **24:** 41–52.

Kettle EH, 1919, See Report 1919.

Kim K-H, Fekety R et al., 1981, Isolation of *Clostridium difficile* from the environment and contacts of patients with antibiotic-associated colitis, *J Infect Dis*, **143:** 42–50.

King A, Phillips I, 1986, The comparative in-vitro activity of perfloxacin, *J Antimicrob Chemother*, **17, Suppl. B:** 1–10.

King A, Rampling A et al., 1984, Neutropenic enterocolitis due to *Clostridium septicum* infection, *J Clin Pathol*, **37:** 335–43.

Knutsdon L, 1983, Postoperative gas gangrene in abdomen and in extremity, *Acta Chir Scand*, **149:** 567–71.

Koransky JR, Stargel MD, Dowell VR Jr, 1979, *Clostridium septicum* bacteremia. Its clinical significance, *Am J Med*, **66:** 63–6.

de Kruif PH, Bollman JL, 1917, The toxin of *Bacillus welchii*. The mechanism of infection with *B. welchii*, *J Infect Dis*, **21:** 588–99.

Kyriakis SC, Sarris K et al., 1995, The effect of salinomycin on the control of *Clostridium perfringens* type A infection in growing pigs, *J Vet Med Ser B*, **42:** 355–9.

Larson HE, Borriello SP, 1988, Infectious diarrhea due to *Clostridium perfringens*, *J Infect Dis*, **157:** 390–1.

Larson HE, Borriello SP, 1990, Quantitative study of antibiotic-induced susceptibility to *Clostridium difficile* enterocecitis in hamsters, *Antimicrob Agents Chemother*, **34:** 1348–53.

Larson HE, Price AB, Borriello SP, 1980, Epidemiology of experimental enterocecitis due to *Clostridium difficile*, *J Infect Dis*, **142:** 408–13.

Larson HE, Parry JV et al., 1977, Undescribed toxin in pseudomembranous colitis, *Br Med J*, **1:** 1246–8.

Larson HE, Price AB et al., 1978, *Clostridium difficile* and the aetiology of pseudomembranous colitis, *Lancet*, **1:** 1063–6.

Larson HE, Barclay FE et al., 1982, Epidemiology of *Clostridium difficile* in infants, *J Infect Dis*, **146:** 727–33.

Laszlow G, Elo G, 1983, The risk of malignant edema following lower limb amputation for ischemic gangrene, *Arch Orthop Trauma Surg*, **102:** 49–50.

Latta RM, 1951, Management of battle casualties from Korea, *Lancet*, **1:** 228–31.

Lawrence G, 1979, The pathogenesis of pig-bel in Papua New Guinea, *P N G Med J*, **22:** 39–49.

Lawrence G, Cooke R, 1980, Experimental pigbel: the production and pathology of necrotising enteritis due to *Clostridium welchii* type C in the guinea-pig, *Br J Exp Pathol*, **61**: 261–71.

Lawrence G, Walker PD, 1976, Pathogenesis of enteritis necroticans in Papua New Guinea, *Lancet*, **1**: 125–6.

Lawrence G, Shann F et al., 1979a, Prevention of necrotising enteritis in Papua New Guinea by active immunisation, *Lancet*, **1**: 227–30.

Lawrence G, Walker PD et al., 1979b, The occurrence of *Clostridium welchii* type C in Papua New Guinea, *P N G Med J*, **22**: 69–73.

Levett PN, 1985, Effect of antibiotic concentration in a selective medium on the isolation of *Clostridium difficile* from faecal specimens, *J Clin Pathol*, **38**: 233–4.

Lewis VL, Myers MB et al., 1978, Early diagnosis of crepitant gangrene caused by *Bacteroides melaninogenicus*, *Plast Reconstr Surg*, **62**: 276–9.

Libby JM, Donta ST, Wilkins TD, 1983, *Clostridium difficile* toxin A in infants, *J Infect Dis*, **148**: 606.

Lindberg RB, Wetzler TF et al., 1955, The bacterial flora of battle wounds at the time of primary debridement. A study of the Korean battle casualty, *Ann Surg*, **141**: 369–74.

Lindner JGEM, Plantema FHF et al., 1978, Quantitative studies of the vaginal flora of healthy women and of obstetric and gynaecological patients, *J Med Microbiol*, **11**: 233–41.

Linsey D, 1959, Gas gangrene. Clinical influences from experimental data, *Am J Surg*, **97**: 592–592.

Lorber B, 1995, Gas gangrene and other clostridium related diseases, *Principles and Practice of Infectious Diseases*, 5th edn, eds Mandell GL, Bennett JE, Dolin R, Churchill-Livingstone, New York, 2182–95.

Lorimer JW, Eidus LB, 1994, Invasive *Clostridium septicum* infection in association with colorectal carcinoma, *Can J Surg*, **37**: 245–9.

Lowry KF, Curtis GM, 1947, Diagnosis of clostridial myositis, *Am J Surg*, **74**: 752–7.

Lyerly DM, Sullivan NM, Wilkins TD, 1983, Enzyme-linked immunosorbent assay for *Clostridium difficile* toxin A, *J Clin Microbiol*, **17**: 72–8.

Lyerly DM, Saum KE et al., 1985, Effects of *Clostridium difficile* toxins given intragastrically to animals, *Infect Immun*, **47**: 349–52.

Lyerly DM, Barroso LA et al., 1992, Characterization of a toxin A-negative, toxin B-positive strain of *Clostridium difficile*, *Infect Immun*, **60**: 4633–9.

McClean D, Rogers HJ, 1944, Detection of bacterial enzymes in infected tissues, *Lancet*, **2**: 434–6.

McClean D, Rogers HJ, Williams BW, 1943, Early diagnosis of wound infection with special reference to gas gangrene, *Lancet*, **1**: 355–60.

McFarland LV, Surawicz CM, Stamm WE, 1990, Risk factors for *Clostridium difficile* carriage and *C. difficile*-associated diarrhea in a cohort of hospitalized patients, *J Infect Dis*, **162**: 678–84.

McFarland LV, Mulligan ME et al., 1989, Nosocomial acquisition of *Clostridium difficile* infection, *N Engl J Med*, **320**: 204–10.

Macfarlane MG, Datta N, 1954, Observations on the immunological and biochemical properties of liver mitochondria with reference to the action of *Clostridium welchii* toxin, *Br J Exp Pathol*, **35**: 202.

Macfarlane RG, MacLennan JD, 1945, The toxaemia of gas-gangrene, *Lancet*, **2**: 328–31.

MacLennan JD, 1943a, Streptococcal infection in muscle, *Lancet*, **1**: 582–4.

MacLennan JD, 1943b, Anaerobic infections of war wounds in the Middle East, *Lancet*, **2**: 63–6, 94–9, 123–6.

MacLennan JD, 1962, The histotoxic clostridial infections of man, *Bacteriol Rev*, **26**: 177–276.

MacLennan JD, Macfarlane RG, 1945, Toxin and anti-toxin studies of gas-gangrene in man, *Lancet*, **2**: 301–5.

Martin PK, Naylor RD, 1994, A latex agglutination test for the qualitative detection of *Clostridium perfringens* epsilon toxin, *Res Vet Sci*, **56**: 259–61.

Martin WJ, Gardner M, Washington JA, 1972, In vitro antimicrobial susceptibility of anaerobic bacteria isolated from clinical specimens, *Antimicrob Agents Chemother*, **1**: 148–58.

Matheson JM, 1968, Infection in missile wounds, *Ann R Coll Surg Engl*, **42**: 347–66.

Mattia AR, Doern GV et al., 1993, Comparison of four methods in the diagnosis of *Clostridium difficile* disease, *Eur J Clin Microbiol Infect Dis*, **12**: 882–6.

Memorandum, 1943, *War Memoranda of the Medical Research Council*, London, 2nd edn, No. 2, HMSO, London.

Merson MH, Dowell VR, 1973, Epidemic, clinical and laboratory aspects of wound botulism, *N Engl J Med*, **289**: 1005–10.

Millar JS, 1981, The surgical treatment of enteritis necroticans, *Br J Surg*, **68**: 481–2.

Millar WM, 1932, Gas gangrene in civil life, *Surg Gynecol Obstet*, **54**: 232–8.

Mitchell TJ, Ketley JM et al., 1986, Effect of toxin A and B of *Clostridium difficile* on rabbit ileum and colon, *Gut*, **27**: 78–85.

Mitchell TJ, Ketley JM et al., 1987, Biological mode of action of *Clostridium difficile* toxin A: a novel enterotoxin, *J Med Microbiol*, **23**: 211–19.

Morton A, 1967, Testicular gas gangrene after hernia repair with cord division, *Med J Aust*, **2**: 605–8.

Mulier T, Morgan M, Fabry G, 1993, *Clostridium septicum* gangrene complicating a closed femoral fracture, *Acta Orthop Belg*, **59**: 416–19.

Mulligan ME, 1988, General epidemiology, potential reservoirs and typing procedures, Clostridium difficile: *its Role in Intestinal Disease*, eds Rolfe RD, Finegold SM, Academic Press, San Diego, 229–56.

Mulligan ME, George WL et al., 1980, Epidemiological aspects of *Clostridium difficile*-induced diarrhea and colitis, *Am J Clin Nutr*, **33**: 2533–8.

Murrell TGC, 1967, Pig-bel: epidemic and sporadic necrotising enteritis in the highlands of New Guinea, *Aust Ann Med*, **16**: 4–10.

Murrell TGC, Roth L, 1963, Necrotising jejunitis: a newly discovered disease in the highlands of New Guinea, *Med J Aust*, **1**: 61–9.

Murrell TGC, Egerton JR et al., 1966a, The ecology and epidemiology of the pig-bel syndrome in man in New Guinea, *J Hyg*, **64**: 375–96.

Murrell TGC, Roth L et al., 1966b, Pig-bel: enteritis necroticans. A study in diagnosis and management, *Lancet*, **1**: 217–22.

Narayan AS, Rao RN, 1970, Unusual enteritis in Manipal, India, *Int J Surg*, **53**: 357–62.

Narula A, Khatib R, 1985, Characteristic manifestations of *Clostridium* induced spontaneous gangrenous myositis, *Scand J Infect Dis*, **17**: 291–4.

Norgaard N, Gehrchen PM et al., 1993, Spontaneous intrahepatic gas gangrene, *Eur J Surg*, **159**: 253–5.

North JP, 1947, Clostridial wound infections and gas gangrene. Arterial damage as a modifying factor, *Surgery*, **21**: 364–72.

Oakley CL, 1954, Gas gangrene, *Br Med Bull*, **10**: 52–8.

Ogilvie WH, 1944, *Forward Surgery in Modern War*, Butterworth, London.

Olubunmi PA, Taylor DJ, 1985, *Clostridium perfringens* type A in enteric diseases of the pig, *Trop Vet*, **3**: 28–33.

Owen-Smith MS, Matheson JM, 1968, Successful prophylaxis of gas gangrene of the high-velocity missile wound in sheep, *Br J Surg*, **55**: 36–9.

Parker MT, 1967, Clostridial sepsis, *Br Med J*, **2**: 698.

Pashby NL, Bolton RP, Sherriff RJ, 1979, Oral metronidazole in *Clostridium difficile* colitis, *Br Med J*, **1**: 1605–6.

Patterson M, Rosenbaum HD, 1952, Enteritis necroticans, *Gastroenterology*, **21**: 110–18.

Pelfrey TM, Turk RP et al., 1984, Surgical aspects of *Clostridium septicum* septicemia, *Arch Surg*, **119**: 546–50.

Perkins SE, Fox JG et al., 1995, Detection of *Clostridium difficile* toxins from the small intestine and caecum of rabbits with naturally acquired enterotoxaemia, *Lab Anim Sci*, **45**: 379–84.

Plimpton NC, 1964, *Clostridium perfringens* infection, *Arch Surg*, **89**: 499–507.

Prescott JF, Sivendra R, Barnum DA, 1978, The use of bacitracin in the control of experimentally induced necrotic enteritis in chickens, *Can Vet J*, **19**: 181–7.

Price AB, 1984, The pathology of antibiotic-associated colitis, *Antibiotic associated Diarrhoea and Colitis*, ed. Borriello SP, Martinus Nijhoff, Boston, 134–49.

Price AB, Davies DR, 1977, Pseudomembranous colitis, *J Clin Pathol*, **30**: 1–12.

Price EH, Borriello SP et al., 1990, *Clostridium difficile* and severe enterocolitis in three infants, *Clinical and Molecular Aspects of Anaerobes*, ed. Borriello SP, Wrightson Biomedical, Petersfield, 75–9.

Princewell TJT, Agba MI, 1982, Examination of bovine faeces for the isolation and identification of *Clostridium* species, *J Appl Bacteriol*, **52**: 97–102.

Pujari BD, Deodhare SG, 1980, Necrotising enteritis, *Br J Surg*, **67**: 254–6.

Pyrtek LJ, Bartus SH, 1962, *Clostridium welchii* infection complicating biliary-tract surgery, *N Engl J Med*, **266**: 689–93.

Reigler M, Sedivy R et al., 1995, *Clostridium difficile* toxin B is more potent that toxin A in damaging colonic epithelium in vitro, *J Clin Invest*, **95**: 2004–11.

Reiner L, Schlesinger MJ, Miller GM, 1952, Pseudomembranous colitis following aureomycin and chloramphenicol, *Arch Pathol*, **54**: 39–67.

Report, 1919, *Special Report Series, Medical Research Council*, London, No.39, HMSO, London.

Report, 1994a, Report of the PHLS *Clostridium difficile* working group, *PHLS Microbiol Dig*, **11**: 22–4.

Report, 1994b, *The Prevention and Management of* Clostridium difficile *Infection*, BAPS, Lancashire.

Richardson SA, Brookfield DSK et al., 1981, Pseudomembranous colitis in a 5 week old infant, *Br Med J (Clin Res Ed)*, **283**: 1510.

Rifkin GD, 1980, Neutropenic enterocolitis and *Clostridium septicum* infection in patients with agranulocytosis, *Arch Intern Med*, **140**: 834–5.

Rifkin GD, Fekety FR et al., 1977, Antibiotic-induced colitis. Implication of a toxin neutralised by *Clostridium sordellii* antitoxin, *Lancet*, **2**: 1103–6.

Riley TV, Adams JE et al., 1991, Gastrointestinal carriage of *Clostridium difficile* in cats and dogs attending veterinary clinics, *Epidemiol Infect*, **107**: 659–65.

Robbins M, Marais R et al., 1987, The in-vitro activity of doxycycline and minocycline against anaerobic bacteria, *J Antimicrob Chemother*, **20**: 379–82.

Robb-Smith AHT, 1945, Tissue changes induced by *Cl. welchii* type A filtrates, *Lancet*, **2**: 362–8.

Robertson M, Keppie J, 1941, In-vitro production of toxin from strains of *Cl. welchii* recently isolated from war wounds and air raid casualties, *J Pathol Bacteriol*, **53**: 95–104.

Roding B, Groeneveld PHA, Boerema I, 1972, Ten years experience in the treatment of gas gangrene with hyperbaric oxygen, *Surg Gynecol Obstet*, **134**: 579–85.

Roggentin P, Hobrecht R et al., 1991, Application of sialidase antibodies for the diagnosis of clostridial infections, *Clin Chim Acta*, **196**: 97–106.

Roggentin P, Kleineidam RG et al., 1993, An immunoassay for the rapid and specific detection of three sialidase-producing clostridia causing gas gangrene, *J Immunol Methods*, **157**: 125–33.

Rooney J, Shepherd A, Suebu A, 1979, *Clostridium welchii* type C antitoxin in the treatment of 'pig-bel' (enteritis necroticans): a controlled trial in Papua New Guinea, *P N G Med J*, **22**: 57.

Rose HD, 1979, Gas gangrene and *Clostridium perfringens* septicemia associated with the use of an indwelling radial artery catheter, *Can Med Assoc J*, **121**: 1595–6.

Rosenblatt JE, 1984, Antimicrobial sensitivity testing of anaerobic bacteria, *Rev Infect Dis*, **6, Suppl. 1**: S242–8.

Rudge FW, 1993, The role of hyperbaric oxygen in the treatment of clostridial myonecrosis, *Milit Med*, **158**: 80–3.

Rutala WA, Gergen MF, Weber DJ, 1993, Inactivation of *Clostridium difficile* spores by disinfectants, *Infect Control Hosp Epidemiol*, **14**: 36–9.

Savage GM, 1974, Lincomycin and clindamycin: their role in chemotherapy of anaerobic and microaerophilic infections, *Infection*, **2**: 152–9.

Schellenberg D, Bonington A et al., 1994, Treatment of *Clostridium difficile* diarrhoea with brewer's yeast, *Lancet*, **343**: 171–2.

Schwan A, Sjolin S et al., 1984, Relapsing *Clostridium difficile* enterocolitis cured by rectal infusion of normal faeces, *Scand J Infect Dis*, **16**: 211–15.

Scopes JW, Smith MF, Beach RC, 1980, Pseudomembranous colitis and sudden infant death, *Lancet*, **1**: 1144.

Seal DV, Borriello SP et al., 1987, Treatment of relapsing *Clostridium difficile* diarrhoea by administration of a non-toxigenic strain, *Eur J Clin Microbiol*, **6**: 51–3.

Sekabunga JG, 1966, Jejunal enteritis. Surgical aspects, *East Afr Med J*, **43**: 541.

Selwyn S, 1980, *The Beta-lactam Antibiotics: Penicillins and Cephalosporins in Perspective*, Hodder and Stoughton, London.

Seppälä K, Hjelt L, Sipponen P, 1981, Colonoscopy in the diagnosis of antibiotic-associated colitis. A prospective study, *Scand J Gastroenterol*, **16**: 465–8.

Severin WPJ, de la Fuente AA, Stringer MF, 1984, *Clostridium perfringens* type C causing necrotising enteritis, *J Clin Pathol*, **37**: 942–4.

Shouler PJ, 1983, The management of missile injuries, *J R Nav Med Serv*, **69**: 80–4.

Skiles MS, Covert GK, Fletcher SH, 1978, Gas producing clostridial and non-clostridial infections, *Surg Gynecol Obstet*, **147**: 65–7.

Smith F, 1969, Surgical aspects of enteritis necroticans in the highlands of New Guinea, *Aust NZ J Surg*, **38**: 199–205.

Smith LDS, 1949, Clostridia in gas gangrene, *Bacteriol Rev*, **13**: 233–54.

Smith LDS, Gardner MV, 1949, Occurrence of vegetative cells of *Clostridium perfringens* in soil, *J Bacteriol*, **58**: 407–8.

Smith LDS, George RL, 1946, The anaerobic bacterial flora of clostridial myositis, *J Bacteriol*, **51**: 271–9.

Spencer RC, 1991, Anaerobic bacteraemia, *Anerobes in Human Disease*, eds Duerden BI, Drasar BS, Wiley Liss, New York, 324–42.

Staempfli HR, Prescott JF, Brash ML, 1992, Lincomycin-induced severe colitis in ponies: association with *Clostridium cadaveris*, *Can J Vet Res*, **56**: 168–9.

Staneck JL, Washington JA, 1974, Antimicrobial susceptibilities of anaerobic bacteria: recent clinical isolates, *Antimicrob Agents Chemother*, **6**: 311–15.

Stevens DL, Laine BM, Mitten JE, 1987, Comparison of single and combination antimicrobial agents for prevention of experimental gas gangrene caused by *Clostridium perfringens*, *Antimicrob Agents Chemother*, **31**: 312–16.

Stevens DL, Maier KA, Mitten JE, 1987a, Comparison of clindamycin, rifampin, teracycline, metronidazole and penicillin for efficacy in prevention of experimental gas gangrene due to *Clostridium perfringens*, *J Infect Dis*, **155**: 220–8.

Stevens DL, Maier KA, Mitten JE, 1987b, Effect of antibiotics on toxin production and viability of *Clostridium perfringens*, *Antimicrob Agents Chemother*, **31**: 213–18.

Stevens DL, Musher DM et al., 1990, Spontaneous non-traumatic gangrene due to *Clostridium septicum*, *Rev Infect Dis*, **12**: 286–96.

Stevens DL, Bryant AE et al., 1993a, Role of theta toxin, a sulfhydryl-activated cytolysin in the pathogenesis of clostridial gas gangrene, *Clin Infect Dis*, **16, Suppl. 4**: S195–9.

Stevens DL, Bryant AE et al., 1993b, Evaluation of therapy with hyperbaric oxygen for experimental infection with *Clostridium perfringens*, *Clin Infect Dis*, **17**: 231–7.

Stock AH, 1947, Clostridia of gas gangrene and local infections during the Italian campaign, *J Bacteriol*, **54**: 169–74.

Strawitz JG, Wetzler TF et al., 1955, The bacterial flora of healing wounds, *Surgery*, **37**: 400–8.

Struble AL, Tang YJ et al., 1994, Faecal shedding of *Clostridium difficile* in dogs: a period prevalence survey in a veterinary hospital, *J Vet Diagn Invest*, **6**: 342–7.

Struelens MJ, Maas A et al., 1991, Control of nosocomial transmission of *Clostridium difficile* based on sporadic case surveillance, *Am J Med*, **91, Suppl. 3B**: 138S–44S.

Surawicz CM, McFarland LV et al., 1989, Treatment of recurrent *Clostridium difficile* colitis with vancomycin and *Saccharomyces boulardii*, *Am J Gastroenterol*, **84**: 1285–7.

Sussman M, 1958, A description of *Clostridium histolyticum* gas gangrene in the Epidemics of Hippocrates, *Med Hist*, **2**: 226.

Sutter VL, Finegold SM, 1976, Susceptibility of anaerobic bacteria to 23 antimicrobial agents, *Antimicrob Agents Chemother*, **10**: 736–52.

Tabaqchali S, Wilks M, 1992, Epidemiological aspects of infections caused by *Bacteroides fragilis* and *Clostridium difficile*, *Eur J Clin Microbiol Infect Dis*, **11**: 1049–57.

Taylor DJ, Estrada Correa A, 1988, Avoparcin in the prevention of enterotoxigenic *C. perfringens* type A infections and diarrhoea in pigs, *Proc Int Pig Vet Soc*, **10**: 139.

Taylor GW, 1960, Preventive use of antibiotics in surgery, *Br Med Bull*, **16**: 51–4.

Teasley DG, Gerding DN et al., 1983, Prospective randomised trial of metronidazole versus vancomycin for *Clostridium difficile*-associated diarrhoea and colitis, *Lancet*, **2**: 1043–6.

Tedesco FJ, 1984, Antibiotics associated with *Clostridium difficile* mediated diarrhoea and/or colitis, *Antibiotic associated Diarrhoea and Colitis*, ed. Borriello SP, Martinus Nijhoff, Boston, 3–8.

Tedesco FJ, Barton RW, Alpers DH, 1974, Clindamycin-associated colitis, *Ann Intern Med*, **81**: 429–33.

Tedesco FJ, Gordon D, Fortson WC, 1985, Approach to patients with multiple relapses of antibiotic-associated pseudomembranous colitis, *Am J Gastroenterol*, **80**: 867–8.

Tedesco FJ, Gurwith M et al., 1978, Oral vancomycin for antibiotic-associated pseudomembranous colitis, *Lancet*, **2**: 226–8.

Teo WS, Balasubramanian P, 1983, Gas gangrene after intramuscular injection of adrenaline, *Clin Orthop*, **174**: 206–7.

Testore GP, Pantosti A et al., 1988, Evidence for cross-infection in an outbreak of *Clostridium difficile*-associated diarrhoea in a surgical unit, *J Med Microbiol*, **26**: 125–8.

Thadepalli H, Chan WH et al., 1978, Microflora of the cervix during normal labor and the puerperium, *J Infect Dis*, **137**: 568–72.

Thom S, 1993, A role for hyperbaric oxygen in clostridial myonecrosis, *Clin Infect Dis*, **17**: 238.

Thomas CG, Keleher MF, McKee AP, 1951, Botulism, complication of *Clostridium botulinum* wound infection, *Arch Pathol*, **51**: 623–8.

Thoresby FP, 1966, 'Cavitation'. The wounding process of the high velocity missile, a review, *J R Army Med Corps*, **112**: 89–99.

Thoresby FP, Darlow HM, 1967, The mechanisms of primary infection of bullet wounds, *Br J Surg*, **54**: 359–61.

Thoresby FP, Matheson JM, 1967a, Gas gangrene of the high velocity missile wound. I. An experimental comparison of surgical treatment methods, *J R Army Med Corps*, **113**: 31–6.

Thoresby FP, Matheson JM, 1967b, Gas gangrene of the high velocity missile wound. II. An experimental study of penicillin prophylaxis, *J R Army Med Corps*, **113**: 36–9.

Thoresby FP, Watts JC, 1967, Gas gangrene in the high-velocity missile-wound, *Br J Surg*, **54**: 25–9.

Triadafilopoulos G, Pothoulakis C et al., 1987, Differential effects of *Clostridium difficile* toxins A and B on rabbit ileum, *Gastroenterology*, **93**: 273–9.

Tucker KD, Wilkins TD, 1991, Toxin A of *Clostridium difficile*

binds to human carbohydrate antigens I, X and Y, *Infect Immun*, **59**: 73–8.

Turner FP, 1964, Fatal *Clostridium welchii* septicemia following cholecystectomy, *Am J Surg*, **108**: 3–7.

van Unnik AJM, 1965, Inhibition of toxin production by *Clostridium perfringens* in vitro by hyperbaric oxygen, *Antonie van Leeuwenhoek J Microbiol Serol*, **31**: 181–6.

Unsworth IP, 1973, Gas gangrene in New South Wales, *Med J Aust*, **1**: 1077–87.

Uzal FA, Belak K et al., 1992, Bacillary haemoglobinuria diagnosis by the peroxidase antiperoxidase technique, *J Vet Med Ser B*, **39**: 595–8.

Valentine JC, 1957, Gas gangrene septicaemia due to carcinoma and muscular trauma, *Br J Surg*, **44**: 630–2.

Viscidi RP, Bartlett JG, 1981, Antibiotic-associated pseudomembranous colitis in children, *Pediatrics*, **67**: 381–6.

Walker PD, 1985, Pig-bel, in, *Clostridia in Gastrointestinal Disease*, ed. Borriello SP, CRC Press, Boca Raton, FL, 93–115.

Walker PD, Foster WH et al., 1979, Development, preparation and safety testing of a *Clostridium welchii* type C toxoid. I. Preliminary observations in man in Papua New Guinea, *J Biol Stand*, **7**: 315–23.

Walters BAJ, Stafford R et al., 1982, Contamination and cross-infection with *Clostridium difficile* in an intensive care unit, *Aust NZ J Med*, **12**: 255–8.

Warren CPW, Mason BJ, 1970, *Clostridium septicum* infection of the thyroid gland, *Postgrad Med J*, **46**: 586–8.

Watt B, Brown FV, 1986, Is ciprofloxacin active against clinically important anaerobes?, *J Antimicrob Chemother*, **17**: 605–13.

Weinberg M, Séguin P, 1918, *La Gangrène Gazeuse*, Paris.

Weinstein L, Barza MA, 1973, Gas gangrene, *N Engl J Med*, **289**: 1129–31.

Welch TP, Sumitswan S, 1975, Acute segmental ischaemic enteritis in Thailand, *Br J Surg*, **62**: 716–19.

Wells AD, Fletcher MS et al., 1985, Clostridial myositis of the psoas complicating percutaneous nephrostomy, *Br J Surg*, **72**: 582.

Wexler HM, Finegold SM, 1985, In-vitro activity of imipenem against anaerobic bacteria, *Rev Infect Dis*, **7, Suppl. 3**: S417–25.

Wheatley PR, 1967, Research on missile wounds – the Borneo operations January 1962–June 1965, *J R Army Med Corps*, **113**: 18–25.

Wierup M, 1977, Equine intestinal clostridiosis and acute disease in horses associated with high intestinal counts of *Clostridium perfringens* type A, *Acta Vet Scand Suppl*, **62**: 1–182.

Wilcox MH, Spencer RC, 1992, *Clostridium difficile* infection: responses, relapses and reinfections, *J Hosp Infect*, **22**: 85–92.

Willey S, Bartlett JG, 1979, Cultures for *Clostridium difficile* in stools containing a cytotoxin neutralised by *Clostridium sordellii* antitoxin, *J Clin Microbiol*, **10**: 880–4.

Willis AT, 1969, *Clostridia of Wound Infection*, Butterworth, London.

Willis AT, 1977, *Anaerobic Bacteriology: Clinical and Laboratory Practice*, 3rd edn, Butterworth, London.

Willis AT, 1985, Host factors predisposing to anaerobic infections, *Scand J Infect Dis Suppl*, **46**: 18–26.

Willis AT, 1988, Historical aspects, Clostridium difficile: *its Role in Intestinal Disease*, eds Rolfe RD, Finegold SM, Academic Press, San Diego, 15–28.

Willis AT, 1991, Gas gangrene and clostridial cellulitis, *Anerobes in Human Disease*, eds Duerden BI, Drasar BS, Wiley Liss, New York, 299–323.

Willis AT, Phillips KD, 1988, *Anaerobic Infections: Clinical and Laboratory Practice*, Public Health Laboratory Service, London.

Wright DH, Stanfield IP, 1967, Enteritis necroticans in Uganda, *J Pediatr*, **71**: 264–8.

Wright GP, 1950, *Cl. welchii* infections as problems in bacterial intoxication, *Proc R Soc Med*, **43**: 886.

Wright GP, Hopkins SJ, 1946, Fixation of *Cl. welchii* toxins by skin cells, *J Pathol Bacteriol*, **58**: 573–5.

Yudis M, Zucker S, 1967, *Clostridium welchii* bacteremia: a case report with survival and review of the literature, *Postgrad Med J*, **43**: 487–9.

Zamecnik PC, Folch J, Brewster LE, 1945, Protection of animals against *Cl. welchii* (type A) toxin by injection of certain purified lipids, *Proc Soc Exp Biol Med*, **60**: 33–9.

Zamecnik PC, Nathanson IT, Aub JA, 1947, Physiologic action of *Clostridium welchii* (type A) toxins in dogs, *J Clin Invest*, **26**: 394–410.

Zeissler J, Rassfeld-Sternberg L, 1949, Enteritris necroticans due to *Clostridium welchii* type F, *Br Med J*, **1**: 267–9.

TETANUS

S M Finegold

Tetanus is a toxin mediated, infective disease resulting from the contamination of a wound or raw surface, or, more rarely, from the parenteral injection of substances contaminated with tetanus bacilli. It is characterized by a series of tonic reflex muscular spasms superimposed upon muscular rigidity. The wounds most commonly implicated are those of the legs, followed by those of hands, arms and neck; in as many as 20% of cases there may be no history of injury and no detectable wound. The frequency with which the masseter muscles are affected has given rise to the popular term 'lockjaw'. In newborn infants the cut surface of the umbilical cord may afford an entrance for the bacilli, giving rise to neonatal tetanus, and in women rare cases of tetanus occur shortly after childbirth, as the result of infection in the genital tract. A small proportion of cases are attributable to growth of tetanus bacilli in an ear affected by chronic otitis media. Infections of the face or head give rise to a peculiar form – cephalic tetanus – characterized by facial paralysis and dysphagia.

1 HISTORY

Tetanus was described by Hippocrates approximately 30 centuries ago. Over the years, it has been documented as a scourge of child-bearing women, newborn babies, and wounded soldiers. In the eighteenth century, one of every 6 infants born in the Rotunda Hospital in Dublin died of tetanus neonatorum.

The impact of the disease can be appreciated from the vivid description by Aretaeus around the second or third century AD (Adams 1856):

Tetanus, in all its varieties, is a spasm of an exceedingly painful nature, very swift to prove fatal, but neither easy to be removed... There is a pain and tension of the tendons and spine, and of the muscles connected with the jaws and cheek; for they fasten the lower jaw to the upper, so that it could not easily be separated even with levers or a wedge. But if one, by forcibly separating the teeth, pour in some liquid that patients do not drink it but squirt it out, or retain it in the mouth, or it regurgitates by the nostrils; for the isthmus faucium is strongly compressed, and the tonsils being hard and tense, do not coalesce so as to propel that which is swallowed. The face is ruddy and of mixed colors, the eyes almost immovable, or are rolled about with difficulty; strong feeling of suffocation; respiration bad, distension of the arms and legs; subsultus of the muscles; the countenance variously distorted; the cheeks and lips tremulous; the jaw quivering, and the teeth rattling, and in certain rare cases even the ears are thus affected. I myself have beheld this and wondered! The urine is retained, so as to induce strong dysuria, or passes spontaneously from contraction of the bladder. These symptoms occur in each variety of the spasms.

But there are peculiarities in each; in Tetanus there is tension in a straight line of the whole body, which is unbent and inflexible; the legs and arms are straight.

Opisthotonos bends the patient backward, like a bow, so that the reflected head is lodged between the shoulder-blades; the throat protrudes; the jaw sometimes gapes, but in some rare cases it is fixed in the upper one; respiration stertorous; the belly and chest prominent, and in these there is usually incontinence of urine; the abdomen stretched, and resonant if tapped; the arms strongly bent back in a state of extension; the legs and thighs are bent together, for the legs are bent in the opposite direction to the hams.

But if they are bent forwards, they are protuberant at the back, the loins being extruded in a line with the back, the whole of the spine being straight; the vertex prone, the head inclining towards the chest; the lower jaw fixed upon the breast bone; the hands clasped together, the lower extremities extended; pains intense; the voice altogether dolorous; they groan, making deep moaning. Should the mischief then seize the chest and the respiratory organs, it readily frees the patient from life; a blessing this, to himself, as being a deliverance from pains, distortion, and deformity; and a contingency less than usual to be lamented by the spectators, were he a son or a father. But should the powers of life still stand out, the respiration, although bad, being still prolonged, the patient is not only bent up into an arch but rolled together like a ball, so that the head rests upon the knees, while the legs and back are bent forwards, so as to convey the impression of the articulation of the knee being dislocated backwards.

An inhuman calamity! an unseemly sight! a spectacle painful even to the beholder! an incurable malady! owing to the distortion, not to be recognized by the dearest friends; and hence the prayer of the spectators, which formerly would have been reckoned not pious, now becomes good, that the patient may depart from life, as being a deliverance from the pains and unseemly evils attendant on it. But neither can the physician, though present and looking on, furnish any assistance, as regards life, relief from pain or from deformity. For if he should wish to straighten the limbs, he can only do so by cutting and breaking those of a living man. With them, then, who are overpowered by this disease, he can merely sympathise. This is the great misfortune of the physician.

In the early nineteenth century, Sir Charles Bell, a Scottish surgeon, made a drawing of a British soldier who had been wounded during the Peninsular War in Spain. This is shown in Fig. 36.1. Also early in the nineteenth century, Brodie proposed that curare in conjunction with artificial ventilation might be useful for managing tetanus and Sewell used curare for farm animals with tetanus. Curare was first used for tetanus in humans in the late 1850s in the USA and in Europe.

The nature of tetanus remained uncertain until, in 1884, Carle and Rattone demonstrated its transmissibility to animals. Nicolaier (1884, 1886) found that the inoculation of soil into mice, guinea pigs or rabbits was frequently followed by a disease closely simulating human tetanus. In the pus at the site of inocu-

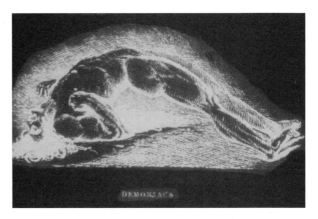

Fig. 36.1 Bell's portrait of a soldier with tetanus; note muscle rigidity and opisthotonus and the striking risus sardonicus.

lation, besides cocci and other organisms, he noticed long, thin bacilli. Though unable to isolate the organism in pure culture, he grew it in deep coagulated serum for 7 generations, and reproduced the disease by injection of the last culture. In animals dying of the experimental disease Nicolaier was unable to find the bacilli microscopically except in the local lesion and, occasionally, in the sciatic nerve sheath and spinal cord. Their limited distribution led him to suggest that the organisms multiplied locally and produced a strychnine-like poison which, on absorption, produced the disease. Rosenbach (1886–87) observed a similar bacillus with a round terminal spore in a human case of tetanus, and the pus proved infective to animals. The final demonstration of the aetiological role of the tetanus bacillus was furnished in 1889 by Kitasato who was able to isolate *Clostridium tetani* in pure culture by first heating pus to 80°C for 45–60 min to destroy non-sporing organisms, plating the purulent material out on gelatin, and incubating in an atmosphere of hydrogen. In 1890, Faber confirmed the theory of Nicolaier by reproducing the disease in experimental animals injected with filtrates of cultures of the organism, thus demonstrating that a cell-free toxin was responsible for the manifestations of the disease. The discovery of tetanus antitoxin was made by Behring and Kitasato, also in 1890. In 1920, Glenny and Ramon independently discovered that the toxin could be made harmless by treating it with formaldehyde to yield a toxoid; this toxoid could still stimulate antibody formation.

Bjornboe, Ibsen and Johnson mentioned involvement of the autonomic nervous system in tetanus in 1954 and the first major report of this issue was by Kerr and colleagues in 1968.

2 AETIOLOGY

C. tetani (Figs 36.2 and 36.3) is a slender gram-positive obligately anaerobic bacillus measuring about 0.5 by 2.5–5.0 μm; as with other clostridia, cells may be gram-variable or even gram-negative. It bears round terminal spores that give the organism a drumstick or

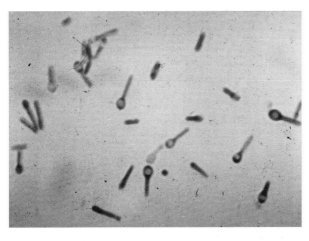

Fig. 36.2   Gram stain of a culture of *C. tetani*; original magnification × 1000. (Reproduced with permission from Bleck TP, 1991b, Tetanus, *Infections of the Central Nervous System*, eds Scheld WM, Whitley RJ, Durack DT, Raven Press, New York).

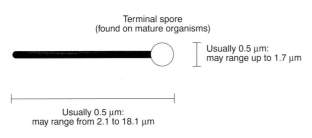

Terminal spore
(found on mature organisms)

Usually 0.5 μm:
may range up to 1.7 μm

Usually 0.5 μm:
may range from 2.1 to 18.1 μm

Fig. 36.3   Schematic diagram of a mature *C. tetani* bacillus, showing the squash-racket morphology. (Reproduced with permission from Bleck TP, 1991b, Tetanus, *Infections of the Central Nervous System*, eds Scheld WM, Whitley RJ, Durack DT, Raven Press, New York).

tennis (or squash) racket appearance. Early spores are oval and subterminal. The spores are very resistant to a variety of deleterious agents including most disinfectants and extremes of temperature. They resist boiling water at neutral pH for several minutes; some strains survive boiling for some hours. Culture in semi-solid glucose medium encourages sporulation. On solid media, colonies spread early as fine feathery projections at the edge of a delicate film of growth. Motility is rather sluggish although there are numerous peritrichous flagella.

The tetanus bacillus displays little biochemical activity. It is typically non-saccharolytic and is weakly proteolytic, hydrolysing gelatin but not other proteins in laboratory tests. Gelatin liquefaction may take 2–4 days or much longer. *C. tetani* is lecithinase-negative and lipase-negative. Many strains produce indole, but often only after 2 days. Hydrogen sulphide is not produced. The organism does not reduce nitrates and is negative in the sulphite reduction test. A neuraminidase is produced. Major end products of metabolism are acetic, propionic and butyric acids and butanol. Haemolysis is noted on blood agar which on occasion can be neutralized by tetanus antitoxin; this is not a reliable test for *C. tetani*. Initially, the colonies are α-

haemolytic; later they are β-haemolytic. Tetanolysin is the responsible haemolysin.

Maximum yields of toxin occur in the stationary phase of growth and very little toxin is released into the medium until the cells are lysed. Phages have been demonstrated in *C. tetani* but they are not involved in toxin production.

It is difficult to distinguish between *C. tetani* and *Clostridium cochlearium* except by DNA sequence differences and the fact that the latter organism is non-toxigenic.

3   EPIDEMIOLOGY

Tetanus spores are rather widespread in the environment (e.g. soil, animal faeces, surfaces of carpets, etc.) so that any breach in the skin (such as wounds, burns, animal or human bites, and even insect bites) (Tonge 1989) may result in inoculation of the spores into the host. Since 7–21% of tetanus cases in most series are cryptogenic, even trivial and unremembered trauma may admit enough spores to cause the disease (Adams 1968). Lesions of the gastrointestinal tract occasionally are implicated as the source of tetanus, particularly in rural environments where the carriage rate of *C. tetani* may be 20 times higher than in urban dwellers (Heare and Shabot 1990). Tetanus bacilli have been recovered from the external auditory canal and it is thought that otogenic tetanus does occur in relation to ear infection.

The recorded prevalence of tetanus bacilli in various parts of the environment depends, of course, on the sensitivity of the method of detection used. Sanada and Nishida (1965) found that the lower the degree of preheating of a soil suspension the greater was the isolation rate of tetanus bacilli and the higher the toxicity of the strains isolated. The most toxic strains were cultivated from soil heated to 60°C for 10 min, and the least toxic from soil heated to 100°C for 30 min.

Nicolaier (1884) demonstrated the presence of tetanus bacilli in 12 of 18 samples of earth, and other workers have subsequently reported comparable findings (see Smith 1984). The organism is commonly found in soil samples all over the world. Surveys in Japan, Canada, Brazil and the USA reveal a soil positivity rate of 30– 42%. Bulloch and Cramer (1919) concluded that the ionizable calcium salts of soil were an important factor in promoting tetanus in soil-contaminated wounds. They noted that calcium salts were more abundant in cultivated than in waste soil and that tetanus was far commoner at the beginning of World War I, when the fighting was mainly on the highly cultivated soil of Flanders, than towards the end, when the soil had largely become waste.

Toledo and Veillon (1891) demonstrated the presence of *C. tetani* in horse and cow dung. Nobel (1915) found it in 18% of 61 samples of horse faeces, but not in 20 samples of cow faeces. Other figures include 30% of 23 samples of guinea pig faeces (Sanfelice 1893) and 17% of 200 samples from London horses (Fildes 1925). Kerrin (1929), in an examination of between 21 and 141 faecal samples from each of several species, obtained the following approximate percentages of positive results: horse, 15; cow, 5; sheep, 27; dog, 46; rat, 37; and hen, 18. About half the strains were atoxic. The presence of the bacillus in faeces, and consequently in manure, may account for the greater prevalence of the organism in cultivated than in uncultivated soils.

In 1898 Pizzini demonstrated the presence of *C. tetani* in human faeces; he found it in 3 of 10 samples from ostlers, and in 2 of 90 samples from peasants. From these results, it has been generally assumed that contact with horses strongly predisposes to the carrier condition in man, but it is doubtful that this assumption is justified. In Great Britain, Tulloch (1919–20) found the bacillus in 5 of 31 specimens of human faeces, and Fildes (1925) only twice in 200 specimens. Others have failed to find it in 304 (Kerrin 1928, 1929), 50 (Scheunemann 1931) and 92 (Bandmann 1953) samples. On the other hand, Bauer and Meyer (1926) in California found it in 24.6% of 487 specimens of faeces. Bandmann (1953) summarized earlier investigations in which the human faecal carrier rates were between 0 and 40% (see also Lowbury and Lilly 1958).

It is uncertain whether the tetanus bacillus multiplies in the human and animal intestine or is an organism of passage, having been ingested in food. Other clostridia are able to thrive in the intestine, and there are reports that small amounts of antitoxin may be found in the serum of some animals and in man (Smith 1984). Even if proliferation and toxin release does occur in the alimentary tract, tetanus, unlike botulism, does not arise as a result of absorption from the intestine.

The bacilli were found in the dust of British surgical operating theatres (Robinson, McLeod and Downie 1946, Sevitt 1949), and with some consistency both in the air of a city hospital and in that of operating theatres ventilated by a system that took in air from the hospital corridors (Lowbury and Lilly 1958).

Contamination by factory and warehouse dust of fibres used in surgical dressings constitutes a special hazard (see, e.g., Report 1959). The bacilli also occur in raw catgut used for surgical sutures (Mackie, McLachan and Anderson 1929, Cuboni 1957). In postoperative tetanus the spores may be derived either from infected catgut, imperfectly sterilized instruments or dressings, plasters and talcum powders, or some other source such as the contaminated air of the operating room as well as, in unusual circumstances, from the bowel.

Among the small number of cases reported in recent years (Fig. 36.4), older women figure prominently, often having received a trivial gardening wound. Athletes who get injuries from shoe spikes are also candidates for tetanus; injuries on playing fields have been shown to be a factor in the risk of tetanus in males aged 15–44 years. The incidence is higher in the non-white than white population of the USA, probably owing to greater exposure and lower immunization rates. Men are less likely to be susceptible (Gergen et al. 1995), the distribution of cases between the sexes depending largely on occupational habits and the active immunization of men in the armed forces. Most cases of tetanus and most deaths in the USA in 1989 and 1990 occurred in persons 60 years of age or older (Fig. 36.5) (Gergen et al. 1995).

In agricultural countries the rural population suffers more than the urban, and more in the summer than the winter. Infections of the legs and feet are liable to occur in heavily manured areas. Those addicted to narcotic drugs are at an increased risk from tetanus; of 142 cases in New York in 1955–65, no fewer than 102 were in addicts (Cherubin 1967).

Portals of entry into the body for *C. tetani* are numerous, but the most common are traumatic and surgical wounds (about 65% of cases) and the umbilical stump after childbirth. The wound is often a minor one such as a wood or metal splinter or a thorn. Chronic skin ulcers account for 5% of cases (Sanford 1995). A significant number of cases of tetanus are cryptogenic.

In the developing countries neonatal tetanus may be responsible for 20–30% of the cases and 70% of deaths (Figs 36.6 and 36.7); this form of tetanus is extremely rare in countries where good hygiene is practised in midwifery. Ritual practices of placing soil or cow dung on the umbilical cord may play a role (Traverso et al. 1989), but most cases probably relate to failure to use good aseptic technique in cutting the umbilical cord and dressing the stump. The longer the cord, the lower the risk of neonatal tetanus; cleanliness of the environment and of the clothes of the patient and the mother are also important (Schofield, Tucker and Westbrook 1961).

4 INCIDENCE

Throughout the world, approximately one million cases of tetanus (about 18 per 100 000 population) occur each year. During the period 1985 through 1990, in the USA there were approximately 60 cases reported annually (Centers for Disease Control 1990, LaForce 1990, Prevots et al. 1992). In 1994, only 36 cases of tetanus were reported in the USA (Sanford 1995). It is estimated that the actual number of cases is at least double the number reported (Gergen et al. 1995). The annual incidence rate from 1985 to 1990 was about 0.02 per 100 000 population. Of the total of 365 cases reported in that 6 year period, only one was neonatal tetanus. In the developing world, neonatal cases account for half the total cases reported (neonatal tetanus is the second leading cause of vaccine-preventable deaths in the world, next to measles, accounting for more than 600 000 reported deaths annually) (Begue and Lindo-Soriano 1991). Neonatal tetanus is endemic in 90 countries throughout the world and in some of these countries it accounts for one-half of the neonatal mortality and one-fourth of infant mortality (Whitman et al. 1992). Approximately 70% of the total cases in the above-mentioned 6 year period in the USA occurred in persons 50 years old

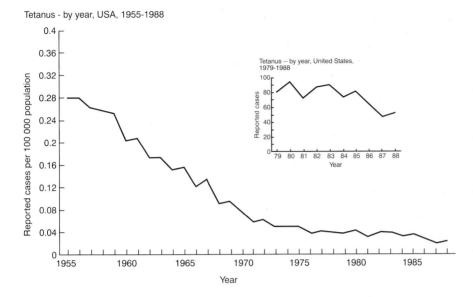

Tetanus - by year, USA, 1955-1988

Tetanus -- by year, United States, 1979-1988

Fig. 36.4 Tetanus, by year; USA, 1955–88. (Reproduced with permission from *Morbid Mortal Weekly Rep* 1988, **37** (54): 39).

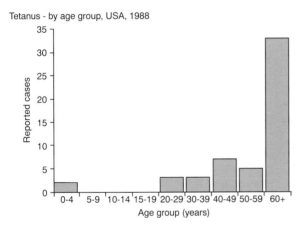

Tetanus - by age group, USA, 1988

Fig. 36.5 Tetanus, by age group; USA, 1988. (Reproduced with permission from *Morbid Mortal Weekly Rep* 1988, **37** (54): 39).

or older. The risk of acquiring tetanus in individuals over 80 years of age was more than 10 times the risk in persons aged 20–29 years.

The number of deaths attributable to tetanus throughout the world is declining for a number of reasons that vary in importance in different countries: improved living standards, urbanization, better hygiene especially in relation to childbirth, increasing use of active immunization, and more effective treatment. Nevertheless, tetanus is still responsible for many deaths in parts of Africa, Asia and Central and South America; in these regions neonatal tetanus is common (Veronesi 1965, Vaishnava and Goyal 1966). In the USA, Europe and other developed parts of the world, tetanus is comparatively rare.

There is an important consequence of the undernotification of cases. Deaths of patients from tetanus, or from associated causes (see Galbraith, Forbes and Tillett 1981), are recorded and counted; because of undernotification, however, the fatality rate gives a misleading impression of the quality of man-

agement of the disease. In Britain, the case-fatality rate of tetanus was stated to be 10% in one report (Edmondson and Flowers 1979). The actual numbers of cases of tetanus may therefore be estimated by multiplying by 10 the total number of deaths from tetanus or associated causes. One reservation should be added, namely, that the figure for the overall case-fatality rate in the USA in 1985 and 1986 was 31% (42% for patients >50 years and 5% for those aged under 50). If, as Galbraith, Forbes and Tillett (1981) have shown, the highest death rate and highest incidence occur in the elderly age groups, the application of a 10% case-fatality ratio to the British data may overestimate the number of cases.

5 INCUBATION PERIOD

The incubation period of tetanus (the time from spore inoculation to the first symptom) is commonly 7–10 days, but it may range from 2 to 30 days. It is typically shorter after head and face wounding than after injury to the leg and foot, and is often 7 days or less in neonatal tetanus (Patel and Mehta 1963). In 10–30% of cases the disease has no obvious cause and the incubation period is therefore in doubt. Prophylactic antitoxin treatment after a wound, when it does not prevent the disease completely, may increase the length of the incubation period. Thus, in World War I the incubation period in patients treated in hospitals in Britain lengthened from 11.8 days in 1914 to 50 days in 1918–19 (Bruce 1920).

6 PERIOD OF ONSET

This period, important to distinguish from the incubation period, is the time from the first symptom to the first reflex spasm. Regardless of the clinical type of tetanus, the shorter the period of onset the poorer the prognosis.

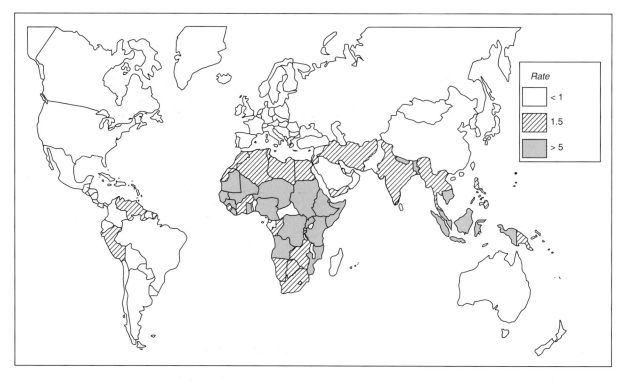

Fig. 36.6   Estimated neonatal tetanus mortality rates (per 1000 live births), 1991. (Reproduced with permission from Whitman et al. 1992).

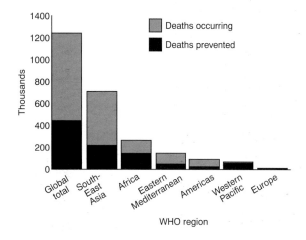

Fig. 36.7   Estimated neonatal tetanus deaths occurring and prevented, developing countries, 1991. (Reproduced with permission from Whitman et al. 1992).

7   TETANUS TOXIN

C. tetani produces a potent neurotoxin, 'tetanospasmin'. Strains vary from completely non-toxigenic to very highly toxigenic. In vitro, maximum yields of toxin are produced after the growth phase, and little toxin is released before the bacterial cells lyse. Tetanus (and botulinum) neurotoxins are the most potent toxins known; their potency is primarily due to their absolute neurospecificity. These toxins are metalloproteases that enter nerve cells and block neurotransmitter releases.

The toxin is a protein (MW c. 150 kDa), occurring in the 'intracellular form' as a single chain. The 'extracellular form' is produced by proteolytic cleavage and comprises a heavy chain (105 kDa) and an aminoterminal light chain (55 kDa) linked by a disulphide bond. Fragment C, the 50 kDa carboxy-terminal portion of the heavy chain, has ganglioside binding and protein binding activities. The light chain, a zinc-dependent protease, mediates the blockade of inhibitor release from neurons by proteolysis of synaptobrevin (VAMP), a constitutive small-vesicle protein. The release of the inhibitory mediators γ-aminobutyric acid (GABA) and glycine is prevented, thus allowing uncontrolled stimulation of the muscles. This mechanism of action will be detailed further later in this chapter. Toxigenesis is plasmid mediated. Various bacterial and animal proteases cleave tetanus toxin; clostridial proteases cleave it within residues 445–461 which is part of a disulphide loop formed by C-438 and C-466 (Figs 36.8 and 36.9) (Krieglstein et al. 1991). This region contains 2 Arg residues but does not contain a recognition site for furin. Purified clostridial protease cleaved a Glu-Asn and then an Ala-Ser bond, whereas other proteases such as trypsin cleaved at positions expected for their established specificities. The entire 3945 nucleotide sequence of the toxin gene has been determined and the correct 1315 amino acid sequence of the toxin molecule has been deduced.

Type B botulinum toxin is almost homologous to tetanus toxin in light chain amino acid sequence and is identical to tetanus toxin in its site of enzymatic action. As a result, immunization with tetanus toxoid may prevent type B infant botulism or reduce its severity (Schechter and Arnon 1995).

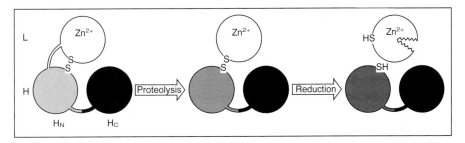

Fig. 36.8 Scheme of the activation mechanism of the neurotoxins responsible for tetanus and botulism. The toxin is produced as a single polypeptide chain of 150 kDa which is later cleaved at a single site by tissue or bacterial proteases. The toxin is depicted as a tripartite structure with the different domains connected by exposed protease-sensitive loops on the basis of biochemical and structural data. The 2 chains are held together by a single interchain disulphide bond, which has to be reduced to free the Zn^{2+} endopeptidase activity of the light chain (L). The H_C domain of the H chain is mainly responsible for the neurospecific binding, whereas the H_N domain appears to be involved in the neuronal penetration of the L chain. (Reproduced with permission from Montecucco and Schiavo 1993).

```
        ┌─A
         ↑ 10            20          30          40          50          60
N- MPITINNFRY  SDPVNNDTII  MMEPPYCKGL  DIYYKAFKIT  DRIWIVPERY  EFGTKPEDIN

        70          80          90          100         110         120
PPSSLIEGAS  EYYDPNYLRT  DSDKDRFLQT  MVKLFNRIKN  NVAGEALLDK  IINAIPYLGN

        130         140         150         160         170         180
SYSLLDKFDT  NSNSVSFNLL  EQDPSGATTK  SASMLTNLIIF  GPGPVLNKNE  VRGIVLRVDN

        190         200         210         220         230         240
KNYFPCRDGF  GSIMQMAFCP  EYVPTFDNVI  ENITSLTIGK  SKYFQDPALL  LMHELIHVLH

        250         260         270         280         290         300
GLYGMQVSSH  EIIPSKQEIY  MQHTYPISAE  ELFTFGGQDA  NLISIDIKND  LYEKTLNDYK

        310         320         330         340         350         360
AIANKLSQVT  SCNDPNIDID  SYKQIYQQKY  QFDKDSNGQY  IVNEDKFQIL  YNSIMYGFTE

        370         380         390         400         410         420
IELGKKFNIK  TRLSYFSMNH  DPVKIPNLLD  DTIYNDTEGF  NIESKDLKSE  YKGQNMRVNT

        430         440         450     ┌─B    470         480
NAFRNVDGSG  LVSKLIGLCK  KIIPPTNIRE  NLYNRTASLT  DLGGELCIKI  KNEDLTFIAE
                            └ ─ ─ ─ ─ ─ ─ S-S ─ ─ ─ ─ ─ ─ ┘

        490         500         510         520         530         540
KNSFSEEPFQ  DEIVSYNTKN  KPLNFNYSLD  KIIVDYNLQS  KITLPNDRTT  PVTKGIPYAP

        550         560         570         580         590         600
EYKSNAASTI  EIHNIDDNTI  YQYLYAQKSP  TTLQRITMTN  SVDDALINST  KIYSYFPSVI

        610         620         630         640         650         660
SKVNQGAQGI  LFLQWVRDII  DDFTNESSQK  TTIDKISDVS  TIVPYIGPAL  NIVKQGYEGN

        670         680         690         700         710         720
FIGALETTGV  VLLLEYIPEI  TLPVIAALSI  AESSTQKEKI  IKTIDNFLEK  RYEKWIEVYK

        730         740         750         760         770         780
LVKAKWLGTV  NTQFQKRSYQ  MYRSLEYQVD  AIKKIIDYEY  KIYSGPDKEQ  IADEINNLKN

        790         800         810         820         830         840
KLEEKANKAM  ININIFMRES  SRSFLVHQMI  NEAKKQLLEF  DTQSKNILMQ  YIKANSKFIG

        850         860  ┌─C  870       880         890         900
ITELKKLESK  INKVFSTPIP  FSYSKNLDCW  VDNEEDIDVI  LKKSTILNLD  INNDIISDIS

        910         920         930         940         950         960
GFNSSVITYP  DAQLVPGING  KAIHLVNNES  SEVIVHKAMD  IEYNDMFNNF  TVSFWLRVPK

        970         980         990         1000        1010        1020
VSASHLEQYG  TNEYSIISSM  KKHSLSIGSG  WSVSLKGNNL  IWTLKDSAGE  VRQITFRDLP

        1030        1040        1050        1060        1070        1080
DKFNAYLANK  WVFITITNDR  LSSANLYING  VLMGSAEITG  LGAIREDNNI  TLKLDRCNNN

        1090        1100        1110        1120        1130        1140
NQYVSIDKFR  IFCKALNPKE  IEKLYTSYLS  ITFLRDFWGN  PLRYDTEYYL  IPVASSSKDV

        1150        1160        1170        1180        1190        1200
QLKNITDYMY  LTNAPSYTNG  KLNIYYRRLY  NGLKFIIKRY  TPNNEIDSFV  KSGDFIKLYV

        1210        1220        1230        1240        1250        1260
SYNNNEHIVG  YPKDGNAFNN  LDRILRVGYN  APGIPLYKKM  EAVKLRDLKT  YSVQLKLYDD

        1270        1280        1290        1300        1310
KNASLGLVGT  HNGQIGNDPN  RDILIASNWY  FNHLKDKILG  CDWYFVPTDE  GWTND -C
```

Fig. 36.9 Amino acid sequence of tetanospasmin: A, origin of the light chain; B, origin of the amino portion of the heavy chain (H_1); C, origin of the carboxy portion of the heavy chain (H_2). The N-terminal methionine is removed during processing of the toxin and the amino acids are numbered starting with the adjacent proline. The disulphide bond connecting the light and heavy chains is illustrated (from cysteine 438 to cysteine 466). A second disulphide bond, connecting cysteine 1076 and cysteine 1092, is not shown. (Reproduced with permission from Matsuda 1989. Additional information from Bergey et al. 1989).

Tetanus can be reproduced by the injection of pure cultures or of toxin into mice, rats, guinea pigs, rabbits, goats, sheep, horses, monkeys and other animals. Cats and dogs are more resistant; birds and cold-blooded animals are highly resistant. The most susceptible animal, calculated on the amount of toxin per g of body weight necessary to cause fatality, is the horse. This species is about 12 times as susceptible as the mouse; the guinea pig is 6 times and the monkey 4 times as susceptible as the mouse (Sherrington 1917). On the other hand, the rabbit is twice, the dog 50 times, the cat 600 and the hen 30 000 times as resistant as the mouse (Kitasato 1891). These figures are approximations only (for other estimates, see Wright 1955).

Toxin is equally active by the intramuscular and subcutaneous routes; much smaller doses are effective on injection into nerve trunks or the spinal cord. The injection of an effective dose (e.g. 0.5 ml of a 2–4 day culture of a toxigenic strain in cooked meat broth) intramuscularly or subcutaneously into the hind limb of a mouse lateral to the base of the tail produces a typical sequence of signs, the severity and time-course of which are dose-dependent and can serve as a crude index of the amount of toxin injected:

1 The limb shows slight stiffness within a day.
2 A limp develops, but the limb is still used.
3 The limb is paralysed, but can still be passively moved.
4 The tail curves towards the side of the injection and the limb becomes fixed in spastic paralysis.
5 Generalized convulsions occur.
6 The animal dies.

Tetanospasmin is highly toxic (MLD c. 130 ng) when introduced into or elaborated in the tissues of man. It is not toxic by the oral route.

A second toxin, tetanolysin, is of uncertain significance in human disease. Tetanolysin is an oxygen-sensitive haemolysin that is related functionally and serologically to streptolysin O. Purified tetanolysin has a molecular mass of 48 ± 3 kDa. Injection into various animal species produced pulmonary oedema, intravascular haemolysis, and cardiotoxicity but it is questionable whether this toxin plays any role in *C. tetani* infections.

8 PATHOGENESIS AND PATHOPHYSIOLOGY

Vaillard and Rouget in 1892 found that when tetanus cultures were heated to 65–67°C for 30 min to destroy the vegetative bacilli and the toxin, the toxin-free spores remaining could be injected in large numbers into a guinea pig without giving rise to the disease. The spores did not germinate in the tissues, but were rapidly taken up by the phagocytes; in 2 or 3 days they were completely ingested. When, however, the spores were protected from the phagocytes by being wrapped in filter paper, they germinated and gave rise to fatal tetanus. The same results were obtained by injury at the site of injection sufficient to cause necrosis or effusion of blood; and by injecting a second bacterial species, particularly an aerobic one. Spores germinated in damaged tissue, but not in clean, aseptic wounds. These observations on the activation of otherwise innocuous toxin-free spores were extended by several workers. It was found that tetanus occurred in guinea pigs challenged simultaneously with washed spores and either staphylococcal culture or quinine. When the spores were given 9–30 days before the adjuvant, only 2 of 20 animals died. Clearly, spores can remain dormant in tissues, including phagocytes (Vaillard and Rouget 1892), for considerable periods.

Dormancy was evident in soldiers wounded during the 1914–18 war. The organism was frequently found in the wounds of men with no symptoms of the disease. Thus of 100 soldiers without tetanus, Tulloch (1919–20) found *C. tetani* in 19. Tetanus sometimes did not develop for weeks or months after a wound had healed, and might then appear suddenly after an operation, perhaps on another part of the body. There are instances of tetanus developing up to 14 years after the presumed introduction of the spores into the tissues.

Tulloch (1919–20) activated toxin-free spores in vivo by injecting them with tissue poisons such as lactic acid, saponin and trimethylamine; toxic filtrates of *C. perfringens* and *Clostridium septicum* were particularly effective activators.

Bulloch and Cramer (1919) made the important discovery that the injection of small quantities of ionizable calcium salts together with toxin-free spores invariably led to the development of tetanus. They obtained the same result when washed bacilli – but not spores – and the salt were injected into different sites. The lesion occurred at the site of injection of the salt. There the organisms were present in large numbers and were not ingested by phagocytes; at the other injection site the bacilli underwent lysis and rapid phagocytosis. Phagocytosis of spores could not, however, be the sole cause of non-germination, because it was always incomplete. The spores germinated only when necrotic areas were produced by the injection of soil or calcium chloride. The calcium ions did not alter the virulence of the bacteria or the potency of the toxin, but damaged the tissues at the site of injection, breaking down their immunity. The effect of soil was lost if its content of calcium salts was removed by precipitation.

The effect of many of the agents that activate tetanus spores is referable to the induction in the tissues of an anaerobic focus of low oxidation–reduction (O–R) potential. It appears that spores germinate in tissues in which, by reasons of necrosis, the O–R potential is decreased to a sufficiently low point (Fildes 1927, Russell 1927). This view is consistent with the inability of tetanus spores to germinate in a medium at pH 7.0–7.6 unless the potential is decreased to Eh +0.1 volt or less. The Eh of the subcutaneous tissue of the guinea pig is higher than this, but when it is lowered by holding the animals in an atmosphere containing only 7% instead of the normal

21% oxygen, spores will often germinate in vivo, under the influence of only mild activating agents (Knight and Fildes 1930, Campbell and Fildes 1931).

Growth of the bacilli in a necrotic, anaerobic lesion may be rapid; from lesions produced in mice by the injection of about 4000 spores in calcium chloride solution, of which about 1000 remained at the injection site, Smith and MacIver (1974) recovered 1.7×10^5 colony-forming units after 18 h and 6.8×10^6 after 24 h. They estimated that 2 MLD of toxin were probably formed as early as 7 h after the spore challenge. The growing bacilli may increase the extent of the anaerobic focus; in guinea pigs Smith and MacIver (1969) found that anaerobic lesions produced by calcium chloride became about 10 times larger in volume when spores were also injected.

We conclude that when tetanus spores are introduced into a wound by contamination with soil, horse faeces, or other material, their fate depends largely on the presence or absence of certain accessory factors. Many of these have been described: notably trauma, haemorrhage, tissue necrosis, and foreign bodies; chemicals such as lactic acid, colloidal silicic acid, and ionizable calcium salts; substances such as the toxins of *C. septicum* and *C. perfringens*; and infection by other microbes. The presence of a suitable accessory factor enables the spores to germinate and multiply in the tissues; it is probable that this action is dependent on the production of necrosis with a sufficiently low oxidation–reduction potential to permit the spores to germinate. A similar local debilitating action by gelatin, vaccine lymph, antitoxin sera and bacterial vaccines is probably the reason for the tetanus that follows the injection of these substances (Smith 1908).

8.1 Tetanus toxin

The means by which tetanus toxin, elaborated in a small, localized wound, gives rise to clinical tetanus has been studied for about a century.

Evidence slowly accumulated that the main site of action of the neurotoxin is the central nervous system to which the toxin gains access by ascending the motor nerves (see review by Mellanby and Green 1981). However, toxin is not delivered directly to the central nervous system by the bloodstream, because to produce fatal tetanus in experimental animals more toxin is required by the intravenous than by the subcutaneous route; and with a given dose of toxin, the incubation period can be longer after the intravenous injection.

Transmission of toxin to the central nervous system along motor nerves was suggested as early as 1890 by the work of Bruschettini (1890, 1892) who observed that toxin injected into the muscle in rabbits could be recovered from the motor nerves supplying the surrounding area. Toxin given into the sciatic nerve is readily detected in the spinal cord. Gumprecht reported in 1894 that local tetanus (see section 9.2, p. 704) was stopped by division of the motor nerve. Likewise it does not develop in a denervated limb (Couermont and Doyon 1899). It can be produced by the injection of a very small and otherwise ineffective

dose of toxin directly into the sciatic nerve (Tizzoni and Cattani 1890, Meyer and Ransom 1903).

Ascent of toxin may be blocked by prior injection of antitoxin into the motor nerve or by sclerosis of the motor nerve. Sclerosis of the nerve by tincture of iodine prevents the spasticity that follows distal but not proximal injection of toxin (Teale and Embleton 1919–20, Baylis et al. 1952b). As a rule, the smaller the animal and the less the distance the toxin has to travel along the nerves, the shorter is the incubation period. In the mouse, for example, it is about 12 h, in the rabbit 18–36 h, in the dog 36–48 h and in the horse 5 days (Meyer and Ransom 1903). The dose of toxin administered is also a determining factor. The larger the dose, the shorter is the incubation period. Wright, Morgan and Wright (1950) induced strabismus, torticollis, salivation and bradycardia by the careful injection of toxin into either the facial, vagus, or hypoglossal nerves – an observation best explained by the central action of toxin on neighbouring bulbar nuclei. Local tetanus in a limb can be abolished by barbiturate anaesthesia, probably because it acts within the central nervous system (Wright, Morgan and Wright 1952). Schellenberg and Matzke (1958) reported that in parabiotic rats local tetanus could be produced in one of the rats when toxin was injected into the hind limb of the other, provided a crossed regenerated nerve was present.

The development of tetanus in one limb, after injection of toxin into it, is usually followed by local tetanus of the opposite limb (Sawamura 1909), suggesting spread of toxin from the anterior horn of one side to that of the other in the segment of cord affected. With larger doses of toxin, there is a gradual ascent of spasticity, first of the muscles of the back, then of the forelimbs and neck. That this is due to movement of toxin up the spinal cord is evident from the results of transection of the cord, whereby the spasm is limited to musculature enervated below the level of transection (Meyer and Ransom 1903, Firor, Lamont and Shumacker 1940, Friedemann, Hollander and Tarlov 1941, Baylis et al. 1952a). In various animal species, including the donkey, in which, as in man, descending tetanus occurs, Kryzhanovsky and his colleagues (see Kryzhanovsky 1966, 1973) studied the spread of toxin at intervals during the course of experimental intoxication of mice by excising pieces of nerve and titrating their toxin content. In an extensive series of experiments they demonstrated that toxin ascended the nerves, both in ascending and descending tetanus, reaching the grey matter of the ventral horns of the spinal cord by way of the ventral roots.

Meyer and Ransom (1903) suggested that the part of the nerve through which toxin was transmitted was the axis cylinder. This view became generally accepted (Wright 1955) and, after 2 decades of conflicting evidence, more recent work with toxin labelled with ^{125}I provided support for the axonal hypothesis (Price et al. 1975, Price, Griffin and Peck 1977). Toxin seems to be taken up only through the neuromuscular nerve endings. It is generally agreed that intra-axonal transport is an important route for the movement of molecules along nerves. The toxin is transported along α but not γ motor fibres (see Strick et al. 1976); the reason for the association of toxin with only α fibres is not known. Evidence of the importance of the axonal route is strong, although it is still not accepted by all workers.

Tetanus in man is usually descending in character, that is, stiffness begins in the head and neck and spreads down the body. A similar form of tetanus is produced in the experimental animal by intravenous injection of toxin and it is presumed that in man toxin is transmitted via the bloodstream to the bulbar motor nuclei. The means by which the blood-borne toxin reaches the central nervous system has been debated. Wright (1955) suggested that local capillary permeability, in the areae postremae in the fourth ventricle, for example, permitted transport of toxin into the brain, but Fedinec (1967) in experiments with tritium-labelled toxin found no supportive evidence. An alternative explanation depends upon the uptake of toxin from the blood and tissue fluids by motor-nerve endings all over the body (Stöckel, Schwab and Thoenen 1975); the onset of symptoms first in the head and neck is then accounted for by the shorter length of the cephalic nerves. The work of Kryzhanovsky and his colleagues, already referred to, provided much evidence to support the latter hypothesis, and Habermann and Dimpfel (1973) found that labelled toxin was not detected in the central nervous system of rats until 6 h after intravenous injection, by which time the concentration in the plasma had fallen sharply. Moreover, the pontine and post-pontine brain stem, from which nerves V–XII arise, were much richer in toxin than the region from which the smaller nerves III and IV arise. Stöckel and his colleagues provided evidence against direct blood–brain passage of toxin by the observation that, in rats given an injection of labelled toxin intramuscularly, toxin appeared in the bloodstream and capillaries in the whole spinal cord, but no label could be detected in the nervous tissue adjacent to these blood vessels.

Wasserman and Takaki reported in 1898 that toxin was absorbed and rendered non-toxic by a suspension of brain tissue but not by liver, kidney, or spleen. The toxin receptor in the nervous system was eventually identified (van Heyningen 1959, van Heyningen and Miller 1961) as a ganglioside which, extracted from beef brain, could fix toxin at an estimated ratio of 1 mole of toxin to 2 moles of ganglioside. It was later reported that it was the heavy chain of the toxin molecule that became bound to the ganglioside (van Heyningen 1976). Tetanus toxin also binds to preparations of synaptosomal membranes, which have been shown to contain gangliosides (Habermann 1976). Toxin also binds to the plasma membrane of thyroid cells, probably through the ganglioside receptors for thyrotropic hormone, which competitively inhibit toxin fixation by the membrane (Ledley et al. 1977); this may account for the state resembling acute thyroid overactivity which sometimes is seen in cases of human tetanus. Cultured neuronal cells from the central nervous system also bind toxin, apparently through long-chain ganglioside receptors (Dimpfel, Huang and Halbermann 1977, Mirsky et al. 1978). Two binding sites have been distinguished on differentiating mouse-neuroblastoma cells in culture. One accepts toxin, but not toxoid, with a resulting contraction of neuron-like processes formed by the cells in culture; this effect is not inhibited by treatment of the cells with neuraminidase or β-galactosidase, both of which modify membrane gangliosides. The second receptor binds both toxin and toxoid but with no visible morphological effect; ganglioside will inhibit the binding of toxoid. The receptor through which toxin mediates its neurological effects may not be the ganglioside (Zimmerman and Piffaretti 1977).

The cell intoxication by tetanus toxin is a 4 step process: cell binding, internalization, membrane translocation and target modification in the cytosol (Montecucco and Schiavo 1994). Receptors for the toxin are located on the motor neuron plasmalemma at the neuromuscular junction; these receptors have very high affinity for the toxin. Although presynaptic gangliosides bind the toxin avidly, it is uncertain that they are the actual receptors (Bleck 1991a). The toxin then moves laterally to bind a protein receptor prior to internalization. The toxin is internalized inside vesicles of unknown nature and is no longer susceptible to neutralization by antitoxin; it is internalized at the neuromuscular junction but moves in retrograde fashion along the axon. It is discharged in the intersynaptic space and enters the inhibitory interneurons; it is confined to a very limited space where it reaches much higher concentrations than at the neuromuscular junction. Tetanus toxin is felt to cross the vesicle membrane following acidification of the lumen and subsequent transition to an acid conformation that can insert in the lipid bilayer and translocate the L chain. Indirect evidence indicates that an intracellular low pH step is required for intoxication; bafilomycin A1, a specific inhibitor of the vacuolar-type ATPase proton pump, protects spinal neurons from tetanus toxin. The intracellular activity of tetanus toxin is due to its L domain. The toxin activity is dependent on the zinc molecule bound to the L chain. The intraneuronal target that is cleaved is synaptobrevin (VAMP, vesicle-associated membrane protein, Fig. 36.10); the cleavage of a fragment from the N-terminal and the cytoplasm-facing end of the protein (Hausinger, Volknandt and Zimmermann 1995) leads to a sustained blocking of neurotransmitter release. Inactivation of transmitter release occurs after calcium entry during depolarization (Bleck 1991a). The intraneuronal activity of the toxin is inhibited by highly specific inhibitors of zinc endopeptidases (Montecucco and Schiavo 1993). The long duration of tetanus poisoning may relate to persistence of toxin in the intracellular location because of a scarcity of free cytosolic proteases (Erdal et al. 1995).

Recent studies suggest that the toxin has a general effect on cell secretory function and that the restriction of its activity to neuronal cells reflects the distribution of its ganglioside receptors (Collee and van Heyningen 1991).

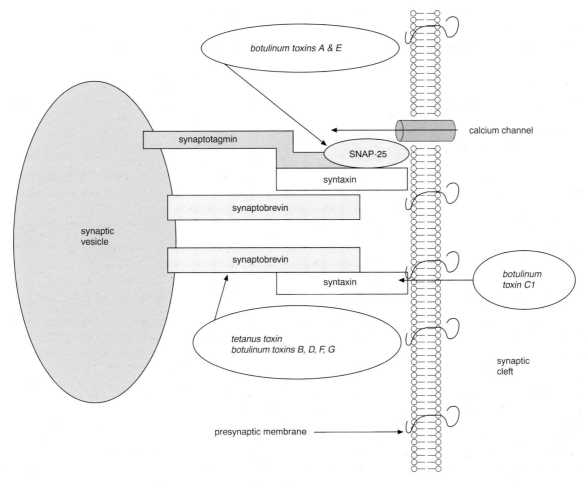

Fig. 36.10 Schematic representation of the proteins involved in synaptic vesicle docking and release, especially those involved in the action of clostridial toxins (reproduced with permission from Bleck TP, Brauner JS, 1997, Tetanus, *Infections of the Central Nervous System*, 2nd edit., eds Scheld WM, Whitley RJ, Durack DT, Raven Press, New York).

In addition to its principal effect on the central nervous system, tetanus toxin may also cause flaccid paralysis by affecting neuromuscular transmission (Abel 1934). Indeed, when toxin is prevented from reaching the central nervous system in the rabbit, paralytic signs develop (Miyasaki et al. 1967). Ambache, Morgan and Payling-Wright (1948a, 1948b) induced non-spastic paralysis of the iris by the injection of crude toxin into the rabbit eye. The affected iris would not respond to stimulation of the oculomotor nerve but contracted in response to the local injection of acetylcholine. The effect was probably due to tetanospasmin, as a non-spasmogenic fraction left after absorption of toxin with ganglioside had no activity on the iris (Mellanby, Pope and Ambache 1968). It was deduced that the toxin impeded the release of acetylcholine at the local nerve endings. Toxin causes flaccid paralysis in goldfish, an animal as sensitive as the mouse to tetanus toxin, apparently as a result of blockage of neuromuscular transmission presynaptically; miniature junction potentials in nerve-muscle preparations from pectoral fins partly paralysed with toxin were reduced in frequency but not in amplitude, implying that postsynaptic sensitivity to acetylcholine was unaffected

(Diamond and Mellanby 1971, Mellanby and Thompson 1972).

In summary, local and 'ascending' tetanus from locally injected toxin is produced by toxin absorbed at the motor nerve endings and carried to the anterior horn cells, where, by interfering at the synaptic junctions with the inhibitory neurons governing the generation of motor impulses (Fig. 36.11), it permits motor hyperactivity and hence spasticity in the appropriate muscles. In 'descending' tetanus the toxin appears to reach the brain stem from the bloodstream also by ascending the motor nerves, the onset of symptoms in the head and neck being accounted for by the shorter length of the nerves supplying those areas. Toxin spreads from the infected site by diffusing into adjacent muscle, by transport by lymphatics (from which it enters the bloodstream), or by passage through the nerves. The toxin attaches to a receptor on the nerve ending and a portion of the bound toxin is taken into the nerve cell, passing on to the central nervous system (spinal cord and brain stem extracellular space) by retrograde passage through the nerve axons (at a rate of 75–250 mm per day). The process of the toxin moving from the infected or contaminated site to the

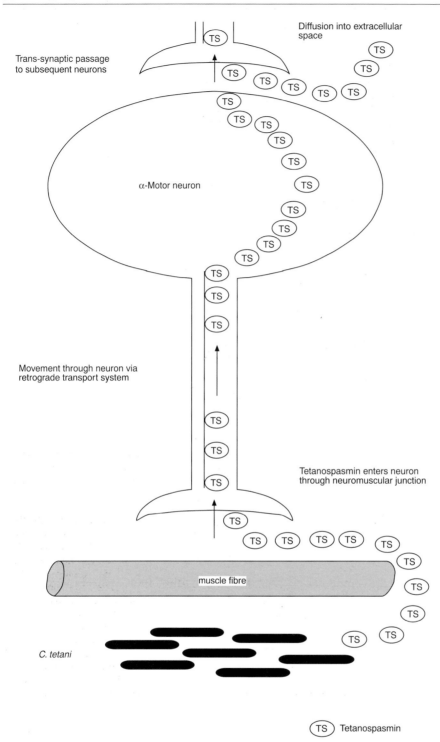

Trans-synaptic passage to subsequent neurons

Diffusion into extracellular space

α-Motor neuron

Movement through neuron via retrograde transport system

Tetanospasmin enters neuron through neuromuscular junction

muscle fibre

C. tetani

TS Tetanospasmin

Fig. 36.11 Tetanospasmin diffuses from the site of introduction to the α motor neuromuscular junction. It moves via the retrograde transport system to the cell body, from which it diffuses out into the synapses and extracellular space within the spinal cord or brain stem. (Reproduced with permission from Bleck TP, 1991b, Tetanus, *Infections of the Central Nervous System*, eds Scheld WM, Whitley RJ, Durack DT, Raven Press, New York).

spinal cord takes 2–14 days (Sanford 1995). The toxin acts by blocking inhibitory synapses of the spinal cord motor neurons, preventing release of inhibitory mediators (GABA and glycine) and thus allowing uncontrolled stimulation of the muscles (Fig. 36.12). Once inside the presynaptic terminal, the toxin prevents release of neurotransmitters for at least several weeks and probably permanently; clinical recovery from tetanus probably requires development of new synapses to replace those that have been inactivated. Though a local action of toxin on myoneural junc-

tions may occur, central action of the toxin appears to account for most of the manifestations of natural and experimental tetanus.

9   CLINICAL PICTURE

Tetanus clinically is classified into 4 principal types – generalized, local, cephalic and neonatal tetanus – primarily related to the site of action of the toxin, at the neuromuscular junction in some cases and in cen-

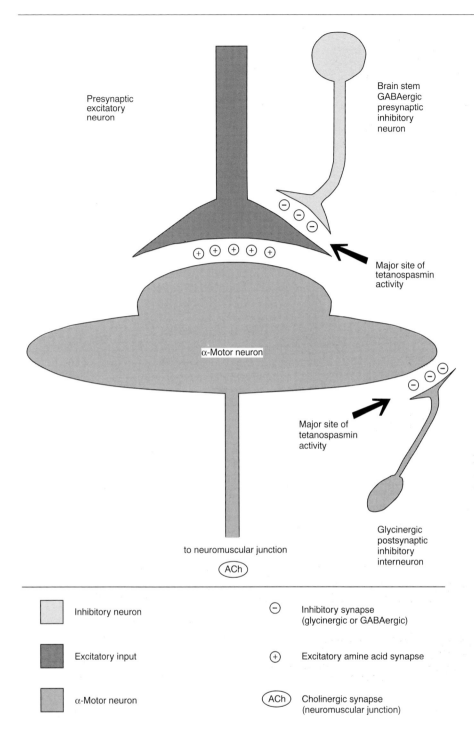

Presynaptic
excitatory
neuron

Brain stem
GABAergic
presynaptic
inhibitory
neuron

Major site of
tetanospasmin
activity

α-Motor neuron

Major site of
tetanospasmin
activity

to neuromuscular junction

ACh

Glycinergic
postsynaptic
inhibitory
interneuron

Inhibitory neuron

Excitatory input

α-Motor neuron

⊖ Inhibitory synapse
(glycinergic or GABAergic)

⊕ Excitatory amine acid synapse

ACh Cholinergic synapse
(neuromuscular junction)

Fig. 36.12 Sites of synaptic activity of TS. The major effects are at the synapse of the α motor neuron with (1) the glycinergic interneuron, and with (2) the brain stem GABA-ergic neuron. The toxin can also inhibit the release of other transmitters, including those of excitatory amino acid synapses and of the neuromuscular junction. (Reproduced with permission from Bleck TP, 1991b, Tetanus, *Infections of the Central Nervous System*, eds Scheld WM, Whitley RJ, Durack DT, Raven Press, New York).

tral inhibitory systems in others. For further details on the clinical picture, beyond that which will be presented here, and for further detail on tetanus generally, the reader is referred to the outstanding monograph by Bleck (1991a).

9.1 Generalized tetanus

This is the most common form of tetanus, at least in adults. Three striking elements seen in most patients are trismus (lockjaw), risus sardonicus and opisthotonus (Fig. 36.13). The principal problems or potential problems are airway obstruction, diaphragmatic

compromise, and dysfunction of the autonomic nervous system. Since the toxin already in the α motor neurons is inaccessible to antitoxin, the disease progresses for 10–14 days after antitoxin is administered.

Trismus is due to rigidity of the masseter muscles and, of course, limits the patient's ability to open the mouth. It is the most common symptom but back or shoulder stiffness may precede it. Risus sardonicus (a 'sneering grin') may be subtle and recognized only by family or close friends. Abdominal rigidity is commonly present at the time of onset of the disease. With severe tetanus, all muscles contract, with the stronger muscles overpowering the weaker. The patient is

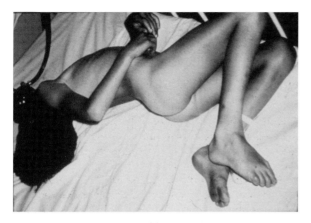

Fig. 36.13 Young boy with tetanus, opisthotonus. (Courtesy of Professor Trevor Willis).

afebrile, rational and anxious. The generalized tetanic spasm, so characteristic of the disease, is dramatic, resembling decorticate posturing. Weinstein's description (1973) of this is excellent: 'a sudden burst of tonic contraction of muscle groups causing opisthotonus, flexion and adduction of the arms, clenching of the fists on the thorax, and extension of the lower extremities'. These spasms are extremely painful and there is no associated loss of consciousness, points crucial in the differential diagnosis of decorticate posturing and of an epileptic seizure. Although epilepsy can be induced with tetanus toxin in experimental animals, true epilepsy occurs in tetanus only when there has been severe hypoxic brain damage.

Airway obstruction during spasms is common and may lead to apnoea, especially when the diaphragm and abdominal musculature are involved. Diaphragmatic or vocal cord paralysis may occur. Autonomic nervous system involvement, with hypersympathetic activity, is typically noted toward the end of the first week of illness; this appears to be mediated by disinhibition of sympathetic neurons in the intermediolateral cell columns. Features of this type of involvement include labile hypertension, tachycardia, cardiac arrhythmias, peripheral vascular constriction, profuse sweating, fever, increased carbon dioxide output, increased levels of plasma catecholamines and increased urinary catecholamine excretion, and, at times, hypotension. The catecholamine picture is similar to that noted in phaeochromocytoma patients and a cardiomyopathy may be seen in both conditions. Parasympathetic function may be disrupted as well, leading to bradycardia, hypotension and even asystole. Gastric emptying may be disturbed.

9.2 Local tetanus

Localized tetanus is manifested by rigidity of the muscles at or near a site of injury. The involved muscles may include the prime movers, agonists, antagonists and fixators. This condition may become stable and chronic (for months) and then resolve spontaneously, but most often it progresses to generalized tetanus. Neuromuscular transmission may be affected, leading to weakness as well as rigidity. Partial immunity may be responsible for the localized form of the disease and thus prevent progression to generalized tetanus.

9.3 Cephalic tetanus

This is a form of localized disease that affects the face, most often the muscles innervated by the lower cranial nerves. Cephalic tetanus makes up only 1% of all cases of tetanus, but 17% of cases related to injuries of the head or face (Mohapatra et al. 1993). Initially, the cranial nerve abnormalities may be unilateral. Peripheral facial nerve weakness, related to neuromuscular junction blocking, is usually present and is typically the initial event noted. Dysphagia may also occur. When the muscles mediating extraocular movement are involved, 'ophthalmoplegic tetanus' results.

9.4 Neonatal tetanus

This form of the disease has 2 prerequisities: a mother lacking in immunity and contamination of the umbilical stump with tetanus spores. Although certain obstetrical practices in some cultures may be responsible, most cases are related to unsterile equipment or dressings. The most common presentation is weakness and inability to suck, usually noted during the second week of life. Later, classical findings of tetanus such as rigidity, spasms and opisthotonus are seen. A hypersympathetic state is commonly seen and often leads to the death of the infant with neonatal tetanus. The prognosis generally is grim. Developmental retardation is common in survivors.

9.5 Complications of tetanus

Hypoxia is one of the more common complications of tetanus, despite the general availability of intensive care units in developed countries; it is due to delay or inadequate treatment of respiratory problems. Cardiovascular problems related to hypersympathetic activity are still seen. Other complications include phrenic and laryngeal nerve palsies, other mononeuropathies, rhabdomyolysis, acute renal failure, myositis ossificans circumscripta, and vertebral compression fractures. Serious psychological after effects are seen in 40% of patients and many patients feel that their general health has worsened after recovery from tetanus (Luisto 1989).

10 TETANUS IN ANIMALS

Mammals vary in their susceptibility to tetanus; some, such as the mouse, the monkey, and the horse, are highly susceptible; others, such as the dog and cat, much less so. Most birds and cold-blooded animals are extremely resistant. Examination of the blood of susceptible and partly susceptible animals shows that, though most cattle contain more than 1/500 unit of antitoxin per ml, no antitoxin is present in the blood of dogs, pigs, monkeys, or rodents. Sheep and goats may contain small quantities (Coleman and Meyer 1926, Coleman 1931, Ramon and Lemétayer 1934, 1935), and also horses in some countries.

The frequent presence of antitoxin in the blood of ruminants may be causally associated with the comparative resistance of these animals to tetanus. It is suggested that in ruminants tetanus bacilli multiply and form toxin in the digestive reservoirs which precede the true stomach, and that the toxin so formed, partly modified perhaps by the products of bacterial fermentation, is absorbed and gives rise to antitoxin. Examination of the blood of naturally resistant species has proved it to be devoid of antitoxin (Vaillard 1892). In some, it may be due to a failure of toxin to reach susceptible nerve tissue. Thus, in the susceptible rabbit a large intravenous dose of toxin disappears from the blood within a day (Marie 1897), but it persists in the blood of the insusceptible hen for several days (Vaillard 1892). The natural disease attacks horses more frequently than other animals, and is especially common in warm and tropical countries. In northern Europe the incidence is low; thus during 1899–1908 in the Prussian Army the annual average number of equine cases was only 0.6 per 1000 (Hutyra and Marek 1912). Tetanus occurs less frequently in cattle, sheep and goats, though it is not uncommon in ewes after parturition and in lambs after docking and castration. It is less common in the pig and uncommon in the dog. Infection occurs by contamination of wounds of skin, or of raw surfaces; nails in the hoof, castration, tail docking, harness galling, bone fractures, and imperfect treatment of the navel at birth seem to be responsible for the majority of cases.

Prophylactic injection of equine antitoxin is recommended in operations on the horse. A dose of not less than 3000 units is recommended. The passive immunity so conveyed lasts longer in the horse than in other animals because the antibodies are homologous, and are therefore destroyed more slowly. The recommended prophylactic dose for pigs, calves and sheep is not less than 500 units, and for piglets, lambs and dogs, not less than 250 units.

Buxton and Glenny (1921) actively immunized horses with 3 injections, at intervals of 3 days, of a toxin–antitoxin mixture. A month later the animals withstood 2000 guinea pig MLD of crude toxin (see also Glenny, Hamp and Stevens 1932).

Tetanus toxoid is an effective prophylactic in the horse and other domestic animals. Two doses of 1–2 ml of purified toxoid adsorbed with aluminium phosphate, 4 weeks or more apart, provide a satisfactory immune response without side effects; reactions to less pure toxoids may be troublesome in thoroughbred horses. Lambs and sheep respond satisfactorily to tetanus toxoid (Adey, Oxer and Kennedy 1939), which may be given as a component of a multiple clostridial vaccine adsorbed with alum (Sterne et al. 1962); it has also been given in Freund's incomplete adjuvant, the water-in-oil emulsion being injected intraperitoneally (Thomson et al. 1969).

In horses, the therapeutic effect of antitoxin is dubious (Mohler and Eichhorn 1911). A dose of not less than 10 000 units followed by daily injections of 1–3 million units has been recommended.

11 DIAGNOSIS

The diagnosis of tetanus must be made clinically and depends on clinical awareness. Absence of a precipitating wound does not exclude the diagnosis. Patients without an apparent source of infection or wound contamination should be questioned and examined for parenteral drug abuse, otitis media or externa, rectal or vaginal instrumentation, recent intramuscular injections, and minor surgical procedures. Laboratory confirmation is often difficult, because the site of infection may be very small or inapparent.

Microscopic examination should be made, where possible, of pus or necrotic material in the wound, and special note taken of bacilli with round, terminal spores. The presence of 'drumstick' bacilli is not, however, pathognomonic of infection with *C. tetani* (see e.g. Boyd and MacLennan 1942). The organisms may be present in such small numbers that they are overlooked.

Cultural methods have also been recommended (see Willis 1969). The pus or wound scrapings, or tissue taken from a necrotic focus in the wound, should be plated on blood agar for anaerobic incubation and seeded into one or more bottles of cooked-meat medium. One bottle should be incubated unheated and the remainder after heating to 80°C in a water bath for various times from 5 to 20 min with the aim of killing non-sporing bacilli and leaving tetanus spores unharmed. Enrichment of the wound specimen in broth containing 1:100 000 crystal violet is said to be effective (Gilles 1937), and ascorbic acid polymyxin thioglycollate broth has also been used for this purpose (Wetzler, Marshall and Cardella 1956). The inoculated liquid media are incubated at 37°C and subcultured on half of a blood agar plate daily for at least 4 days. The plates are incubated anaerobically and examined for the swarming edge of growth of *C. tetani*. Colonies on blood agar are 4–6 mm in diameter, flat, translucent and grey with a matte surface and are surrounded by a narrow zone of β-haemolysis. The colony margins are irregular and rhizoid. The incubated cooked-meat broths should also be heated at 80°C and samples plated at short time intervals. A blood agar plate containing 4% agar to minimize swarming, one half of which has been treated with antitoxin, may be seeded on each half with growth presumed to be *C. tetani* and incubated for 2 days at 37°C. Colonies haemolytic on the untreated half, but not on the antitoxin half, are almost certainly toxigenic *C. tetani* (Lowbury and Lilly 1958). However, it should be appreciated that clinical decisions should not be based on culture results since valuable time would be lost, cultures are not uncommonly negative, recovery of the organism in an immune host is of no meaning, and some strains of *C. tetani* are non-toxigenic.

The toxigenicity of the bacilli is confirmed by demonstrating the production of tetanospasmin in a toxin–antitoxin neutralization test. Two mice, one unprotected and the other given, 1–2 h earlier, a subcutaneous or intraperitoneal injection of 1000 units of tetanus antitoxin, are challenged by a subcutaneous injection in the hind leg of 0.5 ml of a 48 h cooked-meat broth culture of the isolate mixed with 2% calcium chloride. The protected mouse remains well; the unprotected animal shows typical ascending tetanus.

A protective titre of antibody to tetanus toxin measured by immunoassay or haemagglutination may be helpful in excluding the diagnosis, but it usually takes several days to get the results of such tests. Furthermore, there are some reports of localized tetanus, and even generalized tetanus, in patients with titres of antibody that were supposedly protective.

Electrophysiological studies of patients with localized tetanus are said to give characteristic results that would be helpful diagnostically (Woo, Yu and Huang 1988).

The differential diagnosis of tetanus includes strychnine poisoning, dystonic reactions to neuroleptic drugs (these typically involve torticollis and often protrusion of the tongue as well as oculogyric crises), hysteria or psychiatric disorders, hypocalcaemic or alkalotic tetany, the stiff man syndrome, status epilepticus, meningitis, dental or other infection leading to trismus, and dislocation of the mandible with simulated trismus. Rapid improvement of symptoms following intravenous benztropine or diphenhydramine indicate a dystonic reaction to a drug. The cerebrospinal fluid is normal in tetanus (although elevation of the protein level may be seen). Strychnine acts as a direct antagonist at the glycine receptor and thus produces the same lack of presynaptic inhibition seen in generalized tetanus. Lack of abdominal rigidity between spasms is probably more common in strychnine poisoning. Serum and urine should be examined for the presence of strychnine in suspected cases. Even when strychnine intoxication is likely, it would be wise to continue to consider the diagnosis of tetanus.

12 THERAPY

The clinical management of tetanus depends on:

1 the neutralization of any unfixed toxin by antitoxin
2 the control of further bacterial proliferation and toxin production by antimicrobial therapy
3 wound toilet, excision of infected or devitalized tissue, and removal of foreign bodies and
4 the provision of constant nursing care and supportive treatment, supplemented as necessary by anticonvulsive therapy and, in severe cases, by neuromuscular block with curare accompanied by tracheostomy and intermittent positive-pressure ventilation (see Ellis 1963, Laurence and Webster 1963, Smythe, Bowie and Voss 1974, Collee and van Heyningen 1991).

Airway and ventilatory control are critical. Tetanus requires the ultimate in intensive care. Any patient, regardless of age or severity of tetanus, has a chance for full recovery if management is optimal. In one study, patients over 70 years of age fared as well as those under 70; this emphasizes the importance of aggressive care in the intensive care unit setting, no matter how old the patient (Jolliet et al. 1990). Antispasticity drugs, particularly benzodiazepines, play an important role. Autonomic dysfunction is increasingly recognized as a serious problem; it can usually be managed by labetalol, clonidine, morphine, or epidural anaesthesia It is important to remember to actively immunize all tetanus patients upon recovery to prevent recurrence. Remarkable quantities of protein and carbohydrate are required to maintain a positive nitrogen balance because of the muscle activity and excessive autonomic output. There is no evidence that corticosteroid therapy is beneficial in tetanus and it certainly might lead to complications.

12.1 Immunotherapy

Antitoxin neutralization of toxin that has not yet entered the nervous system shortens the course of tetanus and probably reduces its severity. Human tetanus immunoglobulin (HTIG) is the preferred antitoxin preparation and should be given as soon as possible after the patient's spasms are controlled. Effectiveness of antitoxin was demonstrated in the studies of Blake et al. (1976). A dose of 500 IU is as effective as the much larger doses originally recommended. It should be given as a single intramuscular injection; the HTIG preparations currently available in the USA cannot be given intravenously or intrathecally. Intravenous administration is probably preferable to intramuscular in areas where the HTIG is suitable for IV use. Intrathecal therapy has also been considered desirable (Gupta et al. 1980) but a meta-analysis of reports of such therapy by Abrutyn and Berlin (1991) concluded that such therapy is not of proven benefit. In a few cases of tetanus, there has been a recurrence of spasms within a few days after an initial response to antitoxin. A further dose of antitoxin may be of value in such cases (Passen and Andersen 1986).

12.2 Management of portal of entry

The first doses of antitoxin and antimicrobial drugs and control of the patient's spasms should precede surgical debridement of the wound. Surgery should be performed under local anaesthesia.

The course of tetanus is not influenced by wound care and surgery does not affect the need for antitoxin.

12.3 Antimicrobial therapy

C. tetani is susceptible in vitro to a number of antimicrobial agents including penicillins, cephalosporins, penems, erythromycin and other macrolides, metronidazole and tetracycline. Although antimicrobials may be considered of questionable value in a disease process that is an intoxication, penicillin has been recommended by many in the field. However, it must be kept in mind that penicillin is a centrally acting GABA antagonist (Clarke and Hill 1972) and it might therefore act in concert with tetanus toxin to worsen the hypertonic symptoms and perhaps decrease the efficacy of benzodiazepines. A study by Ahmadsyah and Salim (1985) compared metronidazole 2 g per day orally to procaine penicillin (4.5 million units i.m. per day); the metronidazole-treated patients showed significantly less progression of their disease, shorter hospitalization period, and higher survival rate. This might mean that metronidazole was better than penicillin or, alternatively, that penicillin was detrimental. Metronidazole (and clindamycin) were shown to suppress toxin synthesis in *C. perfringens* in an experimental model of gas gangrene (Stevens, Laine and Mitten 1987); they might do this with *C. tetani* as well. In any case, antimicrobial therapy must never be used as a substitute for antitoxin therapy and proper wound care.

12.4 Control of airway and ventilation

The airway must be protected from the beginning because it frequently becomes occluded during tetanic spasms. An endotracheal tube may be placed with the patient under sedation and neuromuscular blockade (it is wise to place a soft feeding tube into the stomach via the oesophagus at the same time). Tracheostomy will not uncommonly be required later as the endotracheal tube itself may serve as a stimulus for further spasms. Careful pulmonary hygiene and management of ventilation will help minimize the incidence of pneumonia and pneumothorax, common problems in these patients.

12.5 Antispasticity agents

Benzodiazepines are the agents of choice for control of rigidity and spasms in tetanus patients; these drugs are GABA agonists and therefore indirectly antagonize the effect of toxin. These drugs, however, do not restore glycinergic inhibition. The greatest experience is with diazepam, but lorazepam may be more desirable because of its longer duration of action. Very large doses may be required and parenteral preparations contain propylene glycol which may lead to metabolic acidosis. Use of a feeding tube for administration of these agents avoids this problem. Another approach is to use midazolam by continuous intravenous infusion at a rate of 5–15 mg h^{-1} (it has a short half-life); this compound does not require propylene glycol as a solvent. Withdrawal symptoms may follow discontinuation of benzodiazepines, so doses should be tapered over a period of 2 weeks. Tachyphylaxis may lead to increased dosage requirements over time. Just enough benzodiazepine compound should be given to prevent spasms and induce adequate sedation. Intrathecal baclofen, a GABA agonist, is another

therapeutic option but has no advantages over the benzodiazepines, except in less developed countries since it may reduce the need for mechanical ventilation. There may be a place for propofol, a nonbarbiturate sedative, but it should not be used as a single agent because it does not have GABA agonist activity.

If GABA agonists cannot control the effects of tetanus, neuromuscular junction blockade is necessary. Vecuronium (by constant infusion) or pancuronium (by intermittent injection) are effective for this purpose. Patients should also receive sedation while getting neuromuscular blockade; this is important to keep them from perceiving their situation and to help blot out the memory of what they have been going through. Autonomic signs cannot be relied on to indicate inadequate sedation because patients may also have sympathetic (and sometimes parasympathetic) dysfunction; accordingly, electroencephalographic monitoring is necessary.

12.6 Autonomic nervous system dysfunction

The therapy of choice for the hypersympathetic signs and symptoms of tetanus is combined α- and β-adrenergic nervous system blockade with labetalol. β-Adrenergic blockade should not be used alone because of the risk of hypertension. Clonidine is a useful alternative to labetalol and morphine can be effective. Epidural anaesthesia is also effective.

Hyperfunction of the parasympathetic nervous system is rare. It may lead to bradycardia or asystole in which case a pacemaker may be required.

13 PROPHYLAXIS

The prevention of tetanus depends primarily on immunization and on prompt and adequate attention to wounds. Hygienic precautions in midwifery are important in the prevention of neonatal tetanus (see Woodruff et al. 1984). Tetanus occurring in children and adults in the general population can be largely controlled by an effective programme of active immunization. In the immunocompetent host, tetanus is an 'inexcusable disease' (Edsall 1976). Active immunization with toxoid is one of the most effective preventive measures in medicine and passive immunization is now readily carried out with human tetanus immunoglobulin.

Specific prophylactic measures include the use of tetanus antitoxin and tetanus toxoid. The administration of antibiotics does not replace adequate surgical toilet but may sometimes be a useful adjunct.

13.1 Principles of management of tetanus-prone wounds

The clinical features of tetanus-prone wounds are shown in Table 36.1.

Table 36.1 Clinical features of tetanus-prone wounds

Clinical features	Tetanus-prone wounds	Non-tetanus-prone wounds
Age of wound	>6 h	≤6 h
Configuration	Stellate wound, avulsion, abrasion	Linear wound
Depth	>1 cm	≤1 cm
Mechanism of injury	Missile, crush, burn, frostbite	Sharp surface (e.g. knife, glass)
Signs of infection	Present	Absent
Devitalized tissue	Present	Absent
Contaminants (dirt, faeces, soil, saliva)	Present	Absent
Denervated and/or ischaemic tissue	Present	Absent

Reprinted from Edlich et al., 1986, with permission.

The perfusion and oxygenation of tissue adjacent to a wound are likely to be impaired for some days and the O–R potential (Eh) within a wound is reduced until healing is established. The impaired oxygenation is exacerbated by the presence of a foreign body or of devitalized tissue. The growth of aerobic and facultative organisms within the wound makes additional demands on the oxygen supply, further reducing the Eh and encouraging the germination of anaerobic spores with toxin production. Wounds requiring special attention are lacerations, stabs, bites (animal and human), wounds that are deep and penetrating, and those that receive delayed attention or are heavily contaminated with agricultural or horticultural materials or soil. In general such wounds should not be sutured; packing, with consequently delayed primary closure, or grafting may be preferable, and frequent follow-up inspection is necessary. Prompt and thorough surgical attention is of paramount importance. Foreign materials and devitalized tissues must be removed and the wound edges excised if the tissues are not viable.

Immune status should be determined if possible, but when a patient is unconscious and there are no records or other reliable data it is advisable to assume that immunity is lacking. Protective immunity depends upon a full course of adsorbed tetanus toxoid (TT) completed or boosted within the previous 5–10 years. If the patient has received a full course of tetanus toxoid or a booster toxoid injection within the previous 5 years, a further toxoid injection should not be given unless the risk of tetanus is assessed as high; unnecessary TT injections may lead to painful local reactions. If 5–10 years have elapsed since the last full course of tetanus toxoid or booster injection, a further booster injection of adsorbed toxoid is advisable. If the patient has not been immunized, or if the matter is in doubt, the first dose of a full course of adsorbed toxoid injections should be given immediately, along with an injection of antitoxin. The prophylactic dose of HTIG is 250 units intramuscularly. Adsorbed tetanus toxoid should be given at the same time as HTIG to start a course of active immunization in a non-immune patient. The toxoid should be given with a separate syringe and injected into a contralateral site. The second and third injections of adsorbed toxoid are given at monthly intervals.

The recommendations of the US Advisory Committee on Immunization Practices for tetanus prophylaxis in routine wound management are noted in Table 36.2.

13.2 Natural immunity

Mammals vary in their susceptibility to tetanus (see below). There is no evidence (see Lahiri 1939) that small amounts of naturally acquired antitoxin (Matzkin and Regev 1985) are protective in man. Indeed, a lethal dose of toxin may be much less than an effective immunizing dose, and patients who survive tetanus are not naturally protected against a further challenge.

Table 36.2 Summary of recommendations of Advisory Committee on Immunization Practices for tetanus prophylaxis in routine wound management – United States, 1991

History of adsorbed tetanus toxoid (doses)	Clean, minor wounds		All other wounds[a]	
	Td[b]	TIG	Td[b]	TIG
Unknown or <3	Yes	No	Yes	Yes
≥3[c]	No[d]	No	No[e]	No

[a]Such as, but not limited to, wounds contaminated with dirt, faeces, soil, saliva; puncture wounds; avulsions; and wounds resulting from missiles, crushing, burns, and frostbite.
[b]For children <7 years old, DTP (DT, if pertussis vaccine is contraindicated) is preferred to tetanus toxoid alone. For persons ≥7 years of age, Td is preferred to tetanus toxoid alone. Diphtheria and tetanus toxoids and acellular pertussis vaccine (DTaP) may be used instead of DTP for the fourth and fifth doses.
[c]If only 3 doses of *fluid* toxoid have been received, then a fourth dose of toxoid, preferably an adsorbed toxoid, should be given.
[d]Yes, if more than 10 years since last dose.
[e]Yes, if more than 5 years since last dose. (More frequent boosters are not needed and can accentuate side effects.)
Reprinted from Prevots et al., 1992, with permission.

13.3 Preparation and specification of tetanus antitoxin

Owing to its exceptional potency, tetanus toxin cannot readily be used in the preparation of antitoxin. Many substances have been used to detoxify the toxin without destroying its immunogenicity.

Detoxification with formaldehyde (Descombey 1924) is now widely used. Usually about 0.4% of formol is added to the toxin and the mixture is incubated at 37–39°C until it is sufficiently detoxified. The toxoid is commonly adsorbed with an aluminium salt to increase its antigenic efficacy (see Glenny et al. 1926). After inducing substantial immunity with formol toxoid, immunization of the horse may be completed with crude toxin to yield serum containing as many as 1000 units of antitoxin per ml.

Human antitetanus immunoglobulin has largely replaced horse serum antitoxin for tetanus prophylaxis because it has the considerable advantages of a longer half-life and freedom from the risks of adverse reactions and of early elimination. It is obtained by separating the IgG fraction from the plasma of immunized volunteers who are free from evidence of hepatitis, HIV or other transmissible infection, usually by cold-ethanol fractionation, and is commonly provided at a concentration of 250 units of antitoxin in an injection volume of 1.0 ml.

The **specification** of the potency of tetanus antitoxin, whether of animal or human origin, is made in terms of a stable, standard antitoxin to which is assigned an arbitrary figure expressed as units.

In 1928, the Permanent Commission on Standardization of the League of Nations recommended the US National Institutes of Health (NIH) standard (Roseneau and Anderson 1908) as the international standard preparation. Although this recommendation was adopted, the international unit was made equal not to the established NIH unit but to one-half this unit, with the result that for many years the international unit (1928) was in conflict with the NIH unit. This discrepancy was resolved in 1950 by the Expert Committee on Biological Standardization of the World Health Organization, which doubled the size of the international unit. The international unit (1950) is now equal to the NIH unit (Report 1950) and, as defined in 1969 by the WHO Expert Committee on Biological Standardization, is the activity contained in 0.03384 mg of the second international standard for tetanus antitoxin (Spaun and Lyng 1970).

Antitoxin titrations are carried out by comparing the amount needed to protect mice against a fixed test dose of toxin with the amount of standard antitoxin needed to give the same degree of protection. A convenient test dose of toxin is the smallest quantity which, mixed with one international unit of the standard antitoxin (or a fraction of one unit), causes clearly recognizable paralysis within 4 days but does not cause significant suffering; mild but definite paralysis of the hind leg is suitable for this purpose. This Lp dose of toxin is preferable to the L + dose, i.e., that which kills the animal by the fourth day, as it minimizes the illness to which the mice are subjected (Mussett and Sheffield 1976, *British Pharmacopoeia* 1980).

Comparative assays in a number of institutions show that, provided one specimen of toxin is employed in the assay of antitoxin in terms of the standard, similar results are obtained by different workers. The toxic filtrates commonly used for assay, however, vary greatly with the strain of *C. tetani* and the medium selected for its growth. Even when the greatest care is taken in the selection of the test toxin,

in the technique of administration, and in the choice of strain, there are qualitative as well as quantitative differences among antitoxins that may vitiate the assay (Report 1938, Smith 1938, Ipsen 1940–41, Hornibrook 1952). The relative potency of 2 antitoxins may vary with the species of animal used in the test (Smith 1943–44) or with the route of administration of the toxin–antitoxin mixtures (Friedemann and Hollander 1943). The change of potency ratio with change of the biological system used for an assay indicates a heterogeneity of some kind in the materials used. In this case we may postulate heterogeneity of the antibodies, either in reactivity (see e.g. Cinader and Weitz 1953) or in specificity. The specificity of the antibody may vary because molecules of toxin vary, or because the antibodies are specific only for portions of the toxin molecule. Nagel and Cohen (1973) described 4 different antigenic determinants on both toxin and formol toxoid, and all of the corresponding 4 antitoxins were capable of neutralizing toxin in vivo. Antibodies to tetanus toxin are able to neutralize even though they do not bind to the ganglioside-binding site of the toxin (Kryzhanovsky 1973).

The potency of unrefined antitoxins may be measured by flocculation methods analogous to the Ramon titration of diphtheria antitoxin (see e.g. Goldie, Parsons and Bowers 1942), but proteolytically refined antitoxins may not flocculate satisfactorily.

Antitoxin may also be assayed in vitro by agglutination of tanned red cells coated with toxoid (Fulthorpe 1957, 1958), by the enzyme-linked immunosorbent assay (Voller, Bidwell and Bartlett 1976) and, in screening assays, by immunodiffusion methods (Eldridge and Entwhistle 1975, Winsnes 1979). Immunoelectrophoresis methods (Wiseman and Gascoigne 1977) have been used to select donors for the preparation of human tetanus antitoxin. However, such tests do not always precisely reflect neutralizing activity, probably owing to avidity effects as well as to the existence of different antigenic determinants on the toxin molecule.

The half-life of homologous human antitoxin in man is longer than that of heterologous antitoxin, approximately 28 days; consequently, a given period of passive protection can be secured with a smaller dose. Although immunoglobulin allotypes occur, immune elimination does not appear to have been reported.

The minimum concentration of antitoxin in the serum that is adequate to provide immunity is uncertain but a figure of 0.01 unit ml^{-1} is often accepted (McComb and Dwyer 1963, Adams, Laurence and Smith 1969, Smith 1969). Thus, when a population of women immunized during pregnancy had a mean serum antitoxin concentration of 0.01 unit ml^{-1}, tetanus neonatorum in their babies was prevented (MacLennan et al. 1965). Similar studies in Colombia suggested that the immunity threshold may be less than 0.01 unit ml^{-1} (Newell et al. 1971), but mild tetanus has been described in patients known to have had concentrations greater than 0.01 unit ml^{-1} in their serum (Goulon et al. 1972, Berger et al. 1978). Moreover, although the neutralizing capacity of antitoxin is considerable – 250 units has the capacity to neutralize in vitro about 30 million minimal lethal doses for the mouse – passive immunity is less protective than active immunity (d'Antona and Valensin 1937). Probably 0.01 unit ml^{-1} of serum should be regarded as the minimum protective concentration in passive immunity, but for patients with severe, soiled wounds, prophylactic doses of antitoxin larger than usual should be considered.

13.4   Antitoxin prophylaxis

Passive immunization with horse-derived antitoxin, coupled with surgical debridement of the wound, was the standard method for prevention of tetanus for a long time. It was used extensively for the wounded in World War I and, for those who have not been actively immunized, is still being used in some countries where human antitoxin is not available. The aim is to provide a protective amount of antitoxin in the serum of the injured person until toxin production in a wound is likely to have ceased.

A dose of 250 units of human antitoxin should provide protection for about 4 weeks in adults (Rubbo 1966), including the severely injured; but in extensively burned patients this dose may be insufficient (Lowbury et al. 1978). The suggested indications for passive immunization of injured persons who are not known to be actively immune are: wounds over 6 h old; infected wounds; wounds through skin contaminated with soil, street mud or dust, animal faeces and the like; deep wounds, including puncture wounds; wounds with devitalizing tissue damage; and wounds that cannot be closed (Parish, Laurent and Moynihan 1957, Smith, Laurence and Evans 1975). In the case of severe wounds and especially burns, the systemic dose may be doubled or tripled. A portion of the dose may be injected around the wound.

Animal experiments clearly establish the value of prophylactic antitoxin. In man the evidence is indirect and often equivocal in that it is not always possible to exclude other causes for the effects attributed to antitoxin:

1   The prophylactic injection of antitoxin within a few hours of wounding appears to diminish greatly the chances of tetanus.
2   When it does not prevent the development of tetanus, antitoxin appears to lengthen the incubation period. Since the passive immunity conferred by a single dose of antitoxin lasts only some 2–3 weeks, it is possible that late developing tetanus in some injured persons who receive antitoxin is due to tetanus bacilli in the wound becoming effectively toxigenic after passive immunity has waned; this might be prevented by repeated doses of antitoxin.
3   Tetanus developing in persons who have received a prophylactic injection appears to be less likely to be fatal than in uninoculated persons (Bruce 1920).
4   Among all patients with tetanus, the percentage in whom the disease became generalized fell from 98.9 in 1914 to 83.5 in 1918 (Bruce 1920). This may be attributed partly to the more general and effective use of antitoxin prophylactically and partly to improved diagnosis of local tetanus.

Suggestive evidence is also provided by Bazy (1914). Of 200 soldiers with similar wounds, 100 were not given antitoxin, for unspecified reasons, and 18 of these patients developed tetanus. In the 100 who were given antitoxin only one case occurred, on the day after injection.

Lucas and Willis (1965) reported that, when horse serum was replaced by antibiotic prophylaxis for injured patients attending a casualty department in Ibadan, Nigeria, the incidence of tetanus among them rose from 2.3 to 7.8 cases per 10 000 patients, and the rate fell to 2.4 cases when there was a return to the use of antiserum.

13.5   Reactions to antitoxin

The use of human antitoxin in place of horse serum has largely overcome the danger of serious reactions to passive tetanus prophylaxis. Mild local reactions sometimes follow intramuscular injection, and a few instances of severe generalized reactions have been reported (Glaser and Wyss-Souffront 1961, Mackenzie and Vlahcevic 1974).

Passive immunization with heterologous antibody (usually of equine origin) has the disadvantage that persons receiving it for the first time may become sensitized and have immediate or delayed types of allergic reactions to a subsequent injection of the same proteins. Similar reactions may occur in persons already sensitized. The incidence of local and general reactions to horse antitoxin has been variously estimated at 5–50%, the variation reflecting differences in the criteria used for defining a reaction, the thoroughness of follow-up, the purity of the antitoxin used, and the differences in the populations studied.

Before injecting the full dose of heterologous antitoxin, it is wise to test the patient's reactivity. The type of test that provides the best indicator of a potential reaction to the full dose is uncertain. An intradermal, conjunctival or subcutaneous test can be used. Laurent and Parish (1958) distrust the intradermal reaction. They have often injected a full dose of serum without ill effect when the test has been positive, and they have known of fatal cases of anaphylactic shock when it has been negative. They regard the reaction to a subcutaneous trial injection of 0.2 ml of serum as giving a more certain indication of the possibility of the reaction most to be feared – acute anaphylaxis.

13.6   Simultaneous active and passive immunization

The simultaneous injection of tetanus toxoid and antitoxin is of value to begin the active immunization in a wounded person. The antitoxin may interfere with the response of the body to the toxoid – the so-called blanketing effect. This has been demonstrated in the guinea pig (see Smith 1964), but in man, provided adsorbed toxoid is used, the objection is primarily of theoretical interest. Though the serum may delay somewhat the response to toxoid given simultaneously, the ultimate immunity after the second and third doses appears to be the same as after the administration of toxoid alone (Bergentz and Philipson 1958, Tasman and Huygen 1962, Fulthorpe 1965, Züst 1967). There is now ample evidence to support the soundness and wisdom of the procedure, both with equine and human antitoxin. In practice, various doses of toxoid and antitoxin are given. Toxoid, adsorbed on to aluminium hydroxide or aluminium phosphate, is generally injected in a dose of 5–20 Lf (flocculation units) into one arm, and 250 units of tetanus immunoglobulin injected into the other (Suri and Rubbo 1961, McComb and Dwyer 1963, Smith et al. 1963, Levine et al. 1966, Züst 1967). The subsequent injections of toxoid are given at the usual intervals. Ideally, simultaneous immunization should ensure a continuous immunity – passive replaced by active – from the time of injection, but this is difficult to secure. Cohen and Leussink (1973) examined the effect of different adsorbed toxoids in small groups of subjects given 250 units of human antitoxin in a different limb. Vaccine that contained 5 Lf of toxoid resulted, 3 weeks after simultaneous immunization, in titres of antitoxin higher than those produced by vaccine containing 10 Lf; this was attributed to the capacity of the toxoid to bind the passive antitoxin. In patients suffering from tetanus and treated with a large dose of antitoxin, active immunization should be deferred for 3 or 4 weeks.

13.7 Active immunization

Since the demonstration of the antitoxigenic value of toxoid (formaldehyde-treated toxin; Descombey 1924) and of toxoid precipitated with alum (Bergey 1934), aluminium hydroxide or phosphate (Tasman and van Ramshorst 1952), or calcium phosphate (Relyveld et al. 1969), these agents have been widely tested in man. Owing to the low incidence of tetanus in peace-time, the efficacy of active immunization has been for the most part judged by the antitoxin response in the inoculated subject, but evidence from World War II showed that it was highly effective in preventing tetanus. There were 2.7 million admissions to US Army hospitals for wounds and injuries during that war. There were only 12 cases of tetanus, 5 with fatal outcome; only 4 of the 12 patients had received the complete basic series of immunizations for tetanus, including a reinforcement dose at 6–12 months. By contrast, during the siege and liberation of Manila in 1945, among 12 000 civilian casualties there were at least 473 cases of tetanus.

A reduction in the incidence of tetanus associated with the introduction of active immunization is reported for a number of civilian communities (Edsall 1959, Ebisawa and Fukutomi 1979, Christenson and Böttiger 1987, Simonsen, Bloch and Heron 1987); this is, at least in part, attributable to immunization. Details on the preparation and control of tetanus toxoid preparations are provided by Wirz, Gentili and Collotti (1990).

13.8 Tetanus toxoid

Formol toxoid is produced from the tetanus toxin released by the bacilli in liquid culture in large-capacity fermenters (Hepple 1968). The choice of medium and of the strain of *C. tetani* used is important, to ensure both a high yield of toxin and freedom from protein in the final product, which might lead to hypersensitivity reactions.

The finding of recombinant tetanus toxin derivatives of fragment C that are immunogenic but do not bind neuronal cells would seem to offer important prospects for a new vaccine (Figueiredo et al. 1995).

13.9 Immunization course

The basic course for immunization adopted in many countries consists of 3 spaced injections. Although a slow antitoxin response usually follows after one injection of adsorbed toxoid and 2 injections suffice to induce a satisfactory immunity, the third injection is usually advised to ensure a long-lasting immunity. The course adopted for the immunization of infants in some countries, the USA and Canada for example, comprises 4 injections of combined diphtheria, tetanus and pertussis vaccine, 3 doses being given at intervals of 4–8 weeks and the fourth dose about 1 year after the third (Centers for Disease Control 1977, National Advisory Committee on Immunization 1979). Even preterm babies respond satisfactorily to tetanus toxoid immunization, starting at 3 months of age (Conway et al. 1987).

There is little doubt that the injection into man of 2–3 doses of toxoid at properly spaced intervals raises the antitoxin content of the blood within a few weeks to prophylactic concentrations. It is noteworthy that in both animals and man the antigenic stimulus of an infection with tetanus is insufficient to induce either a primary antitoxin response, or secondary responsiveness to toxoid. The same observation has been made in relation to diphtheria.

The duration of immunity provided by the basic course of immunization can be long lasting (Trinca 1967), and may be lifelong (Rubbo 1966), though necessarily becoming weaker. The duration is likely to be greater after the use of toxoids of high Lf and aluminium adjuvant content (Trinca 1965, White et al. 1969, MacLennan et al. 1973). Other forms of tetanus toxoid are less immunogenic and should not be used. Since toxoids in use in different countries may differ in these attributes, as well as in the number and spacing of the injections, results from different studies cannot be strictly compared, but numerous observations have shown that even after 10 years the antitoxin content of the serum is usually above that generally accepted as indicative of immunity, namely 0.01 unit ml^{-1} (see Simonsen, Kjeldsen and Heron 1984).

After primary immunization, circulating antitoxin falls gradually for about 10 years and then remains more or less stationary. However, there is variability in the response to primary and secondary immunization in different subjects (see MacLennan et al. 1973). Thus, among the 191 children studied by Scheibel and her colleagues (1966) about 12 years after primary immunization with 3 doses of adsorbed toxin, although most were immune with a mean serum antitoxin of 0.45 unit ml^{-1}, 4.2% had less than 0.01 unit ml^{-1}. The recommendations of the Advisory Committee on Immunization Practices (ACIP) and of the

American Academy of Pediatrics are for 5 immunizations by the age of 6 years with a booster dose at adolescence; this would seem to be a better standard than the current US requirement for 3 immunizations for entry into school. Combined diphtheria–tetanus–pertussis vaccine is used for children up to the age of 7 years. Patients over the age of 7 should receive tetanus–diphtheria vaccine. Poor response has been associated with a particular immunoglobulin allotypic marker (Schanfield, Wells and Fudenberg 1979). The proportion of unsatisfactory responders is liable to be greater after the use of plain toxoid. Thus White and his colleagues (1969) found that 12 of 91 adults immunized with 3 spaced doses of plain toxoid had less than 0.01 unit of antitoxin in their sera 2–4 years after immunization, compared with only 1 of 80 subjects who had had adsorbed toxoid.

The response of the immune mechanism to a reinforcing dose of toxoid in a subject conditioned by primary immunization is striking. Within 3–4 days the antitoxin content of the serum rises and within 10 days often reaches a titre far higher than after primary immunization. Regamey and Schlegel's (1951) observations are reproduced in Table 36.3. The capacity to respond to a single booster dose may persist for at least 30 years after a primary course of adsorbed toxoid (Simonsen, Kjeldsen and Heron 1984). The response to a reinforcing dose is said to vary directly with the preinjection titre (Gottlieb et al. 1964). There appears to be no difference in the rapidity with which an antitoxin response can be detected after a reinforcing dose of plain or adsorbed toxoid (Trinca 1965). Adults who received a partial series earlier in life need only complete the course of immunizations rather than begin again (Gardner and Schaffner 1993).

In view of these considerations there seems little justification for giving repeated reinforcing injections as a routine. The current US Advisory Committee for Immunization Practices (ACIP) recommendation of giving a booster dose of toxoid to adults every 10 years should suffice to keep the antibody content well above the minimal protective concentration. Sanford (1995) feels that hospitals should immunize all adult patients with tetanus and diphtheria toxoids unless there is proof of immunization within the preceding 10 years or a definite contraindication. A reinforcing dose may be required after an injury that might lead to tetanus, but in view of the increasing number of reports of adverse reactions a reinforcing dose is not generally advisable within one year (Report 1972a) or 5 years (Report 1972b, Smith, Laurence and Evans 1975) of a previous injection.

Limited in vitro data suggest that tetanus toxoid administration may provoke activation of latent HIV infection (Margolick et al. 1987) but there is no clinical evidence to indicate that patients with HIV infection should not receive toxoid when indicated. However, one of the immunological consequences of HIV infection is that there is a loss of responsiveness to soluble antigens such as tetanus toxoid (Fuchs et al. 1990); therefore, HIV-infected patients may not achieve immunity. Both HIV-1 and HIV-2 interfere in vitro with proliferation of T lymphocytes specific for tetanus toxin (Chirmule, Saxinger and Pahwa 1989) so that even prior adequate immunizations may not protect them. On the other hand, Opravil et al. (1991) found relatively good baseline levels of antibody and responses to booster immunization in 10 HIV-infected patients, 4 with AIDS. Administration of a monoclonal antibody recognizing the leucocyte common antigen CD45 augments the response of peripheral blood mononuclear cells to tetanus toxoid in vitro (Harris et al. 1990) so similar in vivo manipulation might be beneficial. Further data are reviewed by Pinching (1991).

Patients with humoral immunodeficiencies may have a less than satisfactory response to tetanus toxoid (Webster et al. 1984, Shackelford et al. 1990). Among patients who were seropositive to tetanus before bone marrow transplant, 51% had lost their seropositivity by one year after transplant and 100% by 2 years (Ljungman et al. 1990); reimmunization of 21 patients with 3 doses of toxoid led to seropositivity that was maintained for at least 2 years in all patients.

13.10 Serosurveys of immunity to tetanus

The third National Health and Nutrition Examination Survey conducted in the USA from 1988 to 1991 on over 13 000 individuals over 6 years of age provides data on the prevalence of protective levels of tetanus antibody and identifies groups susceptible to tetanus (Gergen et al. 1995). A solid-phase immunoassay in which the level of antitoxin considered likely to be

Table 36.3 Showing the duration of responsiveness to reinforcing doses of tetanus toxoid induced by 3 primary injections

Years since primary inoculations	Number of subjects tested	Mean number of antitoxin units ml^{-1} of serum at the stated time (days) after reinforcing dose			
		0	4	6	8
1	26	0.70	1.27	9.9	18.9
2–3	10	0.52[a]	2.55	39.6	69.4
4–7	6	0.55	1.32	17.6	63.4
8–9	10	0.22	0.74	25.1	86.0
10	8	0.28	0.63	16.5	90.0

[a]Minimum individual serum antitoxin in this group, 0.0075; in all other groups minima were 0.035 or more.
After Regamey and Schlegel (1951).

protective is 0.15 IU ml^{-1} (considerably higher than the 0.01 IU ml^{-1} determined by a neutralization assay in animals) was used. Over all, 69.7% of the population had protective levels of tetanus antibody. The level was over 80% for persons between 6 and 39 years of age but began to fall sharply at age 40 and was only 27.8% in individuals 70 years of age or older. Non-Hispanic whites had the highest rate of immunity (72.7%), followed by non-Hispanic blacks (68.1%), and then Mexican Americans (57.9%). Poverty was associated with a lower rate of immunity except among non-Hispanic blacks. Birth outside the USA and lower educational status were associated with lower rates of immunity. Males had a higher rate of immunity than females and men who were veterans of military service had a higher rate than other men. Children aged 6 years had an immunity rate of 96%; children 7–9 years, 90%; and children 10–16 years, 80%. There was little difference between children of different racial or ethnic backgrounds. A survey of US travellers gave similar results with regard to older individuals and women having lower titres of tetanus antibody than others (Hilton et al. 1991).

A survey of tetanus immunization status and response to a booster dose of toxoid in an emergency department geriatric population was carried out by Gareau et al. (1990). Of 80 patients, 36 (45%) had inadequate titres at presentation. Only 5 patients could give a definite history of adequate immunization in the past. Response to a booster dose was disappointing; 15 of 34 patients who returned for follow-up 14 days later did not demonstrate a rise in antibody titre. Those who did not seroconvert were significantly older than those who did. More disturbing are data provided in the CDC's *Morbidity and Mortality Weekly Report* for August 8, 1991 in which it was indicated that 58% of tetanus patients with acute injuries did not seek medical care for their injuries and of those who did, 81% did not receive tetanus prophylaxis as recommended by ACIP guidelines (Centers for Disease Control 1991).

13.11 The assay of tetanus toxoid

The specification of fluid tetanus toxoid for use in man is based on the antigenic response in guinea pigs. British regulations, for instance, require that not fewer than 9 guinea pigs are given injections of 5 times the human dose; the vaccine satisfies the requirements if, after 6 weeks, at least two-thirds of the guinea pigs contain 0.05 or more unit of antitoxin per ml of blood serum (*British Pharmacopoeia* 1980). In many countries, plain fluid toxoid is no longer used. The *European Pharmacopoeia*, for example, includes a monograph only for adsorbed toxoid, the potency of which is controlled in terms of International Units by comparison with the International Standard for Tetanus Toxoid (adsorbed). The vaccine is required to possess a minimum potency of not less than 40 units per human dose determined by comparing its ability to immunize mice or guinea pigs with that of the International Standard (van Ramshorst, Sundaresan and Out-

schoorn 1972, Mussett and Sheffield 1973, *European Pharmacopeia* 1977). The potency of adsorbed toxoids determined in mice or guinea pigs has been found to reflect immunizing potency in man. Potency assay of fluid toxoid in mice is less consistent than that of adsorbed toxoid (Cohen, van Ramshorst and Tasman 1959, Scheibel et al. 1968).

The Lf value of a toxoid preparation is not a reliable guide to its antigenicity, mainly because flocculation zones are multiple, and single zones can normally be obtained only with adsorbed sera. With a suitable reference preparation the Lf value can be of use, however, in controlling the purity of tetanus vaccine (Spaun and Lyng 1970, Sheffield et al. 1979). The *European Pharmacopoeia* (1977) and the World Health Organization (1964) requirements specify a minimum acceptable purity for the toxoid of 500 Lf mg^{-1} of protein nitrogen. A purity of over 1000 Lf mg^{-1} of protein nitrogen can readily be secured by salting out with ammonium sulphate.

13.12 Reactions to tetanus toxoid

Purified fluid tetanus toxoid, prepared with protein-free media, is one of the least irritating of vaccines. The primary series of injections seldom causes trouble. In a study of 209 casualty patients at Sheffield only 5 delayed reactions were noted, 3 local and 2 general (Cox, Knowelden and Sharrard 1963). But with repeated reinforcing doses allergy is liable to develop and increase in intensity until injections are followed by severe local and sometimes general reactions (Schneider 1964, Edsall et al. 1967). Very occasionally an anaphylactic reaction occurs in a sensitized subject (Fardon 1967). It is wise to watch all persons for 10 min after injection. Adsorbed toxoid is more irritant. Mahoney, Aprile and Moloney (1967), for example, reported 16% of delayed local reactions after its use. White and his colleagues (1973) reported that among a factory population local reactions occurred in 0.3% of adults after the first injection of the primary course of adsorbed toxoid, in 2.7% after the second dose, and in 7.5% after the third. The rate was 1.6% after post-injury reinforcing doses.

Reactions are more frequently seen in females than males, and are more likely to follow subcutaneous than intramuscular injections (Relihan 1969). Side effects may have become commoner owing to the increasing use of active immunization, especially of reinforcing doses after injury. Although adsorbed toxoid is more liable to cause reactions (Collier, Polakoff and Mortimer 1979), it is more effective, both for primary immunization and for reinforcement of existing immunity. The frequency of reactions is greater when vaccines containing a higher Lf content are used. As with diphtheria, low-dose adsorbed toxoid containing, for example, 1 Lf of antigen, has been found to minimize reactions to reinforcing doses while stimulating a satisfactory antibody response (McComb and Levine 1961, Trinca 1963). Care should be taken to keep tetanus toxoid at a low temperature; if kept for long at

37°C it may regain part of its toxicity (Akama et al. 1971).

Local reactions to purified toxoid are probably the result of an immunologically mediated reaction to the toxoid antigen itself rather than to impurities in the vaccine. Thus, reactors usually have a high titre of serum antitoxin, or respond rapidly to the vaccine (Edsall et al. 1967). Positive skin tests, with the characteristics of delayed-type hypersensitivity, to highly purified toxoid may be found in reactors who do not respond to control tests with purified medium (White et al. 1973); IgE responses occur to reinforcing doses of toxoid (Nagel et al. 1977). However, adjuvants contribute to local reactions and merthiolate sensitivity sometimes plays a part (Hansson and Möller 1971). Toxoid has been reported to increase anti-A and anti-B antibodies, due to the presence of traces of blood group antigens in the vaccine. The immunization of pregnant women with the aim of preventing neonatal tetanus may, therefore, increase the risk of haemolytic disease in the newborn, although no published reports of such a side effect have been made (Gupte and Bahtia 1979). Rare cases of peripheral neuropathy resembling the Guillain–Barré syndrome have been described (Holliday and Bauer 1983).

13.13 Effect of simultaneous immunization with other antigens

It is convenient to mix toxoid with enteric vaccines, pertussis vaccine, diphtheria toxoid or other antigens. The response to toxoid is enhanced by the presence of pertussis vaccine. Scheibel (1944) recorded a depression of the antigenic potency of both diphtheria and tetanus toxoids (adsorbed by $Al(OH)_3$) when they were injected together into guinea pigs. Barr and Llewellyn-Jones (1953) observed a depression of the response when toxoid and enteric vaccines were given in certain proportions to guinea pigs. This occurred especially in animals that had had primary inoculations with the enteric vaccine and in which the secondary response to the vaccine 'crowded out' the response to toxoid. A similar crowding out of primary responses to tetanus toxoid by secondary responses to diphtheria toxoid was observed in children, though not to the extent of diminishing the secondary responsiveness to later injections of tetanus toxoid (Chen et al. 1956, 1957). In man, enteric vaccines are reported to have either no effect (Hegyessey, Bozsoky and Schulek 1956), or a definite adjuvant effect, on toxoid simultaneously administered with them (Ikic 1958). Multiple immunizing antigens should not be given without considering the nature and proportions of the different antigens in the mixture and the immune state of the subject. The frequency of reactions to the diphtheria component of combined diphtheria and tetanus toxoids has led, in the USA, to the use in adults of a combined preparation containing the normal amount of tetanus toxoid and a reduced amount of diphtheria toxoid (Report 1972b). A combined preparation of enteric vaccines with fluid tetanus toxoid has also been found

effective in stimulating a satisfactory antitoxin response when given in an intradermal dose of 0.1 ml containing 2 Lf (Barr, Sayers and Stamm 1959), though the response to the enteric components has not been subjected to clinical trial of the protective effect.

13.14 Community immunization strategy

Formerly, active immunization was confined mainly to the military. The wisdom of immunizing the entire population is now realized, however, and most countries include tetanus toxoid in the vaccines routinely offered to children. The immunization of adults should be directed especially to those at increased risk, such as agricultural, industrial and road workers, persons with chronic ulcers of the lower limbs, and injured patients. Despite such efforts, many people will remain unprotected.

Pregnant women should be immunized, to protect the infant against neonatal tetanus by placentally transmitted maternal antitoxin rather than the mother against puerperal tetanus. Two spaced doses of adsorbed toxoid should be given during pregnancy, if possible before the sixth month (Report 1967). Good results have been reported with a single dose of calcium phosphate-adsorbed vaccine containing 30 Lf of toxoid (Kielmann and Vohra 1977).

14 Prognosis

Prognosis depends on a number of factors such as age, sex, general physique, type and severity of wound, length of incubation period (Table 36.4), receipt of prophylactic antitoxin, the stage at which treatment is begun, the time interval between first symptoms and admission to hospital, and the standard of available treatment – especially in severe cases, which demand curarization and artificial respiration (Cole 1940, Adams, Laurence and Smith 1969, Smythe, Bowie and Voss 1974, Armitage and Clifford 1978). Observations made on large series of patients suggest that the type of injury and its site do not influence the mortality, except in uterine infections and neonatal tetanus, in which the case-fatality rate in the absence of modern methods of treatment may be as high as 90% (Adams and Morton 1955, Patel, Mehta and Modi 1965, Adams 1968). The portal of entry may be an important factor; associated with a poor prognosis are burns, surgical procedures, compound fractures, septic abortions, and intramuscular injections. Narcotic addicts develop very severe tetanus (Cherubin 1968), perhaps because of large inocula of organisms. Fever and tachycardia, related to autonomic dysfunction rather than infection, are dismal signs (Bleck 1991a).

The death rate, apart from that in the newborn, tends to be low in children and to rise later. In England and Wales, the USA and Japan, 50% of the deaths are in persons aged 45 years or over; this may be due partly to the failure of elderly persons to have

Table 36.4 Tetanus mortality in relation to incubation period

Type of tetanus	Number of cases	Incubation period	Case-fatality rate (%)
Adult	2497	0–7 days	52.5
		More than 7 days	32.2
Neonatal	956	0–8 days	60.7
		More than 8 days	19.0

See Patel, Mehta and Modi (1965), Adams (1968).

received immunization. Case fatality is 42% for patients over 50 years of age and 5% for those under 50 (LaForce 1990). There is good evidence that the shorter the incubation period, the worse is the prognosis (see Table 36.4) (see Bruce 1920); according to Cole (1940) and numerous subsequent observers, the period of onset is the more reliable index, this period being defined as the time between appearance of the first symptom of the disease and the first reflex spasms, i.e. convulsive spasms superimposed on the underlying tonic rigidity. From their analysis of the data on 1385 patients treated in India with antitoxin but without curarization, Armitage and Clifford (1978) conclude that the probability of death is separately related to the period of onset, the interval between first symptoms and admission to hospital –

long periods being associated with better prognosis – and the severity of illness on admission. The case-fatality rate was 51% when the period on onset was less than 10 h, and 15% when it was greater than 72 h. Tetanus in patients with reflex spasms but whose illness was judged on admission to be mild had a fatality rate of 26%; when the illness was severe it was 73%. In patients who do not have reflex spasms the prognosis is more favourable. In the days before antiserum was used, the case-fatality rate was about 85% (Bruce 1920). With full modern treatment, including paralysis by curare, positive-pressure ventilation and antitoxin therapy, the case-fatality rate can be reduced to 10% (Smythe, Bowie and Voss 1974, Edmondson and Flowers 1979).

REFERENCES

Abel JJ, 1934, On poisons and diseases and some experiments with the toxin of the bacillus tetani, *Science*, **79:** 63–70, 121.

Abrutyn E, Berlin JA, 1991, Intrathecal therapy in tetanus. A meta-analysis, *JAMA*, **266:** 2262–7.

Adams EB, 1968, The prognosis and prevention of tetanus, *S Afr Med J*, **42:** 739–43.

Adams EB, Laurence DR, Smith JWG, 1969, *Tetanus*, Blackwell Scientific Publications, Oxford.

Adams F (ed. and transl.), 1856, Aretaeus, On tetanus, *The Extant Works of Aretaeus, the Cappadocian*, Sydenham Society, London, as reproduced in Major RH, 1932, *Classic Descriptions of Disease*, C C Thomas, Springfield, IL.

Adams JQ, Morton RF, 1955, Puerperal tetanus, *Am J Obstet Gynecol*, **69:** 169–73.

Adey CW, Oxer DT, Kennedy M, 1939, The efficacy of sero-vaccination of lambs against tetanus, *Aust Vet J*, **15:** 205–9.

Ahmadsyah I, Salim A, 1985, Treatment of tetanus: an open study to compare the efficacy of procaine penicillin and metronidazole, *Br Med J*, **291:** 648–50.

Akama K, Ito A et al., 1971, Reversion of toxicity of tetanus toxoids, *Jpn J Med Sci Biol*, **24:** 181–2.

Ambache N, Morgan RJ, Payling-Wright G, 1948a, Action of tetanus toxin on acetylcholine and cholinesterase contents of rabbit's iris, *J Physiol (Lond)*, **107:** 45–53.

Ambache N, Morgan RJ, Payling-Wright G, 1948b, Action of tenanus toxin on acetylcholine and cholinesterase contents of rabbit's iris, *Br J Exp Pathol*, **29:** 408–18.

d'Antona D, Valensin M, 1937, Súperoproté de l'immunité antitétanique active sur l'immunité passive, *Rev Immunol Paris*, **3:** 437.

Armitage P, Clifford R, 1978, Prognosis in tetanus: use of data from therapeutic trials, *J Infect Dis*, **138:** 1–8.

Bandmann F, 1953, Zum nachweis von tetanusbacillen im darm von ulcus-und carcinomtragern. Experimentellse untersuchungen, *Z Hyg Infektionskr*, **136:** 559.

Barr M, Llewellyn-Jones M, 1953, Some factors influencing the response of animals to immunisation with combined prophylactics, *Br J Exp Pathol*, **34:** 12–22.

Barr M, Sayers MHP, Stamm WP, 1959, Intradermal T.A.B.T. vaccine for immunisation against enteric, *Lancet*, **1:** 816–17.

Bauer JH, Meyer KF, 1926, Human intestinal carriers of tetanus spores in California, *J Infect Dis*, **38:** 295–305.

Baylis JH, Joseph J et al., 1952a, The effect of transection on the ascent of tetanus toxin on the rabbit's spinal cord, *J Pathol Bacteriol*, **64:** 47–52.

Baylis JH, Mackintosh J et al., 1952b, The effect of sclerosis of the nerve trunk on the ascent of tetanus toxin in the sciatic nerve of rabbits and on the development of local tetanus, *J Pathol Bacteriol*, **64:** 33–45.

Bazy M, 1914, Note statistique sur le tétanois, *C R Soc Biol*, **159:** 794–8.

Begue RE, Lindo-Soriano I, 1991, Failure of intrathecal tetanus antitoxin in the treatment of tetanus neonatorum, *J Infect Dis*, **164:** 619–20.

Behring E, Kitasato S, 1890, Ueber das zustandekommen der diptherie-immunitaet und theiren, *Dtsch Med Wochenschr*, **16:** 1113–14.

Bergentz SE, Philipson L, 1958, Studies on combined tetanus prophylaxis in humans, *Acta Chir Scand*, **116:** 58–67.

Berger SA, Cherubin CE et al., 1978, Tetanus despite preexisting antitentanus antibody, *JAMA*, **240:** 769–70.

Bergey DH, 1934, Active immunization against tetanus infection with tetanus toxoid, *J Infect Dis*, **55:** 72–8.

Bergey GK, Habig WH et al., 1989, Proteolytic cleavage of tetanus toxin increases activity, *J Neurochem*, **53:** 155–61.

Bjornboe M, Ibsen B, Johnson S, 1954, Tetanus. A case treated with artificial respiration during 17 days, *Dan Med Bull*, **1:** 129–31.

Blake PA, Feldman RA et al., 1976, Serologic therapy of tetanus in the United States 1965–1971, *JAMA*, **236:** 42–4.

Bleck TP, 1991a, Tetanus: pathophysiology, mangement, and prophylaxis, *Dis Mon*, **37:** 545–603.

Bleck TP, 1991b, Tetanus, *Infections of the Central Nervous System*, eds Scheld WM, Whitley RJ, Durack DT, Raven Press, New York.

Boyd JSK, MacLennan JD, 1942, Tetanus in the Middle East. Effects of active immunisation, *Lancet*, **2**: 745–9.

British Pharmacopoeia, 1980 II, HMSO, London, 879.

Bruce D, 1920, Tetanus. Analysis of 1458 cases, which occurred in home military hospitals during the years 1914–1918, *J Hyg*, **19**: 1–32.

Bruschettini A, 1890, Sulla diffusione nell' organismo del veleno de tetano, *Rif Med*, **6**: 1346.

Bruschettini A, 1892, Ricerche batteriologiche, *Rif Med*, **8**: 256.

Bulloch WE, Cramer W, 1919, On a new factor in the mechanism of bacterial infection, *Proc R Soc Lond [Biol]*, **90**: 513–29.

Buxton JB, Glenny AT, 1921, The active immunisation of horses against tetanus, *Lancet*, **2**: 1109.

Campbell JA, Fildes P, 1931, Tetanus; effect of oxygenation of tissue fluids in controlling infection by *B. tetani*, *Br J Exp Pathol*, **12**: 77–81.

Carle A, Rattone G, 1884, Studio experimentale sull' eziologia del tetano, *GAcadMedTorino*, **32**: 174.

Centers for Disease Control, 1977, Diphtheria and tetanus toxoids and pertussis vaccine, *Morbid Mortal Weekly Rep*, **26**: 401–2.

Centers for Disease Control, 1990, Tetanus – United States, 1987 and 1988, *JAMA*, **263**: 1192–5.

Centers for Disease Control, 1991, Diphtheria, tetanus, and pertussis: recommendations for vaccine use and other preventive measures. Recommendations of the Immunization Practices Advisory Committee, *Morbid Mortal Weekly Rep*, **10**: 1–28.

Chen BL, Chou CT et al., 1956, Studies on diphtheria–pertussis tetanus combined immunization in children. I Heterologous interference of pertussis agglutinin and tetanus antitoxin response by pre-existing latent diphtheria immunity, *J Immunol*, **77**: 144–55.

Chen BL, Chou CT et al., 1957, III. Immune responses after the booster vaccination, *J Immunol*, **79**: 393–400.

Cherubin CE, 1967, Urban tetanus. The epidemiologic aspects of tetanus in addicts in New York City, *Arch Environ Health*, **14**: 802–8.

Cherubin CE, 1968, Clinical severity of tetanus in narcotic addicts in New York City, *Arch Intern Med*, **121**: 156–8.

Chirmule N, Saxinger C, Pahwa S, 1989, Influenzas of related retroviruses on lymphocyte functions, *FEMS Microbiol Immunol*, **1**: 271–8.

Christenson B, Böttiger M, 1987, Epidemiology and immunity to tetanus in Sweden, *Scand J Infect Dis*, **19**: 429–35.

Cinader B, Weitz R, 1953, The interaction of tetanus toxin and antitoxin, *J Hyg*, **51**: 293–310.

Clarke G, Hill RG, 1972, Effects of a focal penicillin lesion on responses of rabbit cortical neurones to putative neurotransmitters, *Br J Pharmacol*, **44**: 435–41.

Cohen H, Leussink AB, 1973, Passive–active immunization of man with human tetanus immunoglobulin and adsorbed toxoids of different origin, *J Biol Stand*, **1**: 313–20.

Cohen H, van Ramshorst JD, Tasman A, 1959, Consistency in potency assay of tetanus toxoid in mice, *Bull W H O*, **20**: 1133–50.

Cole L, 1940, The prognosis of tetanus, *Lancet*, **1**: 164–8.

Coleman GE, 1931, Intestinal carriers of *Cl. tetani* and immunity. Tetanus IX, *Am J Hyg*, **14**: 515–25.

Coleman GE, Meyer KF, 1926, Study of tetanus agglutinins and antitoxin in human serums, *J Infect Dis*, **39**: 332.

Collee JG, van Heyningen S, 1991, Systemic toxigenic diseases (tetanus, botulism), *Anaerobes in Human Disease*, eds Duerden BI, Drasar BS, John Wiley & Sons, New York, 372–94.

Collier LH, Polakoff S, Mortimer J, 1979, Reactions and antibody responses to reinforcing doses of adsorbed and plain tetanus vaccines, *Lancet*, **1**: 1364–8.

Conway SP, James JR et al., 1987, Immunisation of the preterm baby, *Lancet*, **2**: 1326.

Couermont J, Doyon M, 1899, *Le Tetanos*, Baillière, Tindall and Cox, Paris, 53.

Cox CA, Knowelden J, Sharrard WJW, 1963, Tetanus prophylaxis, *Br Med J*, **2**: 1360–6.

Cuboni E, 1957, Il bacillo del teano nella corda di budello o catgut grezzo [The tetanus bacillus in cords of intestine or raw catgut], *Boll Ist Sieroter Milan*, **36**: 1–14.

Descombey P, 1924, L'anatoxine tétanique, *C R Soc Biol*, **91**: 239–41.

Diamond J, Mellanby JM, 1971, The effect of tetanus toxin in the goldfish, *J Physiol (Lond)*, **215**: 727–41.

Dimpfel W, Huang RTC, Halbermann E, 1977, Gangliosides in nervous tissue cultures and binding of 125 I-labelled tetanus toxin, a neuronal marker, *J Neurochem*, **29**: 329–34.

Ebisawa I, Fukutomi K, 1979, Attempts at distinguishing vaccine-related from spontaneous decline of tetanus mortality, *Jpn J Exp Med*, **49**: 131–8.

Edlich RF, Wilder BJ et al., 1986, Quality assessment of tetanus prophylaxis in the wounded patient, *Am Surg*, **52**: 544–7.

Edmondson RS, Flowers MW, 1979, Intensive care in tetanus: management, complications, and mortality in 100 cases, *Br Med J*, **1**: 1401–4.

Edsall G, 1959, Specific prophylaxis of tetanus, *JAMA*, **171**: 417–27.

Edsall G, 1976, The inexcusable disease, *JAMA*, **235**: 62–3.

Edsall G, Elliott MW et al., 1967, Excessive use of tetanus toxoid boosters, *JAMA*, **202**: 17–19.

Eldridge PL, Entwhistle CC, 1975, Routine screening of donor plasma suitable for the preparation of antitetanus immunoglobulin, *Vox Sang*, **28**: 62–5.

Ellis M, 1963, Human antitetanus serum in the treatment of tetanus, *Br Med J*, **1**: 1123–6.

Erdal E, Bartels F et al., 1995, Processing of tetanus and botulinum A neurotoxins in isolated chromaffin, *Naunyn Schmiedebergs Arch Pharmakol*, **351**: 67.

European Pharmacopoeia, 1977, Suppl. to vol. III, Maisonneuve S.A., France, 174.

Faber K, 1890, *Om Tetanus som Infektionssygdom*, Thesis, Copenhagen.

Fardon DE, 1967, Unusual reactions to tetanus toxoid, *JAMA*, **199**: 125–6.

Fedinec AA, 1967, Absorption and distribution of tetanus toxin in experimental animals, *Principles on Tetanus: Proceedings of an International Conference on Tetanus*, ed. Eckmann L, Huber, Berne, 169–75.

Figueiredo D, Turcotte C et al., 1995, Characterization of recombinant tetanus toxin derivatives suitable for vaccine development, *Infect Immun*, **63**: 3218–21.

Fildes P, 1925, Tetanus I. Isolation, morphology and cultural reactions of *B. tetani*, *Br J Exp Pathol*, **6**: 62.

Fildes P, 1927, Conditions under which tetanus spores germinate in vivo, *Br J Exp Pathol*, **8**: 387–93.

Firor WM, Lamont A, Shumacker HB, 1940, Studies on the cause of death in tetanus, *Ann Surg*, **111**: 246–74.

Friedemann U, Hollander A, 1943, Studies of tetanal toxin. I. Qualitative differences among various toxins revealed by bioassays in different species and by different routes of injection, *J Immunol*, **47**: 23–8 .

Friedemann U, Hollander A, Tarlov IM, 1941, Investigations on the pathogenesis of tetanus III, *J Immunol*, **40**: 325–64.

Fuchs D, Shearer GA et al., 1990, Increased serum neopterins in patients with HIV-1 infection is correlated with reduced in vitro interleukin-2 production, *Clin Exp Immunol*, **80**: 44–8.

Fulthorpe AJ, 1957, Tetanus antitoxin titration by haemagglutination, *J Hyg*, **55**: 382–401.

Fulthorpe AJ, 1958, Tetanus antitoxin titration by haemagglutination at a low level of test, *J Hyg*, **56**: 183–9.

Fulthorpe AJ, 1965, The influence of mineral carriers on the simultaneous active and passive immunization of guinea-pigs against tetanus, *J Hyg*, **63**: 243–62.

Galbraith NS, Forbes P, Tillett H, 1981, National surveillance of tetanus in England and Wales 1930–79, *J Infect*, **3**: 181–91.

Gardner P, Schaffner W, 1993, Immunization of adults, *N Engl J Med*, **328**: 1252–8.

Gareau AB, Eby RJ et al., 1990, Tetanus immunization status and immunologic response to a booster in an emergency department geriatric population, *Ann Emerg Med*, **19**: 1377–82.

Gergen PJ, McQuillan GM et al., 1995, A population-based serologic survey of immunity to tetanus in the United States, *N Engl J Med*, **332**: 761–6.

Gilles EC, 1937, Satisfactory method of isolating tetanus organisms from mixed material, *Am J Hyg*, **26**: 394.

Glaser J, Wyss-Souffront WA, 1961, Alleged anaphylactic reactions to human gamma-globulin, *Pediatrics*, **28**: 367–76.

Glenny AT, Hamp AG, Stevens MF, 1932, Protection of horses against tetanus by active immunisation with alum toxoid, *Vet J*, **88**: 90.

Glenny AT, Pope CA et al., 1926, Immunological notes, *J Pathol Bacteriol*, **29**: 31–40.

Goldie H, Parsons CH, Bowers MS, 1942, Titration of tetanal toxins, toxoids, and antitoxins with the flocculative test, *J Infect Dis*, **71**: 212–19.

Gottlieb S, McLaughlin FX et al., 1964, Long-term immunity to tetanus – a statistical evaluation and its clinical implications, *Am J Public Health*, **54**: 961–71.

Goulon M, Girard O et al., 1972, Les anticorps antitétaniques. Titrage avant sero-anatoxinotherapie chez 64 tétaniques, *Nouv Presse Méd*, **1**: 3049–50.

Gumprecht F, 1894, Zur pathogenese des tetanus, *Dtsch Med Wochenschr*, **20**: 546.

Gupta PS, Kapoor R et al., 1980, Intrathecal human tetanus immunoglobulin in early tetanus, *Lancet*, **2**: 439–40.

Gupte SC, Bhatia HM, 1979, Anti-A and anti-B titre response after tetanus toxoid injections in normal adults and pregnant women, *Indian J Med Res*, **70**: 221–8.

Habermann E, 1976, Affinity chromatography of tetanus toxin, tetanus toxoid, and botulinum A toxin on synaptosomes, and differentiation of their acceptors, *Naunyn Schmiedebergs Arch Pharmakol*, **293**: 1–9.

Habermann E, Dimpfel W, 1973, Distribution of 125 I-tetanus toxin and 125 I-toxoid in rats with generalized tetanus, as influenced by antitoxin, *Naunyn Schmiedebergs Arch Pharmakol*, **276**: 327–40.

Hansson H, Möller H, 1971, Cutaneous reactions to merthiolate and their relationship to vaccination with tetanus toxoid, *Acta Allergol (Copenh)*, **26**: 150–6.

Harris PE, Strba-Cechova K et al., 1990, Amplification of T cell blastogenic responses in healthy individuals and patients with acquired immune deficiency syndrome, *J Clin Invest*, **85**: 746–56.

Hausinger A, Volknandt W, Zimmermann H, 1995, Calcium-dependent endogenous proteolysis of the vesicle proteins synaptobrevin and synaptotagmin, *Neuroreport*, **6**: 637–41.

Heare BR, Shabot JM, 1990, Tetanus associated with carcinoma of the rectum, *Am J Gastroenterol*, **85**: 105–6.

Hegyessey G, Bozsoky S, Schulek E, 1956, A study of the immunity against tetanus toxin following the use of a combined typhoid–tetanus vaccine, *Br J Exp Pathol*, **37**: 300–5.

Hepple JR, 1968, Large scale production of *Clostridium tetani* toxin, *Chem Ind*, **21**: 670–4.

van Heyningen S, 1976, Binding of ganglioside by the chains of tetanus toxin, *FEBS Lett*, **68**: 5–7.

van Heyningen WE, 1959, Tentative identification of the tetanus toxin receptor in nervous tissue, *J Gen Microbiol*, **20**: 310–20.

van Heyningen WE, Miller PA, 1961, The fixation of tetanus toxin by ganglioside, *J Gen Microbiol*, **24**: 107–19.

Hilton E, Singer C et al., 1991, Status of immunity to tetanus, measles, mumps, rubella, and polio among U.S. travelers, *Ann Intern Med*, **115**: 32–3.

Holliday PL, Bauer RB, 1983, Polyradiculoneuritis secondary to immunization with tetanus and diphtheria toxoids, *Arch Neurol*, **40**: 56–7.

Hornibrook JW, 1952, The avidity of test toxins in relationship to tetanus antitoxin titrations, *J Lab Clin Med*, **40**: 58–66.

Hutyra F, Marek J, 1912, *Special Pathology and Therapeutics of the Diseases of Domestic Animals*, Baillière, Tindall and Cox, London.

Ikic D, 1958, Amount of A.U. (antitoxic unit) in subjects vaccinated with P.T.A.P. tetanus prophylactic, *Acta Med Iugosl*, **12**: 179–85.

Ipsen J, 1940–41, Comparison of tetanus test toxins prepared by 7 institutes from same strain and by same method. Progress report on production of tetanus test toxin, *Bull Health Organ League Nations*, **9**: 447–51, 452–75.

Jolliet P, Magnenat J-L et al., 1990, Aggressive intensive care treatment of very elderly patients with tetanus is justified, *Chest*, **97**: 702–5.

Kerr JH, Corbett JL et al., 1968, Involvement of the sympathetic nervous system in tetanus. Studies on 82 cases, *Lancet*, **2**: 236–41.

Kerrin JC, 1928, Incidence of *B.tetani* in human faeces, *Br J Exp Pathol*, **9**: 69–71.

Kerrin JC, 1929, Distribution of *B.tetani* in intestines of animals, *Br J Exp Pathol*, **10**: 370–3.

Kielmann AA, Vohra SR, 1977, Control of tetanus neonatorum in rural communities – immunization effects of high-dose calcium phosphate-absorbed tetanus toxoid, *Indian J Med Res*, **66**: 906–16.

Kitasato S, 1889, Ueber den tetanusbacillus, *Z Hyg Infektionskr*, **7**: 225–34.

Kitasato S, 1891, Experimentelle untersuchungen uber das tetanusgift, *Z Hyg Infektionskr*, **10**: 267–305.

Knight BCJG, Fildes P, 1930, CLXV. Oxidation–reduction studies in relation to bacterial growth. III. The positive limit of oxidation–reduction potential required for the germination of *B.tetani* spores in vitro, *Biochem J*, **24**: 1496–502.

Krieglstein KG, Henschen AH et al., 1991, Limited proteolysis of tetanus toxin. Relation to activity and identification of cleavage sites, *Eur J Biochem*, **202**: 41–51.

Kryzhanovsky GN, 1966, *Tetanus*, State Publishing House, Moscow.

Kryzhanovsky GN, 1973, The mechanism of action of tetanus toxin: effect on synaptic process and some particular features of toxin binding by the nervous tissue, *Naunyn Schmiedebergs Arch Pharmakol*, **276**: 247–50.

LaForce FM, 1990, Adult immunizations: are they worth the trouble?, *J Gen Intern Med*, **5**: S57–61.

Lahiri DC, 1939, Absence of specific antitoxin in persons exposed to risk of tetanus infection, *Indian J Med Res*, **27**: 581.

Laurence DR, Webster RA, 1963, Pathologic physiology, pharmacology, and therapeutics of tetanus, *Clin Pharmacol Ther*, **4**: 36–72.

Laurent LJM, Parish HJ, 1958, Intradermal tests for serum sensitivity, *Lancet*, **2**: 376.

Ledley FD, Lee G et al., 1977, Tetanus toxin interactions with thyroid plasma membranes. Implications for structure and function of tetanus toxin receptors and potential pathophysiological significance, *J Biol Chem*, **252**: 4049–55.

Levine L, McComb J et al., 1966, Active–passive tetanus immunization. Choice of toxoid, dose of tetanus immune globulin and timing of injections, *N Engl J Med*, **274**: 186–90.

Ljungman P, Wiklund-Hammarsten M et al., 1990, Response to tetanus toxoid immunization after allogeneic bone marrow transplantation, *J Infect Dis*, **162**: 496–500.

Lowbury EJL, Lilly HA, 1958, Contamination of operating-theatre air with *Cl. tetani*, *Br Med J*, **2**: 1334–6.

Lowbury EJL, Kidson A et al., 1978, Prophylaxis against tetanus in non-immune patients with wounds: the role of antibiotics and of human antitetanus globulin, *J Hyg*, **80**: 267–74.

Lucas AO, Willis AJP, 1965, Prevention of tetanus, *Br Med J*, **2**: 1333–6.

Luisto M, 1989, Outcome and neurological sequelae of patients after tetanus. *Acta Neurol Scand*, **80**: 504–11.

McComb JA, Dwyer RC, 1963, Passive–active immunization with tetanus immune globulin (human), *N Engl J Med*, **268**: 857–62.

McComb JA, Levine L, 1961, Adult immunization. II Dosage reduction as a solution to increasing reactions to tetanus toxoid, *N Engl J Med*, **265:** 1152–3.

MacKenzie DL, Vlahcevic LR, 1974, Lithium toxicity enhanced by diuresis (letter), *N Engl J Med*, **290:** 749.

Mackie TJ, McLachan DGS, Anderson EJM, 1929, *Report to Department of Health for Scotland*, HSMO, Edinburgh.

MacLennan R, Schofield F et al., 1965, Immunization against neonatal tetanus in New Guinea. Antitoxin response of pregnant women to adjuvant and plain toxoids, *Bull W H O*, **32:** 683–97.

MacLennan R, Levine L et al., 1973, The early primary immune response to absorbed tetanus toxoid in man: a study of the influence of antigen concentration, carrier concentration, and sequence of dosage on the rate, extent, and persistence of the immune response to one and to two doses of toxoid, *Bull W H O*, **49:** 615–26.

Mahoney LG, Aprile MA, Moloney PJ, 1967, Combined active–passive immunization against tetanus in man, *Can Med Assoc J*, **96:** 1401–4.

Margolick JB, Volkman DJ et al., 1987, Amplification of HTLV-III/LAV infection by antigen-induced activation of T cells and direct suppression by virus of lymphocyte blastogenic responses, *J Immunol*, **138:** 1719–23.

Marie A, 1897, Recherches sur la toxine tétanique, *Ann Inst Pasteur (Paris)*, **11:** 591–9.

Matsuda M, 1989, The structure of tetanus toxin, *Botulinum Neurotoxin and Tetanus Toxin*, ed. Simpson LL, Academic Press, San Diego, 78.

Matzkin PH, Regev S, 1985, Naturally acquired immunity to tetanus toxin in an isolated community, *Infect Immun*, **48:** 267–8.

Mellanby J, Green J, 1981, How does tetanus toxin act?, *Neuroscience*, **6:** 281–300.

Mellanby J, Pope D, Ambache N, 1968, The effect of the treatment of crude tetanus toxin with ganglioside cerebroside complex on sphincter paralysis in the rabbit's eye, *J Gen Microbiol*, **50:** 479–86.

Mellanby J, Thompson PA, 1972, The effect of tetanus toxin at the neuromuscular junction in the goldfish, *J Physiol (Lond)*, **224:** 407–19.

Meyer H, Ransom F, 1903, Untersuchungen ueber den tetanus, *Arch Pathol Pharmacol*, **49:** 363–416.

Mirsky R, Wendon LMB et al., 1978, Tetanus toxin: a cell surface marker for neurones in culture, *Brain Res*, **148:** 251–9.

Miyasaki S, Okada K et al., 1967, [On the mode of action of tetanus toxin in rabbit. I. Distribution of tetanus toxin in vivo and development of paralytic signs under some conditions], *Jpn J Exp Med*, **37:** 217–25.

Mohapatra MK, Das C et al., 1993, Two cases of cephalic tetanus, *Trop Doct*, **23:** 44–5.

Mohler JR, Eichhorn A, 1911, *28th Annual Report of the Bureau of Animal Industry*, US Department of Agriculture (Washington, DC), 185.

Montecucco C, Schiavo G, 1993, Tetanus and botulism neurotoxins: a new group of zinc proteases, *Trends Biochem Sci*, **18:** 324–7.

Montecucco C, Schiavo G, 1994, Mechanism of action of tetanus and botulinum neurotoxins, *Mol Microbiol*, **13:** 1–8.

Mussett MV, Sheffield F, 1973, A collaborative investigation of methods proposed for the potency assay of adsorbed diphtheria and tetanus toxoids in the *European Pharmacopeia*, *J Biol Stand*, **1:** 259–83.

Mussett MV, Sheffield F, 1976, A collaborative investigation of a potency assay for adsorbed tetanus vaccines based on the protection of mice from tetanic paralysis, *J Biol Stand*, **4:** 141–8.

Nagel J, Cohen H, 1973, Studies on tetanus antitoxins. II. Demonstration of at least four antitoxins of different specificity in antitoxic sera, *J Immunol*, **110:** 1388–95.

Nagel J, Svec D et al., 1977, IgE synthesis in man. I. Development of specific IgE antibodies after immunization with tetanus–diphtheria (TD) toxoids, *J Immunol*, **118:** 334–41.

National Advisory Committee on Immunization, 1979, *A Guide to Immunization for Canadians*, Laboratory Centre for Disease Control, Ottawa, Canada.

Newell KW, LeBlanc DR et al., 1971, The serologic assessment of a tetanus toxoid field trial, *Bull W H O*, **45:** 773–85.

Nicolaier A, 1884, Ueber infectiosen tetanus, *Dtsch Med Wochenschr*, **10:** 842–4.

Nicolaier A, 1886, *Jahresbericht Fortschr Lehre Pathog Mikroorganismen*, **2:** 270.

Nobel W, 1915, Experimental study of the distribution and habitat of the tetanus bacillus, *J Infect Dis*, **16:** 132–41.

Opravil M, Fierz W et al., 1991, Poor antibody response after tetanus and pneumococcal vaccination in immunocompromised HIV-infected patients, *Clin Exp Immunol*, **84:** 185–9.

Parish HJ, Laurent LJM, Moynihan NH, 1957, Notes on prevention of tetanus in injured persons, *Br Med J*, **1:** 639–40.

Passen EL, Andersen BR, 1986, Clinical tetanus despite a 'protective' level of toxin-neutralizing antibody, *JAMA*, **255:** 1171–3.

Patel JC, Mehta BC, 1963, Tetanus. A study of 2,007 cases, *Indian J Med Sci*, **17:** 791–811.

Patel JC, Mehta BC, Modi KN, 1965, *Proceedings of the First International Conference on Tetanus, Bombay, 1963*, 181.

Pinching AJ, 1991, Antibody responses in HIV infection, *Clin Exp Immunol*, **84:** 181–4.

Pizzini L, 1898, *Zentralbl Bakteriol Parasitenkd Infektionskr Hyg*, **24:** 890.

Prevots R, Sutter RW et al., 1992, Tetanus surveillance – United States 1989–1990, *Morbid Mortal Weekly Rep*, **41:** 1–9.

Price DL, Griffin JW, Peck K, 1977, Tetanus toxin: evidence for binding at presynaptic nerve endings, *Brain Res*, **121:** 379–84.

Price DL, Griffin JW et al., 1975, Tetanus toxin: direct evidence for retrograde intraaxonal transport, *Science*, **188:** 945–7.

Ramon G, Lemétayer E, 1934, Sur l'immunité antitétanique naturellement acquise chez quelques espèces de ruminants, *C R Soc Biol*, **116:** 275.

Ramon G, Lemétayer E, 1935, Recherches sur l'immunité antitétanique naturellement acquise chez l'homme et chez différentes espèces animales en particulier chez les ruminants, *Rev Immunol*, **1:** 209.

van Ramshorst JD, Sundaresan TK, Outschoorn AS, 1972, International collaborative studies on potency assays of diphtheria and tetanus toxoids, *Bull W H O*, **46:** 262–76.

Regamey RH, Schlegel HJ, 1951, L'immunité antitétanique dans les 10 ans qui suivent l'immunisation de base [Anti-tetanus immunity in the ten years following basic immunization], *Schweiz Z Allg Pathol Bakteriol*, **14:** 550.

Relihan M, 1969, Reactions to tetanus toxoid, *J Irish Med Assoc*, **62:** 430–4.

Relyveld EH, Martin R et al., 1969, [Calcium phosphate as adjuvant in vaccinations in man], *Ann Inst Pasteur (Paris)*, **116:** 300–6.

Report, 1938, *Bulletin of the Health Organization of the League of Nations*, **7:** 713.

Report, 1950, Expert Committee on Biological Standardization. Report on the third session, *W H O Tech Rep Ser*, **2**.

Report, 1959, Occurrence of tetanus spores in materials used for dressing wounds, *Br Med J*, **1:** 1150–4.

Report, 1967, *Principles on Tetanus: Proceedings of an International Conference on Tetanus*, ed. Eckmann L, Huber, Berne, 576.

Report, 1972a, *Immunization against Infectious Disease*, Department of Health and Social Security, HMSO, London.

Report, 1972b, *Morbid Mortal Weekly Rep*, **21:** 5.

Robinson DT, McLeod JW, Downie AW, 1946, Dust in surgical theatres as possible source of postoperative tetanus, *Lancet*, **1:** 152–4.

Rosenbach J, 1886–87, Zur Aetiologie des Wundstarrkrampfes beim Menchen, *Arch Klin Chir*, **34:** 306–17.

Rubbo SD, 1966, New approaches to tetanus prophylaxis, *Lancet*, **2:** 449–53.

Russell DS, 1927, Tetanus. V. The local fate of tetanus spores inoculated into guinea pigs, *Br J Exp Pathol*, **8**: 377.

Sanada I, Nishida S, 1965, Isolation of *Clostridium tetani* from soil, *J Bacteriol*, **89**: 626–9.

Sanfelice F, 1893, Untersuchungen uber anaerobe Mikroorganismen, *Z Hyg Infektionskr*, **14**: 339–92.

Sanford JP, 1995, Tetanus – forgotten but not gone, *N Engl J Med*, **332**: 812–13.

Sawamura S, 1909, *Arbeiten aus dem Institut für Infektionskrankheiten Bern*, **4**: 1.

Schanfield MS, Wells JV, Fudenberg HH, 1979, Immunoglobulin allotypes and response to tetanus toxoid in Papua, New Guinea, *J Immunogenet*, **6**: 311–15.

Schechter R, Arnon SS, 1995, Immunization against tetanus associated with a decreased risk of acquiring type B infant botulism, *ASM First International Conference on Molecular General Pathogenesis, Tucson, Arizona*, Clostridium Poster A2.

Scheibel I, 1944, Experimental studies on active immunization with combined diphtheria–tetanus vaccine, *Acta Pathol Microbiol Scand*, **21**: 130–41.

Scheibel I, Bentzon MW et al., 1966, Duration of immunity to diphtheria and tetanus after active immunization, *Acta Pathol Microbiol Scand*, **67**: 380–92.

Scheibel I, Chen B-L et al., 1968, Human response to four tetanus vaccines with differing potency when assayed in animals, *Acta Pathol Microbiol Scand*, **73**: 115–28.

Schellenberg DB, Matzke HA, 1958, Development of tetanus in parabiotic rats, *J Immunol*, **80**: 367–73.

Scheunemann K, 1931, Untersuchungen uber das vorkommen von tetanusbazillen im stuhl nicht, *Arch Hyg Bakteriol*, **105**: 287–99.

Schneider CH, 1964, Reactions to tetanus toxoid: a report of five cases, *Med J Aust*, **2**: 303–5.

Schofield FD, Tucker VM, Westbrook GR, 1961, Neonatal tetanus in New Guinea: effect of active immunization in pregnancy, *Br Med J*, **2**: 785–9.

Sevitt S, 1949, Source of two hospital-infected cases of tetanus, *Lancet*, **2**: 1075–8.

Shackelford PG, Granoff DM et al., 1990, Subnormal serum concentrations of IgG2 in children with frequent infections associated with varied patterns of immunologic dysfunction, *J Pediatr*, **116**: 529–38.

Sheffield F, Baldwin PW et al., 1979, The British reference preparation for tetanus antitoxin for the flocculation test, *J Biol Stand*, **7**: 301–6.

Sherrington CS, 1917, Observations with antitetanus serum in the monkey, *Lancet*, **2**: 964–6.

Simonsen O, Bloch AV, Heron I, 1987, Epidemiology of tetanus in Denmark 1920–1982, *Scand J Infect Dis*, **19**: 437–4.

Simonsen O, Kjeldsen K, Heron I, 1984, Immunity against tetanus and effect of revaccination 25–30 years after primary vaccination, *Lancet*, **2**: 1240–2.

Smith JWG, 1964, Simultaneous active and passive immunization of guinea-pigs against tetanus, *J Hyg*, **62**: 379–88.

Smith JWG, 1969, Diphtheria and tetanus toxoids, *Br Med Bull*, **25**: 177–82.

Smith JWG, 1984, Tetanus, *Topley and Wilson's Principles of Bacteriology, Virology and Immunity*, vol. 3, 7th edn, eds Parker MT, Collier LH, Edward Arnold, London, 345–68.

Smith JWG, Laurence DR, Evans DG, 1975, Prevention of tetanus in the wounded, *Br Med J*, **3**: 453–5.

Smith JWG, MacIver AG, 1969, Studies in experimental tetanus infection, *J Med Microbiol*, **2**: 385–93.

Smith JWG, MacIver AG, 1974, Growth and toxin production of tetanus bacilli in vivo, *J Med Microbiol*, **7**: 497–504.

Smith JWG, Evans DG et al., 1963, Simultaneous active and passive immunization against tetanus, *Br Med J*, **1**: 237–8.

Smith ML, 1938, Standardization of tetanus antitoxin; factors influencing the assay, *Q Bull Health Organ League Nations*, **7**: 739–69.

Smith ML, 1943–44, Note on complexity of tetanus toxin, *Q Bull Health Organ League Nations*, **10**: 104–12.

Smith T, 1908, Some neglected facts in the biology of the tetanus bacillus; their bearing on the safety of the so-called biological products, *Trans Chicago Pathol Soc*, **7**: no. 4.

Smythe PM, Bowie MD, Voss TJV, 1974, Treatment of tetanus neonatorum with muscle relaxants and intermittent positive-pressure ventilation, *Br Med J*, **1**: 223–6.

Spaun J, Lyng J, 1970, Replacement of the international standard for tetanus antitoxin and the use of the standard in the flocculation test, *Bull W H O*, **42**: 523–34.

Sterne M, Batty I et al., 1962, Differences between alpha and gamma motoneurons labelled with horseradish peroxidase by retrograde transport, *Vet Rec*, **74**: 909.

Stevens DL, Laine BM, Mitten JE, 1987, Comparison of single and combination antimicrobial agents for prevention of experimental gas gangrene caused by *Clostridium perfringens*, *Antimicrob Agents Chemother*, **31**: 312–16.

Stöckel K, Schwab M, Thoenen H, 1975, Comparison between the retrograde axonal transport of nerve growth factor and tetanus toxin in motor, sensory and adrenergic neurons, *Brain Res*, **99**: 1–16.

Strick PL, Burke RE et al., 1976, Differences between alpha and gamma motoneurons labeled with horseradish peroxidase by retrograde transport, *Brain Res*, **113**: 582–8.

Suri JC, Rubbo SD, 1961, Immunization against tetanus, *J Hyg*, **59**: 29–48.

Tasman A, Huygen FJA, 1962, Immunization against tetanus of patients given injections of antitetanus serum, *Bull W H O*, **26**: 397–407.

Tasman A, van Ramshorst JD, 1952, On the preparation and properties of a new tetanus-prophylactic, the 'tetanmus P.T.', *Antonie van Leeuwenhoek J Microbiol Serol*, **18**: 357–63.

Teale FH, Embleton D, 1919–20, Studies in infection. II The paths of spread of bacterial exotoxins with special reference to tetanus toxin, *J Pathol Bacteriol*, **23**: 50–68.

Thomson RD, Batty I et al., 1969, The immunogenicity of a multicomponent clostridial oil emulsion vaccine in sheep, *Vet Rec*, **85**: 81–4.

Tizzoni G, Cattani G, 1890, Untersuchungen uber das Tetanusgift, *Arch Pathol Pharmakol*, **27**: 432.

Toledo S, Veillon A, 1891, *Zentralbl Bakteriol Parasitenkd Infektionskr Hyg*, **9**: 18.

Tonge BL, 1989, Tetanus from chigger flea sores (letter), *J Trop Pediatr*, **35**: 94.

Traverso HP, Kahn AJ et al., 1989, Ghee applications to the umbilical cord: a risk factor for neonatal tetanus, *Lancet*, **1**: 486–8.

Trinca JC, 1963, Active tetanus immunization: effect of a reduced reinforcing dose of adsorbed toxoid on the partly immunized reactive patient, *Med J Aust*, **2**: 389–92.

Trinca JC, 1965, Active immunization against tetanus: the need for a single all-purpose toxoid, *Med J Aust*, **2**: 116.

Trinca JC, 1967, Problems in tetanus prophylaxis: the immune patient, *Med J Aust*, **2**: 153–5.

Tulloch WJ, 1919–20, Studies on the prophylaxis and treatment of tetanus. II. Studies pertaining to treatment, *J Hyg*, **18**: 103.

Vaillard L, 1892, Sur quelques points concernant l'immunité contre le tétanos, *Ann Inst Pasteur (Paris)*, **6**: 224–32.

Vaillard L, Rouget J, 1892, Contribution à l'étude du tétanos (2 e mémoire), *Ann Inst Pasteur (Paris)*, **6**: 385–435.

Vaishnava H, Goyal RK, 1966, Prevention of tetanus (letter), *Br Med J*, **2**: 466–7.

Veronesi R, 1965, Epidemiology of tetanus in Brazil, *J Hyg Epidemiol Microbiol Immunol*, **9**: 421–33.

Voller A, Bidwell DE, Bartlett A, 1976, *Protides of the Biological Fluids*, 24th Colloquium, Bruges, 1975, Pergamon Press, Oxford, 751–8.

Wassermann A, Takaki T, 1898, Ueber tetanusantitoxische Eigenschaften des normalen Centralnervensystems, *Berl Klin Wochenschr*, **35**: 5.

Webster ADB, Latif AAA et al., 1984, Evaluation of test immunisation in the assessment of deficiency syndromes, *Br Med J*, **288:** 1864–6.

Weinstein L, 1973, Tetanus, *N Engl J Med*, **289:** 1293–6.

Wetzler TF, Marshall JD, Cardella MA, 1956, Rapid isolation of clostridiums by selective inhibition of aerobic flora, *Am J Clin Pathol*, **26:** 418–21.

White WG, Barnes GM et al., 1969, Duration of immunity after active immunisation against tetanus, *Lancet*, **2:** 95–6.

White WG, Barnes GM et al., 1973, Reactions to tetanus toxoid, *J Hyg*, **71:** 283–97.

Whitman C, Belgharbi L et al., 1992, Progress towards the global elimination of neonatal tetanus, *World Health Stat Q*, **45:** 248–56.

Willis AT, 1969, *Clostridia of Wound Infection*, Butterworths, London, 385–461.

Winsnes R, 1979, Quantification of tetanus antitoxin in human sera. I. Counter-immuno-electrophoresis, *Acta Pathol Microbiol Scand Sect B*, **87:** 191–5.

Wirz M, Gentili G, Collotti C, 1990, *Bacterial Vaccines*, ed. Mizrahi A, Alan R Liss, Inc., New York, 35.

Wiseman JC, Gascoigne ME, 1977, Screening of blood donors for the detection of antitetanic antibodies suitable for the production of human antitetanus immunoglobulin, *J Clin Pathol*, **30:** 177–80.

Woo E, Yu YL, Huang CY, **1988:** Local tetanus revisited, *Electromyogr Clin Neurophysiol*, **28:** 117–22.

Woodruff AW, El Bashir EA et al., 1984, Neonatal tetanus: mode of infection, prevalance, and prevention in southern Sudan, *Lancet*, **1:** 378–9.

World Health Organization, 1964, Annex I. Requirements for diphtheria toxoid and tetanus toxoid. (Requirements for biological substances no. 10), *W H O Tech Rep Ser*, **293:** 25.

Wright EA, Morgan RS, Wright GP, 1950, Tetanus intoxication of the brain stem in rabbits, *J Pathol Bacteriol*, **62:** 569–83.

Wright EA, Morgan RS, Wright GP, 1952, The site of action of the toxin in local tetanus, *Lancet*, **2:** 316–19.

Wright GP, 1955, The neurotoxins of *Clostridium botulinum* and *Clostridium tetani*, *Pharmacol Rev*, **7:** 413–65.

Zimmerman JM, Piffaretti J-Cl, 1977, Interaction of tetanus toxin and toxoid with cultured neuroblastoma cells, *Naunyn Schmiedebergs Arch Pharmakol*, **296:** 271–7.

Züst B, 1967, [Simultaneous prophylaxis against tetanus with tetanus vaccine and human anti-tetanus globulin], *Z Immunitätsforsch Allergie Klin Immunol*, **132:** 261–75.

Chapter 37

BOTULISM

E A Johnson and M C Goodnough

1 INTRODUCTION

Botulism is a rare paralytic disease resulting from the action of neurotoxins produced by members of the genus *Clostridium* (Prazmowski 1880). Food-borne botulism results from the ingestion of neurotoxin preformed in foods. Botulism can also occur from the growth and toxin production by *Clostridium botulinum* in the intestine (infant botulism and adult intestinal botulism) and in wounds (wound botulism). Although botulism is extremely rare compared to many other microbial diseases, the disease has long fascinated physicians and scientists because of the peculiar symptoms and relatively high fatality rate of affected humans and animals. Human botulism outbreaks can have dramatic impact on communities in which they occur (Dolman 1964), and outbreaks of animal botulism have periodically devastated populations of domestic and wild animals (Table 37.1) (Smith 1977, Eklund and Dowell 1987).

The outstanding property of *C. botulinum* is its ability to synthesize a neurotoxin of extraordinary potency. Botulinum neurotoxins comprise a family of pharmacologically similar toxins that bind to peripheral cholinergic synapses and block acetylcholine release at neuromuscular junctions. Botulinum poisoning results in a characteristic flaccid paralysis that may affect all peripheral motoneurons. Botulinum neurotoxins are classified into 7 serotypes (A, B, C_1, D, E, F and G) on the basis of neutralization of toxicity by type-specific antibodies (Bowmer 1963, Gimenez and Gimenez 1995). These neurotoxins are the most poisonous substances known and the human lethal dose has been estimated at c. 1 ng kg^{-1} (Schantz and Sugiyama 1974, Gill 1982). Animals vary in susceptibility to botulinum toxin with humans, horses and guinea pigs among the most sensitive to botulinum toxin; rats and carrion-eating birds such as vultures are relatively resistant.

2 MILESTONES IN THE UNDERSTANDING OF BOTULISM

Most of the clostridia range from strict anaerobes to aerotolerant; most species thrive only when oxygen is present in low levels in their growth environment. Anaerobic bacteria were discovered by Pasteur during investigations of butyric acid fermentation (Willis 1969). Pasteur was able to isolate an organism he termed *Vibrion butyrique*, which is now referred to as *Clostridium butyricum*, the type species of the genus *Clostridium*. The genus *Clostridium* was first proposed by Winslow et al. (Willis 1969) and adopted in the first edition of *Bergey's Manual of Determinative Bacteriology* in 1923. Besides being obligately anaerobic, the clostridia have the notable property of forming endospores which are resistant to physical and chemical stresses. Endospores were discovered independently by Ferdinand Cohn and Robert Koch in 1876, soon after Pasteur had made microbiology famous (Keynan and Sandler 1983).

Although anecdotal evidence suggests that botulism occurred in ancient cultures (Smith 1977), the disease was first described in Germany by Muller (1735–93) and by the poet and noted physician Justinius Kerner (1786–1862) (Dewberry 1950). The disease became known as Kerner's disease (Meyer 1956). In Germany, insufficiently smoked sausages ('blood sausages') caused 174 cases and 71 deaths in a disease characterized by muscle paralysis and suffocation. The disease became known as sausage 'botulus' poisoning. In 1822, Kerner showed experimentally that poison developed within the sausage and that exclusion of

Table 37.1 Epidemiological features of botulism in humans and animals

Type	Discovered by	Animal species mainly affected	Common vehicles	Main geographical occurrence
A	Burke 1919	Humans, occasionally chickens, mink, cattle	Vegetables, fruits, meat, fish	World wide, common in Western USA, Russia, China
B	Burke 1919, van Ermengem 1896	Humans, horses, cattle	Vegetables, fruits, meats, fish	World wide, common in Europe (Poland, Germany, France, Italy, Spain, Norway, others), Russia, Canada
C_α	Bengston 1923	Waterfowl, chickens, turkeys, pheasants, other birds, occasionally dogs	Dead marsh vegetation	North and South America, Africa, Australia
C_β	Seddon 1922	Cattle, horses, sheep, mink, ferrets	Forage, carrion	UK, USA, Japan, Australia
D	Theiler et al. 1927	Cattle, horses	Carrion	South Africa, Australia
E	Gunnison, Cummings and Meyer 1936	Humans, fish, occasionally mink, waterfowl	Fish, marine mammals	World wide, Japan, Canada, USA, USSR, occasionally Europe
F	Dolman and Murakami 1961	Humans (rare)	Meats	Denmark, California
G	Gimenez and Ciccarelli 1970	None known	NA	Argentina, Switzerland

air was required for poison formation (Dickson 1918). Kerner isolated a fatty substance from decomposed sausages that produced symptoms of botulism and death in animals, which he suggested as the toxic agent. Liebig (1843 cited in Dewberry 1950) suggested that the disease was due to a 'ferment', and Heller (1853) suggested that a microscopic vegetative mould was responsible for the disease (Dickson 1918). A theory was also advanced that botulism was caused by putrefactive amines, but these substances failed to produce the disease in animals. Nauwerck in 1886 (cited in Dickson 1918) suggested that the toxic compounds were of bacterial origin and he isolated 3 bacilli from sausage that were proteolytic and putrefactive. Following the investigations in Germany, a disease with similar symptoms was recorded in Russia and Denmark from the consumption of fish ('ichthyism').

Although numerous theories were proposed for the cause of botulism, its nature remained obscure until investigations by the Belgian microbiologist Emile Pierre van Ermengem (Fig. 37.1).

In 1895, van Ermengem isolated an anaerobic bacillus from a ham implicated in a botulism outbreak. He showed that, on culturing, the bacillus produced a very potent toxin that was released into the medium. His success was a triumph and representative of the sophisticated nature of bacteriology in Europe at the time. van Ermengem was uniquely qualified to elucidate the aetiology of paralytic botulism: he had been

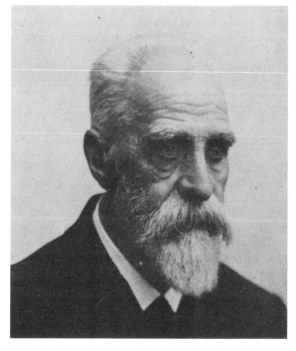

Fig. 37.1 Prof Emile Pierre Van Ermengem (1851–1932), University of Ghent.

a student of the eminent physiologists Bernard and Ranvier and had also trained with Robert Koch (Bulloch 1938). van Ermengem clearly established the aetiology of botulism by isolation of 'Bacillus botulinus' from the ham and the spleens and large intestines of persons who had died from the food poisoning. Kempner (1897) subsequently showed that van Ermengem's cultures produced a substance that on injection in an inactive form gave rise to antitoxin in the blood of goats. This was the first evidence that antitoxin to botulinum toxin could neutralize toxicity and prevent death.

van Ermengem's and Kempner's seminal investigations established several principles of botulism that remain valid today:

1 food-borne botulism is an intoxication and not an infection by *Clostridium botulinum*
2 the toxin is produced in food by a specific organism 'Bacillus botulinus'
3 the toxin is resistant to digestive enzymes
4 the toxin is labile to heat and alkali but is stable in acidic conditions
5 the toxin is not produced in food with sufficient salt or acid
6 *C. botulinum* produces heat-resistant endospores
7 animals vary in their susceptibility to botulinum toxin and
8 animals can develop immunity to the botulinum toxins by exposure to inactive toxin or toxoid.

Subsequent outbreaks of botulism indicated that there were at least 2 types of *C. botulinum*, designated A and B (Smith 1977). In the 1920s, Bengston (1923, 1924) isolated *C. botulinum* from fly larvae (*Lucilia caesar* and *Lucilia sericata*) that produced a botulinum neurotoxin antigenically distinct from types A and B. She noted that chickens which ate these fly larvae died of a paralytic disease characterized by inability to keep their head erected ('limber neck'). In the 1920s, a toxigenic organism was isolated from diseased cattle that resembled the fly larvae strains but which had antigenic differences (Seddon 1922). These antigenic strains were designated type C. An organism was isolated in 1927 in South Africa from cattle carcasses which produced a serologically distinct toxin from the previously described types. It was designated type D (Smith 1977). Type E was isolated from canned fish in Russia (Gunnison, Cummings and Meyer 1936), and has been frequently isolated from marine and freshwater sediments. Type F *C. botulinum* was initially reported in Copenhagen, Denmark in 1958 from home-made liver paste implicated in an outbreak involving 5 persons, 3 of whom had severe botulism and one of whom died (Moeller and Scheibel 1960). The properties of *C. botulinum* type F were described by Dolman and colleagues (Dolman and Murakami 1961). Gimenez and Ciccarelli (1970) reported another distinct serotype from soil, which was designated type G. This is the only serotype not implicated in human or animal botulism. In recent years, organisms have been isolated that produce more than one serotype of botulinum toxin, or that carry genes for unexpressed toxin genes (Hatheway 1995). Organisms resembling *Clostridium baratii* and *C. butyricum*, producing botulinum-like toxins, have been isolated from infants with botulism (Hatheway 1995). Although these clostridia differ widely in phenotypic and genetic relatedness, they all have the common property of producing a characteristic neurotoxic protein.

3 CLINICAL ASPECTS

Since botulinum neurotoxin is responsible for the clinical symptoms, food-borne, infant, and wound botulism are clinically similar. The hallmark symptomatology of botulism poisoning is a progressive descending symmetrical paralysis initially affecting musculature innervated by cranial nerves (Dickson 1918) (Fig. 37.2).

The symptomatology, diagnosis and medical treatment of botulism has been periodically reviewed (Koenig 1971, Hughes et al. 1981, Tacket and Rogawski 1989, Cherington 1990). Botulism caused by food poisoning generally has an incubation period of 12–36 h following consumption of a toxic food. The incubation period is shorter when more toxin is consumed and the fatality rate of 'index' cases is higher (Woodruff et al. 1992). Type B food-borne botulism may have a much longer onset time of several days to a few weeks in mild cases (Koenig 1971, St Louis et al. 1988, Woodruff et al. 1992). Patients with botulism may initially have gastrointestinal symptoms such as nausea, vomiting, abdominal cramps and diarrhoea (Hughes et al. 1981), but these signs may not be

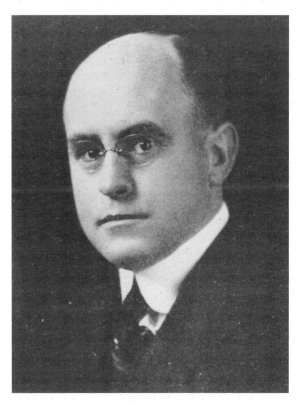

Fig. 37.2 Prof E Dickson (1881–1939), Stanford University.

caused by botulinum toxin since they are not observed in infant or in wound botulism. Constipation, indicated by not passing a stool in 3 days or longer, is commonly observed in infant botulism (Arnon 1995) and occasionally in food-borne botulism (Hughes et al. 1981).

After absorption into the blood the neurotoxin binds to motoneurons and causes flaccid muscle paralysis. Among the first indications of botulism are generalized fatigue and muscular weakness. These are soon followed by disturbances in ocular function, including blurred and double vision, and the pupils become enlarged and unresponsive to light. As intoxication proceeds, weakness and drooping of the eyelids and facial muscles becomes noticeable, speech becomes slurred, and eventual loss of speech ensues. Paralysis of pharyngeal and laryngeal muscles causes difficulty in swallowing and breathing, giving a sensation of suffocation and throat constriction, and regurgitation of food through the nose may be observed. Sputum is often thick and tenacious and thickly coats the tongue. Paralysis of the muscles of the face and neck gives the patient a dull appearance and he becomes unresponsive to stimuli. The inability of the patient to express discomfort can cause hysterical attacks and mental depression. Humans with mild cases of botulism also exhibit poor co-ordination of the arms and legs. Autonomic symptoms of botulism, such as numbness, dizziness, dry mouth, and impairment of salivary and lacrimal secretions, may persist for months (Jenzer et al. 1975). In severe cases extreme muscular weakness leaves the patient unable to raise the head, arms, or legs. The patient becomes gradually weaker, fatigued, and finally death occurs, generally by respiratory failure or possibly by cardiac dysfunction (Lamanna, el-Hage and Vick 1988). Since botulinum toxin primarily affects motor nerves, sensory responses, mental function and conciousness are usually present throughout the illness until the onset of respiratory failure and death. The requirement for intubation and ventilatory support is an indicator of the severity of the disease. Woodruff et al. (1992) found that intubation was necessary for 67% of patients with type A botulism, 52% with type B, and 39% with type E. Of patients that were intubated, 72% involved single case illnesses, whereas only 54% were intubated from outbreak-associated illness. This suggests that patients with mild cases of botulism are often not hospitalized and these cases remain undiagnosed.

Convalescence and recovery from food-borne botulism is generally prolonged, requiring several weeks to months. A retrospective review of cases in the USA found a mean of 58 days of mechanical ventilation for type A, and 26 days for type B (Colice 1987). Recovery of speech and the ability to swallow recurs relatively early. Muscular weakness, vertigo and constipation may persist for several months. The visual disturbances and ability to defecate freely are the last to regain function. Some patients continue to experience weakness, fatigue and symptoms of impaired autonomic nervous system dysfunction, such as dry mouth, consti-

pation, and impotence, even after 1–2 years following the onset of botulism (Colebatch et al. 1989, Cherington 1990).

Although the disease is largely understood, significant mortality (c. 7%) is still associated with food-borne intoxication in the USA. The lethal dose of botulinum toxins in humans is debatable and depends on the individual, the quantity of food and alcohol in the stomach, and the source and serotype of toxin (Schantz and Johnson 1992). Accidental cases of human botulism from ingestion of toxin-contaminated foods showed symptoms of botulism and occasional death from as little as 0.1–1 µg of toxin (100–1000 ng or 3000–30 000 mouse LD50 doses) (Meyer and Eddie 1951, Schantz and Sugiyama 1974). The assumed lethality for humans is c. 1 ng kg^{-1} which is close to the lethal dose of various animals (Gill 1982). Toxins in culture supernatants or preformed in foods are toxic to humans, monkeys, mice, chickens, turkeys and pheasants (Smith 1977, Gill 1982). Toxicity varies according to the serotype, species of animal, and the route of administration (oral, intraperitoneal, or intravenous routes).

Patients with botulism experience varying degrees of illness and are rendered helpless to different extents. Many patients are unable to see because of diplopia and inability to raise their eyelids. Others exhibit difficulty in eating and drinking and with autonomic signs. Still others are admitted to intensive care units and experience difficulty in breathing and require intubation and respiratory assistance. Disease sequelae including infectious diseases such as pneumonia are not uncommon. Communication is disabled by the inability to speak or to write due to ventilatory support and extreme weakness. Agitation, depression and anxiety are common among patients with botulism (Cohen and Anderson 1986).

Infant botulism differs from food-borne and wound botulism in the ages of the affected individuals and because it nearly always begins with severe constipation of 3 days or more that precedes neurological signs by one or more days (Arnon 1995). After initial constipation, the characteristic flaccid paralysis affects the baby's musculature in the head, neck and upper regions of the body. Symptoms include dilated and sluggish response of pupils to light, ptosis of facial muscles, impaired sucking and poor feeding, inability to swallow, a feeble cry, lethargy, generalized weakness, and apathy. Paralysis may gradually become more severe with the baby unable to hold its head erect, increased weakness in extremities, and gradual or abrupt cessation in respiratory ability (Fig. 37.3).

Infant botulism can be difficult to recognize because of the inability of babies to communicate their symptoms and, because it is uncommon, infant botulism is often initially misdiagnosed. Botulism can be misdiagnosed for other neurological diseases such as myasthenia gravis, Guillain–Barré syndrome, tick paralysis, drug reactions, stroke, or viral and bacterial infections of the nervous system. A careful assessment of the progression of clinical signs (L'Hommedieu and Polin 1981) and electrophysiological examination

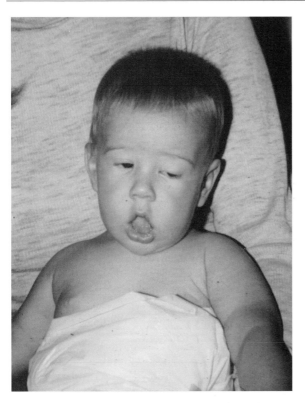

Fig. 37.3 Infant botulism. (Courtesy of Stephen S Arnon, California Department of Health Services, Berkeley, CA).

(Gutierrez, Bodensteiner and Gutmann 1994) can assist in recognizing infant and adult forms of botulism.

As with food-borne botulism, infant botulism varies in severity from mild ptosis and rapid recovery to severe paralysis requiring extended hospitalization. The current clinical picture is composed from those babies showing paralysis of sufficient severity to require hospitalization (Arnon 1995). At the most severe end of the clinical spectrum, babies manifest respiratory difficulties as soon as 5 h after the first neurological effects are recognized (Thompson et al. 1980). It is likely that a fulminant lethal infant botulism occurs in a limited proportion of the infant botulism cases; this severe infant botulism and rapid death may be one cause of sudden infant death syndrome (SIDS) (Arnon 1995). Muscle strength generally returns in 4–8 weeks in the reverse order of occurrence (L'Hommedieu and Polin 1981). Of the classic symptoms, constipation is typically the last to disappear.

Recovery from botulism depends on renewal of neural activity. Although not proved, sprouting from poisoned nerve trunks and formation of new myoneural junctions is required for recovery. This process of renewed neurotransmission requires several weeks to months for completion. Similar to food-borne botulism, infant botulism caused by type A botulinum neurotoxin is often the most severe in symptoms and time required for patient recovery. In California, the mean hospital stay for patients with type A infant botulism was 5.6 weeks, whereas the mean hospital stay for babies with type B infant botulism was 3.7 weeks. For-

tunately, death in hospitalized cases has been rare and babies recover completely with no permanent weakness or neurological abnormalities. When death or chronic morbidity has occurred, it has usually resulted from infections or other secondary complications.

4 DIAGNOSIS AND TREATMENT

4.1 Diagnosis

The diagnosis of botulism relies primarily on assessment of clinical symptoms of the patients and, for food-borne incidents, on the clustering of cases involving a small group of people, often a family or group of friends, who have eaten the same food. For many botulism cases, routine laboratory studies are of no aid in establishing a diagnosis (Koenig 1971). The detection of botulinum toxin in the blood, gastric aspirate and food provides confirmation of botulism. Botulinum toxin has been detected in 60–70% of human patients with type E botulism in large outbreaks or endemic regions (Sebald and Saimot 1973, Barrett 1991). Botulinum toxin is detected less often in type A cases, probably because type A toxin binds more rapidly to motoneurons. Isolation of *C. botulinum* from a suspect food, from faeces of infants, or from wounds provides supporting evidence for the diagnosis of botulism but does not give confirmation since spores are found in the faeces of healthy individuals and from foods (Hatheway 1988).

4.2 Detection of neurotoxin

Following enrichment and isolation of pure cultures from foods or clinical specimens, the identification of botulinogenic clostridia initially involves the demonstration of botulinum neurotoxin by bioassay in animals (Schantz and Kautter 1978, Hatheway 1988, Solomon, Rhodehamel and Kautter 1995). Foods, blood (serum) and stools should also be examined for the presence of botulinum toxin (Solomon, Rhodehamel and Kautter 1995). For toxin assay, centrifuged supernatant from TPGY (trypticase peptone, glucose, yeast extract medium) 5–7 days old, or cooked meat broths, is injected intraperitoneally into mice and the animals observed for signs of botulism periodically for up to 4 days. Symptoms of botulism usually are observed within 24 h and manifest as reduced mobility, ruffling of fur, laboured breathing, contraction of abdominal muscles, followed rapidly by convulsions and death. Animals showing these signs within 2–24 h of injection usually die within 48 h. The presence of botulinum activity is confirmed by neutralization with antitoxin and identified to serotype by neutralization with a type-specific antitoxin (Hatheway 1988, Gimenez and Gimenez 1995, Solomon, Rhodehamel and Kautter 1995).

Complications are often encountered in the mouse assay for botulinum toxin, particularly deaths caused by non-botulinum interfering agents. Fatalities occurring in less than 2 h or after 48 h should be considered suspect and the assay should be repeated. Fatalities from *Clostridium tetani* or other clostridia may be encountered if soil or sediment samples are being examined. With foods or clinical specimens, non-botulinum deaths from infection or endotoxins may occur. These non-specific deaths often take place within a few hours of injection and mice do not exhibit the typical signs of botulism. Generally, it is possible to dilute out the non-specific interfering agent using a gelatin-phosphate buffer to an end point where the non-specific deaths are eliminated. Occasionally, a specimen or culture fluid will contain more than one serotype of botulinum toxin. Cultures which produce type C_1 neurotoxin also produce type D neurotoxin in small amounts and can also produce C_2 toxin. There are also occasional reports of strains that produce 2 toxin types, of which one is at much higher titre than the other. When 2 toxin types are present in the sample being analysed, it is necessary to neutralize the toxicity with a combination of monovalent antitoxins. Since botulinum toxins are extremely labile to heat (Woodburn et al. 1979), heating with loss of activity can also support the view that mice fatalities are caused by a heat-labile protein toxin. Non-proteolytic strains of *C. botulinum* produce botulinum toxins in a less active, unnicked form. These can be activated by a protease such as trypsin to achieve full toxicity. In certain foods, trypsinization can produce peptides exhibiting toxicity in mice; the activation reaction should be stopped by adding soybean trypsin inhibitor after 30–60 min.

Botulinum toxins can be quantitatively titred by determining the dose required to kill 50% of a population of test animals. This quantity, defined as 1 LD50, is a statistical measurement based on the number of animals in each test group and the susceptibility of the test animals to the toxin. Quantitation is usually done with 5–10 animals per dilution and the results plotted logarithmically with % death on the vertical axis and dilution on the horizontal axis. The point at which the line connecting the % death at each dilution crosses 50% is the dilution that contains 1 LD50 per injection volume (Schantz and Kautter 1978). From this curve the number of LD50 in the original sample is calculated. This method is both expensive, due to the number of animals used, and time-consuming. For these reasons other methods of detecting botulinum toxin have been devised.

An alternative method of determining the quantity of active botulinum toxin in a sample is the intravenous time-to-death method of Boroff and Fleck (1966). This method involves injection of a sample into the tail vein of an immobilized mouse. The time-to-death is noted and converted to the number of intraperitoneal LD50 using a standard curve prepared using the dilution to extinction method of Schantz and Kautter (1978). The method is fast and relatively accurate ($\pm 20\%$). Drawbacks to this method are the preparation of the standard curve and the need for a higher level of technical expertise. The method is only applicable when the quantity of toxin injected is within the linear portion of the standard curve: ($1 \times$ 10^6)–(5×10^3) LD50 per ml of type A toxin. Standard curves are required for each serotype of toxin since the time to death differs for each.

A number of immunological methods have been developed (Notermans and Nagel 1989) but few are used routinely. These immunological methods have the drawback of lack of sensitivity, expense, cross-reactions between different serotypes, and the detection of biologically inactive botulinum toxin. The immunological method that appears most practical is the enzyme-linked immunosorbent assay (ELISA). The various ELISA methods use an antibody or series of antibodies specific for a given toxin serotype to capture and label the toxin. An ELISA using snake venom as part of an amplification system to detect botulinum toxins has been developed and has been reported to detect c. 10 pg of neurotoxin or about 1 mouse LD50 (Doellgast et al. 1993). It is unlikely that immunological assays will completely replace the mouse assay.

4.3 Treatment

Treatment of all forms of botulism requires rapid and meticulous supportive and respiratory care. Admission to intensive care units and careful attention to airway sufficiency is of high priority. Intubation with mechanical ventilation, and nasogastric feeding are required in severe cases. Rapid administration of trivalent botulinum antitoxin is of value in decreasing morbidity and mortality from botulism (Tacket et al. 1984). In the USA, patients may be administered multivalent botulism equine antitoxin intravenously [approximately 10 000 International Units (IU) each of type A, B and E antitoxins] as soon as a diagnosis is made. The product is available through government public health departments. One IU neutralizes 10 000 mouse LD50s (types A and B) and 1000 LD50s (type E), which is sufficient to neutralize toxic doses encountered in human botulism. The antitoxin has a half-life in the serum of 5–7 days (Hatheway et al. 1984). It is necessary to administer antitoxin as soon as a diagnosis is confirmed since the antibodies probably do not neutralize neurotoxin that has bound to motoneurons, and certainly not toxin that has been internalized within the nerve by endocytosis. Antitoxin would thus not improve symptoms present at the time of administration, but may stop progression of the paralysis (Hatheway 1995). Over a period of 11 years, equine antitoxin has led to hypersensitivity reactions in about 9% of treated patients (Black and Gunn 1980). It would be useful to produce a supply of antitoxin from human donors or to produce 'humanized' animal antibodies by available molecular biology techniques. A clinical trial underway in California is designed to evaluate the use of botulism immune globulin (BIG) from human donors for infant botulism (Frankovich and Arnon 1991, Arnon 1995).

The fatality rate in the USA from food-borne botulism has decreased from 65% for the period 1899–1949 to 25% for the period 1950–77. Good supportive and ventilatory care and diagnosis of milder cases were probably mostly responsible for the drop in fatality rate during this period, but administration of anti-toxin was also helpful. During the period 1978–93, the fatality rate from food-borne botulism dropped to c. 7% (Centers for Disease Control 1979, 1991–1995, Rhodehamel 1992). This encouraging trend in survival was probably improved by rapid diagnosis, further improved supportive care in intensive care units, rapid administration of trivalent antitoxin, and prevention of secondary infections. Patients given trivalent antitoxin within 24 h of onset of type A botulism had a shorter course of illness but the same fatality rate as those who received antitoxin later (Tacket et al. 1984). These results suggest that antitoxin treatment can be beneficial if administered rapidly. Aminoglycoside antibiotics are to be avoided in the treatment of secondary infections since they can potentiate muscle paralysis (L'Hommedieu and Polin 1981).

Since botulism occurs rarely in humans, it is not practical to routinely immunize human populations. Natural immunity has not been observed in humans, even in individuals who have experienced repeated botulism or in infants continuously exposed to toxin over several weeks in cases of infant botulism. The dose of toxin required to elicit an antibody response is not known, but is probably much higher than the lethal dose. Increasing numbers of humans have developed antibodies when injected periodically for the treatment of neuromuscular disorders (Borodic et al. 1996). Humans who routinely handle botulinum toxins can be effectively immunized by pentavalent toxoid available from the CDC and other international governmental agencies. Vaccines are commercially produced for the immunization of domestic animals such as mink, horses and cattle.

It is noteworthy that 3 cases of botulism occurred in laboratory workers in Germany who administered powdered type A toxin to laboratory animals (van Holzer 1962). This appears to be the only report of botulism from a laboratory accident and it emphasizes the care needed when working with botulinum toxins; aerosols can be formed in laboratory equipment such as centrifuges and scrupulous attention should be paid to laboratory practices when working with *C. botulinum* and its toxins. All materials suspected of containing botulinum toxin should be handled with maximum precaution and only by experienced personnel who have been immunized with pentavalent toxoid. Extreme caution should be taken to avoid contact of toxic materials with the eyes, mouth, or nasal mucosa. Centrifugation and other laboratory procedures that can generate aerosol should be performed only in sealed, non-breakable containers (stainless steel or plastic ware).

5 EPIDEMIOLOGY

5.1 Food-borne botulism

Food-borne botulism occurs in clustered geographical regions of the world (Fig. 37.4) (Hauschild 1993). In most countries it is quite rare, although, like other food-borne diseases, the actual incidence of botulism is undoubtedly greater than reported. Many mild cases are probably not diagnosed and patients are not admitted for treatment or reported. Botulism may be misdiagnosed as another neurological disorder. Even so, the characteristic and often severe symptoms of botulism and careful records of release of antitoxin for treatment probably make botulism one of the most accurately reported food-borne diseases.

Through his thorough ecological surveys and study of *C. botulinum*, Meyer (1956) (Fig. 37.5) concluded that the risk of botulism is greater in regions that have a high telluric incidence of type A, B and E spores. The primary regions of the world with reports of human food-borne botulism are East Asia (China, Japan), North America, certain countries in Europe (Poland, Germany, France, Italy, Spain, Portugal, Denmark, and Norway), the Middle East (Iran), Latin America, Russia and South Africa (Hauschild 1992). Human botulism is rare in the UK, although notable outbreaks, including the Loch Maree tragedy (Leighton 1923), the Birmingham incident (Ball et al. 1979), and the hazelnut yoghurt outbreak (O'Mahony et al. 1990), have attracted much attention. Human botulism is also rare in Africa, Australia, Israel, Taiwan, Greece, New Zealand, India, Mexico and several South American countries (Hauschild 1992).

Botulism is endemic in certain regions of the USA, particularly the Pacific Coast states and Alaska. Botulism outbreaks in the USA reached a peak during the 1930s and then declined due to energetic preventive measures in the commercial canned food industry and the development of guidelines for home canning (Meyer 1956). From 1899 to 1949, there were 1281 cases and 830 deaths, from 1950 to 1977, 678 cases and 169 deaths, and from 1978 to 1993, 423 cases and 31 deaths in the USA (Centers for Disease Control 1991–1995, Rhodehamel, Reddy and Pierson 1992). Foods involved in mainland USA botulism are usually home-canned fruits and vegetables. Of 182 outbreaks identified with foods during 1971–89, 137 were caused by fruits and vegetables, 15 by meats, 13 by fish, and 17 by other foods including mixed vehicles. In the USA, approximately 60% of food-borne botulism cases have been caused by type A toxin, 18% by type B, and 22% by type E (Hatheway 1995). In Alaska, fermented meats and fish accounted for 98% of the outbreaks, most involving type E botulinum toxin (Wainwright et al. 1988, Barrett 1991). Botulism may unexpectedly occur with advances in food handling and changes in preservation practices. Poor process control and maintenance of chilled distribution of smoked whitefish from the Great Lakes resulted in a resurgence of botulism in the 1960s (Foster et al. 1965). In the 1970s, changes in packaging procedures and underprocessing led to botulinum toxin production by *C. botulinum* in canned mushrooms prepared by 7 USA commercial producers (Lynt, Kautter and Read 1975). Production of foods with minimal or no preservatives and relying primarily on refrigeration for controlling *C. botulinum* has led to outbreaks of botulism (Hutchinson 1992, Rhodehamel, Reddy and Pierson 1992). Increased

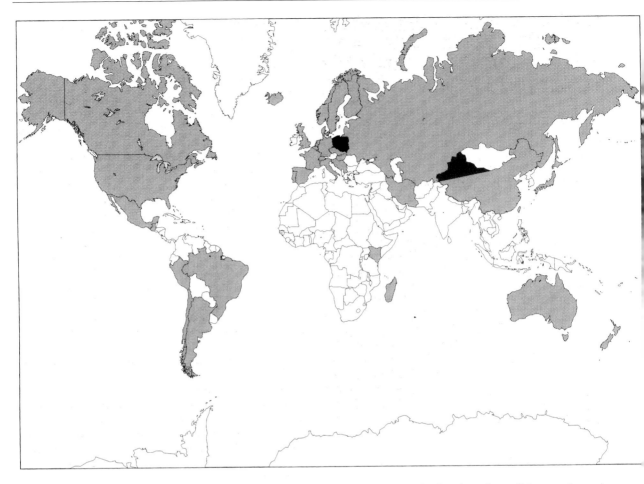

Fig. 37.4 Food-borne botulism in regions of the world. The highest incidence (Poland and northern China are shown in black), countries with reported botulism in grey, and those without reported food-borne botulism are white. (Adapted from the data of Hauschild 1993).

consumption of foods in food service establishments in the USA have had an impact on food-borne disease (Hedberg, MacDonald and Osterholm 1994), including botulism (MacDonald, Cohen and Blake 1986). Several outbreaks of botulism involving commercially processed or restaurant-prepared foods have occurred in various regions of the world (Table 37.2).

Although food-borne botulism is rare, the consequences of botulism outbreaks are extremely serious and it is vital that the food industry process and formulate minimally processed foods to prevent growth and toxin formation by *C. botulinum*. Outbreaks of botulism involving commercial foods or foods prepared in restaurants have generated considerable publicity and expense. The average cost of a botulism case due to a commercially processed food has been estimated to be as high as 30 million USA dollars when issues related to hospital costs, lost productivity and legal expenses are considered (CAST 1994).

In Canada, during the period 1961–89, 87% of botulism cases occurred in northern native Canadian communities. As in Alaska, type E botulinum toxin was involved and the prevalent foods included home fermented meats from marine mammals, fish, or vegetables (Hauschild 1992). The practice of holding meats at ambient temperatures until a desired flavour

and texture is achieved allows *C. botulinum* type E to produce toxin. The largest outbreak in the history of Canada occurred in 1985 and the food vehicle was chopped garlic in oil (St Louis et al. 1988). Canada and the USA have made efforts to reduce the incidence of botulism by encouraging strict adherence to temperature control by processors, distributors, retailers and in restaurants (Rhodehamel 1992), acidifying or providing other *C. botulinum* inhibitory conditions in foods that receive minimal processing. Currently, there is concern of botulism from minimally processed refrigerated foods, restaurant-prepared foods, vacuum-packaged or modified atmosphere packaged foods, and sous-vide products (Rhodehamel 1992).

Botulism is relatively common on the Asian continent. Botulism was first documented in China in 1949 and *C. botulinum* was isolated from botulinogenic food in 1958 (Ying and Shuyan 1986). From 1958 through 1983, 986 outbreaks occurred in China affecting 4377 individuals. The majority of cases have occurred in the northern provinces of Xinjiang (81.3%), Qinghai (3.4%), Xizang (4.5%), Shandong (5.6%) and Hebei (1.9%). The epidemiology of botulism is unique in China compared with other areas of the world; 824 outbreaks (86% of total diagnosed) have been caused

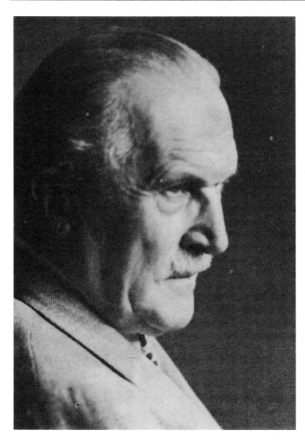

Fig. 37.5 Prof Karl F Meyer (1884–1974), Hooper Foundation, University of California at San Francisco.

by bean products, most (74%) by improperly fermented bean curd. Botulism occurs mainly in the winter and early spring when vegetables are scarce and home-made fermented foods are commonly prepared. During 1958–83, type A botulism accounted for 93.4%, type B for 5.0%, mixtures of types A and B for 0.4%, and type E for 1.0% of the botulism cases in China. The incidence of botulism in China has decreased considerably since 1974 because of education of households, advice to food manufacturing plants, inclusion of 10% salt in bean curd fermentations, and heating of foods prior to consumption (Ying and Shuyan 1986).

The majority of botulism cases in Japan occur in the northern prefectures of Hokkaido, Akita, Aomora and Iwate (Iida 1970). Nearly all cases are caused by fish or fermented fish products, particularly izushi, and involve type E toxin (Iida 1970, Hauschild 1992). Type E spores are common in the soils and sediments of Hokkaido and Tohoku, and they readily contaminate fish. Prominent symptoms of type E botulism in Japan are dysfunction of salivary secretion and retention of urine. These symptoms have not been reported as frequently in types A and B human botulism. The case-fatality rate has decreased over time since type E antitoxin was distributed and communities were advised about the preparation of izushi. In 1984, an outbreak of type A botulism occurrred in Japan, involving 36 cases with 11 deaths. The causative food was vacuum-packaged 'Karashi-Renkon' (deep-fried mustard-stuffed lotus root). Normally, this food is heated by residents but it was eaten unheated by tourists who were presented with the product as a souvenir

Table 37.2 Outbreaks of food-borne botulism from commercial foods or restaurant prepared foods

Food product	Year	Location	Toxin type	No. cases	No. deaths	Reference
Canned peppers	1977	USA	B	58	0	Terranova et al. 1978
Canned Alaskan salmon	1978	UK	E	4	2	Ball et al. 1979
Kapchunka (salt-cured, uneviscerated whitefish)	1981	USA	B	1	0	Rhodehamel, Reddy and Pierson 1992
Beef pot pie	1982	USA	A	1	0	Centers for Disease Control 1983
Sauteed onions	1983	USA	A	28	1	MacDonald et al. 1985
Karahi-renkon (vacuum-packed, deep-fried, mustard-stuffed, lotus root)	1984	Japan	A	36	11	Otofuji, Tokiwa and Takahashi 1987
Chopped garlic-in-oil	1985	Canada	B	36	0	St Louis et al. 1988
Kapchunka	1987	USA/Israel	E	8	2	Slater et al. 1989 Telzak et al. 1990
Chopped garlic-in-oil	1989	USA	A	3	0	Morse et al. 1990
Hazelnut yoghurt	1989	UK	B	27	1	O'Mahony et al. 1990
Faseikh (salted fish)	1991	Egypt	E	92	20	Weber et al. 1993
Cheese sauce	1993	USA	A	5	1	Townes et al. 1996
Skordalia (Greek salad with baked potato)	1994	USA	A	19	0	F Angulo (CDC) personal communication

(Hayashi, Sakaguchi and Sakaguchi 1986, Otofuji, Tokiwa and Takahashi 1987).

In most countries botulism is regionally distributed and is associated mostly with home-prepared foods. Outbreaks of fish-related botulism, 'ichthyism', in Russia were reported in 1927 (Dewberry 1950), and were caused by eating sturgeon or improperly prepared caviar (Smith and Sugiyama 1988). Botulism in Russia and the Ukraine has mostly been caused by salted, dried or smoked fish (Dolman 1964), though home-cured hams, preserved wild mushrooms, and stuffed eggplant have also been food vehicles involving type A and B botulinum toxins (Smith and Sugiyama 1988).

In Europe, most outbreaks of botulism are caused by improperly canned or cured meats such as hams or sausages. Non-proteolytic strains producing type B toxin are most commonly responsible for toxin production. Poland has experienced more botulism than any other nation; most (92%) outbreaks occurred in rural areas through consumption of improperly canned or preserved meats, 7% from fish products. Botulism has occurred in Germany more often than other European countries except Poland (Smith and Sugiyama 1988). The usual vehicle is improperly preserved meats and type B botulinum toxin is usually involved. In France, botulism has occurred periodically, the usual vehicle being home-cured ham (Roblot et al. 1994). Type B toxin was responsible for 97% of the diagnosed cases. Botulism, usually caused by type B botulinum toxin, has sporadically been reported in Italy and Spain, usually from home-canned vegetables or home-preserved vegetables in oil. Botulism in Scandinavia is generally caused by improperly preserved fish and involves type E toxin.

Botulism is comparatively rare in the UK. In 1922, the famous Loch Maree tragedy caused 8 illnesses and 8 deaths from the consumption of sandwiches prepared with wild duck paste. As a result of this outbreak, the Ministry of Health made arrangements for a supply of botulinum antitoxin to be available at various locations. In 1989, the UK observed its largest botulism outbreak in its history (Critchley, Hayes and Issacs 1989). Until this outbreak, there had been only 18 cases reported since the 8 fatal ones in Loch Maree. The vehicle in the 1987 incident was hazelnut yoghurt. The hazelnut puree, added to the yoghurt, had been underprocessed and allowed *C. botulinum* type B to grow and produce toxin. Rapid diagnosis and action by the health authorities prevented additional cases by the commercial product.

Food-borne botulism has also been recorded sporadically in various other countries throughout the world (Smith and Sugiyama 1988, Hauschild 1992). Argentina and Mexico are the only countries in Central and South America that have reported significant numbers of botulism cases. Reports of human botulism are rare in African countries (Hauschild 1992). The first human outbreak in Africa was reported in 1979 and was caused by type A toxin in sour milk (Smith, Timms and Refai 1979). A second outbreak was attributed to consumption of termites, a cultural cuisine. The termites had been kept in a sealed bag for 3 days, which probably promoted growth of *C. botulinum* (Knightingale and Ayim 1980). From 1942 to 1984, only 5 outbreaks of botulism were reported in Australia, 4 associated with vegetables and one with canned tuna (Hauschild 1992).

The majority of food-borne botulism cases have been reported from the northern hemisphere (Hauschild 1992). Types A and B botulinum toxins are responsible for botulism in the more temperate regions, those from type E in colder regions. It seems paradoxical that botulism by proteolytic strains of *C. botulinum* types A and B occurs mostly in vegetables, whereas non-proteolytic type B mostly causes botulism in proteinaceous foods such as meats (Hatheway 1995). This pattern may be due to the heat resistance of spores from proteolytic strains, which survive the heating processes of home canning, whereas the non-proteolytic spores are killed. Botulism by non-proteolytic type B is usually associated with minimally processed foods that are not heated prior to consumption. A final preventive measure that prevents botulism is the heating of foods before eating as all serotypes of botulinum toxin are extremely labile to heat and are inactivated by treatment at 60–100°C for 10 min (Woodburn et al. 1979). Seasonal occurrence of outbreaks is associated with cultural customs of preserving foods. The low frequency of botulism in many countries is related to the density of *C. botulinum* spores in the environment and in foods, to hygienic practices in food production, and to cooking foods prior to consumption.

5.2 Wound botulism

Wound botulism is the counterpart of tetanus and results from botulinum toxin produced from *C. botulinum* infecting a wound. Wound botulism is the rarest form of botulism; only about 80 cases have been reported in the USA since its discovery in 1943 (Davis, Mattman and Wiley 1951). Most cases involve type A botulinum toxin, due in part because about half the USA cases have occurred in California, where type A spores are prevalent. Since wound botulism is so rare, misdiagnosis and delay in treatment have been reported (Burningham et al. 1994). Symptoms of wound botulism are similar to those of food-borne botulism and manifest as a symmetrical descending paralysis starting in the ocular region. The case-fatality rate has been c. 15%. Wound botulism is suspected following trauma or a superficial wound without obvious infection and no history of consumption of botulinogenic food. Wound botulism in the USA has recently been associated with intranasal use of cocaine and subcutaneous injection of heroin (MacDonald, Cohen and Blake 1986, Elston, Wang and Loo 1991). Since 1991, 32 laboratory confirmed cases of wound botulism in California were diagnosed as injecting drug users (Centers for Disease Control 1991–1995). An unfortunate case of wound botulism was also reported in a boy of 5 years who died from toxin produced in a tooth abscess (Weber et al. 1993). Five cases of wound botulism have been reported from France, Italy, Australia and China (Hatheway 1995). *C. botulinum* has been demonstrated recently to infect intestinal lesions, particularly following surgery (Chia et al. 1986, McCroskey et al. 1991). Botulinum toxin is produced in these intestinal lesions and absorbed into the blood.

The rare occurrence of wound botulism in non-immunized humans compared with tetanus suggests that *C. botulinum* is less infective when compared with *C. tetani*. Spores of type A and B *C. botulinum* and *C. tetani* were isolated from 18.5 and 30% of soil samples in the USA (Smith 1978) and the incidence of spores does not explain the different infectious ability. The explanation apparently involves unidentified virulence factors present in *C. tetani*, allowing the invasion and growth within human tissues. Tetanus spores will germinate in human and animal tissues of sufficiently low oxidation–reduction potential and produce a large population of vegetative cells in 6–24 h (Fildes 1927, Smith and MacIver 1974). *C. botulinum* spores germinated but apparently failed to outgrow after subcutaneous injection or tissue implantation in mice (Suzuki et al. 1971, Suzuki and Grecz 1972). Injection of rat caecal contents together with *C. botulinum* type A spores (Joiner et al. 1980) allowed germination and outgrowth of *C. botulinum* spores, suggesting that nutritional requirements or host defences may limit the growth of *C. botulinum* in wound infections (Dezfulian and Bartlett 1985). *C. botulinum* can also infect wounds but toxin production is impaired or toxin is inactivated (Hall 1945). Although vast numbers of neonatal tetanus annual fatalities occur world wide (Stanfield and Galazka 1985), neonatal botulism is unreported and apparently quite rare.

5.3 Infant botulism

Infant botulism is the paralytic syndrome resulting from botulinum neurotoxin produced in the intestinal tract of infants (and also susceptible children and adults). Ingested spores of *C. botulinum* germinate, outgrow in the large intestine and produce botulinum toxin. Infant botulism was recognized in 1976 in California in 2 cases that occurred within 4 months of each other (Pickett et al. 1976). In the same year, Midura and Arnon (1976) isolated and identified *C. botulinum* and demonstrated botulinum toxin in the faeces of infants with botulism. Infant botulism is now the most common cause of botulism in the USA and also has been demonstrated in other countries (Fig. 37.6).

As of January 1994, 1270 hospitalized cases of infant botulism had been reported world wide and 1206 (95%) occurred in the USA (Paisley, Lauer and Arnon 1995); about half the cases were from California. It is likely that infant botulism is often unrecognized and not reported (Cochran and Appleton 1995). Infant botulism has also been reported from various countries world wide, including Argentina (23 cases), Australia (11 cases), Japan (10 cases), the UK (6 cases), Canada (4 cases) and one case each in Chile,

former Czechoslovakia, France, Spain, Sweden, Switzerland and Taiwan (Dodds 1993). Within the USA, infant botulism occurs in clustered geographical regions. The highest incidence has been reported from California, Colorado, Delaware, Hawaii, Utah and Pennsylvania (Arnon 1995). The clustered geographical occurrence of infant botulism is not understood, but may be associated with the distribution of *C. botulinum* spore type and prevalence in the environment. This distribution has been demonstrated in the USA, where the majority of type B cases are reported from the eastern states, and most type A cases from California. The environment, soils, dust and surfaces of foods harvested from soils are probably the main sources of spores in infant botulism. The only known food source is honey (Hauschild et al. 1988, Fenicia et al. 1993, Arnon 1995). The *C. botulinum* spore type contaminating honey will depend on the geographical source and whether the honey is blended before marketing. Although infant botulism is very rare in the UK, efforts are underway to label jars of honey with the statement that it should not be fed to infants under one year of age. In several infant botulism cases, *C. botulinum* spores were isolated from honey fed to infants who contracted botulism, and the spore type has in all cases examined matched the toxin type found in the baby's faeces (Arnon 1995). With education of physicians and parents not to feed honey to babies less than one year of age, the number of honey-related cases has diminished.

Proteolytic strains of *C. botulinum* have been responsible for almost all cases of reported infant botulism, and all but 7 of almost 1300 reported cases have resulted from botulinum neurotoxin type A or B. Type F infant botulism caused by toxigenic *C. baratii* was reported from New Mexico in 1979 (Hoffmann et al. 1982). This case appeared to be an anomaly until 1987 when type F intestinal botulism was reported in an adult in Georgia, and the organism responsible was identified as *C. baratii* (McCroskey et al. 1991). A second case of *C. baratii* infant botulism was reported in 1995 (Paisley, Lauer and Arnon 1995). Like the first type F case, the onset time was very rapid, and the patients were quite young, 9 and 14 days of age, respectively. Type C infant botulism was reported in Japan (Oguma et al. 1990), 2 type E cases from Italy (Aureli et al. 1986), and 3 cases by type Bf in the USA (Arnon 1995).

Although infant botulism has been reported in babies up to 12 months of age, 95% of cases have been reported from babies less than 6 months old. The youngest cases reported were 6 and 8 days of age, respectively, and the oldest 363 days (Arnon 1995). Infant botulism shows a peak in incidence in children 2–6 months of age, and the age-at-onset distribution shows a close match to the SIDS. A proportion of SIDS cases may be the fatal result of a rapid onset, fulminant form of botulism (Arnon 1995). Breast feeding appears to slow the development of the disease (Arnon et al. 1982) and has been considered a risk factor but may actually delay the disease for a sufficient period so that the babies can be hospitalized

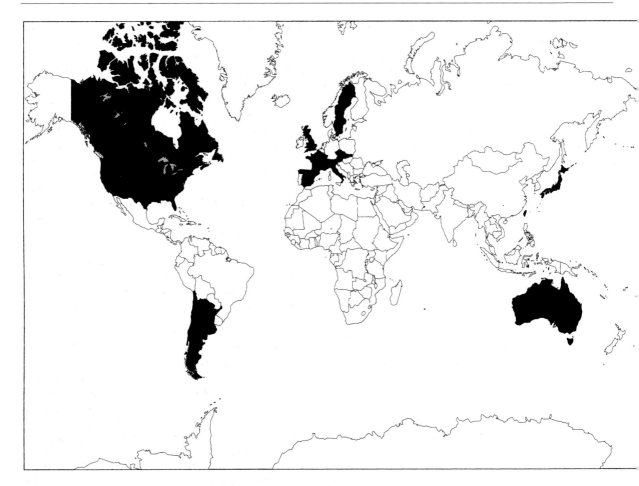

Fig. 37.6 Countries throughout the world with reported infant botulism (shown in black).

and receive supportive care. All fulminant cases of infant botulism where the children died before hospitalization were formula fed. The case-fatality rate of infant botulism in the USA is less than 2%, but infants are hospitalized for several weeks. Boys and girls are equally susceptible and all major racial and ethnic groups are affected.

Intestinal infections by *C. botulinum* with accompanying in vivo botulinum toxin production has occurred in adults, particularly in individuals who have undergone intestinal surgery (Chia et al. 1986, Freedman et al. 1986, McCroskey and Hatheway 1988). Conditions associated with intestinal surgery, such as lesions in the intestine and antibiotic treatment, causing alterations in the microflora could predispose humans to colonization by *C. botulinum*. The use of intense immunosuppression and bowel sterilizing regimens in a 3-year-old girl with neuroblastoma were postulated to enable colonization by *C. botulinum* types A and B with ensuing infant botulism (Shen et al. 1994). Infections by *C. botulinum* in adults have been supported by the finding of botulinum toxin and organisms in the faeces over a period of several months (McCroskey and Hatheway 1988, McCroskey et al. 1991, Hatheway 1995). Most patients with food-borne botulism in the USA are treated with trivalent antitoxin. It is not practical to monitor the serum for

the presence of toxin. In France, Sebald and Saimot (1973) found type B toxin in serum from individuals for up to 122 days after the ingestion of toxic food. Relatively mild and progressive development of botulism occurred over several weeks in patients who had eaten chopped garlic in oil containing type B toxin and organisms (St Louis et al. 1988). These observations suggest that *C. botulinum* type B could colonize the intestine of adults and continuously produce toxin over several weeks to months. These examples involved type B botulinum toxin. *C. botulinum* type B may have a greater abililty than type A to colonize the intestinal tract, which could help explain why more than 50% of the infant botulism cases in the USA involve type B, although type A food-borne botulism is 3 times more prevalent than type B.

5.4 Animal botulism

Animal botulism is the most prevalent type of botulism world wide and has caused enormous losses of wild and domestic animals. Botulism has considerable economic importance in cattle, chickens, turkeys, geese, mink and sheep (Meyer 1956, Eklund and Dowell 1987, Smith and Sugiyama 1988). Vertebrates vary considerably in their susceptibility to botulism (Gunnison and Meyer 1930, Gill 1982). Humans, horses and guinea pigs are among the most susceptible animals to oral exposure of botulinum toxins. Certain animals are relatively resistant to botulinum toxins, including vultures (Kalmbach 1939), dogs and rats. Many of these animals consume rotting vegetation or carrion. Resistance is probably due in most cases to the instability of botulinum toxin in the gut or its inability to enter into the blood, although vultures and possibly other animals possess substances in their blood that neutralize botulinum toxin (Kalmbach 1939). The oral dose for animals and humans varies considerably among individuals as well as between species and is difficult to quantitate since it is influenced by a number of factors, such as the amount of food present in the stomach. The ranges of susceptibility to botulinum toxins are smaller when the toxins are injected intraperitoneally, intravenously, or subcutaneously. Only twice the quantity of type B toxin was needed to kill guinea pigs orally as by subcutaneous injection, 10 times as much for mice, and 5 times as much for rabbits (Gunnison and Meyer 1930). The signs and symptoms of animal botulism are similar to human disease and typically involve sudden weakness, loss of muscle control and tremors, recumbency and eventually death. The clinical diagnosis of botulism in animals is confirmed by detection of botulinum toxin in serum, faeces or both serum and faeces.

Botulism in cattle, referred to as lamsietke in South Africa or forage poisoning in the USA, usually results from ingestion of preformed toxin (Smith and Sugiyama 1988). Growth of *C. botulinum* in the feed silage or supplementation of feeds with animal products such as ensiled poultry litter (Jean et al. 1995) can lead to intoxication. Cattle botulism is associated with phosphorus deficiency in the soil. Botulinum types B, C and D have been responsible for intoxications. Type B poisoning is most common in the USA and Europe, whereas types C and D predominate in Australia and South Africa. Type A botulism was reported for the first time recently in cattle (zebu, *Bos indicus*) raised in Brazil for meat production (Schocken-Iturrino et al. 1990). Botulism in sheep resembles the disease of cattle, and is mostly a problem in Australia and South Africa (Smith and Sugiyama 1988).

Horses are among the most sensitive of animals to botulinum toxin types B, C and D (Swerczek 1980a, 1980b, Kinde et al. 1991). Botulism in horses manifests as sudden generalized weakness, diminished pupillary eye response, severe tremors of the fore and hind limbs, eventual recumbency, laborious breathing, and death. Generally, toxin is produced by *C. botulinum* in the intestinal tract of horses, and thus resembles infant botulism (Swerczek 1980a, 1980b). Toxic infections in horses has been referred to as 'shaker foal syndrome'. Autopsy specimens have revealed intestinal lesions that may provide a suitable environment for the multiplication of *C. botulinum*. Horse botulism can also be caused by ingestion of preformed toxin. Feed containing animal carrion and water harbouring cat or rodent carcasses have caused equine botulism

(Kinde et al. 1991). Therapy for botulism in horses is similar to that in other animals: stall rest, antitoxin in the early stages of the disease, no treatment with aminoglycosides or metronidazole, oral alimentation and respiratory assistance (Whitlock 1996).

Botulism is a considerable problem in the domestic farming of mink, primarily because mink farmers often feed their animals raw and partially decomposed meat or fish. Mink are voracious eaters and can consume several hundred grams of foods each day. Even low levels of toxin in food are suffcient to cause botulism since botulinum toxin accumulates over a suitable period. Most mink botulism is usually caused by type C botulinum toxin, although types A and E have been reported to cause intoxications. Type C toxoids are commercially available for immunizing minks. Botulism has also been observed in other domestic and zoo animals such as dogs, monkeys, turtles and fish. The animals vary in their sensitivity to toxin, and may be quite resistant to certain serotypes and sensitive to others. Dogs seem to be most susceptible to type C toxin (Barsanti et al. 1978, Smith and Sugiyama 1988), monkeys to type A and B, turtles to type C, and fish to type E (Smith and Sugiyama 1988).

Among all phyla of animals, birds experience the largest outbreaks and botulism probably causes the most casualties of microbial diseases afflicting birds (Eklund and Dowell 1987). Almost every family of birds seems susceptible to botulism (Jensen and Price 1987) except for carrion eating types such as vultures. Avian botulism has been reported from all continents except the Antarctic and is generally caused by type C botulinum toxin. Occasional outbreaks have involved types D and E botulinum toxins (Smith and Sugiyama 1988). Large outbreaks due to botulism have been reported in chickens, ducks, pheasants, pelicans, gulls, flamingos, swans, and numerous other species of wild water fowl including endangered species such as the bald eagle and peregrine falcon (Jensen and Price 1987). Most birds seem to acquire botulism through the consumption of preformed toxin, often from the consumption of invertebrates such as fly larvae (maggots) within decomposing dead carcasses.

6 AETIOLOGY

The genus *Clostridium* consists of gram-positive, anaerobic, spore-forming bacilli that obtain energy for growth by fermentation. The genus *Clostridium* is a large and diverse group of prokaryotes and more than 100 species have been assigned to it (Cato, George and Finegold 1986, Hippe, Andreesen and Gottschalk 1992). Over all, the genus *Clostridium* has a wide range of G + C content of 22–55 mol%, whereas the toxigenic species have a much narrower range of G + C content of 24–29 mol% (Hatheway 1990). The clostridia have common phenotypic properties that currently define the genus. Designation of a bacterial isolate in the genus *Clostridium* depends on the presence of 4 primary phenotypic characters (Hippe, Andreesen and Gottschalk 1992):

1 the presence of endospores
2 an anaerobic energy metabolism not involving electron transport with oxygen as an acceptor
3 inability to reduce sulphate to sulphide and
4 a cell wall having a gram-positive structure and positive gram staining reaction in the early stages of growth.

The peptidoglycan of neurotoxigenic clostridia that have been examined is linked by *meso*-diaminopimelic acid (Cummins and Johnson 1971, Schleifer and Kandler 1972, Weiss, Schleifer and Kandler 1981).

The diversity of organisms presently classified as *Clostridium* clearly indicates the genus is in need of taxonomic restructuring (Cato and Stackenbrandt 1989). There has been a proposal to reclassify *Clostridium* into 5 new genera and 11 new species combinations (Collins et al. 1994). Classification based on genetic and protein relatedness may be good indicators of the evolutionary relationships of bacterial groups (Goodfellow and O'Donnell 1993), but it is often not practical to use these methods for routine and rapid identification of pathogenic organisms, including clostridia that produce botulinum neurotoxin. Most investigators will continue to classify clostridia that produce botulinum toxin into only a few species (Table 37.3) because of the characteristic mode of action and medical importance of the neurotoxins.

The standard method for the identification of botulinogenic organisms is the neutralization of neurotoxicity with specific antitoxins (Hatheway 1988, Gimenez and Gimenez 1995). For many years, all organisms that produced botulinum neurotoxin were classified in the species *C. botulinum*. This classification has expanded to include strains of *C. butyricum* (Aureli et al. 1986) and *C. baratii* that produce botulinum neuro-

toxins (Hall et al. 1985, Suen et al. 1988a, 1988b, McCroskey et al. 1991, Paisley, Lauer and Arnon et al. 1995). The species *Clostridium argentinense* has been used for clostridia that produce type G neurotoxin as well as non-toxigenic strains previously identified as *Clostridium subterminale* and *Clostridium hastiforme* (Suen et al. 1988b). These organisms have ≥75% DNA homology to the DNA of the *C. argentinense* type strain, similar fatty acid profiles (Ghanem et al. 1991) and staining patterns by multilocus enzyme electrophoresis (Altwegg and Hatheway 1988, Bories et al. 1993). Clostridia that produce botulinum toxin are closely related to various species of non-toxigenic clostridia by taxonomic criteria (Table 37.3).

7 STRUCTURE, GENETICS AND PHARMACOLOGY OF BOTULINUM NEUROTOXINS

The clostridia produce more kinds of toxins than any other genus of bacteria (van Heyningen 1950); more than 20 toxins have been identified (Hatheway 1990). Of the 84 genera listed in the latest edition of *Bergey's Manual of Systematic Bacteriology* (Cato, George and Finegold 1986), at least 15 are known to produce toxins. Toxins produced by *C. botulinum*, *C. argentinense*, special strains of *C. butyricum*, *C baratii*, *C. tetani* and possibly *Clostridium perfringens* cause intoxications of the nervous system. Many of the clostridia are pathogenic for humans or animals through the production of toxins. The genetic information for toxin formation may be encoded on extrachromosomal elements or prophage DNA, and may be unstable and present on transferable genetic elements (Zhou, Sugiyama and Johnson 1993, Hauser et al. 1995, Johnson 1997).

C. botulinum produces 7 immunologically distinct neurotoxins. These toxins are of extraordinary potency and are considered to be the most poisonous substances known, having a toxicity of ≤1 ng kg^{-1} of body weight. Botulinum neurotoxins are entirely responsible for all the clinical symptoms of botulism. The characteristic flaccid paralysis of botulism results from the toxin-induced block of acetylcholine release at the neuromuscular junction (Montecucco and Schiavo 1995).

Botulinum neurotoxins are produced in culture media and in foods as aggregates of neurotoxin and non-toxic proteins that are non-covalently associated into protein complexes (Schantz 1964, Sugii and Sakaguchi 1975, Sugiyama 1980, Sakaguchi 1983, Inoue, Fujinaga and Watanabe 1996). These complexes have been referred to as progenitor toxins and the neurotoxin obtained through chromatographic separation from the other associated proteins of the complex as derivative toxin. Toxin complexes are described as M for medium (235–400 kDa), L for large (450–500 kDa), and LL for very large (900 kDa). These toxin complexes vary in size from c. 900 kDa for type A LL toxin complex to c. 300 kDa for the type B M complex and type E complex, to 235 kDa for type F M complex (Table 37.4) (Schantz 1964, Kitamura,

Table 37.3 Clostridia producing botulinum neurotoxins

Organism	Botulinum neurotoxin types	Related non-toxigenic clostridial species
Group I *C. botulinum*	A, B, F	*C. sporogenes*, *C. putrificum*
Group II *C. botulinum*	B, E, F	Non-toxigenic derivatives of type B, E (no species designation)
Group III *C. botulinum*	C$_1$, D	*C. novyi*, *C. oedematiens*
Group IV *C. botulinum*	G	*C. subterminale*, *C. hastiforme*
Toxigenic *C. baratii*	F	Typical *C. baratii* strains
Toxigenic *C. butyricum*	E	Typical *C. butyricum* strains

Sakaguchi and Sakaguchi 1969, Kozaki, Sakaguchi and Sakaguchi 1974, Ohishi and Sakaguchi 1974).

According to Sugii and Sakaguchi (1977), during culture the proportions of the different toxin complexes are dependent on the growth medium, particularly the concentration of iron. Some of the non-toxic proteins associated with the various toxin complexes have haemagglutinating abilities (Sugiyama 1980, Somers and DasGupta 1991). In particular, non-neurotoxic fractions of the L complexes of type A, B, C and D have been shown to have haemagglutinating activity. Haemagglutinin fractions isolated from the different serotypes show some serological cross-reactivity. Non-toxic fractions from type A and B serotypes cross-react (Goodnough et al. 1993) as do non-toxic fractions from types E and F. The non-toxic fractions of types C_1 and D are antigenically identical as determined by Ouchterlony diffusion (Sakaguchi et al. 1974). The non-toxic complexing proteins have been demonstrated to be essential for stabilization of the neurotoxin during passage through the digestive tract (Ohishi and Sakaguchi 1974, Sakaguchi, Ohishi and Kozaki 1981). Pure neurotoxin has a peroral LD50 about 100–1000 times lower than that of toxin complex on a weight basis (Sakaguchi 1983, Ohishi 1984). The complexing proteins probably protect the labile neurotoxin molecule from proteolytic cleavage and other types of inactivation by enzymes present in the gut.

The neurotoxin component of the toxin complexes is absorbed from the intestine into the blood, where it binds with high specificity to motoneurons. Biologically active neurotoxin of *C. botulinum* is a dichain molecule of approximately 150 kDa. The fully active toxin molecule is composed of 2 fragments or chains that are termed the heavy chain (c. 100 kDa) and a light chain (c. 50 kDa) that are covalently connected by a disulphide bond. Although *C. botulinum* produces 7 serologically distinct neurotoxins, there are many similarities among the different serotypes. They are all produced as single polypeptide chains of about 150 kDa and undergo proteolytic cleavage to generate the fully active dichain molecule. In all cases, the dichain molecules are composed of a light chain of about 50 kDa and a heavy chain of about 100 kDa connected by a disulphide bridge. All serotypes of botulinum toxin as well as tetanus toxin have been shown to be zinc endopeptidases (Schiavo and Monteccuco 1995). The genes encoding all 7 serotypes of botulinum neurotoxin have been sequenced and the amino acid homology has been shown to be between 30 and 60%

Table 37.4 Molecular sizes of various *C. botulinum* toxin complexes

Toxin type	Sedimentation coefficient	c. M_r (kDa)
LL A	19S	900
L A, B, D	16S	450–500
M A, B, C_1, D, E, F	10–12S	235–350

(Campbell, Collins and East 1993, Popoff and Eklund 1995). The region of highest homology is approximately in the middle of the light chain. This region has been shown in every instance to code for xxHxLEHhLxh where the histidines in the sequence are believed to be co-ordinated with one Zn^{2+} atom. This zinc binding motif is characteristic of metalloproteases (Rawlings and Barrett 1995).

Three functional domains have been identified in botulinum neurotoxins (Montecucco and Schiavo 1995). The carboxyl terminus of botulinum heavy chain is responsible for receptor binding on the neuronal cell surface. After binding, the light chain and a portion of the heavy chain are endocytosed. The light chain is then released into the cytosol of the cell via a translocation event through the phospholipid vesicle membrane. This translocation event is facilitated by a sequence of amino acids within the N-terminal region of the heavy chain. The L chains of the various neurotoxins cleave proteins in the cytosol that are required for exocytosis of neurotransmitter. This cleavage is believed to be mainly responsible for inhibition of release of neurotransmitter and the resulting flaccid paralysis. However, botulinum toxins undoubtedly have secondary effects such as release of neuropeptides, stimulation of nerve growth, and other pharmacological actions. The pharmacology of the botulinum neurotoxins has been studied in depth during the past decade and several excellent reviews have recently been published (Montecucco 1995, Montecucco and Schiavo 1995).

8 USE OF BOTULINUM TOXIN IN MEDICINE

Interest gradually waned in botulism after the 1930s as botulism in foods came under control. However, 3 important discoveries sparked a renewed interest in botulism and botulinum toxin. The first was a series of outbreaks of type E botulism that occurred in the USA due to the consumption of commercially packaged smoked whitefish and outbreaks in certain other commercial foods. The second was the discovery of infant botulism in the 1970s. The third, the development of botulinum toxin to treat humans who suffer from dystonias and hyperactive muscle disorders, had an even greater impact.

Botulinum toxin is increasingly being used to treat humans suffering from neurological diseases characterized by hyperactive muscle activity (Schantz and Johnson 1992, Jankovic and Hallett 1994, Moore 1995). In December 1989 the USA Food and Drug Administration licensed botulinum toxin as an orphan drug for the treatment of the human muscle disorders strabismus, hemifacial spasm and blepharospasm in patients 12 years of age and older, by direct injection of the toxin into the hyperactive muscle. Botulinum toxin is being used for the treatment of an increasing number of dystonias, movement disorders, cosmetic problems, and pain disorders, all which have been notoriously difficult to treat by existing therapies. The use of the toxin for human treatment came about over 25 years ago through the collaborative research efforts of Alan B Scott and Edward J Schantz in the USA (Schantz and Johnson 1992). The key properties of botulinum toxin as a drug is its high specificity for motoneurons, its very high toxicity, which enables the injection of extremely low quantities, thereby avoiding

side effects and an immunological response, and its long (several months) duration of action. The treatment of neurological disorders with botulinum toxin has opened a new field of investigation on the application of the toxin to nerve and muscle tissue in the human body.

REFERENCES

Altwegg M, Hatheway CL, 1988, Multilocus enzyme electrophoresis of *Clostridium argentinense* (*Clostridium botulinum* type G) and phenotypically similar asaccharolytic clostridia, *J Clin Microbiol*, **26**: 2447–9.

Arnon SS, 1995, Botulism as an intestinal toxemia, *Infections of the Gastrointestinal Tract*, eds Blaser MJ, Smith PD et al., Raven Press, New York, 257–71.

Arnon SS, Damus K et al., 1982, Protective role of human milk against sudden death from infant botulism, *J Pediatr*, **100**: 568–73.

Aureli P, Fenicia L et al., 1986, Two cases of type E infant botulism caused by neurotoxigenic *Clostridium butyricum* in Italy, *J Infect Dis*, **154**: 207–11.

Ball AP, Hopkinson RB et al., 1979, Human botulism caused by *Clostridium botulinum* type E: the Birmingham outbreak, *Q J Med*, **191**: 473–91.

Barrett DH, 1991, Endemic foodborne botulism: clinical experience, 1973–1986 at Alaska Native Medical Center, *Alaska Med*, **33**: 101–8.

Barsanti JA, Walser M et al., 1978, Type C botulism in American foxhounds, *J Am Vet Med Assoc*, **172**: 809–13.

Bengston IA, 1923, Toxin-producing anaerobe isolated from fly larvae, *Public Health Rep*, **37**: 164–70.

Bengston IA, 1924, Studies on organisms as causative factors in botulism, *Hyg Lab Bull*, **136**: 1–96.

Black RE, Gunn RA, 1980, Hypersensitivity reactions associated with botulinal antitoxin, *Am J Med*, **69**: 567–9.

Bories PN, Antoniotti C et al., 1993, Use of electrophoretic polymorphisms of esterases for differentiation of *Clostridium argentinense* strains, *J Clin Microbiol*, **31**: 157–9.

Borodic G, Johnson E et al., 1996, Botulinum toxin therapy, immunologic resistance, and problems with available materials, *Neurology*, **46**: 26–9.

Boroff D, Fleck U, 1966, Statistical analysis of a rapid in vivo method for the titration of the toxin of *Clostridium botulinum*, *J Bacteriol*, **92**: 1580–1.

Bowmer EJ, 1963, Preparation and assay of the international standards for *Clostridium botulinum* types A, B, C, D and E antitoxins, *Bull WHO*, **29**: 701–9.

Bulloch W, 1938, *The History of Bacteriology*, Oxford University Press, Oxford, reprinted 1979 by Dover Publications, Inc., New York.

Burke GS, 1919, Notes on *Bacillus botulinus*, *J Bacteriol*, **4**: 555–65.

Burningham MD, Walter FG et al., 1994, Wound botulism, *Ann Emerg Med*, **24**: 1184–7.

Campbell K, Collins M, East A, 1993, Nucleotide sequence of the gene coding for *Clostridium botulinum* (*Clostridium argentinense*) type G neurotoxin: genealogical comparison with other clostridial neurotoxins, *Biochim Biophys Acta*, **1216**: 487–91.

CAST (Council for Agricultural Science and Technology), 1994, *Foodborne Pathogens: Risks and Consequences*, Council for Agricultural Science and Technology, Ames, IA.

Cato EP, George WL, Finegold SM, 1986, The genus *Clostridium*, *Bergey's Manual of Systematic Bacteriology*, vol. 2, eds Sneath HA, Mair NS et al., Williams & Wilkins, Baltimore, 1141–200.

Cato EP, Stackenbrandt E, 1989, Taxonomy and phylogeny, *Clostridia*, Biotechnology Handbooks, vol. 3, eds Minton NP, Clarke DJ, Plenum Press, New York, 1–26.

Centers for Disease Control, 1979, *Botulism in the United States*,

1899–1977, Handbook for epidemiologists, clinicians, and laboratory workers, US Department of Health, Education, Welfare, Public Health Service, Centers for Disease Control, Atlanta, GA.

Centers for Disease Control, 1983, Botulism and commercial pot pie – California, *Morbid Mortal Weekly Rep*, **28**: 73–5.

Centers for Disease Control, 1991–1995, *Annual Summaries of Diseases in the United States*, Centers for Disease Control, Atlanta, GA.

Cherington M, 1990, Botulism, *Semin Neurol*, **10**: 27–31.

Chia JK, Clark JB et al., 1986, Botulism in an adult associated with food-borne intestinal infection with *Clostridium botulinum*, *N Engl J Med*, **315**: 239–41.

Cochran DP, Appleton RE, 1995, Infant botulism – is it that rare?, *Dev Med Child Neurol*, **37**: 274–8.

Cohen RE, Anderson DL, 1986, Botulism: emotional impact on patient and family, *J Psychosom Res*, **30**: 321–6.

Colebatch JG, Wolff AH et al., 1989, Slow recovery from severe foodborne botulism, *Lancet*, **1**: 1216–17.

Colice GL, 1987, Prolonged intubation versus tracheostomy in the adult, *J Intensive Care Med*, **2**: 85–102.

Collins MD, Lawson PA et al., 1994, The phylogeny of the genus *Clostridium*: proposal of five new genera and eleven new species combinations, *Int J Syst Bacteriol*, **44**: 812–26.

Critchley EM, Hayes PJ, Issacs PE, 1989, Outbreak of botulism in north west England and Wales, *Lancet*, **2**: 849–53.

Cummins CS, Johnson JL, 1971, Taxonomy of the clostridia: wall composition and DNA homologies in *Clostridium butyricum* and other butyric acid-producing clostridia, *J Gen Microbiol*, **67**: 33–46.

Davis JB, Mattman LH, Wiley AB, 1951, *Clostridium botulinum* in a fatal wound infection, *JAMA*, **146**: 646–8.

Dewberry EB, 1950, *Food Poisoning. Its Nature, History and Causation Measures for its Control*, Leonard Hill Limited, London.

Dezfulian M, Bartlett JG, 1985, Kinetics of growth and toxigenicity of *Clostridium botulinum* in a model of wound botulism, *Infect Immun*, **49**: 452–4.

Dickson EC, 1918, *Botulism. A Clinical and Experimental Study*, Monograph No. 8 of the B Rockefeller Inst Med Res Monogr. No. 8, Waverly Press, William & Wilkins, Baltimore.

Dodds KL, 1993, Worldwide incidence and ecology of infant botulism, Clostridium botulinum. *Ecology and Control in Foods*, eds Hauschild AHW, Dodds KL, Marcel Dekker, New York, 105–17.

Doellgast G, Triscott M et al., 1993, Sensitive enzyme-linked immunosorbent assay for detection of *Clostridium botulinum* neurotoxins A, B, and E using signal amplification via enzyme-linked coagulation assay, *J Clin Microbiol*, **31**: 2402–9.

Dolman CE, 1964, Botulism as a world health problem, *Botulism. Proceedings of a Symposium*, eds Lewis KH, Casse K Jr, US Department of Health, Education, and Welfare, Cincinnati, Ohio, 5–30.

Dolman CE, Murakami L, 1961, *Clostridium botulinum* type F with recent observations on other types, *J Infect Dis*, **109**: 107–28.

Eklund MW, Dowell VR Jr, 1987, Avian Botulism. An International Perspective, Charles C Thomas, Springfield, IL.

Elston HR, Wang M, Loo LK, 1991, Arm abscesses caused by *Clostridium botulinum*, *J Clin Microbiol*, **29**: 2678–9.

van Ermengem EP, 1897, Ueber einen neuen anaeroben *Bacillus* und seine Beziehungen zum Botulismus, *Z Hyg Infektionskr,* **26:** 1–56.

Fenicia L, Ferrini AM et al., 1993, A case of infant botulism associated with the feeding of honey in Italy, *Eur J Epidemiol,* **9:** 671–3.

Fildes P, 1927, Tetanus. VI. The conditions under which tetanus spores germinate *in vivo, Br J Exp Pathol,* **8:** 387.

Foster EM, Deffner JS et al., 1965, *Clostridium botulinum* food poisoning, *J Milk Food Technol,* **28:** 86–91.

Frankovich TL, Arnon SS, 1991, Clinical trial of botulism immune globulin for infant botulism, *West J Med,* **154:** 103.

Freedman M, Armstrong RM et al., 1986, Botulism in a patient with a jejunoileal bypass, *Ann Neurol,* **20:** 641–3.

Ghanem FM, Ridpath AC et al., 1991, Identification of *Clostridium botulinum, Clostridium argentinense,* and related organisms by cellular fatty acid analysis, *J Clin Microbiol,* **29:** 1114–24.

Gill DM, 1982, Bacterial toxins: a table of lethal amounts, *Microbiol Rev,* **46** 86–94.

Gimenez DF, Ciccarelli AS, 1970, Another type of *Clostridium botulinum, Zentrabl Infektionskr Hyg Abt I Orig,* **215:** 221–4.

Gimenez DF, Gimenez JA, 1995, The typing of botulinal neurotoxins, *Int J Food Microbiol,* **27:** 1–9.

Goodfellow M, O'Donnell AG, 1993, Roots of bacterial systematics, *Handbook of New Bacteria Systematics,* eds Goodfellow M, O'Donnell AG, Academic Press, London, 3–54.

Goodnough MC, Hammer B et al., 1993, Colony immunoblot assay of botulinal toxin, *Appl Environ Microbiol,* **59:** 2339–42.

Gunnison JB, Cummings JR, Meyer KF, 1936, *Clostridium botulinum* type E, *Proc Soc Exp Biol Med,* **35:** 278–80.

Gunnison JB, Meyer KF, 1930, Susceptibility of monkeys, goats, and small animals to oral administration of botulinum toxin, types B, C, and D, *J Infect Dis,* **46:** 335–40.

Gutierrez AR, Bodensteiner J, Gutmann L, 1994, Electrodiagnosis of infant botulism, *J Child Neurol,* **9:** 362–6.

Hall IC, 1945, The occurrence of *Bacillus botulinum,* types A and B, in accidental wounds, *J Bacteriol,* **50:** 213–17.

Hall JD, McCroskey LM et al., 1985, Isolation of an organism resembling *Clostridium barati* which produces type F botulinal toxin from an infant with botulism, *J Clin Microbiol,* **21:** 545–5.

Hatheway CL, 1988, Botulism, *Laboratory Diagnosis of Infectious Diseases. Principles and Practice. Vol. I. Bacterial, Mycotic and Parasitic Diseases,* eds Balows A, Hausler WJ, Jr et al., Springer-Verlag, New York, 111–33.

Hatheway CL, 1990, Toxigenic clostridia, *Clin Microbiol Rev,* **3:** 66–98.

Hatheway CL, 1995, Botulism: the present status of the disease, *Clostridial Neurotoxins,* ed. Montecucco C, Springer, Berlin, 55–75.

Hatheway CL, Snyder JD et al., 1984, Antitoxin levels in botulism patients treated with trivalent equine botulism antitoxin to toxin types A, B, and E, *J Infect Dis,* **150:** 407–12.

Hauschild AHW, 1992, Epidemiology of human and foodborne botulism, Clostridium botulinum. *Ecology and Control in Nature,* eds Hauschild AHW, Dodds KL, Marcel Dekker, Inc., New York, 69–104.

Hauschild AHW, Hilsheimer R et al., 1988, *Clostridium botulinum* in honey, syrups, and dry infant cereals, *J Food Prot,* **51:** 892–4.

Hauser D, Gibert M et al., 1995, Botulinal toxin genes, clostridial neurotoxin homology and genetic transfer in *Clostridium botulinum, Toxicon,* **33:** 515–26.

Hayashi K, Sakaguchi S, Sakaguchi G, 1986, Primary multiplication of *Clostridium botulinum* type A in mustard-miso stuffing of 'karashi-renkon' (deep-fried mustard-stuffed lotus root), *Int J Food Microbiol,* **3:** 311–20.

Hedberg CW, MacDonald KL, Osterholm MT, 1994, Changing epidemiology of food-borne disease: a Minnesota perspective, *Clin Infect Dis,* **18:** 671–82.

van Heyningen WE, 1950, *Bacterial Toxins,* Blackwell Scientific Publications, Oxford.

Hippe H, Andreesen JR, Gottschalk G, 1992, The genus *Clostridium* – nonmedical, *The Prokaryotes,* vol. 2, 2nd edn, eds Balows A, Truper HG et al., Springer-Verlag, New York, 1800–66.

Hoffmann RE, Pincomb BJ et al., 1982, Type F infant botulism, *Am J Dis Child,* **136:** 270–1.

van Holzer E, 1962, Botulisms durch Inhalation, *Med Klin,* **57:** 1735–8.

Hughes JM, Blumenthal JR et al., 1981, Clinical features of types A & B food-borne botulism, *Ann Intern Med,* **95:** 442–5.

Hutchinson DN, 1992, Foodborne botulism. New techniques for preserving foods bring the need for greater awareness of the risks, *Br Med J,* **305:** 264–5.

Iida H, 1970, Epidemiological and clinical observations of botulism outbreaks in Japan, *Proceedings of the First US – Japan Conference on Toxic Microorganisms,* ed. Herzberg M, US Government Printing Office, Washington, DC, 357–9.

Inoue K, Fujinaga Y, Watanabe T, 1996, Molecular composition of *Clostridium botulinum* progenitor toxins, *Infect Immun,* **64:** 1589–94.

Jankovic J, Hallett M, 1994, *Therapy with Botulinum Toxin,* Marcel Dekker, New York.

Jean D, Fecteau G et al., 1995, *Clostridium botulinum* type C intoxication in feedlot steers being fed ensiled poultry litter, *Can Vet J,* **36:** 626–8.

Jensen WI, Price JI, 1987, The global importance of type C botulism in wild birds, *Avian Botulism. An International Perspective,* eds Eklund MW, Dowell VR Jr, Charles C Thomas, Springfield, IL, 33–54.

Jenzer G, Mumenthaler M et al., 1975, Autonomic dysfunction in botulism B: a clinical report, *Neurology,* **25:** 150–3.

Johnson EA, 1997, Extrachromosomal virulence determinants in the clostridia, *Molecular Genetics and Pathogenesis of the Clostridia,* eds Rood J, Songer G et al., Academic Press, London, in press.

Joiner KA, Gelfand JA et al., 1980, Host factors in abscess formation, *J Infect Dis,* **142:** 40–9.

Kalmbach ER, 1939, American vultures and the toxin of *Clostridium botulinum, J Am Vet Med Assoc,* **94:** 187–91.

Kempner W, 1897, [Further contributions to the knowledge of meat poisoning. The antitoxin to botulism], *Z Hyg Infektionskr,* **26:** 481–500 (German).

Keynan A, Sandler N, 1983, Spore research in historical perspective, *The Bacterial Spore,* vol. 2, 2nd edn, eds Hurst A, Gould GW, Academic Press, London, 1–48.

Kinde H, Bettey RL et al., 1991, *Clostridium botulinum* type-C intoxication associated with consumption of processed alfalfa hay cubes in horses, *J Am Vet Med Assoc,* **199:** 742–6.

Kitamura M, Sakaguchi S, Sakaguchi G, 1969, Significance of 12S toxin of *Clostridium botulinum* E, *J Bacteriol,* **98:** 1173–8.

Knightingale KW, Ayim EN, 1980, Outbreak of botulism in Kenya after ingestion of white ants, *Br Med J,* **281:** 1682–3.

Koenig MG, 1971, The clinical aspects of botulism, *Neuropoisons. Their Pathophysiological Actions. Vol. 1. Poisons of Animal Origin,* ed. Simpson LL, Plenum Press, New York, 283–301.

Kozaki S, Sakaguchi S, Sakaguchi G, 1974, Purification and some properties of progenitor toxins of *Clostridium botulinum* type B, *Infect Immun,* **10:** 750–6.

Lamanna CA, el-Hage N, Vick JA, 1988, Cardiac effects of botulinal toxin, *Arch Int Pharmacodyn Ther,* **293:** 69–83.

Leighton GR, 1923, *Botulism and Food Preservation (The Loch Maree Tragedy),* W Collins & Sons, London.

L'Hommedieu CL, Polin RA, 1981, Progression of clinical signs in severe infant botulism, *Clin Pediatr,* **20:** 90–5.

Lynt RK, Kautter DA, Read RB Jr, 1975, Botulism in commercially canned foods, *J Milk Food Technol,* **38:** 546–50.

McCroskey LM, Hatheway CL, 1988, Laboratory findings in four cases of adult botulism suggest colonization of the intestinal tract, *J Clin Microbiol,* **26:** 1052–4.

McCroskey LM, Hatheway CL et al., 1991, Type F botulism due to neurotoxigenic *Clostridium botulinum* from an unknown source in an adult, *J Clin Microbiol,* **29:** 2618–20.

MacDonald KL, Cohen ML, Blake PA, 1986, The changing epidemiology of adult botulism in the United States, *Am J Epidemiol*, **108:** 150–6.

MacDonald KL, Spengler RF et al., 1985, Type A botulism from sauteed onions: clinical and epidemiologic observations, *JAMA*, **253:** 1275–8.

Meyer KF, 1956, The status of botulism as a world health problem, *Bull W H O*, **15:** 281–98.

Meyer KF, Eddie B, 1951, Perspectives concerning botulism, *Z Hyg*, **133, Suppl.:** 255–63.

Midura TF, Arnon SS, 1976, Identification of *Clostridium botulinum* and its toxins in feces, *Lancet*, **2:** 934–6.

Moeller V, Scheibel I, 1960, Preliminary report on the isolation of an apparently new type of *Clostridium botulinum*, *Acta Pathol Scand*, **48:** 80.

Montecucco C, 1995, *Clostridial Neurotoxins*, Springer, Berlin.

Montecucco C, Schiavo G, 1995, Structure and function of tetanus and botulinum neurotoxins, *Q Rev Biophys*, **28:** 423–72.

Moore P, 1995, *Handbook of Botulinum Toxin Therapy*, Blackwell Science, Oxford.

Morse EL, Pickard LK et al., 1990, Garlic-in-oil associated botulism: episode leads to product modification, *Am J Public Health*, **80:** 1372–3.

Notermans S, Nagel J, 1989, Assays for botulinum and tetanus toxins, *Botulinum Neurotoxin and Tetanus Toxin*, ed. Simpson LL, Academic Press, San Diego, 319–31.

Oguma K, Yokota K et al., 1990, Infant botulism due to *Clostridium botulinum* type C, *Lancet*, **336:** 1449–50.

Ohishi I, 1984, Oral toxicities of *Clostridium botulinum* type A and B toxins from different strains, *Infect Immun*, **43:** 487–90.

Ohishi I, Sakaguchi G, 1974, Purification of *Clostridium botulinum* type F progenitor toxin, *Appl Environ Microbiol*, **28:** 923–8.

O'Mahony M, Mitchell E et al., 1990, An outbreak of foodborne botulism with contaminated hazelnut yogurt, *Epidemiol Infect*, **104:** 389–95.

Otofuji T, Tokiwa H, Takahashi K, 1987, A food-poisoning incident caused by *Clostridium botulinum* toxin A in Japan, *Epidemiol Infect*, **99:** 167–72.

Paisley JW, Lauer BA, Arnon SS, 1995, A second case of infant type F botulism caused by *Clostridium baratii*, *Pediatr Infect Dis J*, **14:** 912–14.

Pickett J, Berg B et al., 1976, Syndrome of botulism in infancy: clinical and electrophysiologic study, *N Engl J Med*, **295:** 770–2.

Popoff MR, Eklund MW, 1995, Tetanus and botulinum neurotoxins: genetics and molecular mode of action, *Molecular Approaches to Food Safety. Issues Involving Toxic Microorganisms*, eds Eklund M, Richards J, Alaken, Fort Collins.

Prazmowski A, 1980, Unterschung uber die Entwickelungsgeschichte und Ferment-wirking einiger Bacterien-Arten, *Inaug. Diss. Hugo Voigt*, Leipzig, Germany, 1–58.

Rawlings ND, Barrett AJ, 1995, Evolutionary families of metallopeptidases, *Methods Enzymol*, **248:** 183–228.

Rhodehamel EJ, 1992, FDA's concern with sous vide processing, *Food Technol*, **46:** 73–6.

Rhodehamel EJ, Reddy NR, Pierson MD, 1992, Botulism: the causative agent and its control in foods, *Food Control*, **3:** 125–43.

Roblot P, Roblot F et al., 1994, Retrospective study of 108 cases of botulism in Poitiers, France, *J Med Microbiol*, **40:** 379–84.

Sakaguchi G, 1983, *Clostridium botulinum* toxins, *Pharmacol Ther*, **19:** 165–94.

Sakaguchi G, Ohishi I, Kozaki S, 1981, Purification and oral toxicities of *Clostridium botulinum* progenitor toxins, *Biomedical Aspects of Botulism*, Academic Press, New York, 21–34.

Sakaguchi G, Sakaguchi S et al., 1974, Cross reaction in reversed passive hemagglutination between *Clostridium botulinum* type A and type B toxins and its avoidance by the use of anti-toxic component immunoglobulin isolated by affinity chromatography, *Jpn J Med Sci Biol*, **27:** 161–72.

Schantz E, 1964, *Botulism. Proceedings of a Symposium*, eds Lewis

KH, Casse K Jr , US Department of health, Education, and Welfare, Public Health Service, Cincinnati, Ohio, 91–104.

Schantz EJ, Johnson EA, 1992, Properties and use of botulinum toxin and other microbial neurotoxins in medicine, *Microbiol Rev*, **56:** 80–92.

Schantz EJ, Kautter DA, 1978, Standardized assay for *Clostridium botulinum* toxins, *J Assoc Off Anal Chem*, **61:** 96–9.

Schantz EJ, Sugiyama H, 1974, Toxic proteins produced by *Clostridium botulinum*, *J Agric Food Chem*, **22:** 26–30.

Schiavo G, Montecucco C, 1995, Tetanus and botulinum neurotoxins: isolation and assay, *Methods Enzymol*, **248:** 643–52.

Schleifer KH, Kandler O, 1972, Peptidoglycan types of bacterial cell walls and their taxonomic implications, *Bacteriol Rev*, **36:** 407–77.

Schocken-Iturrino RP, Avila FA et al., 1990, First case of type A botulism in zebu (*Bos indicus*), *Vet Rec*, **126:** 217–18.

Sebald M, Saimot G, 1973, Toxémie botulique. Intérêt de sa mise en évidence dans le diagnostic du botulisme humain de type B, *Ann Microbiol (Inst Pasteur)*, **124A:** 61–9.

Seddon HR, 1922, Bulbar paralysis in cattle due to the action of a toxigenic bacillus with a discussion on the relation of the condition to forage poisoning (botulism), *J Comp Pathol Ther*, **35:** 147–90.

Shen W-PV, Felsing N et al., 1994, Development of infant botulism in a 3-year-old female with neuroblastoma following autologous bone marrow transplantation: potential use of human botulism immune globulin, *Bone Marrow Transplant*, **13:** 345–7.

Slater PE, Addiss DG et al., 1989, Foodborne botulism: an international outbreak, *Int J Epidemiol*, **18:** 693–6.

Smith DH, Timms GL, Refai M, 1979, Outbreak of botulism in Kenyan nomads, *Ann Trop Med Parasitol*, **73:** 145–8.

Smith JWG, MacIver AG, 1974, Growth and toxin production of tetanus bacilli in vivo, *J Med Microbiol*, **7:** 497–504.

Smith LDS, 1977, *Botulism. The Organism, its Toxins, the Disease*, 1st edn, Charles C Thomas, Springfield, IL.

Smith LDS, 1978, The occurrence of *Clostridium botulinum* and *Clostridium tetani* in the soil of the United States, *Health Lab Sci*, **15:** 74–80.

Smith LDS, Sugiyama H, 1988, *Botulism. The Organism, its Toxins, the Disease*, 2nd edn, Charles C Thomas, Springfield, IL.

Solomon HM, Rhodehamel EJ, Kautter DA, 1995, *Clostridium botulinum*, *FDA Bacteriological Analytical Manual*, 8th edn, US Food and Drug Administration, Washington, DC, 17.01–17.10.

Somers E, DasGupta BR, 1991, *Clostridium botulinum* types A, B, C1, and E produce proteins with or without hemagglutinating activity: do they share common amino acid sequences and genes?, *J Protein Chem*, **10:** 415–25.

St Louis ME, Shaun HS et al., 1988, Botulism from chopped garlic: delayed recognition of a major outbreak, *Ann Intern Med*, **108:** 363–8.

Stanfield JP, Galazka A, 1985, Neonatal tetanus – an underreported scourge, *World Health Forum*, **6:** 127–9.

Suen JC, Hatheway CL et al., 1988a, Genetic confirmation of identities of neurotoxigenic *Clostridium barati* and *Clostridium butyricum* implicated as agents of infant botulism, *J Clin Microbiol*, **26:** 2191–2.

Suen JC, Hatheway CL et al., 1988b, *Clostridium argentinense* sp. nov.: a genetically homogenous group composed of all strains of *Clostridium botulinum* type G and some nontoxigenic strains previously identified as *Clostridium subterminale* or *Clostridium hastiforme*, *Int J Syst Bacteriol*, **38:** 375–81.

Sugii S, Sakaguchi G, 1975, Molecular construction of *Clostridium botulinum* type A toxins, *Infect Immun*, **12:** 1262–70.

Sugii S, Sakaguchi G, 1977, Botulinogenic properties of vegetables with special reference to the molecular size of the toxin in them, *J Food Safety*, **1:** 53–65.

Sugiyama H, 1980, *Clostridium botulinum* neurotoxin, *Microbiol Rev*, **44:** 419–48.

Suzuki JB, Grecz N, 1972, Electron microscopy and leukocyte

interaction with spores of *Clostridium botulinum* type A, *Can J Microbiol*, **18:** 1651.

Suzuki JB, Booth R et al., 1971, Pathogenesis of *Clostridium botulinum* type A. Study of in vivo toxin release by implantation of diffusion chambers containing spores, vegetative cells and free toxin, *Infect Immun*, **3:** 659.

Swerczek TW, 1980a, Experimentally induced toxicoinfectious botulism in horse and foals, *Am J Vet Res*, **41:** 348–9.

Swerczek TW, 1980b, Toxicoinfectious botulism in foals and adult horses, *J Am Vet Med Assoc*, **176:** 217–20.

Tacket CO, Rogawski MA, 1989, Botulism, *Botulinum Neurotoxin and Tetanus Toxin*, ed. Simpson LL, Academic Press, San Diego, CA, 351–78.

Tacket CO, Shandera WX et al., 1984, Equine antitoxin use and other factors that predict outcome in type A foodborne botulism, *Am J Med*, **76:** 794–8.

Telzak EE, Bell EP et al., 1990, An international outbreak of type E botulism due to uneviscerated fish, *J Infect Dis*, **161:** 340–2.

Terranova W, Breman JG et al., 1978, Botulism type B: epidemiologic aspects of an extensive outbreak, *Am J Epidemiol*, **108:** 150–6.

Theiler A, Viljoen PR et al., 1927, Lamsiekte (parabotulism) in cattle in South Africa. 12th Report, *Director of Vet Ed Res*, **12:** 821013–61.

Thompson JA, Glasgow LA et al., 1980, Infant botulism: clinical spectrum and epidemiology, *Pediatrics*, **66:** 936–42.

Townes JM, Cieslak PR et al., 1996, An outbreak of type A botulism associated with a commerial cheese sauce, *Ann Intern Med*, **125:** 558–63.

Wainwright RB, Heyward WL et al., 1988, Food-borne botulism in Alaska, 1947–1985: epidemiology and clinical findings, *J Infect Dis*, **157:** 1158–62.

Weber JT, Goodpasture HC et al., 1993, Wound botulism in a patient with a tooth abscess: case report and review, *Clin Infect Dis*, **16:** 635–8.

Weiss N, Schleifer KH, Kandler O, 1981, The peptidoglycan types of Gram-positive anaerobic bacteria and their taxonomic implications, *Rev Inst Pasteur (Lyon)*, **14:** 3–12.

Whitlock RH, 1996, Botulism type C – experimental and field cases in horses, *Vet Clin North Am Equine Pract*, **18:** 11–17.

Willis AT, 1969, *Clostridia of Wound Infection*, Butterworths, London.

Woodburn MJ, Somers E et al., 1979, Heat inactivation rates of botulinum toxins A, B, E and F in some foods and buffers, *J Food Sci*, **44:** 1658–61.

Woodruff BA, Griffin PM et al., 1992, Clinical and laboratory comparison of botulism from toxin types A, B, and E in the United States, 1975–1988, *J Infect Dis*, **166:** 1281–6.

Ying S, Shuyan C, 1986, Botulism in China, *J Infect Dis*, **8:** 984–90.

Zhou Y, Sugiyama H, Johnson EA, 1993, Transfer of neurotoxigenicity from *Clostridium butyricum* to a nontoxigenic *Clostridium botulinum* type E-like strain, *Appl Environ Microbiol*, **59:** 3825–31.

Zhou Y, Sugiyama H et al., 1995, The genes for the *Clostridium botulinum* type G toxin complex are on a plasmid, *Infect Immun*, **63:** 2087–91.

Infections due to non-sporing anaerobic bacilli and cocci

S D Allen and B I Duerden

1 INTRODUCTION

The non-sporing anaerobic bacteria include the numerically predominant members of the indigenous microbiota of humans and animals. Although evidence for the pathogenic potential of these microorganisms existed by the turn of this century, many problems connected with anaerobic methodology, classification and the tendency for anaerobes to cause polymicrobial infections gave rise to scepticism about their role in diseases. Interest in the clinical importance of the non-sporing anaerobes was rekindled about 25 years ago, coinciding with outstanding improvements in anaerobic systems and media for cultivation, better procedures for characterization, taxonomy, nomenclature, and methods for identification. It was fortuitous that these developments in anaerobic bacteriology coincided with the discovery of antimicrobial agents (e.g. metronidazole, clindamycin and others) having excellent activity against the anaerobes. Thus, with the hope of better treatment outcomes among the incentives, there was an explosion of clinical studies in the 1970s and 1980s which established, or re-established, the important and perhaps forgotten role of these bacteria in life-threatening illnesses.

1.1 Historical considerations

Historically, the existence of 'animalcules' that could live in the absence of air was first demonstrated in 1680 by Leeuwenhoek (Dobell 1960), but it was not until 1861, when Pasteur discovered that butyric fermentation (in absence of oxygen) was caused by an anaerobic sporeformer, now called *Clostridium butyricum*, that the role of anaerobes in diseases could be investigated. Pasteur used the terms 'aérobies' and 'anaérobies' for organisms that could live with or without atmospheric oxygen, and discovered the concept of 'anaerobiosis' (Sonnenwirth 1972). Subsequently, various non-sporing anaerobes, as well as clostridia, were cultivated from humans and animals with naturally occurring diseases, and from the normal flora of mucous membrane surfaces and the skin (Sonnenwirth 1972). Some of the most noteworthy studies in the 1890s were by Veillon (1893) and Veillon and Zuber (1897, 1898) who isolated non-sporing anaerobic bacteria from cases of appendicitis, bacteraemia, bartholinitis, chronic otitis media, peritonitis, periurethral suppurative inflammation, pyogenic arthritis, septic thrombophlebitis, and abscesses of the brain, lung, abdomen and pelvis. The organisms isolated included *Bacillus* (*Bacteroides*) *fragilis*, *Bacillus fusiformis* (apparently *Fusobacterium nucleatum*), *Staphylococcus parvulus* (*Veillonella parvula*), *Bacillus* (*Clostridium*) *perfringens*, *Bacillus ramosus* (*Clostridium ramosum*) (Finegold 1994); now, a century later, these are still among the most frequently encountered species.

During the early 1900s through the early 1960s, many important studies of non-sporing anaerobes and anaerobic infections were made by workers from around the world, especially by Robertson, Prévot, Smith, Hungate, Rosebury, Beerens and Tahon-Castel, and many others (Willis 1969, Finegold 1977, 1993a). Particularly noteworthy were the important observations of 2 American surgeons, Altemeier (1938) and Meleney (1948), on the role of non-sporing anaerobes in polymicrobial surgical infections. During the 1940s–1960s, however, interest in the non-sporing anaerobes declined at a time coinciding with the availability of penicillin G, the tetracyclines and chloramphenicol (Finegold 1993a). At the same time, anaerobic methodology was often considered too complex and was avoided in many hospital laboratories. The clinician treated empirically without reliance on anaerobe identification or antimicrobial susceptibility data.

Through the years, advancement in our knowledge about the role of anaerobic bacteria in diseases has been closely linked to anaerobic methodology. Systems for anaerobic cultivation have generally depended upon the removal of oxygen or oxygen tension and the maintenance of a reduced oxidation–reduction potential or Eh (Allen, Siders and Marler 1985). Pasteur was able to establish anaerobic conditions by boiling liquid culture media to remove the adsorbed oxygen. From 1861 to 1915, various containers, flasks, evacuation devices, inert gases, and liquid media, with or without boiling, or reducing agents in the media or chambers, were used. Prior to 1915, the most widely used anaerobic systems for cultivation were deep fluid and shake cultures that had been boiled, then cooled before inoculation (Sonnenwirth 1972). In 1916, the introduction of an anaerobic jar technique by McIntosh and Fildes, which permitted surface cultivation and facilitated studies of isolated colonies, was a significant improvement. A modified jar technique used in the USA until the mid-1960s, the Brewer jar, depended upon evacuation of the atmosphere from the jar with a vacuum pump, the addition of hydrogen back into the jar, and an electrically heated catalyst to catalyse the removal of the remaining oxygen by union with hydrogen to form water. Fear of the hydrogen exploding when the jar was connected to an electrical outlet deterred many laboratory workers from attempting to isolate anaerobes on solid media (Sonnenwirth 1972). Instead, undue reliance was often placed on the use of liquid media (e.g. fluid thioglycollate) to attempt to isolate anaerobes. This was especially problematic because most anaerobe infections other than bacteraemia are mixed infections; thus, broth cultures tended to become overgrown with the most rapidly growing facultatively anaerobic bacteria. The introduction of relatively simple jar techniques, based on the use of 'cold catalyst' active at room temperature without heating, and self-contained, disposable H_2–CO_2 generators (Brewer and Allgeier 1966) was a major breakthrough that greatly simplified the task of working with anaerobes in the clinical laboratory (Allen, Siders and Marler 1985).

Although the necessity for special apparatus and media to cultivate bacteria that can not tolerate oxygen, or are killed by it, is well known, the extent of the difficulty that obtaining and maintaining anaerobes in pure culture has always posed is probably not as widely appreciated (Willis 1969). Not only did this problem plague the early workers, thus leading to confusion in the literature about anaerobe infections, but the bacteriological characterization of anaerobes in mixed cultures that were assumed to be pure probably contributed to the creation of fallacious classification schemes and new species that were not justified (Willis 1969). Another problem in these mixed infections is that species present in small numbers can easily be missed. The use of modern, nutritionally adequate selective media and non-selective plating media has contributed greatly to a better understanding of these polymicrobial infections (Shapton and Board 1971, Dowell et al. 1977, Sutter et al. 1985). Controversy continues about the clinical relevance of how far to go with the identification of anaerobes in mixed infections (Allen, Siders and Marler 1995). In a mixed intra-abdominal infection, for example, should all isolates be identified and tested for susceptibility to antimicrobial agents (Wilson and Hopkins 1995)? Should only one, 2, or 3 species from a specimen that yielded 6, 8, 10 or more different organisms be identified? Or, in the setting of perforated or gangrenous appendicitis, should the clinician simply treat the patient with empirical antibiotics and surgical measures alone and not depend upon anaerobic bacteriology culture data, as some have suggested (Dougherty et al. 1989)? There is far from unanimous agreement on this issue, which has continued, at least in part, because of the historical technical problems confounding the anaerobic bacteriology of wounds and abscesses.

The renewed interest in anaerobic infections during the late 1960s and 1970s was driven by improvements in anaerobic culture methodology, a better, more orderly taxonomic classification, and the availability of several new antibiotics that were highly active against the anaerobes (Bartlett 1992, Finegold 1995a). During the past 3 decades, numerous investigators have firmly established the role of anaerobes in infections involving virtually all anatomical systems of the body. Although the pathogenic potential of many species of anaerobes has been documented, there is concern that we could again enter an era such as was experienced during the first two-thirds of the twentieth century, a time in which clinical anaerobic bacteriology was almost nonexistent and interest in the anaerobes was lacking (Finegold 1993a). Long-standing concerns about costs, particularly now in the era of managed care, have put a damper on the work being done in clinical microbiology laboratories. Some clinical microbiology laboratories have severely restricted the use of anaerobic cultures (i.e. blood cultures), unless specifically requested by the clinician, or they use inadequate identification schemes, and put such low priority on accuracy and turn around time for reporting, that the results received by the clinician have little value. Clinicians, thus, may feel compelled to treat empirically with the most expensive, broad spectrum drugs, which needlessly increase hospital costs and promote the development of increasing resistance in some anaerobes (Finegold 1993b).

2 EPIDEMIOLOGY

2.1 Habitats

Anaerobic bacteria are ubiquitous in the soil and in aquatic environments. In humans and animals, they reside on mucous membranes and the skin, and are prevalent in the oral cavities and gastrointestinal tracts where they reside as part of the indigenous microbiota. The anaerobic microbiota of humans is discussed extensively in Volume 2, Chapter 11, in an excellent review by Hentges (1993), and in some classic monographs (Rosebury 1962, Hentges 1983, Rowland 1988, Hill and Marsh 1989). The vast majority of infections involving non-sporing anaerobic bacteria originate from the flora within the patient's own oral cavity, gastrointestinal tract, genitourinary tract or skin (Finegold 1977), and are termed 'endogenous' infections. On the other hand, exogenous infections, involving anaerobes from sources outside the host, include the toxin-mediated clostridium diseases which are discussed in detail elsewhere (e.g. botulism, tetanus, *C. perfringens* food-borne illness and pig bel). Exogenous infections involving non-sporing anaerobes include bite wounds (human or animal) and sexually transmitted infections (Finegold 1977).

Although the number of anaerobe species encountered in the indigenous microbiota is large, relatively few species are isolated with any frequency from properly selected and collected specimens from humans with anaerobic infections. Some non-sporing members of the indigenous flora that are common and/or important in diseases include the following: species of the *Bacteroides fragilis* group, and of the genera *Prevotella* and *Porphyromonas*; *Fusobacterium nucleatum*, *Fusobacterium necrophorum*, *Fusobacterium mortiferum* and *Fusobacterium varium*; *Peptostreptococcus* species (in particular, *Peptostreptococcus magnus*, *Peptostreptococcus asaccharolyticus*, *Peptostreptococcus anaerobius* and *Peptostreptococcus micros*), *Veillonella parvula*, and certain gram-positive bacilli (e.g. *Actinomyces israelii*, *Actinomyces naeslundii*, and *Actinomyces odontolyticus*, *Bifidobacterium dentium*, *Eubacterium lentum*, *Propionibacterium propionicus* and *Propionibacterium acnes*).

Strict obligate anaerobes, such as *Clostridium novyi* type B and *Clostridium haemolyticum* (Loesche 1969), sometimes cause disease in domestic animals, but they seldom do so in humans (Smith and Williams 1984). Most of the anaerobes associated with infections in animals and humans are moderate obligate anaerobes (Loesche 1969, Allen, Siders and Marler 1985). Several strict obligate anaerobes, including *Treponema denticola*, *Succinivibrio dextrinosolvens*, *Butyrivibrio fibrisolvens*, *Desulfovibrio desulfuricans* and *Selenomonas ruminatum*, are encountered in the normal flora but are rarely associated with disease (Dowell 1977).

Some of the better known non-sporing anaerobic bacteria that cause diseases in animals include *Fusobacterium necrophorum* (bovine and ovine foot-rot, bovine liver abscesses and calf diphtheria), the pigmented *Prevotella–Porphyromonas* group (foot-rot in cattle), *Dichelobacter nodosus* (foot-rot in cattle), *Treponema hyodysenteriae* (swine dysentery) and *Actinomyces bovis*. The latter species, which causes actinomycosis in cattle ('lumpy jaw' and other manifestations), sheep, elk and probably other animals, is covered in Chapter 39.

2.2 Incidence

The frequency of recovery of anaerobes from clinical specimens has been reported from several institutions. Stokes (1958) recovered anaerobes from 10.5% of 4737 specimens. At the Mayo Clinic in the early 1970s, anaerobes were isolated from 49% of the total 14 839 specimens that yielded any bacteria (Martin 1974). At the University of Cincinnati, between 1960 and 1974, 58.5% of 689 specimens yielding bacteria contained anaerobes (Holland, Hill and Altemeier 1977). Between 1973 and 1985 at 2 military hospitals, anaerobes were isolated from 28.1% of 15 844 clinical specimens (Brook 1989). In the author's laboratory in 1992 (Allen, Siders and Marler 1995), anaerobes were recovered from 35% of the 568 wound and abscess specimens that yielded any micro-organisms. Several variables affect the reliability of these data. Anaerobe infections tend to be overlooked and underdiagnosed by some clinicians and are also subject to a number of variables within the laboratory, including failure to use appropriate selective and non-selective plating media, the tendency to overlook anaerobes in mixed culture, errors in characterization, and misidentification of isolates (Finegold 1990, Summanen et al. 1993). The frequency of recovering anaerobes varies considerably in specimens collected from different anatomical regions (see sections 7.1–7.9, pp. 757–763). The incidence of anaerobes in infections of humans has been reviewed extensively in the classic monograph by Finegold (1977) and elsewhere (Allen, Siders and Marler 1985, Finegold, George and Mulligan 1986, Finegold and George 1989, Bartlett 1992, Finegold 1995a).

Infections involving non-sporing anaerobes are not related to season or geographical location and they are common in both males and females. As is true for infections involving aerobic or facultatively anaerobic micro-organisms, extremes of age predispose to anaerobic infections. Although infections involving non-sporing anaerobes (e.g. septicaemia) are commonly documented after the patient has been hospitalized for at least 3 days and therefore might be considered 'nosocomial', they are not usually contagious.

3 PATHOGENESIS

In general, many infections involving non-sporing anaerobes arise close to the mucous membranes of the mouth, lower gastrointestinal tract and genital tract; they often follow surgical or accidental trauma (e.g. perforation of the bowel) which allows the flora to gain entrance into normally sterile tissue. When the mucosal barrier or skin is penetrated, multiplication of aerobic or facultatively anaerobic micro-organisms in the newly infected site tends to lower the oxidation–

reduction potential (Eh), resulting in a tissue environment favourable for subsequent anaerobic growth. Whether or not clinical manifestations of an anaerobic infection occur depends upon an interplay of host factors, the number of anaerobes introduced into the site ('inoculum'), and the micro-organisms involved. In addition, anaerobic infections tend to arise where dead or damaged tissue with a poor blood supply produces a low Eh, low oxygen tension, or both.

3.1   Predisposing factors

Numerous host factors predispose to infections with non-sporing anaerobes (Finegold 1993b). These include diabetes mellitus, chronic alcoholism, loss of consciousness with aspiration of gastric contents and oropharyngeal flora into the lower respiratory tract, cirrhosis, underlying malignant disease, immuno-suppression, receipt of cytotoxic drugs, obstruction (e.g. intestinal, biliary, tracheobronchial, urinary tract, fallopian tube, or vascular), burns, cold, shock with resultant vascular compromise (e.g. intestinal ischaemia), the presence of a foreign body (e.g. bullet in the abdomen), or calcium salts in tissue, injection of adrenaline into tissue, neutropenia, splenectomy, hypogammaglobulinaemia, collagen vascular diseases, therapy with corticosteroids or antimicrobial agents not active against anaerobes. Patients with diabetes mellitus are at particular risk for the development of severe, necrotizing mixed anaerobic infections of the lower extremities and diabetic foot ulcer-related anaerobic osteomyelitis (Wheat et al. 1986). Patients debilitated by neoplasms of the lung, colon, uterus and other malignant diseases, may be at risk for infection because of obstruction, tumour necrosis and tissue hypoxia, or may be immunocompromised and neutropenic because of damage to their bone marrow from radiation, chemotherapy or metastatic neoplasm. Profoundly neutropenic bone marrow transplant patients with mucositis of the oral cavity, who are receiving quinolones, sulphamethoxazole–trimethoprim or other antibiotics, may develop bacteraemia with species of *Fusobacterium*, *Leptotrichia*, *Capnocytophaga*, or non-sporing anaerobic gram-positive bacteria that are resistant to these compounds (Allen et al. 1996). Patients with AIDS are at risk for the development of severe gingivitis and periodontal disease (Lucht, Heimdahl and Nord 1991, Moore et al. 1993), as well as chronic sinusitis involving anaerobes (Tami 1995).

3.2   Pathology and cellular response to anaerobes

Mixed infections involving non-sporing anaerobes are characterized by purulent inflammation, which may be localized (e.g. in an abscess) or not (e.g. in cellulitis or fasciitis), and necrosis. Grossly, pus received in the laboratory from these infections usually has a strikingly acrid odour, and is often thick, creamy, pinkish-tan, sanguinolent, or brownish. An abscess, the pathological hallmark of this kind of pyogenic infection, is a focal accumulation of purulent exudate, within tissue, an organ or a restricted space. Histologically with H & E and Gram's stains, abscesses involving anaerobes are often indistinguishable from those not involving anaerobes; they vary in size from microscopic to several centimetres. Large abscesses may contain several hundred millilitres of exudate. The centre of an abscess typically contains necrotic inflammatory cells, necrotic tissue cells and nuclear debris; it is usually surrounded by an intense band of neutrophils. Outside this zone is often a region containing dilated small blood vessels, in which fibroblast proliferation and collagen formation variably occur. With time, there may be replacement of the neutrophils with macrophages and the abscess may become walled off. On the other hand, the infection may not remain localized and may extend to adjacent tissues, sometimes with gas formation (e.g. as in crepitant cellulitis). Undrained abscesses may become the source from which anaerobes enter the bloodstream. When this happens, a devastating sequence of events sometimes follows, characterized by septic shock and metastatic infections in distant organs. Even with prompt surgical intervention and treatment with appropriate antibiotics, death is often the final outcome in patients with anaerobic bacteraemia.

3.3   Virulence

Among the indigenous flora, certain species of potentially pathogenic non-sporing anaerobes become pathogenic when they are no longer confined to their natural habitat. Characteristics of the pathogenic non-sporing anaerobes include:

1   the ability to tolerate or adapt to the pathogenic ecosystem in which they reside and interact synergistically with other bacteria
2   the ability to adhere to host cells and invade tissues
3   the ability to produce toxins, enzymes or other factors that damage host cells and tissues and
4   the ability to produce surface structures and/or soluble metabolic products that protect against the host's defences.

ABILITY TO OVERCOME LIMITING FACTORS IN THE ECOSYSTEM

As mentioned previously, anaerobic bacteria vary in their ability to tolerate or to multiply in the presence of oxygen (Loesche 1969, Allen, Siders and Marler 1985). It has been hypothesized that superoxide dismutase (SOD) may act as a virulence factor, enabling potentially pathogenic anaerobes to survive in oxygenated tissue sites until conditions (e.g. a sufficiently low oxygen tension or Eh) become favourable for them to multiply (Tally et al. 1977). The production of SOD has been demonstrated in *Bacteroides fragilis*, *Bacteroides thetaiotaomicron*, *Bacteroides vulgatus*, *Bacteroides distasonis*, *Bacteroides ovatus* and in several other moderate obligate anaerobes that are commonly isolated from human infected sites (Carlsson, Wrethen and Beckman 1977, Tally et al. 1977). A good correlation has been demonstrated between the level of SOD produced and the oxygen tolerance of anaerobic bacteria (Tally et al. 1977). Thus, extremely oxygen-sensitive anaerobes that are rarely, if ever, encountered in infections of humans, appear not to produce SOD. Although catalase has long been postulated to be a virulence factor of anaerobes, evidence for a consistent correlation between catalase production, the decomposition of peroxides or H_2O_2, and oxygen tolerance is lacking.

MICROBIAL SYNERGY

Synergistic interactions between bacteria undoubtedly play an important role in the pathogenesis of polymicrobial infections. Synergistic bacterial infections result when 2 or more bacterial species produce an infection that could not be produced by any of the individual species alone (Bjornson 1982). Altemeier reported a good correlation between the severity of peritonitis following acute perforated appendicitis and the number of intestinal bacterial species present within the exudate (Altemeier 1941). Many investigators have suggested that aerobic or facultatively anaerobic organisms aid anaerobes in mixed surgical infections by using oxygen and decreasing the *Eh* (Roberts 1969). In abscesses of rats inoculated subcutaneously with faecal material, the *Eh* on day 7 of −113 mV was sufficiently low for anaerobes to grow (Onderdonk et al. 1979). Other limiting factors, such as changes in pH produced during the growth of one species, may affect the growth of others (Rotstein, Pruett and Simmons 1985).

Nutritional synergism involves the production of a growth factor by one organism that is needed by another, and this has been studied in several experimental animal models (Rotstein, Pruett and Simmons 1985). In one series of studies, vitamin K was found to be an important growth factor for pigmented, asaccharolytic organisms formerly called '*Bacteroides melaninogenicus*' (probably *Porphyromonas* species) that were isolated from human gingival scrapings (Gibbons and MacDonald 1960). In an experimental mixed infection model involving guinea pigs, neither the pigmented anaerobe by itself nor a mixture of bacteria without the pigmented strain produced infection. Abscesses or necrotic lesions were produced if the pigmented anaerobe plus a facultatively anaerobic diphtheroid were included in the inoculum. Apparently, the diphtheroid was able to satisfy the vitamin K requirement of the pigmented anaerobe. Although the pigmented anaerobe produced collagenase and other enzymes in vitro, the role of these enzymes in the pathogenesis of these infections is not clear.

Roberts (1967, 1969) investigated 'foot abscesses' in sheep, which are produced synergistically by the combination of *F. necrophorum* and *Actinomyces pyogenes* (formerly *Corynebacterium pyogenes*). *A. pyogenes* was found to produce a heat-labile factor which stimulated the growth of *F. necrophorum*. In addition, *F. necrophorum* produces a leucocidin that probably protected *A. pyogenes*, as well as itself, from killing by leucocytes.

Meleney's synergistic gangrene, which involved *Staphylococcus aureus* and an anaerobic or microaerophilic streptococcus that had been isolated from a wound infection, is another classic example of bacterial synergy (Brewer and Meleney 1926). When injected together subcutaneously into guinea pigs or other animals, a spreading, gangrenous infection was produced, wheras neither isolate produced infection by itself. Subsequently, the synergistic interaction could be explained by the finding that *S. aureus* produced a heat-labile growth factor that stimulated growth of the anaerobic streptococcus (Mergenhagen, Thonard and Scherp 1958). It was suggested, but not proven, that hyaluronidase produced by the *S. aureus* may have contributed to tissue invasion by the anaerobic streptococcus.

Another kind of bacterial interaction within mixed infections is the protection of a susceptible organism from antimicrobial activity by another that is resistant. Using a mixed infection model in mice, Hackman and Wilkins (1975) demonstrated that *B. fragilis* protected *F. necrophorum* from penicillin in vivo. By contrast, a pure culture infection involving *F. necrophorum* alone was successfully treated with penicillin. *B. fragilis* also protected *F. necrophorum* in vitro. The protection phenomenon is probably best explained by the production of β-lactamase by *B. fragilis*. This phenomenon is of considerable clinical interest in that β-lactamase activity has been demonstrated in about 60–90% of *B. fragilis* isolates (Hecht, Malamy and Tally 1989).

For additional information on microbial synergy readers are referred to reviews by Roberts (1969), Mackowiak (1978), Bjornson (1982), Rotstein, Pruett and Simmons (1985), Brook (1986) and Gharbia and Shah (1993b).

ADHERENCE AND INVASION

Adherence to epithelial surfaces is of fundamental importance in the colonization of the animal host by indigenous flora, and plays a key pathogenetic role in many infectious diseases (Savage 1985). Considerable work has been done on the adherence of oral anaerobic gram-negative bacilli in relation to periodontal disease. *Prevotella melaninogenica*, *Porphyromonas asaccharolytica* (or other species resembling it), and *Porphyromonas gingivalis* all were reported to adhere in vitro to human crevicular epithelium from the oral cavity, and they all adhered to the surfaces of a number of gram-positive bacteria (Slots and Gibbons 1978, Okuda, Slots and Genco 1981). The capacity to agglutinate red blood cells (RBCs) is commonly investigated as one way to measure adherence of bacteria. *P. gingivalis* was the only species that agglutinated human RBCs strongly (Slots and Gibbons 1978). The other 2 species did not agglutinate human RBCs, but agglutinated RBCs from various animals. The adherence of these bacteria to crevicular epithelial cells is probably mediated by fimbriae (or pili), but a haemagglutinin on its surface, and not fimbriae, mediates the agglutination of human RBCs by *P. gingivalis* (Okuda and Takazoe 1974, Slots and Gibbons 1978, Hofstad 1992). In addition, *F. nucleatum* adheres to crevicular epithelium and agglutinates human RBCs through a lectin mediated mechanism involving galactose-containing receptor sites (Falkler and Burger 1981, Duerden 1994). The ability of oral anaerobes to adhere to one another and form coaggregates may also contribute to the pathogenesis of mixed dental–oral infections (Gharbia and Shah 1993b, Duerden 1994).

The role of adherence to host cell surfaces in the pathogenesis of infections involving *B. fragilis* remains uncertain. *B. fragilis*, but not other members of the *B. fragilis* group, possesses a haemagglutinin (Vel et al. 1986). Lectin-like adhesions that attach to D-glucosamine and D-galactosamine have been described; *B. fragilis* strains were more adhesive than other members of the group (Rogemond and Guinet 1986). Fimbriae have been demonstrated in some *B. fragilis* strains and such strains adhere better than others to epithelial cells; they are also more sensitive to phagocytosis by PMNs (Pruzzo, Dainelli and Ricchetti 1984). The role of *B. fragilis* fimbriae in haemagglutination is not clear; neither is their role in adherence or pathogenesis of disease (Hofstad 1992). Onderdonk et al. (1978) found that capsulate strains of *B. fragilis* adhered better to rat peritoneal mesothelium than did non-capsulate strains. It has been suggested that adherence to host cells by *Bacteroides* spp. and *Fusobacterium* spp. may be a first step in invasion (Onderdonk et al. 1978, Kanoe and Iwaki 1987, Styrt and Gorbach 1989a, 1989b).

A different view on the ability of *B. fragilis* to adhere to cell surfaces has been discussed (Botta et al. 1994). It was observed previously that *B. vulgatus*, followed by *B. thetaiotaomicron* and *B. distasonis*, were far more common in human faecal samples than either *B. ovatus* or *B. fragilis* (Moore and Holdeman 1974, Holdeman, Good and Moore 1976). Many investigators have assumed, perhaps falsely, that the frequencies of these species in faeces must be similar to those within the intestinal tract. In order to explain why *B. fragilis* is involved in infections so much more frequently, it was reasoned that some virulence factor (i.e. namely its capsule) is produced by *B. fragilis* but not by the other members of the *B. fragilis* group. A study by Namavar et al. (1989), in which quantitative cultures were done on faeces obtained preoperatively and on colonic biopsy specimens obtained at operation from 10 patients with colon cancer, indicated that the relative frequency of *B. fragilis* was 4% in faeces compared to 43% in the colonic mucosal biopsies. *B. fragilis* was reported to be the most prevalent species of the group within the colonic mucosal tissue. The prevalence of *B. vulgatus* was 45% in the faeces compared to 26% in the colonic biopsies. Based on these findings, it was hypothesized that the adherence of *B. fragilis* to the colonic mucosa could be part of the explanation why *B. fragilis* is more common in infections than in the faecal flora (Namavar et al. 1989). More recently, Poxton and colleagues reported different findings based on quantitative cultures of colonoscopic biopsy samples from the proximal colon and rectum of 12 patients (6 of whom had ulcerative

colitis) (Poxton et al. 1997). The percentages of the different *Bacteroides* spp. isolated from colonic mucosal samples by Poxton et al., especially with regard to *B. fragilis* and *B. vulgatus*, were different from those reported by Namavar et al. (1989). In the study by Poxton and associates (1997), the fluid diet and laxatives received by patients prior to colonoscopy were probably less disruptive to the mucosa-associated microflora than would be the preoperative dietary restrictions, antibiotics, bowel cleansing, operative techniques of surgeons, specimen selection, collection and transport, and other variables that could influence microbiological studies of colonic specimens removed at operation. As was noted above, operative specimens were studied by Namavar et al. (1989). Much more work is needed to answer the question of whether *B. fragilis* adheres to or associates closely with the colonic mucosal epithelium in vivo.

Invasiveness is not a characteristic feature of most non-sporing anaerobes, with the exception of *F. necrophorum*. Pure cultures of *F. necrophorum* are pathogenic for rabbits and mice. Intraperitoneal or intravenous inoculation into rabbits causes death with intense inflammation, exudate and coagulative necrosis; subcutaneous injection into the lower lip gives rise to labial necrosis and death in 4–12 days. Subcutaneous inoculation into mice produces spreading necrotic lesions, and death after about 12 days; the minimum infecting dose may be greatly reduced by the presence of other bacteria, including *A. pyogenes* or *Escherichia coli* (Smith et al. 1989). The specific factors involved in invasion by *F. necrophorum* are not clear; a variety of toxic components probably contribute to its virulence.

TOXINS, ENZYMES OR OTHER FACTORS THAT DAMAGE HOST CELLS AND TISSUES

Since the mid-1980s, strains of *B. fragilis* that produce an enterotoxin have been implicated as causes of diarrhoeal illness in lambs, calves, piglets, foals and infant rabbits (Border et al. 1985, Myers et al. 1985, 1989, Myers and Shoop 1987, Myers, Shoop and Byars 1987). The isolation of enterotoxigenic *B. fragilis* from humans (both children and adults) with diarrhoea was first reported in 1987 (Myers et al. 1987). Since then, it has been implicated epidemiologically as an important cause of acute diarrhoea in Apache children in Arizona (Sack et al. 1992) and in children older than one year in Bangladesh (Sack et al. 1994). A tissue culture assay developed in 1992, using a human colon carcinoma cell line (HT-29), greatly facilitated studies of the enterotoxin (Weikel et al. 1992). The enterotoxin was purified from culture supernatants and found to be a zinc-dependent metalloprotease, called a metzincin, of c. 20 kDa (Van Tassell, Lyerly and Wilkins 1992, Moncrief et al. 1995). Subsequently, the purified enterotoxin was shown to cause significant tissue damage and to elicit a significant fluid accumulation in lamb, rabbit and rat ligated intestinal loops (Obiso et al. 1995). In addition, it was found to act as a cytotoxin in HT-29 cells by reversibly modifying the actin cytoskeleton (Donelli, Fabbri and Fiorentini 1996). Much remains to be learned about the role of the *B. fragilis* enterotoxin in diarrhoea of animals and humans, especially related to the epidemiology, diagnosis, clinical and pathological features of the illness produced.

B. fragilis also produces a number of extracellular or membrane-associated enzymes that may act as toxins or aggressins and thus contribute to virulence. They include collagenase and other proteases, fibrinolysin, haemolysin, neuraminidase, phosphatase, DNAase, hyaluronidase and chondroitin sulphatase (Rudek and Haque 1976). These enzymes are active against many components of mammalian tissue and may play a role in the tissue damage and necrosis that is characteristic of infections involving *Bacteroides* spp. Heparinase activity has been demonstrated in *B. ovatus* and *B. thetaiotaomicron*; reports of heparinase activity in *B. fragilis* have not been substantiated (Steffen and Hentges 1981).

Many enzymes are also produced by a number of species of pigmented *Prevotella* and *Porphyromonas* (Steffen and Hentges 1981, Sundqvist, Carlsson and Hanstrom 1987, Gharbia and Shah 1993a, Duerden 1994). The virulence characteristics of *P. gingivalis* have been the subject of detailed investigations and it has been shown to have greater potential capacity for tissue damage than any other pigmented species of *Prevotella* and *Porphyromonas*. It is strongly proteolytic, producing protease with trypsin-like activity (Tsutsui et al. 1987); Grenier and Mayrand (1987) have shown that proteolytic enzymes are secreted in extracellular vesicles. *P. gingivalis* degrades a range of plasma proteins: albumin, haemopexin, haptoglobin and transferrin (Carlsson, Hofling and Sundqvist 1984); IgM and IgG, and the complement components C3 and C5 (Sundqvist et al. 1984, 1985); fibrinogen (Lantz et al. 1986); and secretory IgA (Sato et al. 1987). It is the only oral pigmented anaerobic gram-negative bacillus that produces a true collagenase that degrades active collagen (Sundqvist, Carlsson and Hanstrom 1987), most other species being capable of attacking only partly denatured collagen (Mayrand and Grenier 1985). The collagenase is a sulphydryl enzyme that is sensitive to H_2O_2 (Sundqvist, Carlsson and Hanstrom 1987). *P. gingivalis* also produces hyaluronidase and chondroitin sulphatase. Phospholipase A, produced by *Prevotella intermedia* and *P. melaninogenica*, may disrupt epithelial cells (Bulkacz et al. 1985).

F. necrophorum produces several potent exotoxins or exoenzymes. These include a lipase, haemolysin, DNAase, protease, a cytoplasmic toxin and a leucocidin that inhibits phagocytosis by polymorphonuclear leucocytes (Roberts 1967, 1970, Langworth 1977).

SURFACE STRUCTURES AND/OR SOLUBLE METABOLIC PRODUCTS

The majority of fresh clinical isolates of *B. fragilis* have been reported to be encapsulated and, with the exception of *B. distasonis*, the other species of the *B. fragilis* group are also encapsulated (although less frequently than *B. fragilis* in some studies) (Babb and Cummins 1978, Burt et al. 1978, Lindberg et al. 1979, Brook, Myhal and Dorsey 1992). Various workers have found

that the capsule is essential for virulence in experimental animals. Onderdonk et al. (1977) found that only capsulate strains of *B. fragilis* produced intraperitoneal abscesses in rats and that partly purified capsular material alone produced sterile abscesses, as did mixtures of capsular material or killed capsulate strains with non-capsulate strains. Their initial work was done with mixed infections involving *B. fragilis* and enterobacteria; subsequently they showed that capsulate strains alone could cause abscesses (Onderdonk et al. 1984). Brook (1987) found that capsulate strains were of greater virulence for mice than non-capsulate strains, causing bacteraemia and metastatic abscesses more readily. However, Rotstein et al. (1987) found that the capsule was not essential for the virulence of *B. fragilis* in mixed infections of the rat peritoneal cavity. In addition to inducing abscess formation, other roles in pathogenicity have been ascribed to the capsule. There is evidence that the capsule of some strains of *B. fragilis* confers resistance to phagocytosis and intracellular killing. Clinical isolates of *B. fragilis* were found to be ingested and killed by polymorphonuclear leucocytes (PMNs) only after opsonization by serum factors (Casciato et al. 1975, Bjornson, Altemeier and Bjornson 1976). In addition, increased resistance to the bactericidal action of serum, to phagocytosis and intracellular killing by PMNs (Reid and Patrick 1984), and to phagocytosis by macrophages, has been reported for capsulate strains (Rodloff et al. 1986).

B. fragilis has been found to inhibit the phagocytosis of aerobic or facultative organisms in mixed cultures, explaining perhaps why treatment of mixed infections with agents active against anaerobes alone is often successful (Ingham et al. 1977). Culture filtrates and an outer-membrane preparation of *B. fragilis* were found to inhibit both the chemotactic response of PMNs to *E. coli* components and the phagocytosis and killing of *E. coli* by both PMNs and macrophages (Namavar et al. 1987).

Capsulate strains of pigmented *Prevotella* and *Porphyromonas*, and anaerobic gram-positive cocci isolated from clinical materials have also been observed (Brook 1986, Brook, Myhal and Dorsey 1992). The role of capsules in these organisms has not been examined in as much detail as that of the *B. fragilis* capsule, but Brook et al. (1983) found that the presence of a capsule in species of *Prevotella* and *Porphyromonas* was related to the ability to produce abscesses in experimentally infected mice. He found that when, in the course of mixed infections, non-capsulate strains acquired the ability to produce capsules, they also acquired the ability to cause abscesses.

LIPOPOLYSACCHARIDE

Ingham et al. (1981) found that *B. fragilis*, by reacting in vitro with the serum necessary for opsonization, protected both itself and certain facultative anaerobes from being killed by PMNs but not from phagocytosis; Connolly, McLean and Tabaqchali (1984) reported that whole *B. fragilis* or capsular polysaccharide alone inhibited the bactericidal activity of both serum and

PMNs. An explanation for this is provided by the report of Jones and Gemmell (1986), which showed that *B. fragilis* absorbed the opsonic capacity of serum, thus reducing the phagocytosis of enterobacteria by inhibiting the classical pathway of complement opsonization. The effect appeared to be mediated by *B. fragilis* lipopolysaccharide (LPS), because treatment of serum with the LPS inhibited the phagocytic uptake of *Proteus mirabilis* by PMNs but treatment with capsular material had no effect (Jones and Gemmell 1986). On the other hand, Connolly, McLean and Tabaqchali (1984) found that the LPS had no effect on the bactericidal action of serum or PMNs.

It was thought until recently that the LPS of *Bacteroides*, *Prevotella* and *Porphyromonas* did not contain keto-deoxyoctonate (KDO), and that it lacked the classical endotoxic activity of enterobacterial LPS (Duerden 1994). It is now known that KDO is produced by these species, but that it is detectable only after acid extraction. Most gram-negative anaerobic bacilli express less endotoxic activity than do enterobacteria (Duerden 1994). Bjornson (1984) found that *B. fragilis* LPS activated Hageman factor, initiating the intrinsic pathway of coagulation. Thus, it is possible that LPS may contribute to the local thrombophlebitis and subsequent septic embolization and metastatic abscesses that occur in *B. fragilis* infections.

The cell wall LPS of *F. necrophorum* contains KDO and has strong endotoxic properties, which resemble those of enterobacterial endotoxin. It is lethal for mice, rabbits and chicken embryos, and produces localized and generalized Shwartzman reactions in rabbits (Duerden 1990).

Metabolic products may also contribute to the resistance of *B. fragilis* to PMN activity. Eftimiadi et al. (1987) found that short-chain fatty acids produced by *B. fragilis* and other *Bacteroides* spp. inhibited neutrophil chemotaxis, reduced chemiluminescence emission when PMNs were mixed with bacteria, prevented lysosomal enzyme release and caused evagination of the cell surface. Among the metabolic products, succinate has been shown to inhibit the respiratory burst of PMNs by reducing the intracellular pH, thus preventing postphagocytic intracellular killing (Rotstein, Nasmith and Grinstein 1987). *B. fragilis* itself does not stimulate chemotaxis and Namavar et al. (1984, 1987) found that culture filtrates and outer-membrane preparations, but not LPS, inhibited chemotaxis of PMNs in response to enterobacterial chemotactic factors.

3.4 Host defences

Non-sporing anaerobic bacteria, like many of the 'pyogenic' facultative anaerobes that are often mixed with them in polymicrobial wound and abscess infections, survive and multiply outside of phagocytic cells as extracellular parasites. Once ingested by phagocytic cells, they are usually killed rapidly (Bjornson 1990). The *B. fragilis* group are susceptible to the bactericidal activity of serum (Casciato et al. 1979), which is mediated by complement (Sundqvist and Johansson 1982). Through activation of serum complement,

PMNs and monocytes are attracted to the *B. fragilis* LPS; this is mediated by complement component C5a during activation of either the classical or the alternate pathway of complement (Bjornson 1990). Phagocytic ingestion and killing of the bacteria by PMNs is facilitated by deposits of C3 (complement) fragments and serum antibodies on the bacteria (Bjornson 1990). *B. fragilis* and *F. mortiferum* are readily killed by PMNs under either aerobic or anaerobic conditions (Mandell 1974, Bjornson, Altemeier and Bjornson 1976, Vel et al. 1984), but the killing of *P. acnes* by PMNs occurred much more slowly under anaerobic conditions than under aerobic conditions (Thore, Lofgren and Tarnvik 1983). Opsonophagocytic killing of *B. fragilis* by PMNs was found to be inhibited by capsules (Simon et al. 1982). On the other hand, phagocytosis was enhanced by fimbriae (or pili) on unencapsulated strains (Pruzzo, Dainelli and Ricchetti 1984). Resistance to encapsulated *B. fragilis* in an intra-abdominal abscess model involved T cell-dependent immunity; however, resistance against bacteraemia involved humoral immunity (circulating antibody and complement) (Onderdonk et al. 1982). In addition to the inhibition of PMN functions by succinate from encapsulated and non-encapsulated strains, there is evidence that macrophage functions may also be inhibited by *B. fragilis* (Bjornson 1989). The subject has been reviewed by Bjornson (1989, 1990).

4 PATHOGENIC ANAEROBIC GRAM-NEGATIVE, NON-SPORING BACILLI

Anaerobic gram-negative bacilli are capable of causing infections in all anatomical regions. They are especially common in dental and oral infections, in infections involving the lungs and pleura, abdominal cavity, female genital tract, and in infections involving the skin, soft tissue and bones (Finegold and George 1989). The clinical clues to most infections involving *Bacteroides*, *Prevotella*, *Porphyromonas* and *Fusobacterium* spp. are indistinguishable clinically from those involving other non-sporing anaerobes. They include the presence of an infection site near a mucosal surface, foul-smelling purulent exudate, tissue necrosis, gas in tissue, infection in patients with risk factors or predisposing factors to anaerobe infections (e.g. a history of underlying malignancy, intra-abdominal or pelvic surgery) and other clinical features (Finegold, George and Mulligan 1986).

The *B. fragilis* group are the anaerobes most frequently involved in infections, accounting for about 25% of all the anaerobes recovered from properly selected and collected clinical specimens (Koneman et al. 1992). They also have the distinction of being the anaerobes that are most resistant to antimicrobial agents (Finegold 1989a, 1995b). The other species of the group are isolated much less often from infections than are *B. fragilis*. They include *B. thetaiotaomicron*, which is a significant member of the faecal flora but is isolated about 4 times less often than *B. fragilis* from infections (Werner and Pulverer 1971, Werner 1974, Holland, Hill and Altemeier 1977, Duerden 1980a). Nevertheless, *B. thetaiotaomicron* is more resistant than *B. fragilis* to antimicrobial agents (e.g. clindamycin, β-lactams and various cephalosporins) and is recovered from >10% of infections yielding the *B. fragilis* group. Although the remaining species in the *B. fragilis* group (e.g. *Bacteroides vulgatus*, *Bacteroides distasonis*, *Bacteroides ovatus*, *Bacteroides uniformis*, *Bacteroides caccae*, *Bacteroides merdae*, *Bacteroides stercoris*, and *Bacteroides eggerthii*) are isolated less frequently from infections, they also are more resistant to antimicrobial agents than *B. fragilis*, and are isolated occasionally from patients with clinically significant anaerobic bacteraemia (Allen et al. 1996). Their clinical significance should be determined on a patient-by-patient basis. At times, they are part of a mixed flora from a patient with a catastrophic breakdown of the gut mucosal barrier, or they could be a sign of gross faecal contamination during specimen collection. *Bacteroides ureolyticus* (which is more closely related to the genus *Campylobacter* and awaiting transfer from the genus *Bacteroides*) is a significant pathogen in superficial necrotizing lesions and in genital infections.

Pigmented species of *Prevotella* and *Porphyromonas*, referred to in many reports as 'pigmented *Bacteroides* spp.', or as '*B. melaninogenicus*' in the past, have often been identified in human infections, though much less frequently than *B. fragilis* (Burdon 1928, Heinrich and Pulverer 1960). They are rarely found in pure culture. Precise identification of the pigmented species is not to be found in the earlier reports; however, Heinrich and Pulverer (1960) regarded *B. melaninogenicus* as asaccharolytic and '*B. asaccharolyticus*' (now *Porphyromonas asaccharolytica* in part) was the commonest pigmented species and the second most common species in Duerden's (1980a) series, being associated particularly with necrotic lesions and abscesses. The asaccharolytic and pigmented *P. gingivalis* has been associated with severe forms of periodontal disease.

F. necrophorum was once fairly common in serious infections of humans. It is sensitive to penicillin and many other antibacterial agents and has been encountered much less frequently since the advent of antibiotics. Although now overshadowed by *B. fragilis*, it can cause serious or fatal disease, including lung abscesses, septicaemia and infections of the central nervous system (Finegold 1977).

4.1 *Bacteroides* species

BACTEROIDES FRAGILIS

B. fragilis accounts for more than 50% of all clinically significant isolates of *Bacteroides* species, and is more pathogenic than the other species of the group (Werner and Pulverer 1971, Werner 1974, Holland, Hill and Altemeier 1977, Duerden 1980a). Infections with *B. fragilis* usually originate from the lower gastrointestinal tract and, when the source of infection is the appendix, colon or rectum, about 60% of all significant anaerobic isolates and more than 75% of the

B. fragilis group isolates consist of *B. fragilis*. Most *Bacteroides* strains in the normal faecal flora belong to the *B. fragilis* group, but *B. vulgatus* and *B. thetaiotamicron* are present in the largest numbers, *B. fragilis* being greatly outnumbered. *B. fragilis* is commoner than any other species in the relatively small number of infections in which a gram-negative anaerobic bacillus is present alone.

BACTEROIDES UREOLYTICUS

B. ureolyticus was first isolated from abscesses, principally of the buccal region (Eiken 1958); most subsequent reports have described strains isolated from fairly superficial soft tissue infections, usually mixed (Khairat 1967, Schroter and Stawru 1970). *B. ureolyticus* is not a major component of the normal flora. It appears to be of pathogenic significance in ulcerative or gangrenous lesions of the groin, perineum and scrotum, in similar lesions associated with peripheral vascular disease, and in some cases of paronychia; although never isolated in pure culture from these lesions, it appears to be one of the main components responsible for the tissue damage. It is often isolated from the deep active areas of the lesions in mixed culture with anaerobic gram-positive cocci, a combination that may produce a form of synergic gangrene (Duerden, Bennett and Faulkner 1982). *B. ureolyticus* has also been associated with non-gonococcal, non-chlamydial, non-mycoplasmal urethritis (Fontaine et al. 1984); the urethritis isolates have been shown to be indistinguishable from *B. ureolyticus* isolates from other sources (Fontaine et al. 1986, Taylor, Costas and Owen 1987).

BACTEROIDES GRACILIS

Now called *Campylobacter gracilis*, *B. gracilis* was originally considered an obligately anaerobic gram-negative bacillus; it, like *B. ureolyticus*, is now known to be a micro-aerophile (Vandamme et al. 1995). It is a corroding species that appears similar to *B. ureolyticus* but does not produce urease. A member of the human oral microflora (Tanner et al. 1981, Kononen, Jousimies-Somer and Asikainen 1994, Kononen et al. 1994), there have been few clinical reports of its role in disease (Lee et al. 1993). Johnson et al. (1985) found that corroding strains were isolated from 7.5% of all anaerobe-positive cultures; 71 of 100 isolates survived for identification and 23 were *C. gracilis*. Most (83%) were from serious visceral or head and neck infections, particularly with pleuropulmonary involvement; one-third of the strains were resistant to penicillin.

4.2 *Prevotella* species

Species of the genus *Prevotella* (referred to as the *Bacteroides melaninogenics-oralis* group in the previous edition of this text) that are part of the normal flora of the gingival crevice and the vagina also cause infections related to these sites. However, the classification of this group has undergone major changes in recent years (see Volume 2, Chapter 58) (Shah and Collins

1990, Shah and Gharbia 1993a, 1993b, Jousimies-Somer 1995, Shah et al. 1995). Most clinical studies have not kept pace with the changing taxonomy, and data are lacking regarding the clinical significance of some of the more recently named species. Until the 1980s most clinical reports of *B. melaninogenicus* infections were based upon the isolation of pigment-producing strains and there is still little information on the specific role of the newly defined species in particular infections. Pigmented species (previously all described as *B. melaninogenicus*) and non-pigmented species (loosely identified as '*B. oralis*') in this group play an important role in oral infections, including periodontal disease and gingivitis, periapical abscesses, and soft tissue infections of the head and neck. Tissue destruction, especially in the gums, may result from the action of a variety of virulence factors produced by these species (see section 3.3, p. 746). Tissue destruction, especially in the gums, may result from the action of a variety of exoenzymes or toxins, particularly proteolytic enzymes, produced by these species. *Prevotella intermedia/Prevotella nigrescens* (Shah and Gharbia 1992) is more strongly proteolytic than the other pigmented species and is the species most commonly associated with oral infections, particularly dental abscesses. It degrades haemopexin (but not albumin, haptoglobin or transferrin) and human IgG and complement factor C3; *P. melaninogenica* is only weakly (or non-) proteolytic (Duerden 1983, Carlsson, Hofling and Sundqvist 1984, Sundqvist et al. 1985). Thrombosis of local vessels occurs commonly.

Some strains of *Prevotella* hydrolyse dextran (Staat, Gawronski and Schachtele 1973, Holbrook and McMillan 1977); this may be significant in the development of dental plaque and periodontal disease. The predominant bacteria in early plaque are dextran-producing streptococci; colonization by *Prevotella* spp. follows and leads to periodontal disease (Hardie 1974). These species are also important pathogens in chronic lung infections such as lung abscess and in cerebral abscesses secondary to lung infections or to chronic otitis media and mastoiditis. The non-pigmented species *P. oris* and *P. buccae*, previously classified as '*B. ruminicola* subsp. *brevis*' and probably reported generally as '*B. oralis* group', are recognized as significant pathogens in infections of the upper body. Holdeman et al. (1982) identified isolates mostly from periodontitis and from infections of bone and soft tissue around the mouth. Johnston et al. (1987) re-identified strains of '*B. ruminicola*' isolated between 1976 and 1986. Of 152 isolates 72 (55 *P. buccae* and 17 *P. oris*) had survived storage. The most common sources were anaerobic pleuropulmonary infections (29.2%) and suppurative lesions of the head and neck (27.8%). All 76 strains had been part of a mixed flora and 32% were resistant to penicillin. Haapasalo (1986) found non-pigmented *Bacteroides* spp. in 35 of 62 necrotic root-canal infections; 15 isolates were *P. buccae*, 12 *P. oris*, 7 *P. oralis* and one was not identified; most were from acute infections and formed part of a mixed flora but were not as a rule found with *P. gingivalis* or *Porphyromonas endodontalis*.

Among the non-oral species of *Prevotella*, *Prevotella bivia*, a normal vaginal commensal, may cause uterine and pelvic infection with abscess formation and bacteraemia in the puerperium or after surgical treatment of the female reproductive tract. McGregor et al. (1986) found that most strains produced collagenase.

4.3 *Porphyromonas* species

PORPHYROMONAS ASACCHAROLYTICA

Formerly *Bacteroides asaccharolyticus* (Shah and Collins 1988), this pigmented, non-fermentative species is a commensal of the lower gastrointestinal tract. It is commonly isolated from infections of, or originating from, the appendix, colon, rectum and perianal area, where it is usually present with *B. fragilis*. It may also be of pathogenic significance in the ulcers and gangrene of patients with peripheral vascular disease and diabetes (Peromet et al. 1973, Duerden 1980a) and in ulcerative lesions of the perineum and genitalia (Duerden 1980a, Masfari, Kinghorn and Duerden 1983, Masfari et al. 1985). *P. asaccharolytica* is rarely isolated in pure culture, but there is strong evidence that it is the main pathogenic component in mixtures with aerobic and facultative species of generally low virulence. Its pathogenicity may be due in part to a small capsule and extracellular slime. The characteristic production of a foul odour and necrotic tissue is probably due to extracellular enzymes or toxins and, in particular, to vigorous proteolytic activity.

PORPHYROMONAS GINGIVALIS

Oral strains of pigmented asaccharolytic, anaerobic gram-negative bacilli associated with destructive periodontitis are assigned to *P. gingivalis* (formerly *Bacteroides gingivalis*) (Shah and Collins 1988). It is found irregularly and in only small numbers in the normal gingival flora but is implicated in the pathogenesis of periodontal disease. It can be isolated in large numbers from periodontal pockets in patients with generalized juvenile periodontitis or advanced destructive adult periodontitis with bone loss (Coykendall, Kaczmarek and Slots 1980, Slots 1982, 1986). Its virulence characters have been discussed in a previous section (see section 3.3, p. 746).

In experimental infections in mice, *P. gingivalis* is more virulent than other oral *Prevotella* and *Porphyromonas* spp., producing skin lesions (van Steenbergen et al. 1982a) and bone resorption (Roeterink, van Steenbergen and de Graaff 1985). Culture filtrates contain a heat-stable substance of 3.5 kDa that is cytotoxic for Vero cells (van Steenbergen et al. 1982b); *P. asaccharolytica* was less cytotoxic, and *P. melaninogenica* non-toxic, in parallel tests. The LPS from *P. gingivalis* is very potent in promoting bone resorption in organ cultures (Millar et al. 1986) and similar preparations inhibit fibroblast growth (Larjava et al. 1987).

PORPHORYMONAS ENDODONTALIS

P. endodontalis (formerly *Bacteroides endodontalis*) (Shah and Collins 1988), the third pathogenic, pigmented, asaccharolytic species encountered in humans, has been isolated from patients with root-canal (i.e. endodontal) infections with periapical destruction and submucous abscesses (van Winkelhoff, Carlee and de Graaff 1985). It was found to be the second commonest species of *Prevotella* or *Porphyromonas* in dental abscesses after *P. intermedia* (van Winkelhoff, Carlee and de Graaff 1985), and Haapasalo et al. (1986) found that *P. endodontalis* and *P. gingivalis* were the commonest anaerobes in apical periodontitis.

4.4 Fusobacteria

FUSOBACTERIUM NUCLEATUM

F. nucleatum is the most commonly encountered species of *Fusobacterium* in properly selected and collected human clinical materials (Allen, Siders and Marler 1985). *F. nucleatum*, along with species of *Prevotella* and *Porphyromonas*, are the organisms most frequently involved in anaerobic pleuropulmonary infections (Marina et al. 1993). Attention has focused on its involvement in life-threatening systemic infections in haematological patients with neutropenia and mucositis following chemotherapy (Landsaat et al. 1995). Fusiform organisms have been associated with gingivitis and periodontal disease since the first reports of Plaut (1894) and Vincent (1896). *F. nucleatum* is the predominant fusobacterium in the oral flora and is found in significantly increased numbers in acute necrotizing ulcerative gingivostomatitis and in destructive periodontal disease (Savitt and Socransky 1984); however, its role in the pathogenesis of these dental/oral diseases remains uncertain. Adhesion to oral epithelial cells (Gibbons and Houte 1975) and to a galactose-containing receptor on some oral bacteria and human erythrocytes (Falkler and Burger 1981) have been described. In 1990, Dzink, Sheenan and Socransky proposed, on the basis of electrophoretic patterns of whole cell proteins and DNA homology studies, that *F. nucleatum* be subdivided into 3 new subspecies. In 1992, Gharbia and Shah proposed that 2 additional subspecies be recognized (see Volume 2, Chapter 58). At present, these subspecies are not readily differentiated in the clinical laboratory using traditional phenotypic methods, and their clinical significance is unclear.

FUSOBACTERIUM NECROPHORUM

Fusiform organisms described under a variety of names (e.g. *Sphaerophorus necrophorus*, *Sphaerophorus funduliformis* and *Sphaerophorus pseudonecrophorus*), but now recognized as *F. necrophorum*, are responsible for certain necrotic lesions in animals, including liver and other soft tissue abscesses in cattle (Kanoe, Nouka and Toda 1984), calf diphtheria (Loeffler 1884), labial necrosis in rabbits (Schmorl 1891), and foot-rot of sheep and cattle (Langworth 1977). It also causes severe necrotic infections in humans, including lung abscesses with septicaemia (Cohen 1932), hepatic abscess (Beaver, Henthorne and Macy 1934), puerperal fever (Harris and Brown 1927), tonsillar and pharyngeal infections (Hansen 1950), oropharyngeal infection accompanied by septicaemia, with secondary septic thrombophlebitis of the internal jugular vein and septic emboli with metastatic abscesses most frequently in the lungs and large joints (Lemierre 1936, Moreno et al. 1989, Sinave, Hardy and Fardy 1989), chronic otitis media and mastoiditis with septicaemia and brain abscess, and lesions associated with ulcerative colitis (Dack, Dragstedt and Heinz 1936).

The pathogenicity of *F. necrophorum* appears to be related to endotoxin and exotoxins (see section 3.3, p. 746). The organism is still isolated occasionally from serious, deep-seated infections of humans, and it is not unusual to isolate it in pure culture from soft tissue lesions (Smith and Williams 1984). *F. necrophorum* was divided into 3 biovars (A, B and C), and subsequently a new species, *Fusobacterium pseudonecrophorum*, was proposed for *F. necrophorum* biovar C (Shinjo, Hiraiwa and Miyazato 1990). *F. pseudonecrophorum* is not pathogenic for mice. In 1991, Shinjo, Fujisawa and Mitsuoka proposed that *F. necrophorum* biovars A and B be renamed *F. necrophorum* subsp. *necrophorum* and *F. necrophorum* subsp. *funduliforme*, respectively. Following intraperitoneal injection of mice with *F. necrophorum* subsp. *necrophorum*, the mice die with diffuse liver abscesses, whereas *F. necrophorum* subsp. *funduliforme* produces a few focal abscesses in their livers, but does not kill the mice (Shinjo, Fujisawa and Mitsuoka 1991).

FUSOBACTERIUM MORTIFERUM

Also called *Sphaerophorus ridiculosus*, *Sphaerophorus necroticus* and *Sphaerophorus freudenii* in the past, *F. mortiferum* is a member of the intestinal tract flora and urogenital tract flora of humans (Smith and Williams 1984). Several patients with infections involving *F. mortiferum* have been reviewed elsewhere (George et al. 1981). Included have been isolates from patients with purulent meningitis, maxillary sinusitis, pleuropulmonary infection, intra-abdominal infection, cholangitis, penile ulceration, perineal abscess and diabetic foot infection (George et al. 1981). Although Smith and Williams (1984) concluded that there is 'no clear evidence that this organism is pathogenic in either animals or man', it has been isolated from a number of compromised patients with bacteraemia, suggesting at least that it is probably an opportunistic pathogen that participates in mixed infections (Felner and Dowell 1971). In addition, *F. mortiferum* is of interest because it is resistant to certain antimicrobial agents. Occasional strains are relatively resistant to β-lactam agents such as penicillin G, certain cephalosporins, erythromycin and tetracycline (George et al. 1981). Chloramphenicol, clindamycin and metronidazole are highly active against this species.

FUSOBACTERIUM VARIUM

Also known previously by other names, *F. varium* has been isolated from the faeces of humans, cats, roaches, termites and rodents (Smith and Williams 1984). It has been recovered from a variety of clinical infections, including conjunctivitis, intraocular infection, pyogenic oral infection, osteomyelitis, cholecystitis and intra-abdominal infections (George et al. 1981). *F. varium* is considered to be pathogenic and is more resistant to antimicrobial agents than other fusobacteria. Resistance to penicillin G, certain cephalosporins, clindamycin, erythromycin and tetracycline in isolates of *F. varium* is relatively common (George et al. 1981). Chloramphenicol and metronidazole have remained active against this species.

FUSOBACTERIUM ULCERANS

This species has been isolated from tropical ulcers in various countries and shown to be distinct from other *Fusobacterium* spp. It appears to be a constant and significant feature of the mixed flora of these lesions (Adriaans and Drasar 1987).

Additional information on *Fusobacterium* spp. and infections has been reviewed elsewhere (George et al. 1981, Finegold and George 1989, Brook 1993, 1994).

4.5 Other recently named anaerobic gram-negative, non-sporing bacilli

BILOPHILA WADSWORTHIA

B. wadsworthia was first isolated from patients with gangrenous and perforated appendicitis (Baron et al. 1989). Subsequent isolates have been recovered from patients with bacteraemia (Kasten, Rosenblatt and Gustafson 1992, Bernard et al. 1994) and a variety of other infections, including acute cholecystitis, liver abscess, bartholinitis, necrotizing fasciitis (Fournier's gangrene), a scrotal abscess, diabetic foot ulcer, decubitus ulcer, mandibular osteomyelitis, osteomyelitis of the knee, axillary hidradenitis suppurativa, thoracic empyema and other infections, almost always as a part of a mixed infection (Baron et al. 1992, Finegold et al. 1992, Summanen et al. 1995). It has also been recovered from faeces and occasionally from saliva and the vagina, as a member of the normal flora (Baron et al. 1992). The majority of isolates have been reported to produce β-lactamase and interpreted to be resistant to penicillins; however, they are susceptible to imipenem, cefoxitin, ticarcillin, and other agents resistant to β-lactamase (Summanen, Wexler and Finegold 1992). In addition, some strains are resistant to clindamycin (Summanen et al. 1995). Although the pathogenicity of *B. wadsworthia* is not clearly established, it has been suggested that the organism is probably important in certain polymicrobial infections (Baron et al. 1992, Summanen et al. 1995).

SUTTERELLA WADSWORTHENSIS

Recently named in honour of V Sutter, this species resembles *Campylobacter gracilis*; it has been isolated from appendices and abdominal fluid. Its clinical significance remains to be determined. Wexler et al. (1996) reported that the organism was resistant to metronidazole and that it grew in the presence of 6% oxygen on brucella agar (without blood) supplemented with formate and fumarate; it did not grow if blood was added. Special media and growth conditions are required for its primary isolation.

DICHELOBACTER NODOSUS

Previously called *Bacteroides nodosus*, this species is an animal pathogen implicated as the major cause of foot-rot in sheep (Dewhirst et al. 1990, La Fontaine and Rood 1990, Piriz et al. 1992). Foot-rot is a mixed infection in which *A. pyogenes* and *F. necrophorum* are other important contributors (Roberts 1969). The virulence of *D. nodosus* is associated with the production of pili and with proteolytic activity; most virulent strains possess elastase activity but keratinolysis has not been demonstrated. Correlation between pilation or proteolytic activity and virulence is not clearcut (Stewart et al. 1986).

5 ANAEROBIC COCCI

Compared with the anaerobic gram-negative bacilli, the anaerobic gram-positive, non-sporing bacilli and the clostridia, the anaerobic cocci generally rank second only to the anaerobic gram-negative bacilli in terms of their frequency of isolation from infected sites of humans. The anaerobic cocci, including all gram-positive and gram-negative isolates, accounted for c. 28% of the total 5400 anaerobes isolated at the Indiana University Medical Center (IUMC) (Koneman et al. 1992). Over three-quarters of the anaerobic cocci are from mixed infections. Their frequency of isolation from properly collected clinical specimens suggests that these bacteria must be at least potentially pathogenic for humans. On the other hand, they are encountered in the indigenous flora of the oral cavity, gastrointestinal tract, genitourinary tract and skin in sufficient concentrations that it is easy to think of them as contaminants or as not having a significant role in the pathogenesis of the infections from which they are isolated (Smith and Williams 1984). In fact, a limited number of species appear to be opportunistic pathogens that play an important role in many kinds of infections. The anaerobic cocci have not received nearly as much attention from microbiologists or clinicians as have species of *Bacteroides*, *Prevotella*, *Porphyromonas*, *Fusobacterium* or the clostridia; thus, far less is known about their pathogenic potential or virulence properties (Smith and Williams 1984).

Only certain anaerobic or micro-aerophilic species of the genera *Peptostreptococcus*, *Streptococcus*, *Gemella*, *Staphylococcus* and *Veillonella* are commonly isolated from properly collected specimens from patients with diseases, although species of other genera of anaerobic cocci (e.g. *Acidaminococcus*, *Coprococcus*, *Megasphaera*, *Peptococcus*, *Ruminococcus* and *Sarcina*) are part of the normal flora (Finegold 1977, Dowell and Allen 1981, Koneman et al. 1992). Anaerobic gram-positive cocci accounted for 89%, and anaerobic gram-negative cocci (*Veillonella parvula*) 11% of 1485 isolates of anaerobic cocci recovered from properly collected human clinical materials in the Anaerobe Laboratory at IUMC (Koneman et al. 1992). Accordingly, the gram-positive species isolated most frequently were *Peptostreptococcus magnus* (21% of all anaerobic cocci),

P. asaccharolyticus (17%), *Peptostreptococcus prevotii* (14%), *P. anaerobius* (10%), *P. micros* (9%), *Streptococcus intermedius* (5%), *Staphylococcus saccharolyticus* (1.5%) and *Gemella morbillorum* (1.2%). This list of commonly isolated species is similar, but not identical to, lists of anaerobic cocci most frequently isolated from clinical specimens which have been reported from other clinical laboratories (Pien, Thompson and Martin 1972, Holland, Hill and Altemeier 1977, Brook 1988b). Among the species involved in infections of humans, *P. magnus* was not only the most frequent at the Mayo Clinic, but was isolated as the only organism (in pure culture) from a relatively large number of patients with clinically significant infections (Bourgault, Rosenblatt and Fitzgerald 1980). It appeared to be particularly important in patients who had septic arthritis, chronic osteomyelitis and severe soft tissue infections.

Severe infections involving synergistic mixtures of anaerobic cocci plus other bacteria have been clearly documented (Altemeier 1938, Meleney 1948) (see section on 'Microbial synergy', p. 747). Anaerobic cocci have been recovered from infections of all major organs.

6 ANAEROBIC GRAM-POSITIVE NON-SPORING BACILLI

The anaerobic gram-positive non-sporing bacilli are part of the normal flora of humans and other animals, although some species inhabit other environments, including water and soil. The species that cause disease are normally found on various mucous membrane surfaces (e.g. of the mouth, intestines and urogenital tract) or skin; however, some species are found in the normal flora only, and probably are harmless saprophytes, not capable of causing disease (Allen 1985). Those that cause infections appear to be opportunistic pathogens (Smith and Williams 1984). All of these bacteria are gram-positive or gram-variable and rod-shaped, but are often highly pleomorphic. Though the majority are obligate anaerobes and it is common to think of them all as 'anaerobic', a number of the species grow in a 5–10% CO_2–air incubator; thus, some are actually facultatively anaerobic and some are micro-aerophilic. All of them grow slowly, the majority requiring at least 2–3 days to form colonies on anaerobic blood agar; some, such as *A. israelii*, require 2 weeks or more of incubation before colonies are large enough to be seen (Allen 1985).

Approximately 1190 (22%) of the 5400 anaerobes isolated during a recent period of 3 years at IUMC were anaerobic gram-positive, non-sporing bacilli (Koneman et al. 1992); thus, this group is less common than the anaerobic cocci. The frequencies of isolation of the genera within this group (from properly collected human clinical materials) were as follows: *Propionibacterium* (57% of all anaerobic gram-positive, non-sporing bacilli), *Eubacterium* (23%), *Lactobacillus* (13%), *Bifidobacterium* (4%) and *Actinomyces* (3%). In the clinical laboratory, *Propionibacterium* is the most

commonly encountered genus of this group, and *Actinomyces* is the least common. *Actinomyces* spp. and *P. propionicus*, which have the potential to cause actinomycosis, are discussed in Chapter 39 and Volume 2, Chapter 20.

6.1 *Propionibacterium acnes*

In the clinical microbiology laboratory, nearly all of the *Propionibacterium* isolates are *P. acnes*. An especially prominent member of the normal microflora of the skin, but also found in the conjunctival sac, nasopharynx, oral cavity, gastrointestinal tract and genitourinary tract, *P. acnes* is often, but not always, a contaminant of blood cultures and other body fluid specimens that are obtained by penetrating the skin. *P. acnes* must be differentiated from *Listeria monocytogenes* and even *A. israelii*, which it sometimes resembles morphologically (Allen 1985).

The presence of *P. acnes* in the hair follicle–sebaceous gland apparatus is probably important in the pathogenesis of acne vulgaris, although the mechanism has not been fully determined. When injected intradermally into laboratory animals, *P. acnes* produces moderate to severe inflammation (Smith and Williams 1984). Within the follicles, *P. acnes* produces enzymes including a lipase that probably hydrolyses triglycerides in sebum and frees certain fatty acids that might act as irritants to induce inflammation (Smith and Williams 1984). With the rupture of the follicular walls and spread of inflammation into the surrounding dermis, erythematous papules, pustules and cysts characteristic of inflamed acne lesions are produced (Greer 1985). Although the quantity of sebum may be related to androgen stimulation of sebaceous glands (at least in part), sebum from which the free fatty acids have been removed is no longer inflammatory. In addition, other factors which might be important in the inflammatory response involved in acne include the activation of complement, production of serum-independent PMN chemotactic factors and the stimulation of lysosomal enzyme release from PMNs by *P. acnes* (Brook and Frazier 1991). Whatever the mechanisms involved, success in treatment of acne vulgaris has been correlated with decreasing the amount of sebum produced, decreasing the amount of hyperkeratosis within the follicular ducts and decreasing the numbers of *P. acnes* within the follicles (Hirschmann and Feingold 1992). In the treatment of patients with acne vulgaris, reduction of the density of *P. acnes* can be achieved with oral antibiotics (e.g. tetracycline), topical antibiotics (e.g. erythromycin or clindamycin), or other topical antibacterial agents such as benzoyl peroxide (Hirschmann and Feingold 1992, Tunkel 1995).

P. acnes has also been encountered in a variety of other clinical conditions. It has been implicated in several cases of endocarditis, with or without prosthetic valves (Felner and Dowell 1970, Felner 1974), central nervous system shunt infections and immune complex glomerulonephritis (Beeler et al. 1976), chronic meningitis (French et al. 1974), brain abscess (Heineman and Braude 1963, Mathisen et al. 1984), subdural empyema (Kaufman, Miller and Steigbel 1975, Yoshikawa, Chow and Guze 1975), contact lens-associated conjunctivitis (Brook 1988a), endophthalmitis (Friedman, Peyman and May 1978), dental/oral infections (Goldberg 1971), pleuropulmonary infections (Finegold and Bartlett 1975), septic arthritis (Yocum et al. 1982), osteomyelitis (Newman and Mitchell 1975) and a number of other infections (Dowell, Stargel and Allen 1976, Brook and Frazier 1991). The most common predisposing factors or conditions in patients with *P. acnes* infections were the presence of foreign bodies, diabetes mellitus and prior surgery or other trauma (Brook and Frazier 1991).

6.2   *Eubacterium* species

Species of *Eubacterium* are commonly isolated from wounds and abscesses from a variety of locations, especially from dental/oral, abdominal, obstetric/gynaecological and genitourinary sites, though they are infrequently implicated in serious infections (Brook and Frazier 1993). Most isolates are from mixed infections. During 1990 through 1995 at IUMC, only 7 isolates of *Eubacterium* spp. were recovered from blood cultures in the author's laboratory (Allen et al. 1996). The species most frequently identified are *Eubacterium limosum* and *E. lentum*; only a few others are encountered in the clinical laboratory with any frequency (Koneman et al. 1992). Three species described in 1980 by Holdeman et al., *Eubacterium timidum*, *Eubacterium brachy* and *Eubacterium nodatum*, were isolated originally from subgingival materials collected from patients with moderate and severe periodontitis. Subsequently, Hill and colleagues isolated these species from several clinical settings or infected sites, including brain abscess, osteomyelitis of the mandible, abscesses and other soft tissue infections of the head and neck, pleuropulmonary specimens, and intra-abdominal/pelvic infections. *E. nodatum*, rather than *Actinomyces* spp., was isolated from a few patients suspected clinically of having cervicofacial actinomycosis ('lumpy jaw') and from several patients with intrauterine contraceptive devices (IUCDs) (Hill, Ayers and Kohan 1987). Hill (1992) pointed out that *E. nodatum* forms branching rods, thus resembling *Actinomyces* spp. morphologically, and that it can be mistaken for species of *Actinomyces* in a Papanicolaou-stained smear, particularly from patients with IUCDs.

6.3   *Bifidobacterium* species

Rarely encountered in properly collected human clinical materials, the only known species of *Bifidobacterium* believed to have pathogenic potential is *B. dentium* (previously called *B. eriksonii* and *Actinomyces eriksonii*) (Allen 1985). It is part of the normal flora of the oral cavity and gastrointestinal tract and has been found in mixed infections involving the lower respiratory tract (Thomas, Sodeman and Bentz 1974).

6.4   *Lactobacillus* species

Lactobacilli are commonly encountered in the clinical laboratory, but usually as commensals or contaminants. Most grow on agar plating media aerobically, but grow better under anaerobic conditions; thus, the majority are aerotolerant anaerobes. *Lactobacillus catenaforme* is an example of an obligately anaerobic species that may be isolated from human clinical materials. In humans, lactobacilli normally inhabit the mouth, gastrointestinal tract and vagina. The appelation 'Doderlein's bacillus' has been used vaguely to describe a variety of gram-positive rods that occur in the human vagina. These organisms have included *Lactobacillus acidophilus*, *Lactobacillus casei*, *Lactobacillus fermentum*, *Lactobacillus leichmanii*, *Lactobacillus jensenii*, *Lactobacillus plantarum*, *Lactobacillus cellobiosus* and bifidobacteria (Smith and Williams 1984, Koneman et al. 1992). Identification of lactobacilli to the species level is often not relevant to patient management because they usually are of little clinical significance. Nevertheless, *Lactobacillus* spp. have been implicated rarely in patients with clinically significant bacteraemia, pneumonia, endocarditis and meningitis, and in patients with focal infections (Sharpe, Hill and Lapage 1973, Rahman 1982, Sussman et al. 1986). Lactobacilli are commonly resistant to vancomycin, in contrast to many other genera and species of gram-positive bacteria that are inhibited by it. Agents that are highly active against lactobacilli include penicillin, gentamicin, minocycline, chloramphenicol and imipenem (Swenson, Facklam and Thornsberry 1990).

6.5   *Mobiluncus* species

Mobiluncus spp. have been isolated from the vaginas of many women with bacterial vaginosis. However, its pathogenetic role in this condition is not clear. Evidence for the pathogenic potential of *Mobiluncus* spp., cited by Hillier and Moncla (1995), is based in part on its isolation (rarely) from non-genital sites, most often mixed with species of *Prevotella* and *Peptostreptococcus*. In addition, *Mobiluncus* spp. has been isolated from endometrial aspirates of women with pelvic inflammatory disease and from chorioamnionic materials from placentas of women with preterm deliveries (Hillier and Moncla 1995).

7   INFECTIONS IN HUMANS CAUSED BY NON-SPORING ANAEROBES

Increased clinical and laboratory awareness of anaerobes, proper selection, collection and rapid transportation of appropriate specimens to the laboratory, and good anaerobic methodology have shown that anaerobic bacteria are common pathogens. The portal of entry of these organisms is often the mucous membranes of the mouth, lower gastrointestinal tract and female genital tract; and the species isolated vary with the site of infection. Many originate from the indigenous flora of the large intestine, but all anatomical regions are susceptible to infection with the non-sporing anaerobic gram-negative and gram-positive bacilli and anaerobic cocci.

7.1 Anaerobic bacteraemia

During the 1970s and 1980s, the percentage of bacteraemias caused by anaerobic bacteria ranged from about 5% to 15% in a number of medical centres (Wilson et al. 1972, Sonnenwirth 1983, Finegold, George and Mulligan 1986, Strand and Shulman 1988). Several reports from the USA and Europe in the late 1980s and 1990s, however, have documented lower percentages of blood cultures yielding anaerobes (e.g. ≤5%) (Dorsher et al. 1991, Murray, Traynor and Hopson 1992, Gomez et al. 1993, Siboni, Graversen and Olsen 1993, Arpi et al. 1995). Earlier treatment of anaerobic infections with antimicrobial agents active against anaerobes and the widespread prophylactic administration of antibiotics preoperatively by surgeons may have contributed to this decline (Dorsher et al. 1991, Finegold 1995a), although the blood culture system used by the laboratory might be another significant variable (Allen et al. 1996). With the exclusion of *P. acnes*, which usually is considered to be a contaminant, about one-half to two-thirds or more of the isolates from patients with clinically significant anaerobic bacteraemia are anaerobic gram-negative bacilli. More than three-quarters of the anaerobic gram-negative bacilli are usually *B. fragilis* group species, and *B. fragilis* accounts for one-half to two-thirds of these isolates. The next most common group is usually the clostridia (c. 10–25% of isolates), followed by the anaerobic cocci (c. 4–12% of isolates) and the anaerobic gram-positive non-sporing bacilli (c. 3–9% of isolates) (Dorsher, Wilson and Rosenblatt 1989, Allen et al. 1996). In recent years, perhaps reflecting changes in patient populations or blood culture technology, more unusual anaerobes, such as *F. mortiferum*, *Lactobacillus* spp., *Leptotrichia buccalis*, *Actinomyces* spp., *Bifidobacterium* spp., *Lactobacillus* spp. and *Sarcina ventriculi*, have been isolated from blood cultures whereas fewer isolates of *F. necrophorum* and *Eubacterium* spp. are now being seen (Allen et al. 1996). *Anaerobiospirillum succiniciproducens*, an unusual anaerobe that is spiral-shaped with bipolar tufts of flagella, was documented to cause bacteraemia in at least 22 patients from 15 states. This organism was believed to have contributed to the death of 7 of these patients; much remains to be learned about the epidemiology, pathogenesis and treatment of this unusual kind of anaerobic bacteraemia (McNeil, Martone and Dowell 1987).

A report from the laboratory indicating the presence of anaerobic bacteria in one or more blood cultures should prompt the clinician to search for the underlying source of the organism(s). Guidance is provided in an excellent monograph on anaerobic infections in general by Finegold, George and Mulligan (1986) who reviewed the portals of entry for 855 episodes of anaerobic bacteraemia. Accordingly,

the portal of entry was the gastrointestinal tract in 52%, female genital tract in 20%, lower respiratory tract in 6%, ear, sinus and pharyngeal area in c. 5%, and the skin and soft tissue in c. 8%. In addition, transient and insignificant bacteraemia involving anaerobes often follows dental manipulation in patients with periodontal disease (Francis and de Vries 1968); it may also result from the insertion of instruments into the gastrointestinal and genitourinary tracts (LeFrock et al. 1973, Chow and Guze 1974). Significant bacteroides bacteraemia may, however, indicate serious underlying diseases (Felner and Dowell 1971, Chow and Guze 1974), usually intra-abdominal abscesses and peritonitis, less often septic abortion and puerperal infection, and occasionally pleuropulmonary infections, brain abscess, chronic otitis media and decubitus or varicose ulcers. Anaerobic bacteraemia is sometimes the first manifestation of a malignant tumour of the colon, rectum or cervix. In the pre-antibiotic era, necrotic tonsillitis caused by *F. necrophorum* often resulted in bacteraemia, often with a devastating outcome.

B. fragilis is the most common cause of bacteraemia arising from intra-abdominal sepsis; *Fusobacterium* spp., especially *F. nucleatum*, may be involved in bacteraemia that arises from oral or upper respiratory tract infection (Allen et al. 1996). Not infrequently, anaerobes may be isolated from patients who have polymicrobial bacteraemia (Hermans and Washington 1970, Wilson et al. 1972, Bouza et al. 1985). *B. fragilis* and *E. coli* or other bacteria often occur together, and in such instances demonstration of the anaerobe may necessitate the use of a selective medium (Von Graevenitz and Sabella 1971).

The clinical features of anaerobic bacteraemia may include fever, chills, peripheral leucocytosis, anaemia and disseminated intravascular coagulation (Finegold, George and Mulligan 1986). By themselves, these features are not distinguishable from those of bacteraemia involving facultative anaerobes. Septic shock sometimes occurs in bacteroides bacteraemia; this complication has been much less common in bacteroides than in enterobacterial bacteraemia (Wilson et al. 1967). Suppurative thrombophlebitis (particularly of the pelvic veins in women), complicated by thromboemboli with metastatic infection, and hyperbilirubinaemia are more specific clues tending to suggest bacteroides bacteraemia, but these are not seen with any frequency (Finegold 1995a).

Mortality associated with anaerobic bacteraemia is usually in the range of 15–35% (Finegold, George and Mulligan 1986), but it depends on the underlying cause; it has varied from 1–2% in patients with septic abortion or puerperal sepsis (Smith, Southern and Lehmann 1970) to more than 70% in patients with malignant tumours (Kagnoff, Armstrong and Blevins 1972).

Endocarditis caused by non-sporing anaerobes is rare. Masri and Grieco (1972) reviewed 27 cases and found pre-existing heart damage in 60%. Most patients had underlying bacteroides infections and the mortality was 36%. Felner (1974) reported similar findings in a review of 22 cases.

7.2 Infections of the central nervous system

Anaerobes, particularly gram-negative anaerobic bacilli and anaerobic or micro-aerophilic cocci, are the commonest cause of brain abscesses, especially those originating from chronic otitis media, mastoiditis and sinusitis (Heineman and Braude 1963, Ingham, Slekon and Roxby 1977). They are found less often in other infections of the central nervous system. Reports of isolated cases have been reviewed by Finegold (1977).

Brain abscesses due to non-sporing anaerobic bacteria may arise from infection at adjacent sites, or by metastatic spread from suppurative lesions elsewhere. Cholesteatoma is an important predisposing factor. Abscesses secondary to chronic otitis media and mastoiditis – the most important primary causes – usually affect the temporal lobes of the cerebrum, the cerebellum being the second most common site. Infection occurs by direct extension, often with localized osteomyelitis; thrombosis or thrombophlebitis of the lateral sinus is a recognized complication. Abscesses of the frontal lobe occasionally occur as a result of chronic sinusitis. Dental infections, oral infections and abscesses may also give rise to brain abscesses, either by direct extension or via the bloodstream. Abscesses of the frontal lobe occasionally follow penetrating injuries of the orbit and sinuses.

Metastatic brain abscesses are not uncommon complications of anaerobic pleuropulmonary infections. They tend to be multiple and usually occur at the junction of the grey and white matter. The frontal, parietal and occipital lobes are most commonly affected; metastatic abscesses of the temporal lobe and cerebellum are rare. It was once thought that metastatic spread from pleuropulmonary infections occurred via the spinal venous system, with the assistance of the increased intrathoracic pressure produced by coughing, but serial arteriographic studies show that the areas first affected are those supplied by the middle cerebral artery, especially on the right side (Prolo and Hanbery 1968). This indicates that the infection spreads through the arterial system by septic emboli from pulmonary thrombophlebitis. There is a possibility that previous cerebral haemorrhage or infarction may predispose to brain abscess (Heineman and Braude 1963).

The micro-organisms isolated from brain abscesses vary with the source of infection (Finegold 1977). Species of *Prevotella*, *Porphyromonas* and *Fusobacterium*, especially *F. nucleatum*, are frequently isolated from the mixed flora of abscesses secondary to otitis media and sinusitis; *B. fragilis* is relatively common in this setting. Brain abscesses arising by direct extension usually yield more than one pathogen; *Bacteroides*, *Prevotella*, *Porphyromonas* and *Fusobacterium* spp. are the commonest and most significant organisms, but facultatively anaerobic, though capnophilic *Streptococcus* spp. and

enterobacteria such as *Proteus* spp. are often found (Ingham, Slekon and Roxby 1977). In metastatic brain abscesses complex mixtures of organisms are uncommon. *Fusobacterium* spp. are generally the cause of abscesses secondary to pleuropulmonary infections; *B. fragilis* is rare. Species of *Prevotella*, *Porphyromonas*, *Fusobacterium* and *Actinomyces* are often present in metastatic abscesses secondary to dental or oral infection.

Meningitis is not commonly caused by anaerobes; most such cases are associated with extradural, subdural or brain abscesses, but some are associated with chronic otitis media and mastoiditis. Anaerobes from the sinuses, mouth and lungs are rarely involved unless access to the meninges has been made by trauma or surgical interference. *Fusobacterium* spp. are the commonest anaerobic pathogens in meningitis; *B. fragilis* may also be found (Duerden 1990).

Subdural empyema usually originates from sinusitis, often of the frontal sinus; trauma, surgical interference and otitis media play only a small role. Gram-positive cocci, including facultative or micro-aerophilic streptococci, are prominent in infections originating from the frontal sinus, but *Prevotella* spp., *Porphyromonas* spp., *B. fragilis* and *Fusobacterium* spp. are also frequently implicated. The pathogenesis and bacteriology of extradural empyema – a less dangerous disease – are the same as for brain abscesses and meningitis.

7.3 Oral and dental infections

The vast majority of odontogenic infections (e.g. infections of the dental pulp and root canals, dentoalveolar abscesses, osteomyelitis of the jaw, periodontal disease and perimandibular space infections) involve anaerobic bacteria derived from the oral flora. The clinical features of these infections vary with the anatomical sites and tissues involved (Newman and Goodman 1989, Tanner and Stillman 1993). Infections of the dental pulp and root canals may result in dentoalveolar abscesses with purulent necrosis of the surrounding tissue and bone. When chronic, the abscesses are often referred to as pyogenic granulomas. They may affect adjacent teeth and cause osteomyelitis of the jaw. Large abscesses may discharge spontaneously (Hardie 1974). Species of *Bacteroides*, *Prevotella*, *Porphyromonas*, *Fusobacterium* and *L. buccalis* have been reported to be the most significant organisms. Van Winkelhoff et al. (1985) described a fastidious, pigmented and asaccharolytic organism, *P. endodontalis*, in infected root canals, particularly those with periapical osteitis and abscess.

The treatment of dentoalveolar infection often necessitates tooth extraction. The post-extraction syndrome, dry socket, is the result of infection, leading to localized osteomyelitis and necrosis of the surrounding tissue. Such infections sometimes occur in previously clean sockets and are painful and foul smelling. The presence of fusiform bacilli and spirochaetes may simulate Vincent's angina; other oral anaerobes are also present. Pigmented gram-negative bacilli and *Fusobacterium* spp., especially *F. nucleatum*, have a particularly important role in the osteomyelitis and cellulitis of the jaw and surrounding tissues that may result from compound fractures, tooth extraction and dentoalveolar abscess (Heinrich and Pulverer 1960).

Acute necrotizing ulcerative gingivostomatitis – otherwise known as ANUG, Vincent's angina, Plaut–Vincent's infection, trench mouth and fusospirochaetosis – was one of the first anaerobic infections to be recognized (Plaut 1894, Vincent 1896). It is associated with poor environmental conditions, malnutrition, debility and poor oral hygiene, such as are common in wartime, and is characterized by pain, haemorrhage, a foul odour, destruction of the interdental papillae, inflammation, recession of the gingival margin, and the formation of a pseudomembrane. It is generally accepted that ANUG is a synergic infection with a fusobacterium and a large coarse spirochaete. The fusiform organism may be *L. buccalis* – probably the present designation of Vincent's bacillus (see Volume 2, Chapter 62) – but other workers believe *F. nucleatum* to be the significant fusiform organism in ANUG (Willis 1977, Moore, Ranney and Holdeman 1982); the spirochaete is *Treponema vincentii*. These organisms are present in the exudate and pseudomembrane; diagnosis is made by direct microscopy. There is evidence that species of *Prevotella*, *Porphyromonas* or both are essential components of the infection and may be the main cause of the tissue damage and necrosis (Kaufman et al. 1972, Hardie 1974, Slots 1982).

The microbiology and pathogenesis of periodontal diseases has attracted considerable interest during the past 2–3 decades. Pigmented anaerobic gram-negative bacilli have long been associated with periodontal disease (Burdon 1928). They are found infrequently and in low numbers in plaque in the absence of such disease and are rare in children, even in those with juvenile periodontal disease, in which *Actinobacillus actinomycetemcomitans* predominates (Slots 1982, Savitt and Socransky 1984). However, they are present in most cases of advanced periodontal disease in adults, where they may account for up to 30% of the cultivable flora (Slots 1982). *P. gingivalis* is associated with the rapidly progressive ('early-onset') adult form of periodontal disease, in which there is extensive alveolar bone destruction, and with generalized juvenile periodontitis (Coykendall, Kaczmarek and Slots 1980, Slots 1982, Savitt and Socransky 1984). It is not found in chronic adult periodontal disease, in which various gram-negative anaerobes are present. *Bacteroides forsythus* also appears to be important in periodontal diseases in which there is active, destructive, progression (Dzink, Socransky and Haffajee 1988, Moore et al. 1991). *P. intermedia* is found in gingivitis (Slots 1982), in advanced periodontitis with inflamed gingiva, and in deep but relatively inactive pockets. A current summary listing of species strongly associated with active periodontitis follows: *Campylobacter* (*Wolinella*) *recta*, *F. nucleatum*, *P. micros*, *P. anaerobius*, *P. gingivalis*, *E. nodatum*, *E. timidum*, *E. brachy*, *Eubacterium alactolyticum*, *Fusobacterium alocis*, *Treponema socranskii* subspp. *socranskii*, *Selenomonas sputigena*, *B. forsythus*, and *A. actinom-*

ycetemcomitans (Dzink, Socransky and Haffajee 1988, Moore et al. 1991, Tanner and Stillman 1993). Species associated with refractory periodontal diseases (characterized by a lack of response to therapy) include the following: *B. forsythus*, *P. melaninogenica*, *C. recta*, *S. intermedius*, *P. intermedia*, *P. gingivalis*, *A. actinomycetemcomitans* and *Eikenella corrodens* (Tanner and Stillman 1993). Additional information on periodontal diseases has been reviewed elsewhere (Newman and Goodman 1989, Tanner and Stillman 1993).

The bacteraemia that often follows extraction of the teeth may, on rare occasion, lead to endocarditis caused by oral anaerobes or streptococci (Okell and Elliott 1935, Pressman and Bender 1944, Khairat 1966). Likewise, the lungs may suffer from the effect of dental sepsis, the result being necrotizing pneumonia, empyema and abscess formation caused by aspiration of these same organisms, occasionally including *B. fragilis*. Dentoalveolar and periodontal infection may spread directly or by the bloodstream to cause retropharyngeal abscesses, osteomyelitis, extradural and subdural abscesses, and brain abscesses, with or without meningitis. Brain abscesses derived from oral sources usually have a mixed bacterial flora. *Actinomyces* spp. and streptococci are common components, but species of *Prevotella*, *Porphyromonas*, or *Fusobacterium* are almost always present; *B. fragilis* occurs occasionally.

7.4 Infections of the respiratory tract

Anaerobes can infect all sites within the upper and lower respiratory tract. Plaut–Vincent's angina has long been known to cause painful ulcerating lesions of the throat and tonsils, (Plaut 1894, Vincent 1896). A severe infection (Lemierre's disease or 'necrobacillosis'), with peritonsillar cellulitis, abscess formation and thrombophlebitis of the internal jugular vein caused by *F. necrophorum*, frequently leads to bacteraemia, pulmonary emboli and sometimes to death (Aoki et al. 1993, Ieven et al. 1993, Goyal et al. 1995, De Sena et al. 1996). Numerous anaerobes, especially species of *Bacteroides*, *Fusobacterium*, *Prevotella* and anaerobic cocci, are found in other peritonsillar and retropharyngeal abscesses, and in chronic tonsillitis; such infections produce foetid breath (Brook, Yocum and Shah 1980, Brook, Yocum and Friedman 1981, Nord 1995).

In the pre-antibiotic era *F. necrophorum* was a common cause of acute otitis media, mastoiditis and sinusitis, sometimes with fulminant bacteraemia. Anaerobes are now uncommon in acute cases, but in the chronic forms of these diseases anaerobic cocci, the pigmented *Prevotella*, *Porphyromonas*, *Bacteroides* and *Fusobacterium* spp. are often found. Rist (1901) considered anaerobes to be the cause of all cases of chronic otitis media; a mixed flora is usually present, but anaerobic cocci and gram-negative anaerobes often predominate. Quantitative studies have shown that anaerobes are present in c. 50% of cases of chronic suppurative otitis media at counts of c. 10^9 ml^{-1} (Sweeney, Picozzi and Browning 1982, Busch

1984). Serious complications may occur; thus, Guillemot (1899) and Rist (1901) reported cases of pulmonary gangrene secondary to chronic otitis media. Local osteomyelitis, soft tissue abscesses and bacteraemia with widespread metastatic infection are also not uncommon. The most serious complication is brain abscess, sometimes with meningitis, subdural or extradural empyema, and intracranial thrombophlebitis. Anaerobes are usually present in chronic sinusitis (Nord 1995).

Anaerobic infections of the lung and pleural space are sufficiently common in the USA to suggest that anaerobes are second only to the pneumococcus as causes of pneumonia in hospital patients (Bartlett and Finegold 1974, Bartlett 1987, 1993, Marina et al. 1993), but this is not true of Great Britain. This discrepancy may be real or due to differences in laboratory methods or to the greater use of aspiration techniques for obtaining specimens in the USA. The source of infection is the patient's mouth and upper respiratory tract. Sputum specimens are unsuitable for diagnosis because they are contaminated with the oropharyngeal flora. Satisfactory specimens from cases of empyema can be obtained by thoracentesis, but for pulmonary specimens percutaneous transtracheal aspiration (Bartlett, Rosenblatt and Finegold 1973), needle biopsy (Beerens and Tahon-Castel 1965), or collection of specimens through a fibreoptic bronchoscope with a protected brush (Bartlett 1987) is necessary.

Guillemot, Hall and Rist (1904) found that empyema fluid from patients with putrid pleurisy contained few aerobes but many anaerobes, which resembled those of the normal oral flora. Aspiration and pneumonia lead to empyema. The incidence of lung abscesses and empyema is increased by the presence of periodontal disease, peritonsillar infections and chronic otitis media or sinusitis, and is low in edentulous patients.

Anaerobic pleuropulmonary infection can be divided into 4 categories: aspiration pneumonia, necrotizing pneumonia, lung abscess and empyema (Bartlett and Finegold 1972). The pathogenesis and source of infection are the same for each category. Anaerobic aspiration pneumonia without necrosis or abscess formation is easily overlooked because of the absence of foul pus and tissue necrosis. It is an acute illness which responds rapidly to appropriate treatment (Bartlett and Finegold 1974). Necrotizing pneumonia is characterized by suppuration, with areas of necrosis and cavity formation. It usually affects one segment or lobe but may spread rapidly through the lung, destroying the tissue and leaving only putrid sloughs; the x-ray findings are characteristic and the disease is associated with a high mortality. It was called pulmonary gangrene by the early workers, who recognized the role of anaerobes in its pathogenesis (Guillemot, Halle and Rist 1904, Rona 1905). Lung abscess is a predominantly anaerobic infection; the mechanism of infection is aspiration, but the infection is localized. It is often a complication of bronchial obstruction, e.g. by a tumour or enlarged lymph nodes; the lung becomes infected by organisms from the upper respiratory tract. There is usually a low-grade fever with anaemia and weight loss; tissue destruction is seen on x-ray as a cavity partly filled with fluid. The copious sputum is putrid and the patient has halitosis. Cerebral abscess is a serious complication of lung abscess, resulting from pulmonary thrombophlebitis, bacteraemia and septic emboli. Empyema is almost invariably associated with underlying parenchymal disease, but is occasionally secondary to subphrenic abscesses. Anaerobes are the predominant pathogens (Bartlett et al. 1974). The empyema fluid is usually purulent and often foul; it may be loculated and difficult to drain, but drainage is an essential part of treatment.

Prevotella spp., *F. nucleatum* and *Peptostreptococcus* spp. predominate in anaerobic pleuropulmonary infections (e.g. aspiration pnumonia, lung abscess and necrotizing pneumonia); *B. fragilis* is found in only a minority of these conditions (Bartlett, Sutter and Finegold 1974, Marina et al. 1993). In a retrospective review of cases of anaerobic empyema at the Wadsworth Anaerobic Bacteriology Laboratory (Los Angeles), the most common anaerobe isolates (in order of occurrence) were *F. nucleatum*, the *Prevotella oris–buccae* group, the *B. fragilis* group, pigmented *Prevotella* spp., *Peptostreptococcus* spp., *Eubacterium* spp., *Lactobacillus* spp., *Actinomyces* spp. and *Clostridium* spp. (Civen et al. 1995). *F. necrophorum* is less common now than formerly but is occasionally responsible for severe pleuropulmonary infections with abscess formation, empyema and bacteraemia (Bartlett, Sutter and Finegold 1974). Anaerobes are also responsible in part for the progressive damage and destruction that occur in bronchiectatic cavities. Species of *Prevotella* and *F. nucleatum*, from the oral flora, are the commonest species isolated. *B. fragilis* is found in a significant minority of these cases.

7.5 Abdominal and perineal infections

Anaerobic bacteria, especially *Bacteroides* spp., are the predominant pathogens in infections associated with surgery, injury, perforation or other underlying abnormality of the gastrointestinal tract (Gorbach and Bartlett 1974, Gorbach, Thadepalli and Norsen 1974). Infection with *Bacteroides* spp. is most common after surgical treatment or perforation of the large intestine; it is less common after surgical treatment of the upper gastrointestinal tract, where contamination with anaerobes from the normal gut flora is less.

The normal stomach and upper small intestine generally contain few bacteria, but they become colonized by faecal bacteria, including those of the *B. fragilis* group, when their normal anatomy and physiology are altered (Drasar and Hill 1974). *B. fragilis* is a minor but significant cause of postoperative wound infection, peritonitis and the intra-abdominal abscesses that follow perforation or surgical operations. Normal gastric acidity provides a barrier between the bacterial populations of the mouth and the large intestine. The normal flora of the oesophagus is derived from the mouth, but most organisms are destroyed when they enter the stomach. Any disturbance of acid production results in colonization of the stomach by oral bacteria, including species of *Prevotella*, and these are found in wound infections, peritonitis and empyemas after surgical treatment or perforation of the oesophagus and stomach (Duerden 1980b), and also in peritonitis secondary to perforation of duodenal ulcers. These infections are usually mixed and the *Prevotella* spp. are present in association with other oral organisms such as non-β and α-haemolytic streptococci and anaerobic cocci.

The most common bacteroides infections are wound infections, intra-abdominal abscesses and peritonitis associated with the appendix or large intestine. Finegold (1977) found that anaerobes, mainly the *B. fragilis* group, were associated with 86% of intra-abdominal infections. *B. fragilis* is the most significant pathogen in the majority of wound infections after surgical treatment of the appendix or large intestine (Leigh, Simmons and Norman 1974, Swenson et al. 1974, Willis 1975, 1977, Willis et al. 1976). Similarly, the *B. fragilis* group are almost always associated with peritonitis and intra-abdominal abscesses (e.g. subphrenic, pelvic and paracolic) resulting from perforation of the large intestine.

The importance of anaerobes as the cause of peritonitis and abscesses in appendicitis was recognized by Veillon and Zuber (1898); gram-negative anaerobic bacilli were the predominant pathogens in 21 of their 22 cases of suppurative appendicitis and appendix abscess. Altemeier (1938) isolated gram-negative anaerobic bacilli from 96 of 100 cases of peritonitis associated with acute perforated appendicitis. Bornstein et al. (1964) found that 25% of bacteroides infections were associated with the appendix. Felner and Dowell (1971) found that 10% of a series of 250 cases of bacteroides bacteraemia originated from appendiceal lesions. Leigh, Simmons and Norman (1974) isolated *Bacteroides* spp. from 78% of 322 swabs taken at appendectomy, and from 90% of the infectious complications of those operations. Willis et al. (1977) found that the incidence of post-appendectomy sepsis varied from 4% for normal appendices to 77% for gangrenous or perforated appendices; and *Bacteroides* spp. were the main pathogens.

Similar infections result from surgical treatment or perforation of the colon. Diverticulosis is a common non-infectious disease but *Bacteroides* spp. are almost invariably present in the infections that arise when diverticulitis leads to diverticular and paracolic abscesses and peritonitis. These infections frequently give rise to bacteraemia; 6–10% of bacteroides bacteraemias originate from diverticulitis (Felner and Dowell 1971, Wilson et al. 1972). There is also a close association between abdominal infections with *Bacteroides* spp. and a carcinoma of the colon or rectum. Peritonitis, intra-abdominal abscesses and wound infections are common complications of the surgical treatment of these tumours. Bacteroides bacteraemia, peritonitis, or abscess formation may on occasion be the first manifestation of the malignancy (Finegold

1977). Perirectal and perianal abscesses frequently yield mixtures of anaerobes in which *Bacteroides* spp. predominate (Finegold 1977).

B. fragilis is the predominant pathogen in 60–70% of abdominal infections and *P. asaccharolytica* is the next most common species. *B. thetaiotamicron* is about 4 times less common than *B. fragilis*; other members of the *fragilis* group are isolated infrequently (Werner and Pulverer 1971, Werner 1974, Holland, Hill and Altemeier 1977, Polk and Kasper 1977, Duerden 1980a). *B. fragilis* is found in at least 60% of perianal and perirectal abscesses; *P. asaccharolytica* is important but less common and rarely present alone. *B. ureolyticus* is rarely isolated from abdominal infections but occurs more commonly in perianal abscesses and other perineal infections (Henriksen 1948, Duerden, Bennett and Faulkner 1982).

7.6 Liver and biliary tract infections

Liver abscesses are generally polymicrobial, but anaerobes, particularly *Bacteroides* spp. and anaerobic cocci (Sabbaj, Sutter and Finegold 1972, Sabbaj 1984) often predominate. The source of infection is usually the faecal flora and the route the portal venous system. Colorectal malignancy, ulcerative colitis, Crohn's disease and intraperitoneal abscesses following perforation of the large intestine are common underlying diseases and blunt abdominal trauma is also an important cause. Consequently the causative organism of hepatic abscess is usually *B. fragilis*; *F. necrophorum* occasionally occurs. *Bacteroides* spp. may be found in hepatic amoebic abscesses (Legrand and Axisa 1905, May, Lehmann and Sanford 1967) and hydatid cysts of the liver (Deve and Guerbet 1907); they may cause the first clinical signs of disease. Bacteroides bacteraemia is a common complication of liver abscess; bacteraemia was present in a series of 5 cases, diagnosed only at autopsy (Sabbaj, Sutter and Finegold 1972). Liver abscess and bacteraemia due to *B. fragilis* sometimes occur in liver transplant patients (Fulginiti et al. 1968).

Faecal bacteroides are responsible for only a minority of cases of cholangitis and cholecystitis. They may be isolated from the bile and the gall bladder wall of patients with biliary obstruction.

7.7 Infections of the female genitourinary tract

Anaerobic bacteria are part of the normal vaginal flora (see Volume 2, Chapter 11) and may be the principal pathogens in serious infections of the female genital tract that sometimes follow surgical interference or accompany other diseases (Ledger, Sweet and Headington 1971, Gorbach and Bartlett 1974, Willis 1977). Species of *Peptostreptococcus*, *Prevotella* (*P. bivia* and *P. disiens* in particular) and *Porphyromonas* are the most frequently isolated anaerobes (Garber and Chow 1989). *E. nodatum*, which can be mistaken in Papanicolaou-stained smears for *Actinomyces* spp., appears to be common in patients with IUCDs (Hill

1992). The relatively high frequencies of *B. fragilis* in these infections, reported during the 1970s, were probably based mostly on incorrect identifications (Bartlett 1992). Anaerobes are frequently implicated in infections of the uterus and pelvis, such as endometritis, pyometra, parametritis, salpingitis, tubal, tubo-ovarian and ovarian abscesses, pelvic cellulitis and abscesses, chorioamnionitis, intrauterine sepsis, post-abortal and puerperal infections, and wound infections and abscesses incidental to gynaecological surgical treatment; they are also found in vulvovaginal infections such as abscesses of the vaginal wall, vulva and Bartholin's and Skene's glands. Many infections may be complicated by peritonitis, pelvic, ovarian and broad-ligament abscesses, pelvic thrombophlebitis, bacteraemia with metastatic abscesses, and cellulitis or abscess formation in the perineum, groin or abdominal wall.

Most cases of septic abortion are due to anaerobes (Rotheram and Schick 1969, Thadepalli, Gorbach and Keith 1973, Rotheram 1974). Patients suffer from fever, uterine tenderness and a foul-smelling cervical discharge. Most respond well to uterine evacuation and antimicrobial therapy effective against anaerobes. Complications (see above) are less common now than in the pre-antibiotic era. Fortunately, the greatly feared clostridial myonecrosis and 'septico-toxaemia' is now only a rare complication of abortions (Garber and Chow 1989). Puerperal infections, caused as a rule by anaerobic gram-negative bacilli, often in association with anaerobic or micro-aerophilic cocci, present with signs and symptoms that are similar to those of septic abortion (Pearson and Anderson 1970, Thadepalli, Gorbach and Keith 1973). Early rupture of the membranes, prolonged labour and postpartum haemorrhage are predisposing factors. Pearson and Anderson (1970) found that bacteria from the normal vaginal flora caused amnionitis in about 10% of deliveries; most such infections were apparently insignificant, but there seemed to be an association with perinatal mortality (Pearson and Anderson 1967). Gibbs et al. (1987) found antibodies to *P. bivia* in the serum of women with intra-amniotic infection. In more severe infections there is also an endometritis, which may spread to produce parametritis, pelvic abscess and peritonitis. These infections produce fever, lower abdominal tenderness and a foul lochial discharge.

In bacterial (anaerobic) vaginosis, a common abnormality in sexually active women, *P. bivia*, *P. disiens*, *Porphyromonas* spp., *Mobiluncus* spp. and *Peptostreptococcus* spp. are major components, along with *Gardnerella vaginalis* and genital mycoplasmas (Spiegel 1991). There is a 'fishy odour' and non-purulent vaginal discharge with a raised pH (>5), but no inflammation; microscopy reveals few lactobacilli but many small gram-positive (*G. vaginalis*) and gram-negative (*Prevotella* and *Porphyromonas* spp.) bacilli and gram-negative curved rods (*Mobiluncus* spp.), and epithelial cells coated with these bacteria ('clue cells') (Spiegel 1991). The normal lactate content of secretions is reduced, succinate is increased (Spiegel et al. 1980), and amines are present (Spiegel 1991); succinate and amines are products of anaerobic metabolism. Although the pathogenesis of bacterial vaginosis is not entirely clear, it involves changes within the indigenous microbiota with replacement of normal lactobacilli by a mixed anaerobe overgrowth and resultant metabolic activity. This condition responds well to metronidazole and, alternatively, to clindamycin (Spiegel 1991). It has been reported that bacterial vaginosis increases the patient's risk for upper genital tract infections including pelvic inflammatory disease, postpartum endometritis, post-hysterectomy vaginal-cuff cellulitis, post-abortion pelvic inflammatory disease, and amniotic fluid infection or chorioamnionitis (Eschenbach et al. 1975, Eschenbach 1993). An especially important finding is the association between bacterial vaginosis and premature delivery of low birth weight infants (Hillier et al. 1995).

Urinary tract infection

Enterobacteria, or coliforms, from the faecal flora are the common cause of infection of the urinary tract in women. Although anaerobes outnumber coliforms in the faecal flora by a factor of 10^3 (Drasar and Hill 1974), and form part of the normal urethral flora, they are not responsible for primary infection of the urinary tract. Possibly the Eh and the dissolved O_2 concentration in urine are too high for anaerobes to become established. However, anaerobes may enter the urine and behave as pathogens in obstructive pyonephrosis, renal or perirenal abscesses, para- or periurethral cellulitis or abscesses, Cowperitis, prostatitis and prostatic abscesses (Duerden 1990).

7.8 Skin and soft tissue infections

Anaerobic bacteria from mucous membranes cause wound infections after surgical treatment or accidental injury. Human and animal bite wounds usually become infected with the person's or animal's oral flora; cellulitis and abscesses are common in such bite-wound infections (Linscheid and Dobyns 1975, Goldstein, Citron and Finegold 1984, Goldstein 1992, Goldstein, Pryor and Citron 1995). Other lesions include cellulitis, gangrene and abscesses. Infections are generally mixed, but anaerobes play a major part in the tissue destruction and necrosis. Non-sporing anaerobes play an important role in Meleney's synergistic gangrene and necrotizing fasciitis.

Necrotic and gangrenous lesions of the face and neck are often caused by anaerobes from the oral flora. Many such infections are associated with periodontal disease, dental abscesses or tooth extraction. Cancrum oris in poorly nourished and debilitated children starts at a mucocutaneous junction and spreads to large areas of the face (Emslie 1963). It is one manifestation of the disease noma. It occurs most commonly around the mouth but may also affect the nose, ear, vulva, prepuce or anus. The destructive process, which is associated with a foul odour, also affects periosteum and bone, with sequestrum formation. The gums and cheeks are destroyed, the teeth fall out and there may be almost complete destruction of the face before death; before the antibiotic era, the mortality was 70–100%. Predisposing factors include systemic disease, chronic infections and infestations, malnutrition and poor oral hygiene. Noma is usually regarded as a fusospirochaetal synergistic infection, but there is evidence that pigmented *Prevotella* or *Porphyromonas* spp. may play an important role (Kaufman et al. 1972).

A similar disease known as **Fournier's gangrene** or **necrotizing dermogenital infection** affects the perineum, groin, vulva, scrotum and penis. It may be a manifestation of noma, usually taking the form of a spreading anaerobic cellulitis and necrotizing fasciitis. It may follow surgical operations on the groin, perineum or lower abdomen and begins as a wound infection; other cases begin as minor lesions of the genitalia. In males, a tight prepuce and poor genital hygiene predispose to balanitis that may spread to surrounding areas. The necrotic lesions extend rapidly and may cover huge areas of the abdominal wall, loin, buttocks and thighs. Without antibiotic therapy and extensive debridement the mortality is high. Infection is always mixed. Anaerobic or micro-aerophilic cocci, *Bacteroides* spp. and *Fusobacterium* spp. have all been isolated; *P. asaccharolytica* and *B. ureolyticus* are particularly associated with necrotizing, ulcerative lesions of the genitalia (Duerden, Bennett and Faulkner 1982, Masfari, Kinghorn and Duerden 1983, Masfari et al. 1985).

Elsewhere in the body, non-sporing anaerobes are found in large numbers in infected pilonidal cysts or abscesses, and sebaceous cysts (Bornstein et al. 1964, Pien, Thompson and Martin 1972). The pus is usually foul and also often contains low-grade pathogens such as micrococci and diphtheroids. Paronychia is caused by pigmented anaerobic gram-negative bacilli and *Fusobacterium* spp., often of oral origin, and sometimes by *B. ureolyticus*. In one study, anaerobes were found in 73% of cases of paronychia in children (Brook 1981).

In varicose or decubitus ulcers, and in gangrenous diabetic ulcers, the superficial areas are colonized by bacteria that are aerobic and facultatively anaerobic, but heavy growth of anaerobes regularly occurs when specimens taken from the depth of the lesions are cultivated (Galpin et al. 1976, Wheat et al. 1986). Some lesions progress to osteomyelitis; several workers have reported bacteroides bacteraemia, sometimes fatal, associated with decubitus ulcers (Felner and Dowell 1971). Various gram-negative anaerobic bacilli have been isolated, but several reports have recognized the special role of *P. asaccharolytica*, or strains of '*B. melaninogenicus*' that were probably *P. asaccharolytica* (Peromet et al. 1973, Duerden 1980a), and *B. ureolyticus* (Duerden, Bennett and Faulkner 1982).

Breast abscesses that occur in the puerperium are usually caused by *S. aureus*, but pigmented anaerobic gram-negative bacilli, *B. ureolyticus*, *Fusobacterium* spp. and occasionally *B. fragilis* have been isolated, particularly from recurrent abscesses of the subareolar region (Pearson 1967).

7.9 Bone and joint infections

Osteomyelitis due to anaerobes arises either by spread from an adjacent lesion or by haematogenous infection. The bones most commonly infected are the mastoid and ethmoid; the infection arises from chronic otitis media, mastoiditis and sinusitis. The maxilla and mandible become infected as a consequence of dental or periodontal disease, and sometimes as the result of tooth extraction or other trauma. The causative organisms include species of anaerobic cocci, *Fusobacterium*, *Prevotella*, *Porphyromonas* and occasionally *B. fragilis*.

Elsewhere in the body, *Peptostreptococcus* spp., *P. asaccharolytica*, *B. fragilis* and *Prevotella* spp. cause chronic osteomyelitis with the formation of sequestra and sinuses containing foul pus. Osteomyelitis of the foot and leg often arises by spread from adjacent lesions in soft tissue, especially in diabetics. There appears to be an association between anaerobic infections of bones and diabetes mellitus, alcoholism, and drug addiction (Ziment, Miller and Finegold 1967, Ziment, Davis and Finegold 1969, Pearson and Harvey 1971). A few reports, most from the pre-antibiotic era, describe purulent arthritis due to haematogenous infection with *F. necrophorum*.

8 DIAGNOSIS OF NON-SPORING ANAEROBE INFECTIONS

8.1 Selection, collection and transport of specimens

This first (and probably most important) step in good, clinically relevant anaerobic bacteriology requires close communication between the microbiology staff, the clinician, the nursing staff, and other paramedical personnel. The laboratory should provide the operating rooms, emergency rooms, nursing stations, or other appropriate locations with anaerobic transport containers and instructions to be used by the clinicians and nurses who have the responsibility for collecting the specimens and transporting them to the laboratory as rapidly as possible (Dowell 1975).

The selection of clinical specimens to collect and dispatch to the laboratory for anaerobic cultures is a decision to be made by the clinician with responsibility for the patient. Almost as important as decisions of what to collect are decisions about **what not to collect**. Although anaerobes might be present on the surface of a superficial skin lesion, documenting the anaerobic flora colonizing it would not be clinically useful. The **timing** of specimen collection is also important. For example, the bacteriology of acute perforated appendicitis has been documented in numerous reports (Stone 1976, Bennion et al. 1990). Initial antimicrobial treatment, by necessity, is empirical; culture results performed routinely on individual patients who show a good clinical response seldom influence clinical management (Dougherty et al. 1989). On the other hand, the results of detailed anaerobic and aerobic bacteriological studies may be very important when patients develop serious complications (e.g. generalized peritonitis, intra-abdominal abscess, bacteraemia) (Finegold 1995a, Wilson and Hopkins 1995). It is essential that specimens be collected from active sites of infection without contamination by the normal flora. Because anaerobic and aerobic bacteria of the indigenous microbiota are present in high numbers on mucous membrane surfaces and the skin, a wide variety of specimens that are predictably contaminated with these bacteria are unacceptable for culture and should not be submitted to the laboratory (Dowell 1975). The laboratory work-up of extraneous normal flora is costly in terms of wasted laboratory resources (labour and supplies) and prolongs reporting time, and the results are likely to mislead the clinician (Allen, Siders and Marler 1995).

Materials that are virtually always unacceptable for the culture of non-sporing anaerobes, and should be rejected if received by the laboratory, include:

1 swabs from the mouth, throat, nasopharynx, periurethral area, vagina, endocervix, rectum, or a skin surface
2 surface swabs of decubitus ulcers, eschars of burns, encrusted material overlying wounds and abscesses, or sinus tracts
3 dry swabs
4 expectorated or induced sputum, materials suctioned from an endotracheal tube, bronchial washings, or bronchoalveolar lavage fluid
5 gastric contents, small bowel contents (except in blind-loop and similar syndromes), faeces, colostomy stomata, colocutaneous fistulae, or other materials contaminated with intestinal contents
6 materials adjacent to mucous membranes or skin that have not been decontaminated properly and
7 voided urine (Allen, Siders and Marler 1985).

Acceptable specimens for isolation of non-sporing anaerobes include:

1 purulent exudate aspirated from an abscess
2 tissue (e.g. biopsy, surgically removed, or autopsy)
3 body fluids other than urine (e.g. pericardial, pleural, peritoneal, synovial, blood)
4 direct fine needle aspirates of lung, other organs and tissues
5 transtracheal aspirates
6 bronchoscopic specimens obtained with a protective, double-lumen catheter (Allen and Siders 1982) and
7 'sulphur granules' from patients suspected of having actinomycosis (Allen, Siders and Marler 1985).

The most reliable specimens are samples of infected tissue, either excised or obtained by biopsy. Pus or exudate aspirated from the depths of an open lesion or from a closed lesion is also appropriate and always preferable to a swab. Swabs are far less satisfactory because they are easily contaminated, tend to dry out, are likely to expose anaerobes to too much oxygen, and only a small (and often inadequate) volume of material can be collected with them. Thus, if it is

necessary to sample an open wound or an ulcerated area, a biopsy of its base or margin (i.e. 'its leading edge') or, alternatively, a deep aspirate should be collected only after careful debridement and careful surface decontamination with povidone-iodine (Allen, Siders and Marler 1985).

Ideally, a tissue biopsy or excised tissue sample should be transported to the laboratory in a loosely sealed tube or vial within a sealed, gas-impermeable anaerobic bag (Finegold 1995a). Such bags with anaerobic gas generators are commercially available (Koneman et al. 1992, Summanen et al. 1993). Most clinically significant anaerobes are fairly aerotolerant (Tally et al. 1975), but they may be killed in transit by prolonged exposure to air, or by desiccation, which can be prevented by the use of a transport medium (Mena et al. 1978). Specimens should be transported to the laboratory quickly. Attebery and Finegold (1969) recommended the use of tubes containing an atmosphere of O_2-free CO_2 and such containers are now commercially available. Bartlett et al. (1976) reported good results with pus held in closed containers at room temperature for up to 48 h. For reviews of methods see Citron (1984), Allen, Siders and Marler (1985), Wren (1991), Koneman et al. (1992), Summanen et al. (1993).

8.2 Direct examination

Direct microscopy may reveal pleomorphic gramnegative forms consistent with *B. fragilis* or the thin, pointed filaments of *F. nucleatum* (Koneman et al. 1992). *Capnocytophaga* spp. (see Volume 2, Chapter 58) also form fusiform rods, and can be morphologically similar to *F. nucleatum*. *Capnocytophaga* spp. have been implicated in some forms of periodontal disease and may cause sepsis in patients with malignancy (e.g. leukaemia, lymphoma, multiple myeloma, endometrial carcinoma) and granulocytopenia (often with oral ulcerations) (Koneman et al. 1992). The presence of large numbers of fusobacteria and coarse spirochaetes in a Giemsa-stained smear from an ulcer of the mouth would be consistent with Vincent's angina, or other fusospirochaetal infections. A relatively large, straight or slightly curved rod with both ends, or only one end pointed, that inhabits the human oral cavity is *L. buccalis* (see Volume 2, Chapter 62) (Smith and Williams 1984). Gram-positive, non-sporing rods with branching could be species of *Actinomyces*, *Eubacterium*, *Propionibacterium*, *Bifidobacterium*, *Nocardia*, or *Mycobacterium* (e.g. *Mycobacterium fortuitum*). Of these examples, only *Nocardia* or *Mycobacterium* spp. would be acid-fast using a modified Kinyoun stain (Koneman et al. 1992). Tiny, round, gram-negative cocci might be *Veillonella* spp.

Direct examination of specimens by gas-liquid chromatography (Gorbach et al. 1976, Phillips, Tearle and Willis 1976), can be highly useful when applied to positive blood cultures, particularly when direct gramstained smears are also prepared and examined (Koneman et al. 1992). Species that are aerobic and facultatively anaerobic produce only acetic acid; the demonstration of other short-chain fatty acids, such as butyric acid or propionic acid, suggests that anaerobes such as *Fusobacterium* spp. or *Propionibacterium* spp. are present. However, the method does not provide a specific diagnosis when applied to pus.

DNA probes have been developed for some of the important pathogenic non-sporing anaerobes, and may provide rapid and specific identification of isolates and, possible, direct detection in biological samples (Phillips 1990, Hofstad 1994); for example, Roberts et al. (Roberts et al. 1985, Roberts, Moncla and Kenny 1987) have reported reliable identification of pigmented *Prevotella* spp. by dot-blot hybridization with chromosomal DNA probes. Love, Bailey and Bastin (1992) have described a dot-blot hybridization assay using chromosomal DNA probes for the specific identification of *Porphyromonas* spp. isolated from cats. Dix et al. (1990) have developed oligodeoxynucleotide probes for the identification of various periodontal bacteria including *A. actinomycetemcomitans*, *P. gingivalis*, *P. intermedia*, *B. forsythus*, *E. corrodens*, *F. nucleatum*, *Haemophilus aphrophilus*, *S. intermedius* and *C. recta*. Shah et al. (1995) have described 16S ribosomal RNA probes that were highly specific for oral strains of *P. intermedia* and *P. nigrescens*. In addition, Bolstad and Jensen (1993) have developed polymerase chain reaction (PCR)-amplified non-radioactive probes for the identification of *F. nucleatum*.

9 SELECTION OF ANTIMICROBIAL AGENTS

In general, the successful management of patients with anaerobic infections requires treatment with appropriate antimicrobial agents, often in combination with surgical intervention. Thus, antimicrobial agents alone may not be sufficient; the removal of anaerobic bacteria may require drainage of abscesses or other accumulations of pus, the debridement of a wound or elimination of dead tissue, the removal of foreign bodies or other surgical measures (Finegold 1977).

The initial selection of antimicrobial agents for patients who have anaerobic infections is usually made empirically, and not based on the results of in vitro susceptibility testing, although direct microscopic examination of material collected from the patient may influence therapeutic decisions (Finegold and Wexler 1988). Information used in selecting agents for therapy includes the anatomical location (e.g. intra-abdominal) and nature of the infectious process, the clinician's experience, and published literature regarding the types of micro-organisms commonly encountered in the clinical setting, any known predisposing factors (such as a recent history of trauma to the abdomen), the patient's condition (e.g. critically ill, febrile and in shock), and, if available, the results of direct microscopic examination of a gram-stained smear. The clinician is also guided by published susceptibility patterns (e.g. hospital, local community, various medical centres in other geographical areas)

and by clinical treatment reports in the literature (Finegold 1989b, 1995a, Cuchural et al. 1992, Hecht, Osmolski and O'Keefe 1993, Aldridge et al. 1994, Marshall et al. 1995). A problem confronting clinicians who see patients with polymicrobial anaerobic–aerobic infections is that the complex mixtures of organisms involved necessitates a relatively slow turnaround time for culture results to become available (Finegold and Wexler 1988). Many of the non-sporing anaerobes require a full 48–72 h of incubation, compared with the usual 18–24 h (or less) required for aerobic and facultatively anaerobic bacteria to form readily visible colonies. Probably an even more practical explanation for the prolonged time to complete the anaerobe culture work is the time required to separate each of the colony types from a complex mixture of organisms, get them into pure cultures, and then to proceed with identification and susceptibility testing. Regardless of the identification methods used (rapid or conventional), additional time for adequate inoculum preparation is required. If in vitro susceptibility testing is done, another 48 h of incubation time is required. Thus, it can take several days to a week or more to receive the final report from the bacteriology laboratory.

Unfortunately, the increasing resistance of anaerobes to antimicrobial agents is becoming a significant problem, with multiple mechanisms of resistance being encountered, similar to the situation with aerobic and facultatively anaerobic bacteria (Finegold 1988, Hecht, Malamy and Tally 1989, Rosenblatt 1989, Rosenblatt and Brook 1993). Connected with this problem are technical problems and issues related to the performance and interpretation of in vitro susceptibility tests on anaerobic bacteria, and the ability of these tests to predict in vivo responses. Addressing these and other issues in the USA, the National Committee for Clinical Laboratory Standards (NCCLS) Working Group on Anaerobic Susceptibility Testing recommended that 'susceptibility testing of anaerobes be done only to: determine patterns of susceptibility of anaerobes to new antimicrobial agents; monitor susceptibility patterns periodically in various centers in the US and in other countries; monitor susceptibility patterns periodically in local communities and hospitals; and to assist in the management of infection in individual patients by performing susceptibility tests as needed' (NCCLS 1993). Their last recommendation would be applied to: a particular organism or species that is known to be resistant; instances of treatment failure and persistence of infection; situations in which the antimicrobial agent is likely to play a pivotal role in determining outcome; difficulties in selecting antibiotics empirically based on precedent; severe infections, and infections requiring long-term therapy. Thus, susceptibility testing of anaerobes should be done on isolates from infections such as brain abscess, osteomyelitis, joint infections, endocarditis, infections involving prosthetic devices, and recurrent or refractory bacteraemia (NCCLS 1993). The question of what organisms to test is also potentially difficult to answer, particularly when dealing with complex mixed infections. In general, organisms that are virulent or commonly resistant to antibiotics (or both) should be tested; these include the *B. fragilis* group, *Prevotella*, *Porphyromonas*, certain *Fusobacterium* spp., *B. wadsworthia*, '*B. gracilis*' (now *C. gracilis*), and certain clostridia (e.g. *C. perfringens*, *C. ramosum* and *C. septicum*) (NCCLS 1993).

Activities of various antimicrobial agents against anaerobes are summarized in Table 38.1. Most members of the *B. fragilis* group (>75%) produce β-lactamase and are resistant to penicillin G and certain other β-lactam agents (Finegold 1989b). Interestingly, β-lactamase production was also demonstrated in

about 55–65% of pigmented and non-pigmented *Prevotella* spp., some *Porphyromonas* strains and in >40% of *Fusobacterium* spp., including many strains of *F. nucleatum*, *F. mortiferum*, *F. varium* and even some strains of *F. necrophorum* (Appelbaum, Spangler and Jacobs 1990); the significance of these results is not clear, however, since >45% of the non-*B. fragilis* group strains that produced β-lactamase were susceptible to amoxycillin, and >90% were susceptible to ticarcillin. Whereas certain drugs are active against >95% of all anaerobes (including ampicillin–sulbactam, chloramphenicol and imipenem), a number of other drugs are not nearly so predictable in their

Table 38.1 Activity of antimicrobial agents against anaerobes[a]

Antimicrobial agents	Exceptions or comment
Active[b] versus ≥95% of all clinically significant anaerobes including *B. fragilis* group	
Chloramphenicol	10% of *Lactobacillus* spp. resistant
Imipenem	Only **rare** strains of *B. fragilis* group resistant
Ampicillin–sulbactam	14% of *B. distasonis* and 6% of pigmented *Prevotella* spp. resistant
Piperacillin–tazobactam	1 of 8 strains of *Actinomyces* spp. resistant
Ticarcillin–clavulanate	24% of *B. distasonis*, 6% of pigmented *Prevotella* spp., 6% of *P. bivia/P. disiens* and 26% of *P. anaerobius* strains resistant
Metronidazole	6% of pigmented *Prevotella*, 9% of *Eubacterium*, 75% of *Actinomyces*, 87% of *Propionibacterium* spp. and 10% of *P. magnus* strains were resistant
Active versus 89% of all clinically significant anaerobes including *B. fragilis* group	
Cefoxitin	Only 8% of *B. fragilis* strains were resistant, but 14% *B. thetaiotaomicron*, 9% *B. vulgatus*, 19% *B. distasonis*, 20% *B. ovatus* and 13% of *B. uniformis* strains were resistant; **no** strains of *Prevotella*, *Porphyromonas*, or *Fusobacterium* spp. were resistant; occasional strains of *Actinomyces* and *Eubacterium*, and 79% of lactobacilli were resistant, as were 70% of *C. difficile* and 68% of *C. innocuum* strains
Active versus only 78% of the *B. fragilis* group, but active versus 95% of all other anaerobes	
Clindamycin	13% of *B. fragilis*, 37% *B. thetaiotaomicron*, 31% *B. vulgatus*, 19% *B. distasonis*, 28% *B. ovatus* and 29% of *B. uniformis* strains were resistant; in addition, 14% of the *Prevotella oralis* group, 1 of 6 *F. varium*, 2 of 8 *Actinomyces* spp., strains and 9% *C. perfringens*, 9% *C. ramosum*, 16% *C. difficile* and 11% of strains of *P. magnus* were resistant
Active versus only 71% of *B. fragilis* group, but active versus >90% of all other anaerobes	
Piperacillin	23% of *B. fragilis*, 27% *B. thetaiotaomicron*, 48% *B. vulgatus*, 62% *B. distasonis*, 28% *B. ovatus* and 29% of *B. uniformis* strains were resistant
Poor activity versus *B. fragilis* group; variable activity versus other anaerobes	
Cefotetan	39% of *B. fragilis* group resistant, including 17% *B. fragilis*, 67% *B. thetaiotaomicron*, 31% *B. vulgatus*, 90% *B. distasonis*, 77% *B. ovatus* and 42% strains of *B. uniformis*; not as active as penicillin G versus anaerobic gram-positive non-sporing rods and cocci
Ceftriaxone, cefoperazone, and cefotaxime	Less active than cefotetan versus *B. fragilis* group; less active than penicillin G versus other anaerobes in general
Penicillin G	95% of the *B. fragilis* group, 18% of pigmented *Prevotella*, 39% *P. bivia/disiens*, 7% *P. oralis* group, 7% *F. nucleatum*, occasional strains of *Actinomyces* and *Eubacterium* spp., 15% *C. clostridiiforme*, 23% *P. anaerobius*, 7% *P. prevotii* and 11% of *Veillonella* strains were resistant
Active versus almost all gram-positive anaerobes, inactive versus gram-negative anaerobes	
Vancomycin	Most lactobacilli are resistant

[a]Based on data from testing 1535 anaerobe isolates from clinical specimens at the Indiana University Medical Center Anaerobe Laboratory, November 1995 through May 1996. The numbers of isolates tested included 562 *B. fragilis* group, 58 *Prevotella* spp., 45 *Fusobacterium* spp., 356 anaerobic cocci (274 gram-positive and 82 *Veillonella* spp.), 284 anaerobic non-sporing gram-positive bacilli and 230 isolates of clostridia.
[b]Breakpoints were based on the following reference: (NCCLS 1994). Microbroth dilution methods were used in accordance with the following reference: (NCCLS 1993).

activities. For example, piperacillin (by itself without tazobactam), the second and third generation cephalosporins, and clindamycin may or may not be active against many isolates of the *B. fragilis* group (Wexler 1991, 1993). In addition, species of the group other than *B. fragilis* are generally more resistant to these drugs than is *B. fragilis* itself. Metronidazole remains active against nearly all anaerobic gram-negative bacilli, but 75% of *Actinomyces* spp., >15% of *Eubacterium* spp., >85% of *Propionibacterium* spp., >95% of *Lactobacillus* spp., and 10% of *P. magnus* strains tested in the author's laboratory are resistant.

10 PREVENTION

Some strategies used to prevent anaerobic infections, particularly in the surgical patient, include those that are also used in the treatment of anaerobic infections; these include debridement and cleansing of wounds, removal of foreign bodies, the maintenance of good haemostasis or the re-establishment of good circulation, and the use of good surgical technique (e.g. delayed closure as indicated) (Finegold 1995a). Other measures for prevention include showering prior to surgery, the use of antibiotics prophylactically in intra-abdominal operations (e.g. antibiotic bowel preparation prior to colon surgery), the use of antibiotics during dental surgery to reduce the incidence of bacteraemia, the use of hydrogen peroxide, iodophors or other germicides in wound care, the prevention of aspiration of gastric and oropharyngeal contents, the avoidance of prolonged operations, the avoidance of prolonged labour, and the use of gentle, careful technique during colonoscopy (Finegold 1977).

11 ANIMAL INFECTIONS CAUSED BY GRAM-NEGATIVE ANAEROBIC BACILLI

Infections occur in cattle, sheep, goats, pigs, rabbits, cats and wild animals, and cause serious economic loss. The organism most commonly responsible is *F. necrophorum*, which produces tissue necrosis and abscess formation, accompanied by a putrid odour. Initiation of infection usually requires a minor injury to the skin or mucosa. Bacteraemia may occur and result in widespread metastatic abscesses. Unlike most infections in humans, animal infections usually occur as primary diseases rather than as secondary complications (Duerden 1990).

11.1 Calf diphtheria

This disease, first associated with '*Bacillus necrophorus*' (*F. necrophorum*) by Loeffler in 1884, is a necrotizing infection of the oral mucosa, tongue, pharynx and larynx. It occurs in calves of all ages and in cattle up to the age of 2 or more years. There is a false membrane, which may extend from the throat down into the trachea, but which more commonly occurs in patches, firmly adherent to underlying, circumscribed and indurated swellings. Initiation of infection prob-

ably requires some minor damage to the mucosa; the organism then proliferates in the damaged mucosa and spreads to the submucosa and muscle. The disease may be fatal. Necrotic material sometimes obstructs the larynx and causes asphyxiation. Smaller amounts of necrotic material may be aspirated and cause lung abscesses or pneumonia (Langworth 1977). *F. necrophorum* can be isolated in culture and seen in smears prepared from the lesions; it forms characteristic long wavy rows of bacilli in the deeper layers of the membrane. Untreated animals usually die within 5 days from asphyxia, bronchopneumonia or toxaemia.

11.2 Liver abscess

Liver abscesses or necrotic focal hepatitis caused by *F. necrophorum* result in serious economic losses in cattle. The disease also occurs in sheep but rarely affects other farm animals. The abscesses are often multiple. *F. necrophorum* is the predominant organism seen in smears prepared from the lesions, and is consistently isolated from the pus (Feldman, Hester and Wherry 1936, Madin 1949). The encapsulated abscesses are usually discovered at slaughter. Most cattle in areas where there is a high incidence of abscesses have antibodies to *F. necrophorum* (Feldman, Hester and Wherry 1936). Kanoe, Nouka and Toda (1984) found that 314 (15%) of 2036 slaughtered cattle examined in Japan had liver abscesses and 58 (3%) had abscesses at other sites: lung 21, abdomen 32, others 5; most were caused by *F. necrophorum*. Of the cattle with extrahepatic abscesses, 19 also had liver abscesses. The factors that predispose to abscess formation have not been clearly established. *F. necrophorum* is thought to reach the liver via the portal circulation from the rumen owing to some alteration in the mucosal protective mechanism (e.g. ulceration) (Madin 1949, Duerden 1990). Abscesses are more common in animals on artificial feeds or concentrates than in those on pasture. Jensen and Mackey (1974) noted that the change from grazing to a high-concentrate diet resulted in increased acid production by the rumen flora which sometimes led to ulceration. Metallic foreign bodies in the bovine stomach may also cause ulceration. Liver abscesses have been reproduced experimentally in cattle and sheep by the intraportal injection of *F. necrophorum* (Duerden 1990).

11.3 Foot-rot

Foot-rot is an infection of the hooves and surrounding tissues in ungulates, and is a major cause of lameness in cattle and sheep (Jensen and Mackey 1974); it also affects goats, pigs and deer. The disease is a bacterial dermatitis; infection begins with superficial necrosis of the skin of the interdigital space and spreads rapidly to the dermis, adjacent skin and hoof margin; there is a foul discharge of pus and necrotic tissue, and the horn may separate. The disease may be mild or debilitating, and may require surgical interference. *F. necrophorum* and *D. nodosus* are considered to be the major pathogens in the mixed flora of these conditions.

F. necrophorum is implicated in most forms of foot-rot (Langworth 1977) but is only one constituent of a mixed infection; the disease is a synergic infection (see section on 'Microbial synergy', p. 747). Ovine interdigital dermatitis can be reproduced by placing pads soaked with *F. necrophorum* on scarified interdigital skin (Parsonson, Egerton and Roberts 1967). *F. necrophorum* is also implicated in foot-rot of cattle, possibly in association with several other species. Berg and Loan (1975) isolated *F. necrophorum* and '*B. melaninogenicus*' from 8 cases of bovine foot-rot. The application of mixed inocula of the 2 species to scarified interdigital skin produced lesions typical of foot-rot.

D. nodosus appears to be the main cause of foot-rot in sheep and goats (Egerton and Parsonson 1966, Wilkinson, Egerton and Dickson 1970, Stewart and Elleman 1987). It is the constant component of the mixed flora of lesions. Pure cultures introduced into scarified skin under conditions appropriate for the development of foot-rot cause typical, severe lesions. *D. nodosus* vaccines (see below) are both curative and prophylactic (Stewart and Elleman 1987). In combination with *F. necrophorum* it causes an infection of the hoof and underlying tissues (in cattle) which may result in the detachment of the hoof. It has been isolated from some cases of foot-rot in cattle in Australia (Egerton and Parsonson 1966, Wilkinson, Egerton and Dickson 1970), Holland (Duerden 1990) and Great Britain (Thorley, Calder and Harrison 1977).

Predisposing factors for the development of foot-rot in any species of animal are unhygienic conditions such as damp soil or litter underfoot and prior injury to the foot (Duerden 1990). Experimental infections can be established only after scarification or similar minor injury to the interdigital skin (Parsonson, Egerton and Roberts 1967, Berg and Loan 1975). *F. necrophorum* can survive in damp soil for several months (Garcia, Neil and McKay 1971), but material from affected feet does not remain infective under saprophytic conditions for more than a week. The disease may be eradicated from a farm by segregation and treatment of infected animals, and removal of uninfected animals to pasture where infection has not occurred in the previous 2–3 weeks. Good foot hygiene must be maintained. Treatment consists of surgical toilet, topical application of antimicrobial substances and sometimes antibiotics injected parenterally. Egerton and Roberts (1971) found that a vaccine composed of *D. nodosus* killed by formalin and emulsified in Freund's incomplete adjuvant gave substantial protection against experimental infections in sheep; it gave partial protection under field conditions (Egerton and Morgan 1972). Vaccines containing pili from *D. nodosus*, or *D. nodosus* pili expressed in recombinant *Pseudomonas aeruginosa*, are protective and therapeutic (Stewart and Elleman 1987).

11.4 Broken mouth

This form of chronic destructive periodontal disease in ruminants such as sheep is, like periodontal disease in humans, associated with the proliferation of anaerobic bacteria in deep gingival pockets. Animal strains similar to *P. gingivalis* are found in sheep; like human strains, they are strongly proteolytic and produce a protease with trypsin-like activity (Friksen et al. 1987). Parent et al. (1986) found that human and animal serotypes of *P. gingivalis* were distinguishable by crossed immunoelectrophoresis.

11.5 Labial necrosis of rabbits

Schmorl (1891) first described this disease in an outbreak among his laboratory rabbits. It is caused by *F. necrophorum* and the disease is characterized by a dark bluish-red swelling of the underlip that spreads along the ventral aspect of the jaw and throat, and in about 8 days reaches the base of the neck. By the fifth day there is a watery nasal discharge and the animal is febrile. It dies in an emaciated condition with considerable dyspnoea. At postmortem examination the underlip is seen to be converted into a yellowish-white, compact, bacon-like, necrotic mass, which may extend to the bone. The cervical glands are swollen, juicy and greyish-red; sometimes they show small caseous foci. There is a bloody, slightly turbid exudate in the pleural and pericardial cavities; sometimes there are a few pneumonic areas in the lung. The viscera appear normal. *F. necrophorum* can be isolated from the necrotic tissue and from the exudates.

11.6 Subcutaneous abscesses in cats

Anaerobic bacteria are the commonest cause of subcutaneous abscesses in cats. These abscesses are often encountered in small-animal veterinary practice and are the result of bites sustained in fights. A mixture of bacterial species is isolated from the foul pus of most abscesses but the majority of strains are anaerobes. Love et al. (1979) found that 66% of their anaerobic isolates were gram-negative bacilli. The commonest species in their study of 36 abscesses were *B. fragilis*, '*B. asaccharolyticus*', *F. nucleatum*, '*B. melaninogenicus*' and *F. necrophorum*.

REFERENCES

Adriaans B, Drasar BS, 1987, The isolation of fusobacteria from tropical ulcers, *Epidemiol Infect*, **99**: 361–72.

Aldridge KE, Gelfand M et al., 1994, A five-year multicenter study of the susceptibility of the *Bacteroides fragilis* group isolates to cephalosporins, cephamins, penicillins, clindamycin, and metronidazole in the United States, *Diagn Microbiol Infect Dis*, **18**: 235–41.

Allen SD, 1985, Gram-positive, nonsporeforming anaerobic bacilli, *Manual of Clinical Microbiology*, 4th edn, eds Lennette EH, Balows A et al., American Society for Microbiology, Washington, DC, 461–72.

Allen SD, Siders JA, 1982, An approach to the diagnosis of anaerobic pleuropulmonary infections, *Clinics in Laboratory Medicine*, ed. Winn WC, 285–303.

Allen SD, Siders JA, Marler LM, 1985, Isolation and examination of anaerobic bacteria, *Manual of Clinical Microbiology*, 4th edn, eds Lennette EH, Balows A et al., American Society for Microbiology, Washington, DC, 413–43.

Allen SD, Siders JA, Marler LM, 1995, Current issues and problems in dealing with anaerobes in the clinical laboratory, *Clin Lab Med*, **15**: 333–64.

Allen SD, Siders JA et al., 1996, Anaerobic bacteremia: a 24 year survey revealing new trends in species isolated in the '90's, *Anaerobe Society of the Americas Congress on Anaerobic Bacteria and Anaerobic Infections*, Chicago, IL.

Altemeier WA, 1938, The bacterial flora of acute perforated appendicitis with peritonitis: a bacteriologic study based upon one hundred cases, *Ann Surg*, **107**: 517–28.

Altemeier WA, 1941, The pathogenicity of the bacteria of appendicitis peritonitis, *Ann Surg*, **114**: 158–9.

Aoki M, Noble RC et al., 1993, Lemierre's syndrome caused by *Fusobacterium necrophorum*: a case report, *J Ky Med Assoc*, **91**: 141–2.

Appelbaum PC, Spangler SK, Jacobs MR, 1990, Beta-lactamase production and susceptibilities to amoxicillin, amoxicillin–clavulanate, ticarcillin, ticarcillin–clavulanate, cefoxitin, imipenem, and metronidazole of 320 non-*Bacteroides fragilis* Bacteroides isolates and 129 fusobacteria from 28 U.S. centers, *Antimicrob Agents Chemother*, **34**: 1546–50.

Arpi M, Renneberg J et al., 1995, Bacteremia at a Danish university hospital during a twenty-five-year period (1968–1992), *Scand J Infect Dis*, **27**: 245–51.

Attebery HR, Finegold SM, 1969, Combined screw-cap and rubber-stopper closure for Hungate tubes (pre-reduced anaerobically sterilized roll tubes and liquid media), *Appl Microbiol*, **18:** 558–61.

Babb JL, Cummins CS, 1978, Encapsulation of *Bacteroides* species, *Infect Immun*, **19:** 1088–91.

Baron EJ, Summanen P et al., 1989, *Bilophila wadsworthia*, gen. nov. and sp. nov., a unique gram-negative anaerobic rod recovered from appendicitis specimens and human faeces, *J Gen Microbiol*, **135:** 3405–11.

Baron EJ, Curren M et al., 1992, *Bilophila wadsworthia* isolates from clinical specimens, *J Clin Microbiol*, **30:** 1882–4.

Bartlett JG, 1987, Anaerobic bacterial infections of the lung, *Chest*, **91:** 901–9.

Bartlett JG, 1992, Infections caused by anaerobic bacteria, *Infectious Diseases*, Gorbach SL, Bartlett JG, Blacklow NR, WB Saunders Company, Philadelphia, 1555–68.

Bartlett JG, 1993, Anaerobic bacterial infections of the lung and pleural space, *Clin Infect Dis*, **16:** S248–55.

Bartlett JG, Finegold SM, 1972, Anaerobic pleuropulmonary infections, *Medicine (Baltimore)*, **51:** 413–50.

Bartlett JG, Finegold SM, 1974, Anaerobic infections of the lung and pleural space, *Am Rev Respir Dis*, **110:** 56–77.

Bartlett JG, Rosenblatt JE, Finegold SM, 1973, Percutaneous transtracheal aspiration in the diagnosis of anaerobic pulmonary infection, *Ann Intern Med*, **79:** 535–40.

Bartlett JG, Sutter VL, Finegold SM, 1974, Anaerobic pleuropulmonary disease: clinical observations and bacteriology in 100 cases, *Anaerobic Bacteria: Role in Disease*, eds Balows A, Dehaan RM et al., Charles C Thomas, Springfield, IL.

Bartlett JG, Gorbach SL et al., 1974, Bacteriology and treatment of primary lung abscess, *Am Rev Respir Dis*, **109:** 510–18.

Bartlett JG, Sullivan-Sigler N et al., 1976, Anaerobes survive in clinical specimens despite delayed processing, *J Clin Microbiol*, **3:** 133–6.

Beaver DC, Henthorne JC, Macy JW, 1934, Abscesses of the liver caused by *Bacteroides funduliformis*. Report of two cases, *Arch Pathol*, **17:** 493.

Beeler BA, Crowder JG et al., 1976, *Propionibacterium acnes*: pathogen in central nervous system shunt infection, *Am J Med*, **61:** 935–8.

Beerens H, Tahon-Castel M, 1965, *Infections Humaines à Bactéries Anaérobies Non-toxigènes*, Presses Académies Européenes, Bruxelles.

Bennion RS, Thompson JE et al., 1990, Gangrenous and perforated appendicitis with peritonitis: treatment and bacteriology, *Clin Ther*, **12:** 31–44.

Berg JN, Loan RW, 1975, *Fusobacterium necrophorum* and *Bacteroides melaninogenicus* as etiologic agents of foot rot in cattle, *Am J Vet Res*, **36:** 1115–22.

Bernard D, Verschraegen G et al., 1994, *Bilophila wadsworthia* bacteremia in a patient with gangrenous appendicitis, *Clin Infect Dis*, **18:** 1023–4.

Bjornson AB, 1989, Host defense mechanisms against nonspore-forming anaerobic bacteria, *Anaerobic Infections in Humans*, eds Finegold SM, George WL, Academic Press, Orlando, FL, 97–110.

Bjornson AB, 1990, Role of humoral factors in host resistance to the *Bacteroides fragilis* group, *Rev Infect Dis*, **12:** S161–8.

Bjornson AB, Altemeier WA, Bjornson HS, 1976, Comparison of the in vitro bactericidal activity of human serum and leukocytes against *Bacteroides fragilis* and *Fusobacterium mortiferum* in aerobic and anaerobic environments, *Infect Immun*, **14:** 843–7.

Bjornson HS, 1982, Bacterial synergy, virulence factors, and host defense mechanisms in the pathogenesis of intraabdominal infections, *Topics in Intraabdominal Surgical Infection*, ed. Simmons RL, Appleton-Century-Crofts, Norwalk, CT, 65–78.

Bjornson HS, 1984, Activation of Hageman factor by lipopolysaccharides of *Bacteroides fragilis*, *Bacteroides vulgatus*, and *Fusobacterium mortiferum*, *Rev Infect Dis*, **6:** S30–3.

Bolstad AI, Jensen HB, 1993, Polymerase chain reaction-amplified nonradioactive probes for identification of *Fusobacterium nucleatum*, *J Clin Microbiol*, **31:** 528–32.

Border M, Firehammer BD et al., 1985, Isolation of *Bacteroides fragilis* from the feces of diarrheic calves and lambs, *J Clin Microbiol*, **21:** 472–3.

Bornstein DL, Weinberg AN et al., 1964, Anaerobic infections – review of current experience, *Medicine (Baltimore)*, **43:** 207–32.

Botta GA, Arzese A et al., 1994, Role of structural and extracellular virulence factors in gram-negative anaerobic bacteria, *Clin Infect Dis*, **18:** S260–4.

Bourgault AM, Rosenblatt JE, Fitzgerald RH, 1980, *Peptococcus magnus*: a significant human pathogen, *Ann Intern Med*, **93:** 244–8.

Bouza E, Reig M et al., 1985, Retrospective analysis of two hundred and twelve cases of bacteremia due to anaerobic microorganisms, *Eur J Clin Microbiol*, **4:** 262–7.

Brewer GE, Meleney FL, 1926, Progressive gangrenous infection of the skin and subcutaneous tissues following operation for acute perforative appendicitis, *Ann Surg*, **84:** 438–50.

Brewer JH, Allgeier DL, 1966, Safe self-contained carbon dioxide–hydrogen anaerobic system, *Appl Microbiol*, **14:** 985–8.

Brook I, 1981, Bacteriologic study of paronychia in children, *Am J Surg*, **141:** 703–5.

Brook I, 1986, Encapsulated anaerobic bacteria in synergistic infections, *Microbiol Rev*, **50:** 452–7.

Brook I, 1987, Bacteraemia and seeding of capsulate *Bacteroides* spp. and anaerobic cocci, *J Med Microbiol*, **23:** 61–7.

Brook I, 1988a, Presence of anaerobic bacteria in conjunctivitis associated with wearing contact lenses, *Ann Ophthalmol*, **20:** 397–9.

Brook I, 1988b, Recovery of anaerobic bacteria from clinical specimens in 12 years at two military hospitals, *J Clin Microbiol*, **26:** 1181–8.

Brook I, 1989, Anaerobic bacterial bacteremia: 12-year experience in two military hospitals [see comments], *J Infect Dis*, **160:** 1071–5.

Brook I, 1993, Infections caused by beta-lactamase-producing *Fusobacterium* spp. in children, *Pediatr Infect Dis J*, **12:** 532–3.

Brook I, 1994, Fusobacterial infections in children, *J Infect*, **28:** 155–65.

Brook I, Frazier EH, 1991, Infections caused by *Propionibacterium* species, *Rev Infect Dis*, **13:** 819–22.

Brook I, Frazier EH, 1993, Significant recovery of nonsporulating anaerobic rods from clinical specimens, *Clin Infect Dis*, **16:** 476–80.

Brook I, Myhal LA, Dorsey CH, 1992, Encapsulation and pilus formation of *Bacteroides* spp. in normal flora abscesses and blood, *J Infect*, **25:** 251–7.

Brook I, Yocum P, Friedman EM, 1981, Aerobic and anaerobic bacteria in tonsils of children with recurrent tonsillitis, *Ann Otol Rhinol Laryngol*, **90:** 261–3.

Brook I, Yocum P, Shah K, 1980, Surface vs core-tonsillar aerobic and anaerobic flora in recurrent tonsillitis, *JAMA*, **244:** 1696–8.

Brook I, Gillmore JD et al., 1983, Pathogenicity of encapsulated *Bacteroides melaninogenicus* group, *B. oralis* and *B. ruminicola* subsp. *brevis* in abscesses in mice, *J Infect*, **7:** 218–26.

Bulkacz J, Schuster GS et al., 1985, Phospholipase A activity of extracellular products from *Bacteroides melaninogenicus* on epithelium tissue cultures, *J Periodont Res*, **20:** 146–53.

Burdon KL, 1928, *Bacterium melaninogenicum* from normal and pathological tissues, *J Infect Dis*, **42:** 161–71.

Burt S, Meldrum S et al., 1978, Colonial variation, capsule formation, and bacteriophage resistance in *Bacteroides thetaiotaomicron*, *Appl Environ Microbiol*, **35:** 439–43.

Busch DF, 1984, Anaerobes in infections of the head and neck and ear, nose, and throat, *Rev Infect Dis*, **6:** S115–22.

Carlsson J, Hofling JF, Sundqvist GK, 1984, Degradation of albumin, haemopexin, haptoglobin and transferrin, by black-pigmented *Bacteroides* species, *J Med Microbiol*, **18:** 39–46.

Carlsson J, Wrethen J, Beckman G, 1977, Superoxide dismutase in *Bacteroides fragilis* and related *Bacteroides* species, *J Clin Microbiol*, **6:** 280–4.

Casciato DA, Rosenblatt JE et al., 1975, In vitro interaction of *Bacteroides fragilis* with polymorphonuclear leukocytes and serum factors, *Infect Immun*, **11:** 337–42.

Casciato DA, Rosenblatt JE et al., 1979, Susceptibility of isolates of *Bacteroides* to the bactericidal activity of normal human serum, *J Infect Dis*, **140:** 109–13.

Chow AW, Guze LB, 1974, Bacteroidaceae bacteremia: clinical experience with 112 patients, *Medicine (Baltimore)*, **53:** 93–126.

Citron DM, 1984, Specimen collection and transport, anaerobic culture techniques, and identification of anaerobes, *Rev Infect Dis*, **6:** S51–8.

Civen R, Jousimies-Somer H et al., 1995, A retrospective review of cases of anaerobic empyema and update of bacteriology, *Clin Infect Dis*, **20:** S224–9.

Cohen J, 1932, The bacteriology of abscess of the lung and methods for its study, *Arch Surg*, **24:** 171–88.

Connolly JC, McLean C, Tabaqchali S, 1984, The effect of capsular polysaccharide and lipopolysaccharide of *Bacteroides fragilis* on polymorph function and serum killing, *J Med Microbiol*, **17:** 259–71.

Coykendall AL, Kaczmarek FS, Slots J, 1980, Genetic heterogeneity in *Bacteroides asaccharolyticus* (Holdeman and Moore 1970) Finegold and Barnes 1977 (approved lists, 1980) and proposal of *Bacteroides gingivalis* sp. nov. and *Bacteroides macacae* (Slots and Genco) comb. nov., *Int J Syst Bacteriol*, **30:** 559–64.

Cuchural GJ Jr, Snydman DR et al., 1992, Antimicrobial susceptibility patterns of the *Bacteroides fragilis* group in the United States, 1989, *Clin Ther*, **14:** 122–36.

Dack GM, Dragstedt LR, Heinz TE, 1936, *Bacterium necrophorum* in chronic ulcerative colitis, *JAMA*, **106:** 7–10.

De Sena S, Rosenfeld DL et al., 1996, Jugular thrombophlebitis complicating bacterial pharyngitis (Lemierre's syndrome), *Pediatr Radiol*, **26:** 141–4.

Deve F, Guerbet M, 1907, Suppuration gazeuse spontanée d'un kyste hydatique du foie. Présence exclusive de germes anaérobies, *C R Soc Biol (Paris)*, **63:** 305–7.

Dewhirst FE, Paster BJ et al., 1990, Transfer of *Kingella indologenes* (Snell and Lapage 1976) to the genus *Suttonella* gen. nov. as *Suttonella indologenes* comb. nov.; transfer of *Bacteroides nodosus* (Beveridge 1941) to the genus *Dichelobacter* gen. nov. as *Dichelobacter nodosus* comb. nov.; and assignment of the genera *Cardiobacterium*, *Dichelobacter*, and *Suttonella* to Cardiobacteriaceae fam. nov. in the gamma division of Proteobacteria on the basis of 16S rRNA sequence comparisons, *Int J Syst Bacteriol*, **40:** 426–33.

Dix K, Watanabe SM et al., 1990, Species-specific oligodeoxynucleotide probes for the identification of periodontal bacteria, *J Clin Microbiol*, **28:** 319–23.

Dobell C, 1960, *Antony van Leeuwenhoek and His 'Little Animals'*, Dover, New York.

Donelli G, Fabbri A, Fiorentini C, 1996, *Bacteroides fragilis* enterotoxin induces cytoskeletal changes and surface blebbing in HT-29 cells, *Infect Immun*, **64:** 113–19.

Dorsher CW, Wilson WR, Rosenblatt JE, 1989, Anaerobic bacteremia and cardiovascular infections, *Anaerobic Infections in Humans*, eds Finegold SM, George WL, Academic Press, San Diego, CA, 289–310.

Dorsher CW, Rosenblatt JE et al., 1991, Anaerobic bacteremia: decreasing rate over a 15-year period, *Rev Infect Dis*, **13:** 633–6.

Dougherty SH, Saltzstein EC et al., 1989, Perforated or gangrenous appendicitis treated with aminoglycosides. How do bacterial cultures influence management?, *Arch Surg*, **124:** 1280–3.

Dowell VR Jr, 1975, Wound and abscess specimens, *Clinical Microbiology. How to Start and When to Stop*, ed. Balows A, Charles C Thomas, Springfield, IL, 70–81.

Dowell VR Jr, 1977, *Clinical Veterinary Anaerobic Bacteriology*, DHEW, PHS, Centers for Disease Control, Atlanta, GA.

Dowell VR Jr, Allen SD, 1981, Anaerobic bacterial infections, *Diagnostic Procedures for Bacterial, Mycotic, and Parasitic Infections*, 6th edn, eds Balows A, Hausler WJ, American Public Health Association, Washington, DC, 171–213.

Dowell VR Jr, Stargel MD, Allen SD, 1976, *Propionibacterium acnes*, *ASCP Check Sample*, 1–23.

Dowell VR Jr, Lombard GL et al., 1977, *Media for Isolation, Characterization, and Identification of Obligately Anaerobic Bacteria*, Centers for Disease Control, Atlanta, GA.

Drasar BS, Hill MJ, 1974, *Human Intestinal Flora*, Academic Press, London.

Duerden BI, 1980a, The identification of gram-negative anaerobic bacilli isolated from clinical infections, *J Hyg*, **84:** 301–13.

Duerden BI, 1980b, The isolation and identification of *Bacteroides* spp. from the normal human gingival flora, *J Med Microbiol*, **13:** 89–101.

Duerden BI, 1983, Bacteroidaceae – *Bacteroides*, *Fusobacterium* and *Leptotrichia*, *Topley and Wilson's Principles of Bacteriology, Virology and Immunity*, 7th edn, eds Wilson G, Miles AA, Parker MT, Edward Arnold, London, 114–36.

Duerden BI, 1990, Infections due to gram-negative non-sporing anaerobic bacilli, *Topley and Wilson's Principles of Bacteriology, Virology and Immunity*, vol. 3, 8th edn, eds Parker MT, Collier LH, BC Decker, Philadelphia/Edward Arnold, London, 287–305.

Duerden BI, 1994, Virulence factors in anaerobes, *Clin Infect Dis*, **18:** S253–9.

Duerden BI, Bennett KW, Faulkner J, 1982, Isolation of *Bacteroides ureolyticus* (*B. corrodens*) from clinical infections, *J Clin Pathol*, **35:** 309–12.

Dzink JL, Sheenan MT, Socransky SS, 1990, Proposal of three subspecies of *Fusobacterium nucleatum* Knorr 1922: *Fusobacterium nucleatum* subsp. *nucleatum* subsp. nov., comb. nov.; *Fusobacterium nucleatum* subsp. *polymorphum* subsp. nov., nom. rev., comb. nov.; and *Fusobacterium nucleatum* subsp. *vincentii* subsp. nov., nom. rev., comb. nov., *Int J Syst Bacteriol*, **40:** 74–8.

Dzink JL, Socransky SS, Haffajee AD, 1988, The predominant cultivable microbiota of active and inactive lesions of destructive periodontal diseases, *J Clin Periodontol*, **15:** 316–23.

Eftimiadi C, Buzzi E et al., 1987, Short-chain fatty acids produced by anaerobic bacteria alter the physiological responses of human neutrophils to chemotactic peptide, *J Infect*, **14:** 43–53.

Egerton JR, Morgan IR, 1972, Treatment and prevention of footrot in sheep with *Fusiformis nodosus* vaccine, *Vet Rec*, **91:** 453–7.

Egerton JR, Parsonson IM, 1966, Isolation of *Fusiformis nodosus* from cattle, *Aust Vet J*, **42:** 425–9.

Egerton JR, Roberts DS, 1971, Vaccination against ovine footrot, *J Comp Pathol*, **81:** 179–85.

Eiken M, 1958, Studies on an anaerobic, rod shaped, Gram-negative microorganism: *Bacteroides corrodens* n. sp., *Acta Pathol Microbiol Scand*, **43:** 404–16.

Emslie RD, 1963, Cancrum oris, *Dent Pract*, **13:** 481–95.

Eschenbach DA, 1993, Bacterial vaginosis and anaerobes in obstetric-gynecologic infection, *Clin Infect Dis*, **16:** S282–7.

Eschenbach DA, Buchanan TM et al., 1975, Polymicrobial etiology of acute pelvic inflammatory disease, *N Engl J Med*, **293:** 166–71.

Falkler WA Jr, Burger BW, 1981, Microbial surface interactions: reduction of the haemagglutination activity of the oral bacterium *Fusobacterium nucleatum* by absorption with *Streptococcus* and *Bacteroides*, *Arch Oral Biol*, **26:** 1015–25.

Feldman WH, Hester HR, Wherry FP, 1936, The occurrence of *Bacillus necrophorus* agglutinins in different species of animals, *J Infect Dis*, **59:** 159–70.

Felner JM, 1974, Infective endocarditis caused by anaerobic bacteria, *Anaerobic Bacteria: Role in Disease*, eds Balows A, Dehaan RM et al., Charles C Thomas, Springfield, IL, 345–52.

Felner JM, Dowell VR Jr, 1970, Anaerobic bacterial endocarditis, *N Engl J Med*, **283:** 1188–92.

Felner JM, Dowell VR Jr, 1971, '*Bacteroides*' bacteremia, *Am J Med*, **50:** 787–96.

Finegold S, Summanen P et al., 1992, Clinical importance of *Bilophila wadsworthia*, *Eur J Clin Microbiol Infect Dis*, **11**: 1058–63.

Finegold SM, 1977, *Anaerobic Bacteria in Human Disease*, Academic Press, New York.

Finegold SM, 1988, Susceptibility testing of anaerobic bacteria, *J Clin Microbiol*, **26**: 1253–6.

Finegold SM, 1989a, Mechanisms of resistance in anaerobes and new developments in testing, *Diagn Microbiol Infect Dis*, **12**: 117S–20S.

Finegold SM, 1989b, Therapy of anaerobic infections, *Anaerobic Infections in Humans*, eds Finegold SM, George WL, Academic Press, New York, 793–818.

Finegold SM, 1990, Anaerobes: problems and controversies in bacteriology, infections, and susceptibility testing, *Rev Infect Dis*, **12**: S223–30.

Finegold SM, 1993a, A century of anaerobes: a look backward and a call to arms, *Clin Infect Dis*, **16**: S453–7.

Finegold SM, 1993b, Host factors predisposing to anaerobic infections, *FEMS Immunol Med Microbiol*, **6**: 159–63.

Finegold SM, 1994, Review of early research on anaerobes, *Clin Infect Dis*, **18**: S248–9.

Finegold SM, 1995a, Anaerobic bacteria: general concepts, *Mandell, Douglas and Bennett's Principles and Practice of Infectious Diseases*, 4th edn, eds Mandell GL, Bennett JE, Dolin R, Churchill Livingstone, New York, 2156–73.

Finegold SM, 1995b, Overview of clinically important anaerobes, *Clin Infect Dis*, **20**: 205–7.

Finegold SM, Bartlett JG, 1975, Anaerobic pleuropulmonary infections, *Cleve Clin J Med*, **42**: 101–11.

Finegold SM, George WL (eds), 1989, *Anaerobic Infections in Humans*, Academic Press, San Diego.

Finegold SM, George WL, Mulligan ME, 1986, *Anaerobic Infections*, Year Book Medical Publishers, Chicago and London.

Finegold SM, Wexler HM, 1988, Therapeutic implications of bacteriologic findings in mixed aerobic–anaerobic infections, *Antimicrob Agents Chemother*, **32**: 611–16.

Fontaine EA, Borriello SP et al., 1984, Characteristics of a gram-negative anaerobe isolated from men with non-gonococcal urethritis, *J Med Microbiol*, **17**: 129–40.

Fontaine EA, Bryant TN et al., 1986, A numerical taxonomic study of anaerobic gram-negative bacilli classified as *Bacteroides ureolyticus* isolated from patients with non-gonococcal urethritis, *J Gen Microbiol*, **132**: 3137–46.

Francis LE, de Vries JA, 1968, Therapeutics and the management of common infections, *Dent Clin North Am*, 243–55.

French RS, Ziter FA et al., 1974, Chronic meningitis caused by *P. acnes*. A potentially important clinical entity, *Neurology*, **24**: 624–8.

Friedman E, Peyman GA, May DR, 1978, Endophthalmitis caused by *Propionibacterium acnes*, *Can J Ophthalmol*, **13**: 50–2.

Friksen KW, Tagg JR et al., 1987, Black-pigmented *Bacteroides* associated with broken-mouth periodontitis in sheep, *J Periodont Res*, **22**: 156–9.

Fulginiti VA, Scribner R et al., 1968, Infections in recipients of liver homografts, *N Engl J Med*, **279**: 619–26.

Galpin JE, Chow AW et al., 1976, Sepsis associated with decubitus ulcers, *Am J Med*, **61**: 346–50.

Garber GE, Chow AW, 1989, Female genital tract infections, *Anaerobic Infections in Humans*, eds Finegold SM, George WL, Academic Press, New York, 429–53.

Garcia MM, Neil DH, McKay KA, 1971, Application of immuno-fluorescence to studies on the ecology of *Sphaerophorus necrophorus*, *Appl Microbiol*, **21**: 809–14.

George WL, Kirby BD et al., 1981, Gram-negative anaerobic bacilli: their role in infection and patterns of susceptibility to antimicrobial agents. II. Little-known *Fusobacterium* species and miscellaneous genera, *Rev Infect Dis*, **3**: 599–626.

Gharbia SE, Shah HN, 1992, *Fusobacterium nucleatum* subsp. *fusiforme* subsp. nov. and *Fusobacterium nucleatum* subsp. *animalis*

subsp. nov. as additional subspecies within *Fusobacterium nucleatum*, *Int J Syst Bacteriol*, **42**: 296–8.

Gharbia SE, Shah HN, 1993a, Hydrolytic enzymes liberated by black-pigmented Gram-negative anaerobes, *FEMS Immunol Med Microbiol*, **6**: 139–46.

Gharbia SE, Shah HN, 1993b, Interactions between black-pigmented Gram-negative anaerobes and other species which may be important in disease development, *FEMS Immunol Med Microbiol*, **6**: 173–8.

Gibbons RJ, Houte JV, 1975, Bacterial adherence in oral microbial ecology, *Annu Rev Microbiol*, **29**: 19–44.

Gibbons RJ, MacDonald JB, 1960, Hemin and vitamin K compounds as required factors for the cultivation of certain strains of *Bacteroides melaninogenicus*, *J Bacteriol*, **80**: 164–70.

Gibbs RS, Forman J et al., 1987, Detection of serum antibody response to *Bacteroides bivius* by enzyme-linked immunosorbent assay in women with intraamniotic infection, *Obstet Gynecol*, **69**: 208–13.

Goldberg MH, 1971, *Corynebacterium*: an oral-systemic pathogen. Report of cases, *J Oral Surg*, **29**: 349–51.

Goldstein EJ, 1992, Bite wounds and infection [see comments], *Clin Infect Dis*, **14**: 633–8.

Goldstein EJ, Citron DM, Finegold SM, 1984, Role of anaerobic bacteria in bite-wound infections, *Rev Infect Dis*, **6**: S177–83.

Goldstein EJ, Pryor EP 3rd, Citron DM, 1995, Simian bites and bacterial infection, *Clin Infect Dis*, **20**: 1551–2.

Gomez J, Banos V et al., 1993, Clinical significance of anaerobic bacteremias in a general hospital. A prospective study from 1988 to 1992, *Clin Investig*, **71**: 595–9.

Gorbach SL, Bartlett JG, 1974, Anaerobic infections, *N Engl J Med*, **290**: 1177–84, 237–45, 289–94.

Gorbach SL, Thadepalli H, Norsen J, 1974, Anaerobic micro-organisms in intraabdominal infections, *Anaerobic Bacteria: Role in Disease*, eds Balows A, Dehaan RM et al., Charles C Thomas, Springfield, IL, 399–407.

Gorbach SL, Mayhew JW et al., 1976, Rapid diagnosis of anaerobic infections by direct gas–liquid chromatography of clinical specimens, *J Clin Invest*, **57**: 478–84.

Goyal M, Sharma R et al., 1995, Unusual radiological manifestations of Lemierre's syndrome: a case report, *Pediatr Radiol*, **25**: S105–6.

Greer KE, 1985, Contemporary therapy for acne: what, when and how to prescribe, *Postgrad Med*, **77**: 241–6.

Grenier D, Mayrand D, 1987, Functional characterization of extracellular vesicles produced by *Bacteroides gingivalis*, *Infect Immun*, **55**: 111–17.

Guillemot L, Halle J, Rist E, 1904, Recherches bactériologiques et expérimentales sur les pleurésies putrides, *Arch Med Exp Anat Pathol*, **16**: 571–640.

Guillemot LD, 1899, *Recherches sur la Gangrène Pulmonaire*, thesis, Faculté de Médecine de Paris, Paris.

Haapasalo M, 1986, *Bacteroides buccae* and related taxa in necrotic root canal infections, *J Clin Microbiol*, **24**: 940–4.

Haapasalo M, Ranta H et al., 1986, Black-pigmented *Bacteroides* spp. in human apical periodontitis, *Infect Immun*, **53**: 149–53.

Hackman SS, Wilkins TD, 1975, In vivo protection of *Fusobacterium necrophorum* from penicillin by *Bacteroides fragilis*, *Antimicrob Agents Chemother*, **7**: 698–703.

Hansen A, 1950, *Nogle Undersogelsen over Gramnegative Anaerobe Ikkesporedannende Bacterier isolerede fra Peritonsilloere Abscesser bos Mennesker*, Munksgaard, Copenhagen.

Hardie JM, 1974, Anaerobes in the mouth, *Infection with Non-sporing Anaerobic Bacteria*, eds Phillips I, Sussman M, Churchill Livingstone, Edinburgh, 99–130.

Harris JW, Brown JH, 1927, Description of a new organism that may be a factor in the causation of puerperal infection, *Bull Johns Hopkins Hosp*, **40**: 203–10.

Hecht DW, Malamy MH, Tally FP, 1989, Mechanisms of resistance and resistance transfer in anaerobic bacteria, *Anaerobic Infections in Humans*, eds Finegold SM, George WL, Academic Press, New York, 755–69.

Hecht DW, Osmolski JR, O'Keefe JP, 1993, Variation in the susceptibility of *Bacteroides fragilis* group isolates from six Chicago hospitals, *Clin Infect Dis*, **16**: S357–60.

Heineman HS, Braude AI, 1963, Anaerobic infection of the brain, *Am J Med*, **35**: 682–97.

Heinrich S, Pulverer G, 1960, Uber den Nachweis des *Bacteroides melaninogenicus* in Krankheitsprozessen bei Mensch and Tier, *Z Hyg*, **146**: 331–40.

Henriksen SD, 1948, Studies in Gram-negative anaerobes. II. Gram-negative anaerobic rods with spreading colonies, *Acta Pathol Microbiol Scand*, **25**: 368–75.

Hentges DJ, 1983, *Human Intestinal Microflora in Health and Disease*, Academic Press, New York.

Hentges DJ, 1993, The anaerobic microflora of the human body, *Clin Infect Dis*, **16**: S175–80.

Hermans PE, Washington JA 2d, 1970, Polymicrobial bacteremia, *Ann Intern Med*, **73**: 387–92.

Hill GB, 1992, *Eubacterium nodatum* mimics *Actinomyces* in intrauterine device-associated infections and other settings within the female genital tract, *Obstet Gynecol*, **79**: 534–8.

Hill GB, Ayers OM, Kohan AP, 1987, Characteristics and sites of infection of *Eubacterium nodatum, Eubacterium timidum, Eubacterium brachy*, and other asaccharolytic eubacteria, *J Clin Microbiol*, **25**: 1540–5.

Hill MJ, Marsh PD, 1989, *Human Microbial Ecology*, CRC Press, Boca Raton, FL.

Hillier SL, Moncla BJ, 1995, *Peptostreptococcus, Propionibacterium, Eubacterium*, and other nonsporeforming anaerobic gram-positive bacteria, *Manual of Clinical Microbiology*, 6th edn, eds Murray PR, Baron EJ et al., ASM Press, Washington, DC, 587–602.

Hillier SL, Nugent RP et al., 1995, Association between bacterial vaginosis and preterm delivery of a low-birth-weight infant. The Vaginal Infections and Prematurity Study Group, *N Engl J Med*, **333**: 1737–42.

Hirschmann JV, Feingold DS, 1992, Normal cutaneous flora and infections they cause, *Infectious Diseases*, eds Gorbach SL, Bartlett JG, Blacklow NR, WB Saunders, Philadelphia, 1066–9.

Hofstad T, 1992, Virulence factors in anaerobic bacteria, *Eur J Clin Microbiol Infect Dis*, **11**: 1044–8.

Hofstad T, 1994, Utility of newer techniques for classification and identification of pathogenic anaerobic bacteria, *Clin Infect Dis*, **18**: S250–2.

Holbrook WP, McMillan C, 1977, The hydrolysis of dextran by gram negative non-sporing anaerobic bacilli, *J Appl Bacteriol*, **43**: 369–74.

Holdeman LV, Good IJ, Moore WE, 1976, Human fecal flora: variation in bacterial composition within individuals and a possible effect of emotional stress, *Appl Environ Microbiol*, **31**: 359–75.

Holdeman LV, Cato EP et al., 1980, Descriptions of *Eubacterium timidum* sp. nov., *Eubacterium brachy* sp. nov., and *Eubacterium nodatum* sp. nov. isolated from human periodontitis, *Int J Syst Bacteriol*, **30**: 163–9.

Holdeman LV, Moore WEC et al., 1982, *Bacteroides oris* and *Bacteroides buccae*: new species from human periodontitis and other human infections, *Int J Syst Bacteriol*, **32**: 125–31.

Holland JW, Hill EO, Altemeier WA, 1977, Numbers and types of anaerobic bacteria isolated from clinical specimens since 1960, *J Clin Microbiol*, **5**: 20–5.

Ieven M, Vael K et al., 1993, Three cases of *Fusobacterium necrophorum* septicemia, *Eur J Clin Microbiol Infect Dis*, **12**: 705–6.

Ingham HR, Slekon JB, Roxby CM, 1977, Bacteriological study of otogenic cerebral abscesses: chemotherapeutic role of metronidazole, *Br Med J*, **2**: 991–3.

Ingham HR, Sisson PR et al., 1977, Inhibition of phagocytosis in vitro by obligate anaerobes, *Lancet*, **2**: 1252–4.

Ingham HR, Sisson PR et al., 1981, Phagocytosis and killing of bacteria in aerobic and anaerobic conditions, *J Med Microbiol*, **14**: 391–9.

Jensen R, Mackey DR, 1974, *Diseases of Feedlot Cattle*, Lea & Febiger, Philadelphia.

Johnson CC, Reinhardt JF et al., 1985, *Bacteroides gracilis*, an important anaerobic bacterial pathogen, *J Clin Microbiol*, **22**: 799–802.

Johnston BL, Edelstein MA et al., 1987, Bacteriologic and clinical study of *Bacteroides oris* and *Bacteroides buccae*, *J Clin Microbiol*, **25**: 491–3.

Jones GR, Gemmell CG, 1986, Effects of *Bacteroides asaccharolyticus* cells and *B. fragilis* surface components on serum opsonisation and phagocytosis, *J Med Microbiol*, **22**: 225–9.

Jousimies-Somer HR, 1995, Update on the taxonomy and the clinical and laboratory characteristics of pigmented anaerobic gram-negative rods, *Clin Infect Dis*, **20**: S187–91.

Kagnoff MF, Armstrong D, Blevins A, 1972, *Bacteroides* bacteremia. Experience in a hospital for neoplastic diseases, *Cancer*, **29**: 245–51.

Kanoe M, Iwaki K, 1987, Adherence of *Fusobacterium necrophorum* to bovine ruminal cells, *J Med Microbiol*, **23**: 69–73.

Kanoe M, Nouka K, Toda M, 1984, Isolation of obligate anaerobic bacteria from bovine abscesses in sites other than the liver, *J Med Microbiol*, **18**: 365–9.

Kasten MJ, Rosenblatt JE, Gustafson DR, 1992, *Bilophila wadsworthia* bacteremia in two patients with hepatic abscesses, *J Clin Microbiol*, **30**: 2502–3.

Kaufman DM, Miller MH, Steigbel NH, 1975, Subdural empyema: analysis of 17 recent cases and review of the literature, *Medicine (Baltimore)*, **54**: 485–98.

Kaufman EJ, Mashimo PA et al., 1972, Fusobacterial infection: enhancement by cell free extracts of *Bacteroides melaninogenicus* possessing collagenolytic activity, *Arch Oral Biol*, **17**: 577–80.

Khairat O, 1966, The non-aerobes of post-extraction bacteremia, *J Dent Res*, **45**: 1191–7.

Khairat O, 1967, *Bacteroides corrodens* isolated from bacteraemias, *J Pathol Bacteriol*, **94**: 29–40.

Koneman EW, Allen SD et al., 1992, *Color Atlas and Textbook of Diagnostic Microbiology*, 4th edn, JB Lippincott Co., Philadelphia, 1154.

Kononen E, Jousimies-Somer H, Asikainen S, 1994, The most frequently isolated gram-negative anaerobes in saliva and subgingival samples taken from young women, *Oral Microbiol Immunol*, **9**: 126–8.

Kononen E, Asikainen S et al., 1994, The oral gram-negative anaerobic microflora in young children: longitudinal changes from edentulous to dentate mouth, *Oral Microbiol Immunol*, **9**: 136–41.

La Fontaine S, Rood JI, 1990, Evidence that *Bacteroides nodosus* belongs in subgroup gamma of the class Proteobacteria, not in the genus *Bacteroides*: partial sequence analysis of a *B. nodosus* 16S rRNA gene, *Int J Syst Bacteriol*, **40**: 154–9.

Landsaat PM, van der Lelie H et al., 1995, *Fusobacterium nucleatum*, a new invasive pathogen in neutropenic patients?, *Scand J Infect Dis*, **27**: 83–4.

Langworth BF, 1977, *Fusobacterium necrophorum*: its characteristics and role as an animal pathogen, *Bacteriol Rev*, **41**: 373–90.

Lantz MS, Rowland RW et al., 1986, Interactions of *Bacteroides gingivalis* with fibrinogen, *Infect Immun*, **54**: 654–8.

Larjava H, Uitto VJ et al., 1987, Inhibition of gingival fibroblast growth by *Bacteroides gingivalis*, *Infect Immun*, **55**: 201–5.

Ledger WJ, Sweet RL, Headington JT, 1971, *Bacteroides* species as a cause of severe infections in obstetric and gynecologic patients, *Surg Gynecol Obstet*, **133**: 837–42.

Lee D, Goldstein EJ et al., 1993, Empyema due to *Bacteroides gracilis*: case report and in vitro susceptibilities to eight antimicrobial agents, *Clin Infect Dis*, **16**: S263–5.

LeFrock JL, Ellis CA et al., 1973, Transient bacteremia associated with sigmoidoscopy, *N Engl J Med*, **289**: 467–9.

Legrand H, Axisa E, 1905, Ueber Anaerobien im eiter Dysenterischer Leber- und Gehirn-abscesse in Aegypten, *Dtsch Med Wochenschr*, **31**: 1959–60.

Leigh DA, Simmons K, Norman E, 1974, Bacterial flora of the appendix fossa in appendicitis and postoperative wound infection, *J Clin Pathol*, **27**: 997–1000.

Lemierre A, 1936, On certain septicaemias due to anaerobic organisms, *Lancet*, **1**: 701–3.

Lindberg AA, Berthold P et al., 1979, Encapsulated strains of *Bacteroides fragilis* in clinical specimens, *Med Microbiol Immunol*, **167**: 29–36.

Linscheid RL, Dobyns JH, 1975, Common and uncommon infections of the hand, *Orthop Clin North Am*, **6**: 1063–104.

Loeffler F, 1884, Untersuchungen uber die Bedeutung der Mikroorganismen fur die Entstehung der Diphtherie beim Menschen, bei der Taube und beim Kalbe, *Mitt a d Kais Ges Sndhtsamte*, **2**: 421–99.

Loesche WJ, 1969, Oxygen sensitivity of various anaerobic bacteria, *Appl Microbiol*, **18**: 723–7.

Love DN, Bailey GD, Bastin D, 1992, Chromosomal DNA probes for the identification of asaccharolytic anaerobic pigmented bacterial rods from the oral cavity of cats, *Vet Microbiol*, **31**: 287–95.

Love DN, Jones RF et al., 1979, Isolation and characterisation of bacteria from abscesses in the subcutis of cats, *J Med Microbiol*, **12**: 207–12.

Lucht E, Heimdahl A, Nord CE, 1991, Periodontal disease in HIV-infected patients in relation to lymphocyte subsets and specific micro-organisms, *J Clin Periodontol*, **18**: 252–6.

McGregor JA, Lawellin D et al., 1986, Protease production by microorganisms associated with reproductive tract infection, *Am J Obstet Gynecol*, **154**: 109–14.

McIntosh J, Fildes P, 1916, A new apparatus for the isolation and cultivation of anaerobic micro-organisms, *Lancet*, **1**: 768–70.

Mackowiak PA, 1978, Microbial synergism in human infections (parts one and two), *N Engl J Med*, **298**: 21–6, 83–7.

McNeil MM, Martone WJ, Dowell VR Jr, 1987, Bacteremia with *Anaerobiospirillum succiniciproducens*, *Rev Infect Dis*, **9**: 737–42.

Madin SH, 1949, A bacteriologic study of bovine liver abscesses, *Vet Med*, **44**: 248–51.

Mandell GL, 1974, Bactericidal activity of aerobic and anaerobic polymorphonuclear neutrophils, *Infect Immun*, **9**: 337–41.

Marina M, Strong CA et al., 1993, Bacteriology of anaerobic pleuropulmonary infections: preliminary report, *Clin Infect Dis*, **16**: S256–62.

Marshall SA, Aldridge KE et al., 1995, Comparative antimicrobial activity of piperacillin–tazobactam tested against more than 5000 recent clinical isolates from five medical centers. A reevaluation after five years, *Diagn Microbiol Infect Dis*, **21**: 153–68.

Martin WJ, 1974, Isolation and identification of anaerobic bacteria in the clinical laboratory. A 2-year experience, *Mayo Clin Proc*, **49**: 300–8.

Masfari AN, Kinghorn GR, Duerden BI, 1983, Anaerobes in genitourinary infections in men, *Br J Vener Dis*, **59**: 255–9.

Masfari AN, Kinghorn GR et al., 1985, Anaerobic bacteria and herpes simplex virus in genital ulceration, *Genitourin Med*, **61**: 109–13.

Masri AF, Grieco MH, 1972, *Bacteroides* endocarditis: report of a case, *Am J Med Sci*, **263**: 357–67.

Mathisen GE, Meyer RD et al., 1984, Brain abscess and cerebritis, *Rev Infect Dis*, **6**: 101–6.

May RP, Lehmann JD, Sanford JP, 1967, Difficulties in differentiating amebic from pyogenic liver abscess, *Arch Intern Med*, **119**: 69–74.

Mayrand D, Grenier D, 1985, Detection of collagenase activity in oral bacteria, *Can J Microbiol*, **31**: 134–8.

Meleney FL, 1948, *Treatise on Surgical Infections*, Oxford University Press, New York.

Mena E, Thompson FS et al., 1978, Evaluation of Port-A-Cul transport system for protection of anaerobic bacteria, *J Clin Microbiol*, **8**: 28–35.

Mergenhagen SE, Thonard JC, Scherp HW, 1958, Studies on synergistic infections. I. Experimental infections with anaerobic streptococci, *J Infect Dis*, **103**: 33–44.

Millar SJ, Goldstein EG et al., 1986, Modulation of bone metabolism by two chemically distinct lipopolysaccharide fractions from *Bacteroides gingivalis*, *Infect Immun*, **51**: 302–6.

Moncrief JS, Obiso R Jr et al., 1995, The enterotoxin of *Bacteroides fragilis* is a metalloprotease, *Infect Immun*, **63**: 175–81.

Moore LV, Moore WE et al., 1993, Periodontal microflora of HIV positive subjects with gingivitis or adult periodontitis, *J Periodontol*, **64**: 48–56.

Moore WE, Holdeman LV, 1974, Human fecal flora: the normal flora of 20 Japanese-Hawaiians, *Appl Microbiol*, **27**: 961–79.

Moore WE, Moore LH et al., 1991, The microflora of periodontal sites showing active destructive progression, *J Clin Periodontol*, **18**: 729–39.

Moore WEC, Ranney RR, Holdeman LV, 1982, Subgingival microflora in periodontal disease: cultural studies, *Host–Parasite Interactions in Periodontal Diseases*, eds Genco RJ, Mergenhagen SE, American Society for Microbiology, Washington, DC, 13–26.

Moreno S, Altozano JG et al., 1989, Lemierre's disease: postanginal bacteremia and pulmonary involvement caused by *Fusobacterium necrophorum*, *Rev Infect Dis*, **11**: 319–24.

Murray PR, Traynor P, Hopson D, 1992, Critical assessment of blood culture techniques: analysis of recovery of obligate and facultative anaerobes, strict aerobic bacteria, and fungi in aerobic and anaerobic blood culture bottles, *J Clin Microbiol*, **30**: 1462–8.

Myers LL, Shoop DS, 1987, Association of enterotoxigenic *Bacteroides fragilis* with diarrheal disease in young pigs, *Am J Vet Res*, **48**: 774–5.

Myers LL, Shoop DS, Byars TD, 1987, Diarrhea associated with enterotoxigenic *Bacteroides fragilis* in foals, *Am J Vet Res*, **48**: 1565–7.

Myers LL, Shoop DS et al., 1985, Association of enterotoxigenic *Bacteroides fragilis* with diarrheal disease in calves, *J Infect Dis*, **152**: 1344–7.

Myers LL, Shoop DS et al., 1987, Isolation of enterotoxigenic *Bacteroides fragilis* from humans with diarrhea, *J Clin Microbiol*, **25**: 2330–3.

Myers LL, Shoop DS et al., 1989, Diarrheal disease caused by enterotoxigenic *Bacteroides fragilis* in infant rabbits, *J Clin Microbiol*, **27**: 2025–30.

Namavar F, Verweij-Van Vught AM et al., 1984, Polymorphonuclear leukocyte chemotaxis by mixed anaerobic and aerobic bacteria, *J Med Microbiol*, **18**: 167–72.

Namavar F, Verweij-Van Vught AM et al., 1987, Effect of *Bacteroides fragilis* cellular components on chemotactic activity of polymorphonuclear leukocytes towards *Escherichia coli*, *J Med Microbiol*, **24**: 119–24.

Namavar F, Theunissen EB et al., 1989, Epidemiology of the *Bacteroides fragilis* group in the colonic flora in 10 patients with colonic cancer, *J Med Microbiol*, **29**: 171–6.

NCCLS, 1993, *Methods for Antimicrobial Susceptibility Testing of Anaerobic Bacteria. Approved Standard*, 3rd edn, National Committee for Clinical Laboratory Standards, Villanova, PA.

NCCLS, 1994, *Performance Standards for Antimicrobial Susceptibility Testing; Fifth Informational Supplement*, National Committee for Clinical Laboratory Standards, Villanova, PA.

Newman JH, Mitchell RG, 1975, Diphtheroid infection of the cervical spine, *Acta Orthop Scand*, **46**: 67–70.

Newman MG, Goodman AD, 1989, Oral and dental infections, *Anaerobic Infections in Humans*, eds Finegold SM, George WL, Academic Press, New York, 233–61.

Nord CE, 1995, The role of anaerobic bacteria in recurrent episodes of sinusitis and tonsillitis, *Clin Infect Dis*, **20**: 1512–24.

Obiso RJ Jr, Lyerly DM et al., 1995, Proteolytic activity of the *Bacteroides fragilis* enterotoxin causes fluid secretion and intestinal damage in vivo, *Infect Immun*, **63**: 3820–6.

Okell CC, Elliott SD, 1935, Bacteremia and oral sepsis with

special reference to the aetiology of subacute endocarditis, *Lancet,* **2:** 869–72.

Okuda K, Slots J, Genco RJ, 1981, *Bacteroides gingivalis, Bacteroides asaccharolyticus,* and *Bacteroides melaninogenicus* subspecies: cell surface morphology and adherence to erythrocytes and human buccal epithelial cells, *Curr Microbiol,* **6:** 7–12.

Okuda K, Takazoe I, 1974, Haemagglutinating activity of *Bacteroides melaninogenicus, Arch Oral Biol,* **19:** 415–16.

Onderdonk AB, Kasper DL et al., 1977, The capsular polysaccharide of *Bacteroides fragilis* as a virulence factor: comparison of the pathogenic potential of encapsulated and unencapsulated strains, *J Infect Dis,* **136:** 82–9.

Onderdonk AB, Moon NE et al., 1978, Adherence of *Bacteroides fragilis* in vivo, *Infect Immun,* **19:** 1083–7.

Onderdonk AB, Kasper DL et al., 1979, Experimental animal models for anaerobic infections, *Res Infect Dis,* **1:** 291–301.

Onderdonk AB, Markham RB et al., 1982, Evidence for T cell-dependent immunity to *Bacteroides fragilis* in an intraabdominal abscess model, *J Clin Invest,* **69:** 9–16.

Onderdonk AB, Shapiro ME et al., 1984, Use of a model of intraabdominal sepsis for studies of the pathogenicity of *Bacteroides fragilis, Rev Infect Dis,* **6:** S91–5.

Parent R, Mouton C et al., 1986, Human and animal serotypes of *Bacteroides gingivalis* defined by crossed immunoelectrophoresis, *Infect Immun,* **51:** 909–18.

Parsonson IM, Egerton JR, Roberts DS, 1967, Ovine interdigital dermatitis, *J Comp Pathol,* **77:** 309–13.

Pearson HE, 1967, *Bacteroides* in areolar breast abscesses, *Surg Gynecol Obstet,* **125:** 800–6.

Pearson HE, Anderson GV, 1967, Perinatal deaths associated with bacteroides infections, *Obstet Gynecol,* **30:** 486–92.

Pearson HE, Anderson GV, 1970, *Bacteroides* infections and pregnancy, *Obstet Gynecol,* **35:** 31–6.

Pearson HE, Harvey JP Jr, 1971, *Bacteroides* infections in orthopedic conditions, *Surg Gynecol Obstet,* **132:** 876–80.

Peromet M, Labbe M et al., 1973, [Anaerobic germs isolated from decubitus ulcers], *Acta Clin Belg,* **28:** 117–21.

Phillips I, 1990, New methods for identification of obligate anaerobes, *Rev Infect Dis,* **12:** S127–32.

Phillips KD, Tearle PV, Willis AT, 1976, Rapid diagnosis of anaerobic infections by gas–liquid chromatography of clinical material, *J Clin Pathol,* **29:** 428–32.

Pien FD, Thompson RL, Martin WJ, 1972, Clinical and bacteriologic studies of anaerobic gram-positive cocci, *Mayo Clin Proc,* **47:** 251–7.

Piriz S, Valle J et al., 1992, Microbiological study of foot-rot in lambs: isolation, elastolytic activity and antimicrobial susceptibility, *Zentralbl Veterinarmed [B],* **39:** 181–6.

Plaut HC, 1894, Studien zur bakteriellen Diagnostik der Diphtherie und Angienen, *Dtsch Med Wochenschr,* **20:** 920–3.

Polk BF, Kasper DL, 1977, *Bacteroides fragilis* subspecies in clinical isolates, *Ann Intern Med,* **86:** 569–71.

Poxton IR, Brown R et al., 1997, Mucosa-associated bacterial flora of the human colon, *J Med Microbiol,* **46:** 85–91.

Pressman RS, Bender IB, 1944, Effect of sulfonamide compounds on transient bacteremia following extraction of teeth, *Arch Intern Med,* **74:** 346–53.

Prolo DJ, Hanbery JW, 1968, Secondary actinomycotic brain abscess: isolation of a new species and review, *Arch Surg,* **96:** 58–64.

Pruzzo C, Dainelli B, Ricchetti M, 1984, Piliated *Bacteroides fragilis* strains adhere to epithelial cells and are more sensitive to phagocytosis by human neutrophils than nonpiliated strains, *Infect Immun,* **43:** 189–94.

Rahman M, 1982, Chest infection caused by *Lactobacillus casei* ss *rhamnosus, Br Med J (Clin Res Ed),* **284:** 471–2.

Reid JH, Patrick S, 1984, Phagocytic and serum killing of capsulate and non-capsulate *Bacteroides fragilis, J Med Microbiol,* **17:** 247–57.

Rist E, 1901, Neue Methoden und neue Ergebnisse im gebiete der Bacteriologischen untersuchung gangranoser und fotider Eiterungen, *Zentralbl Bakteriol Parasitenkd Infektionskr,* **30:** 287–305.

Roberts DS, 1967, The pathogenic synergy of *Fusiformis necrophorus* and *Corynebacterium pyogenes.* I. Influence of the leucocidal exotoxin of *F. necrophorus, Br J Exp Pathol,* **48:** 665–73.

Roberts DS, 1969, Synergic mechanisms in certain mixed infections, *J Infect Dis,* **120:** 720–4.

Roberts DS, 1970, Toxic, allergenic and immunogenic factors of *Fusiformis necrophorus, J Comp Pathol,* **80:** 247–57.

Roberts MC, Moncla B, Kenny GE, 1987, Chromosomal DNA probes for the identification of *Bacteroides* species, *J Gen Microbiol,* **133:** 1423–30.

Roberts MC, Hillier SL et al., 1985, Comparison of gram stain, DNA probe, and culture for the identification of species of *Mobiluncus* in female genital specimens, *J Infect Dis,* **152:** 74–7.

Rodloff AC, Becker J et al., 1986, Inhibition of macrophage phagocytosis by *Bacteroides fragilis* in vivo and in vitro, *Infect Immun,* **52:** 488–92.

Roeterink CH, van Steenbergen TJ, de Graaff J, 1985, Histopathological changes in the hind foot of the mouse induced by black-pigmented *Bacteroides* strains, *J Med Microbiol,* **20:** 355–61.

Rogemond V, Guinet RM, 1986, Lectinlike adhesins in the *Bacteroides fragilis* group, *Infect Immun,* **53:** 99–102.

Rona S, 1905, Zur Atiologie und Pathogenese der Plaut-Vincentschen Angina, der Stomakace, der Stomatitis gangraenosa idiopathica, beziehungsweise der Noma, der Stomatitis mercurialis gangraenosa und der Lungengangran, *Arch Dermatol Syph,* **74:** 171–202.

Rosebury T, 1962, *Microorganisms Indigenous to Man,* McGraw-Hill, New York.

Rosenblatt JE, 1989, Susceptibility testing of anaerobic bacteria, *Clin Lab Med,* **9:** 239–54.

Rosenblatt JE, Brook I, 1993, Clinical relevance of susceptibility testing of anaerobic bacteria, *Clin Infect Dis,* **16:** S446–8.

Rotheram EB Jr, 1974, Septic abortion and related infections of pregnancy, *Anaerobic Bacteria: Role in Disease,* eds Balows A, Dehaan RM et al., Charles C Thomas, Springfield, IL, 369–78.

Rotheram EB Jr, Schick SF, 1969, Nonclostridial anaerobic bacteria in septic abortion, *Am J Med,* **46:** 80–9.

Rotstein OD, Nasmith PE, Grinstein S, 1987, The *Bacteroides* byproduct succinic acid inhibits neutrophil respiratory burst by reducing intracellular pH, *Infect Immun,* **55:** 864–70.

Rotstein OD, Pruett TL, Simmons RL, 1985, Mechanisms of microbial synergy in polymicrobial surgical infections, *Rev Infect Dis,* **7:** 151–70.

Rotstein OD, Pruett TL et al., 1987, The role of *Bacteroides* encapsulation in the lethal synergy between *Escherichia coli* and *Bacteroides* species studied in a rat fibrin clot peritonitis model, *J Infect,* **15:** 135–46.

Rowland IR, 1988, *Role of the Gut Flora in Toxicity and Cancer,* Academic Press, New York.

Rudek W, Haque RU, 1976, Extracellular enzymes of the genus *Bacteroides, J Clin Microbiol,* **4:** 458–60.

Sabbaj J, 1984, Anaerobes in liver abscess, *Rev Infect Dis,* **6:** S152–6.

Sabbaj J, Sutter VL, Finegold SM, 1972, Anaerobic pyogenic liver abscess, *Ann Intern Med,* **77:** 627–38.

Sack RB, Myers LL et al., 1992, Enterotoxigenic *Bacteroides fragilis*: epidemiologic studies of its role as a human diarrhoeal pathogen, *J Diarrhoeal Dis Res,* **10:** 4–9.

Sack RB, Albert MJ et al., 1994, Isolation of enterotoxigenic *Bacteroides fragilis* from Bangladeshi children with diarrhea: a controlled study, *J Clin Microbiol,* **32:** 960–3.

Sato M, Otsuka M et al., 1987, Degradation of human secretory immunoglobulin A by protease isolated from the anaerobic periodontopathogenic bacterium, *Bacteroides gingivalis, Arch Oral Biol,* **32:** 235–8.

Savage DC, 1985, Effects on host animals of bacteria adhering to epithelial surfaces, *Bacterial Adhesion: Mechanisms and*

Physiological Significance, eds Savage DC, Fletcher M, Plenum Press, New York, 437–63.

Savitt ED, Socransky SS, 1984, Distribution of certain subgingival microbial species in selected periodontal conditions, *J Periodont Res*, **19**: 111–23.

Schmorl G, 1891, Ueber ein pathogenes Fadenbacterium (*Streptothrix cuniculi*), *Dtsch Z Thiermed*, **17**: 375–408.

Schroter G, Stawru J, 1970, The role of *Bacteroides corrodens* Eiken 1958 within the tonsil flora, *Z Med Mikrobiol Immunol*, **155**: 241–7.

Shah HN, Collins DM, 1988, Proposal for re-classification of *Bacteroides asaccharolyticus*, *Bacteroides gingivalis*, and *Bacteroides endodontalis* in a new genus, *Porphyromonas*, *Int J Syst Bacteriol*, **38**: 128–31.

Shah HN, Collins DM, 1990, *Prevotella*, a new genus to include *Bacteroides melaninogenicus* and related species formerly classified in the genus *Bacteroides*, *Int J Syst Bacteriol*, **40**: 205–8.

Shah HN, Gharbia SE, 1992, Biochemical and chemical studies on strains designated *Prevotella intermedia* and proposal of a new pigmented species, *Prevotella nigrescens* sp. nov., *Int J Syst Bacteriol*, **42**: 542–6.

Shah HN, Gharbia SE, 1993a, Ecophysiology and taxonomy of *Bacteroides* and related taxa, *Clin Infect Dis*, **16**: S160–7.

Shah HN, Gharbia SE, 1993b, Proposal of a new species *Prevotella nigrescens* sp. nov. among strains previously classified as *Pr. intermedia*, *FEMS Immunol Med Microbiol*, **6**: 97.

Shah HN, Collins MD et al., 1995a, Reclassification of *Bacteroides levii* (Holdeman, Cato, and Moore) in the genus *Porphyromonas*, as *Porphyromonas levii* comb. nov., *Int J Syst Bacteriol*, **45**: 586–8.

Shah HN, Gharbia SE et al., 1995b, Oligonucleotide probes to the 16S ribosomal RNA: implications of sequence homology and secondary structure with particular reference to the oral species *Prevotella intermedia* and *Prevotella nigrescens*, *Oral Dis*, **1**: 32–6.

Shapton DA, Board RG, 1971, *Isolation of Anaerobes*, Academic Press, London.

Sharpe ME, Hill LR, Lapage SP, 1973, Pathogenic lactobacilli, *J Med Microbiol*, **6**: 281–6.

Shinjo T, Fujisawa T, Mitsuoka T, 1991, Proposal of two subspecies of *Fusobacterium necrophorum* (Flugge) Moore and Holdeman: *Fusobacterium necrophorum* subsp. *necrophorum* subsp. nov., nom. rev. (ex Flugge 1886), and *Fusobacterium necrophorum* subsp. *funduliforme* subsp. nov., nom. rev. (ex Halle 1898), *Int J Syst Bacteriol*, **41**: 395–7.

Shinjo T, Hiraiwa K, Miyazato S, 1990, Recognition of biovar C of *Fusobacterium necrophorum* (Flugge) Moore and Holdeman as *Fusobacterium pseudonecrophorum* sp. nov., nom. rev. (ex Prevot 1940), *Int J Syst Bacteriol*, **40**: 71–3.

Siboni A, Graversen K, Olsen H, 1993, Significant decrease of gram-negative anaerobic bacteremia in a major hospital from 1967–73 to 1981–89: an effect of the introduction of metronidazole?, *Scand J Infect Dis*, **25**: 347–51.

Simon GL, Klempner MS et al., 1982, Alterations in opsonophagocytic killing by neutrophils of *Bacteroides fragilis* associated with animal and laboratory passage: effect of capsular polysaccharide, *J Infect Dis*, **145**: 72–7.

Sinave CP, Hardy GJ, Fardy PW, 1989, The Lemierre syndrome: suppurative thrombophlebitis of the internal jugular vein secondary to oropharyngeal infection, *Medicine (Baltimore)*, **68**: 85–94.

Slots J, 1982, Importance of black-pigmented bacteroides in human periodontal disease, *Host–Parasite Interactions in Periodontal Diseases*, eds Genco RJ, Mergenhagen SE, American Society for Microbiology, Washington, DC, 27–45.

Slots J, 1986, Virulence factors of the bacteria that cause periodontal diseases, *Compend Contin Educ Dent*, **7**: 665–8, 70.

Slots J, Gibbons RJ, 1978, Attachment of *Bacteroides melaninogenicus* subsp. *asaccharolyticus* to oral surfaces and its possible role in colonization of the mouth and of periodontal pockets, *Infect Immun*, **19**: 254–64.

Smith GR, Till D et al., 1989, Enhancement of the infectivity of *Fusobacterium necrophorum* by other bacteria, *Epidemiol Infect*, **102**: 447–58.

Smith JW, Southern PM Jr, Lehmann JD, 1970, Bacteremia in septic abortion: complications and treatment, *Obstet Gynecol*, **35**: 704–8.

Smith LDS, Williams BL, 1984, *The Pathogenic Anaerobic Bacteria*, 3rd edn, Charles C Thomas, Springfield, IL.

Sonnenwirth AC, 1972, Evolution of anaerobic methodology, *Am J Clin Nutr*, **25**: 1295–8.

Sonnenwirth AC, 1983, Bacteremia – extent of the problem through three decades, *Bacteremia: Laboratory and Clinical Aspects*, eds Balows A, Sonnenwirth AC, Charles C Thomas, Springfield, IL, 3–8.

Spiegel CA, 1991, Bacterial vaginosis, *Clin Microbiol Rev*, **4**: 485–502.

Spiegel CA, Amsel R et al., 1980, Anaerobic bacteria in non-specific vaginitis, *N Engl J Med*, **303**: 601–7.

Staat RH, Gawronski TH, Schachtele CF, 1973, Detection and preliminary studies on dextranase-producing microorganisms from human dental plaque, *Infect Immun*, **8**: 1009–16.

van Steenbergen TJ, Kastelein P et al., 1982a, Virulence of black-pigmented *Bacteroides* strains from periodontal pockets and other sites in experimentally induced skin lesions in mice, *J Periodont Res*, **17**: 41–9.

van Steenbergen TJ, dan Ouden MD et al., 1982b, Cytotoxic activity of *Bacteroides gingivalis* and *Bacteroides asaccharolyticus*, *J Med Microbiol*, **15**: 253–8.

Steffen EK, Hentges DJ, 1981, Hydrolytic enzymes of anaerobic bacteria isolated from human infections, *J Clin Microbiol*, **14**: 153–6.

Stewart DJ, Elleman TC, 1987, A *Bacteroides nodosus* pili vaccine produced by recombinant DNA for the prevention and treatment of foot-rot in sheep, *Aust Vet J*, **64**: 79–81.

Stewart DJ, Peterson JE et al., 1986, The pathogenicity and cultural characteristics of virulent, intermediate and benign strains of *Bacteroides nodosus* causing ovine foot-rot, *Aust Vet J*, **63**: 317–26.

Stokes EJ, 1958, Anaerobes in routine diagnostic cultures, *Lancet*, **1**: 668–70.

Stone HH, 1976, Bacterial flora of appendicitis in children, *J Pediatr Surg*, **11**: 37–42.

Strand CL, Shulman JA, 1988, *Bloodstream Infections: Laboratory Detection and Clinical Considerations*, ASCP Press, Chicago.

Styrt B, Gorbach SL, 1989a, Recent developments in the understanding of the pathogenesis and treatment of anaerobic infections (2), *N Engl J Med*, **321**: 240–6.

Styrt B, Gorbach SL, 1989b, Recent developments in the understanding of the pathogenesis and treatment of anaerobic infections (2), *N Engl J Med*, **321**: 298–302.

Summanen P, Wexler HM, Finegold SM, 1992, Antimicrobial susceptibility testing of *Bilophila wadsworthia* by using triphenyltetrazolium chloride to facilitate endpoint determination, *Antimicrob Agents Chemother*, **36**: 1658–64.

Summanen P, Baron EJ et al., 1993, *Wadsworth Anaerobic Bacteriology Manual*, 5th edn, Star Publishing, Belmont, CA.

Summanen PH, Jousimies-Somer H et al., 1995, *Bilophila wadsworthia* isolates from clinical specimens, *Clin Infect Dis*, **20**: S210–11.

Sundqvist G, Carlsson J, Hanstrom L, 1987, Collagenolytic activity of black-pigmented *Bacteroides* species, *J Periodont Res*, **22**: 300–6.

Sundqvist G, Johansson E, 1982, Bactericidal effect of pooled human serum on *Bacteroides melaninogenicus*, *Bacteroides asaccharolyticus* and *Actinobacillus actinomycetemcomitans*, *Scand J Dent Res*, **90**: 29–36.

Sundqvist G, Carlsson J et al., 1985, Degradation of human immunoglobulins G and M and complement factors C3 and C5 by black-pigmented *Bacteroides*, *J Med Microbiol*, **19**: 85–94.

Sundqvist GK, Carlsson J et al., 1984, Degradation in vivo of the

C3 protein of guinea-pig complement by a pathogenic strain of *Bacteroides gingivalis*, *Scand J Dent Res*, **92**: 14–24.

Sussman JI, Baron EJ et al., 1986, Clinical manifestations and therapy of *Lactobacillus* endocarditis: report of a case and review of the literature, *Rev Infect Dis*, **8**: 771–6.

Sutter VL, Citron DM et al., 1985, *Wadsworth Anaerobic Bacteriology Manual*, 4th edn, Star Publishing, Belmont, CA.

Sweeney G, Picozzi GL, Browning GG, 1982, A quantitative study of aerobic and anaerobic bacteria in chronic suppurative otitis media, *J Infect*, **5**: 47–55.

Swenson MM, Facklam RR, Thornsberry C, 1990, Antimicrobial susceptibility of vancomycin-resistant *Leuconostoc*, *Pediococcus* and *Lactobacillus* species, *Antimicrob Agents Chemother*, **34**: 543–9.

Swenson RM, Lorber B et al., 1974, The bacteriology of intra-abdominal infections, *Arch Surg*, **109**: 398–9.

Tally FP, Stewart PR et al., 1975, Oxygen tolerance of fresh clinical anaerobic bacteria, *J Clin Microbiol*, **1**: 161–4.

Tally FP, Goldin BR et al., 1977, Superoxide dismutase in anaerobic bacteria of clinical significance, *Infect Immun*, **16**: 20–5.

Tami TA, 1995, The management of sinusitis in patients infected with the human immunodeficiency virus (HIV), *Ear Nose Throat J*, **74**: 360–3.

Tanner A, Stillman N, 1993, Oral and dental infections with anaerobic bacteria: clinical features, predominant pathogens, and treatment, *Clin Infect Dis*, **16**: S304–9.

Tanner ACR, Badger S et al., 1981, *Wolinella* gen. nov. *Wolinella succinogenes* (*Vibrio succinogenes* Wolin et al.) comb. nov., and description of *Bacteroides gracilis* sp. nov. *Wolinella recta* sp. nov., *Campylobacter concicus* sp. nov., and *Eikenella corrodens* from humans with periodontal diseases, *Int J Syst Bacteriol*, **31**: 432–45.

Taylor AJ, Costas M, Owen RJ, 1987, Numerical analysis of electrophoretic protein patterns of *Bacteroides ureolyticus* clinical isolates, *J Clin Microbiol*, **25**: 660–6.

Thadepalli H, Gorbach SL, Keith L, 1973, Anaerobic infections of the female genital tract: bacteriologic and therapeutic aspects, *Am J Obstet Gynecol*, **117**: 1034–40.

Thomas AV, Sodeman TH, Bentz RR, 1974, *Bifidobacterium* (*Actinomyces*) *eriksonii* infection, *Am Rev Respir Dis*, **110**: 663–8.

Thore M, Lofgren S, Tarnvik A, 1983, Oxygen and serum complement in phagocytosis and killing of *Propionibacterium acnes*, *Acta Pathol Microbiol Immunol Scand Sect C*, **91**: 95–100.

Thorley CM Mc, Calder HA, Harrison WJ, 1977, Recognition in Great Britain of *Bacteroides nodosus* in foot lesions of cattle, *Vet Rec*, **100**: 387.

Tsutsui H, Kinouchi T et al., 1987, Purification and characterization of a protease from *Bacteroides gingivalis* 381, *Infect Immun*, **55**: 420–7.

Tunkel AR, 1995, Topical antibacterials, *Mandell, Douglas and Bennett's Principles and Practice of Infectious Diseases*, eds Mandell GL, Bennett JE, Dolin R, Churchill Livingstone, New York, 381–9.

Van Tassell RL, Lyerly DM, Wilkins TD, 1992, Purification and characterization of an enterotoxin from *Bacteroides fragilis*, *Infect Immun*, **60**: 1343–50.

Vandamme P, Daneshvar MI et al., 1995, Chemotaxonomic analyses of *Bacteroides gracilis* and *Bacteroides ureolyticus* and reclassification of *B. gracilis* as *Campylobacter gracilis* comb. nov., *Int J Syst Bacteriol*, **45**: 145–52.

Veillon A, 1893, Sur un micrococque anaérobie trouvé dans des suppurations fétide, *C R Soc Biol (Paris)*, **45**: 807–9.

Veillon A, Zuber A, 1897, Sur quelques microbes strictement anaérobies et leur role dans la pathologie humaine, *C R Soc Biol (Paris)*, **49**: 253–5.

Veillon A, Zuber A, 1898, Sur quelques microbes strictement anaérobies et leur role en pathologie, *Arch Med Exp Anat*, **10**: 517–45.

Vel WA, Namavar F et al., 1984, Killing capacity of human polymorphonuclear leukocytes in aerobic and anaerobic conditions, *J Med Microbiol*, **18**: 173–80.

Vel WA, Namavar F et al., 1986, Haemagglutination by the *Bacteroides fragilis* group, *J Med Microbiol*, **21**: 105–7.

Vincent H, 1896, Sur l'étiologie et sur les lésions anatomo-pathologiques de la pourriture d'hôpital, *Ann Inst Pasteur*, **10**: 488–510.

Von Graevenitz A, Sabella W, 1971, Unmasking additional bacilli in gram-negative rod bacteremia, *J Med*, **2**: 185–91.

Weikel CS, Grieco FD et al., 1992, Human colonic epithelial cells, HT29/C1, treated with crude *Bacteroides fragilis* enterotoxin dramatically alter their morphology, *Infect Immun*, **60**: 321–7.

Werner H, 1974, Differentiation and medical importance of saccharolytic intestinal *Bacteroides*, *Arzneimittelforschung*, **24**: 340–3.

Werner H, Pulverer G, 1971, Occurrence and clinical significance of suppuration inducing *Bacteroides* and *Sphaerophorus* species, *Dtsch Med Wochenschr*, **96**: 1325–9.

Wexler HM, 1991, Susceptibility testing of anaerobic bacteria: myth, magic, or method?, *Clin Microbiol Rev*, **4**: 470–84.

Wexler HM, 1993, Susceptibility testing of anaerobic bacteria – the state of the art, *Clin Infect Dis*, **16**: S328–33.

Wexler HM, Reeves D et al., 1996, *Sutterella wadsworthensis* gen. nov., sp. nov., bile-resistant microaerophilic *Campylobacter gracilis*-like clinical isolates, *Int J Syst Bacteriol*, **46**: 252–8.

Wheat LJ, Allen SD et al., 1986, Diabetic foot infections: bacteriologic analysis, *Arch Intern Med*, **146**: 1935–40.

Wilkinson FC, Egerton JR, Dickson J, 1970, Transmission of *Fusiformis nodosus* infection from cattle to sheep, *Aust Vet J*, **46**: 382–4.

Willis AT, 1969, *Clostridia of Wound Infection*, Butterworths, London.

Willis AT, 1975, A view of bacteroides, *J Antimicrob Chemother*, **1**: 254–5.

Willis AT, 1977, *Anaerobic Bacteriology: Clinical and Laboratory Practice*, 3rd edn, Butterworths, London.

Willis AT, Ferguson IR et al., 1976, Metronidazole in prevention and treatment of bacteroides infections after appendectomy, *Br Med J*, **1**: 318–21.

Willis AT, Ferguson IR et al., 1977, Metronidazole in prevention and treatment of bacteroides infections in elective colonic surgery, *Br Med J*, **1**: 607–10.

Wilson RF, Chiscano AD et al., 1967, Some observations on 132 patients with septic shock, *Anesth Analg*, **46**: 751–63.

Wilson SE, Hopkins JA, 1995, Clinical correlates of anaerobic bacteriology in peritonitis, *Clin Infect Dis*, **20**: S251–6.

Wilson WR, Martin WJ et al., 1972, Anaerobic bacteremia, *Mayo Clin Proc*, **47**: 639–46.

van Winkelhoff AJ, Carlee AW, de Graaff J, 1985, *Bacteroides endodontalis* and other black-pigmented *Bacteroides* species in odontogenic abscesses, *Infect Immun*, **49**: 494–7.

van Winkelhoff AJ, de Graaff J, 1983, Vancomycin as a selective agent for isolation of *Bacteroides* species, *J Clin Microbiol*, **18**: 1282–4.

van Winkelhoff AJ, van Steenbergen TJ et al., 1985, Further characterization of *Bacteroides endodontalis*, an asaccharolytic black-pigmented *Bacteroides* species from the oral S cavity, *J Clin Microbiol*, **22**: 75–9.

Wren MWD, 1991, Laboratory diagnosis of anaerobic infection, *Anaerobes in Human Disease*, eds Duerden BI, Drasar BS, John Wiley & Sons, New York, 180–96.

Yocum RC, McArthur J et al., 1982, Septic arthritis caused by *Propionibacterium acnes*, *JAMA*, **248**: 1740–1.

Yoshikawa TT, Chow AW, Guze LB, 1975, Role of anaerobic bacteria in subdural empyema. Report of four cases and review of 327 cases from the English literature, *Am J Med*, **58**: 99–104.

Ziment I, Davis A, Finegold SM, 1969, Joint infection by anaerobic bacteria: a case report and review of the literature, *Arthritis Rheum*, **12**: 627–35.

Ziment I, Miller LG, Finegold SM, 1967, Nonsporulating anaerobic bacteria in osteomyelitis, *Antimicrob Agents Chemother*, **7**: 77–85.

Chapter 39

ACTINOMYCOSES, ACTINOBACILLOSIS AND RELATED DISEASES

K P Schaal

1 INTRODUCTION

Actinomycosis, actinobacillosis, actinomycetoma and nocardiosis are unrelated diseases in terms of aetiology, epidemiology and treatment but there are good reasons for dealing with them together. They have a common history and nomenclatural origins, and similar clinical and pathological pictures. The taxonomic relationships between some of their causative agents are also similar (see also Volume 2, Chapters 20 and 21).

The history of actinomycoses dates back to the early days of bacteriology. In 1877, the German veterinarian Otto Bollinger found that the tumorous lesions of a chronically destructive disease of the jaws of cattle, which had been thought of as a kind of sarcoma, contained small, opaque, yellowish, granular particles. Because their structure resembled a cluster of crystals these were called 'Drusen', and they were composed of finely filamentous, branching, fungus-like structures subsequently characterized as being gram-positive. The botanist Carl O Harz (1877) considered it to be a new mould and proposed the genus and species designation *Actinomyces bovis* (ray fungus, from Greek aktis = ray; mykes = fungus) referring to the striking radial arrangement of filaments in the granules. He also introduced the term 'actinomycosis' for the animal disease.

The first detailed description of similar pathological conditions in man was published by the Berlin surgeon James Israel in 1878. Some 10 years later it was realized that the most characteristic human pathogens, now called *Actinomyces israelii* or *Actinomyces gerencseriae*, and the animal pathogen *A. bovis* were anaerobes or at least facultatively anaerobic capnophils (Bujwid 1889, Mosselman and Lienaux 1890). Only several decades later it was accepted that the causative agents of human and bovine actinomycoses were separate species, that they were true, but filamentous, bacteria and not fungi, and that they were the first representatives of a large and heterogeneous group of the bacterial kingdom now called Actinomycetales or simply 'actinomycetes'.

Lignières and Spitz (1902) described a new disease in cattle in Argentina that clinically and pathologically mimicked bovine actinomycosis. The organisms cultured from the respective lesions were tiny, short, gram-negative bacterial rods and differed markedly from *A. bovis*. Because of the similarities between the clinical pictures of the 2 diseases the pathogen was at first named 'l'actinobacille' and then validly designated *Actinobacillus lignieresii* (Brumpt 1910).

Before the anaerobic nature of the causative agents of human and bovine actinomycoses had been appreciated, many attempts were made to grow the organisms aerobically. In an extensive study of human and bovine cases of actinomycosis Bostroem (1891) isolated filamentous micro-organisms on aerobic gelatin or agar media, which he regarded as the pathogen, which he called '*Actinomyces bovis*'. He observed an awn of grain at the centre of an actinomycotic lesion and he cultured analogous aerobic filamentous microbes from grasses, grains and other vegetable materials. Bostroem therefore concluded that grasses or grains were the exogenous sources of actinomycotic infections and that chewing grasses or grains could give rise to actinomycotic lesions. This belief continued even after Naeslund (1925, 1931) had shown that *A. israelii* was a member of the indigenous human oral microflora that did not occur in the environment, so that the source of actinomycoses was always endogenous.

This was also due in part to the fact that towards the end of the last century several authors identified pathogenic aerobic actinomycetes similar to the agents of actinomycosis and the isolates of Bostroem. Nocard (1888) described an aerobic filamentous micro-organism from 'farcin du boeuf', a disease of cattle on Guadeloupe Island; it was named *Nocardia farcinica* by Trevisan (1889). A similar branching bacterium was cultured from a human lung infection by Eppinger (1891) and it was subsequently designated *Nocardia asteroides* by Blanchard (1896). Yet another filamentous branching bacterium at first labelled '*Streptothrix madurae*' was isolated by Vincent (1894) from the tumorous lesions of a disease in India and called Madura foot. This organism was later named '*Nocardia madurae*' and is now known as *Actinomadura madurae* (Lechevalier and Lechevalier 1970).

Numerous additional genera and species of aerobic and anaerobic actinomycetes have been described since Bollinger's report. Most are harmless inhabitants of various environmental habitats or the body surfaces of man and animals, and some play or may play a role as human or animal pathogens. This is true not only for several members of the traditional genera *Actinomyces* and *Nocardia*, but also for species of the genera *Bifidobacterium*, *Propionibacterium*, *Oerskovia*, *Gordona*, *Rhodococcus*, *Tsukamurella*, *Actinomadura*, *Nocardiopsis*, *Streptomyces*, *Dermatophilus*, *Thermoactinomyces*, *Saccharopolyspora* (*Faenia*), *Saccharomonospora* and *Thermomonospora*. Despite the growing spectrum of actinomycete pathogens, it does not make good sense to introduce, in addition to actinomycosis, nocardiosis, dermatophilosis, numerous further aetiological designations such as propionibacteriosis, rhodococcosis, tsukamurellosis and so forth. On the other hand, for the sake of clarity it is not wise to use the term actinomycosis for any type of actinomycete infection, as was common practice in the past. Similarly, the term nocardiosis covers neither all types of nocardial infections nor the infections caused by other aerobic actinomycetes. Thus, the classical disease designations actinomycosis and nocardiosis should be reserved for specific, clinically and aetiologically well characterized disease entities.

2 DISEASES CAUSED BY FERMENTATIVE ACTINOMYCETES

Carbohydrate fermenting anaerobic or capnophilic actinomycetes are aetiologically involved in a variety of different diseases in humans and animals. Among these, actinomycosis is the most characteristic disease entity. Additional illnesses that may be caused by fermentative actinomycetes are dental caries and periodontal disease, lacrimal canaliculitis and other eye infections, infections associated with the use of intra-uterine contraceptive devices and vaginal pessaries, and various non-specific inflammatory processes in humans, as well as mastitis, peritonitis, pleuritis, septic abortion, abscesses and various suppurative lesions in animals.

2.1 Actinomycoses

Actinomycosis is a subacute to chronic, granulomatous disease that usually gives rise to suppuration and abscess formation, tends to produce draining sinus tracts, and occurs in man and animals. In addition to the classical pathogens *A. bovis* and *A. israelii*, a variety of other fermentative actinomycetes may produce actinomycotic lesions. The majority of these agents belong to the genus *Actinomyces*, but a few are members of the genera *Propionibacterium* or *Bifidobacterium*. Furthermore, essentially all the typical actinomycotic lesions contain bacteria in addition to the pathogenic actinomycetes. Thus, the term 'actinomycosis' defines a polyaetiological inflammatory infection, rather than a disease attributable to a single pathogen. In order to avoid the introduction of additional or complementary aetiological designations and to remain linguistically and bacteriologically correct, it is appropriate to refer to this group of closely related inflammatory processes as 'actinomycoses' in the plural (Schaal and Beaman 1984, Schaal 1996).

HUMAN ACTINOMYCOSES

In spite of considerable similarities in pathology, pathogenesis and epidemiology, human and animal actinomycoses differ from each other in several important respects. Different actinomycete species are responsible for human and animal infections, and bone involvement is rare in man but usual in animals (Slack and Gerencser 1975).

Clinical manifestations

The initial actinomycotic lesion develops preferentially in tissue adjacent to the mucous membranes that are the natural habitats of the causative agents. The sites of predilection are cervicofacial, thoracic and abdominal. Rarely, skin, bone, or central nervous system may also be involved (Slack and Gerencser 1975, Pulverer and Schaal 1984, Schaal and Beaman 1984, Schaal and Pulverer 1984, Schaal 1996). Once the pathogens are established in tissue, the infection tends to progress slowly without regard to natural organ limits. Haematogenous spread is occasionally observed so that the central nervous system (brain abscess) or natural cavities (empyema) may be involved. There is a characteristic tendency to remission and exacerbation of symptoms with and without antibiotic treatment. Since human actinomycoses are endogenous infections, it is difficult or impossible to define an incubation period. It is believed to take about 4 weeks until the first clinical symptoms appear but numerous reports suggest that it may also be much longer or considerably shorter.

Cervicofacial actinomycoses The vast majority of actinomycotic infections involve the face, neck or both face and neck, the so-called cervicofacial area (data collected in Germany; see Table 39.1), but the figures appear to be different in other geographical areas, in particular from the USA (see section on 'Epidemiology', p. 781).

Actinomycotic lesions are often preceded by a history of dental decay, tooth extraction, jaw fracture, periodontal abscess, penetration of the mucosa by foreign bodies (bone splinters, fish bones, awns of grass or grain) or tonsillar suppuration. Trauma and local or general predisposing conditions are not necessarily present or may be overlooked.

The cervicofacial sites primarily involved in 317 patients were tissue adjacent to the body of the mandible (53.6%), cheek (16.4%), chin (13.3%), submaxillary ramus and angle (10.7%), maxilla (5.7%) and the mandibular joint (0.3%) (Herzog 1981). Other sites that may occasionally be affected are neck, mastoid, sinuses, parotid gland, thyroid gland, tongue, lips, nasal septum and ears (Slack and Gerencser 1975, Kingdom and Tami 1994). Direct invasion of the bone and regional lymph nodes is very rare, but periostitis may develop and post-traumatic osteomyelitis with the presence of fermentative actinomycetes is not uncommon (11.7% of the cases reported by Herzog 1981).

Primary actinomycotic cervicofacial lesions present either as acute, predominantly odontogenic abscesses, as highly acute forms of cellulitis of the floor of the mouth, or as slowly emerging, hard, reddish or livid inflammatory infiltrations (Lentze 1969, Pulverer and Schaal 1978, Schaal 1979, 1981, 1996). Whereas the latter are usually painless, the more acute infections are painful and both may lead to lockjaw when localized in the masseteric area or near the temporomandibular joint.

Surgical incision and drainage are sufficient in only a few cases to initiate rapid and complete healing. Acute and particularly chronic cases tend not to heal without specific antibiotic therapy. At best there is temporary regression of symptoms and relapses are common after weeks or months. The longer both forms of actinomycosis persist, the more they develop analogous and very characteristic late symptoms. These include regression and cicatrization of central suppurative foci, progression of hard, painless, livid infiltrations at the periphery, formation of multiple areas of liquefaction and development of draining sinus tracts (Fig. 39.1). The latter emerge spontaneously or follow surgical incision and, together with the multiple abscesses, form a multilocular system of cavities in the affected tissue which responds poorly to conventional treatment including administration of 'standard' antibiotics and shows a pronounced tendency to recur after temporary spontaneous regression of the inflammatory symptoms. Without treatment or with inappropriate treatment, cervicofacial actinomycoses progress slowly, even across organ borders, and may become life-threatening by extension to the cranial cavity, the mediastinum or by invasion of the bloodstream (Herzog et al. 1984).

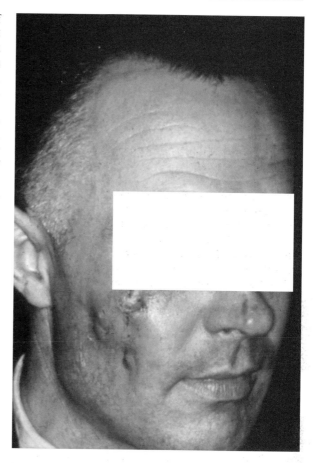

Fig. 39.1 Cervicofacial actinomycosis in a male patient age 45 years with multiple fresh and older abscesses, fistulation through non-healing incision wounds, and central scar formation.

Sinus discharge and pus from abscesses are usually yellowish and thick to serous and often contain the particles originally called 'Drusen' but now more usually referred to as 'sulphur granules'.

Thoracic actinomycoses It remains to be clarified whether there may be regional or continental differences in the incidence of the various forms of human actinomycoses. However, thoracic manifestations occur more rarely than the cervicofacial form (Table 39.1). The former usually follow aspiration of material from the oral cavity, such as dental plaque or calculus, tonsillar crypt contents, or a foreign body contaminated with oral flora including the pathogenic actinomycetes. Occasionally, this form of disease develops by local descent of a cervicofacial actinomycotic infection, by perforation of the diaphragm from an abdominal lesion, or by haematogenous spread from any distant focus (Slack and Gerencser 1975).

Primarily thoracic actinomycoses may present as a mediastinal tumour or a bronchopneumonic infiltrate, necrotizing pneumonia or lung abscess (Slack and Gerencser 1975, Schaal and Beaman 1984, Morris and Sewell 1994). Radiographs show single dense or multiple spotted shadows in which cavitations may develop (Fig. 39.2). In more advanced cases the main

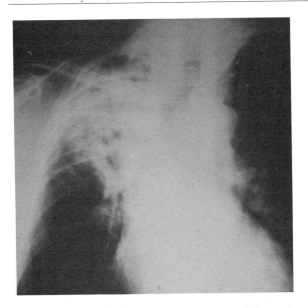

Fig. 39.2 Radiograph of pulmonary actinomycosis in a male patient age 62 years with spotted shadows in the upper field of the right lung. The patient had been treated for advanced bronchial carcinoma until a huge subcutaneous abscess developed on the right shoulder from which *A. israelii* and a characteristic concomitant flora were cultured.

symptoms are chest pain, fever, cough with or without sputum and weight loss, but haemoptysis is unusual. During its further course, the infection may progress to pleural empyema, pericarditis, or involvement of the chest wall. If diagnosis is delayed or treatment is inadequate, late symptoms may include extensive subcutaneous chest wall and paravertebral or psoas abscesses that may occasionally point in the groin and discharge pus with large amounts of sulphur granules.

Abdominal actinomycoses Actinomycotic infections of the abdominal organs and the anorectal area are uncommon (Table 39.1). Their development is associated with acute visceral perforation (appendicitis, diverticulitis, cryptitis, various ulcerative diseases) and surgical or accidental trauma, including injury by ingested bone splinters or fish bones.

Table 39.1 Localization of human actinomycoses[a]

Body site involved	Cases	
	Number	%
Cervicofacial area	3249	97.6
Thoracic organs including chest wall	43	1.3
Abdominal organs including small pelvis	22	0.7
Extremities, skin	9	0.3
Brain	4	0.1
Blood[b]	2	0.06
Totals	3329	100.0

[a]Data collected at the Institute of Hygiene, University of Cologne, 1969–84, and at the Institute for Medical Microbiology and Immunology, University of Bonn, 1984–95.
[b]Blood cultures in patients with signs of septicaemia.

Another source of pelvic and abdominal actinomycete infections has recently been identified. In 10–20% of women with intrauterine contraceptive devices (IUCDs) or vaginal pessaries the uterus and the cervical canal are colonized by a mixed bacterial flora that includes potentially pathogenic fermentative actinomycetes (Gupta, Hollander and Frost 1976, Gupta, Erozan and Frost 1978, Eibach et al. 1989, 1992, Schaal and Lee 1992, Chatwani and Amin-Hanjani 1994) and other predominantly anaerobic bacteria (Schaal and Lee 1992). They are present in only minute numbers or not at all in women who do not use these devices. Rarely, this colonization may serve as initial focus for the development of invasive genital or pelvic actinomycoses and may even induce metastatic hepatic or cranial actinomycotic abscesses (Gupta, Erozan and Frost 1978).

The initial symptoms of abdominal actinomycoses are usually mild and non-specific. They include fever, malaise, weakness and pain that increase slowly but progressively. More advanced cases predominantly present as slowly growing tumours that mimic malignant processes, such as carcinoma of the stomach, colon, rectum, the anorectal area or the uterine cervix (Stein and Schaal 1984, Schaal 1985b, Ewig et al. 1993, Alvarado-Cerna and Bracho-Riquelme 1994, Skoutelis et al. 1995). Large subcutaneous abscesses, extensive livid indurations, or draining fistulae that discharge sulphur granules are often the first indication of the nature of the disease (Schaal and Beaman 1984). Without effective treatment abdominal actinomycoses may extend to any adjacent tissue or organ including liver, spleen, kidney, fallopian tubes, ovaries, uterus, testes, bladder, rectum, or abdominal wall (Slack and Gerencser 1975, Khalaff, Srigley and Klotz 1995, Müller-Holzner et al. 1995).

Actinomycoses of the central nervous system Actinomycoses of the brain and the spinal cord are very rare, possibly because of the more effective treatment now available which protects from haematogenous spread or direct extension of the infection (Table 39.1). These mechanisms are predominantly responsible for the development of the CNS involvement, especially when the primary lesion is located in the lungs or in abdominal organs (Slack and Gerencser 1975, Jamjoom, Jamjoom and al-Hedaithy 1994).

The principal manifestation of CNS actinomycoses is brain abscess. The symptoms depend on localization and they result from growth and displacement as well as tissue destruction. Common symptoms are headache, raised intracranial pressure, focal seizures, hemiparesis, aphasia, ataxia and abnormal reflexes (Slack and Gerencser 1975).

Actinomycoses of bone and skin In contrast to certain animals, osseous involvement is rare in human actinomycoses (Table 39.1). It usually results from direct extension of the infection from an adjacent soft tissue focus. This leads to periostitis, which stimulates new bone formation that is visible upon radiography. More advanced cases present as localized areas of bone destruction surrounded by increased bone density; mandible, ribs and spine are most frequently involved. Actinomycotic infections of other bones have been described, but usually not confirmed by bacteriological culture.

Cutaneous actinomycoses are extremely rare (Table 39.1). They mostly result from wounds contaminated with saliva or dental plaque material, either by human bites or as a consequence of fist-fight traumata. Haematogenous spread to the skin may also occur. The clinical picture of cutaneous or wound actinomycoses is very similar to that of the cervicofacial form.

Epidemiology

The bacterial species that may be cultured from human actinomycotic lesions belong essentially to the resident or transient indigenous microflora of the human mucous membranes. Thus, apart from 'punch actinomycoses' after human bites or fist-fight injuries, the disease is always endogenous in origin and is therefore subject to neither epidemic outbreaks nor transmission in the usual sense. Sporadic actinomycoses occur world wide.

The incidence of actinomycotic processes, however, appears to vary from continent to continent, from country to country, or even from region to region, possibly reflecting varying standards of dental care and differences in the amount and types of antibiotics used. Such factors may explain the lower absolute and relative incidence of cervicofacial actinomycoses in the USA compared with Europe, but not the apparently higher prevalence of thoracic and abdominal infections on the North American continent.

On the basis of histological findings, Hemmes (1963) calculated an incidence of actinomycotic infections in the Netherlands of 1 per 119 000 inhabitants per year. For the Cologne area of Germany up to 1969, Lentze (1969) reported a morbidity rate of 1 per 83 000. This incidence for 1970–85 was recalculated and found to range from 1 per 40 000 (acute and chronic cases together) to 1 per 80 000 (solely chronic cases) per year (Schaal 1979). This is considerably higher than the prevalence reported from other German regions and from other European countries. These differences are difficult to explain but may be related to local variations in diagnostic efficiency rather than to true epidemiological differences.

It has long been known (Slack and Gerencser 1975, Pulverer and Schaal 1978, Schaal 1981, Schaal and Beaman 1984) that characteristic actinomycoses occur 2.5–3.0 times more often in males than in females. Schaal and Pulverer (1984) assumed that this sex ratio was chiefly attributable to the uneven distribution of *A. israelii* infections, which at that time included *A. israelii* and *A. gerencseriae* infections. However, a more detailed analysis (Schaal and Lee 1992) appears to indicate that several species such as *A. israelii*, *A. gerencseriae*, *Actinomyces naeslundii*, *Actinomyces viscosus*, *Propionibacterium propionicum* and *Corynebacterium matruchotii* may contribute to this gender ratio when only characteristic actinomycotic abscesses or empyemas are included in the evaluation.

Furthermore, the epidemiological data appear to show that the uneven sex distribution of the disease is restricted to sexually mature patients. Before puberty and in the climacteric, actinomycoses appears to be evenly distributed

between the sexes (Pulverer and Schaal 1978, Schaal 1981). This suggests that the disease can occur in all age groups (Slack and Gerencser 1975, Pulverer and Schaal 1978, Schaal 1981). Among the author's patients, the youngest one was 1.5 months and the oldest one 89 years old. Nevertheless, the highest incidence of actinomycosis has been observed in males of 21–40 years and in females aged 11–30 years (Pulverer and Schaal 1978, Schaal 1981, 1992, Schaal and Beaman 1984).

Pathology and pathogenesis

The initial stage of the acute disease is an inflammatory process that leads to abscess formation or, if chronic, to simultaneous connective tissue proliferation and formation of multiple small abscesses. More advanced processes are characterized by cicatricial tissue in the centre with granulation tissue at the periphery, the latter interspersed with multiple suppurative foci or cavities and 3-dimensional reticulated sinus tracts. Rarely, when bone is involved osteoclastic and osteoblastic changes may be present.

Sulphur granules can be found embedded in the suppurative foci. They may also be present in abscess contents or sinus discharges in about 25% of the cases and are of great diagnostic importance. The granules are up to 1 mm in diameter and visible to the eye. They are yellowish to reddish to brownish particles that, when derived from human infections, exhibit a cauliflower-like appearance under the microscope at low magnifications (Fig. 39.3, see also plate 39.3). Under the microscope after gentle pressure between slide and cover-slip they are composed of varying numbers of spherical segments that represent filamentous actinomycete microcolonies formed in vivo and account for the cauliflower-like structure of the whole particle. The latter is surrounded by tissue reaction material, especially polymorphonuclear granulocytes.

Completely crushed and gram-stained granules at high magnification reveal that the material consists of clusters of gram-positive, interwoven branching filaments with regularly arranged peripheral hyphae. The stained smears may also contain a variety of other gram-positive and gram-negative rods and cocci that represent the concomitant flora, and numerous leucocytes. Predominantly in tissue sections, and less frequently in purulent discharge, the tips of peripheral filaments in the granule are covered by a club-shaped layer of hyaline material which may aid in the differentiation of actinomycotic sulphur granules from similar particles of various other microbial and non-microbial origin. In haematoxylin–eosin stained tissue sections, when properly in focus, the clubs are eosinophilic at high magnification and have a basically stained filament at their centre. It must be emphasized that the term 'sulphur granules' relates only to the yellow colour of the particles and not to a high sulphur content.

The principal natural habitat of all the fermentative actinomycetes pathogenic to humans is the oral cavity of healthy adults where they occur in considerable numbers. In the digestive and genital tracts, however, they appear to be present only sporadically or in low numbers. The same is true for the oral cavity of babies before teething and of edentulous adults. This may explain the preference of the disease for the cervico-facial area and the comparatively low incidence in very young and very old patients.

The low incidence of the disease as compared with the universal occurrence in human adults of its causative agents is apparently due to requirements for tissue invasion that are more complex than a simple integumental defect. Such conditions consist of local host tissue alterations at the site of entry rather than defective function of the general immune system. In this respect, an indispensable prerequisite for the establishment of fermentative actinomycetes in the host tissues is a negative redox potential on which the pathogenic actinomycetes and many accompanying bacteria depend. Such a local reduction of oxygen tension may be due either to impaired blood circulation resulting from circulatory or vascular disease, crush injury or foreign bodies, or to the reducing and necrotizing capacity of other simultaneously present microbes.

These so-called 'concomitant microbes' are predominantly bacteria that act as the trigger of the actinomycotic process by producing anaerobic conditions. In addition, they amplify the relatively low invasive power of the pathogenic fermentative actinomycetes by providing aggressive enzymes, such as hyaluronidases, and toxins. Thus, actinomycoses are almost always synergistic mixed infections in which the actinomyetes are the specific component, the so-called 'guiding' organisms, responsible for the course and delayed symptoms of the disease. The species composition of the concomitant flora varies from case to case, but it is always present, and is often responsible for the initial clinical picture and for some complications.

The species of fermentative actinomycetes that are able to produce typical actinomycotic lesions in humans are summarized in Table 39.2. *A. israelii* and *A. gerencseriae* have been identified most frequently, but the frequency of the latter is an underestimate because it has only been routinely separated from *A. israelii* since 1987. The third pathogen to be able to produce human actinomycoses is *P. propionicum* but it is not frequently encountered. Previously classified as 'Arachnia propionica' (Schaal 1986), it has recently been transferred to the genus *Propionibacterium* on the basis of 16S rRNA sequence similarities (Charfreitag, Collins and Stackebrandt 1988). It was not always easy to decide whether the other actinomycetes mentioned in Table 39.2 are significant pathogens or members of a mixed bacterial flora without special significance.

The concomitant actinomycotic flora may consist of aerobic as well as anaerobic species. In more than 50 % of the cases examined by the author, the concomitant organisms consisted exclusively of anaerobes (Table 39.3). In the remaining cases, strict anaerobes and facultative anaerobes or aerobes were found. On average, 2–4 concomitant species were present, but on occasion up to 10 may be encountered.

Among the aerobic concomitants (Table 39.3) coagulase-negative staphylococci, *Staphylococcus aureus*, α-haemolytic and β-haemolytic streptococci were the most prevalent. The anaerobic and capnophilic concomitant flora is far more diverse and numerous. Particularly pronounced synergistic interactions seem to exist between *A. israelii* and *A. gerencseriae*, and *Actinobacillus* (*Haemophilus*) *actinomycetemcomitans*. The name of the latter organism, which refers to its characteristic association with the actinomycetes, is often responsible for a particularly chronic course of the disease and for treatment failures. It may sustain the inflammatory process with similar symptoms even after chemotherapy has eliminated the actinomycete. Other common actinomycete companions are black pigmented Bacteroidaceae (*Prevotella* spp., *Porphyromonas* spp.), non-pigmented *Prevotella* and *Bacteroides* spp., fusobacteria, so-called micro-aerophilic streptococci that belong chiefly to the species *Streptococcus anginosus* (*milleri*), propionibacteria and *Eikenella corrodens* (Table 39.4).

Little is known about the humoral and cellular immune responses of patients suffering from actinomycosis. Antibodies against fermentative actinomycetes may be demonstrated in human sera by various techniques, including immunofluorescence methods and immunoassays. Most of these antibodies react more actively with antigens from *A. naeslundii* and *A. viscosus* than with those from *A. israelii*, *A. gerencseriae*, or *P. propionicum*. Furthermore, they are mostly related to periodontal disease and only rarely to previous or existing invasive actinomycotic infection. Thus, it appears that the antibody response to naturally occurring human actinomycoses is either insignificant or only sporadic. Furthermore, the antibodies probably have no protective effect against actinomycosis and their presence is no indication of a self-limiting tendency of the disease.

It has, however, long been known (Lentze 1938) that the immune system of patients with actinomycosis can be stimulated by the injection of formalin-killed cells or cell extracts of pathogenic actinomycetes. This may lead to the formation of antibodies that can be measured by methods such as complement fixation. More importantly, however, the immune response of patients after the injection of *Actinomyces* antigens is evident as the so-called focal reaction. This is a temporary exacerbation of the inflammatory reaction after the initial injections of the antigen. After repeated injections, the immune response helps to overcome the disease. These observations form the basis for the vaccine treatment of actinomyosis that was in use before antimicrobial therapy (Lentze 1938, 1969).

Diagnosis

The diagnosis of human actinomycoses is chiefly based upon the isolation and identification of the causative agents because symptoms are often misleading and histopathology and serology lack specificity and sensitivity.

The presence of sulphur granules that occasionally gives the pus an appearance of semolina soup should initiate a search for actinomycetes. However, since only 25% of samples of actinomycotic pus contain

Table 39.2   Species of fermentative actinomycetes isolated from human actinomycotic lesions[a]

Species/groups identified	Specimens derived from					
	Actinomycotic lesions		IUCD-associated conditions		Eye, tear organs	
	n^a	%	n	%	n	%
Actinomyces israelii[b]	1009	73.3	62	54.4	13	13.3
A. gerencseriae[b]	28	2.0	8	7.0	11	11.2
A. naeslundii	94	6.8	7	6.1	16	16.3
A. viscosus	68	4.9	19	16.7	19	19.4
A. odontolyticus	19	1.4	3	2.6	12	12.2
A. meyeri	8	0.6	4	3.5	0	0.0
A. georgiae[c]	2	0.2	0	0.0	0	0.0
A. neuii[c]	2	0.2	0	0.0	0	0.0
Propionibacterium propionicum	46	3.3	5	4.4	16	16.3
Bifidobacterium dentium	5	0.4	3	2.6	2	2.2
Corynebacterium matruchotii	12	0.9	0	0.0	2	2.2
Rothia dentocariosa	5	0.4	1	0.6	5	5.1
Not identified under routine conditions	78	5.7	2	2.0	2	2.0
Totals	1376	100.0	114	100.0	98	100.0

[a]Data collected at the Institute of Hygiene, University of Cologne, 1969–84, and at the Institute for Medical Microbiology and Immunology, Univeristy of Bonn, 1984–95.
[b]Differentiation between *A. israelii* and *A. gerencseriae* was not performed routinely before 1987.
[c]Recently described new species.

Table 39.3   Aerobically grown micro-organisms associated with fermentative actinomycetes in human clinical specimens

Species/groups identified	Specimens derived from					
	Cervicofacial actinomycoses		IUCD-associated conditions		Eye, tear organs	
	n^a	%	n	%	n	%
No aerobic growth	1509	47.2	26	32.1	2	6.7
Coagulase-negative staphylococci	891	27.9	12	14.8	12	40.0
Staphylococcus aureus	405	12.7	5	6.2	3	10.0
α-Haemolytic streptococci	357	11.2	9	11.1	14	46.8
β-Haemolytic streptococci	157	4.9	9	11.1	4	13.3
Streptococcus pneumoniae	0	0.0	0	0.0	3	10.0
Enterococci	0	0.0	13	16.1	0	0.0
Cutaneous corynebacteria	0	0.0	3	3.7	3	10.0
Haemophilus spp.[b]	3	0.1	1	1.2	4	13.3
Enterobacteriaceae	81	2.5	11	13.6	2	6.7
Gardnerella vaginalis	0	0.0	5	6.2	0	0.0
Non-fermenters	6	0.2	0	0.0	2	6.7
Yeasts	3	0.1	0	0.0	0	0.0
Total number of cases	3197	100.0	81	100.0	30	100.0

[a]n, number of isolates/cases; the percentage is related to the totals given in the bottom line.
[b]Other than *Actinobacillus (Haemophilus) actinomycetemcomitans*.
Modified from Schaal and Lee (1992).

these granules, their absence does not exclude a diagnosis of actinomycosis.

Collection and transport of specimens   Specimens suitable for the bacteriological diagnosis of human actinomycoses are pus, sinus discharge, bronchial secretions, granulation tissue and biopsy specimens. During sample collection, precautions must be taken against contamination with the indigenous mucosal flora. Whenever possible, pus or tissue should be obtained by transcutaneous puncture or transcutaneous needle biopsy.

For the diagnosis of thoracic actinomycoses, bronchial secretions should be obtained by transtracheal aspiration. Sputum is inappropriate because it usually contains oral actinomycetes, including the pathogenic

Table 39.4 Anaerobically grown micro-organisms associated with fermentative actinomycetes in human clinical specimens

Species/groups identified	Specimens derived from					
	Cervicofacial actinomycoses		IUCD-associated conditions		Eye, tear organs	
	n^a	%	n	%	n	%
Actinobacillus actinomycetemcomitans	731	22.9	2	2.5	0	0.0
Micro-aerophilic streptococci[b]	937	29.3	18	22.2	6	20.0
Peptostreptococcus spp.	583	18.2	2.4	29.6	1	3.3
Black pigmented Bacteroidaceae	1204	37.7	47	58.0	4	13.3
Non-pigmented *Bacteroides/Prevotella* spp.	446	14.0	56	69.1	6	20.0
Fusobacterium spp.	1040	32.5	18	22.2	4	13.3
Leptotrichia buccalis	653	20.4	2	2.5	1	3.3
Eikenella corrodens	527	16.5	38	46.9	0	0.0
Capnocytophaga spp.	14	0.4	5	6.2	1	3.3
Campylobacter/Selenomonas spp.	1	0.1	3	3.7	0	0.0
Propionibacterium spp.[c]	974	30.5	20	24.7	9	30.0
Bifidobacterium spp.[d]	2	0.1	1	1.2	2	6.7
Lactobacillus spp.	17	0.5	34	42.0	1	3.3
Total number of cases	3197	100.0	81	100.0	30	100.0

[a]n, number of isolates/cases; the percentage is related to the totals given in the bottom line.
[b]Streptococci that grow best under increased CO_2 concentration.
[c]Other than *P. propionicum.*
[d]Other than *B. dentium.*
Modified from Schaal and Lee (1992).

species. Transthoracic percutaneous needle biopsy or percutaneous puncture of suspected abdominal abscesses is often the only means of obtaining satisfactory samples for diagnosis.

The transport of specimens to the bacteriological laboratory should be expeditious. If a prolonged transportation is unavoidable, a reducing medium such as one of the modifications of Stewart's transport medium should be used, though fermentative actinomycetes are less susceptible than strict anaerobes to oxidative damage.

Microscopic examination of specimens When sulphur granules are present, they allow a rapid and comparatively reliable tentative diagnosis after inspection of a slide under a cover-slip at low magnification ($\times 100$) after embedding in a drop of 1% methylene blue. Actinomycete sulphur granules appear as cauliflower-like particles with an unstained centre and a blue periphery in which leucocytes and short filaments, possibly with clubs, radiate from the centre of the granule (Fig. 39.3, see also plate 39.3). Gram-stained smears of the granules obtained by crushing between 2 slides reveal characteristic filamentous, branched, gram-positive structures that represent the pathogenic actinomycetes, and a variety of other gram-negative and gram-positive bacteria that indicate the presence of concomitant bacteria. Demonstration of the latter is necessary to distinguish actinomycotic sulphur granules from granules formed by various aerobic actinomycetes (*Nocardia, Actinomadura, Streptomyces*) that never contain a concomitant flora. By means of direct or indirect fluorescent antibody techniques, it may be possible without culture to identify to species level the actinomycete present in the granule. The antigenetic heterogeneity of the causative agents of actinomycosis may, however, lead to the correct diagnosis being missed.

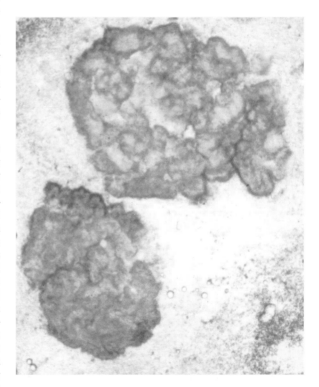

Fig. 39.3 Micrograph ($\times 400$) of 2 sulphur granules showing the typical cauliflower-like structure. The granules are surrounded by a thick layer of inflammatory cells, in particular polymorphonuclear granulocytes. See plate 39.3 for colour.

Bacteriological culture To obtain reliable results, it is indispensable to use transparent culture media so that the plates can be checked microscopically for characteristic filamentous colonies, and to incubate the cultures for at least 14 days. Cultures can be examined every 2–3 days without disturbing the anaerobic conditions if the method of Fortner (1928) is used to obtain a low oxygen tension. If anaerobic jars or chambers are used, 2 or 3 sets of culture media should be inoculated simultaneously and examined for actinomycete growth after 3, 7 and 14 days. Since removal of the plates from anaerobiosis usually inhibits further growth of the organisms, prolonged incubation requires that anaerobic conditions remain undisturbed.

Preliminary results of culture may be obtained after 2–3 days when characteristic spider-like microcolonies of *A. israelii*, *A. gerencseriae* or *P. propionicum* may be visible under the microscope. Confirmation of tentative microscopical or early cultural diagnoses by definitive identification of the pathogenic species may take 14 days or longer. This is indispensable to distinguish reliably between relevant fermentative actinomycetes and morphologically similar contaminants derived from the mucous membranes of the patient and similar aerobic actinomycetes of the genera *Nocardia*, *Actinomadura* and *Streptomyces*. Detailed bacteriological analysis of the concomitant flora may be helpful for the choice of appropriate antibiotic therapy.

Molecular techniques, such as gene probes or the polymerase chain reaction (PCR), to detect pathogenic fermentative actinomycetes in clinical specimens or the identification of clinical isolates are being developed and may allow more rapid diagnosis in the future.

Serological diagnosis Actinomycotic infections do not necessarily stimulate detectable humoral immune responses. Nevertheless, various serological techniques, including counter-immunoelectrophoresis, crossed immunoelectrophoresis, immunofluorescence, enzyme immunoassays, and agglutination and complement fixation tests, have been used to detect diagnostically relevant antibodies. None of these methods with any of a large variety of antigen preparations has provided satisfactory results, because of problems with sensitivity and specificity (Holmberg, Nord and Wadström 1975, Holmberg 1981, Persson and Holmberg 1985).

Treatment

Incision of actinomycotic lesions and drainage of pus have always formed the basis of treatment. However, it is well known that even radical surgery often only results in temporary cure of symptoms and may be followed by one or more relapses. Attempts in the past to overcome these difficulties by the application of substances such as iodides, thymol, copper sulphate, hydrogen peroxide, silver nitrate, and arsenicals, have not improved results. Only vaccination by subcutaneous injection of killed *Actinomyces* cells (heterovaccine of Lentze 1938) has been shown to be effective.

The treatment of actinomycoses was greatly improved when sulphonamides and penicillins became available. Pencillin G was active against the pathogenic actinomycetes in vitro and effective against the disease in vivo. Since many patients respond insufficiently or not at all to penicillin G, it was recommended that treatment should be with large doses of penicillin G for at least 3 months and up to 12–18 months (Harvey, Cantrell and Fisher 1957).

A poor response to penicillin G is often due to concomitant bacteria that are penicillin-resistant. Furthermore, drugs poorly penetrate the chronically indurated tissue of actinomycotic lesions and sulphur granules. Finally, *A. actinomycetemcomitans* is usually resistent to narrow spectrum penicillins although it does not produce a β-lactamase. Thus, penicillin G is effective only when *A. actinomycetemcomitans* is not present and when the concomitant flora does not contain any producer of β-lactamases.

Aminopenicillins are slightly more active than narrow spectrum penicillins against the pathogenic actinomycetes and they inhibit growth of *A. actinomycetemcomitans*. Since they are not resistant to β-lactamases, organisms that produce it may impair their therapeutic efficiency. This is rarely the case in cervicofacial actinomycoses, but in thoracic and especially abdominal infections β-lactamase producers are common. Current treatment schemes therefore include drugs effective against actinomycetes and potential β-lactamase producers such as *S. aureus*, gram-negative anaerobes, and, in cases of abdominal actinomycoses, Enterobacteriaceae.

Current recommendations for the antibiotic treatment of human actinomycoses are as follows: for cervicofacial actinomycoses, amoxycillin plus clavulanic acid or possibly ampicillin plus sulbactam are the treatment of choice. The initial dose is 3×2 g amoxycillin plus 3×0.2 g clavulanic acid per day for 1 week, and 3×1 g amoxycillin plus 3×0.1 g clavulanic acid per day for another week. Rarely, chronic cervicofacial infections may require up to 4 weeks of treatment. The regimen may suffice for thoracic actinomycoses, but the high dose continued for 3–4 weeks is recommended. In advanced chronic pulmonary cases an increased dose of ampicillin may be necessary to increase tissue levels and, depending on the concomitant flora, an aminoglycoside may be necessary if resistant Enterobacteriaceae such as *Klebsiella* spp. or *Enterobacter* spp. are present. The latter is generally the case in abdominal actinomycosis. The treatment of choice for these infections is a combination of amoxycillin and clavulanic acid with metronidazole (or clindamycin) for strict anaerobes plus tobramycin or gentamicin. Imipenem may be a suitable alternative but it has only rarely been used for actinomycotic infections (Edelmann et al. 1987).

It should be noted that neither metronidazole nor clindamycin can be used to treat actinomycotic infections without added antimicrobial agents, especially aminopenicillins, because clindamycin is almost ineffective against *A. actinomycetemcomitans* (Niederau et al. 1982, Schaal 1983, Schaal et al. 1984) and metronidazole is not active against the pathogenic actinomycetes (Schaal and Pape 1980, Niederau et al.1982). Patients allergic to penicillin may be treated with tetracyclines or cephalosporins instead of aminopenicillins, but the clinical efficacy of these drugs is much less than that of aminopenicillins or the combination of aminopenicillins with β-lactamase inhibitors.

Prognosis

Before the introduction of modern antibiotics the prognosis was uncertain to unfavourable. Even today, patients who have been inadequately treated may continue to suffer from actinomycosis for many years and may die from the disease or its complications. This is especially true for thoracic and abdominal infections, which are often diagnosed at a late stage. Provided the diagnosis is established early and antibiotic treatment is adequate, the prognosis of the cervicofacial and cutaneous actinomycotic infections is generally good. Thoracic, abdominal and systemic manifestations, however, remain serious and require energetic treatment.

2.2 Other infections caused by fermentative actinomycetes

Several other diseases may be due to fermentative actinomycetes but they differ significantly from typical actinomycotic lesions in terms of clinical picture, prognosis and treatment; they should not be subsumed under the term 'actinomycosis'. Nevertheless, some of them are clearly more important than actinomycosis from both medical and economic points of view.

Lacrimal canaliculitis and other eye infections

A common, non-invasive disease caused by fermentative actinomycetes is lacrimal canaliculitis with and without conjunctivitis. It is usually characterized by yellowish to brownish concretions within the canaliculus (Fig. 39.4, see also plate 39.4) and by pus in the inner corner of the eye. The most important actinomycetes involved are *P. propionicum, A. viscosus* and *A. israelii* (see Table 39.2). Less frequently, *A. naeslundii, A. gerencseriae,* and *Actinomyces odontolyticus* may be isolated (Schaal and Lee 1992). Concomitant bacteria are often, but not always, present. Their species composition is shown in Tables 39.3 and 39.4. Apart from the occurrence of *Streptococcus pneumoniae* or *Haemophilus influenzae* in the eye and *A. actinomycetemcomitans* in cervicofacial specimens, the concomitant flora at both sites is very similar.

Besides lacrimal canaliculitis, eye infections due to fermentative actinomycetes may also present as conjunctivitis, keratitis, dacryocystitis, hordeolum and even periorbital abscess or granuloma and intraocular infection (Schaal 1986, Schaal and Lee 1992). The specific diagnosis of lacrimal canaliculitis and other actinomycete eye infections is by the bacteriological procedures mentioned above. Removal of the lacrimal concretions that are usually present in canaliculitis and local application of antibiotics almost always result in prompt cure when the condition is localized non-invasive disease. Invasive infections (abscesses, granulomas, intraocular infections) require systemic treatment with suitable antibacterial drugs.

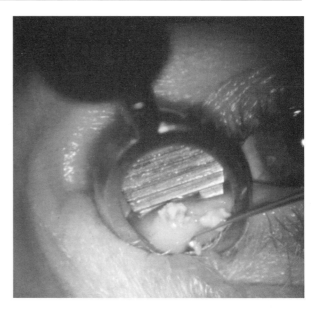

Fig. 39.4 Lacrimal concretions consisting chiefly of branched actinomycete filaments that appear in the aperture of the lacrimal duct on pressure. See plate 39.4 for colour.

IUCD-associated conditions

As we have seen in relation to abdominal actinomycoses (see section on 'Abdominal actinomycoses', p. 780), the uterus and cervical canal of women with intrauterine contraceptive devices (IUCDs) or vaginal pessaries is frequently colonized by a complex bacterial flora that consists of fermentative actinomycetes and various other aerobic and anaerobic bacteria (Eibach et al. 1989, Schaal and Lee 1992). These microbes are particularly abundant along the thread of the IUCD within the cervical canal and they closely resemble the characteristic polymicrobial flora of actinomycotic lesions. The predominant actinomycete under these circumstances is *A. israelii; A. viscosus* is also comparatively common and other species have occasionally been identified (see Table 39.2).

The concomitant flora in these cases is very similar, but not identical, to that of cervicofacial actinomycoses (see Tables 39.3 and 39.4). Of the aerobic bacteria (Table 39.3) enterococci, Enterobacteriaceae and *Gardnerella vaginalis* are found alone or more frequently in IUCD specimens. As far as anaerobes and capnophils (Table 39.4) are concerned, the much lower frequency of *A. actinomycetemcomitans* and the even lower frequency of fusobacteria in IUCD specimens should be noted, whereas non-pigmented species of *Bacteroides* and *Prevotella, E. corrodens* and lactobacilli are isolated more frequently from IUCD specimens than from cervicofacial actinomycoses.

The presence of fermentative actinomycetes and characteristic concomitant bacteria on the intrauterine contraceptive device and in the cervical canal is not necessarily associated with symptoms and is not an indication of invasive actinomycotic infection that needs specific treatment. However, about 28% of the patients with actinomycetes in the cervical canal or on the IUCD exhibit signs of infection of the lower genital tract and another 26% have infection of the upper genital tract (Eibach et al. 1989, 1992). Symptoms, such as fever, pain or vaginal discharge, usually disappear within 4–8 weeks after removal of the IUCD at least in lower genital tract infections.

When a typical actinomycotic flora is found on an IUCD or in the cervical canal, use of the IUCD should be discontinued until the flora has disappeared as shown by bacteriological examinations of cervical swabs. After the flora has returned to normal, intrauterine contraceptive devices can be used again without increased risk of genital actinomycosis.

FURTHER SUPPURATIVE HUMAN INFECTIONS

Fermentative actinomycetes may cause other nonspecific inflammatory processes. These include pharyngitis, otitis, urethritis, funisitis (Wright et al. 1994), cutaneous and subcutaneous suppurative lesions, abscesses with or without an associated mixed anaerobic flora, empyema and septicaemia (Schaal 1986).

These infections may be due to 'classical' *Actinomyces* spp., such as *A. naeslundii*, *A. viscosus*, *A. odontolyticus* and *Actinomyces meyeri*. However, several other *Actinomyces* spp. and *Arcanobacterium haemolyticum* also appear to be important. These *Actinomyces* spp. are *Actinomyces pyogenes* as well as the new taxa *Actinomyces neuii* subsp. *neuii*, *Actinomyces neuii* subsp. *anitratus* (Funke et al. 1994), *Actinomyces bernardiae* (Funke et al. 1995), *Actinomyces radingae* and *Actinomyces turicensis* (Wüst et al. 1995).

3 DISEASES CAUSED BY ACTINOMYCETES WITH AN OXIDATIVE CARBOHYDRATE METABOLISM

Aerobic actinomycetes with an oxidative type of carbohydrate metabolism constitute a large and very heterogeneous group of filamentous bacteria (see also Volume 2, Chapter 21). They are widely distributed in nature, in particular in the soil, and many play a significant role in the turnover of organic matter. Only a few of these free-living organisms have gained medical importance as infective agents or as sources of potent allergens.

Depending on the actinomycete species involved, its portal and mechanism of entry, and the host's immune status, aerobic actinomycetes may produce a variety of diseases in man and animals. Furthermore, it has only recently been appreciated that these microbes may cause human nosocomial infections such as catheter-associated sepsis or postoperative wound infections. The most common pathogens responsible for these diseases belong to the genera *Nocardia* and *Actinomadura* but other actinomycete genera such as *Amycolatopsis*, *Gordona*, *Nocardiopsis*, *Pseudonocardia*, *Rhodococcus*, *Saccharothrix*, *Streptomyces* and *Tsukamurella* may also occasionally be isolated from clinical specimens and they may be aetiologically relevant (Schaal and Lee 1992, McNeil and Brown 1994).

3.1 Nocardial infections

Infections due to *Nocardia* spp. occur in both humans and animals. As far as human infections are concerned, it does not seem appropriate to use the aetiological term 'nocardiosis' for all forms of disease that may be produced by pathogenic nocardiae. Differences in aetiology, clinical picture, treatment and prognosis favour a differentiation into 2 subgroups, namely nocardiosis *sensu stricto* and actinomycetoma. The latter, which may also be called actinomycete mycetoma, is a clinically well defined disease entity with a heterogeneous aetiology that may not only be caused by *Nocardia* but also by *Actinomadura* and *Streptomyces* spp.

HUMAN NOCARDIOSES

The definition of human nocardiosis, though primarily aetiological, is also clinical and pathological. Its potential causative agents are *Nocardia asteroides*, *Nocardia farcinica*, *Nocardia nova*, *Nocardia brasiliensis*, *Nocardia pseudobrasiliensis* (Ruimy et al 1996), *Nocardia otitidiscaviarum* and *Nocardia transvalensis*. Considerable uncertainty continues about the taxonomic status of *N. asteroides*, *N. farcinica* and *N. nova* and this affects their identification (Yano, Imaeda and Tsukamura 1990). Until recently, these organisms were included in *N. asteroides*, but they could be separated from *N. asteroides sensu stricto* by numerical taxonomic and molecular techniques (McNeil and Brown 1994). Thus, it is still difficult to assess the extent to which *N. farcinica* and *N. nova* are involved in human infections although at least the latter can reliably be identified (Miksits et al. 1991, Beaman et al. 1992, Schaal and Lee 1992).

Clinical manifestations

Apart from actinomycetoma, 5 basic forms of human nocardiosis may be recognized (Beaman and Beaman 1994):

1 pulmonary nocardiosis
2 systemic nocardiosis, involving 2 or more body sites
3 nocardiosis of the central nervous system
4 extrapulmonary nocardiosis and
5 cutaneous, subcutaneous and lymphocutaneous nocardiosis.

This subdivision is more detailed than that proposed by Schaal and Beaman in 1984 but is justified from a clinical, therapeutic and prognostic viewpoint.

Pulmonary nocardiosis *Nocardia* cells may become air-borne from their natural habitats in the soil or on vegetable material by mycelial fragmentation either as such or on dust particles. Thus, pulmonary infections result mainly from inhalation of these infective propagules into the lungs. Infections have been reported but are rare after haematogenous spread from the oral cavity or gastrointestinal tract after ingestion of contaminated food, or after accidental inoculation (e.g. by drug addicts) into the bloodstream, or by traumatic introduction into the tissues (Beaman and Beaman

1994). Inhalation of reproductive nocardial cells does not always lead to progressive pulmonary disease. Apart from their transient presence in the airways shortly after inhalation of contaminated dust, it has also been claimed that pathogenic nocardiae may colonize or subclinically infect the respiratory system (Beaman and Beaman 1994, McNeil and Brown 1994). There remains considerable uncertainty about the frequency with which such colonization or subclinical infection occurs.

Apart from systemic immunosuppression impaired local pulmonary defence mechanisms may predispose to the development of nocardiosis. These include chronic bronchitis and emphysema, asthma, bronchiectasis and alveolar proteinosis, but invasive pulmonary infection may also occur in patients without a local or systemic defect of the defence mechanisms.

The clinical presentation of the disease is very variable. Most frequently, subacute or chronic, often necrotizing, pneumonia is seen, often associated with cavitation or abscess formation. In severely immunocompromised patients, the disease may manifest itself as an acute fulminating necrotizing pneumonitis that may lead to death before the diagnosis has been established. Pulmonary nocardiosis may also present as slowly emerging single or multiple pulmonary nodules or a parietal pneumonia with empyema. Common complications include pleural effusion, empyema, pericarditis, mediastinitis, superior vena cava obstruction and occasionally chest wall abscesses. Haematogenous dissemination is characteristic and may lead to systemic nocardiosis, including nocardiosis of the central nervous system.

Patients with pulmonary nocardiosis are usually ill

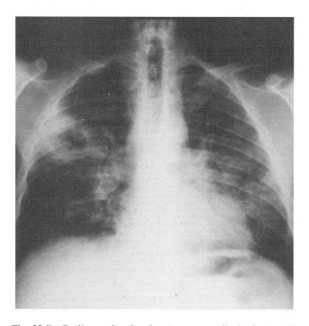

Fig. 39.5 Radiograph of pulmonary nocardiosis due to *N. farcinica* in a patient age 49 years with chronic lymphatic leukaemia. The radiograph shows pneumonic infiltration in both lungs and a large cavity in the right midfield. The patient was successfully treated with a combination of amoxycillin, clavulanic acid and amikacin.

and have symptoms such as fever, night sweats, weight loss, productive cough and possibly haemoptysis. There may be preceding or accompanying empyema and pleuritic chest pain may be a major complaint.

Radiographic findings are usually non-specific and include localized infiltrates that often appear as cuneiform shadows in the right midzone, irregular nodules, cavitations within nodules or infiltrates (Fig. 39.5), pleural effusions, and enlarged hilar nodes. Multiple nodules, abscesses, miliary lesions, diffuse interstitial infiltrations, and subpleural plaques are less commonly seen.

Systemic nocardiosis Nocardial infections at any site may invade the circulation and metastasize to other organs. Occasionally, the organisms may become blood-borne by traumatic inoculation with contaminated materials such as thorns, wood splinters and bullets, by accidental inoculation with contaminated syringes or injection needles in drug addicts, or after insect or animal bites.

By definition, systemic or disseminated nocardiosis is diagnosed if lesions are present in 2 or more sites. Any anatomical location may be involved; the central nervous system and especially the brain are the most frequently involved non-pulmonary sites. Cerebral nocardiosis, in particular nocardial brain abscess, is an important cause of cerebral space-occupying processes. Common locations to which the infection may also disseminate are the kidneys, spleen, liver, subcutaneous tissues and the eye. In the eye the retina is usually affected. Rarely, nocardial metastases are found in bone, joints, heart or skin.

At most of the above sites, exept the eye, abscess formation is the common manifestation of disseminated nocardiosis. Thus, its symptoms depend on the size and location of the abscess and the pain due to inflammation and the displacement of neighbouring tissues.

Nocardiosis of the central nervous system (CNS) Nocardial infections of the central nervous system is one of the systemic forms and often follows pulmonary nocardiosis. Among 1050 cases from the literature analysed by Beaman and Beaman (1994), 22.7% involved the central nervous system, and 44% of patients with disseminated nocardiosis had CNS infections. In 38.2% of cases there was nocardial infection of the CNS without evidence of infection elsewhere. CNS nocardiosis may therefore occur as a primary infection. Furthermore, 42% of the patients studied were previously healthy individuals without apparent predisposing factors. *Nocardia* spp. are therefore primary pathogens of the CNS and especially the brain.

The onset of nocardiosis of the CNS is often insidious and even larger lesions may remain silent. They usually present as abscesses and, more rarely, as granulomas and only occasionally as meningitis.

Brain abscesses and granulomas may be acute with rapid extension, but usually the disease progresses slowly over a period of months to years (Beaman and Beaman 1994). Since CNS infections alone often do not result in fever or alterations of the leucocyte count, they are often misdiagnosed as tumours. Symptoms depend on the localization of the lesion. Occasionally, the spinal cord alone is affected.

Extrapulmonary nocardiosis It is a matter of dispute whether extrapulmonary nocardial infections, such as cutaneous, subcutaneous and lymphocutaneous processes and CNS infections, should be regarded as a separate category, as suggested by Beaman and Beaman (1994).

Extrapulmonary infections may be found in the bone, eyes, heart, joints and kidneys. Ocular nocardial infections with retinal involvement may occur in the course of disseminated nocardiosis. Primary ocular infections usually follow traumatic or, rarely, surgical inoculation with pathogenic nocardiae, with resulting keratitis and ultimately, endophthalmitis. Improperly sterilized soft contact lenses are a less common source of exogenous nocardial infections. Nocardial keratitis may mimic non-infectious inflammatory eye disease, with serious complications if steroids are prescribed.

Nocardial infections of the joints, presenting as septic arthritis are increasing in incidence (Beaman and Beaman 1994). The same may be true for nocardial pericarditis and endocarditis. Endocarditis of an aortic valve prosthesis, successfully treated with imipenem and amikacin and by valve replacement, has been reported (Ertl, Schaal and Kochsiek 1987, Schaal and Lee 1994).

Localized cutaneous, subcutaneous and lymphocutaneous nocardiosis Apart from the involvement of the cutaneous and subcutaneous tissues in the course of disseminated nocardiosis, primary cutaneous and subcutaneous nocardial infections may be encountered. These usually follow traumatic inoculation of pathogenic nocardiae into the skin through puncture wounds, insect bites, animal scratches, or dog bites (Beaman and Beaman 1994). Since *Nocardia* spp. are ubiquitous in the soil, such infections must be common but cutaneous nocardiosis is rare, indicating that these infections are frequently subclinical or undiagnosed, because they are self-limiting and resemble other skin infections.

The primary response to the introduction of the pathogenic nocardiae into the skin is cellulitis or pyoderma from which an abscess may develop. Pustules or slowly expanding nodules may also be seen. All these manifestations resemble infections due to other pyogenic bacteria, except that nocardial infections tend to be more indolent.

Nocardiae may spread through the lymphatics to the regional lymph nodes with the characteristic clinical picture of lymphocutaneous nocardiosis. An almost identical syndrome may result from infection with the fungus *Sporothrix schenckii* (sporotrichosis) and lymphocutaneous nocardial infections are often referred to as sporotrichoid nocardiosis.

Epidemiology

There remains considerable uncertainty about the morbidity, mortality and epidemiology of nocardial infections. This is chiefly due to lack of national and international reporting systems. A still incomplete view of the impact of nocardial infections has been emerging from an analysis of the literature (Beaman and Beaman 1994, McNeil and Brown 1994), surveys by the Infectious Disease Society of America (Beaman et al. 1976), and evaluation of data accumulated in reference laboratories (Beaman et al. 1976, Boiron et al. 1992, Schaal and Lee 1992).

Three major factors apparently influence the epidemiology of nocardial infections. These are the distribution of potentially pathogenic *Nocardia* spp. in the environment, the opportunistic nature of many nocardial infections, and the observation that some species may be nosocomial pathogens.

Pathogenic nocardiae are inhabitants of soil, surface waters and various vegetable materials, but little is known about their population density in different geographical locations and soil types. Indirect evidence indicates that certain *Nocardia* spp. such as *N. asteroides*, *N. farcinica* and *N. otitidiscaviarum* occur world wide in the environment whereas *N. brasiliensis* appears to be restricted to tropical and subtropical zones. Thus, *N. brasiliensis* infections prevail in the southern part of North America, in Central and South America and in Australia. *N. brasiliensis* infection may exceptionally be acquired in temperate zones outside these areas and some of these infections can be related to unusual sources of the organism such as the mould of tropical indoor plants such as cacti (Neubert and Schaal 1982).

It is almost impossible to assess the incidence of human nocardial infections. In the USA between 1972 and 1974 the annual incidence was estimated as 500–1000 (Beaman et al. 1976). Data from the German Reference Laboratory for Actinomycetes for the period from 1979 to 1991 suggest a morbidity rate from nocardial infections of at least 50–100 per year (Schaal and Lee 1992).

Nocardiae are often opportunistic pathogens that affect immunocompromised persons, but amongst 1000 cases reported in the literature 384 had no predisposing factors (Beaman and Beaman 1994) and similar observations have been made in Germany (Schaal and Lee 1992).

Predisposing factors for nocardial infections include alcohol abuse, alveolar proteinosis, neoplasms, diabetes mellitus, Hodgkin's disease, sarcoidosis, systemic lupus erythematosus, tuberculosis and AIDS (Schaal and Lee 1992, Beaman and Beaman 1994, McNeil and Brown 1994). Organ transplantation and long-term administration of corticosteroids are other predisposing factors. Localized cutaneous, subcutaneous, or lymphocutaneous nocardioses do not depend on predisposing factors and occur in otherwise healthy individuals.

As for actinomycoses, nocardial infections are more common in males than in females with a sex ratio that ranges from 2.8:1 to 1.5:1, but this is not the case in AIDS (Schaal and Lee 1992, Beaman and Beaman 1994).

The epidemiology of nocardial infections in AIDS patients is different from that in patients with other underlying diseases but it is unknown how common nocardiosis is in AIDS because there may be geographical differences in the incidence of nocardiosis in AIDS patients (Beaman and Beaman 1994). This was assumed for different parts of the USA but it may be true world wide. Nocardiosis may also be difficult to recognize and diagnose in HIV-infected persons.

Disseminated nocardiosis is a malignant infection with high mortality, which has fallen since 1980. The mortality rate in patients without predisposing factors was about half that in patients with such factors; it was more than 50% in those with systemic or CNS infection whereas it was less than 20% in those with localized pulmonary or extrapulmonary disease (Beaman and Beaman 1994).

Although nocardiosis is a sporadic, environmentally acquired and predominantly opportunistic infection, pathogenic *Nocardia* spp. may also be responsible for nosocomial outbreaks.

Houang et al. (1980) described an outbreak of nocardiosis due to *N. asteroides* in a renal transplant unit in the UK and concluded that nocardiosis might be a transmissible disease, as did Cox and Hughes (1975) who observed temporal and spacial clustering in 3 immunocompromised patients. Further evidence for nosocomial transmission has been reported in heart transplant patients (Krick, Stinson and Remington 1975, Simpson et al. 1981) and in patients with chronic liver disease and after liver transplantation (Sahathevan et al. 1991). In this as well as in another report (Baddour et al. 1986) exposure to dust from construction activities was considered a possible risk factor. This is in agreement with observations that demolition work may produce dust highly contaminated with viable *Nocardia* cells (Schaal 1991). Temporal and spacial clustering of *N. farcinica* postoperative infections has been observed in a hospital setting in relation to cardiac and vascular surgery (Schaal 1991, Schaal and Lee 1992). The source of the pathogens could not be identified but the isolates had a characteristic antibiotic sensitivity pattern and belonged to a single type as defined by pulse field gel electrophoresis (Blümel and Schaal, unpublished observations). A strain with the same characteristics was isolated on settle plates in a store room in the operating suite. The strain responsible for the outbreak, which lasted for several years, probably had a common source and was not transmitted from patient to patient.

Pathology and pathogenesis

Since nocardial infections may be suppurative or granulomatous or a mixture of both, the histopathological appearance of the lesions is very variable. Abscesses and pure granulomas may be seen but the host response often becomes mixed (Beaman and Beaman 1994). Granule formation is not characteristic of any type of human nocardiosis but is usual in actinomycetoma.

Since pathogenic nocardiae occur mainly in the environment, human nocardiosis is always exogenous in origin. Suggestions that commensal nocardiae from the airways cause endogenous infections (McNeil and Brown 1994) are not convincing. The isolation of pathogenic *Nocardia* spp. from sputum or bronchial secretions in the absence of pulmonary disease indicates short-term contamination or subclinical infection (Beaman and Beaman 1994) rather than long-term colonization.

The pathogenicity of the various *Nocardia* spp. mentioned above shows certain species-specific differences. Pulmonary, systemic, CNS and extrapulmonary nocardioses are predominantly caused by *N. asteroides*, *N. farcinica*, possibly *N. pseudobrasiliensis* and occasionally *N. nova*, *N. brasiliensis*, *N. otitidiscaviarum* and *N. transvalensis* (Weinberger et al. 1995).

Considerable uncertainty remains about the clinical importance of *N. farcinica*. In their literature analysis Beaman and Beaman (1994) found only 13 cases of *N. farcinica* infection in 1050 cases, whereas Schaal and Lee (1992) found 60.3% of nocardial infections were due to this organism. It is quite clear that problems of identification affected the results obtained by Beaman and Beaman (1994), but regional differences may have been responsible for the discrepancy.

Superficial cutaneous and subcutaneous infections are caused mainly by *N. brasiliensis*, as well as by *N. otitidiscaviarum* and *N. transvalensis* (Clark et al. 1995). These infections may occasionally also be due to *N. asteroides*, *N. farcinica* and *N. nova*. *Nocardia brevicatena* has been isolated from the respiratory tract, but its aetiological role in human infections has not been established.

Host response

The host–parasite relationship in nocardial infections has been reviewed by Beaman and Beaman (1994). Attempts have been made to detect antibodies to *Nocardia* spp. that could be used for diagnostic purposes. There is little unequivocal information on the diagnostic relevance of these antibody tests. Kjelstrom and Beaman (1993) developed a panel of serological tests for the recognition of nocardial infections using an ELISA of cytoplasmic, culture filtrate and cord factor antigens, an immunofluorescence assay against whole cells, and a Western blot analysis of secreted protein antigens. This panel of tests suggested a correlation between the occurrence of antibodies and nocardial infections if clinical and other factors were taken into account (Beaman and Beaman 1994).

Animal studies show that macrophages, T cells, and cell mediated immunity play an important role in host resistance to nocardial infection. Macrophages phagocytose nocardial cells and, depending on the virulence of the individual strain, kill many of the ingested organisms. A proportion of less virulent strains may survive as L forms within the phagocyte, whereas more virulent strains multiply inside the macrophage and nocardial filaments may finally grow through the cell membrane (Beaman and Beaman 1994). T lymphocytes may either activate macrophages and stimulate a cellular immune response or they may be directly involved in killing nocardiae.

Diagnosis

Reliable diagnosis of nocardiosis is possible only by the isolation of the causative organism from suitable clinical specimens, including sputum, bronchial washings, exudate, pus, cerebrospinal fluid, blood, urine and biopsy or autopsy materials. Although pathogenic nocardiae are rather resistent, specimens should be transported to the laboratory rapidly because the slowly growing nocardiae are readily overgrown by contaminants. Refrigeration is not advisable because certain *Nocardia* strains do not survive low temperatures well.

With suitable staining, such as a modification of the gram stain or silver impregnation, microscopic examination of sputum, pus specimens or tissue sections may reveal filamentous branching bacteria. Microscopy does not differentiate between fermentative and oxidative actinomycetes. Speciation is possible only by cultural methods and may in future become possible by molecular methods.

For blood, cerebrospinal fluid and empyema exudates any general purpose medium incubated at $36 \pm 1°C$ is suitable for the isolation of *Nocardia* spp. Solid media should be transparent, such as brain–heart infusion agar, so that growth can be observed microscopically at an early stage. Selective medium should be used for specimens likely to contain indigenous flora of the mucous membranes (e.g. sputum, bronchial secretions, urine, autopsy material) (Gordon and Hagan 1936, Schaal 1972) to reduce the risk of the overgrowth of the slow-growing nocardiae by contaminants.

The identification of nocardiae to the species level requires the chemotaxonomic, carbon source utilization and hydrolysis tests (Schaal 1984, 1985a). The reliable identification of *N. asteroides sensu stricto, N. farcinica* and *N. nova* is particularly difficult because they share many phenotypic characters. Differences in antibiotic susceptibility may facilitate the recognition of these species (Wallace et al. 1983, 1988, 1990).

Although attempts have been made to develop reliable serological diagnostic procedures to recognize nocardial infections, no single or combination of tests has proved satisfactory (Beaman and Beaman 1994, McNeil and Brown 1994). Attempts have been made to use specific DNA probes for rapid identification of suspected *N. asteroides* isolates (Brownell and Belcher 1990). The diagnostic value of such probes is limited because *N. asteroides* is a heterogeneous species that requires a large panel of probes to identify all its members. The same is true for PCR techniques and identification of the amplified DNA by specific probes, restriction enzyme fingerprinting, and sequencing.

Treatment

The appropriate agents for the treatment of the nocardioses remains controversial because of the problems of susceptibility testing of these organisms and because controlled clinical trials are lacking. Recommendations are based on a limited number of cases. Nevertheless, detailed in vitro and animal studies with the *N. asteroides* complex (Schaal, Schütt-Gerowitt and Goldmann 1986) are directly applicable to human infections (Stasiecky et al. 1985, Ertl, Schaal and Kochsiek 1987, Ruppert et al. 1988, Krone et al. 1989). The pathogenic nocardiae show considerable

differences in sensitivity pattern (Wallace et al. 1983, 1988, 1990) and there may be geographical differences in susceptibility; this appears to be the case for *N. asteroides, N. farcinica* and *N. nova*. Exceptionally, European strains *N. asteroides* and *N. farcinica* are susceptible to sulphonamides or sulphamethoxazole–trimethoprim, which are used in the USA. Only *N. brasiliensis* is usually susceptible to these drugs.

The treatment of choice for nocardioses due to *N. asteroides* and *N. farcinica* is high doses of imipenem and amikacin. The daily dose of imipenem should not be less than 4 g and that of amikacin should be adjusted on the basis of serum levels. Some strains of the *N. asteroides* complex are also sensitive to amoxycillin plus clavulanic acid and this combination may be used when the strain is poorly sensitive to imipenem. *N. brasiliensis, N. otitidiscaviarum* and *N. transvalensis* may not respond as well to this treatment because of resistance to either or both of imipenem and amoxycillin–clavulanic acid. Resistance to amikacin, however, is rarely seen in pathogenic nocardiae and it should always be part of combination therapy. Sulphonamides, sulphamethoxazole–trimethroprim and tetracyclines, especially minocycline, are effective drugs against these infections (Schaal, Schütt-Gerowitt and Goldmann 1986, Naka et al. 1995). Whereas sulphonamides, if effective at all, may require 12 months or more to effect a cure in *N. asteroides* and *N. farcinica*, imipenem or amoxycillin–clavulanic acid plus amikacin usually lead to improvement within a week and cure within 4–6 weeks. If relapses occur after antimicrobial therapy, particularly in lung or brain abscess, or prosthetic valve endocarditis, surgery should be considered.

3.2 Actinomycetoma

Actinomycetoma is a chronic, localized, slowly progressive disease due to a variety of different aerobic actinomycetes. The infection usually begins at the site of a puncture wound by a thorn or splinter. Mycetomas usually involve the lower limbs, but may also involve the hands, arms and even the back, shoulders and head. Whereas actinomycetoma of the foot (Madura foot) can be due to minor injuries, that of the back and shoulders in farm workers has been related to carrying soil-contaminated sacks. These infections are common in rural developing countries and are related to walking barefoot, farm work practices and occurrence in the soil of the agents of actinomycetoma, though *Actinomadura pelletieri* has been isolated only from clinical specimens.

The incubation period ranges from one week to several months, when a painless nodule appears at the site of injury. The nodule slowly increases in size, becomes soft, and may finally discharge pus through a small sinus. The lesion is surrounded by a cellular infiltrate and chronic inflammation, from which multiple secondary nodules form that also develop sinuses.

The infection usually remains localized and progresses by direct extension. This may lead to involvement of tissues such as muscle and bone. The resulting osteomyelitis is associated with periostitis and cavities within the affected bone.

Granules are characteristic of the sinus discharge. In contrast to the sulphur granules of actinomycosis, actinomycetoma granules consist only of colonies of the infecting agent surrounded by inflammatory cells but without concomitant organisms. The granules differ in size, texture and colour depending on the actinomycete species present, so assisting microbiological diagnosis.

The spectrum of agents of actinomycetoma include not only pathogenic *Nocardia* spp. but also pathogenic members of the genera *Actinomadura*, *Streptomyces* and *Nocardiopsis* (see also Volume 2, Chapter 21). These commonly include *N. brasiliensis*, *A. madurae*, *A. pelletieri* and *Streptomyces somaliensis*. *N. asteroides*, *N. otitidiscaviarum* and *N. transvalensis* are infrequent agents of actinomycetoma (McNeil and Brown 1994, Mirza and Campbell 1994). The role of *N. farcinica*, *N. nova* and *Nocardiopsis dassonvillei* remains to be clarified.

Some of these species differ in their geographical soil distribution. Thus, in southern North America, South America, Mexico and Australia *N. brasiliensis* is the most common cause of actinomycetoma. *Actinomadura* infections have been reported in particular from Central and South America and South East Asia. *S. somaliensis* and *Actinomadura* spp. predominate in Africa and the former has also been reported from Venezuela (Serrano et al. 1986).

The diagnosis of actinomycetoma is based on the isolation and identification of the causative organisms. In the search for a diagnosis, 2 points should be noted:

1 Actinomycetomas are indistinguishable from similar disease due to true fungi (eumycetoma). Gram-stained smear of sinus discharge may distinguish between actinomycetoma and eumycetoma on the basis of the morphology of the mycelia of actinomycetes and fungi.
2 The granules produced by various aerobic actinomycetes may show differences that are evident by direct observation.

Nocardial granules are usually less than 1 mm in diameter, soft and lobulated and are white to yellowish. *A. madurae* produces large granules 1–5 mm in diameter that are soft, serpiginous or lobulated and white to yellowish or pinkish to reddish. *A. pelletieri* particles are 0.3–0.5 mm in diameter and rarely reach 1 mm; they are soft, finely denticulate or irregularly spherical, deep red or occasionally yellowish to pinkish. *S. somaliensis* forms larger granules 1–2 mm in diameter that are hard, round to oval, dense and homogeneous, yellow to brown to black.

The causative agents of actinomycetoma can be isolated and identified using the same media and procedures as for *Nocardia* spp. *Actinomadura* spp., however, even on subculture often grow poorly on routine media.

Treatment of actinomycetoma can be difficult and the mortality may reach 50% or more. The problems of treatment reside not only in possible resistance to various antibiotics but also their penetration into infected tissue. Nocardial actinomycetomas respond to the same drugs as those recommended for nocardiosis (see section 3.1, p. 787). Actinomycetoma due to *N. brasiliensis* should be treated with sulphonamides or sulphamethoxazole–trimethoprim, possibly combined with an aminoglycoside. Those due to *Actinomadura* spp. or *S. somaliensis* may also respond to sulphonamides with or without trimethoprim. However, susceptibility testing shows that at least *A. madurae* is always sensitive to amikacin and imipenem (McNeil et al. 1992). Tetracyclines, such as doxycycline and minocycline, are alternatives.

3.3 Other diseases caused by aerobic actinomycetes

Several other infections may be caused by aerobic actinomycetes (see also Volume 2, Chapter 21). These belong to the genera *Actinomadura*, *Streptomyces* and to *Rhodococcus*, *Gordona*, *Tsukamurella*, *Pseudonocardia* and *Amycolatopsis*.

INFECTIONS OTHER THAN ACTINOMYCETOMA CAUSED BY *ACTINOMADURA* AND *STREPTOMYCES* SPP.

A. madurae (11.5%) and *N. asteroides* (26.8%) were found by McNeil et al. (1990) among 366 isolates of aerobic actinomycetes and the majority of the former were from sputum. These data differ considerably from those of Schaal and Lee (1992), who found that *Actinomadura* was very uncommon. There have been few recent reports on *Actinomadura* infections other than actinomycetoma. These include peritonitis in patients undergoing chronic ambulatory peritoneal dialysis, wound infection after hysterectomy and pneumonia in AIDS patients (McNeil and Brown 1994). All of these infections were due to *A. madurae* and none to *A. pelletieri*.

S. somaliensis has long been regarded as the only pathogen in the genus *Streptomyces*. Another species, '*Streptomyces paraguayensis*', reported to cause actinomycetoma, is of doubtful taxonomic significance. It has only recently been appreciated that *Streptomyces* spp. other than *S. somaliensis* may occur in clinical specimens and the majority of these belong to the *Streptomyces griseus* group (Mishra, Gordon and Barnett 1980, Schaal and Lee 1992). Many of these must be regarded as contaminants without aetiological significance, but they have on occasion been isolated from pericarditis, septicaemia, lung infections, brain abscess, and cervical lymphadenitis in an AIDS patient (McNeil and Brown 1994).

INFECTIONS CAUSED BY *RHODOCOCCUS* SPP.

The genus *Rhodococcus* has changed in its species composition since its definition by Goodfellow and Alderson (1977) and, apart from *Rhodococcus equi*, other *Rhodococcus* spp. may occasionally be isolated from clinical specimens and some of these may be opportunist pathogens. All *Rhodococcus* spp. are widely distributed in nature, especially in soil, water and lake and river sediments. *Rhodococcus rhodnii* has been isolated from the intestine of the reduviid *Rhodnius prolixus* where it may be a symbiont.

Rhodococcus equi infections

Under its previous name, 'Corynebacterium equi', R. equi was known as an important animal pathogen. In herbivorous animals it causes pneumonia in foals and ulcerative lymphangitis in cattle, whereas in swine it causes lymphadenitis, but it may also occur as a commensal on the tonsils (McNeil and Brown 1994). Though not present in the majority of stables, R. equi is endemic in some or causes sporadic infections of horses in others. R. equi infections are diagnosed by culture from tracheal aspirates or other specimens and, when the lungs are involved, by radiography. Treatment is with rifampicin or erythromycin.

R. equi has recently been recognized as a potential human pathogen, mainly as a cause of invasive pneumonia in severely immunocompromised patients. Infection occurs by inhalation of contaminated environmental dust. The clinical presentation is usually non-specific and invasive diagnostic procedures may be necessary. In AIDS patients, cavity formation, pleuritis and bacteraemia are common and there may be dissemination with involvement of the brain, liver, or skin.

Cutaneous infections due to R. equi are rare but may also occur in non-immunocompromised patients (Müller et al. 1988). A disseminated R. equi infection in a HIV-infected patient first presented as a mycetoma of the foot (Antinori et al. 1992).

Bacteraemia due to R. equi usually follows pulmonary infection but may be a complication of chronic leg ulcers. Recently, R. equi, or a phenotypically related Rhodococcus sp., was described as the cause of bacteraemia in a patient receiving long-term parenteral nutrition through a central venous catheter (McNeil and Brown 1994).

Sulphamethoxazole–trimethoprim, doxycycline, erythromycin, imipenem and amikacin have been used to treat R. equi infections. R. equi is susceptible to a wide range of antimicrobial drugs, but occasionally resistant strains may be encountered. Striking discrepancies in the sensitivity test results that are not readily explicable have been reported by different authors. Furthermore, since R. equi is an intracellular pathogen there may be discrepancies between in vitro and in vivo susceptibility. At present no optimal antimicrobial treatment for R. equi infections has been defined but combinations of erythromycin plus rifampicin, minocyline plus rifampicin, or erythromycin plus minocycline and high doses of imipenem plus amikacin appear to be most promising in human infections.

HUMAN INFECTIONS CAUSED BY OTHER *RHODOCOCCUS* SPP.

Little is known about the role of other Rhodococcus spp. as human pathogens. The few available reports suggest that infections due to Rhodococcus spp. other than R. equi are rare. Isolated reports state that Rhodococcus rhodochrous and Rhodococcus erythropolis may, rarely, cause skin and other infections in humans with and without predisposing factors. A case of endophthalmitis has been reported due to Rhodococcus luteus (synonym of Rhodococcus fascians) and Rhodococcus erythropolis after lens implantation (von Below et al. 1991).

Infections caused by *Gordona* spp.

The genus Gordona was reintroduced by Stackebrandt, Smida and Collins (1988) on the basis of its 16S rRNA sequence. It currently comprises 7 species, 3 of which, Gordona aichiensis, Gordona bronchialis and Gordona sputi, may be encountered in clinical specimens. Rarely, Gordona terrae and Gordona rubropertincta have been reported from human infections.

The most common manifestations of Gordona infections are subacute to chronic pulmonary inflammatory processes that may be confused with tuberculosis. The major pathogen in these infections is G. bronchialis, but G. rubropertincta has been documented in an immunocompetent female patient age 29 years (Hart et al. 1988). The pathogenic role of G. sputi has not been established but it has been observed in the sputum of patients with chronic pulmonary disease.

G. terrae was reported in patients with long-term indwelling central venous catheters and a nosocomial outbreak of sternal wound infections in patients after coronary artery bypass has been attributed to G. bronchialis (Richet et al. 1991).

Doxycycline in combination with rifampicin has been successfully used to treat Gordona infections.

Infections due to *Tsukamurella* spp.

The genus Tsukamurella was created by Collins et al. (1988) for bacteria previously designated as 'Corynebacterium paurometabolum', 'Gordona aurantiaca', or 'Rhodococcus aurantiacus'. A second species, Tsukamurella wratislaviensis (Goodfellow et al. 1991), should probably be reclassified into another genus; however, Yassin et al. (1995, 1996) described 2 new Tsukamurella spp. from human clinical specimens that were named Tsukamurella inchonensis and Tsukamurella pulmonis. A third new species has been designated Tsukamurella tyrosinosolvens (Yassin et al., unpublished observations). The latter 3 species were isolated from the sputum of patients with lung disease or from blood cultures of patients with septicaemia or catheter-associated sepsis. The lung infections were difficult to differentiate from tuberculosis and infections due to ubiquitous mycobacteria. Cultures of these organisms may be confused with rapidly growing mycobacteria both microscopically and chemotaxonomically. Similar infections due to T. paurometabola have been reported but this species grows best at temperatures below 37°C.

These infections have been successfully treated with sulphamethoxazole–trimethoprim or imipenem plus amikacin, but not with antituberculous drugs.

INFECTIONS CAUSED BY *AMYCOLATOPSIS* AND *PSEUDONOCARDIA* SPP.

Amycolatopsis orientalis subsp. orientalis is the only species of the genus that has been associated with human disease. It has been isolated from cerebrospinal fluid and other specimens, but detailed information about its pathogenicity is not available. The same is true for Pseudonocardia autotrophica (Warwick et al. 1994), which was known as 'Nocardia autotrophica' or 'Amycolata autotrophica'. It has been isolated from the cerebrospinal fluid of a patient with meningitis, from a leg wound, and from blood of a patient with sepsis associated with bone marrow hypoplasia (McNeil and Brown 1994).

INFECTIONS CAUSED BY *OERSKOVIA* SPP.

Oerskovia spp. differ from all the other actinomycetes discussed in this chapter in that they produce motile elements by mycelium fragmentation and in that their glucose metabolism is both oxidative and fermentative. The taxonomic relevance of the genus *Oerskovia* has been questioned recently as a result of 16S rRNA sequence analysis, which indicated that the oerskoviae should be transferred to the genus *Cellulomonas* (Stackebrandt, Hariger and Schleifer 1980). Since this is uncertain and because of nomenclatural problems with *Oerskovia xanthineolytica*, which may be a synonym of *Cellulomonas cellulans*, the old designations are retained here.

Oerskovia turbata and *Oerskovia xanthineolytica* have been isolated from various clinical specimens. In particular, *O. turbata* was recovered from heart valves and heart tissue. Oerskoviae have also been isolated from blood, urine, sputum, lung and wound exudates, tear duct material, cerebrospinal fluid, liver tissue, and granulomas. In many of the cases reported by Sottnek et al. (1977) the aetiological relevance of the organisms was uncertain, but there are documented cases of endocarditis in a patient with heart valve replacement and of pyonephrosis in an immunocompromised patient (Reller et al. 1975, Cruickshank, Gawler and Shalson 1979). Successful treatment has been reported only with vancomycin in a patient with catheter-associated sepsis and in patients with bacteraemia associated with cirrhosis. The use of penicillin, rifampicin, sulphamethoxazole–trimethoprim combined with ampicillin and amoxycillin in meningitis and endocarditis was not effective, though in vitro susceptibility had been demonstrated (McNeil and Brown 1994). *Oerskovia* infections related to indwelling prosthetic devices usually resolve after removal of the devices.

3.4 Dermatophilosis

Dermatophilosis or streptothrichosis is an exudative, pustular dermatitis of world-wide distribution. It primarily affects cattle, sheep and horses and occasionally many other domestic and feral animals (Gordon 1964, Weber 1978, McNeil and Brown 1994). Humans are usually only involved after contact with infected animals or contaminated animal products.

The causative agent of dermatophilosis is *Dermatophilus congolensis*, which has a unique life cycle and a characteristic morphology. In early growth stages it forms filamentous, branched structures that, on further incubation, fragment transversally in at least 2 longitudinal planes to form packets of coccoid cells, which develop into motile spores.

HUMAN DERMATOPHILOSIS

Human *Dermatophilus* infections are characterized by multiple pustules, furuncles or desquamative eczema of the hands or forearms (Gordon 1964). Crateriform keratolysis (pitted keratolysis) has also been reported (Weber 1978). The infection is usually self-limiting and heals spontaneously after 2–3 weeks.

EPIDEMIOLOGY

D. congolensis has been isolated only from diseased animals or humans and its natural habitat is unknown given the sporadic occurrence of the disease. Contaminated soil may be the source of this actinomycete. Direct transmission from diseased to healthy humans and animals appears to be the usual route of infection.

DIAGNOSIS AND TREATMENT

D. congolensis may be present at any developmental stage in clinical materials but the appearance of branched filaments devided both transversally and longitudinally is observed most frequently and is pathognomonic. To demonstrate these structures, wet mounts or methylene blue- or Giemsa-stained smears are recommended; gram-stained smears are not suitable.

Since human infections are self limiting, treatment is not indicated. Animal infections have been treated successfully with penicillin G plus streptomycin (Weber 1978).

4 DISEASES CAUSED BY *ACTINOBACILLUS* SPECIES

4.1 Human *Actinobacillus* infections

The human pathogens of the genus *Actinobacillus* are *A. actinomycetemcomitans*, *Actinobacillus hominis* and *Actinobacillus ureae*. Infections due to *Actinobacillus lignieresii*, *Actinobacillus equuli* and *Actinobacillus suis* have occasionally also been described but the characters used to identify these species have often appeared not to have been sufficient (Mannheim, Fredericksen and Mutters 1992).

INFECTIONS DUE TO *ACTINOBACILLUS ACTINOMYCETEMCOMITANS*

A. actinomycetemcomitans was first described by Klinger (1912) as a characteristic and common member of the synergistic flora of human actinomycotic infections. It is the most characteristic but not the most common concomitant bacterium in 23–25% of cervicofacial actinomycosis (Pulverer and Schaal 1984, Schaal and Pulverer 1984, Schaal and Lee 1992). When this organism is present, actinomycosis takes a particularly chronic course and is difficult to treat. Therapy with penicillin G, to which *A. actinomycetemcomitans* is resistant, often results in treatment failure due to the persistence of this organism even though the pathogenic actinomycete has been eliminated.

A. actinomycetemcomitans is a member of the normal oral flora of healthy humans but it also plays an important part in the pathogenesis of periodontal disease. The organism is present in about 50% of periodontitis lesions in adults. More important, however, is its aetiological involvement in juvenile periodontitis in which it is the main pathogen. Furthermore, *A. actinomycetemcomitans* is in some cases the sole pathogen in endocarditis, abscesses of the internal organs and cutaneous infections associated with intravenous heroin abuse.

Apart from penicillin G and other narrow spectrum penicillins, *A. actinomycetemcomitans* is susceptible to a variety of antibacterial drugs. Ampicillin and amoxycillin are particularly active in vitro and in vivo and are the drugs of choice for treatment.

INFECTIONS DUE TO *ACTINOBACILLUS HOMINIS* AND *ACTINOBACILLUS UREAE*

A. hominis and *A. ureae* (previously *Pasteurella ureae*) have been isolated from the sputum and tracheal secretions of patients suffering from chronic airway infections. Furthermore, *A. hominis* may cause pneumonia and *A. ureae* purulent meningitis. They are upper respiratory tract commensals and are usually opportunistic pathogens.

5 ACTINOMYCETES AS ALLERGENS

Actinomycetes are important allergens that may be responsible for hypersensitivity reactions in the respiratory tract of both man and animals. In humans the allergic diseases induced by actinomycetes are mainly occupational. The most common of these conditions is usually referred to as farmer's lung and similar illnesses may also occur in domestic animals (Schaal and Beaman 1984).

5.1 Hypersensitivity diseases in humans

Apart from farmer's lung disease, similar occupational hypersensitivity diseases are known under the designations bagassosis, mushroom-worker's lung, byssinosis and humidifier fever. These conditions develop when actinomycete spores (conidia) are inhaled and induce hypersensitivity reactions in the lungs. Because of the small size of the conidia they usually reach the alveoli and give rise to the syndrome of allergic alveolitis or hypersensitivity pneumonitis. The hypersensitivity reactions to the actinomycete particles are of the delayed type (Lacey 1981).

CLINICAL PICTURE

The hypersensitivity reaction to actinomycete spores presents as interstitial pneumonitis and is difficult to differentiate from similar conditions of other aetiologies. In its acute phase, the disease shows delayed-onset symptoms such as dyspnoea, fever, restrictive ventilatory defects, malaise, weight loss and radiographic changes. After repeated exposure to the allergen pulmonary fibrosis may develop. If antigen exposure is low, progressive destruction of the lungs may occur insidiously.

EPIDEMIOLOGY

Farmer's lung has been reported from most parts of Europe, the USA and Canada. Its incidence is higher in areas of high rainfall than in drier regions (Burke et al. 1977, Lacey 1981). The other forms of hypersensitivity pneumonitis induced by actinomycetes are restricted to the environment where their growth occurs. Humidifier fever due to allergens other than actinomycetes is associated with particular ventilation and heating systems (Schaal and Beaman 1984).

PATHOLOGY AND PATHOGENESIS

The first symptoms occur at least 4 h after exposure, reach their maximum within 12 h, and resolve after 24–26 h. Histopathologically, the hypersensitivity reaction is characterized by an alveolar mononuclear infiltrate with large numbers of plasma cells and a granulomatous bronchiolitis.

Since actinomycete conidia are usually less than 1 μm in diameter, they are able to penetrate the alveoli where they are deposited. For sensitization a single heavy exposure is more important than constitutional predisposition and such heavy exposures arise when actinomycetes, especially thermophilic species, have multiplied to large numbers in agricultural products, such as hay, grain, cotton, or sugar-cane bagasse and also in mushroom compost or humidifier water. The spores (conidia) produced by these organisms easily become detached and are launched into the air when the substrate on which they have grown is disturbed. Especially under indoor conditions such air-borne spores may reach concentrations sufficiently high to cause hypersensitivity reactions.

The most important agent of farmer's lung disease is *Saccharopolyspora rectivirgula* (Korn-Wendisch et al. 1989). Other thermophilic bacteria that have been implicated as aetiological agents of farmer's lung are *Thermoactinomyces vulgaris*, *Saccharomonospora viridis*, *Thermoactinomyces dichotomicus* and *Thermoactinomyces thalpophilus*. All of these organisms are able to grow heavily in self-heated hay.

Bagassosis is induced by inhalation of dust from stored sugar-cane bagasse. *Thermoactinomyces sacchari* is the most important species able to grow abundantly in bagasse and the most important cause of the disease. Several thermophilic actinomycetes, in particular *Thermomonospora* spp., are associated with mushroom-worker's lung, humidifier fever and byssinosis.

TREATMENT AND PROPHYLAXIS

The principal measure to prevent hypersensitivity pneumonitis is to identify the source and nature of the allergen and avoid further contact with it. Corticosteroids may also be necessary for symptomatic treatment.

Other preventive strategies are aimed at reducing the concentration of actinomycete conidia in the air. This can be done by preventing mould growth in agricultural products, which usually have a low water content, by increasing this or by adding chemical preservatives such as propionic acid. Alternatively, measures can be taken to prevent the workers from inhaling the allergens by installation of ventilation systems to remove the spores or by the use of masks with filters. If ventilation systems are themselves the source of the allergens, steam humidification can be used and efforts made to keep the ventilation ducts dry (Schaal and Beaman 1984).

REFERENCES

Alvarado-Cerna R, Bracho-Riquelme R, 1994, Perianal actinomycosis: a complication of a fistula-in-ano, *Dis Colon Rectum*, **37:** 378–80.

Antinori S, Esposito R et al., 1992, Disseminated *Rhodococcus equi* infection initially presenting as foot mycetoma in an HIV-positive patient, *AIDS*, **6:** 740–2.

Baddour L, Baselski VS et al., 1986, Nocardiosis in recipients of renal transplants: evidence for nosocomial acquisition, *Am J Infect Control*, **14:** 214–19.

Beaman BL, Beaman LV, 1994, *Nocardia* species: host–parasite relationships, *Clin Microbiol Rev*, **7:** 213–64.

Beaman BL, Burnside J et al., 1976, Nocardial infections in the United States, 1972–1974, *J Infect Dis*, **134:** 286–9.

Beaman BL, Boiron P et al., 1992, *Nocardia* and nocardiosis, *Med Vet Mycol*, **30, Suppl. 1:** 317–31.

van Below H, Wilk M et al., 1991, *Rhodococcus luteus* and *Rhodococcus erythropolis* chronic endophthalmitis after lens implantation, *Am J Ophthalmol*, **112:** 596–7.

Blanchard R, 1896, Parasites végetaux à l'exclusion des bactéries, *Trâité de Pathologie Générale*, vol. II, ed. Bouchard C, G Masson, Paris, 811–932.

Boiron P, Provost F et al., 1992, Review of nocardial infections in France 1987–1990, *Eur J Clin Microbiol Infect Dis*, **11:** 709–14.

Bollinger O, 1877, Über eine neue Pilzkrankheit beim Rinde, *Zentralbl Med Wiss*, **15:** 481–5.

Bostroem E, 1891, Untersuchungen über die Aktinomykose des Menschen, *Beitr Pathol Anat Allg Pathol*, **9:** 1–240.

Boué D, Armau E, Tiraby G, 1987, A bacteriological study of rampant caries in children, *J Dent Res*, **60:** 23–8.

Brownell GH, Belcher KE, 1990, DNA probes for the identification of *Nocardia asteroides*, *J Clin Microbiol*, **28:** 2082–6.

Brumpt E, 1910, *Précis de Parasitologie*, Masson and Co., Paris, 849.

Bujwid O, 1889, Über die Reinkultur des *Actinomyces, Zentralbl Bakteriol Parasitenkd Infektionskr*, **6:** 630–3.

Burke GW, Carrington CB et al., 1977, Allergic alveolitis caused by home humidifiers, *JAMA*, **238:** 2705–8.

Charfreitag O, Collins ND, Stackebrandt E, 1988, Reclassification of *Arachnia propionica* as *Propionibacterium propionicus* comb. nov., *Int J Syst Bacteriol*, **38:** 354–7.

Chatwani A, Amin-Hanjani S, 1994, Incidence of actinomycosis associated with intrauterine devices, *J Reprod Med*, **39:** 585–7.

Clark MN, Braun DK et al., 1995, Primary cutaneous *Nocardia otitidiscaviarum* infection: case report and review, *Clin Infect Dis*, **20:** 1266–70.

Collins MD, Smida J et al., 1988, *Tsukamurella* gen. nov. harbouring *Corynebacterium paurometabolum* and *Rhodococcus aurantiacus*, *Int J Syst Bacteriol*, **38:** 385–91.

Cox F, Hughes WT, 1975, Contagious and other aspects of nocardiosis in the compromised host, *Pediatrics*, **55:** 135–8.

Cruickshank JG, Gawler AH, Shalson C, 1979, *Oerskovia* species: rare opportunistic pathogens, *J Med Microbiol*, **12:** 513–15.

Edelmann M, Cullmann W et al., 1987, Treatment of abdomino-thoracic actinomycosis with imipenem, *Eur J Clin Microbiol*, **6:** 194–5.

Eibach HW, Bolte A et al., 1989, Klinische Relevanz und pathognomonische Bedeutung der Aktinomyzetenbesiedlung von Intrauterinpessaren, *Geburtshilfe Frauenheilkd*, **49:** 972–6.

Eibach HW, Neuhaus W et al., 1992, Clinical relevance and pathognomonic significance of actinomycotic colonization of intrauterine pessaries, *Int J Feto-Maternal Med*, **5:** 40–2.

Eppinger H, 1891, Über eine neue pathogene *Cladothrix* und eine durch sie hervorgerufene Pseudotuberculosis (*Cladotrichica*), *Beitr Pathol Anat Allg Pathol*, **9:** 287–328.

Ertl G, Schaal KP, Kochsiek K, 1987, Nocardial endocarditis of an aortic valve prosthesis, *Br Heart J*, **57:** 384–6.

Ewig S, Schaal KP et al., 1993, 42jähriger Patient mit Fieber und einem palpablen abdominellen Tumor, *Internist*, **34:** 59–62.

Fortner J, 1928, Ein einfaches Plattenverfahren zur Züchtung strenger Anaerobier, *Zentralbl Bakteriol Parasitenkd Infektionskr Hyg Abt 1*, **108:** 155–9.

Funke G, Stubbs S et al., 1994, Assignment of human-derived CDC group 1 coryneform bacteria and CDC group 1-like bacteria to the genus *Actinomyces* as *Actinomyces neuii* subsp. *neuii* sp. nov., subsp. nov., and *Actinomyces neuii* subsp. *anitratus* subsp. nov., *Int J Syst Bacteriol*, **44:** 167–71.

Funke G, Pasqual-Ramos C et al., 1995, Description of human-derived Centres for Disease Control coryneform group 2 bacteria as *Actinomyces bernardiae* sp. nov., *Int J Syst Bacteriol*, **45:** 57–60.

Goodfellow M, Alderson G, 1977, The actinomycete genus *Rhodococcus*. A home for the rhodochrous complex, *J Gen Microbiol*, **100:** 99–122.

Goodfellow M, Cakrzewska-Czerwinska J et al., 1991, Polyphasic taxonomic study of the genera *Gordona* and *Tsukamurella* including the description of *Tsukamurella wratislaviensis* sp. nov., *Zentralbl Bakteriol Parasitenkd Infektionskr*, **275:** 162–78.

Gordon MA, 1964, The genus *Dermatophilus*, *J Bacteriol*, **88:** 509–22.

Gordon RE, Hagan WA, 1936, A study of some acid-fast actinomycetes from soil with special reference to pathogenicity for animals, *J Infect Dis*, **59:** 200–6.

Gupta PK, Erozan YS, Frost JK, 1978, Actinomycetes and the IUD: an update, *Acta Cytol*, **22:** 281–2.

Gupta PK, Hollander DH, Frost JK, 1976, Actinomycetes in cervico vaginal smears. An association with IUD usage, *Acta Cytol*, **20:** 295–7.

Hart DHL, Peel MM et al., 1988, Lung infection caused by *Rhodococcus*, *Aust N Z J Med*, **18:** 790–1.

Harvey JC, Cantrell JR, Fisher AM, 1957, Actinomycosis: its recognition and treatment, *Ann Intern Med*, **46:** 868–85.

Harz CO, 1877–78, *Actinomyces bovis*, ein neuer Schimmel in den Geweben des Rindes, *Jahresber Königl Centralen Thierarzneischule München*, **5:** 125–40.

Hemmes GD, 1963, Enige bevindingen over actinomycose, *Ned Tijdschr Geneeskd*, **107:** 193.

Herzog M, Pape HD et al., 1984, Metastasierende Aktinomykose, *Fortschritte der Kiefer- und Gesichtschirurgie. Vol. 29. Septische Mund-Kiefer-Gesichtschirurgie*, eds Pfeifer G, Schwenzer N, Georg Thieme, Stuttgart, New York, 157–8.

Herzog S, 1981, *Retrospektive Untersuchung zur Klinik, Therapie und Bakteriologie der cervicofacialen Aktinomykosen an der Zahn- und Kieferklinik der Universität zu Köln von 1952–1975: Auswertung der Aufzeichnungen von 317 Patienten*, MD Thesis, Köln.

Holmberg K, 1981, Immunodiagnosis of human actinomycosis, *Actinomycetes. Proceedings of the 4th International Symposium on Actinomycete Biology*, eds Schaal KP, Pulverer G, Gustav Fischer, Stuttgart, New York, 259–61.

Holmberg K, Nord CE, Wadström T, 1975, Serological studies of *Actinomyces israelii* by crossed immuno-electrophoresis. Standard antigen–antibody system for *A. israelii*, *Infect Immun*, **12:** 387–97.

Houang ET, Lovett IS et al., 1980, *Nocardia asteroides* infection – a transmissible disease, *J Hosp Infect*, **1:** 31–40.

Israel J, 1878, Neue Beobachtungen auf dem Gebiet der Mykosen des Menschen, *Arch Pathol Anat Physiol Klin Med*, **74:** 15–53.

Jamjoom AB, Jamjoom ZA, al-Hedaithy SS, 1994, Actinomycotic

brain abscess successfully treated by burr hole aspiration and short course antimicrobial therapy, *Br J Neurosurg*, **8:** 545–50.

Khalaff H, Srigley JR, Klotz LH, 1995, Recognition of renal actinomycosis: nephrectomy can be avoided, *Can J Surg*, **38:** 77–9.

Kingdom TT, Tami TA, 1994, Actinomycosis of the nasal septum in a patient infected with the human immunodeficiency virus, *Otolaryngol Head Neck Surg*, **111:** 130–3.

Kjelstrom JA, Beaman BL, 1993, Development of a serologic panel for the recognition of nocardial infections in a murine model, *Diagn Microbiol Infect Dis*, **16:** 291–301.

Klinger R, 1912, Untersuchungen über menschliche Aktinomykose, *Zentralbl Bakteriol Parasitenkd Infektionskr Abt 1*, **62:** 191–200.

Korn-Wendisch F, Kempf A et al., 1989, Transfer of *Faenia rectivirgula* Kurup and Agre 1983 to the genus *Saccharopolyspora* Lacey and Goodfellow 1975, elevation of *Saccharopolyspora hirsuta* subsp. *taberi* Labeda 1987 to species level, and emended description of the genus *Saccharopolyspora*, *Int J Syst Bacteriol*, **39:** 430–41.

Krick JA, Stinson EB, Remington JS, 1975, Nocardia infection in heart transplant patients, *Ann Intern Med*, **82:** 18–26.

Krone A, Schaal KP et al., 1989, Nocardial cerebral abscess cured with imipenem/amikacin and enucleation, *Neurosurg Rev*, **12:** 333–40.

Lacey J, 1981, Air-borne actinomycete spores as respiratory allergens, *Zentralbl Bakteriol Mikrobiol Hyg Abt 1*, **Suppl. 11:** 243–50.

Lechevalier HA, Lechevalier MP, 1970, A critical evaluation of the genera of aerobic actinomycetes, *The Actinomycetales*, ed. Prauser H, VEB Gustav Fischer, Jena, 393–405.

Lentze F, 1969, Die Aktinomykose und die Nocardiosen, *Die Infektionskrankheiten des Menschen und ihre Erreger*, vol. 1, 2nd edn, eds Grumbach A, Bonin O, Georg Thieme, Stuttgart, 954–73.

Lentze FA, 1938, Zur Bakteriologie und Vakzinetherapie der Aktinomykose, *Zentralbl Bakteriol Parasitenkd Infektionskr Hyg Abt 1*, **141:** 21–36.

Lignières J, Spitz G, 1902, L'actinobacillose, *Bull Mém Soc Centr Méd Vét*, **20:** 487–535 and 546–65.

McNeil MM, Brown JM, 1994, The medically important aerobic actinomycetes: epidemiology and microbiology, *Clin Microbiol Rev*, **7:** 357–417.

McNeil MM, Brown JM et al., 1990, Comparison of species distribution and antimicrobial susceptibility of aerobic actinomycetes from clinical specimens, *Rev Infect Dis*, **12:** 778–83.

McNeil MM, Brown JM et al., 1992, Nonmycetomic *Actinomadura madurae* infection in a patient with AIDS, *J Clin Microbiol*, **30:** 1008–10.

Mannheim W, Frederiksen W, Mutters R, 1992, Pasteurellaceae, *Mikrobiologische Diagnostik*, ed. Burkhardt F, Georg Thieme, Stuttgart, New York, 163–73.

Miksits K, Stoltenburg G et al., 1991, Disseminated infection of the central nervous system caused by *Nocardia farcinica*, *Nephrol Dial Transplant*, **6:** 209–14.

Mirza SH, Campbell C, 1994, Mycetoma caused by *Nocardia transvalensis*, *J Clin Pathol*, **47:** 85–6.

Mishra SK, Gordon RE, Barnett DA, 1980, Identification of nocardiae and streptomycetes of medical importance, *J Clin Microbiol*, **11:** 728–36.

Morris JF, Sewell DL, 1994, Necrotizing pneumonia caused by mixed infection with *Actinobacillus actinomycetemcomitans* and *Actinomyces israelii*: case report and review, *Clin Infect Dis*, **18:** 450–2.

Mosselman G, Lienaux E, 1890, L'actinomycose et son agent infecteur, *Ann Med Vét*, **39:** 409–26.

Müller F, Schaal KP et al., 1988, Characterization of *Rhodococcus equi*-like bacterium isolated from a wound infection in a non-compromised host, *J Clin Microbiol*, **26:** 618–20.

Müller-Holzner E, Ruth NR et al., 1995, IUD-associated pelvic actinomycosis: a report of 5 cases, *Int J Gynecol Pathol*, **14:** 70–4.

Naeslund C, 1925, Studies of actinomyces from the oral cavity, *Acta Pathol Microbiol Scand*, **2:** 110–40.

Naeslund C, 1931, Experimentelle Studien über die Ätiologie und Pathogenese der Aktinomykose, *Acta Pathol Microbiol Scand*, **8, Suppl. 6:** 1–156.

Naka W, Miyakawa S et al., 1995, Unusually located lymphocutaneous nocardiosis caused by *Nocardia brasiliensis*, *Br J Dermatol*, **132:** 609–13.

Neubert U, Schaal KP, 1982, Sporotrichoide Infektion durch *Nocardia brasiliensis*, *Hautarzt*, **33:** 548–52.

Niederau W, Pape W et al., 1982, Zur Antibiotikabehandlung der menschlichen Aktinomykosen, *Dtsch Med Wochenschr*, **107:** 1279–83.

Nocard E, 1888, Notes sur la maladie des boeufs de la Guadeloupe connue sous le nom de farcin, *Ann Inst Pasteur (Paris)*, **2:** 293–302.

Persson E, Holmberg K, 1985, Study of precipitation reactions to *Actinomyces israelii* antigens in uterine secretions, *J Clin Pathol*, **38:** 99–102.

Pulverer G, Schaal KP, 1978, Pathogenicity and medical importance of aerobic and anaerobic actinomycetes, *Zentralbl Bakteriol Parasitenkd Infektionskr Hyg Abt 1*, **Suppl. 6:** 417–27.

Pulverer G, Schaal KP, 1984, Medical and microbiological problems in human actinomycoses, *Biological, Biochemical and Biomedical Aspects of Actinomycetes*, eds Ortiz-Ortiz L, Bojalil LF, Yakoleff V, Academic Press, Orlando, New York, London, 161–70.

Reller LB, Maddoux GL et al., 1975, Bacterial endocarditis caused by *Oerskovia turbata*, *Ann Intern Med*, **83:** 664–6.

Richet HM, Craven PC et al., 1991, A cluster of *Rhodococcus* (*Gordona*) *bronchialis* sternal-wound infections after coronary-artery bypass surgery, *N Engl J Med*, **324:** 104–9.

Ruimy R, Riegel P et al., 1996, *Nocardia pseudobrasiliensis* sp. nov., a new species of *Nocardia* which groups bacterial strains previously identified as *Nocardia brasiliensis* and associated with invasive disease, *Int J Syst Bacteriol*, **46:** 259–64.

Ruppert S, Reinold HM et al., 1988, Erfolgreiche antibiotische Behandlung einer pulmonalen Infektion mit *Nocardia asteroides* (Biovarietät A3), *Dtsch Med Wochenschr*, **113:** 1801–5.

Sahathevan M, Harvey FAH et al., 1991, Epidemiology, bacteriology and control of an outbreak of *Nocardia asteroides* infection in a liver unit, *J Hosp Infect*, **18, Suppl. A:** 473–80.

Schaal KP, 1972, Zur mikrobiologischen Diagnostik der Nocardiose, *Zentralbl Bakteriol Parasitenkd Infektionskr Hyg Abt 1 A*, **220:** 242–6.

Schaal KP, 1979, Die Aktinomykosen des Menschen: Diagnose und Therapie, *Dtsch Ärztebl*, **31:** 1997–2006.

Schaal KP, 1981, Actinomycoses, *Rev Inst Pasteur Lyon*, **14:** 279–88.

Schaal KP, 1983, Anaerobierinfektionen in der operativen Medizin, *Immun Infekt*, **11:** 153–68.

Schaal KP, 1984, Laboratory diagnosis of actinomycete diseases, *The Biology of the Actinomycetes*, eds Goodfellow M, Mordarski M, Williams ST, Academic Press, London, New York, San Francisco, 425–56.

Schaal KP, 1985a, Identification of clinically significant actinomycetes and related bacteria using chemical techniques, *Chemical Methods in Bacterial Systematics*, eds Goodfellow M, Minikin DE, Academic Press, Orlando, New York, London, 359–81.

Schaal KP, 1985b, Die Aktinomykosen des Menschen, *Internist Welt*, **8:** 32–8.

Schaal KP, 1986, Genus *Arachnia* Pine and Georg 1969, 269 and genus *Actinomyces* Harz 1877, 133, *Bergey's Manual of Systematic Bacteriology*, vol. 2, eds Sneath PHA, Mair NS et al., Williams & Wilkins, Baltimore, London, Los Angeles, Sydney, 1332–42 and 1383–418.

Schaal KP, 1991, Medical and microbiological problems arising from air-borne infection in hospitals, *J Hosp Infect*, **18, Suppl. A:** 451–9.

Schaal KP, 1992, The genera *Actinomyces*, *Arcanobacterium*, and

Rothia, The Prokaryotes. A Handbook on the Biology of Bacteria: Ecophysiology, Isolation, Identification, Applications, 2nd edn, eds Balows A, Trüper HG et al., Springer, New York, Berlin, Heidelberg, 850–905.

Schaal KP, 1996, Actinomycoses, *Oxford Textbook of Medicine,* 3rd edn, eds Weatherall DJ, Ledingham JGG, Warrell DA, Oxford University Press, Oxford, New York, Tokyo, 680–6.

Schaal KP, Beaman BL, 1984, Clinical significance of actinomycetes, *The Biology of the Actinomycetes,* eds Goodfellow M, Mordarski M, Williams ST, Academic Press, London, New York, San Francisco, 389–424.

Schaal KP, Lee HJ, 1992, Actinomycete infections in humans: a review, *Gene,* **115:** 201–11.

Schaal KP, Pape W, 1980, Special methodological problems in antibiotic susceptibility testing of fermentative actinomycetes, *Infection,* **8, Suppl. 2:** 176–82.

Schaal KP, Pulverer G, 1984, Epidemiologic, etiologic, diagnostic, and therapeutic aspects of endogenous actinomycete infections, *Biological, Biochemical, and Biomedical Aspects of Actinomycetes,* eds Ortiz-Ortiz L, Bojalil LF, Yakoleff V, Academic Press, Orlando, New York, London, 13–32.

Schaal KP, Schütt-Gerowitt H, Goldmann A, 1986, *In vitro* and *in vivo* studies on the efficacy of various antimicrobial agents in the treatment of human nocardiosis, *Biological, Biochemical, and Biomedical Aspects of Actinomycetes, Part B,* eds Szabó G, Biró S, Goodfellow M, Akadémiai Kiadó, Budapest, 619–33.

Schaal KP, Herzog M et al., 1984, Kölner Therapiekonzepte zur Behandlung der menschlichen Aktinomykosen von 1952–1982, *Fortschritte der Kiefer- und Gesichtschirurgie. Vol. 29. Septische Mund-Kiefer-Gesichtschirurgie,* eds Pfeifer G, Schwenzer N, Georg Thieme, Stuttgart, New York, 151–6.

Serrano JA, Beaman BL et al., 1986, Histological and ultrastructural studies of human actinomycetomas, *Biological, Biochemical and Biomedical Aspects of Actinomycetes,* eds Szabó G, Biró S, Goodfellow M, Akadémiai Kiadó, Budapest, 647–62.

Simpson GL, Stinson EB et al., 1981, Nocardial infections in the immunocompromised host: a detailed study in a defined population, *Rev Infect Dis,* **3:** 492–507.

Skoutelis A, Panagopoulos C et al., 1995, Intramural gastric actinomycosis, *South Med J,* **88:** 647–50.

Slack JM, Gerencser MA, 1975, *Actinomyces, Filamentous Bacteria,* Burgess, Minneapolis, Minnesota.

Sottnek FO, Brown JM et al., 1977, Recognition of *Oerskovia* species in the clinical laboratory: characterization of 35 isolates, *Int J Syst Bacteriol,* **27:** 263–70.

Stackebrandt E, Hariger M, Schleifer KH, 1980, Molecular genetic evidence for the transfer of *Oerskovia* species into the genus *Cellulomonas, Arch Microbiol,* **127:** 179–85.

Stackebrandt E, Smida J, Collins M, 1988, Evidence of phylogenetic heterogeneity within the genus *Rhodococcus:* revival of the genus *Gordona (Tsukamura), J Gen Microbiol,* **35:** 364–8.

Stasiecki P, Diehl V et al., 1985, Neue erfolgreiche Therapie bei systemischen Infektionen mit *Nocardia asteroides, Dtsch Med Wochenschr,* **110:** 1733–7.

Stein E, Schaal KP, 1984, Die Aktinomykosen. Das Krankheitsbild aus heutiger Sicht, *Zentralbl Haut-Geschlechtskr,* **150:** 183–7.

Trevisan V, 1889, *I Generi e le Specie delle Batteriacee,* Zanaboni and Gabuzzi, Milan, 9.

Vincent H, 1894, Études sur le parasite du pied le Madura, *Ann Inst Pasteur,* **8:** 129–51.

Wallace RJ Jr, Wiss K et al., 1983, Differences in susceptibility to aminoglycoside and beta-lactam antibiotics and their potential use in taxonomy, *Antimicrob Agents Chemother,* **23:** 19–21.

Wallace RJ Jr, Steele LC et al., 1988, Antimicrobial susceptibility patterns of *Nocardia asteroides, Antimicrob Agents Chemother,* **32:** 1776–9.

Wallace RJ Jr, Tsukamura M et al., 1990, Cephotaxime-resistant *Nocardia asteroides* strains are isolates of the controversial species *Nocardia farcinica, J Clin Microbiol,* **28:** 2726–32.

Warwick S, Bowen T et al., 1994, A phylogenetic analysis of the family Pseudonocardiaceae and the genera *Actinokineospora* and *Saccharothrix* with 16S rRNA sequences and a proposal to combine the genera *Amycolata* and *Pseudonocardia* in an emended genus *Pseudonocardia, Int J Syst Bacteriol,* **44:** 293–9.

Weber A, 1978, Zur Dermatophilose bei Tier und Mensch, *Münch Tierärztl Wochenschr,* **91:** 341–5.

Weinberger M, Eid A et al., 1995, Disseminated *Nocardia transvalensis* infection resembling pulmonary infarction in a liver transplant recipient, *Eur J Clin Microbiol Infect Dis,* **14:** 337–41.

Wright JR Jr, Stinson D et al., 1994, Necrotizing funisitis associated with *Actinomyces meyeri* infection: a case report, *Pediatr Pathol,* **131:** 927–34.

Wüst J, Stubbs S et al., 1995, Assignment of *Actinomyces pyogenes*-like (CDC coryneform group E) bacteria to the genus *Actinomyces* as *Actinomyces radingae* sp. nov. and *Actinomyces turicensis* sp. nov., *Lett Appl Microbiol,* **20:** 76–81.

Yano L, Imaeda T, Tsukamura M, 1990, Characterization of *Nocardia nova, Int J Syst Bacteriol,* **40:** 170–4.

Yassin AF, Rainey FA et al., 1995, *Tsukamurella inchonensis* sp. nov., *Int J Syst Bacteriol,* **45:** 522–7.

Yassin AF, Rainey FA et al., 1996, *Tsukamurella pulmonis* sp. nov, *Int J Syst Bacteriol,* **46:** 429–36.

Chapter 40

ANTHRAX

C P Quinn and P C B Turnbull

1 INTRODUCTION

1.1 History

The extensive history associated with anthrax dating back to about 1250 BC has been well reviewed in previous editions of this publication and elsewhere (Klemm and Klemm 1959, Dirckx 1981, Christie 1987). Classical writings reveal that anthrax was well known to the Greeks and Romans and from early records it appears several pandemics have occurred in Europe and Russia from mediaeval times to the mid-1800s. By the time it was realized in the late 1800s that a single agent was responsible for the different syndromes, the disease had acquired a host of 'colourful' names in addition to anthrax, such as black bain/bane, Bradford disease, malignant pustule/carbuncle (Fig. 40.1), rag picker's disease, Siberian plague, wool sorter's disease and numerous equivalents in other languages.

Anthrax also played a lead role in the history of microbiology, being the disease on which much of the original work on bacterial diseases and vaccines was done in the nineteenth century and from which many of the well known principles of pathogenic microbiology, including Koch's postulates, were derived (Parvizpour 1978, Choquette and Broughton 1981).

1.2 Importance of the disease

Anthrax, primarily a disease of herbivores, has declined strikingly in its importance throughout the world as a result of:

1 the successful development of a highly efficacious livestock vaccine by Sterne (1937), the use of which became and remains to this day the most important of all control measures

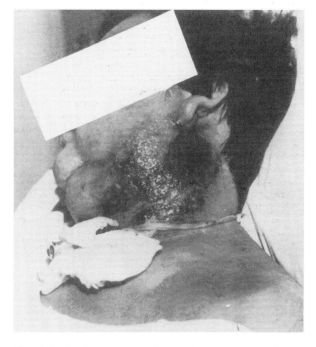

Fig. 40.1 'Malignant pustule' in an abattoir worker. Despite the name, the lesion is not malignant, nor is there pus unless secondarily infected. Note the need for tracheotomy; one of the dangers of facial or neck lesions is compression of the trachea as a result of the extensive oedema which is a primary characteristic of anthrax. This case was described by Darlow and Pride (1969).

2 improved understanding and practice of industrial hygiene and
3 the availability of antibiotics.

The result has been that physicians and clinical laboratories in developed regions of the world encounter the disease or its causative agent only rarely nowadays and notifications of human cases are infrequent in most of the countries that maintain and publish good epidemiological records. In countries that also have good public health organizations the main source of anthrax lies in animal products imported from regions of the world in which the disease is still enzootic.

None the less anthrax is of continuing world-wide importance. It remains prevalent in many less well developed parts of the world and medical and veterinary authorities in areas in which the disease is not endemic must be constantly on the alert for the arrival of *Bacillus anthracis* from endemic areas in imported products of animal origin. *B. anthracis* is exceedingly difficult to eradicate from an affected region and, even in areas considered non-endemic, outbreaks in livestock can occur following disturbance of soil in the vicinity of sites where anthrax carcasses were buried many years or decades previously when the areas were endemic. In wild animals, which for obvious reasons are difficult to vaccinate, anthrax is a major cause of mortality and a threat to endangered species in enzootic areas (Pienaar 1967, Ebedes 1976).

B. anthracis has acquired some notoriety as a potential agent of biological warfare (Manchee et al. 1981, 1994) and the Sverdlovsk incident in 1979 (Meselson et al. 1994) became the stimulus for a considerable research thrust into numerous aspects of the disease in the 1980s. The Gulf War in 1991 heightened the awareness of the possibility that *B. anthracis* could be used as a biological weapon (Friedlander et al. 1993) and served as a renewed stimulus to anthrax research.

2 ANTHRAX IN ANIMALS

2.1 Host range in livestock and wildlife

Few animal species are completely resistant to anthrax. Before an effective veterinary vaccine became available in the late 1930s, it was one of the foremost causes of heavy losses in cattle, sheep and goats throughout the world. This remains the case in affected regions of developing countries that lack an efficient vaccination policy. Reports collated in the 1988–94 *FAO-WHO-OIE Animal Health Yearbooks* show that, in fact, very few countries claim to be completely unaffected. The disease remains common in southern and eastern Europe, including several regions of the Russian sphere of influence. In Australia, sporadic outbreaks continue to occur annually. The disease is now rare in the USA and Canada, but in several countries of Africa and Asia, including several provinces of China, it ranges from common to enzootic.

As reviewed in the previous edition of this publication (Turnbull 1990), anthrax remains a major cause of death in wild herbivores in Africa, Asia, and to a lesser extent, the continents of America, Australasia and Europe. From time to time, a major outbreak in one or another species greatly reduces the population of that species in an area. Anthrax is, in fact, one of nature's main culling agents in such areas. Such losses, however, may have unexpected reper-

cussions for wildlife management and conservation. For example, in the Etosha National Park outbreaks in Namibia, the surfeit of wildebeest and zebra carcasses led to increased numbers of lions and hyenas which subsequently turned to other prey such as giraffe, kudu, gemsbok and eland, thereby reducing their numbers (Berry 1981). Even a few deaths from a disease such as anthrax are, of course, of great significance in a rare species such as the black rhinoceros.

As discussed in more detail in the previous edition of this work, carnivores and birds are generally regarded as highly resistant to anthrax, but numerous cases of predators and scavengers succumbing to the disease are on record. A comparison of the relative frequency of anthrax in lions in the Kruger National Park, South Africa, where anthrax is sporadic, with the Etosha National Park where anthrax is enzootic but where there are no cases on record of anthrax occurring in lions, indicates that in the Etosha, the carnivores are dependent on exposure-induced immunity to protect them from the disease. This is supported by serology (Turnbull et al. 1992).

2.2 Epizootiology

In developed countries, outbreaks of anthrax in livestock can on occasion be attributed directly to the importation of contaminated foodstuffs, or to the effluent from industries that process imported material (Van Ness 1971, Hugh-Jones and Hussaini 1974), but the epizootiology of natural enzootic anthrax is not yet well understood.

In domestic and wild herbivores an outbreak of anthrax usually tends to affect one species more than others; in both animals and man only a proportion of those exposed are usually affected. New South Wales, Australia, for example, has been broadly divided into a northern zone in which bovine and ovine anthrax occur with equal frequency, and a southern zone where bovine anthrax is 4 times as common as ovine, with death rates in cattle 13 times greater than in sheep (Wise and Kennedy 1980). In the Etosha National Park, Namibia, peak anthrax mortalities in the plains ungulates and elephants occur at different times of the year. During a pandemic of anthrax in swine in 1951–52 in midwest USA, cattle and other livestock on the numerous farms involved were not affected (Stein and Stoner 1952a, 1952b). There are numerous examples of epizootics in wildlife affecting one species while other equally susceptible species with apparently equal chances of exposure are relatively or completely unaffected.

At present it is not possible to attribute these phenomena definitely to factors such as variation in the strain of *B. anthracis* or in the condition of the host, or to geological, climatic or terrestrial differences. Most reports appear to confirm an association between enzootic anthrax and soil alkalinity (or low acidity) and warm ambient temperatures, but there is conflicting information on the importance of rainfall and moisture and it is not yet possible to predict the likelihood of an outbreak in an enzootic area.

In Britain, once the influence of the winter use of imported feed supplements had been removed in the 1960s, the incidence of anthrax in livestock became evenly distributed throughout summer and winter (Hugh-Jones and Hussaini 1974).

Ebedes (1976) has reviewed how in South Africa, where in bygone days anthrax was a common disease of domestic livestock, cases occurred during both wet and dry seasons and as often on arid land as on marshy veld. In the Kruger National Park (also South Africa), however, outbreaks occurred during or towards the end of the dry season and major epidemics were preceded by unusually heavy rain (Pienaar 1967).

In the Etosha National Park, the plains ungulates tend to be affected mostly towards the end of the rainy season (March–April), while elephant mortalities peak at the end of the dry season (November) (Lindeque and Turnbull 1994). The large epizootic in Lake Manyara National Park, Tanzania, also began after a long dry season (Prins and Weyerhaeuser 1987).

In Cyprus, where anthrax was once common in livestock, the disease occurred throughout the year but reached a peak in the dry season (Polydorou 1983). In the USA (Saulmon 1972, cited by Ebedes 1976), outbreaks were usually preceded by warm rainy periods.

In New South Wales, Australia, with its different patterns of anthrax in the north and south, outbreaks in the northern zone were more common during the hotter months in years that were drier than normal, but they often occurred after 12 weeks of high humidity; in the southern zone, outbreaks tended to occur mainly in seasons with above-average rainfall (Wise and Kennedy 1980). In Victoria, Australia, some but not all outbreaks occurred at the end of particularly dry seasons (Flynn 1968–69).

The apparent conflict in the evidence concerning the relation of rainfall or drought to the occurrence of anthrax may exist because the influence of climate is exerted in ways that differ according to geographical location. In Europe before World War II, the importation of untreated feed supplements led to a high incidence of anthrax in winter. In arid regions of the world, the dry season is a time of overgrazing, of close cropping to soil level, of competition for available food and water, of crowding of animals around water holes, and of increased stress and reduced bodily condition, this being aggravated in wildlife by the restriction of natural migration routes as a result of farming and territorial fencing. Wise and Kennedy (1980) proposed that the different patterns of anthrax in the northern and southern regions of New South Wales could be attributed partly to different management practices and partly to the natural differences in behaviour and feeding between cattle and sheep. Moro (1967) noted that in Peru anthrax occurred in livestock kept at altitudes below, but not above, 2000 m.

2.3 Forms of anthrax and symptomatology in animals

Because animals usually acquire anthrax by the ingestion of contaminated substances (feed, grass, water, or infected carcasses), they suffer most commonly from the gastrointestinal form of the disease. Cutaneous anthrax probably does occur on occasion through the bite of bloodsucking flies or via a wound or abrasion. It is even conceivable that the disease is acquired by inhalation, for example in elephants taking dust baths.

In herbivores, which are generally highly susceptible to anthrax, the disease frequently runs a hyperacute course and signs of illness may be absent until shortly, sometimes as little as an hour, before death. The animal then appears toxaemic and, occasionally after mild seizures, becomes comatose and dies. The severe mucosal congestion and endothelial cell breakdown that occurs in the final stages frequently leads to haemorrhage from the mouth, nares and anus, a highly pathognomonic sign. Milk may become bloodstained. Occasionally a less acute form occurs, running a course lasting 2–3 days, during which time the animal may appear at first depressed or excited, and then toxaemic, before death supervenes.

In an infected herd of herbivores, only a proportion develop clinical disease and serological evidence of mild or symptomless infection in domesticated and wild herbivores has been reported (Turnbull et al. 1992). Local lesions analogous to the eschar in humans are rare in animals, probably because:

1 infection by the cutaneous route is rare and
2 death in at least the more susceptible species intervenes before such lesions can manifest themselves.

In the more resistant species such as pigs and dogs, infection acquired by ingestion tends to become localized in the regional lymph nodes. In pigs there appear to be 2 manifestations of anthrax acquired by ingestion, the pharyngeal form and the intestinal form. The pharyngeal form, common in the days when pigs were fed food waste which included meat and bones from animal carcasses (which from time to time inadvertently included anthrax carcasses), is characterized by ulcerative stomatitis, laryngitis and markedly oedematous swelling of the throat region, sometimes mechanically restricting respiration, feeding and drinking. The infection is largely limited to the cervical and pharyngeal lymph glands. The clinical signs of the intestinal form are less obvious with digestive disturbance, such as anorexia, vomiting, diarrhoea, sometimes bloody, or constipation. The infection is most apparent in the mesenteric lymph glands. Occasionally, the disease may be fatal but bacteraemia may not be detectable. More often the animal will probably recover.

2.4 Diagnosis in animals

Sudden death in an animal without prior symptoms should lead to suspicion of anthrax, and bloody fluid exuding from the nose and mouth or anus of the dead animal is particularly suggestive. If anthrax is suspected, the carcass should not be opened; contamination of the environment with spilled body fluids, and subsequent spore formation, are thus avoided. Since a characteristic of anthrax is that, at death, the blood clots poorly or not at all, it is usually easy to withdraw a drop of blood from the vein of a reasonably fresh carcass and to make a smear of this. (The traditional instruction to take ear clippings dates from the days when disposable syringes and needles were unavailable.) If anthrax was not suspected and the carcass opened, dark unclotted blood and strikingly enlarged haemorrhagic spleen should alert the investigator. Petechial haemorrhages may be visible throughout the organs. The intestinal mucosa is often dark red and oedematous, with areas of necrosis.

Blood films should be dried, fixed immediately by heat or immersion for 1 min in absolute alcohol, and stained with polychrome methylene blue, which, after 30 s, is washed off into hypochlorite solution. When the slide is dry, it should be examined microscopically (Fig. 40.2) for the characteristic deep blue, square-ended bacilli surrounded by the well demarcated pink capsule ('M'Fadyean reaction') (M'Fadyean 1903).

At the time of death, the blood of highly susceptible species generally contains $>10^8$ bacilli ml^{-1}; these can be cultured readily on nutrient agar if the animal has not been treated with antibiotics.

Some variation in diagnostic signs is found among

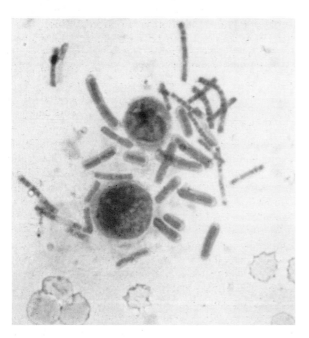

Fig. 40.2 Capsulated *Bacillus anthracis* cells around 2 blood mononuclear cells. Polychrome methylene blue stained blood smear from a guinea pig that died of anthrax (M'Fadyean stain). The cells, occasionally single but usually in short chains of 2 to a few cells and frequently square-ended ('boxcar' shaped), are blue-black; the surrounding capsule is pink. Oil immersion (×100) objective. Note that smears of artificially grown *B. anthracis* would show the cells in endless strings and, unless cultured under special conditions, lacking any capsule.

different species. In horses, the intestine and parenchymatous organs may be much less obviously affected than in sheep and cattle and the subcutaneous and intramuscular tissues may be oedematous (Whitford 1987). In pigs, terminal bacteraemia is very limited and the bacilli are unlikely to be seen in M'Fadyean-stained blood smears. When cervical oedema is present, fluid from the enlarged mandibular and suprapharyngeal lymph nodes should be examined microscopically for the M'Fadyean reaction. In porcine intestinal anthrax, which may be obvious only at necropsy, the bacilli are usually visible in stained smears made from mesenteric lymph nodes or may be cultured from these and from the mesenteric fluid. In carnivores, severe inflammation of the tongue, throat, stomach and intestines may be found; occasionally the lips, gums and jowls are also affected.

In wildlife, if the carcass is relatively fresh, polychrome methylene blue-stained blood smears are again appropriate for diagnosis. In older carcasses, *B. anthracis* can often be cultured from pieces of skin or other tissues left on the bones, but often the best approach is to culture the soil contaminated by the haemorrhagic exudations from the mouth, nose, or anus at death or spilt when the carcass was opened by scavengers (Lindeque and Turnbull 1994). The anthrax bacilli within the unopened carcass, unable to sporulate in the absence of oxygen, are destroyed by the putrefactive processes and therefore, in severely decomposed carcasses, may not be revealed by smears or culture. Ascoli in 1911 devised an immunoprecipitin test to detect residual anthrax antigens in tissues in which it was no longer possible to demonstrate the organism microscopically or by culture. It appears this is still used in parts of eastern Europe and the Middle East. The basis of the test is serum from an animal hyperimmunized with attenuated anthrax spores. The availability of the purified antigens of anthrax toxin has made possible the replacement of the Ascoli test by specific and sensitive enzyme immunoassays, capable of detecting microgram quantities of antigen in leached extracts of animal tissues. Although this is done as an occasional academic exercise at present, rapid on-site diagnostic or detection kits based on this principle and using monoclonal antibodies to epitopes of the protective antigen and lethal factor components of the anthrax toxin (see section 6.1, p. 810), and possibly other antigens, are expected to be available within the foreseeable future. Enzyme immunoassays based on purified toxin antigens are also available for the serological confirmation of infection in animals that survive the disease (Turnbull et al. 1992).

2.5 Transmission in animals

Herbivores, which play the central role in anthrax epizootics, generally acquire the disease by ingesting spores from the soil. As death approaches, the soil is further contaminated by haemorrhagic effusions from the nostrils, mouth and anus. The blood at death carries from 10^8 to $>10^9$ bacilli ml^{-1} and, on exposure to the oxygen in air, these rapidly sporulate. Recent ecological studies (Lindeque and Turnbull 1994) have shown, however, that the normal biological principle of 'many formed, few survive' pertains and that anthrax spore counts in soil contaminated with such blood range from nil to about 10^6 spores per gram with about 80% having counts of <1000 spores per gram.

In the wild in some parts of the world, conditions of calcium or phosphorus deficiency exist and the resulting osteophagia may also play a role in the transmission of anthrax (Sterne 1959, Ebedes 1976).

Biting flies have long been considered capable of transmitting anthrax. Budd (1863) cites Bourgeois as saying 'I have seen, in one case, the disease caused by the puncture of a gadfly that came out of a fleece of wool'. A case reported by Holgate and Holman in 1949 was associated with numerous flea bites. Tabanids were incriminated in anthrax transmission in India (Rao and Mohiyudeen 1958) and stable flies (*Stomoxys* spp.) and horse flies (Tabanidae) were thought by Davies (1983) to have played a major role in the large epidemic in Zimbabwe in 1979–80. The ability of biting flies and mosquitoes to transmit the disease has been confirmed in the laboratory (Schuberg and Boing 1913, cited without reference by McKendrick 1980, Sen and Minett 1944, Turell and Knudson 1987).

Most cases of anthrax, however, are caused by spores in soil or, possibly, water. The usual cycle of infection consists of:

1 uptake of the spores by the animal during feeding or drinking
2 entry of the spores through a lesion at some point along the gastrointestinal tract and carriage to the regional lymph nodes and beyond
3 multiplication in the lymph nodes and spleen
4 endothelial breakdown of vessels and sudden release of bacilli and toxin leading rapidly to death
5 shedding of vegetative bacilli by the dying or dead animal
6 sporulation on exposure to the oxygen in the air and
7 infection of a further animal by the spores, which may in the meantime have been widely dispersed by fomites or by the wind.

Scavengers feeding on an infected carcass may deposit *B. anthracis* spores elsewhere. The transient carriage of anthrax spores in scavengers that have fed on anthrax carcasses has been well documented (Choquette and Broughton 1981, Lindeque and Turnbull 1994). The unsporulated anthrax bacilli present in unopened carcasses die out rapidly as putrefaction proceeds, the precise rate depending on temperature (Christie 1987). When conditions are not conducive to immediate sporulation, the bacilli appear to die rapidly, even in aquatic environments (Lindeque and Turnbull 1994). It therefore seems unlikely that vegetative forms ingested by scavengers will survive passage through the intestinal tract.

The epizootiological importance, particularly in the past, of imported animal foodstuffs or fertilizers and of the contamination of rivers or pastures with industrial waste from the processing of animal products, has already been mentioned. These sources of infection continue to cause occasional episodes of anthrax in livestock in developed countries.

3 PERSISTENCE IN THE ENVIRONMENT

The ability of *B. anthracis* spores to survive in the environment for long periods is the subject of frequent observations in the literature, but there are actually few well documented studies of this. Jacotot and Virat (1954) found that anthrax spores prepared by Pasteur in 1888 were still viable 68 years later. On the other hand, canvas squares heavily inoculated in 1907 with spores and stored in a laboratory cupboard had become sterile 22 years later (Graham-Smith 1930). The survival of anthrax spores in dry soil held in the laboratory for 60 years was noted by Wilson and Russell (1964). On Gruinard Island, off the coast of Scotland, the soil was still heavily contaminated >40 years after bombs containing *B. anthracis* spores were detonated there in 1942–43 (Manchee et al. 1994). Bones recovered during archaeological excavations at Parfuri in the Kruger National Park in 1970 and estimated by carbon dating to be 200 ± 50 years old, are reported to have yielded *B. anthracis* on culture (de Vos et al. 1990). We recently isolated *B. anthracis* from roof insulation material in London's Kings Cross Station which presumably dated from the construction of that building some 110 years ago. Similarly, we have recently been involved in a land contamination problem in a field in the west of England resulting from the burial of the carcass of a bullock that died of anthrax and was buried there some 50 years ago.

The influence of soil type, which, of course, varies greatly in its content of moisture and organic matter, pH and other physical and chemical parameters, has been demonstrated (Lindeque and Turnbull 1994). Much cited is the hypothesis of Van Ness (1971) that 'suitable soils can maintain an organism–spore–organism cycle for years without infecting livestock', but our own experimental data (Bowen and Turnbull 1992, Lindeque and Turnbull 1994) lead us to believe that the nutritional level required for multiplication of germinated spores is far higher than is likely to be found in normal environments and that, should germination occur, the likely outcome is death of the emergent bacillus. Thus we believe that microcycling of *B. anthracis* in the environment is probably very rare and, in fact, the highly conserved nature of the species as a whole may be attributable to the dependence of the organism on an animal host for multiplication and the long time intervals that frequently occur between 2 opportunities to multiply, i.e. between 2 consecutive infections. The vegetative forms are also somewhat protected within the animal host from factors which influence DNA variation, such as DNA transforming events and exposure to phage. The opportunities for

DNA variation in *B. anthracis* would, therefore, appear to be very infrequent compared to most other bacteria.

Other factors in addition to nutritional levels undoubtedly play a role in the observed persistence of *B. anthracis* in the environment. Whether the spores attempt to germinate probably depends on moisture level, pH and temperature as well as on nutrients and germinants present. The long survival of spores in bones at Parfuri and in the Kings Cross roof space material may be related to the very dry conditions there (annual rainfall at Parfuri is 300–350 mm); on Gruinard Island, it was probably a combination of low pH (c. 4.3) and low ambient temperatures that suppressed germination of the spores. In the field in the west of England, it may have been simply the low ambient temperature of the soil (<10°C). Spore dormancy is a complex phenomenon, however, and it is doubtful whether a state of complete dormancy ('zero metabolism') ever occurs (Gould 1977).

The conditions conducive to germination of bacterial spores are also complex and beyond the scope of this chapter. Suffice it to say that they vary from species to species and are not well characterized for *B. anthracis*. The proportion of the spore population that will germinate, and the rate at which it will do so, are influenced by temperature, pH, moisture, the presence or absence of oxygen and carbon dioxide, and the presence of any germination stimulant. Furthermore, these factors may affect each other; for example, the rate and yield of germination may be influenced by temperature in a manner that varies with pH. Figures given for various mesophilic *Bacillus* spp., in particular *Bacillus cereus* (Sussman and Halvorson 1966), suggest that *B. anthracis* spores will not germinate at a pH of <5, a temperature of <8°C, a relative humidity of <96%, or an Eh of <0.3 V. Titball and Manchee (1987) confirmed that at 9°C germination of spores of the Vollum strain of *B. anthracis* was slight and that the optimum germination temperature, in the presence of the germination stimulant L-alanine, was 22°C.

The rate and extent of sporulation by vegetative cells shed from infected animals is also affected by environmental conditions. Lindeque and Turnbull (1994) found good survival with a high percentage of sporulation by the *B. anthracis* in blood from victims of anthrax when seeded into samples of sandy-type soil in the Etosha National Park whereas survival and consequent sporulation was poor in representative samples of karstveld soils from the Park. It did not appear that pH was the factor responsible for these differences.

4 ANTHRAX IN MAN

4.1 Susceptibility to anthrax. Data for risk assessments

As stated in the introduction (section 1, p. 799), anthrax is primarily a disease of herbivores; humans are incidental hosts and, in comparison with herbivores, are fairly resistant to the disease. Evidence for this comes from data on exposure versus infection and mortality rates in persons employed in high risk occupations, and on information extrapolated from monkeys.

In the early years of this century, before antibiotics or vaccines were available and when factory hygiene was relatively basic, workers in high risk industrial occupations (wool, hair, meat, bonemeal, leather processing) were exposed to substantial numbers of anthrax spores on a daily basis. In Britain, in the 13 year period 1899 through 1912, there were 354 cases of anthrax in such industries (Anon 1918). Although the number of exposed persons is not known, it must have been many thousands, illustrating that anthrax cases were few in relation to exposure. In 4 mills in the USA studied by Brachman et al. (1962), in which unvaccinated workforces varying in size from 148 to 655 were 'chronically exposed to anthrax', annual case rates were only 0.6–1.4%. Dahlgren et al. (1960), by means of air-sampling techniques, estimated that in one mill, the workers inhaled between 600 and 1300 spores during an 8 h shift without ill effect. Carr and Rew (1957) recovered *B. anthracis* from the nose and pharynx of 14 of 101 healthy unvaccinated workers in 2 goat-hair mills.

The low infectivity of the spores for man is borne out by other observations. For example, after large epizootics in wild animals in the Kruger National Park, Pienaar (1967) noted that 'of the large teams of workmen ... employed for tracking down and burning carcasses of animals which died of anthrax, none contracted the disease although ... definitely exposed'. Many villagers were known to have eaten meat from hippopotamus carcasses at the time of the large epizootic in the Luangwa River, Zambia, in 1987 but there was not a single case of human anthrax on record (Turnbull et al. 1991). The experience in other wildlife reserves is similar, although occasional human cases have occurred (Pyper and Willoughby 1964, Pienaar 1967).

In the absence of extensive data on exposure versus case rates in humans, the susceptibility of humans to anthrax has, for the most part, to be assessed from information from animal tests. The published information on infectious and lethal doses in humans and animals has been comprehensively collated by Watson and Keir (1994). If it is assumed that the data from monkeys are the most relevant to humans, the inhalation LD50s on record range from 4130 to 760 000 spores. Having larger body weights and being, it is believed, rather more resistant to anthrax than the types of monkeys tested, humans would be expected to have higher infective doses by this route. This is probably true also for infection through ingestion of the organism or its spores; even in areas of the world where meat from anthrax carcasses is consumed on a fairly regular basis, case rates are very low.

It probably does not take many spores to initiate a cutaneous infection given that the spores reach an appropriate infection site (cut, abrasion, etc.); Watson and Keir suggest that 10 spores constitutes a conservative estimate of the cutaneous infectious dose in humans. However, the opportunity for spores to reach such sites is generally very low in at-risk occupations where appropriate clothing, dressing of wounds and other hygienic procedures are standard.

4.2 Epidemiology

Human anthrax is traditionally classified into:

1 'non-industrial', occurring in butchers, farmers, knackers, pathologists and veterinarians, as a result of close contact with infected animals and
2 'industrial', occurring in those employed in the processing of wool, hair, hides, bones or other animal products.

The non-industrial version, which usually manifests itself as cutaneous anthrax (see section on 'Cutaneous anthrax', p. 806), results from handling infected carcasses and tends to be seasonal, reflecting the seasonal incidence of anthrax in the country from which the carcasses originated. Insect transmitted anthrax also takes the cutaneous form. Intestinal anthrax resulting from the consumption of infected meat also belongs to the non-industrial category.

The industrial form also most commonly manifests itself as cutaneous anthrax but has a far higher chance of taking the pulmonary manifestation as a result of the inhalation of spore-laden dust or other aerosols. Of the 354 cases of industrial anthrax recorded in Britain from 1899 through 1912, before the availability of vaccines and antibiotics, 36 (10.2%) were 'internal' (which almost certainly means pulmonary) (Anon 1918). Between 1961 and 1980, of 122 occupationally exposed persons with anthrax in Britain, only one pulmonary case was recorded (Communicable Disease Surveillance Centre 1982).

Anthrax is no longer common in western developed countries. The decline in incidence in these countries is probably due, at least in part, to:

1 the use of a successful vaccine in animals, resulting in a reduction of the contaminated animal products of industrial importance
2 improvement in the sterilization of imported materials of animal origin
3 the use of man-made alternatives to animal products
4 the increased use of vaccines in workers at risk and
5 improved factory hygiene (see also section 1.2, p. 799).

The disease in humans is still prevalent in many parts of Africa, South East Asia, China, Central America, the Indian subcontinent and certain regions of eastern and southern Europe, the Middle East, the Russian Federation and South America (FAO-WHO-OIE 1988–94).

TRANSMISSION

Man almost invariably acquires anthrax directly or indirectly from infected animals, but exceptions have been recorded on rare occasions. An unqualified nursing orderly in Zimbabwe acquired an anthrax lesion on his finger as a result of removing dressings from an anthrax patient (personal visit to St Luke's Hospital, Lupane, Zimbabwe). Communal loofahs appeared to be a means of person-to-person spread in Gambia (Heyworth et al. 1975). Lalitha et al. (1988) recorded an anthrax 'abscess', which developed at the site of an antibiotic injection.

Laboratory-acquired infections have been reported, though not in recent years (Collins 1990/91). A substantial outbreak of anthrax in April 1979 in the city of Sverdlovsk (now Yekaterinburg) in the Urals resulted from the accidental release of spores from a military microbiology facility (Meselson et al. 1994). Official reports put the number of cases at 96 with 64 deaths.

In the pulmonary form of industrial anthrax, spores in dust clouds created from the handling of dry hides, skins, wool, bonemeal and the like are inhaled by the workers. In cutaneous anthrax, the infection occurs via a small cut or abrasion. As a result, and as noted as long ago as 1863 (Budd 1863), exposed regions of the body are most frequently affected and the site of infection often reflects the occupation of the patient. Workers who carry hides or carcasses on their shoulders are prone to infection on the back of the neck. Handlers of other animal products tend to be infected on the arms or wrists, and occasionally the hands. Most lesions are found on the face, head and neck (Figs 40.1 and 40.3); less often affected are the arms, and still less the trunk and lower limbs (Martin 1975, Parvizpour 1978, Davies 1983, Kobuch et al. 1990).

The ability of biting flies to transmit anthrax (see section 2.5, p. 802) also applies to humans (Fig. 40.4).

In some developing countries, the value of meat from animals that have died unexpectedly outweighs the perceived risks of contracting anthrax; this has in the past, and continues to result in the intestinal form of the disease (Pienaar 1967, Hughes 1973, Jena 1980, Davies 1982, Kobuch et al. 1990, Anon 1994a).

4.3 The clinical disease

Anthrax takes one of 3 forms. The cutaneous form is acquired through a lesion in the skin, the intestinal form through a lesion on the mucosa of the gastrointestinal tract, and the pulmonary form by inhalation. Cutaneous anthrax accounts for 95–99% of human cases. All 3 forms are potentially fatal but the cutaneous type is often self-limiting. Data from preantibiotic and vaccine days indicate that 10–20% of untreated cutaneous cases might be expected to result in death (Anon 1918). Nowadays suitable treatment is available almost anywhere in the world and fatalities from cutaneous anthrax are very rare. The characteristic eschar or carbuncle is surrounded by an oedematous zone, which may extend some distance from the lesion. The main dangers are meningitis or cellulitis and, when the lesion is on the face or neck, obstruction of the airways by compression from the oedematous swelling (Figs 40.1, 40.4, 40.5).

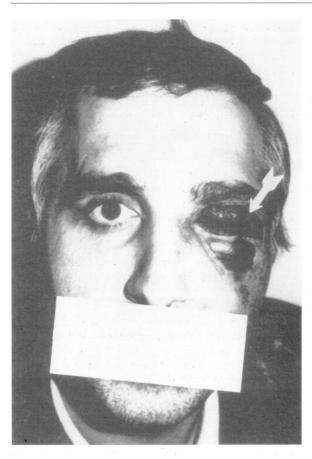

Fig. 40.3 The characteristic eschar in a case of infection of the eyelid (from Doganay 1986, with permission).

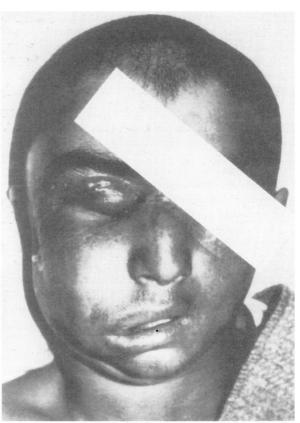

Fig. 40.5 Lesion on the eyelid (from Doganay 1986, with permission).

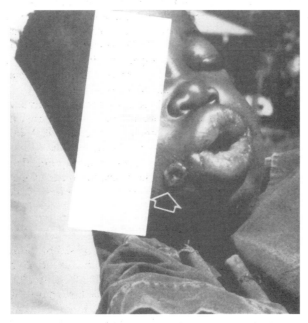

Fig. 40.4 Extensive facial oedema around anthrax infection sites. A presumed fly-bite lesion (from Parry, Turnbull and Gibson 1983, with permission). Photograph by JCA Davies.

The intestinal and pulmonary forms are regarded as being more often fatal than cutaneous anthrax but this is because they frequently go unrecognized until it is too late for effective treatment. It is not known how often low-grade intestinal or pulmonary anthrax ends in recovery, because the nature of the disease is such that a search for the bacilli in faeces or sputum is unlikely to be undertaken. However, the results of serological studies on workers in goat-hair processing mills in the 1950s led experts at the time to conclude that mild or inapparent anthrax infection occurred in those chronically exposed to spores (Brachman et al. 1960, Norman et al. 1960).

CUTANEOUS ANTHRAX

The period between infection via a cut, abrasion or insect bite and the first appearance of a small pimple or papule is usually 2–3 days, although published reports include incubation times as short as half a day (Salmon 1896) and as long as 19 days (Abdenour et al. 1987).

A ring of vesicles develops around the central papule over the next 24 h and as the lesion develops (Fig. 40.6), the central papule ulcerates and dries to form the eschar, which turns black and enlarges to cover the vesicles as these dry up. Pus is present only if the lesion is secondarily infected by pyogenic organisms. The lesion may remain small (c. 2 cm in diameter) but occasionally becomes very extensive (>10 cm)

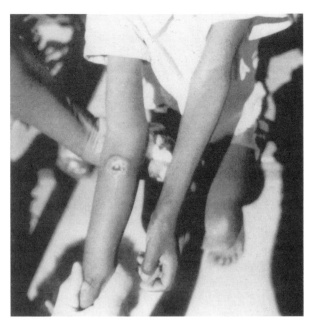

Fig. 40.6 Ring of vesicles surrounding the developing eschar in an early anthrax lesion. Note the oedema along the entire length of the affected arm.

(Fig. 40.7). It is always surrounded by oedema. By the fifth or sixth day it has become a thick black eschar firmly adherent to the underlying tissues.

In uncomplicated cutaneous anthrax, the bacilli remain localized to the lesion. Adenitis of the regional lymph nodes is not uncommon but lymphangitis, if it occurs, may indicate secondary infection of the lesion. Fever is generally mild or absent unless secondary infection has occurred. The eschar begins to resolve about 10 days after the appearance of the initial papule. Resolution is slow, 2–6 weeks regardless of treatment (Turner 1980), but usually complete. Scarring is frequently minimal and surgical intervention is only

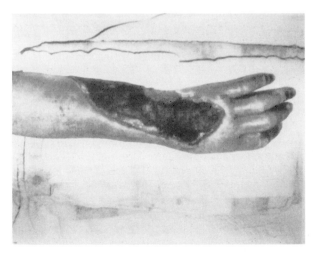

Fig. 40.7 An extensive eschar. The lesion is not painful unless secondarily infected. In the case of smaller lesions, with treatment, resolution is usually complete; surgical intervention would be necessary with a lesion of this size, however (from Doganay 1986, with permission).

necessary when this affects a function, such as movement of an eyelid (Martin 1975, Christie 1987, Kobuch et al. 1990, Doganay et al. 1994), or if the lesion was exceptionally large, when skin grafting may be called for (Martin 1975). The oedema may be very persistent, but there is no pus and neither the eschar nor the surrounding swelling should be incised as this may result in an intractable sinus (Christie 1987, Dr AO Pugh, personal communication, 1987).

In cases that become septicaemic, a feeling of chilliness, headache, anorexia and nausea may herald a rapid and fatal illness, in which the temperature rises to 38.9–40°C and then may fall to below normal within a few hours. The patient becomes irreversibly toxaemic and shocked; dyspnoea, cyanosis and collapse precede death.

In patients who become secondarily infected, gangrene is an occasional complication (Christie 1987).

INTESTINAL ANTHRAX

In this form of the disease the anthrax lesions develop on the mucosa of the intestine after the ingestion of *B. anthracis* spores in meat from an animal that has died of anthrax. Few countries outside Africa or Asia have any recorded cases of this form of the disease and its occurrence in temperate zones appears to be unrecorded. The characteristic eschar occurs most commonly on the wall of the terminal ileum or caecum (Nalin et al. 1977, Whitford 1987); the oropharynx, stomach, duodenum and upper ileum are occasionally affected (Christie 1987, Kobuch et al. 1990). The lesion may appear gangrenous, extensive regions of the intestine and mesentery may be oedematous, and the mesenteric lymph nodes may be enlarged. Early symptoms range from mild gastrointestinal disturbance to nausea, vomiting, anorexia, fever, abdominal pain and bloody diarrhoea (Ndyabahinduka et al. 1984); sometimes there is tenderness in the right upper and lower quadrants. According to Jena (1980) a watery diarrhoea, resembling that of cholera, may occur on occasion.

The incubation period, as in cutaneous anthrax, is 2–5 days. If an early diagnosis is made the disease can be cured (Jena 1980, Ndyabahinduka et al. 1984), but because of the difficulty in identifying cases early enough, this form of anthrax is fatal more often than is cutaneous anthrax. In fatal cases, the onset of malaise is sudden; shock, collapse and death follow within a few hours.

PULMONARY ANTHRAX

This form of anthrax is almost always caused by industrial exposure to spores, although the outbreak in Sverdlovsk, referred to earlier, resulting from accidental release of spores from a military facility is a notable exception. Illness begins insidiously, often 2–5 days after exposure, with mild fever, fatigue, malaise, myalgia and non-productive cough. Moist râles are heard on auscultation of the chest. This mild initial phase, which lasts 2 to a few days, is terminated by the sudden onset of acute illness characterized by acute dyspnoea and subsequent cyanosis. The patient appears moribund with accelerated pulse and respiration and may vomit or cough up a little blood. The temperature may be elevated or, if shock has set in, subnormal. Moist crepitant râles and signs of pleural effusion result from the internal oedema. Terminally, the pulse becomes accelerated and feeble; the dyspnoea, cyanosis, temperature changes and disorientation are quickly followed by coma and death (Albrink et al. 1960, Plotkin et al. 1960, Enticknap et al. 1968, Christie 1987).

The fulminant disease is usually fatal, but successful treatment has been recorded (Plotkin et al. 1960). It is likely that mild infection and recovery can occur and go unrecognized.

ANTHRAX MENINGITIS

Meningitis can develop as a sequel in any of the forms of anthrax. Observations in the first half of this century indicated that, in the majority of cases, anthrax meningitis was secondary to cutaneous anthrax; in about 25% it was secondary to inhalation anthrax, while in 10% of cases, no primary focus could be found. The last were termed 'primary anthrax meningitis' (Haight 1952).

Anthrax meningitis cannot be differentiated clinically from other forms of meningitis unless evidence of one of the other forms of the disease is also present. Trismus appears to be a characteristic feature and signs of cerebral irritation are present in 50% of cases (Lalitha et al. 1990). The clinical signs of meningitis and the appearance of blood in the cerebrospinal fluid are followed rapidly by loss of consciousness and death (Haight 1952, Drake and Blair 1971, Tahernia and Hashemi 1972, Koshi et al. 1981, Levy et al. 1981, Lalitha et al. 1990); the prognosis in this form of anthrax is grave. Currently anthrax meningitis is reported with some frequency in Tamilnadu province, south India (Anon 1994b, George et al. 1994).

4.4 Diagnosis in man

The well developed lesion of cutaneous anthrax is readily recognized by its central eschar, ring of vesicles and accompanying oedema. In the early stages the papule may be mistaken for a boil, but the absence of pain, the lack of pus, and the extensive oedema with a consideration of the patient's occupation, together should raise suspicion of anthrax. The differential diagnosis (Christie 1987) should include boil, primary syphilitic chancre, erysipelas, glanders, plague, orf, vaccinia and tropical ulcer.

Smears of fluid from the early anthrax papule may be stained with polychrome methylene blue and examined microscopically for the presence of the pink-staining capsule (M'Fadyean reaction); material from the same site may be cultured. In older lesions the eschar should be lifted with forceps and fluid for a smear, culture or both obtained by means of a capillary tube. Despite its inflamed appearance, the lesion is not painful unless secondarily infected. Diagnosis of the pulmonary and intestinal forms is likely to be missed unless circumstances suggest that exposure to air-

borne spores or contaminated food respectively may have taken place.

In uncomplicated cutaneous anthrax, the erythrocyte sedimentation rate may be somewhat elevated. The white cell count is usually normal, but there may be a mild neutrophil leucocytosis, of the order of 10 000–13 000 WBC mm^{-3} (Martin 1975, Turner 1980). Even in the acute stages of more severe forms of the disease, leucocytosis is moderate with a slight shift to the left. Haemoglobin concentration, pulse rate and blood pressure remain normal till the final stages of the systemic illness (Plotkin et al. 1960, Jena 1980). In the meningitic form, the cerebrospinal fluid (CSF) contains red and white blood cells, the protein content is raised and the sugar content depressed, and anthrax bacilli can be readily demonstrated (George et al. 1994, see also Walker, Lincoln and Klein 1967 for CSF changes in infected rhesus monkeys and in those given injections of cell-free toxin).

Enzyme immunoassays for the serological confirmation of infection based on the purified protective antigen and lethal factor components of the anthrax toxin provide good supplementary diagnostic aids, although early antibiotic treatment may result in a weak or undetectable antibody response (Turnbull et al. 1992). Ideally 2 or more serum samples should be collected 2–4 weeks apart for demonstration of rising titres; if only one sample is taken, it will be of greater diagnostic reliability if collected more than a week after onset of symptoms.

4.5 Age and sex

We have not seen reports indicating that the occurrence of naturally acquired anthrax in humans is related to age or sex although it was noted in the Sverdlovsk outbreak, and regarded as unexplained, that none of the patients was younger than 24 (Meselson et al. 1994). As reviewed elsewhere (Lindeque and Turnbull 1994), various reports exist of a susceptibility bias towards adult males in a variety of other animal species. The results of a study on the topic by Weinstein (1938) indicated that differences could not be readily attributed to the circulating sex hormones.

5 BACTERIOLOGY

B. anthracis is gram-positive, non-motile, aerobic, facultatively anaerobic and spore-forming. The vegetative form is a square-ended rod, 1–1.5 μm by 5–8 μm. In infected blood or tissue the rods are frequently present in short chains and are surrounded by polypeptide capsule visible under the microscope when stained with polychrome methylene blue (M'Fadyean reaction) or highlighted with India ink (Turnbull et al. 1993). In stained smears made from colonies on nutrient agar plates, they are seen in long chains and there is no capsule unless the medium contained bicarbonate (approximately 0.7%) or serum (approximately 5%) and was incubated under 5–10%

CO_2 (a candle jar works well) (Carman, Hambleton and Melling 1985, Turnbull et al. 1993).

Because sporulation occurs only under aerobic conditions, spores are not seen in blood smears taken from animals within a few hours of death. Once the resting vegetative cell is exposed to air, sporulation occurs, at a rate that depends on temperature and other environmental conditions. The spore is visible by phase-contrast microscopy or in stained preparations as an oval body placed centrally or subterminally within the bacillus and not distending the cell. In contrast to the vegetative cell, the spore is highly resistant to heat, cold, ultraviolet light, desiccation, high and low pH, chemical disinfectants and the metabolic products of other bacteria.

Provided that antibiotic treatment has not been given, no difficulty should be encountered in isolating *B. anthracis* at death from animals or humans that have died from anthrax, or during life from cutaneous lesions. On the other hand, *B. anthracis* in animal hair or hide, bonemeal and soil may be difficult to detect within the background of other *Bacillus* spp. commonly present. In our experience, the most reliable method involves the use of the selective polymyxin–lysozyme–EDTA–thallous acetate (PLET) agar (Knisely 1966). Specimens (1 to a few grams for light materials such as dust; 50–150 g for heavy materials such as soils) should be emulsified in 1–2 volume equivalents of sterile water. These should then be heat shocked at 62.5°C for 15 min and 1:10, 1:100 and 1:1000 dilutions in sterile water prepared. Aliquots, approximately 100 ml and 250 ml of each dilution, should then be spread on blood agar and PLET plates respectively. Typical *B. anthracis* colonies are then looked for on the blood plates after overnight incubation at 37°C and after 36–48 h at 37°C on the PLET plates. There may be occasions when it is thought necessary to prepare the dilutions and to subculture them before as well as after the heat treatment.

Subsequent confirmation of identity can be carried out by tests for lack of haemolysis and motility, diagnostic phage and penicillin sensitivity and capsule production. Possession of the virulence factors, toxin and capsule can now be tested for, both phenotypically and by polymerase chain reaction (PCR). The topic of isolation and confirmation of identity of *B. anthracis* is covered more fully elsewhere (Turnbull et al. 1993, Turnbull and Kramer 1995).

6 PATHOGENESIS AND VIRULENCE FACTORS

As a consequence of the extensive and intensive research conducted into the pathogenesis of anthrax during the post-war period and up until the 1960s, 2 unique virulence factors of anthrax pathogenesis have been identified; a γ-linked poly-D-glutamic acid capsule and a tripartite protein toxin. Of these, the toxin has received by far the greatest attention and elucidation of its mode of action has generated extensive coverage in scientific literature. Conversely, investigation of the capsule and other potential virulence factors has received much less attention. As a consequence, the role of the capsule in pathogenesis is not fully understood. That it is an essential virulence factor is not in doubt but it is a poor immunogen and in the absence of toxin appears to have no value as a protective agent in vaccine formulation (Ivins and Welkos 1988). Its poor antigenicity may be a consequence of its polymeric structure although Makino et al. (1988) have used anti-capsule antisera for the study of capsule gene expression. Little is known about the capsule polymer and thus far research has failed to elucidate its full, and critical, role in pathogenesis beyond that of being an antiphagocytic barrier (Zwartou and Smith 1956, Keppie, Harris-Smith and Smith 1963). Bacterial polysaccharides from other genera, however, are capable of downregulating antibody responses by their effect on populations of suppressor T lymphocytes (Taylor and Bright 1989) and it is possible that the glutamic acid polymer (or other cell-associated antigens) of *B. anthracis* has a similar function.

The toxic effects of cell-free extracts from cutaneous anthrax lesions have been observed as early as 1904 following the use of oedema fluid as a vaccine (Watson et al. 1947, Lincoln and Fish 1970). However, it was not until 1954 that Smith and Keppie showed conclusively that death in anthrax was caused primarily by an intoxication resulting from a bacteraemia. This group, monitoring a developing bacteraemia in guinea pigs, demonstrated that if the bacteraemia was aborted with streptomycin before reaching a critical level the infection could be eliminated and the animals survived. However, if this critical level of micro-organisms was exceeded before antibiotic administration, the animals died despite clearing the bacteraemia. Prior to this it had been held that death was due to capillary blockage, hypoxia and depletion of nutrients by the exceedingly large number of bacilli. That anthrax toxin has a 3 component nature was demonstrated by Stanley and Smith (1961) but it was some years before each of the components, oedema factor (EF), protective antigen (PA) and lethal factor (LF), were fully purified and characterized. Although many aspects of the pathology of anthrax remain unresolved, such as the relationship between toxin production, the onset of bacteraemia and the pathological features visible in the lymph nodes and the spleen, the volume of data concerning function and macromolecular structure of the toxin components is continuously expanding. That such a relationship exists is clear from the protection afforded by PA in vaccinated animals (see section 8.1, p. 814). Studies in primates indicate that the toxin also depresses electrical activity in the cerebral cortex; this affects the respiratory centre and may thereby contribute to anoxia, cardiac collapse, shock and sudden death (Walker, Lincoln and Klein 1967).

6.1 Anthrax toxin components

Protective antigen (PA)

It was not until 1982 that the first understanding of the nature of the toxin components began to unfold. PA had for some time been known to be the pivotal protein in the pathogenesis of anthrax toxin and indeed derived its name from recognition of this fact (Watson et al. 1947). Its prerequisite presence or inclusion in any preparation that provides immunity to the disease serves to underline this (see section 8.1, p. 814). Animal and cell culture experiments have indicated that EF and LF compete for available PA (Ezzell, Ivins and Leppla 1984), prompting the hypothesis that PA might bind to a cell surface receptor and so initiate a toxin internalization event by which EF and LF gain entry to the cytosol of susceptible target cells (Leppla, Ivins and Ezzell 1985). Subsequent developments in anthrax toxin research revealed that cell-bound PA is proteolytically cleaved from an 83 kDa species (PA83) at the target cell to generate a biologically active 63 kDa (PA63) molecule for which both LF and EF compete and to which they both bind with high affinity (Leppla, Friedlander and Cora 1988). The protease activation site in PA83 is defined by the sequence -R-K-K-R- at residues 164–167 of the mature polypeptide (Singh, Chaudhary and Leppla 1989). This sequence is susceptible to a range of proteases including trypsin and the furin-type enzymes (Gordon and Leppla 1994, Gordon et al. 1995). It has been reported that the activated PA63 forms heptamers at reduced pH and that it is probably a high molecular weight species of PA + EF (oedema toxin) or PA + LF (lethal toxin) that undergoes internalization (Milne et al. 1994). No biological activity has, as yet, been assigned to the residual 20 kDa fragment (PA20) nor has the stoichiometry of the PA–EF/LF interaction been established. However, this sequence of events describing PA receptor interaction, proteolytic activation with subsequent EF/LF binding and internalization has now become the accepted model of anthrax toxin activity at the target cell (Fig. 40.8). This toxin is thus considered to fit the accepted binary toxin model which describes the activity of several other bacterial protein toxins (Friedlander et al. 1993).

Oedema factor (EF)

In terms of elucidation of the underlying mechanisms of toxin activity at the cellular level, initial attention focused on the EF component as it had been surmised that the oedema-producing effect may be due to elevated intracellular cyclic adenosine monophosphate (cAMP) levels, an effect similar to that stimulated by cholera toxin (CT) or *Escherichia coli* heat labile toxin (LT). This hypothesis was subsequently confirmed using EF in Chinese hamster ovary (CHO) cell assays (Leppla 1982). Bacterial toxins CT and LT exert their action indirectly by inducing irreversible conformational changes in membrane-bound guanidine diphosphate (GDP)-binding proteins. This in turn stimulates constitutive adenylate cyclase activity (Gill

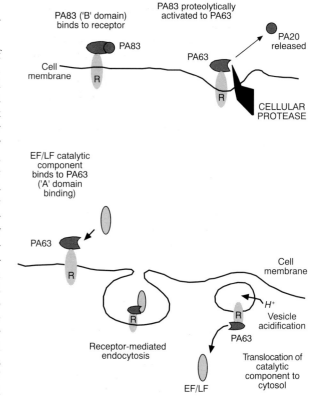

Fig. 40.8 Schematic diagram of the accepted model for anthrax toxin interaction at the cell surface and its subsequent internalization via an acidic endosome. The full length protective antigen (PA83) first binds to a receptor (R) at the cell surface where it is proteolytically cleaved to the receptor-bound PA63 form and the PA20 fragment is released. PA63, which may form heptamers, possesses a high affinity binding site for which the lethal factor (LF) and oedema factor (EF) catalytic components compete. The PA63 complexed to the catalytic component undergoes receptor mediated internalization and translocation into the cytosol via an acidic endosome.

and Coburn 1987). EF, however, was itself shown to be an adenylate cyclase and, perhaps more remarkably, calmodulin-dependent, and hence only functional in eukaryotic cells (Leppla 1982, Leppla, Ivins and Ezzell 1985). (Calmodulin is the major intracellular calcium receptor in eukaryotic cells.) The only other bacterium known to produce a calmodulin-dependent adenylate cyclase is *Bordetella pertussis*. Antigenic cross-reaction between the *B. anthracis* and the *B. pertussis* adenylate cyclases has been demonstrated (Mock et al. 1988) and 3 conserved regions of amino acid and nucleotide homology in the 2 molecules have now been reported (Escuyer et al. 1988, Robertson 1988). However, the overall sequences have little homology and the enzymes would also appear to have different mechanisms of cell internalization; cell entry by EF is blocked by a range of inhibitors of receptor mediated endocytosis whereas cell entry by pertussis adenylate cyclase is not (Gordon, Leppla and Hewlett 1988). Escuyer et al. (1988) and Robertson (1988) have identified putative calmodulin-binding regions of each molecule; these exhibit a high degree of DNA homology and the pertussis enzyme has been shown to cross-react immunologically with rat brain adenylate cyclases which are also calmodulin-dependent (Escuyer et al. 1988).

O'Brien et al. (1985) demonstrated that combinations of PA + EF suppressed polymorphonuclear leucocyte (PMN) activity and inhibited phagocytosis of *B. anthracis* cells. Wade et al. (1985) have also shown that, unlike other cAMP-forming toxins, PA + EF (oedema toxin) enhances the migration of stimulated PMNs; this was also true of PA + LF (lethal toxin).

LETHAL FACTOR (LF)

The binary combination of PA + LF (lethal toxin) is lethal to laboratory animals and lyses certain eukaryotic cell lines, specifically those of monocyte/macrophage lineage (Friedlander 1986). It is considered to be the cause of death in a fatal anthrax infection as a consequence of its cytokine stimulatory and cytotoxic effects on peripheral macrophages (Hanna, Acosta and Collier 1993). LF has recently been demonstrated to contain one or more Zn^{2+}-binding amino acid motifs, one of which is characteristic of the thermolysin family of zinc-dependent metalloproteases (Klimpel, Arora and Leppla 1994, Kochi et al. 1994). Although no substrate has yet been identified for this putative protease, mutational analysis of the catalytic domain of LF has confirmed the relevance of these motifs in an in vitro macrophage lysis assay (Quinn et al. 1991, Klimpel, Arora and Leppla 1994). When the lethal toxin (PA + LF) is administered intravenously to laboratory animals, specifically Fischer 334 rats, death ensues within 60–90 min and is characterized by severe pulmonary oedema (Singh, Chaudhary and Leppla 1989). Although useful for quantifying LF and PA, this assay yields no constructive information on the cellular and molecular mechanisms involved in toxicity and the putative enzymatic substrate of the lethal toxin complex remains unknown (Friedlander 1986). The enigmatic lethal factor thus remains an intriguing aspect of anthrax toxin research. The rat-lethality bioassay developed in the 1960s (Singh, Chaudhary and Leppla 1989) has now been superseded by an in vitro macrophage lysis assay as a convenient and sensitive procedure for the detection of lethal toxin activity (Friedlander 1986, Quinn et al. 1991). Accordingly it has now been shown that anthrax lethal toxin activity in J774A.l macrophage-like cells is calcium-dependent, is preceded by an influx of extracellular calcium and has an absolute requirement for protein synthesis (Bhatnagar and Friedlander 1994). These in vitro observations have now also been directly linked with the in vivo lethality of the disease anthrax by macrophage depletion and replacement studies. In these experiments Hanna, Acosta and Collier (1993) demonstrated that laboratory mice were rendered insensitive to anthrax lethal toxin by specifically depleting their native macrophage population by silica injection. Sensitivity to the toxin could be restored by coinjection of lethal toxin with a toxin-sensitive

monocyte/macrophage cell line, RAW 264, the implication from these data being that macrophages mediate the action of lethal toxin in vivo. Further observations were that levels of toxin sublytic to macrophages were capable of stimulating production of interleukin-1 (IL-1) and tissue necrosis factor α (TNF-α) and this was considered a significant correlation with the characteristic symptoms of secondary shock observed in an anthrax fatality (Hanna, Acosta and Collier 1993).

Studies on sensitive macrophages in vitro have demonstrated that LF causes membrane leakage prior to macrophage lysis and that small ions can pass through the cell membrane in an ATP-independent manner (Hanna, Kochi and Collier 1992). The lethal effect on macrophages in vitro has also been demonstrated to be calcium-dependent insofar as lysis is preceded by a large influx of extracellular calcium (Ca^{2+}). Chelators of Ca^{2+} such as EGTA, or agents that block calcium channels, such as verapamil or nitrendipine, can protect macrophages from the lytic effect of the toxin (Bhatnagar et al. 1989). The lytic effect has also a requirement for concomitant protein synthesis, inhibition of which not only protects the cells in vitro but also abrogates the Ca^{2+} influx (Bhatnagar and Friedlander 1994). Furthermore, macrophages are protected in vitro by osmotic stabilization, indicating that lysis is probably the direct result of the unregulated cation pulse; removal of the osmotic support allows the Ca^{2+} influx to proceed and the cells are lysed (Bhatnagar and Friedlander 1994). With such recent and rapid developments in LF activity analysis, it is surely inevitable that the underlying mechanisms of anthrax fatal intoxication are close to being resolved.

6.2 The genetics of virulence

Both the major virulence factors of *B. anthracis* have been shown to be plasmid mediated. The genes for each of the toxin components are located on a single high molecular weight 176 kb plasmid designated pX01 (Mikesell et al. 1983) and the genes coding for capsule expression, polymerization and transport to the external surface of the cell are located on a separate 90 kb plasmid, pX02 (Green et al. 1985, Uchida et al. 1985). A wild-type strain may be differentially or fully cured of these plasmids by extended incubation at 43°C (pX01 curing) or by culture in the presence of novobiocin (pX02 curing) or both. Strains cured of one or both plasmids are avirulent or of reduced virulence and, where animal vaccination is practised, toxigenic, non-capsulated strains form the basis of current live spore vaccines (Turnbull 1991) (see section 8.1, p. 814). Strains cured of the toxin plasmid pX01 but retaining the ability to produce capsule have residual pathogenicity for certain strains of inbred mice (Welkos, Vietri and Gibbs 1993). An interesting observation with respect to the plasmid profile of *B. anthracis* is that, unlike the phylogenetically related species *Bacillus cereus* and *Bacillus thuringiensis* which present a very heterogeneous plasmid content, *B.*

anthracis isolates of both clinical and environmental origin contain only the 2 virulence plasmids (unpublished observations). Whether this reflects an incompatibility with promiscuous plasmids, an environmental selection pressure for only these 2 plasmids, or merely reflects an artefact of the isolation procedure is not known at present.

The structural genes for each of the toxin components have been cloned (Vodkin and Leppla 1983, Robertson and Leppla 1986, Mock et al. 1988, Todd-Tippetts and Robertson 1988) and sequenced (Escuyer et al. 1988, Robertson 1988, Robertson, Todd-Tippetts and Leppla 1988, Welkos et al. 1988, Bragg and Robertson 1989) and comparative analysis has shown that the 5′ regions of the LF and EF genes (*lef* and *cya* respectively) share areas of high nucleotide homology (Escuyer et al. 1988, Robertson 1988, Bragg and Robertson 1989). This is also reflected in their deduced amino-terminal amino acid sequences and is indicative of a common PA-binding and cell internalization domain (Bragg and Robertson 1989, Quinn et al. 1991). The *lef* gene also contains a region having perhaps 4 repeats of 19 nucleotides which are similarly reflected in the amino acid composition of the mature protein (Bragg and Robertson 1989). The function of these repeats is as yet undetermined, but it has been proposed that they may be involved in calcium binding (Lowe, Salter and Avina 1990). Mutations in this region destabilize the LF protein which probably indicates an important structural role for this region (Quinn et al. 1991). The structure–function relationships of the 3 toxin components are illustrated in Fig. 40.9.

Both toxin and capsule expression in vitro have been demonstrated to be modulated by ambient CO_2 levels or medium hydrogen carbonate (HCO_3^-). It is now understood that the expression of the *pag* gene is under the control of medium HCO_3^- at the transcriptional level by elements also on the pX01 plasmid (Bartkus and Leppla 1989) and a *trans*-acting positive regulator for *pag* expression, *atxA*, has recently been identified and cloned (Uchida et al. 1993). Other reports indicate that this *trans*-acting gene product can activate transcription from one of 2 promoters at the *pag* gene and indeed Sirard, Mock and Fouet (1994) have indicated that all 3 genes of the anthrax toxin complex (*pag*, *lef* and *cya*) are co-ordinately regulated by both HCO_3^- and temperature and may share a common activating element.

Capsule production is only observed in vitro in atmospheres of 5–20% CO_2 or in serum or whole blood. The capsule encoding region of pX02 has also been cloned, mapped and sequenced (Uchida et al. 1987, Makino et al. 1988, 1989). The genes essential for capsule formation have been shown to encode 3 membrane-associated enzymes mediating the polymerization of D-glutamic acid via the cell membrane. Unlike the toxin genes, however, these elements are not functional when subcloned into *B. subtilis*, nor do they appear to have any DNA sequence homology with the capsule producing species *Bacillus subtilis* (natto) and *Bacillus megaterium* although the capsular

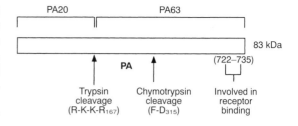

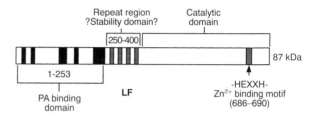

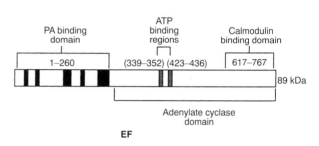

Fig. 40.9 Schematic block diagrams of the 3 polypeptide components of anthrax toxin. Protective antigen (PA) is an 83 kDa polypeptide which cleaves discretely with trypsin and chymotrypsin at the amino acid residues illustrated. The C-terminal residues are considered to be important in receptor binding. Lethal factor (LF) is an 87 kDa polypeptide and is the catalytic component of anthrax lethal toxin. The amino-terminal domain contains 254 amino acid residues and displays regions of sequence identity/homology with the oedema factor (EF). This region facilitates binding to PA. Amino acids 250–400 comprise a region of at least 4 imperfect repeats which are predicted to form α helices. The function of this domain is unclear. Amino acids 401–776 comprise the catalytic domain. This region contains at least one zinc-binding motif which appears to be involved in the LF lytic effect in monocytes in vitro. Oedema factor (EF) is an 89 kDa polypeptide. The amino-terminal 260 amino acid residues are functionally analogous to residues 1–254 of LF and constitute the PA binding domain. The catalytic adenylate cyclase domain forms the remainder of the molecule with the ATP-binding motifs at amino acid positions 339–352 and 423–436 respectively and the calmodulin-binding domain formed by residues 617–767.

materials exhibit a level of immuno-cross-reaction (Makino et al. 1989). Surprisingly, the same authors report that *B. anthracis* capsule material could be expressed in *E. coli* (Uchida et al. 1993). In common with *pag*, the regulation of capsule expression is modulated by a *trans*-acting element, in this case on pX02. As stated above, this regulation of capsule synthesis and the role it plays in the expression of virulence is not understood (Vietri et al. 1995).

7 PATHOLOGY

Most of the detailed studies on the pathology of anthrax were done in the 1940s, 1950s and 1960s with the principal aim of understanding the disease in humans. Mostly guinea pigs, rabbits and monkeys were used. Authors of those years were in universal agreement that anthrax bacilli multiply more rapidly in the lymph nodes than in other tissues and that the nodes act as centres for the proliferation and dissemination of the bacilli leading to septicaemia and death. The earliest histological changes in the lymph nodes and spleen are necrosis of germinal centres with the nodes becoming oedematous and haemorrhagic and the veins and capillaries becoming filled with thrombi composed of leucocytes, platelets, fibrin and bacteria as infection proceeds.

The eschar of cutaneous anthrax is an area of coagulative necrosis and the vesicles in the surrounding zone are filled with clear or bloody fluid. The outer zone of oedema may distend or fragment the connective tissues (Christie 1987). Cromartie, Bloom and Watson (1947) found that, for 2–4 h after the subcutaneous injection of spores, germination and the proliferation of capsulated bacilli proceeded in the intercellular fluids of all animal species studied, both susceptible and resistant. The affected areas became infiltrated with fluid, and dilation and congestion of small blood vessels with extravasation of red blood cells and small areas of haemorrhage occurred in the centre of the lesion. Margination and diapedesis of polymorphonuclear leucocytes and swelling of the endothelial cells occurred in the capillaries. Mononuclear phagocytes and fibrin deposits appeared and the efferent lymphatics became dilated.

In susceptible animals (mice, guinea pigs and rabbits) there was continued proliferation of the bacilli in the lesion to the point of death with, in the terminal stages, extensive fragmentation of the connective tissue, oedema, fibrin deposits, haemorrhage and infiltration by small numbers of polymorphs and mononuclear phagocytes, many of which appeared to be dead. Oedema fluid accumulated between the underlying muscle bundles, some of which showed necrosis and haemorrhage. The bacilli were visible in foci surrounded by large areas of oedematous tissue in which organisms could not be seen. Bloom, Watson and Cromartie (1947) showed that phagocytosis was minimal.

In resistant animals (rats, pigs and dogs), after 4 h the *B. anthracis* cells appeared to lose their capsules and proliferation ceased. Over the next 70 h, the bacterial cells died, disintegrated and disappeared. The initial tissue reaction was minimal, but by 26 h the lesion had become infiltrated with polymorphs and mononuclear cells, many appearing dead. By 72 h, the epidermis in the centre of the lesions was necrotic and the surrounding tissues contained masses of dead leu-

cocytes. At 10 days, the appearance of dense fibrous tissue in the dermis and subcutaneous tissue, and epithelial regeneration indicated that resolution of the lesions was occurring. Bloom, Watson and Cromartie (1947) claimed to have partly identified the substance responsible for the observed destruction of *B. anthracis* in the tissue.

When, in aerosol infection studies, pigs and dogs, representing more resistant hosts, were compared with sheep and rhesus monkeys as representative of the more susceptible hosts, discrete, intensely haemorrhagic and cellular lesions surrounded by dense masses of fibrin were seen in the lungs of the pigs and dogs but not in the sheep and monkeys. This was interpreted as demonstrating an ability on the part of the more resistant animals to 'wall off' the invading organisms into local foci of infection and was seen to explain the lack of systemic infection (Gleiser 1967, Gleiser, Gochenour and Ward 1968).

Gleiser (1967) found that, in rhesus monkeys inoculated subcutaneously with *B. anthracis*, the local (axillary) lymph nodes became haemorrhagic and oedematous and, microscopically, showed necrosis of lymphatic elements, monocytic and neutrophilic infiltration of varying intensity, necrosis of blood vessel walls, and phagocytosis of the bacilli. Lymph nodes more distal to the site of infection were affected to a varying extent and the spleen was frequently enlarged; microscopically, the spleen was depopulated of lymphoid elements but contained much necrotic cellular debris and masses of bacilli.

In pulmonary anthrax in monkeys, the inhaled spores apparently did not germinate in the lungs (Young, Zelle and Lincoln 1946, Barnes 1947) but were ingested by motile macrophages which carried them through the undamaged epithelium to the lymphatics. Germination began on the way to or on arrival at the tracheobronchial lymph nodes, and the vegetative cells freed from the phagocytes then proliferated (Ross 1957). The infection spread through the efferent lymph duct into the bloodstream. Some of the bacteria reached the peribronchial lymph nodes within 15 min of inhaling the spores (Young, Zelle and Lincoln 1946). Clearance from the lung was apparently inefficient, however, and Henderson, Peacock and Belton (1956) found that, in rhesus monkeys protected from contracting anthrax by combined penicillin and vaccine prophylaxis after exposure to single spore clouds, 15–20%, 2% and 0.5–1% of the spores remained in the lungs at 42, 50 and 75 days respectively after exposure; even after 100 days trace levels of spores were present. This has recently been confirmed in similar work in which the last anthrax death in a group of rhesus monkeys exposed to anthrax spores by the aerosol route and maintained on doxycycline for 30 days after exposure occurred on day 58 (Friedlander et al. 1993). Henderson, Peacock and Belton (1956) were of the opinion that the spores did not germinate in the lung in life, although, once the lungs were macerated in a tissue grinder, they would start to do so unless held at <4°C.

The lymphatics act in a manner analogous to continuous culture (Trnka et al. 1958 cited by Lincoln et al. 1961), continuously feeding the bloodstream with vegetative bacilli. Initially these were filtered out by the spleen and other parts of the reticuloendothelial system, but during the final 10–14 h the degree of bacteraemia doubled in c. 50 min in mice and guinea pigs, 95 min in sheep and 115 min in rats (Keppie, Smith and Harris-Smith 1955, Trnka et al. 1958 cited by Lincoln et al. 1961, Lincoln et al. 1961). In the terminal stages in monkeys infected by the respiratory route, the intrathoracic lymph nodes and spleen showed changes similar to those seen in the local lymph nodes of animals infected subcutaneously (Gleiser 1967). Oedema of the mediastinum with some haemorrhage occurred; microscopically, the tissue contained granular non-cellular eosinophilic material and a heterogeneous population of neutrophils, eosinophils and macrophages. Pulmonary oedema and haemorrhages were observed. The principal lesion in the cardiovascular system was necrosis of the walls of small blood vessels commensurate with the characteristic terminal haemorrhage.

8 PREVENTION AND TREATMENT

8.1 Vaccines

Pasteur's vaccine (Pasteur 1881), based on a culture of *B. anthracis* that had been reduced in virulence by passage at 42–43°C for several days (it is now realized that he was curing the cultures of their toxin plasmid), was used to good effect for several decades, but its efficacy was limited and its residual virulence made it unsuitable for use in certain animal species. It was finally superseded by Sterne's attenuated live spore vaccine based on a strain of *B. anthracis* ($34F_2$) which had lost its ability to produce the capsule during culture on 50% horse serum nutrient agar with incubation under a 30% CO_2 atmosphere for 24 h (Sterne 1937). Spores of this strain suspended in 0.5% saponin in 50% glycerol–saline remain the active ingredient of livestock vaccine in most countries of the world today (Turnbull et al. 1993).

The Sterne vaccine, however, retains a low degree of virulence for certain species of domesticated and laboratory animals and, as a result, is regarded in western developed countries as unsuitable for human use. Analogous live spore human vaccines are used, however, in Russia and China (Turnbull et al. 1993). Elsewhere, the only available human vaccines are the US vaccine consisting of an alhydrogel-adsorbed culture filtrate of a non-capsulating, non-proteolytic derivative (V770-NP1-R) of *B. anthracis* strain V770 and the UK vaccine, which is an alum-precipitated culture filtrate of the Sterne strain ($34F_2$) (Turnbull et al. 1993).

It is difficult to assess accurately the contribution made by human vaccine to the declining incidence of anthrax in those whose occupations expose them to risk. However, the study in goat-hair processing mills referred to earlier (Brachman et al. 1962) was carried

out at a time when vaccination of the workers was first being introduced and it was possible to compare case rates in vaccinated and unvaccinated workers; the data indicated a 92.5% degree of effectiveness. Brachman et al. (1960) had already noted from their investigation of the outbreak of pulmonary anthrax in one such mill that 'the vaccine does appear to be effective'. The administration of the human vaccine is impracticable in endemic regions or outside the context of industrial or other specific occupational risks; in endemic areas, emphasis should be placed on vaccinating livestock. The duration of protection afforded by the human and animal vaccines is a subject of some uncertainty. Tests in animals showed that protection from PA-based vaccines had fallen significantly 14 months after completion of the initial series of vaccine injections but that a 6 month booster resulted in good protection at 14 months (Turnbull et al. 1990). At present, on empirical grounds, boosters are administered to human vaccinees 6 months after the initial series of 3 doses and annually thereafter.

The recommendation for livestock vaccination is annual administration of the live spore vaccine as a result of observations made by Sterne (1959), but there is little firm information on the duration of protection afforded by the veterinary vaccine, although, in one study in guinea pigs, protection fell from 87% to 40% over the period 3–16 weeks after vaccination (Berendt et al. 1985, Ivins and Welkos 1988). The spore vaccine is administered to animals in a single dose; it is recognized in the field that it is possible to halt an outbreak in livestock within about 2 weeks by vaccinating.

The protective antigen (PA) component of the toxin was well named by its early proponents (see section 6, p. 809) and has proved to be the essential component in vaccines for inducing protective immunity, although appropriate presentation to the immune system by means of good adjuvants is important to inducing good protection. Tests in animals indicate that large doses of purified PA alone or with poor supplementary adjuvant may produce high antibody titres but only poor protective immunity, whereas good protection can be induced with much lower doses when combined with a suitable adjuvant even though lower antibody titres result (Ivins and Welkos 1988, Turnbull et al. 1988, Ivins et al. 1992, 1995). LF, EF and the various somatic antigens of *B. anthracis* appear capable of inducing relatively low degrees of protection.

The improved understanding of PA and adjuvants, together with revolutionary ideas being explored in the field of vaccines as a whole over the past decade, have led to a variety of suggestions for improving anthrax vaccines. As reviewed elsewhere (Ivins and Welkos 1988, Turnbull 1991, Ivins et al. 1992, 1995) these range from subunit formulations consisting of purified PA mixed with an effective adjuvant, through live vaccines comprising mutant strains which are avirulent but fully immunogenic, and recombinant vaccines in which another host expresses the PA as well as acting as an adjuvant, to oral vaccines consisting of either a suitable recombinant organism, such as a salmonella, or microencapsulated PA. In all these approaches, the aim remains to deliver PA to the vaccinee in such a way as to induce maximal protective immunity, which probably means by inducing the optimal cellular immune response. So far, however, the regulatory and financial obstacles to taking promising formulations to clinical trials and beyond have prevented any of them progressing beyond the developmental stage.

8.2 Treatment

B. anthracis is susceptible to a wide range of antibiotics and, in many parts of the world, penicillins remain the antimicrobials of choice. Penicillin-resistant isolates have only been reported on 3 or 4 occasions but no tendency to acquire penicillin resistance has been described. Cutaneous lesions become sterile within 24–48 h of commencement of therapy but, because the lesion continues to progress through its cycle of development and resolution, case reports often record that treatment was continued for many days.

If the isolate is reported as resistant to penicillin, or the patient is hypersensitive to penicillin, a wide range of alternative choices exists from among the aminoglycosides, macrolides, quinolones and tetracyclines. Chloramphenicol is also a satisfactory alternative. In veterinary circles some dissatisfaction has been expressed with the effectiveness of tetracyclines.

Antibiotics are not active against the spore forms of *B. anthracis* and it appears that inhaled spores do not germinate in the lung and are only cleared from there slowly (Henderson, Peacock and Belton 1956, Friedlander et al. 1993). Consequently, when substantial exposure to aerosolized spores is suspected, it may be considered prudent to administer an antibiotic prophylactically for several weeks in parallel with vaccine so that the exposed person is protected while vaccine-induced immunity develops.

In pre-antibiotic days, serum therapy using, for example, hyperimmune horse serum was a common approach to treating anthrax and apparently achieved varying degrees of success. It seems it is still used in China (Dong 1990) and Russia. With the availability of plasmapheresis techniques, γ-globulin from a vaccinated person conceivably could provide a modern life-saving version of serum therapy in an emergency.

The massive oedema of anthrax may be life-threatening through obstruction of the trachea or larynx (see Fig. 40.1). Early tracheotomy (before the trachea becomes hard to locate) may be advisable. Steroid administration is frequently reported but few comment retrospectively on its value. Kobuch et al. (1990) considered it to have no value and abandoned it as a treatment. Recalling that the swelling is due to toxin-induced oedema rather than an inflammatory response, it is probably logical that the benefits of steroids may be minimal.

REFERENCES

Abdenour D, Larouze B et al., 1987, Familial occurrence of anthrax in Eastern Algeria, *J Infect Dis*, **155**: 1083–4.

Albrink WS, Brosks SM et al., 1960, Human inhalation anthrax: a report of three fatal cases, *Am J Pathol*, **36**: 457–71.

Anon, 1918, Precautions for preventing danger of infection from anthrax in the manipulation of wool, goat hair, and camel hair, *Report of the Departmental Committee on Anthrax*, **3**: 116.

Anon, 1994a, Memorandum from a WHO meeting on anthrax control and research, *Bull W H O*, **72**: 13–22.

Anon, 1994b, Epidemic of human anthrax in the twin districts from January to September 1994, *North Arcot Ambedkar and Tiruvannamalai Sambuvarayar Districts Health Information* Network (NATH1), **11**: 4–7.

Ascoli A, 1911, Die Präzipitindiagnose bei Milzbrand, *Zentralbl Bakteriol I Abt Orig*, **58**: 63–70.

Barnes JM, 1947, The development of anthrax following the administration of spores by inhalation, *Br J Exp Pathol*, **28**: 385–94.

Bartkus JM, Leppla SH, 1989, Transcriptional regulation of the protective antigen gene of *Bacillus anthracis*, *Infect Immun*, **57**: 2295–300.

Berendt R, Jemski J et al., 1985, The use of toxin components for the immunoprophylaxis of inhalation anthrax, *Abstracts of the Annual Meeting of the American Society for Microbiology*, **1**: 85.

Berry HH, 1981, Abnormal levels of disease and predation as limiting factors for wildebeest in the Etosha National Park, *Madoqua*, **12**: 242–53.

Bhatnagar R, Friedlander AM, 1994, Protein synthesis is required for expression of anthrax lethal toxin cytotoxicity, *Infect Immun*, **62**: 2958–62.

Bhatnagar R, Singh Y et al., 1989, Calcium is required for the expression of anthrax lethal toxin activity in the macrophage like cell line J774A.1, *Infect Immun*, **57**: 2107–14.

Bloom WL, Watson DW, Cromartie WJ, 1947, Studies on infec-

tion with *Bacillus anthracis*. IV. Preparation and characterization of an anthracidal substance from various animal tissues, *J Infect Dis*, **80**: 41–52.

Bowen JE, Turnbull PCB, 1992, The fate of *Bacillus anthracis* in unpasteurised and pasteurised milk, *Lett Appl Microbiol*, **15**: 224–7.

Brachman PS, Plotkin SA et al., 1960, An epidemic of inhalation anthrax: the first in the twentieth century. (II) Epidemiology, *Am J Hyg*, **72**: 6–23.

Brachman PS, Gold H et al., 1962, Field evaluation of a human anthrax vaccine, *Am J Public Health*, **52**: 632–45.

Bragg TS, Robertson DL, 1989, Nucleotide sequence and analysis of the lethal factor gene (*lef*) from *Bacillus anthracis*, *Gene*, **81**: 45–54.

Budd W, 1863, Observations on the occurrence of malignant pustule in England illustrated by numerous fatal cases, *Assoc Med J*, **1**: 85, 110, 159, 237.

Carman JA, Hambleton P, Melling J, 1985, *Bacillus anthracis, Isolation and Identification of Micro-organisms of Medical and Veterinary Importance*, Society for Applied Bacteriology Technical Series 21, eds Collins CH, Grange GM, Academic Press, London, 207–14.

Carr EA, Rew RR, 1957, Recovery of *Bacillus anthracis* from the nose and throat of apparently healthy workers, *J Infect Dis*, **100**: 169–71.

Choquette LPE, Broughton E, 1981, Anthrax, *Infectious Diseases of Wild Mammals*, 2nd edn, Iowa State University Press, Ames, Iowa, 288–96.

Christie AB, 1987, Anthrax, *Infectious Diseases: Epidemiology and Clinical Practice*, 4th edn, Churchill Livingstone, Edinburgh, 983–1003.

Collins CH, 1990/91, Carbuncles and coal, *MLW*, December/January: 44–5.

Communicable Disease Surveillance Centre, 1982, Anthrax surveillance 1961–80, *Br Med J*, **284**: 204.

Cromartie WJ, Bloom WL, Watson DW, 1947, Studies on infection with *Bacillus anthracis* I. A histopathological study of skin lesions produced by *B. anthracis* in susceptible and resistant animal species, *J Infect Dis*, **80:** 1–13.

Dahlgren CM, Buchanan LM et al., 1960, *Bacillus anthracis* aerosols in goat hair processing mills, *Am J Hyg*, **72:** 6–23.

Darlow HM, Pride NB, 1969, Serological diagnosis of anthrax, *Lancet*, **2:** 430–1.

Davies JCA, 1982, A major epidemic of anthrax in Zimbabwe, *Cent Afr J Med*, **28:** 291–8.

Davies JCA, 1983, A major epidemic of anthrax in Zimbabwe, *Cent Afr J Med*, **29:** 8–12.

Dirckx JH, 1981, Virgil on anthrax, *Am J Dermatopathol*, **3:** 191–5.

Doganay M, 1986, *Proceedings of the 22nd Turkish Microbiology Congress*, Publication No. 7, Turkish Microbiology Society, Istanbul, 25–40.

Doganay M, Aygen B et al., 1994, Temporal artery inflammation as a complication of anthrax, *J Infect*, **28:** 311–14.

Dong SL, 1990, Progress in the control and research of anthrax in China, *Salisbury Med Bull (Special Suppl)*, **68:** 104–5.

Drake DJ, Blair AW, 1971, Meningitic anthrax, *Cent Afr J Med*, **17:** 97.

Ebedes H, 1976, Anthrax epozoötics in Etosha National Park, *Madoqua*, **10:** 99–118.

Enticknap JB, Galbraith NS et al., 1968, Pulmonary anthrax caused by contaminated sacks, *Br J Ind Med*, **25:** 72–4.

Escuyer V, Duflot E et al., 1988, Structural homology between virulence-associated bacterial adenylate cyclases, *Gene*, **71:** 293–8.

Ezzell JW, Ivins BE, Leppla SH, 1984, Immunoelectrophoretic analysis, toxicity, and kinetics of *in vitro* production of the protective antigen and lethal factor components of *Bacillus anthracis* toxin, *Infect Immun*, **45:** 761–7.

FAO-WHO-OIE, 1988–94, Anthrax reports from FAO and OIE for 1988–94, *FAO-WHO-OIE Animal Health Yearbook*, FAO, Rome.

Flynn DM, 1968–69, Anthrax in Victoria, *Victorian Vet Proc*, 32–3.

Friedlander AM, 1986, Macrophages are sensitive to anthrax lethal toxin through an acid-dependent process, *J Biol Chem*, **261:** 7123–6.

Friedlander AM, Welkos SL et al., 1993, Postexposure prophylaxis against experimental inhalation anthrax, *J Infect Dis*, **167:** 1239–42.

George S, Mathai D et al., 1994, An outbreak of anthrax meningoencephalitis, *Trans R Soc Trop Med Hyg*, **88:** 206–7.

Gill DM, Coburn J, 1987, ADP-ribosylation by cholera toxin: functional analysis of a cellular system that stimulates the enzymatic activity of cholera toxin fragment A_1, *Biochemistry*, **26:** 6364–71.

Gleiser CA, 1967, Pathology of anthrax infection in animal hosts, *Fed Proc*, **26:** 1518–21.

Gleiser CA, Gochenour WS, Ward MK, 1968, Pulmonary lesions in dogs and pigs exposed to a cloud of anthrax spores, *J Comp Pathol*, **78:** 445–9.

Gordon VM, Leppla SH, 1994, Proteolytic activation of bacterial toxins: role of bacterial and host cell proteases, *Infect Immun*, **62:** 333–40.

Gordon VM, Leppla SH, Hewlett EL, 1988, Inhibitors of receptor-mediated endocytosis block the entry of *Bacillus anthracis* adenylate cyclase toxin but not that of *Bordetella pertussis* adenylate cyclase toxin, *Infect Immun*, **56:** 1066–9.

Gordon VM, Klimpel KR et al., 1995, Proteolytic activation of bacterial toxins by eukaryotic cells is performed by furin and by additional cellular proteases, *Infect Immun*, **63:** 82–7.

Gould GW, 1977, Recent advances in the understanding of resistance and dormancy of bacterial spores, *J Appl Bacteriol*, **42:** 297–309.

Graham-Smith GS, 1930, The longevity of dry spores of *B. anthracis*, *J Hyg*, **30:** 213–15.

Green BD, Battisti L et al., 1985, Demonstration of a capsule plasmid in *Bacillus anthracis*, *Infect Immun*, **49:** 291–7.

Haight TH, 1952, Anthrax meningitis: review of literature and report of two cases with autopsies, *Am J Med Sci*, **224:** 57–69.

Hanna PC, Acosta D, Collier RJ, 1993, On the role of macrophages in anthrax, *Proc Natl Acad Sci USA*, **90:** 10198–201.

Hanna PC, Kochi S, Collier RJ, 1992, Biochemical and physiological changes induced by anthrax lethal toxin in J774 macrophage-like cells, *Mol Biol Cell*, **3:** 1269–77.

Henderson DW, Peacock S, Belton FC, 1956, Observations on the prophylaxis of experimental pulmonary anthrax in the monkey, *J Hyg*, **54:** 28–36.

Heyworth B, Ropp ME et al., 1975, Anthrax in the Gambia: an epidemiological study, *Br Med J*, **4:** 79–82.

Holgate JA, Holman RA, 1949, Diagnosis and treatment of cutaneous anthrax, *Br Med J*, **2:** 575–9.

Hughes MH, 1973, Anthrax, *Br Med J*, **1:** 488–9.

Hugh-Jones ME, Hussaini SN, 1974, An anthrax outbreak in Berkshire, *Vet Rec*, **94:** 228–32.

Ivins B, Fellows P et al., 1995, Experimental anthrax vaccines: efficacy of adjuvants combined with protective antigen against an aerosol *Bacillus anthracis* spore challenge in guinea pigs, *Vaccine*, **13:** 1779–84.

Ivins BE, Welkos SL, 1988, Recent advances in the development of an improved human anthrax vaccine, *Eur J Epidemiol*, **4:** 12–19.

Ivins BE, Welkos SL et al., 1992, Immunization against anthrax with *Bacillus anthracis* protective antigen combined with adjuvants, *Infect Immun*, **60:** 662–8.

Jacotot H, Virat B, 1954, La longevité des spores de *B. anthracis* (premier vaccin de Pasteur), *Ann Inst Pasteur*, **87:** 215–17.

Jena GP, 1980, Intestinal anthrax in man: a case report, *Cent Afr J Med*, **26:** 253–4.

Keppie J, Harris-Smith PW, Smith H, 1963, The chemical basis of the virulence of *Bacillus anthracis*. IX: Its aggressins and their mode of action, *Br J Exp Pathol*, **44:** 446–53.

Keppie J, Smith H, Harris-Smith PW, 1955, The chemical basis of the virulence of *Bacillus anthracis*. III: The role of the terminal bacteraemia in death of guinea-pigs from anthrax, *Br J Exp Pathol*, **36:** 315–22.

Klemm DM, Klemm WR, 1959, A history of anthrax, *J Am Vet Med Assoc*, **135:** 458–62.

Klimpel KR, Arora N, Leppla SH, 1994, Anthrax toxin lethal factor contains a zinc metalloprotease consensus sequence which is required for lethal toxin activity, *Mol Microbiol*, **13:** 1093–100.

Knisely RF, 1966, Selective medium for *Bacillus anthracis*, *J Bacteriol*, **92:** 784–6.

Kobuch WE, Davis J et al., 1990, A clinical and epidemiological study of 621 patients with anthrax in western Zimbabwe, *Salisbury Med Bull (Special Suppl)*, **68:** 34–8.

Kochi SK, Schiavo G et al., 1994, Zinc content of the *Bacillus anthracis* lethal factor, *FEMS Microbiol Lett*, **124:** 343–8.

Koshi G, Lalitha MK et al., 1981, Anthrax meningitis, a rare clinical entity, *J Assoc Physicians India*, **29:** 59–62.

Lalitha MK, Anandi V et al., 1988, Primary anthrax presenting as an injection 'abscess', *Indian J Pathol Microbiol*, **31:** 254–6.

Lalitha MK, Anandi V et al., 1990, Unusual forms of anthrax – a clinical problem, *Salisbury Med Bull (Special Suppl)*, **68:** 38–40.

Leppla SH, 1982, Anthrax toxin edema factor: a bacterial adenylate cyclase that increases cyclic AMP concentrations in eukaryotic cells, *Proc Natl Acad Sci USA*, **79:** 3162–6.

Leppla SH, Friedlander AM, Cora EM, 1988, Proteolytic activation of anthrax toxin bound to cellular receptors, *Bacterial Protein Toxins*, Gustav Fischer, Stuttgart, 111–12.

Leppla SH, Ivins BE, Ezzell JW, 1985, Anthrax toxin, *Microbiology – 1985*, American Society for Microbiology, Washington, DC, 63–6.

Levy LM, Baker N et al., 1981, Anthrax meningitis in Zimbabwe, *Cent Afr J Med*, **27:** 101–4.

Lincoln RE, Fish DC, 1970, *Microbial Toxins III*, 1st edn, eds Montie TC, Kadis S, Ajl SJ, Academic Press, New York, 361–414.

Lincoln RE, Rhian MA et al., 1961, *Spores II*, 1st edn, Burgess, Minneapolis, MN, 255–73.

Lindeque PM, Turnbull PCB, 1994, Ecology and epidemiology of anthrax in the Etosha National Park, Namibia, *Onderstepoort J Vet Res*, **61**: 71–83.

Lowe JR, Salter O, Avina JA, 1990, Abstract B320, *Abstracts of the American Society of Microbiology*, American Society for Microbiology, Washington, DC.

McKendrick DRA, 1980, Anthrax and its transmission to humans, *Cent Afr J Med*, **26**: 126–9.

Makino S, Sasakawa C et al., 1988, Cloning and CO$_2$-dependent expression of the genetic region for encapsulation from *Bacillus anthracis*, *Mol Microbiol*, **2**: 371–6.

Makino S, Uchida I et al., 1989, Molecular characterization and protein analysis of the *cap* region, which is essential for encapsulation in *Bacillus anthracis*, *J Bacteriol*, **171**: 722–30.

Manchee RJ, Broster MG et al., 1981, *Bacillus anthracis* on Gruinard island, *Nature (London)*, **294**: 254–5.

Manchee RJ, Broster MG et al., 1994, Formaldehyde solution effectively inactivates spores of *Bacillus anthracis* on the Scottish island of Gruinard, *Appl Environ Microbiol*, **60**: 4167–71.

Martin GHB, 1975, *Cutaneous Anthrax in Rural Ethiopia. A Study of One Hundred Consecutive Cases; Clinical Features and Epidemiology*, MD thesis, Dundee.

Meselson M, Guillemin J et al., 1994, The Sverdlovsk anthrax outbreak of 1979, *Science*, **266**: 1202–8.

M'Fadyean J, 1903, A further note with regard to the staining reaction af anthrax blood with methylene-blue, *J Comp Pathol*, **16**: 360–1.

Mikesell P, Ivins BE et al., 1983, Evidence for plasmid mediated toxin production in *Bacillus anthracis*, *Infect Immun*, **39**: 371–6.

Milne JC, Furlong D et al., 1994, Anthrax protective antigen forms oligomers during intoxication of mammalian cells, *J Biol Chem*, **269**: 20606–12.

Mock M, Labruyère E et al., 1988, Cloning and expression of the calmodulin-sensitive *Bacillus anthracis* adenylate cyclase in *Escherichia coli*, *Gene*, **64**: 277–84.

Moro M, 1967, Influence of altitude in the incidence of anthrax in Peru, *Fed Proc*, **26**: 1503.

Nalin DR, Sultana B et al., 1977, Survival of a patient with intestinal anthrax, *Am J Med*, **62**: 130–2.

Ndyabahinduka DGK, Chu IH et al., 1984, An outbreak of human gastrointestinal anthrax, *Ann Ist Super Sanita*, **20**: 205–8.

Norman PS, Ray JG et al., 1960, Serologic testing for anthrax antibodies in workers in a goat hair processing mill, *Am J Hyg*, **72**: 32–7.

O'Brien J, Friedlander A et al., 1985, Effects of anthrax toxin components on human neutrophils, *Infect Immun*, **47**: 306–10.

Parry JM, Turnbull PCB, Gibson RJ, 1983, *A Colour Atlas of Bacillus Species*, Wolfe Medical Publications, London, 272 pp.

Parvizpour D, 1978, Human anthrax in Iran. An epidemiological study of 468 cases, *Int J Zoon*, **5**: 69–74.

Pasteur L, 1881, De l'attenuation des virus et de leur retour à la virulence, *C R Acad Sci Agric Bulg*, **92**: 429–35.

Pienaar U de V, 1967, Epidemiology of anthrax in wild animals and the control of anthrax epizoötics in the Kruger National Park, South Africa, *Fed Proc*, **26**: 1496–502.

Plotkin SA, Brachman PS et al., 1960, An epidemic of inhalation anthrax, the first in the twentieth century, *Am J Med*, **29**: 992–1001.

Polydorou K, 1983, The campaign against anthrax, *World Anim Rev*, **April–June**: 41–5.

Prins HHT, Weyerhaeuser FJ, 1987, Epidemics in populations of wild ruminants: anthrax and impala, rinderpest and buffalo in Lake Manyara National Park, Tanzania, *OIKOS*, **49**: 28–38.

Pyper JF, Willoughby L, 1964, An anthrax outbreak affecting man and buffalo in the North-West Territories, *Med Serv J*, **20**: 531–40.

Quinn CP, Singh Y et al., 1991, Functional mapping of the anthrax toxin lethal factor by in-frame insertion mutagenesis, *J Biol Chem*, **266**: 20124–30.

Rao NSK, Mohiyudeen S, 1958, Tabanus flies as transmitters of anthrax – a field of experience, *Indian Vet J*, **35**: 348–53.

Robertson DL, 1988, Relationships between the calmodulin-dependent adenylate cyclases produced by *Bacillus anthracis* and *Bordetella pertussis*, *Biochem Biophys Res Commun*, **157**: 1927–32.

Robertson DL, Leppla SH, 1986, Molecular cloning and expression in *Escherichia coli* of the lethal factor gene of *Bacillus anthracis*, *Gene*, **44**: 71–8.

Robertson DL, Todd-Tippetts M, Leppla SH, 1988, Nucleotide sequence of the *Bacillus anthracis* edema factor gene (*cya*): a calmodulin-dependent adenylate cyclase, *Gene*, **73**: 363–71.

Ross JM, 1957, The pathogenesis of anthrax following the administration of spores by the respiratory route, *J Pathol Bacteriol*, **73**: 485–94.

Salmon DE, 1896, *US Department of Agriculture, Bureau of Animal Industry, Special Report on Diseases of the Horse*, Government Printing Office, Washington, DC, 526–30.

Sen SK, Minett FC, 1944, Experiments on the transmission of anthrax through flies, *Indian J Vet Sci Anim Husb*, **14**: 149–59.

Singh Y, Chaudhary VK, Leppla SH, 1989, A deleted variant of *Bacillus anthracis* protective antigen is non-toxic and blocks anthrax toxin action *in vivo*, *J Biol Chem*, **264**: 19103–7.

Sirard JC, Mock M, Fouet A, 1994, The three *Bacillus anthracis* toxin genes are coordinately regulated by bicarbonate and temperature, *J Bacteriol*, **176**: 5188–92.

Smith H, Keppie J, 1954, Observations on experimental anthrax: demonstration of a specific lethal factor produced *in vivo* by *Bacillus anthracis*, *Nature (London)*, **173**: 869–70.

Stanley JL, Smith H, 1961, Purification of factor I and recognition of a third factor of the anthrax toxin, *J Gen Microbiol*, **26**: 49–66.

Stein CD, Stoner MG, 1952a, Anthrax in livestock during the first quarter of 1952 with special reference to outbreaks in swine in the midwest, *Vet Med*, **47**: 274–9.

Stein CD, Stoner MG, 1952b, Anthrax in livestock during 1951 and comparative data on the disease from 1945 through 1951, *Vet Med*, **47**: 315–20.

Sterne M, 1937, The effects of different carbon dioxide concentrations on the growth of virulent anthrax strains, *Onderstepoort J Vet Sci Anim Ind*, **9**: 49–67.

Sterne M, 1959, Anthrax, *Infectious Diseases of Animals*, vol. 1, eds Stableforth AW, Galloway IA, Butterworths, London, 16–52.

Sussman AS, Halvorson HO, 1966, *Spores. Their Dormancy and Germination*, Harper and Row, New York, 193–215.

Tahernia AC, Hashemi GH, 1972, Survival in anthrax meningitis, *Pediatrics*, **50**: 329–33.

Taylor CE, Bright R, 1989, T-cell modulation of the antibody response to bacterial polysaccharide antigens, *Infect Immun*, **57**: 180–5.

Titball RW, Manchee RJ, 1987, Factors affecting the germination of spores of *Bacillus anthracis*, *J Appl Bacteriol*, **62**: 269–73.

Todd-Tippetts M, Robertson DL, 1988, Molecular cloning and expression of the *Bacillus anthracis* edema factor toxin gene: a calmodulin-dependent adenylate cyclase, *J Bacteriol*, **170**: 2263–6.

Turell MJ, Knudson GB, 1987, Mechanical transmission of *Bacillus anthracis* by stable flies (*Stomoxys calcitrans*) and mosquitoes (*Aedes aegypti* and *Aedes taeniorhynchus*), *Infect Immun*, **55**: 1859–61.

Turnbull PCB, 1990, Anthrax, *Topley and Wilson's Principles of Bacteriology, Virology and Immunity*, vol. 3, 8th edn, eds Smith GR, Easman CSF, Edward Arnold, London, 365–79.

Turnbull PCB, 1991, Anthrax vaccines: past, present and future, *Vaccine*, **9**: 533–9.

Turnbull PCB, Kramer JM, 1995, *Manual of Clinical Microbiology*, 6th edn, eds Murray PR, Baron EJ et al., ASM Press, Washington, DC, 349–56.

Turnbull PCB, Leppla SH et al., 1988, Antibodies to anthrax

toxin in humans and guinea pigs and their relevance to protective immunity, *Med Microbiol Immunol*, **177**: 293–303.

Turnbull PCB, Quinn CP et al., 1990, Protection conferred by microbially-supplemented UK and purified PA vaccines, *Salisbury Med Bull (Special Suppl)*, **68**: 89–91.

Turnbull PCB, Bell RHV et al., 1991, Anthrax in wildlife in the Luangwa Valley, Zambia, *Vet Rec*, **128**: 399–403.

Turnbull PCB, Doganay M et al., 1992, Serology and anthrax in humans, livestock and Etosha National Park wildlife, *Epidemiol Infect*, **108**: 299–313.

Turnbull PCB, Böhm R et al., 1993, *Guidelines for the Surveillance and Control of Anthax in Humans and Animals*, World Health Organization, Geneva. WHO/Zoon/93.170.

Turner M, 1980, Anthrax in humans in Zimbabwe, *Cent Afr J Med*, **26**: 160–1.

Uchida I, Sekizaki T et al., 1985, Association of the encapsulation of *Bacillus anthracis* with a 60 megadalton plasmid, *J Gen Microbiol*, **131**: 363–7.

Uchida I, Hashimoto K et al., 1987, Restriction map of a capsule plasmid of *Bacillus anthracis*, *Plasmid*, **18**: 178–81.

Uchida I, Hornung JM et al., 1993, Cloning and characterization of a gene whose product is a *trans*-activator of anthrax toxin synthesis, *J Bacteriol*, **175**: 5329–38.

Van Ness GB, 1971, Ecology of anthrax, *Science*, **172**: 1303–07.

Vietri NJ, Marrero R et al., 1995, Indentification and characterization of a *trans*-activator involved in the regulation of encapsulation by *Bacillus anthracis*, *Gene*, **152**: 1–9.

Vodkin MH, Leppla SH, 1983, Cloning of the protective antigen gene of *Bacillus anthracis*, *Cell*, **34**: 693–7.

de Vos V, 1990, The ecology of anthrax in the Kruger National Park, South Africa, *Salisbury Med Bull (Special Suppl)*, **68**: 19–23.

Wade BH, Wright GG et al., 1985, Anthrax toxin components stimulate chemotaxis of human polymorphonuclear neutrophils (42078), *Proc Soc Exp Biol Med*, **179**: 159–62.

Walker JS, Lincoln RE, Klein F, 1967, Pathophysiological and biochemical changes in anthrax, *Fed Proc*, **26**: 1539–44.

Watson A, Keir D, 1994, Information on which to base assessments of risk from environments contaminated with anthrax spores, *Epidemiol Infect*, **113**: 479–90.

Watson DW, Cromartie WJ et al., 1947, Studies on infection with *Bacillus anthracis*. III. Chemical and immunological properties of the protective antigen in crude extracts from skin lesions of *Bacillus anthracis*, *J Infect Dis*, **80**: 28–40.

Weinstein L, 1938, The prophylaxis of experimental anthrax infection with various hormone preparations, *Yale J Biol Med*, **11**: 369–92.

Welkos SL, Vietri NJ, Gibbs PH, 1993, Non-toxigenic derivatives of the Ames strain of *Bacillus anthracis* are fully virulent for mice: role of plasmid pXO2 and chromosome in strain-dependent virulence, *Microb Pathog*, **14**: 381-8.

Welkos SL, Lowe JR et al., 1988, Sequence and analysis of the DNA encoding protective antigen of *Bacillus anthracis*, *Gene*, **69**: 287–300.

Whitford HW, 1987, *A Guide to the Diagnosis, Treatment and Prevention of Anthrax*, World Health Organization, Geneva. WHO/Zoon/87.163.

Wilson JB, Russell KE, 1964, Islolation of *Bacillus anthracis* from soil stored 60 years, *J Bacteriol*, **87**: 237–8.

Wise GA, Kennedy DJ, 1980, Anthrax in sheep and cattle. Some new thoughts from observations in south-western NSW, *NSW Vet Proc*, 55–9.

Young GA, Zelle MR, Lincoln RE, 1946, Respiratory pathogenicity of *Bacillus anthracis* spores. I. Methods of study and observations on pathogenesis, *Infect Dis*, **79**: 233–46.

Zwartou H, Smith H, 1956, Polyglutamic acid from *Bacillus anthracis* grown *in vivo*: structure and aggressin activity, *Biochem J*, **63**: 437–42.

Chapter 41

BRUCELLOSIS

M J Corbel and A P MacMillan

1 INTRODUCTION

A type of fever characterized by fairly regular remissions or intermissions has been recognized along the Mediterranean littoral since the time of Hippocrates. Many names have been applied to it, often relating to localities in which it was particularly prevalent; Malta fever, Mediterranean fever, Gibraltar or Rock fever, and undulant fever are probably the best known. The cause of this disease was obscure until 1887 when Bruce reported numerous small coccal organisms in stained sections of spleen from a fatally infected soldier and isolated an identical organism in culture from spleen tissue of 4 other soldiers. This bacterium, which he named *Micrococcus melitensis*, produced a remittent fever in inoculated monkeys; one animal died from the infection and the organism was recovered in pure culture from the liver and spleen. Later, Wright and Smith (1897) described an agglutination test for detecting antibodies to *M. melitensis* in the serum of humans and animals. With this test Zammit (1905) detected infection in Maltese goats and, with others, showed the goat to be the natural host of *M. melitensis*; man became infected by the consumption of raw milk or cheese (Report 1905–7, Horrocks and Kennedy 1906).

Alice C Evans (1918a) drew attention to the similarity between *M. melitensis* and the organism described by Bang (1897) as the cause of contagious abortion of cattle. Her observations were confirmed by others, and Meyer and Shaw (1920) proposed the generic name *Brucella* for the 2 organisms, in honour of Sir David Bruce. The possible pathogenicity of the second organism, *Brucella abortus*, for humans was suggested by Evans (1918b) and confirmed by others, including Bevan (1921–22).

Subsequently, a third species, *Brucella suis*, was identified as a cause of epizootic abortion of swine in the USA (Traum 1914) and later implicated as an agent of brucellosis in humans (Huddleson 1943). A variant of *B. suis* was shown to cause genital infections and abortion of swine in Europe (Thomsen 1934) but, unlike the American strains, has rarely been implicated as a cause of disease in man. Strains of *Brucella* from cases of undulant fever in the arctic regions of North America were initially suspected of being *B. melitensis* (Toshach 1963) but later shown to be identical with an organism causing brucellosis in reindeer and caribou in the tundra regions of Alaska, Canada and the USSR. This organism was named *Brucella rangiferi tarandi* (Davydov 1961) but was subsequently reclassified as a fourth biogroup of *B. suis* (Jones 1967). A fifth biogroup of *B. suis*, occurring in rodents in the Caucasian region of the USSR (Vershilova et al. 1983), has been implicated in laboratory-acquired infections but is otherwise of unknown significance in human disease.

A fourth species, *Brucella neotomae*, was isolated by Stoenner and Lackman (1957) from desert wood rats in Utah but has not been found elsewhere.

Brucella ovis was identified almost simultaneously by Simmons and Hall (1953) in Australia and Buddle and Boyes (1953) in New Zealand as the cause of contagious epididymitis of rams. This organism also sometimes causes abortion in ewes and systemic disease in young lambs. It shows a high degree of host specificity for sheep, but serological evidence suggests that it may infect humans (Gavrilov et al. 1972).

Brucella canis was first described as a cause of abortion in beagles in the USA (Carmichael and Bruner 1968). It was subsequently shown to infect dogs in many other countries, irrespective of breed, and was identified as an occasional cause of brucellosis in humans (Schoenemann, Lütticken and Scheibner 1986, Carmichael 1990). Distinctive *Brucella* strains have been isolated from marine mammals in both the

UK (Ross et al. 1994) and the USA (Ewalt et al. 1994). Some heterogeneity exists between isolates, and different biogroups appear to infect cetaceans and seals. Initial observations indicate a low pathogenicity for sheep but a human case of laboratory-acquired infection has occurred (MacMillan, unpublished observations).

All these organisms are closely related, and genetic evidence suggests that they should be regarded as variants of a single species (Verger et al. 1985). This matter is discussed in Volume 2, Chapter 35. Regardless of the infecting species, cases of brucellosis in humans have many features in common, but the severity of disease and the occurrence of complications vary to some extent with the organism responsible. In general, *B. melitensis* produces the severest and most acute human infections. Biogroups 1 and 3 of *B. suis* may produce severe acute infections but have a particular tendency to cause chronic suppurative lesions affecting the skeletal system. *B. abortus* and *B. canis* tend to produce a milder disease, with a higher proportion of subacute and subclinical infections. Indeed, human disease caused by *B. canis* has been diagnosed only infrequently, but serological studies suggest that exposure to infection is common in some populations (Monroe et al. 1975). Brucella infections of animals are dealt with at some length, because of their impact on humans in terms of zoonotic infections and economic loss.

2 *BRUCELLA* INFECTIONS OF HUMANS

2.1 Epidemiology

Most cases of human brucellosis are caused by *B. melitensis* and their geographical distribution follows very closely the distribution of ovine and caprine brucellosis. In Europe, the highest prevalence of human brucellosis occurs in the countries of the Iberian peninsula and the Mediterranean littoral. France, Greece, Italy, Portugal, Spain and Turkey account for most cases but the infection is also present in Albania and is occasionally reported from countries of the former Yugoslavia (Report 1986a).

In the past, *B. abortus* accounted for most cases in northern Europe; because of the successful eradication or control of bovine brucellosis, however, the human cases now seen are increasingly due to *B. melitensis* infections acquired in other countries.

Human brucellosis, mainly caused by *B. melitensis*, is also prevalent on the southern and eastern edges of the Mediterranean basin, particularly in Tunisia, Libya, Egypt, Israel, Lebanon and Syria, and in the Arabian Peninsula and Iran. In Kuwait and Saudi Arabia, the prevalence in the human population has increased as a result of attempts to develop intensive livestock production units against a background of infection in the indigenous animal population (Report 1986a, Mousa et al. 1988). The introduction of measures for the control of the disease in animals

has been followed by a decline in the number of human cases in recent years.

The disease is also common in many parts of North, Central and South America, particularly in Mexico, Argentina, Brazil, Colombia, Ecuador and Peru. Most reported cases are caused by *B. melitensis*, but *B. abortus* accounts for some. Infections caused by *B. suis*, mainly of biogroup 1, are common in Argentina, Brazil and Colombia (Lopez-Merino 1989). Brucellosis is seen infrequently in Canada and the USA, but is common in Mexico in humans, livestock and other animals.

B. abortus and *B. melitensis* infections in humans are widespread in many African countries, but the true prevalence is unknown. *B. melitensis* infection is common in some areas of the Indian subcontinent and was formerly prevalent in Mongolia and northern China but has declined as a result of the intensive vaccination of sheep and goats. *B. abortus* and *B. suis* infection are widespread in many Asian countries but the true prevalence of human brucellosis in this region is unknown.

SOURCES AND TRANSMISSION

Brucellosis is a zoonosis and, with few exceptions, infections in humans result from direct or indirect contact with animal sources. Rare instances of person-to-person transmission have been recorded, either in circumstances implicating sexual contact (Goossens et al. 1983, Stantić-Pavlinić, Cec and Mehle 1983, Mantur, Mangalgi and Mulimani 1996), or by the transfer of tissue, including blood and bone marrow (Naparstek, Block and Slavin 1982). Laboratory-acquired brucellosis, a much greater problem, has been caused by *B. melitensis*, *B. abortus*, *B. suis* and *B. canis* as a result of accidental ingestion, inhalation, infection and mucosal and skin contamination. Circumstantial evidence implicates exposure to infectious aerosols generated during the manipulation of cultures as one of the most common sources of laboratory infection. Several studies have suggested that in the past, brucellosis was acquired in the laboratory more frequently than any other bacterial disease (Pike 1978, Collins 1983). In Britain, the Advisory Group on Dangerous Pathogens has classified *Brucella* as a pathogen requiring containment at the level of Category 3 (Report 1994). Recommendations for appropriate precautions to be taken when handling *Brucella* cultures have been made (Corbel et al. 1979, Report 1986b).

Most cases of infection caused by *B. abortus*, *B. melitensis*, *B. suis* and *B. canis* arise from occupational or domestic contact with infected animals or with an environment contaminated by their discharges. Farmers and their families, abattoir workers, butchers and veterinarians are particularly at risk. Infected animals that have recently aborted or given birth present the greatest hazard; infection may occur through ingestion or inhalation, or by contamination of the conjunctiva or skin with discharges. *B. abortus* 'strain 19' and *B. melitensis* 'Rev 1' – 2 live vaccine strains – retain virulence for humans, and infections have resulted from accidental exposure to them (Sadusk, Browne and Born 1957, Olle Goig and Canela Soler 1987).

The main source of infection for the general population is dairy produce prepared from infected milk. *B. melitensis* presents the greatest hazard. The milk of infected sheep and goats may contain large numbers of viable organisms, which become concentrated in products such as soft cheeses. Indeed, soft cheese has been recognized as a major vehicle of infection in the Mediterranean region, the Middle East and Latin America (Eckman 1975, Sabbaghian 1975, Al-Dubooni, Al-Shirkat and Nagi 1986, Report 1986a).

B. melitensis may be transmitted from infected sheep and goats to cattle kept in contact with them. Camels, which are susceptible to *B. abortus* and *B. melitensis*, can be infected in the same way; their milk is an important source of infection for humans in Middle Eastern countries and in Mongolia (Report 1971).

Cattle infected with *B. abortus* probably present the greatest hazard to humans through direct contact after calving or abortion, or at slaughter. This is reflected in the occupational nature of the disease in Britain and other developed countries (Buchanan et al. 1974b, Report 1980). Of the 494 cases reported in the period 1956–61 to the Public Health Laboratory Service in England and Wales, 69% were in males and 71% in the 10–50 year age group. Farm and dairy workers, abattoir workers, butchers and veterinary surgeons accounted for a disproportionate number of male cases whereas housewives and schoolchildren predominated among the female cases. Dalrymple-Champneys (1960) attributed about 80% of non-occupational cases to the consumption of raw milk and cream. At that time at least 5% of herd samples of raw milk were infected with *B. abortus* (Report 1961). Cases among the non-occupationally exposed population were confined to those who drank Tuberculin Tested or other types of raw milk. They were virtually non-existent in urban populations supplied with pasteurized milk. After the introduction of eradication measures for bovine brucellosis, the disease in the general population declined rapidly. Of 419 cases reported in the period 1975–79, only 13 were attributed to the consumption of raw milk, the remainder being occupational in origin (Report 1980). By 1984 the decline was greater still and even occupationally acquired cases were rare.

Serological surveys have indicated that even in populations consuming raw milk, the number of cases of clinical brucellosis is small in proportion to the number of persons with antibodies to *B. abortus*. This indicates that *B. abortus* has a high infectivity for humans but is less virulent than some other types (for further information on latent or subclinical infections see previous editions of this book).

Infection caused by *B. suis* biogroups 1 and 3 has a much more limited distribution than that caused by *B. abortus* and *B. melitensis*. It is essentially an occupational disease of slaughterers and meat packers, who handle carcasses of infected pigs, and hence affects mainly adult males (Hendricks 1955). It was formerly common in the USA, especially in the middle-western states, but has declined dramatically as a result of the virtual eradication of the disease from the pig population. Epidemiological studies made when the infection was common showed that only a minority of those exposed developed overt as opposed to a subclinical infection (see Hardy et al. 1931, Hardy, Jordan and Borts 1932, Huddleson, Johnson and Hamann 1933, Heathman 1934, Buchanan et al. 1974a). The organism gains entry via the conjunctiva, abraded skin, respiratory tract or by ingestion (Hendricks et al. 1962, Buchanan et al. 1974a). The disease is often prolonged and debilitating, with a tendency to produce severe complications. Occasionally *B. suis* infects cattle, causing milk-borne outbreaks in the general population (Borts et al. 1943). This is not uncommon in Argentina, Brazil and Colombia, where *B. suis* infection of humans is prevalent. The disease also occurs in the South Pacific region and in southern China. Occasional cases contracted from feral pigs occur in the southern USA and in Australia (Crichton and Medveczky 1987).

B. suis biogroup 2 has rarely been implicated in human brucellosis. *B. suis* biogroup 4 infects wild and farmed reindeer and associated human populations in Alaska, northern Canada and Russia (Huntley, Philip and Maynard 1963, Meyer 1964); clinically and epidemiologically the infection is similar to that caused by *B. abortus* and by *B. melitensis*. *B. suis* biogroup 5 has been implicated in a laboratory-acquired infection but the relevance of the natural infection for man is unknown.

B. canis has been implicated as a cause of brucellosis in humans, the manifestations being similar to those resulting from infection with *B. abortus*, *B. melitensis* and *B. suis*, but the disease is usually mild (Polt et al. 1982). Serological studies suggest that subclinical infection is common in some populations (Monroe et al. 1975). For details of early studies on the epidemiology of Mediterranean fever and other forms of brucellosis see the previous editions of this book, Report (1905–7) and Williams (1989).

2.2 Pathogenesis

Brucellae enter the body via the alimentary tract, conjunctival mucosa, respiratory tract, or skin. At or near the site of entry they are likely to be ingested by either mononuclear or polymorphonuclear leucocytes. However, virulent brucellae can depress chemotaxis and phagocytosis by polymorphonuclear leucocytes (Ocon et al. 1994). Phagocytosis is facilitated by pre-existing antibodies but is not dependent upon them (Canning, Deyoe and Roth 1988). A lectin which binds to receptors on the cell membrane of the B lymphocyte has been identified on the surface of brucella cells (Bratescu, Mayer and Teodorescu 1981). This or a similar component may also promote endocytosis of brucellae by other cell types.

Virulent brucellae have the capacity to survive in both polymorphonuclear and mononuclear phagocytes. In both types, the organisms release soluble factors distinct from LPS that inhibit phagolysosome fusion (Frenchick, Markham and Cochrane 1985). They also inactivate the myeloperoxidase–hydrogen peroxide–halide systems by releasing adenine and guanosine monophosphate which prevent degranulation (Bertram, Canning and Roth 1986, Canning, Roth and Deyoe 1986). These or similar factors are probably responsible for inhibiting the oxidative burst (Kreutzer, Dreyfus and Robertson 1979). Purines are also implicated in the suppression of production of tumour necrosis factor α (TNF-α) by monocytes (Caron et al. 1994). This is a major factor in determining the capacity of virulent brucellae to survive in monocytes.

It is evident that the O chain of smooth-type LPS plays a role in intracellular survival as smooth strains generally survive much more effectively than rough variants (Kreutzer and Robertson 1979). However, its precise role is unclear. Other factors that contribute to intracellular survival by protecting the bacteria from hydrogen peroxide and superoxide include catalase (Fitzgeorge, Solotorovsky and Smith 1965) and copper–zinc superoxide dismutase. Strains deficient in the latter produced 10-fold lower splenic counts in experimental infections in mice (Tatum et al. 1992).

Macrophage activation plays a key role in determining the outcome of brucella infection and interferon-γ (IFN-γ) is essential for this process (Cheers and Pagram 1979, Stevens, Pugh and Tabatabai 1992, Zhan and Cheers 1993). However, activation alone is not effective in eliminating the infection (Jones and Winter 1992). In contrast to some other bacteria, in which iron depletion inhibited in vivo growth, iron-saturated transferrin is reported to promote the elimination of brucellae from infected macrophages by catalysing the formation of hydroxyl radical (Jiang and Baldwin 1993).

After phagocytosis, brucellae probably multiply in the lymph nodes draining the site of entry. Subsequently, as the bacteria are released from the dying cells that they have parasitized, they enter the blood and produce the bacteraemia that normally accompanies the acute febrile phase of the disease. Bacteraemia varies in degree with the severity of the disease but is likely to be sustained during the early phase of the acute disease, becoming intermittent as this passes. From the blood, the organisms are distributed throughout the reticuloendothelial system and may be present in large numbers in the liver and spleen. They may also localize in many other sites including the joints, heart, kidneys, central nervous system and genital tract. The nature of the lesions produced depends to some extent upon the type of infecting organism. Thus, *B. abortus* strains produce more typically a granulomatous reaction (Young 1979). *B. suis* strains are often associated with chronic suppurative lesions, especially in the joints and spleen (Spink 1956).

Antibodies to the brucella LPS develop within a few days of the onset of the acute phase or, in subacute cases, may precede the onset of symptoms. Cell mediated responses to brucella antigens may develop in parallel with or independently of the antibody response. Some patients remain anergic throughout the disease whereas others develop cell mediated responses but do not produce antibodies; both antibodies and cell mediated immune responses develop in most patients. The cell mediated response, particularly the production of activated mononuclear phagocytes, is probably largely instrumental in promoting recovery from the disease (Serre et al. 1987, Baldwin and Winter 1994).

The mechanisms whereby the clinical effects of the disease are produced, particularly the fever, asthenia and depression of the central nervous system, are not clearly understood. Endotoxin and hypersensitivity to brucella antigens have been invoked to explain them; similar effects have been produced by partly purified fractions containing these antigens (Abernathy and Spink 1958). Such preparations are capable of releasing cytokines, including interferons and TNF-α (cachectin) from mononuclear cells (Berman and Kurtz 1987). The physiological effects of these mediators are remarkably similar to many of the clinical manifestations of brucellosis.

2.3 Clinical manifestations

Acute or subacute disease follows an incubation period which can vary from 1 week to 6 or more months. In most patients for whom the time of exposure can be identified, the incubation period is between 2 and 6 weeks. The length of the incubation period may be influenced by many factors, including the virulence of the infecting strain, the size of the inoculum, the route of infection, and the resistance of the host. *B. melitensis* infections are likely to be manifested as acute disease of sudden onset; infections caused by the other species are often subacute, with an insidious onset and prolonged and indeterminate incubation period. Acute brucellosis is characterized by an intermittent fever with a maximum temperature that usually lies within the range 38–41°C but is sometimes substantially higher; hyperpyrexia, which occurs in some cases, is a significant cause of death. Typically, the body temperature is often near normal during the early part of the day but rises sharply during the late afternoon or evening; this is accompanied by chills, shivering, malaise, nausea and extreme fatigue. After reaching its peak the temperature shows a rapid fall, accompanied by profuse sweating. The temperature rises may follow a regular pattern, especially early in the disease, but increasingly long intervals between them may occur later. The characteristic undulant fever is most likely to be seen in untreated cases in which the disease has persisted for some time. For a description of the clinical manifestations of undulant fever see Dalrymple-Champneys (1960) and Hughes (1897).

The febrile phase is associated with anorexia, weakness, severe fatigue and loss of weight which may be rapid and substantial. Headache is a frequent symptom as are muscular and joint pains. Objective physical signs other than fever are few in uncomplicated cases. About two-thirds of patients with *B. melitensis* infection have enlargement of the liver, spleen and superficial lymph nodes, sometimes accompanied by transient jaundice, whereas only about one-third of patients with *B. abortus* or *B. suis* infection have splenomegaly and fewer have perceptible enlargement of the liver. A cough sometimes accompanies the acute disease and gastrointestinal disturbance is not uncommon in brucellosis resulting from ingestion of infected foods or milk. Most patients with acute brucellosis will recover from the physical effects of the disease in 1–3 months, but subjective symptoms may persist for much longer. The untreated disease is, however, associated with significant mortality. In *B. melitensis* infections, the case-fatality rate has been estimated as between 2 and 5%, but in infections caused by other species it is substantially lower. Death may result from hyperpyrexia, severe toxaemia, endocarditis, meningoencephalitis, or other serious complications. In some patients, especially those untreated, the acute or subacute disease may persist or recur for 6 months or more, the disease then being regarded as 'chronic'. Complications, which may develop during the acute or chronic stages, affect most frequently the bones and joints, cardiovascular system, central nervous system, genitourinary tract and reticuloendothelial system (see Spink 1956, Dalrymple-Champneys 1960, Young 1983, Young and Corbel 1989, Madkour 1989).

About 10% of patients develop bone or joint complications usually spondylitis or arthritis of the hip, knee, ankle or sacroiliac joints. Paravertebral abscess is fairly frequently associated with spondylitis; osteomyelitis of the cranium, ribs or limb bones has also been reported. Reactive arthritis may follow acute or chronic brucellosis; in patients of European origin, an association with HLA-B27 antigen has been observed (Hodinka et al. 1978), but no such association has been found in patients of ethnic groups in which this antigen is rare (Alarcon et al. 1981).

Nearly all patients with brucellosis experience non-specific symptoms referable to the central nervous system, including headache, irritability, loss of concentration, insomnia, anxiety and depression. In some 3–5% of patients with *B. melitensis* infection but fewer with infection caused by other types, neurobrucellosis may develop as a result of invasion of the central nervous system. Meningitis and meningoencephalitis are the usual manifestations of this, but polyradiculoneuritis and meningomyelitis may also occur (Bashir et al. 1985, Shakir 1986). Neurobrucellosis requires prompt and vigorous treatment with tetracycline, rifampicin and streptomycin if death or permanent disability is to be avoided (Shakir et al. 1987, Al-Deeb and Madkour 1989).

Thrombophlebitis and endocarditis are the most frequent cardiovascular complications of brucellosis. Endocarditis causes a high proportion of the fatalities in brucellosis, especially that caused by *B. abortus* and *B. suis*, and requires vigorous and sustained antibiotic treatment and cardiac surgery.

Epididymo-orchitis, which is the commonest genitourinary complication in the male, may be acute or chronic. Brucellosis in pregnancy may result in abortion; the bacteria have been isolated from the placenta and fetal membranes (Poole, Whitehouse and Gilchrist 1972, Young 1983). There is little indication, however, that *Brucella* spp. have a specific tropism for the human placenta, like that seen in ungulate species. Many pregnant patients with acute brucellosis have proceeded to term even without antibiotic treatment (Williams 1973).

Other complications include a diffuse or focal hepatitis, which may be accompanied by acute inflammatory changes and parenchymal degeneration or may be granulomatous. The former are said to be frequent in *B. melitensis* infection whereas *B. abortus* and *B. suis* are more commonly associated

with granuloma formation (Young 1995). Hepatic and splenic abscesses may also develop, especially in patients with *B. suis* infection.

There is some confusion over the nature of chronic brucellosis. This term should be reserved for disease that has persisted for 6 months or longer, with or without complications but with objective evidence of brucella infection as the cause. In practice, such evidence may be difficult to obtain. Blood culture is usually unsuccessful in the chronic phase. Culture of bone marrow or material removed surgically from localized lesions may be more successful. Serological tests are frequently unhelpful, but radioimmunoassay and enzyme immunoassay are reported to be useful (Parratt et al. 1977, Magee 1980, Araj et al. 1986a, 1986b). The use of polymerase chain reaction (PCR) may offer a means of detecting infection in some of these cases (Fekete et al. 1990, Matar, Khreissir and Abodnoor 1996). However, the selection of appropriate primers is crucial and this procedure is not without its pitfalls. It has yet to be fully evaluated in chronic brucellosis. Illness associated with non-specific symptoms but no physical signs, and a history of occupational or other exposure to *Brucella*, is often diagnosed as chronic brucellosis. Not surprisingly, it usually responds poorly to specific treatment.

2.4 Diagnosis

The variable symptoms, the paucity of distinctive physical signs and the occurrence of subclinical and atypical infections make the clinical diagnosis of brucellosis in humans particularly difficult. Bacteriological and serological examination are usually essential for confirmation of the diagnosis but even these tend to give unsatisfactory results in the chronic phase of the disease. Brucellosis should always be considered as a possible cause of pyrexia of undetermined origin, and of any acute or chronic inflammatory disease that presents diagnostic difficulty. A history of occupational or environmental exposure to possible sources of infection may assist diagnosis. No specific biochemical changes are associated with the disease. Mild leucopenia with a relative lymphocytosis, sometimes accompanied by a secondary anaemia and thrombocytopenia, is a common finding in acute or subacute brucellosis. The erythrocyte sedimentation rate is usually in the normal range except in severe cases.

Cultural examination

Isolation of a *Brucella* sp. is the most certain means of reaching a diagnosis. It is most likely to be successful during the acute phase of infection caused by *B. melitensis* or *B. suis* but is less successful with *B. abortus* infections. Samples of any body fluid, or of tissue collected surgically or at necropsy, may be cultured. Blood is the material most commonly examined, but bone marrow may be more likely to give positive results (Gotuzzo et al. 1986). Blood cultures are best performed on samples collected during the pyrexial phase, preferably while the temperature is rising. The isolation rate is improved if several samples are taken over a period of 24 h. At least 3–5 ml should be inoculated into 20–100 ml of serum dextrose broth, tryptone soya broth or trypticase–soy broth and incubated at 37°C in air enriched with CO_2 5–10%. If desired, a replicate sample may be incubated in air or anaerobically. If an anticoagulant is needed during transport of the specimen, trisodium citrate or preservative-free heparin should be used. Blood clot may also be cultured but should be homogenized first. There is some evidence that buffy coat samples are more likely than whole blood to give positive results.

Selective media are not necessary for the culture of human blood samples taken with aseptic precautions but should be used if samples of excreta or contaminated tissues are to be examined. The liquid media recommended above can be made selective by the addition of an antibiotic mixture containing: amphotericin B 1 mg l^{-1}, bacitracin 25 mg l^{-1}, cycloheximide 100 mg l^{-1}, d-cycloserine 100 mg l^{-1}, nalidixic acid 5 mg l^{-1}, polymyxin B 6 mg l^{-1}, and vancomycin 20 mg l^{-1}. This antibiotic mixture is suitable for most strains of *B. abortus*, *B. melitensis* and *B. suis*. It may be inhibitory, however, for strains of *B. abortus* biogroups 2, 3 and 4 and some strains of *B. melitensis*, *B. canis* and *B. ovis*. For these organisms media may be made selective by adding an antibiotic mixture of vancomycin 3 mg l^{-1}, sodium colistimethate 7.5 mg l^{-1}, nitrofurantoin 10 mg l^{-1}, and nystatin 12 500 units (Brown, Ranger and Kelley 1971).

When liquid media are used for enrichment or primary isolation, subcultures should be made every 3–5 days on to a suitable solid medium such as heated blood agar or serum dextrose agar, which is then incubated at 37°C in air enriched with CO_2 5–10%. The need for frequent subculture can be avoided by use of a 2-phase system (Castañeda 1947) in which both solid and liquid media are contained within the same bottle. Even with this system, subcultures to fresh solid medium should be made immediately growth appears, to minimize the dissociation of smooth cultures to the non-smooth colonial phase. This procedure is capable of achieving isolation rates of up to 85% from patients with acute *B. melitensis* infection. This rate may be improved if the blood, bone marrow or other tissue suspensions are treated by the lysis-concentration method of Finegold et al. (1969) combined with centrifugation rather than filtration (Kolman et al. 1991). Because many patients may have received prior treatment with inappropriate antibiotics that inhibit but do not kill brucellae, all cultures should be incubated for at least 6 weeks, with frequent subculture, before they are discarded as negative. Rapid growth detection methods such as the Bactec or BACT/ALERT systems may also increase the sensitivity of isolation when combined with the lysis-concentration method (Kolman et al. 1991, Solomon and Jackson 1992) but samples should not be discarded as negative without subculture.

The PCR using a 223 bp region of the 31 kDa surface protein of *B. abortus* has given promising results in the diagnosis of both acute and chronic relapsing brucellosis (Matar, Khreissir and Abodnoor 1996). The procedure merits further evaluation, particularly for assessment of patients who have received antibiotics or have suspected chronic brucellosis.

SEROLOGICAL TESTS

Most patients with acute brucellosis produce antibodies of the IgM isotype within a few days of onset of the disease. These antibodies are rapidly followed and superseded by IgG, and to a lesser extent IgA, antibodies. Maximum titres are reached in the third or fourth week of disease and then slowly decline; however, antibodies usually persist throughout the active phase of the disease and in some cases for long after. In subacute or chronic brucellosis this pattern is generally not seen, the serological response consisting of a sustained production of IgG and sometimes IgA antibodies (Araj et al. 1986a, Serre et al. 1987, Ariza et al. 1992). IgE antibodies to *Brucella* spp. have also been observed in some brucellosis patients, but their clinical significance is uncertain (Escande and Serre 1982). These patterns are of diagnostic relevance because antibodies of the IgA, IgG and IgM isotypes vary considerably in their activity in different serological tests.

Numerous serological procedures have been tried in the diagnosis of human brucellosis but few have achieved lasting application. Until recently, the most widely used was the standard tube-agglutination test (SAT). In many laboratories this has now been superseded by the rose bengal plate test and enzyme-linked immunosorbent assay (ELISA). Other useful tests include the 2-mercaptoethanol agglutination test; the complement fixation test; and the Coombs antiglobulin test and radioimmunoassay (Buchanan et al. 1974b, Diaz, Maravi Poma and Rivero 1976, Magee 1980, Araj et al. 1986a, Report 1986b, Diaz and Moriyon 1989). The SAT should be performed with a standardized suspension of heat-killed smooth brucella cells in saline containing phenol 0.5%. Incubation may be at 37°C or 50°C for 18 h. There is some advantage in performing parallel tests with suspensions of smooth biogroup 1 strains of *B. abortus* and *B. melitensis*, but these must be properly standardized. The use of both detects infection caused by M antigen-dominant strains more readily than *B. abortus* antigen alone. It does not, as commonly supposed, identify the infecting strain, because both *B. abortus* and *B. melitensis* biogroups share similar antigenic structures. In many countries the agglutinating suspensions are standardized against the International Standard for *Brucella abortus* antiserum, a practice to be recommended as it permits comparison of tests performed by different laboratories and on different occasions within a single laboratory (see pages 831 and 832). Microagglutination procedures are also available (Baum et al. 1995). If infection by *B. canis* or another non-smooth brucella is suspected, a stable suspension of the appropriate type must be used. Recommendations have been made for the preparation of such suspensions (Report 1986b).

Most patients with acute brucellosis develop agglutinin titres of 640 or more by the end of the third or fourth week of illness. These tend to decline fairly rapidly once the acute phase is over, and may become low within 3 months. Rising titres or titres that decline after appropriate antibiotic treatment indicate recent active infection.

The interpretation of stable titres in the low or intermediate range (20–160) is difficult. In symptomless patients they probably indicate past or latent infection. In patients with symptoms suggestive of brucellosis they may indicate active infection, especially if there is no history of occupational or other previous exposure to infection. In patients with a history of prolonged exposure, titres of this magnitude are common even in the absence of disease and reliance cannot be placed upon agglutination tests alone. In such patients, low agglutinin titres should be investigated by testing with additional procedures such as ELISA and Western blotting. PCR may also be useful in such cases but has received limited evaluation (Matar, Khreissir and Abodnoor 1996). The absence of agglutinins does not exclude brucellosis, as many cases have been recorded in which a positive blood culture was obtained despite a negative agglutination reaction (Gilbert and Dacey 1932, Heathman 1934).

Prozones sometimes occur in the agglutination test. They have been attributed to antibody excess (Serre, Dana and Roux 1970) or to blocking of agglutinins by non-agglutinating IgG or IgA isotypes (Heremans, Vaerman and Vaerman 1963, Wilkinson 1966). This emphasizes the need to use more than one serological test for diagnosis. Of the various rapid slide or plate agglutination tests for brucella antibodies, the most effective is the rose bengal plate or card test. This uses as antigen a dense suspension of smooth brucella cells stained with rose bengal and suspended in an acid buffer. The test discriminates against agglutinins of low avidity and is not subject to prozones. It compares favourably with the SAT in specificity and for detecting antibodies in human sera (Buchanan et al. 1974b, Diaz et al. 1976, Cernyševa, Knjazeva and Egorova 1977) and is useful for detecting antibodies in cerebrospinal fluid in cases of neurobrucellosis (Diaz et al. 1978).

Buchanan et al. (1974b) concluded that the complement fixation and 2-mercaptoethanol tests were the most accurate indicators of active disease. On the grounds of technical convenience the latter was preferred; it has also been used to assess the response to treatment (Buchanan and Faber 1980). The Coombs antiglobulin test and the complement fixation test tend to become positive later in the course of the disease than the agglutination test and are likely still to be reactive in the chronic phase (Kerr et al. 1967, 1968, Robertson et al. 1980). Unfortunately the titres observed at this stage are often no greater than those of symptomless patients with a history of either occupational exposure to *Brucella* or of acute infection with recovery. For this reason Farrell, Robertson and Hinchcliffe (1975) concluded that the diagnosis of chronic brucellosis had to be based on clinical symptoms. Because these are largely subjective, however, it is desirable to obtain objective evidence of infection, and some progress has been made through the use of enzyme-labelled antibody assays.

Magee (1980) concluded that enzyme-labelled antibody assays were as sensitive as radioimmunoassay and could as easily be made specific for immunoglobulin isotypes. He identified 4 classes of sera:

1 those from acute cases with very high concentrations of IgG antibody and moderate ones of IgM and IgA
2 those from chronic cases having high concentrations of IgG but not IgM or IgA antibodies
3 those with low residual titres of IgG, probably representing past infection and
4 those with little or no brucella-specific antibody.

These results are broadly consistent with those of Lindberg and colleagues (1982) who found that patients in the acute stage had high IgM and rising titres of IgG antibodies to *B. abortus* LPS antigen, whereas those in the chronic stage had raised titres of IgG antibody alone. Araj et al. (1986a) also concluded that enzyme immunoassay was an effective method for diagnosing acute and chronic brucellosis; and it was useful for detecting antibodies in the cerebrospinal fluid of patients with neurological complications (Araj et al. 1986b).

Immunoblotting against extracts of *Brucella* cells or purified protein antigens has been reported to differentiate active disease from past exposure to infection (Goldbaum et al. 1993).

All serological tests for brucellosis that are based on detection of antibodies to the LPS antigen of smooth strains are subject to interference from antibodies produced in response to bacteria with structurally related antigens. These include *Escherichia coli* O:157 (Stuart and Corbel 1982), *Francisella tularensis* (Francis and Evans 1926), *Stenotrophomonas maltophilia* (Corbel, Stuart and Brewer 1984), *Salmonella* serotypes of Kauffmann–White group N (Corbel 1975), *Vibrio cholerae* (Wong and Chow 1937, Feeley 1969) and *Yersinia enterocolitica* O:9 (Ahvonen, Janssen and Aho 1969). With the exception of *F. tularensis*, in which the cross-reacting antigen has not been fully characterized, these cross-reactions result from antibodies evoked by epitopes containing 4-amino-4,6-dideoxymannose (perosamine) (Redmond 1979, Bundle et al. 1987). That produced in response to *Y. enterocolitica* O:9 is the most complete as its polysaccharide O chain is almost identical with that of strains of *Brucella* in which the A antigen dominates (Caroff et al. 1984a, 1984b). Antibodies produced in response to *Y. enterocolitica* O:9 react in agglutination, antiglobulin, immunofluorescence, complement fixation and immunoprecipitation tests with brucella antigens (Corbel and Cullen 1970). Various attempts have been made to devise tests that distinguish brucellosis and yersiniosis, but none is entirely satisfactory (Corbel and Cullen 1970, Diaz and Dorronsoro 1971, Mittal and Tizard 1981, Corbel, Stuart and Brewer 1984). The cross-reactions produced by other bacteria are usually less troublesome than those produced by *Y. enterocolitica*, but diagnostic problems have been caused by *E.coli* O:157 (Notenboom et al. 1987), *F. tularensis* (Foshay 1950, Behan and Klein 1982) and by vaccination with *V. cholerae* (Eisele et al. 1946). For further discussion see Corbel (1985a).

TESTS FOR CELL MEDIATED IMMUNITY

Cell mediated immunity is believed to play a major role in recovery from infection with *Brucella*. Most patients show evidence of a cell mediated immune response to brucella antigens as the disease progresses from the acute phase to either recovery or the chronic disease (Serre 1989). There is usually a delayed-hypersensitivity type reaction to the intradermal injection of 0.05–0.1 ml of a suitable preparation of antigen. Such a reaction usually manifests itself within 6–24 h as a slightly raised, sometimes tender, erythematous plaque 2–6 cm or more in diameter. Occasionally much more severe local reactions accompanied by slight fever and malaise develop. False positive reactions generally appear rapidly and disappear within 24 h. Delayed reactions of the type sometimes encountered in tuberculosis have been reported; in these an inflammatory response develops in recently infected patients at the site of an intradermal test performed weeks previously.

Numerous antigen preparations, referred to collectively as 'brucellins', by analogy with tuberculin, have been employed in such tests. They range from culture supernates such as 'abortin' (M'Fadyean and Stockman 1909) or 'melitin' (Burnet 1922) to extracts prepared by physical disruption of cells or by chemical fractionation, including acid or alkaline hydrolysis (for a detailed description see Alton and Jones 1967). Such preparations are poorly defined, of variable composition and often contain LPS antigen which stimulates an antibody response in the recipient and interferes with the interpretation of subsequent serological tests. No reference preparations exist and there are no agreed standard doses; consequently the interpretation of results is difficult. Because of these problems there have been moves towards the development of a defined non-antigenic preparation based on the extraction procedure of Bhongbhibhat, Elberg and Chen (1970). Such a preparation ('Brucellin INRA') has been widely used in France in a screening test for animal brucellosis (Report 1986b).

In general, the intradermal test with brucellin is analogous to the tuberculin test in that it demonstrates previous exposure to infection without clearly indicating its significance. Some patients with high antibody titres react weakly or negatively to brucellin, whereas those without antibodies sometimes react strongly. Provided that a LPS-free preparation is available, the test may be of value in distinguishing between brucellosis and infections caused by bacteria that share antigenic determinants with the brucella O chain. However, it is not recommended as a routine procedure for the diagnosis of active brucellosis.

In vitro tests, based on cell mediated immunity, for the diagnosis of brucellosis in humans include the macrophage migration-inhibition test, the leucocyte-lysis test and the lymphocyte-stimulation test (Peraldi et al. 1976, Report 1986b). All require freshly collected cells, are difficult to standardize, and have yet to be evaluated with well defined antigenic preparations. They cannot be recommended for diagnostic purposes.

2.5 Prophylaxis

The ideal method of prevention, namely the avoidance of direct or indirect contact with infected animals or their products, is usually unattainable for those at risk through occupational exposure. The hazards can be reduced, however, by working practices that minimize the risk of skin or mucosal contamination or the inhalation of infectious aerosols. Adequate protective clothing, including impermeable gloves, should be worn by persons handling animals that have recently aborted or given birth; particular care should be taken when disposing of placental and fetal material. The latter should be incinerated or buried in quicklime and any part of the premises contaminated by discharges should be thoroughly decontaminated with an approved agricultural disinfectant used at the recommended concentration. Specific recommendations have been made for hygienic measures to be adopted by those concerned with the husbandry and slaughter of animals (Report 1986b), and by laboratory workers (Alton, Jones and Pietz 1975, Corbel et al. 1979, Report 1986b).

Most cases of non-occupational brucellosis, which result from the consumption of dairy or other animal products, could be eliminated by adequate heat treatment (pasteurization, boiling or sterilization) of milk, and the thorough cooking of meat products.

No satisfactory vaccine exists for the prevention of human brucellosis. Two attenuated vaccines used in animals, *B. abortus* strain 19 and *B. melitensis* Rev 1, retain virulence for humans and are therefore unacceptable. *B. abortus* strain 19-BA, a more attenuated variant of strain 19, has been used in the former USSR and China to vaccinate populations at high risk of infection from *B. melitensis* (Vershilova 1961). The vaccine is given by the intradermal route, usually by scarification, and is said to produce severe reactions only rarely. The immunity produced is, however, of short duration and where there is a high risk of infection, annual booster doses are required. Repeated doses of these vaccines are apparently associated with an increasing risk of hypersensitivity reactions. Other attenuated strains of *B. abortus* or *B. melitensis* have been used in China, but precise information on their safety and efficacy is lacking. Attempts have been made to produce vaccines from purified fractions of *Brucella*. A peptidoglycan fraction (Lopez-Merino et al. 1976), used in France (Bentejac et al. 1984), is apparently intended to give a minimal degree of protection which will be reinforced by subclinical infection. Its protective value is probably limited, and cases of acute brucellosis have occurred in recipients. Epidemiological evidence and the histories of cases of laboratory-acquired infection indicate that even attacks of clinical brucellosis give only incomplete protection against reinfection, particularly by strains of high virulence.

This suggests that a safe and effective vaccine against human brucellosis will be difficult to produce.

2.6 Treatment

Brucella strains are susceptible to a wide range of antibiotics in vitro, but few have proved effective in the treatment of brucellosis. Of agents subjected to clinical evaluation, the tetracyclines have emerged as the most effective group. In the past the recommended treatment for all forms of brucellosis in adults was tetracycline given orally to a total daily dose of 1–2 g for a minimum of 6 weeks. In severe infections or in those accompanied by localized lesions, this was supplemented by streptomycin in intramuscular doses of 1 g daily for the first 2–3 weeks. Rifampicin has been shown to exert strong inhibitory and bactericidal activity against *Brucella* strains in vitro (Corbel 1976) and was effective in both experimental infections (Philippon et al. 1977) and clinical studies (Bertrand et al. 1979). It has proved useful against brucellosis in young children (Llorens-Terol and Busquets 1980) and is the antibiotic of choice for brucellosis in pregnancy.

The regimen recommended by the World Health Organization consists of rifampicin 600–900 mg and doxycycline 200 mg, both taken as a single daily dose for a minimum of 6 weeks (Report 1986b). The superiority of this over tetracycline in combination with streptomycin has been questioned (Ariza et al. 1985). Strains of *Brucella* resistant to rifampicin have been reported to emerge during treatment (Rautlin de la Roy et al. 1986). Mousa and colleagues (1988) concluded that a combination of tetracycline, streptomycin and rifampicin gave the best results for severe infections. Later studies suggest that combinations of streptomycin and tetracycline, rifampicin and doxycycline or rifampicin and ofloxacin give comparable results provided that treatment is sufficiently prolonged (Ariza et al. 1985, Akova et al. 1993).

Alternatives to these regimens include co-trimoxazole 2–3 g daily for at least 6 weeks. However, relapses after this treatment are common and it is not recommended except when rifampicin and tetracyclines cannot be used. Moxalactam together with chloramphenicol has been used successfully in the treatment of human infection caused by *B. canis* (Tosi and Nelson 1982) and, together with rifampicin and gentamicin, for brucella endocarditis. Gentamicin alone has been recommended as an alternative treatment for uncomplicated brucellosis (Wundt 1982).

For the treatment of brucellosis with complications, modifications of the standard regimens have been used. A combination of rifampicin 600–900 mg daily and tetracycline 2 g daily orally for 8–12 weeks, supplemented with intramuscular streptomycin 1 g per day for the first 6 weeks, has been recommended for patients with meningoencephalitis (Shakir 1986). Similar schedules have been used for brucella endocarditis, usually in conjunction with surgical treatment of the heart valves.

The response of chronic brucellosis to treatment is much less satisfactory than that of the acute disease. This is attributable in part to the vague symptoms, difficulty in diagnosis, and irreversible changes in musculoskeletal tissues. Repeated courses of antibiotic therapy may alleviate symptoms in some cases but in the majority they do not. Immunostimulant therapy with levamisole has been claimed to benefit such patients (Thornes 1977), but objective evidence from properly controlled trials is lacking. Treatment with immunosuppressive agents has also been tried (Thornes et al. 1982) but is difficult to justify in a non-lethal disease; the administration of anti-inflammatory agents may produce symptomatic relief in some patients although the effects are likely to be temporary. Antigen therapy is potentially hazardous and is not now recommended (Report 1986b).

3 BRUCELLA INFECTIONS OF CATTLE

Brucella infection of cattle is also known as contagious abortion, Bang's disease, avortement épizoötique (French) and seuchenhaftes Verwerfen (German). This is an acute contagious disease characterized by an inflammatory response affecting cells of the reticuloendothelial system and of the placenta during pregnancy, and culminating in the death and expulsion of the fetus, usually between the fifth and eighth months of gestation. Localization also occurs in the mammary gland, and large numbers of organisms are excreted in the milk. In the male the organism localizes in the seminal vesicles and testes, leading to an acute or chronic inflammatory process and excretion in the semen.

Confirmation of the infectious nature of contagious abortion was provided in 1878 by Lehnert (quoted by Stableforth 1959), who transmitted the disease by inoculating pregnant cattle intravaginally with placental material and vaginal discharges from aborting animals. Woodhead et al. (1889) also reported transmission not only by the intravaginal route but also by the subcutaneous injection of placental material; however, they failed to isolate a causal organism.

In 1897 Bang, assisted by Stribolt, demonstrated microscopically a small gram-negative bacillus in the exudate of a cow with impending abortion and isolated an organism (Bang's *Bacillus abortus*) in pure culture. The intravaginal inoculation of pregnant heifers with this organism caused them to abort, and the same bacillus was recovered from each animal. Bang's work was confirmed by Preisz (1903) and Nowak (1908) in Europe, M'Fadyean and Stockman (1909) in Great Britain and MacNeal and Kerr (1910) in the USA. Schroeder and Cotton (1911) isolated the organism from the milk of an infected cow; this led to the recognition of its importance as a human pathogen and of its route of transmission to humans.

3.1 **Epidemiology**

Brucellosis in cattle occurs world wide except in those countries from which it has been eradicated. Biogroups of *B. abortus* are usually responsible, but *B. melitensis* infections also occur in regions where the organism causes widespread disease in sheep and goats. This appears to be an increasing problem. *B. suis* infections have also been reported especially in South America and in Australia (Cook and Noble 1984). All 3 bacterial species produce similar clinical manifestations (Philippon, Renoux and Plommet 1970), but Norton and Thomas (1979) claim that infections caused by *B. suis* tend to be self-limiting in cattle.

Before eradication, *B. abortus* biogroup 1 predominated in Britain, Canada, Australia and New Zealand, and biogroup 3 in the Netherlands and Belgium. In predominantly cattle areas of the former Soviet Union most bovine isolates were of biogroups of *B. abortus* whereas in predominantly sheep areas most cattle isolates were of biogroups of *B. melitensis* (Morgan 1982, Verger and Grayon 1984). *B. abortus* biogroups 1 and 4 predominate in Latin America and biogroups 3 and 6 in many African and some Asian countries.

Biotyping can be useful in tracing sources of infection in areas in which multiple biogroups occur. In practice, usually one biogroup predominates, most commonly biogroup 1 or 3. Attempts have been made to subtype strains in their biogroups. Antibiotic resistogram typing distinguished 8 subgroups for *B. abortus* biogroup 1 strains isolated in Britain over a period of 40 years (Corbel 1989). Genetic methods based on polymorphism of selected genes may also be useful for this purpose but have not been evaluated on a field scale (see Volume 2, Chapter 35). However, polymorphism of the 25 kDa, 36 kDa and *dnak* genes allows the differentiation of various subtypes within species and should improve the epidemiological value of *Brucella* typing (Cloeckaert et al. 1995, 1996).

Britain was declared 'Officially Brucellosis-Free' in 1981 after an eradication campaign which started as a voluntary 'Accredited Herds Scheme' in 1967 (Morgan and Richards 1974). Other countries from which the disease has been eradicated include Norway, Sweden, Finland, Denmark, Germany, Belgium, the Netherlands, Switzerland, Austria, Czech Republic, Slovakia, New Zealand and Canada. In some other countries (e.g. France and Italy) eradication is being actively pursued. In the USA and Australia, the disease in cattle has been eradicated from most areas, but a few persistent foci remain. It was formally under control in the western part of the former USSR but the current situation is uncertain.

The disease is, however, assuming greater importance in developing countries, especially in the tropics. In large organized farms, whether populated by indigenous or imported cattle, prevalence is sometimes high. *B. abortus* biogroup 1 is the organism most commonly isolated from such herds. However, in indigenous cattle kept in small dispersed herds, and in nomadic or semi-nomadic herds, biogroup 3 is most frequently isolated. For reviews see Jansen and Müller (1982), Blajan (1984) and Matyas and Fujikura (1984).

There is a need for definitive information on the prevalence of the disease based on carefully planned surveys that take into account herd size, method of management, use of vaccines, and possible access to wild animal reservoirs of infection.

SOURCES OF INFECTION AND METHOD OF SPREAD

Cattle constitute the main reservoir of *B. abortus*, and animals from infected herds form the commonest source of infection for clean herds. Elk and bison are reported to act as a reservoir in certain regions of the USA.

Clean herds are most commonly infected by the introduction of pregnant, recently aborted, or recently calved animals with brucellosis. Equally dangerous are animals in the incubation stage of the disease which do not yet react to diagnostic tests. Because the incubation period may vary from months to years, it is dangerous to purchase animals that are of unknown origin or have been shown on only one occasion to be serologically negative. The disease can also be introduced via food or water contaminated with discharges, or by spreading contaminated slurry. The practice of sharing veterinary and other equipment, and the movement of vehicles from an infected to a clean farm are potential dangers.

After the work of Bang it was concluded that the disease was venereal, being spread largely during service. There is now extensive epidemiological and experimental evidence that sexual transmission does not readily occur when 'clean' heifers are served by an infected bull. However, the disease can be spread by artificial insemination, particularly when infected semen is deposited directly into the uterus (Bendixen and Blom 1947). Even one animal infected in this way may lead to unsuspected and rapid transmission within a clean herd. If one animal in a herd becomes infected, the other cows and heifers must be regarded as a potential danger to other herds.

Calves may be more resistant to infection than sexually mature and pregnant animals. The tissues of newborn calves from infected dams contain large numbers of viable organisms; this often leads to pneumonitis and the shedding of brucellae in the faeces. It was at one time believed, on epidemiological and experimental evidence, that such calves rid themselves of infection within some months of the cessation of exposure to infected milk and other sources of brucellae. It is now known (Manthei 1950, Plommet et al. 1971, Lapraik et al. 1975, Plommet and Plommet 1975, Crawford, Huber and Sanders 1986) that some calves born to infected dams retain infection into adult life. Such animals often become serologically negative once maternally derived antibodies have disappeared; they remain so until after calving or abortion when they become serologically positive. The extent to which congenitally or neonatally acquired infections persist into adult life is not known. Persistent infection was reported by Crawford, Huber and

Sanders (1986) in 2 of 37 parturient heifers weaned from serologically positive dams. Such latent infections complicate control of the disease because of the long incubation period and negative serological reactions. Heifers that are to be retained in the herd should be tested repeatedly until they calve, to avoid the subsequent appearance of clinical disease.

Ticks, mosquitoes and flies can become carriers and transmit the disease (Tovar 1947, Rementsova 1962). The organism may persist in ticks for many months, and flies feeding on contaminated materials and discharges may transmit infection via the conjunctiva.

ROUTE OF INFECTION

The early work on transmission was based on introducing infective material into the vagina, or into the preputial cavity of bulls that were then used to mate 'clean' heifers soon afterwards (Bang 1897, M'Fadyean and Stockman 1909, Huddleson 1921). Transmission occurred irregularly.

Probably the most common means of infection is by the ingestion of contaminated material, the organisms entering the tissues in the mandibulopharyngeal region and subsequently reaching the local lymph nodes. After multiplying there, they spread to the rest of the body haematogenously.

Experimentally, cattle are readily infected via the conjunctival sac, a route that has been used extensively in vaccine trials (McEwen, Priestley and Paterson 1939, Manthei 1950, Stableforth 1959). With a virulent strain, more than 90% of susceptible cattle can be infected in this way. Brucellae can also penetrate unbroken or abraded skin leading to infection and abortion in pregnant animals (Bang and Bendixen 1932, Cotton, Buck and Smith 1933). Because infected cattle excrete large numbers of brucellae in milk, it has been postulated that transmission to other cattle can occur during milking (Kerr and Rankin 1959, Anderson et al. 1962). Laboratory experiments (Morgan 1968) and field experience (Leech et al. 1964) suggest, however, that this does not occur commonly. Infection may also be caused by the inhalation of contaminated dust particles.

COURSE OF THE DISEASE IN A HERD

The incubation period, defined as the time between exposure to *B. abortus* and either abortion or the appearance of a significant serological response, is very variable; it depends on factors that include the age, the stage of pregnancy and the degree of resistance of the animal (naturally or artificially induced), and the virulence and dose of the infecting strain, as well as the route of infection. Usually a significant serological response is the first detectable evidence of infection but not infrequently abortion occurs some 2–3 weeks earlier. Exposure early in pregnancy or before pregnancy usually results in a protracted incubation period. Thomsen (1937) reported that the incubation period (to abortion) varied inversely with the gestational period that had already elapsed at the time of exposure. The incubation period thus varied from 200 days when exposure occurred in the first month of pregnancy to 60 days when it occurred at 6 months.

When the disease is introduced into a previously uninfected herd, one or a few animals may abort after a varying period. Depending on the stage of gestation of the animals in the rest of the herd and the extent of contamination, further abortions may or may not immediately occur. Sooner or later however, an 'abortion storm' takes place, affecting within a year 50% or more of the pregnant females. Non-pregnant animals are just as vulnerable to infection, the organism becoming localized in various lymph nodes. When such animals become pregnant the placenta and fetus are infected during the periodic bacteraemias that occur, and abortion follows after a long incubation period. Most abortions take place in the fifth to eighth months of pregnancy and most cows abort once only; but some abort a second or even a third time (Manthei and Carter 1950). After abortion and subsequent apparently normal calvings, large numbers of brucellae are shed in the placenta and vaginal discharge and excretion may persist for some weeks, exceptionally for up to 6 months or even 2 years (the longest period reported).

Retention of the placenta commonly follows abortion and may lead to secondary bacterial infection. A catarrhal or purulent endometritis may follow, possibly accompanied by extensive damage to the uterus and fallopian tubes and the formation of adhesions that lead to sterility. Irrespective of whether the placenta is retained, there is often a brownish mucopurulent discharge lasting for 1 or 2 weeks after abortion.

In older animals, especially native cattle in tropical regions, hygromas often develop, mainly on the hind limbs (Thienpont et al. 1961). *B. abortus* biogroup 3 and occasionally biogroup 1 have been isolated from joint fluids.

Some infected animals may abort more than once, but most conceive normally (Baker and Faull 1967). However, Manthei and Carter (1950) and Boyd and Reed (1960) reported some interference with conception. Gestation usually proceeds to, or almost to, full term.

The subsequent abortion history of the herd depends on the method of management; susceptible cows, purchased or reared as replacements, may abort when brought into contact with the main herd. In later years the disease becomes chronic with few abortions occurring except in heifers.

Most infected animals excrete brucellae in the milk. The numbers vary from day to day, but excretion continues throughout all lactations for the lifetime of the animal, the right hind quarter being most frequently responsible (Doyle 1935, Nelson et al. 1966). Brucellae may also be isolated from milk secretions of infected unbred animals (Manthei 1950).

In the bull, acute infections are characterized by epididymitis and orchitis, the testes often becoming enlarged and painful. Later they become smaller because of the contraction of fibrous tissue. Large numbers of organisms are excreted in the semen, especially in the early acute stage.

3.2 Pathogenesis

Brucellae first penetrate the mucosa or skin and are then ingested by various phagocytic cells, a process possibly facilitated by a lectin-like substance on the bacterial surface (Bratescu, Mayer and Teodorescu 1981). Fully virulent brucellae survive and multiply in mononuclear and polymorphonuclear cells and are transported to the draining lymph nodes where they cause hyperplasia and acute inflammation (Payne 1960a). Spread from these nodes occurs via the blood to other lymph nodes and the reticuloendothelial cells. In pregnant animals the placenta and mammary gland are also invaded. During this phase repeated episodes of bacteraemia occur from foci within the reticuloendothelial system.

During haematogenous spread, extracellular organisms are exposed to the normal antibacterial defence mechanisms, which include exposure, before phagocytosis, to specific antibody and to a non-immunoglobulin brucellacidal protein found in normal bovine serum (Macrae and Smith 1964, Smith and Fitzgeorge 1964). After phagocytosis, organisms are exposed to intracellular bactericidal mechanisms, including hydrogen peroxide and superoxide formation and halogenation by the myeloperoxidase–hydrogen peroxide–halide system (Canning, Deyoe and Roth 1988). These bactericidal processes can, however, be suppressed or avoided by virulent strains by the elaboration of virulence factors. Thus the organism persists within the host cells even in the face of high concentrations of circulating antibodies (Smith and Fitzgeorge 1964, Olitzki 1970, Bertram, Canning and Roth 1986).

In infected calves, brucellae are fewer in number, are not so widely disseminated in the body, and elicit less inflammatory response than in pregnant cows (Payne 1960b). In experimentally infected cows, 90% of the organisms are found in fetal cotyledons, chorion and purulent fetal fluids (Smith et al. 1961), a predilection attributed to the presence in these tissues of i-erythritol (Pearce et al. 1962, Williams, Keppie and Smith 1962) which stimulates the growth of *Brucella* both in vitro and in vivo. i-Erythritol is preferentially utilized by *Brucella* (Anderson and Smith 1965) and its parenteral administration to calves and guinea pigs increases the severity of infection. The substance is found in normal and infected placentas of cattle, sheep, goats and pigs and in the seminal vesicles of the male of these species. It is not present in human, rabbit, rat or guinea pig placenta, although these can become infected, with subsequent abortion.

The fulminating placental infection leads to abortion followed by a further heavy bacteraemia and a consequent increase in serum antibody. Brucellae can sometimes be isolated from the placenta of animals that possess no serum antibody; in most such animals antibody titres become detectable within 14 days of abortion. The mechanism of abortion is still unclear.

It is suggested that brucella endotoxin promotes production of fetal cortisol. This depresses progesterone production and increases oestrogen synthesis by the placenta. This hormonal shift is associated with increased prostaglandin 2α production by the endometrium and results in premature expulsion of placenta and fetus (Samartino and Enright 1993).

The organisms are widely disseminated in lymph nodes and other tissues, their persistence and localization being similar in artificially and naturally infected animals (Doyle 1935, Lambert et al. 1961). The udder and supramammary, retropharyngeal and iliac lymph nodes are the most commonly infected sites. The rate of isolation from these sites tends to remain constant for at least 4 years and then declines somewhat but has been known to persist for 11 years (Manthei and Carter 1950). Isolation from the uterus of non-pregnant animals is unusual except in recently calved cattle. Vaginal shedding can persist for up to a month after parturition and occasionally for as long as 2 years (Manthei and Carter 1950). Isolation before calving has been reported infrequently (Fitch, Boyd and Bishop 1938), but Philippon, Renoux and Plommet (1970) isolated *B. abortus* from the vagina of non-pregnant heifers from the 39th day after experimental infection via the conjunctival route, and of 70% of pregnant animals from the 11th day.

The numbers of organisms in the milk vary from a few hundred to 200 000 per ml. The count tends to be highest immediately after calving and then to decline or become intermittent; it becomes more consistent and abundant towards the end of lactation when the milk yield is reduced (Morgan 1968). Bacteraemia is a periodic feature of the disease and is detected most readily soon after exposure. Isolations, albeit intermittent, have been made after a period of 30 months (Fitch, Bishop and Kelley 1936, Fitch, Boyd and Bishop 1938, Manthei 1950).

The pathogenesis in bulls is generally similar to that in the female, but the seminal vesicles and testes are affected, according to Smith et al. (1962) because of the presence of i-erythritol. The numbers of organisms in the semen vary greatly (100–50 000 per ml; Thomsen 1943, Lambert, Manthei and Deyoe 1963) between bulls and between various ejaculates of the same bull, being highest in the early acute phase of the disease. Later, excretion may cease altogether.

Morbid anatomy

In the pregnant cow the disease is essentially a necrotizing placentitis and ulcerative endometritis. The placental cotyledons are swollen, necrotic and covered with a yellowish or brownish sticky exudate which often extends into the depths of the crypts (Bang 1897, M'Fadyean and Stockman 1909). Many cotyledons, however, appear normal; the intercotyledonary placenta and umbilical cord may also be affected, often appearing thickened, opaque and leathery. In the early stage of infection the lymph nodes are enlarged and hyperplastic (Payne 1959, 1960a, 1960b).

Despite the excretion of the large number of organisms in milk, the disease seldom, if ever, causes clinical mastitis but the somatic cell count may be increased (Roguinsky, Fensterbank and Phillippon 1972). The presence of other mammary disease, especially subacute infection with *Staphylococcus aureus*, may mask changes due to *B. abortus*.

In the bull, brucellae become preferentially established in seminal vesicles and testes (Lambert, Manthei and Deyoe 1963). Lesions progress from an acute inflammatory response to areas of chronic interstitial inflammation and necrosis which may coalesce or become surrounded by fibrous tissue (Bendixen and Blom 1948, McCaughey and Purcell 1973).

3.3 Diagnosis

The following factors contribute to the complexity of the diagnosis of bovine brucellosis: absence of clinical signs, other than abortion; the variable incubation period; the high proportion of inapparent infections; the degree of resistance, either natural or resulting from vaccination; the presence of natural or nonspecific agglutinins. Diagnosis should be based upon the disease history of the herd, epidemiological observations, tests for serum antibody and cell mediated immunity, and the demonstration of the causal organism; these must all be considered together (Morgan 1982, Report 1986b).

DEMONSTRATION OF THE CAUSAL ORGANISM

This is the definitive method of diagnosis. Brucellae can be demonstrated in fetal tissues and stomach contents, placental cotyledons, vaginal discharges, colostrum, milk, semen and tissues collected post mortem (especially supramammary, iliac and retropharyngeal lymph nodes, udder, testes and seminal vesicles).

The procedures include cultural examination, animal inoculation and microscopical examination of stained preparations. Detection of brucella DNA either directly or after amplification by the PCR is also feasible (Fekete et al. 1990). Because of the danger of human infection, appropriate safety precautions must be taken when handling potentially infected material.

Selective media have been devised which support the growth even of fastidious strains of *B. abortus*, such as those of biogroup 2, from a small inoculum. Various antimicrobial substances are added to a basal medium of serum dextrose agar (see section on 'Cultural examination', p. 823, and Corbel et al. 1979, Morgan 1982, Report 1986b, Alton et al. 1988). Adequately dried plates should be inoculated with fresh and cleanly collected material. Plates should be examined after 2 or 3 days of incubation at 37°C in an atmosphere containing CO_2 5–10%, preferably in a purpose-built CO_2 incubator. Preliminary identification is based on colonial appearance, examination of gram-stained smears, and serological methods. Subcultures should be made for final identification in a specialized laboratory. A biphasic medium (p. 824) containing agents to inhibit the growth of contaminants gives an improved isolation rate, mainly because a larger inoculum can be used (Corner, Alton and Iyer 1985).

Biological examination can be made by inoculating 2–3 guinea pigs or mice subcutaneously with suitably prepared specimens. When the animals are killed

4–6 weeks later the spleen and lymph nodes are cultured and the serum is tested for antibodies. Material should be examined both culturally and biologically as often only one method gives a positive result. Milk can be used as an alternative (Report 1986a).

Stained smears of fetal stomach contents, cotyledons, milk vaginal mucus and semen may be examined microscopically. Besides being gram-negative, brucellae resist decolorization by weak acids. This property, which is made use of in Koester's modified staining method (Christofferson and Ottosen 1941) and in the modified Ziehl–Neelsen method (Stamp et al. 1950), is also possessed by *Coxiella burnetii* and *Chlamydia* spp. Immunospecific staining by antibody labelled with an enzyme or a fluorescent dye offers few practical advantages over tinctorial staining for routine screening of material (Report 1986b), but sensitive enzyme immunoassays have been developed for the detection of traces of brucella antigen (Perera, Creasy and Winter 1983). The use of PCR for detection of brucella DNA has considerable potential value (Fekete et al. 1990).

SEROLOGICAL EXAMINATIONS

Numerous serological tests are available for demonstrating brucella antibodies in such diverse materials as serum, milk, whey, vaginal mucus, semen and muscle juice. They include agglutination in tubes or on plates, with various antigens and diluents, complement fixation, antiglobulin, fluorescent-antibody, and indirect-haemagglutination or haemolysis tests; and enzyme-labelled and radioimmunoassays. Other variations include the pretreatment of serum with heat or disulphide-bond reducing agents (Morgan 1982). The aim has been to increase sensitivity and specificity in order to detect early and chronic infections and to distinguish antibodies resulting from infection from those produced by vaccination.

When a herd is under investigation, individual animals will be at different stages of infection and of pregnancy and will also differ in their immunity to brucellae, so that no single serological test can be expected to identify every infected animal. The existing battery of tests, properly conducted, standardized and interpreted, has been very successful in many countries in controlling and eradicating the disease. The rules for interpretation must take into account the disease situation nationally as well as the criteria laid down for the movement of animals across national boundaries; tests that do not command international recognition have limited value. Large numbers of samples, often repeated, have to be collected, necessitating close co-operation between farmers, field and laboratory staff, and trained epidemiologists.

Tests on serum

The **SAT**, first introduced by Wright and Smith (1897), has been widely used for diagnosis and for the control of the international movement of animals. If the antigen preparation has been standardized against the International Standard for Anti-*B. abortus* Serum, antibody concentrations can be expressed in International Units per ml rather than as titres, which vary according to the sensitivity of the antigen (Stableforth 1936, Report 1986b).

In Britain the antigen is standardized to give 50% (++) agglutination at a final dilution of 1 in 640 of the International Standard Serum. A 50% (++) agglutination at a 1 in 10 dilution of test serum represents 15.5 IU ml⁻¹; ++ at a 1 in 20 dilution represent 31 IU, and so on. A Working Standard Serum, calibrated against the International Standard, must also be included with each day's batch of tests. In the European Union (EU), animals in 'Officially Brucellosis-Free' herds must pass the serum agglutination test with a result of <30 IU ml⁻¹. In EU 'Brucellosis-Free' herds, allowance is made for the use of vaccines by stating the results of the complement fixation test for sera with antibody concentrations of 30–80 IU ml⁻¹ (EEC Directive No. 71/285 of 19 July 1970 and subsequent amendments). In the USA also, allowance is made for the use of S19 vaccine (Report 1971).

The SAT has numerous disadvantages and is now only recommended when alternative procedures are not available. It is often the last of all available tests to detect diagnostic antibody concentrations in the incubative stages of the disease and after abortion. In the chronic stage, agglutinins have often disappeared whereas other tests remain positive. There are many reports of infected animals that give less than diagnostically significant results in the SAT. For example, Alton, Jones and Pietz (1975) reported that 11% and 4% of culturally positive cattle possessed antibody concentrations of <100 and <30 IU respectively. The test also detects non-specific agglutinins and cross-reacting antibodies. The former may include immunoglobulins of the bovine IgM and IgG1, but not the IgG2 or IgA isotypes (Nielsen et al. 1981). These bind to a receptor on the brucella cell surface through their Fc region; this interaction can be blocked by ethylenediaminetetraacetic acid (EDTA) or structurally similar compounds (Nielsen and Duncan 1982). Performance of the SAT in a diluent containing 1 mM EDTA will eliminate such reactions (MacMillan and Cockrem 1985). Heat- and acid-labile agglutinating activity has been associated with poorly defined heat- and acid-labile serum components (macroglobulins and microglobulins; Hess and Roepke 1951, Rose, Roepke and Briggs 1964, see also review by Corbel 1985a). Cross-reacting antibodies are produced in response to bacteria with perosamine in the cell wall (Bundle et al. 1987). *E. coli* O:157, a cause of mastitis, is probably the most frequently identified cause of cross-reactions in cattle sera. *Salmonella* strains of Kauffmann–White group N, *S. maltophilia* and *Y. enterocolitica* O:9 are also potential causes of false positive reactions (see p. 825; also Corbel, Stuart and Brewer 1984, Corbel 1985a). Supplementary procedures (the heat treatment of serum, and the use of disulphide-bond reducing agents, ethacridine lactate and acidified antigens) have been used to improve the specificity and sensitivity of the agglutination test.

The **rose bengal** (or Card or Buffered Brucella Antigen) **plate (RBP) test** was initially introduced in the USA when agglutinins produced as a result of vaccination were found to be more acid-labile than those arising from field infection. The test has been evaluated and used in many countries (Morgan 1982). The antigen is stained with rose bengal dye and suspended in buffer at pH 3.65. At this pH the activity of IgM is much reduced and most of the activity in this test, as in the complement fixation test (Corbel 1972) is mediated through the IgG1 isotype. The test was officially introduced in Britain in 1970 as a screening test for sera, those giving positive reactions being further subjected to the agglutination and complement fixation tests (Morgan and Richards 1974). The test is believed to be oversensitive, especially when vaccination has been widely used. An automated system capable of testing 1200 samples per hour has been used in Britain (Gower et al. 1974).

The **complement fixation (CF) test** was long regarded as the most specific and sensitive of the routine tests. However, comparable or even greater sensitivity and specificity can now be achieved with enzyme immunoassay. When the vaccination status of the animals is known the CF test is of great value in distinguishing between reactions caused by vaccination and infection (Rice et al. 1952, Bürki 1963). In calves vaccinated with *B. abortus* strain 19 when 90–120 days old, agglutinin titres reach their maximum after 2–3 weeks and usually decline to 'pass' concentrations (<100 IU ml⁻¹) by 18 months of age. The CF test becomes 'negative' (<14 International CF Units) much earlier, usually within 6 months of vaccination. In adult animals exposed to infection the CF test becomes positive at the same time as, or slightly before, the agglutination test. As the disease progresses, agglutinins decline or even disappear, but complement-fixing antibodies persist at diagnostic concentrations, the test rarely becoming negative. The CF test is mediated through the IgG1 isotype, any IgM activity being lost during the preliminary heat treatment of the serum. The test is useful in both early and chronic disease and in identifying vaccinal reactions when the date of vaccination is known.

As a result of an international collaborative assay (Morgan, Davidson and Hebert 1973) the WHO Expert Committee on Biological Standardization concluded that the Second International Standard Serum was suitable for standardizing the CF test and assigned to each millilitre 1000 IU of complement-fixing activity (and 1000 IU of agglutinating activity). In the EU the German National Standard Serum has been adopted for both the agglutination and CF tests. Its activity was defined as 1000 EEC complement-fixing units per ampoule (Davidson and Hebert 1978).

In Europe the CF test has been used extensively, the antigen being standardized to give 50% fixation of complement at a dilution of 1 in 200 of the Second International Standard Serum. In non-vaccinated animals antibody concentrations of ≤10 icftu ml⁻¹ are accepted as a 'pass' and ≥20 icftu ml⁻¹ as a 'fail'; animals with concentrations of between 10 and 20 icftu ml⁻¹ are retested.

The **antiglobulin test** for non-agglutinating antibodies was used as an adjunct to the SAT and CF tests. It was useful in the early stages of the disease but not in vaccinated herds because reactions due to vaccination persist for many years. The method was recommended by Cunningham and O'Connor (1971) and Nicoletti (1977) in the form of the so-called anamnestic test, in which the serum was examined immediately before and 6 weeks after an injection of 45/20 adjuvant vaccine (p. 834). The anamnestic test has been used successfully on range cattle in Australia.

An **indirect haemolysis test** (Plackett, Cottew and Best 1976) with erythrocytes sensitized by alkali-activated LPS antigen was devised to overcome the prozone phenomenon that occurs in the CF tests as a result of blocking by IgG2 isotype (Plackett and Alton 1975). This and the antiglobulin test are now rarely used.

A **CF test** with a rough antigen was devised by Miller, Kelly and Roerink (1976) to identify animals vaccinated with the 45/20 adjuvant vaccine. Corbel and Bracewell (1976) concluded that it could not be relied upon to exclude infected animals.

ELISAs have been adopted for routine testing of bovine sera in Canada in place of the CF test (Nielsen et al. 1992) and evaluated extensively in the USA, Australia and the UK (Heck et al. 1984, Sutherland, Evans and Bathgate 1986, MacMillan et al. 1990). These tests can be at least as sensitive and specific as the CF test and are readily modified to detect specific immunoglobulin isotypes to a range of different antigens. These assays, which detect antibodies that persist for long periods after vaccination, are at their maximum value towards the end of an eradication programme (Hornitzky and Pearson 1986). Similarly, radioimmunoassays for measuring IgG1 and IgG2 (but not IgM) isotypes have been used for distinguishing infected from vaccinated animals (Chappell et al. 1976).

Milk tests

Because milk and whey samples are easily obtained, they have been widely used for testing herds or individual animals for antibody. The major immunoglobulin isotypes in serum are also present in milk. Concentrations of IgG1 are high in mammary secretion during the colostral phase, at which time its concentration in serum falls.

The **milk ring test (MRT)**, first described in Germany by Fleischhauer (1937), is routinely used as a periodic test for brucellosis-free herds and in identifying infected herds. In Britain, samples (churn or bulk tank) from all milking animals on farms that sell milk commercially are tested monthly. One drop (0.03 ml) of stained brucella antigen, standardized against the International Standard Serum, is added to 1 ml of whole milk that has been kept refrigerated overnight after collection; tests are read after incubation for 1 h at 37°C. A positive reaction is indicated by a stained cream layer over a white column of milk. Freshly collected milk should not be used and excessive shaking or heating adversely affects the test. As a herd test it has the disadvantage that non-lactating animals such as heifers and dry cows are necessarily excluded. Lauwers (1966) found that 86.8% of herds that gave

3 positive MRTs at intervals of 1 month contained reactors; but 97% of those that gave 3 negative results contained none. With the increasing size of dairy herds and the use of bulk tanks, doubt has been expressed as to whether the MRT would remain sufficiently sensitive; accordingly it has been proposed that the size of the milk sample should be increased to 2 or 3 ml but that the volume of antigen should remain unchanged at 0.03 ml (Pietz 1977). In herds from which brucellosis had been eradicated during the national campaign in Britain, the monthly MRT was found to give the first indication of infection (Morgan 1977).

The MRT can be used on milk from individual animals, but the results, which may be influenced by mastitis or by recent vaccination with strain 19, are not always reliable. It is essential to use a sample of milk obtained from all 4 quarters of the udder. The stronger the MRT reaction the more likely that brucellae can be isolated on culture (Leech et al. 1964).

The **milk ring dilution test**, in which the milk to be examined is diluted in MRT-negative milk, can be used for individual animals. Reactions at dilutions 1 in 10 or greater are likely to be due to infection. Milk and whey can also be subjected to tube agglutination and complement fixation tests as well as to enzyme immunoassays (Forschner and Bunger 1986). Recent studies suggest that the latter are more effective than the MRT for the examination of bulk tank samples. The specificity of both tests was about 99% but the ELISA detected the entry of brucellosis into a herd from 15 days to 6 months before the MRT (Botton et al. 1990).

An **intradermal test** for delayed hypersensitivity, with a refined protein antigen (Brucellin INRA; Fensterbank 1984), is affected by recent vaccination and is probably useful only as a herd test. MacDiarmid (1988) concluded, however, that despite its low sensitivity the test would be more effective than either the CF test or slaughterhouse examination for routine surveillance of beef herds. An in vitro assay of cell mediated immunity based on production of IFN-γ appears to offer a rapid and convenient alternative to intradermal testing (Weynants et al. 1995). It is also reported to differentiate animals responding serologically to cross-reacting antigens from those infected with *Brucella*.

3.4 Prevention and control

No reliable cure for bovine brucellosis has yet been devised. Tetracycline alone (Fensterbank 1976) or in combination with streptomycin (Nicoletti et al. 1985) or delivered in liposomes may modify the course of the disease. Effective control, however, must depend on minimizing by sanitary methods the factors responsible for spread of the disease, and on vaccination.

Prevention of transmission within the herd must include: the identification and slaughter of known infected animals; the isolation of all animals that have recently calved or aborted, or are about to abort; the cleansing and disinfection of the quarantine area before other animals are reintroduced; the safe disposal of all products of abortion, including fetuses, by deep burial under a covering of lime; the purchase of herd replacement from disease-free sources; and the isolation of pregnant replacement animals until they have calved and passed a serological test.

The prevention of transmission to contiguous herds necessitates the restriction of movement of animals and the quarantine of all purchased animals, especially those pregnant and those that have recently calved. All abortions must be reported to the appropriate authority for investigation.

Prevention and control are therefore best conducted on an area or country basis. National campaigns are accompanied by effective information and advice to farmers and veterinary surgeons; by the use of national rules governing diagnosis, vaccination, surveillance, and the movement of animals; and by the compulsory slaughter of infected and in-contact animals, with compensation.

Where the prevalence of brucellosis is high, the widespread use of a licensed vaccine, together with general control measures (above) aimed at preventing transmission, is likely to be highly effective and to reduce the prevalence to a level at which eradication by test and slaughter can be embarked upon.

Strain 19 vaccine (Buck 1930) is widely used in cattle. It is a living vaccine prepared from a smooth-intermediate attenuated strain of *B. abortus*. Its attenuated virulence is stable even after repeated passages in vivo. When properly manufactured from recognized seed material (Report 1986b, Alton et al. 1988) it completely protects 65–75% of animals, the remainder being partly protected. In the USA, it was shown that strain 19 persisted in only 2 in 100 000 vaccinated calves, and there was no evidence of spread to in-contact animals (Jones and Berman 1976). When used in pregnant animals it may cause abortion. Use of the vaccine was shown by Bracewell and Corbel (1980) to be associated with an arthropathy in a small percentage of animals, usually affecting one or both femorotibial joints. The arthropathy is reported to result from immune complex formation (Corbel et al. 1989a, 1989b). One dose of vaccine given in calfhood protects animals for at least 5 pregnancies (Manthei, Mingle and Carter 1951), and revaccination is not necessary.

A programme in which at least 70% of eligible animals are vaccinated over a number of years is more likely to be successful than erratic or low use of vaccine (Jones and Berman 1976). A small dose [(3 × 10^8)–(3 × 10^9) organisms] of S19 vaccine produces, with fewer serological complications, an immunity as good as that given by the standard dose (8 × 10^{10}). Vaccination via the conjunctival sac also produces a satisfactory immunity with little or no detectable serological response (Plommet and Plommet 1975).

B. abortus 45/20 vaccine, which contains killed organisms and adjuvant (Roerink 1967) is prepared from a rough strain (McEwen 1940). There are conflicting reports of its efficacy, but when prepared from reliable seed material, 2 doses given 6–8 weeks apart provide protection comparable with that given by

strain 19 (Ray 1976). Its use is not advocated for calves under 6 months of age. Care should be taken to ensure freedom from smooth LPS antigen. The use of this vaccine has declined in recent years and it is no longer recommended. Attempts have been made to develop alternatives that produce effective immunity without seroconversion in diagnostic tests. One such vaccine is a live preparation of *B. abortus* strain RB51. This is derived from a rough mutant of a rifampicin-resistant strain which does not synthesize the LPS O chain. Extensive studies have been conducted in laboratory animals and cattle. These have confirmed its genetic stability, low residual virulence and lack of agglutinogenicity. Initial studies on protection in cattle have been promising (Tobias, Schurig and Cordes 1992, Cheville et al. 1993). The vaccine is now officially approved for use in the USA.

For further information on control and eradication, see Hugh-Jones, Ellis and Felton (1975), Morgan (1982) and Report (1986b). Other causes of abortion in cattle include *Leptospira*, *Salmonella*, *Campylobacter*, fungi, *Chlamydia* and certain viruses (see Laing, Morgan and Wagner 1988).

4 BRUCELLA INFECTIONS OF SHEEP AND GOATS

The disease in sheep and goats has been closely connected with the disease in humans ever since the work of Zammit (1905) and Horrocks (1905) established that goats could act as carriers of the organism isolated by Bruce from a fatal human case. The economic importance of the disease lies in abortion and reduced milk yield and, in humans, in the serious illness that it causes through contact with infected animals or their products.

Brucellosis occurs widely in sheep and goats, especially in the Mediterranean area, the Middle East, and parts of the former Soviet Union, Republic of Mongolia and .China. It also occurs in Central and South America but not in Australia, New Zealand or northern Europe (Jansen and Müller 1982, Matyas and Fujikura 1984). It also occurs in Africa but to an unknown extent.

4.1 Epidemiology

The disease is almost invariably caused by a member of one of the 3 biogroups of *B. melitensis*. Geographical, epidemiological and pathological differences are not specifically related to any biogroup. Sporadic ovine and caprine infections with *B. abortus* may occur through contact with infected cattle (Allsup 1969); such infections do not appear to spread, but exceptions have been reported in the USA (Luchsinger and Anderson 1979). Sheep and goats are susceptible to artificial infection with *B. abortus*, the clinical and pathological features being similar to those in cattle (Molello et al. 1963, Anderson, Meador and Cheville 1986). Infection caused by *B. suis* has also been reported (Paolicchi, Terzolo and Campero 1993).

According to Alton (1985) all breeds of goat are highly susceptible to *B. melitensis*, whereas different breeds of sheep vary greatly, the fat-tailed Awasi and Kurdi breeds being the most susceptible.

SOURCE OF INFECTION AND METHOD OF SPREAD

Sheep and goats form the most important reservoir of infection, and spread between flocks or countries is closely related to the movement of infected animals. The practice of allowing sheep and goats from different flocks to graze together during the day and penning them together at night favours the spread of the disease and makes control and eradication difficult. Indirect spread through contaminated food, water and equipment also occurs.

Infection usually enters via the nasopharynx, after the ingestion of contaminated material or as a result of inhaling contaminated dust. Experimentally, animals can be readily infected via the conjunctival sac, a method widely used for the reproduction of the disease in vaccine evaluation trials (Elberg 1981). When pregnant or non-pregnant goats were placed in contact with aborting donors, 85–89% of them became infected (Alton 1985). Similar results in fat-tailed sheep were reported by Jones, Entessar and Ardalan (1964). Infection in male animals produces orchitis and epididymitis, but venereal spread is believed to be uncommon. Pathogenesis closely resembles that in cattle (p. 830). Penetration of the mucosa or skin is followed by multiplication within macrophages of the regional lymph nodes, bacteraemia and invasion of the placenta and fetus in pregnant animals. Abortion usually occurs in the last 2 months of pregnancy but less frequently than in cattle. In sheep, abortion rates may be as low as 5–15%. When abortion has occurred subsequent parturitions are associated with heavily infected vaginal discharges that persist for 2–3 months in goats and for a somewhat shorter period in sheep (Entessar et al. 1967), but recurrent abortion in individual animals occurs less commonly than in cattle.

Infection leads to colonization of the udder and its associated lymph nodes, with massive excretion in the milk. In sheep and goats secretion of the organism in the milk often ceases and the animals appear to recover completely; in other cases the disease becomes chronic and persists for years.

In non-pregnant animals the organism persists in the cells of the reticuloendothelial system. Viable kids born of infected dams may already be infected at the time of birth. Generally, however, they lose such infections within a few months. It is not known whether kids or lambs that acquire infection at or shortly after birth retain it into adult life.

The pathological changes are similar to those in cattle with *B. abortus* infection, viz. necrotizing placentitis and ulcerative endometritis in the female, and focal inflammation of the testes and seminal vesicles in the male (see Hellmann 1982).

4.2 Diagnosis

The methods used are similar to those for bovine brucellosis, but there are added difficulties:

1. in some animals the infection disappears but in others it becomes chronic and difficult to demonstrate serologically
2. some vaccines induce persistent antibodies and
3. individual animals, and hence their vaccination status, are difficult to identify.

The organism can be isolated from products of abortion, vaginal discharges and milk, and from tissues (especially the udder and lymph nodes) obtained post mortem. Isolates of *B. melitensis* from goats' milk and from supramammary lymph nodes, but not from other tissues, are often in the rough phase on primary isolation (Alton 1960). The bacteriological procedures have been described by Corbel (1985b). Selective media applicable to the isolation of *B. abortus* are suitable although the medium of Brown, Ranger and Kelley (1971) may be more sensitive. The staining techniques described earlier are applicable. Negative cultural results obtained from tissues and fluids collected from the living animal are often not supported by the examination of material collected post mortem. Methods based on detection of brucella DNA have potential for the diagnosis of *B. melitensis* infection but require validation.

Serological tests are based on those developed for cattle. The serum agglutination test, with 5% saline as diluent in order to avoid the prozone phenomenon, has a low specificity and sensitivity and is also seriously affected by the use of vaccines. The antiglobulin test was found to be positive in 70% of infected animals (Ünel, Williams and Stableforth 1969). The complement fixation test with sera inactivated at 62°C for 30 min is also valuable, particularly where vaccination of young animals is practised (Alton 1990); complement-fixing titres produced by vaccination in lambs and kids decline much more rapidly than those produced by infection. The rose bengal test, preferably with an antigen preparation consisting of bacterial cells 5% in buffer, is useful (Trap and Gaumont 1976) in selecting sera to be examined further by the agglutination, complement fixation and antiglobulin tests (Farina 1985); a proportion of culturally positive animals, however, give a negative result. Recent studies suggest that enzyme immunoassay is superior to all of these tests in specificity and sensitivity (Blasco et al. 1994).

Samples of milk, which are readily obtained from flock or milk-collecting depots, may be examined by the MRT but agglutinates appear either as a coloured ring in the cream layer or as a deposit at the bottom of the tube.

The **intradermal test for delayed hypersensitivity** is a reliable flock test where vaccination is not practised. 'Brucellin fraction F' or 'Brucellin INRA' may be used (Report 1986b). The INRA brucellin, a protein-rich LPS free allergen prepared from rough *B. melitensis* (Jones, Diaz and Taylor 1973), has been widely evaluated in France (Fensterbank 1985). In sheep a dose of 50 μg in 0.5 ml is injected into the lower eyelid and the results are read by comparison with the uninoculated eyelid 48 h later. In goats the skin of the neck can be used. The test detects some infected but serologically negative animals and positive reactions are also produced in some uninfected but vaccinated animals.

4.3 Prevention and control

The choice of method depends on the prevalence of infection and the resources available. In areas of low prevalence the best method is to slaughter whole flocks, with compensation, and to repopulate with animals from brucellosis-free flocks after disinfection and cleansing (Hellman 1982). Where the prevalence in sheep and goats is high, control must be based on the use of sanitary measures to reduce exposure, and on vaccination to increase resistance, the objective being to reduce the prevalence to a point at which eradication by test and slaughter is feasible.

Strain 19 vaccine, though valuable in cattle, has given disappointing results in sheep and goats. The living Rev 1 vaccine (Elberg 1981) is the vaccine of choice. Its attenuated virulence is stable, but abortion may occur if the vaccine is given to pregnant animals, and the organisms may be excreted in the milk. Rev 1, being a smooth strain, gives rise to antibodies indistinguishable from those arising from field infection. Consequently its use is recommended at a standard dose of 10^9 cells in lambs and kids aged 3–6 months. When used in this way, antibodies, especially those detected by the CF test, disappear after about a year. The resulting immunity is virtually lifelong. Field experience of the vaccine is often difficult to evaluate (Alton 1990) but it has led to a dramatic fall in the number of human cases of brucellosis. To reduce interference with the interpretation of serological tests, the dose of vaccine can be reduced to 5×10^4 cells, or the conjunctival route can be used (Fensterbank 1985). The vaccine must be prepared from reliable seed material and subjected to safety and potency tests (Report 1986b).

In China, vaccine prepared from *B. suis* strain 2 and given orally has reduced the prevalence of ovine and caprine brucellosis (Xie 1986). However, in an experimental study, strain 2 was much less effective than Rev 1 in protecting pregnant ewes against a virulent *B. melitensis* challenge (Verger et al. 1995). In a field trial in Libya, strain 2 vaccine was safer but gave only 53% protection in sheep and 71% protection in goats (Mustafa and Abusowa 1993). It was ineffective in protecting rams against *B. ovis* infection (Blasco et al. 1993).

For major reviews of *B. melitensis* see Hellmann (1982), Verger and Plommet (1985), Report (1986b) and Alton (1990). Other causes of abortion in sheep or goats include *Campylobacter*, *Salmonella*, *Listeria*, *Toxoplasma* and *Chlamydia* spp. (Laing, Morgan and Wagner 1988).

4.4 Ram epididymitis caused by *Brucella ovis*

An acute infectious disease characterized by epididymitis and reduced fertility in rams was described in New Zealand by Buddle and Boyes (1953) and in Australia by Simmons and Hall (1953). It has since been reported in the USA, South Africa, France, Germany, Spain, Eastern Europe, parts of South America, and elsewhere. The causal organism, *B. ovis*, differs in many characters from the other 'species' of *Brucella* (see Volume 2, Chapter 35), being in the non-smooth (rough) phase even on primary isolation (Meyer 1982). The disease differs in many respects from that caused in sheep by *B. melitensis*. Rams are much more susceptible than ewes and are responsible for maintaining the disease. Experimentally, rams can be infected by the conjunctival, preputial, intranasal and rectal routes; under natural conditions rams are infected by mating and by contact with infected ewes or rams (Plant, Eamens and Seaman 1986). Infection is followed by a bacteraemic phase resulting in infection of the spleen, kidney (with excretion in the urine), lymph nodes and genital organs, especially the seminal vesicles, ampullae, testes and tail of the epididymis.

In ewes, infection may spread to the placenta and cause abortion, usually in the third month of pregnancy; more commonly, however, the placentitis interferes with fetal nutrition, leading to the birth of abnormally small lambs and consequent losses. In infected flocks, lamb yields sometimes drop from 100 to 25%. Up to 15% of lambs born alive die within the first 6 weeks of life and 20% of the ewes may remain barren (Snowdon 1958).

Transmission between ewes is rare and ewes play little part in maintaining the disease. In rams, infection results in striking changes in semen quality, including reduced sperm output and motility (Afzal 1985). There is also a striking IgA response in the accessory sex glands, especially in the ampullae (Foster et al. 1988).

The organism can be isolated on selective media from semen, products of abortion, and milk (Lee, Cargill and Atkinson 1985). It can also be demonstrated microscopically in semen by tinctorial or fluorescent-antibody staining methods. Serological methods in which *B. ovis* is used as the antigen preparation include the agglutination, antiglobulin, complement fixation, gel-diffusion and passive haemagglutination tests, and enzyme immunoassays (Corbel, Redwood and Gill 1979, Lee, Cargill and Atkinson 1985). The complement fixation test with soluble antigen and cold fixation is one of the more specific and sensitive tests but gives some false negative and false positive results (Plant, Eamens and Seaman 1986). In experimentally infected rams, Corbel and Lander (1982) found the antiglobulin test with *B. ovis* antigen to be the most sensitive serological method. Ficapal et al. (1995) concluded that the enzyme immunoassay was not more sensitive or more specific than the complement fixation test. However, it is more convenient to use.

CONTROL AND ERADICATION

Control is based on immunization or on the test and slaughter of infected rams; stud rams should be purchased only from accredited sources. The Rev 1 live vaccine and a vaccine consisting of killed *B. ovis* cells incorporated in adjuvant give good protection and have been widely used in New Zealand. The use of either vaccine interferes with the interpretation of serological tests. Subcellular vaccines based on hot saline extracts have demonstrated efficacy in a mouse model of *B. ovis* infection, especially when combined with a saponin adjuvant. Interestingly, antibodies contributed more to protection than cell mediated responses (Jiménez de Bagués et al. 1994). For further information see Meyer (1982) and Blasco (1990).

5 *BRUCELLA* INFECTIONS OF PIGS

The disease in pigs, which is invariably caused by members of biogroups 1, 2 or 3 of *B. suis*, is characterized in the female by abortion, stillbirth and the production of weak offspring, and in the male by orchitis and infertility. The disease caused by *B. suis* biogroup 1 was first described by Traum (1914) in the USA and has since been found in Central and South America, southern China and in feral pigs in Australia. *B. suis* biogroup 3 occurs mainly in North America and South East Asia, and biogroup 2 in Europe, where infection is maintained in the wild hare (*Lepus europaeus*) (Hellmann 1982, Report 1986b). The disease does not exist in Britain. Members of biogroups 1 and 3 produce infections of similar severity (Deyoe 1967, 1968). Biogroup 2 strains sometimes cause miliary lesions in the genital tract (Thomsen 1934). Where it occurs, the disease, causing abortion in the female and infertility and impotence in the male, is of considerable economic importance. In some countries the importation and overcrowding of highly susceptible breeding stock has led to severe outbreaks (Report 1986b). The organism causes a serious disease in humans.

The disease is most commonly introduced into a clean herd by an infected boar; large numbers of organisms are excreted in the semen, and the disease is easily transmitted to the female by natural service or by artificial insemination. Infected carrier sows may also introduce the disease. Up to 10% of young pigs may become infected by contact with the dam or ingestion of infected milk; such animals, of both sexes, retain infection until they become sexually mature. The disease can also be introduced via contaminated bedding and food, and by transient contact with other infected animals, for example at shows (Deyoe and Manthei 1976). Transmission to domestic pigs from hares has been reported in Denmark (Bendtsen 1960) and Germany (Fenske and Pulst 1973, Dedek 1983). Feral pigs may also transmit infection.

5.1 Pathogenesis and course of the disease in the herd

Pigs of all ages and of both sexes are susceptible to infection, which is usually acquired by ingestion or venereally. Multiplication in the lymph nodes is followed by a bacteraemia (Hutchings 1950, Deyoe 1967) and localization in other lymph nodes, genital organs, mammary glands, bones, joints, kidneys and brain. Some animals, particularly young stock, may recover spontaneously. Abscesses occur frequently, particularly in bones and joints. Osteomyelitis and discospondylitis may result in hind limb lameness or paralysis.

In the boar, lesions are found in the testes, particularly in the epididymides and seminal vesicles. They consist of foci of caseous or liquefactive necrosis surrounded by accumulations of epithelial cells, lymphocytes and macrophages, and by a fibrous capsule (Jubb, Kennedy and Palmer 1985). Fertility is often reduced and the animals may become impotent.

In sexually mature females the consequences of infection depend on the stage of gestation at the time of exposure. Infection acquired from the boar at mating does not interfere with fertilization or implantation but results in abortion from about the third week of pregnancy. In such circumstances the first indication of infection in a herd is given by sows that return to oestrus some 5–8 weeks after service. Not all sows served by an infected boar become infected (Deyoe and Manthei 1976).

Exposure during early pregnancy often results in abortion after about 33 days; when exposure occurs late in pregnancy the dam may give birth to a normal full-term litter or to a litter containing a mixture of mummified fetuses and stillborn or weak piglets. Late abortions are accompanied by a copious sanguineous or purulent vaginal discharge. Endometritis is a characteristic feature, especially after infection with *B. suis* biogroup 2, resulting in the so-called 'miliary brucellosis'. Sows mated soon after abortion may fail to breed, but those given a period of sexual rest usually conceive and carry their litter to full term. In a small proportion of infected sows, however, the disease persists indefinitely, providing a reservoir of infection. Non-pregnant animals are equally susceptible to infection, which produces a subacute or chronic endometritis and salpingitis (Deyoe 1967). In small herds, after the initial returns to service and the abortions, the disease becomes self-limiting, but in larger herds it becomes endemic and symptoms appear in newly introduced animals.

5.2 Diagnosis

A herd history of reproductive inefficiency must be supported by isolating *B. suis* from the products of abortion, vaginal discharges, milk, semen and material collected post mortem. Care is required because human infection can be serious and debilitating. The selective media described for *B. abortus* are suitable for *B. suis*, and isolates should be sent to a specialist laboratory for confirmation of identification. Material may also be injected into guinea pigs or mice or examined microscopically.

Serological tests, although widely used, present particular problems, partly because non-specific and cross-reacting antibodies occur frequently in pig sera. No single test will detect all infected animals; many false positive reactions occur, especially in the serum-agglutination test. The rose bengal test is favoured for screening large numbers of sera. The complement fixation test, which is also widely used, gives closely similar results (Deyoe and Manthei 1976). The intradermal test for delayed hypersensitivity, based on the use of a protein extract (Bhongbhibhat, Elberg and Chen 1970), is an accurate method for individual animals and herds. Enzyme immunoassay has received limited evaluation but appears promising.

5.3 Prevention and control

There is no effective vaccine for pigs. The *B. suis* strain 2 vaccine, studied in China, protects pigs infected by most routes but not by natural service (Xie 1986).

Test and slaughter, the only effective measures, have been used successfully in Denmark and the former Czechoslovakia; in the USA the reactor rate has been reduced to 0.03%, the majority of the nation's pigs now being found in states that are 'validated brucellosis-free' (Nelson, Huber and Essey 1986). Strategies include the slaughter of the whole herd followed by repopulation with 'clean' animals after disinfection and cleansing; the slaughter of adult pigs and retention of recently weaned animals for repopulation; and serological testing, removal of reactors, and retesting until all animals are serologically negative (Report 1986b). Facilities for isolating sows at parturition and for isolating purchased animals are essential. The use of 'communal' boars must be avoided and all animals with signs of reproductive disease must be removed.

Pigs can be experimentally infected with *B. abortus*, but the disease is self-limiting (Stuart, Corbel and Brewer 1987). Other causes of reproductive disorders in pigs have been reviewed by Wrathall (1975), Hellmann (1982) and Laing, Morgan and Wagner (1988).

6 *BRUCELLA* INFECTIONS OF DOGS

Infections caused by *B. abortus*, *melitensis* and *suis* have been known in dogs and wild Canidae for many years, abortion in pregnant animals being a prominent feature in addition to a variety of other clinical signs. Transmission to other animals, including humans, occurs only rarely. However, Canidae sometimes play a mechanical role in transmission by carrying infected fetuses and placentas across farm boundaries.

In 1966, Carmichael isolated an organism, subsequently named *B. canis*, from cases of abortion in beagles in the USA (Carmichael and Bruner 1968). The disease, which can occur in any breed, has since been described in stray and domestic dogs in many parts of the world (see Weber 1982) but not in Britain, Australia or New Zealand.

Clinical manifestations of *B. canis* infection vary greatly, and inapparent infections are not uncommon. The main signs are abortion (usually after 45–55 days of gestation), early embryonic death, and epididymitis with scrotal dermatitis; infertility occurs in both males and females. Many organisms are shed in the placenta and vaginal discharges. The organisms are present in the semen in large numbers for 1–2 months after initial infection, and then intermittently for over a year.

Infection results from ingestion or venereal transmission. There is a bacteraemia that may last for 5 years or longer, with a local or generalized lymphadenopathy (Carmichael, Zoha and Flores-Castro 1984a, 1984b); discospondylitis of the lumbar vertebrae and recurrent uveitis have also been reported (Henderson et al. 1974). Infected dogs usually lose their bacteraemia after about a year, but the organism may persist in lymphatic tissue and the male genital organs; during this phase serological titres wane.

In infected male dogs an immune response against spermatozoal antigens develops. Most animals show intense phagocytosis of sperm heads and head-to-head agglutination of sperm; antibodies that agglutinate normal canine spermatozoa are found both in serum and seminal plasma (George and Carmichael 1984). Male infertility is mediated by isoimmune reactions resulting from increased non-specific phagocytic activity of inflammatory cells attached to sites of brucella growth in the epididymis (Carmichael and George 1976, Serikawa et al. 1984).

6.1 Diagnosis

Abortion, early embryonic loss, failure to conceive and, in the male, infertility suggest *B. suis* infection but this diagnosis must be supported by the isolation of *B. canis* from the placenta, fetuses, vaginal discharges or semen, especially in the early stage of the disease. Because of the prolonged bacteraemia, blood cultures are often successful during the first 2 years of infection (Carmichael, Zoha and Flores-Castro 1984a).

In serological tests either *B. canis* or *B. ovis* may be used as the antigen. A tube-agglutination test and a plate test with rose bengal antigen buffered at pH 7 have been widely used (Carmichael and George 1976). The results are negative in the early and in the late chronic stages of the disease; positive results must be confirmed by isolating the organism. Canine sera contain non-specific and cross-reacting antibodies, and improvements in specificity have been obtained by pretreating with 0.2 M mercaptoethanol (Badakhsh, Carmichael and Douglas 1982). The use of antigen in buffer at pH 8.9 reduces the adverse effects produced by non-specific agglutinins and haemolysed erythrocytes (Report 1986b). These difficulties may also be overcome by the use of enzyme immunoassay with purified antigens (Serikawa et al. 1989). The use of non-mucoid *B. canis* strains for antigen preparation further improves specificity (Mateu-de-Antonio, Martin and Soler 1993).

6.2 Control

There is no satisfactory vaccine (Carmichael, Zoha and Flores-Castro 1984b) and treatment with minocycline combined with streptomycin is not always successful. Control in breeding kennels depends on strict sanitary procedures, serological testing, culture and the removal of infected animals.

There are a number of recorded cases of transmission of infection to humans from dogs, and serological evidence of infection is not uncommon. The manifestations of the disease in humans are mentioned earlier in this chapter. For further reviews see Weber (1982) and Laing, Morgan and Wagner (1988).

7 *BRUCELLA* INFECTIONS OF OTHER ANIMAL SPECIES

7.1 Horses

Horses, which are generally considered to be relatively resistant to brucella infection, invariably become infected by contact with infected animals of other species, usually cattle. Infected horses have on rare occasions been implicated as a source of infection for cattle (White and Swett 1935). Infections are usually caused by biogroups of *B. abortus* and less frequently by *B. melitensis* and *B. suis* (McNutt and Murray 1924). Cook and Kingston (1988) described a case of *B. suis* infection in a horse in Australia, believed to have been caused by contact with feral pigs.

Many horses with high titres of antibody show no symptoms; in other cases, infection becomes generalized, causing stiffness, lethargy and fever. The organism has a predilection for the bursae, tendons, joints and muscles; 'fistulous withers' (suppurative spinous bursitis) and 'poll evil' (suppurative atlantal bursitis) are common clinical features (Fitch, Delez and Boyd 1930) and the organism can be readily isolated from the bursal fluid (Denny 1972, 1973). Infection may occasionally cause abortion. The disease is commoner in country than in town horses. Experimentally, horses can be infected by mouth or by parenteral routes, but it has proved difficult to reproduce 'fistulous withers' and 'poll evil'. In the work reported by MacMillan et al. (1982) and MacMillan and Cockrem (1986), infected mares produced normal foals at full term and *B. abortus* could not be isolated from the products of parturition; spread to in-contact susceptible cattle did not occur.

Diagnosis is based on the isolation of the organism from local lesions or on serological test, including the agglutination, antiglobulin, complement fixation and rose bengal plate tests. Non-specific agglutinins are common in horse sera and the serum-agglutination test gives equivocal results. The antiglobulin test is the most sensitive, especially in the chronic stage of infection (McCaughey and Kerr 1967). Strain 19 vaccine injected into infected horses results in a febrile reaction within 12 h with patchy sweating, and raised pulse and respiratory rates. Severe inflammation occurs at the site of injection after 24–48 h, gradually resolving by 96 h.

Killed *B. abortus* vaccine has been used therapeutically, especially for fistulous withers and poll evil; 2 or 3 injections of 10 ml are given subcutaneously at intervals of 10 days. Surgical intervention, together with a 3 week course of treatment with antimicrobial agents (usually trimethoprim with sulphadiazine), has also been used.

The separation of horses from infected cattle and infected materials is the best means of prevention. The number of cases in Britain has fallen since the eradication of the disease in cattle.

7.2 Camels

Both one-humped (*Camelus dromedarius*) and 2-humped (*Camelus bactrianus*) camels are susceptible to brucellosis, usually acquired through contact with infected large and small ruminants. Cases have been reported from western Asia, Mongolia and Africa, and infection usually results in abortion with excretion of the organism in genital discharges, urine and milk. Little is known regarding transmission within the camel herd or of the relation between brucellosis in camels and other ruminants.

Diagnosis is based on the isolation of the causal organism and on serological tests, particularly the complement fixation test with sera that have been inactivated at 60–62°C for 30 min. Diagnostic criteria are usually based on those accepted for cattle.

Brucellosis also occurs in llamas and other small camelids in some South American countries. For further review see Rutter and Mack (1963) and Report (1971, 1986b).

7.3 Wildlife

Brucellosis is endemic in caribou and domesticated reindeer (*Rangifer tarandus*) in arctic areas of Alaska, Canada and the former USSR, where it is caused by *B. suis* biogroup 4. Infection with *B. melitensis* has been reported from China. The disease is accompanied by abortion, retained placenta and metritis in the female, and orchitis and epididymitis in the male. In both sexes, abscess formation in joints and internal organs is frequent. Isolation of the organism proves the best evidence of infection in a herd. Infected animals often fail to react to serological tests (Report 1986b). *B. abortus* infection affects elk in parts of the USA, without apparently being transmitted to nearby herds of cattle.

Buffaloes, saiga, antelopes and yaks are all susceptible to brucellosis. The infecting strains are said to be those that affect nearby cattle and sheep, and the disease is similar to that in cattle. The ethacridine lactate (Rivanol) plate agglutination test is reported to be more specific than the complement fixation test for diagnosis in buffaloes (Nicoletti 1992). Brucellosis in the North American bison is endemic in areas of the USA, the biogroups being the same as in cattle. Brucella antibodies have been detected in sera from

African Bovidae including eland, impalas, gazelles, topi and wildebeeste. Feral swine are infected with *B. suis* in Australia, the USA and parts of Europe. Foxes are susceptible, and an epizootic in mink, characterized by abortion, was described by Pritchard et al. (1971) in animals fed infected bovine fetuses.

The European hare (*Lepus europaeus*) is susceptible to infection, especially with *B. suis* biogroup 2, and sometimes transmits the disease to domestic animals, especially pigs. Rats, mice and cats are generally resistant to natural infection. However, the desert woodrat (*Neotoma lepida*) is susceptible to infection with *B. neotomae* (Stoenner et al. 1959, Weber 1982); bank voles (*Clethrionomys* spp.) have been infected experimentally with *B. abortus* (Redwood and Corbel 1985), but badgers (*Meles meles*) developed only localized infections (Corbel et al. 1983).

There is some uncertainty regarding the susceptibility of fowl to brucellosis; early reports indicated that they were susceptible (Emmel and Huddleson 1930), but more recent reports (Kumar et al. 1984) suggests the opposite. A natural case of fowl brucellosis was described by Angus, Brown and Gue (1971), *B. abortus* biogroup 4 being isolated from both the fowl and in-contact cattle.

The recent isolation of *Brucella* strains from marine mammals including seals, sea otters, dolphins and porpoises extends the host range of the group into a new environment (Foster et al. 1996). It is not clear if these infections, which are caused by at least 2 distinct biogroups (see Volume 2, Chapter 35), are associated with disease in their hosts. Seroconversion rates >10% have been observed in seal populations from some areas. It is not known if the *Brucella* strains were acquired from terrestrial sources or were already present in the ancestral populations of these animals when they adopted a marine habitat.

Brucellae have been isolated from a wide range of wildlife including ticks and insects (Tovar 1947), but the isolates have often shown atypical properties. The role, if any, of these insects in the perpetuation and transmission of disease is unknown. For further reviews see Thorpe et al. (1965), Khoch and Davydov (1968), Morgan (1970) and Davis (1990).

For further information on brucellosis see Stableforth (1959), Verger and Plommet (1985), Report (1986b), Alton et al. (1988), Madkour (1989), Young and Corbel (1989), Adams (1990), Nielsen and Duncan (1990), Blobel and Schliesser (1991) and Corbel and MacMillan (1996).

REFERENCES

Abernathy RS, Spink WW, 1958, Studies with brucella endotoxin in humans: the significance of the susceptibility to endotoxin in the pathogenesis of brucellosis, *J Clin Invest*, **37:** 219–31.

Adams LG (ed.), 1990, *Advances in Brucellosis Research*, Texas A and M University Press, Austin, Texas.

Afzal M, 1985, Ultrastructural changes in sperm from rams with epididymitis, *Aust Vet J*, **62:** 391–2.

Ahvonen P, Janssen E, Aho K, 1969, Marked cross-agglutination between brucellae and a subtype of *Yersinia enterocolitica*, *Acta Pathol Microbiol Scand*, **75:** 291–5.

Akova M, Uzun Ö et al., 1993, Quinolones in the treatment of human brucellosis: comparative trial of oxfloxacin–rifampin versus doxycycline–rifampin, *J Antimicrob Chemother*, **37:** 1831–4.

Alarcon GS, Bocanegra TS et al., 1981, Reactive arthritis associated with brucellosis: HLA studies, *J Rheumatol*, **8:** 621–5.

Al-Deeb S, Madkour MM, 1989, Neurobrucellosis, *Brucellosis*, ed. Madkour MM, Butterworths, London, 160–79.

Al-Dubooni HM, Al-Shirkat SAR, Nagi NA, 1986, Brucellosis in children in Iraq, *Ann Trop Paediatr*, **6:** 271–4.

Allsup TN, 1969, Abortion in sheep associated with *Brucella abortus* infection, *Vet Rec*, **84:** 104–8.

Alton GG, 1960, The occurrence of dissociated strains of *Brucella melitensis* in the milk of goats in Malta, *J Comp Pathol*, **70:** 10–17.

Alton GG, 1985, The epidemiology of *Brucella melitensis* in sheep and goats, Brucella melitensis, eds Verger JM, Plommet M, Martinus Nijhoff, Dordrecht, 187–96.

Alton GG, 1990, *Brucella melitensis*, *Animal Brucellosis*, eds Nielsen K, Duncan JR, CRC Press, Boca Raton, FL, 383–409.

Alton GG, Jones LM, 1967, *Laboratory Techniques in Brucellosis*, Monograph Series No. 55, WHO, Geneva.

Alton GG, Jones LM, Pietz DE, 1975, *Laboratory Techniques in Brucellosis*, 2nd edn, Monograph Series No. 55, WHO, Geneva.

Alton GG, Jones LM et al., 1988, *Techniques for the Brucellosis Laboratory*, INRA, Paris.

Anderson JD, Smith H, 1965, The metabolism of erythritol by *Brucella abortus*, *J Gen Microbiol*, **38:** 109–24.

Anderson RK, Pietz DE et al., 1962, Epidemiological studies of bovine brucellosis in problem herds in Minnesota, *Proceedings of the 66th Annual Meeting of the US Livestock Sanitary Association*, Washington, DC, 109–18.

Anderson TD, Meador VP, Cheville NF, 1986, Pathogenesis of placentitis in the goat inoculated with *Brucella abortus*. I. Gross and histologic lesions, *Vet Pathol*, **23:** 219–26.

Angus RD, Brown GM, Gue CS, 1971, Avian brucellosis. A case report of natural transmission from cattle, *Am J Vet Res*, **32:** 1609–12.

Araj GF, Lulu AR et al., 1986a, Evaluation of ELISA in the diagnosis of acute and chronic brucellosis in human beings, *J Hyg Camb*, **97:** 457–69.

Araj GF, Lulu AR et al., 1986b, Rapid diagnosis of neurobrucellosis by ELISA, *J Neuroimmunol*, **12:** 173–82.

Ariza J, Gudiol F et al., 1985, Comparative trial of rifampin–doxycycline versus tetracycline–streptomycin in the therapy of human brucellosis, *Antimicrob Agents Chemother*, **28:** 548–51.

Ariza J, Pellicer T et al., 1992, Specific antibody profile in human brucellosis, *Clin Infect Dis*, **14:** 131–40.

Badakhsh FF, Carmichael LE, Douglas JA, 1982, Improved rapid slide agglutination test for presumptive diagnosis of canine brucellosis, *J Clin Microbiol*, **15:** 286–9.

Baker JR, Faull WB, 1967, Brucellosis in a large dairy herd, *Vet Rec*, **81:** 560–4.

Baldwin CL, Winter AJ, 1994, Macrophages and *Brucella*, *Immunol Ser*, **60:** 363–80.

Bang B, 1897, The etiology of epizootic abortion, *J Comp Pathol*, **10:** 125–49.

Bang O, Bendixen HC, 1932, Traenger Kastningsbakterien ind gennem normal Hud, og er dette en vigtig Smittvej vld Kraegets smitsomme Kastning?, *Medlemsblad Danske Dyrlaegeforening*, **15:** 1–11.

Bashir R, Al-Kawi MZ et al., 1985, Nervous system brucellosis: diagnosis and treatment, *Neurology*, **35:** 1576–81.

Baum M, Zarnir O et al., 1995, Comparative evaluation of microagglutination test and serum agglutination test as supplementary diagnostic tests for brucellosis, *J Clin Microbiol*, **33:** 2166–70.

Behan KA, Klein GC, 1982, Reduction of *Brucella* species and

Francisella tularensis cross-reacting agglutinins by dithiothreitol, *J Clin Microbiol*, **16:** 756–7.

Bendixen HC, Blom E, 1947, Investigations on brucellosis in the bovine male with special regard to spread of the disease by artificial insemination, *Vet J*, **103:** 337–45.

Bendixen HC, Blom E, 1948, Undersogelser over ForeKomsten a brucellose hos tyre specielt med Henblik paa Betydningen und den kunstige insemination, *Maanedsskrift Dyrlaeger*, **59:** 61–140.

Bendtsen H, 1960, Porcine brucellosis. Second report on the fifth outbreak of porcine brucellosis in Denmark, *Nord VetMed*, **12:** 343–63.

Bentejac MC, Biron G et al., 1984, Vaccination contre la brucellose humaine. Bilan sur une periode de 4 ans, *Dev Biol Stand*, **56:** 531–5.

Berman DT, Kurtz RS, 1987, Relationship of biological activities to structures of *Brucella abortus* endotoxin and LPS, *Ann Inst Pasteur (Paris)*, **138:** 98–101.

Bertram TA, Canning PC, Roth JA, 1986, Preferential inhibition of primary granule release from bovine neutrophils by a *Brucella abortus* extract, *Infect Immun*, **52:** 285–92.

Bertrand A, Roux J et al., 1979, Traitement de la brucellose par la rifampicine. Résultats préliminaires, *Nouv Presse Med*, **8:** 3635–9.

Bevan LEW, 1921–22, Infectious abortion of cattle and its possible relation to human health, *Trans R Soc Trop Med Hyg*, **15:** 215–31.

Bhonghibhat N, Elberg SS, Chen MJ, 1970, Characterization of *Brucella* skin-test antigens, *J Infect Dis*, **122:** 70–82.

Blajan L, 1984, La contribution de l'OIE à la lutte contre les brucelloses animal au plan mondial. III International Symposium on Brucellosis, *Dev Biol Stand*, **56:** 21–40.

Blasco JM, 1990, *Brucella ovis, Animal Brucellosis*, eds Nielsen K, Duncan JR, CRC Press, Boca Raton, FL, 351–82.

Blasco JM, Marin C et al., 1993, Efficacy of *Brucella suis* strain 2 vaccine against *Brucella ovis* in rams, *Vaccine*, **11:** 1291–4.

Blasco JM, Marin C et al., 1994, Evaluation of serological and allergic tests for diagnosing *Brucella melitensis* infection in sheep, *J Clin Microbiol*, **32:** 1835–40.

Blobel H, Schliesser T (eds), 1991, *Handbuch der Bakteriellen Infektionen bei Tieren (I)*, 2nd edn, Gustav Fischer Verlag, Jena.

Borts IH, Harris DM et al., 1943, A milk borne epidemic of brucellosis, *JAMA*, **121:** 319–22.

Botton Y, Thiange P et al., 1990, Diagnosis of bovine brucellosis by enzyme immunoassay of milk, *Vet Microbiol*, **24:** 73–80.

Boyd H, Reed HCB, 1960, Investigation into the incidence and causes of infertility in dairy cattle. *Brucella abortus* and *Vibrio fetus* infections, *Vet Rec*, **72:** 836–46.

Bracewell CD, Corbel MJ, 1980, An association between arthritis and persistent serological reactions to *Brucella abortus* in cattle from apparently brucellosis-free herds, *Vet Rec*, **106:** 99–101.

Bratescu A, Mayer EP, Teodorescu M, 1981, Binding of bacteria from the genus *Brucella* to human B lymphocytes, *Infect Immun*, **31:** 816–21.

Brown GM, Ranger CR, Kelley DJ, 1971, Selective media for the isolation of *Brucella ovis*, *Cornell Vet*, **61:** 265–80.

Bruce D, 1887, Note on the discovery of a micro-organism in Malta Fever, *Practictioner*, **39:** 161–70.

Buchanan TM, Faber LC, 1980, 2-Mercaptoethanol brucella agglutination test: usefulness for predicting recovery from brucellosis, *J Clin Microbiol*, **11:** 691–3.

Buchanan TM, Hendricks SI et al., 1974a, Brucellosis in the United States 1960–1972. An abattoir-associated disease. Part II. Epidemiology and evidence for acquired immunity, *Medicine (Baltimore)*, **53:** 427–39.

Buchanan TM, Sulzer CR et al., 1974b, Brucellosis in the United States 1960–1972. An abattoir-associated disease. Part II. Diagnosis aspects, *Medicine (Baltimore)*, **53:** 415–25.

Buck JM, 1930, Studies of vaccination during calfhood to prevent bovine infectious abortion, *J Agric Res*, **41:** 667–89.

Buddle MB, Boyes BW, 1953, A brucella mutant causing genital disease of sheep in New Zealand, *Aust Vet J*, **29:** 145–53.

Bundle DR, Czerwonogrodzky JW et al., 1987, The lipopolysaccharides of *Brucella abortus* and *B. melitensis*, *Ann Inst Pasteur (Paris)*, **138:** 92–8.

Bürki F, 1963, Emploi de l'épreuve de déviation du complément pour distinguer les animaux infectés de brucellose de ceux qui ont vaccinés contre la maladie, *Bull Off Int Epiz*, **60:** 419–32.

Burnet E, 1922, Diagnostic de la fièvre méditeranéene par intra-dermo réaction. Action du filtrat de culture du *M. melitensis*, *Arch Inst Pasteur Afrique Nord*, **2:** 187–201.

Canning PC, Deyoe BL, Roth JA, 1988, Opsonin-dependent stimulation of bovine neutrophil oxidative metabolism by *Brucella abortus*, *Am J Vet Res*, **49:** 160–3.

Canning PC, Roth JA, Deyoe BL, 1986, Release of 5′-guanosine monophosphate and adenine by *Brucella abortus* and their role in the intracellular survival of the bacteria, *J Infect Dis*, **154:** 464–70.

Carmichael LE, 1990, *Brucella canis, Animal Brucellosis*, eds Nielsen K, Duncan JR, CRC Press, Boca Raton, FL, 335–50.

Carmichael LE, Bruner DW, 1968, Characteristics of a newly recognised species of *Brucella* responsible for infectious canine abortions, *Cornell Vet*, **58:** 579–92.

Carmichael LE, George LW, 1976, Canine brucellosis: newer knowledge. II International Symposium on Brucellosis, Rabat, Morocco, 1975, *Dev Biol Stand*, **31:** 237–47, Discussion 247–50.

Carmichael LE, Zoha SJ, Flores-Castro R, 1984a, Problems in the serodiagnosis of canine brucellosis: dog responses to cell wall and internal antigens of *Brucella canis*. III International Symposium on Brucellosis, *Dev Biol Stand*, **51:** 371–83.

Carmichael LE, Zoha SJ, Flores-Castro R, 1984b, Biological properties and dog response to a variant (M-) strain of *Brucella canis*, *Dev Biol Stand*, **51:** 649–56.

Caroff M, Bundle DR et al., 1984a, Structure of the O-chain of the phenol-phase soluble cellular lipopolysaccharide of *Yersinia enterocolitica* serotype O:9, *Eur J Biochem*, **139:** 195–200.

Caroff M, Bundle DR et al., 1984b, Antigenic S-type lipopolysaccharide of *Brucella abortus* 1119-3, *Infect Immun*, **46:** 384–8.

Caron E, Peyrard T et al., 1994, Live *Brucella* spp. fail to induce tumour necrosis factor alpha excretion upon infection of U937-derived phagocytes, *Infect Immun*, **62:** 5267–74.

Castañeda MR, 1947, A practical method for routine blood cultures in brucellosis, *Proc Soc Exp Biol Med*, **64:** 114–15.

Cernyševa MI, Knjazeva EN, Egorova LS, 1977, Study of the plate agglutination test with Rose Bengal antigen for the diagnosis of human brucellosis, *Bull W H O*, **55:** 669–74.

Chappell RJ, Williamson P et al., 1976, Radioimmunoassay for antibodies against *Brucella abortus*; a new serological test for bovine brucellosis, *J Hyg*, **77:** 369–76.

Cheers C, Pagram P, 1979, Macrophage activation during experimental murine brucellosis; a basis for chronic infection, *Infect Immun*, **23:** 197–205.

Cheville NF, Stevens MG et al., 1993, Immune responses and protection against infection and abortion in cattle experimentally vaccinated with mutant strains of *Brucella abortus*, *Am J Vet Res*, **54:** 1591–7.

Christoffersen PA, Ottosen HE, 1941, Recent staining methods, *Skand Vet Tidskr*, **31:** 599–607.

Cloeckaert A, Verger J-M et al., 1995, Restriction site polymorphism of the genes encoding the major 25 kDa and 36 kDa outer membrane proteins of *Brucella*, *Microbiology*, **141:** 2111–21.

Cloeckaert A, Salih-Alj Debarrh H et al., 1996, Polymorphism at the *dnak* locus of *Brucella* species and identification of a *Brucella melitensis* species-specific marker, *J Med Microbiol*, **45:** 200–13.

Collins CH, 1983, *Laboratory-acquired Infections*, Butterworths, London.

Cook DR, Kinston GC, 1988, Isolation of *Brucella suis* biotype 1 from a horse, *Aust Vet J*, **65**: 162–3.

Cook DR, Noble JW, 1984, Isolation of *Brucella suis* from cattle, *Aust Vet J*, **61**: 263–4.

Corbel MJ, 1972, Identification of the immunoglobulin class active in the Rose Bengal plate test for bovine brucellosis, *J Hyg Camb*, **70**: 779–95.

Corbel MJ, 1975, The serological relationship between *Brucella* spp., *Yersinia enterocolitica* serotype 1X and *Salmonella* serotypes of Kauffmann–White Group N, *J Hyg*, **75**: 151–71.

Corbel MJ, 1976, Determination of the *in vitro* similarity of *Brucella* strains to rifampicin, *Br Vet J*, **132**: 266–75.

Corbel MJ, 1985a, Recent advances in the study of brucella antigens and their serological cross-reactions, *Vet Bull*, **55**: 927–42.

Corbel MJ, 1985b, Bacteriological procedures in the diagnosis of *Brucella melitensis* infection, *Brucella melitensis*, eds Verger JM, Plommet M, Martinus Nijhoff, Dordrecht, 105–22.

Corbel MJ, 1989, Brucellosis: epidemiology and prevalence worldwide, *Brucellosis: Clinical and Laboratory Aspects*, eds Young EJ, Corbel MJ, 25–40.

Corbel MJ, Bracewell CD, 1976, The serological response to rough and smooth *Brucella* antigens in cattle vaccinated with *Brucella abortus* strain 45/20 adjuvant vaccine, *Dev Biol Stand*, **31**: 351–7.

Corbel MJ, Cullen GA, 1970, Differentiation of the serological response to *Yersinia enterolitica* and *Brucella abortus* in cattle, *J Hyg Camb*, **68**: 519–30.

Corbel MJ, Lander KP, 1982, Observations on the serological diagnosis of *Brucella ovis* infection in sheep, *WHO Brucellosis Document*, WHO/BRUC/82/373, WHO, Geneva.

Corbel MJ, MacMillan AP, 1996, Bovine brucellosis, *OIE Manual of Standards for Diagnostic Tests and Vaccines*, OIE, Paris.

Corbel MJ, Redwood DW, Gill KPW, 1979, *Diagnostic Procedures for Non-smooth* Brucella *Strains*, MAFF, London.

Corbel MJ, Stuart FA, Brewer RA, 1984, Observations on serological cross-reactions between smooth *Brucella* species and organisms of other genera, *Dev Biol Stand*, **56**: 341–8.

Corbel MJ, Bracewell CD et al., 1979, *Identification Methods for Microbiologists*, 2nd edn, Academic Press, London and New York.

Corbel MJ, Morris JA et al., 1983, Response of the badger (*Meles meles*) to infection with *Brucella abortus*, *Res Vet Sci*, **34**: 296–300.

Corbel MJ, Stuart FA et al., 1989a, Arthropathy associated with *Brucella abortus* strain 19 vaccination in cattle. I. Examination of field cases, *Br Vet J*, **145**: 337–46.

Corbel MJ, Stuart FA et al., 1989b, Arthropathy associated with *Brucella abortus* strain 19 vaccination in cattle. II. Experimental studies, *Br Vet J*, **145**: 347–55.

Corner LA, Alton GG, Iyer H, 1985, An evaluation of a biphasic medium for the isolation of *Brucella abortus* from bovine tissues, *Aust Vet J*, **62**: 187–9.

Cotton WE, Buck JM, Smith HE, 1933, Studies of the skin as a portal of entry of *Brucella abortus* in pregnant cattle, *J Am Vet Med Assoc*, **83**: 91–100.

Crawford RP, Huber JD, Sanders RB, 1986, Brucellosis in heifers weaned from seropositive dams, *J Am Vet Med Assoc*, **189**: 547–9.

Crichton R, Medveczky NE, 1987, The identity, distribution, and epizootiological significance of *Brucella* isolates in Australia, 1981 to 1985, *Aust Vet J*, **64**: 48–52.

Cunningham B, O'Connor M, 1971, The use of killed 45/20 adjuvant vaccine as a diagnostic agent in the final stages of the eradication of brucellosis. The clearance of brucellosis from problem herds by interpretation of anamnestic serological responses, *Vet Rec*, **89**: 680–6.

Dalrymple-Champneys W, 1960, Brucella *Infection and Undulant Fever in Man*, Oxford University Press, London.

Davidson I, Hebert CN, 1978, International standard for anti-*Brucella abortus* serum: comparison of the complement-fixing activity of the first and second International Standards and the EEC Standard, *Bull W H O*, **56**: 123–7.

Davis DS, 1990, Brucellosis in wildlife, *Animal Brucellosis*, eds Nielsen K, Duncan JR, CRC Press, Boca Raton, FL, 323–34.

Davydov NN, 1961, [Properties of *Brucella* isolated from reindeer], *Tr Inst Eksp Vet*, **27**: 24–31.

Dedek J, 1983, [Epidemiology of brucellosis in swine, particularly reservoirs of *Brucella suis*], *Monatshefte VetMed*, **38**: 852–6.

Denny HR, 1972, Brucellosis in the horse, *Vet Rec*, **90**: 86–91.

Denny HR, 1973, A review of brucellosis in the horse, *Equine Vet J*, **5**: 121–5.

Deyoe BL, 1967, Pathogenesis of three strains of *Brucella suis* in swine, *Am J Vet Res*, **28**: 951–7.

Deyoe BL, 1968, Histopatholgic changes in male swine with experimental brucellosis, *Am J Vet Res*, **29**: 1215–20.

Deyoe BL, Manthei CA, 1976, Brucellosis, *Diseases of Swine*, 4th edn, eds Dunne HW, Leman AD, Iowa State University Press, Ames, IA, 492–515.

Diaz R, Dorronsoro I, 1971, Contribucíon al diagnóstico serológico de brucelosis y yesiniosis I. Utilidad de la reactíon de precipitación en gel, *Rev Clin Esp*, **121**: 367–72.

Diaz R, Maravi-Poma E, Rivero A, 1976, Comparison of counter-immunoelectrophoresis with other serological tests in the diagnosis of human brucellosis, *Bull W H O*, **53**: 417–24.

Diaz R, Moriyon I, 1989, Laboratory techniques in the diagnosis of human brucellosis, *Brucellosis: Clinical and Laboratory Aspects*, eds Young EJ, Corbel MJ, CRC Press, Boca Raton, FL, 73–83.

Diaz R, Maravi-Poma E et al., 1978, Rose Bengal plate agglutination and counter-immunoelectrophoresis test on spinal fluid in the diagnosis of *Brucella* meningitis, *J Clin Microbiol*, **7**: 236–7.

Doyle TM, 1935, The distribution of *Brucella abortus* in the body of 'carrier' cows, *J Comp Pathol*, **48**: 192–217.

Eckman MR, 1975, Brucellosis linked to Mexican cheese, *JAMA*, **232**: 636–7.

Eisele CW, McCullough NB et al., 1946, Development of *Brucella* agglutination in humans following vaccination for cholera, *Proc Soc Exp Biol Med*, **61**: 89–91.

Elberg SS, 1981, Rev 1 *Brucella melitensis* vaccine. Part II 1968–1980, *Vet Bull*, **51**: 67–73.

Emmel MW, Huddleson IF, 1930, *Brucella* disease in the fowl, *J Am Vet Med Assoc*, **76**: 449–52.

Entessar F, Ardalan A et al., 1967, Effect of living Rev 1 vaccine in producing long term immunity against *Brucella melitensis* infection in sheep in Iran, *J Comp Pathol*, **77**: 367–76.

Escande A, Serre A, 1982, IgE antiBrucella antibodies in the course of human brucellosis and after specific vaccination, *Int Arch Allergy Appl Immunol*, **68**: 172–5.

Evans AC, 1918a, Further studies on *Bacterium abortus* and related bacteria. III. A comparison of *Bacterium abortus* with *Bacterium bronchisepticus* and with the organism that causes Malta Fever, *J Infect Dis*, **22**: 580–93.

Evans AC, 1918b, Further studies on *Bacterium abortus* and related bacteria. III. *Bacterium abortus* and related bacteria in cows milk, *J Infect Dis*, **23**: 354–72.

Ewalt DR, Payeur JB et al., 1994, Characteristics of a *Brucella* species from a bottlenose dolphin (*Tursiops truncatus*), *J Vet Diagn Invest*, **6**: 448–52.

Farina R, 1985, Current serological methods in *Br. melitensis* diagnosis, *Brucella melitensis*, eds Verger JM, Plommet M, Martinus Nijhoff, Dordrecht, 139–46.

Farrell ID, Robertson L, Hinchcliffe PM, 1975, Serum antibody response in acute brucellosis (human), *J Hyg Camb*, **74**: 23–8.

Feeley JC, 1969, Somatic O antigen relationship of *Brucella* and *Vibrio cholerae*, *J Bacteriol*, **99**: 645–9.

Fekete A, Bantle JA et al., 1990, Rapid sensitive detection of *Brucella abortus* by polymerase chain reaction without extraction of DNA, *Biotech Technol*, **4**: 31–4.

Fenske G, Pulst H, 1973, [Epidemiological significance of brucellosis in hare and wild boar], *Monatshefte VetMed*, **28:** 537–41.

Fensterbank R, 1976, Traitement des vaches atteintes de brucellose ancienne par l'oxytetracycline, *Ann Rech Vet*, **7:** 231–40.

Fensterbank R, 1984, La diagnostic allergique des brucelloses animales. III International Symposium on Brucellosis, *Dev Biol Stand*, **56:** 401–5.

Fensterbank R, 1985, Allergic diagnosis of brucellosis, *Brucella melitensis*, eds Verger JM, Plommet M, Martinus Nijhoff, Dordrecht, 167–71.

Ficapal A, Alonso-Urmeneta B et al., 1995, Diagnosis of *Brucella ovis* infection of rams with an ELISA using protein G as conjugate, *Vet Rec*, **137:** 145–7.

Finegold SM, White ML et al., 1969, Rapid diagnosis of bacteraemia, *Appl Microbiol*, **18:** 458–63.

Fitch CP, Bishop LM, Kelly MD, 1936, The isolation of *Brucella abortus* from the bloodstream of cattle, *Proc Soc Exp Biol Med*, **34:** 696–8.

Fitch CP, Boyd WL, Bishop LM, 1938, A study of the vaginal content of pregnant Bang-infected cows for the presence of *Brucella abortus*, *J Am Vet Med Assoc*, **92:** 171–7.

Fitch CP, Delez AL, Boyd WL, 1930, Preliminary report on the relation of *Bact. abortus* Bang to fistulae, poll-evil and other suppurations of horses, *J Am Vet Med Assoc*, **76:** 17–24.

Fitzgeorge RB, Solotorovsky M, Smith H, 1963, The relation between resistance to hydrogen peroxide and virulence in brucellae, *J Pathol Bacteriol*, **89:** 745–7.

Fleischhauer G, 1937, Die *Abortus*-Bang-Ring-probe (ABR) zur Festellung von bangverdächtigen Vollmilchproben, *Berl Tierarztl Wochenschr*, **53:** 527–8.

Forschner E, Bunger I, 1986, [Detection of antibodies against *Brucella abortus* in farm bulk milk samples by ELISA], *Dtsch Tierarztl Wochenschr*, **93:** 269–73.

Foshay L, 1950, Tularaemia, *Annu Rev Microbiol*, **4:** 313–30.

Foster G, Jahans KL et al., 1996, Isolation of *Brucella* species from cetaceans, seals and an otter, *Vet Rec*, **158:** 583–6.

Foster RA, Ladds PW et al., 1988, Immunoglobulins and immunoglobulin-containing cells in the reproductive tracts of rams naturally infected with *Brucella* ovis, *Aust Vet J*, **65:** 37–40.

Francis E, Evans AC, 1926, Agglutination, cross-agglutination and agglutination absorption in tularaemia, *Public Health Rep*, **41:** 1273–95.

Frenchick PJ, Markham RJF, Cochrane AH, 1985, Inhibition of phagosome and lysosome fusion in macrophages by soluble extracts of virulent *Brucella abortus*, *Am J Vet Res*, 332–5.

Gavrilov PP, Bzhevskaya AN et al., 1972, K epizootologii zabolevaniya, vyzyvaemogo *Br. ovis*, *Veterinariia*, **7:** 55–7.

George LW, Carmichael LE, 1984, Antisperm responses in male dogs with chronic *Brucella canis* infections, *Am J Vet Res*, **45:** 274–81.

Gilbert R, Dacey HG, 1932, The isolation of an organism of the *abortus-melitensis* group from a blood clot, the serum of which failed to give agglutination with *B abortus*, *J Lab Clin Med*, **17:** 345–6.

Goldbaum FA, Leoni J et al., 1993, Characterization of an 18-kilodalton *Brucella* cytoplasmic protein which appears to be a serological marker of active infection of both human and bovine brucellosis, *J Clin Microbiol*, **31:** 2141–5.

Goossens H, Marcelis L et al., 1983, *Brucella melitensis*: person to person transmission?, *Lancet*, **1:** 773.

Gotuzzo E, Carillo C et al., 1986, An evaluation of diagnostic methods for brucellosis – the value of bone marrow culture, *J Infect Dis*, **153:** 122–5.

Gower SGM, Wright EC et al., 1974, An automated Rose Bengal agglutination test using the ADAM system, *Vet Rec*, **95:** 544–7.

Hardy AV, Jordan CF, Borts IH, 1932, A further study of *Brucella* infection in Iowa, *Public Health Rep*, **47:** 187–93.

Hardy AV, Jordan CF et al., 1931, *Undulant Fever with Special Reference to a Study of Brucella Infection in Iowa*, National Institutes of Health Bulletin No. 158, NIH, Bethesda, MD.

Heathman LS, 1934, A survey of workers in packing plants for evidence of *Brucella* infection, *J Infect Dis*, **55:** 243–65.

Heck FC, Nielsen KH et al., 1984, Sensitivity of serological methods for detecting antibody in vaccinated and nonvaccinated *Brucella*-infected cows, *Aust Vet J*, **61:** 265–6.

Hellmann E, 1982, *Brucella melitensis*, Handbuch der bakteriellen Infektionen bei Tieren, eds Blobel H, Schliesser T, Gustav Fischer, Jena, 214–60.

Henderson RA, Hoerlein BF et al., 1974, Discospondylitis in three dogs infected with *Brucella canis*, *J Am Vet Med Assoc*, **165:** 451–5.

Hendricks SL, 1955, Epidemiology of human brucellosis in Iowa, *Am J Public Health*, **45:** 1282–8.

Hendricks SL, Borts IH et al., 1962, Brucellosis outbreak in an Iowa packing house, *Am J Public Health*, **52:** 1166–78.

Heremans JF, Vaerman JP, Vaerman C, 1963, Studies on the imune globulins of human serum. II. A study of the distribution of anti-*Brucella* and anti-diphtheria antibody activities among gamma-ss, gamma IM and gamma IA globulin fractions, *J Immunol*, **91:** 11–17.

Hess WR, Roepke MH, 1951, A non-specific *Brucella* agglutinating substance in bovine serum, *Proc Soc Exp Biol Med*, **77:** 469–72.

Hodinka L, Gömör B et al., 1978, HLA-B27-associated spondyloarthritis in chronic brucellosis, *Lancet*, **1:** 499.

Hornitzky M, Pearson J, 1986, The relationship between the isolation of *Brucella abortus* and serological status of infected, non-vaccinated cattle, *Aust Vet J*, **63:** 172–4.

Horrocks WH, 1905, *Report of the Commission on Mediterranean Fever*, part 3, Harrison and Sons, London, 84.

Horrocks WH, Kennedy JC, 1906, Goats as a means of propagation of Mediterranean Fever, *Report of the Commission on Mediterranean Fever*, part IV, Harrison and Sons, London, 37–69.

Huddleson IF, 1921, Studies in infectious abortion, *J Am Vet Med Assoc*, **58:** 524–31.

Huddleson IF, 1943, *Brucellosis in Man and Animals*, Commonwealth Fund, New York.

Huddleson IF, Johnson HW, Hamann EE, 1933, A study of *Brucella* infection in swine and employees of packing houses, *J Am Vet Med Assoc*, **83:** 16–30.

Hughes L, 1897, *Mediterranean, Malta or Undulant Fever*, Macmillan, London.

Hugh-Jones MW, Ellis PR, Felton MR, 1975, *An Assessment of the Eradication of Bovine Brucellosis in England and Wales*, Study no. 19, University of Reading, Berkshire.

Huntley BE, Philip RN, Maynard JR, 1963, Survey of brucellosis in Alaska, *J Infect Dis*, **112:** 100–6.

Hutchings LM, 1950, *Swine Brucellosis*, American Association for the Advancement of Science, Washington, DC, 188–97.

Jansen S, Müller W, 1982, [Worldwide distribution of brucellosis. Epidemiological trends in 1967–1979], *Tierärztl Umschau*, **37:** 564–70.

Jiang X, Baldwin CL, 1993, Iron augments macrophage-mediated killing of *Brucella abortus* alone and in conjunction with interferon-γ, *Cell Immunol*, **148:** 397–407.

Jiménez de Bagués MP, Elzer PH et al., 1994, Protective immunity to *Brucella ovis* in BALB/C mice following recovery from primary infection or immunization with subcellular vaccine, *Infect Immun*, **62:** 632–8.

Jones LM, 1967, Report to the International Committee on Nomenclature of Bacteria by the Sub-Committee on Taxonomy of Brucellae, *Int J Syst Bacteriol*, **17:** 371–5.

Jones LM, Berman DT, 1976, Studies of *Brucella* lipopolysaccharides. II International Symposium on Brucellosis, *Dev Biol Stand*, **31:** 62–7.

Jones LM, Diaz R, Taylor AG, 1973, Characterisation of allergens prepared from smooth and rough strains of *Brucella melitensis*, *Br J Exp Pathol*, **54:** 492–508.

Jones LM, Entessar F, Ardalan A, 1964, Comparison of living vaccines in producing immunity against natural *Brucella melit-*

ensis infection in sheep and goats in Iran, *J Comp Pathol,* **74:** 17–30.

Jones SM, Winter AJ, 1992, Survival of virulent and attenuated strains of *Brucella abortus* in normal and gamma interferon-activated vaccine peritoneal macrophages, *Infect Immun,* **60:** 3011–14.

Jubb KVF, Kennedy PC, Palmer N, 1985, The female genital system, *Pathology of Domestic Animals,* vol. 3, 3rd edn, Academic Press, New York, 409–59.

Kerr WR, Rankin J, 1959, The spread of brucellosis within herds – the milk problem, *Vet Rec,* **71:** 178–9.

Kerr WR, Payne DJH et al., 1967, Immunoglobulin class of *Brucella* antibodies in human sera, *Immunology,* **13:** 223–5.

Kerr WR, McCaughey WJ et al., 1968, Techniques and interpretation in the serological diagnosis of brucellosis in man, *J Med Microbiol,* **1:** 181–93.

Khoch AA, Davydov NN, 1968, [Characteristics of *Brucella* strains isolated from animals in the Yakutsk ASSR (with reference to *B rangiferi*)], *Veterinariia,* **4:** 14.

Kolman S, Maayan MC et al., 1991, Comparison of the Bactec and lysis concentration method for recovery of *Brucella* species from clinical specimens, *Eur J Clin Microbiol Infect Dis,* **10:** 647–8.

Kreutzer DL, Dreyfus LA, Robertson DC, 1979, Interaction of polymorphonuclear leukocytes with smooth and rough strains of *Brucella abortus, Infect Immun,* **23:** 737–42.

Kreutzer DL, Robertson DC, 1979, Surface macromolecules and virulence in intracellular parasitism: comparison of cell envelope components of smooth and rough strains of *Brucella abortus, Infect Immun,* **23:** 819–28.

Kumar S, Kulshrestha RC et al., 1984, Brucellosis in poultry – an experimental study, *Int J Zoonoses,* **11:** 133–8.

Laing JA, Morgan WJB, Wagner WC (eds), 1988, *Fertility and Infertility in Veterinary Practice,* 4th edn, Baillière Tindall, London.

Lambert G, Manthei CA, Deyoe BL, 1963, Studies on *Brucella abortus* infection in bulls, *Am J Vet Res,* **24:** 1152–7.

Lambert G, Amerault TE et al., 1961, Further studies on the persistence of *Brucella abortus* infection in cattle, *Proc 64th Annu Meet US Livestock Sanit Assoc, Charleston, SC,* 109–17.

Lapraik RD, Brown DD et al., 1975, Brucellosis: a study of five calves from reactor dams, *Vet Rec,* **97:** 52–4.

Lauwers H, 1966, [The ring test, slow agglutination and complement fixation tests in the organized eradication of bovine brucellosis], *Vlaams Diergeneeskd Tijdschrift,* **38:** 326–38.

Lee K, Cargill C, Atkinson H, 1985, Evaluation of an enzyme linked-immunosorbent assay for the diagnosis of *Brucella ovis* infection in rams, *Aust Vet J,* **62:** 91–3.

Leech FB, Vessey MP et al., 1964, *Animal Disease Surveys,* No. 4, MAFF, HMSO, London.

Lindberg AA, Haeggman S et al., 1982, Enzyme immunoassay of the antibody responses to *Brucella* and *Yersinia enterocolitica* O9 infections in humans, *J Hyg (Lond),* **88:** 295–307.

Llorens-Terol J, Busquets RM, 1980, Brucellosis treated with rifampicin, *Arch Dis Child,* **55:** 486–8.

Lopez-Merino A, 1989, Brucellosis in Latin America, *Brucellosis: Clinical and Laboratory Aspects,* eds Young EJ, Corbel MJ, CRC Press, Boca Raton, FL, 151–61.

Lopez-Merino A, Asselineau J et al., 1976, Immunization by an insoluble fraction extracted from *Brucella melitensis:* immunological and chemical characterization of the active substances, *Infect Immun,* **13:** 311–21.

Luchsinger DW, Anderson RH, 1979, Longitudinal studies of naturally acquired *Brucella abortus* infection in sheep, *Am J Vet Res,* **40:** 1307–12.

McCaughey WJ, Kerr WR, 1967, The Coombs' or antiglobulin test in the horse, *Vet Rec,* **81:** 542.

McCaughey WJ, Purcell DA, 1973, Brucellosis in bulls, *Vet Rec,* **93:** 336–7.

MacDiarmid SC, 1988, Future options for brucellosis surveillance in New Zealand beef herds, *NZ Vet J,* **36:** 39–42.

McEwen AD, 1940, The virulence of *Brucella abortus* for laboratory animals and pregnant cattle, *Vet Rec,* **52:** 97–106.

McEwen AD, Priestley FW, Paterson AD, 1939, An estimate of a suitable infective dose of *Brucella abortus* for immunization tests on cattle, *J Comp Pathol,* **52:** 116–28.

M'Fadyean J, Stockman S, 1909, *Report of the Departmental Committee to enquire into Epizootic Abortion,* Appendix to part 1, HMSO, London.

MacMillan AP, Cockrem DS, 1985, Reduction of non-specific reactions to the *Brucella abortus* serum agglutination test by the addition of EDTA, *Res Vet Sci,* **38:** 288–91.

MacMillan AP, Cockrem DS, 1986, Observations on the long term effects of *Brucella abortus* infection in the horse, including effects during pregnancy and lactation, *Equine Vet J,* **18:** 388–90.

MacMillan AP, Baskerville A et al., 1982, Experimental *Brucella abortus* infection in the horse: observations during the three months following inoculation, *Res Vet Sci,* **33:** 351–9.

MacMillan AP, Greiser-Wilke I et al., 1990, A competition enzyme immunoassay for brucellosis diagnosis, *Dtsch Tierärztl Wochenschr,* **97:** 83–5.

MacNeal WJ, Kerr JE, 1910, *Bacillus abortus* of Bang, the cause of contagious abortion in cattle, *J Infect Dis,* **7:** 469–75.

McNutt SH, Murray C, 1924, *Bacterium abortum* (Bang) isolated from the fetus of an aborting mare, *J Am Vet Med Assoc,* **65:** 215–16.

Macrae RM, Smith H, 1964, The clinical basis of the virulence of *Brucella abortus.* VI. Studies on immunity and intracellular growth, *Br J Exp Pathol,* **45:** 595–603.

Madkour MM (ed.), 1989, *Brucellosis,* Butterworths, London.

Magee JT, 1980, An enzyme-labelled immunosorbent assay for *Brucella abortus* antibodies, *J Med Microbiol,* **13:** 167–72.

Manthei CA, 1950, Brucellosis in cattle, *Brucellosis: a Symposium,* American Association for the Advancement of Science, Washington, DC, 172–87.

Manthei CA, Carter RW, 1950, Persistence of *Brucella abortus* infection in cattle, *Am J Vet Res,* **11:** 173–80.

Manthei CA, Mingle CK, Carter RW, 1951, Duration of immunity to brucellosis induced in cattle with Strain 19 vaccine, *Proc Am Vet Med Assoc,* **88:** 128–42.

Mantur BG, Mangalgi SS, Mulimani M, 1996, *Brucella melitensis* – a sexually transmissible agent, *Lancet,* **347:** 1763.

Matar FM, Khreissir IA, Abodnoor AM, 1996, Rapid laboratory confirmation of human brucellosis by PCR analysis of a target sequence on the 31-kilodalton *Brucella* antigen DNA, *J Clin Microbiol,* **34:** 477–8.

Mateu-de-Antonio EM, Martin M, Soler M, 1993, Use of indirect enzyme-linked immunosorbent assay with hot saline solution extracts of a variant (M⁻) strain of *Brucella canis* for diagnosis of brucellosis in dogs, *Am J Vet Res,* **54:** 1043–6.

Matyas Z, Fujikura T, 1984, Brucellosis as a world problem. III International Symposium on Brucellosis, *Dev Biol Stand,* **56:** 3–20.

Meyer KF, Shaw EB, 1920, Comparison of the morphologic, cultural and biochemical characteristics of *Brucella abortus* and *Brucella melitensis.* Studies on the genus *Brucella* Nov. Gen. I., *J Infect Dis,* **27:** 173–84.

Meyer ME, 1964, Species identity and epidemiology of *Brucella* strains isolated from Alaskan Eskimos, *J Infect Dis,* **114:** 169–73.

Meyer ME, 1982, *Brucella ovis, Handbuch der bakteriellen Infektionen bei Tieren,* eds Blobel H, Schliesser T, Gustav Fischer, Jena, 309–28.

Miller JK, Kelly JI, Roerink JHG, 1976, A complement fixation method for quantitative differentiation of reactions to 45/20 vaccine and brucella infection, *Vet Rec,* **98:** 210–15.

Mittal KR, Tizard IR, 1981, Serological cross-reactions between *Brucella abortus* and *Yersinia enterocolitica* serotype O9, *Vet Bull,* **51:** 501–5.

Molello JA, Jensen R et al., 1963, Placental pathology III. Placental lesions of sheep experimentally infected with *Brucella abortus*, *Am J Vet Res*, **24**: 915–22.

Monroe PW, Silberg SL et al., 1975, Sero-epidemiological investigation of *Brucella canis* antibodies in different human population groups, *J Clin Microbiol*, **2**: 382–6.

Morgan WJB, 1968, *Some Diseases of Animals Communicable to Man in Britain*, ed. Graham-Jones O, Pergamon Press, Oxford, 263–73.

Morgan WJB, 1970, Reviews of the progress of dairy science. Section E. Diseases of dairy cattle. Brucellosis, *J Dairy Res*, **37**: 303–60.

Morgan WJB, 1977, The national brucellosis programme of Britain, *Brucellosis: an International Symposium*, eds Crawford RP, Hidalgo RJ, A and M University Press, Austin, Texas, 378–88.

Morgan WJB, 1982, *Brucella abortus, Handbuch der bakteriellen Infektionen bei Tieren*, eds Blobel H, Schliesser T, Gustav Fischer, Jena, 53–213.

Morgan WJB, Davidson I, Hebert CN, 1973, The use of the second International Standard for anti-*Brucella abortus* serum in the complement-fixation test, *J Biol Stand*, **1**: 43–61.

Morgan WJB, Richards RA, 1974, The diagnosis, control and eradication of bovine brucellosis in Great Britain, *Vet Rec*, **94**: 510–17.

Mousa ARM, Elhag KM et al., 1988, The nature of human brucellosis in Kuwait: study of 379 cases, *Rev Infect Dis*, **10**: 211–17.

Mustafa AA, Abusowa M, 1993, Field oriented trial to the Chinese *Brucella suis* strain 2 vaccine on sheep and goats in Libya, *Ann Rech Vet*, **24**: 422–9.

Naparstek E, Block CS, Slavin S, 1982, Transmission of brucellosis by bone marrow transplantation, *Lancet*, **1**: 574–5.

Nelson CJ, Huber JD, Essey MA, 1986, *Proc 90th Annu Meet U S Anim Health Assoc, Kentucky*, 177.

Nelson CJ, Anderson RK et al., 1966, Epizootologic factors of bovine brucellosis: comparative bacteriologic studies of infected herds, *Am J Vet Res*, **27**: 1515–20.

Nicoletti P, 1977, Use of 45/20 bacterin to detect latent infection in brucellosis, *Bovine Brucellosis: an International Symposium*, eds Crawford RP, Hidalgo RJ, A & M University Press, Austin, Texas, 72–8, discussion 79–99.

Nicoletti P, 1992, An evaluation of serologic tests used to diagnose brucellosis in buffaloes (*Butalus tubalis*), *Trop Anim Health Prod*, **24**: 40–4.

Nicoletti P, Milward FW et al., 1985, Efficacy of long-acting oxytetracycline alone or combined with streptomycin in the treatment of bovine brucellosis, *J Am Vet Med Assoc*, **187**: 493–5.

Nielsen K, Duncan JR, 1982, Demonstration that nonspecific bovine *Brucella abortus* agglutinin is EDTA-labile and not calcium-dependent, *J Immunol*, **129**: 366–9.

Nielsen K, Duncan JR (eds), 1990, *Animal Brucellosis*, CRC Press, Boca Raton, FL.

Nielsen K, Duncan JR et al., 1981, Relationship of humoral factors (antibody and complement) to immune responsiveness, resistance and diagnostic serology, *Adv Exp Med Biol*, **137**: 367–89.

Nielsen KH, Gall D et al., 1992, *Enzyme Immunoassay: Application to Diagnosis of Bovine Brucellosis*, Agriculture Canada Monograph, Agriculture Canada, Nepean, Ontario.

Norton JH, Thomas AD, 1979, *Brucella suis* infection in pregnant cattle, *Aust Vet J*, **55**: 525–7.

Notenboom RH, Borczyk A et al., 1987, Clinical relevance of a serological cross-reaction between *Escherichia coli* O157 and *Brucella abortus*, *Lancet*, **2**: 745.

Nowak J, 1908, Le bacille de Bang et sa biologie, *Ann Inst Pasteur (Paris)*, **22**: 541–56.

Ocon P, Reguera JM et al., 1994, Phagocytic cell function in active brucellosis, *Infect Immun*, **62**: 910–14.

Olitzki A, 1970, Immunization procedures in domestic animals and their results, *Immunobiological Methods in Brucellosis Research*, nos 8 and 9, S Karger, Basel, 213–72.

Olle Goig JE, Canela-Soler J, 1987, An outbreak of *Brucella melit-*

ensis infection by airborne transmission among laboratory animals, *Am J Public Health*, **77**: 335–8.

Paolicchi FA, Terzolo HR, Campero CM, 1993, Isolation of *Brucella suis* from the semen of a ram, *Vet Rec*, **132**: 67.

Parratt D, Nielson KH et al., 1977, Radioimmunoassay of IgM, IgG, and IgA *Brucella* antibodies, *Lancet*, **1**: 1075–8.

Payne JM, 1959, The pathogenesis of experimental brucellosis in the pregnant cow, *J Pathol Bacteriol*, **78**: 447–63.

Payne JM, 1960a, The bacteriology of experimental infection of the rats' placenta, *J Pathol Bacteriol*, **80**: 205–13.

Payne JM, 1960b, The pathogenesis of experimental brucellosis in virgin heifers with and without continuous progesterone treatment, *J Endocrinol*, **20**: 345–56.

Pearce JH, Williams AE et al., 1962, The chemical basis of the virulence of *Brucella abortus*, II. Erythritol, a constituent of bovine foetal fluids which stimulates the growth of *Brucella abortus* in bovine phagocytes, *Br J Exp Pathol*, **43**: 31–7.

Peraldi M, Lopez A et al., 1976, [Lymphoblastic transformation by *Brucella* fractions in humans with brucellosis and in those vaccinated with PI vaccine], *Dev Biol Stand*, **31**: 157–64.

Perera VY, Creasy MT, Winter AJ, 1983, Nylon bead enzyme-linked immunosorbent assay for detection of sub-picogram quantities of *Brucella* antibodies, *J Clin Microbiol*, **18**: 601–8.

Philippon A, Renoux G, Plommet M, 1970, Brucellose bovine expérimentale. III. Excrétion vaginale de *Brucella abortus* avant et après la rinse bas, *Ann Rech Vet*, **1**: 215–24.

Philippon A, Renoux G, Plommet M, 1972, Brucellose bovine expérimentale. XI. Infection par *Brucella melitensis*, *Ann Rech Vet*, **3**: 13–22.

Philippon AM, Plommet MG et al., 1977, Rifampin in the treatment of experimental brucellosis in mice and guinea pigs, *J Infect Dis*, **136**: 482–8.

Pietz D, 1977, *Brucella* antigens and serologic test results, *Bovine Brucellosis: an International Symposium*, eds Crawford RP, Hidalgo RJ, A & M University Press, Texas, USA, 49–60, discussion 79–99.

Pike RM, 1978, Past and present hazards of working with infectious agents, *Arch Pathol Lab Med*, **102**: 333–6.

Plackett P, Alton GG, 1975, A mechanism for prozone formation in the complement fixation test for bovine brucellosis, *Aust Vet J*, **51**: 374–7.

Plackett P, Cottew GS, Best SJ, 1976, An indirect haemolysis test (IHLT) for bovine brucellosis, *Aust Vet J*, **52**: 136–40.

Plant JW, Eamens GJ, Seaman JT, 1986, Serological, bacteriological and pathological changes in rams following different routes of exposure to *Brucella ovis*, *Aust Vet J*, **63**: 409–12.

Plommet M, Plommet AM, 1975, Vaccination against bovine brucellosis with a low dose of strain 19 administered by the conjuctival route. I. Protection demonstrated in guinea pigs, *Ann Rech Vet*, **6**: 345–56.

Plommet M, Renoux G et al., 1971, Transmission congénitale de la brucellose bovine d'une génération à l'autre, *Bull Acad Vet Fr*, **44**: 53–9.

Polt SS, Dismukes WE et al., 1982, Human brucellosis caused by *Brucella canis*: clinical features and immune response, *Ann Intern Med*, **97**: 717–19.

Poole PM, Whitehouse DB, Gilchrist MM, 1972, A case of abortion consequent upon infection with *Brucella abortus* biotype 2, *J Clin Pathol*, **25**: 882–4.

Preisz H, 1903, Der Bacillus des seuchenhaften Verwerfens, *Zentralbl Bakteriol Parasitenkd Infektionskr Hyg*, **33**: 190–6.

Pritchard WD, Hagen KW et al., 1971, An epizootic of brucellosis in mink, *J Am Vet Med Assoc*, **159**: 635–7.

Rautlin de la Roy YM, Grignon B et al., 1986, Rifampicin resistance in a strain of *Brucella melitensis* after treatment with doxycycline and rifampicin, *J Antimicrob Chemother*, **18**: 648–9.

Ray WC, 1976, An assessment of investigations conducted in the UK on *Brucella abortus* strain 45/20 bacterins. II International Symposium on Brucellosis, Rabat, Morocco, 1975, *Dev Biol Stand*, **31**: 335–42.

Redmond JW, 1979, The structure of the O-antigenic side chain of the lipopolysaccharide of *Vibrio cholerae* 569B (Inaba), *Biochim Biophys Acta*, **584**: 346–52.

Redwood DW, Corbel MJ, 1985, *Brucella abortus* infection in the bank vole (*Clethrionomys glareolus*), *Br Vet J*, **141**: 397–400.

Rementsova MM, 1962, *[Brucellosis of Wild Animals]*, Alma-Ata, Akademiya Nauk Kazakhskoi SSR. [see *Vet Bull* 1963, 33: abstract 775].

Report, 1905–7, *Mediterranean Fever Commission*, Harrison and Sons, London.

Report, 1961, *Monthly Bulletin of the Ministry of Health and Public Health Laboratory Service*, **20**: 33.

Report, 1971, *Joint FAO/WHO Expert Committee on Brucellosis, 5th Report*, World Health Organization Technical Report Series No. 464, World Health Organization, Geneva.

Report, 1980, Human and bovine brucellosis in Britain, *Br Med J*, **1**: 1458.

Report, 1986a, *La Rage et la Brucellose dans le Bassin Méditerranéen et la peninsule arabe*, Collection Fondation Marcel Mérieux, Lyon.

Report, 1986b, *Joint FAO/WHO Expert Committee on Brucellosis, 6th Report*, World Health Organization Technical Report Series No. 740, World Health Organization, Geneva.

Report, 1994, *Categorization of Pathogens according to Hazard and Categories of Containment*, Advisory Committee on Dangerous Pathogens 3rd Interim Issue 1994, HMSO, London.

Rice CE, Boulanger P et al., 1952, The conglutination complement-fixation test as a supplementary method of detecting activity with *Brucella abortus* antigens, *Can J Comp Med Vet Sci*, **16**: 348–56.

Robertson L, Farrell ID et al., 1980, *Benchbook on* Brucella, Public Health Laboratory Service, Monograph Series no. 14, HMSO, London.

Roerink JHG, 1967, Investigation into the usefulness of the non-agglutogenic *Brucella abortus* adjuvant vaccine Duphavac NA in the control of bovine brucellosis, *Vet Rec*, **80**: 727–3.

Roguinsky M, Fensterbank R, Phillippon A, 1972, Influence de l'infection brucellique de la mamelle sur la teneur en cellules du lait, *Ann Rech Vet*, **3**: 449–57.

Rose JE, Roepke MH, Briggs DR, 1964, Physicochemical properties of nonspecific bovine seroagglutinins for *Brucella abortus*, *Am J Vet Res*, **25**: 118–21.

Ross HM, Foster G et al., 1994, *Brucella* species infection in sea-mammals, *Vet Rec*, **134**: 359.

Rutter TE, Mack R, 1963, Diseases of camels. Part 1: Bacterial and fungal diseases, *Vet Bull*, **33**: 119–24.

Sabbaghian H, 1975, Fresh white cheese as a source of *Brucella* infection, *Public Health*, **89**: 165–9.

Sadusk JF, Browne AS, Born JL, 1957, Brucellosis in man, resulting from *Brucella abortus* (Strain 19) vaccine, *JAMA*, **164**: 1325–7.

Samartino LE, Enright FM, 1993, Pathogenesis of abortion of bovine brucellosis, *Comp Immunol Microbiol Infect Dis*, **16**: 95–101.

Schoenemann J, Lütticken R, Scheibner E, 1986, [*Brucella canis* infection in a human], *Dtsch Med Wochenschr*, **111**: 20–2.

Schroeder EC, Cotton WE, 1911, *28th Annual Report of the Bureau of Animal Industry*, US Department of Agriculture, Washington, DC, 139.

Serikawa T, Takada H et al., 1984, Multiplication of *Brucella canis* in male reproductive organs and detection of autoantibody to spermatozoa in canine brucellosis. III International Symposium on Brucellosis, *Dev Biol Stand*, **56**: 295–305.

Serikawa T, Iwaki S et al., 1989, Purification of a *Brucella canis* cell wall antigen by using immunosorbent columns and use of the antigen in enzyme-linked immunosorbent assay for specific diagnosis of canine brucellosis, *J Clin Microbiol*, **27**: 837–42.

Serre A, 1989, Immunology and pathophysiology of human brucellosis, *Brucellosis: Clinical and Laboratory Aspects*, eds Young EJ, Corbel MJ, CRC Press, Boca Raton, FL, 85–95.

Serre A, Dana M, Roux J, 1970, Nature des anticorps bloquants dans la brucellose humaine, *Pathol Biol*, **18**: 367–74.

Serre A, Bascoul S et al., 1987, Human immune response to *Brucella* infection, *Ann Inst Pasteur (Paris)*, **138**: 113–17.

Shakir RA, 1986, Neurobrucellosis, *Postgrad Med J*, **62**: 1077–9.

Shakir RA, Al-Din AS et al., 1987, Clinical categories of neuro-brucellosis. A report on 19 cases, *Brain*, **110**: 213–23.

Simmons GC, Hall WTK, 1953, Epididymitis of rams. Preliminary studies on the occurrence and pathogenicity of a *Brucella*-like organism, *Aust Vet J*, **29**: 33–40.

Smith H, Fitzgeorge RB, 1964, The chemical basis of the virulence of *Brucella abortus*. V. The basis of intracellular survival and growth in bovine phagocytes, *Br J Exp Pathol*, **45**: 174–86.

Smith H, Keppie J et al., 1961, The chemical basis of the virulence of *Brucella abortus*. I. Isolation of *Br. abortus* from bovine foetal tissue, *Br J Exp Pathol*, **42**: 631–7.

Smith H, Keppie J et al., 1962, The chemical basis of the virulence of *Brucella abortus*. IV. Immunogenic products from *Brucella abortus* given *in vivo* and *in vitro*, *Br J Exp Pathol*, **43**: 538–48.

Snowdon WA, 1958, Opening of discussion, *Aust Vet J*, **34**: 417–23.

Solomon HM, Jackson D, 1992, Rapid diagnosis of *Brucella melitensis* in blood: some operational characteristics of the BACT/ALERT, *J Clin Microbiol*, **30**: 222–4.

Spink WW, 1956, *The Nature of Brucellosis*, University of Minnesota Press, Minneapolis.

Stableforth AW, 1936, A *Br. abortus* suspension of uniform agglutinability standardized by means of a dry stable standard anti-*abortus* serum, *J Comp Pathol*, **49**: 251–62.

Stableforth AW, 1959, Brucellosis, *Infectious Diseases of Animals: Diseases due to Bacteria*, vol. 1, eds Stableforth AW, Galloway IA, Butterworths, London, 53–159.

Stamp JT, McEwen AD et al., 1950, Enzootic abortion in ewes. I. Transmission of the disease [Possible rickettsial infection], *Vet Rec*, **62**: 251–4.

Stantić-Pavlinić M, Cec V, Mehle J, 1983, Brucellosis in spouses and the possibility of interhuman infection, *Infection*, **11**: 313–14.

Stevens MG, Pugh GW, Tabatabai LB, 1992, Effects of gamma interferon and indomethacin in preventing *Brucella abortus* infections in mice, *Infect Immun*, **60**: 4407–9.

Stoenner HG, Lackman DB, 1957, A new species of *Brucella* isolated from the desert wood rat, *Neotoma lepida* Thomas, *Am J Vet Res*, **18**: 947–51.

Stoenner HG, Holdendried R et al., 1959, The occurrence of *Coxiella burnetti*, *Brucella*, and other pathogens among fauna of the Great Salt Lake desert in Utah, *Am J Trop Med Hyg*, **8**: 590–6.

Stuart FA, Corbel MJ, 1982, Identification of a serological cross-reaction between *Brucella abortus* and *Escherichia coli* O:157, *Vet Rec*, **110**: 202–3.

Stuart FA, Corbel MJ, Brewer RA, 1987, Experimental *Brucella abortus* infection in pigs, *Vet Microbiol*, **14**: 365–79.

Sutherland SS, Evans RJ, Bathgate J, 1986, Application of an enzyme-linked immunosorbent assay in the final stages of a bovine brucellosis eradication programme, *Aust Vet J*, **63**: 412–15.

Svetic A, Jian YC et al., 1993, *Brucella abortus* induces a novel cytokine gene expression pattern characterized by elevated IL-10 and IFN-γ in CD4+ T cells, *Int Immunol*, **5**: 877–83.

Tatum FM, Detilleux PG et al., 1992, Construction of Cu-Zn superoxide dismutase deletion mutants of *Brucella abortus*: analysis of survival in vitro in epithelial and phagocytic cells and in vivo in mice, *Infect Immun*, **60**: 2863–9.

Thienpont D, Vandervelden M et al., 1961, L'Hygroma brucellique: l'aspect clinque caractéristique de la brucellose bovine au Rivanda – Burundi, *Rev Elev Med Vet Pays Trop*, **14**: 257–66.

Thomsen A, 1934, Brucella *Infection in Swine*, Levin & Munksgaard, Copenhagen.

Thomsen A, 1937, On the occurrence of copulation infection among cattle with infectious abortion, *J Comp Pathol*, **50:** 1–9.

Thomsen A, 1943, Does the bull spread infectious abortion in cattle? Experimental studies from 1936–1942, *J Comp Pathol*, **53:** 199–211.

Thornes RD, 1977, Chronic human brucellosis and anti-anergic treatment with levamisole, *Vet Rec*, **101:** 27–30.

Thornes RD, Early AM et al., 1982, Chronic brucellosis – clinical response to reduction of suppressor T lymphocytes by cyclophosphamide/prednisolone, *Irish Med J*, **75:** 423–4.

Thorpe BD, Sidwell RW et al., 1965, Brucellosis in wildlife and livestock of West Central Utah, *J Am Vet Med Assoc*, **146:** 225–32.

Tobias L, Schurig GG, Cordes DO, 1992, Comparative behaviour of *Brucella abortus* strains 19 and RB51 in the pregnant mouse, *Res Vet Sci*, **53:** 179–83.

Toshach S, 1963, Brucellosis in the Canadian Arctic, *Can J Public Health*, **54:** 271–5.

Tosi MF, Nelson TJ, 1982, *Brucella canis* infection in a 17 month-old child successfully treated with moxalactam, *J Pediatr*, **101:** 725–7.

Tovar PM, 1947, Infection and transmission of *Brucella* by ecto-parasites, *Am J Vet Res*, **8:** 138–40.

Trap D, Gaumont AJR, 1976, Le diagnostic sérologique de la brucellose bovine et ovine par l'épreuve à l'antigène tamponné, *Bull Mens Soc Vet Prat France*, **60:** 301–8.

Traum JE, 1914, *Report of the Chief of the Bureau of Animal Husbandry*, US Department of Agriculture, Washington, DC, 30.

Ünel S, Williams CF, Stableforth AW, 1969, Relative value of the agglutination test, complement fixation test and Coombs (antiglobulin) test in the detection of *Brucella melitensis* infection in sheep, *J Comp Pathol*, **79:** 155–9.

Verger JM, Grayon M, 1984, [Characteristics of 273 strains of *Brucella abortus* of African origin], *Dev Biol Stand*, **56:** 63–71.

Verger JM, Plommet M (eds), 1985, *Brucella melitensis*, A Seminar in the CEC Programme of Co-ordination of Research on Animal Pathology, held in Brussels on 14–15 November 1984, Martinus Nijhoff, Dordrecht.

Verger JM, Grimont F et al., 1985, *Brucella*, a monospecific genus as shown by deoxyribonucleic acid hybridization, *Int J Syst Bacteriol*, **35:** 292–5.

Verger JM, Grayon M et al., 1995, Comparison of the efficacy of *Brucella suis* strain 2 and *Brucella melitensis* Rev 1 live vaccines against a *Brucella melitensis* experimental infection in pregnant ewes, *Vaccine*, **13:** 191–6.

Vershilova PA, 1961, The use of live vaccine for vaccination of human beings against brucellosis in the USSR, *Bull W H O*, **24:** 85–9.

Vershilova PA, Liamkin G I et al., 1983, *Brucella* strains from mouse-like rodents in South Wartan USSR, *Int J Syst Bacteriol*, **33:** 399–400.

Weber A, 1982, I. *Brucella neotomae* II. *Brucella canis*, *Handbuch der bakteriellen Infektionen bei Tieren*, vol. 4, eds Blobel H, Schliesser T, VEB Gustav Fischer Verlag, Jena, 293–308, 329–69.

Weynants V, Godfroid J et al., 1995, Specific borne brucellosis diagnosis based on in vitro antigen-specific gamma interferon production, *J Clin Microbiol*, **33:** 706–12.

White GC, Swett PP, 1935, Bang's disease infection transmitted to a dairy herd by horses, *J Am Vet Med Assoc*, **87:** 146–50.

Wilkinson PC, 1966, Immunoglobulin patterns of antibodies against *Brucella* in man and animals, *J Immunol*, **96:** 457–67.

Williams AE, Keppie J, Smith H, 1962, The chemical basis of the virulence of *Brucella abortus*. III. Foetal erythritol a cause of the localization of *Brucella abortus* in pregnant cows, *Br J Exp Pathol*, **43:** 530–7.

Williams E, 1973, Brucellosis, *Br Med J*, **1:** 791–3.

Williams E, 1989, The Mediterranean Fever Commission: its origin and achievements, *Brucellosis: Clinical and Laboratory Aspects*, eds Young EJ, Corbel MJ, CRC Press, Boca Raton, FL, 11–23.

Wong DH, Chow CH, 1937, Group agglutinins of *Brucella abortus* and *Vibrio cholerae*, *Chin Med J*, **52:** 591–4.

Woodhead GS, Aitken AP et al., 1889, Epizootic abortion: second report of a committee appointed by the Highland and Agricultural Society of Scotland, *J Comp Pathol*, **2:** 97–105.

Wrathall AE, 1975, *Reproductive Disorders in Pigs*, Review Series No. 11, Commonwealth Bureau of Animal Health, Farnham Royal, Bucks.

Wright AE, Smith F, 1897, On the application of the serum test to the differential diagnosis of typhoid and Malta fever, *Lancet*, **1:** 656.

Wundt W, 1982, Brucellose des Menschen, *Handbuch der bakteriellen Infektionen bei Tieren*, vol. 4, eds Blobel H, Schliesser T, VEB Gustav Fischer Verlag, Jena, 408–65.

Xie X, 1986, Orally administrable brucellosis vaccine: *Brucella suis* strain 2 vaccine, *Vaccine*, **4:** 212–16.

Young EJ, 1979, *Brucella melitensis* hepatitis: the absence of granulomas, *Ann Intern Med*, **91:** 414–15.

Young EJ, 1983, Human brucellosis, *Rev Infect Dis*, **5:** 821–42.

Young EJ, 1995, An overview of human brucellosis, *Clin Infect Dis*, **21:** 283–90.

Young EJ, Corbel MJ (eds), 1989, *Brucellosis: Clinical and Laboratory Aspects*, CRC Press, Boca Raton, FL.

Zammit T, 1905, A preliminary note on the examination of the blood of goats suffering from Mediteranean Fever, *Report of the Commission on Mediterranean Fever*, part III, Harrison and Sons, London, 83.

Zhan Y, Cheers C, 1993, Endogenous gamma interferon mediates resistance to *Brucella abortus* infection, *Infect Immun*, **61:** 4899–901.

LEPTOSPIROSIS

S Faine

1 INTRODUCTION

1.1 General

Leptospirosis is an ubiquitous zoonosis, caused by infection with a spirochaete of the genus *Leptospira*. Infections have been described in all types of warm-blooded vertebrates. Mammals, marsupials and possibly birds can be infected in natural conditions, while all can be infected experimentally. Further studies of leptospirosis in cold-blooded vertebrates are required. Acute leptospirosis ranges in severity from subclinical to fatal. Animals (but seldom humans) that survive acute infection may become chronic carriers, maintaining reservoirs of leptospires in their kidneys or genital tracts. Leptospires excreted from the kidneys in urine infect other animals of the same or a different type, which then may become carriers, completing an epidemiological cycle. Humans, infected through direct or indirect contact with infected animals, are accidental and end hosts from whom transmission does not proceed further; human-to-human transmission is extremely rare, but congenital transplacental infection can occur. Among domesticated animals, genital carriers are known to transmit leptospirosis venereally, and transplacental infection is important. Alexander (1991), Watt (1992), Faine (1994a, 1994b, 1996), Torten and Marshall (1994) and Farrar (1995) have recently written major reviews.

The principles that govern the development, course and management of leptospirosis are the same in all animals. The clinical manifestations, severity and progress, and epidemiological consequences of leptospirosis differ according to the nature of the infecting leptospire, and the biology, habits and habitat of the animal species. The risks and consequences of leptospirosis for humans are determined by sociogeograph-ical considerations. It is especially hard to control transmission of leptospirosis to humans because it is a zoonosis affecting people whose lives are inextricably connected with wild or domesticated animals.

1.2 History

The classical description of leptospirosis is that of Weil's disease, a dramatic acute febrile and sometimes epidemic illness characterized by jaundice, splenomegaly and nephritis. Weil's description was by no means the first. His and other contemporary descriptions of leptospirosis as a distinct disease entity were based on clinical observations and antedated the discovery of the infectious agent by about 30 years. Meanwhile the disease was confused with yellow fever when a spirochaete was observed, but not isolated, in a tissue section from the kidney of a patient whose diagnosis was yellow fever but who had probably died of leptospirosis. Confusion persisted until the viral origin of yellow fever was established. The spirochaetal aetiology, clinical features, pathology, immune response and immunotherapy of leptospirosis were described in Japan in 1915 (Inada et al. 1916) about the same time as a similar discovery was made in Europe (Uhlenhuth and Fromme 1915). Both recognized non-icteric and milder clinical forms. The spirochaetes they both described were forms of *Leptospira interrogans* serovars *icterohaemorrhagiae* or *copenhageni*, both rat-borne. Leptospirosis in dogs was known clinically from the middle of the nineteenth century, but its cause was not known until the aetiology of Weil's disease in humans was recognized. During the 1920s to 1950s the milder forms of leptospirosis, the numerous related but distinct serotypes and the occupational relationships were elucidated in Japan, Indonesia and Germany. The significance for domesticated animals other than dogs was highlighted by work from the USA in the 1950s and 1960s, followed by the development of veterinary vaccines for serovar *pomona* at first, followed by others. In the 1970s and 1980s the ubiquitous distribution of hardjo infections in cattle and in humans involved with them were recognized. Redefinition of the occupational risks to people, clarification of the means of transmission, especially through genital carriers among animals, and improved methods for diagnosis offered by blood culture and ELISA, were the main advances. Ideas about pathogenesis, virulence, immunity and vaccine protection were refined as a result of better understanding of the microbiology of leptospires and the immunological responses in infection by them. Antibiotic therapy with penicillin coupled with modern, general diagnostic and clinical management reduced the fatality rate where these measures were available. The history of leptospirosis was reviewed in detail by Faine (1994a) and the history of the bacteria *Leptospira* by Faine (1994a; see Volume 2, Chapter 57).

2 DESCRIPTION OF THE DISEASE

General and universally applicable principles govern the mode of infection, mechanism of production of lesions, clinical features, potential outcomes, mechanisms of immunity, transmission and management. The balance of biological and ecological factors affecting the animal species, including humans, in their surroundings, determines the responses in individuals or groups. These will be indicated where appropriate to explain the differences encountered in various circumstances. Severe forms, caused (but not exclusively) by serovars *australis, autumnalis, bataviae, copenhageni, icterohaemorrhagiae, javanica,* or *lai,* are frequently fatal if untreated; their main features are jaundice, haemorrhage, potentially fatal kidney and liver failure, meningitis and a myriad of other symptoms. Some patients may have very mild anicteric and non-haemorrhagic symptoms of an infection by a serovar that can otherwise cause a severe infection. Mild forms of leptospirosis range from a febrile incapacitating illness lasting 10–20 days, comprising severe muscle pains, meningism and mild renal incapacity, to an imperceptible subclinical infection. Examples of serovars that usually cause a mild type of leptospirosis are *ballum, hardjo, grippotyphosa, pomona* and *tarassovi.*

2.1 Pathogenesis

THE AETIOLOGICAL AGENTS AND THEIR ENVIRONMENTAL ORIGINS

The aetiological agents of leptospirosis are pathogenic leptospires, which are small thin motile helical bacteria (Faine 1994a; see Volume 2, Chapter 57). Their primary source is the surface of the renal tubules in the kidney of an excreting carrier animal known variously as a 'carrier' or 'excretor'. Carrier animals pass urine containing leptospires into the surroundings, contaminating soil, ground water, or mud. Leptospires survive in moist environments at temperatures from about freezing to about 40°C. They are aquatic bacteria at home in a wet or moist environment; they die when they dry under normal environmental conditions.

PATHOGENIC MECHANISMS AND VIRULENCE

Portals of entry

Leptospires enter a fresh host from urine, water, soil or mud, by penetrating small sometimes invisible abrasions in skin or body surfaces, possibly also by inhalations of aerosols containing leptospires in microscopic droplets, and possibly through the conjunctival sac. They are believed not to penetrate skin unless it is abraded, sodden or waterlogged. Drinking or inhalation of contaminated water following immersion has caused leptospirosis. Infection via dust or in dry circumstances is unknown. Leptospires in maternal blood can infect a fetus. There is no clear evidence that the portal of entry affects the outcome. The sources of leptospires in the environment and their methods of transmission and entry to fresh animals or people are discussed below.

Entry into the host

A very small number of leptospires (1–10) can cause a fatal infection in a susceptible animal. Once in the body leptospires spread rapidly; they can be found in the bloodstream minutes after subcutaneous or intramuscular injection and almost immediately after intraperitoneal injection. Motility may play a part in their spread as the leptospires are more motile in a viscous environment, such as exists in body fluids, than they are in watery fluids.

Survival and growth

Microbiological and immunological factors affect the survival of leptospires in the body. IgM antibodies whose original stimulants are unknown react with one or more surface antigens of the non-pathogenic species *Leptospira biflexa* and with avirulent individual leptospires among those that penetrated the integument. Acting together with complement components and lysozyme (muramase) in the plasma, the IgM lyses the leptospires; the fragments are phagocytosed in the reticuloendothelial system. Virulent leptospires are not affected, and survive and grow in the body. An acute inflammatory reaction does not occur at the site of inoculation, possibly because the inocula in nature are small and the leptospires move away from the site rapidly; there is no localization of infection. If leptospires are artificially localized by injecting intradermally in a guinea pig a very large number (e.g. 10^9–10^{10}) in a small volume of 0.1 ml, a typical inflammatory reaction ensues, regardless of whether the leptospires were *L. biflexa* or virulent or avirulent pathogens. Thus failure to localize and proliferate at the site of inoculation prevents one of the significant general body defences against infection.

The body environment is very different from the wet soil or water or urine from which the invading leptospires have come. There is a large increase in salt concentration and osmotic pressure. Virulent pathogenic leptospires can survive at 37°C in culture media made isotonic with NaCl, final concentration 0.85%, where avirulent leptospires and non-pathogens die. Recently isolated pathogenic leptospires will grow after adaptation at 37°C (their usual and optimum growth temperature in the laboratory is 28–30°C). Growth at 37°C is associated with the development of heat shock proteins similar to those produced by many bacteria

(Hsp60, regulated by a *GroEL* gene). There is no evidence for nutritional selection in vivo. Chemotaxis of virulent leptospires towards haemoglobin has been reported.

A latent period, corresponding to the incubation period in clinical leptospirosis, occurs after infection or experimental inoculation, during which leptospires multiply in the body without causing major subjective or objective ill effects. Microscopic lesions and objective evidence of infection (fever, nitrogen retention) appear 3–10 days after experimental infection in hamsters or guinea pigs, inversely related to the number of leptospires inoculated, and consistent with the clinical incubation period. The growth rate in the body corresponds to a doubling time of 6–8 h. A 10-fold increase in numbers thus takes about a day. Experimentally, lesions appear when there is a threshold number of about 10^8 leptospires in the body and death occurs when there are about 10^{10} leptospires; there is a steady rate of logarithmic growth during this time in the absence of an immune response from the animal. Given that in nature inocula may be very small, these growth rates and incubation times are consistent with clinical and epidemiological outcomes.

Lesions and their cause

In mammals, marsupials and susceptible birds (chick embryos) the primary lesion in leptospirosis is disruption of the integrity of the cell membrane of the endothelial cells lining small blood vessels in all parts of the body. Capillary leakage and haemorrhages result, whose secondary effects, in turn, depend on the structure and anatomical relationships of the tissue or organ. These effects can be attributed to the action of a glycolipoprotein (GLP) toxin of leptospires, whose activity is mediated by its unusual long-chain fatty acids. Hypothetically, these may be intercalated into the cell membrane and act as competitive inhibitors of naturally occurring long-chain fatty acids, leading to membrane disruption and leakage of cytoplasmic constituents and cell death. There is evidence for the accumulation of GLP in affected tissues in leptospirosis. GLP is different from leptospiral lipopolysaccharide (LPS) in its composition and properties (Vinh et al. 1986a, 1986b, Alves et al. 1992). LPS has a chemical structure and ultramicroscopic appearance similar to that of other gram-negative bacteria, but it is not toxic and very feebly pyrogenic. Its sugar link may be different in different species of *Leptospira*, but in *Leptospira interrogans* the ketodeoxyoctulonate (KDO) link may be substituted at the C4 or C5 positions, or both. LPS plays a vital part in immunity but not in toxicity (Vinh et al. 1986b, 1989, Midwinter et al. 1994).

Vascular endothelial damage

The widespread petechial haemorrhages are apparent in all organs and tissues, but are most prominent in those where there is movement that stretches blood vessels, particularly the lungs, omentum and pericardium. Gross bleeding and large haematomata can be found. Gross pulmonary haemorrhages are characteristic of infections with serovar *lai* in China and Korea.

Ischaemia from damage to blood vessels in the renal cortex leads to renal tubular necrosis, particularly of the proximal convoluted tubules. The resulting anatomical damage causes renal failure that can be fatal. The symptom complexes of the various forms of leptospirosis can be attributed to the amount of blood vessel damage in different organs. Liver cell necrosis caused by ischaemia and destruction of hepatic architecture leads to the characteristic jaundice of the severe type of leptospirosis. Blood clotting mechanisms are affected by the liver failure, aggravating the haemorrhagic tendencies. There may also be thrombocytopenia. Leptospires accumulate in areas of haemorrhage, presumably having entered with the blood.

Clearance from the bloodstream

An immunologically competent host is not immunologically idle while these events take place. Leptospiral LPS antigens are recognized and processed to stimulate the development of IgM able to bind specifically to LPS epitopes characteristic for the serovar involved in the infection. The IgM opsonizes the leptospires so that fixed and free phagocytes engulf them in both the reticuloendothelial organs (liver, spleen, lungs, lymph nodes) and areas of haemorrhage or tissue damage where they have invaded. The effect is rapid clearance of circulating leptospires from the bloodstream, an event of prognostic and diagnostic importance. Once clearance has occurred, further and new damage will cease and recovery will commence, within the capacity of the person or animal to recover destroyed structure and function of organs and tissues. Kidney and liver tissue will regenerate provided there is sufficient function or clinical support to keep the patient alive. Similarly, myocardial damage, if not fatal, may or may not be reversible. Animals or people that survive are immune to infection with the same or related serovars. Immunity to initial infection is specific to the infecting leptospire or related strains, and may be passively transferable by convalescent or immune serum. Immunologically experienced animals or people, immunized by prior clinical or subclinical infection or immunization, use the already available specific antibodies to opsonize leptospires and clear them from the bloodstream as soon as they invade.

PERSISTENCE OF LEPTOSPIRES IN TISSUES

Leptospires are able to persist in some anatomically localized and immunologically privileged sites after antibody and phagocytes have cleared leptospires from all other sites. There is no evidence of nutritional tissue tropism. In some organs leptospires enter with extravasations of blood during the initial period of haemorrhage and vascular damage, but cannot move out once vascular endothelial integrity returns.

Renal carriers

The most significant site of persistence is the renal tubule. Leptospires appear in the kidney 2–4 weeks after acute infection, attached to and interdigitated in the brush border of the proximal renal tubular epithelial cells. There may be very dense clumps and bundles. The amount of reaction in the tissue ranges from none at all, to heavy scarring visible on the external surface as well as in histological preparations (Fig. 42.1). Since the presence of even large numbers of leptospires is not necessarily accompanied by scarring, it is reasonable to infer that the scarring results from the process of repair of the tissue and does not occur in response to the presence of the leptospires. In some animals, notably dogs and pigs, severe scarring is common in the kidneys following recovery from acute leptospirosis. Furthermore, a pale, contracted granular kidney, characteristic of chronic nephritis and accompanied by uraemia, is a sequel to infection in some animals.

Animals may excrete leptospires intermittently or regularly for periods of months or years, or for their lifetimes. Excretion rates may vary both between animals and in the same animal from time to time, from very few to 10^8 ml^{-1} of urine. Specific urinary immunoglobulins are found in urine, probably produced in the kidney. Humans do not remain carriers for long. In vegetarians or others whose urine remains alkaline, excretion may continue for weeks to months, but a prolonged renal carrier condition indicating colonization of renal tubules has not been recorded (Spinu et al. 1963). Generally the urine is free of leptospires at the time of clinical recovery.

Other sites

Leptospires enter the brain and can often be found there, perhaps indefinitely, after infection. The anterior chamber of the eye is invaded by leptospires during acute infection, but they are trapped there and cannot move out after the local vasodilation and inflammation subside. Antibody from the circulation can enter, however, and cause an acute hypersensitivity uveitis. In horses the outcome can be a condition known as 'moon blindness'. Similar sequestration can occur in the uterus and appendages in sheep and in the seminal tract in rams and boars. The mechanisms and details of localization are unclear (Watt 1990, Faine 1994a).

THE IMMUNE RESPONSE TO INFECTION

Clearance

The rate of development and timing of the appearance of the opsonizing IgM antibody is critical for the outcome. The larger the initial antigen load (that is, the size of the inoculum), the faster and sooner antibody will appear. An immunologically immature host will not make IgM at all and will be highly susceptible, as are neonatal guinea pigs and hamsters until their B cell system matures. Neonatal mice, on the other hand, are born immunologically more mature and can be infected only in the first few days after birth. Animals whose B cell immunity is suppressed with cyclophosphamide are highly susceptible, comparable with neonatal guinea pigs. T cell deficient nude mice are similar to conventional mice in their susceptibility, confirming that immunity to acute infection is B cell dependent. Cellular immunity does develop, in some animals more than others. However, the pathogenic development of leptospirosis precludes cellular immune mechanisms from a role in resistance to initial infection.

Antigens

The main, if not only, antigens involved in immunity are epitopes of the side chains of the LPS. The extent of cross-immunity between strains depends on which and how many epitopes are shared and whether they are all available, reflected in how closely they are related in serological classification by microscopic agglutination tests (MAT) that utilize LPS epitopes. In practice, there is cross-immunity mainly between members of the same serogroup, irrespective of genospecies.

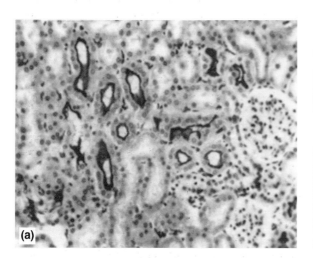
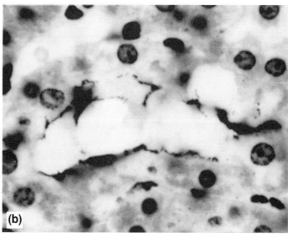

Fig. 42.1 Histological sections of the kidney of a rat carrier of leptospires identified as *L. interrogans* serovar *copenhageni*. The renal tubules are lined with a mat of darkly stained leptospires. Silver stain and haematoxylin and eosin: (a) × 100; (b) × 650. (From front cover, *The Medical Journal of Australia* 1983; Vol 1: 443. Reprinted with permission, Faine 1983, 1994a).

2.2 Modes of transmission

The reservoirs of leptospires in the organs of infected animals, from which they infect fresh hosts by direct or indirect means of transmission, are the sources of leptospirosis. Implications and control of these means of transmission are discussed elsewhere (section 3, p. 857). Humans are infected almost exclusively from sources originating in animals. Direct transmission of leptospirosis between humans is extremely rare (Fig. 42.2).

Most commonly encountered leptospires are transmitted directly from the urine of a renal excretor to another animal or person, from an acutely infected mother to her fetus, or from a chronically infected genital carrier during mating. People in selected occupations who handle infected organs or tissues can get leptospirosis from them. Indirect transmission by water, soil, mud or similar vehicles contaminated with pathogenic and virulent leptospires is common and frequent. The infection can develop at a site remote from the source. Epidemiological implications and control are discussed elsewhere (section 3, p. 857 and section 9, p. 865).

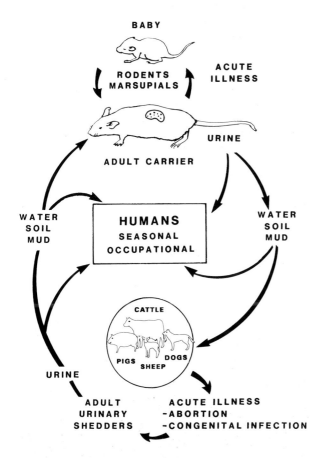

Fig. 42.2 Epidemiological cycles of leptospirosis. Leptospires are excreted in the urine of maintenance (reservoir) animals. The urine infects other animals by either direct entry or contaminated water. Humans are accidental hosts. (Reprinted with permission from Faine S, 1994a, *Leptospira* and Leptospirosis. Copyright Faine S).

2.3 Clinical manifestations

LEPTOSPIROSIS IN HUMANS

Recent reviews of leptospirosis in humans include those by Watt (1992), Faine (1994a, 1994b, 1996) and Farrar (1995).

The clinical manifestations of leptospirosis range from the imperceptible, recognized by seroconversion without illness, to severe, potentially fatal renal and liver failure accompanied by gross haemorrhage and jaundice. The presentation and outcome depend largely on the serovar of *Leptospira*. Since most strains of leptospires have been typed only by serology and not by genospecies it is not yet possible to decide whether species rather than other factors determines the clinical type of illness. In general 2 types of clinical disease can be recognized. The relatively mild type, seldom fatal in the absence of underlying renal deficiency, is short-lived, self-limiting and rarely icteric. It may result from infection with one of several serovars prominent throughout the world, including *ballum, hardjo, grippotyphosa, pomona* and *tarassovi*. The severe type of leptospirosis may be caused by serovars of the serogroup Icterohaemorrhagiae (notably *copenhageni* and *icterohaemorrhagiae*), and serovars *australis, autumnalis, bataviae, lai, pyrogenes* or related serovars in their serogroups. Some serovars almost never cause the severe type of illness. Infections with other serovars may frequently cause the most severe type of leptospirosis, but cases with mild manifestations are common. Patients with mild, non-icteric symptoms of 'severe'-type leptospirosis often do not seek medical care and are not correctly diagnosed when they do. Consequently the appearance of jaundice is not a good basis for classification of leptospirosis and statistics quoting proportions of cases with jaundice or other symptoms are usually meaningless. Similarly, mortality rates need to be scrutinized for validity.

The clinical picture in animals is similar to that in humans, modified according to the nature of the animal and its environment and the infecting type of leptospire (see section on 'Non-human leptospirosis', p. 855) (Torten and Marshall 1994).

Incubation period and onset

The incubation period, measured by experimental infection, epidemiological inferences and study of exposure incidents is usually 5–14 days, ranging from 2 to 30 days or reputedly in some publications, longer. A very sudden onset of severe headache, muscle pains and fever (38–40°C, with rigors and sweats), sometimes with red eyes (not conjunctivitis but conjunctival vasodilation), photophobia or neck stiffness, is common to all types. The muscles of the back and calves are often extremely tender. There may be a skin rash, a flushed appearance and a transient rash on the palate, and vomiting. These initial symptoms coincide with the 'septicaemic' or 'leptospiraemic' phase, lasting about 4–7 days. Symptoms resembling gastroenteritis have been described in children with leptospirosis. Leptospires circulate in the blood and can be found in the urine and sometimes in cerebrospinal fluid at this stage.

Acute leptospirosis

In mild-type leptospirosis the symptoms may then subside or continue for some days, or develop into a non-fatal 'aseptic' meningitis. Acute abdominal pains and muscle pains occur, as may ecchymotic skin rashes over the calves and elsewhere. Renal insufficiency occurs universally but seldom requires treatment unless renal function was previously inadequate. Patients usually improve to return to normal health within 3–6 weeks. Sequelae include psychiatric illness (depression, psychoses), prolonged listlessness and joint pains lasting for weeks to months. Antibiotic treatment reduces the clinical severity and duration of leptospirosis.

Patients who develop 'severe'-type leptospirosis progress from the leptospiraemic phase to the next phase, the 'tissue' or 'immune' phase, either immediately and imperceptibly, or after a brief improvement lasting 1–3 days. The fever recurs, rising quickly to 40°C or more, and the patient deteriorates rapidly as renal failure leads to uraemia and oliguria; jaundice may appear clinically or subclinically and haemorrhages may develop rapidly throughout the body. Adult respiratory distress syndrome and haemoptysis are common in infection with some serovars. The spleen and liver may be enlarged and myocarditis, meningitis and a range of other signs may develop. Treatment with high doses of penicillin at any stage can help prevent death, together with adequate supportive symptomatic treatment to compensate for renal, hepatic or myocardial failure. Patients recover if irreversible damage to vital organs is prevented (Watt et al. 1988b, 1989, 1990, O'Neil, Rickman and Lazarus 1991).

Clinical laboratory tests indicate an invariable, if transient, rise in blood urea and creatinine; in severe cases there may be very high levels. Interstitial nephritis is found if there is a renal biopsy. Urine contains erythrocytes, leucocytes, granular casts and sometimes pigment casts in the leptospiraemic phase. Serum bilirubin may rise to very high levels, but aminotransferase levels are variable. High bilirubin and normal aminotransferase suggests leptospirosis rather than hepatitis.

Diagnosis

The diagnosis of leptospirosis can easily be overlooked because the symptoms and presentation are not specific for the disease. Experienced clinicians in endemic areas, familiar with the disease, may make clinical judgements based on the symptoms, clinical laboratory findings and local epidemiology. Otherwise microbiological laboratory confirmation is required (see section 7, p. 861). There are typical foci of degenerative change in striated muscle, associated with leptospires, especially in biopsies of the gastrocnemius muscle (Fig. 42.3).

The differential diagnosis in the initial stages of the mild type includes influenza, Q fever (where that is a tenable alternative), viral meningitis and acute glomerulonephritis. Hepatitis, yellow fever (where prevalent), hantavirus and other haemorrhagic fevers, dengue, septicaemia or malaria may resemble the severe forms of leptospirosis.

Leptospirosis in pregnancy

Congenital leptospirosis, (reviewed by Faine 1994a), may affect the fetus if the mother is infected in pregnancy. In the first trimester, in humans (or the equivalent stage in animals), the fetus usually aborts, perhaps as much from the effects of the high fever as from leptospirosis. In later months the fetus may die from placentitis or systemic infection severe enough to kill it; the pathology and symptoms are similar to those in an adult and the fetus, if sufficiently immunologically mature, can develop antibodies. A congenital infection was reported where an apparently healthy child was born with leptospirosis contracted late in the mother's pregnancy; it recovered after treatment (Gsell et al. 1971).

Fatal leptospirosis

There is almost no information about pathological changes seen at autopsy of patients with the mild types of leptospirosis because they do not die from it. Diagnostic renal biopsies, usually taken too late to demonstrate leptospires by staining, show an interstitial nephritis with severe tubular degeneration. In tissues removed surgically on account of pain or haemorrhage there are characteristic extravasations of blood and associated non-specific inflammation. In severe cases, death usually occurs from renal failure, with associated liver failure and myocarditis. Death from massive pulmonary haemorrhage can also occur. The postmortem findings are severe jaundice staining all tissues and patches of haemorrhage in the skin, abdominal muscles, peritoneum, omentum and intestines. The spleen may or may not be enlarged. The liver varies in size but may be very yellow and soft. The kidneys are swollen and yellow, with prominent cortical blood vessels. There are usually haemorrhages in the lungs, prominent on the pleural surface, and on the pericardium and pleura. Similar florid pictures are seen in veterinary practice in domesticated animals and in experimental animals (Faine 1994a).

Chronic leptospirosis in humans

Humans do not usually become chronic renal carriers or excretors, but chronic headaches, fatigue or psychiatric disturbances may persist for months or years after leptospirosis. The link with leptospiral infection is not always clear but possible continuing localized infection cannot be ignored. Postmortem diagnosis is excluded because patients do not die and invasive procedures cannot be justified for diagnosis. Paralyses can persist following peripheral neuritis. Chronic eye infections (uveitis, chronic inflammation, cataract) occur, in which leptospires can be isolated from the anterior chamber of the eye (Alexander et al. 1952, Watt 1990) or identified with PCR (Mérien et al. 1993).

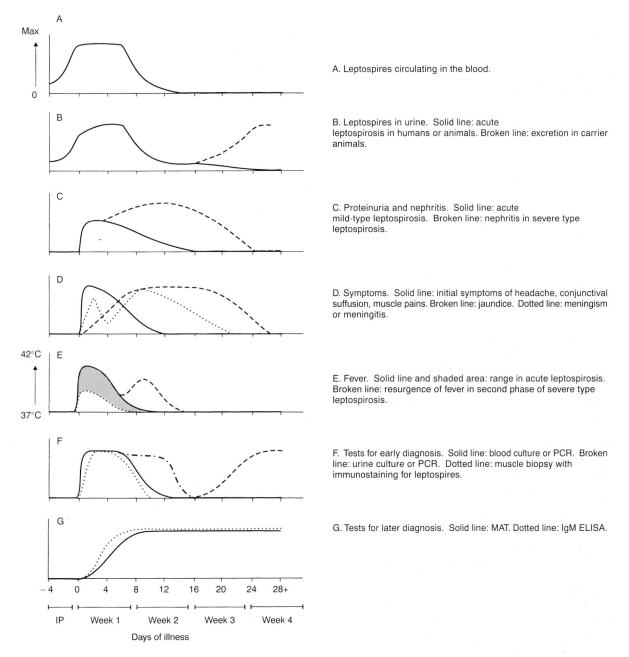

A. Leptospires circulating in the blood.

B. Leptospires in urine. Solid line: acute leptospirosis in humans or animals. Broken line: excretion in carrier animals.

C. Proteinuria and nephritis. Solid line: acute mild-type leptospirosis. Broken line: nephritis in severe type leptospirosis.

D. Symptoms. Solid line: initial symptoms of headache, conjunctival suffusion, muscle pains. Broken line: jaundice. Dotted line: meningism or meningitis.

E. Fever. Solid line and shaded area: range in acute leptospirosis. Broken line: resurgence of fever in second phase of severe type leptospirosis.

F. Tests for early diagnosis. Solid line: blood culture or PCR. Broken line: urine culture or PCR. Dotted line: muscle biopsy with immunostaining for leptospires.

G. Tests for later diagnosis. Solid line: MAT. Dotted line: IgM ELISA.

Fig. 42.3 Synopsis of clinical and diagnostic events in leptospirosis. y-Axis: arbitrary units 0–maximum, except for fever (E), scale 37–42°C. The y-axis reflects the amount of reaction that might be anticipated, not the frequency of its occurrence. IP, incubation period.

NON-HUMAN LEPTOSPIROSIS

Leptospirosis in animals has been reviewed recently by Ellis (1990), Faine (1994a) and Torten and Marshall (1994). The clinical manifestations of leptospirosis in animals are important to humans inasmuch as they depend on domesticated animals for food supplies and as beasts of burden. In some societies illness in their animals is a significant economic threat. Leptospirosis in humans and domesticated animals can come from diseased peridomestic rodents or marsupials, or from diseased wild animals for whose ecology it is also intrinsically important. Clinically apparent leptospirosis will be observed usually only in animals of economic importance where they are close to humans in and around homes or farms, or in pet animals. Listlessness, anorexia, immobility and fever are early signs, common to all animals but not pathognomonic for leptospirosis. Effects related to loss of productivity are often the first indications. They are failure to thrive, low weight gain, abortion or apparent infertility and poor milk quality or quantity. Isolated or epidemic cases of febrile jaundice, abortion, redwater in calves, or milk drop or discoloration in cows, sheep or goats, may first draw attention to the presence of acute leptospirosis. The descriptions here are necessarily brief and extreme. In any animal the signs may be less severe, ranging down to the point of being insignificant, so that the acute illness is clinically inapparent or subclinical.

Cattle, sheep, goats and other ungulates

The serovars causing acute infections throughout the world include *hardjo* (*hardjobovis*), *pomona* and *grippotyphosa*, although many others have been recorded. In addition to the signs above, the conjunctivae may be red and anaemia and diarrhoea occur. 'Redwater' (discoloured urine, from pink to dark brown, indicating acute nephritis) is seen in calves and young animals with pomona infections, accompanied by anaemia, bleeding and jaundice. Encephalitis may occur. Death from renal or hepatic failure may occur in 3–10 days, while survivors may develop chronic nephritis with poor renal function (seen as urine with low specific gravity) and excrete leptospires. There are white spots and scars on the kidneys. Animals may also become genital carriers. An outcome in pregnant cows is abortion or stillbirth, 1–3 weeks after the acute illness. The fetus, which may be jaundiced, and the placenta are highly infectious when fresh.

Pigs

Swine leptospirosis is important throughout the world because pigs are a major source of food and are often farmed in close proximity to humans. In commercial intensive pig breeding an epidemic of leptospirosis can be very expensive. The main serovars causing leptospirosis in pigs are *pomona, tarassovi, grippotyphosa, bratislava, sejroe, canicola* and *icterohaemorrhagiae* or *copenhageni*. The latter 2 usually originate from rodent infestation of the pig territory; the others are transmitted mainly between pigs, sometimes by genital carriers, usually through infected urine from excretors. Abortions or stillbirths, or congenital infection apparent at birth may be the first signs. Usually the young pigs are affected; the signs are weakness, red eyes, jaundice, anorexia and fever, with convulsions, followed by renal failure. Survivors may fail to thrive or may become carriers and excretors, or both (Ellis et al. 1985, Ellis 1991, Torten and Marshall 1994).

Dogs and cats

Serovars *canicola* (transmitted between dogs) and *icterohaemorrhagiae* (mainly transmitted from rodents to dogs) are important causes of canine leptospirosis throughout the world except Australia and New Zealand, where canicola infections are not found. Acute leptospirosis, commencing with vomiting, fever and red eyes, progresses to nephritis (arched back, immobility, blood-stained urine and faeces), dehydration and frequently, death within 4 days. Rapid collapse and death within hours characterizes a 'peracute' form of icterohaemorrhagiae infection. Feline leptospirosis is reported rarely and is clinically similar to the canine form. Dogs that survive are often renal excretors and a risk to humans close to them. Vaccination of domestic dogs is obligatory in most parts of the world.

Horses

Epidemic or isolated cases of leptospirosis, frequently due to infection with serovar *pomona*, have occurred in horses, often as congenital infections of foals, or presenting as stillbirths or abortions. The clinical picture is essentially the same as in cattle. A form of chronic recurrent eye infection (uveitis) called 'periodic ophthalmia' or 'moon blindness' may develop 2–8 months later in survivors (Poonacha et al. 1993).

Non-human primates

The clinical picture has been described in captive animals for both experimental and natural infections acquired from rodents. It is similar to that in humans (Marshall et al. 1980, Baulu, Everard and Everard 1987, Perolat et al. 1991).

Rodents and marsupials

Guinea pigs and hamsters, and some marsupials, are extremely susceptible to infection with leptospires of several serovars. Most of our understanding of the course and mechanisms of leptospirosis originates in laboratory studies in these animals. Rats and mice, on the other hand, are notoriously common and important carriers and excretors of serovars causing severe forms of leptospirosis in humans and animals but they are susceptible to infection in the laboratory only in the first few days after birth (see section 2, p. 850 and section 4, p. 859). The clinical manifestations and course of leptospirosis in guinea pigs and hamsters are very well documented, reviewed by Faine (1994a). Briefly, the signs are ruffled fur, immobility, red eyes and fever commencing about 1–3 days after inoculation, depending on the serovar and the size and virulence of the inoculum. Bloody diarrhoea, red urine, jaundice and convulsions may occur, corresponding to haemorrhages and nephritis. Death occurs in 3–7 days. The picture in neonatal mice is the same, but they become resistant to infection about 10 days after birth. The same picture is seen in feral rodents or marsupials in captivity.

Birds

Chick embryos can be infected by chorioallantoic (CA), or amniotic or yolk sac inoculation of 9–12 day eggs. Following CA inoculation, haemorrhages can be seen on the CA membrane in 3–7 days. The embryo and membranes develop haemorrhages and jaundice and the embryo may die. If it does not, it may hatch jaundiced and leptospires may circulate in the blood. It is not known whether adult birds in nature are susceptible to infection and have endemic leptospirosis (Faine 1994a).

Poikilothermic animals

Leptospirosis in poikilothermic animals has been reviewed by Minette (1983). Leptospires have been isolated from the kidneys of frogs, and fish were experimentally infected without evidence of illness (Maestrone and Benjaminson 1962). Leptospires of serovar *bim*, a common cause of leptospirosis in Barbados, were isolated there from toads (Gravekamp et al. 1991). The roles, if any, of these animals in the transmission of leptospirosis needs elucidation.

3 EPIDEMIOLOGY

Leptospirosis is a world-wide zoonosis; human sources are exceedingly rare. It is an axiom that the only people who get leptospirosis are those in direct or indirect contact with infected animals, and a corollary that those with no contact will not be exposed to risk. Similarly, an animal can acquire leptospirosis only from a source in another animal. Since the aetiological agents, sources and means of transmission are similar and comparable in all parts of the world, the geographical distribution of leptospirosis is determined by sociogeographical factors, summarized below, that mediate exposure to the sources (excretor animals and their urine).

3.1 Sources and spread of leptospirosis

FINDING ANIMAL SOURCES

The main elements in identifying the sources of clinically apparent infections are accurate and prompt diagnosis of illness in humans and animals, followed by identification of the infecting serovar. There may be precise information about recent contacts or risks involving particular suspect animals or exposure in particular situations. Local epidemiological knowledge may guide a search for domesticated, peridomestic or wild animals infected with the same serovar.

MEANS OF SPREAD BETWEEN ANIMALS AND TO HUMANS

Urine

Among rodents, direct contact with parental urine can infect very young animals in the nest, soon after birth. Freshly shed urine is a major means of infection of people who handle animals as an occupation or hobby. Urine splash and aerosol are believed to be the major means of infection of dairy farmers and milkers and also of cross-infection to other cattle. Transporters of animals, swineherds and stablehands are occupationally at risk from contact with urine. Direct infection from urine occurs wherever exposed food scraps, rubbish, or food stores are contaminated by rodents. It is a recognized risk among food industry workers (fish processors, restaurant workers) and sewer workers whose workplace is contaminated with fresh urine from excretor rodents, among veterinarians and their assistants, zoologists trapping rodents, or anyone else handling fresh contaminated urine (including children or their parents mopping up urine from dogs). There are extremely rarely recorded examples of leptospires transmitted directly between humans by urine, because humans are seldom carriers and their hygienic habits generally prevent transmission (Spinu et al. 1963).

Other direct contacts

Humans or animals may be infected by direct contact with infected tissues or organs. Occupational infections of humans from these sources occur in meatworkers (abattoir workers, meat processors and meat transporters), veterinarians, meat inspectors and farmers, and breeders and handlers of laboratory rodents.

Leptospirosis can be spread among animals by sexual contacts with genital carriers or by the use of contaminated semen for artificial insemination of animals. Transplacental infection of the fetus in pregnant animals is an important cause of loss of productivity in animal husbandry. Infection early in pregnancy results in placentitis, fetal haemorrhages, renal and liver failure, disrupted development and fetal death with consequent abortion. Leptospirosis late in pregnancy can cause abortion or stillbirth, or a congenitally infected offspring that fails to thrive, depending on the animal species, the type of leptospira and the stage of pregnancy. The conception products are heavily loaded with leptospires and are highly infectious when fresh (Ellis et al. 1985, Cousins et al. 1989, Ellis, Montgomery and McParland 1989, Poonacha et al. 1993). Transplacental infection during pregnancy in humans is well documented (Faine and Valentine 1984, Faine 1994a) and transmission by breast milk has been recorded (Bolin and Koellner 1988).

Survival of leptospires in the environment

Indirect spread can occur when leptospires remain viable long enough in aqueous surroundings for them to infect new hosts. Leptospires can survive and remain infectious for hours or days in soil, stable effluent, diluted milk (milking shed sluicings), sewage and mud (Faine 1994a; see Volume 2, Chapter 57). They can persist in soils and water apparently indefinitely, depending on acidity and soil type. It is unclear whether pathogenic leptospires grow, as well as persist, in soil and surface waters. Leptospires survive in chilled or frozen meat and meat products; kidneys sold in butcher shops for human consumption may contain viable, infectious leptospires (Peet et al. 1983).

Water

In all means of indirect transmission, urine containing leptospires contaminates ground water, flowing through to puddles or into the soil. Leptospires flow eventually into swamps, streams and rivers, in whose waters people or animals can be infected. Sometimes streams and rivers are contaminated by urine from excretor animals living in or on their banks. Generally, relatively stagnant waters, attractive to wildlife, or used by animals for drinking, are likely to be contaminated. In some areas such places are also attractive to humans as sources of water for drinking, bathing or washing clothes, for camping or for water sports that include immersion (swimming, diving, kayaking, water skiing) (Katz, Manea and Sasaki 1991). Fast flowing major rivers are also sources of leptospirosis in all climates, hazardous for local residents and visitors and for recreational white-water rafters. Wading through swamps (military activities, hunting, angling or ecotourism), rice planting and harvesting, fish farming and other agricultural activities in wet conditions are risks wherever urine from excretor animals has contaminated the environment. Other wet hazardous environments include sewers, drains, caves and mines; people working in or visiting these places are at risk. The animal sources in some of these situations are not always easily discernible.

Soil and mud

Urine from excretor animals finds its way into ground water and soaks into soil or mud. Leptospirosis has been transmitted in soil samples sent for laboratory analysis a very long distance from the source and site of contamination.

Detecting leptospires in environmental specimens

Detecting leptospires in inevitably contaminated environmental specimens of mud, soil, water or effluents is difficult. Culture is virtually impossible because of the gross contamination. Water can be filtered through a 0.22 μm membrane; leptospires will pass through. Mud and soil are agitated and homogenized in sterile water and allowed to settle. The supernatant is treated as a water sample. Immunofluorescence has been used to identify leptospires in samples of soil and mud. As always in immunostaining, the serovar or serogroup must be known or multivalent primary antibodies or mixtures must be used. In situations where such animal experimentation is justified and permitted, water and similar samples may be injected intraperitoneally into a guinea pig, in which signs of leptospirosis may develop, indicating infection with a pathogenic leptospire, that can then be cultured from the animal's tissues (Faine 1982).

LABORATORY INFECTIONS

Leptospires are relatively safe to work with in the laboratory. The usual containment measures and bacteriological precautions are sufficient. Leptospirosis is not air-borne and leptospires do not survive drying in spillages. They are very susceptible to soaps, detergents and disinfectants of all types. Unsuspected sources of laboratory infections include laboratory rats and mice (serovars *ballum, copenhageni, icterohaemorrhagiae* are reported most often) and primary tissue cultures of kidney cells from monkeys, dogs, pigs or calves, used in virology and vaccine production.

3.2 Distribution of leptospirosis and leptospires

Leptospirosis occurs everywhere but is reported only where there are knowledgeable physicians and veterinarians and epidemiologists supported by expert and specialist microbiological services. Statistics based on inaccurate diagnosis are virtually of no value.

SURVEILLANCE

Surveillance statistics are usually based on serological studies of human or animal populations. There are 2 sorts of surveillance. One sort is screening to see if leptospirosis is present in a group; the information is used for planning programmes to look for clinical cases and their animal origins. Serological tests on representative samples of the population are performed using antigens of serospecificity corresponding to those known or assumed to be prevalent. The broader the specificity of the tests the better; one is fishing with a net to see what is present. In the second sort of surveillance, where the animal sources and their serovars are known, a more precise study can be made – fishing with a hook – to find sera that react only with the serovars under study. This will provide information about the numbers of people or animals at risk from the serovar and animal sources in question, to allow planning of preventive measures. In an area where there is endemic leptospirosis and an underlying low level of seroreactivity to many serovars, information about the prevalence of leptospirosis (required for rational planning of immunization with serospecific vaccines) can come only from specific tests for a particular serovar or group of serovars identified with an animal source.

Validity of statistics

Global statistics of leptospirosis are not available and would be unreliable if they were because so much of it occurs where diagnosis and reporting are inadequate. The World Health Organization recommends that leptospirosis should be a notifiable disease. The main sources of statistics of the incidence of human leptospirosis in any location are hospital admissions and notifications from diagnostic microbiology laboratories or medical practitioners. Hospital admission statistics can be expected to be based on reasonably accurate diagnoses but will only include patients sick enough to need hospital care. They will also be biased towards the perceptions of clinical presentations like jaundice, meningitis, myocarditis and will ignore the mild forms. Practitioner notifications can rise dramatically once they recognize local occurrences, often stimulated by an epidemic that is correctly diagnosed. An indication of prevalence of current or past infection can be gained from serological surveys of populations of people or animals or both. In some places leptospirosis occurs almost exclusively in an identified section of the population exposed to animals and thus to the risk of infection. Examples are rural, rather than urban, populations in societies where rodent control is adequate in cities. In a further refinement of statistics, defined occupational groups (e.g. dairy farmers and abattoir workers) may account for nearly all the cases among the rural population. Incidence figures should then be expressed not as a proportion of the total population but as a proportion of the population at risk, in whom the incidence may be many times more than in the total population (see section 3.3).

3.3 Occupational and sociogeographical factors

This section explores the questions 'who gets leptospirosis?' and 'why, rather than how, do they get it?'. The key to the answer is social organization. The factors determining who is exposed to risks of leptospirosis are: proximity to animals likely to be excretors, numbers of animals, numbers of leptospires excreted and volume of urine, amount and nature of direct contact with animal urine or infected animals, amount of indirect contact with contaminated waters and duration of exposure. Many of these factors are mediated in turn by geography, climate, occupation, lifestyle, society and beliefs and expectations (Fig. 42.4). For example, there will be no leptospirosis among urban people who do not come into contact with animals or wet conditions, but they may be at risk if involved in travel, water sports, military activity or civil emergencies where they can be exposed to water contaminated with rodent urine, or if their job is meat inspector at an abattoir. Farmers whose animals are vaccinated and free of leptospirosis, in a wealthy community with good affordable veterinary services, run a low risk. In an Asian village where people plant rice, are constantly immersed in water and mud invariably contaminated with rodent urine and keep pigs peridomestically, leptospirosis is endemic; the population develops an underlying level of immunity to prevalent serovars. Rodent populations thrive in good harvest years, build up a large population reservoir of infected animals, and contaminate crops at the time they are harvested by hand. The new wave of leptospirosis will become epidemic if it is due to a serovar that was previously unknown locally or was recently quiescent; there will be a pool of newly susceptible people without immunity to that serovar (Fig. 42.4).

The lifestyle of most people is dictated by geographic and consequent climatic conditions, determining occupations, crops, animal husbandry, outdoor activities and proximity to wildlife. In addition to these factors, societal organization and beliefs decide the nature and organization of housing, proximity and relationships to animals (including peridomestic rodents), availability and quality of medical and veterinary services and expectations of those services. In societies where febrile illnesses are common and expectations or availability of medical services are low, leptospirosis may be only one of several diseases, some of them more widespread and serious (e.g. malaria), contributing to endemic ill health. Changes in social organization such as urbanization, clearing forests, changing crop patterns, or damming inland waterways can have very large beneficial or detrimental effects on risks of leptospirosis (Fig. 42.4).

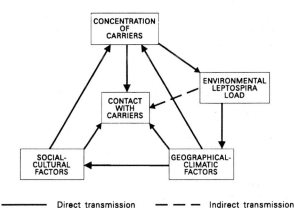

Fig. 42.4 Interplay of determinants in the epidemiology of leptospirosis. Direct or indirect contact with leptospires is essential for the development of leptospirosis in a person or animal. The interplay of factors affecting risks is represented by the arrows. (From Faine 1994a).

Some examples of sociogeographical influences from experiences on the east coast of Australia illustrate some of these principles. The climate ranges from tropical and subtropical in the north to temperate and cool in the south. Severe, frequently fatal leptospirosis due to serovars of the Australis, Autumnalis, Icterohaemorrhagiae and Pyrogenes serogroups was recognized among workers cutting sugarcane by hand in the tropical areas in the 1930s. The reservoirs were numerous species of native rodents and marsupials, living in burrows and among the debris in the cane fields. Burning of the cane fields to drive out the wildlife and dry the surface of the fields before harvest was enforced by law to reduce the incidence of fatal leptospirosis. By the 1980s sugar-cane was harvested mechanically and very few workers were employed in cane harvesting, none of them cutting by hand. Leptospirosis of the 1930s pattern disappeared; cane is no longer burnt before harvest. A different type of leptospirosis is now seen, mild leptospirosis due to *L. borgpetersenii* serovar *hardjo* (hardjobovis) that affects workers in a relatively new dairy cattle industry. More recently, more severe infections of cattle and humans with serovar *zanoni* have appeared, probably contracted by rodent or marsupial invasion of the farm environments. In the temperate dairy-farming areas of the state of Victoria, in the south, hardjo infections were diagnosed in the 1980s among farmers previously thought to encounter epidemics of influenza every year. Leptospirosis here is a disease of the wet spring and early summer, disappearing in the winter. In 1992, a wet year, there were 65 clinical cases diagnosed in a population at risk of about 5000, in a period of 4 months, corresponding to a very high annual incidence of 13 per 1000 in the population at risk. Ninety-three cases were reported for the whole of the state. Related to the total state population of about 3.5 million, about 3 million of them urban with no notifications, the incidence of leptospirosis is 93 in 3.5 million, or about 3 per 100 000 and the disease appears to be epidemiologically insignificant. In 1994, a very dry year, only about one-third of the 1992 numbers were diagnosed (Midwinter and Faine 1995).

4 HOST RESPONSE

Antibodies are produced early after infection. They are important for serological diagnosis as well as for recovery from infection and for immunity to reinfection. Serological tests are the main methods used for diagnosis (see section 7, p. 861) because leptospires are hard to see and slow to culture in the laboratory; special skills, equipment and culture media are needed to recognize and grow leptospires.

The main tests for antibodies to leptospires are the microscopic agglutination test (MAT) (read microscopically under darkfield), using a live standardized culture of leptospires as the antigen suspension, and an ELISA test, using as antigen either a sonicate of leptospires or, more commonly, boiled leptospires. In ELISA tests it is easy to determine the responding immunoglobulin (Ig) class. In all tests, the serovar-specific antigens are LPS epitopes. The MAT is more sensitive; it can detect very small amounts of Ig. The height of the titre varies according to the serovar. Titres of 800–3000 are common maxima for hardjo infection in humans, while titres of 5000–10 000 are recorded for icterohaemorrhagiae infections. Maximum titres are achieved in 2–3 weeks after infection, but some slow responders will not produce significant titres for 4–5 weeks.

The nature of the Ig and its duration in the circulation differ according to animal species. In humans, individuals differ in their responses. Usually IgM is detectable within 10 days after infection, most commonly within a week, but sometimes the appearance of antibody is delayed. In some humans, IgG never appears; in others, the initial response detected may be IgG. It is estimated that specific IgG persists after a single episode of infection for 0.5–20 years or longer, depending on the height of the initial response (Chapman et al. 1991, Lupidi et al. 1991, Palit et al. 1991). In many populations of humans and animals, continuous exposure to reinfection maintains titres at high levels indefinitely without clinical illness. Surveys of the prevalence of persistent titres can be used to estimate the prevalence of infections in a population (Palit et al. 1991).

5 CELLULAR RESPONSE

Leptospires spread throughout the body immediately on entry. The reason that they are not localized is that probably there is too small a concentration of them at the site of entry to elicit an inflammatory response before they move away. For the same reason there is no inflammatory reaction to the presence of leptospires in tissues. Whatever reaction there is late in infection results from cellular and tissue damage. Disintegrated individual leptospires are opsonized and phagocytosed before specific immunoglobulins appear, in 3–10 days. Leptospires may be killed and are opsonized, by specific immunoglobulins directed at epitopes of the LPS, before phagocytosis, appearing as spherical degeneration forms inside phagocytes of all types (Faine, 1994a; see Volume 2, Chapter 57). The immune response to leptospires is entirely B cell mediated both in initial infection and in the immediate response to reinfection with the same or similar serovars. Immature animals that cannot mount a B cell response are susceptible until the B cell system matures. There are differences in susceptibility to leptospirosis among animal species; young guinea pigs are more susceptible than mice. The difference is due to the different rates of postnatal maturation of their B cell mediated immune systems. Athymic nude mice respond to leptospiral infection in the same way as immunologically intact mice (Faine 1994a). A patient with AIDS reacted to leptospiral infection in the same way as an immunologically intact person (Neves et al. 1994).

In some animals, notably pigs and dogs, and experimentally infected mice, gross scarring and chronic inflammation may be found in the kidneys of carrier and excretors, sometimes accompanied by renal insufficiency. There is no evidence that the scarring is related to the large numbers of leptospires that can be visualized in the renal tubules, which are histologically normal in appearance. Rather, it may be a consequence of the previous damage to the renal tissue and

of an autoimmune reaction to tissue components or to leptospires that penetrate into the renal tissue (van den Ingh and Hartman 1986). Cellular immunity can be demonstrated in some animals after leptospiral infection, but there is no evidence that it operates, rather than antibody-mediated immunity, to prevent either initial or subsequent infections. Hypersensitivity to leptospiral antigens accounts for the chronic uveitis persisting after leptospirosis (Barkay and Garzozi 1984). The specific immune protective epitopes of leptospires are complexes of oligosaccharides including phosphorylated sugars and amino sugars in the LPS side chains (Jost, Adler and Faine 1989, Midwinter et al. 1994, Vinh et al. 1994).

6 AETIOLOGY

6.1 The genus *Leptospira*

Leptospirosis in humans or in animals is caused by infection with one of the thin helical bacteria that belong to the genus *Leptospira*, referred to generally as leptospires. Leptospires stain gram-negative although they can barely be seen by the usual microscopic methods; they are motile and easily visualized by darkfield microscopy. They are about 10–20 μm long and 0.5 μm in diameter. On electron microscopy, all comprise a helical body of about 0.5 μm width and a coil amplitude of 0.10–0.15 μm. A single flagellum inserted at an origin near each end is inserted through the helix. It is similar to gram-negative bacterial flagella. The helix contains cytoplasmic and genetic elements and ribosomes, within a cell wall resembling that of gram-negative bacteria. An outer envelope surrounds the cell wall. Leptospires contain a high lipid content, attributable to lipopolysaccharide (LPS) in the outer envelope. The LPS is an important antigen for immunity and diagnosis. There are 7 genospecies, *L. borgpetersenii*, *L. inadai*, *L. interrogans*, *L. kirschneri*, *L. noguchii*, *L. santarosai* and *L. weilii*, that are morphologically indistinguishable from one another and from several species of a similar genus of non-pathogenic leptospires, *L. biflexa*. Leptospires are aerobic bacteria that require long-chain fatty acids for respiration and growth. These fatty acids are also toxic (lytic) for leptospires and must be available in a non-toxic form, usually bound to an adsorbent such as serum albumin or charcoal. Growth, optimal in rate at 28–30°C, is slow; the doubling time in culture or in an animal is about 6–8 h. Liquid media are usually used for culture because growth in solid media is relatively slower to observe and not always achieved. Greywhite colonies are small at first, then expand in the medium to form subsurface circular rings up to several centimetres in diameter. Sometimes they remain discrete and fluffy. A fuller description of leptospires can be found in Volume 2, Chapter 57 and in a recent complete review (Faine 1994a).

6.2 The world-wide distribution of the aetiological agent and its relationships to its natural hosts

Leptospires are distributed throughout the world as possibly the most widespread zoonosis (Torten and Marshall 1994). There is an apparent geographical distribution of species; *L. santarosai* and *L. noguchii* strains occur almost exclusively in the Americas, while *L. weilii* occurs almost only in Europe and Asia. Several serovars appear in more than one species of leptospire. All leptospirosis arises from reservoirs of infectious leptospires residing in the renal tubules of carrier animals, which may be feral, peridomestic or domesticated. The leptospires are excreted in urine contaminated surface waters and soil, whence they pass on to new hosts.

There is a long and well documented association of certain serovars almost exclusively with particular host species in nature. These host species may be widely or narrowly distributed in the world. There is no clear biological basis for these relationships, which may also reflect chance ecological and geographic proximity of leptospires and potential host species. Nevertheless, some careful ecological studies showed that a serovar from a single reservoir animal species failed to infect other animal species sharing their habitat, contrary to other experience where cross-species infection occurs. Certain animal species cannot be infected with particular serovars; there is no common laboratory animal susceptible to lethal infection with *L. borgpetersenii* serovar *hardjo* (hardjobovis) and most cannot be made carriers. The roles of leptospiral characteristics related to their species rather than their serovars have yet to be explored. Generally speaking, rodent-borne serovars may cause either relatively mild leptospirosis in humans (serovars *ballum, grippotyphosa, hardjo, pomona*) or severe types (serovars *australis, bataviae, copenhageni, icterohaemorrhagiae, javanica*), while serovars indigenous in cattle, dogs or pigs cause only mild-type leptospirosis in humans (*canicola, grippotyphosa, hardjo, pomona, tarassovi*) but can be lethal to young animals, especially, in their reservoir hosts. (For further discussion, including contrary views, see Torten 1979 and Torten and Marshall 1994). The natural geographical distribution of host species is determined by climatic and territorial associations that evolved with changes to the earth throughout its history. The interventions of humans in the last few thousand years led to a change in distributions of animal hosts and the evolution of new relationships between leptospires and new hosts species in new habitats. Humans can become accidental hosts where they intrude into the natural environment.

7 LABORATORY DIAGNOSIS

Laboratory participation in the diagnosis is mandatory because the clinical picture is not specific in either humans or animals. Even where leptospirosis is endemic and well recognized the existence of other similar infections can confuse diagnosis. Unlike the conventional approach to the diagnosis of bacterial infections, it is not appropriate to diagnose leptospirosis by examining directly a stained specimen of pus or exudates and culturing them to look for colonies as an aid to identification of the aetiological agent. Special microscopic methods are required for visualization. Leptospires grow slowly and are cultivated only in liquid media, for practical purposes, at 28–30°C. The requirements and methods for diagnosis are similar in human and veterinary medicine. Differences are indicated where they are significant. Diagnosis is reviewed by Alexander (1991), Faine (1994a) and Torten and Marshall (1994).

Direct methods of diagnosis (microscopy, culture) including molecular methods, are important but limited. In non-endemic areas the diagnosis of leptospirosis may not be considered until the patient's illness has progressed to a point where direct methods are no longer valuable. The only means of confirming the diagnosis would then be serological (see Fig. 42.3).

7.1 Direct diagnostic methods

MICROSCOPY

Direct microscopic observation is used to look for leptospires in body fluids or environmental specimens, to check whether cultures have grown, to identify organisms in culture, and to read microscopic agglutination tests. Darkfield microscopy is the usual method, but immunostaining is useful in special circumstances mentioned below (see section on 'Immunostaining', p. 862). Electron microscopy is not used for routine tests.

Darkfield and phase contrast

Leptospires are seen as thin, bright, actively motile rods, moving with characteristic rapid spinning and jerking motility. One or both ends appear to be bent in a loop and appear to be hooked at times when movement slows or stops. Phase contrast microscopy is not used for routine purposes.

A low-power, small numerical aperture (n. a.) darkfield condenser (n. a. about 0.8) and a compatible, long working-distance objective (preferably × 20 magnification) are used with a × 10 eyepiece. An intense source of parallel light must be used and the microscope must have screws or another device for centring the condenser. The light path must be accurately aligned and the condenser focused on the plane of the object to be viewed. A drop of fluid to be examined is placed on a very clean thin slide; dirt, grease or scratches on the slide diffract light and create glare and a grey rather than black background. A thin, very clean coverglass is placed over the drop. A coverglass is not necessary or desirable for rapid examination of cultures or agglutinations, but it is essential for examination at higher objective magnifications, with shorter working distances. Oil-immersion high n. a. objectives and condensers are used only to confirm morphological details or for research; they are an impediment to routine work with wet preparations.

Immunostaining

Immunostaining can be used to find leptospires where they are scarce, or where there is extraneous material that precludes the use of darkfield microscopy, as in tissue sections or smears, or in environmental specimens. Staining with immunofluorescence is most easily visible, but immunoperoxidase and immunogold are preferred by some because fluorescence equipment is not required. Any immunostain requires a primary antibody specific for the serovar being sought, on its own or in a pool or composite mixture of antibodies to different serovars. Too many varieties in a pool will dilute any one, so high-titre antisera conjugates are required. Double staining with different fluorochrome conjugates can detect either or both of 2 serovars simultaneously.

CULTURE

Diagnostic specimens suitable for culture include blood, CSF, urine, tissue biopsies and postmortem tissue fragments, including renal cortex to identify renal carriers. Blood culture in the acute stages and urine culture are advocated for the isolation and identification of the infecting serovar. They should be attempted wherever possible (see Fig. 42.3).

Media and cultural conditions

Fluid media are used for primary culture. Greater yields and faster growth are usually obtained in Tween–albumin (oleate–albumin) media such as EMJH (Ellinghausen, McCullough, Johnson, Harris) (Faine 1994a) than in media containing rabbit serum, 8–10% v/v. The former are available commercially. Media with special supplements have been used to isolate fastidious leptospires from animal tissues, especially serovar *bratislava* from pigs (Ellis et al. 1985). Media with actidione, rifampicin, neomycin or other inhibitors have been used for primary isolation from contaminated sources, but leptospires growing in these media must be subcultured quickly into media without antibiotics to preserve their viability.

A pipette is used to inoculate media. Extreme care in aseptic technique is essential because antibiotics are not used to protect against laboratory contamination. Cultures are incubated at 28–30°C for up to 4 weeks before discarding, and examined daily for birefringent swirling growth, using oblique light against a dark background. Suspicious growth is confirmed by darkfield, recalling that fibrin threads can look like leptospires, even to experienced observers. Growth is never heavily turbid; if it is, one should suspect contamination with other bacteria. Maximum density occurs in 3–10 days, but may be delayed much longer. Subcultures are made into fluid medium when growth is detected, both to maintain viability and as a precaution against contamination by slow-growing micro-organisms. Subculture to solid media is not used routinely, except to check for contaminants. Non-pathogenic filter-passing leptospiral contaminants have been encountered where water or utensils that were not sterilized by heat were used for preparing media. Attempts can be made to purify contaminated cultures by several means. The contaminated culture can be filtered through a cellulose filter of average pore diameter (APD) 0.22 μm; leptospires pass the filter and will grow from the filtrate. A point in the centre of a plate of solid medium can be inoculated; the leptospires migrate out in a circle and can be subcultured free of contaminants from the centrifugally advancing ring of growth.

A mouse, guinea pig or hamster can be injected intraperitoneally with the contaminated culture and bled by heart puncture under anaesthetic about 20–60 min after injection. The leptospires enter the circulation rapidly, in advance of any other bacteria, and can be grown from the heart blood.

Identification of isolates

The questions to be asked are: is it a *Leptospira*, is it a pathogen, what serovar and serogroup, and what species, type or subgroup? Leptospires are identified by morphology and growth characteristics. Non-pathogens will grow at lower temperatures of 11–13°C, grow in 8-azaguanine or 2,6-diaminopurine and produce lipases. No pathogen has all of these attributes. A battery of reference antisera is the first requirement for serotyping. Pools of sera whose components are representative of the known serogroups are used to agglutinate the new isolate. The components of a reactive group of antisera are then tested individually until one is found that agglutinates the new isolate to the titre of the antiserum, perhaps uniquely; low-titre cross-reactions are common. Identification beyond this presumptive level is done only in reference laboratories. It is necessary to prepare a rabbit antiserum to the isolate and to use one or more reference strains of the suspected serovar and their antisera. The antisera to the new and the reference strains are cross-absorbed and retitrated. The strains are considered to belong to the same serovar if the residual titre is less than 10% of the original titre. Batteries of monoclonals, that will react in a pattern characteristic of a serovar, can also be used (Dikken and Kmety 1978, Korver et al. 1988, Alexander 1991, Faine 1994a).

Serovar-specific probes for use with PCR are being developed and are available for some serogroups in random amplified polymorphic DNA fingerprinting (RAPD) (Ralph et al. 1993, Gerritsen et al. 1995). Molecular methods that correlate less precisely with serovar include analysis and comparisons of patterns after electrophoresis of DNA on gels (restriction length fragment polymorphism, RFLP). Fatty acid methyl ester (FAME) profiles analysed by gas chromatography can also be used for the chemotaxonomic identification of leptospires (Cacciapuoti, Ciceroni and Attard-Barbini 1991, Ellis 1995).

The leptospiral species is determined by DNA–DNA homology as the reference method (Yasuda et al. 1987, Ramadass et al. 1992). Comparable results can be achieved by the simpler pulse-field electrophoresis analysis of *Not*I digests, mapped restriction site polymorphism PCR (MRSP) and arbitrarily primed PCR (APPCR) (Ralph et al. 1993).

MOLECULAR METHODS FOR DIAGNOSIS OF LEPTOSPIROSIS

Direct PCR on specimens of body fluids enables rapid specific and direct diagnosis, at least in the early and convalescent stages of infection (van Eys et al. 1989, Mérien et al. 1992, 1993, Gravekamp et al. 1993). The reaction detects leptospiral DNA in the specimen, down to extremely small amounts equivalent to the DNA content of about 10 leptospires, or less. Some tests use serovar-specific probes. The oligonucleotide composition of various primers have been published and the subject is developing rapidly at the time of writing. It is not clear how long leptospiral DNA persists in the body after infection; some publications suggest that it is for much longer than is assumed. At present molecular diagnosis with PCR is not seen to be suitable for diagnosis in the later or convalescent stages of leptospirosis, or for retrospective diagnosis.

7.2 Serological and other indirect methods

Tests on patients' or animals' sera for antibodies to leptospires are used as the main means of diagnosis. Within the limits of cross-reactions between serovars, serological tests can be a guide to the infecting serovar; this information is an advantage for prognosis and epidemiology. The infecting serovar cannot be identified reliably as the serovar to which the patient's serum reacts with the highest titre. Serological tests do not react until a few days after infection, but reactions persist for months or years. Persistent antibodies allow retrospective diagnosis, including confirmation for workers compensation or similar legal purposes that a previous illness was leptospirosis. People or animals exposed regularly to one or more forms of leptospirosis retain antibodies at a relatively low level indefinitely, confusing the diagnosis of a fresh illness that might be leptospirosis and affecting the interpretation of further serological results. In all tests using agglutination or antibodies involved in agglutination, including ELISA tests, the significant reacting epitopes of the leptospires are oligosaccharides that are part of the LPS.

TESTS AND INTERPRETATIONS

The tests used most widely are microscopic agglutination tests (MAT) and ELISA. ELISA derivatives such as immunoblots are useful (Watt et al. 1988a) but are mainly used for experimental purposes. Macroscopic agglutination on slides is used by some as a preliminary screening test; it should not be used for final diagnosis. Other tests such as complement fixation, immune haemolysis or haemagglutination, latex particle agglutination and platelet adhesion are of historical interest only, although some continue to use the first 2.

MICROSCOPIC AGGLUTINATION TEST (MAT)

The MAT is slow, tedious, potentially biohazardous, painstaking and subjective, but very sensitive and reliable when used by skilled people. Preparation for it requires the meticulous curating of a collection of strains used alive as antigen suspensions in the tests, their regular subculture and quality control for authenticity, purity, agglutination and skilled educated personnel. A recent advance is the use of standardized preparations of dried leptospires available to accredited diagnostic laboratories from a central reference laboratory. The test is performed by titrating dilutions of antisera, usually in several rows in parallel in a microtitration tray, in doubling dilutions starting from a 2-fold or a 10-fold dilution. An equal volume of antigen is added to each dilution and the tray incubated covered at room temperature or 30°C or 37°C (the temperature is not critical) for 2 h. The antigen is a live culture, standardized for density, of a leptospiral serovar representative of a serogroup. Each serogroup

prevalent locally should be represented. Reference laboratories may test sera against all serogroups where the serogroup is not known. After incubation a drop of each well is taken out with a loop, placed on a slide and checked microscopically under darkfield for agglutination. The end point is 50% agglutination, assessed visually and semiquantitatively by comparison with dilutions of the antigen without sera.

Interpretation of diagnostic MAT

In a non-endemic area a level of antibodies, however low, may signify leptospirosis in the first week of a clinically compatible illness. The titre will rise in a second specimen taken after 3–7 days. If the titre remains below 100, even on repeated testing, it may be assumed that it was due to previous leptospirosis unrelated to the current illness. A titre of 400–800 is considered to be significant for an initial infection, rising to 1000–10 000 in later sera. A single titre of 400 or more, or a 4-fold rise in titre between 2 tests, is diagnostic in the presence of a clinical illness compatible with leptospirosis. In endemic areas, MAT titres from previous infections with the same or different serovars may persist in people or animals. A diagnosis of leptospirosis will be confirmed if the titre rises on retesting, but will be negated if it is unchanged, assuming that the infecting serovar was included among the antigens for the MAT. A check-list for diagnosis was published (Faine 1982, 1994a). A high starting dilution of 1 in 100 is sometimes used in endemic areas because most people or animals will have low-level titres not related to the current illness. Only high or rising titres are considered clinically significant for diagnosis. This reasoning is fallacious in non-endemic areas, where the lowest starting dilutions should be used. Even the lowest titre in a serum taken early in the illness can be an important pointer to justify treatment as leptospirosis; in a patient with acute leptospirosis the titre will have risen sometimes dramatically, on retesting after 2–3 days.

ENZYME-LINKED IMMUNOSORBENT ASSAYS (ELISA) AND THEIR INTERPRETATION

Serological diagnosis of leptospirosis, type unspecified, as early in the illness as possible, is advantageous. Serovar-unspecified diagnosis of leptospirosis can be accelerated by using an ELISA test directed specifically at IgM. IgM ELISA-reactive antibodies appear a day or so earlier than those detectable by MAT, in some laboratories. IgG or unspecified class Ig ELISA tests are also valuable for diagnosis but they sometimes react only at a late stage. The tests can be done by any laboratory able to perform ELISA tests if the antigens and conjugates are available. Sera either may be titrated, or tested at one or more recommended dilutions. The test system must be sensitive enough to detect the relatively small amount of antibody found early. If it is not, it can mislead diagnosis; MAT, which is often more sensitive, would be better. There is often poor correlation between ELISA and MAT results on sera of individuals. The reference standard is MAT (Terpstra 1992).

ELISA tests are evaluated by calibration with a batch of sera known to be reactive or not reactive to MAT; serospecificity is not involved directly. A 'positive' ELISA means that the serum reacts at a level consistent with titres to MAT in leptospirosis patients. ELISA results may be expressed as 'positive' or 'negative', based on optical density readings of fixed dilutions, or as 'reactive' at a certain titre. In either case the effect is the same.

7.3 Screening tests and surveillance

Serological tests are used for surveillance to ascertain how many people or animals in a population have had leptospirosis and to what serovars they react. Epidemiological needs decide who or which animals to test and which serovars should be represented in the tests. Either MAT or ELISA may be used; the former is more labour-intensive. Slide agglutination tests are not recommended. Most information is obtained by starting with a low serum dilution for MAT, or including low-level ELISA reactions, because the aim is to detect, not to exclude, reactors. Reactors can be grouped later by level of reaction, serovar reactivity and personal or epidemiological criteria.

7.4 Summary of diagnostic tests and when to use them

SPECIMENS TO COLLECT AND TEST EARLY IN THE ILLNESS

The terms 'early', 'late' and 'onset' need to be defined in leptospirosis in 2 different but overlapping time-scales, the pathogenic and the clinical. The pathogenic time-scale dates from the moment of infection and includes the incubation period. The usual, clinical, time-scale refers to the onset of symptoms as the beginning of illness. The time taken for a patient to get medical advice and management depends on social as much as medical factors, as does a decision to treat a patient in hospital or a clinic rather than at home, or indeed, at all. The value of diagnostic tests depends on the pathogenic stage of illness. Tests suitable for a febrile leptospiraemic patient a day or 2 after the onset of headache and myalgia are likely to be inappropriate, perhaps useless for a patient not admitted to hospital until in terminal renal and hepatic failure, 7 days after the onset of symptoms, but still regarded as an acute case diagnosed relatively early. Nevertheless, a timetable of useful tests can be compiled (see Fig. 42.3).

In the first 7–10 days or so, during the fever and leptospiraemia, leptospires can be found in blood, urine, CSF, pleural or peritoneal fluid and sometimes in acute exudates into joints. They are not found in faeces, or in sputum except in massive haemoptysis. In congenital maternally transmitted infection the placenta and fetal membranes contain leptospires.

Direct microscopic examination of blood is rarely productive; it is not recommended, but direct PCR is valuable. Urine must be alkaline, or passed after alkalinization of the patient. It may be centrifuged and examined by darkfield, or the sediment cultured, or both. Leptospires can usually be grown in blood culture, taking 5–10 ml aseptically and inoculating volumes of not more than 0.5 ml into volumes of 5–10 ml EMJH or other medium containing sodium polyanethane sulphonate (Liquoid®) 0.5–1.0%, with β-lactamase if the patient has been treated with penicillin. CSF may be examined microscopically or cultured like blood. In all cases fibrin threads may resemble leptospires and trap the uncritical observer. Examination of specimens for leptospires by microscopy or culture should be repeated throughout the febrile period. Immunofluorescence staining and PCR are also most likely to be positive at this time. A serum sample for MAT also should be taken as soon as possible as a baseline for interpreting the titre in subsequent tests. It usually will be negative, in non-endemic areas, until the second week. Examination of the first serum sample should not be delayed until a paired specimen taken later is available; a reaction at the earliest time is useful for guiding management.

SPECIMENS TO TEST LATER

Blood for serology and tissues for examination

During and after the second week of illness, the main specimen to take is blood for serology. Blood culture is unlikely to grow leptospires, especially in the third week or later. Leptospires are sparse, if present, in urine during the second to third week. They are unlikely to be found in CSF after the first 7–10 days, even in meningitic patients, but the CSF may react in MAT. In fatal cases leptospires can be found in tissues during weeks 2–3; characteristic leptospiral shapes, degeneration forms and amorphous antigenic material can be stained by immunofluorescence in liver, kidneys, areas of haemorrhage and other sites. PCR-based diagnostic methods should be useful at this stage. Tissue removed for biopsy should be tested for leptospires by culture in the first 10 days and by immunostaining at any time. Urinary antibody can be found sometimes in animals after this time; its presence may be correlated with excretion.

Congenital and fetal leptospirosis

Aborted material will contain leptospires at the time of fetal death, but they will deteriorate and be non-viable, and even invisible, as tissues autolyse. Particularly in veterinary practice it may be impossible to visualize leptospires in fetal membranes and tissues on account of delays and contamination before examination. Culture in media for fastidious leptospires containing inhibitors of bacterial growth can help isolate the causal leptospires in animal abortions. Leptospires can be seen microscopically in the lesions of placentitis and in the fetus in late human congenital infection and cultured from these sites where examinations can be made under ideal conditions.

Examination of urine in carrier and excretor animals

Urine samples can be obtained by standard veterinary

clinical methods; the diuretic drug frusemide (furosemide) may be administered to promote urination. Darkfield examination is useful only where there are many leptospires. Cultures in selective media containing actidione and other inhibitors of bacterial growth are recommended (see section 7.1, p. 861). It is hard to find very small numbers of leptospires microscopically or by culture, but PCR methods in development offer promise.

Examination of kidneys from suspected carriers

Animal kidneys for examination should be excised aseptically at autopsy if possible. Slaughterhouse kidneys should be chilled and removed in a clean container. Kidneys from dead animals in the field may be autolysed and contaminated; the chances of finding leptospires are small, although PCR methods may help.

The kidneys are observed by eye for surface changes, such as scars, white or grey spots and general size and appearance. Dull, pale, granular, shrunken kidneys are seen in animals with gross nephritis. Scars and inflammation may be visible on the cut surface. Leptospires may be found by microscopy or culture. Scarred areas in or near the cortex are excised for histological examination. Clumps of leptospires can be seen lining groups of renal tubules at the corticomedullary junction, in histological sections stained by immunofluorescence of silver deposition, examined with a × 40 or similar dry objective. Where there are few leptospires, not in easily visible clumps, they may be detected with an oil-immersion × 60 or × 100 objective (see Fig. 42.1). Various methods have been recommended for culturing carrier kidneys, all requiring the exposure and sampling of the corticomedullary area. They include scraping with a serrated scraper, slicing with a scalpel or razor blade, and taking plugs of tissue with a Pasteur pipette. The kidneys of small rodents can be ground in a sterile tube with a plunger, with a little sterile phosphate buffered saline, pH 7.2, or culture medium. The contents are allowed to settle after the plunger is withdrawn and the supernatant examined microscopically and cultured. The volume of material added to the culture tube must be small (0.1 ml of tissue is suggested) because too much autolysing tissue in the culture medium will make it anaerobic and stop leptospires from growing.

8 GENERAL APPROACHES TO TREATMENT

8.1 General medical treatment and management

General supportive measures are vital. In humans, in the early stages and in mild leptospirosis, alleviation of the muscle pains, headaches and fever is essential, as are fluids to correct dehydration from vomiting. Symptomatic treatment is required for renal and liver failure, myocarditis, meningitis and pulmonary symptoms and haemorrhages elsewhere.

8.2 Antibiotic therapy and chemoprophylaxis

Leptospirosis in all its forms is amenable to treatment with antibiotics. Leptospires are susceptible in laboratory tests to all clinically useful antibiotics except chloramphenicol and rifampicin. Leptospires are not usually cultivated and tested for susceptibility in individual cases. Resistance in clinical use has not been reported, although, rarely, failures of treatment have been suggested. The antibiotics most usually recommended are penicillin, in high doses, unless the patient is hypersensitive to penicillin, in which case erythromycin is used. Tetracyclines are used, but have disadvantages and are contraindicated in people with renal insufficiency, children and in pregnancy. Doxycycline is recommended for treatment (McClain et al. 1984) and short-term chemoprophylaxis (Takafuji et al. 1984). Penicillin should be administered as early as possible, during the leptospiraemic phase, parenterally in very ill patients. No antibiotic can reverse the destructive effects of leptospirosis in tissues and organs, but penicillin was found to have beneficial effects, reducing mortality and duration of illness in severe leptospirosis, when given intravenously at even a late stage (Watt et al. 1988b). Antibiotic treatment may be accompanied by a Jarisch–Herxheimer reaction (a transient increase in fever and severity of symptoms immediately following treatment), which does not contraindicate continued administration of antibiotics (Friedland and Warrell 1991, Vaughan et al. 1994).

ANTIBIOTIC TREATMENT OF CARRIER ANIMALS

Streptomycin and dihydrostreptomycin treatment can eradicate leptospires from renal carrier cattle and pigs. Penicillin is also effective but not used because of the risks of antibiotic residues remaining in milk or meat. Antibiotic treatment is expensive and reserved for situations where it is economically justifiable. Semen used for artificial insemination may be treated with streptomycin and penicillin to protect recipient animals from the potential transmission of leptospirosis.

8.3 Immunotherapy

In the days before antibiotics immunotherapy with animal antisera was used. More recently it was used in some countries, but there is no indication for it and every reason to condemn it.

9 PREVENTION AND TRANSMISSIBILITY

Prevention of leptospirosis in all situations is not possible because it is widespread in so many animals and places all over the world. The best that can be done is to limit the effects of leptospirosis on humans and the animals they depend on. To do this one has to find the sources, contain them and eliminate them or their effects. More detailed recommendations for control programmes have been published (Faine 1982, 1994a).

9.1 Identification of sources

The first step in control is to recognize and understand the problem. Indications that leptospirosis occurs come from correctly diagnosed sick people or animals, or from surveys. All of these depend on accurate laboratory studies, for which the first requirement is laboratory expertise and quality assurance. Hospital, clinic or practitioner records can point to known or suspected leptospirosis. Clusters of cases can suggest a common source; a similar infection in several children who all swam in a stagnant river pool at the same time is an easy clue. The prevalent serovar or serovars can likewise suggest animal reservoirs. A history of contact with animals may not be obvious to the patient or relatives, especially where infection has occurred remote from the animal source, from surface waters, or during occupational or recreational travel or pursuits. Where contact with peridomestic and feral animals is part of the way of life, no particular animal can be incriminated unless the leptospires are isolated and their serovars matched with those of the suspected source animal; molecular epidemiology for leptospirosis is in its infancy.

9.2 Principles of prevention

CONTAINMENT

Containment implies a notional barrier around sources of leptospirosis, particularly infected animals and contaminated wet areas. Where people or animals must be exposed to risk, a mental (educational), physical or spatial barrier can be interposed.

Avoidance and education

The way to avoid leptospirosis is to keep away from animals and areas that may be contaminated by their urine. This advice is relevant for people in cities where there is good rodent and canine control, whose occupational, leisure or travel activities do not involve them in direct or indirect contact with potential animal reservoirs. In most of the world, especially where people live closely associated with their animals in village communities in rural settings, this counsel of perfection is not appropriate. The main measures to protect them are education, rodent control, protective clothing where acceptable and appropriate, and immunization.

Similar principles apply to the protection of animals. Cattle and pigs in herds known to be free of leptospirosis can be protected from infection by screening fresh animals to be added to the herds and ensuring total rodent control. Mass serological screening of animals before transport between locations is used widely. Attempts to develop and maintain leptospirosis-free herds have been unsuccessful in the long term. Immunization is discussed below (see section on 'Active protection – immunization and chemoprophylaxis', p. 867).

Leptospirosis is part of the ecology of wildlife; human intervention is not required. Changes in the environment resulting from human activities, such as construction of dams, drainage of swamps, or destruction of forests, can alter the ecological balance between animals and the landscape, affecting the equilibria of animal populations and leptospirosis. Insofar as these population changes may impinge on risks to humans or domesticated animals, they are significant for the epidemiology of animal and human leptospirosis.

Awareness of leptospirosis can prevent it. People whose occupations, travel or hobbies involve risks should know of the disease and how to avoid it. The main groups at risk are dairy farmers and milkers (especially those working in shallow trenches in 'herring-bone'-type milking sheds), at risk from hardjo infections transmitted from cows; abattoir workers, meat inspectors, veterinarians and transporters in meat industries; people who work habitually in wet occupations (rice farmer, sugar-cane harvesters, drainers, sewer workers, miners); and adventure travellers (cave exploration, white-water rafting, water sports) and military or civil emergency personnel. People should be aware of the dangers and dissuaded from swimming in rivers or pools known to be contaminated. Education through industry or community self-help groups can raise awareness and prevent infections in humans and the animals they keep. Medical and veterinary professional groups are not immune to the need for special education about leptospirosis. The most compelling advocates for the control of leptospirosis are people who have been patients themselves.

Rodent control

Even in urban centres civil emergencies that break drains and sewers, from which rats and effluent emerge, break the spatial barrier between them and urban dwellers. Rat control in and around food storage and preparation areas, crops, stables, milking sheds, intensive animal production installations and dwellings is difficult but will remove a major source of leptospirosis for humans and domesticated animals. Rodent and marsupial carriers intermingle with domesticated animals in field grazing conditions. Managing the domesticated animals out of the range of the wildlife perimeter, if feasible, can provide a dubious barrier.

Treatment of carriers

Antibiotic treatment of carriers is successful (Gerritsen et al. 1994) but considered to be expensive, often limited in application to breeding stock. Proof of success is difficult when leptospires are excreted irregularly and sometimes in very small numbers.

Protective clothing and occupational hygiene

An effective but controversial method of protection for humans is the wearing of protective clothing, controversial because of its cost and because it is usually uncomfortable and unacceptable in the hot climatic or workplace environments where it is needed. Protective equipment for most industries includes rubber or other impermeable knee-high boots, impermeable aprons and gloves and face masks or eye protection. Smoking while working should be prohibited. Cuts and scratches should be covered. The principle is to protect skin from wet conditions contaminated with urine or effluent.

ACTIVE PROTECTION – IMMUNIZATION AND CHEMOPROPHYLAXIS

Immunization of animals

The purposes of immunization of domesticated food and breeding animals are to protect them from leptospirosis so that productivity is maximized and to protect humans in contact with the animals. Dogs are immunized to protect them and human contacts. Effective vaccines containing suspensions of killed *L. borgpetersenii* serovar *hardjo* (hardjobovis) and *L. interrogans* serovar *pomona* are widely available commercially. The use of locally prevalent strains is recommended, because there may be differences in cross-immunity between serologically similar strains. Vaccines licensed for use according to international protocols are tested on natural target animals after laboratory tests have been completed. The cultures for vaccines are sometimes grown in protein-free media to minimize reactions to culture medium proteins on repeated vaccination; the recipes for most of these media are commercial secrets or patents. Cattle (*hardjo* and *pomona*) and pigs (*pomona*) are the main target animals. The vaccines are given subcutaneously or intramuscularly in 2 initial doses, one month apart, followed by annual boosters. Herding, labour and vaccine costs for cattle can be substantial. To the extent that vaccination of herds can reduce the number of animals excreting, it is a protective measure for humans exposed to bovine sources of leptospirosis.

Similarly, protection of pigs by reducing the excretor population protects pig farmers and pig meat industry workers. Licensed vaccines are not available for unusual serovars affecting a small population of animals to be immunized.

Immunization of humans

Vaccines composed of killed cultures of leptospires protect people against leptospirosis. Washing or ultrafiltration are used to remove unwanted proteins from the culture medium. Nevertheless, these vaccines may cause side effects ranging from local soreness to fever and incapacity for a few days. Two doses are given subcutaneously, 3–4 weeks apart, followed by annual boosters. Multivalent combinations effective against several serovars are compounded as required by local needs. They are available to selected high-risk groups where the side effects are preferable to severe leptospirosis. In Asia they are used more widely in exposed populations (Chen 1985, 1986, Tang 1991). Work is progressing towards a non-toxic vaccine based on requisite LPS epitopes.

CHEMOPROPHYLAXIS

Doxycycline can prevent leptospirosis if given before and during exposure. Prolonged administration is not recommended.

OCCUPATIONAL HYGIENE

People who have contact with leptospires or animals should be advised how to reduce risks of leptospirosis. All workers employed with hazardous animals should be aware of the risks. Wildlife trappers and zoologists should wear impermeable gloves to protect themselves from urine entering the inevitable scratches on their hands (Looke 1986). Protective clothing should be available to all workers and farmers at risk, and travellers and military personnel as needed. Part of the occupational training should include instruction in how to manage accidents or other emergencies and bites which may enhance the risks of leptospirosis. Laboratory workers should understand the biohazards and be trained to work with cultures and handle laboratory animals safely.

REFERENCES

Alexander AD, 1991, Leptospira, *Manual of Clinical Microbiology*, 5th edn, eds Balows A, Hausler WJ et al., American Society for Microbiology, Washington, 554–9.

Alexander AD, Baer A et al., 1952, Leptospiral uveitis. Report of a bacteriogically verified case, *Ann Ophthalmol*, **48**: 292–7.

Alves VA, Gayotto LC et al., 1992, Leptospiral antigens in the liver of experimentally infected guinea pig and their relation to the morphogenesis of liver damage, *Exp Toxicol Pathol*, **44**: 425–34.

Barkay S, Garzozi H, 1984, Leptospirosis and uveitis, *Ann Ophthalmol*, **16**: 164–8.

Baulu J, Everard COR, Everard JD, 1987, Leptospires in vervet monkeys (*Cercopithecus aethiops sabaeus*) on Barbados, *J Wildl Dis*, **23**: 60–6.

Bolin CA, Koellner P, 1988, Human-to-human transmission of *Leptospira interrogans* by milk, *J Infect Dis*, **158**: 246–7.

Cacciapuoti B, Ciceroni L, Attard-Barbini D, 1991, Fatty acid profiles, a chemotaxonomic key for the classification of strains of the family *Leptospiraceae*, *Int J Syst Bacteriol*, **41**: 295–300.

Chapman AC, Everard COR et al., 1991, Antigens recognized by the human immune response to severe leptospirosis in Barbados, *Epidemiol Infect*, **107**: 143–55.

Chen TZ, 1985, Development and situation of and techniques for production of leptospirosis vaccine in China, *Jpn J Bacteriol*, **40**: 755–62.

Chen TZ, 1986, Development and present status of leptospiral vaccine and technology of production of the vaccine in China, *Ann Immunol Hung*, **26**: 125–51.

Cousins DV, Ellis TM et al., 1989, Evidence for sheep as a maintenance host for *Leptospira interrogans* serovar *hardjo*, *Vet Rec*, **124**: 123–4.

Dikken H, Kmety E, 1978, Serological typing methods of leptospires, *Methods in Microbiology*, vol. 11, eds Bergan T, Norris R, Academic Press, New York, 260–95.

Ellis WA, 1990, Leptospirosis: a review of veterinary aspects, *Ir Vet News*, **12**: 6–12.

Ellis WA, 1991, *Leptospira interrogans* serovar *bratislava* infection in domestic animals, *Leptospirosis. Proceedings of the Leptospirosis*

Research Conference 1990, ed. Kobayashi Y, Hokusen-Sha, Tokyo, 20–33.

Ellis WA, 1995, International Committee on Systematic Bacteriology. Subcommittee on the Taxonomy of *Leptospira*. Minutes of the Meetings, 1 and 2 July 1994, Prague, Czech Republic, *Int J Syst Bacteriol*, **45:** 872–4.

Ellis WA, Montgomery JM, McParland PJ, 1989, An experimental study with a *Leptospira interrogans* serovar *bratislava* vaccine, *Vet Rec*, **125:** 319–21.

Ellis WA, McParland PJ et al., 1985, Leptospires in pig urogenital tracts and fetuses, *Vet Rec*, **117:** 66–7.

van Eys GJJM, Gravenkamp C et al., 1989, Detection of leptospires in urine by polymerase chain reaction, *J Clin Microbiol*, **27:** 2258–62.

Faine S (ed.), 1982, *Guidelines for the Control of Leptospirosis*, WHO Offset Publication No. 67, World Health Organization, Geneva, 1–171.

Faine S, 1983, Is leptospirosis a 'rare' disease?, *Med J Aust*, **1:** 445–6.

Faine S, 1994a, *Leptospira and Leptospirosis*, CRC Press, Boca Raton, FL, USA.

Faine S, 1994b, Leptospirosis, *Infectious Diseases*, 5th edn, eds Hoeprich PD, Jordan MC, Roland AR, Lippincott, Philadelphia, USA, 619–25.

Faine S, 1996, Leptospirosis, *Bacterial Infections of Humans. Epidemiology and Control*, 3rd edn, eds Evans AS, Brachman PS, Plenum Medical, New York, In Press.

Faine S, Valentine R, 1984, Leptospirosis hardjo in pregnancy, *Med J Aust*, **140:** 311–12.

Farrar WE, 1995, Leptospira species (leptospirosis), *Principles and Practice of Infectious Diseases*, vol. 2, 4th edn, eds Mandell GL, Bennett JE, Dolin R, Churchill Livingstone, New York, 2137–41.

Friedland JS, Warrell DA, 1991, The Jarisch–Herxheimer reaction in leptospirosis: possible pathogenesis and review, *Rev Infect Dis*, **13:** 207–10.

Gerritsen MA, Smits MA, Olyhoek T, 1995, Random amplified polymorphic DNA fingerprinting for rapid identification of leptospira of serogroup Sejroe, *J Med Microbiol*, **42:** 336–9.

Gerritsen MJ, Koopmans MJ et al., 1994, Effective treatment with dihydrostreptomycin of naturally infected cows shedding *Leptospira interrogans* serovar *hardjo* subtype hardjobovis, *Am J Vet Res*, **55:** 339–43.

Gravekamp C, Korver H et al., 1991, Leptospires isolated from toads and frogs on the island of Barbados, *Zentrabl Bakteriol Parasitenkd Infektionskr Hyg Abt I Orig*, **275:** 403–11.

Gravekamp C, van de Kemp H et al., 1993, Detection of seven species of pathogenic leptospires by PCR using two sets of primers, *J Gen Microbiol*, **139:** 1691–700.

Gsell HO, Olafsson A et al., 1971, Intrauterine leptospirosis pomona, *Dtsch Med Wochenschr*, **96:** 1263–8.

Inada R, Ido Y et al., 1916, The etiology, mode of infection, and specific therapy of Weil's disease (spirochaetosis icterohaemorrhagica), *J Exp Med*, **23:** 377–402.

van den Ingh TS, Hartman EG, 1986, Pathology of acute *Leptospira interrogans* serotype *icterohaemorrhagiae* infection in the Syrian hamster, *Vet Microbiol*, **12:** 367–76.

Jost BH, Adler B, Faine S, 1989, Experimental immunisation of hamsters with lipopolysaccharide antigens of *Leptospira interrogans*, *J Med Microbiol*, **29:** 115–20.

Katz AR, Manea SJ, Sasaki DM, 1991, Leptospirosis on Kauai: investigation of a common source waterborne outbreak, *Am J Public Health*, **81:** 1310–12.

Korver H, Kolk AHJ et al., 1988, Classification of the icterohaemorrhagiae serogroup by monoclonal antibodies, *Isr J Vet Med*, **44:** 15–18.

Looke DFM, 1986, Weil's syndrome in a zoologist, *Med J Aust*, **144:** 597–601.

Lupidi R, Cinco M et al., 1991, Serological follow-up of patients involved in a localized outbreak of leptospirosis, *J Clin Microbiol*, **29:** 805–9.

McClain JBL, Ballou WR et al., 1984, Doxycycline therapy for leptospirosis, *Ann Intern Med*, **100:** 696–8.

Maestrone G, Benjaminson MA, 1962, Leptospira infection in the gold fish, *Nature (London)*, **195:** 719–20.

Marshall RB, Baskerville A et al., 1980, Benign leptospirosis: the pathology of experimental infections of monkeys with *Leptospira interrogans* serovars *balcanica* and *tarassovi*, *Br J Exp Pathol*, **61:** 124–31.

Mérien F, Amouriaux P et al., 1992, Polymerase chain reaction for detection of *Leptospira* spp. in clinical samples, *J Clin Microbiol*, **30:** 2219–24.

Mérien F, Perolat P et al., 1993, Detection of *Leptospira* DNA by polymerase chain reaction in aqueous humor of a patient with unilateral uveitis, *J Infect Dis*, **168:** 1335–6.

Midwinter A, Faine S, 1995, Leptospirosis in Victoria in 1992 and 1993 – a report from a diagnostic laboratory, *Communicable Dis Intell*, **19:** 32–5.

Midwinter A, Vinh T et al., 1994, Characterization of an antigenic oligosaccharide from *Leptospira interrogans* serovar *pomona* and its role in immunity, *Infect Immun*, **62:** 5477–82.

Minette HP, 1983, Leptospirosis in poikilothermic vertebrates, *Int J Zoonoses*, **10:** 111–21.

Neves ES, Pereira MM et al., 1994, Leptospirosis patient with AIDS: the first case reported, *Rev Soc Bras Med Trop*, **27:** 39–42.

O'Neil KM, Rickman LS, Lazarus AA, 1991, Pulmonary manifestations of leptospirosis, *Rev Infect Dis*, **13:** 705–9.

Palit A, Hosking C et al., 1991, Leptospirosis in dairy farmers of western Victoria, Australia, *Leptospirosis. Proceedings of the Leptospirosis Research Conference, 1990*, ed. Kobayashi Y, Hokusen-Sha Publishing Co., Tokyo, 126–37.

Peet RL, Mercy A et al., 1983, The significance of leptospira isolated from the kidneys of slaughtered pigs, *Aust Vet J*, **60:** 226–7.

Perolat P, Poingt JP et al., 1991, Occurrence of severe leptospirosis in a breeding colony of squirrel monkeys, *Leptospirosis. Proceedings of the Leptospirosis Research Conference 1990*, ed. Kobayashi Y, Hokusen-Sha, Tokyo, 39–41.

Poonacha KB, Donahue JM et al., 1993, Leptospirosis in equine fetuses, stillborn foals, and placentas, *Vet Pathol*, **30:** 362–9.

Ralph D, McClelland M et al., 1993, *Leptospira* species categorized by arbitrarily primed polymerase chain reaction (PCR) and by mapped restriction polymorphisms in PCR-amplified rRNA genes, *J Bacteriol*, **175:** 973–81.

Ramadass P, Jarvis BD et al., 1992, Genetic characterization of pathogenic *Leptospira* species by DNA hybridization, *Int J Syst Bacteriol*, **42:** 215–19.

Spinu I, Topciu V et al., 1963, L'homme comme réservoir de virus dans une épidémie de leptospirose survenue dans la jungle, *Arch Roum Pathol Exp Microbiol*, **22:** 1081–100.

Takafuji ET, Kirkpatrick JW et al., 1984, An efficacy trial of doxycycline chemoprophylaxis against leptospirosis, *N Engl J Med*, **310:** 497–500.

Tang YK, 1991, A field study on the post-inoculation reaction and immunological effects in vaccinated population immunized with 'Zhejiang type-D' leptospiral vaccine, *Chung Hua Liu Hsing Ping Hsueh Tsa Chih*, **12:** 335–8.

Terpstra WJ, 1992, Serodiagnosis of bacterial diseases: problems and developments, *Scand J Immunol*, **36, Suppl 11:** 91–5.

Torten M, 1979, Leptospirosis, *CRC Handbook Series in Zoonoses. Section A. 1. Bacterial, Rickettsial and Mycotic Diseases*, 1st edn, ed. Steele JH, CRC Press, Boca Raton, FL, 363–421.

Torten M, Marshall RB, 1994, Leptospirosis, *Handbook of Zoonoses, Section A: Bacterial, Rickettsial, Chlamydial and Mycotic Diseases*, vol. 1, 2nd edn, ed. Beran GW, CRC Press, Boca Raton, FL, 245–64.

Uhlenhuth P, Fromme W, 1915, Experimentelle Untersuchungen über die sogenannte Weilsche Krankheit (ansteckende Gelbsucht), *Med Klin*, **44:** 1202, 1264, 1296.

Vaughan C, Cronin CC et al., 1994, The Jarisch–Herxheimer reaction in leptospirosis, *Postgrad Med J*, **70:** 118–21.

Vinh T, Adler B, Faine S, 1986a, Glycolipoprotein cytotoxin from

Leptospira interrogans serovar *copenhageni*, *J Gen Microbiol*, **132:** 111–23.

Vinh T, Adler B, Faine S, 1986b, Ultrastructure and chemical composition of lipopolysaccharide extracted from *Leptospira interrogans* serovar *copenhageni*, *J Gen Microbiol*, **132:** 103–9.

Vinh T, Shi M-H et al., 1989, Characterization and taxonomic significance of lipopolysaccharides of *Leptospira interrogans* serovar *hardjo*, *J Gen Microbiol*, **135:** 2663–73.

Vinh T, Faine S et al., 1994, Immunochemical studies of opsonic epitopes of the lipopolysaccharide of *Leptospira interrogans* serovar *hardjo*, *FEMS Immunol Med Microbiol*, **8:** 99–107.

Watt G, 1990, Leptospirosis as a cause of uveitis, *Arch Intern Med*, **150:** 1130.

Watt G, 1992, Leptospirosis, *Curr Opin Infect Dis*, **5:** 659–63.

Watt G, Manoloto C, Hayes CG, 1989, Central nervous system leptospirosis in the Philippines, *Southeast Asian J Trop Med Public Health*, **20:** 265–9.

Watt G, Alquiza LM et al., 1988a, The rapid diagnosis of leptospirosis: a prospective comparison of the dot enzyme-linked immunosorbent assay and the genus-specific microscopic agglutination test at different stages of illness, *J Infect Dis*, **157:** 840–2.

Watt G, Padre LP et al., 1988b, Placebo-controlled trial of intravenous penicillin for severe and late leptospirosis, *Lancet*, **1:** 433–5.

Watt G, Padre LP et al., 1990, Skeletal and cardiac muscle involvement in severe, late leptospirosis, *J Infect Dis*, **162:** 266–9.

Yasuda PH, Steigerwalt AG et al., 1987, Deoxyribonucleic acid relatedness between serogroups and serovars in the family Leptospiraceae with proposals for seven new *Leptospira* species, *Int J Syst Bacteriol*, **37:** 407–15.

SPIROCHAETOSIS

S L Josephson

1 **Relapsing fever**	4	**Swine dysentery**
2 **Animal borreliosis**	5	**Spirillary rat-bite fever**
3 **Intestinal spirochaetosis**		

Spirochaetosis, by definition, refers to infections caused by spirochaetes of the order Spirochaetales. In recent years the term has been expanded to include not only true spirochaetes but also other helical-shaped bacteria. In this chapter, a number of important human and animal spirochaetoses are described, including tick-borne and louse-borne relapsing fever, animal borreliosis, intestinal spirochaetosis, swine dysentery and spirillary rat-bite fever. Some of these illnesses are well known whereas others have only recently been characterized.

1 RELAPSING FEVER

Epidemics of relapsing fever have occurred since ancient times (Bryceson et al. 1970). However, only in the past 125 years have we acquired a detailed understanding of the disease and the means to control it. Historically, epidemics of relapsing fever have resulted in extensive morbidity and mortality. Aggressive public health measures together with improved hygiene and the availability of insecticides and antibiotics have reduced the incidence and mortality rate of relapsing fever in recent years. Relapsing fever is caused by certain species of *Borrelia* (Table 43.1). The *Borrelia* spirochaetes are transmitted to humans either by a soft-bodied tick of the genus *Ornithodoros* or by the body louse, *Pediculus humanus*. Since there are 2 main transmission vectors, relapsing fever has been generically classified as tick-borne and louse-borne. Epidemic outbreaks of louse-borne relapsing fever, although relatively rare, continue in parts of Africa. Furthermore, endemic and sporadic outbreaks of tick-borne relapsing fever continue world wide.

1.1 Description of the disease

Relapsing fever presents as an acute febrile illness with subsequent defervescence and recurrence of symptoms (Southern and Sanford 1969, Bryceson et al. 1970). The severity of the illness can range from mild to life-threatening. Louse-borne relapsing fever is often more severe than the tick-borne variety. Following transmission from vector to man, the *Borrelia* spirochaetes invade the bloodstream where they reproduce and spread throughout the body. The mean incubation period for relapsing fever is approximately 7 days (range of 4 to more than 18 days). An infected individual eventually experiences a rapid onset of high fever accompanied by chills, headache, nausea, vomiting, malaise and myalgia. Tachycardia, arthralgia, abdominal pain and eye pain may also occur. The spleen of the infected individual is usually tender and enlarged. The liver may also be enlarged. At least 7% of patients become juandiced. Respiratory complications, including pneumonia and bronchitis, have been reported but are rare. A case of adult respiratory distress syndrome (ARDS) associated with relapsing fever has been reported (Davis, Burke and Wright 1992). Mucous membrane haemorrhages and neurological manifestations such as meningitis, encephalitis and neuropathy are observed in some cases. Neuropsychiatric symptoms, including insomnia, mental lethargy and psychotic episodes, are common. Approximately 8% of tick-borne and 30% of louse-borne relapsing fever cases manifest neurological signs and symptoms.

The initial signs and symptoms of relapsing fever typically last 3–6 days and end abruptly in a state of crisis. At this stage, the host experiences rapid defervescense. The drop in temperature is accompanied by drenching sweats, intense thirst and weakness. Bradycardia is common. Significant hypotension and shock are uncommon. A local or gen-

Table 43.1 Relapsing fever borreliae, hosts, vectors and distribution

Borrelia	Host	Vector	Distribution
B. caucasica	Rodents, humans	*Ornithodoros verrucosus*	Caucasus
B. crocidurae	Rodents, humans	*Ornithodoros erraticus*	Africa, Near East, Central Asia (small variety)
B. duttonii	Human	*Ornithodoros moubata*	Africa
B. graingeri	Rodents, humans	*Ornithodoros graingeri*	East Africa
B. hermsii	Rodents, humans	*Ornithodoros hermsi*	Western USA, Canada
B. hispanica	Rodents, humans	*Ornithodoros erraticus*	Spain, Portugal, Morocco, Algeria, Tunisia (large variety)
B. latyschewii	Rodents, reptiles, humans	*Ornithodoros tartakovskyi*	Iran, Central Asia
B. mazzotti	Rodents, armadillos, monkeys, humans	*Ornithodoros talaje*	Mexico, Guatemala
B. parkeri	Rodents, humans	*Ornithodorus parkeri*	Western USA
B. persica	Rodents, bats, humans	*Ornithodoros tholozani*	Middle East, Central Asia
B. recurrentis	Humans	*Pediculus humanus*	South America, Europe, Africa, Asia
B. turicatae	Rodents, humans	*Ornithodoros turicata*	USA, Mexico
B. venezuelensis	Rodents, humans	*Ornithodoros rudis*	Central and South America

Adapted from *Bergey's Manual of Determinative Bacteriology* (Holt et al. 1994).

eralized rash, petechial, papular, or macular in nature, develops in up to 28% of cases. Death is most likely to occur at this stage.

The afebrile period prior to relapse lasts approximately 6–9 days. The average number of relapses observed in tick-borne relapsing fever is 3 (range 0–13). With louse-borne relapsing fever, there is usually only a single relapse. Each relapse is characterized by the return of fever and other symptoms. However, the duration and severity of the illness tends to diminish with each relapse.

The estimated case fatality rate when the infection goes untreated is 2–5% for tick-borne relapsing fever and up to 40% for louse-borne relapsing fever. Women who develop relapsing fever during pregnancy usually abort. At least one case of transplacental transmission has been documented (Fuchs and Oyama 1969). In this case, the newborn, who died of meningitis 39 h after birth, had spirochaetes present in the cerebrospinal fluid and splenic lesions at autopsy. The experience with louse-borne relapsing fever in Ethiopia indicates that myocarditis, perhaps associated with cardiac arrhythmia, is a common cause of death (Parry et al. 1970, Judge et al. 1974). Hepatic failure also appears to be a major contributing factor. In terms of the pathology of relapsing fever, the spleen is the most commonly affected organ (Southern and Sanford 1969). Necrotic lesions of the spleen are often detected at autopsy (Judge et al. 1974). Hepatic damage and central nervous system lesions also occur. Spirochaetes have been isolated in culture from brain tissue, cerebrospinal fluid, liver and spleen.

Rodents are the primary vertebrate reservoir for all but one of the *Borrelia* species associated with tick-borne relapsing fever (Table 43.1). The exception, *Borrelia duttonii*, and the agent of louse-borne relapsing fever, *Borrelia recurrentis*, are only known to infect humans in nature. Some species of *Borrelia* that infect rodents occasionally infect other vertebrates. Depending on the species of *Borrelia*, alternative hosts may include bats, armadillos, calves, dogs, foxes, horses, sheep and goats (Felsenfeld 1965). Experimental infections of mice, rats, guinea pigs and monkeys produce illness similar to that seen in humans. Numerous animal studies have yielded a wealth of information about the natural history and pathogenesis of relapsing fever. For example, studies have shown that a single organism is sufficient to cause relapsing fever in mice (Stoenner, Dodd and Larson 1982). The generation time of *Borrelia hermsii* during the logarithmic phase of growth in the blood circulation of a mouse is approximately 3 h. At the peak of spirochaetaemia, 800 000 or more spirochaetes per millilitre may be present in the blood. During the afebrile period prior to relapse, borreliae remain in the circulation but at a low concentration. During relapses, the concentration of spirochaetes circulating in the blood again increases dramatically but to a lesser extent than in the initial attack (Barbour 1990). As with human infection, the spleens of infected animals are usually enlarged. Neurological involvement is also common. *Borrelia* can be found in the brain tissue and organs of infected laboratory mice and rats after spirochaetes have disappeared from the circulation (Southern and Sanford 1969). *Borrelia* can persist in brain tissue for months. The potential neurotropic aspect of relapsing fever has been controversial. In a recent report, *B. hermsii* infection of the brain parenchyma and subarachnoid space of mice was demonstrated conclusively with spirochaetes observed in the brain early in the course of infection (Cadavid, Bundoc and Barbour 1993). The persistence of borreliae in the brains of laboratory animals has been valuable from the standpoint of strain preservation. Investigators have been able to maintain some strains of *Borrelia* in frozen brain tissue for months or years.

1.2 Aetiology

Borrelia, the aetiological agent of relapsing fever, is a helical-shaped, motile bacterium belonging to the order Spirochaetales and the family Spirochaetaceae (Canale-Parola 1984). The various species associated with relapsing fever range in width from 0.2 to 0.5 μm and in length from 3 to 20 μm (Kelly 1984). There are usually 5–7 spirals per organism, each with an amplitude of 1–2 μm. The spirochaete consists of an outer lipid membrane surrounding a coiled protoplasmic cylinder. There may also be a mucoid slime layer exterior to the outer membrane. The protoplasmic cylinder consists of a peptidoglycan cell wall surrounding an inner cell membrane and the cytoplasm. The cytoplasm of *Borrelia* does not contain tubules. Motility is provided by flagella that lie in the periplasmic space between the outer membrane and the protoplasmic cylinder. The flagella are anchored subterminally in the protoplasmic cylinder, have a bipolar distribution and extend from both ends inward along the periplasm and cross one another midway along the length of the organism. The *Borrelia* spp. associated with relapsing fever have between 15 and 30 unsheathed flagella that are structurally similar to the flagella of other eubacteria (Barbour and Hayes 1986). Borreliae are not found free-living in nature. The organisms are micro-aerophilic, possess an iron-containing superoxide dismutase but not peroxidase or catalase, ferment glucose by the Embden–Meyerhof pathway to DL-lactic acid, and have complex nutritional requirements.

The *Borrelia* spirochaete does not tolerate desiccation and survives best at a slightly alkaline pH. In terms of temperature tolerance, the organism remains viable for only a day at room temperature in an aqueous environment (Felsenfeld 1965). When refrigerated, viability can be maintained for weeks or months. Freezing borreliae at −20°C does not promote viability. The organism has been successfully maintained at −70°C for at least 1 year but does not tolerate repeated freeze-thawing.

Historically, the classification of each tick-borne relapsing fever *Borrelia* has been tied to the species of tick involved in transmission. Recently, molecular genetic analysis has shown that at least some of the classifications may not be valid. For example, hybridization experiments and nucleotide sequence analysis of the North American species of relapsing fever *Borrelia* showed that *Borrelia parkeri* and *Borrelia turicatae* are virtually identical but are markedly different from *B. hermsii* (Picken 1992). The differentiation was based on the highly conserved flagellin gene of *Borrelia*.

1.3 Epidemiology

Outbreaks of relapsing fever have occurred on every continent with the possible exception of Australia. Louse-borne relapsing fever tends to be epidemic or endemic whereas tick-borne relapsing fever is endemic or sporadic. Epidemics of louse-borne relapsing fever can be devastating. In this century alone, there have been at least 7 major epidemics with many thousands and perhaps millions of deaths (Bryceson et al. 1970). The incidence of louse-borne relapsing fever decreased dramatically after World War II as living conditions improved world wide. The most recent focus has been in Africa, especially Ethiopia and Sudan. Predisposing factors for an outbreak of louse-borne relapsing fever include war, overcrowding, poor hygiene conditions and malnutrition. The epidemic cycle occurs as follows. The vector, *P. humanus*, becomes infected after ingesting *B. recurrentis* in a blood meal from an infected human host. The organism penetrates the gut wall and then multiplies in the haemolymph. The louse is infected for life (approximately 4–7 weeks) and, unlike the tick, does not pass the infection transovarially to progeny (Felsenfeld 1965). Furthermore, the spirochaete does not enter the salivary glands, ducts, ovaries or eggs. Therefore, spirochaetes cannot be transmitted from the louse to humans via saliva or excrement during a blood meal. Instead, transmission occurs when the infected louse is crushed, releasing contaminated haemolymph. The spirochaetes in the haemolymph then enter the body through the bite wound, abraded skin, conjunctiva or other mucosa (Felsenfeld 1965).

The endemic or sporadic nature of tick-borne relapsing fever is primarily a function of the host–vector relationship (Felsenfeld 1965). The *Ornithodoros* ticks associated with relapsing fever reside in areas such as rodent burrows, caves, earthen-floored dwellings, tree stumps, logs and the crevices of walls. Since humans tend to have limited contact with these habitats, the likelihood of human exposure is predictably low. However, when there is a high prevalence of infection in rodents, an abundance of ticks, and frequent human contact with vector habitats, the infection can become endemic in a human population (Trape et al. 1991). When human exposure does occur, the tick feeds quickly (often less than 30 min). The tick bite is usually not painful and therefore goes unnoticed. The spirochaetes present in tick saliva and coxal fluid enter the human host during the feeding process. A tick becomes infected with *Borrelia* either by feeding on an infected vertebrate host or through vertical transmission from an infected parent. Spirochaetes acquired in a blood meal pass from the midgut of the tick into the haemocoel where the organisms multiply in the haemolymph and spread to various organs, including salivary gland, coxal gland, central ganglion, reproductive organs and malpighian tubules. Transovarial passage of *Borrelia* in some tick species is very efficient. The ticks associated with relapsing fever can live for years without feeding. During periods of starvation, spirochaetes disappear from the haemolymph but persist sometimes for years in the organs. In addition to vector-associated *Borrelia* transmission, there have been several reports of blood transfusion-associated relapsing fever (Nadelman, Wormser and Sherer 1990).

1.4 Host response

With relapsing fever, there is a serotype-specific antibody response directed against the invading *Borrelia*. It has long been hypothesized that relapsing fever borreliae are able to elude immune destruction and ultimately re-emerge by changing antigenically. The intricacies of the host response and antigenic variation in the spirochaete have only recently been elucidated. Studies of relapsing fever in mice and rats have provided valuable information about the dynamics of the host immune response. In mice, the rate of antibody development depends on the number of *Borrelia* inoculated (Stoenner, Dodd and Larsen 1982). With an inoculation of approximately one million spirochaetes, a serotype-specific antibody response is detected approximately 60 h following injection. The elimination of *Borrelia* is mediated by specific antibody and the activity of phagocytes, including polymorphonuclear leucocytes (Spagnuolo et al. 1982, Newman and Johnson 1984). The elimination of spirochaetes is T cell independent. Furthermore, complement mediated lysis and opsonization are not essential for clearance when specific antibody is present, but probably play a role in the non-immune host (Butler 1985). There are indications that humans living where ticks are prevalent may acquire some degree of immunity (Felsenfeld 1965).

Antigenic variation is the defining characteristic of relapsing fever. Stoenner, Dodd and Larsen (1982) detected at least 24 different serotypes among the progeny of a single *B. hermsii* organism inoculated into a mouse. Antigenic conversions occurred spontaneously and constantly, independent of relapses and antibody production. Furthermore, the antigenic changes were reversible. The rate of spontaneous change was estimated to be 10^{-4}–10^{-3} per cell per generation. With relapsing fever, spirochaetaemia persists with relapses occurring when the spirochaete population reaches visually detectable levels. The antibody response of the host results in the destruction of the dominant serotype population. Barbour, Tessier and Stoenner (1982) were able to show that the antigenic determinants of serotype specificity are located on outer-membrane proteins known as variable major proteins or Vmp. At least 24 antigenically distinct serotypes exist, each associated with a different Vmp. Molecular genetic analysis has shown that the *vmp* genes are located on linear plasmids. Only one *vmp* gene at a time is active. All other *vmp*s are silent in terms of transcription. When there is a switch in serotype, a copy of a silent *vmp* gene located on a silent plasmid is transposed to an expression plasmid (Donelson 1995). A second type of activation involving a gene deletion within a linear plasmid has also been described.

1.5 Laboratory

Routine laboratory blood tests such as cell counts, erythrocyte sedimentation rate and haematocrit are not predictive and therefore have minimal value in the diagnosis of relapsing fever (Southern and Sanford 1969). An evaluation of cerebrospinal fluid often shows lymphocytic pleocytosis and elevated protein and, therefore, may be of some diagnostic value.

The examination of peripheral blood collected during an acute febrile episode is the preferred method for diagnosing relapsing fever. The spirochaetes can be detected directly in blood with a darkfield or phase contrast microscope or by examining thick and thin blood smears stained with Giemsa or Wright's stain. Based on previous experience, the spirochaetes will be detected in approximately 70% of cases under these circumstances (Southern and Sanford 1969). Cerebrospinal fluid is examined in a similar manner. Spirochaetes are usually not present in the blood circulation in sufficient quantity during mild infections and the afebrile phase to be detected by microscopy. In addition to direct observation, relapsing fever *Borrelia* can be detected by injecting blood or other biological fluids and tissues into susceptible laboratory animals and then examining blood samples from the inoculated animals daily for the presence of spirochaetes for at least 1 week. With animal inoculations, it is possible to detect *Borrelia* even when the organism is present at low concentration. *Borrelia* can also be propagated in chick embryos (Felsenfeld 1965). In vitro cultivation of relapsing fever *Borrelia* is possible with some but not all species. Kelly (1971) developed a medium capable of supporting the growth of *B. hermsii* through many passages. Kelly's medium was subsequently modified, resulting in BSK, a highly complex liquid medium (Stoenner, Dodd and Larsen 1982, Barbour 1984). Various media formulations have been used to cultivate borreliae from the biological fluids and tissues of animals, humans and ticks. Cultivation has been most successful with tick-borne borreliae. Recently, however, *B. recurrentis* was also recovered, using BSK II medium, from the serum of a patient with louse-borne relapsing fever (Cutler et al. 1994).

Several methods are available for identifying *Borrelia*. Monoclonal antibodies have been used in an immunofluorescence format to detect *B. hermsii* in the blood of infected mice and in the central ganglia of ticks (Schwan et al. 1992). The polymerase chain reaction (PCR) and other techniques of molecular biology are also now being applied to *Borrelia*. Highly conserved regions of the genome such as the flagellin gene have been targeted in an effort to develop a species-specific but inclusive PCR-DNA probe system for the detection of North American tick-borne borreliae (Picken 1992). PCR amplification may be particularly useful for detecting low numbers of the organism in biological fluids and tissues (Cadavid, Bundoc and Barbour 1993).

Various serological tests have been used over the years to detect *Borrelia*-specific complement fixing, bactericidal, immobilizing and agglutinating antibodies (Felsenfeld 1965). However, the antigenic variation associated with relapsing fever makes serodiagnosis difficult. In recent years, the indirect immunofluorescent antibody assay (IFA) technique has supplanted other serological tests. IFA has been used alone and in combination with a Western blot test (Flanigan et al. 1991, Ciceroni et al. 1994). These techniques are effective but require the use of specific *Borrelia* antigens as targets. Unfortunately, not all relapsing fever spirochaetes have been successfully cultivated in vitro. Consequently, the value of serological testing has been severely limited by antigen availability. Both acute and convalescent sera are needed for serodiagnostic testing.

1.6 Treatment

Therapies for relapsing fever include tetracycline, erythromycin, chloramphenicol and penicillin. Penicillin binding proteins have been detected in *B. hermsii* (Barbour, Todd and Stoenner 1982). The administration of a therapeutic dose of antibiotic results in the resolution of symptoms and the disappearance of spirochaetes from the circulation. The fatality rate for treated relapsing fever is less than 5% (Southern and Sanford 1969).

In many cases, antimicrobial therapy results in a Jarisch–Herxheimer (JH) reaction. The JH reaction begins 60–90 min after the initiation of therapy and is characterized by an onset of chills, leucopenia and increases in body temperature, blood pressure and respiratory rate. This is followed 10–30 min later by sustained hypotension (Judge et al. 1974, Seboxa and Rahlenbeck 1995). The recovery period, which may last for hours, begins when the spirochaetes disappear from the circulation. The induced crisis resolves whether or not antibiotic therapy is continued. The JH reaction can be fatal. Case fatality rates have ranged up to 6%. Any antibiotic used clinically can precipitate the reaction. Although the JH reaction has similarities with septic shock, endotoxin has not been detected in relapsing fever *Borrelia*. There is growing evidence that the JH reaction is directly associated with the clearance of spirochaetes from the circulation by phagocytes after antibiotic therapy is started. The clearance of spirochaetes may precipitate the reaction through the action of an endogenous pyrogen and a cytokine cascade consisting of tumour necrosis factor and interleukins 6 and 8 (Negussie et al. 1992).

The use of either tetracycline or erythromycin leads to the rapid elimination of spirochaetes from the circulation without relapse but often results in a severe JH reaction (Butler, Jones and Wallace 1978, Warrell et al. 1983). Penicillin therapy is less likely to produce a severe JH reaction but is also less effective at eliminating the organism and preventing relapse. Furthermore, the use of slow release penicillin may significantly prolong hypotension. In the treatment of louse-borne relapsing fever, investigators have used low dose procaine penicillin therapy to dramatically reduce the likelihood of developing a serious JH reaction (Seboxa

and Rahlenbeck 1995). Unfortunately, nearly half the patients receiving the low dose treatment relapsed. The use of combination therapy with penicillin administered first, followed a day later by a dose of tetracycline, has been evaluated (Salih and Mustafa 1977). Because of the various confounding factors outlined above, there is currently no consensus treatment for relapsing fever.

1.7 Prevention and transmissibility

Epidemics of louse-borne relapsing fever are most likely to occur where there is extreme overcrowding, malnutrition and poor personal hygiene. Steps that can be taken to alleviate these conditions are extremely important for prevention. Once an outbreak of louse-borne relapsing fever begins, the emphasis inevitably switches to antibiotic therapy and the elimination of the transmission vector. The importance of eliminating the vector as well as treating the infection was demonstrated recently in Ethiopia where an outbreak of relapsing fever occurred simultaneously at 2 transit camps (Sundnes and Haimanot 1993). At one camp, affected individuals were treated only with antibiotics whereas at the other camp the treatment regimen included delousing as well as antibiotic therapy. The delousing procedure involved shaving hair, a shower with soap, the boiling of clothing for 30 min, and chemical decontamination of personal belongings with DDT. Over a 20 day period, the frequency of cases increased with antibiotic therapy alone but decreased when both antibiotic treatment and vector control measures were provided. There was a significant correlation between non-deloused patients and new cases of relapsing fever. Pediculicides such as permethrin and lindane can be used to eliminate body lice.

With tick-borne relapsing fever, vector control is more difficult since outbreaks tend to be sporadic and limited in scope and the vector is often widespread. The best way to prevent infection is to avoid contact with the tick vector.

2 ANIMAL BORRELIOSIS

There are 3 species of *Borrelia* that cause significant infections in animals but not in humans. The agents are *Borrelia theileri*, *Borrelia anserina* and *Borrelia coriaceae*.

2.1 Cattle and horse spirochaetosis

The spirochaete *B. theileri* causes a benign illness in cattle, horses and sheep. The organism was initially observed by Theiler (1904) in the blood of cattle in South Africa. In the infected animal, progressive spirochaetaemia develops along with an increasing fever (Brocklesby, Scott and Rampton 1963). The fever usually lasts 1–2 days and ultimately resolves when the spirochaetes disappear from the circulation. The infection has been encountered primarily in South Africa and Australia (Callow 1967).

According to *Bergey's Manual* (Kelly 1984), the *B. theileri* spirochaete is 0.25–0.3 μm wide and 20–30 μm long in cattle and somewhat shorter in horses. The accuracy of this description has been questioned by at least one investigator. Callow (1967) observed average lengths of 12.1 μm (range 9.6–18.9 μm) and 13.2 μm (range 6–19.5 μm), respectively for *B. theileri* in blood smears from Australian and South African cattle. The spirochaetes were described as having 3–7 large wavy spirals. The author suggests that the 20–30 μm measurement, which was taken from a 1903 observation, actually represented an upper limit. The length of the organism is critical since the diagnosis is based on morphology. In vitro cultivation has not been reported. The tick vectors known to transmit *B. theileri* include *Rhipicephalus* spp. and *Boophilus microplus* (Holt et al. 1994).

2.2   Avian spirochaetosis

Avian spirochaetosis, a life-threatening disease of birds including chickens, ducks, turkeys and geese, is caused by *B. anserina*. The primary vectors involved in disease transmission are various species of argasid tick including *Argas miniatus*, *Argas persicus* and *Argas reflexus* (Kelly 1984). There is evidence that *B. anserina* can also be transmitted from one bird to another either by mosquitoes or by ingestion of contaminated bird faeces (Zuelzer 1936, Loomis 1953). The organism was first observed by Sakharoff (1891) in the blood of geese suffering from a febrile illness. Thereafter, the illness was observed in other species of birds at many locations around the world. The characteristic symptoms of avian spirochaetosis include fever, greenish diarrhoea, loss of appetite, listlessness and in some cases weight loss (McNeil, Hinshaw and Kissling 1949). The incubation period is approximately 4 days (range 3–8 days). The spirochaetaemia can be detected in the blood circulation 24–72 h into the infection. The spirochaetes remain in the circulation for approximately 4 days. The mortality rate is often high. Birds that survive the infection develop long-lasting immunity. Investigators have experimentally infected chickens and turkeys in order to study pathogenesis (McNeil, Hinshaw and Kissling 1949, Bandopadhyay and Vegad 1983, 1984). During the course of the disease, birds infected with *B. anserina* develop spirochaetaemia, enteritis, anaemia and splenomegaly. Spirochaetes tend to localize in the spleen, liver, intestine and kidneys. Mobilization of macrophages, phagocytosis of erythrocytes, and extravascular haemolysis occur in the spleen, liver and small intestine even after the disappearance of spirochaetes from blood and tissues. *B. anserina* is only known to infect birds. The inability of the organism to infect rodents and rabbits can actually be used in the identification process.

The *B. anserina* spirochaete is 0.22–0.26 μm wide and 9–21 μm long and has 5–8 loose coils with a wavelength of 1.7 μm (Hovind-Hougen 1995). Motility is provided by 7–8 flagella. The organism can be grown in embryonated duck and chicken eggs and maintained in young ducks and chickens. *B. anserina* has also been cultivated in vitro in BSK liquid medium (Levine et al. 1990).

In terms of treatment, a single dose of 10 000 units of penicillin given intramuscularly was sufficient to cure avian spirochaetosis in turkeys (McNeil, Hinshaw and Kissling 1949). In chickens, penicillin, bacitracin, chloramphenicol, streptomycin, tetracycline, kanamycin, erythromycin and various arsenicals have cured the infection (Packchanian 1960, Stoianove-Zaikova and Doneva 1982). Furthermore, *B. anserina* was recently shown to be susceptible to cefuroxime in vitro (Johnson et al. 1990).

Susceptible hosts can be immunized to prevent avian spirochaetosis. Inactivated vaccines consisting of infected blood, tissues, or isolated spirochaetes have induced nearly complete protection against infection (Packchanian and Smith 1970). Alternatively, Drumev and Stoianova (1976) were able to elicit immunity by giving live *B. anserina* to chickens simultaneously with sodium arsanilate.

2.3   Epizootic bovine abortion

Epizootic bovine abortion (EBA) is an asymptomatic infection of cattle which often results in abortion late in pregnancy. Characteristic lesions of EBA in the fetus include generalized haemorrhage, subcutaneous oedema, ascites and hepatopathy (Howarth, Moulton and Frazier 1956). The disease occurs primarily in the western USA where it has had a significant economic impact. EBA is closely associated with the soft tick *Ornithodoros coriaceus* (Schmidtmann et al. 1976). Investigators have studied the pathogenesis of EBA by exposing pregnant cows to *O. coriaceus* and observing fetuses up to 126 days following exposure. In these experiments, fetuses obtained 50 and 100 days after exposure showed mild to moderate lymphoid and mononuclear cell hyperplasia (Kimsey et al. 1983). However, characteristic lesions of EBA were not detected until at least 100 days after the exposure. With prolonged infection, investigators observed acute vasculitis and acute necrotizing lesions or pyogranulomas in the lymph nodes and spleen of fetuses (Kennedy et al. 1983). The initial steps taken to identify the aetiological agent of EBA focused on chlamydial and viral agents transmitted by *O. coriaceus* (Wada et al. 1976, McKercher et al. 1980). Although the connection between a chlamydia-like agent and EBA initially seemed to be fairly strong, ultimately it could not be confirmed. In 1985, a spirochaete was isolated in BSK II medium from the larval, nymph and adult stages of *O. coriaceus* (Lane et al. 1985). The spirochaete was subsequently identified as a new species of *Borrelia* and officially named *B. coriaceae* (Johnson et al. 1987).

Although *B. coriaceae* has never been isolated directly from cattle, it is considered to be the putative agent of EBA. Spirochaetes morphologically similar to those found in *O. coriaceus* have been detected in the fetal blood of calves with lesions of EBA (Osebold et al. 1986). Osebold and colleagues (1987) subsequently presented data showing that superinfection brought on by repeated exposure to spirochaetes can increase the severity of infection. Furthermore, immunological studies revealed that the quantity of immunoglobulins in the blood of diseased fetuses with spirochaete-like organisms is markedly increased, indicating fetal antibody synthesis (Spezialetti and Osebold 1991). In spite of the mounting evidence indicating a causal relationship between the spirochaete and EBA, a recently developed *B. coriaceae*-specific PCR assay failed to confirm the association (Zingg and LeFebvre 1994). Morphologically, the *B. coriaceae* spirochaete measures 8–10 μm in length and 0.3–0.4 μm in width with 3–5 waves. It has 11–15 overlapping periplasmic flagella (Lane et al. 1985).

3 INTESTINAL SPIROCHAETOSIS

Spirochaetes were first observed in the faeces of humans over 100 years ago (Parr 1923). Since that time, there have been reports linking spirochaetes to various gastrointestinal maladies, including chronic diarrhoea, rectal bleeding and pseudoappendicitis (Henrik-Nielsen et al. 1985). Investigators have also detected spirochaetes in the faeces of apparently healthy individuals. The pathogenic potential of spirochaetes in the gastrointestinal tract remains controversial. Some investigators believe that spirochaetes are no more than commensal colonizers. There is increasing evidence, however, that illness secondary to colonization does occur. The strongest evidence has come from cases of chronic diarrhoea and rectal bleeding in which no enteric pathogens were detected and both the symptoms and spirochaetes disappeared following the administration of appropriate antibiotic therapy (Douglas and Crucioli 1981, Lo, Heading and Gilmour 1994).

3.1 Description of disease

Spirochaetes have been observed in colorectal biopsies and in the appendix. Electron micrographs of tissue sections from infected patients typically show spirochaetes attached to the colonic or rectal epithelium in an end-on arrangement. The organism is often interdigitated between and parallel to the microvilli of the mucosal surface. Significant tissue invasion and inflammation are uncommon. However, there have been reports of indentation of the epithelial cell membrane, blunting and destruction of microvilli, and the presence of spirochaetes within the cytoplasm of cells of the intestinal mucosa, subepithelial macrophages and Schwann cells deep in the lamina propria (Henrik-Nielsen et al. 1985, Rodgers et al. 1986, Lo, Heading and Gilmour 1994). Intestinal spirochaetosis is primarily an infection or infestation of the large intestine. However, the distrubution within the large intestine is not always uniform. For example, Lo and colleagues (1994) recently reported a case of chronic diarrhoea in which spirochaetes were present in biopsies of the proximal colon and caecum but not in biopsies of the distal descending colon, sigmoid colon and rectum. It is not clear whether disease is caused by overgrowth of spirochaetes or some other pathogenic mechanism. Some investigators have suggested that massive colonization may interfere with readsorption.

Intestinal spirochaetosis also occurs in pigs. The infection is characterized by clear mucous diarrhoea, reduced feed conversion efficiency, decreased growth rate, and in some instances mild colitis and punctate haemorrhage of the mucosa (Taylor, Simmons and Laird 1980, Jacques et al. 1989). As in the case of humans, the intestine is heavily colonized with spirochaetes attached in an end-on arrangement to the intestinal mucosa. The illness is distinct from swine dysentery.

3.2 Aetiology

Some cases of human intestinal spirochaetosis have been attributed to colonization by *Brachyspira aalborgi*, a recently characterized intestinal spirochaete. In at least 3 cases, the identification was based solely on morphological characteristics and was not confirmed (Henrik-Nielsen et al. 1985, Rodgers et al. 1986, da Cunha Ferreira et al. 1993). *Brachyspira* is a motile, helical, gram-negative spirochaete with tapered ends. The organism measures 1.7–6 μm in length, 0.2 μm in width, and has 4 flagella inserted at each end and a wavelength of 2 μm (Hovind-Hougen et al. 1982). *B. aalborgi* is described as a non-pathogenic colonizer of the intestinal tract (Henrik-Nielsen et al. 1983).

Lee and Hampson (1994) have identified another spirochaete, unofficially designated as (proposed) genus *Anguillina*, which appears to have a much stronger association with symptomatic intestinal spirochaetosis. Based on miltilocus enzyme analysis, these investigators determined that 71 intestinal spirochaete isolates from symptomatic cases involving Australian aboriginal children, Italian adults, Omani Arabs and homosexual males were all genetically consistent with *Anguillina*. Furthermore, these organisms were closely related to the putative agent of swine spirochaetosis (Lee et al. 1993a, Lee and Hampson 1994). The human isolates, however, were not related to *B. aalborgi* or *Serpulina* spp., including *Serpulina hyodysenteriae*, the aetiological agent of swine dysentery. Fifty-nine porcine isolates associated with intestinal spirochaetosis were also identified as being *Anguillina*. The *Anguillina* spirochaete is 7–11 μm long, 2–3 μm wide, contains 4–6 axial flagella, and has tapered ends. The organism is weakly β-haemolytic on blood agar.

3.3 Epidemiology

Biopsy-proven intestinal spirochaetosis has been reported in children as well as adults (White et al. 1994). The distribution of intestinal spirochaetosis is world wide (Teglbjaerg 1990). In general, reported rates of colonization for intestinal spirochaetes have been around 5% or less. However, the rates are substantially higher in certain groups including Gulf Arabs, Africans, Indians, Australian Aborigines, homosexual men and AIDS patients (Lee and Hampson 1994). Colonization rates as high as 36% have been reported. The source of the spirochaetes colonizing the intestinal tract is unknown.

3.4 Laboratory

Colonizing spirochaetes can be detected in haematoxylin and eosin (H & E) stained thin sections of colon and rectal biopsies. The organisms collectively appear as a light blue, haematoxylin-positive fringe along the brush border of the intestinal mucosa. Silver, Giemsa and periodic acid–Schiff stains have also been used to detect the organism. The diagnosis can be confirmed by using electron microscopy to visualize individual spirochaetes. Transverse sections containing spirochaetes surrounded by microvilli yield a rosette appearance.

Besides direct examination, stool and tissue samples can be cultivated on solid media containing 5–10% blood. Trypticase soy agar supplemented with calf, human, sheep, or horse blood will support growth of the organism. Antibiotics such as spectinomycin, polymyxin B, colistin, vancomycin and rifampicin can be added to the medium to make it selective. The inoculated medium is incubated at 37°C in an anaerobic atmosphere for at least 3–5 days. Biochemical and enzymatic profiles for various intestinal spirochaetes have been published (Hunter and Wood 1979, Taylor, Simmons and Laird 1980, Hovind-Hougen et al. 1982, Jones, Miller and George 1986, Lee et al. 1993b). Recent reports indicate that attempts to culture are not always successful. The most promising method for discriminating various types of intestinal spirochaetes is PCR. Recently, Park and colleagues (1995) used PCR amplification of 16S rDNA to identify *Anguillina* recovered from stool cultures of humans and pigs. *Serpulina* spp. and *B. aalborgi* were not amplified with this procedure.

3.5 Treatment

Neomycin, bacitracin and metronidazole have been used to eradicate intestinal spirochaetes. Treatment is typically administered via the oral route or rectal suppository. It is important to note that there have been treatment failures. Some cases of spirochaete-associated chronic diarrhoea resolve spontaneously without antibiotic treatment.

4 SWINE DYSENTERY

Swine dysentery, a mucohaemorrhagic diarrhoeal disease of swine, was first described by Whiting and colleagues in 1921. The disease occurs world wide and is responsible for significant morbidity and mortality in affected herds. The search for the aetiological agent of swine dysentery was essentially unproductive until 1944 when Doyle discovered an association between a vibrio-like organism and swine dysentery. The organism, later named *Campylobacter (Vibrio) coli*, was isolated in pure culture from the colonic mucosa of dysenteric hogs and then fed to healthy pigs. Most of the inoculated pigs developed diarrhoea similar to but less severe than the diarrhoea observed in typical cases of swine dysentery. Subsequent attempts to confirm a causal relationship between *C. coli* and swine dysentery were unsuccessful.

Nearly 50 years after the disease was first described, Vallejo (1969) speculated that there might be an association between intestinal spirochaetes and swine dysentery after finding a preponderance of spirochaetes among the intestinal contents of pigs with mucohaemorrhagic diarrhoea. The association was supported by electron microscopic observations of spirochaetes in early colonic lesions (Blakemore and Taylor 1970). The aetiology of the swine dysentery was conclusively demonstrated by Taylor and Alexander in 1971 when they induced the disease in specific pathogen free pigs by feeding the animals pure cultures of a spirochaete. The spirochaete associated with the disease was subsequently identified as *Serpulina (Treponema) hyodysenteriae* (Harris et al. 1972).

4.1 Description of disease

Swine dysentery begins with the ingestion of *Serpulina hyodysenteriae*. The incubation period of the disease is usually 10–16 days (Songer and Harris 1978). The disease occurs most often in pigs 10–16 weeks old (Alexander and Taylor 1969). The infected pig experiences a reduction in appetite and the passage of soft, discoloured faeces which may contain streaks of blood and mucus. As the disease progresses the amount of blood and mucus increases, the colour of the watery faeces darkens, and shreds of epithelium may appear. The discharge of faeces is often uncontrolled. The affected pig becomes dehydrated and develops a gaunt appearance. Gross lesions of swine dysentery are confined to the fundus of the stomach and the large intestine. At autopsy, the colonic mucosa is typically eroded and congested. Furthermore, lymph nodes in the affected area may be enlarged.

More detailed descriptions of the interaction between the spirochaete and the colonic mucosa have emerged since the mid-1970s. Glock, Harris and Kluge (1974) observed spirochaetes near the luminal surface before lesions appeared. As lesions developed, numerous spirochaetes were detected at the luminal surface and within the crypts. Degenerative changes in the epithelium, particularly involving the microvilli, first appeared where there was close contact with the spirochaete. Intact spirochaetes were observed in goblet and epithelial cells in the early stage of infection and later in degenerating epithelial cells. In advanced disease, spirochaetes were present in the lamina propria underlying the epithelium. As the epithelium is lost, there tends to be congestion and haemorrhage of vessels in the lamina propria and submucosa (Kinyon, Harris and Glock 1977). The infection usually does not extend beyond the lamina propria. In a subsequent study it was shown that *S. hyodysenteriae* primarily colonizes the mucosa (Kennedy et al. 1988). The spirochaete typically does not attach to the epithelium but instead colonizes the overlying mucous layer and mucus-filled crypts of Lieberkühn. The extensive colonization of the mucosa appears to be the result of a chemotactic response of the spirochaete to colonic mucin (Milner and Sellwood 1994).

In terms of the actual pathogenesis of the infection, recent findings indicate that a cytotoxic haemolysin of *S. hydysenteriae* is a major factor in the disease process (Lysons et al. 1991, Bland, Frost and Lysons 1995). Purified haemolysin injected into ligated loops of the ileum and colon of germ-free pigs produces changes similar to those seen in natural cases of swine dysentery including exfoliation and stunting of absorptive villi and eventually damage to subepithelial myofibroblasts. Lipopolysaccharide (LPS) has also been implicated as a potential pathogenic factor in swine dysentery (Neussen, Joens and Glock 1983).

4.2 Aetiology

Serpulina (Treponema) hyodysenteriae is the recognized aetiological agent of swine dysentery. The spirochaete is 7–9 μm in length and 0.3–0.4 μm in width and has loose, regular, serpentine coils (Holt et al. 1994). It is highly motile and has 8 or 9 endoflagella, inserted at each end of the cell, which extend along the periplasmic space. The spirochaete is gram-negative, obligately anaerobic and weakly fermentative. The enzymatic profile of the organism is available (Hunter and Wood 1979). The organism produces haemolysin which is considered to be an important virulence factor. Three haemolysins encoded by genes *tlyA*, *tlyB* and *tlyC* have been described (ter Huurne et al. 1994).

4.3 Epidemiology

An initial outbreak of swine dysentery is often insidious with only a few animals affected in the beginning (Alexander and Taylor 1969). The disease is transmitted by the faecal–oral route. The susceptibility of pigs within a group is variable and probably dose related. The causative agent, *S. hyodysenteriae*, remains viable in dysenteric pig faeces for 7 days at 25°C (Chia and Taylor 1978). Outbreaks are most common in fattening units but may occur in breeding herds, sows and suckling pigs. In sows, the disease results in decreased fertility and breeding performance and an increase in piglet mortality (van Leengoed et al. 1985). Pigs that develop swine dysentery and recover naturally may become carriers. Songer and Harris (1978) demonstrated transmission of swine dysentery from untreated carriers which had been asymptomatic for up to 70 days. Asymptomatic carriers appear to account for much of the transmission between herds.

Although recovery from swine dysentery does not always result in the immediate elimination of the spirochaete, some level of immunity usually emerges. In a study by Joens, Harris and Baum (1979) untreated survivors of swine dysentery remained resistant to challenge exposures for 16–17 weeks. Furthermore, specific antibody was detected for approximately 8 weeks after the pigs were infected. Dysenteric pigs that are treated with antibiotics often recover but then relapse. The relapse may simply reflect an insufficient stimulation of the immune system rather than resistance of the spirochaete to the antimicrobial agent. In order to contain an outbreak, it is extremely important to institute control measures as early as possible.

Various serological methods including microtitration agglutination and enzyme-linked immunosorbent assays have been used to determine the prevalence of swine dysentery in herds (Egan, Harris and Joens 1983). In one recent survey from Australia, the prevalence ranged from 2.5% to 47.5% (Mhoma, Hampson and Robertson 1992).

4.4 Laboratory

Colonic contents and tissues collected from affected animals should be examined with a phase, darkfield, or, in the case of stained slides, a light microscope for the presence of the *S. hyodysenteriae* spirochaete. Dried smears and tissue sections can be stained with Giemsa, Victoria blue 4-R or silver stain (Harris 1974). The spirochaete can also be detected with *S. hyodysenteriae*-specific fluorescent antibodies (Hunter and Saunders 1977). Gram stain is not recommended. For further identification, specimens are cultivated anaerobically on agar-based or liquid-based media. Liquid media generally consist of a nutrient broth such as brain–heart infusion or trypticase soy broth supplemented with serum and other nutrients (Kunkle, Harris and Kinyon 1986). Since the colonic contents and tissues sent for culture are often contaminated, it is important to use a selective medium. A typical selective medium contains trypticase soy agar supplemented with 5% bovine, sheep, or horse blood and appropriate antibiotics. A recent formulation contains trypticase soy agar supplemented with 5% citrated bovine blood, 5% pig faeces extract and 5 antibiotics including spiramycin, rifampicin, vancomycin, colistin and spectinomycin (Kunkle and Kinyon 1988). The presumptive identification of an *S. hyodysenteriae* isolate requires the presence of characteristic large spirochaetes in stained smears, strong β-haemolysis on blood agar, and characteristic signs and lesions in the affected swine (Olson and Fales 1983).

A definitive identification requires additional testing. *Serpulina innocens*, a non-enteropathogenic intestinal spiro-chaete of swine, is very similar to *S. hyodysenteriae* in appearance. The only significant differential culture characteristic is the weak β-haemolysis of *S. innocens*. Belanger and Jacques (1991) have used haemolysis and a ring phenomenon test together with a spot indole test to rapidly differentiate the 2 species. Several commercial tests have also been used to confirm the identification (Hunter and Wood 1979, Milner et al. 1995). When necessary, enteropathogenicity is confirmed by inoculating an isolate into susceptible pigs or mice and then examining the animals for characteristic pathology (Joens and Kinyon 1980). In addition to the conventional methods described above, investigators have used PCR to detect and identify *S. hyodysenteriae* directly in faecal specimens (Elder et al. 1994).

Isolates of *S. hyodysenteriae* are subdivided according to their LPS serotype (Mapother and Joens 1985). Nine different serotypes are recognized at the present time (Li, Belanger and Jacques 1991). Immunodiffusion, immunoblotting and microagglutination have been used to serotype LPS extracted from the spirochaete (Li et al. 1992, Diarra, Mittal and Achacha 1994). Molecular typing based on either DNA restriction enzyme analysis or multilocus enzyme analysis is rapidly becoming an acceptable alternative to the current methods of identification and characterization (Lee et al. 1993a, Sotiropoulos, Coloe and Smith 1994, Harel and Forget 1995).

4.5 Treatment

Various antimicrobial agents have been evaluated and used in the treatment of swine dysentery and for prophylaxis. The agents are usually administered in either water or feed. Traditional therapies include tylosin and organic arsenical (Alexander and Taylor 1969). Newer agents with demonstrable activity include lincomycin, carbadox, tiamulin, metronidazole, furazolidone, monensin, olaquindox, virginiamycin and terdecamycin (Coulson 1981, Kitai et al. 1987, Ueda and Narukawa 1995).

In addition to antimicrobial agents, dietary zinc has been evaluated as a potential prophylactic agent (Zhang et al. 1995). The results obtained with a mouse model of swine dysentery indicate that dietary supplementation with 6000 mg of zinc per kg of feed significantly reduces the recovery of *S. hyodysenteriae* from infected mice and provides partial protection against the development of caecal lesions. The precise mode of action of the zinc is unknown. However, there have been reports that zinc may negatively regulate haemolysin biosynthesis (Dupont et al. 1994).

4.6 Control and prevention

Recommended control measures include the treatment of diseased animals and the prophylaxis of unaffected animals with appropriate antimicrobial agents, identification and separation of carriers, isolation of new breeding stock, timely removal of waste, and the cleaning and disinfection of pens. Programmes have been instituted in a number of countries to control and, wherever possible, eradicate swine dysentery. In Britain a successful effort was made to maintain, foster and expand disease-free herds (Goodwin and Whittlestone 1984). Alternatively, in Germany the emphasis was placed on eradication of the disease from infected breeding herds through a combination of antimicrobial treatment, extensive cleaning, disinfection and rodent control (Blaha, Erler and Burch 1987). The economic benefit of disease eradication is considerable. The cost of such an effort is rapidly recouped because of improved production and reduced drug usage

(Wood and Lysons 1988). Disease prevention through vaccination has been of limited success. Although various vaccines have been tested, none has elicited complete protection (Hampson, Robertson and Mhoma 1993, Diego et al. 1995).

5   SPIRILLARY RAT-BITE FEVER

Rat-bite fever is an illness characterized by chills, rash and intermittent fever. As the name implies, the disease is primarily associated with the bite of a rat. Two types of rat-bite fever, spirillary and streptobacillary, have been described. Although an association between rodents and disease has existed for centuries, reports of rat-bite fever only began to appear frequently at the beginning of this century. However, by 1916, nearly 100 cases of the illness had been reported from various countries around the world. During that period, considerable progress was made in the search for an aetiological agent. In 1909, Ogata was able to transmit rat-bite fever experimentally by allowing rats to bite guinea pigs (Ishiwara, Ohtawara and Tamura 1917). The guinea pigs went on to develop fever, swelling and congestion at the site of the bite, and swelling of the lymph glands. Several years later, Futaki and colleagues (1916), while studying 2 patients with rat-bite fever, observed spirochaetes in skin excised from a typical exanthem and in fluid and tissue collected from a swollen lymph gland. The inoculation of skin tissue and blood from one of the patients into monkeys, guinea pigs and white rats resulted in disease in all the animals. The association between rats, rat-bite fever and spirochaetes was further supported by Ishiwara, Ohtawara and Tamura (1917). Guinea pigs inoculated by rat bite experienced intermittent fever, swelling and congestion of the bite area, swelling of the subcutaneous lymph nodes, and weight loss. Acute changes in the adrenals and kidneys were also detected. The disease was passed to fresh guinea pigs through subcutaeous or intraperitoneal inoculation of diseased guinea pig tissues or blood. Spirochaetes were detected in blood and tissues of the donors and recipients. Similar results were reported by Futaki and colleagues (1917) who went on to name the aetiological agent *Spirochaeta morsus muris*. The name was later changed to *Spirillum minus* (Robertson 1924). Irrefutable evidence of the association between *S. minus* and rat-bite fever in humans was obtained when 104 patients inoculated with the organism for the treatment of general paresis developed typical rat-bite fever (Brown and Nunemaker 1942).

The aetiological agent of the streptobacillary form of rat-bite fever, which is not dealt with extensively here, was first described by Shottmuller and then Blake (1916) and ultimately named *Streptobacillus moniliformis* (Levaditi, Nicolau and Poincloux 1925). In addition to causing a form of rat-bite fever, *S. moniliformis* is associated with a food-borne illness, Haverhill fever. Although the characteristics of the spirillary and streptobacillary forms of rat-bite fever overlap in some respects, there are substantial differences.

5.1   Description of the disease

The spirillary form of rat-bite fever, also known by its Japanese name sodoku (rat-poison), affects all ages and typically presents as an intermittent relapsing fever often accompanied by a rash and regional lymphadenitis. Various investigators have characterized the disease after reviewing a large number of case reports (Bayne-Jones 1931, Brown and Nunemaker 1942, Watkins 1946, Roughgarden 1965). Spirillary rat-bite fever most often begins with a rat bite although other modes of transmission, including mouse bite, cat scratch, cat bite, or contact with a dog, have been reported. In most cases, the bite wound heals promptly. The incubation period is usually more than 7 days but has ranged from 1 to 36 days. The disease begins with the appearance of a purplish induration, usually without suppuration in the area of the bite wound. Ulceration or eschar can also occur. Along with the changes at the wound site, the patient experiences an onset of moderate to high fever, occasionally with chills. In most cases, a rash appears which has been variously described as dark and purple, purplish-red, red-brown, or bluish-red in colour and maculopapular or roseolar-urticarial in appearance. The rash can be either localized or generalized. After several days, the fever disappears, usually along with the other signs and symptoms of infection. The individual remains asymptomatic for a number of days before relapsing. Each relapse is characterized by the reappearance of fever, inflammation at the wound site, and a rash. The number and frequency of relapses are not at all predictable. The illness may continue for months in untreated patients. Leucocytosis, most often between 10 000 and 20 000 mm^{-3}, and moderate anaemia are common and coincide with fever. Diarrhoea, vomiting and weight loss also occur in some cases.

Complications of spirillary rat-bite fever include nephritis and endocarditis and the estimated death rate is 6.5%. Arthritis, which is a common feature of streptobacillary rat-bite fever, is rarely present in the spirillary form of the disease. Pathology findings obtained at autopsy have included degeneration and necrosis of the liver, splenitis, splenomegaly, subacute endocarditis, hyperaemia of organs, and degeneration of the tubular epithelium of the kidneys.

5.2   Aetiology

The aetiological agent of spirillary rat-bite fever, *S. minus*, is a rigid spiral cell with 2 or 3 turns, blunt or pointed ends, and one or more flagella at each end (Krieg 1984). The cell diameter is approximately 0.2 μm, the length 3–5 μm, and the wavelength 0.8–1.0 μm. The organism is very actively motile. Although *S. minus* was originally designated as a *Spirillum* species, it is actually an unclassified organism. The absence of reproducible in vitro cultivation has made it impossible to obtain a definitive classification.

5.3 Epidemiology

Rats and mice are considered to be the natural reservoir for *S. minus*. However, reports of the incidence of *S. minus*-like organisms in wild rodents have been inconsistent. For example, Joekes (1925) found spirilla in at least 25% of the wild rats examined in London whereas in Japan, the reported incidence in wild rats ranged from 3 to 14% (Futaki et al. 1917, Brown and Nunemaker 1942). Knowles and Das Gupta (1928) found that 22% of rats in Calcutta, India were infected. In North America, the search for the organism in wild rats has been much less successful although it is presumed, based on confirmed cases of spirillary rat-bite fever in the USA, that at least some wild rats carry the organism (Brown and Nunemaker 1942, Beeson 1943). In addition to wild rats, laboratory mice and rats may be naturally infected with *S. minus*. As a result, laboratory workers who handle these animals are at increased risk for contracting rat-bite fever (Anderson, Leary and Manning 1983). It is important to note that, unlike guinea pigs, mice and rats do not develop symptoms when infected with *S. minus* and survive the infection without ill-effect (Ishiwara, Ohtawara and Tamura 1917).

Although mice and rats are known to transmit *S. minus* to humans through their bite, the source of the organism within the rodent is not known with certainty. The organism is typically not found in the mouth and saliva of infected rats (Futaki et al. 1917). There is evidence, however, that the organism is often present in eye exudates of infected rats with keratitis, conjunctivitis, or iritis (Mooser 1924). It is possible that *S. minus* in an eye exudate may drain into the mouth and thereby be available for transmission. In recent years, only a few reports of spirillary rat-bite fever have appeared in the literature (Hinrichsen et al. 1992, Bhatt and Mirza 1992). It is not at all clear whether the low number of cases represents decreased incidence of infection, under-reporting of the illness, or lack of detection of the organism.

5.4 Laboratory

For the laboratory diagnosis of spirillary rat-bite fever, blood is collected from the patient during a febrile episode and submitted for direct examination and intraperitoneal inoculation into mice or guinea pigs. Aspirates and biopsies of the bite wound, regional lymph nodes and skin lesions can also be tested. The blood and aspirates are examined by darkfield or phase contrast microscopy for the presence of *S.*

minus. Giemsa or Wright's stained smears or sections may also reveal the organism. Historically, the best results have been obained with darkfield microscopy. In the case of the animal inoculations, the blood of the patient is injected intraperitonially, usually into 4 different mice. Blood samples are then collected from the tail each day thereafter and examined for the presence of spirilla. Since laboratory rodents may be naturally infected with *S. minus*, the animals that are to be inoculated must be prescreened for the presence of the organism. The animals are usually monitored for at least 3 weeks following inoculation. However, more extensive monitoring may be advisable since in some cases the organism has taken as long as 30 days to appear (Beeson 1943). Three reports of successful in vitro cultivation of *S. minus* have appeared in the literature (Futaki et al. 1917, Joekes 1925, Hitzig and Liebesman 1944). Unfortunately, other investigators have not been able to cultivate the organism using similar methods. Serological testing to detect *S. minus* is not done. However, serological tests for syphilis may be affected by the organism. In fact, approximately 50% of patients with spirillary rat-bite fever have a false positive syphilis serology (Roughgarden 1965).

5.5 Treatment

Penicillin is the drug of choice for treating either spirillary or streptobacillary rat-bite fever. The drug is particularly effective against *S. minus*. Patients suffering from this illness who are treated with penicillin tend to respond in just 1 day (Roughgarden 1965). The value of penicillin was initially demonstrated by Tani and Takano (1958) who tested the effectiveness of various drugs against transfusible agents, including *S. minus*. The data showed that as little as 1000 units of penicillin G added to a *S. minus* suspension is sufficient to prevent transmission of the organism. Furthermore, in one case of spirillary rat-bite fever a dose as small as 24 000 units given daily for 5 days resulted in a prompt and lasting remission (Roughgarden 1965). Because the identity of the agent responsible for rat-bite fever may not be known at the time therapy is initiated, the recommended treatment has to be effective against *S. minus* and *S. moniliformis*. An effective regimen is 400 000–600 000 units of penicillin daily for at least 7 days. In the case of a treatment failure, the dose should be raised to 1 200 000 units daily. Alternative therapeutic agents include tetracycline and streptomycin. In some cases, antimicrobial therapy has resulted in a Jarisch–Herxheimer reaction.

REFERENCES

Alexander TJL, Taylor DJ, 1969, The clinical signs, diagnosis and control of swine dysentery, *Vet Rec*, **85**: 59–63.

Anderson LC, Leary SL, Manning PJ, 1983, Rat-bite fever in animal research laboratory personnel, *Lab Anim Sci*, **33**: 292–4.

Bandopadhyay AC, Vegad JL, 1983, Observations on the pathology of experimental avian spirochaetosis, *Res Vet Sci*, **35**: 138–44.

Bandopadhyay AC, Vegad JL, 1984, Enteritis and green diarrhoea in experimental avian spirochaetosis, *Res Vet Sci*, **37**: 381–2.

Barbour AG, 1984, Isolation and cultivation of Lyme disease spirochetes, *Yale J Biol Med*, **57**: 521–5.

Barbour AG, 1990, Antigenic variation of a relapsing fever *Borrelia* species, *Annu Rev Microbiol*, **44**: 155–71.

Barbour AG, Hayes SF, 1986, Biology of *Borrelia* species, *Microbiol Rev*, **50**: 381–400.

Barbour AG, Tessier SL, Stoenner HG, 1982, Variable major proteins of *Borrelia hermsii*, *J Exp Med*, **156**: 1312–24.

Barbour AG, Todd WJ, Stoenner HG, 1982, Action of penicillin on *Borrelia hermsii*, *Antimicrob Agents Chemother*, **21**: 823–9.

Bayne-Jones S, 1931, Rat-bite fever in the United States, *Int Clin*, **3**: 235–53.

Beeson PB, 1943, The problem of the etiology of rat bite fever: report of two cases due to *Spirillum minus*, *JAMA*, **123**: 332–4.

Belanger M, Jacques M, 1991, Evaluation of the An-Ident System and the indole spot test for the rapid differentiation of porcine treponemes, *J Clin Microbiol*, **29**: 1727–9.

Bhatt KM, Mirza NB, 1992, Rat bite fever: a case report of a Kenyan, *East Afr Med J*, **69**: 542–3.

Blaha T, Erler W, Burch DG, 1987, Swine dysentery control in the German Democratic Republic and the suitability of injections of tiamulin for the programme, *Vet Rec*, **121**: 416–19.

Blake FG, 1916, The etiology of rat-bite fever, *J Exp Med*, **23**: 39–60.

Blakemore WF, Taylor DJ, 1970, An agent possibly associated with swine dysentery, *Vet Rec*, **87**: 59–60.

Bland AP, Frost AJ, Lysons RJ, 1995, Experimental disease. Susceptibility of porcine ileal enterocytes to the cytotoxin of *Serpulina hyodysenteriae* and the resolution of the epithelial lesions: an electron microscopic study, *Vet Pathol*, **32**: 24–35.

Brocklesby DW, Scott GR, Rampton CS, 1963, *Borrelia theileri* and transient fevers in cattle, *Vet Rec*, **75**: 103–4.

Brown TM, Nunemaker JC, 1942, Rat-bite fever: a review of the American cases with reevaluation of etiology; report of cases, *Johns Hopkins Hosp Bull*, **70**: 201–307.

Bryceson ADM, Parry EHO et al., 1970, Louse-borne relapsing fever: a clinical and laboratory study of 62 cases in Ethiopia and a reconsideration of the literature, *Q J Med*, **39**: 129–70.

Butler T, 1985, Relapsing fever: new lessons about antibiotic action, *Ann Intern Med*, **102**: 397–9.

Butler T, Jones PK, Wallace CK, 1978, *Borrelia recurrentis* infection: single-dose antibiotic regimens and management of the Jarisch–Herxheimer reaction, *J Infect Dis*, **137**: 573–7.

Cadavid D, Bundoc V, Barbour AG, 1993, Experimental infection of the mouse brain by a relapsing fever *Borrelia* species: a molecular analysis, *J Infect Dis*, **168**: 143–51.

Callow LL, 1967, Observations on tick-transmitted spirochaetes of cattle in Australia and South Africa, *Br Vet J*, **123**: 492–7.

Canale-Parola E, 1984, Order I. Spirochaetales Buchanan 1917, 163[AL], *Bergey's Manual of Systematic Bacteriology*, eds Krieg NR, Holt JG, Williams & Wilkins, Baltimore, 38–9.

Chia SP, Taylor DJ, 1978, Factors affecting the survival of *Treponema hyodysenteriae* in dysenteric pig faeces, *Vet Rec*, **103**: 68–70.

Ciceroni L, Bartoloni A et al., 1994, Prevalence of antibodies to *Borrelia burgdorferi*, *Borrelia parkeri* and *Borrelia turicatae* in human settlements of the Cordillera Province, Bolivia, *J Trop Med Hyg*, **97**: 13–17.

Coulson A, 1981, Eradication of swine dysentery from closed pig herds, *Vet Rec*, **108**: 503.

da Cunha Ferreira RMC, Phillips AD et al., 1993, Intestinal spirochaetosis in children, *J Pediatr Gastroenterol Nutr*, **17**: 333–6.

Cutler SJ, Fekade D et al., 1994, Successful in-vitro cultivation of *Borrelia recurrentis*, *Lancet*, **343**: 242.

Davis RD, Burke JP, Wright LJ, 1992, Relapsing fever associated with ARDS in a parturient woman: a case report and review of the literature, *Chest*, **102**: 630–2.

Diarra AT, Mittal KR, Achacha M, 1994, Evaluation of microagglutination test for differentation between *Serpulina* (*Treponema*) *hyodysenteriae* and *S. innocens* and serotyping of *S. hyodysenteriae*, *J Clin Microbiol*, **32**: 1976–9.

Diego R, Lanza I et al., 1995, *Serpulina hyodysenteriae* challenge of fattening pigs vaccinated with an adjuvanted bivalent bacterin against swine dysentery, *Vaccine*, **13**: 663–7.

Donelson JE, 1995, Mechanisms of antigenic variation in *Borrelia hermsii* and African trypanosomes, *J Biol Chem*, **270**: 7783–6.

Douglas JG, Crucioli V, 1981, Spirochaetosis: a remediable cause of diarrhoea and rectal bleeding? *Br Med J*, **283**: 1362.

Doyle LP, 1944, A vibrio associated with swine dysentery, *Am J Vet Res*, **5**: 3–5.

Drumev D, Stoianova L, 1976, Effectiveness of sodium arsamilate and its effect on the immunity of hens experimentally infected with *Borrelia anserina*, *Vet Med Nauki*, **13**: 3–10.

Dupont DP, Duhamel GE et al., 1994, Effect of divalent cations on hemolysin synthesis by *Serpulina* (*Treponema*) *hyodysenteriae*: inhibition induced by zinc and copper, *Vet Microbiol*, **41**: 63–73.

Egan IT, Harris DL, Joens LA, 1983, Comparison of the microtitration agglutination test and the enzyme-linked immunosorbent assay for the detection of herds affected with swine dysentery, *Am J Vet Res*, **44**: 1323–8.

Elder RO, Duhamel GE et al., 1994, Rapid detection of *Serpulina hyodysenteriae* in diagnostic specimens by PCR, *J Clin Microbiol*, **32**: 1497–502.

Felsenfeld O, 1965, Borreliae, human relapsing fever, and parasite–host relationships, *Bacteriol Rev*, **29**: 46–74.

Flanigan TP, Schwan TG et al., 1991, Relapsing fever in the US Virgin Islands: a previously unrecognized focus of infection, *J Infect Dis*, **163**: 1391–2.

Fuchs PC, Oyama AA, 1969, Neonatal relapsing fever due to transplacental transmission of *Borrelia*, *JAMA*, **208**: 690–2.

Futaki K, Takaki F et al., 1916, The cause of rat-bite fever, *J Exp Med*, **23**: 249–50.

Futaki K, Takaki I et al., 1917, *Spirochaeta morsus muris*, N.Sp., the cause of rat-bite fever: second paper, *J Exp Med*, **25**: 33–44.

Glock RD, Harris DL, Kluge JP, 1974, Localization of spirochetes with the structural characteristics of *Treponema hyodysenteriae* in the lesions of swine dysentery, *Infect Immun*, **9**: 167–78.

Goodwin RF, Whittlestone P, 1984, Monitoring for swine dysentery: six years' experience with a control scheme, *Vet Rec*, **115**: 240–1.

Hampson DJ, Robertson ID, Mhoma JR, 1993, Experience with a vaccine being developed for the control of swine dysentery, *Aust Vet J*, **70**: 18–20.

Harel J, Forget C, 1995, DNA probe and polymerase chain reaction procedure for the specific detection of *Serpulina hyodysenteriae*, *Mol Cell Probes*, **9**: 111–19.

Harris DL, 1974, Current status of research on swine dysentery, *J Am Vet Med Assoc*, **164**: 809–12.

Harris D, Glock L et al., 1972, Swine dysentery. I. Inoculation of pigs with *Treponema hyodysenteriae* (new species) and reproduction of the disease, *Vet Med Small Anim Clin*, **67**: 61–4.

Henrik-Nielsen R, Lundbeck FA et al., 1985, Intestinal spirochetosis of the vermiform appendix, *Gastroenterology*, **88**: 971–7.

Henrik-Nielsen R, Orholm M et al., 1983, Colorectal spirochetosis: clinical significance of the infestation, *Gastroenterology*, **85**: 62–7.

Hinrichsen SL, Ferraz S et al., 1992, Sodoku – a case report, *Rev Soc Bras Med Trop*, **25**: 135–8.

Hitzig WM, Liebesman A, 1944, Subacute endocarditis associated with infection with *Spirillum*, *Arch Intern Med*, **73**: 415–24.

Holt JG, Krieg NR et al. (eds), 1994, *Bergey's Manual of Determinative Bacteriology*, 9th edn, Williams & Wilkins, Baltimore, 29–33.

Hovind-Hougen K, 1995, A morphological characterization of *Borrelia anserina*, *Microbiology*, **141**: 79–83.

Hovind-Hougen K, Birch-Andersen et al., 1982, Intestinal spirochetosis: morphological characterization and cultivation of the spirochete *Brachyspira aalborgi* gen. nov., sp. nov., *J Clin Microbiol*, **16**: 1127–36.

Howarth JA, Moulton JE, Frazier LM, 1956, Epizootic bovine abortion characterized by fetal hepatopathy, *J Am Vet Med Assoc*, **128**: 441–9.

Hunter D, Saunders CN, 1977, Diagnosis of swine dysentery using an absorbed fluorescent antiserum, *Vet Rec*, **101**: 303–4.

Hunter D, Wood T, 1979, An evaluation of the API ZYM system

as a means of classifying spirochaetes associated with swine dysentery, *Vet Rec*, **104**: 383–4.

ter Huurne AAHM, Muir S et al., 1994, Characterization of three putative *Serpulina hyodysenteriae* hemolysins, *Microb Pathog*, **16**: 269–82.

Ishiwara K, Ohtawara T, Tamura K, 1917, Experimental rat-bite fever: first report, *J Exp Med*, **25**: 45–64.

Jacques M, Girard C et al., 1989, Extensive colonization of the porcine colonic epithelium by a spirochete similar to *Treponema innocens*, *J Clin Microbiol*, **27**: 1139–41.

Joekes T, 1925, Cultivation of the spirillum of rat-bite fever, *Lancet*, **2**: 1225–6.

Joens LA, Harris DL, Baum DH, 1979, Immunity to swine dysentery in recovered pigs, *Am J Vet Res*, **40**: 1352–4.

Joens LA, Kinyon JM, 1980, Differentiation of *Treponema hyodysenteriae* from *T. innocens* by enteropathogenicity testing in the CF1 mouse, *Vet Rec*, **107**: 527–9.

Johnson RC, Burgdorfer W et al., 1987, *Borrelia coriaceae* sp nova: putative agent of epizootic bovine abortion, *Int J Syst Bacteriol*, **37**: 72–4.

Johnson RC, Kodner CB et al., 1990, Comparative in-vitro and in-vivo susceptibilities of the Lyme disease spirochete *Borrelia burgdorferi* to cefuroxime and other antimicrobial agents, *Antimicrob Agents Chemother*, **34**: 2133–6.

Jones MJ, Miller JN, George WL, 1986, Microbiological and biochemical characterization of spirochetes isolated from the feces of homosexual males, *J Clin Microbiol*, **24**: 1071–4.

Judge DM, Samuel I et al., 1974, Louse-borne relapsing fever in man, *Arch Pathol*, **97**: 136–40.

Kelly R, 1971, Cultivation of *Borrelia hermsii*, *Science*, **173**: 443.

Kelly RT, 1984, Genus IV. *Borrelia* Swellengrebel 1907, 582^AL, *Bergey's Manual of Systematic Bacteriology*, eds Krieg NR, Holt JG, Williams & Wilkins, Baltimore, 57–62.

Kennedy MJ, Rosnick DK et al., 1988, Association of *Treponema hyodysenteriae* with porcine intestinal mucosa, *J Gen Microbiol*, **134**: 1565–76.

Kennedy PC, Casaro AP et al., 1983, Epizootic bovine abortion: histogenesis of the fetal lesion, *Am J Vet Res*, **44**: 1040–8.

Kimsey PB, Kennedy PC et al., 1983, Studies on the pathogenesis of epizootic bovine abortion, *Am J Vet Res*, **44**: 1266–71.

Kinyon JM, Harris DL, Glock RD, 1977, Enteropathogenicity of various isolates of *Treponema hyodysenteriae*, *Infect Immun*, **15**: 638–46.

Kitai K, Kashiwazaki M et al., 1987, In vitro antimicrobial activity against reference strains and field isolates of *Treponema hyodysenteriae*, *Antimicrob Agents Chemother*, **31**: 1935–8.

Knowles R, Das Gupta BM, 1928, Rat-bite fever as an Indian disease, *Indian Med Gaz*, **63**: 493–512.

Krieg NR, 1984, Aerobic/microaerophilic, motile, helical/vibrioid Gram-negative bacteria, *Bergey's Manual of Systematic Bacteriology*, eds Krieg NR, Holt JG, Williams & Wilkins, Baltimore, 89.

Kunkle RA, Harris DL, Kinyon JM, 1986, Autoclaved liquid medium for propagation of *Treponema hyodysenteriae*, *J Clin Microbiol*, **24**: 669–71.

Kunkle RA, Kinyon JM, 1988, Improved selective medium for the isolation of *Treponema hyodysenteriae*, *J Clin Microbiol*, **26**: 2357–60.

Lane RS, Burgdorfer W et al., 1985, Isolation of a spirochete from the soft tick, *Ornithodoros coriaceus*: a possible agent of epizootic bovine abortion, *Science*, **230**: 85–7.

Lee JI, Hampson DJ, 1994, Genetic characterization of intestinal spirochaetes and their association with disease, *J Med Microbiol*, **40**: 365–71.

Lee JI, Hampson DJ et al., 1993a, Genetic relationships between isolates of *Serpulina* (*Treponema*) *hyodysenteriae*, and comparison of methods for their subspecific differentiation, *Vet Microbiol*, **34**: 35–46.

Lee JI, McLaren AJ et al., 1993b, Human intestinal spirochetes are distinct from *Serpulina hyodysenteriae*, *J Clin Microbiol*, **31**: 16–21.

van Leengoed LA, Smit HF et al., 1985, Swine dysentery in a sow herd. I. Clinical manifestation and elimination of the disease with a combination of lincomycin and spectinomycin, *Vet Q*, **7**: 146–50.

Levaditi C, Nicolau S, Poincloux P, 1925, Sur le rôle étiologique de *Streptobacillus moniliformis* (nov. spec.) dans l'erythème polymorphe aigu septicémique, *C R Acad Sci*, **180**: 1188–90.

Levine JF, Dykstra MJ et al., 1990, Attenuation of *Borrelia anserina* by serial passage in liquid medium, *Res Vet Sci*, **48**: 64–9.

Li Z, Belanger M, Jacques M, 1991, Serotyping of Canadian isolates of *Treponema hyodysenteriae* and description of two new serotypes, *J Clin Microbiol*, **29**: 2794–7.

Li Z, Jensen NS et al., 1992, Molecular characterization of *Serpulina* (*Treponema*) *hyodysenteriae*, *J Clin Microbiol*, **30**: 2941–7.

Lo TCN, Heading RC, Gilmour HM, 1994, Intestinal spirochetosis, *Postgrad Med J*, **70**: 134–7.

Loomis EC, 1953, Avian spirochetosis in California turkeys, *Am J Vet Res*, **14**: 612–15.

Lysons RJ, Kent KA et al., 1991, A cytotoxic haemolysin from *Treponema hyodysenteriae* – or probable virulence determinant in swine dysentery, *J Med Microbiol*, **34**: 97–102.

McKercher DG, Wada EM et al., 1980, Preliminary studies on transmission of *Chlamydia* to cattle by ticks (*Ornithodoros coriaceus*), *Am J Vet Res*, **41**: 922–4.

McNeil E, Hinshaw WR, Kissling RE, 1949, A study of *Borrelia anserina* infection (spirochetosis) in turkeys, *J Bacteriol*, **57**: 191–206.

Mapother ME, Joens LA, 1985, New serotypes of *Treponema hyodysenteriae*, *J Clin Microbiol*, **22**: 161–4.

Mhoma JR, Hampson DJ, Robertson ID, 1992, A serological survey to determine the prevalence of infection with *Treponema hyodysenteriae* in Western Australia, *Aust Vet J*, **69**: 81–4.

Milner JA, Sellwood R, 1994, Chemotactic response to mucin by *Serpulina hyodysenteriae* and other porcine spirochetes: potential role in intestinal colonization, *Infect Immun*, **62**: 4095–9.

Milner JA, Truelove KG et al., 1995, Use of commercial enzyme kits and fatty acid production for the identification of *Serpulina hyodysenteriae*: a potential misdiagnosis, *J Vet Diagn Invest*, **1995**: 92–7.

Mooser H, 1924, Experimental studies with a spiral organism found in a wild rat, *J Exp Med*, **39**: 589–601.

Nadelman RB, Wormser GP, Sherer C, 1990, Blood transfusion-associated relapsing fever, *Transfusion*, **30**: 380–1.

Negussie Y, Remick DG et al., 1992, Detection of plasma tumor necrosis factor, interleukins 6 and 8 during the Jarisch–Herxheimer reaction of relapsing fever, *J Exp Med*, **175**: 1207–12.

Newman K, Johnson RC, 1984, T-cell-independent elimination of *Borrelia turicatae*, *Infect Immun*, **45**: 572–6.

Nuessen ME, Joens LA, Glock RD, 1983, Involvement of lipopolysaccharide in the pathogenicity of *Treponema hyodysenteriae*, *J Immunol*, **131**: 997–9.

Olson LD, Fales WH, 1983, Comparison of stained smears and culturing for identification of *Treponema hyodysenteriae*, *J Clin Microbiol*, **18**: 950–5.

Osebold JW, Spezialetti R et al., 1986, Congenital spirochetosis in calves: association with epizootic bovine abortion, *J Am Vet Med Assoc*, **188**: 371–6.

Osebold JW, Osburn BI et al., 1987, Histopathologic changes in bovine fetuses after repeated reintroduction of a spirochete-like agent into pregnant heifers: association with epizootic bovine abortion, *Am J Vet Res*, **48**: 627–33.

Packchanian A, 1960, Chemotherapy of *Borrelia anserina* infection (spirochetosis) in chicks with amphomycin, kanamycin, telomycin and tetracycline, *Antibiot Chemother*, **10**: 731–9.

Packchanian A, Smith JB, 1970, Immunization of chicks against avian spirochetosis with vaccines of *Borrelia anserina*, *Texas Rep Biol Med*, **28**: 287–301.

Park NY, Chung CY et al., 1995, Polymerase chain reaction for the identification of human and porcine spirochaetes recovered from cases of intestinal spirochaetosis, *FEMS Microbiol Lett*, **125:** 225–30.

Parr LW, 1923, Intestinal spirochetes, *J Infect Dis*, **33:** 369–83.

Parry EHO, Warrell DA et al., 1970, Some effects of louse-borne relapsing fever on the function of the heart, *Am J Med*, **49:** 472–9.

Picken RN, 1992, Polymerase chain reaction primers and probes derived from flagellin gene sequences for specific detection of the agents of Lyme disease and North American relapsing fever, *J Clin Microbiol*, **30:** 99–114.

Robertson A, 1924, Observation of the causal organism of rat-bite fever in man, *Ann Trop Med Parasitol*, **18:** 157–75.

Rodgers FG, Rodgers C et al., 1986, Proposed pathogenic mechanism for the diarrhea associated with human intestinal spirochetosis, *Am J Clin Pathol*, **86:** 679–82.

Roughgarden JW, 1965, Antimicrobial therapy of ratbite fever; a review, *Arch Intern Med*, **116:** 39–54.

Sakharoff N, 1891, *Spirochaeta anserina* et la septicémie des oies, *Ann Inst Pasteur (Paris)*, **5:** 564–6.

Salih SY, Mustafa D, 1977, Louse-borne relapsing fever. II. Combined penicillin and tetracycline therapy in 160 Sudanese patients, *Trans R Soc Trop Med Hyg*, **71:** 49–51.

Schmidtmann ET, Bushnell RB et al., 1976, Experimental and epizootiologic evidence associating *Ornithodoros coriaceus* Koch (Acari: Argasidae) with the exposure of cattle to epizootic bovine abortion in California, *J Med Entomol*, **13:** 292–9.

Schwan TG, Gage KL et al., 1992, Identification of the tick-borne relapsing fever spirochete *Borrelia hermsii* by using a species-specific monoclonal antibody, *J Clin Microbiol*, **30:** 790–5.

Seboxa T, Rahlenbeck SI, 1995, Treatment of louse-borne relapsing fever with low dose penicillin or tetracycline: a clinical trial, *Scand J Infect Dis*, **27:** 29–31.

Songer JG, Harris DL, 1978, Transmission of swine dysentery by carrier pigs, *Am J Vet Res*, **39:** 913–16.

Sotiropoulos C, Coloe PJ, Smith SC, 1994, Identification and characterization of *Serpulina hyodysenteriae* by restriction enzyme analysis and Southern blot analysis, *J Clin Microbiol*, **32:** 1397–401.

Southern PM, Sanford JP, 1969, Relapsing fever: a clinical and microbiological review, *Medicine (Baltimore)*, **48:** 129–49.

Spagnuolo PJ, Butler T et al., 1982, Opsonic requirements for phagocytosis of *Borrelia hermsii* by human polymorphonuclear leukocytes, *J Infect Dis*, **145:** 358–64.

Spezialetti R, Osebold JW, 1991, Surface markers on bovine fetal lymphocytes and immunoglobulin synthesis in a congenital infection related to epizootic bovine abortion, *Res Vet Sci*, **51:** 239–45.

Stoenner HG, Dodd T, Larsen C, 1982, Antigenic variation of *Borrelia hermsii*, *J Exp Med*, **156:** 1297–311.

Stoianova-Zaikova L, Doneva M, 1982, Blood concentrations and anti-*Borrelia anserina* activity of erythromycin salts in birds, *Vet Med Nauki*, **19:** 97–103.

Sundnes KO, Haimanot AT, 1993, Epidemic of louse-borne relapsing fever in Ethiopia, *Lancet*, **342:** 1113–15.

Tani T, Takano S, 1958, Prevention of *Borrelia duttonii*, *Trypanosoma gambiense*, *Spirillum minus* and *Treponema pallidum* infections conveyable through transfusion, *Jpn J Med Sci Biol*, **11:** 407–13.

Taylor DJ, Alexander TJL, 1971, The production of dysentery in swine by feeding cultures containing a spirochaete, *Br Vet J*, **127:** 58–61.

Taylor DJ, Simmons JR, Laird HM, 1980, Production of diarrhoea and dysentery in pigs by feeding pure cultures of a spirochaete differing from *Treponema hyodysenteriae*, *Vet Rec*, **106:** 326–32.

Teglbjaerg PS, 1990, Intestinal spirochaetosis, *Curr Top Pathol*, **81:** 247–56.

Theiler A, 1904, Spirillosis of cattle, *J Comp Pathol Ther*, **17:** 47–55.

Trape JF, Duplantier JM et al., 1991, Tick-borne borreliosis in West Africa, *Lancet*, **337:** 473–5.

Ueda Y, Narukawa N, 1995, Effect of terdecamycin on experimentally induced swine dysentery in pigs, *J Vet Med Sci*, **57:** 173–6.

Vallejo MT, 1969, Spirochaetales microorganisms: an agent possible associated with swine dysentery, *Vet Rec*, **85:** 562–3.

Wada EM, McKercher DG et al., 1976, Preliminary characterization and pathogenicity studies of a virus isolated from ticks (*Ornithodoros coriaceus*) and from exposed cattle, *Am J Vet Res*, **37:** 1201–6.

Warrell DA, Perine PL et al., 1983, Pathophysiology and immunology of the Jarisch–Herxheimer-like reaction in louse-borne relapsing fever: comparison of tetracycline and slow-release penicillin, *J Infect Dis*, **147:** 898–909.

Watkins CG, 1946, Ratbite fever, *J Pediatr*, **28:** 429–48.

White J, Roche D et al., 1994, Intestinal spirochetosis in children: report of two cases, *Pediatr Pathol*, **14:** 191–9.

Whiting RA, Doyle LP, Spray RS, 1921, Swine dysentery, *Purdue Univ Agric Exp Sta Bull*, **257:** 1–15.

Wood EN, Lysons RJ, 1988, Financial benefit from the eradication of swine dysentery, *Vet Rec*, **122:** 277–9.

Zhang P, Duhamel GE et al., 1995, Prophylactic effect of dietary zinc in a laboratory mouse model of swine dysentery, *Am J Vet Res*, **56:** 334–9.

Zingg BC, LeFebvre RB, 1994, Polymerase chain reaction for detection of *Borrelia coriaceae*, putative agent of epizootic bovine abortion, *Am J Vet Res*, **55:** 1509–15.

Zuelzer M, 1936, *Culex*, a new vector of *Spirochaeta gallinarum*, *J Trop Med Hyg*, **39:** 204.

Chapter 44

PLAGUE

K L Gage

1 INTRODUCTION

Plague is an acute and often fatal bacterial zoonosis that is transmitted primarily by the fleas of commensal rats and other rodents. Although there is some debate about the first recorded instances of plague in humans, few would argue that plague has had a tremendous impact on the course of human history (Zinsser 1934, Tuchman 1978, Gregg 1985, Dennis and Orloski 1995).

Probably the first reliable reports of plague are those from the Plague of Justinian. This outbreak was the first historically documented pandemic of plague and began sometime around 540 AD (Zinsser 1934, Dennis and Orloski 1995). According to Procopius, who was an eyewitness to many of the events he described, Justinian's Plague originated in East Africa, spread down the Nile to Pelusium, and later invaded the great port city of Alexandria (Zinsser 1934). From Alexandria, the disease was carried to the rest of Egypt and to Palestine, and thence to the whole Mediterranean region, first appearing along the coasts and later spreading inland. By most estimates, this pandemic persisted for 50–60 years and caused 40 million deaths, a figure that is even more striking when one considers that the world's population at the time probably only slightly exceeded 260 million persons and was definitely less than 500 million (Fisher and Hoy 1992). Many believe that this pandemic hastened the fall of the Roman Empire and contributed to the ensuing cultural darkness that engulfed Europe until the advent of Charlemagne's reign in 800 AD (Zinsser 1934).

Almost 750 years elapsed before the next pandemic, now aptly named the Black Death, arose from central Asia and killed millions in China, India, the Middle East, North Africa and Europe (Pollitzer 1954). In 1346 AD Europeans began to hear rumours of a terrible disease that had swept the East and was spreading westward into Tartary (Central Asia), India, Persia, Mesopotamia, Syria and elsewhere (Tuchman 1978). The dreadful truth of these stories was revealed in the following year, when Genoese trading ships, returning from the plague-infected Crimea, arrived at the Sicilian port of Messina bearing dead and dying men. Thus, Messina became the first of many European cities to be ravaged over the next few years by the Black Death. By the time the epidemic had peaked a few years later, perhaps one-fourth to one-third of the continent's population had perished. Unlike the first pandemic, which probably was almost entirely flea-borne (bubonic plague), the Black Death also caused explosive outbreaks of primary pneumonic plague, an air-borne form of the disease that can be passed directly from person to person by coughing and is virtually always fatal unless promptly treated with appropriate antibiotics. The epidemic was especially terrible in western Europe, where survivors were left in states of shock and despair. The Black Death's impact, however, lasted far beyond the lives of these survivors and resulted in fundamental changes in medieval European society, including a decline in the influence of the Catholic Church and a serious weakening of the feudal system. According to Tuchman (1978):

> Survivors of the plague, finding themselves neither destroyed nor improved, could discover no Divine purpose in the pain they had suffered. God's purposes were usually mysterious, but this scourge was simply too terrible to be accepted without questioning. If a disaster of such magnitude, the most lethal ever known, was a mere wanton act of God or perhaps not God's work at all, then the absolutes of a fixed order were loosed from their moorings. Minds that opened to admit these questions could never again be shut. Once people envisioned the possibility of change in a fixed order, the end of an age of submission came in sight; the turn to individual conscience lay ahead. To that extent the Black Death may have been the unrecognized beginning of modern man.

The last of the 3 great plague pandemics, usually referred to as the Modern Pandemic, originated in China, perhaps in Yunnan province. Human cases occurred as early as 1866 in the southern Chinese city of Kun-ming, spread to the port of Pei-hai (Pakhoi) in 1882, and eventually appeared in Canton and Hong Kong in 1894 (Gregg 1985). From Hong Kong the disease was carried by ships to Bombay and Calcutta in India and San Francisco in the USA. Soon port cities in Asia, Africa, Australia, North and South America, and Europe were affected and the third pandemic was under way. Before it had run its course, epidemics had occurred in every continent, except Antarctica, and the death toll exceeded 12 million in India and hundreds of thousands elsewhere (Poland, Quan and Barnes 1994). The Modern Pandemic did not produce the tremendous mortality and social chaos associated with the previous 2 pandemics, but it did result in a great expansion in the natural distribution of plague. Many regions of the world that were free of the disease before the last pandemic now have active foci, including North and South America, southern Africa, certain regions of Asia, and the islands of Java and Madagascar (Fig. 44.1) (Pollitzer 1954, Gregg 1985).

Research activities undertaken during the early stages of the Modern Pandemic also resulted in critical scientific discoveries. These included identification of the aetiological agent in Hong Kong in 1894 by Alexandre Yersin (the organism was eventually named *Yersinia pestis* in his honour); incrimination of fleas as vectors of plague by Simond in 1898 and proof of this hypothesis by Liston in 1905; development of a partially effective, heat-killed vaccine by Haffkine in 1896; and, beginning in 1905, a decade of thorough studies by the British Commission for the Investigation of Plague in India that elucidated the roles played by commensal rats (*Rattus rattus* and *Rattus norvegicus*) and their fleas, especially *Xenopsylla cheopis*, in outbreaks of human bubonic plague (Pollitzer and Meyer 1961, Gregg 1985). At present, plague remains a threat in many regions of the world, as indicated by the fact that it is one of only 3 diseases, along with cholera and yellow fever, that are subject to mandatory international reporting and other provisions of the International Health Regulations, including possible quarantine.

2 PATHOGENESIS

Plague is an acute febrile illness that causes high mortality unless promptly diagnosed and treated. All races and ethnic groups are susceptible to infection and typically develop severe illness when infected with *Y. pestis*. Many series of cases from different regions of the world have been reviewed by various authors (Mengis 1962, Caten and Kartman 1968, Reed et al. 1970, Reiley and Kates 1970, Palmer et al. 1971, Butler 1972, Butler et al. 1974, Welty et al. 1985, Crook and Tempest 1992). Other reports have described paediatric plague (Mann, Shandler and Cushing 1982), septicaemic plague (Hull, Montes and Mann 1987), meningeal plague (Martin et al. 1967, Tuan et al. 1971, Butler 1976, Becker et al. 1987), pneumonic plague (Meyer 1961, Trong, Nhu and Marshall 1967), and plague fatalities or autopsied cases (Finegold 1968, Jones, Mann and Braziel 1979). The above studies and others indicate that the common symptoms of plague include fever, headache, chills, myalgia, prostration, malaise, gastrointestinal symptoms and often acute lymphadenopathy (buboes) (Pollitzer 1954, Poland and Barnes 1979, Butler 1984, Poland, Quan and Barnes 1994). The 3 predominant clinical forms are bubonic, septicaemic and pneumonic plague.

Bubonic plague is the most common of the 3 forms and is characterized by the appearance of a swollen lymph node or bubo that ranges in size from a few millimetres to as large as a hen's egg. These buboes, which are often extremely tender and painful, usually develop in the lymph nodes draining the initial site of infection. An inguinal bubo is likely to appear in those persons who are bitten on the leg by an infectious flea, whereas those who contract plague as a result of handling an infected animal are likely to develop an axillary bubo. The 3 most common bubo locations, in descending order, are inguinal, axillary and cervical.

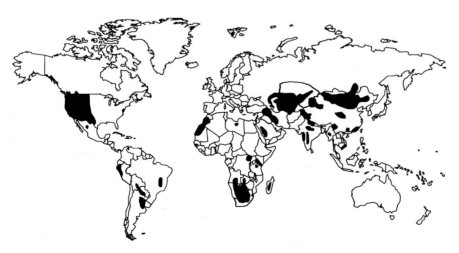

Probable foci

Fig. 44.1 Probable natural foci of plague, compiled from WHO and CDC sources.

Other lymph nodes may be affected but involvement of deeper nodes probably is due to secondary spread of the organism via the bloodstream (Sites and Poland 1972, Poland and Barnes 1979). In most instances, patients develop only a single bubo. Fatality rates for untreated bubonic cases are reported to be 50–60% (Poland and Barnes 1979).

The second most common form of the disease is septicaemic plague, which is characterized by the continuous presence and proliferation of *Y. pestis* in the bloodstream. Septicaemic plague is likely to develop in inadequately treated bubonic cases (secondary septicaemic plague), but also can occur without prior lymphadenopathy (primary septicaemic plague). The latter form is especially dangerous because of the difficulties encountered in rapidly diagnosing human plague in the absence of a bubo. Dissemination of *Y. pestis* via the bloodstream can result in secondary plague pneumonia and, occasionally, meningitis, endophthalmitis and the development of focal abscesses in the liver, spleen, kidneys and lungs (Hull, Montes and Mann 1987, Poland, Quan and Barnes 1994). Small amounts of plague endotoxin may be released into the bloodstream during bacillary growth and larger amounts released from bacteriolysis induced by host immune responses or drug therapy. Although plague endotoxin has been proposed by some to be less potent than the endotoxins produced by other Enterobacteriaceae, it can cause septic shock, multiple organ failure, consumptive coagulopathy, coma and death, if present at sufficiently high concentrations (Butler et al. 1974, 1976, Poland, Quan and Barnes 1994). Septicaemic patients also are at risk of developing adult respiratory distress syndrome. It is not unusual to observe plague bacilli in peripheral blood smears taken from severe cases of septicaemic plague, an observation that is rarely reported for sepsis caused by other gram-negative organisms. The identification of *Y. pestis* bacteria on such smears indicates a grave, but not hopeless, prognosis (Butler et al. 1976, Poland and Barnes 1979). In the USA about 10% of cases do not develop buboes and about 50% of these non-bubo-forming cases die (Poland and Barnes 1979). Elderly persons are reported to be at greatest risk, but septicaemic plague can occur in any age group, especially among persons, such as hunters or trappers, who are likely to cut themselves or introduce *Y. pestis* into cuts or abrasions while handling infected animals (Hull, Montes and Mann 1987, Gage, Montenieri and Thomas 1994). According to Hull, Montes and Mann (1987), most deaths from septicaemic plague occur in persons 30 years of age or younger, perhaps because, unlike the elderly, these individuals are less likely to receive empirical antibiotic treatment.

The least common, but most dangerous, form of the disease is pneumonic plague. In addition to the general symptoms described above, pneumonic plague patients are likely to have cough, dyspnoea and haemoptysis. Pneumonic plague can develop as a complication of inadequately treated septicaemic plague (secondary pneumonic plague) or occur due to the inhalation of infectious materials (primary pneumonic plague). The latter form is usually acquired as a result of close contact (1–2 m) with a pneumonic plague patient who is coughing, but also has occurred when persons were exposed to infectious respiratory droplets from cats with plague pneumonia (Doll et al. 1994, Gage, Montenieri and Thomas 1994). Individuals have also developed primary pneumonic plague as a result of exposure to infectious aerosols or air-borne droplets in laboratory environments (Burmeister, Tiggert and Overholt 1962). Mortality rates for pneumonic plague are very high and probably reach 100% for untreated cases (Poland and Barnes 1979). Persons who survive pneumonic plague occasionally experience cavitation or focal necrosis of lung tissues. Usually these cavitary lesions disappear over time, but at least one patient required surgery more than 2 years after the acute stage of her illness to remove damaged lung tissue (Poland 1989). Radiographic manifestations of 42 plague cases were reviewed by Alsofrom, Mettler and Mann (1981), who reported a high, but not entirely specific, association between bilateral alveolar infiltrates and secondary pneumonic plague.

Other relatively rare complications of plague not mentioned above include pharyngitis and the development of an ulcer at the site where *Y. pestis* first entered the patient's body (usually through a cut or abrasion on the skin or at the site where an infectious flea fed). Plague in pregnant women and a neonate and its successful treatment have also been described (Mann and Moskowitz 1977, Coppes 1980, White 1981, Welty 1985, Wong 1986).

3 DESCRIPTION OF DISEASE IN OTHER HOSTS

The primary vertebrate hosts of *Y. pestis* are certain rodent species, but other mammals become infected and some develop severe illness. Birds and other non-mammalian vertebrates appear to be completely resistant to plague.

The most commonly used animal models are guinea pigs and laboratory mice, but rats, rabbits and non-human primates are also highly susceptible (Pollitzer 1954). Although guinea pigs and mice usually die following infection by virulent *Y. pestis* strains (median lethal dose values of approximately 1–100 organisms), the course of illness differs somewhat in these 2 species (Poland, Quan and Barnes 1994). Mice are more likely than guinea pigs to die within 5 days after exposure to infection and seldom exhibit the characteristic organ pathologies that are commonly observed in infected guinea pigs. The relatively low survival times for infected mice probably reflect their extreme sensitivity to murine toxin, an exotoxin that specifically affects mice and rats (Brubaker 1991). Unlike mice, guinea pigs frequently survive for more than 5 days after being inoculated with low to moderate doses of *Y. pestis*, and often have signs attributable to the pathogenic effects of plague endotoxin, including fever, listlessness and anorexia. Guinea pigs infected by subcutaneous inoculation in the abdominal region often develop inguinal lymphadenopathy within 2–4 days after exposure; those that survive for 5 or more days frequently have swollen lymph nodes (buboes) that may be necrotic. Characteristic organ pathologies are also likely to be apparent at necropsy, including livers that are pale and contain light-coloured necrotic nodules, enlarged, dusky red spleens with necrotic nodules, and lungs that exhibit haemorrhagic lesions, necrotic foci, focal congestion and consolidation (Poland and Barnes 1979). Ulcerations can develop at the site of inoculation and may be surrounded with gelatinous oedema. The hearts, kidneys and brains of infected guinea pigs typically appear normal.

The susceptibilities of different wild rodent species to plague-related mortality vary greatly. Some species, such as the prairie dogs (burrowing squirrel-like rodents belonging to the genus *Cynomys*) of western North America, are extremely susceptible. Epizootics among colonies of these animals spread very quickly and may cause greater than 99% mortality (Barnes 1982). Other rodents, such as kangaroo rats (*Dipodomys* spp.) in North America or some gerbil species of the genus *Meriones* in Asia, can be infected with *Y. pestis* but are relatively resistant and apparently suffer few ill effects. Certain species have both highly susceptible and relatively resistant populations (Hubbert and Goldenberg 1970, Thomas et al. 1988).

Relatively few studies have investigated the course of *Y. pestis* infection in wild rodent hosts, but available evidence indicates that at least some of these animals develop organ pathologies and other signs of infection that are similar to those observed in laboratory animals. McCoy (1911) reported that experimentally infected California ground squirrels (*Spermophilus beecheyi*) developed buboes, splenomegaly and occasionally necrotic nodules in the liver or spleen. Later studies done with the same species (Williams, Moussa and Cavanaugh 1979), and with the closely related rock squirrel (*Spermophilus variegatus*) (Quan et al. 1985), indicate that some of these animals survive high dosages (60 000 or more *Y. pestis*) and others succumb to inoculations containing as few as 10 plague bacilli. Terminally ill rock squirrels and California ground squirrels developed nasal bleeding, petechial haemorrhaging (subcutaneous and cutaneous), splenomegaly, occasional infarctions and abscess formations in spleens, and signs of plague pneumonia.

Naturally occurring plague infections have been reported from many species of mammals other than rodents. Carnivores living in plague-enzootic areas are often found to be seropositive, especially when epizootics have recently occurred in sympatric rodent populations (Barnes 1982). Members of the following carnivore families have been reported to be seropositive: Canidae (dogs, coyotes, foxes), Felidae (cats, bobcats, mountain lions), Procyonidae (raccoons and ring-tailed cats), Mustelidae (weasels, ferrets, skunks, badgers, martens), Ursidae (bears), Viverridae (mongooses) (Davis et al. 1968, Hallett, McNeill and Meyer 1970, Rust et al. 1971b, Barnes 1982, Burdelov 1982, Messick, Smith and Barnes 1983, Zielinski 1984, Clover et al. 1989). With the notable exception of cats and their wild relatives, however, it is rare to observe unusual carnivore mortality during rodent plague epizootics. This has led some to propose that many of these species are relatively resistant to infection. Only a handful of studies have investigated the susceptibilities of carnivores under laboratory conditions. Dogs and coyotes fed *Y. pestis*-infected animal carcasses did not develop obvious signs of illness but did seroconvert following exposure (Rust et al. 1971a, Poland, Quan and Barnes 1994). Although these limited studies indicate that canids are relatively resistant to plague, a survey of veterinary records in the southwest plague focus of the USA suggests that dogs occasionally exhibit signs of illness (Orloski and Eidson 1995). An isolated report of a human case of plague in a

boy who handled a dead coyote that was infected with *Y. pestis* also suggests that some coyotes are susceptible to plague (Von Reyn et al. 1976b).

Occasionally, *Y. pestis* has been identified in dead or sick domestic cats, or in tissue samples taken from bobcats or mountain lions found dead in the wild in western North America (Barnes 1982, Smith, Nelson and Barnes 1984, Tabor and Thomas 1986, CDC unpublished data). Although there are few experimental data on the susceptibility of wild felids, Rust et al. (1971a) reported that each of 5 cats infected by consumption of infected mice (3 cats) or by subcutaneous inoculation (2 cats) exhibited fever, bacteraemia and severe illness. Three of these cats died, including 2 that ingested infected mice and another that was infected by subcutaneous inoculation. Gasper et al. (1993) fed *Y. pestis*-infected mice to 16 cats and reported that 6 (38%) of these animals died. Only 3 of the 16 cats failed to exhibit signs of illness, 75% became bacteraemic, and 56% had lymphadenopathy (primarily submandibular and cervical). Eidson, Thilsted and Rollag (1991) reviewed the clinical and pathological findings for 119 cases of plague in domestic cats in New Mexico, USA and reported that most (53%) infected cats developed bubonic plague. Only 8% were reported to be septicaemic and another 10% developed plague pneumonia. One-third of the cats exhibited a combination of buboes, fever, lethargy and anorexia; 25% had these signs plus abscesses. Among the cats with bubonic plague, 75% had submandibular buboes, which suggests that they contracted plague as a result of consuming infected rodent prey, a finding that agrees with other epidemiological observations (Eidson et al. 1988). Eidson, Thilsted and Rollag (1991) also reported that one-third of the cats in their study died. They believed that this was an underestimation of the true mortality, however, because many animals probably become ill and die without being examined. Other carnivores have been reported to seroconvert, but not die, following experimental infection with *Y. pestis*, including raccoons, skunks, domestic ferrets, Siberian polecats, pine martens and mongooses (Higa, Matsuura and Watanabe 1971, Williams et al. 1991, Poland, Quan and Barnes 1994). There is a single published report of a fatal plague infection in a black-footed ferret (Williams 1994), but additional deaths are known to have occurred at a captive rearing facility, when these endangered animals were mistakenly fed *Y. pestis*-infected prairie dog carcasses (CDC unpublished data).

Mammals other than rodents and carnivores may seroconvert following infection with *Y. pestis*. Some of these animals also have been reported to exhibit moderate to severe illness. For example, non-human primates are highly susceptible and exhibit symptoms and pathologies that are similar to those observed in humans (Pollitzer 1954, Chen and Meyer 1965, 1974, Finegold 1969, Hallet, Isaacson and Meyer 1973, Chen, Elberg and Eisler 1977). Infections have also been reported among artiodactyls (even-toed ungulates), including goats, camels, mule deer, swine, water buffaloes and a prong-horned antelope (Gordon, Isaacson and Taylor 1979, Christie, Chen and Elberg 1980, Thorne et al. 1987, WHO 1991, Poland, Quan and Barnes 1994). Although many of these infections were detected only by serological means, Christie, Chen and Elberg (1980) reported that infected camels and goats exhibited recognizable illness, an observation that agrees with experimental susceptibility studies on camels (Feodorov 1960). Thorne et al. (1987) described plague in a free-ranging mule deer that was noted to be seriously ill just prior to its death. According to Marshall et al. (1972), swine seroconvert following inoculation of *Y. pestis* but do not exhibit obvious signs of illness. Feral hogs living in areas enzootic for plague also have been reported to seroconvert to *Y. pestis* (Clark et al. 1983). Lagomorphs (rabbits and hares) are extremely susceptible to plague and occasionally suffer significant mortality during rodent epizootics (Pollitzer 1954, Von Reyn et al. 1976a). Among the Insectivora, house shrews (*Suncus murinus*) have been reported to be infected and are generally believed to be moderately resistant (Marshall et al. 1967a).

4 AETIOLOGY

Y. pestis is a gram-negative coccobacillus of the family Enterobacteriacae. It is aerobic or facultatively anaerobic, non-motile, non-spore-forming, non-lactose fermenting and grows in a variety of liquid or solid media, including nutrient broth, brain–heart infusion broth, blood agar and unenriched agar (Quan, Barnes and Poland 1981). Growth can occur at temperatures ranging from 4 to 37°C but is optimal at 28°C. Even at optimal temperatures, *Y. pestis* requires 48 h or more to produce non-mucoid, greyish colonies of 1–2 mm in size. When viewed under a stereo microscope, these colonies have a pitted appearance that is reminiscent of hammered copper. Growth in liquid media is flocculent, lacks turbidity and typically occurs on the side of the tube, with characteristic stalactite-like structures projecting downward from the main areas of growth. When stained with Giemsa, Wright's or Wayson's stain, *Y. pestis* exhibits bipolar staining that results in a characteristic 'safety pin' appearance. Unlike other yersiniae, all *Y. pestis* strains are generally believed to belong to a single serotype.

Although well adapted to its complex parasitic lifestyle in mammalian hosts and flea vectors, the plague bacteria cannot survive long under saprophytic conditions, or high temperatures (>40°C), or in desiccating environments. Metabolic studies and other observations indicate that *Y. pestis* has lost the ability to express many metabolic properties or other characteristics exhibited by its congeners, *Yersinia pseudotuberculosis* and *Yersinia enterocolitica* (Brubaker 1991). The latter 2 species differ from *Y. pestis* in their ability to survive for relatively long periods of time under saprophytic conditions (primarily in host faeces) and then proliferate in the digestive tracts of their hosts following transmission via oral routes. Unlike *Y. pseudotuberculosis* and *Y. enterocolitica*, *Y. pestis* is non-motile, lacks hydrophobic sugars in its lipopolysaccharides (has rough lipopolysaccharides (LPS) without extended O-antigen chains), is unable to produce some amino acids and lacks certain enzymes responsible for processing various intermediary molecules in the tricarboxylic acid cycle or other metabolic pathways (Brubaker 1991, Straley and Perry 1995). Apparently, retention of these capabilities is of little selective advantage to *Y. pestis* strains, either because the required metabolites can be obtained from the host or because these factors are not necessary for survival within the mammalian host or flea vector.

Y. pestis also differs from its less pathogenic congeners in a number of other ways, including possession of a greater variety of virulence factors. These unique virulence factors are in most instances important for survival of the plague bacillus in its mammalian hosts and flea vectors. Many of the genes associated with these various factors reside on one or another of the 3 plasmids found in *Y. pestis*. The smallest of these plasmids (c. 9.5 kb) is the pesticin or Pst plasmid, which has genes encoding for a plasminogen activator, a bacteriocin (pesticin) and its corresponding immunity protein, and the production of factors that enhance certain activities associated with other factors encoded on the Lcr plasmid described below (Brubaker 1991). Plasminogen activator (Pla) is responsible for fibrinolytic activities that promote dissemination of *Y. pestis* within the mammalian hosts (Sodeinde et al. 1992). Pla also coagulates rabbit plasma, but not human, mouse, or rat plasma. This coagulase activity, which is higher at 28°C than at 37°C, has not been shown to be significant in mammals, but could have a pulicidal effect (McDonough et al. 1993). Pesticin itself probably plays no direct role in virulence, but loss of sensitivity to this bacteriocin is correlated with a dramatic decrease in the virulence of such *Y. pestis* strains for mice. It is believed that pesticin binds to a receptor site located on a surface protein of *Y. pestis* that is involved in iron uptake and is probably the same receptor used by a *Y. pestis* siderophore (Fetherston, Lillard and Perry 1995). Therefore, loss of pesticin sensitivity presumably correlates to loss of the siderophore binding site and the inability of *Y. pestis* to obtain sufficient iron for growth in the mammalian host environment.

The Lcr (low calcium response) plasmid of *Y. pestis* is approximately 70 kb in size and encodes for gene products involved in the low calcium response of *Y. pestis*. This response is expressed at 37°C in low calcium environments (<2.5 mM Ca^{2+}), such as those encountered within mammalian host phagocytes but not while circulating freely in the bloodstream (Straley and Perry 1995). *Y. pestis* exhibiting the low calcium response, halt stable RNA synthesis, reduce adenylate energy charge, cease cell division and initiate synthesis of Lcr plasmid-encoded virulence factors. The later include *Yersinia* outer-membrane proteins (Yops) and soluble V antigen, both of which are probably essential for survival in phagocytic cells (Brubaker 1991). Fowler and Brubaker (1994) reported that Lcr+ strains can undergo significant cell division in experimental low calcium environments, providing the medium is formulated so that potassium ions are substituted for sodium ions, chloride ions are eliminated, and L-aspartate supplements are added. Growth of these strains could also be enhanced by increasing the amounts of fermentable carbohydrate in the medium. Nakajima and Brubaker (1993) also presented evidence that Lcr+ strains of *Y. pestis* interfere with host production of interferon-γ and tumour necrosis factor α. Lcr− strains are avirulent and do not interfere with production of these cytokines in infected animals.

The third *Y. pestis* plasmid (Tox plasmid) is approximately 110 kb in size and bears genes coding for murine exotoxin (murine toxin) and the F1 capsular antigen (Brubaker 1991, Straley and Perry 1995). Murine exotoxin reportedly functions as an adrenergic antagonist and is unusual in that is highly toxic for mice and rats but is apparently harmless for other mammalian species (Brubaker 1991). Encapsulated (F1 positive) *Y. pestis* strains are reported to be resistant to phagocytosis in the absence of opsonizing antibodies and loss of the F1 capsular antigen significantly reduces the virulence of such *Y. pestis* strains for guinea pigs and rats (Janssen 1963, Brubaker 1991). F1 negative strains retain the capacity to kill mice when inoculated by peripheral routes, but the time required to do so is significantly longer than for encapsulated strains. Rats injected subcutaneously with non-encapsulated (F1 negative) strains do not die, as is typical for rats inoculated with encapsulated strains, but rather develop chronic infections and abscesses on their spleens or livers, or persistent pleural or abdominal buboes that may contain viable *Y. pestis* for a year or longer (Williams and Cavanaugh 1983).

Other virulence factors are encoded by chromosomal genes, including those associated with the LPS production (endotoxin) and pigmentation (haemin storage locus) (Brubaker 1991, Straley and Perry 1995). Strains that are pigment minus are typically avirulent in mammalian hosts and reportedly are incapable of inducing block formation in the flea vector. Another chromosomally encoded gene product, referred to as pH 6 antigen (Psa), is expressed under low pH conditions similar to those found in the phagolysosomes of host phagocytes. This antigen has been proposed to be important for survival of *Y. pestis* within host phagocytes, including polymorphonuclear leucocytes, that are likely to be attracted to the initial site of infection (usually the site of a flea bite) (Straley and Perry 1995).

Devignat (1951) identified 3 biotypes of *Y. pestis* based on the abilities of different strains to ferment glycerol and reduce nitrate. Interestingly, the distribution of the antiqua, mediaevalis, and orientalis biotypes corresponds reasonably well with the presumed origins and distributions of the first, second and third pandemics, respectively (Pollitzer 1954, 1960). Guiyoule et al. (1994) described a ribotyping system that identifies a number of distinct ribotypes and gives results that agree reasonably well with those of Devignat's typing system.

5 HOST RESPONSE

Both humoral and cell mediated immune mechanisms are reported to be important in immunity to plague (Wong and Elberg 1977, Wake, Morita and Wake 1978, Nakajima, Motin and Brubaker 1995). Laboratory animal studies of mice, rats, guinea pigs and monkeys immunized with formalin-inactivated vaccine or live, attenuated vaccine strains expressing F1 antigen, suggest that induction of sufficiently high levels of antibody to the F1 capsular antigen, or the passive transfer of such antibodies to susceptible hosts, is correlated with protection against later subcutaneous challenge inoculations of virulent *Y. pestis* (mimics transmission by flea bite) (Meyer and Foster 1948, Meyer 1970, 1971, Bartelloni, Marshall and Cavanaugh 1973, Hallett, Isaacson and Meyer 1973, Chen, Elberg and Eisler 1976, Williams and Cavanaugh 1979). Passive transfer of sera from humans immunized with killed bacterial vaccine also protected mice, providing the titres of these sera were 1:128 or higher by passive haemagglutination assays (Meyer 1970). More recent studies have indicated that purified preparations of recombinant *Y. pestis* F1 antigen expressed in *E. coli* are capable of protecting mice against challenge by virulent *Y. pestis* (Simpson, Thomas and Schwan 1990). Oyston et al. (1995) also reported that mice could be protected against plague by immunizing these animals with a live recombinant *Salmonella typhimurium aroA* expressing *Y. pestis* F1 antigen.

Although the above cited studies suggest that induction of antibodies to F1 is important for protection against subcutaneous challenge inoculations of *Y. pestis*, the resulting immune response is short-lived and may not protect hosts against air-borne routes of infection. Various other antigens are known to exist and some of these might be protective (Mazza, Karu and Kingsbury 1985, Abath et al. 1991, Motin et al. 1994, Leary et al. 1995). Leary et al. (1995) demonstrated that mice could be protected against challenge with virulent *Y. pestis* by immunization with preparations of a recombinant V antigen of *Y. pestis* that was expressed in *E. coli*. Protected mice developed both high titres to V antigen and a T cell response specific for V antigen.

6 ECOLOGICAL AND EPIDEMIOLOGICAL ASPECTS

Understanding the epidemiology of plague requires a basic knowledge of the natural history of this flea-borne zoonosis. This is no small task, as evidence of *Y. pestis* infection has been identified in over 200 species of mammals belonging to at least 8 different mammalian orders, and in more than 150 species of fleas (Pollitzer and Meyer 1961, Poland and Barnes 1979, Barnes 1982, CDC unpublished data). Most of these mammals and fleas probably are 'accidental' hosts of *Y. pestis* and play only minor roles in the ecology of plague. The true reservoirs of the disease are certain highly to moderately susceptible rodents and their fleas, which maintain *Y. pestis* in ongoing rodent–flea–rodent transmission cycles (Fig. 44.2).

These rodent hosts become bacteraemic when infected with *Y. pestis* and, therefore, serve as sources of infectious blood meals for feeding vector fleas. Rodents also provide adult fleas with blood meals, which are their sole source of nutrition. Undoubtedly, the best known rodent hosts of plague are commensal rats (*R. rattus* and *R. norvegicus*). These animals suffer high mortality during epizootics and are often heavily infested with important flea vectors, including *X. cheopis*, and, in some regions of Africa and South America, *Xenopsylla brasiliensis*. Movement of plague-infected rats and rat fleas from one region to another was the major means by which plague was carried to regions outside its central Asian homeland or, perhaps, the ancient focus in eastern Africa. These invasions of plague-infected rats and rat fleas into previously unaffected areas often cause tremendous die-offs among resident rat populations, as well as bubonic plague epidemics among humans in these areas. Of the 2 commensal rat species mentioned above, the roof or black rat (*R. rattus*) is usually considered to be of greater historical, epidemiological and ecological significance than the Norway or brown rat (*R. norvegicus*). Roof rats have been associated since ancient times with human populations in many regions of Asia, the Middle East and the coast of the Mediterranean Sea. This rat later spread throughout most of Europe during the Middle Ages and eventually reached the New World in the post-Columbian era. Today, roof rats are extremely abundant throughout much of the world, including many areas with natural foci of plague infection. Unlike the roof rat, the Norway rat was not important during the first and

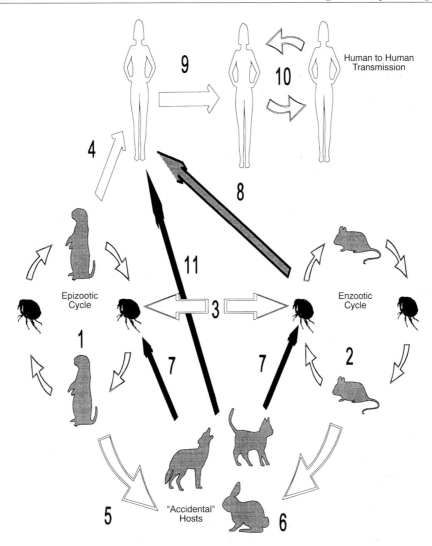

Fig. 44.2 Natural cycle of *Y. pestis*. 1 Epizootic cycle involving commensal rats or wild rodents that are highly susceptible to plague; results in amplification and geographical spread of plague. 2 Enzootic cycle involving moderately resistant enzootic or maintenance hosts; responsible for maintaining plague during interepizootic periods. 3 Transfers of *Y. pestis*-infected fleas from enzootic hosts to epizootic hosts can result in widespread epizootics that threaten other animals and humans; reverse transfers from epizootic to enzootic hosts can result in establishment of new enzootic foci of infection. 4 Transmission of *Y. pestis* to humans via the bites of infectious rodent fleas or via handling of infected epizootic hosts; such transmission can result in epidemics of human bubonic plague when commensal rats are involved. 5 Transmission of *Y. pestis* to non-rodent mammals, including carnivores and lagomorphs, via bites of infectious rodent fleas or consumption of infected epizootic hosts by carnivores. 6 Transmission of *Y. pestis* to non-rodent mammals via bites of infectious rodent fleas or consumption of infected enzootic hosts by carnivores. 7 Transport of infectious rodent fleas by non-rodent mammals, especially carnivores, or by raptorial birds; can result in saltatory spread of plague. 8 Transmission of *Y. pestis* from enzootic hosts to humans, a process that is considered to be relatively unimportant compared to process number 4. 9 Transmission of *Y. pestis* to humans via inhalation of infectious respiratory droplets expelled from coughing patients with secondary pneumonic plague. 10 Continued person-to-person transmission of *Y. pestis* via inhalation of infectious respiratory droplets expelled from persons with primary pneumonic plague. 11 Transmission of *Y. pestis* to humans via direct contact with infected animals or inhalation of infectious respiratory droplets expelled from cats with plague pneumonia; pets also can transport infectious fleas in human habitations.

second pandemics and probably did not spread to the Middle East and Europe until the 1700s. After this time, however, it largely replaced the roof rat in many areas of Europe, and in certain urban and port areas elsewhere in the world (Pollitzer 1961). *R. norvegicus* are more aggressive than *R. rattus* and often displace the latter species from certain ground-level habitats that they prefer, thus forcing *R. rattus*, which are excellent climbers, to occupy attics, trees, or other above-ground and commonly marginal habitats. In general, displacements of *R. rattus* by *R. norvegicus* usually occur in ports and urban sites, but are much less common in the rural areas of many developing countries where the roof rat reigns supreme and plague occurs most frequently. During the last pandemic, Norway rats and roof rats both played significant roles in spreading plague from one region to another and causing increased plague risks for humans. The relative importance of each species, however, varied from place to place, depending on local environmental characteristics (rural versus urban, for example).

Although roof and Norway rats played critical roles in spreading plague around the globe, these animals and their fleas are generally considered to be incapable of maintaining plague continuously in an area without repeated reintroductions of *Y. pestis* from external sources. Most authorities believe that long-term persistence of *Y. pestis* in a given area requires the presence of wild rodent hosts that are both moderately resistant to plague and also infested with species of fleas that are efficient vectors of plague. The areas where plague is maintained in populations of these semi-resistant rodents and their fleas are termed enzootic, wild rodent, or sylvatic foci. The term sylvatic foci is probably the most commonly used of these 3 basically synonymous terms. It is etymologically somewhat of a misnomer, however, as plague usually occurs in semiarid steppe or mountainous regions rather than in heavily forested areas, as implied by the word sylvatic.

Each of the world's major wild rodent plague foci can be distinguished by their distinctive rodent hosts and flea vectors. In western North America, 2 large sylvatic foci (southwest and Pacific Coast plague foci; not distinctly recognizable in Fig. 44.1) exist, along with other smaller and less well characterized areas of infection. In the southwest plague focus the most important hosts are various prairie dogs (primarily *Cynomys gunnisoni*), ground squirrels (*Spermophilus variegatus* and to lesser extents *Spermophilus spilosoma* and *Spermophilus lateralis*), antelope ground squirrels (primarily *Ammospermophilus leucurus*), chipmunks (*Tamias* sp.), wood rats (primarily *Neotoma albigula* and *Neotoma mexicana*), and deer mice (*Peromyscus maniculatus*) and their relatives (other *Peromyscus* spp.) (Barnes 1982, CDC unpublished data). The important rodent hosts in different regions of the Pacific Coast focus include various ground squirrels (primarily *Spermophilus beecheyi*, *Spermophilus beldingi* and *Spermophilus lateralis*), chipmunks (*Tamias amoenus*, *Tamias merriami*, *Tamias quadrimaculatus*, *Tamias siskiyou*, *Tamias sonomae*, *Tamias speciosus* and *Tamias townsendi*), wood rats (*Neotoma fuscipes* and to a lesser extent *Neotoma cinerea*), deer mice (*P. maniculatus*) and voles (primarily *Microtus californicus* and *Microtus montanus*) (Barnes 1982). Hosts in other regions of western North America are less well defined, but *Y. pestis*-infected animals and fleas, and even epizootics, have been reported occasionally from a variety of areas. Among the rodents likely to be important hosts in these other areas are certain ground squirrels, including *Spermophilus elegans* in the central Rocky Mountains, *Spermophilus armatus* in the west-central Rocky Mountains, and *Spermophilus townsendi* in the northern Great Basin region. Similarly, plague occasionally devastates colonies of black-tailed prairie dogs (*Cynomys ludovicianus*) on the Great Plains. A number of epizootics also have occurred in introduced fox squirrel populations in cities in Colorado, Texas, and Wyoming (Barnes 1982, CDC 1994). Evidence of *Y. pestis* infection has also been reported from Mexico and Canada, including the identification of plague in Mexican prairie dogs (*Cynomys mexicanus*) collected in northern Mexico (Varela and Vasquez 1954), and in bushy-tailed wood rats (*N. cinerea*) and Richardson's ground squirrels (*Spermophilus richardsoni*) collected in southwestern Canada (Pollitzer 1960, CDC unpublished data). The distributions and status of natural foci of infection in the latter 2 countries have yet to be determined. Commensal rats are no longer considered to be important hosts of plague in North America, possibly because rat populations that are located near sylvatic foci are infested with very few

fleas (Schwan, Thompson and Nelson 1985, CDC 1994). The primary vectors of plague among wild rodents in North America include various prairie dog fleas (*Opisocrostis* spp.), ground squirrel fleas [*Diamanus montanus* (*Oropsylla montana*), *Thrassis* spp., *Opisocrostis* spp., *Oropsylla idahoensis*, *Hoplopsyllus anomalus*], chipmunk fleas (primarily *Eumolpianus eumolpi*), wood rat fleas (*Orchopeas neotomae*, *Orchopeas sexdentatus* and others), and mouse fleas (*Malaraeus* spp., *Aetheca wagneri*, *Orchopeas leucopus* and others) (Pollitzer 1960, Barnes 1982, CDC unpublished data).

In South America, *Y. pestis* has been reported from a variety of rodent species, including commensal rats, rice rats (*Oryzomys* spp.), cotton rats (*Sigmodon* spp.), South American field mice (*Akodon* spp.), cane mice (*Zygodontomys* spp.), leaf-eared mice (*Phyllotis* spp.), tree squirrels (*Sciurus stramineus*), wild cavies and domestic guinea pigs (family Caviidae, especially the genera *Cavia* and *Galea*) and, perhaps, other wild rodent species or rabbits (*Sylvilagus* spp.) (PAHO 1965). At present, active foci exist in Brazil, Bolivia and along both sides of the Peruvian–Ecuadoran border (Fig. 44.1). The animals most frequently reported to be infected in Brazil include *R. rattus*, *Zygodontomys pixuna* (cane mice), *Bolomys lasiurus* (formerly *Zygodontomys lasiurus*) and species of *Oryzomys* (PAHO 1965, Almeida et al. 1981, de Almeida et al. 1987). The role of commensal rats and domestic guinea pigs needs to be better defined in this Andean focus, but both species are presumed to be important in many situations. The hosts of plague in Bolivia probably include *R. rattus* and *Oryzomys* spp., along with a few other sylvatic rodent species. The primary vectors in South American foci are *X. cheopis* on rats and, in many instances, species of *Polygenis* on wild rodents (PAHO 1965). The wild rodent flea, *Pleochaetis dolens*, has been reported to be a vector in the Peruvian–Ecuadoran focus.

The most important hosts of plague in Africa include multimammate mice (*Mastomys* spp.), unstriped grass mice (*Arvicanthis* spp.), swamp rats (*Otomys* spp.), and members of 2 genera of gerbils (*Tatera* and *Desmodillus*) (Pollitzer and Meyer 1961, Davis 1964, Hallett, McNeill and Meyer 1970, Poland and Barnes 1979). In southern Africa, plague is maintained in wild habitats by transmission between gerbils, *Tatera brantsi*, *Tatera leucogaster* and *Desmodillus auricularis*, and their fleas (primarily *Xenopsylla philoxera*) (Davis 1964, Hallett, McNeill and Meyer 1970). Spring hares (*Pedetes capensis*) also have been suggested to be important hosts in southern Africa (Hallett, McNeill and Meyer 1970, Isaacson and Hallett 1975). During widespread epizootics, plague can spread from gerbil populations to multimammate mice living in fields and in close proximity to human habitations. Infected fleas from multimammate mice may, in turn, pass the infection to commensal rats and rat fleas (primarily *X. brasiliensis*) living on farms and in villages. In Kenya the most important wild rodent hosts are believed to be multimammate mice, unstriped grass rats and swamp rats (Heisch, Grainger and D'Souza 1953). In Tanzania plague infections have been identified in multimammate mice, unstriped grass mice, swamp rats, and groove-toothed cheek rats (*Pelomys* spp.) (Njumwa et al. 1989, Kilonzo 1992). The important vectors in Kenya and Tanzania include *X. cheopis* and *X. brasiliensis* on commensal rats and occasionally wild rodents, and species of *Dinopsyllus* on wild rodents.

The most important plague hosts in the interior of the Eurasian landmass vary from one region to another (Pollitzer 1960, 1966, Pollitzer and Meyer 1961, Poland and Barnes 1979). Gerbils are important hosts in certain central Asian foci, including Iranian Kurdistan (*Meriones persicus*, *Meriones libycus*, *Meriones tristrami* and *Meriones vinogradovi*), the Transcaucasian focus southwest of the Caspian Sea (*Meriones*

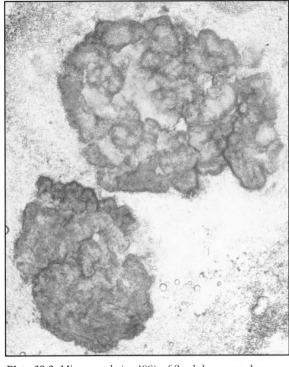

Plate 39.3 Micrograph (x 400) of 2 sulphur granules showing the typical cauliflower-like structure. The granules are surrounded by a thick layer of inflammatory cells, in particular polymorphonuclear granulocytes.

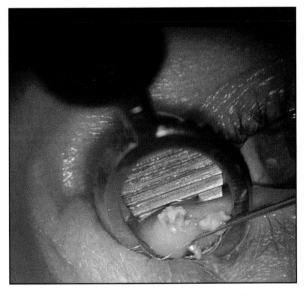

Plate 39.4 Lacrimal concretions consisting chiefly of branched actinomycete filaments that appear in the aperture of the lacrimal duct on pressure.

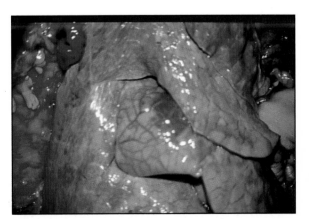

Plate 54.1 Acute contagious bovine pleuropneumonia. Exterior of bovine lung showing distension of the interlobular septa with serous fluid. (Courtesy of Dr R A J Nicholas).

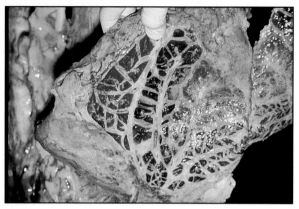

Plate 54.2 Acute contagious bovine pleuropneumonia. Bovine lung cut to show hepatization of lobules with oedema and thickening of interlobular septa giving a 'marbled' appearance. (Courtesy of Dr R A J Nicholas).

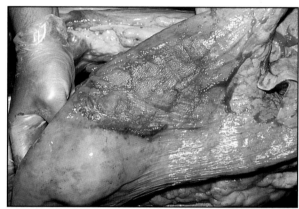

Plate 54.3 Chronic contagious bovine pleuropneumonia. Bovine lung showing point of adhesion of pleural membrane (top) and a sequestrum (bottom). (Courtesy of Dr R A J Nicholas).

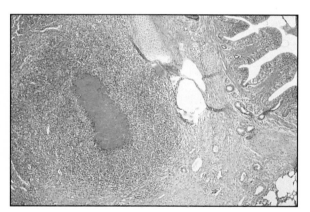

Plate 54.4 *Mycobacterium bovis* infection in a gnotobiotic calf. Section of lung showing an area of coagulative necrosis surrounded by cellular infiltration. Haematoxylin and eosin stain. (Courtesy of Dr C J Howard).

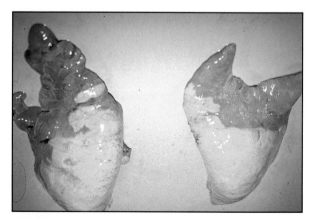

Plate 54.5 Enzootic porcine pneumonia. Affected lungs showing consolidation of the apical lobes. (Courtesy of Dr J R Walton).

erythrourus), the Pre-Caspian focus near the northwestern shores of the Caspian Sea (*Meriones meridianus* and *Meriones tamariscinus*), the central Asiatic plains of the former Soviet Union (*Meriones erythrourus* and *Rhombomys opimus*), Mongolia (*M. meridianus*, *Meriones unguiculatus* and *R. opimus*) and north-central China (*Meriones unguiculatus*). The primary vectors on these gerbils are various sylvatic species of *Xenopsylla* and *Nosopsyllus*, and species of *Coptopsylla* (Pollitzer 1960, 1966). Marmots (*Marmota* spp.) are important hosts in Transbaikalia, high mountain areas in central Asia, and northeast China. Depending on the specific region, the primary vectors on marmots are various species of *Oropsylla*, *Rhadinopsylla*, *Citellophilus*, or *Callopsylla* (Kucheruk 1960, Bibikov 1965, Pollitzer 1966). Various susliks and sisels (ground squirrels of the genus *Spermophilus*, formerly *Citellus*) are known to be infected in other regions, including *Spermophilus dauricus* in north-central China, Transbaikalia and Mongolia, *Spermophilus pallidicaudai* in Mongolia, *Spermophilus fulvus* in the Central Asiatic Plains, and *Spermophilus pygmaeus* in the Pre-Caspian focus and Volgo-Ural area (Pollitzer 1960). The primary vectors on these ground squirrels vary by region and include *Citellophilus tesquorum* and species of *Neopsylla* (Pollitzer 1960). *Y. pestis* has also been identified in Pere David's voles (*Eothenomys* spp.) in south-central China, Brandt's voles (*Microtus brandti*) in north-central China and western Mongolia, and common voles (*Microtus arvalis*) in central Asia and southeast Russia (Pollitzer 1960, Balabkin et al. 1962). *Y. pestis*-infected species of *Amphipsylla* and *Rhadinopsylla* fleas have been collected from species of *Microtus* in Asia.

The primary hosts of plague in Vietnam and Myanmar (Burma) are *R. rattus* (subspecies *diardii*, sometimes referred to as a separate species *Rattis diardi*) and the Polynesian rat, *Rattus exulans* (Marshall et al. 1967a, Cavanaugh et al. 1968a, Cavanaugh, Ryan and Marshall 1969, Velimorovic 1972, Brooks et al. 1977, Thaung 1978). *R. rattus* (subsp. *flavipectus*) is the most important host in nearby southern China. *R. exulans*, like *R. rattus*, is often heavily infested with *X. cheopis* fleas and probably plays an important role in both rural and urban outbreaks in Vietnam (Marshall et al. 1967a, Cavanaugh et al. 1968a, Cavanaugh, Ryan and Marshall 1969). *R. norvegicus* is reported to be an important host of plague in urban areas in Vietnam (Cavanaugh et al. 1968a). Bandicoot rats (*Bandicota indica*) have also been reported to be infected in Vietnam and Myanmar (Cavanaugh et al. 1968b). The above rodents are generally considered to be commensals and are typically found near human dwellings or in fields or other agricultural sites. The primary vector of plague in Vietnam, Myanmar and southern China is *X. cheopis*, but *Xenopsylla astia*, a less efficient vector, also are present on animals in Vietnam and Myanmar (Brooks et al. 1977, Cavanaugh, Ryan and Marshall 1969). True sylvatic plague cycles involving wild rodent species and their fleas have yet to be identified in Vietnam or Myanmar, although Cavanaugh, Ryan and Marshall (1969) reported *Y. pestis* infection in the forest rat, *Rattus nitidus* in Vietnam. The house shrew (*Suncus murinus*), a non-rodent species belonging to the mammalian order Insectivora, has also been suggested by some to be an important host in Vietnam and Myanmar (Marshall et al. 1967a). These shrews live in peridomestic environments, are often infested with *X. cheopis* fleas, and have been reported to be infected with *Y. pestis* or harbour *Y. pestis*-infected fleas (primarily *X. cheopis*).

The Indian gerbil (*Tatera indica*) is generally considered to be the most important sylvatic host on the Indian subcontinent, but *Y. pestis* infections have been identified in a variety of other sylvatic and commensal rodents, including *Rattus* spp., bandicoot rats (*Bandicota bengalensis* and *Bandicota indica*), metads (*Millardia meltada*), Indian field mice (*Mus booduga*), spiny field mice (*Mus platythrix*), Indian bush rats (*Golunda ellioti*) and palm squirrels (*Funambulus* spp.). Most evidence suggests that *Y. pestis* is normally maintained in the Indian countryside by transmission between gerbils and their fleas (primarily *X. astia* and *Nosopsyllus punjabensis*), but can spread from these animals to other rodents, including bandicoot rats and commensal rats living in fields and in villages (Baltazard and Bahmanyar 1960, Pollitzer 1960, Seal 1960).

Polynesian rats (*Rattus exulans*) are generally considered to be the primary hosts of plague in Java. These rats are found primarily in fields but occasionally enter peridomestic environments. *Y. pestis* has also been isolated from commensal rats (*R. rattus diardii*) following epizootics and from fleas taken from white-bellied mountain rats (*Rattus niviventer*), Malayan wood rats (*Rattus tiomanicus*) and house shrews (*S. murinus*). As mentioned above, the latter species is not a rodent, but rather a commensal insectivore that has been proposed to play a role in peridomestic plague in Java (Williams et al. 1980). The primary vectors in Java probably are *X. cheopis* and *Stivalius cognatus*. *X. cheopis* occurs abundantly on *R. rattus diardii* and is often encountered on *R. exulans* and *S. murinus* in plague-affected areas. *S. cognatus* is common on *R. exulans* but also occurs on *R. rattus diardii* and other rodents on the slopes of 2 adjoining volcanoes in the Boyolali district of central Java (Turner, Martoprawiro and Padmowiryono 1974, Williams et al. 1980). This small region and another similar one located on another volcano (Mt Bromo) in eastern Java are believed to be the only areas where plague still exists on this island.

As noted above, each of the world's major plague foci typically has one or more species of rodent that is moderately resistant to plague-related mortality and are important for maintaining *Y. pestis* in that foci. These moderately resistant animals, termed enzootic or maintenance hosts, usually coexist with other species, referred to as epizootic hosts, that are extremely susceptible to plague and die in large numbers during epizootics. Different enzootic host populations often vary greatly in their susceptibility to plague (Poland, Quan and Barnes 1994). Existing evidence suggests that this resistance is inherited rather than acquired and may be the result of selection owing to past exposures of populations to *Y. pestis* infection (Thomas et al. 1988). Members of resistant populations can become infected with *Y. pestis* and serve as sources of infection for feeding fleas, but rarely die of plague. Enzootic hosts typically have shorter life spans (1–2 years) and higher reproductive rates (most are polyoestrous) than epizootic hosts, which results in non-immune juveniles being introduced frequently into populations throughout much of the year, depending on environmental conditions. Because many members of enzootic host populations are resistant to plague-related mortality, it is not unusual to see relatively high percentages of seropositive individuals in plague-enzootic areas (Hudson, Quan and Goldberg 1964).

The primary enzootic hosts in North America are generally believed to be species of voles (*Microtus* spp.) and deer mice and their relatives (*Peromyscus* spp.) (Poland and Barnes 1979). Examples of potential enzootic hosts in other regions of the world include certain gerbil species in Kurdistan (*M. persicus* and *M.*

lybicus), in the southern portions of the Volga-Ural and Trans-Ural areas (*M. meridianus*), in India (*T. indica*), and in southern Africa (*Desmodillus auricularis* and *Tatera brantsi*) (Pollitzer 1960, Davis 1964). Heisch, Grainger and D'Souza (1953) reported that grass rats (*Arvicanthis abyssinicus*) and multimammate mice (*Mastomys natalensis*) populations in Kenya were relatively resistant to infection and, therefore, probably act as 'reservoir' (enzootic) hosts. Such a proposed role for multimammate mice is interesting because populations of these animals in southern Africa are usually considered to be highly susceptible (epizootic hosts). This apparent discrepancy can be explained by the fact that *M. natalensis sensu lato* comprises 2 separate species that are morphologically similar but differ in chromosome number (Isaacson, Taylor and Arntzen 1983). The species of *Mastomys* found in the Kenyan study area of Heisch, Grainger and D'Souza (1953) is still referred to as *M. natalensis* and is relatively resistant to plague infection. Multimammate mice from southern Africa, however, belong to a recently recognized species, *Mastomys coucha*, that is highly susceptible to plague and experiences high mortality during epizootics (Isaacson, Taylor and Arntzen 1983).

Unlike enzootic hosts, epizootic hosts are highly susceptible to plague and usually die following infection with *Y. pestis*. Depending on the species involved, mortality among epizootic hosts can reach approximately 85–99% during epizootics. Compared to enzootic hosts, these animals also have longer life spans (2–3 years or more), lower reproductive rates (many are mono-oestrous), and exhibit much more uniformity between populations with respect to their susceptibility to infection (Poland and Barnes 1979). Epizootic hosts are sometimes referred to as amplifying hosts, in recognition of the important role they play in spreading plague from one area to another during epizootics. Some epizootics have been reported to extend over thousands of square kilometres and involve multiple species of epizootic hosts (Craven et al. 1993). Following widespread epizootics, populations of these animals are likely to decrease to levels that are insufficient for maintaining flea-borne transmission cycles within their populations. Numbers of these animals may remain below pre-epizootic levels for many years, but will eventually recover, as long as adequate habitat and food sources are available. As populations of these animals recover, however, they are increasingly likely to experience other widespread epizootics and subsequent crashes in numbers. These unstable fluctuations in epizootic host numbers and their presumed impact on plague transmission rates have led many authorities to propose that plague cannot persist in areas lacking the more resistant enzootic host species.

Many different species of rodents act as epizootic hosts in various plague foci around the world. In North America, the most important epizootic hosts include prairie dogs, ground squirrels, antelope ground squirrels, chipmunks and wood rats (Barnes 1982). In most instances, these epizootic hosts support dense populations of one or 2 species of fleas that are regionally important plague vectors. Each of these epizootic host–flea 'complexes' can be responsible for extensive amplification of plague epizootics over wide geographical areas during periods when epizootic host populations are high and environmental conditions are favourable for flea reproduction and survival (Barnes 1982). Likely epizootic hosts in central Asia include susliks and sisels, marmots and the highly susceptible gerbil species, *M. tristrami* and *M. vinogradovi* (Pollitzer and Meyer 1961). The primary epizootic hosts in southern China and other regions of South East Asia appear to be *R. rattus* or other species of *Rattus*. In Africa the list of epizootic hosts undoubtedly includes *R. rattus* and multimammate mice, especially *M. coucha*, but the roles played by other species are less clear (Poland and Barnes 1979). Based on the limited evidence available, the most likely epizootic hosts in South America are commensal rats, rice rats, cane mice, cavies and, perhaps, cotton rats (PAHO 1965).

The factors governing the occurrence of epizootics are complex and not completely understood. It is likely that extended periods of favourable weather, including above average rainfall and moderate temperatures, lead to increased food resources for rodents, which, in turn, result in larger rodent populations and increased epizootic risks, especially when the survival of infected fleas is prolonged by relatively mild temperatures and adequate humidity. The likelihood of epizootics can also vary with the seasons. In the USA, most epizootics, as well as most human cases, occur during the summer when certain flea populations peak and rodents are most active. Ambient temperatures also have been proposed to play an important role in affecting the course of epizootics. During the early 1900s, it was observed that the incidence and intensity of rat epizootics (ratfalls) in India, and the epidemics of human bubonic plague associated with these ratfalls, declined dramatically when daily temperatures exceeded 80°F (26.67°C). Similarly, Cavanaugh and Marshall (1972) reported that the number of plague cases in Vietnam decreased rapidly when daily temperatures exceeded 27.5°C. Although favourable weather may increase the likelihood of epizootics among many species, other rodents may be at greatest risk during unfavourable conditions. Severe droughts in southern Africa can force wild rodents, especially gerbils, to leave their homes in the veldt and seek food on farms and in small villages (Isaacson 1983). If these starving rodents are infected with *Y. pestis* or are infested with infected fleas, they can spread their infections to multimammate mice (*M. coucha*) and commensal rats (*R. rattus*) living in these farms and villages. The resulting epizootics among the latter 2 species are likely to result in epidemics of bubonic plague in the area's human population.

Non-rodent species, such as certain even-toed ungulates, insectivores, lagomorphs and carnivores, occasionally become infected with *Y. pestis* but are unlikely to serve as important sources of infection for feeding fleas (Pollitzer and Meyers 1961, Christie 1982, Gage, Montenieri and Thomas 1994, Poland, Quan and Barnes 1994). These animals can, however, play ecologically important roles by serving as temporary flea hosts and as means of transporting infected fleas from one region to another (Gage, Montenieri and Thomas 1994). This is especially true for those carnivore species, such as certain wild members of the dog family (Canidae), that prey on plague-susceptible rodents and are, therefore, likely to encounter and become temporarily infested with *Y. pestis*-infected rodent fleas. As noted above, the insectivore *S. murinus* might represent an exception to the generalization that non-rodent species are unimportant as sources of infection for vector fleas (Marshall et al. 1967b).

6.1 Fleas as vectors of plague

Soon after commensal rat fleas (primarily *X. cheopis*) were identified as the primary vectors of human bubonic plague in India, McCoy (1910) demonstrated that wild rodent fleas (*Diamanus montanus*) were capable of transmitting *Y. pestis* to their natural host, the California ground squirrel (*S. beecheyi*). Since that time more than 150 additional species of fleas, most of which infest wild rodents, have been reported to be naturally infected with *Y. pestis* (Pollitzer and Meyer 1961, CDC unpublished data). Although each of these naturally infected flea species can be thought of as potential transmitters of plague, simply finding *Y. pestis* in a flea species is a poor indicator of its actual importance as a vector. Only those fleas that become 'blocked' after ingesting viable plague bacilli are thought to be efficient vectors of plague (Bacot and Martin 1914).

Microscopical observations of fleas fed on *Y. pestis*-infected animals indicate that plague bacilli begin to multiply in the flea soon after being ingested and eventually form small brown colonies in the proventriculus or midgut of the infected flea (Pollitzer 1954). As these colonies increase in size, they begin to coalesce and form sticky gelatinous masses that adhere to spines in the flea's proventriculus. Eventually these masses become sufficiently large to occlude the gut tract. At this point, the flea is said to be blocked. Because the blood meal cannot pass beyond the blocked proventriculus into the midgut, the flea begins to starve and will attempt to feed repeatedly on almost any available host. As the blocked flea attempts to feed, it regurgitates viable *Y. pestis* and other components of the block in an attempt to clear the obstruction in its gut, thereby resulting in transmission of the plague bacillus to susceptible mammalian hosts.

The blocking process depends, at least in part, on both the characteristics of the plague bacillus and on environmental temperatures. Plague strains that are capable of binding Congo red in culture (pigment-positive strains) are reportedly capable of blocking fleas, whereas pigment-negative strains lack such a capacity (Bibikova 1977, Kutyrev et al. 1992). The pig-

mentation characteristic is indicative of a strain's ability to bind iron-containing haemin to the surface of its cells. Colonies of such pigment-positive strains are more 'sticky' than pigment-negative strains, which, of course, suggests that the former strains are also more likely to form colonies that will adhere to the spines in a flea's proventriculus and thus result in blockage formation, a contention that agrees with microscopical observations (Bibikova 1977). Hinnebusch, Perry and Schwan (1996) have demonstrated recently that a pigmented (*hms* +) *Y. pestis* strain was capable of developing blockages in fleas, while isogenic non-pigmented (*hms* −) mutants failed to do so. The ability of non-pigmented mutants to promote blockage formation could be restored by complementation of these mutants with pHMS1, a low copy number recombinant plasmid containing *hmsHFR* (a combination of 3 genes comprising the haemin storage locus of *Y. pestis*).

Blocking also depends on temperature. Competent vector fleas will become blocked when held at temperatures below 28°C, but fail to do so when incubated at higher temperatures (>28°C) and may actually become cleared of infection (Cavanaugh 1971). Blocking takes 9–26 days at temperatures ranging from approximately 10°C to 26.7°C in *X. cheopis*, but can take as long as 3 weeks to 4 months in some wild rodent fleas (Eskey and Haas 1940). Cavanaugh (1971) proposed that the observed effects of temperature could be explained by an enzyme that acted either as a coagulase at low temperatures (promotes blocking) or as a fibrinolysin at high temperatures (degrades blockages). As noted earlier, the gene encoding this fibrinolytic–coagulase activity is found on the 9.5 kb plasmid of *Y. pestis* and it would be expected that loss of this plasmid would result in the failure of such strains to promote block formation. Hinnebusch and his colleagues, however, recently demonstrated that 2 *Y. pestis* strains that had been cured of their 9.5 kb plasmids were still capable of forming blocks in *X. cheopis* fleas (Hinnebusch, personal communication 1996).

Many species of fleas appear to be incapable of becoming blocked and, therefore, are unlikely to efficiently transmit plague. Nevertheless, some authors have reported transmission by apparently unblocked fleas. In most instances, the limited amounts of transmission that are observed in these experiments probably can be attributed to mechanical transmission (i.e. transmission of *Y. pestis* to susceptible animals via contaminated mouthparts). Available evidence indicates that transmission by such means is very inefficient compared to transmission of plague by blocked fleas and probably becomes important only when the putative mechanical vector exists in high numbers and has frequent opportunities to move quickly from one susceptible host to another. The situation where mechanical transmission is most often suggested to be important involves *Pulex irritans*, the so-called human flea. This flea is widely distributed in human and domestic animal dwellings throughout much of the world, has a very wide host range, has been found to be naturally infected with *Y. pestis*, exists in very high numbers in some human dwellings, and has been implicated on epidemiological grounds as a likely vector in bubonic plague epidemics in Peru, Morocco and Kurdistan (Swellengrebel 1953, Blanc 1956, Baltzard et al. 1960, PAHO 1965, Hopla 1980). Laboratory studies, however, indicate that *P. irritans* is an extremely inefficient vector of *Y. pestis* and that transmission occurs only when susceptible animals are infested with large numbers of fleas that have recently fed on an infected animal (Hopla 1980). Such results are probably best explained by occasional instances of mechanical transmission rather than transmission of *Y. pestis* by blocked *P. irritans*.

The ability of a given species of flea to become blocked is not the only factor determining its importance as a vector of plague. Other characteristics that must be considered include the species of rodents the flea normally infests, its abundance during seasons of peak transmission, its geographical distribution, its ability to survive for a number of days to weeks in off-host environments when normal hosts are absent or die during epizootics (i.e. are relatively resistant to adverse conditions such as low humidity and high temperatures), and its degree of host specificity when normal hosts are absent. The last item can be especially important in determining what other mammals, including humans, are at risk of infection. Highly host-specific fleas might efficiently transmit plague among populations of their preferred hosts or those of closely related hosts, but, in most instances, these fleas are not as likely as less host-specific species to transmit the disease from their normal hosts to other mammalian species, including humans. The Oriental rat flea (*X. cheopis*) and the North American ground squirrel flea (*D. montanus*) are excellent examples of flea vectors that normally infest important epizootic hosts (commensal rats and ground squirrels, respectively) but readily feed on other animals, including humans, after their normal hosts have died during a plague epizootic.

In some instances, a flea species might be a relatively inefficient vector but still play an important role in transmission because of its sheer abundance (Kartman 1957). *Malaraeus telchinum*, a common flea on mice and voles in California, USA, is a poor vector under laboratory conditions, but might be a more important vector under natural conditions than *Hystrichopsylla linsdalei*. The latter flea species shares hosts with the former and is an efficient experimental vector, but is far less abundant than *M. telchinum*.

Survival times for infected fleas also must be considered. *D. montanus* is generally reported to be a less efficient vector than *X. cheopis*, but infected *D. montanus* survive almost 3 times longer than infected *X. cheopis* (47 days versus 17 days) (Eskey and Haas 1940). Although an extreme example, infected prairie dog fleas, living in a cool, high altitude site in Colorado, USA, were recovered from the burrows of their hosts more than one year after these animals had perished during an epizootic (Lechleitner, Tileston and Kartman 1962).

6.2 Epidemiology

According to the latest statistics from the World Health Organization (WHO), a total of 16 312 cases were reported from 21 countries during the period 1979–93 (Table 44.1) (WHO 1995). A few unreported cases also have occurred in Saudi Arabia (Poland, Quan and Barnes 1994). The statistics given in Table 44.1 are undoubtedly an undersestimate of the true number of cases that occurred during this period. These statistics were somewhat dated at the time of publication and do not include the more than 5000 suspect cases that were reported to WHO during the Indian outbreak of 1994. This outbreak included cases of pneumonic plague in the industrial city of Surat and bubonic cases in rural Maharashtra. Although there were serious concerns that persons fleeing Surat might spread the disease to other regions of India or to other countries, this did not occur. Retrospective studies by an international team of experts from WHO, the USA Centers for Disease Control and Prevention, and the Russian Federation indicated that limited pneumonic and bubonic outbreaks did occur in Surat and rural Maharashtra state, respectively. Most of the suspect cases, however, were thought to be due to illnesses other than plague. Regardless of the extent of the outbreak, the appearance of any cases was surprising because plague was believed by some to have disappeared from India after 1966, the last time cases were reported to WHO.

The most common mode of transmission of *Y. pestis* to humans is through the bites of infectious fleas. Transmission can also occur when persons have direct contact with infected animals or inhale infectious respiratory droplets expelled from humans or animals with plague pneumonia. Although certain racial or ethnic groups, such as Native American populations in the American southwest, may experience higher incidences of plague than others, these differences are not believed to be due to inherent variations in susceptibility but rather to higher risks of exposure to infection (Barnes et al. 1988). Increased exposure risks in plague-enzootic areas can be due to many factors, including living in areas that frequently experience rodent epizootics, failing to reduce the amounts of food and shelter available to plague-susceptible rodents in peridomestic environments, or engaging in work- or recreation-related activities that place individuals at relatively high risk of plague exposure (PAHO 1965, Velimirovic 1972, Mann et al. 1979, Barnes et al. 1988, Craven et al. 1993, Gage, Montenieri and Thomas 1994).

Most cases of bubonic plague occur in developing countries and are typically associated with exposures to infectious commensal rat fleas, especially *X. cheopis* or, in some areas, *X. brasiliensis*. Risks of exposure to infectious rat fleas are especially high in plague-affected rural areas of certain developing countries that have large rat populations as a result of poverty and poor sanitation and food storage practices. Epidemics of bubonic plague are most likely to occur among residents of such areas when plague epizootics

Table 44.1 Human plague cases reported to the World Health Organization (1979–93)*

Region	Country	Cases	Deaths
Africa	Angola	27	4
	Botswana	173	12
	Kenya	276	11
	Libya	8	0
	Madagascar	1287	300
	South Africa	19	1
	Uganda	660	48
	Tanzania	4486	367
	Zaire	2161	504
	Zimbabwe	5	3
	Total	9102	1250
Americas	Bolivia	199	27
	Brazil	696	9
	Ecuador	83	3
	Peru	1302	93
	USA	228	33
	Total	2508	165
Asia	China	253	78
	Kazakhstan	10	4
	Mongolia	52	19
	Myanmar	1227	16
	Vietnam	3160	136
	Total	4702	253
	World total	16 312	1668

*Source: WHO 1995.

(ratfalls) result in high mortality among rats and cause their fleas to seek other hosts, such as passing humans.

The risks of rat-associated plague epidemics are relatively low in other foci, however, including those found in the USA or central Asia. Most cases in these areas occur singly, or in small clusters, either as a result of exposures to infectious wild rodent fleas or handling infected animals. In the USA probable modes of transmission were identified for 294 of the 342 cases that occurred during the interval 1970–95 (CDC unpublished data). About 79% of the 294 cases were infected by flea bite, as determined by the presence of an inguinal bubo or recollection of flea bite(s). Probably all of the above flea bite cases were exposed to infectious wild rodent fleas, especially *D. montanus* on rock squirrels, California ground squirrels and, in some areas in the far western USA, golden-mantled ground squirrels. Other ground squirrel or antelope ground squirrel fleas (*Thrassis* spp., especially *Thrassis bacchi*), prairie dog fleas (primarily *Opisocrostis hirsutus*) and, perhaps, chipmunk fleas (primarily *Eumolpianus eumolpi*) are thought to transmit *Y. pestis* to humans occasionally. Another 19% of cases were infected by direct contact with infected animals, including wild rabbits, domestic cats, wild carnivores, prairie dogs and an Abert's squirrel. These contact-associated cases included hunters, trappers and pet owners. Seven cases (2%) were exposed through inhalation of infectious materials. Five of

these 7 primary pneumonic plague cases occurred among cat owners or veterinarians and their staff and resulted from inhalation of infectious respiratory droplets or other air-borne materials from cats with plague pneumonia or, perhaps, oral lesions. The probable source of infection for the other 2 primary pneumonic cases, both of which were fatal, could not be determined. One of these cases occurred in a veterinarian who also could have been exposed to an infected cat. No instances of commensal rat-associated epidemics or direct human-to-human transmission resulting from exposures to persons with pneumonic plague cases have occurred in the USA since the mid-1920s.

Wild rodent fleas undoubtedly transmit *Y. pestis* to humans in other parts of the world, but this can be difficult to verify in areas where infectious commensal rat fleas occur alongside infectious wild rodent fleas. In the majority of these situations it is likely that rat fleas are the most important sources of infection for humans. Wild rodent fleas have been proposed, however, to be important vectors in some Andean areas of South America where commensal rat fleas are rare (PAHO 1965). Humans in these areas are believed to be exposed to infectious wild rodent fleas (*Polygenis litargus* or *Pleochaetis dolens*) while working in fields or sleeping out of doors near these fields. Persons working in these fields might also transport infectious wild rodent fleas into homes. Cases resulting from direct contact with infected animals also occur in a number of countries other than the USA, including northwest and northeast China (marmots), Libya, Saudi Arabia and central Asia (goats, sheep and camels) (Christie, Chen and Elberg 1980, Christie 1982, Shen 1990, Zhu 1993, Poland, Quan and Barnes 1994).

Primary pneumonic plague epidemics are, at present, rare and result from human-to-human transmission via inhalation of infectious respiratory droplets expelled from persons with plague pneumonia. Such outbreaks are especially dangerous because they can spread very quickly and cause high mortality in the absence of appropriate treatment and public health practices. Extensive pneumonic plague outbreaks are believed to have occurred during the Black Death in Europe and during the Modern Pandemic in India and Manchuria (Meyer 1961). The Manchurian epidemic, which occurred in 1910–11, is reported to have caused over 60 000 deaths. The pneumonic outbreak in Surat, India, described above, probably caused fewer than 100 cases. Meyer (1961) described smaller outbreaks in the USA in 1919 (12 cases, not including the index case of secondary plague pneumonia) and 1924 (32 cases). Although the source of infection for the index case could not be determined in the 1924 outbreak, the index case in the 1919 outbreak occurred in a squirrel hunter. Marmot hunters with secondary pneumonic plague were reported to be sources of infection for primary pneumonic plague cases in China (Zhu 1993). Other pneumonic outbreaks have been reported from Ecuador in 1939, Manchuria in 1946, Madagascar in 1958, Vietnam in 1967 and Tanzania in 1968 (Murdock 1940, Meyer

1961, Trong, Nhu and Marshall 1967, Isaacson et al. 1976). Human-to-human spread during pneumonic outbreaks is favoured by crowded conditions and humid, preferably cool, environments (Pollitzer 1954, Meyer 1961). The former increases the degree of contact between infective pneumonic plague patients and potential victims and the latter prolongs the survival of *Y. pestis* in air-borne respiratory droplets or other materials. Individual cases of primary pneumonic plague have also been associated with handling *Y. pestis*-infected cats or working in research laboratories (Burmeister, Tiggert and Overholt 1962, Doll et al. 1994).

7 DIAGNOSIS

Prompt diagnosis and treatment are important for reducing the high fatality rate of plague. Unfortunately, actual confirmation of *Y. pestis* infection requires either isolation and identification of *Y. pestis* in culture or demonstration of a 4-fold change in specific antibodies. Both these processes require considerable time and, in many instances, physicians must base treatment decisions primarily on clinical signs and symptoms. Presumptive identification of plague infection can be made by identifying a single positive sample in a serological test or by identifying plague antigens in patient or animal samples. Immunofluorescence assays are especially effective for rapid (2–3 h), albeit presumptive, identification of *Y. pestis* in tissue, sputum, or bubo aspirate samples. Detection of specific antigens by agglutination assays and enzyme-linked immunosorbent assays has been described but is more time-consuming than immunofluorescence. DNA probes or polymerase chain reaction could also be used for presumptive identification of *Y. pestis*-specific nucleic acids in samples, but these methods are largely restricted to research laboratories and have not received widespread use in clinical laboratories (McDonough et al. 1988, Thomas, McDonough and Schwan 1989, Hinnebusch and Schwan 1993). Identification of bipolar staining bacteria in samples stained with Wayson's or Giemsa increases the suspicion that a patient's illness might be plague, but is not specific and should not be taken as presumptive evidence of infection. Clinical laboratory findings for plague patients include lowered platelet counts, the presence of fibrin split products, and polymorphonuclear leucocytosis (approximately $20\,000$–$25\,000$ mm^{-3}) (Quan, Barnes and Poland 1981).

Recommended diagnostic samples include blood samples for culture and serology, bubo aspirates and sputum cultures for patients with respiratory symptoms. It is generally recommended that at least 4 blood samples be taken in citrated or heparinized tubes at approximately 15–20 min intervals to increase the chances of obtaining isolates from patients with intermittent bacteraemia (Quan, Barnes and Poland 1981). Bubo aspirates can be collected with a syringe that is fitted with a small needle (20–22 gauge) and contains a small amount of sterile saline. After a local anaesthetic has been applied to the region of the bubo, the saline is injected into the bubo. The syringe plunger is then withdrawn so that the syringe fills with a mixture of the saline and material from the bubo. The aspirated material is then applied to paired culture media and incubated at room temperature and 37°C. Pieces of liver, spleen, lung, bone marrow and excised lymph node (bubo) can be obtained for culture and mouse inoculation from fatal cases or animal necropsies. Serum and blood specimens should be kept cold while being held for analysis. If refrigeration is impossible, samples intended for culture can be transported at ambient temperatures in Cary–Blair transport medium. In those situations where refrigeration is unavailable, samples of blood can be collected on special filter paper strips (Nobuto strips) and held at ambient temperature for later serological analysis. This technique requires more involved processing procedures in the laboratory than is the case for actual serum samples but is of great use to those working in remote areas (Wolff and Hudson 1974).

Y. pestis grows well in a variety of media including infusion broth, brain–heart infusion broth, trypticase soy broth or agar, nutrient broth or agar and blood agar. Characteristics of growth in liquid or on solid media were described above (see section 4, p. 889). Susceptible mice are often inoculated subcutaneously with sample materials when it is suspected that these are likely to be grossly contaminated with other microorganisms. Inoculated mice are then monitored and necropsied at death to obtain spleen and liver tissue for culture. Surviving mice can be bled for serology 21 days after inoculation. Specific identification of *Y. pestis* can be made by demonstrating a negative reaction in gram stain, characteristic appearance in culture, production of F1 capsule (usually verified by immunofluorescence), and lysis with specific bacteriophage at both 37°C and 20°C. Biochemical tests are also helpful but often require considerable experience for proper performance and interpretation of results. Serological tests include whole cell agglutination assays, passive haemagglutination assays, latex agglutination assays, and enzyme-linked immunosorbent assays (Quan et al. 1981, Williams et al. 1982, 1986). The serological test most commonly used in public health laboratories is the passive haemagglutination assay. None of these serological tests is currently available from commercial vendors and their performance is generally limited to a handful of public health laboratories that have the necessary reagents.

8 PREVENTION AND TRANSMISSIBILITY

The first step in preventing plague and reducing plague-related mortality is implementation of effective human- and animal-based surveillance programmes. These programmes should be capable of rapidly identifying suspect cases of human plague so that these individuals can be promptly treated and emergency measures can be taken to prevent other persons from acquiring the disease. All suspect cases should be isolated for at least 48 h after treatment begins to reduce risks of human-to-human transmission (pneumonic plague cases should be isolated until sputum cultures are negative). Suspect cases should also be queried about their whereabouts and activities during the incubation period (usually 2–6 days, but rarely as long as 10 days) to determine likely exposure sites or sources of infection. Individuals who have had significant contact with pneumonic plague patients (within 2 m) should be advised of their risks, monitored for illness, and offered prophylactic antibiotic therapy. Those who have had only brief contact at distances of 2 or more metres are unlikely to become infected, but should be informed of their risks and monitored closely during the week following the potential exposure. Surveillance personnel should also perform environmental investigations at likely exposure sites to determine probable sources of infection and assess the potential risks for other persons living in the area. All suspect plague cases should be reported to national health authorities and all laboratory-confirmed cases must be reported through appropriate channels to WHO, Geneva, Switzerland, according to the requirements of the International Health Regulations.

Animal-based surveillance programmes should be capable of monitoring levels of *Y. pestis* infection in mammal and flea populations and rapidly identifying epizootics in important rodent species. Prompt detection of rodent epizootics allows control measures to be implemented before human cases appear. Useful surveillance samples include fleas taken from rodent hosts or their environment, tissue samples collected from rodents or other animals suspected to have died of plague, and serum samples taken from rodents or other animals, especially carnivores. The types of samples collected should be determined by the size of the area to be examined and the goals of the project. Carnivore serosurveillance is especially useful when extensive geographical areas must be surveyed, but follow-up rodent and flea surveillance should be performed in those areas where seropositive carnivores were identified, to determine the actual rodent species involved in local epizootics and the extent of these epizootics (Barnes 1982, Taylor and Pugh 1982).

Other recommended prevention and control measures include public education, avoidance of sick or dead animals, avoidance of areas where epizootics or epidemics have occurred, use of personal protective measures such as insect repellents or insecticide-treated clothing, treatment of pets with insecticides to reduce the risks that these animals will carry infectious fleas into homes, modifying environments near homes or other areas to reduce the amount of food and shelter available to rodents, and treating rodents or their burrows, nests, or runways with insecticides to reduce risks of flea-borne transmission. Rodenticides are also occasionally employed, but these agents should not be applied until an aggressive flea control campaign has been initiated. Killing rodent hosts without first eliminating their fleas is likely to increase human risks as the fleas attempt to find new hosts to replace those killed by rodenticides. A formalin-inactivated vaccine is also available, but its efficacy has not been demonstrated in clinical trials. Indirect evidence suggests that it is effective for reducing risks of flea-borne plague, but the occurrence of cases of pneumonic plague among vaccinated persons suggests that the vaccine might not be effective for preventing plague cases resulting from air-borne transmission (Cohen and Stockard 1967). Vaccination is recommended only for persons, such as research laboratory workers, certain mammalogists, or others, who are repeatedly exposed to high risks of *Y. pestis* infection.

9 TREATMENT

Prompt treatment is extremely important for a successful outcome following infection. Patients whose clinical symptoms and exposure histories are compatible with plague should be treated immediately with appropriate antibiotics because the course of the disease can progress very rapidly and it is often difficult to obtain timely laboratory confirmation of *Y. pestis.* The drug of choice for treating plague is streptomycin, but tetracycline and chloramphenicol have also been used successfully (Poland 1989, Dennis 1996). Chloramphenicol, which can be used in combination with streptomycin, penetrates tissues well and is, therefore, recommended for treating plague meningitis, endophthalmitis, myocarditis and pleuritis. Gentamicin is more readily available than streptomycin and often has been substituted for the latter drug with apparently good results but this has not been verified by clinical studies. The efficacy of doxycycline has also not been investigated, but this antibiotic is often recommended for prophylaxis and probably is as effective as tetracycline. Other antibiotics, such as penicillins, cephalosporins and fluoroquinones, may be bactericidal in vitro but are not considered to be effective in vivo or have produced questionable results (Poland, Quan and Barnes 1994). Regardless of the antibiotic chosen, treatment should be continued for at least 3 days after the patient becomes afebrile and, in most instances, a 10 day course of treatment is recommended. Patients usually show improvement after 2–3 days of treatment, although buboes may continue to increase in size for a few days and remain swollen and tender for many weeks after recovery. These slowly resolving buboes, however, are not indicative of continuing infection (Dennis 1996).

Persons who have been exposed to *Y. pestis* infection can be given prophylactic antibiotics. The drugs of choice for prophylaxis are tetracycline, doxycycline and trimethoprim–sulphamethoxazole (Poland 1989, Dennis 1996). Children under 9 years of age should be given trimethoprim–sulphamethoxazole rather than tetracycline or doxycycline. Persons should continue taking prophylactic antibiotics at the prescribed doses for a period of 7 days after treatment begins.

REFERENCES

de Almeida AMP, Brasil DP et al., Pesquisa de *Yersinia pestis* em roedores e outros pequenos mamiferos nos focos pestosos do nordeste do Brasil no periodo 1966 a 1982, *Rev Saude Publica*, 1987, **21:** 265–7.

Almeida CR, Almeida AR et al., 1981, Plague in Brazil during two years of bacteriological and serological surveillance, *Bull W H O*, **59:** 591–7.

Alsofrom DJ, Mettler FA Jr, Mann JM, 1981, Radiographic manifestations of plague in New Mexico, 1975–1980. A review of 42 proved cases, *Radiology*, **139:** 561–5.

Bacot AW, Martin CJ, 1914, Observations on the mechanism of the transmission of plague by fleas, *J Hyg (Lond)*, **13, Plague suppl. III:** 423–39.

Balabkin AK et al., 1962, The natural plague focus in the Gorny Altai, *Dokl Irkutsk Protivochumn Inst*, **4:** 3–5.

Baltazard M, Bahmanyar H, 1960, Research on plague in India, *Bull W H O*, **23:** 169–215.

Baltazard M, Bahmanyer M et al., 1960, Recherches sur la peste en Iran, *Bull W H O*, **23:** 152–5.

Barnes AM, 1982, Surveillance and control of plague in the United States, *Animal Disease in Relation to Animal Conservation*, Symposia of the Zoological Society of London, Number 50, eds Edwards MA, Mcdonnel U, Academic Press, London, 237–70.

Barnes AM, Quan TJ et al., 1988, Plague in American Indians, 1956–1987, *Morbid Mortal Weekly Rep CDC Surveill Summ*, **37:** 11–16.

Bartelloni PJ, Marshall JD, Cavanaugh DC, 1973, Clinical and serological responses to plague vaccine U.S.P., *Milit Med*, **138:** 720–2.

Becker TM, Poland JD et al., 1987, Plague meningitis – a retrospective analysis of cases reported in the United States, 1970–1979, *West J Med*, **147:** 554–7.

Bibikov DI, 1965, Spatial laws of natural focality of plague in marmots, *Theoretical Questions of Natural Foci of Diseases*, eds Rosicky B, Heyberger K, Czechoslovak Acad Sci, Prague, 83–8.

Bibikova VA, 1977, Contemporary views on the interrelationships between fleas and the pathogens of human and animal diseases, *Annu Rev Entomol*, **22:** 23–32.

Blanc G, 1956, Une opinion nonconformiste sur le mode de transmission de la peste bubonique et septicémique, *Arch Inst Pasteur Maroc*, **3:** 173–349.

Brooks JE, Naing UH et al., 1977, Plague in small mammals and humans in Rangoon, Burma, *Southeast Asian J Trop Med Public Health*, **8:** 335–44.

Brubaker RR, 1991, Factors promoting acute and chronic diseases caused by yersiniae, *Clin Microbiol Rev*, **4:** 309–24.

Burdelov LA, 1982, Experience in the comparative evaluation of the population sensitivity of mammals to the plague microbe based on the results of an epizootiological survey, *Zh Mikrobiol Epidemiol Immunobiol*, **1:** 26–9.

Burmeister RW, Tiggert WD, Overholt EL, 1962, Laboratory-acquired pneumonic plague – report of a case and review of previous cases, *Ann Intern Med*, **56:** 789–800.

Butler T, 1972, A clinical study of bubonic plague, *Am J Med*, **53:** 268–76.

Butler T, 1984, *Plague and other Yersinial Infections*, Plenum Press, New York.

Butler T, Bell WR et al., 1974, *Yersinia pestis* infection in Vietnam. I. Clinical and hematologic aspects, *J Infect Dis*, **129, Suppl.:** S78–84.

Butler T, Levin J et al., 1976, *Yersinia pestis* infection in Vietnam: II. Quantitative blood cultures and detection of endotoxin in the cerebrospinal fluid of patients with meningitis, *J Infect Dis*, **133:** 493–9.

Caten JL, Kartman L, 1968, Human plague in the United States during 1966, case reports, *Southwest Med*, **49:** 102–8.

Cavanaugh DC, 1971, Specific effect of temperature upon transmission of the plague bacillus by the oriental rat flea, *Am J Trop Med Hyg*, **20:** 264–73.

Cavanaugh DC, Marshall JR Jr, 1972, The influence of climate on the seasonal prevalence of plague in the Republic of Vietnam, *J Wildl Dis*, **8:** 85–94.

Cavanaugh DC, Ryan PF, Marshall JD, 1969, The role of commensal rodents and their ectoparasites in the ecology and transmission of plague in Southeast Asia, *Wildl Dis*, **5:** 187–92.

Cavanaugh DC, Dangerfield HG et al., 1968a, Some observations on the current plague outbreaks in the Republic of Vietnam, *Am J Public Health*, **58:** 742–52.

Cavanaugh DC, Hunter DH et al., 1968b, Ecology of plague in Vietnam III. Sylvatic plague; *Bandicota indica*, a transitional species, *Trans R Soc Trop Med Hyg*, **62:** 456.

CDC (Centers for Disease Control and Prevention), 1994, Human plague – United States, 1993–1994, *Morbid Mortal Weekly Rep*, **43:** 242–6.

Chen TH, Elberg SS, Eisler DM, 1976, Immunity in plague: protection induced in *Cercopithecus aethiops* by oral administration of live, attenuated *Yersinia pestis*, *J Infect Dis*, **123:** 302–9.

Chen TH, Elberg SS, Eisler DM, 1977, Immunity in plague: protection of the vervet (*Cercopithecus aethiops*) against pneumonic plague by the oral administration of live attenuated *Yersinia pestis*, *J Infect Dis*, **135:** 289–93.

Chen TH, Meyer KF, 1965, Susceptibility of the langur monkey (*Semnopithecus entellus*) to experimental plague: pathology and immunity, *J Infect Dis*, **115:** 456–64.

Chen TH, Meyer KF, 1974, Susceptibility and immune response to experimental plague in two species of langurs and in African green (grivet) monkeys, *J Infect Dis*, **129, Suppl.:** S46–52.

Christie AB, 1982, Plague: review of ecology, *Ecol Dis*, **1:** 111–15.

Christie AB, Chen TH, Elberg SS, 1980, Plague in camels and goats: their role in human epidemics, *J Infect Dis*, **141:** 724–6.

Clark RK, Jessup DA et al., 1983, Serologic survey of California wild hogs for antibodies against selected zoonotic disease agents, *J Am Vet Med Assoc*, **183:** 1248–51.

Clover JR, Hofstra TD et al., 1989, Serologic evidence of *Yersinia pestis* infection in small mammals and bears from a temperate rainforest of North Coastal California, *J Wildl Dis*, **25:** 52–60.

Cohen RJ, Stockard JL, 1967, Pneumonic plague in an untreated plague-vaccinated individual, *JAMA*, **202:** 365–6.

Coppes JB, 1980, Bubonic plague in pregnancy, *J Reprod Med*, **25:** 91–5.

Craven RB, Maupin GO et al., 1993, Reported cases of human plague infections in the United States, 1970–1991, *J Med Entomol*, **30:** 758–61.

Crook LD, Tempest B, 1992, Plague, a clinical review of 27 cases, *Arch Intern Med*, **152:** 1253–5.

Davis DHS, 1964, Ecology of wild rodent plague, *Ecological Studies in Southern Africa*, ed. Davis DHS, Junk, The Hague, Netherlands, 301–14.

Davis DHS, Heisch RB et al., 1968, Serological survey of plague in rodents and other small mammals in Kenya, *Trans R Soc Trop Med Hyg*, **62:** 838–61.

Dennis DT, 1996, Plague, method of, *Conn's Current Therapy*, ed. Rakel RE, WB Saunders, Philadelphia, 124–6.

Dennis DT, Orloski K, 1995, Plague! *1996 Medical and Health Annual*, Encyclopedia Britannica, Inc., Chicago, IL, 160–91.

Devignat R, 1951, Variétés de l'espèce *Pasteurella pestis*. Nouvelle hypothèse, *Bull W H O*, **4:** 247–63.

Doll J, Zeitz PS et al., 1994, Cat-transmitted fatal pneumonic plague in a person who traveled from Colorado to Arizona, *Am J Trop Med Hyg*, **51:** 109–14.

Eidson M, Thilsted JP, Rollag OJ, 1991, Clnical, clinicopathologic, and pathologic features of plague in cats: 119 cases (1977–1988), *J Am Vet Med Assoc*, **199:** 1191–7.

Eidson M, Tierney LA et al., 1988, Feline plague in New Mexico:

risk factors and transmission to humans, *Am J Public Health*, **78**: 1333–5.

Eskey CR, Haas VH, 1940, Plague in the western part of the United States, *Public Health Bull No. 254*, 1–82.

Feodorov VN, 1960, Plague in camels and its prevention in the USSR, *Bull W H O*, **23**: 275–81.

Fetherston JD, Lillard JW, Perry RD, 1995, Analysis of the pesticin receptor from *Yersinia pestis*: role in iron-deficient growth and possible regulation by its siderophore, *J Bacteriol*, **177**: 1824–33.

Finegold MJ, 1968, Pathogenesis of plague, a review of plague deaths in the United States during the last decade, *Am J Med*, **45**: 549–54.

Finegold MJ, 1969, Pneumonic plague in monkeys – an electron microscopic study, *Am J Pathol*, **54**: 167–85.

Fisher JS, Hoy DR, 1992, *Geography and Development – A World Regional Approach*, 4th edn, ed. Hoy JS, Macmillan Publishing Co., New York, 23–4.

Fowler JM, Brubaker RR, 1994, Physiological basis of the low calcium repsonse in *Yersinia pestis*, *Infect Immun*, **62**: 5234–41.

Gage KL, Montenieri JA, Thomas RE, 1994, The role of predators in the ecology, epidemiology, and surveillance of plague in the United States, *Proceedings of the 16th Vertebrate Pest Conference*, eds Halverson WS, Crabb AC, University of California, Davis, CA, 201–6.

Gasper PW, Barnes AM et al., 1993, Plague (*Yersinia pestis*) in cats: description of experimentally induced disease, *J Med Entomol*, **30**: 20–6.

Gordon DH, Isaacson M, Taylor P, 1979, Plague antibody in large African mammals, *Infect Immun*, **26**: 767–9.

Gregg CT, 1985, *Plague – An Ancient Disease in the Twentieth Century*, revised edn, University of New Mexico Press, Albuquerque, New Mexico, 1–169.

Guiyoule A, Grimont F et al., 1994, Plague pandemics investigated by ribotyping of *Yersinia pestis* strains, *J Clin Microbiol*, **32**: 634–41.

Haffkine WM, 1897, Remarks on the plague prophylactic fluid, *Br Med J*, **1**: 1461.

Hallett AF, Isaacson M, Meyer KF, 1973, Pathogenicity and immunogenic efficacy of a live attenuated plague vaccine in vervetmonkeys, *Infect Immun*, **8**: 876–81.

Hallett AF, McNeill D, Meyer KF, 1970, A serological survey of the small mammals for plague in southern Africa, *S Afr Med J*, **44**: 831–7.

Heisch RB, Grainger WE, D'Souza AM, 1953, Results of a plague investigation in Kenya, *Trans R Soc Trop Med Hyg*, **47**: 503–21.

Higa HH, Matsuura WT, Watanabe WH, 1971, Plague antibody response in the mongoose, *Hawaii Med J*, **30**: 92–4.

Hinnebusch BJ, Perry RD, Schwan TG, 1996, Role of the *Yersinia pestis* hemin storage (*hms*) locus in the transmission of plague in fleas, *Science*, **273**: 367–70.

Hinnebusch J, Schwan TG, 1993, New method for plague surveillance using polymerase chain reaction to detect *Yersinia pestis* in fleas, *J Clin Microbiol*, **31**: 1511–14.

Hopla CE, 1980, A study of the host associations and zoogeography of *Pulex*, *Fleas*, eds Traub R, Starcke H, AA Balkema, Rotterdam, 185–207.

Hubbert WT, Goldenberg MI, 1970, Natural resistance to plague: genetic basis in the vole (*Microtus californicus*), *Am J Trop Med Hyg*, **19**: 1015–19.

Hudson BW, Quan SF, Goldenberg MI, 1964, Serum antibody responses in a population of *Microtus californicus* and associated rodent species during and after *Pasteurella pestis* epizootics in the San Francisco Bay Area, *Zoonoses Res*, **3**: 15–29.

Hull HF, Montes JM, Mann JM, 1987, Septicemic plague in New Mexico, *J Infect Dis*, **155**: 113–18.

Isaacson M, 1983, A review of some recent developments in human plague with special reference to southern Africa, *Ecol Dis*, **2**: 161–71.

Isaacson M, Hallett AF, 1975, Serological studies on human plague in Southern Africa. Part I. Plague antibody levels in

a population during a quiescent and a subsequent active period in an endemic region, *S Afr Med J*, **49**: 1165–8.

Isaacson M, Taylor P, Arntzen L, 1983, Ecology of plague in Africa: response of indigenous wild rodents to experimental plague infection, *Bull W H O*, **61**: 339–44.

Isaacson M, Qhobela QM et al., 1976, Serological studies on human plague in southern Africa. Part II. A bubonic/pneumonic plague epidemic in Lesotho, *S Afr Med J*, **50**: 929–32.

Janssen WA, 1963, The pathogenesis of plague. I. A study of the correlation between virulence and relative phagocytosis resistance of some strains of *Pasteurella pestis*, *J Infect Dis*, **113**: 139–43.

Jones AM, Mann J, Braziel R, 1979, Human plague in New Mexico: report of three autopsied cases, *J Forensic Sci*, **24**: 26–38.

Kartman L, 1957, The concept of vector efficiency in experimental studies of plague, *Exp Parasitol*, **6**: 599–609.

Kilonzo BS, 1992, Observations on the epidemiology of plague in Tanzania during the period 1974–1988, *East Afr Med J*, **69**: 494–9.

Kucheruk VV, 1960, A classification of natural foci of plague in non-tropical Eurasia, *Med Parazitol Parazit Bol*, **29**: 5–15.

Kutyrev VV, Filippov A et al., 1992, Analysis of *Yersinia pestis* chromosomal determinants Pgm⁺ and Pstˢ associated with virulence, *Microb Pathog*, **12**: 177–86.

Leary SE, Williamson ED et al., 1995, Active immunization with recombinant V antigen from *Yersinia pestis* protects mice against plague, *Infect Immun*, **63**: 2854–8.

Lechleitner RR, Tileston JV, Kartman L, 1962, Die-off of a Gunnison's prairie dog colony in central Colorado, *Zoonosis Res*, **1**: 185–99.

Liston WG, 1905, Plague rats and fleas, *J Bombay Nat Hist Soc*, **16**: 253–73.

McCoy GW, 1910, A note on squirrel fleas as plague carriers, *Public Health Rep*, **25**: 465.

McCoy GW, 1911, Studies upon plague in ground squirrels, *Public Health Bull*, **43**: 1–51.

McDonough KA, Schwan TG et al., 1988, Identification of a *Yersinia pestis*-specific DNA probe with potential for use in plague surveillance, *J Clin Microbiol*, **26**: 2515–19.

McDonough KA, Barnes AM et al., 1993, Mutation in the *pla* gene of *Yersinia pestis* alters the course of the plague bacillus-flea (Siphonaptera: Ceratophyllidae) interaction, *J Med Entomol*, **30**: 772–80.

Mann JM, Moskowitz R, 1977, Plague and pregnancy, a case report, *JAMA*, **237 (17)**: 1854–5.

Mann JM, Shandler L, Cushing AH, 1982, Pediatric plague, *Pediatrics*, **69 (6)**: 762–7.

Mann JM, Martone WJ et al., 1979, Endemic human plague in New Mexico: risk factors associated with infection, *J Infect Dis*, **140 (3)**: 397–401.

Marshall JD, Quy DV et al., 1967a, Ecology of plague in Vietnam: commensal rodents and their fleas, *Military Med*, **132**: 896–903.

Marshall JD, Quy DV et al., 1967b, Ecology of plague in Vetnam I. Role of *Suncus murinus*, *Proc Soc Exp Biol Med*, **124**: 1083–6.

Marshall JD, Harrison DN et al., 1972, The role of domestic animals in the epidemiology of plague. III. Experimental infection of swine, *J Infect Dis*, **125**: 556–9.

Martin AR, Hurtado FP et al., 1967, Plague meningitis. A report of three cases in children and review of the problem, *Pediatrics*, **40**: 610–16.

Mazza G, Karu AE, Kingsbury DT, 1985, Immune response to plasmid- and chromosome-encoded *Yersinia* antigens, *Infect Immun*, **48**: 676–85.

Mengis CL, 1962, Plague, *N Engl J Med*, **267**: 543–6.

Messick JP, Smith GW, Barnes AM, 1983, Serologic testing of badgers to monitor plague in southwestern Idaho, *J Wildl Dis*, **19**: 1–6.

Meyer KF, 1961, Pneumonic plague, *Bact Rev*, **25**: 249–61.

Meyer KF, 1970, Effectiveness of live or killed plague vaccines in man, *Bull W H O*, **42**: 653–66.

Meyer KF, 1971, The clinical and immunological response of man to *P. pestis* vaccine, *Proceedings of the Symposium on Bacterial Vaccines*, Yugoslav Academy of Sciences and Arts, Zagreb, 299–312.

Meyer KF, Foster LE, 1948, Measurement of protective serum antibodies in human volunteers inoculated with plague prophylactics, *Stanford Med Bull*, **6**: 75–79.

Motin VL, Nakajima R et al., 1994, Passive immunity to yersiniae mediated by anti-recombinant V antigen and protein A-V antigen fusion peptide, *Infect Immun*, **62**: 4192–201.

Murdock JR, 1940, Pneumonic plague in Ecuador during 1939, *Public Health Rep*, **55**: 2172–8.

Nakajima R, Brubaker RR, 1993, Association between virulence of *Yersinia pestis* and suppression of gamma interferon and tumor necrosis factor alpha, *Infect Immun*, **61**: 23–31.

Nakajima R, Motin VL, Brubaker RR, 1995, Suppression of cytokines in mice by protein A-V antigen fusion peptide and restoration of synthesis by active immunization, *Infect Immun*, **63**: 3021–9.

Njunwa KJ, Mwaiko GL et al., 1989, Seasonal patterns of rodents, fleas, and plague status in the Western Usambara Mountains, Tanzania, *Med Vet Entomol*, **3**: 17–22.

Orloski KA, Eidson M, 1995, *Yersinia pestis* infection in three dogs, *J Am Vet Med Assoc*, **207**: 316–18.

Oyston PC, Williamson ED et al., 1995, Immunization with live recombinant *Salmonella typhimurium* aroA producing F1 antigen protects against plague, *Infect Immun*, **63**: 563–8.

PAHO (Pan American Health Organization), 1965, *Plague in the Americas*, Pan American Health Organization, Pan American Sanitary Bureau, Regional Office of the World Health Organization, Washington, DC, 1–152.

Palmer DL, Kisch AL et al., 1971, Clinical features of plague in the United States: The 1969–1970 epidemic, *J Infect Dis*, **124**: 367–71.

Poland JD, 1989, Plague, *Infectious Disease*, 4th edn, eds Hoeprich PD, Jordan MC, JB Lippincott, Philadelphia, 1296–306.

Poland JD, Barnes AM, 1979, Plague, *CRC Handbook Series in Zoonoses. Section A: Bacterial, Rickettsial, and Mycotic Diseases*, vol. 1, ed. Steele JH, CRC Press, Boca Raton, FL, 515–97.

Poland JD, Quan TJ, Barnes AM, 1994, Plague, *CRC Handbook Series in Zoonoses. Section A: Bacterial, Rickettsial, and Mycotic Diseases*, ed. Beran GW, CRC Press, Boca Raton, FL, 93–112.

Pollitzer R, 1954, *Plague*, World Health Organization, Geneva.

Pollitzer R, 1960, A review of recent literature on plague, *Bull W H O*, **23**: 313–400.

Pollitzer R, 1966, *Plague and Plague Control in the Soviet Union. History and Bibliography through 1964*, Institute of Contemporary Russian Studies, Fordham University, New York.

Pollitzer R, Meyer KF, 1961, *Studies in Disease Ecology*, ed. May JF, Hafner, New York, 433–590.

Quan TJ, Barnes AM, Poland JD, 1981, Yersinioses, *Diagnostic Procedures for Bacterial, Mycotic and Parasitic Infections*, eds Balows A, Hausler WJ, American Public Health Association, Washington, DC, 723–45.

Quan TJ, Barnes AM et al., 1985, Experimental plague in rock squirrels, *Spermophilus variegatus* (Erxleben), *J Wildl Dis*, **21**: 205–10.

Reed WP, Palmer DL et al., 1970, Bubonic plague in the southwestern United States, a review of recent experience, *Medicine (Baltimore)*, **49**: 465–86.

Reiley CG, Kates ED, 1970, The clinical spectrum of plague in Vietnam, *Arch Intern Med*, **126**: 990–4.

Rust JH, Cavanaugh DC et al., 1971a, The role of domestic animals in the epidemiology of plague: I. Experimental infection of dogs and cats, *J Infect Dis*, **124**: 522–6.

Rust JH, Miller BE et al., 1971b, The role of domestic animals in the epidemiology of plague, II. Antibody to *Yersinia pestis* in sera of dogs and cats, *J Infect Dis*, **124**: 527–31.

Schwan TG, Thompson D, Nelson BC, 1985, Fleas on roof rats in six areas of Los Angeles County, California: their potential role in the transmission of plague and murine typhus to humans, *Am J Trop Med Hyg*, **34**: 372–9.

Seal SC, 1960, Epidemiological studies of plague in India. I. The present position, *Bull W H O*, **23**: 283–92.

Shen EL, 1990, Human plague during 1979–1988 in China and strategy of its control, *Chung Hua Liu Hsing Ping Hsueh Tsa Chih*, **11**: 156–9.

Simond PL, 1898, La propagation de la peste, *Ann Inst Pasteur*, **12**: 625–87.

Simpson WJ, Thomas RE, Schwan TG, 1990, Recombinant capsular antigen (fraction 1) from *Yersinia pestis* induces a protective antibody response in BALB/c mice, *Am J Trop Med Hyg*, **43**: 389–96.

Sites VR, Poland JD, 1972, Mediastinal lymphadenopathy in bubonic plague, *Am J Roentgenol Radium Ther Nucl Med*, **116 (3)**: 567–70.

Smith CR, Nelson BC, Barnes AM, 1984, The use of wild carnivore serology in determining patterns of plague activity in rodents in California, *Proc 11th Vertebrate Pest Conf*, **11**: 71–6.

Sodeinde OA, Subrahmanyam YV et al., 1992, A surface protease and the invasive character of plague, *Science*, **258**: 1004–7.

Straley SC, Perry RD, 1995, Environmental modulation of gene expression and pathogenesis in *Yersinia*, *Trends Microbiol*, **3**: 310–19.

Swellengrebel NH, 1953, Researches on ectoparasites of man in the vicinity of Marrakech (Morocco), *Doc Med Geogr Trop*, **5**: 151–6.

Tabor SP, Thomas RE, 1986, The occurrence of plague (*Yersinia pestis*) in a bobcat from the Trans-Pecos area of Texas, *Southwest Naturalist*, **31**: 135–6.

Taylor P, Pugh A, 1982, Plague in Zimbabwe. A review of the situation in 1982, *Cent Afr J Med*, **28**: 249–53.

Thaung U, Kyi KM et al., 1978, An outbreak of plague in Hlegu, Burma in 1977, *Southeast Asian J Trop Med Public Health*, **9**: 390–6.

Thomas RE, McDonough KA, Schwan TG, 1989, Use of DNA hybridization probes for detection of the plague bacillus (*Yersinia pestis*) in fleas (Siphonaptera: Pulicidae and Ceratophyllidae), *J Med Entomol*, **26**: 342–8.

Thomas RE, Barnes AM et al., 1988, Susceptibility to *Yersinia pestis* in the northern grasshopper mouse (*Onychomys leucogaster*), *J Wildl Dis*, **24**: 327–33.

Thorne ET, Quan TJ et al., 1987, Plague in a free-ranging mule deer in Wyoming, *J Wildl Dis*, **23**: 155–9.

Trong P, Nhu TQ, Marshall JD, 1967, A mixed pneumonic bubonic plague outbreak in Vietnam, *Military Med*, **132**: 93–7.

Tuan PD, Dai VQ et al., 1971, Plague meningitis in infants, *Southeast Asian J Trop Med Public Health*, **2**: 403–5.

Tuchman BW, 1978, *A Distant Mirror*, Ballantine Books, New York, 92–125.

Turner RW, Martoprawiro S, Padmowiryono SA, 1974, Dynamics of the plague transmission cycle in central Java (ecology of potential plague flea vectors), *Bull Penelitian Kesehatan, Health Studies Indonesia*, **11**: 15–37.

Varela G, Vasquez A, 1954, Hallazgo de la peste selvatica en la Republica Mexicana. Infeccion natural del *Cynomys mexicanus* (perros llaneros) con *Pasteurella pestis*, *Rev Inst Salub Enferm Trop Mex*, **14**: 219–23.

Velimirovic B, 1972, Plague in southeast Asia – a brief historical summary and present geographical distribution, *Trans R Soc Trop Med Hyg*, **66**: 479–504.

Von Reyn CF, Barnes AM et al., 1976a, Bubonic plague from exposure to a rabbit: a documented case, and a review of rabbit-associated plague cases in the United States, *Am J Epidemiol*, **104**: 81–7.

Von Reyn CF, Barnes AM et al., 1976b, Bubonic plague from direct exposure to a naturally infected wild coyote, *Am J Trop Med Hyg*, **25**: 626–9.

Wake A, Morita H, Wake M, 1978, Mechanisms of long and short term immunity to plague, *Immunology*, **34**: 1045–52.

Welty TK, Grabman J et al., 1985, Nineteen cases of plague in Arizona. A spectrum including ecthyma gangrenosum due to plague and plague in pregnancy, *West J Med*, **142:** 641–6.

White ME, Rosenbaum RJ et al., 1981, Plague in a neonate, *Am J Dis Child*, **135:** 418–19.

WHO (World Health Organization), 1991, Human plague in 1990, *Wkly Epidemiol Rec*, **44:** 321–3.

WHO (World Health Organization), 1995, Human plague in 1993, *Wkly Epidemiol Rec*, **7:** 45–8.

Williams ES, Thorne ET et al., 1991, Experimental infection of domestic ferrets (*Mustela putorius furo*) and Siberian polecats (*Mustela eversmanni*) with *Yersinia pestis*, *J Wildl Dis*, **27:** 441–5.

Williams ES, Mills K et al., 1994, Plague in a black-footed ferret (*Mustela nigripes*), *J Wildl Dis*, **30:** 581–5.

Williams JE, Cavanaugh DC, 1979, Measuring the efficacy of vaccination in affording protection against plague, *Bull W H O*, **57:** 309–13.

Williams JE, Cavanaugh DC, 1983, Chronic infections in laboratory rodents from inoculation of nonencapsulated plague bacilli (*Yersinia pestis*), *Experientia*, **39:** 408–9.

Williams JE, Moussa MA, Cavanaugh DC, 1979, Experimental plague in the California ground squirrel, *J Infect Dis*, **140:** 618–21.

Williams JE, Hudson BW et al., 1980, Plague in Central Java, Indonesia, *Bull W H O*, **58:** 459–65.

Williams JE, Arntzen L et al., 1982, Comparison of passive hemagglutination and enzyme-linked immunosorbent assay for serodiagnosis of plague, *Bull W H O*, **60:** 777–81.

Williams JE, Arntzen L et al., 1986, Application of enzyme immunoassays for the confirmation clinically of suspect plague in Namibia, *Bull W H O*, **64:** 745–52.

Wolff KL, Hudson BW, 1974, Paper-strip blood sampling technique for the detections of antibody to the plague organism, *Appl Microbiol*, **28:** 323–5.

Wong JF, Elberg SS, 1977, Cellular immune response to *Yersinia pestis* modulated by product(s) from thymus-derived lymphocytes, *J Infect Dis*, **135:** 67–78.

Wong TW, 1986, Plague in a pregnant patient, *Trop Doct*, **16:** 187–9.

Yersin A, 1894, La peste bubonique, *Ann Inst Pasteur*, **8:** 666.

Zhu J, 1993, Analysis of human plague episodes in Qinghai from 1958 to 1991, *Chung Hua Liu Hsing Ping Hsueh Tsa Chih*, **14:** 227–30.

Zielinski WJ, 1984, Plague in pine martens and the fleas associated with its occurrence, *Great Basin Naturalist*, **44:** 170–5.

Zinsser H, 1934, *Rats, Lice and History*, Little, Brown, and Company, Boston, 145–9.

Chapter 45

YERSINIAL INFECTIONS OTHER THAN PLAGUE

T J Quan

1 INTRODUCTION

The genus *Yersinia* is classified as genus XI of the family Enterobacteriaceae. As members of this family, the species of *Yersinia* are oxidase-negative, catalase-positive, straight, gram-negative rods (or coccobacilli) $(0.3-1.0) \times (1.0-6.0)$ μm in size, that ferment glucose, are non-acid fast, and do not form endospores. Except for *Yersinia pestis*, the species may be motile at temperatures less than 30°C. With the exception of one biovar of *Y. pestis*, the species are nitratase-positive. The organisms are facultatively anaerobic and predominantly mesophilic though all exhibit growth at lower temperatures (e.g. 0–4°C). Cold enrichment is often employed as a means of recovering enteropathogenic and environmental isolates of *Yersinia enterocolitica* and the closely related congeners. The species are chemo-organotrophic and exhibit respiratory and fermentative metabolism. Acid, but not gas, is produced from D-glucose and other carbohydrates and polyhydroxylalcohols.

Three species are well known pathogens for humans, other mammals and birds: *Y. pestis*, the plague organism (see Chapter 44); *Yersinia pseudotuberculosis* and *Y. enterocolitica*, which cause a variety of gastroenteritis or enteric-type diseases and are occasionally manifested in other disorders. Also, species closely related to *Y. enterocolitica* occasionally have been associated with disease in a variety of hosts, including humans. A fourth species, *Yersinia ruckeri*, causes enteric redmouth disease in fish, especially trout. This last species, however, is probably not a true *Yersinia*.

Although *Y. pestis* grows quite well on many of the media commonly used in initial isolation attempts in the laboratory, extra incubation time (36–48 h) is often required for production of visible colonies. The other species generally form visible colonies in 18–30 h. Optimal growth temperature is 28°C for *Y. pestis* and 26–28°C for the other species. Differentiation of the yersiniae by biochemical tests is summarized in Table 45.1.

2 INFECTIONS WITH *YERSINIA PSEUDOTUBERCULOSIS*

2.1 Description of the disease

PATHOGENESIS

Y. pestis is more pathogenic than other yersiniae and has an untreated case-fatality rate in excess of 65% (Poland, Quan and Barnes 1994). The other agents usually cause less severe disease with lower case-fatality rates but often longer periods of chronic morbidity.

Pathogenicity and virulence in *Y. pestis* are governed by a number of chromosomal determinants and by the activities of 3 separate plasmids; in *Y. pseudotuberculosis* only one plasmid (identical, or closely related, to a *Y. pestis* plasmid) contributes to virulence. This common plasmid is approximately 70 kb (with a molecular weight of c. 42 000 kDa) and encodes for the low calcium response (LCR), producing at least 4 of the *Yersinia* outer-membrane proteins (Yops), and the V and W antigens (Brubaker 1984, 1991, Portnoy et al. 1984, Gemski et al. 1980). The Yops produced by *Y. pestis* are Yop B, C, D, E, F, H, J, K, L, M and N, of which Yop E, H, K, L and M are essential for full virulence.

Table 45.1 Differential characteristics of the yersiniae

Test	Yersinia pestis	Yersinia pseudotuberculosis	Yersinia enterocolitica	Yersinia intermedia	Yersinia fredriksenii	Yersinia kristensenii	Yersinia aldovae	Yersinia mollaretii	Yersinia bercovie	Yersinia rohdei	Yersinia ruckeri
Pathogenic	Yes	Yes	Yes	Opportunistic	Opportunistic	Opportunistic	Opportunistic	Opportunistic	Opportunistic	Opportunistic	Yes–fish
G + C content (%)	46	46.5	48.5 ± 0.5	48.5 ± 0.5	48.0	48.5 ± 0.5	46	50–51	50	48.7–49.4	48.0 ± 0.5
Motility (22°C)	–*	+	+	+	+	–	+	+	+	+	+
Nitrate reductase	V†	+	+	+	+	+	+	+	+	+	+
Urease	–*	+	+	+	+	+	+	+	+	d	–
Simmons citrate	–	–	–	+22°C or –	V	–	d	–	d	+	–
Ornithine decarboxylase	–	–	+	+	+	+	d	+	–	+	+
Acetylmethyl-carbinol (22°C)	–	–	+	+	+	–	+	+	+	+	+
β-Galactosidase	d	d	+	+	+	d	+	+	+	d	d
Indole	–	–	V	+	+	V	–	–	–	–	–
H₂S production	–	–	–	–	–	–	–	–	–	–	–
Aesculin hydrolysis	+	+	V	+	+	–	–	–	–	–	–
Gelatin hydrolysis	–	–	–	–	–	–	–	–	–	–	–
Methyl red	(+)	V	V	+	+	+	(+)	+	V	+	+
Glucose	+	+	+	+	+	+	+	+	+	+	+
Lactose	–	–	–	d	d	–	–	d	–	–	–
Sucrose	–	–	+	+	+	–	–	+	+	+	–

Glycerol	V†	V	+	d	+	d	−	−	−	d	d
α-Methylglucoside	−	−	−	−	−	−	d	−	−	−	−
Cellobiose	−	−*	+	+ (22°C)	+	+	+	+	+	+	−
Melibiose	V	+	−	22°C*	V	−*	−	−	−	d	−
Mucate	−	−	−	V	d	−	d	+	+	−	−
Raffinose	−	−	−	d	d	−	−	−	−	d	−
L-Rhamnose	+	+**	−	d	V	−	−	−	+	−	−
Trehalose	+	+	V	+	+	+	+	+	+	+	+
Sorbose	−	−	V	+	+	d	NR	NR	NR	NR	NR
Sorbitol	d	−*	+	+	+	+	d	+	+	+	d
Arabinose	+	+	+	+	+	+	+	d	+	+	+
Maltose	V	V	+	+	+	−	−	d	+	−	−
D-Xylose	+	+	+	+	+	d	d	d	+	d	+
Mannitol	+	+	+	+	+	+	+	+	+	+	+
Parazinamidase	−	−	V	+	+	+	−	−	V	+	+
Usual habitat	Rodents, other mammals, fleas, humans	Animals, birds, humans	Environmental sources, humans, animals	Water, sewage, fish, rodents, humans	Water, fish, food, animals	Soil, environmental sources, animals	Water, fish, humans	Humans, water, food	Humans, vegetables, soil	Water, dogs, humans	Water, fish, food, animals, humans

*Key test to differentiate species.

†Key test to differentiate biovars.

( ), Delayed reaction; L, late; NR, not reported.

Note: All *Yersinia* spp. are fermentative; negative for H_2S, oxidase, arginine dihydrolase, phenylalanine deaminase, malonate, dulcitol, DNAase (25°C), and pigmentation; all are positive for mannitol and mannose. Motile species have peritrichous flagella and motility is more pronounced at temperatures less than or equal to 30°C. Except for delayed reactions in some *Y. ruckeri*, all species are negative for gelatin hydrolase and lysine decarboxylase.

Data from: Bissett (1981), Brenner (1984, 1992), Clark et al. (1984), Wauters et al. (1988), Bottone (1992), Quan (1992).

In the enteropathogenic *Yersinia*, this 70 kb plasmid also encodes an adhesin, YadA (or YopA, or protein 1). Other Yops expressed by this plasmid are Yop B through J and YopN; again YopE and YopH are required for full virulence (see Table 45.2 for a summary of Yops and their functions) (Brubaker 1991). The Yops are highly conserved in the 3 species of virulent yersiniae and have similiar molecular weights and similiar immunological properties. However, as mentioned by Cornelis et al. (1989), establishment of complete correspondence among the Yops produced by the 3 species cannot be established. It is suspected that loss of Yops contributes to severe reductions in virulence and a substantial increase in the LD50s for mice (Straley and Bowmer 1986, Bolin and Wolf-Watz 1988, Forsberg and Wolf-Watz 1988, Sory and Cornelis 1988, Mulder et al. 1989).

In *Y. pestis* an approximately 10 kb plasmid encodes for the virulence factors: plasminogen activator and post-translational degradation of the Yops, as well as production of the bacteriocin, pesticin. The third plasmid of *Y. pestis* encodes for murine toxin and for the envelope antigen, fraction 1, both of which are unique to *Y. pestis*.

Pathogenicity of *Y. pseudotuberculosis* is partially dependent on the presence of only one of these plasmids, the VW or LCR plasmid. Additional chromosomally controlled virulence factors include production of the protein invasin in the outer membrane, which enables the organism to penetrate host cells (Isberg and Falkow 1985, Cornelis et al. 1989, Brubaker 1991). One case of acute mesenteric lymphadenitis in a human caused by a strain of *Y. pseudotuberculosis* serotype IVA lacking a virulence plasmid was reported by Fukushima et al. (1991); however, it is unclear whether the agent lost the virulence plasmid prior to infection or by laboratory manipulations after its isolation from the patient. The description of the disease was typical for *Y. pseudotuberculosis*.

MODES OF TRANSMISSION

As an infectious agent, *Y. pestis* is typically vector-borne; almost any flea species can occasionally transmit the organism, though some species are more efficient than others and some are more commonly involved in epizootic and epidemic situations. The other species of *Yersinia* do not require the intermediary services of arthropod vectors, usually being transmitted via typical faecal–oral routes or via contaminated water. *Y. pseudotuberculosis* has been recovered on occasion from ectoparasites, including ticks, lice and fleas. Experimental infection with virulent *Y. pseudotuberculosis* killed most lice in 2 days in lethal infections whereas survivors cleared bacteria rapidly (Krynski 1968).

2.2 Clinical manifestations

HUMANS

The spectrum of disease manifestations produced by *Y. pseudotuberculosis* and *Y. enterocolitica* are similiar but they do vary in definite and perceptible ways when examined epidemiologically (Bottone 1992). *Y. pseudotuberculosis* most frequently causes an acute abdominal syndrome marked by mesenteric adenitis (also called pseudoappendicitis) affecting most commonly young males – children and young adults. Terminal ileitis is infrequently seen in *Y. pseudotuberculosis* infection, but is very common and often severe in *Y. enterocolitica* infections. In Finland, among a cluster of 19 cases of serotype III infections the following distribution of signs and symptoms were reported (Tertii et al. 1984):

1 abdominal distress (pain) (14)
2 gastroenteritis (4)
3 pseudoappendicitis (3)
4 fever (11)
5 asymptomatic (2).

Table 45.2 Described *Yersinia* outer-membrane proteins and their functions in the enteropathogenic species

Identity	Molecular weight	Known or inferred role
YadA	160×10^3	Adhesion to (human) epithelial cells; aids intestinal colonization; confers resistance to (Yop1) serum bactericidal activity (Balligand, LaRoche and Cornelis 1985, Heesemann and Gruter 1987, Kapperud et al. 1987)
Required for full virulence:		
YopE (Yop5)	25×10^3	Unclear role; iron metabolism; required for prompt growth in tissues; cytotoxic
YopH (Yop2b)	45×10^3	Inhibition of phagocytosis
Association with virulence suspected but not established:		
YopF	76×10^3	
YopG	58×10^3	Ca^{2+}
YopI	43×10^3	
YopJ	31×10^3	
YopN	34×10^3	Temperature sensor

Sources: Straley and Bowmer (1986), Sample, Fowler and Brubaker (1987), Bolin and Wolf-Watz (1988), Forsberg and Wolf-Watz (1988), Sory and Cornelis (1988), Cornelis et al. (1989), Mulder et al. (1989).

Complications of *Y. pseudotuberculosis* infection occurred in 10 of the 19 patients in this cluster and included erythema nodosum in 6; iritis in 1; Reiter's syndrome or arthritis in 4; and nephritis in 1. Duration of illness ranged from one week to 6 months. Systemic *Y. pseudotuberculosis* infection is rare in humans; enteric infection with haematogenous spread to adjacent (mesenteric) lymphatics apparently is the rule.

NON-HUMAN

Pathogenesis in wild animals is not fully established since most infections are diagnosed post mortem in fatal cases. The diagnosis is estabished by the isolation of the organism from suitable specimens, which may include heart blood, spleen, liver, lymph nodes, other organs and/or faeces. Cold enrichment of cultures may enhance the isolation rates for *Y. pseudotuberculosis* in heavily contaminated specimens. Signs of disease in animals due to pseudotuberculosis infection have been described as involving chronic inappetence; intermittent diarrhoea; lymphadenitis; caseous abscessation resembling tuberculosis of various organs including spleen, liver and lungs; enteritis; and generalized septicaemia. It is important to differentiate the disease caused by *Y. pseudotuberculosis* from that caused by *Corynebacterium pseudotuberculosis*, a gram-positive bacillus; the former is a more common, and more serious, pathogen of man.

ENVIRONMENTAL

Y. pseudotuberculosis is found in a large array of mammalian and avian hosts (and perhaps reptiles). Many of these infections are inapparent or chronic; the infected hosts shed the organisms into the environment over long periods of time. A series of papers by investigators at the Institute Pasteur in Paris, France indicated potential long-term survival of *Y. pestis* in soil contaminated by animal carcasses killed by plague (Karimi 1963, Mollaret et al. 1963). No similiar occurrence of longevity or survival of *Y. pseudotuberculosis* were found. Unpublished observations by this author indicate that this organism, like the plague organism, is quite susceptible to desiccation, suggesting that longevity in an unprotected environment would be limited. A single report has incriminated water as the source of infection of more than 200 humans with *Y. pseudotuberculosis* serotypes 1b and 4b in Japan (Fukushima et al. 1989).

2.3 Epidemiology

Y. pseudotuberculosis causes disease in humans, mammals and birds, often in zoos or other holding areas (Stovell 1963, Bronson, May and Ruebner 1972, Baskin et al. 1977). The species enjoys a fairly broad distribution with certain serotypes or biotypes seemingly more prevalent in certain areas and in certain hosts than others. For example, in North America and Europe the organisms associated with most human infections fall into serotype IA or IB; infection of birds in several North American outbreaks were found to be

of serotype III. In Japan, several outbreaks were associated with serotype IV and V and one outbreak each (each involving more than 60 human patients) were due to serotypes I and III (Tsubokura et al. 1989). Also in Japan, cats have been incriminated as the reservoir of infection for a number of human cases (Fukushima et al. 1989) and as much as 2% of pork products were found contaminated with *Y. pseudotuberculosis* of serotypes VB, IIB, IIC and III (Shiozawa et al. 1988). Japanese investigators have identified the common family dog and cat as potential reservoirs for infection of humans with *Y. pseudotuberculosis* (Fukushima et al. 1989).

Before the recognition and description of serotypes VI, VII and VIII, Wetzler and Hubbert (1968), Wetzler (1970) and others presented lists of diverse animals and birds found naturally infected or susceptible to experimental infection with *Y. pseudotuberculosis* with organisms of each of the various serotypes represented. These lists contained 60 species of 6 orders of wild mammals, and 50 species of 9 orders of wild birds.

The original isolation of the organism now identified as *Y. pseudotuberculosis* by Malassez and Vignal in 1883 was from the internal organs of a laboratory guinea pig. Rodents, both in the wild and in laboratory colonies, continue to be found naturally infected sporadically and may serve as the source of infection of other animals and humans. Other collections of animals, e.g. turkeys, canaries, primate centres (Yerkes Primate Center in Georgia, and the University of California at Davis), The National Zoo in Washington, DC (Baskin et al. 1977) and the Tokyo Zoo (Sasaki et al. 1989), have also experienced occasional epizootics or epornithics. Some limited success in identifying both a wild rodent and a wild bird reservoir of infection was achieved in one of these outbreaks (Baskin et al. 1977).

Among domestic animals, the most commonly infected are pigs – not necessarily diseased (Tsubokura, Itagaki and Kawamura 1970, Toma and Diedrick 1975, Doyle, Hugdahl and Taylor 1981, Shayegani et al. 1981). A survey in Japan revealed that 6.3% of healthy dogs were infected with *Y. pseudotuberculosis* of 5 serotypes as well as 2 strains that were nontypable (Fukushima et al. 1984). Isolates have also been recovered from chickens and geese (Kilian et al. 1962, Borst et al. 1977). Even reptiles have not escaped infection according to Corbel who cited 3 reports of reptilian infection in the previous edition of this text (see Stoll 1965, Mair 1968, Kageruka 1970). According to Lee (1987), *Y. pseudotuberculosis* infection or contamination is uncommon in meat from cattle, pigs, sheep and fowl, in contrast to the quite common presence of *Y. enterocolitica* and *Y. enterocolitica*-like organisms. Shiozawa et al. (1988), however, reported frequent isolation of *Y. pseudotuberculosis* (especially serotypes IVB and VB) in pork and estimated an infection rate of 1–2% for pork in Japan. No estimate of numbers of human cases associated with these contaminated pork products was offered, though a potential for transmission is certainly present to both butchers and food preparers handling the raw meat, as well as to persons ingesting undercooked contaminated pork.

The diversity of hosts that has been described suggests that almost any species may be found harbouring *Y. pseudotuberculosis* naturally if one were to test for its presence in a suitable fashion (Wetzler 1971a, 1971b).

Some serotypes are more commonly involved with infections of different host species. The majority of human and animal infections are of serotype I (both IA and IB). Infections with members of serotypes II and III, respectively, are the next most common. In Australia, *Y. pseudotuberculosis* serotypes I, II and III have been documented as enteropathogens of a variety of ungulates, including sheep, cattle, deer, goats and pigs (Slee and Skilbeck 1992). Serotype I *Y. pseudotuberculosis* (IA and IB) are predominant among isolates of human and animal sources in North America and Europe whereas serotypes IV and V are most common in Japan. For example, Fukushima et al. (1984) reported that 6.3% of 252 dogs studied harboured *Y. pseudotuberculosis* – 4 with type I, 10 with types IV and V, and 2 with untypable isolates.

2.4 Aetiology

Disease attributable to this agent was first described by Malassez and Vignal in 1883; the agent itself was first described bacteriologically by Pfeiffer in 1889 and named *Bacillus pseudotuberculosis rodentium*. Generic assignment to *Pasteurella* was proposed in 1965 by Smith and Thal.

Culturally and biochemically *Y. pseudotuberculosis* is quite similiar to *Y. pestis*, so much so that taxonomists have determined the 2 are simply varieties of the same species and that 'correct nomenclature' is *Yersinia pseudotuberculosis pseudotuberculosis* and *Yersinia pseudotuberculosis pestis*. However, the diseases caused by the 2 organisms are inherently different. The organisms were regarded 'officially' for a brief time as varieties of the same species (Bercovier et al. 1980). This designation was subsequently rejected by the Judicial Commission of the International Committee on Systematic Bacteriology (1985) because 'the use of the name could have serious consequences for human welfare and health'. The Commission did recognize the validity of the evidence indicating the 2 species are closely related.

SEROTYPES OF *YERSINIA PSEUDOTUBERCULOSIS*

Y. pestis has a single serotype, detectable by current tests; the other species produce multiple serotypic antigens. Fraction 1 antigen (the envelope antigen) of *Y. pestis* is an excellent immunogen and very specific. Other somatic antigens of the organism may be shared with *Y. pseudotuberculosis*, other yersiniae and other members of the Enterobacteriaceae. There are 8 major serotypes of *Y. pseudotuberculosis* with 9 subtypes (IA, IB, IIA, IIB, IIC, III, IVA, IVB, VA, VB, VI, VII and VIII) (Tsubokura, Itagaki and Kawamura 1971, Wetzler 1970). Although the serotypes have been designated by the appropriate Roman numeral; recently there has been a trend to use Arabic numerals for these designations.

2.5 Collection of specimens

The best specimens for the recovery of *Y. pseudotuberculosis* are excised tissues such as lymph nodes, pieces of affected ileum or appendix, and occasionally, blood. It is difficult to recover this species from specimens such as stools that are heavily contaminated with other organisms. Use of highly inhibitory agars such as deoxycholate agar or *Salmonella–Shigella* agar might eliminate some of the competing organisms, but they also tend to reduce the recovery rate for *Y. pseudotuberculosis*. Incubation of the specimen in isotonic saline with or without 25 µg ml^{-1} potassium tellurite at 4°C for varying periods of time may increase the success of recovery (Wetzler 1970). Because cold enrichment requires incubation periods that preclude achievement of a rapid diagnosis, direct culture of suitable specimens should be made at the time of receipt in the laboratory on a variety of suitable media followed by close examination for small colonies consistent with *Y. pseudotuberculosis*.

2.6 General approaches to treatment

Kanazawa, Ikemura and Kuramata (1987) showed that *Y. pseudotuberculosis* lacks β-lactamase and is susceptible to penicillins and cephalosporins. Use of penicillins in chemotherapy of yersinal infections should not be based solely on in vitro susceptibility. In vitro susceptibility of *Y. pestis* to penicillin is well known as is the lack of efficacy of penicillin for plague infections in either humans or animals. Wetzler (1970) predicted good efficacy for any broad spectrum antibiotic for the treatment of pseudotuberculosis in highly sensitive hosts or valuable, captive animals. For prophylaxis he suggested the use of sulphonamides and nitrofurans.

2.7 Prevention and transmissibility

Preventive measures similar to those used in the control of any disease transmitted by the faecal–oral route should reduce or eliminate infections with *Y. pseudotuberculosis*. Foods normally eaten raw should be thoroughly washed, and peeled, if possible, prior to ingestion. Meat from animals potentially infected with this organism should be examined for obvious lesions and discarded should such lesions be found (this is especially true for game animals and birds not commercially obtained). Food storage areas and bins should be kept clean and built and maintained in such a manner as to exclude rodents and birds.

Persons who are diagnosed with enteric disease due to *Y. pseudotuberculosis* should refrain from handling foods or preparing meals for others until they have been seen by a physician, placed on a suitable antibiotic for 48 h or more, and are afebrile.

3 INFECTIONS WITH *YERSINIA ENTEROCOLITICA*

3.1 Description of the disease

PATHOGENESIS

Virulence in *Y. enterocolitica* depends on the presence of at least 3 plasmids including the 72 kb low calcium response plasmid present in virulent *Y. pestis* and *Y. pseudotuberculosis*. The other plasmids encode for 8 or more *Yersinia* outer-membrane proteins. One of these Yops, protein 1 ('P1'), is associated with resistance to killing by serum, hydrophobicity, autoagglutination in fluid media, and production of a fibrillar adhesin which enhances attachment of the bacteria to epithelial cells of the host. Many of the other Yops function to inhibit phagocytosis by mammalian hosts (Forsberg, Rosqvist and Wolf-Watz 1994). Yops produced by *Y. enterocolitica* are YadA, Yops B, C, D, E and H. As for *Y. pseudotuberculosis*, YopE and YopH are essential for full virulence in *Y. enterocolitica* (see Table 45.2 for a summary of Yop identities and functions) (Sodeinde et al. 1988, Brubaker 1991). Chromosomally determined virulence factors include production of an invasin similiar to that of *Y. pseudotuberculosis* and of a second factor that allows specific invasion of various cell types (Miller and Falkow 1988).

Experimental infection of rodents and rabbits with *Y. enterocolitica* offers some parallels to the infection in humans (Heesemann, Gaede and Autentrieth 1993). From studies of experimental infections these reseachers were able to determine that M cells in the Peyer's patches were the primary target cells of invading yersiniae and that in the Peyer's patches the bacilli were strictly extracellular. Evidence for an active role of T cells and cytokine-activated macrophages against primary *Yersinia* infection in mice was obtained in a study of adoptive transfer of *Yersinia*-specific T cells and from in vivo neutralization of tumour necrosis factor α and interferon-γ. Only *Y. enterocolitica* O:8 proved arthritogenic in various strains of laboratory rats and was shown to be dependent on T cell depletion.

Y. enterocolitica strains associated with human disease are mainly of serotypes 3 and 9 in Europe but type 8 in North America; in Japan other serotypes are common, but serotype 8 was recognized only as recently as 1990 (Ichinohe et al. 1991). In Australia, *Y. enterocolitica* serotype O:2,3 (and similiar to biotype 5; currently designated serotype O:3) was reported as a common pathogen of sheep and occasionally of cattle (Slee and Skilbeck 1992). New hosts or reservoirs are also being reported. For example, infections have been recognized in birds in Japan (Kato et al. 1985) and Norway (Kapperud and Rosef 1983); in companion animals in Italy (Mingrone et al. 1987) and Japan (Fukushima et al. 1984); in foods and other environmental sources (Botzler 1979, 1987, Aulisio et al. 1983, Moustafa, Ahmed and Marth 1983a, Lee 1987, Kwaga and Iversen 1992).

MODES OF TRANSMISSION

The primary method of transmission for *Y. enterocolitica* is via the faecal–oral route as for *Y. pseudotuberculosis* and may also occasionally involve contaminated water sources (Lassen 1972, Saari and Quan 1976, Saari and Jansen 1977, Wetzler et al. 1978) and contaminated meats (Aulisio et al. 1983) and poultry (DeBoer, Hartog and Oosterom 1982). Uncommon infections have resulted from the transfusion of contaminated units of blood from bacteraemic, though apparently healthy, donors (Jacobs et al. 1989, CDC 1991). Several outbreaks of *Y. enterocolitica* infections have been traced to the consumption of pasteurized milk (Aulisio et al. 1983, Shayegani et al. 1983, Tacket et al. 1984) and chocolate milk (Black et al. 1978) as well as of raw milk and cheese and contaminated foods (Aulisio et al. 1983) and meats (Doyle, Hugdahl and Taylor 1981, Shayegani et al. 1983).

Y. enterocolitica has been recovered from 2 separate pools of fleas collected from rats during plague surveillance studies (CDC Annual Reports 1971, 1972). These 2 isolations of *Y. enterocolitica* were unusual in that:

1 this was the first report of naturally occurring infection of fleas with this agent and
2 the 2 isolates killed laboratory mice after a long holding period of 21 and 22 days, respectively.

Prior to this finding, the gerbil (*Meriones unguiculatus*) was the only experimental animal that was found useful in pathogenetic studies (Wetzler 1965). A significant role of arthropod vectors has not been defined. In addition to the flea pools mentioned above, at least 2 other studies have appeared: one involving lice and one incriminating house flies. Death of experimentally infected lice was slower following infection with *Y. enterocolitica* than with *Y. pseudotuberculosis* but cures were rare (Krynski 1968). Fukushima et al. (1979) suggested a possible role for house flies in the inter-pig transmission of *Y. enterocolitica*, most probably by simple contamination. Studies of vector efficiency for other arthropods apparently have not been common.

Contamination of foodstuffs with *Y. enterocolitica* also poses special hazards. Several outbreaks of gastrointestinal illness were traced to the ingestion of contaminated foods such as raw and pasteurized milk (Moustafa, Ahmed and Marth 1983a, 1983b, Tacket et al. 1984) and tofu (Aulisio et al. 1983).

3.2 Clinical manifestations

HUMAN

In humans, mesenteric adenitis referable to *Y. enterocolitica* is evenly distributed among the sexes of adolescents and young adults. The most common presentation in *Y. enterocolitica* infections, but rare in *Y. pseudotuberculosis* infections, is acute enteritis. This complication is often quite severe, painful and distressing, but is usually self-limiting. In all the presentations mentioned, abdominal lymph nodes are enlarged and may be matted; the intestinal mucosa are often ulcerated and haemorrhagic. Both agents cause signs and symptoms that are easily confused with acute appendicitis and quite a few appendectomies were initiated only to find normal appendices but inflamed mesenteric lymph nodes, or terminal ileitis caused by enteric infection with one agent or the other, or both (Bottone 1992).

Enteric infections may lead to severe complications such as hypokalaemia and flaccid quadriparesis (Orman and Lewis 1989). Other disease presentations less frequently associated with infection with these agents include systemic disorders, focal abscesses of liver, spleen, kidney and lung, myocarditis, pneumonia, meningitis, septicaemia, osteomyelitis; and local manifestations such as cellulitis and wound infections, pustules, conjunctivitis and panophthalmitis (Bottone 1992). Endocarditis (Urbano-Marquez et al. 1983), pericarditis (Lecomte et al. 1989) and osteitis (Fisch et al. 1989) have been reported as sequelae to enteric infection. Lenz, Schulte and Meyer-Sabeller (1984) reported serious complications of *Y. enterocolitica* infection in patients under immunosuppressive therapy. Human infection with *Y. enterocolitica* has been reported as a plague-like disease complete with bubo (Alvin and Middleton 1986). Boelaert et al. (1987) reported *Yersinia* septicaemia in 2 dialysis patients who received treatment with deferoxamine (and 8 others who did not). It was suggested that deferoxamine increased the virulence of the *Yersinia* by acting as a siderophore for organisms not able to synthesize iron-binding compounds. In other cases of yersinial bacteraemia in dialysis patients iron status was not investigated, but immunosuppressive therapy and iron overload may have been predisposing factors. Hepatic abscess and septicaemia due to *Y. enterocolitica* were also reported in one patient who had received long-term iron therapy for chronic anaemia (Leighton and MacSween 1987).

Increasingly, case reports appear in the literature describing 'new' occurrences of disease associated with *Y. enterocolitica*, which only serve to fill lapses in our knowledge of the full spectrum of activities in the organism's repertoire (Anjorin et al. 1979, Fisch et al. 1989, Orman and Lewis 1989). Because of their psychroduric and psychrophilic nature *Y. enterocolitica* organisms pose special hazards when blood donors have a bacteraemia – the organisms can grow during cold temperature storage in the highly nutrient blood unit and cause severe infection in transfusion recipients (Arduino et al. 1989, CDC 1991). Jacobs et al. (1989) reported on the occurrence of an infection traced to transfusion with the blood of a donor who had a history of chronic terminal ileitis but was apparently healthy at the time the blood unit was drawn. Jacobs et al. also reviewed reports of 14 additional transfusion-acquired infections, many of which were quite serious or even fatal. Seven of 10 *Y. enterocolitica* infections associated with blood transfusions in the USA between April 1987 and February 1991 were fatal (CDC 1991). This is perhaps more a result of the weakened condition of the host and concomitant increased susceptiblity to infection with *Y. enterocolitica*.

NON-HUMAN

Fur-farm chinchillas were among the first animals in which an epizootic referable to *Y. enterocolitica* (as now known) was proven (Becht 1963). Since that time recognition of such infections has been made in a wide variety of both wild and domestic animals and, to a lesser degree, of birds.

The progression of infection in naturally infected animals is not documented. Studies of the pathogenesis of experimentally infected animals with organisms of serogroups 8, 3 or 9 (the classic enteropathogens of the species) have shown penetration of the epithelial linings of the intestinal mucosa, including Peyer's patches, followed by invasion of the reticuloendothelial tissue and mononuclear cells. Enterocolitis ensued, characterized by production of small focal ulcerative lesions and abscesses in the mucosa and granulomatous lesions in mesenteric lymph nodes, spleen and liver (Hanski et al. 1991).

ENVIRONMENTAL

Y. enterocolitica and *Y. enterocolitica*-like organisms (or members of the more recently created taxons) are not uncommon contaminants of water supplies and were first reported by Botzler and colleagues (Botzler, Wetzler and Cowan 1968, Botzler et al. 1976) in the USA and by Lassen (1972) and Wauters (1972) in Europe. In 1973, Toma reported the occurrence of *Y. enterocolitica* in water samples in Canada. Highsmith et al. (1977) reported the isolation in 1975 of *Y. enterocolitica* from well waters associated with a number of human cases of gastroenteritis. The strains that were serotypable (5 of 14 isolates) were of types not commonly involved in human disease. Almost every major river in Colorado was found to contain a variety of different serotypes and biotypes of this group of organisms (Saari and Quan 1976). Saari and Jansen (1977) found many Wisconsin streams and rivers contaminated. Wetzler et al. (1978) reported numerous isolates from a variety of water sources and waste waters in Washington State. All of these reports predate the creation of the newer taxons and most of the isolates recovered would probably fit into one or another of the 'environmental' *Yersinia* spp. rather than *Y. enterocolitica sensu stricto*. Barre et al. (1976) first reported soil-derived *Y. enterocolitica* from France. Soil isolates were reported from California in infected wapiti (elk) range and from forest soils in Germany by the same investigator (Botzler 1979, 1987). Three of Botzler's German soil samples also yielded *Y. frederiksenii*. Most German strains were not serotypable using serotyping reagents available at the time; the one *Y. enterocolitica* that could be serotyped was O:6,33, not commonly involved in human infection. The California soil isolates were of serotypes O:4,32; O:5, O:17; and O:20, also uncommon in human infections. Re-evaluation of the biochemical reactions and screening by a current set of serotyping reagents might help in assigning these environmental strains to the correct species. For example, the O:17 isolates would currently be identified as *Y. intermedia* (see section 3.4, p. 913).

3.3 Epidemiology

There have been several large outbreaks of infection following common source exposure to *Y. enterocolitica*; these have been commonly food-borne instances involving milk, pasteurized as well as raw, tofu, or meat, commonly pork (see p. 909). Person-to-person transmission has not been well documented; the major mode of transmission does seem to be the faecal–oral route. Domestic pets are not infrequent hosts and are being increasingly associated with the occurrence of human disease (Gutman et al. 1973, Fantasia et al. 1985, Fukushima et al. 1988).

3.4   Aetiology

Y. enterocolitica (Frederiksen 1964) was originally called *Bacterium enterocoliticum* by Schliefstein and Coleman in 1943 but was also known as *Pasteurella pseudotuberculosis* type B (Dickinson and Mocquot 1961); *Pasteurella* 'X' (Knapp and Thal 1963); and Les Germes X (Mollaret and Chevalier 1964).

Recent specific taxa have been suggested or adopted for former biovars of *Y. enterocolitica* and are shown in Table 45.3.

SEROTYPES OF *Y. ENTEROCOLITICA* (AND RELATED SPECIES)

Serotypes of *Y. enterocolitica* have numbered as many as 54, which, by convention, are designated with Arabic numerals. Some strains exhibit multiple serotypic antigens. Serotyping refinements proceed and with the definition of new species from the heterogenous complex once called *Y. enterocolitica* and '*Y. enterocolitica*-like' organisms, new designations or reassignments will undoubtedly be established. Many isolates have been untypable with the antigenic spectrum available to investigators at the time of testing. Serotyping antigens of *Y. enterocolitica* may exist in the more recently described species.

Serotypes O:3, O:8 and O:9 of *Y. enterocolitica* are most commonly involved in human and animal infections; O:3 and O:9 in Europe and serotype O:8 in North America. These statements, however, do not preclude the occasional isolations of other serotypes from humans or animals.

Wauters et al. (1972) and Wauters (1981) proposed the most widely used antigenic typing scheme for *Y. enterocolitica* that included a total of 50 serogroups. Aleksic and Bockemuhl (1984) proposed a revision of serotyping schemes, merging some serofactors into single factors and eliminating other designations as invalid. Thus, serotype O:1,2,3 was equated to serotype O:3; serotype O:34 was equated to O:10; and serotype O:29 was eliminated. Serogroups O:4,33 and O:17 were found only among *Y. intermedia*; serogroups O:11,23, O:11,24, O:12,25, O:12,26 and O:26 were exclusive to *Y. kristensenii*; and one serofactor, O:16, was found in both *Y. kristensenii* and *Y. frederiksenii*. Other O serogroups were associated with *Y. enterocolitica* – giving a new total of 18 serogroups with 20 O factors. Aleksic and Bockemuhl (1984) continued their revision of the antigenic relationships by examining flagellar (H) antigens. Their study indicated that *Y. enterocolitica* flagellar antigens belonged to groups H:a through H:k, H:m and H:n. Other H antigens were found in other species as follows: l, r, s, and t in *Y. kristensenii*; p in *Y. frederiksenii*; H:q in *Y. intermedia*; H:o was found in *Y. kristensenii*, *Y. frederiksenii* and *Y. intermedia*.

A bacteriophage typing system was suggested by Baker and Farmer (1982) which included patterns for 4 species (*Y. enterocolitica*, *Y. kristensenii*, *Y. frederiksenii* and *Y. intermedia*); the other species had yet to be described. In their scheme, 24 bacteriophages were selected as being the most useful for differentiating strains. More than 90% of the 300 strains were typable with this set. It is probable that some of the untypable bacterial strains represented organisms that would be identified as other species of *Yersinia* with current techniques.

3.5   Collection of specimens

In the case of human or animal infections, stool specimens and tissues such as lymph nodes, pieces of inflamed intestine and appendix often yield isolates of *Y. enterocolitica* but may require cold enrichment. Various cold enrichment techniques have been used to isolate the species; usually incubation at 4°C in isotonic saline is sufficient. Wetzler (1970) suggested incorporation of 25 μg ml^{-1} of potassium tellurite into the isotonic saline used for enrichment. Periodic samplings of the cold enriched suspension on routine enteric media should be done for up to 6 weeks. Food and water samples may be handled by the same technique employing selective enrichment broths containing Irgasan, ticarcillin and potassium chlorate (Wauters et al. 1988). Fukushima (1985) reported favourable recovery rates of a small number of *Y. enterocolitica* and *Y. pseudotuberculosis* strains seeded onto separate meat samples at concentrations ranging from 10 to 10^4 cells per gram of meat. The samples were suspended in saline containing 0.4 M potassium hydroxide and plated on CIN (cefsulodin–Irgasan–novobiocin) agar. Incubation for as little as 1 day at 4°C (as for cold enrichment techniques) in the potassium hydroxide solution, however, inhibited recovery of the organism seeded at any concentration.

3.6   General approaches to treatment

Infections with *Y. enterocolitica* and the related species are generally self-limiting. Effective therapy was achieved with trimethoprim–sulphamethoxazole in treating patients in a small outbreak of enteritis in North Carolina in 1972 (Gutman, Wilfert and Quan 1973). This combination drug was found effective in in vitro tests on virulent *Y. enterocolitica* in several studies (Gutman, Wilfert and Quan 1973, Baker and Farmer 1982, Kanazawa, Ikemura and Kuramata 1987). Other antibiotics to which this species seems susceptible include the

Table 45.3   Specific taxa suggested and/or adopted for former biovars of *Y. enterocolitica*

Suggested taxon	Reference	Group
Yersinia intermedia	Brenner et al. 1980	Rhamnose +, sucrose +, melibiose +, raffinose +
Yersinia frederiksenii	Brenner 1981	Rhamnose +, sucrose +
Yersinia kristensenii	Brenner 1981	Rhamnose −, sucrose −
Yersinia aldovae	Bercovier et al. 1984	Formerly group X2
Yersinia rohdei	Aleksic et al. 1987	Rhamnose +, sucrose −
Yersinia mollaretii	Wauters et al. 1988	Formerly biogroup 3A
Yersinia bercovieri	Wauters et al. 1988	Formerly biogroup 3B

+, positive; −, negative.

aminoglycosides, chloramphenicol, quinolones and tetracycline, and the third generation cephalosporins. Most serotypes of *Y. enterocolitica* possess β-lactamase and are resistant to penicillin, ampicillin, carbenicillin and cephalothin; serotype O:8, however, is susceptible to ampicillin (Cornelis, Wauters and VanderHaeghe 1973, Baker and Farmer 1982, Ahmedy et al. 1985, Kanazawa, Ikemura and Kuramata 1987).

3.7 Prevention and transmissibility

The same precautions discussed for *Y. pseudotuberculosis* (see section 2.7, p. 910) extend to *Y. enterocolitica*, perhaps somewhat more broadly applied due to the increased involvment of the latter with foods (meats, dairy products, others) and environmental reservoirs.

4 INFECTIONS WITH *YERSINIA RUCKERI*

Y. ruckeri is probably not a true *Yersinia* but transfer to another genus has not occurred.

4.1 Disease

Y. ruckeri is a pathogen of fish, primarily trout and other salmonid species. Enteric redmouth disease is systemic and characteristically produces inflammation of the head and mouth, about the vent and at the bases of the fins. Most often it is an acute infection, causing widespread mortality; chronic conditions occur and produce dark discoloration, lethargy and bilateral exophthalmia (Dulin et al. 1977). Young fish seem more susceptible to severe infection as do fat or debilitated fish.

4.2 Aetiology

Y. ruckeri was described in 1966 by Ross, Rucker and Ewing as 'The Redmouth Disease' bacterium, and subsequently as Enteric Redmouth Bacterium, Redvent Bacterium and Hagerman Redmouth Bacterium; it causes disease predominantly in trout and other salmonids. Ewing et al. (1978) proposed the name *Yersinia ruckeri*. The organism has also been recovered from a muskrat, but infections with this agent have not been reported in other species.

4.3 Serotypes and biotypes

Isolates of *Y. ruckeri* are fairly homogenous with only 2 serotypes and 2 biotypes identified to date. Serotype 1 organisms generally are sorbitol-positive and serotype 2 are usually sorbitol-negative, with some exceptions (Stevenson and Daly 1982). Immunization with antigens of one serotype seems to provide some protection against infection with the other serotype (Cipriano and Ruppenthal 1987). Four electrophoreotypes were described by isoenzyme assessment (Schill, Phelps and Pyle 1984) but one of these represented only 2 isolates and each of 2 types were represented by single isolates among the 47 strains studied.

The reservoir of *Y. ruckeri* appears to be chronically infected fish which may account for 2–3% in nature; carrier rates in hatchery fish may be 6% or more (Dulin et al. 1977).

The organism seems adapted to a saphrophytic aquatic lifestyle (McDaniel 1972).

5 OTHER YERSINIAE

The other yersiniae do not generally elicit disease responses, though on occasion they have been recovered from clinical specimens (usually faecal cultures) or from normal, healthy hosts (human and animal). None of the non-*pestis* species has been found to be efficiently transmitted by fleas, ticks, lice, or other arthropods. *Y. intermedia*, *Y. kristensenii*, *Y. fredericksenii* and *Y. rohdei* have all been isolated from specimens of human and animal origin, but their roles in disease production have not been fully elucidated (Shayegani et al. 1981, Aleksic et al. 1987, Punsalang, Edinger and Nolte 1987, Robins-Browne et al. 1991). Identifying characteristics of these species are included in Table 45.1.

6 SEROLOGY AND SEROTYPING

Conventional tests for the serodiagnosis of yersinial infections involve bacterial agglutination tests using paired patient sera and antigens prepared from cultures of the typing strains of the specific bacterial species. Titres in excess of 128 are considered minimal levels of reactivity for single serum specimens; a 4-fold rise in titre between acute and convalescent sera is diagnostic. The convalescent sample should be drawn 14 days after the acute sample, but in suspect *Y. pseudotuberculosis* infections it is important that the second specimen be taken in early convalescence because titres fall rapidly. The antigens used have been either killed, preserved whole cells (least sensitive) or autoclaved spent broths containing lipopolysaccharide antigens. Often antigens have been prepared from cultures isolated from the patient for testing with the patient's sera. If no culture from the patient is available, the sera are titrated against the antigens of the typing kit and assignment of the infection to a serotype is assumed to be that of the antigen providing the strongest reaction. Antigens of the serotyping set may be made more specific by absorbing the preparations with hyperimmune sera (usually rabbit) against other cross-reacting serotypes. Antibodies to serotypes I, III and V *Y. pseudotuberculosis* are quite specific, but antibodies to serotypes II and IV are cross-reactive with *Salmonella* groups B and D (Wetzler 1970, Bottone 1992).

When a culture has been isolated, it may be serotyped by agglutination reactions against hyperimmune, absorbed, rabbit antisera against the serotyping strains of the species of interest.

Monoclonal antibodies prepared against the specific serotypes of the yersiniae are not generally available, but would provide specific reagents for both serodiagnostic tests and serotyping of cultures, using current techniques such as radioimmunoassay and enzyme-linked immunosorbent assays (ELISA). Use of the latter tests have been reported by a number of investigators in defining IgG, IgM and IgA antibody levels with good sensitivity and specificity, but the tests were developed by each investigator and are not as yet available (Cafferty and Buckley 1987, Stahlberg et al. 1987, Granfors et al. 1988, Kaneko and Maruyama 1989).

7 PREVENTION AND TRANSMISSIBILITY OF VARIOUS SPECIES OF THE YERSINIAE

In general, avoidance of direct contact with potential reservoir species and protection of foods from possible rodent or insect infestation or contamination will reduce the potential for infection with any of the enteropathogenic yersiniae. In addition, assurance of adequate water treatment with an appropriate disinfectant such as chlorine or iodine, including provision for adequate residual level throughout the entire distribution system, should prevent water-borne infection.

Persons with occupational or recreational contact with potentially infected animals should avail themselves of appropriate personal protection clothing (especially gloves) when contact is necessary. Hunters who dress their game in the field should examine the viscera for obvious lesions and discard any meat or carcasses with such lesions in such a manner as to prevent spread of the infection.

Rodent-proof construction with adequate maintenance of buildings housing captive animals and birds as well as for human residences or businesses will minimize the potential for transmission of infectious agents from commensal or wild rodent sources. Bird-proof construction would probably be somewhat more problematic, especially for large open-air pens in zoological gardens.

No vaccine is currently available for use in preventing infection with the enteropathogenic yersiniae. A bacterin for use in fish hatcheries to prevent enteric redmouth disease was developed and shown to have some efficacy in preventing outbreaks of *Y. ruckeri* infection among trout fingerlings (Cipriano and Ruppenthal 1987). Prohibition of transfer of fish (in stocking operations) from known contaminated areas to areas not known to be contaminated will help curtail the spread of infection.

8 SPECIMEN COLLECTION AND CULTIVATION

Most isolates of the enteropathogenic yersiniae grow well on many of the commonly used selective media such as MacConkey agar and eosin–methylene blue agar; their growth is often somewhat inhibited or delayed on *Salmonella–Shigella* agar and deoxycholate agar.

Specimens for culture include stool samples for *Y. enterocolitica* and related species (not often useful for *Y. pseudotuberculosis*); blood; tissue biopsy specimens from spleen, liver and lymph nodes.

Cold temperature incubation of stool specimens is recommended for increased success of isolation for *Y.*

enterocolitica. This may be accomplished in tetrathionate broth or selenite F broth or simply in physiological saline or a nutrient broth, all of which are kept in the refrigerator at 4°C for up to 6 weeks with periodic subculturing for recovery of the agents. Among the more commonly used selective media for rapid identification of the *enterocolitica* group of yersiniae are CIN agar developed by Schiemann (1979) and VYE agar (virulent *Y. enterocolitica* agar) developed by Fukushima (1987). *Y. enterocolitica* and closely related species form red colonies on the CIN formulations, the latter medium reportedly allows differentiation between virulent and environmental species of *Yersinia* as well as from other gram-negative enterobacteria. Other differential and selective media have been used to allow recognition of virulent yersiniae: Riley and Toma (1989) formulated a Congo red–magnesium oxalate agar medium to detect virulence-associated calcium dependence and adsorption of the dye, Congo red. Congo red adsorption was shown to be characteristic for virulent but not avirulent *Y. pestis* colonies by Surgalla, Beezley and Albizo (1970). Bhaduri, Conway and Lachica (1987) developed a technique for the in vitro recognition of virulent organisms in which colonies bearing the virulence plasmid differentially bound crystal violet dye. Prolonged contact with the crystal violet may prove lethal to the organisms, so colonies binding the dye should be picked rapidly and diluted in a suitable medium. Other in vitro assays for virulence factors have been described and found to have varying degrees of usefulness, ease of performance and interpretation, etc. (Chang et al. 1984; see Bottone 1992 for a fuller description).

Culture of specimens not grossly contaminated on an enriched medium such as blood agar or brain–heart infusion agar may facilitate recovery of the suspect agent. Recovery (especially of virulent organisms) may also be enhanced if incubation after the first 24 h is conducted at room temperature (24–28°C).

9 INTERACTIONS WITH THE LABORATORY

When infection with one of the yersiniae is suspected, the laboratory should be alerted to the suspect diagnosis and requested to attempt isolation using one or more of the techniques described above. Organisms may be missed if the cultures are inadequately processed. Often the special media are not on hand, or need to be specially prepared. Cold enrichment may allow recovery of the *Y. enterocolitica* and related organisms but may require as much as 6 weeks of incubation before success is realized.

REFERENCES

Ahmedy A, Vidon DJ et al., 1985, Antimicrobial susceptibilities of food-isolated strains of *Yersinia enterocolitica, Y. intermedia, Y. frederiksenii*, and *Y. kristensenii, Antimicrob Agents Chemother,* **28:** 351–3.

Aleksic S, Bockemuhl J, 1984, Proposed revision of the Wauters et al. antigenic scheme for serotyping of *Yersinia enterocolitica, J Clin Microbiol,* **20:** 99–102.

Aleksic S, Steigerwalt AG et al., 1987, *Yersinia rohdei* sp. nov. isolated from human and dog feces and surface water, *Int J Syst Bacteriol,* **37:** 327–32.

Alvin R, Middleton DB, 1986, Plaguelike presentation of *Yersinia enterocolitica* disease, *J Pediatr,* **109:** 79–80.

Anjorin FI, Sturrock RD et al., 1979, *Yersinia enterocolitica* infection from West Africa – a case report, *Trans R Soc Trop Med Hyg,* **73:** 634–5.

Arduino MJ, Bland LA et al., 1989, Growth and endotoxin production of *Yersinia enterocolitica* and *Enterobacter agglomerans* in packed erythrocytes, *J Clin Microbiol,* **27:** 1483–5.

Aulisio CCG, Stanfield JT et al., 1983, Yersinioses associated with tofu consumption: serological, biochemical, and pathogenicity studies of *Yersinia enterocolitica* isolates, *J Food Prot,* **46:** 226–30.

Baker PM, Farmer JJ, 1982, New bacteriophage typing system for *Yersinia enterocolitica, Yersinia kristensenii, Yersinia fredericksenii*, and *Yersinia intermedia*: correlation with serotyping, biotyping, and antibiotic susceptibility, *J Clin Microbiol,* **15:** 491–502.

Balligand G, LaRoche Y, Cornelis G, 1985, Genetic analysis of virulence plasmid from a serogroup 9 *Yersinia enterocolitica* strain: role of outer membrane protein P1 in resistance to human serum and autoagglutination, *Infect Immun,* **48:** 782–6.

Barre N, Louzis C et al., 1976, Premiers isolements de *Yersinia enterocolitica* a partir d'echantillos de sols, *Med Mal Infect,* **6:** 520–1.

Baskin GB, Montali RJ et al., 1977, Yersiniosis in captive exotic mammals, *J Am Vet Med Assoc,* **171:** 908–12.

Becht H, 1963, Untersuchungen uber die Pseudotuberkulose beim Chinchilla, *Dtsch Tierarztl Wochenschr,* **69:** 626.

Bercovier H, Mollaret HH et al., 1980, Intra- and interspecies relatedness of *Yersinia pestis* by DNA hybridization and its relationship to *Yersinia pseudotuberculosis, Curr Microbiol,* **4:** 225–9.

Bercovier H, Steigerwalt AGet al., 1984, *Yersinia aldovae* (formerly *Yersinia enterocolitica*-like group X-2): a new species isolated from aquatic ecosystems, *Int J Syst Bacteriol,* **34:** 166–72.

Bhaduri S, Conway LK, Lachica RV, 1987, Assay of crystal violet binding for rapid identification of virulent plasmid-bearing clones of *Yersinia enterocolitica, J Clin Microbiol,* **25:** 1039–42.

Bissett ML, 1981, Microbiological aspects of *Yersinia pseudotuberculosis, Yersinia enterocolitica*, ed. Bottone EJ, CRC Press, Boca Raton, FL, 31–40.

Black RE, Jackson RJ et al., 1978, Epidemic *Yersinia enterocolitica* infection due to contaminated chocolate milk, *N Engl J Med,* **298:** 76–9.

Boelaert JR, Vanlandgat HW et al., 1987, The role of iron overload in *Yersinia enterocolitica* and *Yersinia pseudotuberculosis* bacteremia in hemodialysis patients, *J Infect Dis,* **156:** 384–7.

Bolin I, Wolf-Watz H, 1988, The plasmid-encoded Yop2b protein of *Yersinia pseudotuberculosis* is a virulence determinant regulated by calcium and temperature at the level of transcription, *Mol Microbiol,* **2:** 237–45.

Borst GHA, Buitelaar M et al., 1977, *Yersinia pseudotuberculosis* in birds, *Tidjschr Diergeneeskd,* **102:** 81–5.

Bottone EJ, 1992, The genus *Yersinia* (excluding *Yersinia pestis*), *The Prokaryotes,* 2nd edn, eds Balows A, Trüper HG et al., Springer-Verlag, New York, 2862–87.

Botzler RG, 1979, Yersiniae in the soil of an infected wapiti range, *J Wildl Dis,* **15:** 529–32.

Botzler RG, 1987, Isolation of *Yersinia enterocolitica* and *Y. fred-eriksenii* from forest soil, Federal Republic of Germany, *J Wildl Dis,* **23:** 311–13.

Botzler RG, Wetzler T, Cowan AB, *Yersinia enterocolitica* and *Yersinia*-like organisms isolated from frogs and snails, *Bull Wildl Dis Assoc,* **4:** 110–15.

Botzler RG, Wetzler T et al., 1976, Yersiniae in pond water and snails, *J Wildl Dis,* **12:** 492–6.

Brenner DJ, 1981, Classification of *Yersinia enterocolitica, Yersinia enterocolitica*, ed. Bottone EJ, CRC Press, Boca Raton, FL, 1–8.

Brenner DJ, 1984, Differentiation of the genus *Yersinia, Bergey's Manual of Determinative Bacteriology*, 8th edn, eds Buchanan RE, Gibbons NE, Williams & Wilkins, Baltimore, MD, 503–6.

Brenner DJ, 1992, Introduction to the Family Enterobacteriaceae, *The Prokaryotes,* 2nd edn, eds Balows A, Trüper HG et al., Springer-Verlag, New York.

Brenner DJ, Ursing J et al., 1980, *Yersinia intermedia*, a new species of Enterobacteriaceae composed of rhamnose-positive, melibiose-positive, raffinose-positive strains (formerly called *Yersinia enterocolitica* or *Yersinia enterocolitica*-like), *Curr Microbiol,* **4:** 207–12.

Bronson RT, May BD, Ruebner BH, 1972, An outbreak of infection by *Yersinia pseudotuberculosis* in non-human primates, *Am J Pathol,* **69:** 289–308.

Brubaker RR, 1984, Molecular biology of the dread Black Death, *ASM News,* **50:** 240–5.

Brubaker RR, 1991, Factors promoting acute and chronic diseases caused by yersiniae, *Clin Microbiol Rev,* **4:** 309–24.

Cafferky MT, Buckley TF, 1987, Comparison of saline agglutination, antibody to human gammaglobulin, and immunofluorescence tests in the routine serological diagnosis of yersiniosis, *J Infect Dis,* **156:** 845–8.

Centers for Disease Control, 1972, Annual Report, 1971, Zoonoses Branch, Division of Vector Borne Diseases, Fort Collins, CO.

Centers for Disease Control, 1991, Update: *Yersinia enterocolitica* bacteremia and endotoxin shock associated with red blood cell transfusions – United States, 1991, *Morbid Mortal Weekly Rep,* **40:** 176–8.

Chang MT, Schink J et al., 1984, Comparison of three tests for virulent *Yersinia enterocolitica, J Clin Microbiol,* **20:** 589–91.

Cipriano RC, Ruppenthal T, 1987, Immunization of salmonids against *Yersinia ruckeri*: significance of humoral immunity and cross-protection between serotypes, *J Wildl Dis,* **23:** 545–50.

Clark WA, Hollis DG et al., 1984, *Identification of Unusual Gram-negative Aerobic and Facultatively Anaerobic Bacteria.* Centers for Disease Control, US Department of Health and Human Services, Atlanta, GA.

Cornelis G, Wauters G, VanderHaeghe H, 1973, Presence de beta-lactamase chez *Yersinia enterocolitica, Ann Microbiol,* **124B:** 139–52.

Cornelis G, Laroche Y et al., 1987, *Yersinia enterocolitica*, a primary model for bacterial invasiveness, *Rev Infect Dis,* **9:** 64–7.

Cornelis GR, Biot T et al., 1989, The *Yersinia* yop regulon, *Mol Microbiol,* **3:** 1455–9.

DeBoer E, Hartog BJ, Oosterom J, 1982, Occurrence of *Yersinia* in poultry products, *J Food Prot,* **45:** 322–5.

Dickinson AB, Mocquot G, 1961, Studies on the bacterial flora of the alimentary tract of pigs. I. Enterobacteriaceae and other Gram-negative bacteria, *J Appl Bacteriol,* **24:** 252–84.

Doyle MP, Hugdahl MB, Taylor SL, 1981, Isolation of virulent *Yersinia enterocolitica* from porcine tongues, *Appl Environ Microbiol,* **42:** 661–6.

Dulin MP, Huddleston T et al., 1977, *Enteric Redmouth Disease,* Contr # 16 Forest, Wildlife, & Range Experiment Station, ID 83843, University of Idaho, Moscow, ID.

Ewing WH, Ross AJ et al., 1978, *Yersinia ruckeri* sp nov., the redmouth (RM) bacterium, *Int J Syst Bacteriol,* **28:** 37–44.

Fantasia M, Grazia Mingrone M et al., 1985, Isolation of *Yersinia enterocolitica* biotype 4 serotype O3 from canine sources in Italy, *J Clin Microbiol*, **22**: 314–15.

Fisch A, Prazuck T et al., 1989, Hematogenous osteitis due to *Yersinia enterocolitica*, *J Infect Dis*, **160**: 554.

Forsberg A, Rosqvist R, Wolf-Watz H, 1994, Regulation and polarized transfer of the *Yersinia* outer proteins (Yops) involved in antiphagocytosis, *Trends Microbiol*, **2**: 14–19.

Forsberg A, Wolf-Watz H, 1988, The virulence protein Yop5 of *Yersinia pseudotuberculosis* is regulated at transcriptional level by plasmid-p1B1-encoded transacting elements controlled by temperature and calcium, *Mol Microbiol*, **2**: 121–33.

Fredricksen W, 1964, A study of some *Yersinia pseudotuberculosis*-like bacteria ('*Bacterium enterocoliticum*' and '*Pasteurella* X', *Proc XIV Scand Congress Pathol Microbiol, Oslo*, 103–4.

Fukushima H, 1985, Direct isolation of *Yersinia enterocolitica* and *Yersinia pseudotuberculosis* from meat, *Appl Environ Microbiol*, **50**: 710–12.

Fukushima H, 1987, New selective agar medium for isolation of virulent *Yersinia enterocolitica*, *J Clin Microbiol*, **25**: 1068–73.

Fukushima H, Ito Y et al., 1979, Role of the fly in the transport of *Yersinia enterocolitica*, *Appl Environ Microbiol*, **38**: 1009–10.

Fukushima H, Nakamura R et al., 1984, Prospective systematic study of *Yersinia* spp. in dogs, *J Clin Microbiol*, **19**: 616–22.

Fukushima H, Gomyoda M et al., 1988, *Yersinia pseudotuberculosis* infection contracted through water contaminated by a wild animal, *J Clin Microbiol*, **26**: 584–5.

Fukushima H, Gomyoda M et al., 1989, Cat-contaminated environmental substances lead to *Yersinia pseudotuberculosis* infection in children, *J Clin Microbiol*, **27**: 2706–9.

Fukushima H, Sato T et al., 1991, Acute mesenteric lymphadenitis due to *Yersinia pseudotuberculosis* lacking a virulence plasmid, *J Clin Microbiol*, **29**: 1271–5.

Gemski P, Lazere J et al., 1980, Presence of a virulence-associated plasmid in *Yersinia pseudotuberculosis*, *Infect Immun*, **28**: 1044–7.

Granfors K, Lahesmaa-Rantala R, Toivanen A, 1988, IgM, IgG, and IgA antibodies in *Yersinia* infection, *J Infect Dis*, **157**: 601–2.

Gutman LT, Wilfert CM, Quan TJ, 1973, Susceptibility of *Yersinia enterocolitica* to trimethoprim-sulfamethoxazole, *J Infect Dis*, **128S**: 538.

Gutman LT, Ottesen EA et al., 1973, An inter-familial outbreak of *Yersinia enterocolitica* enteritis, *N Engl J Med*, **288**: 1372–7.

Hanski C, Naumann M et al., 1991, Humoral and cellular defense against murine infection with *Yersinia enterocolitica*, *Infect Immun*, **59**: 1106–11.

Heesemann J, Gaede K, Autenrieth IB, 1993, Experimental *Yersinia enterocolitica* infection in rodents: a model for human yersiniosis, *APMIS*, **101**: 417–29.

Heesemann J, Gruter L, 1987, Genetic evidence that the outer membrane protein YOP1 of *Yersinia enterocolitica* mediates adherance (sic) and phagocytosis resistance to human epithelial cells, *FEMS Microbiol Lett*, **40**: 37–41.

Highsmith AK, Feeley JC et al., 1977, Isolation of *Yersinia enterocolitica* from well water and growth in distilled water, *Appl Environ Microbiol*, **34**: 745–50.

Ichinohe H, Yoshioka M et al., 1991, First isolation of *Yersinia enterocolitica* serotype O:8 in Japan, *J Clin Microbiol*, **29**: 846–7.

Isberg RR, Falkow S, 1985, Genetic analysis of bacterial virulence determinants in *Bordetella pertussis* and the pathogenic *Yersinia*, *Curr Top Microbiol Immunol*, **118**: 1–11.

Jacobs J, Jamaer D et al., 1989, *Yersinia enterocolitica* in donor blood: a case report and review, *J Clin Microbiol*, **27**: 1119–21.

Judicial Commission of the International Committee on Systematic Bacteriology, 1985, Opinion 60. Rejection of the name *Yersinia pseudotuberculosis* subsp. *pestis* (vanLoghem) Bercovier et al 1981 and conservation of the name *Yersinia pestis* (Lehmann and Neumann) vanLoghem 1944 for the plague bacillus, *Int J Syst Bacteriol*, **35**: 540.

Kageruka P, 1970, [Infections caused by the Malassez and Vignal bacillus (*Y. pseudotuberculosis*) in the annals of the Antwerp Zoo], *Acta Zool Pathol Antverp*, **51**: 3–16.

Kanazawa Y, Ikemura K, Kuramata T, 1987, Drug susceptibility of *Yersinia enterocolitica* and *Yersinia pseudotuberculosis*, Contrib Microbiol Immunol, **9**: 127–35.

Kaneko S, Maruyama T, 1989, Evaluation of enzyme immunoassay for the detection of pathogenic *Yersinia enterocolitica* and *Yersinia pseudotuberculosis* strains, *J Clin Microbiol*, **27**: 748–51.

Kapperud G, Rosef O, 1983, Avian wildlife reservoir of *Campylobacter fetus* subsp. *jejuni*, *Yersinia* spp., and *Salmonella* spp. in Norway, *Appl Environ Microbiol*, **45**: 375–80.

Kapperud G, Namork E et al., 1987, Plasmid-mediated surface fibrillae of *Yersinia pseudotuberculosis* and *Yersinia enterocolitica*: relationship to the outer membrane protein YOP1 and possible importance for pathogenesis, *Infect Immun*, **55**: 2247–54.

Karimi Y, 1963, Conservation naturelle de la peste dans le soil, *Bull Soc Pathol Exot*, **56**: 1183–6.

Kato Y, Ito K et al., 1985, Occurrence of *Yersinia enterocolitica* in wild-living birds and Japanese serows, *Appl Environ Microbiol*, **49**: 198–200.

Kilian JM, Yamamoto R et al., 1962, *Avian Dis*, **6**: 403.

Knapp W, Thal E, 1963, Untersuchungen uber die Kulturlbiochemischen, Serologishen, Tierexperimentellen und Immunologishen Eigenschaften Einer Vorlaussig '*Pasteurella* X' Bekannten Bakterienart, *Zentralbl Bakteriol Parasitenkd Hyg Abt I Orig*, **190**: 472–84.

Krynski S, 1968, Analogies et differences dans l'infection expérimentale du pou par '*Pasteurella pseudotuberculosis*' et *Yersinia enterocolitica*, *International Symposium on* Pseudotuberculosis *Paris 1967*, Karger, Basel, Switzerland, 7–8.

Kwaga JKP, Iversen JO, 1992, Laboratory investigation of virulence among strains of *Yersinia enterocolitica* and related species isolated from pigs and pork products, *Can J Microbiol*, **38**: 92–7.

Lassen J, 1972, *Yersinia enterocolitica* in drinking water, *Scand J Infect Dis*, **4**: 125–7.

Lecomte F, Eustache M et al., 1989, Purulent pericarditis due to *Yersinia enterocolitica*, *J Infect Dis*, **159**: 363.

Lee WH, 1987, An assessment of *Yersinia enterocolitica* and its presence in foods, *J Food Prot*, **40**: 486–9.

Leighton PM, MacSween HM, 1987, *Yersinia* hepatic abscesses subsequent to long term iron therapy, *JAMA*, **257**: 964–5.

Lenz T, Schulte K-L, Meyer-Sabeller W, 1984, *Yersinia enterocolitica* septicemia during long-term immunosuppressive treatment, *J Infect Dis*, **150**: 963.

McDonald DW, 1972, *Hatchery Biologist Quarterly Report, First Quarter 1972*.

Mair N, 1968, *Symp Zool Soc Lond*, **24**: 107.

Malassez L, Vignal W, 1883, Tuberculose zoogloeique (forme ou espèce de tuberculose sans bacilles), *Arch Physiol Norm Pathol*, **2 (3rd ser)**: 369–412.

Miller VL, Falkow S, 1988, Evidence for two genetic loci in *Yersinia enterocolitica* that can promote invasion of epithelial cells, *Infect Immun*, **56**: 1242–8.

Mingrone MG, Fantasia M et al., 1987, Characteristics of *Yersinia enterocolitica* isolated from children with diarrhea in Italy, *J Clin Microbiol*, **25**: 1301–4.

Mollaret HH, Chevalier A, 1964, Contribution à l'Etude d'un Nouveau Groupe de Germes Proches du Bacille de Malassez et Vignal, *Ann Inst Pasteur*, **107**: 121–7.

Mollaret HH, Karimi Y et al., 1963, La peste du fouissement, *Bull Soc Pathol Exot*, **56**: 1186–93.

Moustafa MK, Ahmed AA-H, Marth EH, 1983a, Occurrence of *Yersinia enterocolitica* in raw and pasteurized milk, *J Food Prot*, **46**: 276–8.

Moustafa MK, Ahmed AA-H, Marth EH, 1983b, Behavior of virulent *Yersinia enterocolitica* during manufacture and storage of Colby-like cheese, *J Food Prot*, **46**: 318–20.

Mulder B, Michiels T et al., 1989, Identification of additional virulence determinants on the pYV plasmid of *Yersinia enterocolitica* W227, *Infect Immun*, **57**: 2534–41.

Orman RA, Lewis JB, 1989, Flaccid quadriparesis associated with

Yersinia enterocolitica-induced hypokalemia, *Arch Intern Med*, **149:** 1193–4.

Pfeiffer A, 1889, *Ueber die Bacillare Pseudotuberculosis bei Nagethieren*, Verlag von Georg Thieme, Leipzig.

Poland JD, Quan TJ, Barnes AM, 1994, Plague, *Handbook of the Zoonoses. Part A: Bacterial, Rickettsial, Chlamydial and Mycotic*, 2nd edn, ed. Beran GW, CRC Press, Boca Raton, FL, 93–112.

Portnoy DA, Moseley SL, Falkow S, 1981, Characterization of plasmids and plasmid-associated determinants of *Yersinia enterocolitica* pathogenesis, *Infect Immun*, **31:** 775–82.

Portnoy DA, Wolf-Watz H et al., 1984, Characterization of common virulence plasmids in *Yersinia* species and their role in the expression of outer membrane proteins, *Infect Immun*, **43:** 108–14.

Punsalang A, Edinger R, Nolte FS, 1987, Identification and characterization of *Yersinia intermedia* isolated from human feces, *J Clin Microbiol*, **25:** 859–62.

Quan TJ, 1992, *Yersinia pestis, The Prokaryotes*, vol. 3, 2nd edn, eds Balows A, Trüper HG et al., Springer-Verlag, New York, 2888–98.

Riley G, Toma S, 1989, Detection of pathogenic *Yersinia enterocolitica* by using Congo red-magnesium oxalate agar medium, *J Clin Microbiol*, **27:** 213–14.

Robins-Browne RM, Cianciosi S et al., 1991, Pathogenicity of *Yersinia kristensenii* for mice, *Infect Immun*, **59:** 162–7.

Ross AJ, Rucker RR, Ewing WH, 1966, Description of a bacterium associated with redmouth disease of trout (*Salmo gairdneri*), *Can J Microbiol*, **12:** 763–70.

Saari TN, Jansen GP, 1977, *Waterborne* Yersinia enterocolitica *in Wisconsin*, Abstr Bacteriol Proc, New Orleans, LA.

Saari TN, Quan TJ, 1976, *Waterborne* Yersinia enterocolitica *in Colorado*, Abstr Bacteriol Proc, Atlantic City, NJ.

Sample AK, Fowler JM, Brubaker RR, 1987, Modulation of the low calcium response in *Yersinia pestis* via plasmid–plasmid interaction, *Microb Pathog*, **2:** 443–53.

Sasaki Y, Hayashidani H et al., 1989, Occurrence of *Yersinia enterocolitica* in the Tokyo Tama Zoo, *J Wildl Dis*, **25:** 287–90.

Schiemann DA, 1979, Synthesis of selective agar medium for isolation of *Yersinia enterocolitica*, *Can J Microbiol*, **25:** 1298–304.

Schill WB, Phelps SR, Pyle SW, 1984, Multilocus electrophoretic assessment of the genetic structure and diversity of *Yersinia ruckeri*, *Appl Environ Microbiol*, **48:** 975–9.

Schliefstein J, Coleman MB, 1943, *Bacterium enterocoliticum*, *Annual Report of the Division of Laboratories and Research*, New York State Department of Health, New York, 56.

Shayegani M, DeForge I et al., 1981, Characteristic of *Yersinia enterocolitica* and related species isolated from human, animal, and environmental sources, *J Clin Microbiol*, **14:** 304–12.

Shayegani M, Morse D et al., 1983, Microbiology of a major foodborne outbreak of gastroenteritis caused by *Yersinia enterocolitica* serogroup O:8, *J Clin Microbiol*, **17:** 35–40.

Shiozawa K, Hayashi M et al., 1988, Virulence of *Yersinia pseudotuberculosis* isolated from pork and from the throats of swine, *Appl Environ Microbiol*, **54:** 818–21.

Slee KJ, Skilbeck NW, 1992, Epidemiology of *Yersinia pseudotuberculosis* and *Y. enterocolitica* infections in sheep in Australia, *J Clin Microbiol*, **30:** 712–15.

Smith JE, Thal E, 1965, A taxonomic study of the genus *Pasteurella* using a numerical technique, *Acta Pathol Microbiol Scand*, **64:** 213–23.

Sodeinde OA, Sample AK et al., 1988, Plasminogen activator/coagulase gene of *Yersinia pestis* is responsible for degradation of plasmid encoded outer membrane proteins, *Infect Immun*, **56:** 2743–8.

Sory M-P, Cornelis G, 1988, *Yersinia enterocolitica* O:9 as a potential live oral carrier for protective antibodies, *Microb Pathog*, **4:** 517–29.

Stahlberg TH, Tertti R et al., 1987, Antibody response in *Yersinia pseudotuberculosis* III infection: analysis of an outbreak, *J Infect Dis*, **156:** 388–91.

Stevenson RMW, Daly JG, 1982, Biochemical and serological characteristics of Ontario isolates of *Yersinia ruckeri*, *Can J Fish Aquat Sci*, **39:** 870–6.

Stoll L, 1965, *Proceedings of VII International Symposium on Disease of Zoo Animals*, Zurich–Basel, 135–8.

Stovell PL, 1963, *Epizootiological Factors in Three Outbreaks of Pseudotuberculosis in British Columbia Canaries* (Serinus canarius), MS Thesis, University of British Columbia, Vancouver, British Columbia, Canada.

Straley SC, Bowmer WS, 1986, Virulence genes regulated at the transcriptional level by Ca^{+2} in *Yersinia pestis* include structural genes for outer membrane proteins, *Infect Immun*, **51:** 445–54.

Surgalla MJ, Beezley ED, Albizo JM, 1970, Practical applications of new laboratory methods for plague investigations, *Bull W H O*, **42:** 993–7.

Tacket CO, Narain JP et al., 1984, A multistate outbreak of infections caused by *Yersinia enterocolitica* transmitted by pasteurized milk, *JAMA*, **251:** 483–6.

Tertti R, Granfors K et al., 1984, An outbreak of *Yersinia pseudotuberculosis* infection, *J Infect Dis*, **149:** 245–50.

Toma S, 1973, Survey on the incidence of *Yersinia enterocolitica* infection in Canada, *Appl Microbiol*, **28:** 469–73.

Toma S, Diedrick VR, 1975, Isolation of *Yersinia enterocolitica* from swine, *J Clin Microbiol*, **2:** 478–81.

Tsubokura M, Itagaki K, Kawamura K, 1970, Studies on *Yersinia* (*Pasteurella*) *pseudotuberculosis*. I. Sources and serological classification of the organism isolated in Japan, *Jpn J Vet Sci*, **32:** 227–33.

Tsubokura M, Itagaki K, Kawamura K, 1971, Studies on *Yersinia* (*Pasteurella*) *pseudotuberculosis*. II. A new type of *Y. pseudotuberculosis*, type VI, and subdivision of type V strains, *Jpn J Vet Sci*, **33:** 137–44.

Tsubokura M, Otsuki K et al., 1989, Special features of distribution of *Yersinia pseudotuberculosis* in Japan, *J Clin Microbiol*, **27:** 790–1.

Urbano-Marquez A, Estruch R et al., 1983, Infectious endocarditis due to *Yersinia enterocolitica*, *J Infect Dis*, **148:** 940.

Wauters G, 1972, Souches de *Yersinia enterocolitica* isolées de l'eau, *Rev Ferm Ind Ailment*, **7:** 18.7.

Wauters G, 1981, Antigens of *Yersinia enterocolitica*, Yersinia enterocolitica, ed. Bottone E, CRC Press, Boca Raton, FL, 41–53.

Wauters G, Le Minor L et al., 1972, Supplement au schema antigenique de '*Yersinia enterocolitica*', *Ann Inst Pasteur (Paris)*, **122:** 951–6.

Wauters G, Jannsens M et al., 1988, *Yersinia mollarettii* sp. nov. and *Yersinia bercovieri* sp. nov., formerly called *Yersinia enterocolitica* biogroups 3A and 3B, *Int J Syst Bacteriol*, **38:** 424–9.

Wetzler TF, 1965, *Antigens and Factors affecting Virulence of* Pasteruella pseudotuberculosis *and* Yersinia enterocolitica *with a Description of a New Serofactor and a New Strain*, Dissertation, University of Michigan, Ann Arbor, MI.

Wetzler TF, 1970, Pseudotuberculosis, *Diagnostic Procedures for Bacterial, Mycotic and Parasitic Infections*, 5th edn, eds Bodily HL, Updyke EL, Mason JO, American Public Health Association, New York, 449–68.

Wetzler TF, 1971a, Pseudotuberculosis, *Infectious Diseases of Wild Mammals*, eds Anderson JW, Karstad L, Trainer DO, Iowa State University Press, Ames, IA.

Wetzler TF, 1971b, Pseudotuberculosis, *Infectious and Parasitic Diseases of Wild Birds*, eds Davis JW, Anderson RC et al., Iowa State University Press, Ames, IA.

Wetzler TF, Hubbert WT, 1968, *Pasteurella pseudotuberculosis in North America*, International Symposium on Pseudotuberculosis, Karger, Basel, Switzerland.

Wetzler TF, Rea JT et al., 1978, *Yersinia enterocolitica* in waters and waste waters, Presented at 106th Annual Meeting, American Public Health Association, Los Angeles, CA, October 18, 1978.

Chapter 46

MELIOIDOSIS AND GLANDERS

D A B Dance

1 INTRODUCTION

Melioidosis and glanders are infections caused respectively by 2 closely related gram-negative bacilli, *Burkholderia pseudomallei* and *Burkholderia mallei*. These organisms have previously been classified in various genera (e.g. *Malleomyces*, *Pfeifferella*, *Actinobacillus*, *Bacillus*), and most recently resided in rRNA homology group II of the genus *Pseudomonas*. Yabuuchi et al. (1992) proposed that the group be assigned to a new genus, *Burkholderia*, which now has some 13 member species (see Volume 2, Chapter 47).

Glanders is the 'older' of the 2 diseases, and equine glanders is identifiable in the writings of Aristotle in the fourth century AD. Its communicability to humans was recognized in the early nineteenth century and the causative agent was first isolated by Loeffler and Schütz in 1882 (Loeffler 1886). Melioidosis was first described as a 'glanders-like' illness in Burma 30 years later by Whitmore and Krishnaswami (1912). The subsequent confirmation of the taxonomic relatedness of the 2 organisms vindicated Whitmore's proposal of the specific epithet 'pseudomallei'. The term melioidosis, derived from the Greek μηλίζ (glanders or distemper of asses), was later suggested by Stanton and Fletcher (1921) working in Kuala Lumpur. These days human glanders is extremely rare, whereas melioidosis is increasingly recognized as a cause of morbidity and mortality in the tropics.

MELIOIDOSIS

2 CLINICAL MANIFESTATIONS

The clinical spectrum of *B. pseudomallei* infection is extremely broad and analogous, for example, to the range of disease caused by *Staphylococcus aureus*. Melioidosis has been referred to as 'the remarkable imitator' (Poe, Vassallo and Domm 1971). The majority of infections appear to be subclinical, but melioidosis may run a fulminant, rapidly fatal course, particularly in the immunocompromised. Several attempts have been made to develop a clinical classification of melioidosis, but none is entirely satisfactory. Infections may be acute or chronic, localized or disseminated, but one form of the disease may progress to another and individual patients are often difficult to categorize. Several reviews have summarized the clinical manifestations of melioidosis (Howe, Sampath and Spotnitz 1971, Leelarasamee and Bovornkitti 1989, Punyagupta 1989, Dance 1990).

2.1 Mild and subclinical infections

In endemic areas such as north east Thailand, antibodies to *B. pseudomallei* are found in approximately 80% of children by the time they are 4 years old (Kanaphun et al. 1993), so the majority of infections are presumably mild or asymptomatic. A flu-like illness associated with seroconversion has been reported from Australia (Ashdown et al. 1989).

2.2 Latent infections

In people who have resided in endemic areas for a limited time, the infection may remain latent for more than 20 years before becoming clinically apparent (Mays and Ricketts 1975), giving rise to the nickname 'Vietnamese Time Bomb' (Goshorn 1987). Relapses usually occur at times of intercurrent stress (e.g. other acute infections, burns or trauma, malignancies, diabetes mellitus). The sites and mechanisms of persistence are unknown, although clinically silent, chronic, localized foci of melioidosis in the lung, liver or spleen have been reported in animals, and intracellular survival may play a part. The proportion of seropositive individuals who harbour latent infection, and are therefore at risk of relapse, is also uncertain.

2.3 Clinical disease

Only a small proportion of *B. pseudomallei* infections are sufficiently severe to come to medical attention. The literature is full of individual case reports and case series, of which several may be of interest (Whitmore 1913, Stanton and Fletcher 1932, Everett and Nelson 1975, Rode and Webling 1981, Guard et al 1984, Chaowagul et al. 1989, Punyagupta 1989, Vatcharapreechasakul et al. 1992, Putucheary, Parasakthi and Lee 1992, Kosuwon et al. 1993, Lumbiganon and Viengnondha 1994). Common clinical pictures are summarized below.

SEPTICAEMIC MELIOIDOSIS

Sixty per cent of cases of culture-positive melioidosis have positive blood cultures (Suputtamongkol et al. 1994a). The majority of these present clinically as community-acquired 'sepsis syndrome', with a short history (median 6 days; range 1 day to 2 months) of high fever and rigors (Chaowagul et al. 1989). Only half have evidence of a primary focus of infection, usually in the lung or skin and subcutaneous tissues. Confusion and stupor, jaundice and diarrhoea may also be prominent features. Initial investigations usually reveal anaemia, a neutrophil leucocytosis, coagulopathy and evidence of renal and hepatic impairment. Such patients often deteriorate rapidly, developing widespread metastatic abscesses, particularly in the lungs, liver and spleen, and metabolic acidosis with Kussmaul's breathing. Once septic shock has supervened the mortality approaches 95%, many patients dying within 48 h of hospital admission. Other poor prognostic features include absence of fever, leucopenia, azotaemia, and abnormal liver function tests (Chaowagul et al. 1989).

If the patient survives this acute phase, the manifestations of the multiple septic foci that result from bacteraemic dissemination become prominent. Any site or tissue may be involved, but the commonest foci are in the lungs, liver and spleen, and skin and soft tissues. An abnormal chest x-ray is found in 60–80% of patients, the most common pattern being widespread, nodular shadowing (Fig. 46.1) (Dhiensiri, Puapairoj and Susaengrat 1988, Chaowagul et al. 1989,

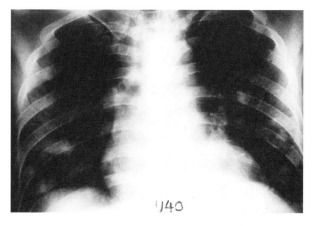

Fig. 46.1 Chest radiograph showing widespread nodular opacities (blood-borne pneumonia) in septicaemic melioidosis. (Reproduced, with permission, from Dance 1996).

Putucheary, Parasakthi and Lee 1992). Liver and splenic abscesses are usually multiple (Fig. 46.2) (Vatcharapreechasakul et al. 1992). Cutaneous pustules or subcutaneous abscesses occur in 10–20% of cases (Chaowagul et al. 1989). Other common sites for secondary lesions include the urinary tract (kidneys and prostate gland), and bones and joints. Involvement of the central nervous system may comprise cerebral abscesses, or a recently described syndrome known as 'neurological melioidosis', characterized by peripheral motor weakness, brain stem encephalitis, aseptic meningitis and respiratory failure, which may be toxin mediated (Woods et al. 1992).

B. pseudomallei bacteraemia may also cause a less fulminant disease. Such patients usually have a swinging fever, often associated with profound weight loss. This presumably reflects overspill from occult or apparent localized foci of infection. Patients with multiple, noncontiguous foci of infection, which probably reflect bacteraemia at some stage, behave similarly.

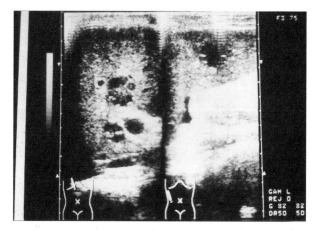

Fig. 46.2 Abdominal ultrasound showing multiple echolucent areas (abscesses) in the liver in septicaemic melioidosis. (Reproduced, with permission, from Dance 1992).

LOCALIZED MELIOIDOSIS

This occurs most frequently in the lung. It may manifest as acute bronchitis or pneumonia, but most often as a subacute cavitating pneumonia accompanied by profound weight loss, which is often confused with tuberculosis or lung abscess (Everett and Nelson 1975) (Fig. 46.3). Relative sparing of the apices and the infrequency of hilar adenopathy may help to distinguish melioidosis from tuberculosis (Dhiensiri, Puapairoj and Susaengrat 1988). Any lung zone may be affected, although there is a predilection for the upper lobes. Complications include pneumothorax, empyema and purulent pericarditis, and ultimately progression to septicaemia.

Acute suppurative parotitis is a characteristic manifestation of melioidosis in children, accounting for approximately one-third of paediatric cases in north east Thailand (Fig. 46.4) (Dance et al. 1989a). The reason for this strong age–site association is unclear. Most cases are unilateral and result in parotid abscesses which require surgical drainage, although they may rupture spontaneously into the auditory canal. Facial nerve palsy and septicaemia are rare complications.

Localized *B. pseudomallei* infection without bacteraemia may affect any other organ. Well described examples include cutaneous and subcutaneous abscesses, lymphadenitis, osteomyelitis and septic arthritis, liver and/or splenic abscesses, cystitis, pyelonephritis, prostatic abscesses, epididymo-orchitis, keratitis and brain abscesses.

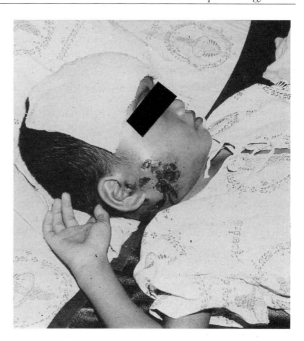

Fig. 46.4 Acute suppurative parotitis with abscess formation, a common manifestation of melioidosis in children. (Reproduced, with permission, from Dance 1992).

3 EPIDEMIOLOGY

3.1 Geographical distribution

The main areas of melioidosis endemicity are South East Asia and northern Australia. Following the early work by Whitmore in Burma and Stanton and Fletcher in the Federated Malay States, further cases were observed in the French and Dutch colonies in South East Asia (now Vietnam, Cambodia and Indonesia) before the Second World War. More cases are currently diagnosed in Thailand than in any other country in the region (Punyagupta 1989). Since 1949, melioidosis has been recognized as endemic in northern Australia (Rode and Webling 1981, Guard et al. 1984). It has been proposed that the organism was introduced to Australia by troops returning from endemic areas at the end of the war (Fournier 1965), but this remains controversial. In recent years it has become clear that the disease is also prevalent in China (Li Li and You-wen 1992), Singapore (Tan, Ang and Ong 1990), and there is mounting evidence that it is underdiagnosed in the Indian subcontinent (Kang et al. 1996), which has been the source of infection for several recent cases diagnosed in Britain.

It is likely that the true distribution of melioidosis extends beyond South East Asia and northern Australia. Sporadic cases have been reported from the Pacific Islands, central Africa, Central and South America and the Caribbean. The disease is probably underdiagnosed in many of these regions, since relatively sophisticated laboratory facilities are necessary to confirm the diagnosis. Furthermore, reports of cases in Iran and an epizootic which occurred in France during the 1970s (Mollaret 1988) have indi-

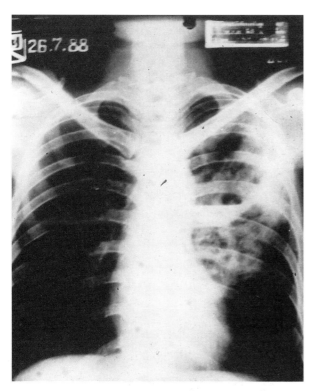

Fig. 46.3 Chest x-ray in pulmonary melioidosis showing a large area of consolidation with cavitation and an air/fluid level. (Reproduced, with permission, from Pitt and Dance 1991).

cated that the disease is not confined to the tropics. The distribution of melioidosis was comprehensively reviewed by Dance (1991).

3.2 Reservoirs and transmission

Stanton and Fletcher (1932) were the first to identify melioidosis in animals. They concluded that the disease was a zoonosis with a reservoir in rodents. However, workers in French Indochina, noticing that the disease was sometimes acquired after contact with muddy water and that wild rats were rarely infected, later proved that *B. pseudomallei* was really an environmental saprophyte, readily isolated from soil and surface water in endemic areas (Chambon 1955). The organism is particularly associated with rice paddy (Strauss et al. 1969), and using selective media it may be recovered from 68–78% of rice fields in Thailand (Nachiangmai et al 1985, Wuthiekanun et al. 1995). The ecology of *B. pseudomallei* is poorly understood. It is thought to persist in deeper clay layers during the dry season, rising to the surface after the annual rains (Thomas, Forbes-Faulkner and Parker 1979). Its presence in greater numbers in the soil of some areas, which presumably depends on a range of chemical (e.g. pH), biological and environmental factors (Kanai and Kondo 1994), may affect the incidence of melioidosis in these areas (Smith et al. 1995a).

Humans and animals are thought usually to become infected by inoculation or contamination of wounds or mucosae with soil or water, although a specific episode of exposure is only identified in approximately 6% of cases (Suputtamongkol et al. 1994a). Aerosols of dust were thought to be a source of infection for helicopter crews during the Vietnam war (Howe, Sampath and Spotnitz 1971), but the role of ingestion and insect vectors in transmission is doubtful. Although melioidosis has been observed in a wide range of animal species (including rodents, primates, sheep and goats, pigs, cattle, horses, deer, dogs and cats, dolphins, koalas, kangaroos, camels, crocodiles and birds), transmission from animals to humans has rarely been reported, and only 2 instances of person-to-person spread have been described (Kunakorn, Jayanetra and Tanphaichitra 1991). Iatrogenic infection from contaminated injections has also been reported occasionally, as have laboratory-acquired infections, resulting in the classification of *B. pseudomallei* as a containment level 3 (Advisory Committee on Dangerous Pathogens 1995; see also Volume 2, Chapter 19) pathogen.

3.3 Descriptive epidemiology

Melioidosis is a disease of people in regular contact with soil and water, such as rice farmers in South East Asia and aboriginals in Australia. In Australia 20–50 human cases are diagnosed annually, whereas several hundred are reported each year in Thailand. Suputtamongkol and colleagues (1994a) reviewed the epidemiology of culture-positive melioidosis seen over a 5 year period in Ubon Ratchatani, north-east Thailand, where melioidosis accounts for 18% of community-acquired septicaemia (Chaowagul et al. 1989). The average annual incidence was 4.4 per 100 000 population, with evidence of space–time clustering. All age groups were affected, with the peak incidence occurring from 40 to 60 years. The male to female ratio was 3:2, and in males aged 60–69 years, the annual incidence approached 30 per 100 000. As observed elsewhere, the disease was markedly seasonal, 75% of cases presenting during the rainy season. Although this pattern suggests that most cases are recently acquired, the incubation period before the onset of clinically apparent melioidosis has varied from 2 days to 26 years, and it is possible that some other seasonal factor precipitates relapses of latent infections. Other risk factors confirmed in this study were occupational exposure to soil and water (81% of cases were rice farmers or their children) and the presence of underlying disease (identified in 53% of cases), particularly diabetes mellitus, which increased the relative risk by up to 100-fold in some population groups.

3.4 Epidemiological typing

To some extent, the study of melioidosis epidemiology has been hampered in the past by the lack of a typing system for *B. pseudomallei*. The species is remarkably homogeneous serologically (Pitt, Aucken and Dance 1992), but French workers have described 2 serotypes (Dodin and Fournier 1970). Several molecular typing techniques are able to discriminate between strains of the organism and are helping to elucidate some of the outstanding epidemiological questions. Examples include ribotyping (Desmarchelier et al. 1993, Lew and Desmarchelier 1993, Sexton et al. 1993, Currie et al. 1994), pulsed field gel electrophoresis (Trakulsomboon, Pitt and Dance 1994), and random amplified polymorphic DNA analysis (Haase et al. 1995).

4 PATHOLOGY AND PATHOGENESIS

The pathogenesis of melioidosis is poorly understood and was until recently relatively little studied. *B. pseudomallei* is a pyogenic organism that causes localized abscesses or granulomata at the site of primary infection, depending on the duration of the lesion, and septicaemia when the bloodstream is invaded. This may in turn lead to seeding and localized foci of infection in other tissues. A high level of bacteraemia (>50 cfu ml^{-1}) is associated with a fatal outcome (Walsh et al. 1995a). The outcome of contact with *B. pseudomallei* presumably depends on the immune system of the host, the virulence of the infecting strain and the size and route of the initial inoculum.

4.1 Histopathology

Lesions of melioidosis are extremely variable in nature and may range from an acute, necrotizing inflammatory process with abscess formation, to chronic granulomatous inflammation; sometimes a mixed picture is seen (Piggott and Hockholzer 1970). Although the process may be difficult to distinguish from other inflammatory conditions, features that may be helpful include the presence of intracellular 'globi' of gramnegative bacilli combined with giant cells in a background of acute necrotizing inflammation (Wong, Putucheary and Vadivelu 1995).

4.2 Bacterial virulence factors

B. pseudomallei possesses a number of characteristics that may contribute to virulence, but the precise role of each of these in natural infections is unclear. Interstrain differences in virulence undoubtedly occur (Miller et al. 1948). Potential virulence factors include: lipopolysaccharide (LPS) (Rapaport, Millar and Ruch 1961, Iwasa et al. 1992); a heat labile, lethal exotoxin (Heckly 1964) with a molecular weight of approximately 31 kDa (Ismail et al. 1987) which appears to act by inhibition of synthesis of macromolecules (Mohamed 1989); haemolysin, lecithinase, lipase and proteases (Ashdown and Koehler 1990); extracellular, capsule-like polysaccharides (Popov, Tikhonov and Kurilov 1994, Steinmetz, Rohde and Brenneke 1995); a siderophore, malleobactin (Yang, Chaowagul and Sokol 1991, Yang, Kooi and Sokol 1993); and acid phosphatase (Kanai and Kondo 1994). There is increasing evidence that *B. pseudomallei* is able to survive intracellularly (Pruksachartvuthi, Aswapokee and Thankerngpol 1990, Jones, Beveridge and Woods 1996), which probably contributes to the recalcitrant nature of melioidosis, its potential for long periods of latency, and its tendency to relapse (Chaowagul et al. 1993, Desmarchelier et al. 1993).

4.3 Host defence

Melioidosis severe enough to be seen in hospital is an opportunistic disease; some 50–70% of patients have an underlying predisposition to infection (Chaowagul et al. 1989, Suputtamongkol et al. 1994a). As has already been noted, diabetes mellitus is particularly important in this regard, and other underlying conditions that have been reported include chronic renal disease, malignancy, immunosuppressive treatment (particularly steroids), liver disease, alcohol or drug abuse, and pregnancy. Little is known about the specific immunological mechanisms responsible for protection, but cell mediated immunity is probably of particular importance. Relapse of latent infection also usually occurs at times when cellular immunity is likely to be suppressed (see above). In this context, it is perhaps surprising that infection with the human immunodeficiency virus does not appear to have predisposed to relapses of latent melioidosis.

5 HOST RESPONSE

The importance of host defences in protecting against melioidosis is discussed above. Once infected, the majority of patients mount a vigorous response. This is presumably usually effective in eliminating infection in view of the frequency of mild or asymptomatic infection. Patients with clinical melioidosis usually have evidence of both humoral and cellular immunity. Most studies show that 90% or more of patients with culture-positive melioidosis have detectable IgG and IgM antibodies at some stage in their illness, and a failure to mount an antibody response has not been correlated with a fatal outcome. Evidence from studies in experimental animals suggests that antibodies to both the exotoxin (Smith et al. 1987) and LPS (Bryan et al. 1994) may be partially protective.

There is also evidence of massive activation of the cellular immune system as witnessed by the presence of high concentrations of urinary neopterin (Brown et al. 1990) and soluble interleukin-2 receptor in patients with melioidosis, although the absence of a rise in soluble CD8 protein implies an impairment of specific T cell immunity (Brown et al. 1991). Cytokine cascades are also activated, and the serum levels of several cytokines, including interferon-γ (Brown et al. 1991), TNF (Suputtamongkol et al. 1992), interleukin-6 and interleukin-8 (Friedland et al. 1992), are correlated with mortality, indicating that they may even play a pathogenic role in the disease.

6 DIAGNOSIS

The protean manifestations of melioidosis make the disease difficult to diagnose on clinical grounds alone. The diagnosis should be considered in any patient who has ever visited an endemic area who presents with septicaemia, abscesses, or chronic suppuration, particularly if there is evidence of an underlying disease such as diabetes mellitus. Specific diagnosis depends on the detection of *B. pseudomallei* or of corresponding antibodies. The laboratory should always be warned if melioidosis is suspected, both to enable appropriate methods and media to be employed and to ensure that appropriate containment measures are taken.

6.1 Microscopy and culture

The organism should be sought in blood, pus, sputum, urine, or any other appropriate specimen. Microscopy of a gram-stained smear may reveal bipolar or unevenly staining gram-negative rods, but this is neither specific nor sensitive. Direct immunofluorescent microscopy may be worthwhile in endemic areas, and has a sensitivity of 73% and a specificity of 99% compared with culture (Walsh et al. 1994). Definitive diagnosis depends on isolation and identification of *B. pseudomallei*, of which asymptomatic carriage has never been reported. The organism grows readily on most laboratory media, although it may take

48 h or more to develop characteristic colonial morphology. The sensitivity of culture from sites with a normal flora may be increased by the use of selective media such as Ashdown's agar (Wuthiekanun et al. 1990), and selective broth pre-enrichment increases the yield still further (Wuthiekanun et al. 1990, Walsh et al. 1995c). In children or others who cannot produce sputum, culture of a throat swab by means of selective techniques has a sensitivity approaching that of sputum culture. Identification of cultures may be conducted with conventional biochemical tests or commercial kits such as the API 20E (Ashdown 1979), Microbact 24E (Thomas 1983), API 20NE (Dance 1989b), or Minitek discs (Ashdown 1992a), although in experienced hands none is more accurate than a few simple tests (colonial appearance on Ashdown's medium, resistance to gentamicin and colistin). More rapid results may be obtained using immunofluorescence (Naigowit et al. 1993), latex agglutination (Smith et al. 1993), or direct agglutination with monoclonal antibodies (Rugdech, Anuntagool and Sirisinha 1995). Identification is, however, often delayed in non-endemic areas, because microbiologists are not familiar with the appearance and characteristics of the organism, which are described in more detail in Volume 2 (see Volume 2, Chapter 47).

6.2 Detection of antigens and nucleic acids

Several rapid diagnostic techniques for the detection of *B. pseudomallei* antigens have been developed (Desakorn et al. 1994, Smith et al. 1995b), but these have suboptimal sensitivity and are not widely available. Tests for the detection of *B. pseudomallei* nucleic acids show promise but await further evaluation (Lew and Desmarchelier 1994, Sermswan et al. 1994, Kunakorn and Markham 1995).

6.3 Detection of antibodies

Several tests have been described for the serodiagnosis of melioidosis, although the nature of the immune response to infection and the antigens involved have been poorly characterized. The test most widely used in endemic areas is an indirect haemagglutination (IHA) test, which detects IgM antibodies to crude heat-stable antigens (probably predominantly LPS) (Ashdown 1987). The test is poorly standardized, and there is considerable inter-laboratory variation between titres that are regarded as positive. Cross-reactions occur with some other organisms such as *Legionella pneumophila* (Klein 1980), and the background seropositivity rate is high in endemic areas, leading to a low specificity (Chaowagul et al. 1989). None the less, a single high titre (>1:40) in someone from a non-endemic area, or a rising titre, may be diagnostically useful. Enzyme-linked immunosorbent assays (ELISA) which detect IgG antibodies appear to give similar results (Ashdown et al. 1989). Assays that detect specific IgM (indirect immunofluorescence, ELISA) correlate better with disease activity (Ashdown

1981, Khupulsup and Petchclai 1986, Ashdown et al. 1989, Kunakorn et al. 1990, 1991) and are thus more useful in endemic areas and in follow-up of patients on treatment. Assays based on more purified antigens are also under development but require further evaluation (Anuntagool, Rugdech and Sirisinha 1993, Wongratanacheewin et al. 1993).

7 CONTROL

Since *B. pseudomallei* is ubiquitous in the environment in endemic areas, it is almost impossible for those whose occupations involve soil and water contact to avoid exposure. It may be worthwhile for those particularly at risk (e.g. diabetics) to avoid rice farming, but the effectiveness of this has not been evaluated. Elimination of the organism from soil with disinfectants was attempted in the French outbreak (Mollaret 1988). No *B. pseudomallei* vaccine has been developed for human use, but experimental vaccines have been used in animals. The organism should be handled in containment level 3 facilities in the laboratory. Patients should ideally be nursed in standard isolation, but person-to-person spread is very rare.

8 TREATMENT

8.1 Supportive treatment

Patients with septicaemic melioidosis usually require aggressive supportive treatment and should ideally be managed in an intensive therapy unit. Particular attention should be paid to correction of fluid volume depletion and septic shock, respiratory and renal failure, and hyperglycaemia or ketoacidosis. Abscesses should, whenever possible, be drained. Corticosteroids are of doubtful benefit, and anti-endotoxin and anti-cytokine antibodies have not yet been evaluated.

8.2 Specific treatment

B. pseudomallei is intrinsically resistant to many antibiotics, including aminoglycosides and early β-lactams (see Volume 2, Chapter 47). Indeed, a complete lack of response to penicillin plus gentamicin, a combination often used for the empirical treatment of septicaemia in the tropics, is characteristic of melioidosis (Chaowagul et al. 1989).

Until the mid-1980s, various empirical combination regimens were used to treat melioidosis, usually including a tetracycline, chloramphenicol and co-trimoxazole. Several recent studies have shown that the mortality of acute severe melioidosis can be substantially reduced by newer β-lactam agents such as ceftazidime or co-amoxiclav, with or without co-trimoxazole (White et al. 1989, Sookpranee et al. 1992, Suputtamongkol et al. 1994b). Ceftazidime is currently the treatment of choice and should be given in full doses (120 mg kg^{-1} per day or a dose appropriately adjusted for renal function) for 2–4 weeks according to the clinical response. The carbapenem antibiotics have some potential advantages over ceftazidime (Smith et al. 1994, 1996, Walsh et al. 1995b) but await further clinical evaluation before they can be recommended as first choice treatment.

On completion of parenteral treatment, prolonged oral antibiotics are needed to prevent relapse, which occurs in up to 23% of patients (Chaowagul et al. 1993), and is commoner in patients with more severe disease. This can be reduced to less than 10% if antibiotics are given for 20 weeks (Rajchanuvong et al. 1995). The combination of chloramphenicol (40 mg kg^{-1} per day), doxycycline (4 mg kg^{-1} per day) and co-trimoxazole (10 mg trimethoprim + 50 mg sulphamethoxazole per kg per day) was associated with a lower relapse rate than co-amoxiclav (60 mg amoxycillin + 15 mg clavulanic acid per kg per day) in the latter study, but this may have been accounted for by differences in compliance and either regimen is probably adequate. Co-amoxiclav is preferable in children and pregnant or lactating women.

In patients with mild localized disease, either of the oral regimens described above may be used, although the optimal agents and duration of treatment remain to be defined. The fluoroquinolones are relatively inactive against *B. pseudomallei* but warrant further evaluation because of their high intracellular concentrations.

8.3 Outcome and follow-up

Even with optimal treatment, the mortality from acute severe melioidosis is high (30–47%). Patients who survive often have chronic morbidity that results both from the disease itself and the underlying conditions. Patients require long-term follow-up to detect relapse. Serial measurements of IgM (Ashdown 1981) or C-reactive protein (Ashdown 1992b) may give an early clue to relapse. Susceptibility tests should be carried out on isolates obtained during or after treatment, since resistance may emerge in 5–10% of cases (Dance et al. 1989c).

GLANDERS

Glanders is a zoonotic disease of equines that may occasionally be transmitted to humans or other animals (sheep, goats, dogs and cats). Traditionally 'glanders', a systemic disease involving the nasal mucosa and lower respiratory tract, has been distinguished from 'farcy', a cutaneous infection with lymphangitis; both are caused by *B. mallei*. In contrast to melioidosis, there has been remarkably little recent work on this disease. The history of glanders has been reviewed by Wilkinson (1981).

9 CLINICAL MANIFESTATIONS

Glanders has a similar range of clinical presentations

to that of melioidosis, as originally observed by Whitmore (1913). Occult infections are probably under-reported. At the other end of the spectrum, glanders may present as overwhelming sepsis resulting in severe toxaemia and widespread abscesses, culminating in delirium, shock and death. The disease may be fatal within days or may persist for many years with remissions and relapses. In reality, the distinction between glanders and farcy is artificial since, as with melioidosis, an acute phase may precede or follow chronic disease and localized cutaneous infection may disseminate or may result from metastatic infection.

Characteristic local manifestations include wound infection and ulceration, lymphangitis with abscesses along the course of lymphatic drainage ('farcy buds'), ulceration of the respiratory (especially nasal) mucosa, polyarthritis, pneumonia and lung abscesses, and nodular abscesses in any site, particularly muscle and subcutaneous tissue. A widespread necrotizing skin eruption has been described as a terminal feature of disseminated glanders. Readers requiring a more detailed description of the manifestations of glanders are referred to the excellent review by Howe (1950).

10 EPIDEMIOLOGY

10.1 Geographical distribution

In the early part of this century, equine glanders was present world wide and was still relatively common in Europe and the USA. More than 200 000 horses were destroyed as a result of glanders during the First World War (Howe 1950). However, no naturally acquired case has been reported in the USA or the UK since 1938, although occasional laboratory-acquired infections have occurred (Howe and Miller 1947). Currently, glanders is still known to occur in parts of the Middle East, Africa and Asia, but the true incidence is uncertain. Occasional cases have arisen amongst carnivora in non-endemic areas, probably through the ingestion of contaminated imported meat (Alibasoglu et al. 1986).

10.2 Reservoirs and transmission

Human glanders, which was rare even when equine glanders was common, is primarily an occupational disease of those in close contact with infected animals. Natural infection is thought usually to result from contamination of wounds, abrasions or mucous membranes. The infectivity by these routes is probably low, although the organism is particularly hazardous to laboratory workers who may acquire infection by inhalation (Howe and Miller 1947). This route may also account for some naturally acquired cases. Person-to-person spread has occurred, so patients require isolation.

B. mallei is more delicate than *B. pseudomallei* and is usually considered to be an obligate parasite. It may, however, survive for up to 4 weeks in water (Howe 1950), although the role of ingestion in human infections is uncertain.

11 PATHOLOGY AND PATHOGENESIS

After inoculation, *B. mallei* establishes local infection, often with ulceration, and may subsequently disseminate via the lymphatics or bloodstream.

11.1 Histopathology

As with melioidosis, the nature of glanders lesions varies according to the duration of infection. Nodular foci of infection range from abscesses with acute inflammation to chronic granulomata with central caseous necrosis (Howe 1950). These lesions are said to be distinguishable from tuberculous granulomata (Zubaidy and Al-Ani 1978). Involvement of small blood vessels and lymphatics with inflammation and endothelial proliferation progressing to subintimal and medial degeneration and thrombosis is characteristic (Howe 1950).

11.2 Bacterial virulence factors

Although interstrain differences in virulence have been reported, the specific virulence factors of *B. mallei* have been little studied. There is some evidence that, like *B. pseudomallei*, *B. mallei* forms an antiphagocytic capsule in vivo (Popov, Tikhonov and Kurilov 1994).

11.3 Host defence

Several animal species are susceptible to experimental glanders, but species vary in their susceptibility to infection, with cattle, pigs, rats and fowl being intrinsically resistant. It is not clear whether underlying diseases render humans susceptible to glanders.

12 HOST RESPONSE

Both humoral and cellular immune responses occur in natural and experimental infections with *B. mallei*, but these have not been well characterized. However, neither natural infection nor immunization induces protection in horses, despite some success with the latter in guinea pigs (Mohler and Eichhorn 1914).

13 DIAGNOSIS

13.1 Culture

As with melioidosis, the clinical manifestations of glanders are rarely pathognomonic. The diagnosis thus hinges on an appropriate history (contact with animals in an endemic area or laboratory exposure) and on isolation and identification of *B. mallei* from an appropriate clinical specimen (e.g. blood, wound swab or pus, sputum) or the detection of specific antibodies. Although *B. mallei* will grow on orthodox media, the laboratory should be alerted if the diagnosis is suspected, both to increase the chances of detection and because, like *B. pseudomallei*, *B. mallei* requires containment level 3 accommodation. Its rarity means that most microbiologists are unfamiliar with its characteristics, and it might easily be overlooked unless sought specifically. Selective techniques have been described (Howe 1950), but recent experience of these is limited. The characteristics of the organism are described in Volume 2 (see Volume 2, Chapter 47).

13.2 Serodiagnosis

Serological tests (complement fixation, bacterial agglutination or haemagglutination, or ELISA), may be available through reference or veterinary laboratories (Verma et al. 1990), but are of little use for the diagnosis of acute cases and may give cross-reactions in patients exposed to *B. pseudomallei*. Skin testing with a crude extract of *B. mallei* (mallein) has been used for screening animals and has been reported to be useful in human glanders, but cannot be recommended because of its unreliability, the risk of adverse reactions, and problems obtaining mallein. As yet no rapid diagnostic tests have been developed.

14 CONTROL

The remarkable decline of glanders has been attributed variously to the compulsory slaughter of infected or seropositive animals, the decreasing use of the horse, and the removal of communal water troughs (Blancou 1994). There is no effective vaccine for either human or animal use, and prevention in those countries where glanders persists will depend on veterinary public health measures and the continued reduction of reliance on the horse as a means of transport.

15 TREATMENT

15.1 Specific treatment

Since most human infections occurred in the pre-antibiotic era, data on treatment are scarce. *B. mallei* is sensitive in vitro to aminoglycosides, tetracyclines, sulphonamides and trimethoprim, but resistant to early β-lactams and colistin (Al-Izzi and Al-Bassam 1989). Sulphonamides in full doses for at least 20 days were effective in curing experimental infections (Miller, Pannell and Ingalls 1948) and have been used successfully to treat human cases (Howe and Miller 1947). Until further data are available, initial treatment for severe glanders should comprise an aminoglycoside (with monitoring of the serum levels), possibly in combination with co-trimoxazole, in doses appropriate to renal function. Mild infections can probably be treated with co-trimoxazole or a tetracycline. Treatment should be continued for at least 3 weeks and probably longer, depending on the patient's response. As with melioidosis, adjunctive supportive therapy, including the drainage of abscesses, may be needed.

15.2 Outcome and follow-up

The mortality of reported cases, many of whom have

not been effectively treated, has been high (over 90%), but this should be reduced if appropriate antibiotics are given. Long-term follow-up to detect relapse should be arranged.

REFERENCES

Advisory Committee on Dangerous Pathogens, 1995, *Categories of Biological Agents according to Hazard and Categories of Containment*, 4th edn, HSE Books, Sudbury, Suffolk.

Alibasoglu M, Yesildere T et al., 1986, Glanders outbreak in lions in the Istanbul zoological garden, *Berl Munch Tierarztl Wochenschr*, **99**: 57–63.

Al-Izzi SA, Al-Bassam LS, 1989, In vitro susceptibility of *Pseudomonas mallei* to antimicrobial agents, *Comp Immunol Microbiol Infect Dis*, **12**: 5–8.

Anuntagool N, Rugdech P, Sirisinha S, 1993, Identification of specific antigens of *Pseudomonas pseudomallei* and evaluation of their efficacies for diagnosis of melioidosis, *J Clin Microbiol*, **31**: 1232–6.

Ashdown LR, 1979, Identification of *Pseudomonas pseudomallei* in the clinical laboratory, *J Clin Pathol*, **32**: 500–4.

Ashdown LR, 1981, Relationship and significance of specific immunoglobulin M antibody response in clinical and subclinical melioidosis, *J Clin Microbiol*, **14**: 361–4.

Ashdown LR, 1987, Indirect haemagglutination test for melioidosis, *Med J Aust*, **147**: 364–5.

Ashdown LR, 1992a, Rapid differentiation of *Pseudomonas pseudomallei* from *Pseudomonas cepacia*, *Lett Appl Microbiol*, **14**: 203–5.

Ashdown LR, 1992b, Serial C-reactive protein levels as an aid to the management of melioidosis, *Am J Trop Med Hyg*, **46**: 151–7.

Ashdown LR, Koehler JM, 1990, Production of hemolysin and other extracellular enzymes by clinical isolates of *Pseudomonas pseudomallei*, *J Clin Microbiol*, **28**: 2331–4.

Ashdown LR, Johnson RW et al., 1989, Enzyme-linked immunosorbent assay for the diagnosis of clinical and subclinical melioidosis, *J Infect Dis*, **160**: 253–60.

Blancou J, 1994, Early methods for the surveillance and control of glanders in Europe, *Rev Sci Tech Off Int Epiz*, **13**: 545–57.

Brown AE, Dance DAB et al., 1990, Activation of cellular immune responses in melioidosis patients as assessed by urinary neopterin, *Trans R Soc Trop Med Hyg*, **84**: 583–4.

Brown AE, Dance DAB et al., 1991, Immune cell activation in melioidosis: increased serum levels of interferon-γ and soluble interleukin-2 receptors without change in soluble CD8 protein, *J Infect Dis*, **163**: 1145–8.

Bryan LE, Wong S et al., 1994, Passive protection of diabetic rats with antisera specific for the polysaccharide portion of the lipopolysaccharide isolated from *Pseudomonas pseudomallei*, *Can J Infect Dis*, **5**: 170–8.

Chambon L, 1955, Isolement du bacille de Whitmore à partir du milieu extérieur, *Ann Inst Pasteur*, **89**: 229–35.

Chaowagul W, White NJ et al., 1989, Melioidosis: a major cause of community-acquired septicemia in northeastern Thailand, *J Infect Dis*, **159**: 890–9.

Chaowagul W, Suputtamongkol Y et al., 1993, Relapse in melioidosis: incidence and risk factors, *J Infect Dis*, **168**: 1181–5.

Currie B, Smith-Vaughan H et al., 1994, *Pseudomonas pseudomallei* isolates collected over 25 years from a non-tropical endemic focus show clonality on the basis of ribotyping, *Epidemiol Infect*, **113**: 307–12.

Dance DAB, 1990, Melioidosis, *Rev Med Microbiol*, **1**: 143–50.

Dance DAB, 1991, Melioidosis: the tip of the iceberg?, *Clin Microbiol Rev*, **4**: 52–60.

Dance DAB, 1992, Melioidosis, glanders and tularaemia, *Med Int*, **107**: 4508–11.

Dance DAB, 1996, Melioidosis, *Manson's Tropical Diseases*, 20th edn, ed. Cook GC, WB Saunders, London and Philadelphia, 927.

Dance DAB, Davis TME et al., 1989a, Acute suppurative parotitis caused by *Pseudomonas pseudomallei* in children, *J Infect Dis*, **159**: 654–60.

Dance DAB, Wuthiekanun V et al., 1989b, Identification of *Pseudomonas pseudomallei* in clinical practice: use of simple screening tests and API 20NE, *J Clin Pathol*, **42**: 645–8.

Dance DAB, Wuthiekanun V et al., 1989c, The antimicrobial susceptibility of *Pseudomonas pseudomallei*. Emergence of resistance in vitro and during treatment, *J Antimicrob Chemother*, **24**: 295–309.

Desakorn V, Smith MD et al., 1994, Detection of *Pseudomonas pseudomallei* antigen in urine for the rapid diagnosis of melioidosis, *Am J Trop Med Hyg*, **51**: 627–33.

Desmarchelier PM, Dance DAB et al., 1993, Relationships among *Pseudomonas pseudomallei* isolates from patients with recurrent melioidosis, *J Clin Microbiol*, **31**: 1592–6.

Dhiensiri T, Puapairoj S, Susaengrat W, 1988, Pulmonary melioidosis: clinical-radiologic correlation in 183 cases from northeastern Thailand, *Radiology*, **166**: 711–15.

Dodin A, Fournier J, 1970, Antigènes précipitants et antigènes agglutinants de *Pseudomonas pseudomallei* (*B. de Whitmore*). I. Complexe thermostable et complexe thermolabile. Typage sérologique, *Ann Inst Pasteur*, **119**: 211–21.

Everett ED, Nelson RA, 1975, Pulmonary melioidosis. Observations in thirty-nine cases, *Am Rev Respir Dis*, **112**: 331–40.

Fournier J, 1965, La mélioïdose et le *B. de Whitmore*. Controverses épidémiologiques et taxonomiques, *Bull Soc Pathol Exot*, **58**: 753–65.

Friedland JS, Suputtamongkol Y et al., 1992, Prolonged elevations of interleukin-8 and interleukin-6 concentrations in plasma and of leukocyte interleukin-8 mRNA levels during septicemic and localized *Pseudomonas pseudomallei* infection, *Infect Immun*, **60**: 2402–8.

Goshorn RK, 1987, Recrudescent pulmonary melioidosis. A case report involving the so-called 'Vietnamese Time Bomb', *Indiana Med*, **80**: 247–9.

Guard RW, Khafagi FA et al., 1984, Melioidosis in far North Queensland. A clinical and epidemiological review of twenty cases, *Am J Trop Med Hyg*, **33**: 467–73.

Haase A, Smith-Vaughan H et al., 1995, Subdivision of *Burkholderia pseudomallei* ribotypes into multiple types by random amplified polymorphic DNA analysis provides new insights into epidemiology, *J Clin Microbiol*, **33**: 1687–90.

Heckly RJ, 1964, Differentiation of exotoxin and other biologically active substances in *Pseudomonas pseudomallei* filtrates, *J Bacteriol*, **88**: 1730–6.

Howe C, 1950, Glanders, *Oxford System of Medicine*, vol. 5, Chapter 8, ed. Christian HA, Oxford University Press, Oxford, 185–202.

Howe C, Miller WR, 1947, Human glanders: report of six cases, *Ann Intern Med*, **26**: 93–115.

Howe C, Sampath A, Spotnitz M, 1971, The pseudomallei group: a review, *J Infect Dis*, **124**: 598–606.

Ismail G, Embi MN et al., 1987, Enzyme immunoassay for the

detection of antibody to *Pseudomonas pseudomallei* endotoxin in mice, *FEMS Microbiol Lett*, **40**: 27–31.

Iwasa S, Petchanchanopong W et al., 1992, Endotoxin of *Pseudomonas pseudomallei* detected by the body-weight decreasing reaction in mice and comparison of it with those of *P. cepacia* and *P. aeruginosa*, *Jpn J Med Sci Biol*, **45**: 35–47.

Jones AL, Beveridge TJ, Woods DE, 1996, Intracellular survival of *Burkholderia pseudomallei*, *Infect Immun*, **64**: 782–90.

Kanai K, Kondo E, 1994, Recent advances in biomedical sciences of *Burkholderia pseudomallei* (basonym: *Pseudomonas pseudomallei*), *Jpn J Med Sci Biol*, **47**: 1–45.

Kanaphun P, Thirawattanasuk N et al., 1993, Serology and carriage of *Pseudomonas pseudomallei*: a prospective study in 1000 hospitalized children in Northeast Thailand, *J Infect Dis*, **167**: 230–3.

Kang G, Rajan DP et al., 1996, Melioidosis in India, *Lancet*, **347**: 1565–6.

Khupulsup K, Petchclai B, 1986, Application of indirect hemagglutination test and indirect fluorescent antibody test for IgM antibody for diagnosis of melioidosis in Thailand, *Am J Trop Med Hyg*, **35**: 366–9.

Klein GC, 1980, Cross-reaction to *Legionella pneumophila* antigen in sera with elevated titers to *Pseudomonas pseudomallei*, *J Clin Microbiol*, **11**: 27–9.

Kosuwon W, Saengnipanthkul S et al., 1993, Musculoskeletal melioidosis, *J Bone Joint Surg [Am]*, **75**: 1811–15.

Kunakorn M, Jayanetra P, Tanphaichitra D, 1991, Man-to-man transmission of melioidosis, *Lancet*, **337**: 1290–1.

Kunakorn M, Markham RB, 1995, Clinically practical seminested PCR for *Burkholderia pseudomallei* quantitated by enzyme immunoassay with and without solution hybridization, *J Clin Microbiol*, **33**: 2131–5.

Kunakorn M, Boonma P et al., 1990, Enzyme-linked immunosorbent assay for immunoglobulin M specific antibody for the diagnosis of melioidosis, *J Clin Microbiol*, **28**: 1249–53.

Kunakorn M, Petchclai B et al., 1991, Gold blot for detection of immunoglobulin M (IgM)- and IgG-specific antibodies for rapid serodiagnosis of melioidosis, *J Clin Microbiol*, **29**: 2065–7.

Leelarasamee A, Bovornkitti S, 1989, Melioidosis: review and update, *Rev Infect Dis*, **11**: 413–25.

Lew AE, Desmarchelier PM, 1993, Molecular typing of *Pseudomonas pseudomallei*: restriction fragment length polymorphisms of rRNA genes, *J Clin Microbiol*, **31**: 533–9.

Lew AE, Desmarchelier PM, 1994, Detection of *Pseudomonas pseudomallei* by PCR and hybridization, *J Clin Microbiol*, **32**: 1326–32.

Li Li, You-wen H, 1992, *Pseudomonas pseudomallei* and melioidosis in China, *Chin Med J*, **105**: 775–9.

Loeffler F, 1886, Die Aetiologie der Rotzkrankheit, *Arb Reichsgesundheitsamte*, **1**: 141–98.

Lumbiganon P, Viengnondha S, 1994, Clinical manifestations of melioidosis in children, *Pediatr Infect Dis J*, **14**: 136–40.

Mays EE, Ricketts EA, 1975, Melioidosis: recrudescence associated with bronchogenic carcinoma twenty-six years following initial geographic exposure, *Chest*, **68**: 261–3.

Miller WR, Pannell L, Ingalls MS, 1948, Experimental chemotherapy in glanders and melioidosis, *Am J Hyg*, **47**: 205–13.

Miller WR, Pannell L et al., 1948, Studies on certain biological characteristics of *Malleomyces mallei* and *Malleomyces pseudomallei*. II. Virulence and infectivity for animals, *J Bacteriol*, **55**: 127–35.

Mohamed R, Nathan S et al., 1989, Inhibition of macromolecular synthesis in cultured macrophages by *Pseudomonas pseudomallei* exotoxin, *Microbiol Immunol*, **33**: 811–20.

Mohler JR, Eichhorn A, 1914, Immunisation tests with glanders vaccine, *J Comp Pathol*, **27**: 183–5.

Mollaret HH, 1988, L'affaire du jardin des plantes ou comment la mélioïdose fit son apparition en France, *Med Mal Infect*, **18**: 643–54.

Nachiangmai N, Patamasucon P et al., 1985, *Pseudomonas pseudo-*

mallei in southern Thailand, *Southeast Asian J Trop Med Public Health*, **16**: 83–7.

Naigowit P, Kurata T et al., 1993, Application of indirect immunofluorescence microscopy to colony identification of *Pseudomonas pseudomallei*, *Asian Pac J Allergy Immunol*, **11**: 149–54.

Piggott JA, Hockholzer L, 1970, Human melioidosis. A histopathologic study of acute and chronic melioidosis, *Arch Pathol*, **90**: 101–11.

Pitt TL, Aucken H, Dance DAB, 1992, Homogeneity of lipopolysaccharide antigens in *Pseudomonas pseudomallei*, *J Infect*, **25**: 139–46.

Pitt TL, Dance DAB, 1991, Melioidosis and *Pseudomonas pseudomallei*, *PHLS Microbiol Dig*, **8**: 127–30.

Poe RH, Vassallo CL, Domm BM, 1971, Melioidosis: the remarkable imitator, *Am Rev Respir Dis*, **10**: 427–31.

Popov SF, Tikhonov NG, Kurilov VY, 1994, Influence of capsule formation in *Pseudomonas pseudomallei* and *Pseudomonas mallei* on their relations with host cells, *Immunol Infect Dis*, **4**: 142–5.

Pruksachartvuthi S, Aswapokee N, Thankerngpol K, 1990, Survival of *Pseudomonas pseudomallei* in human phagocytes, *J Med Microbiol*, **31**: 109–14.

Punyagupta S, 1989, Melioidosis: review of 686 cases and presentation of a new clinical classification, *Melioidosis*, Bangkok Medical Publisher, Bangkok, 217–29.

Putucheary SD, Parasakthi N, Lee MK, 1992, Septicaemic melioidosis: a review of 50 cases from Malaysia, *Trans R Soc Trop Med Hyg*, **86**: 683–5.

Rajchanuvong A, Chaowagul W et al., 1995, A prospective comparison of co-amoxiclav and the combination of chloramphenicol, doxycycline, and co-trimoxazole for the oral maintenance treatment of melioidosis, *Trans R Soc Trop Med Hyg*, **89**: 546–9.

Rapaport FT, Millar JW, Ruch J, 1961, Endotoxic properties of *Pseudomonas pseudomallei*, *Arch Pathol*, **71**: 429–36.

Rode JW, Webling DD'A, 1981, Melioidosis in the Northern Territory of Australia, *Med J Aust*, **1**: 181–4.

Rugdech P, Anuntagool N, Sirisinha S, 1995, Monoclonal antibodies to *Pseudomonas pseudomallei* and their potential for diagnosis of melioidosis, *Am J Trop Med Hyg*, **52**: 231–5.

Sermswan RW, Wongratanacheewin S et al., 1994, Construction of a specific DNA probe for diagnosis of melioidosis and use as an epidemiological marker of *Pseudomonas pseudomallei*, *Mol Cell Probes*, **8**: 1–9.

Sexton MM, Goebel LA et al., 1993, Ribotype analysis of *Pseudomonas pseudomallei* isolates, *J Clin Microbiol*, **31**: 238–43.

Smith CJ, Allen JC et al., 1987, Human melioidosis: an emerging medical problem, *MIRCEN J*, **3**: 343–66.

Smith MD, Wuthiekanun V et al., 1993, Latex agglutination test for identification of *Pseudomonas pseudomallei*, *J Clin Pathol*, **46**: 374–5.

Smith MD, Wuthiekanun V et al., 1994, Susceptibility of *Pseudomonas pseudomallei* to some newer β-lactam antibiotics and antibiotic combinations using time-kill studies, *J Antimicrob Chemother*, **33**: 145–9.

Smith MD, Wuthiekanun V et al., 1995a, Quantitative recovery of *Burkholderia pseudomallei* from soil in Thailand, *Trans R Soc Trop Med Hyg*, **89**: 488–90.

Smith MD, Wuthiekanun V et al., 1995b, Latex agglutination for rapid detection of *Pseudomonas pseudomallei* antigen in urine of patients with melioidosis, *J Clin Pathol*, **48**: 174–6.

Smith MD, Wuthiekanun V et al., 1996, In-vitro activity of carbapenem antibiotics against β-lactam susceptible and resistant strains of *Burkholderia pseudomallei*, *J Antimicrob Chemother*, **37**: 611–15.

Sookpranee M, Boonma P et al., 1992, Multicenter prospective randomized trial comparing ceftazidime plus co-trimoxazole with chloramphenicol plus doxycycline and co-trimoxazole for treatment of severe melioidosis, *Antimicrob Agents Chemother*, **36**: 158–62.

Stanton AT, Fletcher W, 1921, Melioidosis, a new disease of the tropics, *Trans 4th Congr Far Eastern Assoc Trop Med*, **2**: 196–8.

Stanton AT, Fletcher W, 1932, Melioidosis, *Studies from the Institute of Medical Research, Federated Malay States, No. 21*, John Bale & Son and Danielson Ltd, London.

Steinmetz I, Rohde M, Brenneke B, 1995, Purification and characterization of an exopolysaccharide of *Burkholderia* (*Pseudomonas*) *pseudomallei*, *Infect Immun*, **63**: 3959–65.

Strauss JM, Groves MG et al., 1969, Melioidosis in Malaysia. II. Distribution of *Pseudomonas pseudomallei* in soil and surface water, *Am J Trop Med Hyg*, **18**: 698–702.

Suputtamongkol Y, Kwiatkowski D et al., 1992, Tumor necrosis factor in septicemic melioidosis, *J Infect Dis*, **165**: 561–4.

Suputtamongkol Y, Hall AJ et al., 1994a, The epidemiology of melioidosis in Ubon Ratchatani, northeast Thailand, *Int J Epidemiol*, **23**: 1082–90.

Suputtamongkol Y, Rajchanuwong A et al., 1994b, Ceftazidime vs. amoxicillin/clavulanate in the treatment of severe melioidosis, *Clin Infect Dis*, **19**: 846–53.

Tan AL, Ang BSP, Ong YY, 1990, Melioidosis: epidemiology and antibiogram of cases in Singapore, *Singapore Med J*, **31**: 335–7.

Thomas AD, 1983, Evaluation of the API 20E and Microbact 24E systems for the identification of *Pseudomonas pseudomallei*, *Vet Microbiol*, **8**: 611–15.

Thomas AD, Forbes-Faulkner J, Parker M, 1979, Isolation of *Pseudomonas pseudomallei* from clay layers at defined depths, *Am J Epidemiol*, **110**: 515–21.

Trakulsomboon S, Pitt TL, Dance DAB, 1994, Molecular typing of *Pseudomonas pseudomallei* from imported primates in Britain, *Vet Rec*, **135**: 65–6.

Vatcharapreechasakul T, Suputtamongkol Y et al., 1992, *Pseudomonas pseudomallei* liver abscesses: a clinical, laboratory, and ultrasonographic study, *Clin Infect Dis*, **14**: 412–17.

Verma RD, Sharma JK et al., 1990, Development of an avidin-biotin dot enzyme-linked immunosorbent assay and its comparison with other serological tests for diagnosis of glanders in equines, *Vet Microbiol*, **25**: 77–85.

Walsh AL, Smith MD et al., 1994, Immunofluorescence microscopy for the rapid diagnosis of melioidosis, *J Clin Pathol*, **47**: 377–99.

Walsh AL, Smith MD et al., 1995a, Prognostic significance of quantitaive bacteremia in septicemic melioidosis, *Clin Infect Dis*, **21**: 1498–500.

Walsh AL, Smith MD et al., 1995b, Postantibiotic effects and *Burkholderia* (*Pseudomonas*) *pseudomallei*: evaluation of current treatment, *Antimicrob Agents Chemother*, **39**: 2356–8.

Walsh AL, Wuthiekanun V et al., 1995c, Selective broths for the isolation of *Pseudomonas pseudomallei* from clinical samples, *Trans R Soc Trop Med Hyg*, **89**: 124.

White NJ, Dance DAB et al., 1989, Halving the mortality of severe melioidosis by ceftazidime, *Lancet*, **2**: 697–700.

Whitmore A, 1913, An account of a glanders-like disease occurring in Rangoon, *J Hyg*, **13**: 1–34.

Whitmore A, Krishnaswami CS, 1912, An account of the discovery of a hitherto undescribed infective disease occurring among the population of Rangoon, *Indian Med Gaz*, **47**: 262–7.

Wilkinson L, 1981, Glanders: medicine and veterinary medicine in common pursuit of a contagious disease, *Med Hist*, **25**: 363–84.

Wong KT, Putucheary SD, Vadivelu J, 1995, The histopathology of human melioidosis, *Histopathology*, **26**: 51–5.

Wongratanacheewin S, Tattawasart U et al., 1993, Characterization of *Pseudomonas pseudomallei* antigens by SDS-polyacrylamide gel electrophoresis and western blot, *Southeast Asian J Trop Med Public Health*, **24**: 107–13.

Woods ML, Currie BJ et al., 1992, Neurological melioidosis: seven cases from the Northern Territory of Australia, *Clin Infect Dis*, **15**: 163–9.

Wuthiekanun V, Dance DAB et al., 1990, The use of selective media for the isolation of *Pseudomonas pseudomallei* in clinical practice, *J Med Microbiol*, **33**: 121–6.

Wuthiekanun V, Smith MD et al., 1995, Isolation of *Pseudomonas pseudomallei* from soil in north-eastern Thailand, *Trans R Soc Trop Med Hyg*, **89**: 41–3.

Yabuuchi E, Kosako Y et al., 1992, Proposal of *Burkholderia* gen. nov and transfer of seven species of the genus *Pseudomonas* homology group II to the new genus, with the type species *Burkholderia cepacia* (Palleroni and Holmes 1981) comb. nov., *Microbiol Immunol*, **36**: 1251–75.

Yang H, Chaowagul W, Sokol P, 1991, Siderophore production by *Pseudomonas pseudomallei*, *Infect Immun*, **59**: 776–80.

Yang H, Kooi CD, Sokol PA, 1993, Ability of *Pseudomonas pseudomallei* malleobactin to acquire transferrin-bound, lactoferrin-bound, and cell-derived iron, *Infect Immun*, **61**: 656–62.

Zubaidy AJ, Al-Ani FK, 1978, Pathology of glanders in horses in Iraq, *Vet Pathol*, **15**: 566–8.

PASTEURELLOSIS

E J Bottone

1 INTRODUCTION

The genus *Pasteurella*, along with *Actinobacillus* and *Haemophilus*, comprises one of 3 genera in the family Pasteurellaceae. The genus *Pasteurella* was named in honour of Louis Pasteur, subsequent to its establishment. Using phenotypic and genetic analysis, approximately 20 named and unnamed species of *Pasteurella* have been identified, of which *Pasteurella multocida* and *Pasteurella haemolytica* are the most common pathogens causing severe disease and economic loss among cattle, sheep, swine and poultry.

2 HABITAT

Regarded primarily as zoonotic agents with a capability of inducing human infections, pasteurellae, especially *P. multocida*, the genus type species, colonize the mucous membranes of the upper respiratory tract of a wide variety of mammalian and avian species including, but not restricted to, goats, cattle, pigs, turkeys, chickens and especially cats and dogs (Weaver, Hollis and Bottone 1985). Although *P. multocida* and other *Pasteurella* spp. have been recovered from domestic cats and dogs, it is not a cause of spontaneous zoonosis in these animals. In avian species, e.g. chickens and turkeys, however, *P. multocida* causes fowl cholera; in cattle and buffalo a haemorrhagic septicaemia; and in pigs atrophic rhinitis and swine plague (Biberstein 1981). Among the other *Pasteurella* spp. associated with zoonotic infection are *P. haemolytica*, a primary cause of pneumonia in cattle and sheep, often with concomitant septicaemia, especially in lambs under 3 months old. Gangrenous mastitis has also been attributed to *P. haemolytica*. *Pasteurella pneumotropica* is a primary agent of pneumonia in laboratory rodents, especially mice, rats and hamsters. Numerous other *Pasteurella* spp. have been recovered from diverse animal hosts, but they seem to be commensals

in these settings (Table 47.1). Another described species, *Pasteurella caballi*, has been recovered from respiratory and genital tract infections in horses (Sclater et al. 1989) and has been associated with a finger wound in a veterinarian (Bisgaard et al. 1991).

Generally, although *Pasteurella* spp. are inhabitants of the mucous membranes of the respiratory and intestinal tracts of mammals and birds, it is held that infectious complications of these animal species are often precipitated by environmental stress, or prior or concurrent viral or mycoplasma infection (Ciprian et al. 1988). Stress results in diminished superoxide production and chemotactic responsiveness among polymorphonuclear leucocytes (Henricks, Binkhorst and Nijkamp 1987). Under such conditions, host invasion occurs, resulting in a variety of clinical manifestations including pneumonia, abortion, diarrhoea, mastitis, sinusitis and septicaemia (Biberstein 1981). In many animal species, *P. multocida* infection may occur as a septicaemia associated with widespread haemorrhages, but the term haemorrhagic septicaemia is used specifically to denote such primary infection in cattle and buffaloes. Furthermore, there exists a close correlation between the serogroup of *P. multocida*, and the biotype of *P. haemolytica* and their animal host(s), form of disease (Table 47.1), and geographic distribution. *P. multocida* capsular types A and D, for example, are global in distribution and predominate in pasteurellosis of avian species. Serogroup F, a new capsule serogroup of *P. multocida*, has been isolated from turkeys from different areas in the USA (Rimler and Rhoades 1987). The serological classification of *P. multocida* is based on the presence of a specific capsule antigen which renders a serogroup designation, e.g. serogroups A–F (Carter 1962, Rimler and Rhoades 1987), whereas specific somatic antigens render the serotype, e.g. 1–16, within these serogroups. Thus, one may designate a *P. multocida* isolate as serogroup A, serotype 5, or A:5.

Table 47.1 Host range, disease and geographic distribution of principal *Pasteurella* spp.

Species/serotype		Major host(s)	Disease	Geographical distribution
P. multocida				
type A		Cattle	Shipping fever, fibrinous pneumonia	Global
		Deer	Septicaemia	
		Cattle, sheep	Mastitis	
		Poultry	Fowl cholera	
		Swine	Pneumonia	
		Rabbits	'Snuffles', pneumonia	
	B	Camel	Haemorrhagic septicaemia	Sudan
	B:3	Deer	Haemorrhagic septicaemia	United Kingdon
	B:6	Buffalo, cattle	Haemorrhagic septicaemia	South East Africa
	D	Swine	Atrophic rhinitis	Global
		Poultry	Fowl cholera	
	E	Buffalo, cattle	Haemorrhagic septicaemia	Central Africa, Europe, Russia
	F	Turkeys	Normal flora (?)	USA
P. haemolytica				
Biotype	A1	Cattle	Shipping fever, fibrinous pneumonia, mastitis	Global
	A2	Sheep	Pneumonia	
Biotype	T	Sheep	Septicaemia	Global
P. pneumotropica		Rodents	Pneumonia	Global
P. granulomatis		Cattle	Cutaneous lesions	Brazil

3 DISEASES

3.1 *Pasteurella multocida*

CATTLE AND BUFFALO

Haemorrhagic septicaemia of cattle and buffalo is of significant economic loss and occurs predominantly in Asia and Africa (Table 47.1). In Asia, the disease is caused primarily by serogroup B:6 strains which appear to be particularly virulent for buffaloes, mice and rabbits, but rather less virulent for cattle, pigs, sheep, goats and avirulent for chickens. In Central Africa, haemorrhagic septicaemia is usually caused by strains of capsular serogroup E, which has not been encountered elsewhere. Episodes of the disease have also occurred in southern Europe and in Russia. In 1987, Rimler, Rhoades and Jones isolated a strain of capsular serogroup B:3,4 from fallow deer during the first outbreak of haemorrhagic septicaemia in the UK.

Haemorrhagic septicaemia in animals occurs mainly in the rainy season and often appears to be associated with cattle fatigue. Nasopharyngeal carriers provide a source of infection and the portal of entry is probably the tonsillar region; animals can be infected experimentally by means of a nasal spray. Once clinical infection is established, death is almost certain. On bacteriological examination large numbers of pasteurellae are found in saliva, milk, faeces and urine. Blood smears contain large numbers of coccobacilli that exhibit bipolar staining. In the terminal stages the disease bears a resemblance to endotoxic shock. Many animals die within 24 h of the onset of symptoms, but those that live longer may show a variable degree of pneumonia at necropsy. Sometimes oedematous swelling occurs in the region of the throat, neck and brisket due to infiltration of the subcutaneous tissues with a straw-coloured exudate. The main postmortem features are widespread petechial haemorrhages and swollen and congested lymph nodes. There may also be exudates in the serous cavities, oedema in the laryngeal region, and acute gastroenteritis with blood in the intestinal contents. The lungs are often congested with thickened interlobular septa and fibrinous pleurisy.

More than 10% of unvaccinated cattle and buffaloes in India and South East Asia may be immune, and serum from such animals or from artificially immunized animals is capable of affording passive protection to mice against experimental *P. multocida* infection. In areas where the disease is known to occur, vaccination is often routinely used, especially before the beginning of the rainy season. Vaccines consist of formalin-inactivated strains of *P. multocida* isolated from cases of haemorrhagic septicaemia. Protection is thought to last no more than 6–8 months. Nagy and Penn (1976) reported the successful immunization of cattle against haemorrhagic septicaemia by means of capsular antigens of serogroups B and E. Haemorrhagic septicaemia has also occurred in camels (Hassan and Mustafa 1985).

Respiratory infections with *P. multocida* occur in young cattle, especially those kept under intensive systems of husbandry or subjected to stress by fatigue, excitement or fear, irregular feeding or watering, and overcrowding. Such factors are often present in a particularly damaging combination when animals are transported for protracted periods. Such respiratory tract infections induced under stressful conditions of herd transport led to naming the disease 'shipping fever', i.e. the occurrence of pulmonary infections during or shortly after a journey. Whereas *P. multocida* capsular serogroup A and occasionally D are primary incitants, *P. haemolytica* biotype A serotype 1 (A1) is also frequently incriminated (Yates 1982), as are viruses and chlamydia. An extracellular neuraminidase has been found in a *P. multocida* A:3 strain associated with bovine pneumonia that is distinct from the *P. haemolytica* A1 neuraminidase (White et al. 1995) which has also been detected in bovine pneumonia strains (Strauss, Unbehagen and Purdy 1993).

P. multocida and *P. haemolytica* produce a severe fibrinous pneumonia accompanied by thickening of interlobular septa and by fibrinous pleurisy; rarely, septicaemia may also complicate the respiratory course. Carrigan et al. (1991) reported an outbreak of septicaemic illness involving 13 of 100 fallow deer, aged between 6 months and 10 years. All 13 died with pulmonary congestion and oedema and froth-filled airways; fibrinous pneumonia and pleurisy were also present at necropsy in 4 deer. *P. multocida* serogroup A:3,4 was isolated from numerous tissues from 7 of 8 deer.

P. multocida has been reported as a cause of bovine mastitis and has also been isolated from the synovial fluid of calves suffering from polyarthritis. It has also been incriminated as a rare cause of bovine abortion and isolated from calves with meningoencephalitis and from the brains of other animal species. *P. haemolytica* A9, a causative agent of severe mastitis in ewes, and *P. haemolytica* A1 (a cause of bovine pneumonia) have been shown experimentally to produce mastitis in lactating cows, but not lactating mice, rabbits, or sows (Watkins, Scott and Jones 1992). The inoculation of *P. haemolytica* A1 and A9 into lactating mammary glands induced mastitis only in ruminants.

Lechiguana, an unusual cutaneous lesion, has been described in cattle in Brazil (Riet-Cornea et al. 1992). Characterized by large subcutaneous swellings (45 × 50 cm), mainly over the scapula area, the lesions occurred in 18 cattle; aspiration of the lesions grew *P. granulomatis* in 14 cases. Inoculation of an isolate into a steer reproduced the disease. Because of the anatomical distribution of the lesions, the authors concluded that transmission of the infectious agent was mediated through an insect, *Dermatobia hominis*.

SWINE

In swine, *P. multocida* serogroup D, along with *Bordetella bronchiseptica*, is associated with progressive atrophic rhinitis. Characterized by catarrhal rhinitis and hypoplasia of the nasal turbinate bones, this infection often leads to snout deformities. The interactive dynamics of these 2 bacterial species in producing rhinitis mainly in piglets aged 2–5 months is not completely understood. Nevertheless, either intranasal (Dominick and Rimler 1986), or intramuscular (Martineau-Doize, Frantz and Martineau 1990) inoculation of pigs with cell extracts of *P. multocida* serogroup D results in nasal turbinate lesions in conchae cartilage and bone leading to conchae atrophy.

Evidence is beginning to mount in support of the primary role of *P. multocida* in atrophic rhinitis. Two lines of experimental reasoning have shown that the dermonecrotic toxin (DNT) produced by *P. multocida* may be more active in the pathogenesis of atrophic rhinitis in pigs than DNT of *B. bronchiseptica*. Initially, Elias et al. (1990) showed that parenteral administration of DNT from both *P. multocida* and *B. bronchiseptica* to piglets aged 2 weeks produced nasal turbinate lesions whereas administration of DNT only from *P. multocida* induced lesions in piglets aged 7–12 weeks. The authors concluded that DNT of *B. bronchiseptica* differs from that of *P. multocida* in biological properties, although there are some similarities. de Jong and Akkermans (1986) showed that the presence of atrophic rhinitis in swine herds correlated with the presence of toxigenic *P. multocida* and not with *B. bronchiseptica* infection. Furthermore, de Jong, de Wachter and Marcel (1986) showed induction of atrophic rhinitis and protection against atrophic rhinitis in newborn piglets after intramuscular injection into sows of cell-free filtrates and emulsions containing the *P. multocida* DNT.

Further support for the role of toxigenic serogroup D *P. multocida* in atrophic rhinitis may be derived from the epidemiological study of Rutter and colleagues (1984) who showed that in field cases of atrophic rhinitis among 4 pig herds, severe disease was only noted among pigs infected with toxigenic *P. multocida*. In 2 herds with no history of atrophic rhinitis, *B. bronchiseptica* was recovered with non-toxigenic strains of *P. multocida*.

It may well be that the prior or concomitant colonization of the nasal passages by *B. bronchiseptica* facilitates adherence and establishment of colonization by both toxigenic and non-toxigenic strains of *P. multocida* serogroup D; when the former, atrophic rhinitis ensues. Furthermore, a significant role for the dermonecrotic toxin in atrophic rhinitis whether produced by *P. multocida* or non-*multocida* species has been advanced by Kamp, Terlaak and de Jong (1990). From cattle with atrophic rhinitis these authors recovered 4 non-*P. multocida* pasteurellae which produced a dermonecrotic toxin whose toxic affects (haemorrhagic dermonecrosis in guinea pigs, mouse lethality) were neutralized by an antiserum against the purified dermonecrotic toxin of *P. multocida*. Western blot analysis of the bovine strain toxin showed it to be of the same molecular weight as the *P. multocida* dermonecrotic toxin. One can only speculate that perhaps these non-*P. multocida* isolates obtained the genes encoding the dermonecrotic toxin from *P. multocida* by transfection with a bacteriophage or other genetic vector.

POULTRY

Fowl cholera is a disease of domestic poultry and wildfowl in which outbreaks can cause heavy losses on large commercial chicken and turkey farms. The strains of *P. multocida* incriminated in fowl cholera belong mainly to capsular type A, some to capsular type D and others are untypable. *P. multocida* strains isolated from outbreaks of fowl cholera are often of heightened virulence for their avian hosts (Rhoades and Rimler 1990).

The acute epizootic form of fowl cholera is characterized by an incubation period of about 12 h, listlessness and the general symptoms of an acute illness. There may be a discharge from the beak and nostrils and diarrhoea with the passage of bright yellow or green, often blood-stained, faecal material. Death follows in a few hours to 3 days. The main lesions are acute septicaemia, a serofibrinous pericarditis and an acute haemorrhagic enteritis, most noticeable in the duodenum. The disease may also be subacute or chronic, taking the form of nasal catarrh or sinusitis, swelling and oedema of the wattles, or lameness due to arthritis. Coombs and Botzler (1991) correlated the daily activities of wildfowl with avian cholera mortality and proposed that outbreaks and mortality were directly correlated with mean flock size, time spent on land, and time spent grazing on land or in shallow water. Grazing on land may lead to acquisition of *P. multocida* from contaminated environmental sources and flock densities may facilitate transmission. Indeed, using restriction endonuclease analysis (REA), Christiansen et al. (1992) showed the same REA pattern of *P. multocida* isolates from 52 of 80 turkey flocks in which an outbreak had occurred.

Fowl cholera has also been described in Muscovy ducks (*Cairina moschata*) in Okinawa Prefecture in Japan in November 1990 (Nakamine et al. 1992). Fifty of 200 birds succumbed to an acute disease characterized by necrosis with bacterial aggregates in several organs, especially in the liver. *P. multocida* was recovered from all tissues of 2 birds that had expired. Capsular serogroups A:3,4,12 and A:5 were identified which, upon intravenous (10^8 colony-forming units per ml) inoculation into chickens, was lethal. Similarly, Rhoades, Rimler and Bagley (1992) reported an outbreak of fowl cholera involving turkey flocks in Utah. *P. multocida* A:3 and B:4 were isolated; the rarely encountered B:4 capsular group was also virulent upon exposure to pouts. Unusual cutaneous manifestations of fowl cholera have also been described. In one instance (Frame, Clark and Smart 1994), cutaneous lesions vertical and lateral to the tail recurred during outbreaks of fowl cholera, whereas facial cellulitis and cephalic swelling occurred on 7 separate occasions among commercial turkeys during a 2 year period (Jeffrey et al 1993). The lesions were histologically characterized by extensive fibronecrotic inflammation of the deep dermis with perivasculitis and thrombosis. *P. multocida* A was the predominant isolate in both instances.

RABBITS

P. multocida is endemic in many rabbit colonies and may cause 'snuffles' – a chronic respiratory infection that may result in death. The disease is associated with an increase in the normal carrier rate among rabbits, although the susceptibility of individual rabbits varies greatly. In addition to snuffles, *P. multocida* has been associated with acute pneumonia, septicaemia, mastitis, otitis media, encephalitis, abscesses and pyometritis. *P. multocida* capsular serogroups A and D were frequently isolated; somatic type A:12 was particularly common (Percy, Prescott and Bhasin 1984). Transmission of *P. multocida* among rabbits occurs most readily by contact with acutely infected rabbits rather than from rabbits with chronic infection. Air-borne transmission of *P. multocida* to rabbits in adjacent cages appears not to occur (DiGiacomo, Jones and Wathes 1987). Serological surveys of rabbits from colonies reported to have endemic *P. multocida* show 59% conversion rate compared with 7.6% seroconversion among rabbits in colonies reported to be free of *P. multocida* (Zaoutis et al. 1991). These data affirm a correlation between carriage rate and acute infections.

DOGS AND CATS

It has been well established that healthy dogs and cats are major reservoirs for *P. multocida* and other *Pasteurella* spp. In 1955, Smith reported the recovery of *P. multocida* from 10% of nasal swabs and 54% of the tonsils of 111 dogs surveyed. *P. multocida* is also common (50–75%) in the oral cavity of healthy cats (Francis, Holmes and Brandon 1975). In the course of his studies, Smith (1958) reported that dog strains of *P. multocida* (*P. septica* in his article) differed from strains producing disease in cattle, sheep, pigs and poultry in biochemical reactions (maltose fermented but not xylose or mannitol, low pathogenicity for mice and non-capsulated). Furthermore, canine and feline strains often differ from each other; for example, most canine strains are of low virulence for mice whereas feline strains are more virulent when introduced into the mouse peritoneum. This fact may explain that although dogs are most frequently involved in bite wounds, cat bites result in infections 3 times as often (Holmes and Brandon 1965, Francis, Holmes and Brandon 1975). The exact virulence factors accounting for the seeming increased virulence of feline *P. multocida* isolates are unclear and worthy of elucidation, as *P. multocida* in canine and feline hosts does not play an important pathogenic role. Although not indicative of virulence, Oberhofer (1981) showed a 61% correlation between the fermentation patterns (biotype) of feline isolates to cat bite infections whereas such a correlation was absent from dog bite isolates. Oberhofer (1981) identified 2 biotypes (A and B) which indicates a constancy of strains among cats and in turn could also account for the increased incidence of infections subsequent to cat bites if these biotypes were shown to have virulence attributes. In this regard, Müller and Kraseman (1974) showed that there was a difference in mouse virulence of *P. multocida* isolated from dogs and cats as a function of the level of their neuraminidase production. High level producers were more virulent. The recovery of *P. multocida* and *P. pneumotropica* from human and animal sources may be enhanced through the use of a selective medium containing clindamycin, gentamicin, potassium tellurite and amphotericin B in 5% horse blood agar (Knight et al. 1983).

3.2 *Pasteurella haemolytica*

CATTLE AND SHEEP

P. haemolytica is responsible for economically significant morbidity and mortality among cattle and sheep in which it produces pneumonic pasteurellosis in cattle in North America, and pneumonia and septicaemia in sheep. *P. haemolytica* is the most common gram-negative bacterium recovered from tonsils of healthy domestic and Bighorn sheep (Queen, Ward and Hunter 1994).

P. haemolytica is divided into 16 capsular serotypes and 2 biotypes based on sugar fermentation patterns (Table 47.2), e.g. biotype A isolates ferment arabinose and include serotypes 3, 4, 10 and 15, whereas biotype T strains ferment trehalose and include the 12 remaining serotypes. Younan and Fodar (1995) have described a new *P. haemolytica* serotype (A17) isolated from sheep in Syria.

In the acute form of the disease known as enzootic pneumonia of sheep, *P. haemolytica* is invariably present in pneumonic lung tissue in large numbers. Biotype A is almost always responsible and, of all the serotypes, serotype 2 occurs with particular frequency in sheep (Yates 1982), whereas serotype 1 is more common in cattle (Thompson, Benson and Savan 1969). In the few instances in which biotype T is found, either alone or together with biotype A, its presence is probably often the result of septicaemia.

Enzootic pneumonia affects sheep of all ages. Out-breaks, which occur sporadically and unpredictably, are generally considered to be associated with various forms of stress such as fatigue or inclement weather. The predisposing factors are, however, poorly understood. Mortality rarely exceeds 10%, but sheep that recover clinically may remain in poor condition. Postmortem examination of sheep that die from acute infection shows that the anterior lobes of the lungs are most commonly affected. The diseased tissue, which usually contains at least 10^7 viable organisms per gram, is consolidated and, macroscopically, often resembles the liver. The interlobular septa are very obvious and opalescent. The pleura may be thickened; straw-coloured exudate, often containing fibrin, is present in the pleural cavity. Pericarditis and haemorrhages on the heart and serous surfaces are common findings. It would seem that death results not so much from destruction of lung tissue as from the accumulation of bacteria and their toxic products. The abnormal lung tissue contains necrotic areas and alveoli packed with elongated cells.

P. haemolytica produces a variety of factors that may enhance its virulence. Among those that have been identified and have been the subject of intensive investigation are a secreted leucotoxin (Kaehler et al. 1980, Shewen and Wilkie 1982), secreted neuraminidase (Straus, Unbehagen and Purdy 1993) and secreted sialoglycoprotease (Abdullah et al. 1992), along with a capsular polysaccharide (Adlam et al. 1984), outer-membrane proteins (Squire, Smiley and Croskell 1984) and fimbriae (Morck et al. 1989).

The putative role of the heat labile *P. haemolytica* leucotoxin is to destroy ruminant leucocytes (polymorphonuclear leucocytes, lymphocytes,

Table 47.2 Differential characteristics of major zoonotic *Pasteurella* spp.

| Characteristics | **Pasteurella species** | | | |
	multocida	*haemolytica*	*pneumotropica*	*caballi*
Fermentation				
glucose	+	+	+	+ (gas)
maltose	V	+	+	+
sucrose	+	+	+	NA
arabinose	0	+, 0[a]	0	
trehalose	V	0, +[b]		0
lactose	0	+	0	(+)
Indole production	+	0	+	0
Ornithine decarboxylase	+	0	+	V
β-Haemolysis	0	+	0	0
Yellow pigment	0	0	0	+
Growth on				
MacConkey agar	0	+	–	–
Urease	0	0	+	0
Oxidase	+	+	+	+
Catalase	+	+	+	0

[a]Biovar A positive; biovar T negative.
[b]Biovar A negative; biovar T positive.
+, positive; –, negative; V, variable; NA, not available; (+), late positive.

monocytes) at the site of infection in the lung, thereby impairing an immune response and effective inflammatory response (Shewen and Wilkie 1982). Lysis of immune cells also leads to release of toxic enzymes which may destroy lung tissue, leading to the severe necrosis seen in *P. haemolytica* pneumonia. Marked accumulation of bacteria in the pneumonic lung is a direct consequence of impairment of bacterial clearance by lysis of pulmonary macrophages and infiltrating leucocytes. The secreted leucotoxin may induce a transmembrane pore in susceptible leucocytes, resulting in the rapid leakage of intracellular potassium, cell swelling with leakage of larger cytoplasmic components, and osmotic lysis (Clinkenbeard, Mosier and Confer 1989). In recovering animals, leucotoxin-neutralizing antibodies can be demonstrated (Shewen and Wilkie 1983). Leucotoxin negative mutants of *P. haemolytica* are less virulent for goats and cattle in comparison to leucotoxin producing wild-type strains (Petras et al. 1995).

Neuraminidase activity has been demonstrated for *P. haemolytica* A1 strains associated with bovine pneumonia (Straus, Unbehagen and Purdy 1993) and to a lesser degree among sheep isolates of serotype 2 (Frank and Tabatabai 1981). These data suggest that a direct correlation between the level of neuraminidase activity and pneumonic capability may not exist. Nevertheless, as even small quantities of enzymatically active neuraminidase, which acts to cleave surface components off susceptible target cells, may synergistically enhance leucotoxin activity and even expose ligands on cell surfaces, facilitating adherence and colonization through fimbrial attachment (Morck et al. 1989).

The neutral sialoglycoprotease of *P. haemolytica* A1 has been isolated and shown to cleave glycophorin A on human erythrocytes which is O glycosylated (Abdullah et al. 1992). Thus, this secreted enzyme may act in concert with neuraminidase to render cell membranes more vulnerable to leucotoxin attack.

Fimbriae of *P. haemolytica* may aid colonization of the upper respiratory tract of cattle as a prelude to infection. Indeed, Morck et al. (1989) showed through transmission and scanning electron microscopy of lung sections that feedlot cattle suffering from pneumonic pasteurellosis had numerous microcolonies of gram-negative bacteria morphologically consistent with *P. haemolytica*. The dense aggregates of gram-negative coccobacilli were enmeshed through their polysaccharide glycocalyx and through proteinaceous material suggestive of fimbriae. Microcolonies of *P. haemolytica* may well render the constituent members resistant to phagocytosis and other host defences during early phases of infection. Purified fimbriae of *P. haemolytica* are rigid but are devoid of haemagglutinating activity (Potter, Ready and Gilchrist 1988).

The capsule of *P. haemolytica* accounts for serotype designation and mediates several important anti-infection factors such as antiphagocytic activity, resistance to intracellular killing and resistance to complement mediated serum bactericidal activity. The capsule may also have a role in the adherence of *P. haemolytica* to alveolar epithelium (Confer et al. 1990).

Although a brisk antibody response is induced to purified capsule polysaccharide of *P. haemolytica* A1 (Tigges and Loan 1993), capsular polysaccharide administered alone or in combination with recombinant leucotoxin does not protect cattle from subsequent challenge with logarithmic-phase *P. haemolytica* (Conlon and Shewen 1993). Interestingly, 36% of calves immunized with capsular polysaccharide developed anaphylaxis. These data attest to the complexity of the role of the capsule in virulence and to the difficulty in achieving protective immunity.

P. haemolytica lipopolysaccharide is not toxic for bovine leucocytes (Confer and Simmons 1986) but has been shown to induce inflammatory cytokines in bovine alveolar macrophages during the course of bovine pneumonic pasteurellosis (Yoo et al. 1995). Serum antibodies to *P. haemolytica* lipopolysaccharide are induced by the administration of live *P. haemolytica* to calves and confer a degree of resistance to intrapulmonic challenge (Confer, Panciera and Mosier 1986). *P. haemolytica*, both haemolytic and non-haemolytic phenotypes, may be recovered by culture of specimens on a modified Cary and Blair medium (Wild and Miller 1994).

3.3 *Pasteurella pneumotropica*

RODENTS

Pasteurella pneumotropica is a major cause of infectious complications often secondary to viral pneumonia in laboratory rodents, especially mice, rats and hamsters (Carthew and Gannon 1981). Although primary infections, e.g. abscesses (Wilson 1976) and otitis media (Eamens 1984), can occur, secondary opportunistic infections ensue because rodents become colonized with *P. pneumotropica* within 24 h of birth (Mikazuki et al. 1994). In mice 0–15 weeks old, *P. pneumotropica* may be isolated from the upper respiratory and lower intestinal tracts, faeces and the vagina through which newborn mice are colonized. In adult female rats, the vaginal counts of *P. pneumotropica* increase dramatically during oestrus in association with an increase in cornified non-nucleated epithelial cells for which *P. pneumotropica* has a high affinity.

Transmission of *P. pneumotropica* (Yamada, Baba and Arakawa 1983) in mouse colonies may occur through the respiratory route or through contact with contaminated faeces. As colonization occurs shortly after birth, *P. pneumotropica* is often regarded as a latent infection with a propensity for exacerbation under appropriate conditions. Latent infection has also been documented in horses, calves, dogs, humans and other species (Shepherd, Leman and Barnett 1982). *P. pneumotropica* was also isolated from the nasopharynx of 2 of 5 rabbits obtained from a 'Pasteurella-free' production colony in the absence of disease (Kirchner, Magoc and Sidor 1983). Mice latently infected with *P. pneumotropica* develop antibodies to several cell wall antigens which may be detected by an enzyme-linked immunosorbent assay (ELISA) (Manning et al. 1991).

To date, virulence traits of *P. pneumotropica* have not been detected.

3.4 *Pasteurella* infections in humans

P. multocida is the most frequently isolated *Pasteurella* sp. from human infections. As a colonizer of the mucous membranes of the upper respiratory tract of a wide variety of wild and domesticated animals, especially dogs and cats, human exposure to this species is heightened. Whereas most human infections ensue subsequent to traumatic introduction of *P. multocida* through the skin secondary to dog or cat bites or scratch, the spectrum of human infections is not restricted by body compartments or fascial planes (Weber et al. 1984).

Following an animal bite, severe swelling and erythema may surround the traumatized tissue. If the penetrating animal bite has punctured the periosteum, osteomyelitis may result (Fig. 47.1). Complications of animal bites include cellulitis, abscess formation and bacteraemia, leading to metastatic foci in various organs and joints (Table 47.3).

Pulmonary infections in the setting of chronic lung disease is perhaps an underappreciated infectious complication associated with *P. multocida*, often mimicking *Haemophilus influenzae* in presentation. Considering the extent of human exposure to *P. multocida* through contact with domestic aninmals, it is noteworthy that this micro-organism is not a more frequent colonizer of the human upper respiratory tract. In the setting of compromised pulmonary architecture, as may exist in chronic obstructive pulmonary disease, *P. multocida* functions as an opportunistic colonizer of devitalized pulmonary tissue. Pulmonary involvement may range from colonization of the tracheobronchial tree to pneumonia and empyema with concomitant bacteraemia (Table 47.3). Furthermore, *P. multocida* is often present as a mucoid highly encapsulated phenotype when recovered from the respiratory tract of patients with chronic pulmonary disease (Fig. 47.2).

Primary bacteraemia from a point inoculation or transgression across a mucous membrane usually

Table 47.3 Documented human *P. multocida* infections

Local
Skin and bone infections
cellulitis
osteomyelitis
septic arthritis
subcutaneous abscesses
Systemic
Blood and vascular
endocarditis
infected vascular graft pericarditis
mycotic aneurysm
pericarditis
septicaemia
Central nervous system
cerebral abscesses
meningitis
Respiratory
empyema
epiglottitis
lung abscess
pneumonia
pharyngitis
sinusitis
Uncommon
Abdominal
appendicitis
hepatosplenic abscesses
peritonitis
renal abscess
upper genitourinary tract
Ocular
conjunctivitis
corneal ulcer
endophthalmitis

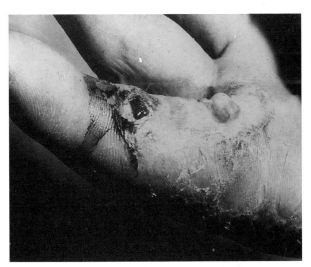

Fig. 47.1 Cellulitis and underlying osteomyelitis of finger caused by *Pasteurella multocida* subsequent to penetrating cat bite.

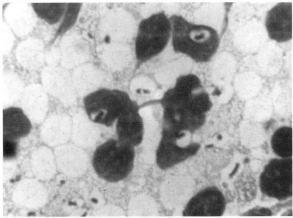

Fig. 47.2 Gram stain smear of purulent pulmonary exudate showing encapsulated diplobacillary forms of *Pasteurella multocida* ($\times$ 535).

occurs mainly in patients with an underlying hepatic dysfunction such as cirrhosis, hepatitis and carcinoma (Weber et al. 1984). Alternatively, *P. multocida* may gain access to the bloodstream through the gastrointestinal tract as suggested by the development of spontaneous bacterial peritonitis in a patient with hepatic cirrhosis (Gerding et al. 1976, Vakil et al. 1984). Two cases of *P. multocida* peritonitis developed in patients undergoing out-patient peritoneal dialysis subsequent to a cat scratch (Paul and Rostand 1987) and cat bite (London and Bottone 1991) to the peritoneal dialysis tubing.

Central nervous system infections have developed following a penetrating cranial dog bite (Klein and Cohen 1978), through contiguity from an infected adjacent site (Larsen, Harris and Holden 1969), and by haematogenous spread from a primary focus. Ocular infections have also occurred secondary to animal contact (Weber et al. 1984). Although most human infections are associated with some form of animal contact, there are numerous instances in which this association cannot be established (Itoh et al. 1980, Hubbert and Rosen 1970). Human infections caused by *P. haemolytica* (cutaneous, endocarditis, septicaemia), *P. dagmatis* (endocarditis, wound infection), *P. pneumotropica* (wounds, bone, joint, septicaemia) and *P. ureae* (meningitis, peritonitis, septicaemia, pneumonia) have also occurred.

REFERENCES

Abdullal KM, Udoh EA et al., 1992, A neutral glycoprotease of *Pasteurella haemolytica* A1 specifically cleaves O-sialoglycoproteins, *Infect Immun*, **60:** 56–62.

Adam C, Knights JM et al., 1984, Purification, characterization and immunological properties of the serotype-specific capsular polysaccharide of *Pasteurella haemolytica* (serotype A1) organisms, *J Gen Microbiol*, **130:** 2415–26.

Biberstein EL, 1981, Haemophilus, Pasteurella, *and* Actinobacillus, eds Kilian M, Fredericksen W, Biberstein EL, Academic Press, London, 61–74.

Bisgaard M, Holtberg O, Frederiksen W, 1991, Isolation of *Pasteurella caballi* from an infected wound on a veterinary surgeon, *APMIS*, **99:** 291–4.

Carrigan MJ, Dawkins HJ et al., 1991, *Pasteurella multocida* septicemia in fallow deer (*Dama dama*), *Aust Vet J*, **68:** 201–3.

Carter GR, 1962, Further observations on typing *Pasteurella multocida* by the indirect hemagglutination test, *Can J Comp Med Vet Sci*, **26:** 238–40.

Carthew P, Gannon J, 1981, Secondary infection of rat lungs with *Pasteurella pneumotropica* after Kilham rat virus infection, *Lab Anim*, **15:** 219–21.

Christiansen KH, Carpenter TE et al., 1992, Transmission of *Pasteurella multocida* on California turkey premises in 1988–89, *Avian Dis*, **36:** 262–71.

Ciprian A, Pijoan C et al., 1988, Mycoplasma hypopneumoniae increases the susceptibility of pigs to experimental *Pasteurella multocida* pneumonia, *Can J Vet Res*, **52:** 434–8.

Clinkenbeard KD, Mosier DA, Confer AW, 1989, Transmembrane pore size and role of cell swelling in cytotoxicity caused by *Pasteurella haemolytica* leukotoxin, *Infect Immun*, **57:** 420–5.

Confer AW, Panciera RJ, Mosier DA, 1986, Serum antibodies to *Pasteurella haemolytica* lipopolysaccharide: relationship to experimental bovine pneumonic pasteurellosis, *Am J Vet Res*, **47:** 1134–8.

Confer AW, Simons KR, 1986, Effects of *Pasteurella haemolytica* lipopolysaccharide or selected functions of bovine leukocytes, *Am J Vet Res*, **47:** 154–7.

Confer AW, Panciera RJ et al., 1990, Molecular aspects of virulence of *Pasteurella haemolytica*, *Can J Vet Res*, **54, Suppl.:** S48–52.

Conlon JA, Shewen PE, 1993, Clinical and serological evaluation of *Pasteurella haemolytica* A1 capsular polysaccharide vaccine, *Vaccine*, **11:** 767–72.

Coombs SM, Botzler RG, 1991, Correlations of daily activity with avian cholera mortality among wildfowl, *J Wildl Dis*, **27:** 543–50.

DiGiacomo RF, Jones CD, Wathes CM, 1987, Transmission of *Pasteurella multocida* in rabbits, *Lab Anim Sci*, **37:** 621–3.

Dominick MA, Rimler RB, 1986, Turbinate atrophy in gnotobiotic pigs intranasally inoculated with protein toxin isolated from type D *Pasteurella multocida*, *Am J Vet Res*, **47:** 1532–6.

Eamens GJ, 1984, Bacterial and mycoplasmal flora of the middle ear of laboratory rats with otitis media, *Lab Anim Sci*, **34:** 480–3.

Elias B, Boros G et al., 1990, Clinical and pathological effects of the dermonecrotic toxin of *Bordetella bronchiseptica* and *Pasteurella multocida* in specific-pathogen-free piglets, *Nippon Juigaku Zasshi*, **52:** 677–88.

Frame DD, Clark FD, Smart RA, 1994, Recurrent outbreaks of a cutaneous form of *Pasteurella multocida* infection in turkeys, *Avian Dis*, **38:** 390–2.

Francis DP, Holmes MA, Brandon G, 1975, *Pasteurella multocida*. Infections after domestic animal bites and scratches, *JAMA*, **233:** 42–5.

Frank GH, Tabatabai LB, 1981, Neuraminidase activity of *Pasteurella haemolytica* isolates, *Infect Immun*, **32:** 1119–22.

Gerding DN, Kham MY et al., 1976, *Pasteurella multocida* peritonitis in hepatic cirrhosis with ascites, *Gastroenterology*, **70:** 413–15.

Hassan AK, Mustafa AA, 1985, Isolation of *Pasteurella multocida* type B from an outbreak of haemorrhagic septicemia in camels in the Sudan, *Rev Elev Med Vet Pays Trop*, **38:** 31–3.

Henricks PA, Binkhorst GJ, Nijkamp FP, 1987, Stress diminishes infiltration and oxygen metabolism of phagocytic cells in calves, *Inflammation*, **11:** 427–37.

Holmes MA, Brandon G, 1965, *Pasteurella multocida* infections in 16 persons in Oregon, *Public Health Rep*, **80:** 1107–12.

Hubbert WT, Rosen MN, 1970, *Pasteurella multocida* infection in man unrelated to animal bites, *Am J Public Health*, **60:** 1109–17.

Itoh M, Tierno PM et al., 1980, A unique outbreak of *Pasteurella multocida* in a chronic disease hospital, *Am J Public Health*, **70:** 1170–3.

Jeffreys JS, Shivaprasad HL et al., 1993, Facial cellulitis associated with fowl cholera in commercial turkeys, *Avian Dis*, **37:** 1121–9.

de Jong MF, Akkermans JP, 1986, Investigation into the pathogenesis of atrophic rhinitis in pigs. I. Atrophic rhinitis caused by *Bordetella bronchiseptica* and *Pasteurella multocida* and the meaning of a thermolabile toxin of *P. multocida*, *Vet Q,* **8:** 204–14.

de Jong MF, de Wachter JC, Marcel GM, 1986, Investigation into the pathogenesis of atrophic rhinitis in pigs. II. AR induction and protection after intramuscular injection of cell-free filtrates and emulsions containing AR toxin of *Pasteurella multocida*, *Vet Q,* **8:** 215–24.

Kachler KL, Markum RJF et al., 1980, Evidence of cytocidal effects of *Pasteurella haemolytica* on bovine peripheral blood mononuclear leukocytes, *Am J Vet Res*, **41:** 1690–3.

Kamp EM, Terlaak EA, de Jong MF, 1990, Atypical *Pasteurella* strains producing a toxin similar to the dermonecrotic toxin of *Pasteurella multocida* subspecies *multocida*, *Vet Rec*, **126:** 434–7.

Kirchner BK, Magoc TJ, Sidor MA, 1983, *Pasteurella pneumotropica* in rabbits from a '*Pasteurella*-free' production colony, *Lab Anim Sci*, **33:** 461–2.

Klein DM, Cohen ME, 1978, *Pasteurella multocida* brain abscess following penetrating cranial dog bite, *J Pediatr*, **92:** 588–9.

Knight DP, Paine JE, Speller DC, 1983, A selective medium for *Pasteurella multocida* and its use with animal and human specimens, *J Clin Pathol*, **36:** 591–4.

Larsen TE, Harris L, Holden FA, 1969, Isolation of *Pasteurella multocida* from an otogenic cerebellar abscess, *Can Med Assoc J*, **101:** 629–30.

London RL, Bottone EJ, 1991, *Pasteurella multocida*: zoonotic cause of peritonitis in a patient undergoing peritoneal dialysis, *Am J Med*, **91:** 202–4.

Manning PJ, DeLong D et al., 1991, An enzyme-linked immunosorbent assay for detection of chronic subclinical *Pasteurella pneumotropica* infection in mice, *Lab Anim Sci*, **41:** 162–5.

Martineau-Doize B, Frantz JC, Martineau GP, 1990, Effects of purified *Pasteurella multocida* dermonecrotoxin on cartilage and bone of the nasal ventral conchae of the piglet, *Anat Rec*, **228:** 237–46.

Mikazuki K, Hirasawa T et al., 1994, Colonization pattern of *Pasteurella pneumotropica* in mice with latent pasteurellosis, *Jikken Dobutsu*, **43:** 375–9.

Morck DW, Olson ME et al., 1989, Presence of bacterial glycocalyx and fimbriae on *Pasteurella haemolytica* in feedlot cattle with pneumonic pasteurellosis, *Can J Vet Res*, **53:** 167–71.

Müller HE, Krasemann C, 1974, Die Virulenz von *Pasteurella multocida*-Stammen und irhe Neuraminadase-Produktion, *Zentralbl Bakteriol [Orig A]*, **229:** 391–400.

Nagy LK, Penn CW, 1976, Protection of cattle against experimental haemorrhagic septicaemia by the capsular antigens of *Pasteurella multocida* types B and E, *Res Vet Sci*, **20:** 249–53.

Nakmine M, Ohshiro M et al., 1992, The first outbreak of fowl cholera in Muscovy ducks (*Cairina moschata*) in Japan, *J Vet Med Sci*, **54:** 1225–7.

Oberhofer TR, 1981, Characteristics and biotypes of *Pasteurella multocida* isolated from humans, *J Clin Microbiol*, **13:** 566–71.

Paul RV, Rostand SG, 1987, Cat-bite peritonitis: *Pasteurella multocida* peritonitis following feline contamination of peritoneal dialysis tubing, *Am J Kidney Dis*, **10:** 318–19.

Percy DH, Prescott JF, Bhasin JL, 1984, Characterization of *Pasteurella multocida* isolated from rabbits in Canada, *Can J Comp Med*, **48:** 162–5.

Petras SF, Chidambaram M et al., 1995, Antigenic and virulence properties of *Pasteurella haemolytica* leukotoxin mutants, *Infect Immun*, **63:** 1033–9.

Potter AA, Ready K, Gilchrist J, 1988, Purification of fimbriae from *Pasteurella haemolytica* A1, *Microb Pathog*, **4:** 311–16.

Queen C, Ward AC, Hunter DL, 1994, Bacteria isolated from nasal and tonsillar samples of clinically healthy Rocky Mountain bighorn and domestic sheep, *J Wildl Dis*, **30:** 1–7.

Rhoades KR, Rimler RB, 1990, Virulence and toxigenicity of capsular serogroup D *Pasteurella multocida* strains isolated from avian hosts, *Avian Dis*, **34:** 384–8.

Rhoades KR, Rimler RB, Bagley RA, 1992, Fowl cholera epornitic: antigenic characterization and virulence of selected *Pasteurella multocida* isolates, *Avian Dis*, **36:** 84–7.

Riet-Correa F, Mendez MC et al., 1992, Bovine focal proliferative fibrogranulomatous panniculitis (lechiguana) associated with *Pasteurella granulomatis*, *Vet Pathol*, **29:** 93–103.

Rimler RB, Rhoades KR, 1987, Serogroup F, a new capsule serogroup of *Pasteurella multocida*, *J Clin Microbiol*, **25:** 615–18.

Rimler RB, Rhoades KR, Jones TO, 1987, Serological and immunological study of *Pasteurella multocida* strains that produced septicaemia in fallow deer, *Vet Rec*, **121:** 300–1.

Rutter JM, Taylor RJ et al., 1984, Epidemiological study of *Pasteurella multocida* and *Bordetella bronchiseptica* in atrophic rhinitis, *Vet Rec*, **115:** 615–19.

Sclater LK, Brenner DJ et al., 1989, *Pasteurella caballi*, a new species from equine clinical specimens, *J Clin Microbiol*, **27:** 2169–74.

Shepherd AJ, Leman PA, Barnett RJ, 1982, Isolation of *Pasteurella pneumotropica* from rodents in South Africa, *J Hyg Lond*, **89:** 79–87.

Shewen PE, Wilkie BN, 1982, Cytotoxin of *Pasteurella haemolytica* acting on bovine leukocytes, *Infect Immun*, **35:** 91–4.

Shewen PE, Wilkie BN, 1983, *Pasteurella haemolytica* cytotoxin neutralizing activity in sera from Ontario beef cattle, *Can J Comp Med*, **47:** 497–8.

Smith JE, 1955, Studies on *Pasteurella septica*. I. The occurrence in the nose and tonsils of dogs, *J Comp Pathol*, **65:** 239–45.

Smith JE, 1958, Studies on *Pasteurella septica*. II. Some cultural and biochemical properties of strains from different host species, *J Comp Pathol*, **68:** 315–33.

Squire PG, Smiley DW, Croskell RB, 1984, Identification and extraction of *Pasteurella haemolytica* membrane proteins, *Infect Immun*, **45:** 667–73.

Straus DC, Unbehagen PJ, Purdy CW, 1993, Neuraminidase production by a *Pasteurella haemolytica* A1 strain associated with bovine pneumonia, *Infect Immun*, **61:** 253–9.

Thompson RG, Benson ML, Savan M, 1969, Pneumonic pasteurellosis of cattle: microbiology and immunology, *Can J Comp Med*, **33:** 194–206.

Tigges MG, Loan RW, 1993, Serum antibody response to purified *Pasteurella haemolytica* capsular polysaccharide in cattle, *Am J Vet Res*, **54:** 856–61.

Vakil N, Adiyody J et al., 1984, *Pasteurella multocida* septicemia and peritonitis in a patient with cirrhosis: case report and review of the literature, *Am J Gastroenterol*, **80:** 565–8.

Watkins GH, Scott MJ, Jones JE, 1992, The effect of inoculation of *Pasteurella haemolytica* into the lactating mammary gland of mice, rats, rabbits, sows, and cows, *J Comp Pathol*, **106:** 221–8.

Weaver RC, Hollis DG, Bottone EJ, 1985, Gram-negative fermentative bacteria and *Francisella tularensis*, *Manual of Clinical Microbiology*, 4th edn, American Society for Microbiology, Washington, DC, 305–29.

Weber DJ, Wolfson JS et al., 1984, *Pasteurella multocida* infections. Report of 34 cases and review of the literature, *Medicine (Baltimore)*, **63:** 133–54.

White DJ, Jolley WL et al., 1995, Extracellular neuraminidase production by a *Pasteurella multocida* A:3 strain associated with bovine pneumonia, *Infect Immun*, **63:** 1703–9.

Wild MA, Miller MW, 1994, Effects of modified Cary and Blair medium on recovery of nonhemolytic *Pasteurella haemolytica* from Rocky Mountain bighorn sheep (*Ovis canadensis canadensis*) pharyngeal swabs, *J Wildl Dis*, **30:** 16–19.

Wilson P, 1976, *Pasteurella pneumotropica* as the causal organism of abscesses in the masseter muscle of mice, *Lab Anim*, **10:** 171–2.

Yamada S, Baba E, Arakawa A, 1983, Proliferation of *Pasteurella pneumotropica* at oestrus in the vagina of rats, *Lab Anim*, **17:** 261–6.

Yates WDG, 1982, A review of infectious bovine rhinotracheitis, shipping fever pneumonia and viral–bacterial synergism in respiratory disease of cattle, *Can J Comp Med*, **46:** 225–63.

Yoo HS, Maheswaran SK et al., 1995, Induction of inflammatory cytokines in bovine alveolar macrophages following stimulation with *Pasteurella haemolytica* lipopolysaccharide, *Infect Immun*, **63:** 381–8.

Younan M, Fodar L, 1995, Characterization of a new *Pasteurella haemolytica* serotype (A17), *Res Vet Sci*, **58:** 98.

Chapter 48

BARTONELLOSIS AND CAT SCRATCH DISEASE

C J Hunter and W A Petri

1 INTRODUCTION

Although cat scratch disease (CSD) has been recognized as a distinct clinical entity with a presumed infectious aetiology for many years, it is only in the last decade that the agents of this disease have been definitively identified and the relationship of this to other related disorders defined. Through the use of molecular techniques the primary agent of CSD, a previously unrecognized gram-negative organism, has been identified and subsequently has been cultured in cell-free media in vitro. Although originally classified as *Rochalimaea henselae*, this and other members of the genus *Rochalimaea* have been reassigned to the genus *Bartonella* based on studies of DNA homology.

Recent work has expanded the spectrum of disease produced by *Bartonella henselae* to include relapsing bacteraemia, bacillary angiomatosis (BA) and bacillary peliosis (BP). These last 2 entities were recognized in the 1980s in patients with acquired immunodeficiency syndrome (AIDS) and have striking similarities to the chronic manifestations of bartonellosis, as described in South America more than 80 years ago. In addition, it is now clear that other species, particularly *Bartonella quintana*, can produce illness that on occasion overlaps the clinical spectrum associated with *B. henselae*. Several excellent reviews have been published (Schwartzman 1992, Thompkins and Steigbigel 1993, Adal, Cockerell and Petri 1994, Hensel and Slater 1995).

2 *BARTONELLA* RELATED DISEASE

2.1 Pathogenesis

The *Bartonella* have limited potential for invasion and low virulence, analogous to organisms of the closely related genus *Brucella*. Infections are produced only after direct inoculation of bacteria through a defect in the integument. In vitro studies have demonstrated low endotoxin potency and diminished induction of neutrophil oxidative metabolism, degranulation and chemotaxis by *B. henselae* compared to *Escherichia coli* (Fumarola et al. 1994). These organisms, like *Brucella*, are considered intracellular pathogens. As is typical for organisms of marginal pathogenicity and the capability for intracellular growth, the clinical spectrum of disease is wide and is greatly influenced by the immune status of the host.

In vitro studies have shown a trypsin sensitive cytosolic factor in *B. henselae*, *B. bacilliformis* and some strains of *B. quintana* which can stimulate proliferation and migration of endothelial cells (Conley, Slater and Hamilton 1994). Species of *Bartonella* are tropic for endothelial and red blood cells. These findings may explain the vasoproliferative histopathological change in some patients with *Bartonella* associated disease and the haemolytic anaemia produced by *B. bacilliformis* (see p. 942).

2.2 Modes of transmission

The *Bartonella* require an ectoparasite for transmission. *B. bacilliformis* is transmitted by a sandfly, *B. quintana* by the body louse (*Pediculus humanus*) and *B. henselae* is most likely transmitted by a cat flea (*Ctenocephalides felis*). The relationship of *B. quintana* with its vector has been studied most extensively. After feeding on bacteraemic humans, the organisms localize to the gastrointestinal tract of lice and can be excreted in the faeces for the duration of the parasite's life without shortening its life span. The bacteria are quite resistant to cold and drying and may remain viable for weeks or months in desiccated lice faeces. Trench fever can be produced by rubbing lice excrement on abraded skin; transmission by lice from person to person has been established under controlled conditions. Direct person-to-person spread has not been documented. The infrequency of *B. quintana* infection in humans other than wartime epidemics may be explained by the apparent absence of an animal reservoir and lack of transovarial passage in lice.

One reservoir for *B. henselae* is the cat. Koehler et al. (1994) found *B. henselae* in blood cultures from 25 of 61 (41%) healthy asymptomatic impounded and domestic cats in the San Francisco Bay area. Some of these animals were bacteraemic over a period of more than a year. Although bacteraemia is not associated with specific illness in cats, regional unexplained lymphadenopathy is common in general veterinary practice (Groves and Harrington 1994). Zangwill et al. (1993) found serological evidence of past infection in 81% of cats of CSD patients compared to 38% of control cats. In unselected populations, <5% of people are seropositive, although 24% of veterinary workers demonstrated antibody production in one study (Carithers 1985). *B. henselae* has been demonstrated in the feline flea by PCR amplification of 16S rRNA (Koehler et al. 1994).

2.3 Clinical manifestations

Cat scratch disease was first recognized in both the United States and France in 1932 (Debré et al. 1950). Most often the disease begins with a papular skin lesion at the site of inoculation 4–6 days after a cat scratch injury to an extremity, or the head and neck. This is followed at an interval of 1–7 weeks by regional, most often cervical, lymphadenopathy which suppurates in the minority of cases. Resolution of signs and symptoms generally occurs in weeks to several months regardless of therapy. Diagnosis has generally relied on a constellation of findings including a history of cat exposure, regional lymphadenopathy, characteristic histopathology and reactivity to skin test antigens prepared from purulent material obtained from lymph nodes of established cases. Currently, specific laboratory tests such as EIA for anti-*B. henselae* antibodies are available for the diagnosis of CSD (see p. 944).

Approximately 10% of persons develop atypical manifestations which include lesions of the liver and spleen which may mimic the clinical presentation of metastatic neoplasm, osteomyelitis, soft tissue abscess, encephalitis, seizure, transverse myelitis and vitritis (Carithers 1985). Despite the sometimes severe nature of the symptoms and signs of atypical CSD, documented cases of significant long-term morbidity are unusual (Revol et al. 1992) and death is rare. In contrast to typical CSD, atypical CSD may respond to therapy.

Originally described by Stoler et al. in 1983, bacillary angiomatosis (BA) and related conditions are manifestations of systemic involvement by *B. henselae* or *B. quintana*, characterized by vasoformative and inflammatory lesions of the skin, subcutis, liver and spleen, occasionally involving lymph nodes, conjunctiva, tracheobroncheal tree and brain (Koehler and Tappero 1993, Cotell and Noskin 1994). The relationship to the agent of CSD was first postulated in 1988 (Koehler et al. 1988, Leboit et al. 1988). The majority of affected persons have established AIDS (average CD4 count 57 mm^{-1}) at the time of diagnosis; however, in one-third it is the initial AIDS-defining illness. A small subset of cases occurs in those immunosuppressed by cancer or organ transplantation therapy and BA is rarely identified in healthy adults without identifiable predisposition (Lucey et al. 1992, Tappero et al. 1993a, 1993b).

B. quintana is responsible for trench fever, which occurred almost exclusively during the first and second world wars. Epidemics involved more than a million soldiers, producing a febrile and often relapsing illness associated with variable morbidity but little or no mortality. Aside from epidemics associated with crowding and poor hygiene, disease due to *B. quintana* has infrequently been identified. Recently, however, this organism has been documented to be an uncommon cause of CSD (Raoult et al. 1994) and BA (Maurin et al. 1994). Additionally, this bacterium has been associated with relapsing bacteraemia in AIDS patients and with bacteraemia in a regional cluster of homeless alcoholic men and a single case of endocarditis (Larson et al. 1994, Drancourt et al. 1995, Spach et al. 1995).

Infection with *B. bacilliformis* is limited to the distribution of its vector, the sandfly, to the Andes mountains and river valleys of Chile, Ecuador and Columbia at elevations of 2000–8000 feet (600–2400 m) and is responsible for 2 clinical syndromes. Oroya fever is characterized by a febrile illness of variable severity and duration, similar to trench fever. A unique feature of this disorder is profound haemolytic anaemia which has been associated with significant morbidity and occasional mortality. Verruga peruana is an indolent chronic form which manifests months after infection with vasoproliferative cutaneous lesions histopathologically similar to those of bacillary peliosis.

A single case report of endocarditis due to *B. elizabethae* has been reported (Daly et al. 1993). *B. vinsonii* has not been associated with human illness.

3 EPIDEMIOLOGY

Two recent studies in the USA have helped define the epidemiology of CSD (Jackson, Perkins and Wenger 1993, Zangwell et al. 1993). These studies, based on diagnoses using clinical, historical and skin test reactivity, showed an incidence of 2–9 cases per 100 000 persons per year in ambulatory care settings. They confirmed the previous association with kittens and minor trauma, the seasonal predominance (autumn) and a wide age range with a peak incidence in the second decade. The seasonal predominance can be explained by the tendency for kittens to be most numerous in the autumn and to be more apt to carry fleas than adult cats. BA is also epidemiologically linked to cat exposure and *Bartonella* species have been identified by culture or molecular techniques in patient tissues, cats and a cat flea. There are, however, some patients with CSD or BA that have no exposure to cats or fleas; therefore an alternative reservoir or vector may exist (Tappero et al. 1993b).

4 HOST RESPONSE

The host response to *Bartonella* infection depends on a number of factors, including the patient's age, immune status, site of inoculation, species of organism and perhaps other as yet unidentified factors. In the most common scenario a healthy child or adult sustains a mild injury while playing with a cat which presumably transmits the organism via saliva or flea excreta. A localized, self-limited inflammatory skin lesion develops with seeding of organisms via lymphatics to regional lymph nodes, producing the clinical picture recognized as CSD for many years. Enlarged lymph nodes demonstrate characteristic histopathological changes characterized by follicular hyperplasia, mixed granulomatous and pyogenic inflammation and stellate microabscesses. Organisms are identified by Warthin–Starry, modified Brown–Hopps (tissue gram) or Giemsa stain in the necrotic zones of lymph nodes in 35–85% of cases (Wear et al. 1983, Min et al. 1994).

In most instances the disease remains localized, or if systemic it is subclinical. Occasionally the organism disseminates haematogenously, producing visceral, central nervous system, ocular or skeletal disease characterized by inflammatory lesions and discomfort or dysfunction. Those with hepatic and splenic involvement often present with prolonged fever, significant constitutional symptoms, mild abdominal pain and radiographically demonstrable lesions. Organisms have been identified in visceral lesions by Warthin–Starry stain (Malatack and Jaffe 1993).

B. henselae, the agent of most CSD, typically produces disseminated disease in immunocompromised adults, resulting in vasoformative inflammatory lesions of the skin, subcutis, viscera, bone and central nervous system (bacillary angiomatosis). In most instances the histopathology findings include vascular proliferation and inflammation. The degree of vascular prolifer-ation may be such that the lesion must be differentiated from vascular neoplasia or Kaposi's sarcoma. In other cases, the vascular lesions consist of large blood-filled spaces that mimic the changes seen with non-infectious peliosis hepatis. In other instances vascular proliferation is scant or absent and inflammation predominates (Slater et al. 1994). In any case, large numbers of extra- and intracellular organisms are generally present. Identical disease can be produced by both *B. henselae* and *B. quintana*. In addition, both organisms have been responsible for relapsing bacteraemic fever in the immunocompromised host without localized disease (Slater et al. 1989, Lucey et al. 1992, Regnery et al. 1992a, Welch et al. 1992). *B. henselae* has been implicated as a cause of encephalopathy in AIDS patients.

B. bacilliformis, although geographically limited, has received increased attention because of the more recently described related organisms. As previously mentioned, this organism produces a spectrum of illness from asymptomatic bacteraemia to indolent disseminated vasoproliferative lesions (verruga peruana) similar to those produced by *B. henselae* (Arias-Stella et al. 1986). Like the lesion of bacillary angiomatosis, the degree of vascular proliferation and inflammation is variable. In contrast to BA, organisms are not readily identifiable in verrugo of *B. bacilliformis* using Warthin–Starry staining but are identified in the extracellular space by electron microscopy. Unlike *B. henselae*, *B. bacilliformis* is able to produce severe systemic manifestations (haemolysis) and disseminates frequently in the immunocompetent host.

5 AETIOLOGICAL AGENTS: *AFIPIA FELIS* AND THE BARTONELLAE

As of 1989, the family Bartonellaceae resided within the order Rickettsiales and contained a single species, *Bartonella bacilliformis* (Brenner et al. 1991b).

Rochalimaea quintana, *R. vinsonii* and the newly identified agents *R. henselae* and *R. elizabethae* phenotypically and genotypically are most closely aligned with *B. bacilliformis*; therefore it has been proposed that all 5 species be classified within the genus *Bartonella* (Brenner et al. 1993). In addition, Brenner suggests the family Bartonellaceae be removed from the order Rickettsiales. The relationship of members of *Bartonella* to each other and the other members of the proteobacteria, including *Afipia felis*, is presented in Fig. 48.1.

CSD was confirmed as an infectious disease in 1983 by Wear and colleagues who demonstrated small pleomorphic bacilli in tissue sections from 29 of 34 lymph nodes using the Warthin–Starry silver stain. The organisms were intracellular, often associated with endothelium and macrophages, limited to areas of inflammation, and identified by antibodies from the sera of convalescent patients. English et al. (1988) published the first report of in vitro propagation of a small gram-negative organism in 10 of 19 lymph nodes. Hyperimmune sera raised to one isolate

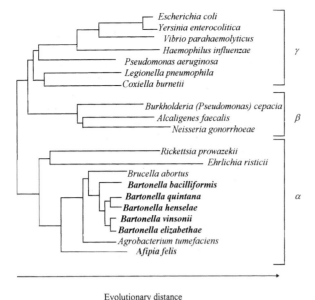

Escherichia coli
Yersinia enterocolitica
Vibrio parahaemolyticus
Haemophilus influenzae
Pseudomonas aeruginosa
Legionella pneumophila
Coxiella burnetii

γ

Burkholderia (Pseudomonas) cepacia
Alcaligenes faecalis
Neisseria gonorrhoeae

β

Rickettsia prowazekii
Ehrlichia risticii
Brucella abortus
Bartonella bacilliformis
Bartonella quintana
Bartonella henselae
Bartonella vinsonii
Bartonella elizabethae
Agrobacterium tumefaciens
Afipia felis

α

Evolutionary distance

Fig. 48.1 Phylogenic relationship of *Bartonella, Afipia* and other proteobacteria. (Adapted from Relman et al. 1992, Brenner et al. 1993).

reacted with the 9 other organisms. Additionally, serum from 19 of 34 patients reacted at titres at least 4-fold higher than negative controls with this same isolate. This unique organism was named *Afipia felis* (Brenner et al. 1991a). Although responsible for some cases of CSD, including some atypical forms (Bernini, Gorczyca and Modlin 1994), the weight of current evidence indicates that the vast majority of CSD is due to *B. henselae.*

B. henselae was first propagated in vitro by Slater in 1989 from febrile immunocompromised patients using blood cultures processed by the lysis-centrifugation technique. Electrophoresis of cell wall proteins and RFLP analysis of DNA revealed unique patterns that were similar, but not identical to those of *B. quintana.* Subsequent publications confirmed this observation and expanded the spectrum of disease produced by this bacterium to include bacillary angiomatosis and bacillary peliosis (Relman et al. 1990, Cockerell et al. 1991, Koehler et al. 1992, Slater, Welch and Min 1992). Comprehensive analysis of blood isolates (Welch et al. 1992) revealed biochemical characteristics, cell wall fatty acid composition and DNA hybridization data which supported the unique character of *B. henselae,* its close phylogenetic relation to *B. quintana* and lack of relatedness to *A. felis.* Additional studies such as 16s rRNA sequencing, RFLP of the citrate synthetase gene, and biochemical profiles have confirmed the unique identity of *B. henselae* (Regnery et al. 1992a, 1992b, 1992c, Welch et al. 1992, Matar et al. 1993). Recognizing the morphological similarity of the organisms seen in tissues of patients with CSD and bacillary angiomatosis, a number of investigators have sought and found strong evidence implicating *B. henselae* in most cases of CSD.

The association of *B. henselae* and cat scratch disease

has been investigated using serum indirect fluorescent antibodies (IFA), enzyme immunoassay (EIA), tissue immunocytochemistry and PCR amplification of 16S rRNA. Slater et al. (1992) established the production of strain-specific antibodies to *B. henselae* and *B. quintana* following experimental infection in mice. A serum IFA assay for *B. henselae* antibody developed at the Centers for Disease Control found titres of 1:64 in 88% of suspected cases of CSD while 94% of controls had titres less than 1:64. A minority of patients also had low titre antibody to *B. quintana* and *A. felis* (Regnery et al. 1992c). A similar assay, developed in France, produced titres at a dilution of 1:50 or greater in one-half to two-thirds of clinically diagnosed cases of CSD. None of the patients demonstrated titres of 1:50 or greater to *A. felis.* None of the negative control group patients was seropositive for either *A. felis* or *B. henselae* (Raoult, Tissot Dupont and Enea-Mutilod 1994). A microtitre plate EIA has also been developed which appears to identify more than 90% of positive cases and does not cross-react with *A. felis* (Barka et al. 1993).

Antibody raised in rabbits to outer-membrane extracts of *B. henselae* identified 13 isolates from blood, cutaneous bacillary angiomatosis, bacillary peliosis and bacillary splenosis. The antiserum showed no cross-reactivity to *A. felis* (Reed et al. 1992). Anderson et al. (1993), using 16s rRNA primers and species-specific oligonucleotide probes, detected DNA of *B. henselae* in lymph node tissue from 21 of 25 patients with CSD. *B. quintana* was not detected. In another PCR hybridization based study, *Bartonella* DNA was amplified from tissue of 96% of patients with skin-test positive CSD and 60% of those diagnosed on clinical criteria. *A. felis* was not detected in either group, although the sensitivity of the assay for this organism was reduced compared to *B. henselae* (Bergmans et al. 1995). DNA of *B. henselae* has been amplified from CSD skin antigen from 4 independent sources (Anderson et al. 1994, Bergmans et al. 1995). Additionally, *B. henselae* has been cultured from lymph node aspirates of 2 patients (Dolan et al. 1993).

6 LABORATORY ISOLATION, IDENTIFICATION AND SUSCEPTIBILITY TESTING

The *Bartonella* are fastidious, slow-growing, haemophilic organisms. *B. henselae* has been successfully cultivated on endothelial cell lines and a number of cell-free media (Koehler et al. 1992, Dolan et al. 1993, Welch et al. 1993). Specimens suitable for culture include blood, skin, lymph node or purulent material from deeper body sites. The majority of blood culture isolates of *Bartonella* have been with the use of the lysis-centrifugation system, resulting in titres of up to 1000 organisms per ml. *B. henselae, B. elizabethae* and *B. quintana* have been recovered from automated broth-based systems; however, because CO_2 production is generally not detected (even with prolonged incubation), samples from automated broth-based systems must be selectively subcultured based on acridine orange screening or blindly subcultured. Tissue homogenates may be directly plated to blood containing media.

Growth is best in Brucella compared to Columbia and brain–heart infusion based broth systems. *B. henselae* has been isolated on anaerobic blood, chocolate and charcoal-yeast extract agars; Columbia, brain–heart infusion or trypticase–soy agar supplemented with 5% sheep blood; and heart infusion agar supplemented with 5% rabbit blood. It appears that the growth-enhancing element of blood are associated with the cell membrane, as the supernatant of lysed red blood cells is suboptimal in promoting growth.

Schwartzman, Nesbit and Baron (1993) evaluated a number of blood-free culture systems and found the growth of *B. henselae* in Brucella broth or agar with 6–8% Fildes' solution and 250 µg of haemin per ml to be equivalent to that seen in blood-supplemented media. This level of haemin supplementation is 6-fold higher than the optimum required to augment growth of *B. quintana*. No unsupplemented agar supported more than minimal growth, nor can the organism be cultivated on MacConkey's, Sabouraud's dextrose, campylobacter or mycobacterium media. The organism requires CO_2, grows best at 30–35°C, and will not grow at 25 or 42°C. Cultures should be plated on media less than 2 weeks old and incubated at 35°C in 5% CO_2 and maintained for 3 weeks or more, as colonies are generally not seen for 5–15 days and may take as long as 7 weeks to appear.

B. henselae produces heterogeneous colonies that may be smooth, or rough resembling a cauliflower, small, grey or white, dry, and adhere to or pit the agar. They may satellite around *Micrococcus* species and *Staphylococcus aureus*. With serial passage, the colonies appear more quickly and lose the rough phenotype. The *Bartonella* are weakly gram-negative, non-acid-fast, pleomorphic, slightly curved rods 0.5 µm in diameter and 1.5–2 µm in length which display twitching motility. *B. henselae* does not appear to have a flagellum although *B. bacilliformis* has a single polar flagellum. Rare filamentous forms measure up to 6 µm. The organisms appear biochemically inert: they do not ferment or oxidize carbohydrates and they fail to react in tests for indole, ornithine decarboxylase, catalase, urease, aesculin hydrolysis, nitrate reduction and oxidase. Of 6 commercial identification systems, the MicroScan rapid anaerobe panel separated *B. henselae* and *B. quintana* with the greatest certainty (Welch et al. 1993).

Of 5 species of *Afipia* identified, only *Afipia felis* has been associated with cat-borne disease; all others have been isolated from wounds or respiratory sources (Brenner et al. 1991a). A single lymph node isolate of *A. felis* (Wear et al. 1983) grown in BHI-Biphasic broth produced 1.5 mm grey-white, opaque, glistening, convex, non-haemolytic colonies in 72 h on blood agar incubated at 32°C. Repeated subculture of this organism and isolates from 9 other patients produced 2 mm, slightly raised, transparent colonies that grew poorly or not at all when passed in hypertonic media.

These investigators believe the small colony variant represents cell wall defective (vegetative) forms. They grow on buffered charcoal yeast extract agar and nutrient broth but not on MacConkey's agar or in high salt media. Growth is best at 25–30°C, is diminished at 35°C and is completely inhibited at 42°C.

Afipia spp. are weakly gram-negative and motile via a single polar flagellum. Unlike *Bartonella*, they are oxidase, urease and catalase (weakly) positive. *Afipia* spp. do not react with the following reactions: H_2S (triple sugar agar and lead acetate strip), indole, citrate, aesculin hydrolysis. They produce acid weakly from D-xylose but not from D-mannitol, maltose, lactose or glucose. Some discriminating features of *Bartonella* and *Afipia* are summarized in Table 48.1.

Data on in vitro susceptibilities are limited and not standardized. Preliminary results suggest that *B. henselae* has favourable MICs to ampicillin, second and third generation cephalosporins, rifampin, tetracycline, chloramphenicol, trimethoprim–sulphamethoxazole, aminoglycosides and macrolides. They are relatively resistant to penicillin G, oxacillin and vancomycin and resistant to first generation cephalosporins (Dolan et al. 1993, Maurin and Raoult 1993). A single isolate of *B. quintana* displayed a similar pattern. An isolate of *B. elizabethae* from blood appeared sensitive to erythromycin, ciprofloxacin, cefoxitin, gentamicin, vancomycin and oxacillin (Daly et al. 1993). *A. felis* is sensitive to aminoglycosides, cefotaxime, cefoxitin and mezlocillin but resistant to ampicillin, cefazolin, cefoperazone, cephalothin, cefamandole, chloramphenicol, clindamycin, erythromycin, nitrofurantoin, penicillin G and tetracycline (Brenner et al. 1991a).

7   TREATMENT AND PREVENTION

Antibiotics appear to have a limited role in CSD. In a retrospective analysis of 268 patients receiving 18 different antibiotics, Margileth (1992) found evidence of efficacy for rifampin, ciprofloxacin, trimethoprim–sulphamethoxazole and gentamicin. This and other studies suggest that antibiotics are indicated in severe or atypical CSD and do little to alter the natural history of typical CSD. In contrast, BA often responds dramatically to antibiotics (erythromycin, azithromycin, rifampin, doxycycline, trimethoprim–sulphamethoxazole), particularly those with good intracellular penetration. Relapses are common and long-term or indefinite therapy may be needed in severely immunocompromised individuals.

8   SUMMARY

The past decade has produced a wealth of information about CSD and organisms of the genus *Bartonella* and has dramatically demonstrated the power of molecular techniques in investigations of infectious diseases. In the coming years the full clinical spectrum, epidemiology, pathogenesis and treatment and prevention strategies for *Bartonella* related disease should be

Table 48.1 Distinguishing features of *Bartonella* and related species

	Cellular fatty acid composition (%)				Biochemical reactions						% 16S rRNA homology *B. henselae*	Hybridization with *B. henselae* (%)	
	C16:1	C16:0	C18:1	C18:0	LYA	PRO	URE	LYAL	TYR	ILE		55°C	70°C
B. henselae	<1	16–22	51–58	18–26	+	+(96%)	−	+	+(40%)	+(40%)	100	92–100	100
B. quintana	<1	20–23	58	16–17	−	+	−	+	−	−	99.1–99.4	56–66	38
B. bacilliformis	18	25	35	7	+	−	−	−			98.5–98.8	43–47	35
B. elizabethae	1	15–18	39–43	8–9		+	−	−			99.2–99.4	49	16
B. vinsonii	2	18	45	9	−	−	−				99.3–99.5	55	29
Brucella sp.	8	24	58	10		+	+				95.7		
A. felis	6–9	3–4	28–43	9–12							90.7	1	1
R. prowazekii											86.3	14	2

Compiled from Slater et al. 1989, Brenner et al. 1991a, 1991b, Regnery et al. 1992a, 1992b, 1992c, Relman et al. 1992, Welch et al. 1992, 1993, Daly et al. 1993, Larson et al. 1994. LYA, lysine-β-naphthylamide (acid); PRO, L-proline-β-naphthylamide–Microscan Rapid Anaerobe Panel, Baxter Diagnostics; URE, urea; LYAL, L-lysyl-L-alanine; TYR, L-tyrosine; ILE, L-isoleucine–Rapid Yeast Identification Panel, Baxter Healthcare Corp.

firmly established. Recognition of cultural requirements, development of economical and commercially available serological and immunocytochemical reagents, and accumulation of biochemical phenotypic data on commercial identification systems should aid in establishing timely and specific diagnoses.

REFERENCES

Adal KA, Cockerell CJ, Petri WA Jr, 1994, Cat scratch disease, bacillary angiomatosis, and other infections due to *Rochalimaea*, *N Engl J Med*, **330**: 1509–15.

Anderson B, Kelly C et al., 1993, Detection of *Rochalimaea henselae* in cat scratch disease test antigens, *J Infect Dis*, **168**: 1034–6.

Anderson B, Sims K et al., 1994, Detection of *Rochalimaea henselae* DNA in specimens from cat scratch disease patients by PCR, *J Clin Microbiol*, **32**: 942–8.

Arias-Stella J, Lieberman PH et al., 1986, Histology, immunohistochemistry, and ultrastructure of the verruga in Carrion's disease, *Am J Surg Pathol*, **10**: 595–610.

Barka NE, Hadfield T et al., 1993, EIA for detection of *Rochalimaea henselae*-reactive IgG, IgM, and IgA antibodies in patients with suspected cat scratch disease, *J Infect Dis*, **167**: 1503–4.

Bergmans AM, Groothedde JW et al., 1995, Etiology of cat scratch disease: comparison of polymerase chain reaction detection of *Bartonella* (formerly *Rochalimaea*) and *Afipia felis* DNA with serology and skin tests, *J Infect Dis*, **171**: 916–23.

Bernini PM, Gorczyca JT, Modlin JF, 1994, Cat scratch disease presenting as a paravertebral abscess. A case report, *J Bone Joint Surg*, **76A**: 1858–63.

Brenner DJ, Hollis DG et al., 1991a, Proposal of *Afipia* gen. nov., with *Afipia felis* sp. nov. (formerly the cat scratch disease bacillus), *Afipia clevelandensis* sp. nov. (formerly the Cleveland Clinic Foundation strain), *Afipia broomeae* sp. nov., and three unnamed genospecies, *J Clin Microbiol*, **29**: 2450–60.

Brenner DJ, O'Conner SP et al., 1991b, Molecular characterization and proposal of a neotype strain for *Bartonella bacilliformis*, *J Clin Microbiol*, **29**: 1299–302.

Brenner DJ, O'Connor SP et al., 1993, Proposals to unify the genera *Bartonella* and *Rochalimaea*, with descriptions of *Bartonella quintana* comb. nov., *Bartonella vinsonii* comb. nov., *Bartonella henselae* comb. nov., and *Bartonella elizabethae* comb. nov., and to remove the family Bartonellaceae from the order Rickettsiales, *Int J Syst Bacteriol*, **43**: 777–86.

Carithers HA, 1985, Cat scratch disease: an overview based on a study of 1,200 patients, *Am J Dis Child*, **139**: 1124–33.

Cockerell CJ, Tierno PM et al., 1991, Clinical, histologic, microbiologic, and biochemical characterization of the causative agent of bacillary (epithelioid) angiomatosis: a rickettsial illness with features of bartonellosis, *J Invest Dermatol*, **97**: 812–17.

Conley T, Slater L, Hamilton K, 1994, *Rochalimaea* species stimulate human endothelial cell proliferation and migration in vitro, *J Lab Clin Med*, **124**: 521–8.

Cotell SL, Noskin GA, 1994, Bacillary angiomatosis, *Arch Intern Med*, **154**: 524–8.

Daly JS, Worthington MG et al., 1993, *Rochalimaea elizabethae* sp. nov. isolated from a patient with endocarditis, *J Clin Microbiol*, **31**: 872–81.

Debré R, Lamy M et al., 1950, La maladie des griffes de chat, *Bull Mem Soc Med Hop Paris*, **166**: 1462.

Dolan MJ, Wong MT et al., 1993, Syndrome of *Rochalimaea henselae* adenitis suggesting cat scratch disease, *Ann Intern Med*, **118**: 331–6.

Drancourt M, Mainardi JL et al., 1995, *Bartonella* (*Rochalimaea*) *quintana* endocarditis in three homeless men, *N Engl J Med*, **332**: 419–23.

English CK, Wear DJ et al., 1988, Cat scratch disease, *JAMA*, **259**: 1347–52.

Fumarola D, Giuliani G et al., 1994, Pathogenicity of cat scratch disease bacilli, *Pediatr Infect Dis J*, **13**: 162–3.

Groves MG, Harrington KS, 1994, *Rochalimaea henselae* infections: newly recognized zoonoses transmitted by domestic cats, *J Am Vet Med Assoc*, **204**: 267–71.

Hensel DM, Slater LN, 1995, The genus *Bartonella*, *Clin Microbiol Newslett*, **17**: 9–14.

Jackson LA, Perkins BA, Wenger JD, 1993, Cat scratch disease in the United States: an analysis of three national databases, *Am J Public Health*, **83**: 1707–11.

Koehler JE, Tappero JW, 1993, Bacillary angiomatosis and bacillary peliosis in patients infected with human immunodeficiency virus, *Clin Infect Dis*, **17**: 612–24.

Koehler JE, LeBoit PE et al., 1988, Cutaneous vascular lesions and disseminated cat scratch disease in patients with the acquired immunodeficiency syndrome (AIDS) and AIDS-related complex, *Ann Intern Med*, **109**: 449–55.

Koehler JE, Quinn FD et al., 1992, Isolation of *Rochalimaea* species from cutaneous and osseous lesions of bacillary angiomatosis, *N Engl J Med*, **327**: 1625–31.

Koehler JE, Glaser CA et al., 1994, *Rochalimaea henselae* infection: a new zoonosis with the domestic cat as reservoir, *JAMA*, **271**: 531–5.

Larson AM, Dougherty MJ et al., 1994, Detection of *Bartonella* (*Rochalimaea*) *quintana* by routine acridine orange staining of broth blood cultures, *J Clin Microbiol*, **32**: 1492–6.

LeBoit PE, Egbert BM et al., 1988, Epithelioid haemangioma-like vascular proliferation in AIDS: manifestation of cat scratch disease bacillus infection? *Lancet*, **1**: 960–3.

Lucey D, Dolan MJ et al., 1992, Relapsing illness due to *Rochalimaea henselae* in immunocompetent hosts: implications for therapy and new epidemiological associations, *Clin Infect Dis*, **14**: 683–8.

Malatack JJ, Jaffe R, 1993, Granulomatous hepatitis in three children due to cat scratch disease without peripheral adenopathy, *Am J Dis Child*, **147**: 949–53.

Margileth AM, 1992, Antibiotic therapy for cat scratch disease: clinical study of therapeutic outcome in 268 patients and a review of the literature, *Pediatr Infect Dis J*, **11**: 474–8.

Matar GM, Swaminathan B et al., 1993, Polymerase chain reaction-based restriction fragment length polymorphism analysis of a fragment of the ribosomal operon from *Rochalimaea* species for subtyping, *J Clin Microbiol*, **31**: 1730–4.

Maurin M, Raoult D, 1993, Antimicrobial susceptibility of *Rochalimaea quintana*, *Rochalimaea vinsonii*, and the newly recognized *Rochalimaea henselae*, *J Antimicrob Chemother*, **32**: 587–94.

Maurin M, Roux V et al., 1994, Isolation and characterization by immunoflourescence, sodium dodecyl-polyacrylamide gel electrophoresis, Western blot, restriction fragment length polymorphism-PCR, 16S rRNA gene sequencing, and pulsed-field gel electophoresis of *Rochalimaea quintana* from a patient with bacillary angiomatosis, *J Clin Microbiol*, **32**: 1166–71.

Min KW, Reed JA et al., 1994, Morphologically variable bacilli of cat scratch disease are identified by immunocytochemical labeling with antibodies to *Rochalimaea henselae*, *Am J Clin Pathol*, **101**: 607–10.

Raoult D, Tissot Dupont H and Enea-Mutillod M, 1994, Positive predictive value of *Rochalimaea henselae* antibodies in the diagnosis of cat scratch disease, *Clin Infect Dis*, **19**: 355.

Raoult D, Drancourt M et al., 1994, *Bartonella* (*Rochalimaea*) *quintana* isolation in patient with chronic adenopathy, lymphopenia and a cat, *Lancet*, **343**: 977.

Reed JA, Brigati DJ et al., 1992, Immunocytochemical identification of *Rochalimaea henselae* in bacillary (epithelioid) angiomatosis, parenchymal bacillary peliosis, and persistent fever with bacteremia, *Am J Surg Pathol*, **16**: 650–7.

Regnery RL, Anderson BE et al., 1992a, Characterization of a novel *Rochalimaea* species, *R. henselae* sp. nov., isolated from blood of a febrile, human immunodeficiency virus positive patient, *J Clin Microbiol*, **30:** 265–74.

Regnery RL, Martin M et al., 1992b, Naturally occurring '*Rochalimaea henselae*' infection in domestic cat, *Lancet*, **340:** 557.

Regnery RL, Olson JG et al., 1992c, Serological response to '*Rochalimaea henselae*' antigen in suspected cat scratch disease, *Lancet*, **339:** 1443–5.

Relman DA, Loutit JS et al., 1990, The agent of bacillary angiomatosis: an approach to the identification of uncultered pathogens, *N Engl J Med*, **323:** 1573–80.

Relman DA, Lepp PW et al., 1992, Phylogenetic relationships among the agent of bacillary angiomatosis, *Bartonella bacilliformis*, and other alpha proteobacteria, *Mol Microbiol*, **6:** 1801–7.

Revol A, Vighetto A et al., 1992, Encephalitis in cat scratch disease with persistent dementia, *J Neurol Neurosurg Psychiatry*, **55:** 133–5.

Schwartzman WA, 1992, Infections due to *Rochalimaea*: the expanding clinical spectrum, *Clin Infect Dis*, **15:** 893–902.

Schwartzman WA, Nesbit CA, Baron EJ, 1993, Development and evaluation of a blood-free medium for determining growth curves and optimizing growth of *Rochalimaea henselae*, *J Clin Microbiol*, **31:** 1882–5.

Slater LN, Welch DF, Min KW, 1992, *Rochalimaea henselae* causes bacillary angiomatosis and peliosis hepatis, *Arch Intern Med*, **152:** 602–6.

Slater LN, Welch DF et al., 1989, A newly recognized fastidious gram negative pathogen as a cause of fever and bacteremia, *N Engl J Med*, **323:** 1587–93.

Slater LN, Coody DW et al., 1992, Murine antibody responses distinguish *Rochalimaea henselae* from *Rochalimaea quintana*, *J Clin Microbiol*, **30:** 1722–7.

Slater LN, Pitha JV et al., 1994, *Rochalimaea henselae* infection in acquired immunodeficiency syndrome causing inflammatory disease without angiomatosis or peliosis: demonstration by immunocytochemistry and corroboration by DNA amplification, *Arch Pathol Lab Med*, **118:** 33–8.

Spach DH, Kanter AS et al., 1995, *Bartonella (Rochalimaea) quintana* bacteremia in inner-city patients with chronic alcoholism, *N Engl J Med*, **332:** 424–8.

Stoler MH, Bonfiglio TA et al., 1983, An atypical subcutaneous infection associated with acquired immune deficiency syndrome, *Am J Clin Pathol*, **80:** 714–18.

Tappero JW, Koehler JE et al., 1993a, Bacillary angiomatosis and bacillary splenitis in immunocompetent adults, *Ann Intern Med*, **118:** 363–5.

Tappero JW, Mohle-Boetani J et al., 1993b, The epidemiology of bacillary angiomatosis and bacillary peliosis, *JAMA*, **269:** 770–5.

Tompkins DC, Steigbigel RT, 1993, Rochalimaea's role in cat scratch disease and bacillary angiomatosis, *Ann Intern Med*, **118:** 388–9.

Wear DJ, Margileth AM et al., 1983, Cat scratch disease: a bacterial infection, *Science*, **221:** 1403–4.

Welch DF, Pickett DA et al., 1992, *Rochalimaea henselae* sp. nov., a cause of septicemia, bacillary angiomatosis, and parenchymal bacillary peliosis, *J Clin Microbiol*, **30:** 275–80.

Welch DF, Hensel DM et al., 1993, Bacteremia due to *Rochalimaea henselae* in a child: practical identification of isolates in the clinical laboratory, *J Clin Microbiol*, **31:** 2381–6.

Zangwill KM, Hamilton DH et al., 1993, Cat scratch disease in Connecticut: epidemiology, risk factors, and evaluation of a diagnostic test, *N Engl J Med*, **329:** 8–13.

Chapter   49

TULARAEMIA

Scott J Stewart

1   INTRODUCTION

Tularaemia is, with rare exception, the only disease produced by the genus *Francisella*. In humans it is an acute febrile infection that exhibits a wide range of clinical manifestations mimicking many other disorders. The disease is most frequently described as sudden onset of flu-like symptoms with fever, chills, prostration and regional lymphadenitis in a patient that has a history of wild animal association or a bite of a blood-sucking insect.

2   DESCRIPTION OF THE DISEASE

Primarily a disease of wild animals, tularaemia is perpetuated by a contaminated environment, cannibalism or acute and chronic carriers. Human infection is considered incidental and is usually the result of interaction with wild animals and their environs. The disease elicits a strong immune reaction that results in a life-long immunity; second infections are extremely rare.

Tularaemia can be found in most countries of the temperate zone in the northern hemisphere between latitudes 30° and 71°. Only a few poorly documented cases have been reported from the southern hemisphere.

An excellent review on the geographical distribution of human tularaemia was published by Hopla (1974).

There are several subspecies that are distinguishable by their virulence, epidemiological behaviour and minor differences in genetic and biochemical characteristics. The 2 principal subspecies of *Francisella tularensis* are: (1) *nearctica* (subspecies *tularensis*) and (2) *holarctica* (subspecies *palaearctica*) (Olsufiev 1970). The disease produced by *F. tularensis* subspecies *tularensis*, which is limited to North America, is a more serious disease lasting several months with a fatality rate of about 5%. This subspecies is usually associated with wild rabbits, sheep and ticks. The disease produced by *F. tularensis* subspecies *palaearctica*, found throughout the Holarctic Region including North America, is milder, frequently subclinical with fatalities almost unknown. It is usually associated with water, beaver, rodents and mosquitoes. A thorough enumeration of the wild animals and vectors reported to harbour *F. tularensis* was published by Bell and Reilly (1981).

During the 1930s there were 1–2 thousand reported cases of tularaemia per year in the United States but there has been a steady decline from 1939 to only a few hundred reported cases annually today. A good description of the history, investigators and the evolution of research on human tularaemia in North America was published by Jellison (1974). Olsufiev and Rudnev (1960) suggested that during the years 1940–48 more than 100 000 cases per year occurred in the Soviet Union.

Known as yato-byo (hare disease) or Ohara's disease for Hirachi Ohara's early studies of human tularaemia, tularaemia in Japan followed a somewhat different trend from the rest of the world. A thorough description of tularaemia as it has evolved in Japan was published by Yoshiro Ohara (1991).

Diagnosis of tularaemia has always been difficult due to its wide range of symptoms. The many countries encompassed in its geography have different diagnostic and reporting procedures. The aetiological agent has been considered a candidate for biological warfare, further compromising the available epidemiological data with political and military considerations (Sterling 1991).

Humans of any age, sex, or race are universally susceptible. Local customs, however, have a dramatic influence on the epidemiology of human tularaemia. In a 6 year study in Hungary, 86% of the reported cases were in adult men. Their unique occupation of hunting wild hamsters for fur placed them at increased risk (Münnich and Lakatos 1979). In the USA the disease has changed from a fall–winter disease of hunters, farmers and trappers to a spring–summer disease of recreationalists exposing themselves to wild animal habitats. In a 5 year study in Arkansas (USA), preschoolchildren, students and retired men comprised more than 40% of the cases, whereas less than 10% were farmers (McChesney and Narain 1983). The annual incidence of tularaemia in humans has declined steadily with the change of culture from rural life, including market hunting and trapping, to an urban one with limited wild animal association. In China where wild rabbits are still commercially hunted and processed for food the association of market hunting and human disease continues (Pang 1987).

3 HISTORY

Human tularaemia was first described as 'hare meat poisoning' by the Japanese physician, Soken Homma, in his 1837 *Manual of Surgery* (Ohara 1954). It was recognized in northern Europe and Asia early in the twentieth century as a nuisance disease among trappers; hence it was called 'trappers' ailment', or 'lemming fever' (Horne 1911). In North America, the severe and sometimes fatal disease known as 'rabbit fever' and 'deer-fly fever' in humans was linked with the 'plague-like disease in ground squirrels' described by McCoy and Chapin in 1912 (Francis 1921). Edward Francis, for whom the genus is named, dedicated his career to describing the clinical manifestations, diagnosis and histopathology of this disease. Indeed, his landmark article 'Tularemia' is considered an excellent description of the disease as it occurs today (Francis 1925).

4 PATHOGENESIS

Infection begins when the organism penetrates the skin. Following an incubation period of 2–10 days, an ulcer forms at the site of penetration, which becomes the local focus of infection and may persist for several months. The organism is transported via the lymphatic system to regional nodes which become inflamed. Sometimes the organism enters the bloodstream, usually for a short duration early in the infection. Occasionally it relocates in one or more organ groups unrelated to the original site. Widespread dissemination and typical endotoxaemia can result. The organism is capable of surviving intracellularly for long periods of time (Boyce 1990).

In northern Europe skin manifestations are seen in 14% of the cases and are 68% female oriented. They range from a papular rash most commonly seen with ulceroglandular tularaemia to erythema nodosum

most commonly associated with pulmonary tularaemia (Syrjälä, Karvonen and Salminen 1984). This phenomenon has not been as well documented in the rest of the world.

5 MODES OF TRANSMISSION

The sources for this disease are extensive. Literally hundreds of species of wild and domestic mammals and several species of birds have been found infected with *F. tularensis*, including common house pets. Dozens of biting and blood-sucking insects have been shown to be vectors. Ticks, mosquitoes and biting flies are the most common arthropod vectors in human disease. In the USA tularaemia is the third most commonly reported tick-borne infection. Association with wild rabbits, hares, beavers and microtine rodents is responsible for large numbers of human infections. Human-to-human transmission, however, is unheard of.

F. tularensis is extremely infectious; 1–10 organisms are considered an infectious dose in humans. Many authors claim it is able to penetrate the intact skin, although 'intact skin' is difficult to prove. Tularaemia has been the first or second leading cause of laboratory acquired bacterial infections in the United States since its recognition in the 1920s (NIH/CDC 1993).

6 CLINICAL MANIFESTATIONS

Several different clinical presentations are exhibited by this disease, making it extremely difficult to diagnose. These variations result mainly from the location of the portal of entry and to a lesser extent to the inoculum, virulence and underlying health of the patient.

6.1 Ulceroglandular

The ulceroglandular form of tularaemia constitutes about 80% of the reported cases in North America and Europe but only about 20% in Japan (Ohara et al. 1991). The ulcer, usually 4–8 mm in diameter, is erythematous, indurated, non-healing and has a punched-out appearance at 1–3 weeks. Ulcers on the upper extremities usually result from exposure to infected mammals and occur mostly on hunters and ranchers. When the initial ulcer appears on the lower extremities, head, neck or back it is usually attributed to the bite of a blood-sucking arthropod such as a tick, deer-fly or a mosquito. The regional lymph nodes enlarge, sometimes exceeding several centimetres in diameter, become quite painful and frequently suppurate, resembling the 'buboes' of bubonic plague. Since many of the symptoms, vectors and endemic areas are identical with that of plague, immediate treatment is essential. A differential diagnosis would eliminate the unnecessary isolation of the patient with tularaemia.

The Japanese variant, *F. tularensis palaearctica japonica*, produces a smaller ulcer which appears to heal faster than the ulcer produced by the *F. tularensis tularensis* found in North America. This may explain the fact that the Japanese report fewer ulceroglandular (20%) than glandular (60%) cases (Ohara et al. 1991).

6.2   Ocular

Ocular tularaemia, most frequently seen by an ophthalmologist, is an uncommon variation of the ulceroglandular form. The conjunctivae, usually infected by rubbing with contaminated fingers, is painfully inflamed with numerous yellowish nodules and pinpoint sized ulcers, described as Parinaud's syndrome (Guerrant et al. 1976). Due to the debilitating pain of this form of infection, the patient usually seeks medical attention before regional lymphadenopathy is evident (Nohinek and Marr 1983). Painful preauricular adenopathy is unique for tularaemia and separates it from cat scratch disease, tuberculosis, sporotrichosis and syphilis (Halperin, Gast and Ferrieri 1985).

6.3   Oropharyngeal

Oropharyngeal tularaemia presents as a sore throat, painful beyond its appearance. The nasal, buccal or pharyngeal area is considered the portal of entry because the classic ulcer is frequently found there. The tonsils become enlarged and covered with a yellow-white pseudo-membrane similar to that described for diphtheria (Ohara 1934). This form of the disease is usually misdiagnosed as an infection of streptococcal or viral origin, delaying specific treatment.

This manifestation is primarily paediatric in the USA (Fulginiti and Hoyle 1966, Parkhurst and San Joaquin 1990), constituting about 1% of the total reported cases. The infection is limited to toddlers and is probably due to their practice of putting things from the ground into their mouths. In Japan this form of the disease, also known as 'tonsillar tularaemia' or 'angina', has increased from <1% in the 1940s to about 15% of total cases today. The wild hare is considered to be the origin but not the direct source due to thorough cooking prior to consumption. It is speculated that the organism is carried to the throat by consuming raw vegetables and perhaps by fish that are prepared with the same utensils or prepared on the same work surfaces that were contaminated by the preparation of the hare (Ohara 1986, Ohara et al. 1991). In Scandinavian countries this clinical presentation is male oriented and associated with aerosols generated in the collection and handling of hay. In Italy this form of the disease occurs in small localized epidemics and is primarily water-borne (Mignani et al. 1988).

6.4   Glandular

Glandular tularaemia is the term used when an ulcer is not found, has been overlooked, or has healed. On occasion patients with unexplained regional lymphadenopathy have undergone lymph node biopsy for a suspected malignancy (Evans et al. 1985). Surgical manipulations of otherwise untreated tularaemic lymph nodes have initiated severe infections due to the release of large numbers of organisms from within the node (Saslaw 1961) but more commonly the nodes have been found to be sterile.

6.5   Typhoidal

Typhoidal or systemic tularaemia is the acute form of infection in which the organism appears to have overrun the host's protective barriers. Usually there is evidence of infection in several organ groups such as concurrent pneumonia, meningitis, hepatitis, carditis and renopathy. This condition is limited to North America and has a mortality rate of 30–60%. The clinical presentation is usually either associated with a massive inoculum or in a patient who is otherwise immunologically compromised. Most laboratory acquired infections are of this type and are considered to be air-borne in origin. The disease appears as an acute septicaemia, lacking the classic external ulcer and lymphadenopathy but commonly presenting with toxaemia, severe headache and a continuous high fever. The patient may be delirious and develop prostration and shock. If suspected, specific antibiotic therapy must be initiated immediately as the course can be so rapidly fulminating that the patient's death may precede a diagnostic workup.

6.6   Pleuropulmonary

Pleuropulmonary tularaemia can result from either inhalation of an infectious aerosol or colonization of the pleural cavity following dissemination via the bloodstream (Rubin 1978). Pulmonary involvement may be unilateral or bilateral with lobar, segmental, or patchy infiltrates. Miliary pattern, cavitation and residual cysts are less common. Hilar lymphadenopathy occurs in about half the cases. Bronchoscopical findings are indistinguishable from tuberculosis or sarcoidosis (Syrjälä et al. 1986). Pericarditis is frequently associated with this form of the disease (Berkman 1980). In northern Europe epidemics of air-borne infections have been reported (Syrjälä et al. 1985) but in North America pleuropulmonary tularaemia is most frequently the result of disease dissemination and not associated with aerosols. This complication appears in about 15% of the ulceroglandular cases late in the infection and presents a poor prognosis (Sanford 1983) and is a common complication in typhoidal tularaemia (Scofield, Lopez and McNabb 1992).

6.7   Gastrointestinal

Gastrointestinal tularaemia is almost always traced to the consumption of contaminated food or water (Amos and Sprunt 1936) and is usually associated with additional abdominal or low back pain and diarrhoea (Hoyte 1988). The course of infection can vary from mild unexplained persistent diarrhoea with no other symptoms to a rapidly fulminating fatal disease. When fatal cases have been autopsied, extensive ulceration throughout the bowel has been found, suggesting a massive inoculum (Simpson 1928). It is interesting to note that ingestion of the less virulent strains found in Europe and Japan result in oropharyngeal rather than the gastrointestinal disease found in North America.

7 COLLECTION OF SPECIMENS

Direct isolation, or evidence of infection, can be achieved by examining ulcer scrapings, lymph node biopsies, respiratory secretions, gastric washings and sputum. In disseminated disease the organism has been found in blood and cerebrospinal fluid. Rarely is the organism observed in urine or faeces.

Collection and processing of specimens suspected of containing *F. tularensis* should be conducted with extreme caution and enhanced biological safety precautions.

8 LABORATORY TESTS

8.1 Serology

Tularaemia is most frequently confirmed by the agglutination test, but unfortunately significant antibody levels for this test do not occur until the about the third week of illness. Such a delay of treatment may allow the disease to become further complicated, increasing the severity and making it more difficult to manage.

A microagglutination test has been described that is about 100-fold more sensitive than the tube agglutination but the reagents are not commercially available (Brown et al. 1980, Sato et al. 1990).

The standard tube agglutination test is still the most commonly used for confirmation of disease. Commercial antigens (BBL 4087, Difco 2240-56-5) are available. A titre of less than 1:20 is not considered significant because non-specific cross-reactions especially with *Brucella* sp. are sometimes found at this level. A 4-fold titre increase between acute and convalescent sera (a span of 2 weeks or more) or a single titre of 1:160 or greater is considered diagnostic. Titres into the thousands are common late in infection and can persist for years at levels of 1:20 to 1:80.

ELISA tests have proved useful for detecting both antibodies and antigens (Tärnvik et al. 1987, Bavanger, Maeland and Naess 1988, Yurov et al. 1991). When using a known antigen and patient sera, this test becomes positive for tularaemia about one week earlier in the infection than other commonly used serological tests (Meshcheryakova and Pavlova 1995). This procedure should be useful in the early differentiation of disease.

8.2 Culture

Bacterial isolation is difficult; in a study of over 1000 human cases, 84% of which were laboratory confirmed by serology, the organism was isolated in slightly more than 10% (Taylor et al. 1991). Biochemical reactions of the isolated organism are of no particular value and do not justify the additional risk to laboratory personnel. A standardized antimicrobial susceptibility test is not useful for *Francisella* because the media commonly used for this assay will not support growth of the organism. Antimicrobial studies have been conducted using a modified Mueller–Hinton broth (Baker, Hollis and Thornsberry 1985).

Conventional microscopy of polychromatic stained tissue smears or sections show the organism occurs singularly and in groups both intra- and extracellularly. Gram stain of biopsy material is of little value as the small, weakly staining organism cannot readily be discerned from the background.

A commercially available indirect fluorescent antibody test can be performed on clinical specimens suspected of containing the organism (BBL Microbiology Systems, Cockeysville, MD, Difco Laboratories, Detroit, MI). False-positive fluorescent antibody staining for *Legionella* has been reported in a specimen harbouring *Francisella* (Roy, Fleming and Anderson 1989). Interestingly, guinea pigs vaccinated with live tularaemia vaccine are protected from challenge with *Legionella* (Konyukhov et al. 1991).

Polymerase chain reaction has been used to demonstrate tularaemia using blood as a source for DNA. The test is about as sensitive as direct culturing but is much faster and safer to perform (Long et al. 1993). PCR could prove effective when other specimens such as ulcer scrapings or biopsies are used.

Radioimmunoprecipitation appears to be at least 1000 times more sensitive than other diagnostic tests in common use for detecting the organism or its antigenic components (Meshcheryakova and Pavlova 1995). The test is fairly complex and incorporates hazardous reagents but still is far safer than handling live cultures. It is suggested that a battery of known antisera with appropriate controls could be used for screening the specimen; a positive result would be conclusive and could be obtained in less than 4 h.

F. tularensis novicida and *F. philomiragia*, first isolated in 1951 and 1959, respectively, are serologically identical with the other subspecies of *F. tularensis* but have been considered non-pathogens for humans until recently. In extremely rare cases these strains produce diseases similar to glandular or typhoidal tularaemia. Growth on MacConkey agar or in nutrient broth containing 6% NaCl will differentiate these from *F. tularensis* subspecies *tularensis* and *palaearctica* (Hollis et al. 1989).

A skin test has been used both for screening and as a diagnostic tool but its potential for complicating subsequent serological studies has stopped its use in most countries.

The leucocyte differential cell count frequently shows atypical lymphocytes suggestive of mononucleosis (Luotonen et al. 1986). C-Reactive protein is elevated usually in relation to the severity of disease but this does not differentiate tularaemia pleuropneumonia from a viral or tubercular infection (Syrjälä 1986). If the liver or the kidneys are involved they will exhibit reduced function according to the severity of disease.

The best that a patient can expect is a physician who suspects tularaemia from a review of recent exposure and present symptoms. Most cases are successfully treated before confirmation of the disease. It is suspected that many cases go undiagnosed because studies of the population at large have revealed a substantial percentage of people with detectable antibody levels for tularaemia with no history of the disease (Philip et al. 1962).

9 TREATMENT

The aminoglycoside antibiotics are the treatment drugs of choice. Streptomycin has been the most frequently used, with defervescence common in 24 h. These agents would be indicated for the potential life-threatening typhoidal infections or others complicated with pleuropneumonia. Streptomycin, however, is no longer registered for general use in Norway and perhaps other European countries (Scheel, Reiersen and Hoel 1992). Amikacin has been shown to be more effective in treating the disease in laboratory animals but no human data are available at this time (Tynkevich, Pavlovich and Ryzhko 1990). Imipenem–cilastatin has been successfully used when the aminoglycosides are contraindicated due to renal complications (Lee, Horowitz and Linder 1991) and the fluoroquinolones have shown promise due to their low toxicity and their potential for oral and topical application (Scheel, Reiersen and Hoel 1992). Chloramphenicol would be the drug of choice for meningeal complications because of its satisfactory penetration of the CNS although it is associated with high relapse rates. Tetracyclines have proved their effectiveness and their low toxicity and oral delivery make them good alternatives to the aminoglycosides even though they are associated with high relapse rates. These treatment problems may be overcome by a longer course of treatment (Enderlin et al. 1994). Except for imipenem, the β-lactams and sulphonamides are considered ineffective (Roy, Fleming and Anderson 1989). Macrolide antibiotics are not recommended (Vasilyev et al. 1989). Surgical drainage of empyemas and abscessed lymph nodes is useful.

10 PREVENTION

Since there is no effective control of this disease in nature, public awareness of the organism's ubiquitous presence and potential for human infection should be maintained. In endemic areas one should avoid handling dead or moribund animals and reduce the possibility of insect bites by wearing protective clothing, using insect repellents and removing ticks promptly. Chlorination of municipal drinking water has virtually eliminated outbreaks from that origin but untreated water still may serve as a source.

An investigational live attenuated vaccine is available which greatly reduces the severity of an infection. It is recommended for persons with a high probability of exposure either to the organism or to infected animals.

REFERENCES

Amos HL, Sprunt DH, 1936, Tularemia. Review of literature of cases contracted by ingestion of rabbit, *JAMA*, **106:** 1078–80.

Baker CN, Hollis DG, Thornsberry C, 1985, Antimicrobial susceptibility testing of *Francisella tularensis* with a modified Mueller–Hinton broth, *J Clin Microbiol*, 212–15.

Bavanger L, Maeland JA, Naess AI, 1988, Agglutinins and antibodies to *Francisella tularensis* outer membrane antigens in the early diagnosis of disease during an outbreak of tularemia, *J Clin Microbiol*, **26:** 433–7.

Bell JF, Reilly JR, 1981, Tularemia, *Infectious Diseases in Wild Animals*, Iowa State University Press, Ames, Iowa, 213–31.

Berkman YM, 1980, Uncommon acute bacterial pneumonias, *Semin Roentgenol*, **15:** 17–24.

Boyce JM, 1990, *Principles and Practice of Infectious Diseases*, 3rd edn, Churchill Livingstone, New York, New York, 1742–6.

Brown SL, McKinney FT et al., 1980, Evaluation of a safranin-O-stained antigen microagglutination test for *Francisella tularensis* antibodies, *J Clin Microbiol*, **11:** 146–8.

Enderlin G, Morales L et al., 1994, Streptomycin and alternative agents for the treatment of tularemia: review of the literature, *Clin Infect Dis*, **19:** 42–7.

Evans ME, Gregory DW et al., 1985, Tularemia: a 30 year experience with 88 cases, *Medicine (Baltimore)*, **64:** 251–69.

Francis E, 1921, A new disease of man, *JAMA*, **78:** 1015–18.

Francis E, 1925, Tularemia, *JAMA*, **84:** 1243–50.

Fulginiti VA, Hoyle C, 1966, Oropharyngeal tularemia, *Rocky Mountain Med J*, **63:** 41–2, 67.

Guerrant RL, Humphries MK Jr et al., 1976, Tickborne oculoglandular tularemia: case report and review of seasonal and vectorial associations in 106 cases, *Arch Intern Med*, **136:** 811–13.

Halperin SA, Gast T, Ferrieri P, 1985, Oculoglandular syndrome caused by *Francisella tularensis*, *Clin Pediatr*, **24:** 520–2.

Hollis DG, Weaver RE et al., 1989, *Francisella philomiragia* comb. nov. (formerly *Yersinia philomiragia*) and *Francisella tularensis* biogroup *novicida* (formerly *Francisella novicida*) associated with human disease, *J Clin Microbiol*, **27:** 1601–8.

Holpa CE, 1974, The ecology of tularemia, *Adv Vet Sci Comp Med*, **18:** 25–53.

Horne H, 1911, En lemen og marsvinpest, *Nord Vet Tidskrift*, **23:** 16–33.

Hoyte RE, 1988, Typhoidal tularemia presenting as enteritis with leukopenia, *Va Med*, **8:** 388–9.

Jellison WL, 1974, *Tularemia in North America 1930–1974*, University of Montana Press, Missoula, Montana, USA, 1–276.

Konyukhov VF, Tartakovsky IS et al., 1991, The nonspecific protection of guinea pigs immunized with a live tularemia vaccine against lung infection by *Legionella pneumophilia*, *Zh Mikrobiol Epidemiol Immunobiol*, **8:** 50–1.

Lee HC, Horowitz E, Linder W, 1991, Treatment of tularemia with imipenem/cilastatin sodium, *South Med J*, **84:** 1277–8.

Long GW, Oprandy JJ et al., 1993, Detection of *Francisella tularensis* in blood by polymerase chain reaction, *J Clin Microbiol*, **31:** 152–4.

Luotonen J, Syrjälä H et al., 1986, Tularemia in otolaryngologic practice. An analysis of 127 cases, *Arch Otolaryngol Head Neck Surg*, **112:** 77–80.

McChesney TC, Narain J, 1983, A five-year evaluation of tularemia in Arkansas, *J Arkansas Med Soc*, **80:** 257–62.

Meshcheryakova IS, Pavlova IP, 1995, Methods of tularemia diagnosis and identification of *F. tularensis*, *First International Conference on Tularemia*, 1st edn, National Defence Research Establishment/Umeå University, Umeå, Sweden, 15.

Mignani E, Palmieri F et al., 1988, Italian epidemic of waterborne tularemia [letter], *Lancet*, **2:** 1423.

Münnich D, Lakatos M, 1979, Clinical, epidemiological and therapeutical experience with human tularemia, *Infection*, **7:** 61–3.

NIH\CDC, 1993, *Biosafety in Microbiological and Biomedical Laboratories*, 3rd edn, US Government Printing Office, Washington, DC, 90–1.

Nohinek B, Marr JJ, 1983, Tularemia: two manifestations in modern man, *Mo Med*, **80:** 687–9, 698.

Ohara H, 1934, Oto-rhino-laryngologia, *Otolaryngology*, **7:** 432–7.

Ohara S, 1954, Studies on Yato-Byo (Ohara's disease, tularemia in Japan) Report I, *Jpn J Exp Med*, **24:** 69–79.

Ohara S, 1986, On 'tularemic angina', *Annu Rep Ohara Hosp*, **29:** 7–11.

Ohara Y, Sato T et al., 1991, Clinical manifestations of tularemia in Japan – analysis of 1,355 cases observed between 1924 and 1987, *Infection*, **19:** 14–17.

Olsufiev NG, 1970, Taxonomy and characteristics of the genus *Francisella Dodofeev*, 1947, *J Hyg Epidemiol Microbiol Immunol*, **14:** 67–74.

Olsufiev NG, Rudnev GP, 1960, *Tularemia*, Publishing House for Medical Literature, Moscow.

Pang ZC, 1987, The investigation of the first outbreak of tularemia in Shandong Peninsula, *Chung Hua Liu Hsing Ping Hsueh Tsa Chih*, **8:** 261–3.

Parkhurst JB, San Joaquin VH, 1990, Tonsillopharyngeal tularemia: a reminder [letter], *Am J Dis Child*, **144:** 1070.

Philip RN, Huntley B et al., 1962, Serological and skin test evidence of tularemia infection among Alaskan Eskimos, Indians and Aleuts, *J Infect Dis*, **110:** 220–30.

Roy TM, Flemming D, Anderson WH, 1989, Tularemic pneumonia mimicking Legionnaires' disease with false-positive direct fluorescent antibody stains for *Legionella*, *South Med J*, **82:** 1429–31.

Rubin SA, 1978, Radiographic spectrum of pleuropulmonary tularemia, *Am J Roentgenol*, **131:** 277–81.

Sanford JP, 1983, Tularemia, *JAMA*, **250:** 3225–6.

Saslaw S, 1961, Tularemia vaccine study, *Arch Intern Med*, **107:** 689–701.

Sato T, Fujita H et al., 1990, Microagglutination test for early and specific serodiagnosis of tularemia, *J Clin Microbiol*, **28:** 2372–4.

Scheel O, Reiersen R, Hoel T, 1992, Treatment of tularemia with ciprofloxacin, *Eur J Clin Microbiol Infect Dis*, **11:** 447–8.

Scofield RH, Lopez EJ, McNabb SJ, 1992, Tularemia pneumonia in Oklahoma, 1982–1987, *J Okla State Med Assoc*, **85:** 165–70.

Simpson WP, 1928, Tularemia (Francis' disease), *Ann Intern Med*, **1:** 1007.

Sterling J, 1991, Gulf War, *Genet Eng News*, **March:** 16–17.

Syrjälä H, 1986, Peripheral blood leukocyte counts, erythrocyte sedimentation rate and C-reactive protein caused by the type B strain of *Francisella tularensis*, *Infection*, **14:** 51–4.

Syrjälä H, Karvonen J, Salminen A, 1984, Skin manifestations of tularemia: a study of 88 cases in northern Finland during 16 years (1967–1983), *Acta Derm Venereol (Stockh)*, **64:** 513–16.

Syrjälä H, Kujala P et al., 1985, Airborne transmission of tularemia in farmers, *Scand J Infect Dis*, **17:** 371–5.

Syrjälä H, Sutinen S et al., 1986, Bronchial changes in airborne tularemia, *J Laryngol Otol*, **100:** 1169–76.

Tärnvik A, Lofgren S et al., 1987, Detection of antigen in urine of a patient with tularemia [letter], *Eur J Clin Microbiol*, **6:** 318–19.

Taylor JP, Istre GR et al., 1991, Epidemiologic characteristics of human tularemia in the southwest-central states, 1981–1987, *Am J Epidemiol*, **133:** 1032–8.

Tynkevich NK, Pavlovich NV, Ryzhko IV, 1990, Comparative study of the effectiveness of amikacin and streptomycin in experimental tularemia, *Antibiot Khimioter*, **8:** 35–7.

Vasilyev NT, Oborin VA et al., 1989, Sensitivity spectrum of *Francisella tularensis* to antibiotics and synthetic antibacterial drugs, *Antibiot Khimioter*, **34:** 662–5.

Yurov SV, Pchilintsev SYu et al., 1991, The use of microdot immunoenzyme analysis with visual detection for the determination of tularemia antibodies, *Zh Mikrobiol Epidemiol Immunobiol*, **3:** 61–4.

BORRELIOSES

R C Johnson

Borrelia are vector-borne, obligate parasites of a wide variety of vertebrates. Among the diseases caused by these spirochaetes are Lyme borreliosis, the relapsing fevers, avian spirochaetosis and possibly epizootic bovine abortion. The borrelioses, with the exception of louse-borne relapsing fever, are tick-transmitted zoonoses. The borreliae have effectively adapted to multiplying in the radically different environments of the poikilothermic arthropod vectors and homeothermic hosts, and some are able to evade the immune response of the host through antigenic variation (for a detailed description of the borreliae see Volume 2, Chapter 56). Interest in the borreliae has been revived with the discovery of *Borrelia burgdorferi sensu lato* as the agent of Lyme borreliosis.

1 LYME BORRELIOSIS

Lyme borreliosis is a zoonosis caused by several closely related genospecies of *B. burgdorferi sensu lato*. These spirochaetes are transmitted by ticks of the *Ixodes ricinus* complex and cause a broad spectrum of clinical syndromes in humans, collectively referred to as Lyme disease or Lyme borreliosis. The chronic dermatological feature of this disease, acrodermatitis chronica atrophicans, was described in Europe during the late 1800s (Pick 1894) and named and further characterized by Herxheimer and Hartmann in 1902. The pathognomonic skin lesion (rash), erythema migrans, of Lyme borreliosis was reported in 1910 by the Swedish dermatologist Afzelius who also suggested it was an infection transmitted by a tick bite. The French physicians Garin and Bujadoux (1922) described the neurological involvement (meningoradiculitis) associated with this infection. Prior to this report the European erythema migrans was recognized as a new syndrome without general constitutional or specific systemic reactions. The first case in the USA of endogenously acquired erythema migrans with neuro-

logical sequelae was reported by Scrimenti in 1970 and was contracted in Wisconsin. An outbreak of an epidemic of oligoarthritis in children and adults occurred in Lyme and adjoining communities in Connecticut. This outbreak of oligoarthritis was thought to be a previously unrecognized clinical entity and was named Lyme arthritis (Steere et al. 1977a). Subsequently, the occurrence of a red skin lesion on these patients and its similarity to the erythema migrans of Europe were noted. Also, in addition to arthritis, some of the patients experienced neurological or cardiac abnormalities. Accordingly, Lyme arthritis was recognized as a complex, multisystem disorder and was renamed Lyme disease (Steere et al. 1977b). See Dammin (1989) for a review of erythema migrans.

Although some of the clinical manifestations of Lyme borreliosis were described in the late 1800s and *Ixodes* ticks were implicated as potential vectors, the aetiological agent remained elusive until 1982. During a survey for tick-borne rickettsiae on Long Island, New York, Burgdorfer made the serendipitous discovery of a spirochaete in the midgut of the deer tick, *Ixodes scapularis* (Burgdorfer et al. 1982). The subsequent isolation of the spirochaete from US patients (Benach et al. 1983, Steere et al. 1983) and European patients (Asbrink, Hederstedt and Hovmark 1984, Pfister et al. 1984) established it as the aetiological agent of Lyme borreliosis. The spirochaete isolated by Burgdorfer was identified as a new species of *Borrelia* and named *B. burgdorferi* in his honour (Johnson et al. 1984) (Fig. 50.1). Recent studies on the classification of *B. burgdorferi* resulted in the identification of 3 closely related genospecies of *Borrelia*, *B. burgdorferi sensu stricto*, *Borrelia garinii* and *Borrelia afzelii*, as agents of Lyme borreliosis (Baranton et al. 1992, Canica et al. 1993, Postic et al. 1994). The generic term *B. burgdorferi sensu lato* (*s.l.*) will be used to refer to the 3 genospecies of *Borrelia* responsible for Lyme borreliosis and *B. burgdorferi* will be used for *B. burgdorferi sensu stricto*.

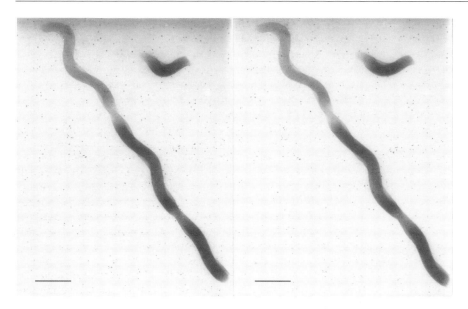

Fig. 50.1 A stereo pair of electron microscopic images of *Borrelia burgdorferi*. Bar denotes 1 μm. (Courtesy of Dr SF Goldstein, University of Minnesota, Minneapolis and Wadsworth Center's Biological Microscopy and Image Reconstruction Facility, Albany, New York).

1.1 Description of the disease

TRANSMISSION AND PATHOGENESIS

The aetiological agents of Lyme borreliosis are transmitted during the feeding of infected ticks of the genus *Ixodes*. The spirochaetes are present and primarily restricted to the midgut of the questing (unfed) tick. These slow-growing spirochaetes have a generation time of 12–24 h in vitro; they are activated by the ingestion of blood by the tick and migrate from the midgut to the salivary glands where they are transmitted to the host via the tick's salivary secretions. *B. burgdorferi s.l.* has successfully adapted to an alternating life in the arthropod vector ticks and mammalian and avian hosts. The Lyme borreliosis spirochaetes are the first tick-borne bacterial pathogens shown to alter the expression of major outer-surface proteins as a prelude to infecting the mammalian host (Fingerle et al. 1995, Schwan et al. 1995). *B. burgdorferi s.l.* in the unfed tick expresses outer-surface protein (Osp) A and no OspC. After attachment to the host and initiation of feeding, the spirochaete begins to express OspC and no longer expresses OspA. Two environmental signals, temperature and nutrients, prompt this change in Osp expression. The temperature of the feeding tick rapidly approximates the body temperature of the host and the spirochaetes are provided blood as a substrate for growth. Schwan et al. (1995) found the spirochaetes express OspC at 32–37°C but not at 24°C; blood was necessary for the expression of this new Osp. Evidence for the expression of OspC and little or no OspA in the mammalian host is provided by analysis of the host antibody response during early Lyme disease. The major antibody response is to OspC with no significant response to OspA (Wilske et al. 1986, Padula et al. 1993, Engstrom, Shoop and Johnson 1995). Antibodies to OspA may be present months to years after disease onset in a limited number of patients (Dressler et al. 1993). The expression of OspC appears to be necessary for *B. burgdorferi s.l.* to be infectious for the mammalian host. Piesman (1993)

found that spirochaete-infected midguts from partially engorged ticks are infectious for mammals whereas spirochaete-infected midguts from unfed ticks are not. Two days or longer are necessary for this change in infectivity to occur.

B. burgdorferi s.l. is very invasive. After entering the bloodstream, the spirochaetes may invade a number of organ systems; they also migrate through the dermis centrifugally from the site of the tick bite. Cell adherence may have a role in the invasiveness of *B. burgdorferi*. In vitro studies have shown that these spirochaetes can adhere to a wide variety of tissue cells (Kurtti et al. 1988, Szczepanski and Benach 1991, Garcia-Monco, Fernandez-Villar and Benach 1989, Hechemy et al. 1989, Thomas and Comstock 1989, Szczepanski et al. 1990) and to extracellular matrices (Szczepanski et al. 1990). The apparent non-specific in vitro adherence of *B. burgdorferi s.l.* to different tissue cell types may be due to adherence to the extracellular matrix.

Following adherence to monolayers of human umbilical vein endothelial cells, *B. burgdorferi* was shown to migrate across the monolayers in the region of the intracellular space (Szczepanski et al. 1990) and penetrate endothelial cells by a transcytotic process (Comstock and Thomas 1989). The invasiveness of the spirochaetes may also be enhanced by a change in the permeability of blood vessels which may be due to the induction of IL-1 formation by *B. burgdorferi s.l.* (Habicht et al. 1985, Habicht, Beck and Benach 1988). *B. burgdorferi* can be found in cerebrospinal fluid of rats 24 h following intravenous injection of spirochaetes. This invasion of the central nervous system was preceded by an alteration of the blood–brain barrier 12 h post-inoculation (Garcia-Monco et al. 1990). Evidence for the early invasion of the central nervous system of Lyme disease patients has also been reported (Garcia-Monco et al. 1990, Luft et al. 1992).

Several characteristics of *B. burgdorferi s.l.* probably play major roles in its ability to disseminate in the host. The internal location of the periplasmic flagella endow borreliae with a unique type of motility that allows them to move effectively in viscous environments such as the extracellular matrices of host tissues (Goldstein, Charon and Kreiling 1994). Although *B. burgdorferi* does not produce any endogenous proteases to degrade the extracellular matrix (Klempner et al. 1995), it does have the ability to bind and activate human plasminogen on its surface (Fuchs et al. 1994, Coleman et al. 1995, Hu et al. 1995, Klempner et al. 1995). Although the spirochaete does not produce a plasminogen activator, an accelerated formation of the bioactive plasmin occurs as the result of the host-derived urokinase-type plasminogen activator (Klempner et al. 1995). OspA was reported to be the primary binding site for plasminogen (Fuchs et al. 1994, Klempner et al. 1995). Subsequently, Hu et al. (1995) established that the primary plasminogen site is a 70 kDa protein rather than OspA. *B. burgdorferi s.l.* can be isolated throughout and beyond the expanding margin of the characteristic erythema migrans skin lesion of early Lyme disease (Berger et al. 1992a). The presence of the host-derived protease on the surface of the spirochaetes could be responsible for both their rapid dissemination in this skin lesion and the relative absence of an acute inflammatory response.

Histopathological and cultural evidence has yielded a paucity of *B. burgdorferi* in lesions from patients with early or late Lyme disease. Since so few spirochaetes are present in patients manifesting the multiple signs and symptoms of this illness, the spirochaetes either form potent toxin(s) or the inflammatory response is a result of amplification by potent host-derived cytokines. The effective resolution of the disease manifestations with appropriate antimicrobial therapy strongly suggests that viable organisms are necessary for the pathology to occur. An extract from *B. burgdorferi* with biological activities similar to those of an endotoxin of gram-negative bacteria was reported (Beck et al. 1985). However, chemical analysis of this extract in another study failed to detect the hydrophobic backbone characteristic of classic lipopolysaccharide (Takayama, Rothenberg and Barbour 1987). The prevailing hypothesis for explaining the pathogenetic activities of *B. burgdorferi* is the release of potent host-derived mediators of inflammation as a result of the interaction of viable spirochaetes with host cells (Schaible et al. 1989, Hurtenbach et al. 1995).

Determinants of *B. burgdorferi* virulence may be associated with extrachromosomal DNA. Virulence (infectivity) of *B. burgdorferi* is lost during in vitro culture (Johnson, Marek and Kodner 1984) and this change in infectivity is associated with the loss of some circular and linear plasmids (Schwan, Burgdorfer and Garon 1988, Simpson, Garon and Schwan 1990). Norris et al. (1992) reported that the non-infective high passage strain B31 lacked the 38 kb linear plasmid encoding the 28 kDa protein OspD which is present in the infectious low passage strain. However, the subsequent examination of the infectivity and the plasmid and polypeptide content of clonal populations of *B. burgdorferi* derived from a common parent strain failed to find a consistent relationship of OspD

with infectivity (Norris et al. 1995). The results of this study suggest that the changes causing decreased infectivity may be more subtle than previously thought.

1.2 Clinical manifestations

Lyme disease is a multisystem infection; although for convenience of discussion the clinical manifestations are commonly described as early localized, early disseminated and late persistent disease, there can be considerable variation for individual presentations (Steere 1989). Prodromal features such as fever, chills, headache, stiff neck, arthralgias, myalgias and lymphadenopathy precede or accompany the more definitive cases of Lyme disease. However, most infections affect one or some combination of 4 organ systems: skin, heart, nervous and musculoskeletal. The first sign of early disease is usually erythema migrans, a minimally symptomatic but pathognomonic rash occurring 3–30 days (median 7 days) following exposure to an infected tick. The skin lesions usually appear as reddish macules that expand centrifugally to diameters of 6–65 cm or greater; the lesions are flat or slightly elevated and vary in size, shape, colour, number, duration and recurrence. It is estimated that erythema migrans may be absent in 20% or more of clinical cases of Lyme disease but clinical studies to validate this estimate are lacking (Nadelman and Wormser 1995). In the untreated patient, the erythema migrans will resolve in an average of 28 days (range, 1 day to 14 months) whereas in the treated patient the lesion will diminish within several days of therapy. The erythema migrans may be difficult to identify, especially if atypical in appearance or if the physician's experience with this disease is limited. The erythema migrans must be distinguished from other dermatological conditions such as hypersensitivity reaction to arthropod bites, streptococcal and staphylococcal cellulitis, plant dermatitis, tinea and granuloma annulare. The erythema migrans lesions may be pruritic or painful but are generally mild.

Primary erythema migrans lesions begin at the site of the tick bite as red macules or papules that expand centrifugally to form a patch with varying intensities of redness or with bands of normal appearing skin (Berger 1984). Sunlight or warming of the skin sometimes makes the erythema migrans more obvious. One study reported that the lesion area expands in area at approximately 20 cm^2 per day and is probably due to the outward movement of the spirochaetes from the tick bite site since they can be isolated from the peripheral and peripheripheral regions of the lesion (Berger et al. 1992a). The shape of the lesion is most commonly round or oval but a variety of forms may occur. Central clearing of the solitary erythema migrans lesion occurs less frequently in the USA (37%) as compared to Europe (80%) and may be due to early initiation of treatment (Nadelman and Wormser 1995). The occurrence of secondary skin lesions also differs in the USA and Europe. The multiple erythema migrans lesions are seen more often in the USA (48%

of patients) but have decreased to less than 25% as a result of early recognition and treatment of Lyme disease. It has been estimated that only 60–80% of patients with clinical Lyme disease have a history of a prior erythema migrans. However, the true incidence remains unknown.

Approximately 20% or more of US patients with erythema migrans fail to develop systemic symptoms that would cause them to see a physician. The remaining 80% of patients with erythema migrans experience a spectrum of systemic symptoms, more pronounced in patients with multiple lesions. The most common systemic symptoms experienced by a series of 79 patients with culture-confirmed infections were: fatigue (54%), mylagia (44%), arthralgia (44%), headache (42%), fever and or chills (39%) and stiff neck (35%). Regional lymphadenopathy (23%) and fever (16%) were the most common objective physical findings (Nadelman and Wormser 1995). In untreated patients, arthritis usually occurs weeks to months (mean 6 months) after resolution of the skin lesion. Cranial nerve abnormalities (facial palsy) and meningitis generally are manifested earlier and may accompany the skin lesion. These early clinical manifestations of Lyme borreliosis usually resolve or improve within weeks to months with or without treatment.

Patients who do not receive treatment during early disease may develop late or persistent disease months to years later despite a strong cellular and humoral response. The isolated migratory musculoskeletal pain in joints, bursae, tendons and muscle that occurred in early disease may, over several years, evolve into intermittent or chronic monoarticular or oligoarticular arthritis. The large joints, especially the knee, are commonly affected. In children the arthritis appears to be milder and may be the only clinical manifestation of the infection (Steere 1995).

Considerable controversy exists concerning the full spectrum of neurological disorders of late or persistent Lyme borreliosis. The most typical neurological disorders associated with early Lyme borreliosis are lymphocytic meningitis, cranial neuritis (especially facial paralysis) and radiculoneuritis (Reik et al. 1979, Pachner and Steere 1985). Radiculoneuritis and cranial neuropathies may also occur in late disease. It has been difficult to document that central nervous system disorders present in late or persistent disease are the result of infection by *B. burgdorferi* (Helprin 1995).

B. burgdorferi s.l. has been isolated or detected in wild animals, domestic animals and birds (Anderson and Magnarelli 1993). Although animals such as deer and reptiles are important hosts in the life cycle of *Ixodes* ticks, *B. burgdorferi* cannot be isolated from these animals (Telford et al. 1988, Lane 1990). However, deer do manifest a strong anti-*B. burgdorferi* antibody response which results from multiple exposures to infected ticks (Gill et al. 1994). Feral animals are not known to suffer any adverse effects of this spirochaetal infection. By contrast, infected domestic animals such as the dog and horse develop signs of Lyme borreliosis.

1.3 Epidemiology

Lyme borreliosis occurs in environments that support competent tick vectors and wildlife reservoir hosts (Table 50.1). These environments are present in large areas of the northern hemisphere. Approximately 10 000 cases of Lyme disease are reported yearly in the USA; they occur primarily in the north central and north east regions and in northern California (Centers for Disease Control and Prevention 1994). The tick vectors are *Ixodes scapularis* for the first 2 locations and *Ixodes pacificus* for the third. Lyme borreliosis occurs in most European countries (Stanek et al. 1988), China (Ai et al. 1988, 1990) and Japan (Kawabata et al. 1987). *I. ricinus* is the major vector in Europe and *Ixodes persulcatus* serves this role in Asia. The tick vectors of Lyme borreliosis share a common life cycle. Upon hatching from eggs, the ticks develop through 3 feeding stages, larvae, nymph, and adult, by parasitizing 3 different host animals. The larval and nymphal stages will parasitize many different small and large animals whereas the adult stage will only feed on medium- and large-sized mammals. The preferred hosts for the subadult ticks are rodents whereas adults tend to feed on deer. Many bird species are parasitized by subadult ticks; this results in the spread of ticks over long distances, especially by migrating birds (Weisbrod and Johnson 1989). Some of the birds are also reservoir competent (Anderson, Magnarelli and Stafford 1990, McLean et al. 1993). The major reservoir competent hosts for the subadult forms of the tick are white-footed mice, *Peromyscus leucopus*, in North America and *Apodemus* species of mice in Europe and Asia. Host blood and tissues containing borreliae are passed into the tick's food canal, formed between the cheliceral sheaths and the dorsum of the hypostome. They are carried through the oesophagus and deposited into the diverticula of the multi-branched midgut where they multiply and invade other tissues of the tick. The borreliae are largely restricted to the midgut after the tick moults to the next developmental stage. When the tick obtains a blood meal, the borreliae begin to multiply and penetrate the midgut into the haemocoel where they invade various tissues including the salivary glands. The borreliae then pass through the salivary ducts and are carried along with salivary secretions through the food canal into host tissues (Ribeiro et al. 1987). The larvae are not considered to be vectors of borreliae due to the near absence of transovarial transmission. In areas endemic for Lyme borreliosis, infection rates are approximately 50% and 25% for unfed adults and nymphs, respectively (Piesman et al. 1986). Most human cases of Lyme borreliosis are acquired during early summer when the nymphal ticks are active. A few cases occur in the fall when adult ticks are questing. The spread of *I. scapularis* into new areas in the northern United States continues to occur (White et al. 1991) and can be rapid and unpredictable (Lastavica et al. 1989). The emergence of Lyme borreliosis as a public health problem in north east and north central United States is directly related to ecological changes

Table 50.1 Characteristics of *Borrelia* species of medical and veterinary significance

Species	Disease	Vector	Geographical distribution
B. recurrentis	Louse-borne relapsing fever	*Pediculus humanus humanus*	World wide
B. hermsii	American tick-borne relapsing fever	*Ornithodoros hermsi*	Western Canada, USA
B. turicatae	American tick-borne relapsing fever	*O. turicata*	Southwestern USA
B. parkeri	American tick-borne relapsing fever	*O. parkeri*	Western USA
B. mazzottii	American tick-borne relapsing fever	*O. talaje*	Southern USA, Mexico, Central and South America
B. venezuelensis	American tick-borne relapsing fever	*O. rudis*	Central and South America
B. duttonii	East African tick-borne relapsing fever	*O. moubata*	Central, eastern, and southern Africa
B. hispanica	Hispano-African tick-borne relapsing fever	*O. erraticus*	Spain, Portugal, Morocco, Algeria, Tunisia
B. crocidurae, B. merionesi, B. microti, B. dipodilli	North African tick-borne relapsing fever	*O. erraticus*	Morocco, Libya, Egypt, Iran, Turkey, Senegal, Kenya
B. persica	Asiatic-African tick-borne relapsing fever	*O. tholozani*	Middle East, Central Asia
B. caucasica	Caucasian tick-borne relapsing fever	*O. verrucosus*	Iraq, southwestern former USSR
B. latyschewii	Caucasian tick-borne relapsing fever	*O. tartakovskyi*	Iraq, Iran, Afghanistan, south central and southwestern former USSR
B. burgdorferi sensu stricto	Lyme borreliosis	*Ixodes scapularis*	Midwestern and eastern USA
		I. pacificus	Western USA
		I. ricinus	Europe
B. garinii	Lyme borreliosis	*I. ricinus*	Europe
		I. persulcatus	Russia, China, Japan
B. afzelii	Lyme borreliosis	*I. ricinus*	Europe
		I. persulcatus	Russia, China, Japan
B. anserina	Avian borreliosis	*Argas persicus* and other *Argas* spp.	Worldwide
B. theileri	Bovine borreliosis	*Rhipicephalus evertsi, Boophilus microplus, B. annulatus, B. decoloratus*	South Africa, Australia, Brazil, Mexico
B. coriaceae	Epizootic bovine abortion (?)	*O. coriaceus*	California

(Spielman et al. 1985). Deforestation during the eighteenth and nineteenth centuries to provide land for agricultural use caused the elimination of deer except for a few isolated areas. This resulted in a corresponding decrease in the *I. scapularis* population and the maintenance of *B. burgdorferi* in the wildlife population. As the use of land for agricultural purposes decreased, reforestation and a dramatic increase in the deer and *I. scapularis* populations ensued. This reestablishment of the wildlife population is responsible for the emergence of Lyme borreliosis as an important public health problem. A similar situation exists in Europe where the deer population that was nearly eliminated during World War II is being restored.

1.4 Diagnosis of Lyme borreliosis

The diagnosis of Lyme borreliosis should be based primarily on the clinical presentation and epidemiological information. However, laboratory tests can be an important adjunct to the diagnosis, especially when the erythema migrans lesion is atypical or lacking. The direct detection of the spirochaete in patients' specimens provides the most definitive diagnosis of infection. Unfortunately, one of the characteristics of Lyme borreliosis is the paucity of spirochaetes in the patient. This, in combination with the requirement for special media, has made isolation a procedure (1) restricted to reference laboratories and (2) a low yield test for most patient specimens. Culture of skin biopsy material from the periphery of the erythema migrans lesion provides the highest yield. Skin biopsy specimens obtained 4 mm inside the erythema migrans margin provide the best specimens for culture with up to 86% of specimens culture-positive (Berger et al. 1992a). Although *B. burgdorferi* is migrating centrifugally from the lesion, isolation success declines to 60% if the skin biopsy is taken 4 mm outside the margin of the erythema migrans. Antimicrobial therapy for only 1 day before obtaining the skin specimen will probably result in negative culture results (Berger et al. 1992a). Adequate antimicrobial therapy will eliminate spirochaetes from the erythema migrans lesion. Skin biopsies obtained from the site of the previously culture-positive region were culture-negative following therapy (Berger et al. 1992b). In contrast to these results, Lyme borreliosis spirochaetes have been isolated from erythema migrans skin biopsies of 2 treated patients in Europe (Preac-Mursic et al. 1989a), suggesting either that the patients were inadequately treated or that some inherent differences exist in these spirochaetes. Antibiotic resistance has not been reported for any of the Lyme disease spirochaetes, even those isolated from patients who did not respond well to therapy (Berger and Johnson 1989). If patients with erythema migrans are not treated, the lesion will eventually resolve. Skin biopsies from the site of the erythema migrans remain culture-positive weeks to years after the lesion resolves (Strle et al. 1995). The propensity for Lyme borreliosis spirochaetes to survive in dermal tissue is exemplified by their isolation from an acrodermatitis chronica atrophicans lesion that had been present for 10 years (Asbrink and Hovmark 1988). The infecting Lyme borreliosis spirochaete was probably *B. afzelii* which is isolated more frequently from chronic skin lesions than *B. burgdorferi* or *B. garinii* (Balmelli and Piffaretti 1995).

Spirochaetes have been isolated from other sites but the yield is very low. Early in the disease *B. burgdorferi* can be isolated from the blood but only 2–7% of specimens are culture-positive. Spirochaetes were cultured from the cerebrospinal fluid of 4 of 38 (11%) clinically selected patients with neuroborreliosis. These 4 patients had pleocytosis in their cerebrospinal fluid and a history of neurological symptoms of only 4–10 days (Karlsson et al. 1990). *B. burgdorferi* has rarely been isolated from synovial fluid specimens (Schmidli et al. 1988).

Another direct method for the detection of the Lyme borreliosis spirochaete is the polymerase chain reaction (PCR). The PCR detects specific target DNA sequences of the spirochaete and may be a promising adjunct to existing diagnostic tests. The PCR is an extremely sensitive assay and can detect the DNA of as few as 1–10 spirochaetes. However, this high level of sensitivity has presented problems with false positive results due to contamination of PCR laboratories or specimens with spirochaetal DNA. When the PCR is conducted by an experienced laboratory the results can be very useful. Goodman et al. (1995) compared culture and PCR for the detection of spirochaetaemia

during early disease. Only 4 of 76 (5.3%) of the blood specimens of erythema migrans patients were culture-positive whereas 14 of the 76 patients (18.4%) had *B. burgdorferi* DNA present in the blood. The plasma was found to be the optimal blood fraction for detection by both culture and PCR. PCR has also demonstrated the intra-articular persistence of *B. burgdorferi* DNA in culture-negative Lyme arthritis; these results suggest that persistent organisms and their components are important in maintaining ongoing immune and inflammatory processes even among some patients treated with antibiotics (Bradley, Johnson and Goodman 1994). At the present time the PCR should be restricted for investigational use since it has not been rigorously evaluated for diagnostic use.

Serology is the most useful laboratory test that is readily available as an adjunct to the clinical diagnosis of Lyme borreliosis. The maximum value of serological results is achieved when they are used in combination with clinical history, patient presentation and an understanding of the antibody response in Lyme borreliosis. Serological testing in Lyme borreliosis can be performed with a high degree of sensitivity and specificity. However, the results have varied between laboratories because testing was not standardized. This lack of standardization resulted in false negative and false positive results.

To minimize these testing discrepancies the Centers for Disease Control and Prevention (CDC) and the Association of State and Territorial Public Health Laboratory Directors (ASTPHLD) recommend that all serum specimens submitted for Lyme borreliosis serology be analysed by a 2 test procedure. The first test is a sensitive screening test (e.g. ELISA or IFA) and all samples judged equivocal or positive should be confirmed by the second test, the Western blot. Specimens that test negative by a sensitive ELISA or IFA need not be tested further (Centers for Disease Control and Prevention 1995).

Patients with Lyme borreliosis usually do not have negative ELISA or IFA results. They can occur when specimens are obtained before the patient has developed a significant antibody response. Approximately one-half of patients that present with erythema migrans will be seronegative. The probability that a patient will be seropositive will increase the longer the erythema migrans has been present and the more marked the clinical manifestations. Both IgM and IgG antibodies are present in early disease. Patients who are reinfected may only have an IgG response in early disease. The initiation of adequate antimicrobial therapy will abort the antibody response in about 20% of patients and these patients will be susceptible to reinfection. The peak antibody response occurs 8–12 days into treatment. Antibody titre cannot be used to monitor a patient's response to therapy. Although most adequately treated patients will have a declining antibody titre, approximately 25% of successfully treated early Lyme disease patients will remain seropositive by ELISA or IFA for at least 1 year after treatment (Engstrom, Shoop and Johnson 1995). If a patient suspected of having Lyme borreliosis is seronegative, a second serum sample should be tested 2 weeks later.

Untreated late Lyme borreliosis patients, particularly those with arthritis, will have a strong antibody response with a predominance of IgG antibody. Treated patients will have slowly decreasing antibody titres. However, these antibodies may persist for years despite successful antibiotic treatment. For neuroborreliosis, testing of the cerebrospinal fluid can be useful because IgM or IgG antibody specific for the spirochaete may be produced intrathecally (Steere et al. 1990).

False negative ELISA or IFA results will occur when the serological assay lacks adequate sensitivity. False positive ELISA or IFA assays can result from overly sensitive tests and in patients with cross-reacting antibodies. These antibodies can occur with certain viral infections such as infectious mononucleosis and bacterial infections such as syphilis and relapsing fever.

The Western blot detects antibodies that are reactive with specific antigens of *B. burgdorferi*. This serological assay is used to confirm borderline (equivocal) and positive serologies obtained by ELISA or IFA. As presently used, the Western blot does not determine antibody concentration (titre); rather, it only determines the presence of *B. burgdorferi* specific antibodies. The Western blot must be used in conjunction with quantitative ELISA or IFA since antibodies can be detected with the Western blot years after treatment (Feder et al. 1992).

The CDC and the ASTPHLD recommend (Centers for Disease Control and Prevention 1995) that for the interpretation of the Western blot an IgM immunoblot be considered positive if 2 of the following 3 bands are present: 24 kDa (OspC), 39 kDa (BmpA) and 41 kDa (Fla) (Engstom, Shoop and Johnson 1995). An IgG immunoblot should be considered positive if 5 of the following 10 bands are present: 18 kDa, 21 kDa (OspC), 28 kDa, 30 kDa, 39 kDa (BmpA), 41 kDa (Fla), 45 kDa, 58 kDa (not GroEL), 66 kDa and 93 kDa (Dressler et al. 1993). Not all strains of *B. burgdorferi* express adequate amounts of immunoreactive proteins of diagnostic importance, especially those that have been passaged many times in culture media. Only strains of *B. burgdorferi* expressing adequate amounts of the proteins of diagnostic importance should be used for the immunoblot (Johnson and Johnson 1996).

1.5 Treatment

Most patients presenting with erythema migrans respond exceptionally well to treatment. In vitro studies of the antimicrobial susceptibility of the Lyme borreliosis spirochaete show them to be susceptible to the macrolides, tetracyclines, semisynthetic penicillins and the late second and third generation cephalosporins (Johnson, Kodner and Russell 1987, Preac-Mursic et al. 1989b, Johnson et al. 1990a, 1990b, Agger, Callister and Jobe 1992, Dever, Jorgensen and Barbour 1993). *B. burgdorferi* was moderately sensitive to penicillin G and chloramphenicol and relatively resistant to the

aminoglycosides, trimethoprim, sulphamethoxazole, quinolines and rifampicin. First generation cephalosporins generally possessed a low level of activity. There is no documented report of the development of antimicrobial resistance in *Borrelia* (Berger and Johnson 1989). Antimicrobials that displayed good in vitro activity against *B. burgdorferi* also had good in vivo activity with the exception of erythromycin (Johnson, Kodner and Russell 1987, Preac-Mursic et al. 1989b, Johnson et al. 1990a, 1990b, Agger, Callister and Jobe 1992, Dever, Jorgensen and Barbour 1993).

Effective oral drugs for treating patients with erythema migrans include amoxycillin, penicillin, tetracycline, doxycycline and cefuroxime axetil (Anonymous 1992, Peter 1994). Studies comparing amoxycillin and doxycycline (Dattwyler et al. 1990) and tetracycline and doxycycline (Nowakowski et al. 1995) found no significant difference in outcome of patients treated with these drugs. A randomized, multicentre, investigator-blinded clinical trial of cefuroxime axetil and doxycycline found the drugs to be equally effective for treatment of patients with erythema migrans and in preventing subsequent development of late Lyme borreliosis (Nadelman et al. 1992). A satisfactory clinical outcome was achieved in 88–93% of patients. A similar clinical trial was conducted comparing amoxycillin and azithromycin. Amoxycillin was found to be significantly more effective than azithromycin in resolving the signs and symptoms of patients with erythema migrans and preventing subsequent relapse (Luft et al. 1996). Patients with early disease with cardiac or neurological manifestations are treated parenterally with ceftriaxone. Cefotaxime and penicillin are alternative and second choice drugs respectively (Anonymous 1992, Peter 1994). Duration of oral and parenteral treatments is 14–30 days depending on the severity of disease. At this time there is no scientific evidence to support long-term oral or parenteral therapy.

I. scapularis, in addition to being the vector for the Lyme borreliosis spirochaetes, may also carry the agents of babesiosis and human granulocytic ehrlichiosis. The possibility of concurrent infection should be considered if patients do not respond to therapy for Lyme borreliosis. In areas where both ehrlichiosis and Lyme disease are present, doxycycline is considered the drug of choice since it is effective against both agents.

1.6 Prevention and transmissibility

Vector-borne diseases are most effectively prevented through vector control. However, ticks are very durable arthropods and effective, practical and environmentally acceptable methods for their control are not presently available (Wilson and Deblinger 1993). *Ixodes* ticks are susceptible to a number of insecticides such as carbaryl, diazinon, chlorpyrifos and cyfluthrin (Curran, Fish and Piesman 1993, Schulze et al. 1994) but the timing of application is critical for maximal effect. Insecticide treatment during the period of nymphal tick activity appears to be effective (Curran, Fish and Piesman 1993). A novel method of tick control, which uses permethrin-treated cotton as a source of nesting for the white-footed mouse, failed to reduce significantly the abundance of infected host-seeking nymphal *I. scapularis* (Daniels, Falco and Fish 1991). Personal protection can be achieved by the wearing of protective clothing, the use of tick or insect repellents (Schreck, Snoddy and Spielman 1986) and daily inspections and removal of attached ticks. The latter is an important means of preventing infection since studies with rodents have shown that effective transmission of spirochaetes does not occur until after 48 h of tick attachment (Piesman 1993).

Passive immunization experiments in the Syrian hamster suggested that a vaccine for Lyme borreliosis was feasible (Johnson, Kodner and Russell 1986a). Antisera received 18 h before syringe challenge with *B. burgdorferi* provided protection from infection. If administration of the antisera was postponed until 17 h after challenge, the protective activity of the antibodies was abrogated (Johnson et al. 1988). Subsequently, a single dose of inactivated whole cell *B. burgdorferi* vaccine provided full protection from infection for animals challenged 30 days post-vaccination (Johnson, Kodner and Russell 1986b). A chemically inactivated whole cell *B. burgdorferi* vaccine has been licensed for use in dogs in the USA (Chu et al. 1992).

Recombinant single-protein vaccines are candidates for the prevention of Lyme borreliosis in humans. The most extensively studied of the recombinant protein vaccines are OspA (Fikrig et al. 1990) and OspC (Preac-Mursic et al. 1992). Prospects for a vaccine to prevent Lyme borreliosis in humans has been reviewed by Wormser (1995). Recombinant OspA vaccines for humans are being tested for efficacy and safety in the USA and Europe. A potential limitation of the OspA and OspC vaccines is the heterogeneity of these proteins in *B. burgdorferi* isolates (Milch and Barbour 1989, Dykhuizen et al. 1993, Wilske et al. 1993a, 1993b). OspA variability is greatest in European strains (Wilske et al. 1993b). Another limitation of the OspA vaccine is the decreased expression of OspA by *B. burgdorferi* in the tick as a prelude to infecting the mammalian host (Fingerle et al. 1995, Schwan et al. 1995). However, this lack of OspA expression in the host may be compensated for by the elimination or reduction of *B. burgdorferi* in ticks after a blood meal containing anti-OspA antibodies (Fikrig et al. 1992). Protective immunity is induced by a *B. burgdorferi* mutant that lacks OspA and OspB (Hughes et al. 1993), indicating other antigens can elicit a protective response. This mutant did contain OspC which is immunogenic (Preac-Mursic 1992) and may be responsible in part for the protective immunity provided by this vaccine preparation.

2   RELAPSING FEVER

Relapsing fever is characterized by the occurrence of one or more relapses after the initial acute febrile illness. The 2 main forms of relapsing fever are louse-borne (epidemic) relapsing fever and tick-borne (endemic) relapsing fever. Most of the basic clinical and epidemiological concepts of louse-borne relapsing fever resulted from its spread and the resulting epidemics during and after World War I. The aetiological agent of louse-borne relapsing fever, *Borrelia recurrentis*, was discovered by Obermeier in 1868 and Mackie (1907) was the first to incriminate the louse as the vector of epidemic relapsing fever. Epidemic relapsing fever occurs in Africa, Europe and Asia. It remains an important public health problem in Ethiopia (Daniel, Beyene and Tessema 1992, Borgnolo et al. 1993). Tick-borne relapsing fever in Africa was probably first described by Livingston in 1857 (Carlisle 1906). The disease is endemic and is present world wide.

2.1   Description of the disease

TRANSMISSION AND PATHOGENESIS

A single species of *Borrelia*, *B. recurrentis*, is the aetiological agent of louse-borne (epidemic) relapsing fever and is transmitted from person to person by the human body louse, *Pediculus humanus humanus*. Following the ingestion of human infective blood, the spirochaetes penetrate the midgut and multiply in the haemolymph. Since other tissues are not infected, the spirochaetes are not present in the saliva or excrement nor transmitted transovarially. Once the louse is infected it remains so for the rest of its life – usually about 3 weeks. Humans are the only host for *B. recurrentis* and are infected as a result of crushing lice. The released infective fluid contaminates the bite site and the spirochaetes penetrate the host tissues.

Various *Borrelia* species cause tick-borne relapsing fever (see Table 50.1) and they were initially identified based on vector specificity. This classification is being re-evaluated using genetic techniques (Hyde and Johnson 1984, Johnson et al. 1987, Schwan et al. 1989). The tick-borne relapsing fever borreliae are transmitted by soft ticks of the genus *Ornithodoros* and the infection is maintained by a variety of rodents (Felsenfeld 1971). The exception to this is *B. duttonii*, whose exclusive mammalian host is humans. Ticks develop a generalized infection and humans are infected by the saliva, coxal fluid or excrement of the feeding tick. Transovarial transmission of borreliae occurs and may be an important mechanism for the maintenance of the spirochaete when the populations of reservoir hosts are low. It is possible for a tick to be infected by more than one species of *Borrelia* and to remain infected for life which may be as long as 5 years.

The internal location of flagella endows the borreliae with a unique type of motility which enhances their invasiveness (Goldstein, Charon and Kreiling 1994) (see Volume 2, Chapter 56). The relapsing fever borreliae invade a number of organ systems and are present in the blood during the febrile episodes with spirochaetaemia levels as high as 100 000 spirochaetes per mm^3 of blood (Bryceson et al. 1970). The spirochaetes disappear from the blood prior to the afebrile periods; their return correlates with a new febrile episode. The disappearance and re-emergence of the spirochaetaemia is due to a mechanism of antigenic variation which closely resembles that of the African trypanosome (Donelson 1995). As the host forms antibodies to the variable major protein expressed on the borrelial outer membrane, that antigenic type is eliminated from the blood and is replaced by a new antigenic type. Although a single cell of *B. hermsii* is capable of producing 40 antigenically distinct types (Plasterk, Simon and Barbour 1985), usually between 3 and 7 febrile episodes are experienced during human infection. The genes encoding these variable outer-membrane lipoproteins are located on the linear plasmids of the relapsing fever borreliae. The mechanism of antigenic variation of the relapsing fever borreliae has been reviewed by Barbour (1990).

The mechanism of pathogenicity of the relapsing fever borreliae is poorly understood. These spirochaetes do not possess any known endotoxin or exotoxin and appear to be predominantly extracellular pathogens. The fever and other pathology associated with these infections is probably due to the induction and release of host-derived cytokines as has been proposed for the Lyme borreliosis spirochaetes. The thrombocytopenia is thought to be due to sequestration of platelets and disseminated intravascular coagulation.

2.2 Clinical manifestations

Louse-borne and tick-borne relapsing fevers have similar clinical manifestations. The bite of an infected louse or tick is followed by an incubation period of 4–18 days. During this time the spirochaetes are multiplying. The doubling time of the spirochaetes in humans is unknown but may be similar to the 4–6 h generation time of *B. hermsii* in experimentally infected mice (Stoenner, Dodd and Larsen 1982). When the spirochaetaemia reaches 10^6–10^8 cells ml^{-1}, there is a sudden onset of shaking, chills, fever, headache and fatigue. Arthralgia, myalgia, anorexia, dry cough and abdominal pain may increase in intensity for several days. After a symptomatic period of 3–7 days, the formation of specific antibodies results in the elimination of detectable spirochaetes from the blood and an afebrile period of a few days to several weeks. Additional relapses of decreasing intensity and duration are frequently experienced with tick-borne relapsing fever but are infrequent in the louse-borne illness.

B. recurrentis has a greater propensity to infect the central nervous system than the tick-borne relapsing fever borreliae (Southern and Sanford 1969, Horton and Blaser 1985). Myocarditis, cerebral haemorrhage and hepatic failure are the most common causes of death. The relapsing fever borreliae, especially *B. recurrentis*, can cross the placenta and cause congenital infection (Barclay and Coulter 1990, Melkert and Stel 1991, Borgnolo et al. 1993).

2.3 Epidemiology

Relapsing fever occurs in the temperate and tropical zones of most areas of the world. Louse-borne relapsing fever is caused by a single species of *Borrelia*, *B. recurrentis*. Humans are the only host for this spirochaete which is transmitted by the body louse. Louse-borne relapsing fever is associated with persons living under crowded, unhygienic conditions that favour infestation with body lice. The last great epidemic was during World War II and was responsible for an estimated 50 000 deaths in North Africa and Europe. Louse-borne relapsing fever is endemic in Ethiopia and outbreaks of the illness continue to occur (Borgnolo et al. 1993, Sundnes and Haimanot 1993).

Tick-borne relapsing fever is a zoonosis caused by a number of *Borrelia* species (Table 50.1). Rodents serve as the maintenance hosts and the borreliae are transmitted to humans by soft ticks of the genus *Ornithodoros*. The intrusion of humans into the habitat of the tick provides the opportunity for disease transmission and they may be carried into human dwellings by rodents in East Africa. Humans appear to serve as the reservoir for *B. duttoni* which is transmitted by the domestic tick *Ornithodoros moubata* (Felsenfeld 1971). Since *Ornithodoros* ticks are largely nocturnal, rapid feeders (5–30 min) and their bite is painless, most patients are not aware of the tick bite. The largest outbreak of tick-borne relapsing fever in the western hemisphere, involving 62 persons residing in log cabins, took place at the northern rim of the Grand Canyon, Arizona, in 1973. Tick-borne relapsing fever is endemic in the northwestern United States but disease recognition remains low. Tick-borne relapsing fever is a greater public health problem in children and pregnant women in Africa. In a single year, 488 children under the age of 15 years and 45 pregnant women with tick-borne relapsing fever were seen at one hospital in Tanzania (Barclay and Coulter 1990).

2.4 Host response

The humoral response of the host plays a major role in providing immunity to infection by the relapsing fever borreliae. The formation of antibodies reactive with the expressed variable major protein are responsible for the elimination of spirochaetes preceding the afebrile intervals and the eventual recovery from this illness (Barbour 1990). The availability of serotype-specific IgM antibodies has confirmed the role of antibodies in the elimination of borreliae from experimentally infected mice (Cadavid, Bundoc and Barbour 1993).

2.5 Diagnosis of relapsing fever

Tick-borne relapsing fever is difficult to diagnose because of its sporadic occurrence and non-specific symptoms. A clinical diagnosis of louse-borne relapsing fever is relatively simple in endemic areas.

A definitive diagnosis of relapsing fever is achieved by demonstration of the borreliae in the blood of febrile patients. This can be accomplished by examining the blood by darkfield illumination or after staining with Wright or Giemsa; inoculation of a susceptible animal and monitoring for spirochaetaemia; and the inoculation of BSK (Barbour–Stoenner–Kelly) medium (Barbour 1984) for the isolation of tick-borne relapsing fever borreliae (Schwan, Burgdorfer and Rosa 1995). The successful in vitro cultivation of *B. recurrentis* has been reported (Cutler et al. 1994).

The borreliae that cause relapsing fever and Lyme disease are antigenically very similar. Antibodies of relapsing fever patients will react strongly in IFA, ELISA and Western blot assays for Lyme disease. However, relapsing fever must be discriminated clinically and epidemiologically since it is very difficult to distinguish serologically. Patients with relapsing fever will frequently have false positive results with the fluorescent treponemal antibody-absorption (FTA-ABS) and microhaemagglutination assay for *Treponema pallidum* (MHA-TP) tests for syphilis. However, these patients will have negative non-treponemal tests such as that of the Venereal Disease Research Laboratory (VDRL). The tick-borne relapsing fever spirochaete *B. hermsii* can be identified with a species-specific monoclonal antibody (Schwan et al. 1992) and DNA hybridization probes can be used to identify the relapsing fever borreliae and differentiate them from *B. burgdorferi* (Schwan et al. 1989).

2.6 Treatment

The in vitro antimicrobial susceptibility of the tick-borne relapsing fever borreliae is the same as *B. burgdorferi* (Johnson 1996); relapsing fever has been successfully treated with tetracycline, doxycyline, chloramphenicol, penicillin, ceftriaxone and erythromycin (Perine and Teklu 1983, Butler 1985, Horton and Blaser 1985). Tetracycline in a single oral dose (500 mg) is the treatment of choice except for children younger than 7–9 years of age and pregnant women. Erythromycin given orally as a single dose is an alternative to tetracycline (Butler, Jones and Wallace 1978). Penicillin G therapy may result in slow clearance of spirochaetes and frequent relapses (Warrell et al. 1983).

Most patients with louse-borne relapsing fever and some with tick-borne relapsing fever will experience a Jarisch–Herxheimer reaction shortly after treatment is initiated. Intensive nursing care and intravenous fluid support may be necessary during the first day of treatment (Butler, Jones and Wallace 1978). The Jarisch–Herxheimer reaction is associated with transient elevation of plasma tumour necrosis factor, interleukin-6 and interleukin-8 concentrations (Negussie et al. 1992). Seboxa and Rahlenbeck (1995) reported that the severity of the Jarisch–Herxheimer reaction can be reduced with low-dose penicillin or tetracycline.

2.7 Prevention

The prevention of relapsing fever is best accomplished by avoidance of the arthropod vectors. Good personal hygiene and delousing procedures when necessary will prevent louse-borne relapsing fever (Sundnes and Haimanot 1993). Reduction of the reservoir of infection is achieved by detection and treatment of cases of this illness. The control of tick-borne relapsing fever is more difficult because of diverse habitats and large geographical areas populated by *Ornithodoros* ticks and the sporadic occurrence of the infection. Dwellings should be rodent proof and personal precautions such as wearing protective clothing and application of tick repellents should be used when in potential habitats of the vector ticks. Vaccines are not available for relapsing fever.

3 BORRELIOSIS IN DOMESTIC ANIMALS

Lyme borreliosis has been reported in cats, dogs, sheep, cattle and horses. The disease has been reported most frequently and described in greatest detail in dogs and horses (Lindenmayer, Weber and Onderdonk 1989, Levy and Dreesen 1992). The signs of the disease in dogs and horses are lameness, arthritis, loss of appetite, fever and fatigue. Amoxycillin and tetracycline are effective antibiotics and a vaccine is available for the prevention of Lyme borreliosis in dogs.

Avian borreliosis is caused by *B. anserina* which is transmitted by species of the soft tick *Argus*. The disease occurs in chickens, ducks, geese and turkeys and can be of considerable economic importance. Birds do not experience relapses of the illness and mammals are resistant to this infection.

B. coriaceae, a new species of *Borrelia* (Johnson et al. 1987), is carried by the soft tick *Ornithodoros coriaceus* (Lane et al. 1985). The spirochaete has been implicated as the agent of epizootic bovine abortion, a disease of major economic importance in California (Lane et al. 1985). However, a recent study failed to establish a definite association of *B. coriaceae* with this disease (Zingg and LeFebvre 1994).

B. theileri causes a mild disease of cattle, horses and sheep in South Africa, South America and Australia. The disease is characterized by 1–2 episodes of fever, weight loss, weakness and anaemia. Species of the hard ticks *Rhipicephalus* and *Boophilus* are vectors for this spirochaete.

REFERENCES

Afzelius A, 1910, Verhandlungen der dermatologischen Gesellschaft zu Stockholm on October 28, 1909, *Arch Dermatol Syph*, **101:** 404.

Agger WA, Callister SM, Jobe DA, 1992, *In-vitro* susceptibilities of *Borrelia burgdorferi* to five oral cephalosporins and ceftriaxone, *Antimicrob Agents Chemother*, **36:** 1788–99.

Ai CX, Wen YX et al., 1988, Clinical manifestations and epidemiological characteristics of Lyme disease in Hailin county, Heilongjiang province, China, *Ann NY Acad Sci*, **539:** 302-13.

Ai CX, Hu RJ et al., 1990, Epidemiological and aetiological evidence for transmission of Lyme disease by adult *Ixodes persulcatus* in an endemic area in China, *Int J Epidemiol*, **19:** 1061–5.

Anderson JF, Magnarelli LA, 1993, Epizootiology of Lyme disease-causing borreliae, *Clin Dermatol*, **11:** 339–51.

Anderson JF, Magnarelli LA, Stafford KC III, 1990, Bird-feeding ticks transstadially transmit *Borrelia burgdorferi* that infect Syrian hamsters, *J Wildl Dis*, **26:** 1–10.

Anonymous, 1992, Treatment of Lyme disease, *Med Lett*, **34:** 95–7.

Asbrink E, Hederstedt B, Hovmark A, 1984, Spirochetal etiology of acrodermatitis chronica atrophicans Herxheimer, *Acta Dermatol Venereol*, **64:** 506–12.

Asbrink E, Hovmark A, 1988, Early and late cutaneous manifestations in *Ixodes*-borne borreliosis, *Ann NY Acad Sci*, **539:** 4–16.

Balmelli T, Piffaretti JC, 1995, Association between different clinical manifestations of Lyme disease and different species of *Borrelia burgdorferi* sensu lato, *Res Microbiol*, **146:** 329–40.

Baranton G, Postic D et al., 1992, Delineation of *Borrelia burgdorferi* sensu stricto, *Borrelia garinii* sp. nov. and group VS461 associated with Lyme borreliosis, *Int J Syst Bacteriol*, **42:** 378–83.

Barbour AG, 1984, Isolation and cultivation of Lyme disease spirochetes, *Yale J Biol Med*, **57:** 521–5.

Barbour AG, 1990, Antigenic variation of a relapsing fever *Borrelia* species, *Annu Rev Microbiol*, **44:** 155–71.

Barclay AJ, Coulter JB, 1990, Tick-borne relapsing fever in Central Tanzania, *Trans R Soc Trop Med Hyg*, **84:** 852–6.

Beck G, Habicht GS et al., 1985, Chemical and biologic characterization of a lipopolysaccharide from the Lyme disease spirochete (*Borrelia burgdorferi*), *J Infect Dis*, **152:** 108–17.

Benach JL, Bosler EM et al., 1983, Spirochetes isolated from the blood of two patients with Lyme disease, *N Engl J Med*, **308:** 740–2.

Berger BW, 1984, Erythema chronicum migrans of Lyme disease, *Arch Dermatol*, **120:** 1017–21.

Berger BW, Johnson RC, 1989, Clinical and microbiologic findings in six patients with erythema migrans of Lyme disease, *J Am Acad Dermatol*, **21:** 1188–91.

Berger BW, Johnson RC et al., 1992a, Cultivation of *Borrelia burgdorferi* from erythema migrans lesions and perilesional skin, *J Clin Microbiol*, **30:** 359–61.

Berger BW, Johnson RC et al., 1992b, Failure of *Borrelia burgdorferi* to survive in the skin of patients with antibiotic-treated Lyme disease, *J Am Acad Dermatol*, **27:** 34–7.

Borgnolo G, Hailu B et al., 1993, Louse-borne relapsing fever: a clinical and an epidemiological study of 389 patients in Asella hospital, Ethiopia, *Trop Geogr Med*, **45:** 66–9.

Bradley JF, Johnson RC, Goodman JL, 1994, The persistence of spirochetal nucleic acids in active Lyme arthritis, *Ann Intern Med*, **120:** 487–9.

Bryceson ADE, Parry EHO et al., 1970, Louse-borne relapsing fever. A clinical and laboratory study of 62 cases in Ethiopia and a reconsideration of the literature, *J Med*, **39:** 129–70.

Burgdorfer W, Barbour AG et al., 1982, Lyme disease – a tick-borne spirochetosis? *Science*, **216:** 1317–19.

Butler T, 1985, Relapsing fever: new lessons about antibiotic action, *Ann Intern Med*, **102:** 397.

Butler T, Jones PK, Wallace CK, 1978, *Borrelia recurrentis* infection: clinical trials of antibiotics and management of the Jarisch-Herxheimer-like reaction, *J Infect Dis*, **137:** 573–7.

Cadavid D, Bundoc V, Barbour A, 1993, Experimental infection of the mouse brain by a relapsing fever *Borrelia* species: a molecular analysis, *J Infect Dis*, **168:** 143–51.

Canica MM, Nato F et al., 1993, Monoclonal antibodies for identification of *Borrelia afzelii* sp. nov. associated with late cutaneous manifestations of Lyme borreliosis, *Scand J Infect Dis*, **25:** 441–8.

Carlisle RJ, 1906, Two cases of relapsing fever; with notes on the occurrence of this disease throughout the world at the present day, *J Infect Dis*, **3:** 233–65.

Centers for Disease Control and Prevention, 1994, Lyme disease – United States, 1993, *Morbid Mortal Weekly Rep*, **43:** 564–72.

Centers for Disease Control and Prevention, 1995, Recommendations for test performance and interpretation from the Second National Conference on Serologic Diagnosis of Lyme disease, *Morbid Mortal Weekly Rep*, **44:** 590–1.

Chu H-J, Chavez LG Jr et al., 1992, Immunogenicity and efficacy study of a commercial *Borrelia burgdorferi* bacterin, *J Am Vet Med Assoc*, **201:** 403–11.

Coleman JL, Sellati TJ et al., 1995, *Borrelia burgdorferi* binds plasminogen, resulting in enhanced penetration of endothelial monolayers, *Infect Immun*, **63:** 2478–84.

Comstock LE, Thomas DD, 1989, Penetration of endothelial cell monolayers by *Borrelia burgdorferi*, *Infect Immun*, **57:** 1626–8.

Curran KL, Fish D, Piesman J, 1993, Reduction of nymphal *Ixodes dammini* (Acari: Ixodidae) in a residential suburban landscape by area application of insecticides, *J Med Entomol*, **33:** 1–7.

Cutler SJ, Fekade D et al., 1994, Successful *in-vitro* cultivation of *Borrelia recurrentis*, *Lancet*, **343:** 242.

Dammin GJ, 1989, Erythema migrans: a chronicle, *Rev Infect Dis*, **11:** 142–51.

Daniel E, Beyene H, Tessema T, 1992, Relapsing fever in children: demographic, social and clinical features, *Ethiop Med J*, **30:** 207–14.

Daniels TJ, Falco RC, Fish D, 1991, Evaluation of host-targeted acaricide for reducing the risk of Lyme disease in southern New York state, *J Med Entomol*, **28:** 537–43.

Dattwyler RJ, Volkman DJ et al., 1990, Amoxycillin plus probenecid versus doxycycline for treatment of erythema migrans borreliosis, *Lancet*, **336:** 1404–6.

Dever LL, Jorgenson JH, Barbour AG, 1993, Comparative *in-vitro* activities of clarithromycin, azithromycin, and erythromycin against *Borrelia burgdorferi*, *Antimicrob Agents Chemother*, **37:** 1704–6.

Donelson JE, 1995, Mechanisms of antigenic variation in *Borrelia hermsii* and African trypanosomes, *J Biol Chem*, **270:** 7783–86.

Dressler F, Whalen JA et al., 1993, Western blotting in the diagnosis of Lyme disease, *J Infect Dis*, **167:** 392–400.

Dykhuizen DE, Polin DS et al., 1993, *Borrelia burgdorferi* is clonal – implications for taxonomy and vaccine development, *Proc Natl Acad Sci USA*, **90:** 10163–7.

Engstrom SM, Shoop E, Johnson RC, 1995, Immunoblot interpretation criteria for serodiagnosis of early Lyme disease, *J Clin Microbiol*, **33:** 419–27.

Feder HM, Gerber MA et al., 1992, Persistence of antibodies to *Borrelia burgdorferi* in patients treated for Lyme disease, *Clin Infect Dis*, **15:** 788–93.

Felsenfeld O, 1971, *Borrelia. Strains, Vectors, Human and Animal Borreliosis*, Warren H. Green, St Louis.

Fikrig E, Barthold SW et al., 1990, Protection of mice against the Lyme disease agent by immunizing with recombinant OspA, *Science*, **250:** 533–6.

Fikrig E, Telford SR 3rd et al., 1992, Elimination of *Borrelia burgdorferi* from vector ticks feeding on OspA-immunized mice, *Proc Natl Acad Sci USA*, **89:** 5418–21.

Fingerle V, Hauser V et al., 1995, Expression of outer surface proteins A and C of *Borrelia burgdorferi* in *Ixodes ricinus*, *J Clin Microbiol*, **33:** 1867–9.

Fuchs H, Wallich R et al., 1994, The outer surface protein A of the spirochete *Borrelia burgdorferi* is a plasmin(ogen) receptor, *Proc Natl Acad Sci USA*, **91:** 12594–8.

Garcia-Monco JC, Fernandez-Villar B, Benach JL, 1989, Adherence of the Lyme disease spirochetes to glial cells and cells of glial origin, *J Infect Dis*, **160:** 497–506.

Garcia-Monco JC, Fernandez-Villar B et al., 1990, *Borrelia burgdorferi* in the central nervous system: experimental and clinical evidence for early invasion, *J Infect Dis*, **161:** 1187–93.

Garin C, Bujadoux C, 1922, Paralysie par les tiques, *J Med Lyon*, **71:** 765–7.

Gill JS, McLean RG et al., 1994, Serological surveillance for the Lyme disease spirochete, *Borrelia burgdorferi*, in Minnesota by using white-tailed deer as sentinel animals, *J Clin Microbiol,* **32:** 444–51.

Goldstein S, Charon NW, Kreiling JA, 1994, *Borrelia burgdorferi* swims with planar waveform similar to that of eukaryotic flagella, *Proc Natl Acad Sci USA,* **91:** 3433–7.

Goodman JL, Bradley JF et al., 1995, Bloodstream invasion in early Lyme disease: results from a prospective, controlled study utilizing the polymerase chain reaction, *Am J Med,* **99:** 6–12.

Habicht GS, Beck G, Benach JL, 1988, The role of interleukin-1 in the pathogenesis of Lyme disease, *Ann NY Acad Sci,* **539:** 80–6.

Habicht GS, Beck G et al., 1985, Lyme disease spirochetes induce human and murine IL-1 production, *J Immunol,* **134:** 3147–54.

Hechemy KE, Samsonoff WA et al., 1989, *Borrelia burgdorferi* attachment to mammalian cells, *J Infect Dis,* **159:** 805–6.

Helprin JJ, 1995, Neuroborreliosis, *Am J Med,* **98 (4A):** 52S–9S.

Herxheimer K, Hartmann K, 1902, Über Acrodermatitis chronic atrophicans, *Arch Dermatol,* **61:** 57–76.

Horton JM, Blaser MJ, 1985, The spectrum of relapsing fever in the Rocky Mountains, *Arch Intern Med,* **145:** 871–5.

Hu LT, Perides G et al., 1995, Binding of human plasminogen to *Borrelia burgdorferi, Infect Immun,* **63:** 3491–6.

Hughes CA, Engstrom SM et al., 1993, Protective immunity is induced by a *Borrelia burgdorferi* mutant that lacks OspA and OspB, *Infect Immun,* **61:** 5115–22.

Hurtenbach U, Museteanu C et al., 1995, Studies on early events of *Borrelia burgdorferi*-induced cytokine production in immunodeficient SCID mice by using a tissue chamber model for acute inflammation, *Int J Exp Pathol,* **76:** 111–23.

Hyde FW, Johnson RC, 1984, Genetic relationship of Lyme disease spirochetes to *Borrelia, Treponema,* and *Leptospira* spp., *J Clin Microbiol,* **20:** 151–4.

Johnson RC, Johnson BBJ, 1996, *Manual of Clinical Laboratory Immunology,* 5th edn, American Society for Microbiology, Washington, DC, in press.

Johnson RC, Kodner CB, Russell ME, 1986a, Passive immunization of hamsters against experimental infection with *Borrelia burgdorferi, Infect Immun,* **53:** 713–14.

Johnson RC, Kodner CB, Russell ME, 1986b, Active immunization of hamsters against experimental infection with *Borrelia burgdorferi, Infect Immun,* **54:** 897–8.

Johnson RC, Kodner CB, Russell ME, 1987, *In-vitro* and *in-vivo* susceptibility of the Lyme disease spirochete, *Borrelia burgdorferi* to four antimicrobials, *Antimicrob Agents Chemother,* **31:** 164–7.

Johnson RC, Marek N, Kodner CB, 1984, Infection of Syrian hamsters with Lyme disease spirochetes, *J Clin Microbiol,* **20:** 1099–101.

Johnson RC, Hyde FW et al., 1984, *Borrelia burgdorferi* sp. nov. etiological agent of Lyme disease, *Int J Syst Bacteriol,* **34:** 496–7.

Johnson RC, Burgdorfer W et al., 1987, *Borrelia coriaceae* sp. nov.: putative agent of epizootic bovine abortion, *Int J Syst Bacteriol,* **37:** 72–4.

Johnson RC, Kodner CB et al., 1988, Experimental infection of the hamster with *Borrelia burgdorferi, Ann NY Acad Sci,* **539:** 258–63.

Johnson RC, Kodner CB et al., 1990a, Comparative *in-vitro* and *in-vivo* susceptibilities of the Lyme disease spirochete *Borrelia burgdorferi* to cefuroxime and other antimicrobial agents, *Antimicrob Agents Chemother,* **34:** 2133–6.

Johnson RC, Kodner CB et al., 1990b, *In-vitro* and *in-vivo* susceptibility of *Borrelia burgdorferi* to azithromycin, *J Antimicrob Chemother,* **25, Suppl. A:** 33–8.

Karlsson M, Hovind-Hougen K et al., 1990, Cultivation of spirochetes from cerebrospinal fluid of patients with Lyme borreliosis, *J Clin Microbiol,* **28:** 473–9.

Kawabata M, Baba S et al., 1987, Lyme disease in Japan and its possible incriminated tick vector, *Ixodes persulcatus, J Infect Dis,* **156:** 854.

Klempner MS, Noring R et al., 1995, Binding of human plasmin-ogen and urokinase-type plasminogen activator to the Lyme disease spirochete, *Borrelia burgdorferi, J Infect Dis,* **171:** 1258–65.

Kurtti TJ, Munderloh UG et al., 1988, *Borrelia burgdorferi* in tick cell culture: growth and cellular adherence, *J Med Entomol,* **25:** 256–61.

Lane RS, 1990, Susceptibility of the Western fence lizard (*Sceloporus occidentalis*) to the Lyme borreliosis spirochete (*Borrelia burgdorferi*), *Am J Trop Med Hyg,* **42:** 75–82.

Lane RS, Burgdorfer W et al., 1985, Isolation of a spirochete from the soft tick, *Ornithodoros coriaceus*: a possible agent of epizootic bovine abortion, *Science,* **230:** 85–7.

Lastavica CC, Wilson ML et al., 1989, Rapid emergence of a focal epidemic of Lyme disease in coastal Massachusetts, *N Engl J Med,* **320:** 133–7.

Levy SA, Dreesen DW, 1992, Lyme borreliosis in dogs, *Canine Pract,* **17, No. 2.**

Lindenmayer M, Weber A, Onderdonk A, 1989, *Borrelia burgdorferi* infection in horses, *J Am Vet Med Assoc,* **194:** 1384.

Luft BJ, Steinman CR et al., 1992, Invasion of the central nervous system by *Borrelia burgdorferi* in acute disseminated infection, *JAMA,* **267:** 1364–7.

Luft BJ, Dattwyler RJ et al., 1996, Azithromycin compared with amoxicillin in the treatment of erythema migrans. A double-blind, randomized, controlled trial, *Ann Intern Med,* **124:** 785–91.

Mackie FP, 1907, The part played by *Pediculus corporis* in the transmission of relapsing fever, *Br Med J,* **2:** 1706–9.

McLean RG, Ubico SR et al., 1993, Isolation and characterization of *Borrelia burgdorferi* from the blood of a bird captured in the Saint Croix river valley, USA, *J Clin Microbiol,* **31:** 2038–43.

Melkert PW, Stel HV, 1991, Neonatal borrelia infections (relapsing fever): a report of 5 cases and review of the literature, *East Afr Med J,* **68:** 999–1005.

Milch LJ, Barbour AG, 1989, Analysis of North American and European isolates of *Borrelia burgdorferi* with antiserum to a recombinant antigen, *J Infect Dis,* **160:** 351–3.

Nadelman RB, Wormser GP, 1995, Erythema migrans and early Lyme disease, *Am J Med,* **98 (4A):** 15S–22S.

Nadelman RB, Luger SW et al., 1992, Comparison of cefuroxime axetil and doxycycline in the treatment of early Lyme disease, *Ann Intern Med,* **117:** 273–80.

Negussie Y, Remick DG et al., 1992, Detection of plasma tumor necrosis factor, interleukins 6 and 8 during the Jarisch-Herxheimer reaction of relapsing fever, *J Exp Med,* **175:** 1207–12.

Norris SJ, Carter CJ et al., 1992, Low-passage-associated proteins of *Borrelia burgdorferi* B31: characterization and molecular cloning of OspD, a surface-exposed, plasmid-encoded lipo-protein, *Infect Immun,* **60:** 4662–72.

Norris SJ, Carter CJ et al., 1995, High- and low-infectivity pheno-types of clonal populations of *in-vitro*-cultured *Borrelia burgdorferi, Infect Immun,* **63:** 2206–12.

Nowakowski J, Nadelman RB et al., 1995, Doxycycline versus tetracycline therapy for Lyme disease, *Ann Intern Med,* **117:** 273–80.

Obermeier O, 1873, Vorkommen feinster, eine Eigenbewgung zeigender Fäden im Blute von Recurrenskranken, *Zentralbl Med Wissensch,* **11:** 145–7.

Pachner AR, Steere AC, 1985, The triad of neurological manifestations of Lyme disease, *Neurology,* **35:** 47–53.

Padula SJ, Sampieri F Dias, et al., 1993, Molecular characterization and expression of p23 (OspC) from a North American strain of *Borrelia burgdorferi, Infect Immun,* **61:** 5097–105.

Perine PL, Teklu B, 1983, Antibiotic treatment of louse-borne relapsing fever in Ethiopia: a report of 377 cases, *Am J Trop Med Hyg,* **32:** 1096–100.

Peter G, 1994, *1994 Red Book: Report of the Committee on Infectious Diseases,* 23rd edn, American Academy of Pediatricians, Elk Grove Village, Illinois, 541–57.

Pfister HW, Einhaupl KM et al., 1984, The spirochetal etiology of lymphocytic meningoradiculitis of Bannwarth (Bannwarth's syndrome), *J Neurol*, **231**: 141–4.

Pick PhJ, 1894, *Über eine neue Krankheit 'Erythromelie'. Verh Ges Dtsch Naturf 66 Verslg Wein*, II, Leipzig, 336.

Piesman J, 1993, Dynamics of *Borrelia burgdorferi* transmission by nymphal *Ixodes dammini* ticks, *J Infect Dis*, **167**: 1082–5.

Piesman J, Donahue JG et al., 1986, Transovarially acquired Lyme disease spirochetes (*Borrelia burgdorferi*) in field-collected larval *Ixodes dammini* (Acari: Ixodidae), *J Med Entomol*, **23**: 219.

Plasterk RHA, Simon MI, Barbour AG, 1985, Transportation of structural genes to an expression sequence on a linear plasmid causes antigenic variation in the bacterium *Borrelia hermsii*, *Nature (London)*, **318**: 257–63.

Postic D, Assous MV et al., 1994, Diversity of *Borrelia burgdorferi* sensu lato evidenced by restriction fragment length polymorphism of rrf (5S)-rrl (23S) intergenic spacer amplicons, *Int J Syst Bacteriol*, **44**: 743–52.

Preac-Mursic V, Weber K et al., 1989a, Survival of *Borrelia burgdorferi* in antibiotically treated patients with Lyme borreliosis, *Infection*, **17**: 355–9.

Preac-Mursic V, Wilske B et al., 1989b, Comparative antimicrobial activity of the new macrolides against *Borrelia burgdorferi*, *Eur J Clin Microbiol Infect Dis*, **8**: 651–3.

Preac-Mursic V, Wilske B et al., 1992, Active immunization with pC protein of *Borrelia burgdorferi* protects gerbils against *B. burgdorferi*, *Infection*, **20**: 342–9.

Reik L, Steere AC et al., 1979, Neurologic abnormalities of Lyme disease, *Neurology*, **35**: 47–53.

Ribeiro JMC, Mather TN et al., 1987, Dissemination and salivary delivery of Lyme disease spirochetes in vector ticks (Acari: Ixodidae), *J Med Entomol*, **24**: 201–5.

Schaible UE, Kramer MD et al., 1989, The severe combined immunodeficiency (scid) mouse: a laboratory model for the analysis of Lyme arthritis and carditis, *J Exp Med*, **170**: 1427–32.

Schmidli J, Hunziker T et al., 1988, Cultivation of *Borrelia burgdorferi* from joint fluid three months after treatment of facial palsy due to Lyme borreliosis, *J Infect Dis*, **158**: 905–6.

Schreck CE, Snoddy EL, Spielman A, 1986, Pressurized sprays of permethrin or DEET on military clothing for personal protection against *Ixodes dammini* (Acari: Ixodidae), *J Med Entomol*, **23**: 396–9.

Schulze TL, Jordan RA et al., 1994, Suppression of *Ixodes scapularis* (Acari: Ixodidae) nymphs in a large residential community, *J Med Entomol*, **31**: 206–11.

Schwan TG, Burgdorfer W, Garon CF, 1988, Changes in infectivity and plasmid profile of the Lyme disease spirochete, *Borrelia burgdorferi*, as a result of *in vitro* cultivation, *Infect Immun*, **56**: 1831–6.

Schwan TG, Burgdorfer W, Rosa PA, 1995, *Manual of Clinical Microbiology*, 6th edn, American Society for Microbiology, Washington, DC, 626–35.

Schwan TG, Simpson WJ et al., 1989, Identification of *Borrelia burgdorferi* and *B. hermsii* using DNA hybridization probes, *J Clin Microbiol*, **27**: 1734–8.

Schwan TG, Gaage KL et al., 1992, Identification of the tick-borne relapsing fever spirochete *Borrelia hermsii* using a species-specific monoclonal antibody, *J Clin Microbiol*, **30**: 790–5.

Schwan TG, Piesman J et al., 1995, Induction of an outer surface protein on *Borrelia burgdorferi* during tick feeding, *Proc Natl Acad Sci USA*, **92**: 2909–13.

Scrimenti RJ, 1970, Erythema chronicum migrans, *Arch Dermatol*, **102**: 104–5.

Seboxa T, Rahlenbeck SI, 1995, Treatment of louse-borne relapsing fever with low dose penicillin or tetracycline: a clinical trial, *Scand J Infect Dis*, **27**: 29–31.

Simpson WJ, Garon CF, Schwan TG, 1990, Analysis of supercoiled circular plasmids in infectious and non-infectious *Borrelia burgdorferi*, *Microb Pathog*, **8**: 109–18.

Southern PM Jr, Sanford JP, 1969, Relapsing fever: a clinical and microbiological review, *Medicine (Baltimore)*, **48**: 129–49.

Spielman A, Wilson ML et al., 1985, Ecology of *Ixodes dammini*-borne human babesiosis and Lyme disease, *Annu Rev Entomol*, **30**: 439.

Stanek G, Pletschette M et al., 1988, European Lyme borreliosis, *Ann NY Acad Sci*, **539**: 274–82.

Steere AC, 1989, Lyme disease, *N Engl J Med*, **321**: 586–96.

Steere AC, 1995, Musculoskeletal manifestations of Lyme disease, *Am J Med*, **98 (4A)**: 44S–51S.

Steere AC, Malawista SE et al., 1977a, Erythema chronicum migrans and Lyme arthritis: the enlarging clinical spectrum, *Ann Intern Med*, **86**: 685–98.

Steere AC, Malawista SE et al., 1977b, Lyme arthritis. An epidemic of oligoarticular arthritis in children and adults in three Connecticut communities, *Arthritis Rheum*, **20**: 7–17.

Steere AC, Grodzicki RL et al., 1983, The spirochetal etiology of Lyme disease, *N Engl J Med*, **308**: 733–40.

Steere AC, Berardi VP et al., 1990, Evaluation of the intrathecal antibody response to *Borrelia burgdorferi* as a diagnostic test for Lyme neuroborreliosis, *J Infect Dis*, **161**: 1203–9.

Stoenner HG, Dodd T, Larson C, 1982, Antigenic variation of *Borrelia hermsii*, *J Exp Med*, **156**: 1297–311.

Strle F, Chen Y et al., 1995, Persistence of *Borrelia burgdorferi* sensu lato in resolved erythema migrans, *Clin Infect Dis*, **21**: 380–9.

Sundnes KO, Haimanot AT, 1993, Epidemic of louse-borne relapsing fever in Ethiopia, *Lancet*, **342**: 1213–15.

Szczepanski A, Benach JL, 1991, Lyme borreliosis: host responses to *Borrelia burgdorferi*, *Microbiol Rev*, **55**: 21–34.

Szczepanski A, Furie MB et al., 1990, Interaction between *Borrelia burgdorferi* and endothelium *in vitro*, *J Clin Invest*, **85**: 1637–47.

Takayama K, Rothenberg RJ, Barbour AG, 1987, Absence of lipopolysaccharide in the Lyme disease spirochete, *Borrelia burgdorferi*, *Infect Immun*, **55**: 2311–13.

Telford SR III, Mather TM et al., 1988, Incompetence of deer as reservoir hosts of the Lyme disease spirochete, *Am J Trop Med Hyg*, **39**: 105–9.

Thomas DD, Comstock LE, 1989, Interaction of Lyme disease spirochetes with cultured eucaryotic cells, *Infect Immun*, **57**: 1324–6.

Warrell DA, Perine PL et al., 1983, Pathophysiology and immunology of Jarisch-Herxheimer-like reaction in louse-borne relapsing fever: comparison of tetracycline and slow-release penicillin, *J Infect Dis*, **147**: 898–909.

Weisbrod AR, Johnson RC, 1989, Lyme disease and migrating birds in the Saint Croix River Valley, *Appl Environ Microbiol*, **55**: 1921–4.

White DJ, Chang HG et al., 1991, The geographic spread and temporal increase of the Lyme disease epidemic, *JAMA*, **266**: 1230–6.

Wilske B, Preac-Mursic V et al., 1986, Immunochemical and immunological analysis of European *Borrelia burgdorferi* strains, *Zentralbl Bakteriol Mikrobiol Hyg Ser A*, **263**: 92–102.

Wilske B, Preac-Mursic V et al., 1993a, Immunological and molecular polymorphisms of OspC, an immunodominant major outer surface protein of *Borrelia burgdorferi*, *Infect Immun*, **61**: 2182–91.

Wilske B, Preac-Mursic V et al., 1993b, An OspA serotyping system for *Borrelia burgdorferi* based on reactivity with monoclonal antibodies and OspA sequence analysis, *J Clin Microbiol*, **31**: 340–50.

Wilson ML, Deblinger RD, 1993, *Ecology and Environmental Management of Lyme Disease*, Rutgers University Press, New Brunswick, 126–56.

Wormser GP, 1995, Prospects for a vaccine to prevent Lyme disease in humans, *Clin Infect Dis*, **21**: 1267–74.

Zingg BC, LeFebvre RB, 1994, Polymerase chain reaction for detection of *Borrelia coriaceae* putative agent of epizootic bovine abortion, *Am J Vet Res*, **55**: 1509–15.

Chapter 51

HAEMOTROPHIC INFECTIONS

T J Cleary

1 INTRODUCTION

This chapter focuses on those bacteria that exhibit a close association with red blood cells in human and animal hosts. These infections are caused by organisms that belong to the genera *Bartonella*, *Haemobartonella*, *Eperythrozoon*, *Anaplasma* and *Aegyptianella*. The eighth edition of *Bergey's Manual of Systematic Bacteriology* (Weiss and Moulder 1984) classified these genera within 2 families of the order Rickettsiales. The family Bartonellaceae contains 2 genera, *Bartonella* and *Grahamella*, which have distinct cell walls and have been cultivated in artificial media (Ristic and Kreier 1984a). *Bartonella bacilliformis* infects humans whereas *Grahamella* species are found in rodents and other small animals; a human infection by *Grahamella* has been reported (Puntaric et al. 1994). The family Anaplasmataceae contains 4 genera, *Anaplasma*, *Aegyptianella*, *Haemobartonella* and *Eperythrozoon*. Characteristics of the group include presence of a cell membrane but no cell wall and these organisms have not yet been grown in vitro (Ristic and Kreier 1984b, Kreier et al. 1991). Organisms within this group commonly infect various animal species, including laboratory animals; human infections have been reported in immuno-compromised patients (Duarte et al. 1992).

Major taxonomic revisions were proposed recently for the family Bartonellaceae. The 16S rRNA sequence analysis of *Bartonella bacilliformis* showed that this organism was aligned with the α_2 subgroup of the purple bacteria (Brenner et al. 1991), class Proteobacteria (Woese 1987). Closely related species within this group include *Rochalimaea quintana* and *Brucella abortus*. Furthermore, 16S rRNA sequence data and DNA hybridization data show that the 4 species of the genus *Rochalimaea* should be reclassified in the genus *Bartonella* and the family Bartonellaceae should be removed from the order Rickettsiales (Brenner et al. 1993). The newly designated species are *B. quintana*, *B. vinsonii*, *B. henselae* and *B. elizabethae*. Additionally,

it has been proposed that the genus *Grahamella* should be unified with the genus *Bartonella* (Birtles et al. 1995). The newly designated species are *B. talpae*, *B. peromysci*, *B. grahamii*, *B. taylorii* and *B. doshiae*.

Although there remains concern about the classification of these organisms, they share features that allow them to be discussed within this chapter. These organisms have been described as bodies in close association with red blood cells in humans and animals suffering from infections in which anaemia may be a prominent feature. The bodies stain readily, demonstrated by Romanowsky-type stains. Table 51.1 lists some of the differential characters of these organisms.

2 BARTONELLOSIS

2.1 The disease

Bartonella bacilliformis is the aetiological agent of bartonellosis, which has been known as Carrion's disease, Oroya fever and verruga peruana. Bartonellosis is a disease of humans that may have 2 distinctive clinical presentations (Weinman 1944a). Oroya fever is the systemic form of disease that presents as an acute febrile illness and may be associated with haemolytic anaemia. Verruga peruana is the cutaneous form of disease and is characterized by the appearance of wart-like eruptions that occur after the primary infection. Lesions may occur after a primary infection regardless of the previous clinical manifestations. Humans are the only reservoir for infection and the organism is transmitted to humans by a sandfly vector (Hertig 1942).

2.2 Pathogenesis

Following the inoculation of organisms from a sandfly, there is an initial multiplication of organisms within the vascular endothelial cells. Once released into the

Table 51.1 Characteristics of *Bartonella bacilliformis* and the family Anaplasmataceae

Character	Bartonella	Haemobartonella	Eperythrozoon	Anaplasma	Aegyptianella
Morphology	Mainly rods; cocci late in infection	Mainly cocci; may occur as branching chains	Mainly ring forms	Mainly cocci	Mainly cocci
Situation	In and on RBC; and in cytoplasma of endothelial cells	Surface of RBC; forms indentations	Surface of RBC; forms indentations	In RBC: form inclusions containing 'initial bodies'	In RBC: form inclusions containing 'initial bodies'
Bacterial species (animal infected)	*B. bacilliformis* (humans)	*H. felis* (cat) *H. canis* (dog) *H. muris* (mice, rat)	*E. ovis* (sheep) *E. suis* (pig) *E. wenyonii* (cattle) *E. coccoides* (mice)	*A. marginale* (cattle) *A. centrale* (cattle) *A. ovis* (sheep/goat)	*A. pullorum* *A. botuliformis* (guinea fowl)
Distribution	Restricted to Andes Mountains area in South America	World wide	World wide	World wide	World wide
Vector	Sandfly	Fleas, ticks, lice	Flies, keds, mosquito, ticks	Ticks, flies, mosquito	Ticks
Growth in vitro	Yes	No	No	No	No

peripheral circulation, the organisms parasitize red blood cells. Electron microscopy studies have demonstrated that the organisms adhere to and penetrate erythrocytes (Cuadra and Takano 1969). Various potential virulence factors have been described for this organism, including bacterial adherence to a glycolipid moiety on the erythrocytes (Walker and Winkler 1981), flagella-based motility factors (Scherer, DeBuron-Connors and Minnick 1993) and the secretion of a polypeptide, referred to as deformin (Xu, Lu and Ihler 1995), which produces morphological changes on the red blood cells. A 2 gene chromosomal locus has been cloned and used to confer the invasive phenotype to non-invasive *Escherichia coli* strains (Mitchell and Minnick 1995). The interplay of these genes and the other virulence factors is under investigation.

Phagocytosis of parasitized erythrocytes by the reticuloendothelial system, particularly by cells in the liver and spleen, accounts for the destruction of red blood cells. Immunological functions may also serve to modulate the illness but eventually the organisms localize in the cutaneous tissue where they continue to proliferate. The verrugas are highly vascular and organisms may be found intracellularly in the endothelial cells or extracellularly in the fibrous interstitium associated with the verruga (Recavarren and Lumbreras 1972).

2.3 Modes of transmission

Bartonellosis is not communicable from human to human. The phlebotomine sandfly, *Lutzomyia*, is responsible for transmission of the organism. Infected individuals act as reservoirs for the organism in nature (Weinman and Pinkerton 1937). Inoculation of individuals with infected blood or skin tissue may result in an infection.

2.4 Clinical manifestations of disease

Clinical manifestations of the disease following an initial infection varies within the susceptible population. Asymptomatic infections do occur; however, most infections are accompanied by fever, malaise, myalgias and arthralgias (Ricketts 1949). The incubation period is approximately 3 weeks. A proportion of these individuals develops a progressive haemolytic anaemia that is characteristic of Oroya fever but the factors that determine the severity of infection are unknown. However, epidemics with a resultant high mortality are more likely to occur in those populations that have had no prior exposure to the organism as compared to those living in endemic areas (Weinman 1944a). In severe cases, 60–90% of the erythrocytes may contain organisms.

If untreated, the cutaneous phase (verruga peruana) follows a primary episode in 1–3 weeks. This form of disease is characterized by red wart-like skin eruptions on any part of the body surface. Initially, a small red papule develops which progressively enlarges to 1–2 cm in the following days to weeks. Verrugas may appear as multiple lesions over the body, as nodular forms of various sizes and shapes, or as ulcerating lesions that represent infection in the deeper tissues (Ricketts 1949). Successive eruptions may occur over a period of 1–3 months and the lesions may be observed in all stages of development. Cutaneous lesions are non-tender but there may be arthralgias and myalgias that accompany the eruptions. These lesions may become secondarily infected with other micro-organisms.

2.5 Epidemiology

The cutaneous form of the disease was recognized long before its association with the bacteraemic phase (Weinman 1944a, Schultz 1968). Names applied to the cutaneous phase reflecting its epidemiological location include warts of the Andes and verruca Peruviana (Peruvian warts). In 1870, while a railroad was being constructed from Lima to Oroya, Peru, many workers developed fever and anaemia. The cause of the illness was unknown, but it acquired the name 'Oroya fever'. After the outbreak, it was noted that cutaneous lesions developed in several individuals recovering from their acute infection. This observation suggested that the 2 features were probably different manifestations of the same illness. Several years later a Peruvian medical student, Daniel Carrion, was intentionally inoculated with a blood sample from a patient with skin lesions and within 21 days he developed the classical manifestations of Oroya fever and eventually died. Alberto Barton, in 1909, described the organisms in erythrocytes from an infected individual but Noguchi and Battistini (1926) were the first to isolate the organism in culture from the blood of a patient with anaemia. The organism was also isolated from a cutaneous lesion on an experimentally infected monkey (Noguchi 1927).

Geographical distribution of the disease is limited to areas where the vector survives in nature. The habitat of the *Lutzomyia* sandfly is in certain valleys in the Andes mountains region of Peru, Ecuador and Colombia (Weinman 1944a, 1981). The vector is not found at elevations above 8000 ft (2400 m) where the temperature is less than 10°C or in arid regions (below 2500 ft; 750 m) where the annual rainfall is low. No other insect vector has been shown to transmit this organism (Weinman and Pinkerton 1937, Hertig 1942). Serological data from individuals who live in the endemic area indicate that a majority has been infected at some time in the past (Knobloch et al. 1985).

2.6 Host response

Overall mortality in untreated Oroya fever is reported to be as high as 40–70%. The high mortality is not necessarily related to the severity of the anaemia associated with the illness, but rather due to complicating infections by other organisms, particularly *Salmonella* species, which may occur in these compromised hosts (Ricketts 1948). Mortality is markedly reduced if individuals are treated with the appropriate antibiotics. Infection can be self-limiting in those individuals who recover from the initial bacteraemic episode without treatment. There is little, if any, mortality associated with the cutaneous form of the illness and the majority of lesions resolve within a few months. Secondary infections may occur in these lesions and lead to delays in healing and even more serious complications. Immunity usually develops following recovery.

2.7 Laboratory identification

Bartonella bacilliformis is a motile, aerobic gram-negative rod (0.2–0.5 μm × 0.3–3 μm). Flagella are only found in culture and appear as a tuft of 1–10 unipolar filaments. The organism can be isolated on a variety of media supplemented with animal sera, blood or a combination of both. Walker and Winkler (1981) demonstrated 2 colony types when they cultured American Type Culture Collection (ATCC 35686 and ATCC 35685) isolates on heart infusion agar supplemented with 10% rabbit serum, 0.1% glucose and 0.5% rabbit haemoglobin. The distinct colony types were designated T1 and T2. Subcultures of each type contained both colony types after 7 days of incubation at 29°C. T1 colonies were small, dark and friable with an entire edge. T2 colonies were larger, lighter in colour and not friable with an irregular edge.

Multiple blood cultures should be obtained during the bacteraemic illness. Recovery of organisms is enhanced by using a lysis–centrifugation method for the processing of blood samples. Biopsy samples of infected tissue should be obtained aseptically and may be placed between moistened, sterile gauze for transport to the laboratory. Blood cultures obtained from patients with the cutaneous form of disease have yielded the organism. Media that have been used for the primary isolations of the organism include a *Leptospira* medium (Noguchi and Battistini 1926) and a triphasic medium originally described by Colichon and colleagues (Kreier et al. 1991). Cultures are incubated at 28°C for 1–2 weeks. The greater the number of infected erythrocytes the less time needed for growth of the organism. Once isolated in the laboratory, the organism can be maintained on blood-containing media such as Columbia agar supplemented with 5% defibrinated sheep blood or enriched chocolate agar. There are no specific biochemical tests for the identification of the organism or its differentiation from other members of the genus (Welch and Slater 1995).

Blood smears may be stained with Wright's or Giemsa's stain for visualization of the organism. Several of the quick staining methods are useful for work in the field. Infected red blood cells may carry more than one organism. During the acute stage of the infection the organism has a rod-shaped appearance. When multiple organisms infect the cell, they may appear in groups or overlaying one another. As the infection develops, the number of infected erythrocytes decreases and the organism appears more coccoid. In stained tissue sections, organisms are found in the cytoplasm of infected cells or extracellularly in the fibrous interstitium of the lesion.

Using a combination of serological tests, Knobloch et al. (1985) showed that approximately two-thirds of individuals tested from *Bartonella* endemic areas in Peru were positive for antibodies. Sera from individuals outside the endemic area and other healthy controls were negative. No cross-reactivity between *B. bacilliformis* and other bacteria was detected. Data from this study demonstrated that the disease is endemic within certain localities and asymptomatic infections occur.

2.8 Diagnosis

The classical form of Oroya fever is easily recognized in the endemic area. Diagnosis is difficult to appreciate in patients who present with a non-specific febrile illness. For health care workers outside the endemic area, a history of travel to the endemic area would aid in diagnosis. Regardless, blood cultures obtained during the acute form of disease should yield the organism; diagnosis of verruga peruana is suggested by the characteristic lesions present on individuals who are from the endemic area and biopsy specimens from representative lesions should be submitted for culture and histological examination. Patients with the cutaneous form of disease should have blood cultures drawn because the organism is present in the blood during this stage of the illness.

2.9 Treatment

Bartonella is susceptible to a variety of antibiotics, including penicillin, tetracycline, streptomycin and chloramphenicol (Cuadra 1986). Within 24 h of the initiation of appropriate therapy there is rapid resolution of fever and a marked decrease in the number of parasitized erythrocytes. Treatment of individuals during this initial, bacteraemic phase of the infection will prevent or markedly reduce the development of the cutaneous form of disease. However, treatment of individuals who present with the cutaneous form of disease does not appear to alter the course of infection.

2.10 Prevention and control

Since a vaccine is not available for immunization, all methods of prevention and control are directed toward measures that reduce the likelihood of vector contact (Weinman 1944b). Insecticides have been effective in the elimination of the sandfly but their use over wide areas has not been practical. Other measures include screening of windows and securing of floors, walls and ceilings to prevent access to the house, use of insect repellent and wearing clothing that protects the body from bites. Because the sandfly feeds during the evening, one effective measure, if possible, is to leave the endemic area during this time.

3 ANAPLASMOSIS

3.1 Aetiological agents

Organisms in the family Anaplasmataceae are obligate parasitic organisms found within or on erythrocytes or free in the plasma of various animal species, including frequently used laboratory animals (Kreier et al. 1991, Woldehiwet and Ristic 1993). Members of the family are found throughout the world. In the natural environment, the organism may be transmitted by arthropods or by contaminated blood-containing tissue. Infection may or may not cause overt disease but usually results in long-term persistence of the agent with concomitant resistance to clinically demonstrable reinfection. Anaemia is the most prominent feature of the clinical disease. An extraerythrocytic stage of disease has not been described. The organisms and the species that they normally infect are listed in Table 51.1.

3.2 The disease

Haemobartonella felis causes a severe anaemia in apparently healthy cats and *H. canis* may be seen in the erythrocytes of splenectomized dogs but appears not to cause disease in healthy animals (Nash and Bobade 1993). Infections in rats by *H. muris* are fairly common but are normally not expressed. A latent infection can be activated by splenectomy and by certain chemical poisons and other infections. *Eperythrozoon ovis* and *E. wenyonii* cause mild anaemia in sheep and cattle, respectively; *E. suis* is responsible for an economically important and sometimes fatal disease of swine (Scott and Woldehiwet 1993). *E. coccoides* will cause overt disease in splenectomized mice. *Anaplasma marginale* and *A. centrale* cause infections in cattle (Wanduragala and Ristic 1993) and it is estimated that they are responsible for 50 000–100 000 cattle deaths per year in the United States (Goodger, Carpenter and Riemann 1979). Infections in sheep and goats are caused by *A. ovis*. *Aegyptianella* species are known to infect birds.

3.3 Pathogenesis

The mechanism(s) responsible for the pathogenesis and pathophysiology of these infections are not understood but they are probably similar to other erythron infections. Members of the genera *Haemobartonella* and *Eperythrozoon* are found on the surface of erythrocytes in folds or indented areas. The organisms do not penetrate red blood cells. The epicellular nature of the infection has been confirmed by scanning and transmission electron microscopy (Venable and Ewing 1968, McKee et al. 1973). Members of the genera *Anaplasma* and *Aegyptianella* form inclusion bodies within erythrocytes that contain the infectious initial bodies.

The sequence of events following entry of the parasite into a susceptible host has been extensively studied in anaplasmosis (Wanduragala and Ristic 1993). Upon entry into the bovine host, *A. marginale* initial bodies invade erythrocytes. Two polypeptides, designated MSP1a and MSP1b, have been isolated and purified from the organism and function as adhesions for receptors on the red blood cells (McGarey et al. 1994). The organism is internalized in a vacuole of host cell origin where it undergoes binary fission, resulting in the formation of marginal bodies containing 8–10 initial bodies. The organisms may invade fresh erythrocytes through intercellular tissue bridges. Under experimental conditions, the prepatent period (interval between exposure and appearance of marginal bodies in the erythrocyte) varies from 24 to 35 days and the animal becomes a symptomless carrier following recovery from the initial disease.

3.4 Modes of transmission

Transmission of infection to susceptible animals may occur by biological and mechanical means. For *Eperythrozoon* and *Haemobartonella* species, various bloodsucking arthropods are implicated in the transmission of organisms by mechanical means. These vectors include fleas, stable flies, keds, mosquito, ticks and lice. Ticks are capable of becoming infected and then transmitting anaplasmosis. It has been shown that after a blood meal the organism is present in the gut and salivary gland (Kocan et al. 1993).

3.5 Clinical manifestations

Disease manifestations caused by these agents varies with the infecting organism and the host animal species. All the agents may cause inapparent infections in their respective host, whereas others may be primary agents of clinical disease. It is known that the likelihood of clinical disease increases in incidence with age. Following recovery from a primary infection, a chronic carrier state usually develops in the animal and recurrent infections may occur in animals that develop unrelated diseases. Infected animals demonstrate fever, anorexia and weight loss because of the severe anaemia that may accompany the disease.

3.6 Epidemiology

For the most part, the agents responsible for these infections are found throughout the world. The organisms survive in the natural environment either in the chronically infected animal or in one or more vectors. The ability of persistently infected animals to serve as disease reservoirs for transmission to vectors has been studied for *A. marginale* (Eriks, Stiller and Palmer 1993). By using nucleic acid probes to quantitate the microbial load, it was found that *Dermacentor andersonii* ticks effectively transmitted the disease from asymptomatic, chronic carriers.

3.7 Laboratory identification

The family Anaplasmataceae contains 4 genera: *Anaplasma*, *Aegyptianella*, *Haemobartonella* and *Eperythrozoon* (see Table 51.1). Organisms within this group contain both DNA and RNA and multiply by binary fission. As yet, they have not been successfully cultivated in vitro. Growth in vivo is inhibited by tetracycline compounds, but not by penicillin or streptomycin.

Blood smears are stained with Romanowsky-type stains. In a recent report, 3 commercially available differential stains, Camco-Quik, Diff-Quik and Wright-Giesma, were evaluated for the detection of intra-erythrocytic parasites in bovine blood smears (Hart et al. 1992). The single step Camco-Quik stain was as good as or better than the other differential stains. In addition, an acridine orange stain has proved useful for the detection of infected erythrocytes (Gainer 1961). The marginal *Anaplasma* body appears as a dense, homogenous, bluish-purple, round-to-oval structure that measures 0.3–1.0 μm in diameter. Within each marginal body are 8–10 subunits known as initial bodies. In some species there are comet-like projections extending from the inclusion body into the cytoplasm. Inclusion bodies are also found in erythrocytes infected by *Aegyptianella* species. *Haemobartonella* organisms occur as small purple to blue staining cocci, rings and rods that are firmly attached to erythrocytes; very few are free in the plasma. Organisms are approximately 0.5 μm in diameter and appear to be partially buried in indented foci on the surface of the erythrocytes. *H. canis* differs from *H. felis* in that it more commonly forms chains extending across the surface of the affected erythrocyte. *Eperythrozoon* organisms appear as blue to pinkish-blue staining parasites usually found as ring forms on the surface of red blood cells or in depressions in the cell surface. Frequently, organisms are found free in the plasma. In Giemsa-stained films they are round and often exhibit a ring form.

Various nucleic acid amplification procedures have been employed for the detection of these organisms (Gwaltney and Oberst 1994, Figueroa and Buening 1995). The use of nucleic acid probes has provided an opportunity to differentiate genetic variability among isolates and to study the transmission of these parasites from various vectors.

3.8 Treatment, prevention and control

The tetracycline family of drugs is most widely used to treat haemotrophic infections. In addition, the organisms are sensitive to organic arsenical compounds. Vaccine preparations are available for the prevention of anaplasmosis. All infections can be prevented by eliminating the biological and mechanical vectors of the disease.

REFERENCES

Birtles RJ, Harrison TG et al., 1995, Proposals to unify the genera *Grahamella* and *Bartonella*, with descriptions of *Bartonella talpae* comb. nov., *Bartonella peromysci* comb. nov., and three new species, *Bartonella grahamii* sp. nov., *Bartonella taylorii* sp. nov., and *Bartonella doshiae* sp. nov., *Int J Syst Bacteriol*, **45:** 1–8.

Brenner DJ, O'Connor SP et al., 1991, Molecular characterization and proposal of a neotype strain for *Bartonella bacilliformis*, *J Clin Microbiol*, **29:** 1299–301.

Brenner DJ, O'Connor SP et al., 1993, Proposal to unify the genera *Bartonella* and *Rochalimaea*, with descriptions of *Bartonella quintana* comb. nov., *Bartonella vinsonii* comb. nov., *Bartonellae henselae* comb. nov., and *Bartonella elizabethae* comb. nov., and to remove the family *Bartonellaceae* from the order *Rickettsiales*, *Int J Syst Bacteriol*, **43:** 777–86.

Cuadra M, 1986, Bartonellosis, *Infectious Diseases and Medical Microbiology*, 2nd edn, eds Braude AI, Davis CE, Fierer J, WB Saunders, Philadelphia, 1219–25.

Cuadra M, Takano J, 1969, The relationship fo *Bartonella bacilliformis* to the red blood cell as revealed by the electron microscope, *Blood*, **33:** 708–16.

Duarte MIS, Oliveira MS et al., 1992, Haemobartonella-like microorganism infection in AIDS patients: ultrastructural pathology, *J Infect Dis*, **165:** 976–7.

Eriks IS, Stiller D, Palmer GH, 1993, Impact of persistent *Anaplasma marginale* rickettsemia on tick infection and transmission, *J Clin Microbiol*, **31:** 2091–6.

Figueroa JV, Buening GM, 1995, Nucleic acid probes as a diagnostic method for tick-borne hemoparasites of veterinary importance, *Vet Parasitol*, **57:** 75–92.

Gainer JH, 1961, Demonstration of *Anaplasma marginale* with the fluorescent dye, acridine orange: comparison with the complement-fixation test and Wright's stain, *Am J Vet Res*, **22:** 882–6.

Goodger WJ, Carpenter T, Riemann M, 1979, Estimation of economic loss associated with anaplasmosis in California beef cattle, *J Am Vet Med Assoc*, **174:** 1333–6.

Gwaltney SM, Oberst RD, 1994, Comparison of an improved polymerase chain reaction protocol and the indirect hemag-glutination assay in the detection of *Eperythrozoon suis* infection, *J Vet Diagn Invest*, **6:** 321–5.

Hart LT, Morris NG et al., 1992, Single-step technique for staining *Anaplasma marginale* in bovine blood smears, *Am J Vet Res*, **53:** 1732–3.

Hertig M, 1942, Phlebotomus and Carrion's disease, *Am J Trop Med*, **22, Suppl.:** 1–80.

Knobloch J, Solano L et al., 1985, Antibodies to *Bartonella bacilliformis* as determined by fluorescence antibody test, indirect haemagglutination and ELISA, *Trop Med Parasitol*, **36:** 183–5.

Kocan KM, Goff WL et al., 1993, Development of *Anaplasma marginale* in salivary glands of male *Dermacentor andersoni*, *Am J Vet Res*, **54:** 107–12.

Kreier JP, Gothe R et al., 1991, The hemotrophic bacteria: the families *Bartonellaceae* and *Anaplasmataceae*, *The Prokaryotes: a Handbook on the Biology of Bacteria: Ecophysiology, Isolation, Identification, Applications*, eds Balows A, Truper HG et al., Springer-Verlag, New York, 3994–4022.

McGarey DJ, Barbet AF et al., 1994, Putative adhesins of *Anaplasma marginale*: major surface polypeptides 1a and 1b, *Infect Immun*, **62:** 4594–601.

McKee AE, Ziegler RF, Giles RC, 1973, Scanning and transmission electron microscopy of *Haemobartonella canis* and *Eperythrozoon ovis*, *Am J Vet Res*, **34:** 1196–201.

Mitchell SJ, Minnick MF, 1995, Characterization of a two-gene locus from *Bartonella bacilliformis* associated with the ability to invade human erythrocytes, *Infect Immun*, **63:** 1552–62.

Nash AS, Bobade PA, 1993, Haemobartonellosis, *Rickettsial and Chlamydial Diseases of Domestic Animals*, eds Woldehiwet Z, Ristic M, Pergamon Press, New York, 89–110.

Noguchi H, 1927, Etiology of Oroya fever. VI. Pathological changes observed in animals experimentally infected with *Bartonella bacilliformis*, *J Exp Med*, **45:** 437–55.

Noguchi H, Battistini TS, 1926, Etiology of Oroya fever. I. Cultivation of *Bartonella bacilliformis*, *J Exp Med*, **43:** 851–64.

Puntaric V, Borcic D et al., 1994, Haemotropic bacteria in man, *Lancet*, **343:** 359–60.

Recavarren S, Lumbreras H, 1972, Pathogenesis of the verruga of Carrion's disease, *Am J Pathol*, **66:** 461–4.

Ricketts WE, 1948, *Bartonella bacilliformis* anemia (Oroya fever). A study of thirty cases, *Blood*, **3:** 1025–49.

Ricketts WE, 1949, Clinical manifestations of Carrion's disease, *Arch Intern Med*, **84:** 751–81.

Ristic M, Kreier JP, 1984a, Family II. *Bartonellaceae* Gieszczykiewicz 1939, 25[al], *Bergey's Manual of Systematic Bacteriology*, vol. 1, eds Krieg NR, Holt JG, Williams and Wilkins, Baltimore, 717–19.

Ristic M, Kreier JP, 1984b, Family III. *Anaplasmataceae* Philip 1957, 980[al], *Bergey's Manual of Systematic Bacteriology*, vol. 1, eds Krieg NR, Holt JG, Williams and Wilkins, Baltimore, 719.

Scherer DC, DeBuron-Connors I, Minnick MF, 1993, Characterization of *Bartonella bacilliformis* flagella and effect of anti-flagellin antibodies on invasion of human erythrocytes, *Infect Immun*, **61:** 4962–71.

Schultz MG, 1968, A history of bartonellosis (Carrion's disease), *Am J Trop Med Hyg*, **17:** 503–15.

Scott GR, Woldehiwet Z, 1993, Eperythrozoonoses, *Rickettsial and Chlamydial Diseases of Domestic Animals*, eds Woldehiwet Z, Ristic M, Pergamon Press, New York, 111–29.

Venable JH, Ewing SA, 1968, Fine-structure of *Haemobartonella canis* (*Rickettsiales: Bartonellacea*) and its relation to the host erythrocyte, *J Parasitol*, **54:** 259–68.

Walker TS, Winkler HH, 1981, *Bartonella bacilliformis*: colonial types and erythrocyte adherence, *Infect Immun*, **31:** 480–6.

Wanduragala L, Ristic M, 1993, Anaplasmosis, *Rickettsial and Chlamydial Diseases of Domestic Animals*, eds Woldehiwet Z, Ristic M, Pergamon Press, New York, 65–87.

Weinman D, 1944a, Bartonella and human bartonellosis, *Trans Am Phil Soc*, **33:** 246–87.

Weinman D, 1944b, Public health aspects of bartonellosis, *Trans Am Phil Soc*, **33:** 339–45.

Weinman D, 1981, Bartonellosis and anemias associated with *Bartonella*-like structures, *Diagnostic Procedures for Bacterial, Mycotic and Parasitic Infections*, 6th edn, eds Balows A, Hausler WJ, American Public Health Association, Inc. Washington, DC, 235–48.

Weinman D, Pinkerton H, 1937, Carrion's disease. IV. Natural sources of bartonella in the endemic zone, *Proc Soc Exp Biol Med*, **37:** 596–8.

Weiss E, Moulder JW, 1984, Order I. *Rickettsiales* Gieszczykiewicz 1939, 25[al], *Bergey's Manual of Systematic Bacteriology*, vol. 1, eds Krieg NR, Holt JG, Williams and Wilkins, Baltimore, 687–8.

Welch DF, Slater LN, 1995, Bartonella, *Manual of Clinical Microbiology*, 6th edn, eds Murray PR, Baron EJ et al., ASM Press, Washington DC, 690–5.

Woese CR, 1987, Bacterial evolution, *Microbiol Rev*, **51:** 221–71.

Woldehiwet Z, Ristic M, 1993, The Rickettsiae, *Rickettsial and Chlamydial Diseases of Domestic Animals*, eds Woldehiwet Z, Ristic M, Pergamon Press, New York, 1–26.

Xu YH, Lu ZY, Ihler GM, 1995, Purification of deformin, an extracellular protein synthesized by *Bartonella bacilliformis* which causes deformation of erythrocyte membranes, *Biochim Biophys Acta*, **1234:** 173–83.

Chlamydial diseases

J Schachter, G L Ridgway and L Collier

1 INTRODUCTION

There are currently 4 species recognized within the genus *Chlamydia*. They resemble each other in their morphology and, most importantly, share a unique mode of replication. They possess a common complement fixing antigen. They differ in their host range and organ specificity. *C. trachomatis* and *C. pneumoniae* have been considered strictly human pathogens without animal reservoirs. However, the recent isolation of organisms similar to *C. trachomatis* from ferrets and swine and reports of *C. pneumoniae*-like organisms from horses and koalas challenge that concept. *C. trachomatis* and *C. pneumoniae* affect mostly the eye, the respiratory and urogenital tracts of man, whereas *C. psittaci* primarily infects birds and mammals, in which it causes a wide range of syndromes, including pneumonitis, polyarthritis, encephalomyelitis and infections of the gut and placenta. *C. psittaci* is a common pathogen in avian species and mammals and, although capable of causing human disease, does so as a zoonosis with very little person-to-person transmission being documented. *C. pecorum*, the fourth species, is not known to infect humans, but is a common pathogen for cattle and sheep, also causing encephalomyelitis, pneumonia and arthritis. The various species of *Chlamydia* are each capable of infecting a wide variety of organs in their naturally occurring hosts and can cause many different diseases. Although specific tissue tropisms have been noted for specific strains, the biological basis for such specificity is unknown.

For useful reviews on chlamydial infection, see the Symposia listed in the references, Storz (1971), Schachter and Dawson (1978), Oriel and Ridgway (1982), Mårdh, Paavonen and Puolakkainan (1989).

2 DISEASES CAUSED BY *C. TRACHOMATIS*

In humans, the syndromes caused by *C. trachomatis* fall into 3 groups, each of which tends to be associated with a particular set of serotypes:

1 trachoma (mainly serotypes A, B, Ba and C)
2 oculogenital and, occasionally, more general infections (mainly serotypes D–K, although serovar B has been recovered from both genital disease and endemic trachoma) and
3 lymphogranuloma venereum (serotypes L1, L2 and L3).

2.1 Trachoma and inclusion conjunctivitis

TRACHOMA

History

Trachoma is one of the earliest recorded diseases. The Ebers papyrus (c.1500 BC) refers to an affliction that was almost certainly trachoma and to its alleviation with copper salts, a form of treatment that persisted well into the twentieth century. Trachoma was familiar to the ancient Greeks and Romans. The name is Greek (τραχῶμα = roughness) and refers to the characteristic conjunctival follicles.

Accounts of military campaigns from the Crusades to the Napoleonic wars refer to severe ophthalmic infections acquired in the Middle East and it is quite possible that trachoma was disseminated to Europe and elsewhere by returning soldiers. The disease did not spread to the general population and eventually disappeared from most of Europe, even before the introduction of specific treatment.

Inclusion conjunctivitis was first recognized in the early years of this century as an infection of infants caused by an agent very similar to that of trachoma, but which is acquired at birth from the maternal genital tract. It was realized later that these neonatal infections represent the tip of a large iceberg of genital tract infections in adults.

Epidemiology of trachoma

Geographical distribution Trachoma is endemic primarily in tropical and subtropical countries; those worst affected are North Africa, the Middle East and the northern part of the Indian subcontinent. The disease is also prevalent in sub-Saharan Africa, the Far East, Australasia and Latin America. Its prevalence and severity vary considerably from country to country and in different areas within the same country. Trachoma is associated with poor living standards and hygiene and thus tends to be more prevalent in rural than in urban settings.

The world-wide prevalence of trachoma is often quoted as 400–500 million cases, but because of the paucity of information from many areas, this figure is a very crude estimate. Only a minority suffer severe visual impairment, but even so the cases in this category must number several million. The epidemiology of trachoma is reviewed by Treharne (1985). For detailed statistics of the prevalence of trachoma see Thylefors et al. (1995).

Mode of spread Trachoma is spread from eye to eye, but the mechanism is not certain and may vary in different circumstances; what evidence there is is largely circumstantial. Flies contaminated with infectious discharges are often blamed, and Jones (1975) showed that fluorescein-stained ocular discharge can be transferred in this way between children in the same household. This mode of transmission is more likely to occur in areas such as North Africa and the Middle East, where ocular discharges are copious because of associated bacterial infections and flies are numerous (p. 979). On the other hand, trachoma is highly prevalent in areas where neither epidemic bacterial conjunctivitis nor fly infestation is serious; in such areas, poor hygiene, close physical contact and infected fomites may be the main factors in transmission. Shared eye cosmetics such as mascara (Thygeson and Dawson 1966) and kohl have also been implicated in the spread of trachoma. The incubation period of naturally acquired trachoma is uncertain since the onset is insidious and it is difficult or impossible to establish the date of contact. In experimental infections of volunteers the incubation period is 2–7 days; on the premise that under natural conditions the inoculum is smaller, it seems reasonable to assume a period of 7–14 days.

Age incidence The higher the prevalence of trachoma in a given community, the younger is the age of onset. Thus in a Gambian village the prevalence was highest (91%) in the 5–9 year age group and thereafter declined to about 50% in those aged more than 20 years (Sowa et al. 1965). In a Tunisian community all children had acquired the infection by the age of 2 years (Dawson et al. 1976).

Clinical features of trachoma

Trachoma was defined by the World Health Organization (1962) as 'a specific communicable keratoconjunctivitis, usually of chronic evolution ... characterized by follicles, papillary hyperplasia, pannus and, in its later stages, cicatrization'.

Conjunctival papillae result from hypertrophy of the normal papillary processes; when numerous, they give the palpebral conjunctiva a reddened, velvety appearance.

Lymphoid follicles with typical germinal centres appear in the palpebral and sometimes in the bulbar conjunctiva as pale round elevations which have been likened to sago grains (Fig. 52.1). Follicles at the limbus are pathognomonic of trachoma, as are the depressed pigmented areas ('Herbert's pits') left on regression.

Corneal lesions mainly affecting the upper segment usually appear early; their subsequent course is variable. Superficial punctate keratitis is usually transient. Pannus (L.= a veil) is a cellular infiltration of the cornea accompanied by new blood vessels growing in from the limbus; gross pannus extending over the pupil may impair vision. Cicatrization of the subepithelial tissues may so distort the lids, particularly the upper, that the border turns inward (entropion) or more rarely outward (ectropion). Entropion results in continual trauma to the cornea by the inwardly directed lashes (trichiasis) and hence in ulceration, opacities and visual impairment. Stenosis of the lacrimal duct may cause xerophthalmia and further corneal damage. On the other hand, the disease often resolves with little or no scarring.

For more detailed descriptions of physical signs see Dawson, Jones and Darougar (1975) and Darougar and Jones (1983).

Clinical classification MacCallan (1936) distinguished 4 stages (Tr I–IV) in the course of trachoma: in brief, they are those of onset, established trachoma, cicatrization and final resolution. This classification was useful, but gave no information about the severity of the infection or the incidence of sequelae, both of which are important in the studies of epidemiology and control. A WHO Expert Committee on Trachoma (World Health Organization 1962) therefore made a

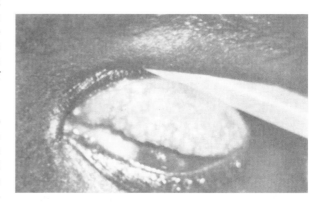

Fig. 52.1 Trachoma stage II, showing severe follicular hyperplasia. (Photograph by the late Josef Sowa).

distinction between the relative intensity and the relative gravity of trachoma; the first term refers to the degree of activity at a given time and the second to the degree of disabling complications and sequelae, or to lesions that, untreated, are liable to lead to such sequelae. Intensity and gravity are not necessarily related, since highly active disease of short duration may have a better outcome than chronic trachoma of low intensity (Assaad and Maxwell-Lyons 1967). Assessments of relative gravity are much the more important for estimating the impact of potentially blinding complications on a community, and the effects of treatment.

Reinfection and reactivation The prolonged course of trachoma in endemic areas has been ascribed to both periodic reinfections and to reactivations; but because the number of chlamydial serotypes is small, the value of change in serotype as a marker of reinfection is limited. Nevertheless, the balance of opinion is toward repeated reinfection rather than reactivation as a factor in chronicity.

Intercurrent eye infections In some areas where trachoma is highly endemic, notably North Africa and the Middle East, outbreaks of bacterial conjunctivitis, especially in the spring and summer, are common. The worst of these are caused by *Haemophilus aegyptius*; infection with *Haemophilus influenzae* and to a lesser extent *Neisseria* spp., *Moraxella* spp. and streptococci and staphylococci also occur. It is generally held that the increased volume of discharge occasioned by such infection assists the spread of trachoma, possibly through the medium of flies; and that repeated bacterial infections increase the severity of trachoma. The possibility of intercurrent eye infections with epidemic viruses such as adenovirus type 8 or enterovirus virus type 70 should be borne in mind.

INCLUSION CONJUNCTIVITIS OF ADULTS
Clinical features

The incubation period is generally between 1 and 2 weeks. The onset is acute, with intense hyperaemia, mucopurulent discharge and follicular hyperplasia. In contrast to trachoma, follicles are more pronounced in the lower lid. Diffuse punctate keratoconjunctivitis may occur some 2–3 weeks after the onset of symptoms. Pannus is unusual, but well documented (Viswalingam, Wishart and Woodland 1983). In the acute phase preauricular lymphadenopathy and upper respiratory symptoms may occur, with involvement of the middle ear. It is usually necessary to enquire directly about genital symptoms, which may be minimal or absent, particularly in women. Untreated, the disease runs a fluctuating course before resolving without conjunctival cicatrization. Corneal clouding (keratitis) may persist.

PATHOLOGY OF CHLAMYDIAL EYE INFECTIONS

Only epithelial cells are parasitized by the infecting agent; inflammatory changes in the subjacent tissues are secondary. The pathological changes in the con-

junctiva can be followed by studying Giemsa-stained scrapings taken at intervals after infection (Collier 1967). The earliest is subepithelial infiltration with neutrophil leucocytes and lymphocytes; the former predominate at first, but within a week or so are largely replaced by lymphocytes; as the follicles mature, lymphoblasts from their germinal centres also appear. Lymphocytes within the follicles are typically B cells, while cytotoxic T cells predominate in the subepithelial spaces between follicles. The nuclei of the epithelial cells become enlarged and eosinophilic and vacuoles appear in the cytoplasm which is shed, giving rise to much basophilic debris; the cause of these degenerative changes is unknown, but may be related to the presence of toxic chlamydial lipopolysaccharide. In trachoma and inclusion conjunctivitis a proportion of the epithelial cells contain the characteristic inclusion bodies (see Volume 2, Chapter 59), which can be stained by Giemsa's method (Fig. 52.2), with Lugol's iodine or by immunofluorescence. Inclusions are often numerous in the early stages, but become progressively more scanty as the disease progresses. The nuclei of the epithelial cells become enlarged and eosinophilic and vacuoles appear in the cytoplasm which is shed, giving rise to much basophilic debris; the cause of these degenerative changes is unknown. Macrophages containing ingested debris ('Leber cells') are often present. These cytological changes persist for long periods in the absence of treatment.

In trachoma, the pathological changes are more pronounced in the upper than in the lower lid, whereas the reverse is true in inclusion conjunctivitis. Limbal follicles occur in trachoma but not in inclusion conjunctivitis; the reason for these differences is unknown. Another striking dissimilarity between the 2 syndromes is the frequency of pannus and scarring in trachoma and their rarity in inclusion conjunctivitis. This may, at least in part, be explicable in terms of reinfection, the opportunities for which are much greater in trachoma, a community disease, than in inclusion conjunctivitis, a sporadic infection of individuals. Experiments in monkeys and observations in

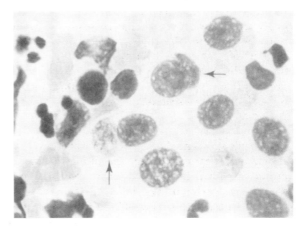

Fig. 52.2 Trachoma: 2 conjunctival inclusions (arrowed). Giemsa stain (× 1000).

the field suggest a similar explanation for the comparative frequency of these potentially blinding complications in areas where trachoma is highly endemic (see, e.g. Grayston et al. 1985). In this hypothesis, reinfections are assumed to result in hypersensitivity to chlamydial antigen with consequent immunopathological damage. There is some evidence that the antigen concerned may be a detergent-soluble substance elaborated by replicating chlamydiae. This material, which has been identified as a member of the heat shock protein family (Hsp60, Morrison et al. 1989) is capable of eliciting an inflammatory reaction when dropped on the conjunctiva of previously infected monkeys or guinea pigs. The prevailing theory is that much of the pathology in diseases caused by *C. trachomatis* is due to delayed hypersensitivity reactions to this antigen.

2.2 Oculogenital and associated infection

History

Within 3 years of the first description of *C. trachomatis* the association of this organism with non-trachomatous infection of the neonatal eye and genital infection in adults was confirmed (Fritsch, Hofstätter and Lindner 1910). However, it was not until the advent of laboratory isolation techniques that the true extent of chlamydial involvement in these syndromes became apparent. The first isolations of *C. trachomatis* from a neonate with inclusion conjunctivitis and from the mother of another such infant were reported by Jones, Collier and Smith (1959). Jones (1964) drew attention to the close association between adult genital infection and adult inclusion conjunctivitis. The spectrum of diseases known to be caused by *C. trachomatis* has been widened to include upper genital tract infection in women, epididymitis in men, reactive arthritis of adults and respiratory infection of the newborn.

Epidemiology

The epidemiology of oculogenital infection by *C. trachomatis* (sometimes termed paratrachoma) differs markedly from that of classical endemic trachoma. Adult inclusion conjunctivitis is primarily a sexually transmitted disease, in contrast to the eye-to-eye spread of trachoma. The former may be acquired by direct or indirect contact with genital secretions from an infected person, or by autoinfection. Inadequate chlorination of swimming baths has in the past been implicated in the transmission of eye infection, presumably from contamination of the water with genital secretions.

Genital infections of men

Non-gonococcal urethritis (NGU)   In most communities, non-gonococcal urethritis (NGU) is far more common than gonococcal urethritis. The incubation period is variable, but is usually between 7 and 14 days after intercourse with an infected partner. Urethral irritation and dysuria are followed by the appearance of a mucopurulent discharge. Microscopy reveals 5 or more polymorphonuclear cells (PMN) per × 1000 field in a gram-stained smear of the discharge, or more than 15 PMN per × 400 field in the spun deposit of a 'first catch' urine sample.

C. trachomatis is the only agent firmly implicated in the causation of NGU. The organism is isolated from 20–30% of cases, compared to 3–5% of matched controls without urethritis (Oriel and Ridgway 1982). *Ureaplasma urealyticum* (see Volume 2, Chapter 34) may account for a minority of cases of NGU. The role of other organisms, including *Mycoplasma genitalium*, *Mycoplasma hominis*, *Bacteroides ureolyticus*, *Herpesvirus hominis*, cytomegalovirus and *Trichomonas vaginalis*, remains to be fully elucidated, but on available evidence these organisms are unlikely to be responsible for more than 10% of NGU.

Post-gonococcal urethritis (PGU)   The persistence or recurrence of symptoms and signs following effective treatment of gonococcal urethritis is almost always due to concurrent infection with an agent or agents of NGU. *C. trachomatis* is isolated from 11–30% of men with gonococcal urethritis and probably accounts for 80–90% of PGU cases (Oriel and Ridgway 1982).

Other infections of the male genital tract   Epididymitis in men under 35 years old is associated with *C. trachomatis* in approximately 50% of cases, compared with 15% of older men (Berger et al. 1978). Diminished fertility is an accepted consequence of epididymitis, but to what extent *C. trachomatis per se* contributes to male infertility is unknown. The role of the organism in acute or chronic prostatitis is more controversial. The balance of evidence suggests that *C. trachomatis* is not causally linked to prostatitis. *C. trachomatis* has been isolated from the rectum of 4–8% of randomly selected homosexual males, most of whom admitted anoreceptive intercourse (Goldmeier 1985). In a group of 288 men with symptoms of proctitis, 12% yielded the organism (Quinn et al. 1981). Three of the isolates were of the L2 serotype and the patients had more severe symptoms than those infected with non-lymphogranuloma venereum serotypes.

Diagnosis can be made by a variety of techniques. For many years, culture was considered the diagnostic test of choice. Antigen detection methods (either direct fluorescent antibody tests or enzyme immunoassay) and nucleic acid detection tests are now more commonly used. Specimens from the urethra require insertion of a swab 3–4 cm, having first removed any excess discharge. There is increasing evidence that urine samples may provide a satisfactory alternative. Polymerase chain reaction (PCR) and ligase chain reaction (LCR) tests for chlamydial DNA may well prove to be suitable techniques for use on urine specimens from men, providing a more acceptable alternative to swab insertion, particularly in asymptomatic men (Jaschek et al. 1993, Chernesky et al. 1994b).

Genital infections of women

Sexually acquired chlamydial infection in women may involve not only the cervix and urethra, but also the endometrium, fallopian tubes and rectum. Extension of infection into the peritoneal cavity may result in perihepatitis.

Lower genital tract infection Chlamydial infection of the cervix is found in 15–30% of women attending clinics for sexually transmitted diseases. Carrier rates for this organism are relatively high in women because up to 70% of the infections may have neither signs nor symptoms of infection. With no obvious need for evaluation or treatment, prevalence increases. Thus, a wide range of infection rates may be found in women having routine pelvic examinations at family planning clinics or settings where they are having annual physical examinations. Lower socioeconomic class and young age are the most readily identifiable risk factors for chlamydial infection. The organism is present in the cervix of over 80% of primary contacts of men with chlamydial urethritis. Some 35–45% of women with cervical gonorrhoea have concurrent chlamydial infection, i.e. approaching twice the prevalence in men with gonorrhoea.

There are few distinctive symptoms or signs. Brunham et al. (1984) demonstrated a relationship between chlamydial infection and mucopurulent cervical discharge in the absence of *Neisseria gonorrhoeae*. Predictive values associating this sign and infection are often less than 30%. An association between chlamydial cervical infection and hypertrophic cervicitis was noted by Rees and colleagues (1977), but there is no evidence that *C. trachomatis* causes the erosion. Cytological changes are non-specific and include degeneration of epithelial cells, an increase in parabasal cells and the presence of polymorphonuclear leucocytes, lymphocytes and large mononuclear cells.

Urethral infection This may occur in the absence of cervical infection in up to one-third of infected women. Although infections with *C. trachomatis* may cause urinary symptoms, its role in the urethral syndrome remains controversial. Stamm et al. (1980) found that 10 of 16 women with abacterial pyuria had *C. trachomatis* infection of the urethra. By contrast, Feldman et al. (1986) found no association between *C. trachomatis* infection and urinary symptoms, pyuria or urethral leucocytosis in a series of 250 women attending a STD clinic. Age and clinic type may bias the presentations.

For diagnosis, cervical specimens are best collected from the squamocolumnar junction after removal of excess exudate. They may be processed by any of the presently available techniques (see section 2.6, p. 985). Few clinics routinely take urethral samples in addition to cervical swabs; consequently the true prevalence of infection will be underestimated. To increase the yield of chlamydiae from the lower genital tract of women, at little additional cost, the pooling of urethral and cervical specimens from a patient has its advocates (e.g. Manuel et al. 1987). It has been demonstrated that LCR tests on urine may be a substitute for cervical specimens (Lee et al. 1995).

C. trachomatis may cause vaginitis in prepubertal girls and also in hysterectomized women. Davies et al. (1978) isolated chlamydiae from Bartholin's ducts in 9 women, of whom 7 had concurrent gonorrhoea. The true prevalence of chlamydial infection at this site is unknown.

Upper genital tract infection Ascending chlamydial infection of the female genital tract has been well reviewed by Mårdh (1987). Chlamydial endometritis does occur. Mid-cycle bleeding is often the only abnormal sign associated with chlamydial infection. The possibility should be considered in the differential diagnosis of irregular menstrual bleeding. Post-vaginal delivery and post-abortal endometritis are well documented.

The association of *C. trachomatis* with salpingitis has been recognized for many years. Less clear are the frequency of a chlamydial aetiology and the interrelationship of *C. trachomatis* with other organisms associated with salpingitis, including *N. gonorrhoeae*, *M. hominis* aerobic and anaerobic bacteria. Mårdh (1987) suggests that 8% of women with cervical chlamydial infection will experience salpingitis as a complication. The organism has been recovered from the fallopian tubes at laparoscopy. Experimental infection of the oviducts of monkeys has provided additional evidence (Weström and Mårdh 1983). Opinions differ as to the relative frequencies of chlamydial and gonococcal salpingitis. This may reflect the milder and more protracted symptoms of the former, the imprecision of clinical diagnosis of salpingitis, or a geographical variation in the distribution of the 2 organisms. Thus, identification rates for *C. trachomatis* vary between 5 and 20% in the USA, to 25–40% in Europe (Mårdh 1987). Bevan, Ridgway and Siddle (1995) recently reported a UK cohort study on 104 laparoscopy confirmed cases of pelvic inflammatory disease. *C. trachomatis* was identified (culture, antigen detection or serology) in 55%.

Characteristically, the patient with chlamydial salpingitis has abdominal pain of longer duration and the ESR is higher than is usual in gonococcal salpingitis. A modest pyrexia is present (rectal temperature 38°C or higher). At laparoscopy, the tubal damage seen may be more severe than expected from the milder onset. Involuntary infertility is an important complication in 12–13% of women following a first attack, rising to 75% after more than 2 episodes (Weström 1975).

Tubal factor infertility may also be more likely after a severe episode than a mild one. Ectopic pregnancy is another common outcome of chlamydial salpingitis, reflecting the subsequent tubal damage. Ectopic pregnancy rates increase 7–10-fold after episodes of salpingitis.

Seroepidemiological studies have shown a very strong association between high levels of antichlamydial antibody and tubal factor infertility and ectopic pregnancy. High levels of antibody are not only seen to be specific for chlamydial major outer membrane protein (MOMP) antigens but also for Hsp60. Many of the women who have tubal damage and high levels of antibody to chlamydia have no prior clinical history of salpingitis. This has led to the concept that a silent salpingitis may occur during what is an apparently uncomplicated chlamydial infection and that this may be more common than clinically apparent salpingitis. Studies by Stacey et al. (1990) and Bevan, Ridgway and Siddle (1995), demonstrating the presence of chlamydial antigen in the fallopian tubes of patients with symptoms of pelvic inflammatory disease (PID), but laparoscopically normal would seem to support this concept.

Extension of infection into the peritoneal cavity results in perihepatitis (Curtis–Fitz-Hugh syndrome), characterized by right hypochondrial pain without derangement of hepatic function. At laparoscopy, thin fibrous adhesions ('violin string') are seen between the fallopian tubes and the liver capsule. A similar condition may occur with non-chlamydial salpingitis.

The role of *C. trachomatis* in abortion, stillbirth and prematurity remains uncertain.

Rectum　Little interest has been shown in rectal chlamydial infection in women. Dunlop et al. (1971) demonstrated the organism in 13 women, none of whom complained of relevant symptoms, although scarring, congestion and a cloudy exudate were seen with an operating microscope. Stamm et al. (1982) reported on 42 women with rectal chlamydial infection. Twelve had symptoms, including rectal discharge, pain and loose stools. All of these women and 7 of 14 asymptomatic women yielded rectal polymorphonuclear leucocytes.

Neonatal and childhood infections

Babies born vaginally to mothers with cervical chlamydial infection are at risk of becoming colonized or infected with the organism. Estimates of the risk are as high as 70%. Conjunctival infection occurs in 30–40% and pneumonia in 10–20% of these babies. Other sites infected (either alone or concurrently) include the middle ear, nasopharynx and the rectum. The association with overt disease at some of these sites is uncertain. Infection of the vagina, rectum and pharynx may be delayed for up to 7 months after birth (Bell et al. 1987). True congenital infection has not been reported.

Ocular infection　Chlamydial infection of the neonate eye is more common than gonococcal ophthalmia. Estimates in the USA range from 1.6% to 12% of neonates (Rapoza et al. 1986). Onset is from 6 to 21 days after birth. Physical signs range from florid conjunctivitis with pronounced conjunctival and periorbital oedema and a purulent or mucopurulent discharge to little more than a 'sticky eye'. Pseudomembranes are seen occasionally. Untreated, the condition resolves over 2–3 months; conjunctival scarring occurs in some cases (Hobson, Rees and Viswalingam 1982). Inclusions are usually numerous and may be found in scrapings from the lower conjunctival fornix.

Pneumonia　This syndrome was described by Schachter et al. (1975) and by Beem and Saxon (1977). Onset occurs characteristically 4–12 weeks after birth. The main features are dyspnoea, a staccato cough and sometimes a nasal discharge. There may be evidence of otitis media. Chest radiography shows hyperexpansion with symmetrical diffuse interstitial and patchy alveolar infiltrates. Significant laboratory findings include eosinophilia and raised immunoglobulin titres. High serum titres of antichlamydial IgM are usually present. Untreated, the disease runs a benign clinical course, leading to apparent recovery. Although the number of children who have had long-term follow-up after an episode of chlamydial pneumonia in infancy is quite small, in one study, two-thirds of them had long-term consequences. Approximately one-third developed asthma, whilst the rest had abnormal respiratory functions tests (Weiss, Newcombe and Beem 1986).

Other infections　Vaginal infection occurred in 8% of 120 infants born to *Chlamydia*-positive mothers in the series followed by Bell et al. (1987). They caution that colonization/infection may persist for more than 2 years, which suggests that detection of chlamydiae has a limited use in the evaluation of suspected sexual abuse in children. The situation is further confused by reports of chlamydial vulvovaginitis in older children.

C. trachomatis may be shed from the rectum in large amounts during the first year of life, particularly from children with pneumonia. Prospective studies show that shedding does not occur before the age of 6–12 weeks, suggesting that the infection is not acquired at birth, but arises from ingestion of organisms derived from ocular or respiratory infection. The long-term sequelae of gastrointestinal infection are unknown.

Sexually acquired reactive arthritis (SARA)

Sexually acquired reactive arthritis (SARA) describes a group of rheumatoid factor negative arthritides, including non-dysenteric Reiter's syndrome, which are apparently associated with genital infection (Keat 1983). Men are 10 times more likely to acquire the disease than women and approximately 1% of men with NGU develop arthritis. Synovitis usually develops within 30 days of symptomatic infection. The classic triad of Reiter's syndrome (arthritis, ocular and genital symptoms) occurs in 30–50% of patients with reactive arthritis. In 50% of patients, the knee is the first site to be involved. Other joints commonly affected are the wrist, ankle and metatarsophalangeal joints. More than one joint is involved in some 90% of patients. There is a strong association with carriage of the histocompatibility antigen HLA-B27. *C. trachomatis* is probably involved as a trigger antigen, resulting in an enhanced immune response in susceptible individuals. Whether viable organisms can be found in the synovium or synovial fluid is controversial. The presence of antigenic components of the organism at these sites is an alternative possibility. Keat et al. (1987) detected chlamydial antigen by immunofluorescence in the synovium or synovial fluid from the knees of 5 of 8 patients with SARA. This finding has been confirmed by several other investigators, but the number of positive cases is low. Chlamydial nucleic acid has also been detected in synovial specimens using a MOMP-based PCR (Taylor-Robinson et al.

1992). It is becoming apparent that reactive arthritis, including SARA, is a response to a number of different infectious agents, of which *C. trachomatis* is one, in genetically predisposed individuals.

Other infections of adults

The involvement of non-LGV strains of *C. trachomatis* in other conditions is less well documented. The association with adult respiratory infection has always been uncertain, and the evidence requires reappraisal in the light of *C. pneumoniae*. Cases of endocarditis (Van der Bel Khan et al. 1978), myocarditis (Ringel et al. 1982) and meningoencephalitis (Myrhe and Mårdh 1981) have been reported. The organism is rarely recovered from bronchiolar specimens from AIDS cases with pneumonia.

2.3 Lymphogranuloma venereum

Lymphogranuloma venereum (LGV) differs considerably from other syndromes caused by *C. trachomatis*; it is caused by members of serotypes L1, L2 and L3, which attack lymphatic and subepithelial rather than epithelial tissues and there may be extensive fibrosis in the later stages. Although less prevalent than other sexually transmitted diseases in industrialized countries, it has a wide geographical distribution, prevalence being highest in the tropics and subtropics.

Clinical features

Transmission occurs by sexual contact; the incubation period is usually 1–3 weeks. In men the primary lesion is a vesicle or ulcer on the penis; rectal infections occur in homosexuals. In women the commonest site is the fourchette. In both sexes the lesion may pass unnoticed. Primary lesions occasionally occur on extragenital sites, for example fingers or tongue. Healing of the primary lesion is rapidly followed by the second stage, which is characterized by swelling of the inguinal lymph nodes. Such swelling occurs more frequently in men than in women. Enlargement of the nodes both above and below the inguinal ligament sometimes results in a characteristic 'groove sign'. The nodes become matted, fluctuant and fixed to the skin; they may break down and discharge through multiple sinuses. Primary vaginal or cervical lesions will result in pelvic lymphadenopathy, which may go undetected. In the acute phase there may be constitutional disturbances such as fever and joint pains. Complications include conjunctival infection and preauricular lymphadenopathy, meningitis, synovitis, pneumonitis and cardiac abnormalities. If untreated, the disease progresses after some years to the third stage, which is usually more serious in women than in men. Ulceration, proctitis, rectal strictures and rectal or rectovaginal fistulae may occur. The vulva may become grossly affected by ulceration and granulomatous hypertrophy ('esthiomène'). Elephantiasis of the vulva or scrotum may also develop.

Diagnosis

Because of the variable physical signs, clinical diagnosis may be difficult. Chancroid in particular, along with syphilis, granuloma inguinale, filariasis, herpes simplex, plague, hernias and malignant disease, all enter into the differential diagnosis; the possibility of simultaneous infections must always be borne in mind.

Serological tests Frei-type skin tests for delayed hypersensitivity to LGV antigen have been superseded by serological methods; microimmunofluorescence (MIF), rather than complement fixation, is now the method of choice. However, even MIF is not wholly specific, since there are cross-reactions between LGV antigens and antibodies to other chlamydiae; nevertheless, if the patient presents early, a rising titre of antibody may provide good confirmatory evidence of infection. More typically, patients with LGV show very high levels of antibody (>1:1000 in the MIF test) which are unusual for males infected with the trachoma biovar. But this may complicate diagnosis for women who more often have high levels of antibody due to PID.

Isolation of LGV agent The organism may be isolated in a suitable cell culture from the primary lesion or from pus aspirated from a suppurating lymph node. LGV agents do not require mechanical assistance (centrifugation) to successfully infect tissue culture cells.

Histology In practice, histological examination is not much used, but in experienced hands may be a useful adjunct to diagnosis. Sections of lymph nodes contain multinucleate giant cells and masses of epithelioid cells, at the centres of which are degenerate polymorphonuclear leucocytes. Gamna–Favre inclusion bodies may be seen within the cytoplasm of mononuclear cells. Giant cells and granuloma formation may be seen at subepithelial levels of infected mucosal sites.

2.4 Mouse pneumonitis

Chlamydiae that produce inclusions that stain for glycogen and that are sensitive to sulphonamides have been isolated from a number of animal species. Some of them are sufficiently different to think they may ultimately be placed in a separate species (mouse pneumonitis agent) whereas others appear virtually identical with *C. trachomatis* strains isolated from humans (ferret). The infection of animals with *C. trachomatis* is important as a possible source of error when attempting animal experiments with isolates from humans. Their presence in a colony should be excluded by macroscopic examination of the lungs and inoculation of material into cell cultures, if necessary after several 'blind' mouse-to-mouse passages by the intranasal route. Testing of experimental animals for antichlamydial antibody should be routine.

2.5 Immune responses to chlamydiae

As with other micro-organisms, the immune responses to *Chlamydia* spp. often differ according to whether they result from infections induced by natural routes, whether in the wild or in the laboratory, or from artificial inoculations of whole organisms or antigens by, for example, parenteral injection. Here, we shall consider primarily responses to infection by natural routes; since there seem to be no fundamental differences in those induced respectively by *C. trachomatis* and *C. psittaci*, we shall consider them together. Because of wide variations in methods, types of chlamydiae and study populations reported by various workers, this short account is necessarily generalized. For reviews see Kunimoto and Brunham (1985) and Jones and Batteiger (1986).

ANTIBODY RESPONSES

Chlamydia spp. specific antibodies of the IgM, IgG and IgA classes appear in both the serum and local secretions, including tear fluid in the case of eye infections; the nature and magnitude of the responses vary with the type and duration of infection.

Antibody classes

Specific IgA (mostly secretory IgA) is more constantly demonstrable in secretions from infected mucous membranes than in serum, whereas the reverse is true of IgM antibody. Some or all of the IgG antibody detectable in secretions may be derived by transudation from the blood. IgM and IgG serum antibody titres are liable to be higher in generalized diseases such as LGV than in localized infections such as trachoma. IgM antibody appears early in the serum, but may persist alongside IgG for relatively long periods, especially if reinfections occur. Individuals with complicated infections tend to have higher levels of antibody (that may persist for many years), than do individuals with uncomplicated localized infections. For example, women with salpingitis have higher levels of antibody when compared with women with cervical infection; and men with epididymitis have high levels of antibody when compared with men with uncomplicated urethritis.

Antibody functions

It is much easier to measure chlamydia-specific antibodies than to define their role in protection and recovery from infection. In the sera of patients with proven chlamydial infections of the genital tract, IgG, IgM and IgA antibodies are directed against the major outer-membrane protein (MOMP) and various other polypeptides of elementary and reticulate bodies (Cevenini et al. 1986). Serotype-specific epitopes on some of these polypeptides (see Volume 2, Chapter 59) elicit neutralizing antibodies which, if produced at mucous surfaces, may play some part in protecting against reinfection, at least in the short term. Antibodies against a variety of specific chlamydial proteins are capable of neutralizing infectivity in cell culture systems, but it has not been possible to relate them to protection against infections in vivo.

CELLULAR RESPONSES

Polymorphonuclear leucocytes

In vitro, these cells readily inactivate chlamydiae (Yong et al. 1982); in vivo their early appearance and comparatively rapid diminution in numbers in the face of persisting infection suggest that their part in the recovery process is limited.

Mononuclear phagocytes

The relation between these cells and chlamydiae is complex. Experiments with mouse peritoneal cells showed that viable elementary bodies (EB) are phagocytosed, but by contrast with what happens in permissive cells, the phagosomes fuse with lysosomes and the EB are degraded with loss of infectivity.

Lymphocytes

Levitt, Danen and Bard (1986) showed that both *C. trachomatis* and *C. psittaci* bind to and cause polyclonal stimulation of murine B lymphocytes in vitro; the effector molecule does not appear to be the lipopolysaccharide, which is common to both species; it may be the major outer-membrane protein. By contrast with B lymphocytes, T cells showed specific clonal stimulation by *C. trachomatis* (serotype L2) with class II HLA restriction (Qvigstad et al. 1985); in these experiments primed blood monocytes served as antigen-presenting cells. The role of T cell mediated cytotoxicity in chlamydial infection may depend upon the chlamydial species.

It has become obvious in a number of experimental systems that resistance to reinfection and the ability to clear primary infection is, in large part, dependent on T cell functions. Both CD4 and CD8 cells have been shown to have a protective role. Earlier reports indicating that there was no cytotoxic action against infected target cells have been shown to have been flawed on technical grounds and specific lysis of chlamydia-infected cells has now been demonstrated. Natural killer cell activity may also play a role (Igietseme et al. 1994).

INTERFERON

The induction of cytokines by infection may play an important role in determining the outcome of chlamydial infection and may be important not only in defensive and protective responses, but in pathogenesis. Interferons are active against chlamydiae and the most important one appears to be interferon-γ (IFN-γ). Chlamydial infections induce the production of IFN-γ and the organisms are sensitive to its action. In the presence of IFN-γ (which acts by depleting tryptophan levels in cells) chlamydial replication is inhibited at the reticulate body stage. This may result functionally in dramatic reduction in chlamydial infection and as some infected cells may be sloughed, the infection may be abrogated. However, the infected cells may also be excreting chlamydial antigen that can induce further sensitization and contribute to pathogenic mechanisms. Thus it is likely that the delayed-type hypersensitivity reactions to *Chlamydia* spp. represent a double-edged sword with both protective and immunopathological implications. Tumour necrosis factor may also play a role, either independently or by enhancing IFN-γ.

Little is known about the respective roles of helper and suppressor T cells in chlamydial infections. Young and Taylor (1984) found that lymphocytes from monkeys repeatedly reinfected with trachoma proliferated weakly in vitro when exposed to *C. trachomatis* antigen. Depletion of suppressor T cells significantly increased proliferation, from which it was inferred that such cells might impair the cell mediated response to infection; but later experiments (Young and Taylor 1986) did not support this supposition. Whittum Hudson et al. (1986) showed by immunohistochemical methods that both T helper and T suppressor/cytotoxic cells, the latter predominating, appeared in large numbers in the conjunctival follicles of monkeys inoculated with *C. trachomatis*. It is clear that the roles of the various T cell subsets also needs further exploration.

There is more evidence, much of it indirect, about the part played by delayed hypersensitivity (DH) in chronic chlamydial infections and re-exposures to chlamydial antigens. The Frei reaction, formerly used to test for LGV infection, depended on a DH response in the skin to injection of antigen. More recently, the cellular infiltration leading to scarring that characterizes many chronic or repeated ocular and genital tract infections has been ascribed by a number of workers to immunopathological mechanisms with a strong DH component. Such a conclusion was reached by, for example, Wang and Grayston (1967) from studies of chronic trachoma in monkeys; by Grayston et al. (1985) from observations of repeated trachoma infections in a human population; and by Watkins and coworkers (1986) from repeated inoculation of the guinea pig eye with *C. psittaci* [Guinea pig inclusion conjunctivitis] (GPIC).

ARTIFICIAL IMMUNIZATION

The wide prevalence of trachoma, its major role as a cause of visual disability and the difficulties of mass treatment have led to several attempts to produce an effective vaccine. The results of experiments in animals (see Symposium 1967, 1971) gave encouraging results, but those of field trials were disappointing (for reviews see Collier 1973 and Schachter and Dawson 1978). In brief, different vaccines either conferred short-term protection, had no discernible effect or were actually deleterious: some appeared to enhance the severity of trachoma in those who subsequently acquired the infection, whereas others increased rather than diminished the attack rate. There seems little doubt that some of these vaccines induced hypersensitivity rather than protection and field trials have been abandoned pending the development of safer antigens for use in man. Using genetic engineering it has been possible to insert chlamydial genes into poliovirus vaccine. By use of serovar-specific portions of the major outer-membrane protein it has been possible to induce neutralizing antibodies in mice and monkeys. Thus, models have been created that allow

for development of vaccines that present potentially protective chlamydial antigens while deleting the sensitizing antigens that may contribute to disease. Such vaccines have been targeted for prevention of pelvic inflammatory disease as well as trachoma. None has been evaluated in humans, but these vaccines have not produced the type of protection that was seen with cruder vaccines in the monkey studies for trachoma vaccine. This subject has been reviewed by Brunham (1994).

The economic loss caused by chlamydiosis of cattle and birds also makes a vaccine desirable: in general *C. psittaci* vaccines seem to have been rather more successful than those against *C. trachomatis* and routine immunization against enzootic abortion of ewes and feline pneumonitis has been available for many years (for review, see Storz 1971). Nevertheless, the evaluation of such vaccines has not always been rigorous and some of those in routine use are not fully effective.

In summary then, the immune responses to chlamydial infections are relatively ineffective in promoting either recovery or immunity to reinfection. On the contrary, cell mediated responses may contribute significantly to tissue damage, especially in chronic or repeated infections.

2.6 Laboratory diagnosis

Infection with *C. trachomatis* may be diagnosed by isolating the organism in cell culture, by direct detection (by microscopy of stained specimens) in clinical material, by detection of specific antigens or genes, or by the use of serological methods.

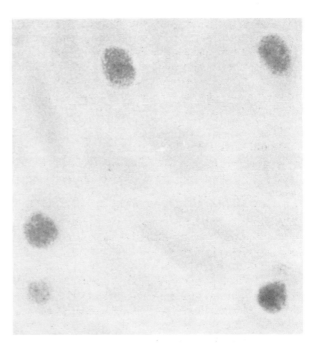

Fig. 52.3 *Chlamydia trachomatis* inclusions in idoxuridine-treated McCoy cells, 45 h after inoculation. Iodine stain (× 670).

CELL CULTURE

Formation of inclusions in cell culture provides the most convenient method for the isolation of *C. trachomatis* from clinical material. The technique involves the inoculation of a suitable cell line (e.g. HeLa 229 or cycloheximide treated McCoy (mouse L) cells), followed by centrifugation and incubation (see Volume 2, Chapter 59). Cell monolayers are fixed and then stained, most commonly by iodine, Giemsa (for dark ground examination) (Figs 52.3, 52.4), or by immunofluorescent antibody stain, with the last being more sensitive.

DIRECT DETECTION OF CHLAMYDIAL ANTIGEN

For over 50 years, the only practical means of identifying *C. trachomatis* in clinical material was the demonstration of inclusions by suitable stains: a method both of low sensitivity and often low specificity. The development of highly specific monoclonal and polyclonal antibodies, with improved immunological techniques, combined with the high cost of a cell culture service resulted in a return to direct methods. The advent of PCR and LCR technology may revolutionize direct detection of the organism in clinical material in the near future.

Papanicolaou staining is a widely used screening technique for cervical dysplasia. It is unreliable for the detection of chlamydial infection; thus Forster et al. (1985) found that only 13% of women cultured positive for *C. trachomatis* had cytological changes consistent with this finding. Furthermore, only 40% of women with cytological changes consistent with chlamydial infection yielded isolates.

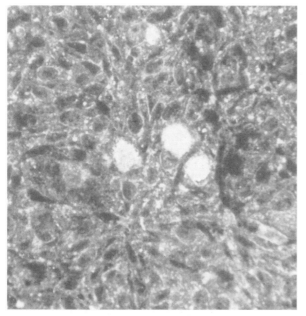

Fig. 52.4 As Fig. 52.3, Giemsa's stain, darkfield illumination (× 670).

Direct immunofluorescence (DIF)

Clinical material can be examined by direct immunofluorescence (DIF) for the presence of elementary bodies. Tam et al. (1982) described a species-specific monoclonal antibody directed against the 40 kDa MW major outer-membrane protein. They described the appearance of elementary bodies, rather than inclusions in DIF-stained smears of clinical material, and concluded that seeking whole inclusions in direct smears was the wrong approach. Previous antibody preparations were of insufficient sensitivity to detect anything other than large inclusions. Since 1982, these findings have been confirmed by many groups, using commercially prepared polyclonal and monoclonal antibodies. Early reports recommended that 10 or more elementary bodies should be observed before the specimen was reported as positive. The sensitivity of the test is, however, reduced if this criterion is used.

The subjectivity of DIF is a cause for concern. On the one hand, smears provide visual confirmation that adequate material has been collected; but this advantage must be balanced against overenthusiastic diagnosis of 'chlamydial' particles. False positives, e.g. with certain strains of *Staphylococcus aureus* (Krech et al. 1985), may also be misleading.

Enzyme immunoassay (EIA)

EIA offers the potential advantages over DIF of objectivity and ease of mechanization. However, the results of studies comparing the reliability of such methods with cell culture are conflicting. For example, Mumtaz et al. (1985) reported a sensitivity for EIA of 92.5% compared with cell culture. In contrast, Taylor-Robinson, Thomas and Osborn (1987) reported a sensitivity for EIA of only 67% compared with cell culture. The specificity of the EIA was 97% and 100% respectively, and the populations studied were comparable.

There are other potential advantages of EIA over DIF. It allows for batch processing, which is more conducive to large-scale screening. EIA tests can be mechanized and results are objective. The best EIAs seem to have a sensitivity similar to that of DIF in expert hands. However, non-culture tests are subject to false positive results. They should therefore be used with caution in low prevalence settings because of the effect of false positive results on the predictive value of a positive result (for example, in a 3% prevalence setting a test with 97% specificity would yield a false positive result rate of 3%, meaning that any positive test result could only have a predictive value for a positive of 50% (Schachter 1985). Blocking assays to confirm positive results have improved specificity of these tests to greater than 99%, so that when confirmatory assays are used, EIA can be performed in low prevalence settings (Moncada et al. 1990). Sensitivity is, however, another issue. Under ideal conditions, both DIF and EIA are less sensitive than culture. Isolation in cell culture is recognized to have a sensitivity of only 75–85%, thus a major proportion of infected individuals will not be detected. DIF and EIA tests perform better in high prevalence settings than in low prevalence populations.

DNA detection

Direct DNA hybridization assays appear to have a sensitivity of the order of 75%, which is similar to that of DIF and EIA. Amplified DNA tests, however, are far more sensitive. Both PCR and LCR have been used for the diagnosis of chlamydial infections (Jaschek et al. 1993, Chernesky et al. 1994a). Commercially available assays target DNA sequences in the chlamydial cryptic plasmid which is present at 7–10 copies per elementary body. These tests are capable of detecting less than one chlamydial particle and are more sensitive than culture. Indeed, these tests are so sensitive, they require a redefinition of the 'gold standard' for diagnostic tests because some infections can only be diagnosed (and confirmed) by using a number of different targets for DNA amplification tests.

DETECTION OF CHLAMYDIAL ANTIBODY

A serological test with a high positive predictive value continues to be elusive. The methods most applicable to *C. trachomatis* infections are immunofluorescence (based on the microimmunofluorescence test of Wang (see Wang and Grayston 1982), immunoperoxidase (Cevenini et al. 1984) or EIA (Ridgway 1986). In general, determination of antibody titres on a single specimen of serum from adults is unhelpful, with the possible exception of cases of pelvic inflammatory disease, epididymitis or LGV. Detection of specific IgM titres in neonates is useful for the diagnosis of chlamydial pneumonitis.

Skin tests

With the possible exception of LGV (see p. 983), the results of skin tests for the diagnosis of *C. trachomatis* infection are so variable as to make them useless. There are currently no commercial sources of Frei test antigen, and 'home brew' tests are inappropriate.

2.7   Prevention and treatment

OCULAR INFECTIONS

Trachoma

The control of endemic trachoma depends on the improvement of living standards, which in itself can significantly reduce the prevalence; on antimicrobial treatment campaigns designed to eliminate ocular infection, both with chlamydiae and with bacteria such as *Haemophilus aegyptius*; and on surgical correction of potentially blinding lid deformities. These aspects are well reviewed in handbooks published by the World Health Organization (1973, 1979). WHO-assisted programmes have resulted in the virtual or complete eradication of trachoma in countries where governmental support has been forthcoming. In less favoured areas where logistic, economical and organizational difficulties are more intractable, trachoma remains a major public health problem.

The planning of any treatment campaign must begin with an evaluation of the prevalence of trachoma and its complications in the various age groups. In areas of high endemicity, specific therapy is given by mass treatment with tetracycline eye ointment or oily suspension; intermittent schedules (e.g. twice daily for 5 consecutive days every 6 months) enable large numbers of persons to be treated by small mobile teams. Where prevalence is lower, selective treatment, e.g. of schoolchildren only, may be employed. Oral therapy with antibiotics is more rapidly effective than topical therapy, but problems of expense, compliance and supervision make it impracticable for mass use. For treatment of active disease in individuals, tetracycline by mouth (250 mg 4 times daily for 3 weeks) may be given. Erythromycin (e.g. erythromycin stearate 500 mg twice daily) is a suitable alternative and should be given to children in preference to tetracycline. Such treatment results in rapid subsidence of inflammation, but follicles may persist for weeks or months after infection is eliminated. Unduly short courses of treatment may result in relapse. More recently, a single oral dose of azithromycin, a long-acting azalide macrolide, has been shown to be effective in the treatment of trachoma (Bailey et al. 1993). It is possible that such an antibiotic may play a role in future trachoma control.

Inclusion conjunctivitis

The association between inclusion conjunctivitis and genital infection both of patient and consort must be borne in mind when considering therapy. Systemic treatment should always be used. Oral tetracyclines or erythromycin for 10–14 days, in the doses given for trachoma, are suitable for adults.

Ophthalmia neonatorum

Credé's silver nitrate drops are of no value in the prophylaxis of chlamydial ophthalmia. The infection responds to oral erythromycin (30–50 mg kg^{-1} day^{-1} for 3 weeks). Topical therapy is unreliable alone and unnecessary in addition to systemic therapy. Furthermore, the use of topical antibiotics will not prevent pharyngeal or pulmonary infection. When present, gonococcal infection should be treated before beginning antichlamydial therapy. Oral erythromycin is also effective against chlamydial pneumonitis. The parents must be referred for investigation for genital tract infection and treatment.

GENITAL INFECTION

Treatment of chlamydial genital infection is always indicated to avoid complications. Because of the possibility of multiple infection, the drug of choice should be effective against other likely pathogens. Tetracyclines are the mainstay of therapy and it appears that, provided treatment is given for not less than 7 days, the dose and duration have little effect on microbiological cure. Tetracycline hydrochloride or oxytetracycline 500 mg 4 times daily, minocycline 100 mg twice daily, or doxycycline 100 mg twice daily are equally effective oral treatments for uncomplicated infection in men and women. As an alternative to tetracyclines, erythromycin (erythromycin stearate 500 mg twice daily for 14 days; Oriel et al. 1977) has proved acceptable. This regimen is likely to be replaced by a single 1 g oral dose of azithromycin, which has been shown to be as effective as the 7 day doxycycline regimen (Martin et al. 1992). In parallel evaluations, success rates of greater than 96% for uncomplicated genital chlamydial infection were obtained with both regimens. Amongst the fluorinated quinolones, only ofloxacin (400 mg twice daily for 7 days) has proved to be clinically reliable to date (Ridgway 1995). Other fluorinated quinolones such as sparfloxacin are undergoing clinical evaluation with encouraging results. Persistent urethritis will develop in 10–15% of men treated for *Chlamydia*-positive NGU, even though cultures for *C. trachomatis* become negative. As with any sexually transmitted disease, the tracing and treatment of contacts is an integral part of the control and prevention of infection. Treatment of PID is more complicated and requires multiple drugs.

Lymphogranuloma venereum

In general, early treatment has the best chance of success; fibrosis and other changes in the later stages make the disease less amenable to medical treatment. Published data on controlled clinical trials are scanty; both sulphonamides and tetracyclines given for at least 3 weeks are effective (Greaves et al. 1957). Rifampicin has been successfully used in at least one study (Menke et al. 1979) and erythromycin may also be useful but has not been extensively evaluated. Rifampicin should be used with caution and as a component of a multidrug regimen, because resistance is easily induced in vitro.

3 DISEASES CAUSED BY *C. PSITTACI*

By contrast with *C. trachomatis*, *C. psittaci* mainly affects birds and non-primate mammals (see review by Storz 1971); infections of man are rare by comparison, but the association between pneumonitis and contact with psittacine birds has long been recognized. The term 'psittacose' (psittacosis) was first used by Morange (1895). Chlamydial infections in other avian species are referred to as 'ornithosis'. Neither term is appropriate for infections of mammals and Storz (1971) suggested 'chlamydiosis' to designate the generalized infections caused by *C. psittaci*. The various syndromes in birds and mammals are associated with particular biogroups that are distinguishable by serological and other methods (see Volume 2, Chapter 59).

3.1 Infections of birds

CLINICAL AND PATHOLOGICAL FEATURES

Infection is usually acquired by the respiratory or oral route but in some species may be transmitted vertically via the egg. Ticks, lice and mites infesting poultry may harbour chlamydiae, but there is no evidence that the organisms replicate within them and their role in transmission is unknown. Inapparent infection is much more common than overt disease, which is often precipitated by stress, e.g. exposure to dampness or overcrowding. The clinical signs may vary in nature and severity from outbreak to outbreak, between species and by age, younger birds being the more severely affected; such signs include loss of condition, diarrhoea, respiratory distress and conjunctivitis. If unchecked, the mortality rate in domestic flocks may reach 30%.

Chlamydiosis of birds is a generalized infection that may affect all the major systems, especially the reticuloendothelial, alimentary and respiratory. At necropsy, the lungs are consolidated; the liver and spleen are enlarged and may be haemorrhagic; serous surfaces are inflamed and covered with exudate; the gut lining is inflamed; and there may be signs of meningoencephalitis. The histological findings include oedema, haemorrhage and extensive infiltration with lymphocytes and histiocytes. In poultry, there may be intercurrent infection with bacteria, e.g. salmonellae and pasteurellae.

CONTROL OF AVIAN CHLAMYDIOSIS

The high prevalence of *C. psittaci* in avian species makes eradication an unrealistic proposition. Strict quarantine procedures should be applied to imported psittacine birds but the high commercial value of some show birds sometimes leads to smuggling. Chlamydiosis in poultry can be minimized by keeping and transporting birds under good conditions. Particularly in the USA, attempts have been made with some success to control the infection in poultry and pet-bird breeding establishments by incorporating tetracycline in the feed. The efficacy of such measures depends on their efficient application and the maintenance of adequate blood concentrations; however, even under the best conditions it would be prudent to regard them as suppressive rather than therapeutic. Furthermore, the use of tetracycline in this way carries the risk of producing antibiotic-resistant bacteria. No effective immunization procedure for birds has as yet been devised. Imported birds must be held in quarantine and undergo a course of tetracycline prophylaxis before they are released into commercial trade.

3.2 Infections of animals

Infections with *C. psittaci*, often inapparent, are widespread in mammalian species; they are of economic importance in farm animals and may also affect pets (for reviews see Meyer 1967, Storz 1971, Wachendörfer and Lohrbach 1980). As in birds, there is a wide range of syndromes.

ENTERIC INFECTIONS

Chlamydiae may be excreted in the faeces of apparently healthy sheep and cattle; overt enteritis is, however, uncommon except as part of a more generalized chlamydiosis. The main importance of such infections is that they disseminate organisms, which may then give rise to more serious disease in animals that ingest or inhale them. Chlamydiae associated with enteric infection in cattle and sheep have recently been consigned to a separate genus; *C. pecorum* (Fukushi and Hirai 1992).

OCULAR AND GENITAL INFECTIONS

Conjunctivitis and keratoconjunctivitis occur in farm and domestic animals, sometimes as part of a more general infection. Murray (1964) isolated a 'guinea pig inclusion conjunctivitis agent' (GPIC agent), which has since been detected in a number of laboratory colonies (see also Volume 2, Chapter 59). In natural infections the clinical signs are inconspicuous, but artificial inoculation results in severe keratoconjunctivitis with many inclusions. Infections induced in the guinea pig eye and genital tract have been used extensively as models for those caused by *C. trachomatis* in man. Feline strains of *C. psittaci* may serve a similar purpose; they may cause persistent follicular keratoconjunctivitis and can be transmitted to newborn kittens by their mothers. These agents occur sporadically in domestic cats and may be endemic in catteries. *C. psittaci* has been isolated from the genital tract of a female cat; infections with features analogous to those caused in man by *C. trachomatis* can be induced by inoculation of the feline eye and genital tract (Kane et al. 1985).

ABORTION

C. psittaci causes ovine and bovine abortion, usually enzootic in character but sometimes occurring in epizootics. Up to 30% of ewes in a flock may be affected. In animals that have aborted, the immune response usually prevents a repetition. In sheep, the most important factor in transmission is the shedding of large numbers of organisms in the products of conception at the time of abortion; the importance of faecal–oral transmission is not clear and the roles of sexually acquired infection and of transmission by arthropods (Meyer 1967) remain uncertain. Abortions usually occur in the final stages of pregnancy and result from placentitis consequent upon haematogenous spread of chlamydiae. The fetus may look more or less normal on external examination; lesions found at necropsy include generalized petechial haemorrhages and lymphadenopathy, focal necrosis of the liver and ascites.

The diagnosis may be confirmed by microscopic or cultural demonstration of chlamydiae in the placenta and fetus. Paired serum samples from both ewes and cows taken at the time of abortion and 2–4 weeks later show rises of 4-fold or more in the titre of antibody. The presence of other pathogens that cause abortion, notably *Brucella abortus* and *Campylobacter fetus*, must be considered.

Control measures include segregation of aborting animals and careful disposal of the products of conception. Chemoprophylaxis with tetracycline has been attempted with varying success. Both live and inactivated vaccines, usually prepared from chick-embryo yolk sacs, have been tried and are available commercially. The results of a number of trials, reviewed by Storz (1971), were variable but suggest that some vaccines confer a moderate degree of protection.

PULMONARY INFECTIONS

Pneumonitis due to *C. psittaci* has been reported in sheep, goats, pigs, cats, mice and other species. Feline pneumonitis (cat distemper) is a highly infectious disease, spread by the respiratory route and characterized by sneezing, coughing, anorexia and mucopurulent discharge from the nose and eyes. Except in kittens and elderly animals it is not usually fatal, but may cause debility lasting for a month or so. Chlamydial pneumonitis is characterized by clearly demarcated reddish-grey areas of consolidation, sometimes affecting a whole lobe or lung. (It should be noted that mouse pneumonitis, p. 983, is caused by *C. trachomatis*.)

OTHER INFECTIONS

Polyarthritis in lambs and calves is a well recognized manifestation of chlamydiosis and is of interest in relation to the pathogenesis of SARA associated with *C. trachomatis* in man (p. 982), although in the animals, a direct infection of the joint is easily shown. Chlamydiosis in various avian and mammalian species may also take the form of encephalomyelitis. In bulls, epididymitis and seminal vesiculitis may impair fertility (Storz et al. 1968). For a review of chlamydial zoonoses, see Wills (1986).

3.3 Infections of man

PSITTACOSIS AND ORNITHOSIS

There is no evidence of any constant difference in the clinical course of infections acquired from psittacine birds and those transmitted from other avian species; the description that follows applies to both types of infection.

Epidemiology

Psittacosis first acquired prominence during the widespread outbreaks in 1929–30, which started in Latin America and thence spread to Europe, affecting about 600 people. This episode originated from parrots sold as pets. Because most if not all avian species may be infected, often subclinically, it follows that persons whose occupation or recreation brings them into continual contact with birds are those at greatest risk. They include poultry farmers and processors, owners of pet shops and of racing pigeons and workers in zoos. In the Faroe Islands, ornithosis was reported in women who pluck and process fulmar petrels for human consumption (Bedson 1940). Serological surveys show that inapparent infections are not uncommon in persons at risk (Meyer and Eddie 1962). There have been a number of cases, some fatal, among laboratory workers handling avian strains of *C. psittaci*. Palmer (1982) described an outbreak of psittacosis among workers in a duck-processing factory and another in veterinarians, both of which appeared to be due to liberation of aerosols during evisceration of the bird.

In man, infection is acquired by the respiratory route; some strains are highly infectious and the disease may be contracted by the most casual contact with a sick bird or its environment. Case-to-case infection is unusual, but may occur with particularly virulent strains. An outbreak of chlamydial pneumonia in the Bayou region of Louisiana was remarkable in that 18 persons became infected by secondary or tertiary spread from a single fatal case, the wife of a trapper. There were 7 more deaths, all in contacts who attended fatal cases during the final 48 h of their illness (Olson and Treuting 1944). The detailed clinical (Treuting and Olson 1944) and pathological (Binford and Hauser 1944) observations on these patients are of considerable interest.

Clinical and pathological features

The incubation period is usually 1–2 weeks, but may be as long as a month. The onset is sometimes insidious with malaise and pains in the limbs, but is more often abrupt, with high fever, rigors and headache. Patients usually have a cough, but sputum is scanty and respiratory distress is unusual except in severe cases. Characteristically, the pulse rate is slow in relation to the temperature; a high rate is held by some to indicate a poor prognosis. Physical signs in the chest are limited with little or no evidence of consolidation and are thus at variance with the extensive signs of pneumonitis seen on radiological examination. Epistaxis is not infrequent and rose spots on the skin, somewhat like those in typhoid, are sometimes seen. The spleen may be enlarged and occasionally there is frank hepatitis with jaundice. Severe cases may be complicated by meningitis or meningoencephalitis, myocarditis and, more rarely, endocarditis. In the acute phase the white cell count is often normal, but leucopenia is evident in about 25% of cases.

In patients who recover without treatment, the infection usually resolves slowly within 2 or 3 weeks, or sometimes longer; chlamydiae may be shed for quite long periods. Severely affected patients may become drowsy or stuporous if the central nervous system is affected. Death is usually the result of cardiovascular and respiratory insufficiency. The disease sometimes has the characteristics of a severe toxaemia. At necropsy, extensive pneumonitis with areas of consolidation is a constant finding. The alveoli are packed with exudate containing erythrocytes, mononuclear cells and polymorphonuclear leucocytes; characteristically, the alveolar cells are swollen. The enlarged spleen shows loss of the normal architecture and areas of focal necrosis may be seen in the liver. There may also be signs of inflammation in the meninges and congestion of the cerebral parenchyma. Hyaline necrosis and haemorrhages in the rectus muscles may occur. Deaths from psittacosis are rare since the advent of antibiotics. Earlier, the death rate was about 20%.

OTHER INFECTIONS

In spite of the wide host range of *C. psittaci*, infection of man from non-avian animals is rare. A case of endocarditis (Regan, Dathan and Treharne 1979) and sporadic cases of conjunctivitis in man caused by the feline

pneumonitis agent have been reported. Johnson (1983) reviewed human infection with the feline pneumonitis agent and with bovine chlamydiae. It is apparent that chlamydial infections of non-avian species are generally of low infectivity to man. There are, however, increasing numbers of reports of abortion in women as a result of contact with sheep infected with the ewe abortion agent. Johnson et al. (1985) described the case of a woman aborting after a mild febrile illness in the 28th week of pregnancy. She became severely ill and *C. psittaci* was isolated from fetal tissue. Chlamydial inclusions were demonstrated by light and electron microscopy.

LABORATORY DIAGNOSIS

Except during an outbreak, diagnosis of *C. psittaci* infections on clinical grounds alone is difficult, especially in the absence of a history of contact with birds. The differential diagnosis must take account of other causes of atypical pneumonia such as *Mycoplasma pneumoniae* infection, Q fever, brucellosis and influenza. The skin rash, when present, may at first suggest typhoid.

Chlamydiae may be isolated from the blood and respiratory secretions, but this should not be attempted in laboratories without adequate facilities for handling dangerous pathogens. The diagnosis is usually made by demonstrating a significant rise in antibody in paired sera taken on admission and 10–20 days later; either the complement fixation or immunofluorescence test may be used. Low titres of antibody (around 16) are not infrequently found in normal persons and are of no diagnostic significance in single samples of serum. A titre of 64 or greater in a single sample is suggestive of active infection and the finding of specific IgM antibody in such a serum is good presumptive evidence of a current or recent infection; even so, it is preferable to obtain evidence of a rise in titre.

The immune response to *C. psittaci* is considered on pp. 988–990.

TREATMENT

The antibiotic of choice is tetracycline in a dose (for adults) of at least 250 mg 4 times a day, continued for at least 3 weeks to avoid relapse. Severely ill patients may need measures for cardiovascular and respiratory support. Erythromycin (500 mg 4 times a day orally) is an alternative therapy.

CONTROL MEASURES

These are directed at preventing the importation of birds by quarantine measures and at avoiding the activation of latent infections by rearing, keeping and transporting birds under satisfactory conditions. Chemoprophylaxis may be useful for controlling infections in commercially reared pet birds, but is less so for poultry. Persons in frequent contact with birds and sheep should be made aware of the signs and risks of infection by publicity channelled through employers, societies and other organizations. In hospitals, person-to-person spread must be prevented by appropriate isolation measures and proper disposal of sputum, which is to be considered highly infective. Reference has already been made to the precautions needed for handling specimens in the laboratory.

4 INFECTIONS WITH *C. PNEUMONIAE* (TWAR AGENTS)

In recent years, evidence has accumulated that atypical chlamydiae known as TWAR (Taiwan Acute Respiratory) strains (see Volume 2, Chapter 59) cause outbreaks of acute infection of the lower respiratory tract in man. These agents form a genetically and serologically homogeneous group which resembles *C. psittaci* more than *C. trachomatis* but which differs sufficiently from both to be classified as a third species of *Chlamydia*, for which the name *C. pneumoniae* was proposed by Grayston et al. (1989a). Their prevalence explains the finding by Darougar and colleagues (1980) of antichlamydial antibody in 24% of male and 14% of female blood donors in London, compared with respective figures of 0.75% and 3% for antibodies to *C. trachomatis*. Similar findings in sera from the UK, Europe and tropical countries were described by Forsey et al. (1986). Outbreaks of acute infection of the lower respiratory tract caused by TWAR agents have been reported from Finland (Saikku et al. 1985) and the USA (Grayston et al. 1986).

C. pneumoniae is distinguished sharply from *C. psittaci* by being spread from man to man and by the fact that as yet no avian or other mammalian host has been identified.

C. pneumoniae is now recognized as a common cause of mild pneumonias in young adults. This has been found to be true in studies of college students and in studies of epidemics among military conscripts. Serious respiratory disease may occur in young children in developing countries and in older debilitated individuals who are hospitalized (see Cook and Honeybourne 1994). Hahn, Dodge and Golubjatnikov (1991) have presented evidence to suggest that repeated or prolonged exposure to *C. pneumoniae* may be causally associated with wheezing, asthmatic bronchitis and adult onset asthma.

The features of the respiratory infections are bronchitis or, more often, pneumonitis, similar to that caused by *Mycoplasma pneumoniae*. They may be severe in the acute phase and tend to follow a relapsing course, with persistent cough. Subclinical infections are probably frequent.

C. pneumoniae may play a role in coronary artery disease (Saikku et al. 1988, 1992). Patients with such conditions have been found to have high levels of antibody to this organism and chlamydial antigens and genes have been detected in involved sites (Kuo et al. 1993).

C. pneumoniae can be isolated in HL and Hep 2 cells more efficiently than in the cell culture system used for isolation of *C. trachomatis* (Cles and Stamm 1990, Wong, Skelton and Chang 1992). The microimmunofluorescence and the complement fixation tests can both play a role in serodiagnosis, with the former being the more sensitive. A complicating feature in serodiagnosis is the fact that it may take months for seroconversion to be demonstrated. IgM antibody is a good indicator of current or recent infection (Saikku et al. 1985).

TREATMENT

Grayston et al. (1989b) found that both tetracycline and erythromycin are effective against *C. pneumoniae* in vitro; they recommended either drug in a dosage of 2 g daily for 10–14 days or 1–1.5 g daily for 21 days, but stated that relapses may occur even after this intensive treatment. The role of newer compounds, such as azithromycin, is under evaluation.

REFERENCES

Assaad FA, Maxwell-Lyons, F, 1967, Application of clinical scoring systems to trachoma research. Conference on Trachoma and Allied Diseases, *Am J Ophthalmol*, **63:** 1327–56.

Bailey RL, Arullendran P et al., 1993, Randomised controlled trial of single-dose azithromycin in treatment of trachoma, *Lancet*, **342:** 453–6.

Bedson SP, 1940, Virus diseases acquired from animals, *Lancet*, **2:** 577–9.

Beem M, Saxon EM, 1977, Respiratory tract colonization and a distinctive pneumonia syndrome in infants infected with *C. trachomatis*, *N Engl J Med*, **296:** 306–10.

Bell TA, Stamm WE et al., 1987, Delayed appearance of *Chlamydia trachomatis* infections acquired at birth, *Pediatr Infect Dis J*, **6:** 928–31.

Berger RE, Alexander ER et al., 1978, *Chlamydia trachomatis* as a cause of acute 'idiopathic' epididymitis, *N Engl J Med*, **298:** 301–4.

Bevan C, Ridgway GL, Siddle N, 1995, Clinical and laparoscopic and microbiological findings in acute salpingitis: report on a United Kingdom cohort, *Br J Obstet Gynaecol*, **102:** 407–14.

Binford CH, Hauser GH, 1944, An epidemic of a severe pneumonitis in the Bayou Region of Louisiana. III. Pathological observations. Report of autopsy on two cases with a brief comparative note on psittacosis and Q fever, *Public Health Rep Washington*, **59:** 1363–73.

Brunham RC, 1994, Vaccine design for the prevention of *C. trachomatis* infection, *Chlamydial Infections*, eds Orfila J, Byrne GI et al., Cambridge University Press, Cambridge, 73–82.

Brunham RC, Paavonen J et al., 1984, Mucopurulent cervicitis – the ignored counterpart in women of urethritis in men, *N Engl J Med*, **311:** 1–6.

Cevenini R, Sarov I et al., 1984, Serum specific IgA antibody to *Chlamydia trachomatis* in patients with chlamydial infections detected by ELISA and an immunofluorescence test, *J Clin Pathol*, **37:** 686–91.

Cevenini R, Rumpianesi F et al., 1986, Class specific immunoglobulin response to individual polypeptides of *Chlamydia trachomatis*, elementary bodies in patients with chlamydial infection, *J Clin Pathol*, **39:** 1313–16.

Chernesky M, Jang D et al., 1994a, Diagnosis of Chlamydia trachomatis infections in men and women by testing first void urine by ligase chain reaction, *J Clin Microbiol*, **32:** 2682–5.

Chernesky M, Lee H et al., 1994b, Diagnosis of *Chlamydia trachomatis* urethral infection in symptomatic and asymptomatic men by tesing first-void urine in a ligase chain reaction assay, *J Infect Dis*, **170:** 1308–11.

Cles LD, Stamm WE, 1990, Use of HL cells for improved isolation and passage of *Chlamydia pneumoniae, J Clin Microbiol,* **28**: 938–40.

Collier LH, 1967, The immunopathology of trachoma: some facts and fancies, *Arch Gesamte Virusforsch,* **22**: 280–93.

Collier LH, 1973, Life at the Border. A review of the work of the MRC Trachoma Unit, *Annu Rep Lister Inst Prev Med,* 1–26.

Cook PJ, Honeybourne D, 1994, *Chlamydia pneumoniae, J Antimicrob Chemother,* **34**: 859–73.

Darougar S, Jones BR, 1983, Trachoma. Chlamydial Disease, ed. Darougar S, *Br Med Bull,* **39**: 117–22.

Darougar S, Forsey T et al., 1980, Prevalence of antichlamydial antibody in London blood donors, *Br J Vener Dis,* **56**: 404–7.

Davies JA, Rees E et al., 1978, Isolation of *C. trachomatis* from Bartholin's ducts, *Br J Vener Dis,* **54**: 409–13.

Dawson CR, Jones BR, Darougar S, 1975, Blinding and non-blinding trachoma: assessment of intensity of upper tarsal inflammatory disease and disabling lesions, *Bull W H O,* **52**: 279–82.

Dawson CR, Daghfous T et al., 1976, Severe endemic trachoma in Tunisia, *Br J Ophthalmol,* **60**: 245–52.

Dunlop EMC, Hare MJ et al., 1971, Chlamydial isolates from the rectum in association with chlamydial infection of the eye or genital tract, *Trachoma and Related Infections caused by Chlamydial Agents,* ed. Nichols RL, Excerpta Medica, Amsterdam, 507–12.

Feldman R, Johnson AL et al., 1986, Aetiology of urinary symptoms in sexually active women, *Genitourin Med,* **62**: 333–41.

Forsey T, Darougar S, Treharne J, 1986, Prevalence in human beings of antibodies to IOL-207, an atypical strain of chlamydia, *J Infect,* **12**: 145–52.

Forster GE, Cookey I et al., 1985, Investigation into the value of Papanicolaou stained cervical smears for the diagnosis of chlamydial cervical infection, *J Clin Pathol,* **38**: 399–402.

Fritsch H, Hofstätter A, Lindner K, 1910, Experimentelle Studien zur Trachomfrage, *Graefes Arch Ophthalmol,* **76**: 547–58.

Fukushi H, Hirai K, 1992, Proposal of *Chlamydia pecorum* sp. nov. for *Chlamydia* strains derived from ruminants, *Int J Syst Bacteriol,* **42**: 306–8.

Goldmeier D, 1985, Proctitis, *Clinical Problems in Sexually Transmitted Diseases,* ed. Taylor-Robinson D, Nijhoff, Dordrecht, 237–83.

Grayston JT, Wang S-P et al., 1985, Importance of reinfection in the pathogenesis of trachoma, *Rev Infect Dis,* **7**: 717–25.

Grayston JT, Kuo CC et al., 1986, A new *Chlamydia psittaci* strain, TWAR, isolated in acute respiratory tract infections, *N Engl J Med,* **315**: 161–18.

Grayston JT, Kuo C-C et al., 1989a, *Chlamydia pneumoniae* sp. nov. for *Chlamydia* sp. strain TWAR, *Int J Syst Bacteriol,* **39**: 88–90.

Grayston JT, Wang S-P et al., 1989b, Current knowledge of *Chlamydia pneumoniae,* strain TWAR, an important cause of pneumonia and other acute respiratory diseases, *Eur J Clin Microbiol Infect Dis,* **8**: 191–202.

Greaves AB, Hillman MR et al., 1957, Chemotherapy in bubonic lymphogranuloma venereum: a clinical and serological evolution, *Bull W H O,* **16**: 277–89.

Hahn DL, Dodge RW, Golubjatnikov R, 1991, Association of *Chlamydia pneumoniae* (strain TWAR) infection with wheezing, asthmatic bronchitis, and adult-onset asthma, *JAMA,* **266**: 225–30.

Hobson D, Rees E, Viswalingam ND, 1982, Chlamydial infections in neonates and older children, *Chlamydial Infections,* eds Mårdh PA, Holmes KK et al., Elsevier, Amsterdam, 128–32.

Igietseme JU, Magee DM et al., 1994, Role for CD8+ T cells in antichlamydial immunity defined by chlamydia-specific T-lymphocyte clones, *Infect Immun,* **62**: 5195–7.

Jaschek G, Gaydos CA et al., 1993, Direct detection of *Chlamydia trachomatis* in urine specimens from symptomatic and asymptomatic men by using a rapid polymerase chain reaction assay, *J Clin Microbiol,* **31**: 1209–12.

Johnson FWA, 1983, Chlamydiosis, *Br Vet J,* **139**: 93–101.

Johnson FWA, Matheson BA et al., 1985, Abortion due to infection with *Chlamydia psittaci* in a sheep farmer's wife, *Br Med J,* **290**: 592–4.

Jones BR, 1964, Ocular syndromes of TRIC virus infection and their possible genital significance, *Br J Vener Dis,* **40**: 3–15.

Jones BR, 1975, The prevention of blindness from trachoma, *Trans Ophthalmol Soc UK,* **95**: 16–33.

Jones BR, Collier LH, Smith CH, 1959, Isolation of virus from inclusion blennorrhoea, *Lancet,* **1**: 902–5.

Jones RB, Batteiger BE, 1986, Human immune response to *C. trachomatis* infections, *Chlamydial Infections,* eds Oriel D, Ridgway G et al., Cambridge University Press, Cambridge, 423–32.

Kane, JL, Woodland RM et al., 1985, Chlamydial pelvic infection in cats: a model for the study of human pelvic inflammatory disease, *Genitourin Med,* **61**: 311–18.

Keat AC, 1983, Reiter's syndrome and reactive arthritis in perspective, *N Engl J Med,* **309**: 1607–15.

Keat AC, 1986, *Chlamydia trachomatis* infection in human arthritis, *Chlamydial Infections,* eds Oriel D, Ridgway G et al., Cambridge University Press, Cambridge, 269–79.

Keat AC, Thomas BJ et al., 1987, *C. trachomatis* and reactive arthritis: the missing link, *Lancet,* **329**: 72–4.

Krech T, Gerhard Fsadni D et al., 1985, Interference of *S. aureus* in the detection of *C. trachomatis* by monoclonal antibodies, *Lancet,* **1**: 1161–2.

Kunimoto D, Brunham RC, 1985, Human immune response and *C. trachomatis* infection, *Rev Infect Dis,* **7**: 665–73.

Kuo CC, Shor A et al., 1993, Demonstration of *Chlamydia pneumoniae* in atherosclerotic lesions of coronary arteries, *J Infect Dis,* **167**: 841–9.

Lee HH, Chernesky MA et al., 1995, Diagnosis of *Chlamydia trachomatis* genitourinary infection in women by ligase chain reaction assay of urine, *Lancet,* **345**: 213–16.

Levitt D, Danen R, Bard J, 1986, Both species of chlamydia and two biovars of *C. trachomatis* stimulate mouse B lymphocytes, *J Immunol,* **136**: 4249–54.

MacCallan AF, 1936, *Trachoma,* Butterworth, London.

Manuel ARG, Veeravahu M et al., 1987, Pooled specimens for *C. trachomatis:* new approach to increase yield and cost efficiency, *Genitourin Med,* **63**: 172–5.

Mårdh PA, 1987, Chlamydial pelvic inflammatory disease, *Chlamydial Infections,* ed. Reeves P, Springer-Verlag, Berlin, 45–55.

Mårdh PA, Paavonen J, Puolakkainan M, 1989, *Chlamydia,* Plenum Medical, New York.

Martin DH, Mroczkowski TF et al., 1992, A controlled trial of a single dose of a azithromycin for the treatment of chlamydial urethritis and cervicitis, *N Engl J Med,* **327**: 921–5.

Menke HE, Schuller JL, Stolz E, 1979, Treatment of lymphogranuloma venereum with rifampicin, *Br J Vener Dis,* **55**: 379–80.

Meyer K, 1967, The host spectrum of psittacosis-lymphogranuloma venereum (PL) agents. Conference on Trachoma and Allied Diseases, *Am J Ophthalmol,* **63**: 1225–46.

Meyer KF, Eddie B, 1962, Immunity against some *Bedsonia* in man resulting from infection and in animals from infection or vaccination, *Ann NY Acad Sci,* **98**: 288–313.

Moncada J, Schachter J et al., 1990, Confirmation assay increases the specificity of the Chlamydiazyme test for *Chlamydia trachomatis* infection of the cervix, *J Clin Microbiol,* **28**: 29–34.

Morange A, 1895, *De la Psittacose, ou Infection Spécial déterminée par des Perruches,* Thesis, Académie de Paris.

Morrison RP, Belland RJ et al., 1989, Chlamydial disease pathogenesis. The 57-kD chlamydial hypersensitivity antigen is a stress response protein, *J Exp Med,* **170**: 1271–84.

Mumtaz G, Mellars BJ et al., 1985, Enzyme immunoassay for the detection of *Chlamydia trachomatis* antigen in urethral and endocervical swabs, *J Clin Pathol,* **38**: 740–2.

Murray ES, 1964, Guinea pig inclusion conjunctivitis virus. I. Isolation and identification as a member of the psittacosis-lymphogranuloma-trachoma group, *J Infect Dis,* **114**: 1.

Myrhe EB, Mårdh PA, 1981, *Chlamydia trachomatis* infection in a patient with meningoencephalitis, *N Engl J Med,* **304**: 910–11.

Olson BJ, Treuting WL, 1944, An epidemic of a severe pneumonitis in the Bayou Region of Louisiana. I. Epidemiology study, *Public Health Rep Washington*, **59:** 1299–311.

Oriel JD, Ridgway GL, 1982, *Genital Infection by* Chlamydia trachomatis, Edward Arnold, London.

Oriel JD, Ridgway GL, Tchamouroff S, 1977, Comparison of erythromycin stearate and oxytetracycline in the treatment of nongonococcal urethritis: their efficacy against *C. trachomatis*, *Scott Med J*, **22:** 375–9.

Palmer SR, 1982, Psittacosis in man – recent developments in the UK: a review, *J R Soc Med*, **75:** 262–7.

Qvigstad E, Skaug K, Hirschberg H, 1985, Characterization of *Chlamydia trachomatis* serotypes by human T-lymphocyte clones, *Scand J Immunol*, **21:** 215–20.

Quinn TC, Goodsell SE et al., 1981, *Chlamydia trachomatis* proctitis, *N Engl J Med*, **305:** 195–200.

Rapoza PA, Quinn TC et al., 1986, Assessment of neonatal conjunctivitis with a direct immunofluorescent monoclonal antibody stain for chlamydia, *JAMA*, **255:** 3369–73.

Rees E, Tait IA et al., 1977, Perinatal chlamydial infection, *Nongonococcal Urethritis and Related Infections*, eds Hobson D, Holmes KK, American Society for Microbiology, Washington DC, 140–7.

Regan RL, Dathan JRE, Treharne JD, 1979, Infective endocarditis with glomerulonephitis associated with cat chlamydia (*C. psittaci*) infection, *Br Heart J*, **42:** 349–52.

Ridgway GL, 1986, The laboratory diagnosis of chlamydial infection, *Chlamydial Infections*, eds Oriel D, Ridgway G et al., Cambridge University Press, Cambridge, 539–49.

Ridgway GL, 1995, Quinolones in sexually transmitted disease, *Drugs*, **49, Suppl 2:** 115–22.

Ringel RE, Brenner JL et al., 1982, Serologic evidence for *C. trachomatis* myocarditis, *Pediatrics*, **70:** 54–6.

Saikku P, Wang SP et al., 1985, An epidemic of mild pneumonia due to an unusual strain of *Chlamydia psittaci*, *J Infect Dis*, **151:** 832–9.

Saikku P, Leinonen M et al., 1988, Serological evidence of an association of a novel chlamydia, TWAR, with chronic coronary heart disease and acute myocardial infarction, *Lancet*, **2:** 983–5.

Saikku, P, Leinonen M et al., 1992, Chronic *Chlamydia pneumoniae* infection as a risk factor for coronary heart disease in the Helsinki Heart Study, *Ann Intern Med*, **116:** 273–8.

Schachter J, 1985, Immunodiagnosis of sexually transmitted disease, *Yale J Biol Med*, **58:** 443–52.

Schachter J, Dawson CR, 1978, *Human Chlamydial Infections*, PSG Publishing Company Inc., Littlejohn, Massachusetts.

Schachter J, Lum L et al., 1975, Pneumonitis following inclusion blennorrhea, *J Pediatr*, **87:** 779–80.

Sowa S, Sowa J et al., 1965, *Trachoma and Allied Infections in a Gambian Village*, Medical Research Council Special Report Series No. 308, HMSO, London.

Stacey C, Munday P et al., 1990, *Chlamydia trachomatis* in the fallopian tubes of women without laparoscopic evidence of salpingitis, *Lancet*, **336:** 960–3.

Stamm WE, Wagner KF et al., 1980, Causes of the acute urethral syndrome in women, *N Engl J Med*, **303:** 409–15.

Stamm WE, Quinn TC et al., 1982, *Chlamydia trachomatis* proctitis, *Chlamydial Infections*, eds Mårdh PA, Holmes KK et al., Elsevier, Amsterdam, 111–18.

Storz J, 1971, *Chlamydia and Chlamydia induced Diseases*, Charles C Thomas, Springfield, IL.

Storz J, Carroll E et al., 1968, Isolation of a psittacosis agent (*Chlamydia*) from semen and epididymis of bulls with seminal vesiculitis syndrome, *Am J Vet Res*, **29:** 459.

Symposium, 1967, Conference on Trachoma and Allied Diseases, *Am J Ophthalmol*, **63:** 1027–657.

Symposium, 1971, *Trachoma and Related Infections caused by Chlamydial Agents*, ed. Nichols RL, Excerpta Medica, London.

Symposium, 1977, *Nongonococcal Urethritis and Related Infections*, eds Hobson D, Holmes KK, American Society for Microbiology, Washington DC.

Symposium, 1982, *Chlamydial Infections*, eds Mårdh PA, Holmes KK et al., Elsevier, Amsterdam.

Symposium, 1983, Chlamydial Disease, ed. Darougar S, *Br Med Bull*, **39:** 107–208.

Symposium, 1985, Infectious Causes of Blindness: I.Trachoma, eds Cook JA, Taylor HR, *Rev Infect Dis*, **7:** 711–86.

Symposium, 1986, *Chlamydial Infections*, eds Oriel D, Ridgway G et al., Cambridge University Press, Cambridge.

Symposium, 1990, *Chlamydial Infections*, eds Bowie WR, Caldwell HD et al., Cambridge University Press, Cambridge.

Symposium, 1994, *Chlamydial Infections*, eds Orfila J, Byrne GI et al., Cambridge University Press, Cambridge.

Tam MR, Stephens RS et al., 1982, Use of monoclonal antibodies to *C. trachomatis* as immunodiagnostic reagents, *Chlamydial Infections*, eds Mårdh PA, Holmes KK et al., Elsevier, Amsterdam, 317–20.

Taylor-Robinson D, Thomas BJ, Osborn MF, 1987, Evaluation of enzyme immunoassay (Chlamydiazyme) for detecting *C. trachomatis* in genital tract specimens, *J Clin Pathol*, **40:** 194–9.

Taylor-Robinson D, Gilroy CB et al., 1992, Detection of *Chlamydia trachomatis* DNA in joints of reactive arthritis patients by polymerase chain reaction, *Lancet*, **340:** 81–2.

Thygeson P, Dawson CR, 1966, Trachoma and follicular conjunctivitis in children, *Arch Ophthalmol (NY)*, **75:** 3–12.

Thylefors AD, Negrel R et al., 1995, Global data on blindness – an update, *Bull W H O*, **73:** 115–21.

Treharne JD, 1985, The community and epidemiology of trachoma. Infectious Causes of Blindness: I. Trachoma, eds Cook JA, Taylor HR, *Rev Infect Dis*, **7:** 760–4.

Treuting WL, Olson BJ, 1944, An epidemic of a severe pneumonitis in the Bayou Region of Louisiana. II. Clinical feature of the disease, *Public Health Rep Washington*, **59:** 1331–50.

Van der Bel Khan JM, Watanakunakorn C et al., 1978, *C. trachomatis* endocarditis, *Am Heart J*, **95:** 627–36.

Viswalingam ND, Wishart MS, Woodland RM, 1983, Adult chlamydial ophthalmia (paratrachoma), *Br Med Bull*, **39:** 123–7.

Wachendorfer G, Lohrbach W, 1980, Neuere Erkenntnisse zur Humanpathogenitat von Saugetierchlamydien, *Berl Münch Tierärztl Wochenschr*, **93:** 248–51.

Wang S P, Grayston JT, 1967, Pannus with experimental trachoma and inclusion conjunctivitis agent infection of Taiwan monkeys. Conference on Trachoma and Allied Diseases, *Am J Ophthalmol*, **63:** 1133–45.

Wang SP, Grayston JT, 1982, Microimmunofluorescence antibody responses in *C. trachomatis* infection, *Chlamydial Infections*, eds Mårdh PA, Holmes KK et al., Elsevier, Amsterdam, 301–16.

Watkins NG, Hadlow WJ et al., 1986, Ocular delayed hypersensitivity: a pathogenetic mechanism of chlamydial conjunctivitis in guinea pigs, *Proc Natl Acad Sci USA*, **83:** 7480–4.

Weiss SG, Newcombe RW, Beem MO, 1986, Pulmonary assessment of children after chlamydial pneumonia of infancy, *J Pediatr*, **108:** 659–64.

Weström L, 1975, Effect of acute pelvic inflammatory disease on fertility, *Am J Obstet Gynecol*, **121:** 707–13.

Weström L, Mårdh PA, 1983, Chlamydia salpingitis. Chlamydial Disease. ed. Darougar S, *Br Med Bull*, **39:** 145–50.

Whittum Hudson JA, Taylor HR et al., 1986, Immunohistochemical study of the local inflammatory response to chlamydial ocular infection, *Invest Ophthalmol Vis Sci*, **27:** 64–9.

Wills JM, 1986, Chlamydia zoonoses, *J Small Anim Pract*, **27, Suppl:** 717–31.

Wong KH, Skelton SK, Chan YK, 1992, Efficient culture of *Chlamydia pneumoniae* with cell lines derived from the human respiratory tract, *J Clin Microbiol*, **30:** 1625–30.

World Health Organization, 1962, *Expert Committee on Trachoma*, Third Report, W H O, Geneva.

World Health Organization, 1971, *World Health Statistical Reports*, 24, No.4, W H O, Geneva.

World Health Organization, 1973, *Field Methods for the Control of Trachoma*, W H O, Geneva.

World Health Organization, 1979, *Guidelines for Programmes for the Prevention of Blindness*, W H O, Geneva.

Yong EC, Klebanoff SJ, Kuo CC, 1982, Toxic effect of human polymorphonuclear leucocytes on *C. trachomatis*, *Infect Immun*, **37:** 422–31.

Young E, Taylor HR, 1984, Immune mechanisms in chlamydial eye infection: cellular immune responses in chronic and acute disease, *J Infect Dis*, **150:** 745–51.

Young E, Taylor HR, 1986, Immune mechanisms in chlamydial eye infections. Development of T suppressor cells, *Invest Ophthalmol Vis Sci*, **27:** 615–19.

Chapter 53

RICKETTSIAL DISEASES

J E McDade

1 INTRODUCTION

Rickettsiae are small, gram-negative, obligate intracellular bacteria. Taxonomically, they are grouped in the family Rickettsiaceae in the order Rickettsiales (Weiss and Moulder 1984). Species in 3 genera (*Rickettsia*, *Coxiella* and *Ehrlichia*) are pathogenic for humans. Common characteristics of rickettsiae include their association with mammals and arthropod vectors (lice, ticks, fleas and mites) as part of their life cycles. Phenotypic criteria have been traditionally used to differentiate genera and species. For example, *Rickettsia* spp. grow within the cytoplasm of host cells, unbounded by membranes, and some species also grow in the nucleus (Fig. 53.1). *Ehrlichia* grow in membrane-lined vacuoles in host cells, and compact clusters of growing micro-organisms comprise mulberry-shaped inclusions (morulae) that typify the genus (Rikihisa 1991) (Fig 53.2). *Ehrlichia* are also distinguished from other rickettsiae by their tropism for host leucocytes. The genus *Coxiella* comprises a single species, *Coxiella burnetii*, which grows in phagolysosomes (Fig. 53.3).

Selected characteristics of *Rickettsia*, *Ehrlichia* and *Coxiella* are presented in Table 53.1.

Members of the genus *Rickettsia* have been divided into 3 groups of antigenically related species: typhus, scrub typhus and spotted fever. The spotted fever group comprises many species, most of which are tick-borne. *Rickettsia akari*, which is transmitted by gamasid mites, is an exception. The scrub typhus group consists of multiple serovars of one species, *Rickettsia tsutsugamushi*; trombiculid mites are both reservoirs and vectors. *Rickettsia prowazekii* and *Rickettsia typhi* (formerly *Rickettsia mooseri*) constitute the typhus group and are transmitted by lice and fleas, respect-

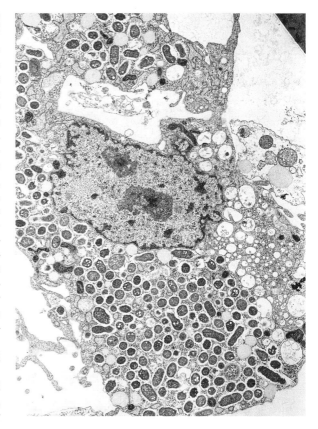

Fig. 53.1 *Rickettsia prowazekii*, the aetiological agent of louse-borne typhus, in cytoplasm of chick embryo cells.

ively. Characteristics of micro-organisms in the 3 serogroups are presented in Table 53.2.

Rickettsial phylogeny and taxonomy have been confounded somewhat in recent years by a lack of uni-

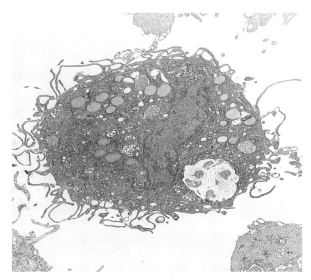

Fig. 53.2 Phagosome containing *E. chaffeensis*, an agent of human ehrlichiosis in the USA.

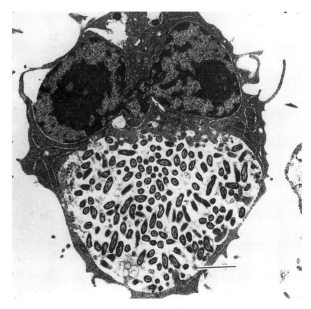

Fig. 53.3 *Coxiella burnetii* in J 774 macrophage cells. Bar = 2 μm. (Reproduced from Baca 1984, with permission of the author and publisher).

form criteria for classification, particularly since molecular techniques have been introduced and used to characterize isolates. DNA–DNA hybridization data, gene sequences for 16S rRNA molecules, restriction fragment length polymorphisms, polyacrylamide gel electrophoresis, reactivity with monoclonal antibodies, and various combinations of these techniques have been used for classification (Myers and Wisseman 1980, Weisburg et al. 1989, Regnery, Spruill and Plikaytis 1991, Manor et al. 1992, Uchida 1993, Kelly et al. 1994, Ohashi et al. 1995). All molecular analyses confirm the appropriateness of generic designations and grouping of pathogenic *Rickettsia* into typhus, scrub typhus and spotted fever groups. However, many isolates of spotted fever group rickettsiae, which

apparently are strains of *Rickettsia conorii*, have been proposed as separate species because they can be distinguished by certain molecular techniques. However, a phylogenetic analysis of the genus *Rickettsia*, performed by sequencing of the gene for 16S rRNA, confirms that such isolates are very closely related and likely are the same species (Roux and Raoult 1995). This chapter will use conventional species designations for *R. conorii* and other rickettsiae, i.e. when attributable diseases are distinct, when isolates have unique phenotypic characteristics or nucleotide sequences for the 16S rRNA gene, or when they exist in distinct geographical areas or ecosystems (Table 53.2).

Multiple species of *Ehrlichia* have been isolated and characterized (Rikihisa 1991). *Ehrlichia canis* is a well known pathogen of dogs; *Ehrlichia phagocytophila*, *Ehrlichia equi* and *Ehrlichia risticii* are pathogenic for domestic animals. *Ehrlichia sennetsu*, which causes a mononucleosis-like disease in Japan, was identified as a human pathogen in the 1950s. Since 1986, 2 additional species of *Ehrlichia* that cause human illness in the USA have been identified: *Ehrlichia chaffeensis* and an unnamed ehrlichia that is closely related to *E. equi* and *E. phagocytophila*. The general properties of ehrlichiae are presented in Table 53.1.

2 MORPHOLOGY

Rickettsia spp. are short, rod-shaped or coccobacillary micro-organisms, approximately 0.8–2.0 μm in length and 0.3–0.5 μm wide; *C. burnetii* is somewhat smaller. Ehrlichiae vary from 0.2 to 1.5 μm in diameter and usually are coccoid or ellipsoid in shape. Rickettsiae do not contain flagella or pili; genetic recombination has not been demonstrated. *Rickettsia* and *Coxiella* are best visualized in infected cells by the Giménez stain (Giménez 1964); Romanowsky's stains, especially Giemsa and Wright stains, are preferred for visualizing *Ehrlichia*. At the untrastructural level, rickettsiae contain chromosomal structures, ribosomes and other subcellular organelles (Silverman and Wisseman 1978). Rickettsiae are surrounded by an outer envelope (cell wall) that is similar to that of other gram-negative bacteria. The cell wall of *Rickettsia* and *C. burnetii* contains lipopolysaccharide (LPS) and its precursor, 2-keto-3-deoxyoctulosonic acid (KDO) (Schramek, Brezina and Tarasevich 1976, Smith and Winkler 1979); it also contains peptidoglycan (Pang and Winkler 1994). *R. tsutsugamushi* is deficient in both LPS and peptidoglycan (Amano et al. 1987), which probably accounts for the thin inner leaflet of its cell wall compared with that of other *Rickettsia* spp. LPS and peptidoglycan are limited in *Ehrlichia* (Rikihisa 1991). Typhus and spotted fever group rickettsiae are surrounded by a polysaccharide slime layer, which is difficult to visualize except with special stains (Silverman et al. 1978).

C. burnetii is unique among the rickettsiae in that it displays an antigenic phase variation that is analogous to the smooth-to-rough variation of certain types of

Table 53.1 General properties of rickettsiae pathogenic for humans

Property	Rickettsia	Coxiella	Ehrlichia
Attributable diseases	Epidemic and murine typhus; scrub typhus; Rocky Mountain spotted fever; various forms of tick typhus; rickettsialpox	Q fever	Sennetsu fever; 2 forms of human ehrlichiosis
Pathogenic species	Many	*Coxiella burnetii*	*E. sennetsu*; *E. chaffeensis* Unnamed species, related to *E. equi* and *E. phagocytophila*
Reservoirs	Mostly small mammals; mites are reservoirs of scrub typhus rickettsia; humans are principal reservoir of *R. prowazekii*	Primarily domestic animals (cattle, goats and sheep)	Uncertain for *E. sennetsu*; deer, dogs and mice have been incriminated as reservoirs in the USA
Vectors	Lice, ticks, fleas, or mites, depending on the aetiological agent	Transmission occurs primarily by aerosol inhalation; ticks are also infected	Ixodid ticks
Stability outside host cell	Unstable	Very stable	Unstable
Replication in host cells	Organisms multiply in cytoplasm or nucleus, unbounded by membranes	Multiplication occurs in phagolysosome of host cells	Form characteristic mulberry-shaped inclusions (morulae) in leucocytes

bacteria (Stoker and Fiset 1956). Phase I antigen is a polysaccharide that is attached as a side chain to the LPS molecule of *C. burnetii*; the polysaccharide is truncated or absent when organisms are in antigenic phase II (Hackstadt et al. 1985). *C. burnetii* exists in antigenic phase I in reservoir animals and changes to phase II when cultured in tissue culture or embryonated eggs.

C. burnetii is the only rickettsia that contains plasmids (Samuel et al. 1983). Functions of the plasmids remain cryptic, but an association of certain plasmids with acute or chronic Q fever has been postulated (Samuel, Frazier and Mallavia 1985). However, more recent characterizations of additional isolates of *C. burnetii* fail to verify a correlation between plasmid type and clinical manifestations of Q fever patients (Stein and Raoult 1993, Thiele and Willems 1994, Valková and Kazár 1995). Endospore formation has been postulated for *C. burnetii* and may explain its stability outside host cells compared with other rickettsiae (McCaul and Williams 1981).

3 REPLICATION

Rickettsia spp. enter host cells by induced phagocytosis, i.e. *Rickettsia* and host cells actively participate in the process (Winkler and Turco 1988). *R. prowazekii* will infect virtually any eukaryotic cell, which indicates that receptor molecules for *Rickettsia* are virtually ubiqui-

tous on host cells. Attachment of *Rickettsia* to the host cell induces phospholipase A activity, which presumably is rickettsial in origin (Silverman et al. 1992). Phospholipase A degrades phospholipids in the host cell membrane; the host cell responds by internalizing the damaged portion of the membrane, and the attached rickettsiae are internalized in the process (Teysseire, Boudier and Raoult 1995). *R. prowazekii* quickly escapes from the phagosome, presumably by continued degradation of phagosomal membranes by phospholipase A.

Rickettsia multiply within the cytoplasm of host cells by binary fission (Ris and Fox 1949, Schaechter, Bozeman and Smadel 1957). The generation time for rickettsial multiplication ranges from approximately 4 to 9 h (Oaks and Osterholm 1969, Wisseman and Waddell 1975). *R. prowazekii* accumulates within the original infected cell until the cell bursts. In contrast, *Rickettsia rickettsii* and *R. typhi* move freely to adjacent cells, following the initial infection (Wisseman and Waddell 1975, Silverman, Wisseman and Waddell 1981). *R. tsutsugamushi* also replicates in the cytoplasm but then moves to the periphery of host cells and becomes encased in a host cell membrane as it buds from the cell surface (Ewing et al. 1978). Intracellular movement of rickettsiae is directed by actin filaments (Schaechter, Bozeman and Smadel 1957, Todd, Burgdorfer and Wray 1983, Teysseire, Chiche-Portiche and Raoult 1992).

Table 53.2 Features of *Rickettsia* species pathogenic for humans

Biogroup and species	Disease(s)	Reservoirs	Distribution of disease	Transmission to humans
Typhus				
R. prowazekii	Louse-borne typhus (epidemic typhus)	Humans	Louse-infested populations, usually highlands of Africa, South America	Infected louse faeces
	Recrudescent typhus (Brill–Zinsser disease)	Humans	World wide	Reactivation of latent infection
	Sylvatic typhus	Flying squirrels (*Glaucomys volans*)	USA	Contact with flying squirrels; mechanism of transfer to humans uncertain
R. typhi (*R. mooseri*)	Murine typhus	Primarily *Rattus* rats	World wide, primarily follows distribution of *Rattus* rats	Infected flea feaces
Spotted fever				
R. rickettsii	Rocky Mountain spotted fever	Ticks, small mammals	Western hemisphere	Tick bite
R. conorii	Tick typhus (also called Mediterranean spotted fever or boutonneuse fever)	Ticks, small mammals	Mediterranean area, Africa, parts of Europe, India	Tick bite
R. sibirica	Siberian tick typhus	Ticks, small mammals	Siberia, Mongolia, parts of Eastern Europe	Tick bite
R. australis	Queensland tick typhus	Ticks, mammals	Australia	Tick bite
R. japonica	Oriental spotted fever	Ticks, small mammals	Japan	Tick bite
R. akari	Rickettsialpox	Mites, mice, voles	USA, Russia, Korea	Mite bite
Scrub typhus *R. tsutsugamushi* (multiple serotypes and strains)	Scrub typhus	Trombiculid mites	Asia, Australia, some Pacific Islands	Chigger bite

Modifications of the basic infectious process occur with *Ehrlichia* and *Coxiella*. Internalized ehrlichiae remain coated by membranes and proliferate in the phagosome of host cells; phagolysosomal fusion is prevented by metabolic activities of the ehrlichiae (Wells and Rikihisa 1988). Host cells infected with ehrlichiae show little cytopathology until the cytoplasm is filled with micro-organisms and the cells burst. *C. burnetii* enters into host cells by phagocytosis; phagosomes containing *C. burnetii* fuse with lysosomes and *C. burnetii* proliferates within the confines of the phagolysosome (Burton, Kordová and Paretsky 1971, Akporiaye et al. 1983). Factors that allow *C. burnetii* to survive in the harsh environment of the phagolysosome have not been determined, but the low pH optimum (4.5) of *C. burnetii* for certain metabolic activities (Hackstadt and Williams 1981) could facilitate survival.

4 METABOLISM

Although rickettsiae are obligate intracellular parasites, they possess considerable metabolic activity, both energy producing and synthetic. Glucose is not metabolized, but rickettsiae can produce ATP by Krebs cycle reactions. Glutamate is the principal energy substrate for *Rickettsia* and *Coxiella*, but glutamine and pyruvate are also metabolized (Weiss and Moulder 1984). Glutamine is preferentially metabolized by ehrlichiae because it penetrates the phagosomal membranes that surround ehrlichiae better than does glutamate (Rikihisa 1991). Independent synthesis of proteins and amino acids occurs if rickettsiae are provided an appropriate combination of metabolic intermediates. *Rickettsia* spp. also incorporate metabolites from the host cell via various transport systems;

for example, carrier mediated transport of lysine, proline, K$^+$, AMP, ATP/ADP and other metabolites has been demonstrated. The ability of *Rickettsia* to exchange ADP for ATP molecules from the host cell provides them with an alternative source of energy. Moreover, *Rickettsia* spp. can regulate their enzymatic activity to optimize that exchange; rickettsial metabolic activity is low when the concentration of host cell ATP is high and available for exchange (Winkler and Turco 1988). The rickettsial genome is relatively small compared with that of eubacteria (approximately 1100 kb) (Eremeeva, Roux and Raoult 1993), which may account for the inability of rickettsiae to grow on artificial or synthetic media.

5 TRANSMISSION, PATHOGENESIS AND CLINICAL MANIFESTATIONS

5.1 *Rickettsia*

Rickettsia spp. are transmitted to the host directly by the bite of vectors (ticks or mites) or when infective faeces from vectors (fleas or lice) contaminates the skin; in the latter situation, scratching facilitates transfer of micro-organisms. Contamination of oropharyngeal mucous membranes by inhalation of aerosolized faeces from fleas or lice may also result in infection. *Rickettsia* spp. invade the capillaries at the site of entry and infect vascular endothelial cells. *Rickettsia* spp. proliferate in vascular endothelial cells, spread to contiguous cells, and produce small foci of infection (Walker, Firth and Edgell 1982). Infection continues to extend centripetally to include arterioles and venules. *Rickettsia* eventually become broadly disseminated in the vascular endothelium of small and large blood vessels. All organs systems may be involved, including the dermis, lungs, heart, kidneys, brain, stomach, liver and intestines (Walker 1995).

The extent of cytopathology varies depending on the infecting species. With *R. prowazekii*, little cytopathology is evident until the cell bursts (Silverman, Wisseman and Waddell 1980). Cells infected with *R. rickettsii* undergo more dramatic changes within the first few days following infection: for example, the rough endoplasmic reticulum dilates; electron-dense material accumulates in the cisternae of smooth membranes; and organized Golgi regions disappear. Eventually plasma membranes lose their integrity, the cytoplasm becomes fragmentated, the nucleus and nucleolus are destroyed, and cells lyse (Silverman and Wisseman 1979, Silverman 1984). The cytopathic effect is thought to be due to peroxidation of membrane lipids by oxygen radicals (Silverman and Santucci 1988). *Rickettsia* do not produce exotoxins, and their limited LPS content is considered inconsequential to the pathogenic process (Kaplowitz et al. 1983).

Direct rickettsial injury to infected endothelial cells and subsequent vasculitis are the underlying pathogenic events of rickettsial infections (Walker and Mattern 1980, Walker 1988). Polymorphonuclear leuco-

cytes, lymphocytes, plasma cells and macrophages surround damaged vasculature. Depending on the extent of vascular damage and inflammation, vasculitis may manifest clinically as meningoencephalitis, interstitial pneumonitis and myocarditis; focal necrosis of the kidney and liver occurs in some patients. Necrosis and swelling of the vascular endothelium result in increased vascular permeability. Extravasation of blood from the microcirculation produces the rash that is characteristic of rickettsial diseases; severe damage to blood vessels can occur with Rocky Mountain spotted fever (RMSF), epidemic typhus, or scrub typhus and result in loss of plasma and electrolytes, hypotension and shock. Deaths are most common when oedema occurs in the brain and lungs. Platelets attach to infected endothelial cells and thrombi are observed in blood vessels. Haemostatic fibrin-platelet plugs abate haemorrhage in seriously ill patients but seldom occlude vessels or cause ischaemic necrosis. Platelets are consumed in this process, but true disseminated intravascular coagulation with hypofibrinogenaemia is unusual (Walker 1995). In vitro, platelets adhere to infected endothelial cells (Silverman 1986), but do not degranulate and release pharmacological mediators. Infected endothelial cells also secrete prostaglandins PGI$_2$ and PGE$_2$ in vitro (Walker et al. 1990). Although these molecules are known to affect vasodilation and vascular permeability, their pathogenic role in patients has not been elucidated.

Because all organ systems are affected by rickettsial infections, patients have common but non-specific clinical manifestations. Signs and symptoms vary, depending on the particular disease and the extent of cellular damage subsequent to infection with respective species; clinical presentation may also vary among individual patients infected with the same microorganism (Sexton and Burgdorfer 1975, Brown et al. 1976, Hattwick, O'Brien and Hanson 1976, Bradford and Hawkins 1977, Helmick, Bernard and d'Angelo 1984, Raoult et al. 1986b, Dumler, Taylor and Walker 1991, Perine et al. 1992, Uchida 1993, Kass et al. 1994). Symptoms usually include fever, headache and myalgias. Conjunctivitis and pharyngitis are common; malaise, anorexia, nausea, vomiting, abdominal pain, diarrhoea, photophobia and cough are noted by some patients. Pneumonia and abnormalities of the central nervous system complicate the clinical course in a small percentage of patients. Thrombocytopenia, low serum sodium levels, and elevated levels of liver enzyme activity are common laboratory abnormalities. Because of the non-specific nature of symptoms, rickettsial diseases are confused with many other bacterial and viral illnesses and other conditions that are prevalent in a given geographical area. Ultimately, clinical diagnosis requires a high index of suspicion by the attending physician; documentation of exposure to ticks or other vectors contributes to the diagnosis.

Rash is characteristic of many rickettsial infections and the type and distribution of rash can help distinguish rickettsial diseases (Walker 1989) (Table 53.3). For example, patients with epidemic typhus, murine typhus, or scrub typhus develop a macular or

Table 53.3 Clinical manifestations of rickettsial diseases

Manifestation	Rocky Mt spotted fever	Tick typhus	Rickett-sialpox	Ehrlichiosis due to *E. chaffeensis*	Human granulocytic ehrlichiosis	Epidemic typhus	Murine typhus	Scrub typhus	Q fever
Severity	Moderate to severe	Moderate to severe	Mild to moderate	Asymptomatic to severe	Moderate to severe	Moderate to severe	Mild to moderate	Moderate to severe	Asymptomatic to chronic
Fever, headache, myalgias Rash	Yes	Yes	Yes	Yes	Yes	Yes	Yes	Yes	Yes
Type of rash	Common Maculo-papular; frequently petechial	Common Maculo-papular; eschar frequently present	Common Vesicular; eschar usually present	Uncommon Maculo-papular	Uncommon Maculo-papular	Common Maculo-papular; petechiae common	Common Maculo-papular	Common Maculo-papular	Uncommon Maculo-papular or purpuric
Location	Extremities including palms and soles; trunk	Lower extremities; palms and soles; trunk	Face, trunk, extremities; eschar common	Trunk, extremities	Trunk, extremities	Trunk, extremities	Trunk, extremities	Trunk, extremities; some have eschar	Trunk
Pneumonia	Uncommon	Uncommon	Uncommon	Uncommon	Uncommon	Uncommon	Uncommon	Uncommon	Common
Thrombocyto-penia	Common	Common	No	Common	Common	Common	Uncommon	Common	Uncommon
Leucopenia	No	No	No	Yes	Yes	No	No	No	No
Case-fatality ratio (%)	3–5	2	0	2–5	7–10	10–50	<1	3–5	<1

maculopapular rash on the trunk that may later spread to the extremities, but rash usually is not found on the face, palms, or soles. By contrast, patients with RMSF first develop rash on the ankles, feet and wrists; the rash may become petechial and spread to other parts of the body, including the palms and soles. Rash in patients with Mediterranean spotted fever (tick typhus) is similar to that found in RMSF; many patients with Mediterranean spotted fever also develop an eschar (a 1 cm focus of epidermal and dermal necrosis) at the site of the tick bite (Walker et al. 1988). Eschars are characteristic of rickettsialpox infections and are frequently found in scrub typhus patients. The vesicular rash of rickettsialpox distinguishes it from other rickettsial infections. Rash is relatively rare in patients with Q fever.

Fatality rates vary among rickettsial diseases (Table 53.3) and are affected by antibiotic therapy. For example, fatality rates for RMSF exceeded 20% in the pre-antibiotic era but the current rate is only 3–5%. Fatality rates exceeding 50% can occur during outbreaks of epidemic typhus, particularly when disease occurs among undernourished or distressed populations and where supportive medical care is generally unavailable. Illness is generally less severe in younger patients. Fatalities are rare in cases of murine typhus. Rickettsialpox is a relatively mild disease and no fatalities have been reported.

5.2 *Ehrlichia*

Sennetsu fever is a mononucleosis-like illness that occurs in Japan. The aetiological agent, *E. sennetsu*, is thought to be transmitted by infected ticks, but the vectors and reservoirs have not been determined. Sennetsu fever is a relatively mild illness and the absence of fatalities has precluded meaningful examination of patient tissues to study pathogenesis. Clinical manifestations include fever, malaise and anorexia. Lymphadenopathy is observed and patients have increased peripheral mononuclear cells and atypical lymphocytes. Otherwise, the disease is unremarkable. *E. sennetsu* has been isolated from blood, bone marrow and lymph nodes of patients (Misao and Kobayashi 1954).

Human ehrlichiosis was first described in the USA in the 1980s (Maeda et al. 1987, McDade 1990). Exposure to ticks has been well documented in these patients, and the organisms are presumed to be transmitted directly by tick bite into dermal blood vessels. Ehrlichiae may be found in bone marrow and in lymphoid, mononuclear and polymorphonuclear leucocytes, indicating that haematopoietic cells are a target of infection. Mechanisms of pathogenesis have not been well described. Endothelial cells of blood vessels are not infected and, unlike the case in rickettsial infections, vasculitis is not observed in ehrlichiosis. Involved organs include liver, spleen, bone marrow and lymph nodes (Dumler and Bakken 1995). Studies of tropical canine pancytopenia, which occurs in dogs infected with *E. canis*, may provide useful correlates (Buhles, Huxsoll and Ristic 1974). Cytopenia in ehrlichiosis patients is probably due to destruction or

sequestration; erythrophagocytosis and leucophagocytosis occur. Infiltration of tissues by histiocytes is common.

In the USA, 2 agents that cause human ehrlichiosis have been identified: *E. chaffeensis* (Anderson et al. 1991) and another, as yet unnamed ehrlichia (herein called the HGE agent) that is closely related to *E. equi* and *E. phagocytophila* (Chen et al. 1994). Most information about human ehrlichiosis in the USA accrues from studies of patients infected with *E. chaffeensis*. Clinical manifestations of human ehrlichiosis vary from asymptomatic to severe, although most cases are symptomatic. Symptoms are similar to those of RMSF and include fever, headache, chills, malaise and myalgias. Thrombocytopenia is observed in most patients and anaemia occurs in about 50% of patients. Most patients also have elevated levels of liver enzyme activity. Leucopenia is common in ehrlichiosis but uncommon in RMSF. Rash occurs in less than half of ehrlichiosis patients; the lack of rash helps distinguish ehrlichiosis from RMSF. Additionally, nausea or vomiting is more common in ehrlichiosis than in RMSF (Fishbein, Dawson and Robinson 1994).

A second form of human ehrlichiosis has recently been described in the USA. It is called human granulocytic ehrlichiosis (HGE) because the aetiological agent is found in patients' polymorphonuclear leucocytes. Clinical manifestations of this illness are generally similar to those of ehrlichiosis due to *E. chaffeensis* infection (Bakken et al. 1994, Dumler and Bakken 1995). Cases of HGE described to date have generally been more severe than ehrlichiosis due to *E. chaffeensis* infection, but the full spectrum of HGE has probably not been elucidated. Ehrlichiosis due to *E. chaffeensis* has been called human monocytic ehrlichiosis because the micro-organisms infect the monocytes of patients. However, *E. chaffeensis* can also be found in lymphocytes and granulocytes, so the term may be inappropriate. Selected characteristics of ehrlichiosis are presented in Table 53.3.

5.3 *Coxiella burnetii*

Patients contract Q fever by inhalation of infectious aerosols. Symptoms vary considerably among patients. Acute Q fever is characterized by fever, chills, headache, fatigue and myalgias. Cough, nausea and sweats are also reported. Hepatomegaly and splenomegaly are common; elevated liver enzymes are observed in most patients. In contrast to common perception, an exanthem may be observed. Pneumonia is an important clinical manifestation but its frequency varies from country to country, presumably due to variation of local strains of *C. burnetii*. However, radiographs are non-specific and similar to those observed in patients with pneumonia caused by viruses, *Mycoplasma*, or *Chlamydia* (Marrie 1990, Raoult and Marrie 1995). A low percentage of patients develop chronic Q fever months to years following the initial infection (Turck et al. 1976, Tobin et al. 1982, Raoult, Raza and Marrie 1990). About two-thirds of all cases of chronic Q fever manifest as endocarditis; underlying heart disease is a predisposing risk factor. Hepatic involvement, thrombocytopenia, anaemia, increased creatinine levels, hypergammaglobulinaemia, circulating immune complexes and presence of autoantibodies are also important diagnostic features of chronic Q fever. Arterial embolism has been documented in patients with Q fever endocarditis; venous thrombi and pulmonary embolisms also occur. Liver involvement includes mononuclear cell infiltration of the portal tracts and prominent sinusoidal Kupffer cells; focal necrosis of parenchymal cells is also noted (Turck et al. 1976).

6 EPIDEMIOLOGY AND NATURAL HISTORY

6.1 *Rickettsia*

Spotted fever group rickettsiae and associated diseases occur throughout much of the world. *R. rickettsii* (RMSF) is most common in the USA, but cases also occur in Central and South America. *R. conorii* (the agent of Mediterranean spotted fever, a form of tick typhus) is found primarily in the Mediterranean basin, the Middle East, the Indian subcontinent, and parts of Africa. Siberian tick typhus (*Rickettsia sibirica* infection) occurs in a broad band that ranges from the Indian subcontinent, across the former Soviet Union to Eastern Europe. Tick typhus also occurs in eastern Australia and Japan and is due to infection with *Rickettsia australis* and *Rickettsia japonica*, respectively.

The epidemiological factors of RMSF and the various forms of tick typhus are similar. Ticks are both reservoirs and vectors of spotted fever group rickettsiae; humans become infected when they intrude on these natural cycles of infection. Cases usually occur sporadically but clusters of RMSF have been reported.

Spotted fever group rickettsiae are maintained in successive generations of tick by transovarial passage; ticks remain infected during all stages of their developmental cycle. Most tick tissues are infected, including the salivary glands; rickettsiae are transmitted to hosts in tick salivary secretions during the feeding process. Rodents and other small mammals are susceptible to spotted fever rickettsiae. Infection of animals is usually asymptomatic, but animals may develop levels of rickettsaemia that last from days to weeks and provide a source of rickettsiae for uninfected ticks (McDade and Newhouse 1986). Several genera of ixodid ticks (e.g. *Dermacentor*, *Ixodes*, *Rhipicephalus* and *Amblyomma*) serve as vectors among animals and to humans, depending on the species of rickettsiae and the particular locality (Hoogstraal 1967, Burgdorfer 1975). RMSF and the various forms of tick typhus are seasonal diseases; most cases occur when tick activity is highest. For example, approximately 90% of cases of RMSF occur between April 1 and September 30. The highest incidence of RMSF is among children younger than 15 years; males are more likely than females to contract RMSF (Hattwick, O'Brien and

Hanson 1976, Dalton et al. 1995). The incidence of RMSF varies over time. For example, in 1980 more than 1000 cases were reported in the USA, but a decade later about 500–600 cases were reported annually. Reasons for variation are unknown but have been a subject of considerable speculation.

Rickettsialpox is typically an urban disease. Relatively few cases have been reported, but rickettsialpox may be confused with chickenpox and probably is greatly under-reported. The aetiological agent, *R. akari*, is transmitted by mites (*Liponyssoides sanguineus*, formerly *Allodermanyssus sanguineus*) that are ectoparasites of domestic mice (*Mus musculus*) (Huebner, Jellison and Pomerantz 1946, Huebner, Jellison and Armstrong 1947). Sporadic cases and outbreaks have been associated with tenements or other multiple family dwellings that are infested with mice. Both mites and mice are infected with *R. akari*, and their relative contributions to maintaining this micro-organism in nature have not been thoroughly evaluated. *R. akari* has also been isolated from voles (*Microtus fortis pelliceus*) in Korea (Jackson et al. 1957) and additional cycles of infection may be operational.

Surveillance for murine typhus is lacking, but it is thought to occur throughout the world with considerable frequency. Cases of murine typhus usually occur in association with commensal rats. *Rattus* rats (*Rattus rattus* and *Rattus norvegicus*) are the primary reservoirs of murine typhus rickettsiae (*R. typhi*) and the oriental rat flea (*Xenopsylla cheopis*) is the principal vector. Warm, humid climates that enhance proliferation of fleas favour this association. However, other reservoir–vector associations have been implicated in the transmission of infection (Traub, Wisseman and Farhang Azad 1978, Azad 1990). For example, cases of murine typhus have occurred in southern California in association with opossums (*Didelphis marsupialis*) and cat fleas (*Ctenocephalides felis*) (Sorvillo et al. 1993). Fleas become infected when feeding on rickettsaemic rats, and *R. typhi* proliferates profusely in midgut cells. *R. typhi* is excreted in flea faeces and contaminates the skin of hosts; scratching of irritated skin at the bite site facilitates infection. Patients may also become infected by inhaling infected flea faeces or when contaminated faeces comes into contact with mucous membranes or the conjunctiva. Laboratory studies indicate that direct transmission of *R. typhi* by flea bite occurs at a low frequency, apparently by regurgitation of the gut contents that contain rickettsiae (Azad and Traub 1989).

Epidemic typhus is unique among rickettsial diseases in that humans are the principal reservoir: infection is transmitted by body lice. The aetiological agent, *R. prowazekii*, proliferates in louse midgut cells; organisms are shed in louse faeces and contaminate the skin. Persons may also become infected by inhaling aerosols of infectious louse faeces. A non-sterile immunity results following epidemic typhus infection and recrudescent typhus (Brill–Zinsser disease) can occur from months to years following the initial infection (Murray et al. 1950). Subsequent outbreaks of louse-borne typhus can occur if a patient with Brill–

Zinsser disease and patient contacts are infested with lice and if generalized immunity is lacking in the local population. Louse-borne typhus occurs primarily in developing countries, usually in highland areas of Africa and Central and South America, where lousiness persists. Although louse-borne typhus occurs sporadically in endemic areas, epidemics are observed periodically, usually in association with famine, war, displacement of personnel, or other events that distress the population.

R. prowazekii has also been isolated from flying squirrels (*Glaucomys volans*) captured in Florida and Virginia (Bozeman et al. 1975). The biological and biochemical properties of *R. prowazekii* isolates from flying squirrels are virtually identical to those of isolates from patients with louse-borne typhus (Woodman et al. 1977). Infection is transmitted among flying squirrels by their lice (*Neohaematopinus sciuropteri*), presumably in a manner analagous to human infection (Bozeman et al. 1981). Sporadic cases of typhus have occurred in the USA among persons who have had exposure to flying squirrels (McDade et al. 1980, Duma et al. 1981). The mode of transmission has not been established with certainty but is presumed to occur by inhalation of aerosolized faeces from infected squirrel lice. Theoretically, outbreaks of louse-borne typhus could originate from such cases, provided that persons who live in areas where flying squirrels are enzootic are infested with body lice.

The epidemiology of scrub typhus is directly related to the ecology and natural history of mites (*Leptotrombidium* spp.), which are both reservoirs and vectors of the aetiological agent, *R. tsutsugamushi*. The endemic area for scrub typhus is widespread and includes central, eastern, and southeastern Asia and countries in the southeastern Pacific. During World War II and the Vietnam conflict, large numbers of cases occurred among troops deployed in tropical and subtropical areas in this region. Small, ground-dwelling mammals, especially wild rats (*Rattus* spp.), are hosts for vector mites but are not thought to be directly involved in transmitting infection. Areas with changing ecology that are marked by transitional or secondary vegetation provide typical habitats for these rodents. Such habitats may range from sandy beaches to alpine areas and disturbed forests and usually are quite focal (Traub and Wisseman 1974). Infection is maintained by transovarial transmission of *R. tsutsugamushi* to the next generation of mites (Urakami et al. 1994). As with most other rickettsioses, humans become infected when they intrude in a habitat that is infested with vectors. Only mites in the larval stage (chiggers) feed on hosts.

6.2 *Ehrlichia*

Nearly 400 cases of ehrlichiosis were reported in the USA in the decade from 1985 through 1994 (Fig. 53.4), mostly attributable to *E. chaffeensis* infection.

Cases have also been reported in Europe (Portugal and Spain) and Africa (Mali). The epidemiology of

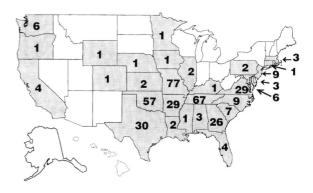

Fig. 53.4 Distribution of human ehrlichiosis in the USA, 1985–94; 386 cases. Data from the Centers for Disease Control and Prevention (CDC).

human ehrlichiosis is similar to that of RMSF. Both RMSF and ehrlichiosis are transmitted by ticks. Like RMSF, most cases of ehrlichiosis occur from April through September when ticks are most active. However, whereas RMSF typically occurs in suburban areas among children, ehrlichiosis occurs most frequently in adults in rural settings. Males are much more likely than females to become infected. Ehrlichiosis caused by *E. chaffeensis* infection occurs primarily in south-central and southeastern states. In contrast, human granulocytic ehrlichiosis (HGE) has been documented primarily in upper midwestern and northeastern states (Bakken et al. 1994, Dumler and Bakken 1995, Fishbein, Dawson and Robinson 1994, Telford et al. 1995, CDC 1995).

Reservoirs and vectors for ehrlichiosis are still under investigation. In the USA, *E. chaffeensis* has been detected in *Amblyomma americanum* (Anderson et al. 1993), and the known distribution of *A. americanum* follows the distribution of cases attributable to *E. chaffeensis* infection. Antibodies to *E. chaffeensis* have been detected in white-tailed deer (*Odocoileus virginianus*) and experimental infectivity studies have verified that deer are susceptible to *E. chaffeensis* (Dawson et al. 1994a, 1994b). Additionally, *E. chaffeensis* has been transmitted experimentally among white-tailed deer by *A. americanum* (Ewing et al. 1995).

Cases of HGE have been linked to exposure to *Ixodes scapularis* and *Dermacentor variabilis* (Bakken et al. 1994). However, cases of HGE have occurred in areas outside the known range of these ticks and other vectors are suspected. A species *of Ehrlichia* that appears identical to the agent of HGE in the USA has been detected in dogs and horses in Sweden (Johannson et al. 1995) and in dogs in the USA (Greig et al. in press). To date, all characterizations of strains of the HGE agent have revealed identical nucleotide sequence data for the 16S rRNA gene, suggesting that the agent of HGE may be distinct from, but closely related to, *E. equi* and *E. phagocytophila*.

6.3 *Coxiella burnetii*

Q fever has been reported on every continent. Unlike other rickettsioses, Q fever is usually transmitted by the inhalation of small particle aerosols that originate from infected animals. Q fever is enzootic among domestic animals, especially sheep, cattle and goats; infected cats have also been reported as sources of infection and other animal reservoirs are known or suspected (Marrie et al. 1988). *C. burnetii* proliferates profusely in the placenta of infected females and is shed at parturition. *C. burnetii* is extremely stable under environmental conditions, is highly infectious, can be broadly disseminated by dust, dried manure, or other materials, and presents an infectious hazard in areas where animal husbandry is practised. Disease occurs sporadically, but outbreaks are common, particularly among abattoir workers. Outbreaks of Q fever have also occurred at research facilities where sheep are utilized as experimental animals (Meikeljohn et al. 1981). Q fever can also be contracted by consumption of raw milk from infected animals (Fishbein and Raoult 1992). Ticks may also be infected with *C. burnetii* but are not thought to be a common source of infection in humans.

7 HOST RESPONSE

Patients who contract rickettsial infections usually develop lifelong immunity to reinfection. Epidemic typhus is the most notable exception. A non-sterile immunity occurs following epidemic typhus infection and recrudescent typhus can occur years later. How *R. prowazekii* persists and whether typhus rickettsiae remain in all patients are not clear. One possibility is that *R. prowazekii* remains sequestered in the lymph nodes of some patients (Price 1955). Multiple scrub typhus infections occur among persons who live in endemic areas because of the antigenic heterogeneity of *R. tsutsugamushi*. Although immunity to the homologous infecting strain is long lasting, immunity to heterologous strains is of short duration and former scrub typhus patients may become infected with different strains at a later time (Elisberg, Campbell and Bozeman 1968). However, repeat infections are much milder than primary infections.

The immune response to rickettsial infections has not been thoroughly described but remains a subject of active investigation. Available evidence indicates that cell mediated immunity is the critical component of the immune response, but the precise sequence of events has not been determined. Characteristic nodules of inflammatory cells (neutrophils, monocytes and mast cells) surround infected endothelial cells in epidemic typhus patients (Wolbach, Todd and Palfrey 1922). Monocytes and macrophages rapidly infiltrate the site of rickettsial replication in guinea pigs that are experimentally infected with *R. typhi* (Murphy, Wisseman and Fiset 1978). Polymorphonuclear leucocytes (PMN) are directed to the site of rickettsial infection by chemotaxis and accumulate there in large numbers (Wisseman and Tabor 1964). However, PMN have a relatively short half-life (1–2 days) and are minimally effective in eliminating rickettsial infection. PMN phagocytize cell-free rickettsiae, but most rickettsiae escape the phagosome and begin replication in the cytoplasm (Wisseman and Tabor 1964, Rikihisa and Ito 1979).

Lymphocyte actvity is central to the immune response to rickettsial infections. Adoptive transfer of spleen cells from immune mice to non-immune mice protects naive animals from infectious challenge. Depletion of T lymphocytes from the spleen cell population significantly reduces the protective effect, whereas depletion of B lymphocytes does not affect protection (Shirai et al. 1976, Crist, Wisseman and Murphy 1984). The susceptibility of T lymphocyte-deficient mice to rickettsial infections confirms the importance of T lymphocytes in the immune response (Kenyon and Pederson 1980, Montenegro, Walker and Hegarty 1984).

Delayed-type hypersensitivity (DTH) reactions have been observed in persons who have recovered from rickettsial infections; both CD4+ and CD8+ T lymphocytes were found in the perivascular mononuclear cell infiltrate (Dumler and Wisseman 1992). When inbred mice are experimentally infected with *R. typhi*, immunity correlates with DTH and lymphoproliferative responses by T lymphocytes (Jerrells and Osterman 1983). Lymphocytes are also cytotoxic for cells that are infected with rickettsiae. Fibroblast cells infected with rickettsiae have rickettsial antigens on their membranes; T lymphocytes from immune mice are cytotoxic for infected fibroblasts in vitro (Rollwagen et al. 1985, Rollwagen, Dasch and Jerrells 1986). Peripheral blood lymphocytes from typhus-immune persons also lyse infected lymphocytes in vitro, provided that effector lymphocytes are prestimulated with rickettsial antigens or interleukin-2. Lymphokine-activated killer cells contain OKT3, OKT4 and OKT8 lymphocyte antigens; antibodies to the OKT3 antigen inhibit the activity of killer cells (Carl and Dasch 1986).

Lymphocytes also produce interferons and other cytokines that augment the immune response to rickettsial infections (Kazár, Krautwurst and Gordon 1971, Nacy, Leonard and Meltzer 1981). Interferons have no direct rickettsiacidal activity, but they inhibit the growth of rickettsiae in non-phagocytic cells such as endothelial cells or fibroblasts; they can also stimulate infected macrophages to kill rickettsiae (Nacy and Meltzer 1979, Turco and Winkler 1983). Interferons may also have a direct cytolytic effect on infected cells (Wisseman and Waddell 1983, Turco and Winkler 1984). Interferon-γ (IFN-γ) is the likely mediator of these functions. The mechanism of action of IFN-γ in rickettsial infections is not known, but the respiratory burst is not involved nor is the receptor for the Fc portion of antibody (Keysary, McCaul and Winkler 1989, Turco, Keysary and Winkler 1989). A combination of IFN-α and IFN-β inhibits the growth of rickettsiae in fibroblast cells (Turco and Winkler 1990). Recombinant tumour necrosis factor α also inhibits rickettsial replication (Geng and Jerells 1994).

Antibody alone does not prevent infection, but it does contribute to the immune response. Antibody provides partial protection to animals that are experimentally infected with rickettsiae, particularly when it is administered prior to infection (Lange and Walker 1984). Antibody-dependent cell mediated cytotoxicity has also been demonstrated in vitro. In the presence of specific antibody, monocytes from non-immune donors lyse macrophage cells that are persistently infected with *C. burnetii*; lysis is mediated by the Fc receptor of monocytes (Koster et al. 1984). Antibody also prepares rickettsiae for phagocytosis and elimination by macrophages. Rickettsiae proliferate freely in the cytoplasm of normal macrophages in vitro, but if rickettsiae are pretreated with immune serum (opsonized), they are phagocytized, incorporated into phagolysosomes and destroyed (Beaman and Wisseman 1976, Nacy and Osterman 1979).

8 SPECIMEN COLLECTION AND DIAGNOSIS

Because patients with rickettsial infections present with non-specific clinical manifestations, laboratory testing is necesssary to confirm a diagnosis. Numerous techniques have been developed and evaluated, but serological testing remains the preferred approach to diagnosis because of its relative ease and simplicity. Newer cultivation techniques may provide acceptable alternatives (Marrero and Raoult 1989). However, neither serology nor isolation allows a diagnosis to be made early enough to affect patient management.

Other diagnostic techniques are less commonplace. For example, rickettsiae can be detected directly in punch biopsies taken from petechiae or macules but false positive results are common (Walker, Cain and Olmstead 1978). Rickettsiae can also be visualized in fixed cutaneous specimens by an indirect immunoperoxidase technique, but this procedure also lacks sensitivity (Dumler et al. 1990). Morulae can be detected in peripheral blood leucocytes of ehrlichiosis patients by light microscopy, but this technique is extremely laborious and also lacks sensitivity (Dumler and Bakken 1995). Rickettsiae can be detected directly in circulating endothelial cells by immunofluorescent staining if cells are first captured and concentrated by antibody-coated immunomagnetic beads (Drancourt et al 1992). This promising procedure provided simple and rapid diagnosis of a group of patients with Mediterranean spotted fever, but it has not been thoroughly evaluated or applied to other rickettsial infections. Rickettsial DNA is readily detected in patients' blood by polymerase chain reaction (PCR) technology (Carl et al. 1990, Anderson et al. 1992) and shows promise as an early diagnostic procedure; however, PCR testing is only available in research laboratories.

9 SEROLOGICAL ASSAYS

The indirect fluorescent antibody (IFA) procedure remains the most widely used technique for the sero-diagnosis of rickettsial diseases, but other techniques have been applied with variable success. Enzyme-linked immunosorbent assays (ELISA) are extremely sensitive, particularly IgM capture assays. Complement fixation (CF), latex agglutination and other techniques have also been used. The choice of technique depends on many factors. Sensitivity, specificity and reproducibility are primary considerations; cost, simplicity and appropriateness for a given setting are also important factors. For example, end points obtained with the IFA technique are subjective, but the IFA procedure is convenient for testing individual specimens. The ELISA technique provides objective end points and allows rapid testing of many specimens. However, rickettsial antigens for use in ELISA testing are extremely expensive to produce and are not readily available. The CF technique is still used but has fallen into disfavour because of its lack of sensitivity. Factors related to serodiagnosis are summarized in Table 53.4.

Diagnostic titres have been determined empirically for most serological procedures (see references in Table 53.4). Fourfold or greater rises in titre remain the mainstay for confirming a diagnosis, but diagnostic titres for single specimens have been also been proposed. Serum specimens collected during the acute and convalescent phases of disease are optimum for serodiagnosis.

Several factors must be considered when interpreting results of serological tests. Isolation of the aetiological agent of human granulocytic ehrlichiosis has only recently been reported; serological testing has been performed with antigens prepared from *E. equi*, a closely related species, which may give unreliable results. Member species in the spotted fever and typhus groups contain common antigens which cross-react with other rickettsiae in the respective groups and preclude identification of the specific aetiological agent. Testing for scrub typhus requires special consideration because of the antigenic heterogeneity of infecting strains (Elisberg, Campbell and Bozeman 1968). Multiple isolates of *R. tsutsugamushi*, including locally circulating strains, should be used as antigens in the diagnostic panel to ensure that antibodies are detected.

Isolation of *Rickettsia* and *Coxiella* provides an alternative to serodiagnosis. Whole blood, collected aseptically during the febrile period and prior to the administration of antibiotics, should be used for rickettsial isolation attempts. Clotted blood is preferred, because it allows removal of serum that may contain neutralizing antibodies. However, processing of clots is laborious and time-consuming and may present an infection hazard. Whole blood containing anticoagulants provides an expedient alternative. In either event, blood for isolation attempts should be stored and shipped frozen ($-20°C$ or colder), unless isolation attempts are undertaken immediately. Fresh tissues, collected post mortem, can also be used for isolation attempts. Small pieces of spleen or lung are preferred specimens, but liver, heart and kidney are also acceptable. Tissue specimens should also be stored and shipped frozen.

Rickettsia and *Coxiella* can be isolated in cell cultures,

Table 53.4 Features of some serological techniques for diagnosis of rickettsial diseases

Technique	Time from onset of disease until diagnostic titres are detected	Antibody persistence	Comment	Selected references
Indirect immunofluorescence	IgM test are positive in 6–10 days; IgG tests are positive in 2–3 weeks	IgM, 10 weeks; IgG approximately 1 year	Currently most widely used technique; relatively sensitive and requires little antigen; can distinguish immunoglobulin isotypes	Ormsbee et al. 1977, Philip et al. 1977, Hechemy et al. 1979, Newhouse et al. 1979, Saunders et al. 1980, Peacock et al. 1983, Dupuis et al. 1985, Kaplan and Schonberger 1986, Dawson et al. 1990
ELISA	≤1 week in many instances, particularly IgM assays	Not thoroughly evaluated; 1 year?	IgM capture assay useful for early diagnosis	Halle, Dasch and Weiss 1977, Dasch, Halle and Bourgeois 1979, Field, Hunt and Murphy 1983, Döller, Döller and Gerth 1984
Complement fixation	3–4 weeks	≥1 year	Lacks sensitivity compared with IFA and ELISA, but is very specific; now used infrequently	Ormsbee et al. 1977, Philip et al. 1977, Newhouse et al. 1979, Dupuis et al. 1985, Kaplan and Schonberger 1986
Latex agglutination	6–10 days	Approximately 8 weeks	Antigen preparation may mask some epitopes; lacks sensitivity for late convalescent phase sera	Hechemy et al. 1980, Kaplan and Schonberger 1986

embryonated hens' eggs, or experimental animals. Isolation from tissues is best performed in experimental animals to minimize or prevent growth of adventitious micro-organisms. Guinea pigs or mice are preferred laboratory animals for isolation attempts, depending on the species to be isolated (Weiss 1981, Marrero and Raoult 1989). Fluorescein-labelled monoclonal antibodies or mono-specific polyvalent antisera can be used to confirm the identify of isolates. However, because such antisera are not readily available, rickettsial isolation is best performed at reference laboratories. To date, *Ehrlichia* have been difficult to isolate (Dawson et al. 1993) and such efforts should also be performed by specialty laboratories.

10 TREATMENT

All rickettsiae are susceptible to antibiotics and prompt administration of appropriate antibiotic therapy is the most effective measure for minimizing disease and preventing fatalities. Early antibiotic therapy is especially important in cases of RMSF, louse-borne typhus, and scrub typhus, in which fulminant disease frequently develops and resists attempts at intervention. Early treatment shortens the course of all rickettsial infections.

Tetracyclines and chloramphenicol remain the drugs of choice for treating rickettsial diseases, although ciprofloxacin has been used successfully to treat patients with Mediterranean spotted fever (Raoult et al. 1986a) and other quinolones have been shown to be effective in vitro (Yeaman, Mitscher and Baca 1987, Raoult et al. 1991). Tetracyclines are generally preferred because they are less likely to produce haematological abnormalities in patients. Moreover, the response to tetracyclines may exceed that to chloramphenicol (Rose 1952, Powell et al. 1962, Sheehy, Hazlett and Turk 1973, Dalton et al. 1995). However, chloramphenicol may be indicated for pregnant women and children less than 8 years of age because tetracycline can depress skeletal growth and discolour teeth in children. Adults should receive 250–500 mg of tetracycline or chloramphenicol every 6 h. Children older than 8 years should receive 5–10 mg kg^{-1} of tetracycline every 6 h, not to exceed 2 g per day. Patients who are unable to take drugs orally should receive treatment intravenously; 2.5–5 mg kg^{-1} of tetracycline or 12.5–25 mg kg^{-1} of chloramphenicol every 6 h is the indicated dosage.

No particular tetracycline is preferred, but long-acting tetracyclines such as doxycycline may have advantages in certain situations. For example, doxycycline would be especially valuable during epidemics of louse-borne typhus, particularly when medical personnel are limited in number and unable to attend to patients on a regular basis. Single dose doxycycline may be as effective as a 10 day course of tetracycline or chloramphenicol for treating epidemic typhus or scrub typhus (Krause et al. 1975, Brown et al. 1978).

Clinical improvement is rapid in properly treated patients. Patients with RMSF who receive antibiotic therapy within 5 days of onset of illness are significantly more likely to survive than patients who are treated subsequently (Kirkland, Wilkinson and Sexton 1995). Defervescence usually begins within 24 h of treatment and temperature returns to normal in 1–4 days. However, because tetracyclines and chloramphenicol are rickettsiostatic and not rickettsiacidal, full recovery depends on the patient mounting an effective immune response. Treatment should continue for 7–10 days, or at least 3 days after patients become completely afebrile. Seriously ill patients should be treated for 2 weeks. Rickettsial infections in immunocompromised patients have rarely been reported; the clinical course remains primarily a matter of speculation, but long-term treatment may be necessary to prevent serious illness and preclude relapses.

Treatment of Q fever merits special consideration, particularly chronic Q fever. Whereas acute Q fever usually resolves uneventfully in 2–3 weeks, even in the absence of antimicrobial therapy, chronic Q fever endocarditis is much more difficult to treat and lifelong administration of antibiotics may be necessary to prevent the recurrence of symptoms. Tetracyclines are usually given in combination with another drug such as rifampicin or trimethoprim–sulphamethoxazole (Turck et al. 1976, Raoult and Marrie 1995). Other combinations have been given.

Resistance to tetracyclines or chloramphenicol has not been observed in rickettsiae. Most rickettsiae are maintained in wildlife or vectors, do not encounter antibiotics during their natural life cycles, and therefore are not subject to typical selection pressures. Utilization of antibiotics in domestic animal feed has not resulted in resistance among isolates of *C. burnetii.*

11 PREVENTION

With the exception of Q fever, vaccines are generally unavailable for rickettsial diseases. Q fever vaccine proved efficacious when administered to abattoir workers in Australia (Marmion et al. 1984) and is appropriate for other at-risk populations. However, Q fever vaccine can cause side effects (sterile abscesses that may require surgical excision) in persons with underlying immunity. Determination of antibody titres to *C. burnetii* and skin tests of potential vaccinees are necessary to identify and exclude persons who might develop untoward side effects after immunization.

Because most rickettsial infections occur when humans intrude on areas infested with reservoir animals and vectors, avoidance of such areas is still the most effective preventive measure. Control of rodent populations is important for preventing murine typhus and rickettsialpox. Rodent trapping and application of rodenticides are useful preventive measures, but depriving rodents of food sources is a more effective long-term prevention strategy. Vector fleas and mites will abandon dead animals and could seek out humans as alternative hosts and increase the risk of infection. Thus, rodent control programmes should be accompanied by the systematic application of appropriate insecticides.

Vector and rodent control are also essential for the prevention of scrub typhus. Disease typically occurs in focal areas with unique ecological features that may be amenable to control efforts. Removal of local vegetation reduces harbourages for rodents and the potential for exposure to vector mites. Treatment of the ground and residual vegetation with insecticides (organophosphates, organochlorines, or carbamates) will also reduce the density of mites. Mitocides (e.g. benzyl benzoate) can be used to impregnate clothing, and mite repellents (e.g. diethyltoluamide) can be applied to the skin. Prophylactic use of doxycycline, administered weekly to exposed persons, has limited effectiveness as a preventive measure. Although prophylaxis was efficacious, symptoms of scrub typhus developed among exposed persons when tetracycline was withdrawn (Twartz et al. 1982).

Theoretically, RMSF, ehrlichiosis and various forms of tick typhus could be prevented by tick reduction programmes. However, because the range of endemic areas is so vast, the cost of integrated control measures may be prohibitive. Wearing clothing that has been treated with permethrin and diethyltoluamide may reduce the frequency of tick bites (Evans, Korch and Lawson 1990). Prompt detection and removal of ticks is a useful and cost-effective preventive measure. Persons who must enter tick-infested areas should wear light coloured clothing to facilitate detection of ticks. Embedded ticks should be removed with curved tweezers by grasping them as close to the skin as possible and pulling up with slow, steady traction (Needham 1985). Careful disinfection of the attachment site with soap and water is also a useful precaution.

Delousing is essential for the control of epidemic typhus. Ideally, louse-infested persons should also be provided with clean clothing and bedding and facilities for bathing. Otherwise, residual insecticides should be applied to patients and their contacts and to their bedding, clothing and living quarters. Malathion has been used effectively for this purpose but other compounds may prove suitable. Resistance to insecticides occurs among lice and susceptibility testing of local lice populations is recommended prior to delousing programmes. Health care workers in the field should wear clothing that is impregnated with repellents and maintain good personal hygiene. Typhus vaccine, made from an attenuated (Madrid-E) strain of *R. prowazekii*, proved efficacious (Fox et al. 1959) but has been unavailable since the early 1980s. Among other factors, concerns that the vaccine strain might spontaneously revert to virulence has discouraged its use.

REFERENCES

Akporiaye ET, Rowatt JD et al., 1983, Lysosomal response of a murine macrophage-like cell line persistently infected with *Coxiella burnetii*, *Infect Immun*, **40:** 1155–62.

Amano K, Tamura A et al., 1987, Deficiency of peptidoglycan and lipopolysaccharide components in *Rickettsia tsutsugamushi*, *Infect Immun*, **55:** 2290–2.

Anderson BE, Dawson JE et al., 1991, *Ehrlichia chaffeensis*, a new species associated with human ehrlichiosis, *J Clin Microbiol*, **29:** 2838–42.

Anderson BE, Sumner JW et al., 1992, Detection of the etiologtic agent of human ehrlichiosis by polymerase chain reaction, *J Clin Microbiol*, **30:** 775–80.

Anderson BE, Sims DG et al., 1993, *Amblyomma americanum*: a potential vector of human ehrlichiosis, *Am J Trop Med Hyg*, **49:** 239–44.

Azad AF, 1990, Epidemiology of murine typhus, *Annu Rev Entomol*, **35:** 553–69.

Azad AF, Traub R, 1989, Experimental transmission of murine typhus by *Xenopsylla cheopis* flea bites, *Med Vet Entomol*, **3:** 429–33.

Baca O, 1994, Q fever, *Microbiology 1984*, ed. Schlesinger D, ASM Press, Washington DC, 269–72.

Bakken JS, Dumler JS et al., 1994, Human granulocytic ehrlichiosis in the upper midwest United States, *JAMA*, **272:** 212–18.

Beaman L, Wisseman CL Jr, 1976, Mechanisms of immunity in typhus infections VI. Differential opsonizing and neutralizing action of human typhus rickettsia-specific cytophilic antibodies in cultures of human macrophages, *Infect Immun*, **14:** 1071–6.

Bozeman FM, Masiello SA et al., 1975, Epidemic typhus rickettsiae isolated from flying squirrels, *Nature (London)*, **255:** 545–7.

Bozeman FM, Sonenshine DE et al., 1981, Experimental infection of ectoparasitic arthropods with *Rickettsia prowazekii* (GvF-16 strain) and transmission to flying squirrels, *Am J Trop Med Hyg*, **30:** 253–63.

Bradford WD, Hawkins HK, 1977, Rocky Mountain spotted fever in childhood, *Am J Dis Child*, **131:** 1228–32.

Brown GW, Robinson DM et al., 1976, Scrub typhus: a common cause of illness in indigenous populations, *Trans R Soc Trop Med Hyg*, **70:** 444–8.

Brown GW, Saunders JP et al., 1978, Single dose doxycycline therapy for scrub typhus, *Trans R Soc Trop Med Hyg*, **72:** 412–16.

Buhles WC Jr, Huxsoll DL, Ristic M, 1974, Tropical canine pancytopenia: clinical, hematologic, and serologic response of dogs to *Ehrlichia canis* infection, tetracylcine therapy, and challenge inoculation, *J Infect Dis*, **130:** 357–67.

Burgdorfer W, 1975, A review of Rocky Mountain spotted fever (tick-borne typhus), its agent, and its tick vectors in the United States, *J Med Entomol*, **12:** 269–78.

Burton PR, Kordová N, Paretsky D, 1971, Electron microscopic studies of the rickettsia *Coxiella burneti*: entry, lysosomal response, and fate of rickettsial DAN in L-cells, *Can J Microbiol*, **17:** 143–50.

Carl M, Dasch GA, 1986, Lymphokine-activated-killer-mediated lysis of cells infected with typhus group rickettsiae can be inhibited by ODT3 monoclonal antibody, *Infect Immun*, **53:** 226–8.

Carl M, Tibbs CW et al., 1990, Diagnosis of acute typhus infection using the polymerase chain reaction, *J Infect Dis*, **161:** 791–3.

CDC, 1995, Human granulocytic ehrlichiosis – New York, 1995, *Morbid Mortal Weekly Rep*, **44:** 593–5.

Chen SM, Dumler JS et al., 1994, Identification of a granulocytotropic *Ehrlichia* species as the etiologic agent of human disease, *J Clin Microbiol*, **32:** 589–95.

Crist AE Jr, Wisseman CL Jr, Murphy JR, 1984, Characteristics of lymphoid cells that adoptively transfer immunity to *Rickettsia mooseri* infection in mice, *Infect Immun*, **44:** 55–60.

Dalton MJ, Clarke MJ et al., 1995, National surveillance for Rocky Mountain spotted fever, 1981–1992: epidemiologic summary and evaluation of risk factors for fatal outcome, *Am J Trop Med Hyg*, **52:** 405–13.

Dasch GA, Halle S, Bourgeois AL, 1979, Sensitive microplate enzyme-linked immunosorbent assay for detection of antibodies against the scrub typhus rickettsiae, *J Clin Microbiol*, **9:** 38–48.

Dawson JE, Fishbein DB et al., 1990, Diagnosis of human ehrlichiosis with the indirect fluorescent antibody test: kinetics and specificity, *J Infect Dis*, **162:** 91–5.

Dawson JE, Candal FJ et al., 1993, Human endothelial cells as an alternative to DH82 cells for isolation of *Ehrlichia chaffeensis*, *E. canis*, and *Rickettsia rickettsii*, *Pathobiology*, **61:** 293–6.

Dawson JE, Childs JE et al., 1994a, White-tailed deer as a potential reservoir of *Ehrlichia* spp., *J Wildl Dis*, **30:** 162–8.

Dawson JE, Stallknecht DE et al., 1994b, Susceptibility of white-tailed deer (*Odocoileus virginianus*) to infection with *Ehrlichia chaffeensis*, the etiologic agent of human ehrlichiosis, *J Clin Microbiol*, **32:** 2725–8.

Döller G, Döller PC, Gerth H-J, 1984, Early diagnosis of Q fever: detection of immunoglobulin M by radioimmunoassay and enzyme immunoassay, *Eur J Clin Microbiol*, **3:** 550–3.

Drancourt M, George F et al., 1992, Diagnosis of Mediterranean spotted fever by indirect immunofluorescence of *Rickettsia conorii* in circulating endothelial cells isolated with monoclonal antibody-coated immunomagnetic beads, *J Infect Dis*, **166:** 660–3.

Duma RJ, Sonenshine DE et al., 1981, Epidemic typhus in the United States associated with flying squirrels, *JAMA*, **245:** 2318–23.

Dumler JS, Bakken JS, 1995, Ehrlichial diseases of humans: emerging tick-borne infections, *Clin Infect Dis*, **20:** 1102–10.

Dumler JS, Taylor JP, Walker DH, 1991, Clinical and laboratory features of murine typhus in South Texas, 1980 through 1987, *JAMA*, **266:** 1365–70.

Dumler JS, Wisseman CL Jr, 1992, Preliminary characterization of inflammatory infiltrates in response to *Rickettsia prowazekii* reinfection in man: immunohistology, *Acta Virol*, **36**: 45–51.

Dumler JS, Gage WR et al., 1990, Rapid immunoperoxidase demonstration of *Rickettsia rickettsii* in fixed cutaneous specimens from patients with Rocky Mountain spotted fever, *Am J Clin Pathol*, **93**: 410–14.

Dupuis G, Péter O et al., 1985, Immunoglobulin responses in acute Q fever, *J Clin Microbiol*, **22**: 484–7.

Elisberg BL, Campbell JM, Bozeman FM, 1968, Antigenic diversity of *Rickettsia tsutsugamushi*: epidemiologic and ecologic significance, *J Hyg Epidemiol Microbiol Immunol*, **12**: 18–25.

Eremeeva ME, Roux V, Raoult D, 1993, Determination of genome size and restriction pattern polymorphism of *Rickettsia prowazekii* and *Rickettsia typhi* by pulsed field gel electrophoresis, *FEMS Microbiol Lett*, **112**: 105–12.

Evans SR, Korch GW, Lawson MA, 1990, Comparative field evaluation of permethrin and DEET-treated military uniforms for personal protection against ticks (Acari), *J Med Entomol*, **27**: 829–34.

Ewing EP Jr, Takeuchi A et al., 1978, Experimental infection of mouse peritoneal mesothelium with scrub typhus rickettsiae: an ultrastructural study, *Infect Immun*, **19**: 1068–75.

Ewing SA, Dawson JE et al., 1995, Experimental transmission of *Ehrlichia chaffeensis* (Rickettsiales: Ehrlichieae) among whitetailed deer by *Amblyomma americanum* (Acari: Ixodidae), *J Med Entomol*, **32**: 368–74.

Field PR, Hunt JG, Murphy AM, 1983, Detection and persistence of specific IgM antibodies to *Coxiella burnetii* by enzyme-linked immunosorbent assay: a comparison with immunofluorescence and complement fixation tests, *J Infect Dis*, **148**: 477–87.

Fishbein DB, Dawson JE, Robinson LE, 1994, Human ehrlichiosis in the United States, 1985 to 1990, *Ann Intern Med*, **120**: 736–43.

Fishbein DB, Raoult D, 1992, A cluster of *Coxiella burnetii* infections associated with exposure to vaccinated goats and their unpasteurized dairy products, *Am J Trop Med Hyg*, **47**: 35–40.

Fox JP, Montoya JA et al., 1959, Immunization of man against epidemic typhus by infection with avirulent *Rickettsia prowazekii* (strain E). V. A brief review and observations during a 3½ year period as to the occurrence of typhus among vaccinated and control populations in the Peruvian Andes, *Arch Inst Pasteur (Tunis)*, **36**: 449–79.

Geng P, Jerrells TR, 1994, The role of tumor necrosis factor in host defence against scrub typhus rickettsiae. Inhibition of growth of *Rickettsia tsutsugamushi*, Karp strain, in cultured murine embryonic cells and macrophages by recombinant tumor necrosis factor-alpha, *Microbiol Immunol*, **38**: 703–11.

Giménez DF, 1964, Staining rickettsiae in yolk-sac cultures, *Tech*, **39**: 135–40.

Greig B, Asanovich KM et al., 1996, Geographic, clinical, serologic, and molecular evidence of granulocytic ehrlichiosis, a likely zoonotic disease, in Minnesota and Wisconsin dogs, *J Clin Microbiol*, **34**: 44–8.

Hackstadt T, Williams JC, 1981, Biochemical stratagem for obligate parasitism of eukaryotic cells by *Coxiella burnetti*, *Proc Natl Acad Sci USA*, **78**: 3240–4.

Hackstadt T, Peacock MG et al., 1985, Lipopolysaccharide variation in *Coxiella burnetii*: intrastrain heterogeneity in structure and antigenicity, *Infect Immun*, **48**: 359–65.

Halle S, Dasch GA, Weiss E, 1977, Sensitive enzyme-linked immunosorbent assay for detection of antibodies against typhus rickettsiae, *Rickettsia prowazekii* and *Rickettsia typhi*, *J Clin Microbiol*, **6**: 101–10.

Hattwick MAW, O'Brien RJ, Hanson BF, 1976, Rocky Mountain spotted fever: epidemiology of an increasing problem, *Ann Intern Med*, **84**: 732–9.

Hechemy KE, Stevens RW et al., 1979, Discrepancies in Weil–Felix and microimmunofluorescence test results for Rocky Mountain spotted fever, *J Clin Microbiol*, **9**: 292–3.

Hechemy KE, Anacker RL et al., 1980, Detection of Rocky Mountain spotted fever antibodies by a latex agglutination test, *J Clin Microbiol*, **12**: 144–50.

Helmick CG, Bernard KW, D'Angelo LJ, 1984, Rocky Mountain spotted fever: clinical, laboratory, and epidemiological features of 262 cases, *J Infect Dis*, **150**: 480–8.

Hoogstraal H, 1967, Ticks in relation to human diseases caused by *Rickettsia* species, *Annu Rev Entomol*, **12**: 377–420.

Huebner RJ, Jellison WL, Armstrong C, 1947, Rickettsialpox – a newly recognized rickettsial disease. V. Recovery of *Rickettsia akari* from a house mouse (*Mus musculus*), *Public Health Rep*, **62**: 777–80.

Huebner RJ, Jellison WL, Pomerantz C, 1946, Rickettsialpox – a newly recognized rickettsial disease. IV. Isolation of a rickettsia apparently identical with the causative agent of rickettsialpox from *Allodermanyssus sanguineus*, a rodent mite, *Public Health Rep*, **61**: 1677–82.

Jackson EB, Danauskas JX et al., 1957, Recovery of *Rickettsia akari* from the Korean vole *Microtus fortis pelliceus*, *Am J Hyg*, **66**: 301–8.

Jerrells TR, Osterman JV, 1983, Parameters of cellular immunity in acute and chronic *Rickettsia tsutsugamushi* infections of inbred mice, *Host Defenses to Intracellular Pathogens*, Plenum Publishing, New York, 355–9.

Johansson KE, Pettersson B et al., 1995, Identification of the causative agent of granulocytic ehrlichiosis in Swedish dogs and horses by direct solid phase sequencing of PCR products from the 16S rRNA gene, *Res Vet Sci*, **58**: 109–12.

Kaplan JE, Schonberger LB, 1986, The sensitivity of various serologic tests in the diagnosis of Rocky Mountain spotted fever, *Am J Trop Med Hyg*, **35**: 840–4.

Kaplowitz LG, Lange JV et al., 1983, Correlation of rickettsial titers, circulating endotoxin, and clinical features in Rocky Mountain spotted fever, *Arch Intern Med*, **143**: 1149–51.

Kass EM, Szaniawski WK et al., 1994, Rickettsialpox in a New York City hospital, 1980 to 1989, *N Engl J Med*, **331**: 1612–17.

Kazar J, Krautwurst PA, Gordon FB, 1971, Effect of interferon and interferon inducers on infections with a nonviral intracellular microorganism, *Rickettsia akari*, *Infect Immun*, **3**: 819–24.

Kelly PJ, Beati L et al., 1994, A new pathogenic spotted fever group rickettsia from Africa, *J Trop Med Hyg*, **97**: 129–37.

Kenyon RH, Pedersen CE Jr, 1980, Immune responses to *Rickettsia akari* infection in congenitally athymic nude mice, *Infect Immun*, **28**: 310–13.

Keysary A, McCaul TF, Winkler HH, 1989, Roles of the Fc receptor and respiratory burst in killing of *Rickettsia prowazekii* by macrophage-like cell lines, *Infect Immun*, **57**: 2390–6.

Kirkland KB, Wilkinson WE, Sexton DJ, 1995, Therapeutic delay and mortality in cases of Rocky Mountain spotted fever, *Clin Infect Dis*, **20**: 1118–21.

Koster FT, Kirkpatrick TL et al., 1984, Antibody-dependent cellular cytotoxicity of *Coxiella burnetii*-infected J774 macrophage target cells, *Infect Immun*, **43**: 253–6.

Krause DW, Perine PL et al., 1975, Treatment of louse-borne typhus fever with chloramphenicol, tetracyline or doxycycline, *East Afr Med J*, **52**: 421–7.

Lange JV, Walker DH, 1984, Production and characterization of monoclonal antibodies to *Rickettsia rickettsii*, *Infect Immun*, **46**: 289–94.

McCaul TF, Williams JC, 1981, Developmental cycle of *Coxiella burnetii*: structure and morphogenesis of vegetative and sporogenic differentiations, *J Bacteriol*, **147**: 1063–76.

McDade JE, 1990, Ehrlichiosis – a disease of animals and humans, *J Infect Dis*, **161**: 609–17.

McDade JE, Newhouse VF, 1986, Natural history of *Rickettsia rickettsii*, *Annu Rev Microbiol*, **40**: 287–309.

McDade JE, Shepard CC et al., 1980, Evidence of *Rickettsia prowazekii* infection in the United States, *Am J Trop Med Hyg*, **29**: 277–84.

Maeda K, Markowitz N et al., 1987, Human infection with

Ehrlichia canis, a leukocytic rickettsia, *N Engl J Med*, **316:** 853–6.

Manor E, Ighbarieh J et al., 1992, Human and tick spotted fever group rickettsia isolates from Israel: a genotypic analysis, *J Clin Microbiol*, **30:** 2653–6.

Marmion BO, Ormsbee RA et al., 1984, Vaccine prophylaxis of abattoir-associated Q fever, *Lancet*, **2:** 1411–14.

Marrero M, Raoult D, 1989, Centrifugation-shell vial technique for rapid detection of Mediterranean spotted fever rickettsia in blood culture, *Am J Trop Med Hyg*, **40:** 197–9.

Marrie TJ, 1990, Acute Q fever, *Q Fever. Vol. I. The Disease*, ed. Marrie TJ, CRC Press, Boca Raton, FL, 125–60.

Marrie TJ, Durant H et al., 1988, Exposure to parturient cats: a risk factor for acquisition of Q fever in maritime Canada, *J Infect Dis*, **158:** 101–8.

Meikeljohn G, Reiner LG et al., 1981, Cryptic epidemic of Q fever in a medical school, *J Infect Dis*, **144:** 107–14.

Misao T, Kobayashi Y, 1954, Studies on infectious mononucleosis (glandular fever). Isolation of etiologic agent from blood, bone marrow, and lymph node of patients with infectious mononucleosis by using mice, *Tokyo Iji Shinshi*, **71:** 683–6.

Montenegro NR, Walker DH, Hegarty BC, 1984, Infection of genetically immunodeficient mice with *Rickettsia conorii*, *Acta Virol (Praha)*, **28:** 508–14.

Murphy JR, Wisseman CL Jr, Fiset P, 1978, Mechanisms of immunity in typhus infection: some characteristics of intra-dermal *Rickettsia mooseri* infection in normal and immune guinea pigs, *Infect Immun*, **22:** 810–20.

Murray ES, Baehr G et al., 1950, Brill's disease, *JAMA*, **142:** 1059–66.

Myers WF, Wisseman CL Jr, 1980, Genetic relatedness among the typhus group of rickettsiae, *Int J Syst Bacteriol*, **30:** 143–50.

Nacy CA, Leonard EJ, Meltzer MS, 1981, Macrophages in resistance to rickettsial infections: characterization of lymphokines that induce rickettsiacidal activity in macrophages, *J Immunol*, **126:** 204–7.

Nacy CA, Meltzer MS, 1979, Macrophages in resistance to rickettsial infection: macrophage activation in vitro for killing of *Rickettsia tsutsugamushi*, *J Immunol*, **123:** 2544–9.

Nacy CA, Osterman JV, 1979, Host defenses in experimental scrub typhus: role of normal and activated macrophages, *Infect Immun*, **26:** 744–50.

Needham GR, 1985, Evaluation of five popular methods for tick removal, *Pediatrics*, **75:** 997–1002.

Newhouse VF, Shepard CC et al., 1979, A comparison of the complement fixation, indirect fluorescent antibody and microagglutination tests for the serological diagnosis of rickettsial diseases, *Am J Trop Med Hyg*, **28:** 387–95.

Oaks SC Jr, Osterholm JV, 1969, The influence of temperature and pH on the growth of *Rickettsia conorii* in irradiated mammalian cells, *Acta Virol (Praha)*, **23:** 67–72.

Ohashi N, Fukuhara M et al., 1995, Phylogenetic position of *Rickettsia tsutsugamushi* and the relationship among its antigenic variants by analyses of 16S rRNA gene sequences, *FEMS Microbiol Lett*, **125:** 299–304.

Ormsbee R, Peacock R et al., 1977, Serologic diagnosis of epidemic typhus fever, *Am J Epidemiol*, **105:** 261–71.

Pang H, Winkler HH, 1994, Analysis of the peptidoglycan of *Rickettsia prowazekii*, *J Bacteriol*, **176:** 923–6.

Peacock MG, Philip RN et al., 1983, Serological evaluation of Q fever in humans: enhanced phase I titers of immunoglobulins G and A are diagnostic for Q fever endocarditis, *Infect Immun*, **41:** 1089–98.

Perine PL, Chandler BP et al., 1992, A clinico-epidemiological study of epidemic typhus in Africa, *Clin Infect Dis*, **14:** 1149–58.

Philip RN, Casper EA et al., 1977, A comparison of serologic methods for diagnosis of rocky Mountain spotted fever, *Am J Epidemiol*, **105:** 56–67.

Powell OW, Kennedy KP et al., 1962, Tetracycline in the treatment of 'Q' fever, *Aust Ann Med*, **11:** 184–8.

Price WH, 1955, Studies on interepidemic survival of louse-borne epidemic typhus fever, *J Bacteriol*, **69:** 106–7.

Raoult D, Marrie T, 1995, Q fever, *Clin Infect Dis*, **20:** 489–96.

Raoult D, Raza A, Marrie TJ, 1990, Q fever endocarditis and other forms of chronic Q fever, *Q Fever. Vol. I. The Disease*, ed. Marrie TJ, CRC Press, Boca Raton, FL, 179–99.

Raoult D, Gallais H et al., 1986a, Ciprofloxacin therapy for Mediterranean spotted fever, *Antimicrob Agents Chemother*, **30:** 606–7.

Raoult D, Weiller PJ et al., 1986b, Mediterranean spotted fever: clinical, laboratory and epidemiological features of 199 cases, *Am J Trop Med Hyg*, **35:** 845–50.

Raoult D, Bress P et al., 1991, In vitro susceptibilities of *Coxiella burnetii*, *Rickettsia rickettsii* and *Rickettsia conorii* to the fluoroquinolone sparfloxacin, *Antimicrob Agents Chemother*, **35:** 88–91.

Regnery RL, Spruill CL, Plikaytis BD, 1991, Genotypic identification of rickettsiae and estimation of intraspecies sequence divergence for portions of two rickettsial genes, *J Bacteriol*, **173:** 1576–89.

Rikihisa Y, 1991, The tribe *Ehrlichieae* and ehrlichial diseases, *Clin Microbiol Rev*, **4:** 286–308.

Rikihisa Y, Ito S, 1979, Intracellular localization of *Rickettsia tsutsugamushi* in polymorphonuclear leukocytes, *J Exp Med*, **150:** 703–8.

Ris H, Fox JP, 1949, The cytology of rickettsiae, *J Exp Med*, **89:** 681–6.

Rollwagen FM, Dasch GA, Jerrells TR, 1986, Mechanisms of immunity to rickettsial infection: characterization of a cytotoxic effector cell, *J Immunol*, **136:** 1418–21.

Rollwagen FM, Bakun AJ et al., 1985, Mechanisms of immunity to infection with typhus rickettsiae: infected fibroblasts bear rickettsial antigens on their surfaces, *Infect Immun*, **50:** 911–16.

Rose HM, 1952, The treatment of rickettsialpox with antibiotics, *Ann NY Acad Sci*, **55:** 1019–26.

Roux V, Raoult D, 1995, Phylogenetic analysis of the genus *Rickettsia* by 16S rDNA sequencing, *Res Microbiol*, **146:** 385–96.

Samuel JE, Frazier ME, Mallavia LP, 1985, Correlation of plasmid type and disease caused by *Coxiella burnetii*, *Infect Immun*, **49:** 775–9.

Samuel JE, Frazier ME et al., 1983, Isolation and characterization of a plasmid from phase I *Coxiella burnetii*, *Infect Immun*, **41:** 488–93.

Saunders JP, Brown GW et al., 1980, The longevity of antibody to *Rickettsia tsutsugamushi* in patients with confirmed scrub typhus, *Trans R Soc Trop Med Hyg*, **74:** 253–7.

Schaechter M, Bozeman FM, Smadel JE, 1957, Study of the growth of rickettsiae II. Morphologic observations of living rickettsiae in tissue culture cells, *Virology*, **3:** 160–72.

Schramek SR, Brezina R, Tarasevich IV, 1976, Isolation of a lipopolysaccharide antigen from *Rickettsia* species, *Acta Virol (Praha)*, **20:** 270.

Sexton DJ, Burgdorfer W, 1975, Clinical and epidemiologic features of Rocky Mountain spotted fever in Mississippi, 1933–1973, *South Med J*, **68:** 1529–35.

Sheehy TW, Hazlett D, Turk RE, 1973, Scrub typhus. A comparison of chloramphenicol and tetracycline in its treatment, *Arch Intern Med*, **132:** 77–80.

Shirai A, Catanzaro PJ et al., 1976, Host defenses in experimental scrub typhus: role of cellular immunity in heterologous protection, *Infect Immun*, **14:** 39–46.

Silverman DJ, 1984, *Rickettsia rickettsii*-induced cellular injury of human vascular endothelium in vitro, *Infect Immun*, **44:** 545–53.

Silverman DJ, 1986, Adherence of platelets to human endothelial cells infected by *Rickettsia rickettsii*, *J Infect Dis*, **153:** 694–700.

Silverman DJ, Santucci LA, 1988, Potential for free radical-induced lipid peroxidation as a cause of endothelial cell injury in Rocky Mountain spotted fever, *Infect Immun*, **56:** 3110–15.

Silverman DJ, Wisseman C Jr, 1978, Comparative ultrastructural study on the cell envelopes of *Rickettsia prowazekii*, *Rickettsia rickettsii*, and *Rickettsia tsutsugamushi*, *Infect Immun*, **21**: 1020–3.

Silverman DJ, Wisseman CL Jr, 1979, In vitro studies of *Rickettsia* host–cell interactions: ultrastructural changes induced by *Rickettsia rickettsii* infection of chicken embryo fibroblasts, *Infect Immun*, **26**: 714–27.

Silverman DJ, Wisseman CL Jr, Waddell A, 1980, In vitro studies of *Rickettsia* host–cell interactions: ultrastructural study by *Rickettsia prowazekii*-infected chicken embryo fibroblasts, *Infect Immun*, **29**: 778–90.

Silverman DJ, Wisseman CL Jr, Waddell A, 1981, *Rickettsiae and Rickettsial Diseases*, eds Burgdorfer W, Anacker RL, Academic Press, New York, 241–53.

Silverman DJ, Wisseman CL Jr et al., 1978, External layers of *Rickettsia prowazekii* and *Rickettsia rickettsii*: occurrence of a slime layer, *Infect Immun*, **22**: 233–46.

Silverman DJ, Santucci LA et al., 1992, Penetration of host cells by *Rickettsia rickettsii* appears to be mediated by a phospholipase of rickettsial origin, *Infect Immun*, **60**: 2733–40.

Smith DK, Winkler HH, 1979, Separation of inner and outer membranes of *Rickettsia prowazekii* and characterization of their polypeptide composition, *J Bacteriol*, **137**: 963–71.

Sorvillo FJ, Gondo B et al., 1993, A suburban focus of endemic typhus in Los Angeles county: association with seropositive domestic cats and opossums, *Am J Trop Med Hyg*, **48**: 269–73.

Stein A, Raoult D, 1993, Lack of pathotype specific gene in human *Coxiella burnetii* isolates, *Microb Pathog*, **15**: 177–85.

Stoker MGP, Fiset P, 1956, Phase variation of the nine mile and other strains of *Rickettsia burneti*, *Can J Microbiol*, **2**: 310–26.

Telford III SR, Lepore TJ et al., 1995, Human granulocytic ehrlichiosis in Massachusetts, *Ann Intern Med*, **123**: 277–9.

Teysseire N, Boudier J-A, Raoult D, 1995, *Rickettsia conorii* entry into vero cells, *Infect Immun*, **63**: 366–74.

Teysseire N, Chiche-Portiche C, Raoult D, 1992, Intracellular movements of *Rickettsia conorii* and *R. typhi* based on actin polymerization, *Res Microbiol*, **143**: 821–9.

Thiele D, Willems H, 1994, Is plasmid based differentiation of *Coxiella burnetii* in 'acute' and 'chronic' isolates still valid? *Eur J Epidemiol*, **10**: 427–34.

Tobin MJ, Cahill N et al., 1982, Q fever endocarditis, *Am J Med*, **72**: 396–400.

Todd WJ, Burgdorfer W, Wray P, 1983, Detection of fibrils associated with *Rickettsia rickettsii*, *Infect Immun*, **41**: 1252–60.

Traub R, Wisseman CL Jr, 1974, The ecology of chigger-borne rickettsiosis (scrub typhus), *J Med Entomol*, **11**: 237–303.

Traub R, Wisseman CL Jr, Farhang-Azad A, 1978, The ecology of murine typhus – a critical review, *Trop Dis Bull*, **75**: 237–317.

Turck WPG, Howitt G et al., 1976, Chronic Q fever, *Q J Med*, **45**: 193–217.

Turco J, Keysary A, Winkler HH, 1989, Interferon-γ- and *Rickettsia*-induced killing of macrophage-like cells is inhibited by anti-rickettsial antibodies and does not require the respiratory burst, *J Interferon Res*, **9**: 615–29.

Turco J, Winkler HH, 1983, Inhibition of the growth of *Rickettsia prowazekii* in cultured fibroblasts by lymphokines, *J Exp Med*, **157**: 974–86.

Turco J, Winkler HH, 1984, Effect of mouse lymphokines and cloned mouse interferon-γ on the interaction of *Rickettsia prowazekii* with mouse macrophage-like RAW264.7 cells, *Infect Immun*, **45**: 303–8.

Turco J, Winkler HH, 1990, Interferon-α/β and *Rickettsia prowazekii*: induction and sensitivity, *Ann NY Acad Sci*, **590**: 168–86.

Twartz JC, Shirai A et al., 1982, Doxycycline prophylaxis for human scrub typhus, *J Infect Dis*, **146**: 811–18.

Uchida T, 1993, *Rickettsia japonica*, the etiologic agent of oriental spotted fever, *Microbiol Immunol*, **37**: 91–102.

Urakami H, Takahashi M et al., 1994, Electron microscopic study of the distribution of the vertical transmission of *Rickettsia tsutsugamushi* in *Leptotrombidium pallidum*, *Jpn J Med Sci Biol*, **47**: 127–39.

Valková D, Kazár J, 1995, A new plasmid (QpDV) common to *Coxiella burnetii* isolates associated with acute and chronic Q fever, *FEMS Microbiol Lett*, **125**: 275–80.

Walker DH, 1988, *Biology of Rickettsial Diseases*, vol. 1, CRC Press, Boca Raton, FL, 115–38.

Walker DH, 1989, *Clinical Dermatology*, vol. 3, JB Lippincott, Philadelphia, 1–17.

Walker DH, 1995, Rocky Mountain spotted fever: a seasonal alert, *Clin Infect Dis*, **20**: 1111–7.

Walker DH, Cain BG, Olmstead PM, 1978, Laboratory diagnosis of Rocky Mountain spotted fever by immunofluorescent demonstration of *Rickettsia rickettsii* in cutaneous lesions, *Am J Clin Pathol*, **69**: 619–23.

Walker DH, Firth WT, Edgell C-JS, 1982, Human endothelial cell culture plaques induced by *Rickettsia rickettsii*, *Infect Immun*, **37**: 301–6.

Walker DH, Mattern WD, 1980, Rickettsial vasculitis, *Am Heart J*, **100**: 896–906.

Walker DH, Occhino C et al., 1988, Pathogenesis of rickettsial eschars: the tache noire of boutonneuse fever, *Hum Pathol*, **19**: 1449–54.

Walker TS, Brown JS et al., 1990, Endothelial prostaglandin secretion: effects of typhus rickettsiae, *J Infect Dis*, **162**: 1136–44.

Weisburg WG, Dobson ME et al., 1989, Phylogenetic diversity of the rickettsiae, *J Bacteriol*, **171**: 4202–6.

Weiss E, 1981, *The Prokaryotes*, Springer-Verlag, Berlin, Heidelberg, 2137–60.

Weiss E, Moulder JW, 1984, *Bergey's Manual of Systematic Bacteriology*, vol. 1, ed. Krieg NR, Williams & Wilkins, Baltimore, London, 687–704.

Wells MY, Rikihisa Y, 1988, Lack of lysosomal fusion with phagosomes containing *Ehrlichia risticii* in P388D₁ cells: abrogation of inhibition with oxytetracycline, *Infect Immun*, **56**: 3209–15.

Winkler HH, Turco J, 1988, *Rickettsia prowazekii* and the host cell: entry growth and control of the parasite, *Curr Top Microbiol Immunol*, **138**: 81–107.

Wisseman CL Jr, Tabor H, 1964, Interaction of rickettsiae and phagocytic host cells. IV. Early cellular response of man to typhus rickettsiae as revealed by the skin window technique, with observations on in vivo phagocytosis, *J Immunol*, **93**: 816–25.

Wisseman CL Jr, Waddell AD, 1975, In vitro studies on rickettsia-host cell interactions: intracellular growth cycle of virulent and attenuated *Rickettsia prowazekii* in chicken embryo cell, *Infect Immun*, **11**: 1391–404.

Wisseman CL Jr, Waddell A, 1983, Interferonlike factors from antigen- and mitogen-stimulated human leukocytes with anti-rickettsial and cytolytic actions on *Rickettsia prowazekii*, *J Exp Med*, **157**: 1780–93.

Wolbach SB, Todd JL, Palfrey FW, 1922, *The Etiology and Pathology of Typhus*, The League of Red Cross Societies, Harvard University Press, Cambridge, MA.

Woodman DR, Weiss E et al., 1977, Biological properties of *Rickettsia prowazekii* strains isolated from flying squirrels, *Infect Immun*, **16**: 853–60.

Yeaman MR, Mitscher LA, Baca OG, 1987, In vitro susceptibility of *Coxiella burnetii* to antibiotics, including several quinolones, *Antimicrob Agents Chemother*, **31**: 1079–84.

Chapter 54

MYCOPLASMA DISEASES

D Taylor-Robinson and J Bradbury

1 Mycoplasma infections in humans	2 Mycoplasma infections in animals

The 5 genera, *Mycoplasma*, *Ureaplasma*, *Acholeplasma*, *Anaeroplasma* and *Asteroplasma*, comprise more than 120 named species (see Volume 2, Chapter 34). Of these, most belong to the genus *Mycoplasma* and are found mainly in the mouth, the upper respiratory tract and the more distal parts of the genital tract of humans and animals; the majority are host-specific. A few cause severe diseases, others are associated with diseases of a less obvious nature, and many appear to be non-pathogenic. Not surprisingly, the pathogenic status of some species is uncertain. The isolation of a mycoplasma from healthy subjects or animals does not prove that it is merely a commensal; conversely, isolation from diseased tissue, particularly when other micro-organisms are present, does not prove pathogenicity. Mycoplasmas of medical importance have, understandably, only rarely been studied in volunteers. On the other hand, mycoplasmas of veterinary importance can be subjected more easily to examination by inoculation of the natural host, although a low degree of pathogenicity may be difficult to demonstrate, especially if its expression depends on a synergic interaction between several micro-organisms, or on ill-defined stress factors. The interpretation of experiments in conventionally reared animals may be complicated by the unknown microbiological status of the host; the use of gnotobiotic animals, on the other hand, raises difficulties by virtue of the host's microbial artificiality.

For a general description of the mycoplasmas see Volume 2, Chapter 34, and for a review of the factors concerned in pathogenicity see Razin (1978) and Razin and Barile (1985).

1 MYCOPLASMA INFECTIONS IN HUMANS

Sixteen different mycoplasmas, 13 species within the genus *Mycoplasma*, 2 in the genus *Acholeplasma* and one in the genus *Ureaplasma*, have been isolated from humans (see Volume 2, Chapter 34), mostly from the oropharynx, but only a few unequivocally cause disease. The diseases attributed to *Mycoplasma* or *Ureaplasma* spp. and the strength of the associations are shown in Table 54.1.

1.1 Respiratory tract infections

COLONIZATION WITHOUT DAMAGE

The species found most commonly in the oropharynx are *Mycoplasma salivarium* and *Mycoplasma orale*. One or other or both species can probably be found as members of the resident flora in all adults; in other words they behave as commensals. They may, however, become involved in chronic disease (see below). Several other mycoplasmas come into the commensal category but are isolated less frequently. These are *Mycoplasma buccale*, *Mycoplasma faucium*, *Mycoplasma lipophilum*, *Mycoplasma primatum*, *Acholeplasma laidlawii* and, in adults, *Ureaplasma urealyticum*. Infrequent detection may be due to uncommon occurrence in the oropharynx or that the preferred habitat is the genital tract, with intermittent or transient presence in the oropharynx after orogenital contact. In addition, some of the mycoplasmas may seem to occur infrequently, simply because they have fastidious nutritional requirements that limit successful culture. In any event, these mycoplasmas should be regarded as commensals unless proved otherwise.

MYCOPLASMAS THAT EXHIBIT SOME SIGNS OF PATHOGENICITY

Mycoplasma hominis

In the 1960s, antibody responses to *M. hominis* (strain

Table 54.1 Diseases attributed to mycoplasmas or ureaplasmas: strength of the association

Disease	Mycoplasma/ureaplasma	Strength of the association
Pneumonia in children and adults	M. pneumoniae	++++
	M. fermentans	+
NGU	M. genitalium	+++
	U. urealyticum	++
Epididymitis	M. hominis; U. urealyticum	+
Pyelonephritis	M. hominis	++
Infection stones	U. urealyticum	++
Pelvic inflammatory disease	M. hominis	+
Postpartum and post-abortion fever	M. hominis	+++
	U. urealyticum	+++
Pneumonia, chronic lung disease in very low birth weight infants	U. urealyticum	++
Arthritis		
In immunocompetent patients	M. fermentans	++
	M. genitalium	+
Sexually acquired reactive	U. urealyticum	++
In hypogammaglobulinaemia and immunosuppressed patients	M. hominis	++++
	U. urealyticum & others	++++
Various conditions in immunosuppressed patients	M. hominis	+++

++++, Overwhelming; +++, strong; ++, moderate; +, weak.

DC63) recovered from the oropharynx were found to develop in some patients with pneumonia. Thus, of 346 patients with pneumonia, 3.2% developed complement-fixing antibody, whereas of 939 patients without respiratory disease only 0.3% did so ($p<0.001$). This prompted a volunteer experiment (Mufson et al. 1965) in which 50 men were given a large number of organisms of strain DC63 into the oropharynx and nose. The organisms were recovered from 42 of the men and 38 developed a 4-fold or greater rise in indirect haemagglutinating antibody. Pharyngitis developed in 25 men, half of whom had cervical adenopathy and one-quarter complained of a sore throat. In addition, pharyngitis occurred more often in men who did not have pre-existing antibody than in those who did, providing further evidence for *M. hominis* as the cause of the pharyngitis. However, subsequent attempts to link this mycoplasma with naturally occurring sore throats in children and adults failed (Mufson 1983), probably because contact with smaller numbers of organisms occurs under natural conditions. None the less, the volunteer study points to the potential pathogenicity of *M. hominis*.

Mycoplasma genitalium

M. genitalium was originally found in the male genitourinary tract (Tully et al. 1981) and then in a small proportion of respiratory tract specimens that also contained *Mycoplasma pneumoniae* (Baseman et al. 1988). The enormous difficulty experienced subsequently in detecting *M. genitalium* by culture in the genitourinary tract was eventually overcome with the development of the polymerase chain reaction (PCR) and this has resulted in it being associated strongly with acute non-gonococcal urethritis (see section on 'Non-gonococcal urethritis, p. 1017). However, use of the PCR has not led to reports that *M. genitalium* exists frequently in the respiratory tract and causes disease. Indeed, the evidence tends to indicate that *M. genitalium* occurs far more often in the genitourinary tract than in the respiratory tract. Nevertheless, because of its known pathogenicity, the potential for *M. genitalium* to cause disease in the respiratory tract should be kept in mind. Furthermore, the close antigenic similarity between *M. genitalium* and *M. pneumoniae* (see p. 1019), means that some caution is necessary when complement fixation or other tests are used to diagnose a *M. pneumoniae* respiratory infection.

Mycoplasma fermentans

M. fermentans was isolated first from the genitourinary tract (Ruiter and Wentholt 1952) and, after its detection in various tissues of AIDS patients (Lo et al. 1989), it was also detected by PCR in the urine of 5%, the blood of 10% and the throat of about 20% of HIV-positive homosexual men, and in about the same proportions of specimens from HIV-negative, mainly homosexual, individuals (Katseni et al. 1993). From the viewpoint of respiratory disease, *M. fermentans* has been recovered from the throats of about 16% of children with community-acquired pneumonia, two-thirds of whom apparently had no other respiratory pathogen (Cassell et al. 1994); the frequency of its occurrence in healthy children is unknown. It has also been detected in a few adults who presented with an acute influenza-like illness, which sometimes deteriorated rapidly with development of an often fatal respiratory distress syndrome (Lo et al. 1993). It is clear that infection and associated disease are not necessarily linked with immunosuppression. Most recently, however, *M. fermentans* has been detected by PCR in bronchoalveolar lavage specimens from 25% of AIDS patients with pneumonia (Ainsworth et al. 1994), but not in such specimens from HIV-negative subjects examined for other reasons. It seems possible, therefore, that under the conditions of such immune dysfunction, *M. fermentans* may behave as an opportunistic pathogen.

Infections caused by *Mycoplasma pneumoniae*

In the late 1930s non-bacterial pneumonia was recognized as distinct from typical lobar pneumonia and the term 'primary atypical pneumonia' (PAP) was coined. In one variety of PAP, in which cold agglutinins often developed, an infectious micro-organism, the 'Eaton agent', was isolated in fertile eggs and was at first thought to be a virus. Serious doubts about this arose when its growth was found to be inhibited by chlortetracycline and gold salts (Marmion and Goodburn 1961) and cultivation on a cell-free agar medium finally established its mycoplasmal nature (Chanock, Hayflick and Barile 1962). Subsequently, it was appropriately named *M. pneumoniae* and its ability to cause respiratory disease was confirmed by numerous studies based on isolation, serology, volunteer inoculation and vaccine protection.

M. pneumoniae occurs world wide and infection is endemic in most areas. It is detected throughout all months of the year, with a slight preponderance in the late summer and early autumn, at least where seasonal climatic changes are striking. Apart from seasonal variation, epidemic peaks have been observed in some countries about every 4–7 years (Taylor-Robinson 1996a). Spread from person to person occurs slowly and is fostered by continual or repeated close contact, for example in a family, rather than by casual contact (Foy 1993). *M. pneumoniae* causes inapparent and mild respiratory tract infections more often than severe disease. It is responsible for only a small proportion of all upper respiratory tract disease and most cases of pneumonia are caused by bacteria or *Chlamydia pneumoniae*. However, in the USA it has been calculated that in a large general population, *M. pneumoniae* accounted for about 15–20% of all pneumonias (Taylor-Robinson 1996a) and in certain groups, for example military recruits, it has been responsible for as much as 40% (Denny, Clyde and Glezen 1971).

Clinical presentation

M. pneumoniae affects children and adults, the consequence of infection depending upon age and immune status (Couch 1990, Foy 1993). Infection is common in children under 5 years of age and it seems that most of the infections are symptomatic, although they tend to be mild and non-pneumonic, usually in the form of coryza and wheezing without fever. Infection rates are greatest in school-aged children and teenagers (5–15 years) and in these groups the risk of an infection that results in pneumonia is maximum (possibly 30% or more); such *M. pneumoniae*-induced disease consti-

tutes about half of all cases of pneumonia. In the 25–45 years age group, the incidence of pneumonia is 5-fold less than at 10 years of age and it diminishes further thereafter; in adults, perhaps only about 5% of *M. pneumoniae* infections manifest as pneumonia. However, when it occurs, the disease in the middle-aged and elderly is often more severe than in the young. The clinical manifestations of pneumonia are often insufficiently distinctive to permit an early definitive diagnosis. Indeed, in mycoplasmal pneumonia, as in other non-bacterial pneumonias, general symptoms such as malaise and headache often precede chest symptoms by 1–5 days, and physical signs such as râles often appear only after radiographic evidence of pneumonia has been obtained (Clyde 1979). X-rays often show patchy opacity, usually of one of the lower lobes. About one-fifth of patients suffer bilateral pneumonia, but pleurisy and pleural effusions are unusual. The course of the disease is variable, but cough, abnormal chest signs and radiographic changes may last for several weeks and relapse is common. In children, a prolonged illness with paroxysmal cough followed by vomiting, simulating the features of whooping cough, may occur. In adults, the more severe disease that occurs in the elderly may be even worse in patients with immunodeficiency (Foy 1993) or sickle cell anaemia, but death is rare.

Extrapulmonary manifestations

Disease caused by *M. pneumoniae* is usually limited to the respiratory tract, but a wide variety of extrapulmonary manifestations may occur during or after the respiratory infection (Murray et al. 1975, Foy 1993). These complications and an estimation of their frequency are shown in Table 54.2. Haemolytic anaemia with crisis is brought about by the development and action of cold haemagglutinins (anti-I antibodies); the organisms apparently alter the I antigen on erythrocytes sufficiently to stimulate an autoimmune response (Feizi 1987). It is possible that neurological and other complications arise in a similar way, but because *M. pneumoniae* has been isolated from cerebrospinal fluid, a direct effect cannot be discounted. Isolation of *M. pneumoniae* from the genital tract is referred to below (see section 1.2, p. 1017).

Histopathological changes

Death attributable to *M. pneumoniae* infection is rare and, therefore, there is little opportunity for postmortem examination. Hence, a picture of the histopathological events that occur in the human respiratory tract as a result of *M. pneumoniae* infection has been derived mainly from experimental infection of small laboratory animals. The pneumonic infiltrate takes the form mainly of a peribronchiolar and perivascular cuffing by lymphocytes, most of which are thymus-dependent; immunosuppressive agents prevent the pneumonia or diminish its severity (Taylor, Taylor-Robinson and Fernald 1974). The development of a cell mediated immune response to *M. pneumoniae* in humans, initiated apparently by a T cell epitope on the adhesin protein P1 (Jacobs, Rock and Dalehite

Table 54.2 Extrapulmonary sequelae of *M. pneumoniae* infection

System	Manifestations	Estimated frequency
Cardiovascular	Myocarditis, pericarditis	<5%
Dermatological	Erythema multiforme; Stevens–Johnson syndrome; other rashes	Some skin involvement in about 25%
Gastrointestinal	Anorexia, nausea, vomiting and transient diarrhoea	Up to 45%
	Hepatitis	?
	Pancreatitis	?
Genitourinary	Tubo-ovarian abscess	Insignificant
Haematological	Cold haemagglutinin production	About 50%
	Haemolytic anaemia	?
	Thrombocytopenia	?
	Intravascular coagulation	Few cases reported
Musculoskeletal	Myalgia, arthralgia	Up to 45%
	Arthritis	?
Neurological	Meningitis, meningoencephalitis, ascending paralysis, transient myelitis, cranial nerve palsy and poliomyelitis-like illness	6–7%
Renal	Acute glomerulonephritis	?

1990), has been shown by positive lymphocyte transformation, macrophage migration-inhibition and delayed hypersensitivity skin tests (Taylor and Taylor-Robinson 1975), and delayed hypersensitivity correlates with disease severity (Mizutani et al. 1971). The initial lymphocyte response is followed by polymorphonuclear leucocytes and macrophages which predominate in the bronchiolar exudate. The rather slow development of these events on primary infection contrasts with the accelerated and often more intense host response seen on reinfection. To a large extent, therefore, *M. pneumoniae* seems to cause pneumonia through an immunopathological process (Fernald 1979). Young children often possess antibody to *M. pneumoniae*, suggesting infection at an early age, and it is tempting to speculate that the pneumonia to which the organism gives rise in older persons is an immunological over-response to reinfection, the lung being infiltrated by previously sensitized lymphocytes.

CHRONIC RESPIRATORY DISEASE

Since mycoplasmal infections of animals are often associated with or are the cause of chronic illnesses, the possible role of mycoplasmas in human chronic respiratory disease, particularly chronic bronchitis, is worthy of consideration.

Mycoplasma pneumoniae infections

There is a tendency for *M. pneumoniae* to persist in the respiratory tract after clinical recovery, as mentioned before, and occasionally the respiratory disease it causes has a protracted course. Furthermore, soon after a *M. pneumoniae* infection, tracheobronchial clearance is very much reduced and slow clearance may persist for many months (Jarstrand, Camner and Philipson 1974). Despite this, however, there is no evidence that *M. pneumoniae* is a primary cause of chronic

bronchitis, or that it is responsible for maintaining chronic disease other than by possibly causing, together with other micro-organisms, some acute exacerbations. Indeed, the isolation of *M. pneumoniae* from some patients with an acute exacerbation of chronic bronchitis, in addition to their having a serological response, suggests that this is the case (Carilli et al. 1964, Hers and Masurel 1967, Cherry et al. 1971). The occurrence of complement-fixing antibody to *M. pneumoniae* more frequently in the sera of patients who suffer from chronic bronchitis than in those of normal subjects (Lambert 1968) is in keeping with this suggestion, although patients with chronic bronchitis sometimes acquire a mycoplasmal infection without an apparent worsening of disease (Mufson et al. 1974).

Other mycoplasmal infections

M. salivarium, *M. orale*, and perhaps other mycoplasmas present in the oropharynx of healthy persons, spread to the lower respiratory tract of some patients suffering from chronic bronchitis (Cherry et al. 1971). There is no evidence that these mycoplasmas, which are regarded as commensals, are a cause of acute exacerbations, but antibody responses to them occur more often in association with such exacerbations than they do at other times (Cherry et al. 1971). This suggests that the organisms are more antigenic during exacerbations, probably because of increased multiplication. As a result of this, it is tempting to conjecture that they participate in tissue damage brought about primarily by viruses and bacteria and in this way play some part in perpetuating a chronic condition.

1.2 Genitourinary infections

Eight *Mycoplasma* spp. (*M. fermentans, M. genitalium, M. hominis, M. penetrans, M. pneumoniae, M. primatum, M. salivarium, M. spermatophilum*) and *Ureaplasma urealyticum* (ureaplasmas) have been isolated from or detected in the human genitourinary tract. The conditions that have or are most likely to have a mycoplasmal aetiology are mentioned briefly and the likely role of *U. urealyticum, M. hominis* and *M. genitalium*, which are the species found most frequently, is summarized in Table 54.1.

Non-gonococcal urethritis (NGU)

Debate about the role of ureaplasmas in NGU has continued since the report of their detection in 1954 (Shepard 1954). However, although still contentious, there is some evidence to implicate these organisms as one of the causes of non-chlamydial acute NGU. This derives from the results of inoculating volunteers and animals, together with serological and differential antibiotic studies (Taylor-Robinson 1985) and observations on immunodeficient patients (Taylor-Robinson, Furr and Webster 1985). The proportion of cases for which ureaplasmas are responsible has not been defined accurately and their occurrence in the urethra of symptomless men suggests that only certain serotypes are pathogenic or that predisposing factors, such as impaired mucosal immunity, exist in those in whom disease develops. The importance of ureaplasmas certainly seems to be less than that of *Chlamydia trachomatis* or *M. genitalium*. Evidence has gradually accrued for the importance of the latter; although isolated with extreme difficulty from the urethra of men with acute NGU (Jensen, Hansen and Lind 1996), it has been detected much more easily by PCR and significantly more often in urethral specimens from such men than from those without urethritis. An antibody response has been detected and the mycoplasma has produced urethritis in subhuman primates, and it is associated with chronic NGU (Taylor-Robinson 1995a, 1996b). Recently, NGU has been associated with bacterial vaginosis, in which *M. hominis* is involved (Taylor-Robinson 1996b). This raises the so far unanswered question as to whether this mycoplasma plays a part in NGU, since it has been isolated from the urethra of about one-fifth of NGU patients and could be implicated either alone or together with other bacteria prominent in bacterial vaginosis. So far, there is no evidence to implicate *M. fermentans* or *M. penetrans* in acute NGU (Deguchi, Gilroy and Taylor-Robinson 1996). In women, there is weak evidence that ureaplasmas may play a role in the urethral syndrome (Stamm et al. 1983), but no evidence, as yet, that *M. hominis, M. genitalium* or other mycoplasmas are involved.

Prostatitis and epididymitis

The occasional apparent response of chronic abacterial prostatitis to tetracycline treatment has led to mycoplasmas being considered as a possible cause. Examination of expressed prostatic secretion may lead to false conclusions because of contamination by organisms from the urethra. Although some workers, who used non-invasive localization procedures, have claimed to have shown an association between ureaplasmas and chronic prostatitis (Brunner, Weidner and Schiefer 1983), others (Doble et al. 1989) have failed to demonstrate mycoplasmas in inflamed prostatic tissue removed without urethral contamination. At present there is no convincing evidence that *M. genitalium, M. hominis* or ureaplasmas cause chronic abacterial prostatitis. In contrast, *M. hominis* has been isolated from a percutaneous epididymal aspirate of a patient with acute non-gonococcal epididymitis (Furness et al. 1974) and ureaplasmas have been found in a similar aspirate from a patient with acute non-chlamydial, non-gonococcal epididymo-orchitis accompanied by a specific ureaplasmal antibody response (Jalil et al. 1988). Thus, it is possible that both micro-organisms occasionally cause this disease in young men.

Urinary infection and calculi

M. hominis has been isolated from the upper urinary tract but only in patients with symptoms of acute infection, many of whom have significant antibody titres (Thomsen 1978). It has been estimated that it probably causes about 5% of cases of acute pyelonephritis, obstruction or 'instrumentation' of the urinary tract serving as predisposing factors. Evidence has not emerged to suggest that ureaplasmas have a similar aetiological role. However, the fact that they produce urease, induce crystallization of struvite and calcium phosphates in urine in vitro, and lead to the production of calculi experimentally in laboratory animals (Texier-Maugein et al. 1987) raises the question of whether they cause calculi in the human urinary tract. The occurrence of ureaplasmas more often in the urine and calculi of patients with infection stones than in those with metabolic stones suggests that they may have a causal role (Grenabo, Hedelin and Pettersson 1988).

Reproductive tract disease in women

M. hominis and to a lesser extent ureaplasmas are found in much larger numbers in the vagina of women suffering from bacterial vaginosis than in healthy persons; together with various bacteria they may contribute to the disease (Taylor-Robinson and Munday 1988). Unlike *M. hominis, M. genitalium* is not associated with bacterial vaginosis (Keane, Gilroy and Taylor-Robinson, unpublished data), but it has been detected in the lower genital tract of 7–20% of women attending sexually transmitted disease clinics (Taylor-Robinson 1995a) and, perhaps not surprisingly, *M. pneumoniae* may be recovered occasionally from this site too (Goulet et al. 1995). However, whether bartholinitis or cervicitis is caused by these mycoplasmas is unknown.

Pelvic inflammatory disease (PID) in affluent societies is caused principally by *C. trachomatis* and, to a far lesser extent, by gonococci. Bacterial vaginosis may lead to PID, and since *M. hominis* organisms increase greatly in number in bacterial vaginosis, they may have a role in PID. The mycoplasma has been isolated from the endometrium, and from the fallopian tubes of about 10% of women with acute salpingitis diagnosed by laparoscopy (Mårdh and Weström 1970a), together with a significant antibody response (Mårdh and Weström 1970b). However, whether it is a cause on its own is still debatable. Although ureaplasmas have also been isolated directly from affected fallopian tubes (Mårdh and Weström 1970a), known pathogens have usually also been present. This, coupled with largely negative serological findings and the failure of ureaplasmas to produce salpingitis in subhuman primates (Taylor-Robinson and Munday 1988), fails to suggest a causal role. On the other hand, antibody responses to *M. genitalium* in some patients with PID (Møller, Taylor-Robinson and Furr 1984) and the production of salpingitis in subhuman primates following inoculation suggest that it may have a role in a small proportion of cases.

INFERTILITY IN WOMEN AND MEN

Because the contribution of *M. hominis* as a cause of salpingitis remains unclear, its true role in infertility as a consequence of tubal damage, or occlusion, or both, is entirely speculative. So, too, is the notion that ureaplasmas play a causal role in involuntary infertility, a possibility that was first raised over 25 years ago. These organisms have been associated with altered sperm motility, but specimens from fertile and infertile subjects contain ureaplasmas with similar frequency, and the results of antibiotic trials do not favour a causal hypothesis (Taylor-Robinson 1986).

1.3 Diseases associated with pregnancy

M. hominis and ureaplasmas have been isolated from the amniotic fluid of women with severe chorioamnionitis who subsequently experienced premature labour (Cassell et al. 1983). Ureaplasmas have been isolated more frequently from spontaneously aborted fetuses and stillborn or premature infants than from deliberately aborted fetuses or normal full term infants (Taylor-Robinson and McCormack 1979). The ability to isolate ureaplasmas from the internal organs of some aborted fetuses, together with some serological responses (Quinn 1986), and an apparent diminished occurrence following antibiotic therapy (Glatt, McCormack and Taylor-Robinson 1990), have been used to support a role for these organisms in abortion. However, pre-term labour and late miscarriage are strongly associated with bacterial vaginosis (Hay et al. 1994) in which *M. hominis* and ureaplasmas contribute to the disturbed microbial flora, so that it is not clear whether they play a part independently in abortion or as part of the abnormal flora.

The belief that *M. hominis* is a cause of post-abortion fever is based on isolation of the micro-organism from the blood of about 10% of affected women, but not from that of aborting afebrile women or normal pregnant women (Taylor-Robinson and Munday 1988). Further, antibody responses to this mycoplasma have been detected in about half of the febrile women but in few of the afebrile ones. *M. hominis* has been isolated also from the blood of about 5–10% of women with postpartum fever, but seldom from the blood of afebrile but otherwise comparable women. Similar observations have been made for ureaplasmas (Eschenbach 1986). Assuming that *M. hominis* and ureaplasmas are isolated in pure culture and not with other micro-organisms involved in bacterial vaginosis, the evidence suggests that both induce the fevers described.

1.4 Diseases of the newborn

An association between genitally associated mycoplasmas, particularly ureaplasmas, and low birth weight, in some but not all populations studied (Taylor-Robinson and Munday 1988) has been supported by serological data (Kass et al. 1981). However, the importance of these micro-organisms *per se* is clouded by the fact that bacterial vaginosis, in which ureaplasmas are implicated, has been shown to be strongly associated with low birth weight (Hillier et al. 1995). Furthermore, a study in which women given erythromycin in the third trimester of pregnancy delivered larger babies than those receiving a placebo (McCormack et al. 1987) has not been supported subsequently by the results of other trials.

M. hominis and ureaplasmas occasionally infect the respiratory tract of the newborn, the organisms sometimes being acquired in utero. In a critical appraisal of 4 cohort studies in which the relationship between ureaplasmas and chronic neonatal lung disease was analysed (Wang et al. 1993a), it was concluded that there was strong but not definitive evidence that ureaplasmas are a cause of such disease and occasionally death in infants weighing less than 1250 g at birth. Indecision will remain until the role of bacterial vaginosis has been resolved. Such premature infants are particularly prone to invasion of the cerebrospinal fluid by both *M. hominis* and ureaplasmas within the first few days of life (Waites et al. 1988). Meningitis may occur, running a mild subclinical course without sequelae, or there may be more severe neurological damage leading to permanent handicap.

1.5 Joint infections

There is evidence that, apart from *C. trachomatis*, ureaplasmas are involved in the aetiology of sexually acquired reactive arthritis. This is based on synovial fluid mononuclear cell proliferation in response to specific ureaplasmal antigens (Horowitz et al. 1994). Furthermore, *M. genitalium* together with *M. pneumoniae* has been found in the joint of a patient with pneumonia and polyarthritis (Tully et al. 1995), and *M. genitalium* has been detected by means of a PCR assay in the joint of a patient with Reiter's disease and also in that of a patient with rheumatoid arthritis (Taylor-Robinson et al. 1994). In the 1970s it was suggested that *M. fermentans* might be a cause of the latter disease but a relationship was never established. Of interest, therefore, has been the detection of *M. fermentans* by PCR in the joints of at least 20% of patients with rheumatoid arthritis and in those of patients with other inflammatory rheumatic disorders (Schaeverbeke et al. 1996; see Table 54.1). The role of ureaplasmas and other mycoplasmas in arthritis occurring in patients with hypogammaglobulinaemia is mentioned below (see section 1.6).

1.6 Infections at other sites and in immunocompromised hosts

Extragenital infections caused by *M. hominis* or urea-plasmas probably occur more often than is realized (Table 54.1) because these micro-organisms are rarely sought routinely. Most extragenital *M. hominis* infections have been discovered fortuitously as a result of growth of the organism on blood agar or in routine blood cultures. Apart from post-abortion and postpartum fever, septicaemia due to *M. hominis* has been demonstrated after injury and after genitourinary manipulations, and the organism has been found in wound infections, brain abscesses and osteomyelitis (Myhre and Mårdh 1983, Glatt, McCormack and Taylor-Robinson 1990).

A small proportion of hypogammaglobulinaemic patients develop suppurative arthritis and myco-plasmas, particularly those in the genitourinary tract, are responsible for at least two-fifths of the cases, being isolated from the joints in the absence of other microbes (Furr, Taylor-Robinson and Webster 1994). In some of the cases due to ureaplasmas, the arthritis has been associated with subcutaneous abscesses, persistent urethritis and chronic urethrocystitis or cystitis (Taylor-Robinson, Furr and Webster 1986).

Patients who have undergone organ transplants, and others receiving immunosuppressive treatment, quite often suffer *M. hominis* septicaemia with arthritis, surgical wound infection, or peritonitis. Sternal-wound infections are particularly common after heart–lung transplantation (Steffensen et al. 1987) and both *M. hominis* and ureaplasmas were isolated from the joint of a patient with polyarthritis receiving immunosuppressive drugs following a kidney allograft (Taylor-Robinson, Furr and Webster 1986).

The notion that mycoplasmas may be important in the pathogenesis of the acquired immune deficiency syndrome (AIDS) arose from the detection of *M. fermentans* in various tissues of patients with AIDS (Lo et al. 1989) and from studies in which various myco-plasmas in cell cultures were shown to influence HIV replication, usually in an enhancing way (Montagnier and Blanchard 1993, Taylor-Robinson et al. 1993). In particular, it has been suggested that *M. fermentans*, and possibly other mycoplasmas, might lead to more rapid development of AIDS and that *M. penetrans* is associated uniquely with HIV positivity and possibly with Kaposi's sarcoma (Wang et al. 1993b). However, *M. fermentans* has been found in peripheral blood leucocytes of HIV-negative individuals as frequently as in those of HIV-positive homosexual men (Katseni et al. 1993) and neither mycoplasma has been found more often in patients who are progressing rapidly to AIDS

than in those who are progressing more slowly (Ainsworth et al. 1996, unpublished data). Thus, convincing evidence for the involvement of these myco-plasmas in the pathogenesis of AIDS has not yet been forthcoming.

1.7 Diagnosis

MYCOPLASMA PNEUMONIAE INFECTION

Laboratory diagnosis of *M. pneumoniae* infection depends on detection of the organism by culture and/or molecular techniques, serological tests or a combination of these. Other micro-organisms capable of giving rise to pneumonic symptoms, such as bacteria, chlamydiae, rickettsiae and viruses, should be excluded. The Edward-type medium (see Volume 2, Chapter 34) employed most often in the past for the isolation of *M. pneumoniae* consists of PPLO broth, horse serum 20% and fresh yeast extract (25% w/v) 10%. A greater chance of isolation, however, is afforded by using the medium (SP4) designed for the isolation of spiroplasmas, which comprises a conventional mycoplasmal broth with fetal calf serum and a tissue-culture supplement (Tully et al. 1979). Both media contain a broad spectrum penicillin, glucose and phenol red as a pH indicator. Fluid medium, inoculated with sputum, throat washing, pharyngeal swab, or other specimen, is incubated at 37°C and a colour change (red to yellow), which occurs usually within 21 days, signals the production of acid due to fermentation of glucose by multiplying organisms. This preliminary indication of the existence of a myco-plasma may be confirmed after subculture to agar medium. Colonies of *M. pneumoniae* develop best in an atmosphere of air–5% CO_2 usually with a 'scrambled egg' rather than the classical 'fried egg' appearance. Colonies of *M. pneumoniae* were formerly believed to be unique in their ability to adsorb erythrocytes but, because those of *M. genitalium* share this property, specific identification must depend on the serological procedures detailed in Volume 2, Chapter 34. The methods used most widely are the inhibition of colony development around discs impregnated with specific antiserum, or the fluorescence of colonies treated with such antiserum labelled with a fluorochrome. The close serological relation between *M. pneumoniae* and *M. genitalium* (Lind et al. 1984) may, however, necessitate the use of several techniques, more than one antiserum, and monoclonal antibodies for Western blotting (Morrison-Plummer et al. 1987). Methods for detecting *M. pneumoniae* antigen in respiratory exudates include the little-used direct immunofluorescence (Hers 1963) and counter immunoelectrophoresis (Wiernik, Jarstrand and Tunevall 1978) techniques, immunoblotting with monoclonal antibodies (Madsen et al. 1988) and several enzyme immunoassays (Taylor-Robinson 1995b). Although these methods may be rapid, lack of sensitivity is a problem with all of them. The same may be said for the commercial DNA probes which has been an obstacle to their widespread use. The PCR assay does not have this drawback and DNA primers specific for *M. pneumoniae* have been developed and used for DNA amplification (Bernet et al. 1989, Jensen et al. 1989). A sensible approach to detection might be to test specimens by both PCR and culture and, if an isolate is required, to continue incubating cultures of those specimens that prove to be PCR-positive.

PCR may eventually take over from other diagnostic procedures. This will be an advance because currently, in view of time constraints and difficulty, culture is avoided in most diagnostic laboratories and reliance is placed on serology. Antibody is detectable by a variety of procedures (Taylor-Robinson 1995b), many of which are unsuitable for routine laboratory use. The complement fixation test (Clyde and Senterfit 1985), however, is widely used, recent infection being indicated by a ≥4-fold rise in antibody titre with a peak at about 3–4 weeks after the onset of infection. Such results are obtained in about 80% of cases. A ≥4-fold fall in antibody titre, perhaps over 6 months, may be helpful but is sometimes difficult to relate to a particular illness. Diagnosis based on testing a single serum sample is always difficult, but an antibody titre of ≥1:64 in a suggestive clinical setting should be sufficient to begin therapy. A ≥4-fold *M. pneumoniae* antibody response or a titre of ≥1:64 in an indirect haemagglutination test, for which kits are available commercially, is diagnostically suggestive in an appropriate clinical setting. A modification of the test (Marmion and Williamson 1993), an IgM antibody capture assay (Coombs et al. 1988), and a commercially available particle agglutination test (Barker, Sillis and Wreghitt 1990) have all been tried. The sensitivity of these tests may be a little greater than noted with the complement fixation test, but the specificity of all tests, including the complement fixation test, is a problem (Jacobs 1993) highlighted by the antigenic cross-reactivity between *M. pneumoniae* and *M. genitalium* (Lind 1982). More specific, perhaps, is the microimmunofluorescence test in which IgM antibody is sought; the presence of this antibody provides some confidence in accurately diagnosing a current or recent infection, but sensitivity is less than that seen with the complement fixation test (Sillis 1990). However, there seems to be no sense in changing from one test to another in search of greater specificity. A sensible and realistic approach to serodiagnosis would seem to be continued use of a familiar test, for example complement fixation, with Western blotting to check specificity in dubious cases (Kenny 1992). In the future, it is possible that a sensitive enzyme immunoassay (Kenny 1992), in which purified P1 adhesin protein provides greater specificity (Jacobs 1993), will find a place. Cold agglutinins, detected by agglutination of O Rh-negative erythrocytes at 4°C, develop in about 50% of patients. They are occasionally induced by other diseases such as paroxysmal haemoglobinuria, tropical eosinophilia, trypanosomiasis, cirrhosis of the liver and haemolytic anaemia, but a titre of ≥1:64 is suggestive of recent infection with *M. pneumoniae*. When the result of the test is negative, it should be repeated after a week or two.

GENITOURINARY TRACT AND OTHER MYCOPLASMAL INFECTIONS

The Edward-type medium described previously (see Volume 2, Chapter 34 and p. 1019) is suitable for most genitally associated mycoplasmas, but for *M. genitalium* SP4 is the medium of choice. As with *M. pneumoniae*, advantage is taken of the metabolic activity of the organisms to detect growth. Clinical material is inoculated in separate vials of liquid medium containing phenol red and either glucose, arginine, or urea, all at 0.1%. *M. genitalium* metabolizes glucose and changes the colour of the medium from red to yellow (Taylor-Robinson et al. 1981, Tully et al. 1981). *M. fermentans* does likewise but in addition converts arginine to ammonia, as do *M. hominis*, *M. primatum* and other arginine-metabolizing mycoplasmas. Ureaplasmas possess a urease which breaks down urea to ammonia. In each case, the pH of the medium increases and there is a colour change from yellow to red. The colour change produced by ureaplasmas occurs usually within 1–2 days, but that brought about by *M. genitalium* may take 50 days or longer. The extreme difficulty of isolating *M. genitalium* has seen the use, with some success, of a strategy involving both cell culture and a liquid medium (Jensen, Hansen and Lind 1996). Subculture from liquid to agar medium results in the formation of colonies about 200–300 μm in diameter by most genitally associated mycoplasmas; those of *M. genitalium* are usually smaller but vary in diameter up to 200 μm. Ureaplasma colonies are small (15–60 μm) but their brown coloration produced on medium containing manganous sulphate or calcium chloride (Shepard and Robertson 1986) makes for easier detection. *M. hominis* organisms, but not ureaplasmas, grow and produce non-haemolytic pinpoint colonies on ordinary blood agar, and they also multiply in most routine blood-culture media; the mycoplasma-inhibitory effect of sodium polyanethol sulphonate, included as an anticoagulant, can be overcome by the addition of gelatin, 1% w/v. Kits designed to isolate and identify *M. hominis* and ureaplasmas are available commercially and successful use has been reported (Renaudin and Bébéar 1990). They may be of particular value when the need for detection arises infrequently. As with *M. pneumoniae*, definitive identification of the genitally associated mycoplasmas is based on the use of one or more serological procedures (see Volume 2, Chapter 34). Inhibition of colonial development around a disc impregnated with specific antiserum ('agar growth inhibition') has been, and still is, a widely used method. There is no doubt, however, that epi-immunofluorescence and immunoperoxidase techniques (Taylor-Robinson 1983), which enable colonies on agar to be identified directly, have the advantage that mixtures of different mycoplasmal species or ureaplasmal serotypes can be detected. Isolation and identification procedures have been discussed in detail elsewhere (Taylor-Robinson and Furr 1981, Taylor-Robinson 1995b, 1996c).

Antigen-detection tests for genitally associated mycoplasmas have never found widespread use because of their inadequate sensitivity. The latter has also seen straightforward DNA probes being abandoned and a move to the use of PCR. DNA primers specific for *U. urealyticum* (Blanchard et al. 1993) and *M. genitalium* (Jensen et al. 1991, Palmer et al. 1991), among others, have been developed and used for DNA amplification by the PCR. The method has proved rapid, specific and sensitive and, in the case of *M. genitalium* in particular, of considerable value diagnostically.

Genitourinary mycoplasmal infections stimulate antibody responses. It would be feasible, therefore, to use them for diagnostic purposes, although this has rarely been done. A $\geq$4-fold rise in antibody titre is required and caution should be exercised in assessing the significance of a high titre in a single sample. The complement fixation test is neither specific nor sensitive. The indirect haemagglutination test also lacks specificity and has been used only rarely, for example in studies of salpingitis (Lind et al. 1985, Lind and Kristensen 1987). Metabolism-inhibition tests have been used to detect antibody responses to *M. hominis* and to the ureaplasmas for epidemiological purposes (Purcell, Chanock and Taylor-Robinson 1969). However, type specificity among the ureaplasmas may lead to false negative results unless a range of serovars is used, as for example was the case in detecting ureaplasmal antibody responses of infants and women who had aborted spontaneously (Quinn et al. 1983). The feasibility of using enzyme immunoassays is apparent because they have been employed to measure antibody responses to *M. hominis* in patients with salpingitis (Miettinen et al. 1983), and to ureaplasmas in patients with NGU (Brown et al. 1983). Furthermore, an enzyme immunoassay based on lipid-associated membrane proteins (LAMP) of *M. penetrans* has been used to measure antibody to this mycoplasma (Wang et al. 1992) and the same method has been applied to detecting antibody to *M. genitalium*. Microimmunofluorescence, which has been used to detect antibody responses to *M. genitalium* in patients with salpingitis (Møller, Taylor-Robinson and Furr 1984) and NGU (Taylor-Robinson, Furr and Hanna 1985), is less subject to exhibiting cross-reactivity with *M. pneumoniae* than is the case with some of the other tests. Western blot analysis is also useful in making the distinction (Morrison-Plummer et al. 1987).

1.8 Treatment

MYCOPLASMA PNEUMONIAE INFECTION

The susceptibility of *M. pneumoniae* and several other mycoplasmas to various antimicrobial agents is dealt with in Volume 2, Chapter 34. In brief, mycoplasmas are indifferent to penicillins, cephalosporins and other antibiotics that affect cell wall synthesis, but they are generally sensitive to antibiotics that inhibit protein synthesis (Taylor-Robinson 1995b). Thus, *M. pneumoniae*, like other mycoplasmas, is sensitive to the tetracyclines and more sensitive to erythromycin than some of the other mycoplasmas of human origin. In the case of pregnant women and children, it is advis-

able to use erythromycin rather than a tetracycline, and the former antibiotic has sometimes proved more effective than a tetracycline in adults. Over all, there should be no concern over therapeutic options because *M. pneumoniae* is also inhibited by the newer macrolides, such as clarithromycin and azithromycin, and the newer quinolones, such as sparfloxacin (Bébéar et al. 1993).

The value of antibiotic therapy in *M. pneumoniae*-induced disease was shown first in a controlled trial of dimethylchlortetracycline undertaken in US marine recruits; the duration of fever, pulmonary infiltration and other signs and symptoms were reduced significantly (Kingston et al. 1961). Subsequently, other trials provided evidence for the effectiveness of various tetracyclines, as well as erythromycin and other macrolides (Shames et al. 1970). It should be noted, however, that antibiotics tend to behave more effectively in planned trials than they do in routine clinical practice, probably because disease has become more established in practice before treatment is instituted. This should not be construed as meaning that antibiotic therapy is not worthwhile, although clinical improvement is not always accompanied by early eradication of the organisms from the respiratory tract (Smith, Friedewald and Chanock 1967). The likely reason for this is that almost all antibiotics only inhibit multiplication of the organisms and do not kill them. The quinolones are an exception, having cidal qualities, although the earlier ones have only moderate activity against *M. pneumoniae* (Bébéar et al. 1993). Failure to kill is also an explanation for clinical relapse in some patients and a plausible reason for recommending a 2–3 week course of antibiotic treatment rather than a shorter course. It is a moot point whether early treatment may prevent some of the complications but, nevertheless, it should commence as soon as possible. If facilities for rapid laboratory diagnosis, namely PCR assay, are not available, confirmation of a *M. pneumoniae* infection inevitably will be slow. In this circumstance, it would seem wise to start antibiotic treatment on the basis of the clinical evidence alone, a cold haemagglutinin or suggestive single serum antibody titre, or both, perhaps providing some diagnostic assurance, despite the drawbacks mentioned previously of attempting to make the diagnosis in this way.

GENITOURINARY INFECTION

The antibiotic susceptibilities of the genitally associated mycoplasmas have been presented before (see Volume 2, Chapter 34, Taylor-Robinson 1995b). Many of the diseases mentioned earlier in this chapter, however, are caused not only by mycoplasmas but also by various other micro-organisms, so that the antibiotic sensitivity of these must also be taken into account. Thus, in the case of NGU, for example, patients should receive a tetracycline that inhibits *C. trachomatis*, *M. genitalium* and ureaplasmas. Doxycycline is often used, given in a dose of 100 mg twice daily for 7 days. However, at least 10% of ureaplasma strains isolated from patients attending sexually transmitted disease clinics are resistant to tetracyclines (Taylor-

Robinson and Furr 1986) and patients who fail to respond should be treated with erythromycin (0.5 g daily for 7 days), to which most tetracycline-resistant ureaplasmas are sensitive. A tetracycline should also be included in the antibiotic armamentarium against PID, so that *C. trachomatis* and *M. hominis* strains are covered. However, an increasing proportion ($\geq 20\%$) of *M. hominis* strains are resistant to tetracyclines (Koutsky et al. 1983) and other antibiotics such as lincomycin or clindamycin may therefore need to be used on occasion (see Volume 2, Chapter 34). Azithromycin, which is being used increasingly to treat NGU and other infections in which *C. trachomatis* may be involved, is active against a wide range of mycoplasmas. If mycoplasma-induced maternal fever occurs after abortion or after vaginal delivery of a live baby and does not subside rapidly, tetracycline treatment should be started, but keeping tetracycline resistance in mind. Erythromycin would be the first choice in neonatal infection.

IMMUNOCOMPROMISED PATIENTS

Treatment of *M. pneumoniae* and other mycoplasmal and ureaplasmal infections in patients who are immunodeficient may prove particularly challenging. Thus, for example, in patients with hypogammaglobulinaemia, *M. pneumoniae* organisms and respiratory disease may persist for many months despite apparently adequate treatment (Taylor-Robinson et al. 1980). Furthermore, treatment of ureaplasma-induced arthritis in such patients with tetracyclines and other antibiotics has sometimes failed even when coupled with anti-inflammatory and gammaglobulin replacement therapy. However, administration of specific mycoplasmal high titre antiserum prepared in an animal (for example, sheep, rabbit) has aided clinical and microbiological recovery in such cases (Furr, Taylor-Robinson and Webster 1994). This is an indication of the important contribution made by the immune system to successful treatment, a view which has been supported by the failure of antibiotic therapy to eliminate mycoplasmas from nude mice in contrast to elimination from their immunocompetent counterparts (D Taylor-Robinson and PM Furr, unpublished data).

1.9 Prevention

MYCOPLASMA PNEUMONIAE-INDUCED DISEASE

It seems that infection with *M. pneumoniae* early in life confers short-lived protection and there is speculation that such infection is then responsible for disease in teenagers and young adults. However, as the population grows older, protection is maintained for longer periods. The attack rate diminishes with increasing age and although known cases of reinfection and disease have been reported (Foy et al. 1977), this is rare in older adults. Over all, the suggestions are that infection with or without disease is protective in later life and that immunization should provide a useful approach to the prevention of infection and disease.

Pulmonary disease induced in hamsters with virulent *M. pneumoniae* organisms given intratracheally protected them against subsequent challenge, whereas hamsters given the organisms parenterally were not protected, despite high titres of serum antibodies (Barile et al. 1988, Ellison, Olson and Barile 1992). This suggests that local, or cell mediated immune mechanisms, or both, in the animal model are involved in the protective response, findings that are in concert with clinical observations. Thus, the presence of humoral antibody to *M. pneumoniae* correlates only partially with protection (McCormick et al. 1974), since infection and the development of pneumonia may occur despite high titres of, for example, serum mycoplasmacidal antibody. Furthermore, resistance of adult volunteers to *M. pneumoniae*-induced disease has been related to the presence of IgA antibody in respiratory secretions (Brunner et al. 1973a). Such antibody could act as a first line of defence by preventing attachment of the organisms to respiratory epithelial cells.

The efficacy of formalin-inactivated *M. pneumoniae* vaccines in preventing pneumonia caused by this mycoplasma was assessed in 11 separate field trials involving more than 40 000 military recruits, university students and institutionalized children over a period of 15 years in the USA (Wenzel et al. 1976, Ellison, Olson and Barile 1992). Seroconversion rates ranged from 0% to 90%, and reduction in naturally occurring disease ranged from 28% to 67%. The failure of killed *M. pneumoniae* vaccines to protect fully may be explained by poor antigenicity of some preparations. However, poor protection associated with the induction of humoral antibody levels that in some cases were similar to those that develop after naturally occurring disease suggests that the failure of such vaccines may be due to their inability to stimulate cell mediated immunity or local antibody production. With this in mind, Brunner and colleagues (1973b) developed temperature-sensitive mutants of *M. pneumoniae* which multiplied at the temperature of the upper respiratory tract, but not at that of the lower tract. Some of these mutants produced pulmonary infection in hamsters without causing pathological changes and in so doing induced significant resistance to challenge with virulent wild-type *M. pneumoniae*. However, the same mutants caused moderately severe bronchitis or pneumonia in volunteers (Ellison, Olson and Barile 1992) so that they were unacceptable for general human use and this approach to vaccination was abandoned. Recombinant DNA vaccines involving the P1 adhesin and other proteins, and a live adenovirus recombinant vaccine developed by cloning a component of the *M. pneumoniae* P1 gene into an adenovirus vector, are new approaches (Ellison, Olson and Barile 1992). Whether they will ever come to fruition in a climate in which *M. pneumoniae* vaccine development is regarded as of low priority because the infection is treatable, is open to question.

2 MYCOPLASMA INFECTIONS IN ANIMALS

The involvement of mycoplasmas in natural and experimentally induced disease has frequently been described in many different animal hosts. This review is confined to natural disease conditions that are clearly caused by mycoplasmas and those in which mycoplasmas play a predisposing or exacerbating role (Table 54.3).

2.1 Cattle

CONTAGIOUS BOVINE PLEUROPNEUMONIA (CBPP)

CBPP is probably the most economically important of all the animal mycoplasmal diseases. It is caused by the small colony (SC) biotype/variant (bovine biotype) of *Mycoplasma mycoides* subsp. *mycoides* which was the first mycoplasma to be cultured in vitro (Nocard et al. 1898). The large colony (LC) biotype of this myco-

Table 54.3 Mollicutes with a role in animal disease[a]

Host		Mollicute species	Disease
Cattle		*M. mycoides* subsp. *mycoides* (SC)	Contagious bovine pleuropneumonia (CBPP)
		M. bovis	Pneumonia, mastitis, arthritis, urogenital infection
		M. dispar	Pneumonia
		Ureaplasma diversum	Vulvitis, reduced fertility?
		M. bovoculi	Role in keratoconjunctivitis
		M. bovigenitalium	Mastitis (occasional)
		M. bovirhinis	Mastitis
		M. californicum	Mastitis
		M. canadense	Mastitis
		M. alkalescens	Mastitis (occasional)
		Bovine group 7	Mastitis, polyarthritis, pneumonia
Sheep/goats	SG	*M. agalactiae*	Contagious agalactia, mastitis, polyarthritis
	SG	*M. capricolum* subsp. *capricolum*	Septicaemia, mastitis, polyarthritis, pneumonia
	G	*M. capricolum* subsp. *capripneumoniae* 'F38'	Contagious caprine pleuropneumonia (CCPP)
	G	*M. mycoides* subsp. *capri*	Pleuropneumonia, septicaemia, arthritis, mastitis
	G(S)	*M. mycoides* subsp. *mycoides* (LC)	Pleuropneumonia, septicaemia, mastitis, polyarthritis, keratoconjunctivitis
	SG	*M. conjunctivae*	Keratoconjunctivitis
	SG	*M. ovipneumoniae*	Pneumonia (with *Pasteurella haemolytica*)
	G	*M. putrefaciens*	Mastitis, arthritis
Pigs		*M. hyopneumoniae*	Enzootic pneumonia of pigs (EPP)
		M. hyorhinis	Polyserositis, arthritis, pneumonia
		M. hyosynoviae	Arthritis in fattening pigs
Chickens/turkeys/ game birds	CTG	*M. gallisepticum*	Respiratory disease, lowered egg production, occasional arthritis
	CTG	*M. synoviae*	Respiratory disease, infectious synovitis
	T	*M. meleagridis*	Airsacculitis, bone deformities, reduced hatchability and growth
	CT	*M. iowae*	Turkey embryo mortality
Rats and mice	R	*M. arthritidis*	Arthritis
	RM	*M. pulmonis*	Murine respiratory mycoplasmosis (MRM), genital disease, arthritis (occasional)
Horse		*M. felis*	Pleuritis
Cat		*M. felis*	Conjunctivitis

[a]Other species of mollicute have been shown to cause disease under experimental conditions (e.g. arthritis after joint inoculation) but those in this table are recognized causes of, or predisposing factors for natural disease conditions.

plasma, which cannot be distinguished serologically from the SC biotype, is found mainly in goats, although it has also been isolated from sheep and cattle. The LC biotype does not cause CBPP and occurs in countries, such as the USA and Australia, that are free of the disease. In addition to these biotypes, there are several other related mycoplasmas of ruminants belonging to the so-called '*mycoides* cluster' (Cottew et al. 1987). Various investigators (for example, Perreau and Bind 1981, Machado and Ferreira 1994, Brandão 1995) have suggested that the host specificity of the bovine and ovine and caprine members of this cluster may not be as strict as was once thought.

CBPP occurs in members of the *Bos* genus, that is mainly bovine and zebu cattle, and also in the water buffalo (*Bubalus bubalis*) in some areas. The American buffalo (*Bison bison*) and the yak are considered susceptible but wild African buffaloes (*Syncerus caffer*) and other wild ruminants are thought not to be susceptible (Jones 1991a).

In the nineteenth century the disease was widespread in Europe, from where it was transmitted by shipment of cattle to various parts of the world including Africa, the USA, Australia and the Middle and Far East. By the turn of the century slaughter policies had resulted in its eradication from a number of countries, including the UK and the USA, but Australia was not declared free until 1973. The disease persists in parts of sub-Saharan Africa, and has recurred in some countries from which it had been eradicated. It also persists in parts of the Middle and Far East (ter Laak 1992, Nicholas and Bashiruddin 1995) and has recently reappeared in several countries within the European Union (the Franco-Spanish border in the 1960s and 1980s, Italy in 1990 and Portugal from 1983 onwards). Strict control measures were successful in France and have reduced the number of outbreaks in the other European Union countries, but there is still concern about spread, particularly since the introduction of less stringent controls on the movement of animals between countries.

Acute CBPP is characterized by fever, respiratory embarrassment, fibrinous interstitial pneumonia and pleurisy (ter Laak 1992) but many animals develop subacute or subclinical forms of the disease. In untreated acute disease there is exudative inflammation of the interlobular lymph vessels and of the alveolar and interstitial tissue of the lungs. Infiltration and distension by serous fluid of the connective tissue layers between the lobules of the lungs give rise to the characteristic 'marbled' appearance (Figs 54.1 and 54.2).

Abundant serofibrinous exudate may accumulate in the pleural cavity. In many animals only one lung may be affected. In animals that are recovering or those with chronic disease, necrotic tissue may become walled off by fibrous tissue (Fig. 54.3). These sequestra can contain viable mycoplasmas for many months and later can break down to transmit the organisms to susceptible animals. In contrast to pneumonic lesions, infection in calves may present as arthritis (Gourlay

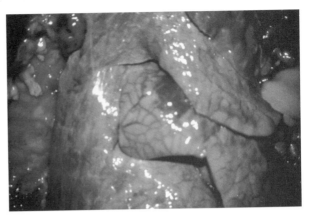

Fig. 54.1 Acute contagious bovine pleuropneumonia. Exterior of bovine lung showing distension of the interlobular septa with serous fluid. (Courtesy of Dr R A J Nicholas). See also Plate 54.1.

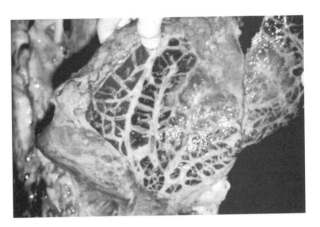

Fig. 54.2 Acute contagious bovine pleuropneumonia. Bovine lung cut to show hepatization of lobules with oedema and thickening of interlobular septa giving a 'marbled' appearance. (Courtesy of Dr R A J Nicholas). See also Plate 54.2.

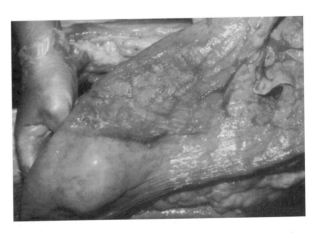

Fig. 54.3 Chronic contagious bovine pleuropneumonia. Bovine lung showing point of adhesion of pleural membrane (top) and a sequestrum (bottom). (Courtesy of Dr R A J Nicholas). See also Plate 54.3.

and Howard 1979), although typical pulmonary lesions have been seen in infected calves in the Iberian peninsula (RAJ Nicholas, personal communication 1995).

The incubation period of CBPP is variable, rarely less than 3 weeks and sometimes more than 3 months. The onset of disease is insidious and within an infected herd the disease may range from hyperacute to subclinical; some cattle may even remain uninfected (Losos 1986). In Africa the mortality may vary from less than 10% to more than 70% and the severity of disease is thought to be affected by husbandry and climate. In Europe very low mortality is reported and most animals have subclinical infection, which is possibly the consequence of the widespread use of antimicrobial agents and accelerated development of a carrier state. A galactan, found in in vitro cultures of the mycoplasma and in the lymph nodes, blood, lung and urine of infected cattle, probably influences the pathogenicity of the organisms (Lloyd, Buttery and Hudson 1971, Buttery, Lloyd and Titchen 1976).

Transmission of the organism usually requires close contact between infected and susceptible cattle and occurs probably by inhalation of infected droplets. The risk of indirect transmission by contamination of the environment is thought to be low. Occasional isolation of the SC biotype has been reported from sheep and goats and the results of limited studies suggest that such isolates may be pathogenic for cattle. However, their importance for transmission is unclear.

Diagnosis can sometimes be made on the basis of clinical signs together with the presence of characteristic postmortem lesions in the lung, although the disease may resemble that produced by *Pasteurella multocida*. Laboratory procedures must be used to detect subacute or symptomless infections. Isolation of *M. mycoides* subsp. *mycoides* can be attempted from live animals using nasal swabbings or discharges, bronchoalveolar or tracheal lavages and blood or pleural fluid collected by puncture from the lower thoracic cavity. From dead animals lung lesions, pleural fluid and local lymph nodes can be cultured (Jones 1991a). The organisms are not difficult to grow as long as the medium is satisfactory but, as with all such investigations, a negative result is not conclusive. Great care should be taken to transport material under conditions that will maintain viability and discourage growth of contaminating bacteria. If a mycoplasma is isolated, identification of the species (see Volume 2, Chapter 34) is essential. Diagnosis in this manner is complicated by the existence of the 2 biotypes, which are not always readily distinguishable by their growth characteristics. Thus DNA detection methods have been developed and include a diagnostic probe which distinguishes the SC from the LC biotype (Taylor, Bashiruddin and Gould 1992a) and also PCR systems which detect the 'mycoides cluster' and which further single out the SC biotype of *M. mycoides* subsp. *mycoides* (Bashiruddin, Taylor and Gould 1994, Dedieu, Mady and Lefevre 1994). These are expected to be useful, particularly in countries that have CBPP-free status but

where the LC biotype is isolated. Sensitive detection methods are still needed for latent carriers.

Other methods that have been used with some success to detect *M. mycoides* subsp. *mycoides* in infected animals are immunofluorescence with smears of pleural fluid and agar gel precipitation to detect the galactan in blood, pleural fluid, lung homogenates or sequestra (Jones 1991a). Both tests require the use of high titre specific antisera. The precipitation test has been modified for rapid field testing (Turner 1962, Provost 1972). Detection of specific serum antibodies is used widely for diagnosis although in the late stages of disease antibodies may be masked by the presence of antigen in the blood. Complement fixation (CF) (Campbell and Turner 1953, Queval, Provost and Villemot 1964) has been the test of choice for many years and is useful on a herd basis, especially during acute infection. However, infection may be missed in the early or later stages of disease or in small groups of animals and false positive reactions sometimes occur. Since vaccinal antibodies are detected for only a relatively short period by using the CF test, it is still useful for diagnosing genuine outbreaks in areas where vaccination is practised. Enzyme-linked immunosorbent assays (ELISAs) have been developed (Onoviran and Taylor-Robinson 1979) but probably require some refining before gaining wide acceptance. A slide agglutination test (Turner and Etheridge 1963) has also been used in the past as a means of rapid screening. Specific agglutinins can be detected in blood or serum but the test lacks sensitivity and can only be used reliably on a herd basis to detect early infection.

Control measures include quarantine, restriction of movement, slaughter and vaccination, depending on whether the disease is endemic or recently introduced. Vaccination is not permitted in many countries. A combination of the above measures was used to eradicate CBPP from Australia but the more recent outbreak in France was controlled by slaughter of infected and contact cattle (Barile et al. 1985). In areas of Africa where CBPP is endemic, a nomadic style of cattle husbandry encourages spread to susceptible animals and is a considerable hindrance to eradication measures. In this situation, for many years vaccination has been the only practical control measure.

Many different vaccines have been described since the last century when crude pleural exudates were inoculated into the tail tip. Today the only ones in common use are prepared from live attenuated *M. mycoides* subsp. *mycoides* SC strains (Jones 1991a). In general, the inactivated vaccines have not been successful because they have given inadequate protection or have produced undesirable side effects (Barile 1985), although Garba et al. (1986) described protection of cattle in a field trial by vaccination with the Gladysdale strain, inactivated and in an oil adjuvant. Attenuated vaccines have been derived from the T1 strain or the KH3J strain by passage through embryonated chicken eggs. The attenuated T1 strain (T1-44) is safe for use in zebu cattle but is too virulent for the more susceptible *Bos taurus* breeds which should be vaccinated with the milder KH3J strain

(Jones 1991a). The minimal recommended dose is 10^7 viable organisms and, to maintain this, vaccine preparations should be lyophilized rather than frozen and should be tested for safety and efficacy. The degree of attenuation of vaccine strains is reflected quantitatively in reduced ability to produce mycoplasmaemia in mice following intraperitoneal injection (Smith 1968, Dyson and Smith 1976). The vaccines are given normally by the subcutaneous route and the duration of effective immunity is at least a year with the T1 vaccine but only 6–8 months with the KH3J strain (Jones 1991a). Treatment of diseased cattle with antimicrobials has been used in the past but with limited success (Brunner and Laber 1985) and, since it may encourage the development of carrier animals, is not now recommended (Sahu and Yedloutschnig 1994). However, antimicrobial agents have been used for animals with severe vaccine reactions.

There are reviews of the early work on CBPP by Turner (1959) and Cottew and Leach (1969) and a more recent review has been compiled by ter Laak (1992). Nicholas and Bashiruddin (1995) have reviewed current information on the causative agent including its phylogeny, structure, molecular features and diagnostic tests.

OTHER MYCOPLASMAL INFECTIONS OF CATTLE

In addition to *M. mycoides* subsp. *mycoides*, at least 16 other mollicute species have been isolated from healthy or diseased cattle, but none produces a disease as well defined as that caused by *M. mycoides* subsp. *mycoides*. The pathogenicity of some is unproven and many are probably harmless commensals (Gourlay and Howard 1979, Howard 1983). The favoured sites are the respiratory and urogenital tracts and the organisms can also localize, sometimes in the mammary glands or in the joints where they may give rise to mastitis or arthritis, respectively. Strictly anaerobic mollicutes of the genera *Anaeroplasma* and *Asteroleplasma* have been isolated from the bovine rumen but appear to be harmless.

Mycoplasma bovis, *Mycoplasma dispar* and *Ureaplasma diversum* are capable of causing subclinical pneumonia in gnotobiotic calves (Gourlay, Thomas and Howard 1976, Howard et al. 1976) and in the field they contribute to the complex aetiology of calf pneumonia (Howard 1983). *M. bovis* is the most invasive and causes a 'cuffing' pneumonia which is characterized by mononuclear cell infiltration in the peribronchial and alveolar regions (Thomas et al. 1986) (Fig. 54.4).

M. dispar, which is often present in healthy calves, can produce an interstitial pneumonia or alveolitis characterized by mononuclear cell infiltration of the alveolar walls. Experimental inoculation of calves with this mycoplasma resulted in infection with impaired tracheobronchial clearance of bacteria (Almeida and Rosenbusch 1994), a phenomenon that may contribute to its involvement in disease. An inactivated multivalent vaccine containing *M. bovis*, *M. dispar*, respiratory syncytial virus and parainfluenza virus type 3 met

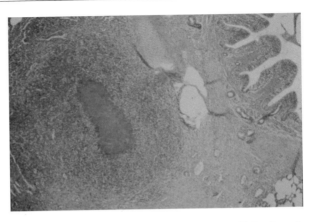

Fig. 54.4   *M. bovis* infection in a gnotobiotic calf. Section of lung showing an area of coagulative necrosis surrounded by cellular infiltration. Haematoxylin and eosin stain. (Courtesy of Dr C J Howard). See also Plate 54.4.

with some success in protecting calves against respiratory disease in field trials (Stott et al. 1987).

Several *Mycoplasma* spp. have been associated with bovine mastitis but *M. bovis* is the most common agent and its association has been reported from many areas of the world. *Mycoplasma canadense* and *Mycoplasma californicum* are also important causes of mastitis in California and certain other areas (Jasper 1994), whereas other species, including *Mycoplasma alkalescens* and *Mycoplasma bovigenitalium* are less commonly involved. The disease is characterized usually by swollen quarters and a sudden fall in milk production followed by discolouration of the milk and the presence of flaky or sandy deposits (Jasper 1979). A strong inflammatory reaction occurs, sometimes with obliteration of the alveoli and milk ducts, and secretion of large numbers of neutrophils in the milk (Jasper, Boothby and Thomas 1987). Although haematogenous spread may account for some mammary infections, most are thought to occur via the teat canal at milking or when cows are being treated for bacterial mastitis during lactation or at drying off (Jasper 1982). Diagnosis of mycoplasmal mastitis is usually by culture of milk samples. An antigen capture ELISA for *M. bovis* in milk has been used to detect subclinical cases (Heller et al. 1993). Antimicrobial therapy is not very successful and such animals may become intermittent shedders. A review of control procedures has been given by Jasper (1994).

The role of mycoplasmas in genital disease of cattle is less easily defined, partly because several mycoplasmas, and also ureaplasmas and acholeplasmas, are common inhabitants of the genital tract of healthy animals. There have been a number of reports implicating *U. diversum* (formerly referred to as T-strain mycoplasma) in granular vulvitis and other reproductive tract abnormalities in the female (Doig, Ruhnke and Palmer 1980, Ruhnke 1994). Its significance in the male is less clear although contaminated semen is an important means of transmission.

Of the other bovine mycoplasmas, those in 'group 7', which is part of the '*mycoides* cluster', have been associated with cases of mastitis, polyarthritis and pneumonia (Cottew and Leach 1969, Alexander et al. 1985) and *Mycoplasma bovoculi* has been incriminated in keratoconjunctivitis together with *Moraxella bovis* (Rosenbusch and Knudtson 1980, Rosenbusch 1983).

2.2 Goats and sheep

Goats and sheep can be infected with a number of different mollicutes including species of *Mycoplasma*, *Acholeplasma*, *Ureaplasma*, *Anaeroplasma* and *Asterole-plasma*. As with cattle, many of these appear to be of little or no pathogenic significance, but some in the genus *Mycoplasma* produce diseases that are well recognized and of considerable economic importance.

CONTAGIOUS CAPRINE PLEUROPNEUMONIA (CCPP) AND DISEASES CAUSED BY RELATED ORGANISMS

The aetiological agent of classical acute CCPP is a mycoplasma originally termed 'F38' (MacOwan and Minette 1976, McMartin, MacOwan and Swift 1980), but which is now classified as *M. capricolum* subsp. *capripneumoniae* due to its close genomic relationship with another caprine mycoplasma, *M. capricolum*, now reclassified as *M. capricolum* subsp. *capricolum* (Bonnet et al. 1993, Leach, Ernø and MacOwan 1993). These organisms belong to the '*mycoides* cluster' referred to above, which also contains the caprine or LC biotype of *M. mycoides* subsp. *mycoides*, as well as *M. mycoides* subsp. *capri*. The latter was earlier, but wrongly, incriminated in CCPP. All of the above-mentioned organisms can cause pneumonia in goats and this, together with their genomic and serological inter-relationships, has presented taxonomic difficulties and has hampered the elucidation of their true aetio-logical roles in disease (Cottew et al. 1987, International Committee on Systematic Bacteriology: Sub-committee on the Taxonomy of Mollicutes 1988, 1991). Diagnosis is greatly complicated by these problems and by the fact that SC strains of *M. mycoides* subsp. *mycoides* are also isolated occasionally from goats and sheep (Cottew 1979, Brandão 1995), although their pathogenic role in these hosts and in cattle needs further elucidation.

Classical CCPP was first described more than 100 years ago (Hutcheon 1881, 1889) and is still of major importance in many countries in Africa and Asia due to the large goat populations in these areas (Jones 1991b). There is no apparent involvement of sheep. The disease is characterized by fever and respiratory distress following an incubation period of approximately 1–4 weeks. There is also inappetance and loss of condition which may progress to prostration and death. The mortality rate may be very high and at postmortem examination interstitial, intralobular oedema, hepatization and fibrinous pleurisy are seen in the lungs. This pneumonia, caused by the F38-like strains, differs from that caused by the *M. mycoides* subsp. *capri* and the LC biotype of *M. mycoides* subsp. *mycoides* in which there is thickening of the interlobular septa (McMartin, MacOwan and Swift 1980, MacOwan 1984,

Jones 1989). Furthermore, disease caused by F38-like strains is normally confined to the lungs, whereas *M. mycoides* subsp. *capri* can also produce mastitis, arthritis and septicaemia, and the LC biotype of *M. mycoides* subsp. *mycoides* generally causes a syndrome which includes mastitis, polyarthritis, keratoconjunctivitis and acute septicaemic death in young animals (MacOwan 1984, Jones 1991b). The LC biotype is a very important pathogen in milk-producing goats in many countries including the USA (DaMassa, Wakenell and Brooks 1992) and sometimes may affect sheep. *M. capricolum* subsp. *capricolum* has also been implicated in pneumonia, but more usually causes septicaemia resulting in severe polyarthritis and mastitis. This mycoplasma may also cause disease in sheep (DaMassa, Wakenell and Brooks 1992).

It is noteworthy that several mycoplasmal species, including the LC biotype of *M. mycoides* subsp. *mycoides*, *M. mycoides* subsp. *capri* and *M. capricolum* subsp. *capricolum*, can be found in the ear canal of healthy goats and may play a role in the epidemiology of these organisms, particularly as isolations have also been made from the associated ear mites (Cottew and Yeats 1981, 1982).

Rapid differential diagnosis of CCPP is essential if sick animals are to be treated successfully (Rurangirwa et al. 1981) or if emergency vaccination programmes are to be implemented (Rurangirwa et al. 1987a). Diagnosis is difficult due to lack of pathognomonic signs, and requires recognition of the causal organism or antibodies to it. This has usually been by isolation and identification techniques, although gel precipitation tests to detect antigens in affected lungs may be feasible (Jones 1991b). The best tissue samples when CCPP is suspected are lung or pleural fluid, but from other conditions milk, joint fluid or eye swabs may also be cultured as appropriate. Identification of isolates by conventional serological methods is complicated by the inter-relationship of the different organisms, and monoclonal antibodies have been used to aid the detection of 'F38' strains (Belton et al. 1994) or to detect the organism directly in infected pleural fluid by an immunobinding assay (Thiaucourt et al. 1994). However, even the monoclonals were not entirely specific for *M. capricolum* subsp. *capripneumoniae*. More recently, DNA technology has paved the way for more satisfactory diagnostic methods. For example, Taylor, Bashiruddin and Gould (1992b) used a gene probe to demonstrate inter-relationships between members of the '*mycoides* cluster' by their hybridization patterns in Southern blots. Since it did not distinguish between the 2 subspecies of *M. capricolum*, a second probe was used to do this. Bascuñana and coworkers (1994) have described a PCR system by which a fragment of the 16S rRNA gene of the '*mycoides* cluster' is amplified and then F38 identified by restriction enzyme analysis. Thus DNA detection methods can be expected to resolve some of the diagnostic problems associated with these mycoplasmas, but it may be several years before they can be used routinely in some countries. Serological tests have been used to detect antibody to members of the '*mycoides* cluster' in goats and sheep, usually complement fixation and passive haemagglutination tests. A latex agglutination test has been developed for rapid detection of antibodies to F38 strains (Rurangirwa et al. 1987b). A blocking ELISA based on a monoclonal antibody has also been described (Thiaucourt et al. 1994).

Live vaccines have been used to protect against CCPP, but later research has concentrated on inactivated products (Rurangirwa 1987a). The inactivated F38 strain vaccine used in Kenya provides protection for more than a year (Rurangirwa et al. 1987c).

CONTAGIOUS AGALACTIA OF SHEEP AND GOATS

Contagious agalactia is an economically important disease of sheep and goats and has been recognized for more than 100 years. The aetiological agent, *Mycoplasma agalactiae*, was first isolated in 1923 by Bridré and Donatien and the disease is now known to occur in many parts of the world including Europe, Asia and Africa and occasionally the USA. It appears, however, to be most common in Mediterranean countries. Despite its name, infection is not restricted to lactating animals and, furthermore, several other mycoplasmal species cause mastitis which can result in agalactia. The condition produced by *M. agalactiae* infection is one of high morbidity but not always high mortality, and disease can range from inapparent to acute or chronic (DaMassa, Wakenell and Brooks 1992). The organism sometimes causes keratoconjunctivitis, a painful arthritis in one or more joints, or both. Lameness is the main manifestation in males and in the ewe signs are usually noted shortly after the onset of lactation and consist of fever and mastitis leading to decreased milk yield. Abortions have also been reported and Hasso, Al-Aubaidi and Al-Darraji (1993) have suggested that pregnancy may be more important than parturition and lactation in acting as an exacerbating factor in infected females. The organisms can be found in the milk, which may contain flaky yellowish clots, and there is a short mycoplasmaemia. Spread occurs mainly by ingestion following excretion into the environment in exudates and from the milk. Although antimicrobial therapy may relieve the mastitis it does not prevent excretion of the mycoplasmas in milk. *M. agalactiae* has also been found in the ear canal of healthy goats and the ear mites therein (Cottew and Yeats 1981, 1982), but the role in the epidemiology of contagious agalactia is not known. Diagnosis has been by conventional means, but DNA detection technology is being developed to provide an additional tool for screening animals for importation into countries which are free of this infection (Tola, Rizzu and Leori 1994). Treatment with antimicrobials may encourage the carrier state and vaccination attempts so far have met with limited success (Nicholas 1995).

The early work on contagious agalactia was reviewed by Cottew and Leach (1969) and diagnostic procedures for *M. agalactiae* and the other caprine–ovine mycoplasmas have been reviewed by Rosendal (1994).

OTHER MYCOPLASMAL INFECTIONS OF GOATS AND SHEEP

Of the other caprine–ovine mycoplasmas, *Mycoplasma putrefaciens*, *Mycoplasma ovipneumoniae* and *Mycoplasma conjunctivae* are all established pathogens. *M. putrefaciens* is the cause of sporadic outbreaks of mastitis and agalactia in goats and has been associated with severe arthritis in these animals (DaMassa et al. 1987). *M. ovipneumoniae*, although prevalent in clinically healthy sheep, can act synergistically with *Pasteurella haemolytica* biotype A serotypes to produce a chronic pneumonia in lambs (Jones and Gilmour 1991). Severe disease associated with *M. ovipneumoniae* was reported in a captive herd of Dall's sheep (Black et al. 1988) and was attributed to exposure to infected domestic sheep followed by environmental and social stress. *M. conjunctivae* is associated with keratoconjunctivitis ('pink eye') in sheep (Jones 1991c) and goats (Baas et al. 1977, Trotter et al. 1977). Spread of the organism is rapid but the disease is often self-limiting and corneal damage due to ulceration is thought to be due to secondary bacterial infection (Egwu et al. 1989).

Three newly identified mycoplasmal species have been found in the external ear canal of goats (DaMassa et al. 1994). The pathogenicity of 2 of them, *Mycoplasma auris* and *Mycoplasma cottewii*, is unknown, but *Mycoplasma yeatsii* has been isolated from the internal organs and milk of mastitic goats in the USA (DaMassa et al. 1991). There is lack of information on the importance of other mollicutes, such as ureaplasmas, that are found in goats and sheep.

2.3 Pigs

Pigs can harbour several mollicute species but only a few of these are known to be pathogenic.

ENZOOTIC PNEUMONIA

This economically important disease is caused by *Mycoplasma hyopneumoniae* (Goodwin, Pomeroy and Whittlestone 1965, Maré and Switzer 1965), a fastidious mycoplasma which was also earlier referred to as *Mycoplasma suipneumoniae*. The disease occurs in all areas of the world where pigs are reared intensively and is exacerbated by poor ventilation and overcrowding. The organism is spread by droplet infection and although carrier animals have been implicated in spread between pigs in close contact, transmission by aerosol from pigs on neighbouring premises seems to be a possibility. The onset of disease tends to be insidious. Animals of all ages are thought to be susceptible but signs are often more obvious in older ones (Whittlestone 1979). The condition is characterized by a chronic non-productive cough, retardation of growth rate and poor feed conversion. Morbidity is high but mortality is generally low, although secondary infection with bacteria or with other mycoplasmas is common. The presence in the UK of swine influenza and porcine reproductive and respiratory syndrome (blue ear disease) has complicated the typical picture of enzootic pneumonia (P Whittlestone, personal communication 1994). In uncomplicated infection, gross lesions are seen most frequently in the anterior lobes of the lungs and are lobular in distribution (Fig. 54.5). Affected lobules appear purple to grey in colour, are often swollen and the airways contain a sticky white exudate (Armstrong 1994). Such lesions are characteristic, but they are not pathognomonic. Histological sections reveal mononuclear cells in large numbers and peribronchial hyperplasia, indicating a significant involvement of the immune response in the development of lesions (Ross 1992). The *M. hyopneumoniae* organisms, which may be present in large numbers in affected lungs, can be recognized by experienced investigators in Giemsa-stained impression smears (Ross and Whittlestone 1983), but they can be identified more specifically by immunofluorescence staining of such smears or sections, or by isolation and subsequent identification. *M. hyopneumoniae* is fastidious and is one of the most difficult of all mycoplasmas to grow and, furthermore, it is often overgrown by *Mycoplasma hyorhinis*, a common inhabitant of the respiratory tract. Another complication is its antigenic (Freeman et al. 1984) and genomic (Stemcke et al. 1992) relationship with *Mycoplasma flocculare*, which also colonizes the respiratory tract. Detection of *M. hyopneumoniae* has therefore been attempted by the use of other methods, such as DNA probes and an antigen capture ELISA and more recently by the PCR, which has been found useful for examining nasal swabs, although for a limited time (Mattsson et al. 1995). A number of serological tests have been used for diagnosing *M. hyopneumoniae* infection, including indirect haemagglutination, complement fixation and agglutination. More recently, emphasis has been placed on producing ELISAs which avoid cross-reactivity with other porcine mycoplasmas. In these, purified or recombinant immunogenic proteins have been used as antigens (Djordjevic et al. 1994, Frey et al. 1994, Futo et al. 1995) or monoclonal antibodies have been used in a blocking technique (Feld et al. 1992, Lepotier et al. 1994). Diagnostic procedures have been reviewed by Ross (1992) and have been presented in some detail by Armstrong (1994).

Tetracyclines have been used to prevent pneumonia, although such prophylaxis does not prevent infection. Other antimicrobial agents such as tylosin tartrate, lincomycin and tiamulin have been used in the feed of infected herds with varying success and the newer quinolone antibiotics are reported to be effective in treating the disease (Ross 1992). Control measures include the provision of good environmental conditions and use of an all-in, all-out production system. Progress can be monitored by examination of lungs at the slaughterhouse. Programmes to develop and maintain *M. hyopneumoniae*-free herds have been implemented in a number of countries and usually commence with hysterectomy- or hysterotomy-derived piglets, which are then reared in isolation and used as a nucleus of mycoplasma-free breeding stock. Success relies on good management and screening for evidence of infection, but breakdowns are not uncommon with air-borne transmission being implicated as one of the main causes (Goodwin 1985, Stark, Keller and Eggenberger 1992). Protective immunity develops following natural infection; vaccination with adjuvanted whole organisms and certain subunit vaccines are reported to reduce disease severity (Ross 1992), although they are not yet in widespread use.

OTHER INFECTIONS OF PIGS

M. hyorhinis is found commonly in the nose and trachea of healthy young pigs and has been implicated as a secondary invader, especially in enzootic porcine pneumonia. Although *M. hyorhinis* is frequently isolated from the lungs of pneumonic pigs, its role as a primary pathogen is unclear (Ross 1992). However, it is associated with outbreaks of polyserositis and arthritis in young animals, localizing in the serous membrane-lined body cavities and the joints. In the field, stress factors, such as other diseases, are thought to predispose to the development of the condition (Friis and Feenstra 1994). Recent work in Japan has implicated *M. hyorhinis* in porcine otitis media, with inflammation of the eustachian tube as the most common manifestation (Morita et al. 1995).

Mycoplasma hyosynoviae is a common inhabitant of the nasopharynx and tonsils of adult pigs (Friis, Ahrens and Larsen 1991) and has been associated with outbreaks of arthritis in a number of countries. A comprehensive account of these and other mycoplasmal infections of pigs has been given by Ross (1992).

2.4 Birds

INFECTIONS OF DOMESTIC POULTRY

Four mycoplasmal species are of economic importance in domestic poultry and of these, *Mycoplasma gallisepticum*, which affects chickens, turkeys and game birds, is the most significant. *Mycoplasma synoviae* also infects these hosts but *Mycoplasma meleagridis* appears to be specific for turkeys. *Mycoplasma iowae* has emerged more recently as a cause of turkey embryo mortality. Acholeplasmas and ureaplasmas have been isolated from birds but their role in disease is uncertain. Strains of the pathogens show variations in virulence and sometimes in their predilection for certain

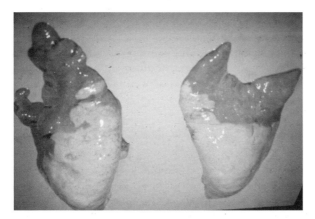

Fig. 54.5 Enzootic porcine pneumonia. Affected lungs showing consolidation of the apical lobes. (Courtesy of Dr J R Walton). See also Plate 54.5.

tissues. In general they inhabit the respiratory and reproductive tracts, but *M. iowae* is unusual in its proclivity also for the alimentary tract (Shah-Majid and Rosendal 1987).

M. gallisepticum plays an important role in chronic respiratory disease (CRD) of chickens, which is of considerable economic significance in broilers in many parts of the world and was the first mycoplasmal disease reported in birds (Nelson 1935). CRD is associated with intensive husbandry and with stress factors such as overcrowding or poor environment (Jordan 1990). Frequently, *M. gallisepticum* acts synergistically with other agents, such as pathogenic strains of *Escherichia coli*, and wild or live vaccine strains of respiratory viruses, such as Newcastle disease or infectious bronchitis virus (Bradbury 1984). The main manifestations are usually a check in growth rate and airsacculitis resulting in condemnation at slaughter, and there may be coughing, tracheal râles and nasal discharge. *M. gallisepticum* can also cause economic loss in laying chickens by reducing egg production, with or without respiratory signs. Turkeys are more susceptible than chickens to *M. gallisepticum*-induced respiratory disease and the organism on its own can cause severe 'infectious sinusitis' characterized by swelling of the infraorbital sinuses and nasal and ocular discharge. Although mortality is usually low the disease may persist as a chronic condition, thus compounding the economic loss.

Field evidence suggests that *M. synoviae* can produce respiratory disease in chickens and turkeys similar to that caused by *M. gallisepticum*, but it is difficult to reproduce experimentally (Bradbury and Levisohn 1995) and, furthermore, the organism can inhabit the respiratory tract of apparently healthy birds for long periods. Thus, it appears that some complicating factor is necessary to trigger disease (Kleven, King and Anderson 1972). The classical manifestation of *M. synoviae* infection, particularly in broilers but also sometimes in older birds and in turkeys, is 'infectious synovitis' (Olson et al. 1956). Swollen hock joints and feet occur, which on further examination show osteoarthritis and tenosynovitis. Sometimes the sternal bursae are swollen with exudate. The incidence of this condition seems to vary with time and may depend partly on the strain of organism and conditions of husbandry.

M. meleagridis affects young turkey poults causing reduced weight gain, airsacculitis and sometimes feathering and skeletal abnormalities (Yamamoto 1991). There are no signs of disease in the infected adult but the organism has a predilection for the oviduct and phallus and, hence may be transmitted to the egg. This can result in death of the embryo or an infected hatched poult which can transmit the organisms to its pen-mates. In the past, *M. meleagridis* was responsible for considerable economic losses due to poor hatchability and the costs of control programmes.

The economic impact of *M. iowae* is on the turkey embryo, causing between 2 and 5% mortality (Kleven 1991). Infected poults may hatch and maintain the infection in the next generation. Experimental infections have resulted in stunting, feathering and skeletal abnormalities not unlike those caused by *M. meleagridis* in poults (Bradbury, Ideris and Oo 1988), but there is very limited evidence for this occurring naturally.

All the avian mycoplasmas mentioned are transmitted through the egg to the next generation and *M. meleagridis* and *M. iowae* are also transmitted venereally in turkeys (Jordan 1990), so that artificial insemination, as practised in the modern turkey industry, aids the spread of both these mycoplasmas. All 4 species can also spread horizontally within a flock, although close contact is thought to be needed. Aerosol spread between flocks has not been documented but is suspected in some cases. Since the organisms have the potential to survive for several days on certain materials such as feathers, fomite spread is also a possibility. The ability of *M. gallisepticum* to survive on the human nasal mucosa for 24 h (Christensen et al. 1994) raises the possibility of transmission by man. Spread of *M. gallisepticum* to commercial flocks from infected game birds released into the wild is also a possibility. There has been little evidence to implicate free-flying birds in spread but recently *M. gallisepticum* has been isolated from house finches with eye lesions (Ley, Berkhoff and McLaren 1996). These ranged from slightly swollen eyelids with a clear ocular drainage to severe swelling with mucoid nasal exudate. In 1995 this condition was reported in at least 21 States in the USA and also in Canada and the implications for valuable commercial poultry flocks were of considerable concern.

Diagnosis of infection by the pathogenic poultry mycoplasmas has traditionally been by antibody detection, supplemented if required by culture and identification of the organisms (Kleven 1994, Jordan, Bradbury and Kleven 1996). Tests for detecting antibodies have included rapid serum agglutination using a stained antigen, haemagglutination inhibition and, more recently, ELISAs, for which several commercial kits are available. None of these is suitable for *M. iowae*, infection with which does not reliably produce a serum antibody response, so that culture has been used for detecting this organism. DNA detection methods, particularly those using PCR amplification, have now been developed for the pathogenic species and commercial kits are available or in preparation.

All 4 pathogenic avian mycoplasmal species have been targets for successful eradication from primary breeding stock. This was feasible because of:

1 the economic advantages for breeders supplying mycoplasma-free stock
2 the efficacy of antimicrobial agents in treating infected hatching eggs
3 the relative ease of maintaining mycoplasmal freedom in a closed flock and
4 the availability of diagnostic techniques to pinpoint infected groups of birds.

Eradication programmes are usually initiated by treating hatching eggs with anti-mycoplasma drugs either by injection or by 'dipping'. Heating of chicken hatching eggs to 45°C for 12–14 h (Yoder 1970) is a useful alternative or adjunct but it causes unacceptably high mortality of turkey embryos and *M. meleagridis* and *M. iowae* can survive the treatment. Since egg treatments are not expected to eliminate mycoplasmas from every egg, the resulting progeny are reared in relatively small groups and monitored frequently for infection; positive groups are discarded from the programme. To prevent venereal spread of mycoplasmas, turkeys can be cultured from the oviduct, cloaca or phallus and excluded from the breeding programme if positive.

Mycoplasmal freedom in commercial stock is best maintained by all-in, all-out systems of husbandry. Infections are treated as appropriate with antimicrobial agents such as tylosin tartrate, tiamulin or the newer fluoroquinolones, but overuse may encourage the development of resistant strains. *M. gallisepticum* vaccines have been produced for protection against loss of egg production in layers kept on large continuous production (multiple-age) sites. Inactivated 'bacterins' and live F strain vaccines have been used in some countries, but live avirulent preparations, such as the 6/85 strain vaccine and the ts-11 temperature-sensitive mutant vaccine (Whithear et al. 1990), are gaining popularity. These appear to protect against reduced egg production and respiratory disease and, unlike the F strain, are not pathogenic for turkeys. In the future, such vaccines may also be used for broilers and turkeys, although eradication of *M. gallisepticum* from breeding flocks should still be the method of control where possible.

OTHER BIRDS

Although ducks, geese and pigeons are known to harbour several mycoplasmas, including apparently host-specific species, little is known of their ability, or otherwise, to produce disease. Likewise, recently described new species from birds of prey are of unknown pathogenicity. Interest in diseases of ostriches has been generated in many countries due to the expansion of commercial farming. This has yielded numerous unclassified mycoplasmal isolates and occasional reports of isolation of one of the poultry pathogens, or of antibody to them. However, the role, if any, of any of these mycoplasmas in disease remains to be established.

Several comprehensive reviews on avian mycoplasmal infections are available, including those by Jordan (1990), Kleven, Rowland and Olson (1991), Yamamoto (1991), Yoder (1991), and Al-Ankari and Bradbury (1996).

2.5   Rats and mice

Rats and mice are the only rodents known to succumb to mycoplasmal disease, the most important pathogen being *Mycoplasma pulmonis* which causes murine respiratory mycoplasmosis (MRM) in both species. The organism is frequently present in clinically normal animals and tends to cause overt disease when there is an increased concentration of ammonia, or a concurrent

infection exists. It is a particular problem in laboratory colonies and the signs of disease are varied and non-specific but include 'snuffling' in rats, 'chattering' in mice and a gradual loss of condition (Davidson et al. 1994). There is also a lack of uniformity in the development of lesions but the main lesions may be acute or chronic and include rhinitis, otitis media, laryngotracheitis and bronchopneumonia. Characteristically there are neutrophils in the airways, hyperplasia of mucosal epithelium and a lymphoid response in the submucosa (Lindsay, Cassell and Baker 1978). *M. pulmonis* can also cause genital tract disease and infection in utero may give rise to vertical transmission and account for the occurrence of the mycoplasma in caesarean-derived animals. Occasionally arthritis occurs.

Mycoplasma arthritidis appears to occur widely in rat and mouse populations and, as its name suggests, has been recognized as a cause of arthritis. However, naturally occurring disease appears to be rare in rats, and not documented in mice, although arthritis caused by experimental inoculation of these rodents, and of rabbits, is well documented (Cole, Washburn and Taylor-Robinson 1985).

Although *Mycoplasma neurolyticum* was named for the 'rolling disease' produced by a neurotoxin in experimentally inoculated rats and mice, this organism has not been implicated in naturally occuring rodent disease for many years and is now considered to be a commensal along with a number of other mycoplasmal species.

Diagnosis of rat and mouse infections can be achieved by the usual methods, but serological screening of laboratory colonies to detect subclinical infections has proved difficult. ELISAs may be of value but there are cross-reactions between *M. pulmonis*, *M. arthritidis* and another rodent mycoplasma, *Mycoplasma muris* (Davidson et al. 1994).

2.6   Other animal species

Numerous mycoplasmas have been isolated from other wild and domesticated mammals in both the presence and absence of disease and there have also been isolations from reptiles and fish. *Mycoplasma felis* is thought to play a role in conjunctivitis in cats (Haesebrouck et al. 1991) and in pleuritis in horses (Ogilvie et al. 1983), but it seems unlikely that mycoplasmas are ever more than secondary 'opportunists' in dogs. Three mycoplasmas, each described as a new species, were isolated from seals with respiratory disease but their role, if any, was probably secondary to viral infections. Recently, mycoplasmas have been implicated as the cause of upper respiratory tract disease in the desert tortoise (Brown et al. 1994) and of polyarthritis in farmed crocodiles (Mohan et al. 1995). The single isolate of *Mycoplasma mobile*, from the gills of a tench, is the only mycoplasma so far to be found in fish and has been shown to cause gill epithelial cell necrosis in vivo and in vitro (Stadtländer et al. 1995).

REFERENCES

Ainsworth JG, Hourshid S et al., 1994, Detection of *Mycoplasma fermentans* in HIV-positive individuals undergoing bronchoscopy, *IOM Letters – Programme and Abstracts, 10th Int Congr of IOM*, **3**: 319–20.

Al-Ankari A-R, Bradbury JM, 1996, *Mycoplasma iowae*: a review, *Avian Pathol*, **25**: 205–29.

Alexander PG, Slee KJ et al., 1985, Mastitis in cows and polyarthritis and pneumonia in calves caused by *Mycoplasma* species bovine group 7, *Aust Vet J*, **62**: 135–6.

Almeida RA, Rosenbusch RF, 1994, Impaired tracheobronchial clearance of bacteria in calves infected with *Mycoplasma dispar*, *J Vet Med Ser B*, **41**: 473–82.

Armstrong CH, 1994, Porcine mycoplasmas, *Mycoplasmosis in Animals: Laboratory Diagnosis*, eds Whitford HW, Rosenbusch RF, Lauerman L, Iowa State University Press, Ames, Iowa, 68–83.

Baas EJ, Trotter SL et al., 1977, Epidemic caprine keratoconjunctivitis: recovery of *Mycoplasma conjunctivae* and its possible role in pathogenesis, *Infect Immun*, **18**: 806–15.

Barile MF, 1985, Immunization against mycoplasma infections, *The Mycoplasmas. Vol. 4. Mycoplasma Pathogenicity*, eds Razin S, Barile MF, Academic Press, New York, 451–92.

Barile MF, Bové JM et al., 1985, Current status on control of mycoplasmal diseases on man, animals, plants and insects, *Bull Inst Pasteur*, **83**: 339–73.

Barile MF, Chandler DKF et al., 1988, Hamster challenge potency assay for evaluation of *Mycoplasma pneumoniae* vaccines, *Infect Immun*, **56**: 2450–7.

Barker CE, Sillis M, Wreghitt TG, 1990, Evaluation of Serodia Myco II particle agglutination test for detecting *Mycoplasma pneumoniae* antibody: comparison with μ-capture ELISA and indirect immunofluorescence, *J Clin Pathol*, **43**: 163–5.

Bascuñana CR, Mattson JG et al., 1994, Characterization of the 16S rRNA genes from *Mycoplasma* sp. strain F38 and development of an identification system based on PCR, *J Bacteriol*, **176**: 2577–86.

Baseman JB, Dallo SF et al., 1988, Isolation and characterization of *Mycoplasma genitalium* strains from the human respiratory tract, *J Clin Microbiol*, **26**: 2266–9.

Bashiruddin JB, Taylor TK, Gould AR, 1994, A PCR-based test for the specific identification of *Mycoplasma mycoides* subspecies *mycoides* SC, *J Vet Diagn Invest*, **6**: 428–34.

Bébéar C, Dupon M et al., 1993, Potential improvements in therapeutic options for mycoplasmal respiratory infections, *Clin Infect Dis*, **17, Suppl.**: 202–7.

Belton D, Leach RH et al., 1994, Serological specificity of a monoclonal antibody to *Mycoplasma capricolum* strain F38, the agent of contagious caprine pleuropneumonia, *Vet Rec*, **134**: 643–6.

Bernet C, Garret M et al., 1989, Detection of *Mycoplasma pneumoniae* by using the polymerase chain reaction, *J Clin Microbiol*, **27**: 2492–6.

Black SR, Barker IK et al., 1988, An epizootic of *Mycoplasma ovipneumoniae* infection in captive Dall's sheep (*Ovis dalli dalli*), *J Wildl Dis*, **24**: 627–35.

Blanchard A, Hentschel J et al., 1993, Detection of *Ureaplasma urealyticum* by polymerase chain reaction in the urogenital tract of adults, in amniotic fluid, and in the respiratory tract of newborns, *Clin Infect Dis*, **17, Suppl.**: 148–53.

Bonnet F, Saillard C et al., 1993, DNA relatedness between field isolates of mycoplasma F38 group, the agent of contagious caprine pleuropneumonia, and strains of *Mycoplasma capricolum*, *Int J Syst Bacteriol*, **43**: 597–602.

Bradbury JM, 1984, Avian mycoplasma infections: prototype of mixed infections with mycoplasmas, bacteria and viruses, *Ann Microbiol (Paris)*, **135A**: 83–9.

Bradbury JM, Levisohn S, 1995, Experimental infections in poultry, *Molecular and Diagnostic Procedures in Mycoplasmology*, vol. 2, eds Tully JG, Razin S, Academic Press, New York, 361–70.

Bradbury JM, Ideris A, Oo TT, 1988, *Mycoplasma iowae* infection in young turkeys, *Avian Pathol*, **17**: 149–71.

Brandão E, 1995, Isolation and identification of *Mycoplasma mycoides* subspecies *mycoides* SC strains in sheep and goats, *Vet Rec*, **136**: 98–9.

Bridré J, Donatien A, 1923, Le microbe de l'agalaxie contagieuse et sa culture in vitro, *C R Acad Sci*, **177**: 841–3.

Brown MB, Cassell CH et al., 1983, Measurement of antibody to *Ureaplasma urealyticum* by an enzyme-linked immunosorbent assay and detection of antibody responses in patients with non-gonococcal urethritis, *J Clin Microbiol*, **17**: 288–95.

Brown MB, Schumacher IM et al., 1994, *Mycoplasma agassizii* causes upper respiratory tract disease in the desert tortoise, *Infect Immun*, **62**: 4580–6.

Brunner H, Laber G, 1985, Chemotherapy of mycoplasma infections, *The Mycoplasmas. Vol. 4. Mycoplasma Pathogenicity*, eds Razin S, Barile MF, Academic Press, New York, 403–50.

Brunner H, Weidner W, Schiefer H-G, 1983, Studies on the role of *Ureaplasma urealyticum* and *Mycoplasma hominis* in prostatitis, *Infect Immun*, **147**: 807–13.

Brunner H, Greenberg HB et al., 1973a, Antibody to *Mycoplasma pneumoniae* in nasal secretions and sputa of experimentally infected human volunteers, *Infect Immun*, **8**: 612–20.

Brunner H, Greenberg HB et al., 1973b, Decreased virulence and protective effect of genetically stable temperature-sensitive mutants of *Mycoplasma pneumoniae*, *Ann NY Acad Sci*, **225**: 436–52.

Buttery SH, Lloyd LC, Titchen DA, 1976, Acute respiratory, circulatory and pathological changes in the calf after intravenous injections of the galactan from *Mycoplasma mycoides* subsp. *mycoides*, *J Med Microbiol*, **9**: 379–91.

Campbell AD, Turner AW, 1953, Studies on contagious pleuropneumonia of cattle. IV. An improved complement-fixation test, *Aust Vet J*, **29**: 154–63.

Carilli AD, Gohd RS et al., 1964, A virologic study of chronic bronchitis, *N Engl J Med*, **270**: 123–7.

Cassell GH, Davis RO et al., 1983, Isolation of *Mycoplasma hominis* and *Ureaplasma urealyticum* from amniotic fluid at 16–20 weeks of gestation: potential effect on outcome of pregnancy, *Sex Transm Dis*, **10, Suppl.**: 294–302.

Cassell GH, Yanez A et al., 1994, Detection of *Mycoplasma fermentans* in the respiratory tract of children with pneumonia, *IOM Letters – Programme and Abstracts, 10th Int Congr of IOM*, **3**: 456.

Chanock RM, Hayflick L, Barile MF, 1962, Growth on artificial medium of an agent associated with atypical pneumonia and its identification as a PPLO, *Proc Natl Acad Sci USA*, **48**: 41–9.

Cherry JD, Taylor-Robinson D et al., 1971, A search for mycoplasma infections in patients with chronic bronchitis, *Thorax*, **26**: 62–7.

Christensen NH, Yavari CA et al., 1994, Investigations into the survival of *Mycoplasma gallisepticum*, *Mycoplasma synoviae* and *Mycoplasma iowae* on materials found in the poultry house environment, *Avian Pathol*, **23**: 127–43.

Clyde WA, 1979, *Mycoplasma pneumoniae* infections of man, *The Mycoplasmas. Vol. 2. Human and Animal Mycoplasmas*, eds Tully JG, Whitcomb RF, Academic Press, New York, 275–306.

Clyde WA, Senterfit LB, 1985, Laboratory diagnosis of mycoplasma infections, *The Mycoplasmas. Vol. 4. Mycoplasma Pathogenicity*, eds Razin S, Barile MF, Academic Press, New York, 391–402.

Cole BC, Washburn LR, Taylor-Robinson D, 1985, Mycoplasma-induced arthritis, *The Mycoplasmas. Vol. 4. Mycoplasma Pathogenicity*, eds Razin S, Barile MF, Academic Press, New York, 107–60.

Coombs RRA, Easter G et al., 1988, Red-cell IgM-antibody capture assay for the detection of *Mycoplasma pneumoniae*-specific IgM, *Epidemiol Infect*, **100**: 101–9.

Cottew GS, 1979, Caprine–ovine mycoplasmas, *The Mycoplasmas*.

Vol. 2. Human and Animal Mycoplasmas, eds Tully JG, Whitcomb RF, Academic Press, New York, 103–32.

Cottew GS, Leach RH, 1969, Mycoplasmas of cattle, sheep and goats, *The Mycoplasmatales and the L-phase of bacteria*, ed. Hayflick L, Appleton-Century-Crofts, New York, 527–70.

Cottew GS, Yeats FR, 1981, Occurrence of mycoplasmas in clinically normal goats, *Aust Vet J*, **57**: 52–3.

Cottew GS, Yeats FR, 1982, Mycoplasmas and mites in the ears of clinically normal goats, *Aust Vet J*, **59**: 77–81.

Cottew GS, Breard A et al., 1987, Taxonomy of the *Mycoplasma mycoides* cluster, *Isr J Med Sci*, **23**: 632–5.

Couch RB, 1990, *Mycoplasma pneumoniae* (primary atypical pneumonia), *Principles and Practice of Infectious Diseases*, 3rd edn, eds Mandell GL, Douglas RG, Bennett JE, Churchill Livingstone, New York, 1446–58.

DaMassa AJ, Wakenell PS, Brooks DL, 1992, Mycoplasmas of goats and sheep, *J Vet Diagn Invest*, **4**: 101–13.

DaMassa AJ, Brooks DL et al., 1987, Caprine mycoplasmosis: an outbreak of mastitis and arthritis requiring the destruction of 700 goats, *Vet Rec*, **120**: 409–13.

DaMassa AJ, Nascimento ER et al., 1991, Characteristics of an unusual mycoplasma isolated from a case of caprine mastitis and arthritis with possible systemic manifestations, *J Vet Diagn Invest*, **3**: 55–9.

DaMassa AJ, Tully JG et al., 1994, *Mycoplasma auris* sp. nov., *Mycoplasma cottewii* sp. nov., and *Mycoplasma yeatsii* sp. nov., new sterol-requiring mollicutes from the external ear canals of goats, *Int J Syst Bacteriol*, **44**: 479–84.

Davidson MK, Davis JK et al., 1994, Mycoplasmas of laboratory rodents, *Mycoplasmosis in Animals: Laboratory Diagnosis*, eds Whitford HW, Rosenbusch RF, Lauerman L, Iowa State University Press, Ames, Iowa, 97–133.

Dedieu L, Mady V, Lefevre PC, 1994, Development of a selective polymerase chain-reaction assay for the detection of *Mycoplasma mycoides* subsp. *mycoides* SC (contagious bovine pleuropneumonia agent), *Vet Microbiol*, **42**: 327–39.

Deguchi T, Gilroy C, Taylor-Robinson D, 1996, Failure to detect *Mycoplasma fermentans*, *Mycoplasma penetrans* or *Mycoplasma pirum* in the urethra of patients with acute nongonococcal urethritis, *Eur J Clin Microbiol Infect Dis*, **15**: 169–71.

Denny FW, Clyde WA, Glezen WP, 1971, *Mycoplasma pneumoniae* disease: clinical spectrum, pathophysiology, epidemiology and control, *J Infect Dis*, **123**: 74–92.

Djordjevic SP, Eamens GJ et al., 1994, An improved enzyme-linked immunosorbent assay (ELISA) for the detection of porcine serum antibodies against *Mycoplasma hyopneumoniae*, *Vet Microbiol*, **39**: 261–73.

Doble A, Thomas BJ et al., 1989, A search for infectious agents in chronic abacterial prostatitis utilising ultrasound guided biopsy, *Br J Urol*, **64**: 297–301.

Doig PA, Ruhnke HL, Palmer NC, 1980, Experimental bovine genital ureaplasmosis. II. Granular vulvitis, endometritis and salpingitis following uterine inoculation, *Can J Comp Med*, **44**: 259–66.

Dyson DA, Smith GR, 1976, Virulence of established vaccine strains and artificially passaged field strains of *Mycoplasma mycoides* subsp. *mycoides*, *Res Vet Sci*, **20**: 185–90.

Egwu GO, Faull WB et al., 1989, Ovine infectious keratoconjunctivitis: a microbiological study of clinically unaffected and affected sheep's eyes with special reference to *Mycoplasma conjunctivae*, *Vet Rec*, **125**: 253–6.

Ellison JS, Olson LD, Barile MF, 1992, Immunity and vaccine development, *Mycoplasmas: Molecular Biology and Pathogenesis*, eds Maniloff J, McElhaney RN et al., American Society for Microbiology, Washington, DC, 491–504.

Eschenbach DA, 1986, *Ureaplasma urealyticum* as a cause of postpartum fever, *Pediatr Infect Dis*, **5, Suppl.**: 258–61.

Feizi T, 1987, Significance of carbohydrate components of cell surfaces, *Autoimmunity and Autoimmune Disease*, Ciba Symposium 129, ed. Evered D, Wiley, Chichester, 43–58.

Feld NC, Qvist P et al., 1992, A monoclonal blocking ELISA detecting serum antibodies to *Mycoplasma hyopneumoniae*, *Vet Microbiol*, **30**: 35–46.

Fernald GW, 1979, Humoral and cellular immune responses to mycoplasmas, *The Mycoplasmas. Vol. 2. Human and Animal Mycoplasmas*, eds Tully JG, Whitcomb RF, Academic Press, New York, 398–423.

Foy HM, 1993, Infections caused by *Mycoplasma pneumoniae* and possible carrier state in different populations of patients, *Clin Infect Dis*, **17, Suppl.**: 37–46.

Foy HM, Kenny GE et al., 1977, Second attacks of pneumonia due to *Mycoplasma pneumoniae*, *J Infect Dis*, **135**: 673–7.

Freeman MJ, Armstrong CH et al., 1984, Serological cross-reactivity of porcine reference antisera to *Mycoplasma hyopneumoniae*, *M. flocculare*, *M. hyorhinis* and *M. hyosynoviae* indicated by the enzyme-linked immunosorbent assay, complement fixation and indirect hemagglutination tests, *Can J Comp Med*, **48**: 202–7.

Frey J, Haldimann A et al., 1994, Immune response against the L-lactate dehydrogenase of *Mycoplasma hyopneumoniae* in enzootic pneumonia of swine, *Microb Pathog*, **17**: 313–22.

Friis, NF, Ahrens P, Larsen H, 1991, *Mycoplasma hyosynoviae* isolation from the upper respiratory tract and tonsils of pigs, *Acta Vet Scand*, **32**: 425–9.

Friis NF, Feenstra AA, 1994, *Mycoplasma hyorhinis* in the etiology of serositis among piglets, *Acta Vet Scand*, **35**: 93–8.

Furness G, Kamat MH et al., 1974, The relationship of epididymitis to gonorrhea, *Invest Urol*, **11**: 312–14.

Furr PM, Taylor-Robinson D, Webster ADB, 1994, Mycoplasmas and ureaplasmas in patients with hypogammaglobulinaemia and their role in arthritis: microbiological observations over 20 years, *Ann Rheum Dis*, **53**: 183–7.

Futo S, Seto Y et al., 1995, Recombinant 46 kilodalton surface antigen (p46) of *Mycoplasma hyopneumoniae* expressed in *Escherichia coli* can be used for early specific diagnosis of mycoplasmal pneumonia of swine by enzyme-linked immunosorbent assay, *J Clin Microbiol*, **33**: 680–3.

Garba SA, Ajayi A et al., 1986, Field trial of inactivated oil-adjuvant Gladysdale strain vaccine for contagious bovine pleuropneumonia, *Vet Rec*, **119**: 376–7.

Glatt AE, McCormack WM, Taylor-Robinson D, 1990, Genital mycoplasmas, *Sexually Transmitted Diseases*, 2nd edn, eds Holmes KK, Mårdh P-A et al., McGraw Hill, New York, 279–93.

Goodwin RFW, 1985, Apparent reinfection of enzootic-pneumonia-free herds: search for possible causes, *Vet Rec*, **116**: 690–4.

Goodwin RFW, Pomeroy AP, Whittlestone P, 1965, Production of enzootic pneumonia in pigs with a mycoplasma, *Vet Rec*, **77**: 1247–9.

Goulet M, Dular R et al., 1995, Isolation of *Mycoplasma pneumoniae* from the human urogenital tract, *J Clin Microbiol*, **33**: 2823–5.

Gourlay RN, Thomas LH, Howard CJ, 1976, Pneumonia and arthritis in gnotobiotic calves following inoculation with *Mycoplasma bovis*, *Vet Rec*, **98**: 506–7.

Gourlay RN, Howard CJ, 1979, Bovine mycoplasmas, *The Mycoplasmas. Vol. 2. Human and Animal Mycoplasmas*, eds Tully JG, Whitcomb RF, Academic Press, New York, 49–102.

Grenabo L, Hedelin H, Pettersson S, 1988, Urinary infection stones caused by *Ureaplasma urealyticum*: a review, *Scand J Infect Dis*, **53, Suppl.**: 46–9.

Haesebrouck F, Devriese LA et al., 1991, Incidence and significance of isolation of *Mycoplasma felis* from conjunctival swabs of cats, *Vet Microbiol*, **26**: 95–101.

Hasso SA, Al-Aubaidi JM, Al-Darraji AM, 1993, Contagious agalactia in goats: its severity as related to the route of infection and pregnancy, *Small Ruminant Res*, **10**: 263–75.

Hay PE, Lamont RF et al., 1994, Abnormal bacterial colonisation of the genital tract and subsequent preterm delivery and late miscarriage, *Br Med J*, **308**: 295–8.

Heller M, Berthold E et al., 1993, Antigen capture ELISA using a monoclonal antibody for the detection of *Mycoplasma bovis* in milk, *Vet Microbiol*, **37**: 127–33.

Hers JF, 1963, Fluorescent antibody techniques in respiratory viral diseases, *Am Rev Respir Dis*, **88**: 316–33.

Hers JF, Masurel N, 1967, Infection with *Mycoplasma pneumoniae* in civilians in the Netherlands, *Ann NY Acad Sci*, **143**: 447–60.

Hillier SL, Nugent RP et al. for the Vaginal Infections and Prematurity Study Group, 1995, Association between bacterial vaginosis and preterm delivery of a low-birth-weight infant, *N Engl J Med*, **333**: 1737–42.

Horowitz S, Horowitz J et al., 1994, *Ureaplasma urealyticum* in Reiter's syndrome, *J Rheumatol*, **21**: 877–82.

Howard CJ, 1983, Mycoplasmas and bovine respiratory disease: studies related to pathogenicity and the immune response – a selective review, *Yale J Biol Med*, **56**: 789–97.

Howard CJ, Gourlay RN et al., 1976, Induction of pneumonia in gnotobiotic calves following inoculation of *Mycoplasma dispar* and ureaplasmas (T-mycoplasmas), *Res Vet Sci*, **21**: 227–31.

Hutcheon D, 1881, Contagious pleuropneumonia in Angora goats, *Vet J*, **13**: 171–80.

Hutcheon D, 1889, Contagious pleuropneumonia in goats at Cape Colony, South Africa, *Vet J*, **29**: 399–404.

International Committee on Systematic Bacteriology: Subcommittee on the Taxonomy of Mollicutes, 1988, Minutes of interim meeting, 25 and 28 August, Birmingham, Alabama, *Int J Syst Bacteriol*, **38**: 226–30.

International Committee on Systematic Bacteriology: Subcommittee on the Taxonomy of Mollicutes, 1991, Minutes of interim meeting, 7 and 8 July 1990, Istanbul, Turkey, *Int J Syst Bacteriol*, **41**: 333–6.

Jacobs E, 1993, Serological diagnosis of *Mycoplasma pneumoniae* infections: a critical review of current procedures, *Clin Infect Dis*, **17, Suppl.**: 79–82.

Jacobs E, Rock R, Dalehite L, 1990, A B-cell-, T-cell-linked epitope located on the adhesin of *Mycoplasma pneumoniae*, *Infect Immun*, **58**: 2464–9.

Jalil N, Doble A et al., 1988, Infection of the epididymis by *Ureaplasma urealyticum*, *Genitourin Med*, **64**: 367–8.

Jarstrand C, Camner P, Philipson K, 1974, *Mycoplasma pneumoniae* and tracheobronchial clearance, *Am Rev Respir Dis*, **110**: 415–19.

Jasper DE, 1979, Bovine mycoplasmal mastitis, *J Am Vet Med Assoc*, **175**: 1072–4.

Jasper DE, 1982, The role of *Mycoplasma* in bovine mastitis, *J Am Vet Med Assoc*, **181**: 158–62.

Jasper DE, 1994, Mycoplasmas and bovine mastitis, *Mycoplasmosis in Animals: Laboratory Diagnosis*, eds Whitford HW, Rosenbusch RF, Lauerman L, Iowa State University Press, Ames, Iowa, 62–7.

Jasper DE, Boothby JT, Thomas CB, 1987, Pathogenesis of bovine mycoplasma mastitis, *Isr J Med Sci*, **23**: 625–7.

Jensen JS, Hansen HT, Lind K, 1996, Isolation of *Mycoplasma genitalium* strains from the male urethra, *J Clin Microbiol*, **34**: 286–91.

Jensen JS, Sondergard-Andersen J et al., 1989, Detection of *Mycoplasma pneumoniae* in simulated clinical samples by polymerase chain reaction, *APMIS*, **97**: 1046–8.

Jensen JS, Uldum SA et al., 1991, Polymerase chain reaction for detection of *Mycoplasma genitalium* in clinical samples, *J Clin Microbiol*, **29**: 46–50.

Jones GE, 1989, *Contagious Caprine Pleuropneumonia*, Technical Series No. 9, Office Internationale des Epizooties, Paris, 1–63.

Jones GE, 1991a, Contagious bovine pleuropneumonia, *OIE Manual of Recommended Diagnostic Techniques and Requirements for Biological Products*, vol. 3, Office Internationale des Epizooties, Paris, A/006/1–12.

Jones GE, 1991b, Contagious caprine pleuropneumonia, *OIE Manual of Recommended Diagnostic Techniques and Requirements for Biological Products*, vol. 3, Office Internationale des Epizooties, Paris, B/027/1–17.

Jones GE, 1991c, Infectious keratoconjunctivitis, *Diseases of Sheep*,

2nd edn, eds Martin WB, Aitken ID, Blackwell Scientific Publications, Oxford, 280–3.

Jones GE, Foggie A et al., 1976, Mycoplasmas and ovine keratoconjunctivitis, *Vet Rec*, **99**: 137–41.

Jones GE, Gilmour JS, 1991, Non-progressive (atypical) pneumonia, *Diseases of Sheep*, 2nd edn, eds Martin WB, Aitken ID, Blackwell Scientific Publications, Oxford, 150–7.

Jordan FTW, 1990, Avian mycoplasmosis, *Poultry Diseases*, 3rd edn, ed. Jordan FTW, Baillière Tindall, London, 74–85.

Jordan FTW, Bradbury JM, Kleven SH, 1996, Avian mycoplasmosis, *OIE Manual of Standards for Diagnostic Tests and Vaccines*, 3rd edn, Office Internationale des Epizooties, Paris, 512–21.

Kass EH, McCormack W et al., 1981, Genital mycoplasmas as a hitherto unsuspected cause of excess premature delivery in the under-privileged, *Clin Res*, **29**: 575A.

Katseni VL, Gilroy CB et al., 1993, *Mycoplasma fermentans* in individuals seropositive and seronegative for HIV-1, *Lancet*, **341**: 271–3.

Kenny GE, 1992, Serodiagnosis, *Mycoplasmas: Molecular Biology and Pathogenesis*, eds Maniloff J, McElhaney RN et al., American Society for Microbiology, Washington, DC, 505–12.

Kingston JR, Chanock RM et al., 1961, Eaton agent pneumonia, *JAMA*, **176**: 118–23.

Kleven SH, 1991, Other mycoplasmal infections, *Diseases of Poultry*, 9th edn, eds Calnek BW, Barnes HJ et al., Iowa State University Press, Ames, Iowa, 231–5.

Kleven SH, 1994, Avian mycoplasmas, *Mycoplasmosis in Animals: Laboratory Diagnosis*, eds Whitford HW, Rosenbusch RF, Lauerman L, Iowa State University Press, Ames, Iowa, 31–8.

Kleven SH, King DD, Anderson DP, 1972, Airsacculitis in broilers from *Mycoplasma synoviae*: effect on air sac lesions of vaccinating with infectious bronchitis and Newcastle virus, *Avian Dis*, **16**: 915–24.

Kleven SH, Rowland GN, Olson NO, 1991, *Mycoplasma synoviae* infection, *Diseases of Poultry*, 9th edn, eds Calnek BW, Barnes HJ et al., Iowa State University Press, Ames, Iowa, 223–31.

Koutsky LA, Stamm WE et al., 1983, Persistence of *Mycoplasma hominis* after therapy: importance of tetracycline resistance and of coexisting vaginal flora, *Sex Transm Dis*, **10, Suppl.**: 374–81.

ter Laak EA, 1992, Contagious bovine pleuropneumonia. A review, *Vet Q*, **14**: 104–10.

Lambert HP, 1968, Antibody to *Mycoplasma pneumoniae* in normal subjects and in patients with chronic bronchitis, *J Hyg (Lond)*, **66**: 185–9.

Leach RH, Ernø H, MacOwan KJ, 1993, Proposal for designation of F38-type caprine mycoplasmas as *Mycoplasma capricolum* subsp. *capripneumoniae* susp. nov. and consequent obligatory relegation of strains currently classified as *M. capricolum* (Tully, Barile, Edward, Theodore, and Ernø 1974) to an additional new subspecies, *M. capricolum* subsp. *capricolum* subsp. nov., *Int J Syst Bacteriol*, **43**: 603–5.

Lepotier MF, Abiven P et al., 1994, A blocking ELISA using a monoclonal antibody for the serological detection of *Mycoplasma hyopneumoniae*, *Res Vet Sci*, **56**: 338–45.

Ley DH, Berkhoff EJ, McLaren JM, 1996, *Mycoplasma gallisepticum* isolated from house finches (*Carpodacus mexicanus*) with conjunctivitis, *Avian Dis*, **40**: 480–3.

Lind K, 1982, Serological cross-reaction between *Mycoplasma genitalium* and *M. pneumoniae*, *Lancet*, **2**: 1158–9.

Lind K, Kristensen GB, 1987, Significance of antibodies to *Mycoplasma genitalium* in salpingitis, *Eur J Clin Microbiol*, **6**: 205–7.

Lind K, Lindhardt BO et al., 1984, Serological cross-reactions between *Mycoplasma genitalium* and *Mycoplasma pneumoniae*, *J Clin Microbiol*, **20**: 1036–43.

Lind K, Kristensen GB et al., 1985, Importance of *Mycoplasma hominis* in acute salpingitis assessed by culture and serological tests, *Genitourin Med*, **61**: 185–9.

Lindsey JR, Cassell GH, Baker HJ, 1978, Diseases due to mycoplasmas and rickettsias, *Pathology of Laboratory Animals*, eds

Benirschke K, Garner FM, Jones TC, Springer-Verlag, New York, 1481–550.

Lloyd LC, Buttery SH, Hudson JR, 1971, The effect of the galactan and other antigens of *Mycoplasma mycoides* var. *mycoides* on experimental infection with that organism in cattle, *J Med Microbiol*, **4:** 425–39.

Lo S-C, Dawson MS et al., 1989, Identification of *Mycoplasma incognitus* infection in patients with AIDS: an immunohistochemical, in situ hybridization and ultrastructural study, *Am J Trop Med Hyg*, **41:** 601–16.

Lo S-C, Wear DJ et al., 1993, Adult respiratory distress syndrome with or without systemic disease associated with infections due to *Mycoplasma fermentans*, *Clin Infect Dis*, **17, Suppl.:** 259–63.

Losos GJ, 1986, Contagious bovine and caprine pleuropneumonia, *Infectious Diseases of Domestic Animals*, Longman Scientific and Technical, Harlow, Essex, 653–92.

McCormack WM, Rosner B et al., 1987, Effect on birth weight of erythromycin treatment of pregnant women, *Obstet Gynecol*, **69:** 202–7.

McCormick DP, Wenzel RP et al., 1974, Relationship of pre-existing antibody to subsequent infection by *Mycoplasma pneumoniae* in adults, *Infect Immun*, **9:** 53–9.

McMartin DA, MacOwan KJ, Swift LL, 1980, A century of classical contagious caprine pleuropneumonia: from original description to aetiology, *Br Vet J*, **136:** 507–15.

MacOwan KJ, 1984, Role of mycoplasma strain F38 in contagious caprine pleuropneumonia, *Isr J Med Sci*, **20:** 979–81.

MacOwan KJ, Minette JE, 1976, A mycoplasma from acute contagious caprine pleuropneumonia in Kenya, *Trop Anim Health Prod*, **8:** 91–5.

Machado M, Ferreira H et al., 1994, Biotype 'large colony'-like strains of *Mycoplasma mycoides* subsp. *mycoides* isolated from bovines, *Rev Port Cienc Vet*, **89:** 94–101.

Madsen RD, Weiner LB et al., 1988, Direct detection of *Mycoplasma pneumoniae* antigen in clinical specimens by a monoclonal antibody immunoblot assay, *Am J Clin Pathol*, **89:** 95–9.

Mårdh P-A, Weström L, 1970a, Tubal and cervical cultures in acute salpingitis with special reference to *Mycoplasma hominis* and T-strain mycoplasmas, *Br J Vener Dis*, **46:** 179–86.

Mårdh P-A, Weström L, 1970b, Antibodies to *Mycoplasma hominis* in patients with genital infections and in healthy controls, *Br J Vener Dis*, **46:** 390–7.

Maré CJ, Switzer WP, 1965, New species: *Mycoplasma hyopneumoniae*, a causative agent of virus pig pneumonia, *Vet Med*, **60:** 841–6.

Marmion BP, Goodburn GM, 1961, Effect of an inorganic gold salt on Eaton's primary atypical pneumonia agent and other observations, *Nature (London)*, **189:** 247–8.

Marmion BP, Williamson J, 1993, Experience with newer techniques for the laboratory detection of *Mycoplasma pneumoniae* infection: Adelaide, 1978–1992, *Clin Infect Dis*, **17, Suppl.:** 90–99.

Mattsson JG, Bergstrom K et al., 1995, Detection of *Mycoplasma hyopneumoniae* in nose swabs from pigs by in vitro amplification of the 16S ribosomal RNA gene, *J Clin Microbiol*, **26:** 213–14.

Miettinen A, Paavonen J et al., 1983, Enzyme immunoassay for serum antibody to *Mycoplasma hominis* in women with acute pelvic inflammatory disease, *Sex Transm Dis*, **10, Suppl.:** 289–93.

Mizutani H, Mizutani H et al., 1971, Delayed hypersensitivity in *Mycoplasma pneumoniae* infections, *Lancet*, **1:** 186–7.

Mohan K, Foggin CM et al., 1995, *Mycoplasma*-associated polyarthritis in farmed crocodiles (*Crocodylus niloticus*) in Zimbabwe, *Onderstepoort J Vet Res*, **62:** 45–9.

Møller BR, Taylor-Robinson D, Furr PM, 1984, Serologic evidence implicating *Mycoplasma genitalium* in pelvic inflammatory disease, *Lancet*, **2:** 1102–3.

Montagnier L, Blanchard A, 1993, Mycoplasmas as cofactors in

infection due to the human immunodeficiency virus, *Clin Infect Dis*, **17, Suppl.:** 309–15.

Morita T, Fukuda H et al., 1995, Demonstration of *Mycoplasma hyorhinis* as a possible primary pathogen for porcine otitis media, *Vet Pathol*, **32:** 107–11.

Morrison-Plummer J, Jones DH et al., 1987, Molecular characterization of *Mycoplasma genitalium* species-specific and cross-reactive determinants: identification of an immunodominant protein of *M. genitalium*, *Isr J Med Sci*, **23:** 453–7.

Mufson MA, 1983, *Mycoplasma hominis*: a review of its role as a respiratory tract pathogen of humans, *Sex Transm Dis*, **10, Suppl.:** 335–40.

Mufson MA, Ludwig WM et al., 1965, Exudative pharyngitis following experimental *Mycoplasma hominis* type 1 infection, *JAMA*, **192:** 1146–52.

Mufson MA, Saxton D et al., 1974, Virus and mycoplasma infections in exacerbations of chronic bronchitis, *Clin Res*, **22:** 646A.

Murray HW, Masur H et al., 1975, The protean manifestations of *Mycoplasma pneumoniae* infection in adults, *Am J Med*, **58:** 229–42.

Myhre EB, Mårdh P-A, 1983, Treatment of extragenital infections caused by *Mycoplasma hominis*, *Sex Transm Dis*, **10, Suppl.:** 382–5.

Nelson JB, 1935, Cocco-bacilliform bodies associated with an infectious fowl coryza, *Science*, **82:** 43–4.

Nicholas RAJ, 1995, Contagious agalactia, *State Vet J*, **5:** 13–15.

Nicholas RAJ, Bashiruddin JB, 1995, *Mycoplasma mycoides* subspecies *mycoides* (small colony variant): the agent of contagious bovine pleuropneumonia and member of the 'Mycoplasma mycoides cluster', *J Comp Pathol*, **113:** 1–27.

Nocard E, Roux E et al., 1898, La microbe de la péripneumonie, *Ann Inst Pasteur (Paris)*, **12:** 240–62.

Ogilvie TH, Rosendal S et al., 1983, *Mycoplasma felis* as a cause of pleuritis in horses, *J Am Vet Med Assoc*, **182:** 1374–6.

Olson NO, Shelton DC et al., 1956, Studies of infectious synovitis in chickens, *Am J Vet Res*, **17:** 747–54.

Onoviran O, Taylor-Robinson D, 1979, Detection of antibody against *Mycoplasma mycoides* subsp. *mycoides* in cattle by an enzyme-linked immunosorbent assay, *Vet Rec*, **105:** 165–7.

Palmer HM, Gilroy CB et al., 1991, Development and evaluation of the polymerase chain reaction to detect *Mycoplasma genitalium*, *FEMS Microbiol Lett*, **61:** 199–203.

Perreau P, Bind JL, 1981, Infection naturelle du veau par *Mycoplasma mycoides* subsp. *mycoides* (biotype chèvre), *Bull Acad Vét France*, **54:** 491–6.

Provost A, 1972, Recherches immunologiques sur la péripneumonie. XIV. Description de deux techniques applicables sur le terrain pour le diagnostic de la maladie, *Rev Elev Méd Vét Pays Trop*, **25:** 475–96.

Purcell RH, Chanock RM, Taylor-Robinson D, 1969, Serology of the mycoplasmas of man, *The Mycoplasmatales and the L-phase of Bacteria*, ed. Hayflick L, Appleton-Century-Crofts, New York, 221–64.

Queval R, Provost A, Villemot JM, 1964, Comparaison de méthodes de déviation du complément utilisées dans l'étude de la péripneumonie bovine, *Bull Epizoot Afr*, **12:** 159–70.

Quinn PA, 1986, Evidence of an immune response to *Ureaplasma urealyticum* in perinatal morbidity and mortality, *Pediatr Infect Dis*, **5, Suppl.:** 282–7.

Quinn PA, Shewchuk AB et al., 1983, Serologic evidence of *Ureaplasma urealyticum* infection in women with spontaneous pregnancy loss, *Am J Obstet Gynecol*, **145:** 245–50.

Razin S, 1978, The mycoplasmas, *Microbiol Rev*, **42:** 414–70.

Razin S, Barile MF (eds), 1985, *The Mycoplasmas. Vol. 4. Mycoplasma Pathogenicity*, Academic Press, New York.

Renaudin H, Bébéar C, 1990, Evaluation des systèmes Mycoplasma PLUS et SIR Mycoplasma pour la détection quantitative et l'étude de la sensibilité aux antibiotiques des mycoplasmes genitaux, *Pathol Biol*, **38:** 431–5.

Rosenbusch RF, 1983, Influence of mycoplasma preinfection on the expression of *Moraxella bovis* pathogenicity, *Am J Vet Res*, **44:** 1621–4.

Rosenbusch RF, Knudtson WU, 1980, Bovine mycoplasmal conjunctivitis: experimental reproduction and characterization of the disease, *Cornell Vet*, **70:** 307–20.

Rosendal S, 1994, Ovine and caprine mycoplasmas, *Mycoplasmosis in Animals: Laboratory Diagnosis*, eds Whitford HW, Rosenbusch RF, Lauerman L, Iowa State University Press, Ames, Iowa, 84–96.

Ross RF, 1992, Mycoplasmal diseases, *Diseases of Swine*, 7th edn, eds Leman Ad, Straw BE et al., Wolfe Publishing Ltd, Ames, Iowa, 537–51.

Ross RF, Whittlestone P, 1983, Recovery of, identification of, and serological response to porcine mycoplasmas, *Methods in Mycoplasmology*, vol. 2, eds Tully JG, Razin S, Academic Press, New York, 115–27.

Ruhnke HL, 1994, Mycoplasmas associated with bovine genital tract infection, *Mycoplasmosis in Animals: Laboratory Diagnosis*, eds Whitford HW, Rosenbusch RF, Lauerman L, Iowa State University Press, Ames, Iowa, 56–62.

Ruiter M, Wenthold HMM, 1952, The occurrence of pleuropneumonia-like organism in fuso-spirillary infections of the human genital mucosa, *J Invest Dermatol*, **18:** 313–25.

Rurangirwa FR, Masiga WN et al., 1981, Treatment of contagious caprine pleuropneumonia, *Trop Anim Health Prod*, **13:** 177–82.

Rurangirwa FR, McGuire TC et al., 1987a, Vaccination against contagious caprine pleuropneumonia, *Isr J Med Sci*, **23:** 641–3.

Rurangirwa FR, McGuire TC et al., 1987b, A latex agglutination test for field diagnosis of contagious caprine pleuropneumonia, *Vet Rec*, **121:** 191–3.

Rurangirwa FR, McGuire TC et al., 1987c, An inactivated vaccine for contagious caprine pleuropneumonia, *Vet Rec*, **121:** 397–402.

Sahu SP, Yedloutschnig RJ, 1994, Contagious bovine pleuropneumonia, *Mycoplasmosis in Animals: Laboratory Diagnosis*, eds Whitford HW, Rosenbusch RF, Lauerman L, Iowa State University Press, Ames, Iowa, 39–50.

Schaeverbeke T, Gilroy CB et al., 1996, *Mycoplasma fermentans*, but not *M. penetrans*, detected by PCR assays in synovium from patients with rheumatoid arthritis and other rheumatic disorders, *J Clin Pathol*, **49:** 824–8.

Shah-Majid M, Rosendal S, 1987, Oral challenge of turkey poults with *Mycoplasma iowae*, *Avian Dis*, **31:** 365–9.

Shames JM, George RB et al., 1970, Comparison of antibiotics in the treatment of mycoplasmal pneumonia, *Arch Intern Med*, **125:** 680–4.

Shepard MC, 1954, The recovery of pleuropneumonia-like organisms from Negro men with and without nongonococcal urethritis, *Am J Syph Gonor Vener Dis*, **38:** 113–24.

Shepard MC, Robertson JA, 1986, Calcium chloride as an indicator for colonies of *Ureaplasma urealyticum*, *Pediatr Infect Dis*, **5, Suppl.:** 349.

Sillis M, 1990, The limitation of IgM assays in the serological diagnosis of *Mycoplasma pneumoniae* infection, *J Med Microbiol*, **33:** 253–8.

Smith CB, Friedewald WT, Chanock RM, 1967, Shedding of *Mycoplasma pneumoniae* after tetracycline and erythromycin therapy, *N Engl J Med*, **276:** 1172–5.

Smith GR, 1968, Factors affecting bacteraemia in mice inoculated with *Mycoplasma mycoides* subspecies *mycoides*, *J Comp Pathol*, **78:** 267–74.

Stadtländer CTK-H, Lotz W et al., 1995, Piscine gill epithelial cell necrosis due to *Mycoplasma mobile* strain 163K: comparison of in-vivo and in-vitro infection, *J Comp Pathol*, **112:** 351–9.

Stamm WE, Running K et al., 1983, Etiologic role of *Mycoplasma hominis* and *Ureaplasma urealyticum* in women with the acute urethral syndrome, *Sex Transm Dis*, **10, Suppl.:** 318–22.

Stark KDC, Keller H, Eggenberger E, 1992, Risk factors for the reinfection of specific pathogen-free pig breeding herds with enzootic pneumonia, *Vet Rec*, **131:** 532–5.

Steffensen DO, Dummar JS et al., 1987, Sternotomy infections with *Mycoplasma hominis*, *Ann Intern Med*, **106:** 204–8.

Stemcke GW, Laigret F et al., 1992, Phylogenetic relationships of three porcine mycoplasmas, *Mycoplasma hyopneumoniae*, *Mycoplasma flocculare*, and *Mycoplasma hyorhinis*, and complete 16S rRNA sequence of *M. flocculare*, *Int J Syst Bacteriol*, **42:** 220–5.

Stott EJ, Thomas LH et al., 1987, Field trial of a quadrivalent vaccine against calf respiratory disease, *Vet Rec*, **121:** 342–7.

Taylor G, Taylor-Robinson D, 1975, The part played by cell-mediated immunity in mycoplasma respiratory infections, *International Symposium on Immunity to Infections of the Respiratory System in Man and Animals*, Dev Biol Standard No. 28, Karger, Basel, 195–210.

Taylor G, Taylor-Robinson D, Fernald GW, 1974, Reduction in the severity of *Mycoplasma pneumoniae*-induced pneumonia in hamsters by immunosuppressive treatment with anti-thymocyte sera, *J Med Microbiol*, **7:** 343–8.

Taylor TK, Bashiruddin JB, Gould AR, 1992a, Application of a diagnostic DNA probe for the differentiation of the two types of *Mycoplasma mycoides* subspecies *mycoides*, *Res Vet Sci*, **53:** 154–9.

Taylor TK, Bashiruddin JB, Gould AR, 1992b, Relationships between members of the *Mycoplasma mycoides* cluster as shown by DNA probes and sequence analysis, *Int J Syst Bacteriol*, **42:** 593–601.

Taylor-Robinson D, 1983, Serological identification of ureaplasmas from humans, *Methods in Mycoplasmology*, vol. 2, eds Tully JG, Razin S, Academic Press, New York, 57–63.

Taylor-Robinson D, 1985, Mycoplasmal and mixed infections of the human male urogenital tract and their possible complications, *The Mycoplasmas. Vol. 4. Mycoplasma Pathogenicity*, eds Razin S, Barile MF, Academic Press, New York, 27–63.

Taylor-Robinson D, 1986, Evaluation of the role of *Ureaplasma urealyticum* in infertility, *Pediatr Infect Dis*, **5, Suppl.:** 262–5.

Taylor-Robinson D, 1995a, The history and role of *Mycoplasma genitalium* in sexually transmitted diseases, *Genitourin Med*, **71:** 1–8.

Taylor-Robinson D, 1995b, *Mycoplasma and Ureaplasma, Manual of Clinical Microbiology*, 6th edn, eds Murray PR, Baron EJ et al., American Society for Microbiology, Washington, DC, 652–62.

Taylor-Robinson D, 1996a, Mycoplasmas and their role in human respiratory tract disease, *Viral and Other Infections of the Human Respiratory Tract*, eds Myint S, Taylor-Robinson D, Chapman and Hall, London, 319–39.

Taylor-Robinson D, 1996b, The history of nongonococcal urethritis, *Sex Transm Dis*, **23:** 86–91.

Taylor-Robinson D, 1996c, Diagnosis of sexually transmitted diseases, *Molecular and Diagnostic Procedures in Mycoplasmology*, vol. 2, eds Tully JG, Razin S, Academic Press, New York, 225–36.

Taylor-Robinson D, Furr PM, 1981, Recovery and identification of human genital tract mycoplasmas, *Isr J Med Sci*, **17:** 648–53.

Taylor-Robinson D, Furr PM, 1986, Clinical antibiotic resistance of *Ureaplasma urealyticum*, *Pediatr Infect Dis*, **5, Suppl.:** 335–7.

Taylor-Robinson D, Furr PM, Hanna NF, 1985, Microbiological and serological study of non-gonococcal urethritis with special reference to *Mycoplasma genitalium*, *Genitourin Med*, **61:** 319–24.

Taylor-Robinson D, Furr PM, Webster ADB, 1985, *Ureaplasma urealyticum* causing persistent urethritis in a patient with hypogammaglobulinaemia, *Genitourin Med*, **61:** 404–8.

Taylor-Robinson D, Furr PM, Webster ADB, 1986, *Ureaplasma urealyticum* in the immunocompromised host, *Pediatr Infect Dis*, **5, Suppl.:** 236–8.

Taylor-Robinson D, McCormack WM, 1979, Mycoplasmas in human genitourinary infections, *The Mycoplasmas. Vol. 2. Human and Animal Mycoplasmas*, eds Tully JG, Whitcomb RF, Academic Press, New York, 307–66.

Taylor-Robinson D, Munday PE, 1988, Mycoplasmal infection of the female genital tract and its complications, *Genital Tract*

Infection in Women, ed. Hare MJ, Churchill Livingstone, Edinburgh, 228–47.

Taylor-Robinson D, Webster ADB et al., 1980, Prolonged persistence of *Mycoplasma pneumoniae* in a patient with hypogammaglobulinaemia, *J Infect*, **2**: 171–5.

Taylor-Robinson D, Tully JG et al., 1981, Urogenital mycoplasma infections of man: a review with observations on a recently discovered mycoplasma, *Isr J Med Sci*, **17**: 524–30.

Taylor-Robinson D, Ainsworth J et al., 1993, Are mycoplasmas involved in the pathogenesis of AIDS? *Retroviruses of Human AIDS and Related Animal Diseases*, 8eme Colloque des Cent Gardes, eds Girard M, Vallette M, Fondation Marcel Mérieux, Lyons, France, 11–16.

Taylor-Robinson D, Gilroy CB et al., 1994, *Mycoplasma genitalium* in the joints of two patients with arthritis, *Eur J Clin Microbiol Infect Dis*, **13**: 1066–9.

Texier-Maugein J, Clerc M et al., 1987, *Ureaplasma urealyticum*-induced bladder stones in rats and their prevention by fluorfamide and doxycycline, *Isr J Med Sci*, **23**: 565–7.

Thiaucourt F, Bölske G et al., 1994, The use of monoclonal antibodies in the diagnosis of contagious caprine pleuropneumonia (CCPP), *Vet Microbiol*, **41**: 191–203.

Thomas LH, Howard CJ et al., 1986, *Mycoplasma bovis* infection in gnotobiotic calves and combined infection with respiratory syncytial virus, *Vet Pathol*, **23**: 571–8.

Thomsen AC, 1978, Mycoplasmas in human pyelonephritis: demonstration of antibodies in serum and urine, *J Clin Microbiol*, **8**: 197–202.

Tola S, Rizzu P, Leori G, 1994, A species-specific DNA probe for the detection of *Mycoplasma agalactiae*, *Vet Microbiol*, **41**: 355–61.

Trotter SL, Franklin RM et al., 1977, Epidemic caprine keratoconjunctivitis: experimentally induced disease with a pure culture of *Mycoplasma conjunctivae*, *Infect Immun*, **18**: 816–22.

Tully JG, Rose DL et al., 1979, Enhanced isolation of *Mycoplasma pneumoniae* from throat washings with a newly modified culture medium, *J Infect Dis*, **139**: 478–82.

Tully JG, Rose DL et al., 1995, *Mycoplasma pneumoniae* and *Mycoplasma genitalium* in synovial fluid isolate, *J Clin Microbiol*, **33**: 1851–5.

Tully JG, Taylor-Robinson D et al., 1981, A newly discovered mycoplasma in the human urogenital tract, *Lancet*, **1**: 1288–91.

Turner AW, 1959, Pleuropneumonia group of diseases, *Infectious Diseases of Animals: Diseases due to Bacteria*, eds Stableforth AW, Galloway IE, Butterworths Scientific Publications, London, 437–80.

Turner AW, 1962, Detection of *Mycoplasma mycoides* antigen and antibody by means of precipitin tests, as aids to diagnosis of bovine contagious pleuropneumonia, *Aust Vet J*, **38**: 335–7.

Turner AW, Etheridge JR, 1963, Slide agglutination tests in the diagnosis of bovine contagious pleuropneumonia, *Aust Vet J*, **39**: 445–51.

Waites KB, Rudd PT et al., 1988, Chronic *Ureaplasma urealyticum* and *Mycoplasma hominis* infections of central nervous system in preterm infants, *Lancet*, **2**: 17–21.

Wang EEL, Cassell GH et al., 1993a, *Ureaplasma urealyticum* and chronic lung disease of prematurity: critical appraisal of the literature on causation, *Clin Infect Dis*, **17, Suppl.**: 112–16.

Wang RY-H, Shih JW-K et al., 1992, High frequency of antibodies to *Mycoplasma penetrans* in HIV-infected patients, *Lancet*, **340**: 1312–16.

Wang RY-H, Shih JW-K et al., 1993b, *Mycoplasma penetrans* infection in male homosexuals with AIDS: high seroprevalence and association with Kaposi's sarcoma, *Clin Infect Dis*, **17**: 724–9.

Wenzel RP, Carven RB et al., 1976, Field trial of an inactivated *Mycoplasma pneumoniae* vaccine. I. Vaccine efficacy, *J Infect Dis*, **134**: 571–6.

Whithear KG, Soeripto et al., 1990, Immunogenicity of a temperature sensitive mutant *Mycoplasma gallisepticum* strain, *Aust Vet J*, **67**: 168–74.

Whittlestone P, 1979, Porcine mycoplasmas, *The Mycoplasmas. Vol. 2. Human and Animal Mycoplasmas*, eds Tully JG, Whitcomb RF, Academic Press, New York, 133–76.

Wiernik A, Jarstrand C, Tunevall G, 1978, The value of immunoelectroosmorphoresis (IEOP) for etiological diagnosis of acute respiratory tract infections due to pneumococci and *Mycoplasma pneumoniae*, *Scand J Infect Dis*, **10**: 173–6.

Yamamoto R, 1991, *Mycoplasma meleagridis* infection, *Diseases of Poultry*, 9th edn, eds Calnek BW, Barnes HJ et al., Iowa State University Press, Ames, Iowa, 212–23.

Yoder HW Jr, 1970, Preincubation heat treatment of chicken hatching eggs to inactivate *Mycoplasma*, *Avian Dis*, **14**: 75–86.

Yoder HW Jr, 1991, *Mycoplasma gallisepticum* infection, *Diseases of Poultry*, 9th edn, eds Calnek BW, Barnes HJ et al., Iowa State University Press, Ames, Iowa, 198–212.

INDEX

Note: Volume numbers are in **bold**. Page numbers in *italics* refer to major discussions. *vs* denotes differential diagnosis or comparisons.

Cross-references from entries for individual species to the entry for that genus are not always inserted, but are assumed.